OPERATIVE TECHNIQUES IN SURGERY

Second Edition

VOLUME TWO

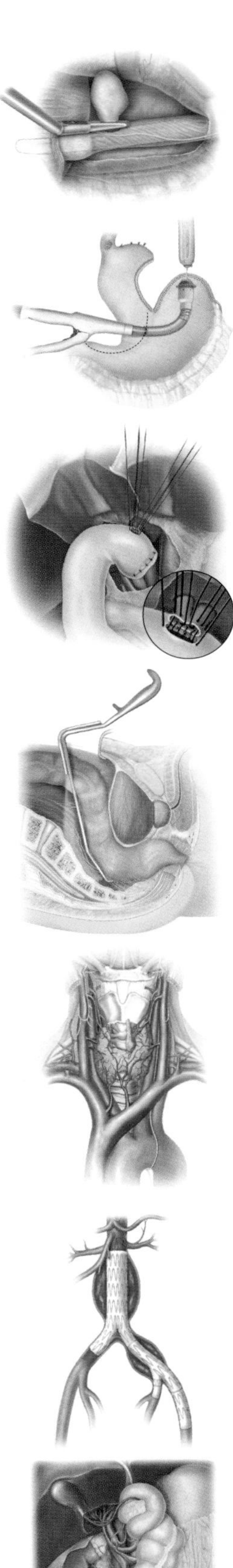

OPERATIVE TECHNIQUES IN SURGERY

Second Edition

VOLUME TWO

Mary T. Hawn, MD, MPH
EDITOR-IN-CHIEF

Emile Holman Professor and Chair
Department of Surgery
Stanford University School of Medicine
Stanford, California

EDITORS

Aurora D. Pryor, MD, MBA, FACS, FASMBS
Professor of Surgery
Bariatric, Foregut and Advanced GI Surgery Department
Stony Brook University Hospital
Stony Brook, New York

Steven J. Hughes, MD
Professor of Surgery
Vice Chair, General Surgery
Chief, Division of Surgical Oncology
University of Florida
College of Medicine
Gainesville, Florida

Daniel Albo, MD, PhD, FACS
Chair, Department of Surgery
The University of Texas Rio Grande Valley (UTRGV) School of Medicine
Harlingen, Texas

Michael S. Sabel, MD, FACS, FSSO
Professor
Department of Surgery
University of Michigan Medical School
Ann Arbor, Michigan

Kellie R. Brown, MD
Professor of Surgery, with Tenure
Division of Vascular and Endovascular Surgery
The Medical College of Wisconsin
Milwaukee, Wisconsin

Amy J. Goldberg, MD, FACS
Interim Dean and Professor of Surgery
Lewis Katz School of Medicine at Temple University
Philadelphia, Pennsylvania

Illustrations by: Body Scientific International, LLC

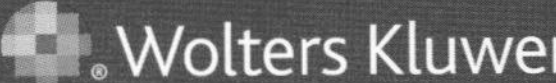

Philadelphia • Baltimore • New York • London
Buenos Aires • Hong Kong • Sydney • Tokyo

Senior Acquisitions Editor: Keith Donnellan
Senior Development Editor: Ashley Fischer
Editorial Coordinator: Erin E. Hernandez
Marketing Manager: Kirsten Watrud
Production Project Manager: Bridgett Dougherty
Manager, Graphic Arts & Design: Stephen Druding
Manufacturing Coordinator: Beth Welsh
Prepress Vendor: TNQ Technologies

9 8 7 6 5 4 3 2 1

Printed in Singapore.

Library of Congress Cataloging-in-Publication Data

ISBN-13: 978-1-975176-46-4

Cataloging in Publication data available on request from publisher.

This work is provided "as is," and the publisher disclaims any and all warranties, express or implied, including any warranties as to accuracy, comprehensiveness, or currency of the content of this work.

This work is no substitute for individual patient assessment based upon healthcare professionals' examination of each patient and consideration of, among other things, age, weight, gender, current or prior medical conditions, medication history, laboratory data and other factors unique to the patient. The publisher does not provide medical advice or guidance and this work is merely a reference tool. Healthcare professionals, and not the publisher, are solely responsible for the use of this work including all medical judgments and for any resulting diagnosis and treatments.

Given continuous, rapid advances in medical science and health information, independent professional verification of medical diagnoses, indications, appropriate pharmaceutical selections and dosages, and treatment options should be made and healthcare professionals should consult a variety of sources. When prescribing medication, healthcare professionals are advised to consult the product information sheet (the manufacturer's package insert) accompanying each drug to verify, among other things, conditions of use, warnings and side effects and identify any changes in dosage schedule or contraindications, particularly if the medication to be administered is new, infrequently used or has a narrow therapeutic range. To the maximum extent permitted under applicable law, no responsibility is assumed by the publisher for any injury and/or damage to persons or property, as a matter of products liability, negligence law or otherwise, or from any reference to or use by any person of this work.

shop.lww.com

MKO822

Contributing Authors

PART 1 OPERATIVE TECHNIQUES IN ESOPHAGEAL AND FOREGUT SURGERY

Roslyn Alexander, DO
Department of Surgery
St. Luke's University Health Network
Bethlehem, Pennsylvania

Evan T. Alicuben, MD
Fellow
Department of Cardiothoracic Surgery
University of Pittsburgh Medical Center
Pittsburgh, Pennsylvania

Yewande R. Alimi, MD, MHS
Assistant Professor
Department of Surgery
Georgetown University School of Medicine
Attending Physician
Department of Surgery
Medstar Georgetown University Hospital
Washington, D.C.

Marco Ettore Allaix, MD, PhD
Associate Professor
Department of Surgical Sciences
University of Torino
Attending Surgeon
Department of Surgery
Citta della Salute e della Scienza di Torino
Torino, Italy

Scott A. Anderson, MD
Associate Professor of Surgery
Division of Pediatric Surgery
Department of Surgery
University of Alabama at Birmingham School of Medicine
Director, ECMO Program
Children's of Alabama
Birmingham, Alabama

Thomas J. Birdas, MD, MBA
Associate Professor
Department of Surgery
Indiana University School of Medicine
Indianapolis, Indiana

Andrew M. Brown, MD
Clinical Assistant Professor of Surgery
Department of Surgery
Lewis Katz School of Medicine at Temple University
Philadelphia, Pennsylvania
General Surgeon
Department of Surgery
St. Luke's University Health Network
Bethlehem, Pennsylvania

John M. Campbell, MD
Department of Surgery
Renaissance School of Medicine at Stony Brook University
Stony Brook University Hospital
Stony Brook, New York

DuyKhanh P. Ceppa, MD
Associate Professor of Surgery
Division of Cardiothoracic Surgery
Department of Surgery
Indiana University School of Medicine
Indianapolis, Indiana

Ernest G. Chan, MD, MPH
Department of Cardiothoracic Surgery
University of Pittsburgh Medical Center
Pittsburgh, Pennsylvania

Mike K. Chen, MD, MBA
Professor and Chief of Pediatric Surgery
Division of Pediatric Surgery
Department of Surgery
University of Alabama at Birmingham School of Medicine
Surgeon-in-Chief
Children's of Alabama
Birmingham, Alabama

Jazmín M. Cole, MD
Assistant Professor
Department of Surgery
Emory University School of Medicine
Emory University Hospital Midtown
Atlanta, Georgia

Jennifer Colvin, MD
Assistant Professor
Department of Surgery
University of Cincinnati
Cincinnati, Ohio

Salvatore Docimo, Jr., DO, FACS, FASMBS
Associate Professor
Department of Surgery
Morsani College of Medicine
University of South Florida
Tampa, Florida

Christopher DuCoin, MD, MPH
Associate Professor of Surgery
Division of GI Surgery
University of South Florida
Chief, Division of Gastrointestinal Surgery
Department of Surgery
Tampa General Hospital
Tampa, Florida

Luke M. Funk, MD, MPH
Associate Professor of Surgery
Department of Surgery
University of Wisconsin-Madison School of Medicine and Public Health
Chief, Division of General Surgery
Department of Surgery
William S. Middleton VA
Madison, Wisconsin

Robert E. Glasgow, MD, MBA, FACS
Professor and Interim Chair
Department of Surgery
University of Utah
Salt Lake City, Utah

Abigail Gotsch, MD
Department of General Surgery
St. Luke's University Health Network
Bethlehem, Pennsylvania

Meredith A. Harrison, MD, FACS
Assistant Professor Thoracic Surgery
Department of General Surgery
St. Luke's University Health Network
Bethlehem, Pennsylvania

Mary T. Hawn, MD, MPH
Emile Holman Professor and Chair
Department of Surgery
Stanford University School of Medicine
Stanford, California

John G. Hunter, M.D., FACS
Professor of Surgery
Oregon Health & Sciences University School of Medicine
Executive Vice President, OHSU
Chief Executive Officer
OHSU Health System
Portland, Oregon

Hope T. Jackson, MD, FACS
Associate Professor of Surgery
Department of Surgery
George Washington University School of Medicine and Health Sciences
Washington, D.C.

Saher-Zahra Khan, MD
Department of Surgery
The Cleveland Clinic Lerner College of Medicine of Case Western University
University Hospitals Cleveland Medical Center
Cleveland, Ohio

Ryan M. Levy, MD, FACS
Assistant Professor of Thoracic Surgery
University of Pittsburgh School of Medicine
Chief of Thoracic Surgery
Department of Cardiothoracic Surgery
University of Pittsburgh Medical Center
Pittsburgh, Pennsylvania

James D. Luketich, MD
Professor of Surgery
Department of Cardiothoracic Surgery
University of Pittsburgh School of Medicine
Chair, Department of Cardiothoracic Surgery
University of Pittsburgh Medical Center
Pittsburgh, Pennsylvania

Jeffrey M. Marks, MD
Professor of Surgery
The Cleveland Clinic Lerner College of Medicine of Case Western University
Director of Surgical Endoscopy
Department of Surgery
University Hospitals Cleveland Medical Center
Cleveland, Ohio

W. Scott Melvin, MD
Vice Chair, Professor of Surgery
Albert Einstein School of Medicine
Montefiore Medical Center
New York, New York

Robert E. Merritt, MD
Division Director of Thoracic Surgery
Department of Surgery
The Ohio State School of Medicine
Thoracic Surgeon
Department of Surgery
The Ohio State University Wexner Medical Center
Columbus, Ohio

Aanuoluwapo Obisesan, MD
Department of Surgery
St. Luke's University Health Network
Bethlehem, Pennsylvania

David D. Odell, MD
Associate Professor of Surgery
Department of Surgery
Feinberg School of Medicine, Northwestern University
Thoracic Surgeon
Northwestern Memorial Hospital
Chicago, Illinois

Brant K. Oelschlager, MD
Chief, General Surgery
Department of General Surgery
University of Washington Medical Center
Seattle, Washington

Gilbert Pan, MS
Boston University School of Medicine
Boston, Massachusetts

Marco G. Patti, MD
Department of Surgery
University of Virginia
Charlottesville, Virginia

Kyle A. Perry, MD, MBA
Professor of Surgery
Department of Surgery
The Ohio State University School of Medicine
Columbus, Ohio

William Richards, MD
Professor and Chair
Department of Surgery
University of South Alabama College of Medicine
Mobile, Alabama

Richard Rieske, MD
Department of Surgery
University of South Alabama College of Medicine
Mobile, Alabama

C. Daniel Smith, MD
Director
Esophageal Institute of Atlanta
Atlanta, Georgia

Ryland S. Stucke, MD
Clinical Instructor
Department of Surgery
Oregon Health & Sciences University School of Medicine
OHSU Adventist Health
Portland, Oregon

Joseph Adam Sujka, MD
Assistant Professor of Surgery
Division of GI Surgery
University of South Florida
Attending Surgeon
Division of GI Surgery
Department of Surgery
Tampa General Hospital
Tampa, Florida

Jordan A. Wilkerson, MD
Thoracic Surgery Fellow
Division of Cardiothoracic Surgery
Department of Surgery
Indiana University School of Medicine
Indianapolis, Indiana

PART 2 OPERATIVE TECHNIQUES IN GASTROINTESTINAL SURGERY

Sherif R.Z. Abdel-Misih, MD
Associate Professor of Surgery
Program Director, General Surgery Residency
Department of Surgery
Renaissance School of Medicine at Stony Brook University
Program Director, General Surgery Residency
Department of Surgery
Stony Brook University Hospital
Stony Brook, New York

Waddah B. Al-Refaie, MD, FACS
John S. Dillon Professor of Surgical Oncology
Department of Surgery
Georgetown University School of Medicine
Regional Chief of Surgical Oncology
Surgical in-Chief, Georgetown Lombardi Comprehensive Cancer Center
MedStar Health
Washington, D.C.

Melissa M. Alvarez-Downing, MD
Assistant Professor
Department of Surgery
Rutgers New Jersey Medical School
Newark, New Jersey

Sullivan A. Ayuso, MD
Department of GI & Minimally Invasive Surgery
Carolinas Medical Center
Charlotte, North Carolina

Xavier Lyndell Baldwin, MD
Post-Doctoral Research Fellow
Department of Surgery
University of North Carolina at Chapel Hill
Department of Surgery
University of North Carolina Hospitals
Chapel Hill, North Carolina

Juan S. Barajas-Gamboa, MD
Postdoctoral Research Fellow
Department of General Surgery
Cleveland Clinic Abu Dhabi
Abu Dhabi, United Arab Emirates

Givi Basishvili, MD
Clinical Assistant Instructor
Renaissance School of Medicine at Stony Brook University
Department of Surgery
Stony Brook University Hospital
Stony Brook, New York

Andrew T. Bates, MD
Assistant Professor
Department of Surgery
Zucker School of Medicine at Hofstra/Northwell
Hempstead, New York
Director, Minimally-Invasive Surgery
Department of Surgery
South Shore University Hospital
Bay Shore, New York

Lucas R. Beffa, MD, FACS
Assistant Professor of Surgery
Digestive Diseases and Surgery Institute
Cleveland Clinic
Cleveland, Ohio

Susan M. Cera, MD, FACS, FASCRS
Colorectal Surgeon
Clinical Associate
Cleveland Clinic Florida
Department of Surgery
Physicians Regional Medical Center
Naples, Florida

Paul D. Colavita, MD, FACS
Associate Professor of Surgery
Department of Surgery
Carolinas Medical Center
Charlotte, North Carolina

Courtney E. Collins, MD, MS
Assistant Professor
Department of Surgery
The Ohio State University School of Medicine
Columbus, Ohio

Tuesday F. A. Cook, MD
Director
Department of Minimally Invasive, Foregut and Bariatric Surgery
Adventist HealthCare Fort Washington Medical Center
Fort Washington, Maryland

Erin E. Devine, MD, PhD
Department of Surgery
Stanford University School of Medicine
Stanford Hospital and Clinics
Stanford, California

Elizabeth A. Dovec, MD, FACS, FASMBS, DBOM
Medical Director and Bariatric Surgeon
Department of Weight Loss and Bariatric Surgery
Digestive Health and Surgery Institute
AdventHealth at Orlando
AdventHealth Medical Group
Orlando, Florida

Sharbel A. Elhage, MD
Department of Surgery
Carolinas Medical Center
Charlotte, North Carolina

Mary T. Hawn, MD, MPH
Emile Holman Professor and Chair
Department of Surgery
Stanford University School of Medicine
Stanford, California

B. Todd Heniford, MD, FACS
Professor of Surgery
Chief, Gastrointestinal and Minimally Invasive Surgery
Chief, Carolinas Hernia Center
Department of Surgery
Carolinas Medical Center
Charlotte, North Carolina

Martin J. Heslin, MD, MSHA
Professor of Surgery
Executive Director Mitchell Cancer Institute
Department of Surgery
University of South Alabama School of Medicine
Mobile, Alabama

David I. Hindin, MD, MS
Surgical Critical Care Fellow
Department of Surgery
Stanford University Hospital
Stanford, California

Charlotte M. Horne, MD
Assistant Professor of Surgery
Department of General Surgery
Pennsylvania State University
Milton S. Hershey Medical Center
Hershey, Pennsylvania

Matthew M. Hutter, MD, MBA, MPH
Professor of Surgery
Harvard Medical School
Director, Codman Center for Clinical Effectiveness in Surgery
Department of Surgery
Massachusetts General Hospital
Boston, Massachusetts

Kamal M.F. Itani, MD
Professor of Surgery
Boston University
Chief of Surgery
Department of Surgery
VA Boston Health Care System
Boston, Massachusetts

Patrick G. Jackson, MD
Professor of Surgery
Department of Surgery
Georgetown University School of Medicine
Chief of General Surgery
MedStar Georgetown University Hospital
Washington, D.C.

Harel Jacoby, MD
Fellow
Department of Advanced Gastrointestinal Surgery
AdventHealth
Tampa, Florida

Kunoor Jain-Spangler, MD
Assistant Professor
Director, Advanced GI/MIS and Bariatric Surgery Fellowships
Department of Surgery
Duke University School of Medicine
Durham, North Carolina

Susan Laura Jao, BA
Renaissance School of Medicine at Stony Brook University
Stony Brook University Hospital
Stony Brook, New York

Shaneeta M. Johnson, MD, MBA, FACS, FASMBS
Professor of Surgery
Chief, Minimally Invasive and Bariatric Surgery
Department of Surgery
Morehouse School of Medicine
Atlanta, Georgia

Matthew Kroh, MD
Professor of Surgery
Vice Chair, Innovation and Technology
Digestive Disease and Surgery Institute
Cleveland Clinic
Cleveland, Ohio

Megan P. Lundgren, MD
Surgical Fellow
Digestive Disease Institute
Cleveland Clinic
Cleveland Ohio

Ugwuji N. Maduekwe, MD, MMSc, MPH
Associate Professor
Division of Surgical Oncology
Department of Surgery
The Medical College of Wisconsin
Milwaukee, Wisconsin

Elizabeth G. McCarthy, MD
MIS/Bariatric Fellow
Department of Surgery
Stony Brook University Hospital
Stony Brook, New York

Ozanan R. Meireles, MD
Assistant Professor of Surgery
Harvard Medical School
Bariatric, Foregut, and Advanced Endoluminal Surgeon
Department of Surgery
Massachusetts General Hospital
Boston, Massachusetts

Marcovalerio Melis, MD, FACS
Associate Professor of Surgery
Division of Surgical Oncology
Zucker School of Medicine at Hofstra/Northwell
Lenox Hill Hospital
Chief, Division of Surgical Oncology
Phelps Hospital
New York, New York

Kelsey B. Montgomery, MD
Department of Surgery
University of Alabama at Birmingham
Birmingham, Alabama

Elliot Newman, MD
Professor of Surgery
Department of Surgery
Zucker School of Medicine at Hofstra/Northwell
Hempstead, New York
Chief of Surgical Oncology
Northwell Cancer Institute at Lenox Hill Hospital
New York, New York

Sean Michael O'Neill, MD, PhD
Clinical Assistant Professor
Department of Surgery
University of Michigan Medical School
Ann Arbor, Michigan
General Surgeon
Department of Surgery
St. Joseph Mercy Chelsea Medical Center
Chelsea, Michigan

David M. Pechman, MD, MBA
Assistant Professor of Surgery
Department of Surgery
Zucker School of Medicine at Hofstra/Northwell
Hempstead, New York
Minimally Invasive and Bariatric Surgeon
Department of Surgery
South Shore University Hospital
Bay Shore, New York

Dana Portenier, MD, FASC, FASMBS
Division Chief, Duke Center for Metabolic and Weight Loss Surgery
Duke University School of Medicine
Durham, North Carolina

John R. Porterfield, Jr., MD, MSPH, FACS
Professor of Surgery
Division of Gastrointestinal Surgery
Department of Surgery
University of Alabama at Birmingham School of Medicine
UAB University Hospital
Birmingham, Alabama

Benjamin Kuttikatt Poulose, MD, MPH
Robert M. Zollinger Lecrone-Baxter Chair
Chief, Division of General and Gastrointestinal Surgery
Department of Surgery
The Ohio State University Wexner Medical Center
Columbus, Ohio

Ajita S. Prabhu, MD, FACS
Associate Professor of Surgery
Department of General Surgery
Cleveland Clinic Foundation
Cleveland, Ohio

Aurora D. Pryor, MD, MBA, FACS, FASMBS
Professor of Surgery
Bariatric, Foregut and Advanced GI Surgery Department
Stony Brook University Hospital
Stony Brook, New York

Carla M. Pugh, MD, PhD, FACS
Thomas Krummel Professor of Surgery
Director of the Technology Enabled Clinical Improvement (T.E.C.I.) Center
Department of Surgery
Stanford University School of Medicine
Stanford, California

Sushanth Reddy, MD
Associate Professor of Surgery
Department of Surgery
University of Alabama at Birmingham School of Medicine
Birmingham, Alabama

John H. Rodriguez, MD, FACS
Assistant Professor of Surgery
Department of Surgery
Cleveland Clinic Lerner College of Medicine
Cleveland, Ohio
Chair, Department of General Surgery
Cleveland Clinic Abu Dhabi
Abu Dhabi, United Arab Emirates

Alexander S. Rosemurgy, II, MD
Professor
Department of Surgery
University of Central Florida
Orlando, Florida
Professor
Department of Surgery
Nova Southeastern University
Fort Lauderdale, Florida

Michael J. Rosen, MD
Professor of Surgery
Cleveland Clinic
Cleveland, Ohio

Amy Rosenbluth, MD
Clinical Assistant Professor of Surgery
Associate Program Director of Surgical Residency
Department of Surgery
Stony Brook University Hospital
Stony Brook, New York

Sharona B. Ross, MD, FACS
Professor
Department of Surgery
University of Central Florida
Orlando, Florida
Director, Minimally Invasive Robotic Surgery and Surgical Endoscopy
Digestive Health Institute Tampa
AdventHealth Tampa
Tampa, Florida

George A. Sarosi, Jr., MD
Robert H. Hux MD Professor
Vice Chair for Education
Department of Surgery
University of Florida College of Medicine
Gainesville, Florida

Samer Sbayi, MD, MBA, FACS
Assistant Professor
Department of General Surgery
Renaissance School of Medicine at Stony Brook University
Director, Emergency General Surgery
Chief, Mastery in General Surgery Fellowship
Deputy Chief Medical Information Officer
Department of General Surgery
Stony Brook University Hospital
Stony Brook, New York

Scott W. Schimpke, MD, FACS
Assistant Professor
Program Director, General Surgery Residency
Associate Program Director, MIS/Bariatric Fellowship
Department of Surgery
Rush University Medical Center
Chicago, Illinois

Eric G. Sheu, MD, PhD
Assistant Professor of Surgery
Harvard Medical School
Associate Program Director, Minimally Invasive and Bariatric Surgery Fellowship
Department of Surgery
Brigham and Women's Hospital
Boston, Massachusetts

John H. Stewart, IV, MD, MBA
Director, LSU NO/LCMC Cancer Center
Professor of Surgery
Department of Surgery
Louisiana State University School of Medicine
New Orleans, Louisiana

Andrew T. Strong, MD
Clinical Associate
Center for Metabolic and Weight Loss Surgery
Duke University Hospital
Durham, North Carolina

Iswanto Sucandy, MD, FACS
Associate Professor of Surgery
Department of Surgery
University of Central Florida
Director, Liver Surgery and Disorders Program
Digestive Health Institute
AdventHealth Tampa
Tampa, Florida

Cameron Syblis, BS
Digestive Health Institute
AdventHealth Tampa
Tampa, Florida

Dana A. Telem, MD, MPH
Lazar J Greenfield Professor of Surgery
Section Chief, General Surgery
Department of Surgery
University of Michigan Medical School
Ann Arbor, Michigan

Jennifer F. Tseng, MD, MPH, FACS
James Utley Professor and Chair of Surgery
Department of Surgery
Boston University School of Medicine
Surgeon-in-Chief
Department of Surgery
Boston Medical Center
Boston, Massachusetts

Anthony M. Villano, MD
Fellow
Department of Surgical Oncology
Fox Chase Cancer Center
Philadelphia, Pennsylvania

Jin Soo Yoo, MD
Associate Professor
Department of Surgery
Duke University School of Medicine
Duke University Health System
Durham, North Carolina

PART 3 OPERATIVE TECHNIQUES IN HEPATO-PANCREATO-BILIARY SURGERY

David B. Adams, MD
Distinguished University Professor Emeritus
Department of Surgery
The Medical University of South Carolina
Charleston, South Carolina

Reid B. Adams, MD
S. Hurt Watts Professor and Chair
Department of Surgery
Chief Medical Officer
University of Virginia Health System
Charlottesville, Virginia

David L. Bartlett, MD
Professor
Department of Surgery
Drexel University College of Medicine
Philadelphia, Pennsylvania
System Chair, AHN Cancer Institute
AHN Surgery Institute
Allegheny Health Network
Pittsburgh, Pennsylvania

Kevin E. Behrns, MD
Professor of Surgery
Department of Surgery
University of Florida College of Medicine
Chief Medical Officer
Department of Surgery
UF Health, The Villages Hospital
The Villages, Florida

Mark Bloomston, MD, FACS, FSSO
Surgical Oncologist
South Florida Surgical Oncology
GenesisCare
Fort Myers, Florida

Richard J. Bold, MD, MBA
Physician-In-Chief
UC Davis Comprehensive Cancer Center
Professor and Chief
Division of Surgical Oncology
Department of Surgery
University of California Davis School of Medicine
Sacramento, California

Morgan M. Bonds, MD
Assistant Professor
Department of Surgery
University of Oklahoma Health Sciences Center
Oklahoma City, Oklahoma

Brian A. Boone, MD, FACS
Assistant Professor
Department of Surgery
Department of Microbiology, Immunology and Cell Biology
West Virginia University
Morgantown, West Virginia

Adam S. Brinkman, MD
Assistant Professor
Pediatric Trauma Director
Pediatric Surgical Critical Care Medical Director
Department of Surgery
American Family Children's Hospital
University of Wisconsin Health
Madison, Wisconsin

Zachary J. Brown, DO
Complex General Surgical Oncology Fellow
Department of Surgical Oncology
The Ohio State University Wexner Medical Center
Columbus, Ohio

Emily F. Cantrell, MD, FACS
Assistant Professor
Division of Acute Care Surgery
Department of Surgery
University of Nebraska Medical Center
Omaha, Nebraska

Hop S. Tran Cao, MD, FACS
Associate Professor
Department of Surgical Oncology
The University of Texas MD Anderson Cancer Center
Houston, Texas

Patrick R. Carney, PhD
Department of Surgery
University of Wisconsin School of Medicine and Public Health
Madison, Wisconsin

Jason A. Castellanos, MD, MS
Assistant Professor of Surgical Oncology
Department of Surgical Oncology
Fox Chase Cancer Center
Philadelphia, Pennsylvania

Eugene P. Ceppa, MD, FACS
Associate Professor
Department of Surgery
Indiana University School of Medicine
Indianapolis, Indiana

Shailendra S. Chauhan, MD
Clinical Associate Professor of Medicine
Department of Gastroenterology and Hepatology
Atrium Health
Charlotte, North Carolina

Jordan M. Cloyd, MD
Assistant Professor
Ward Family Professor of Surgical Oncology
Department of Surgery
The Ohio State Wexner Medical Center
Columbus, Ohio

Charles S. Cox, Jr., MD
George and Cynthia Mitchell Distinguished Chair
Professor of Pediatric Surgery
Department of Pediatric Surgery
McGovern Medical School at University of Texas
UT Health Science Center at Houston
Houston, Texas

Kaitlyn Crespo, BS
Digestive Health Institute
AdventHealth Tampa
University of Central Florida
Tampa, Florida

Mary E. Dillhoff, MD, MS, FACS
Associate Professor
Division of Surgical Oncology
Department of Surgery
The Ohio State University School of Medicine
Columbus, Ohio

Matthew E. Dixon, MD, FACS
Assistant Professor of Surgery
Department of Surgery
Penn State College of Medicine
Hepatopancreatobiliary Surgery
Division of Surgical Oncology
Department of Surgery
Penn State Hershey Medical Center
Hershey, Pennsylvania

Epameinondas Dogeas, MD
Fellow
Division of Surgical Oncology
University of Pittsburgh Medical Center
Pittsburgh, Pennsylvania

Barish H. Edil, MD
John A. Schilling Chair and Professor of Surgery
Department of Surgery
University of Oklahoma Health Sciences Center
Oklahoma City, Oklahoma

Rony Eshkenazy, MD, PhD
Surgeon
Department of Hepato-Biliary and Pancreatic Surgery
Tel Aviv University
Department of Hepato-Biliary and Pancreatic Surgery
Sheba - Tel Hashomer Hospital Medical Center
Ramat-Gan, Israel

William Edward Fisher, MD
Professor and Vice Chair, Clinical Affairs
George L. Jordan, M.D. Chair of General Surgery
Michael E. DeBakey Department of Surgery
Baylor College of Medicine
Vice President
Baylor St. Luke's Medical Center
Texas Medical Center
Houston, Texas

Jared A. Forrester, MD
HPB Fellow
Hepatobiliary and Pancreatic Surgery Program
Providence Cancer Institute
Providence Portland Medical Center
Portland, Oregon

T. Clark Gamblin, MD, MS, MBA, FACS
Professor and Chief of Surgical Oncology
Department of Surgery
The Medical College of Wisconsin
Milwaukee, Wisconsin

Brian S. Geller, MD
Assistant Professor
Department of Radiology
University of Florida College of Medicine
UF Health
Gainesville, Florida

Jon M. Gerry, MD
Associate Program Director HPB Fellowship
Providence Cancer Institute
Providence Portland Medical Center
Portland, Oregon

Ryan T. Groeschl, MD
Hepatopancreatobiliary Surgeon
Department of Surgical Oncology
Essentia Health
Duluth, Minnesota

Julie Gail Grossman, MD
Surgical Oncology Fellow
Department of Surgery
Jackson Memorial Hospital
University of Miami
Miami, Florida

Niraj J. Gusani, MD, MS, FACS, FSSO
Chief, Section of Surgical Oncology
Department of Surgery
Baptist MD Anderson Cancer Center
Jacksonville, FL

Nathania M. Figueroa Guilliani, MD
HPB Fellow
Hepatobiliary and Pancreatic Surgery Program
Providence Cancer Institute
Providence Portland Medical Center
Portland, Oregon

Samuel Han, MD, MS
Assistant Professor
Section of Therapeutic Endoscopy
Division of Gastroenterology, Hepatology, and Nutrition
The Ohio State University Wexner Medical Center
Columbus, Ohio

Alan William Hemming, MD, MSc
Professor
Department of Surgery
University of Iowa
Director Liver Transplantation & HPB Surgery
Department of Surgery
University of Iowa Hospitals & Clinics
Iowa City, Iowa

O. Joe Hines, MD
Professor and Interim Chair
Department of Surgery
David Geffen School of Medicine at UCLA
Los Angeles, California

Steven J. Hughes, MD
Professor of Surgery
Vice Chair, General Surgery
Chief, Division of Surgical Oncology
University of Florida College of Medicine
Gainesville, Florida

Kamran Idrees, MD, MSCI, MMHC, FSSO
Chief, Division of Surgical Oncology and Endocrine Surgery
Ingram Associate Professor of Cancer Research
Department of Surgery
Vanderbilt University Medical Center
Nashville, Tennessee

Saleem Islam, MD, MPH
Professor and Division Chief, Pediatric Surgery
Department of Surgery
University of Florida College of Medicine
Gainesville, Florida

Crystal N. Johnson-Mann, MD
Assistant Professor
Department of Surgery
University of Florida College of Medicine
Gainesville, Florida

Rebecca Y. Kim, MD, MPH
Assistant Professor
Department of Surgery
Huntsman Cancer Institute
University of Utah
Salt Lake City, Utah

Song Cheol Kim, MD, PhD
Professor
Division of Hepatobiliary and Pancreatic Surgery
Department of Surgery
University of Ulsan College of Medicine
Asan Medical Center
Seoul, South Korea

Stephanie S. Kim, MD
Department of Surgery
David Geffen School of Medicine at UCLA
UCLA Medical Center
Los Angeles, California

KMarie King, MD, MS, MBA, FACS
Henry and Sally Schaffer Chair
Department of Surgery
Albany Medical College
Chief of Surgery
Department of Surgery
Albany Medical Center
Albany, New York

Kelly Lynn Koch, MD
Surgical Oncology Fellow
Division of Surgical Oncology
Department of Surgery
University of Miami Sylvester Cancer Center
Jackson Memorial Hospital
Miami, Florida

Shawn D. Larson, MB, ChB, FACS
Associate Professor
Division of Pediatric Surgery
Department of Surgery
University of Florida College of Medicine
Gainesville, Florida

Kenneth K.W. Lee, MD
Jane and Carl Citron Professor of Surgery
Department of Surgery
University of Pittsburgh School of Medicine
Pittsburgh, Pennsylvania

Aijun Li, MD, PhD
Professor
The 2nd Department of Special Therapy
Naval Medical University
Eastern Hepatobiliary Surgery Hospital
Shanghai, China

Tyler John Loftus, MD
Assistant Professor
Department of Surgery
University of Florida College of Medicine
Gainesville, Florida

Thomas K. Maatman, MD
Department of Surgery
Indiana University School of Medicine
Indianapolis, Indiana

Priyadarshini Manay, MBBS
Clinical Associate
Organ Transplant Center
Department of General Surgery
Carver College of Medicine
University of Iowa Hospitals and Clinics
Iowa City, Iowa

David McAneny, MD, FACS
Vice Chair and Professor of Surgery
Department of Surgery
Boston University School of Medicine
Chief Medical Officer
Department of Surgery
Boston Medical Center
Boston, Massachusetts

Sarah Meade, DO
Assistant Professor of Surgery
Department of Surgery
Boston University School of Medicine
Transplant Surgeon
Department of Surgery
Boston Medical Center
Boston, Massachusetts

Nipun B. Merchant, MD
Professor of Surgery
Department of Surgery
University of Miami
University of Miami Hospital
Miami, Florida

Rebecca M. Minter, MD, FACS
A.R. Curreri Professor and Chair
Department of Surgery
University of Wisconsin School of Medicine and Public Health
Madison, Wisconsin

Alicia M. Mohr, MD, FACS, FCCM
Division Chief, Acute Care Surgery
Department of Surgery
University of Florida College of Medicine
Gainesville, Florida

Katherine A. Morgan, MD, FACS
Professor
Director, Division of Gastrointestinal Surgery
Department of Surgery
Medical University of South Carolina
Charleston, South Carolina

Catalina Mosquera, MD
Surgical Oncologist
South Florida Surgical Oncology
GenesisCare
Fort Meyers, Florida

Ido Nachmany, MD
Senior lecturer
Sackler School of Medicine
Tel Aviv University
Chief, Department of Surgery B
Sheba - Tel Hashomer Hospital Medical Center
Ramat-Gan, Israel

Ibrahim Nassour, MD, MSCS
Assistant Professor
Division of Surgical Oncology
Department of Surgery
University of Florida College of Medicine
Gainesville, Florida

Timothy E. Newhook, MD
Assistant Professor
Department of Surgical Oncology
The University of Texas MD Anderson Cancer Center
Houston, Texas

Ankesh Nigam, MD
Associate Professor
Director of Surgical Oncology
Department of Surgery
Albany Medical College
Albany, New York

Alessandro Paniccia, MD
Assistant Professor of Surgery
Department of Surgery
University of Pittsburgh Medical Center
Pittsburgh, Pennsylvania

Georgios Papachristou, MD, PhD
Professor of Medicine
Section of Therapeutic Endoscopy
Division of Gastroenterology, Hepatology, and Nutrition
The Ohio State University Wexner Medical Center
Columbus, Ohio

Alexander A. Parikh, MD, MPH, FACS, FSSO
Professor of Surgery
Chief, Division of Surgical Oncology
Director of Hepatobiliary and Pancreas Surgery
East Carolina University The Brody School of Medicine
Greenville, North Carolina

Timothy M. Pawlik, MD, MPH, MTS, PhD, FACS, FRACS (Hon.)
Professor and Chair
Department of Surgery
The Urban Meyer III and Shelley Meyer Chair for Cancer Research
Professor of Surgery, Oncology, and Health Services Management and Policy
Surgeon in Chief
The Ohio State University Wexner Medical Center
Columbus, Ohio

Niv Pencovich, MD, PhD
Associate Professor
Faculty of Medicine
Attending Surgeon
Department of Surgery B
Sheba - Tel Hashomer Hospital Medical Center
Ramat-Gan, Israel

June S. Peng, MD
Assistant Professor
Division of Surgical Oncology
Department of Surgery
Penn State College of Medicine
Hershey, Pennsylvania

Darren W. Postoak, MD
Assistant Professor
Division of Vascular and Interventional Radiology
Department of Radiology
University of Florida College of Medicine
Gainesville, Florida

Martin D. Rosenthal, MD
Assistant Professor
Director, Abdominal Wall Reconstruction and Intestinal Rehab
Chair, UF Nutrition Committee
Department of Surgery
University of Florida College of Medicine
Gainesville, Florida

Jorge Sanchez-Garcia, MD
Research Fellow
Abdominal Transplant Services
Intermountain Medical Center
Salt Lake City, Utah

Courtney L. Scaife, MD
Professor
Department of Surgery
Huntsman Cancer Institute
University of Utah
Salt Lake City, Utah

Cameron Schlegel, MD
Clinical Instructor
Allegheny Health Network Surgery Institute
Allegheny Health Network
Pittsburgh, Pennsylvania

C. Max Schmidt, MD, PhD, MBA, FACS
Vice Chair and Professor of Surgery
Professor of Biochemistry and Molecular Biology
Indiana University School of Medicine
Chief of Surgery
IU Health University Hospital
Indianapolis, Indiana

Michael Collins Scott, MD, MPH
Department of Surgery
University of Texas Health Science Center
Children's Memorial Hermann Hospital
Houston, Texas

Rebecca A. Snyder, MD, MPH, FACS, FSSO
Assistant Professor
Division of Surgical Oncology
East Carolina University The Brody School of Medicine
Greenville, North Carolina

Ki Byung Song, MD, PhD
Associate Professor
Division of Hepatobiliary and Pancreatic Surgery
Department of Surgery
University of Ulsan College of Medicine
Asan Medical Center
Seoul, South Korea

Iswanto Sucandy, MD, FACS
Associate Professor of Surgery
Department of Surgery
University of Central Florida
Director, Liver Surgery and Disorders Program
Digestive Health Institute
AdventHealth Tampa
Tampa, Florida

Jennifer F. Tseng, MD, MPH, FACS
James Utley Professor and Chair of Surgery
Department of Surgery
Boston University School of Medicine
Surgeon-in-Chief
Department of Surgery
Boston Medical Center
Boston, Massachusetts

Allan Tsung, MD
Professor of Surgery
Chief, Division of Surgical Oncology
Department of Surgery
The Ohio State University School of Medicine
The Ohio State University Wexner Medical Center
Columbus, Ohio

George Van Buren, II, MD
Associate Professor
Department of Surgery
Baylor College of Medicine
Houston Texas

Erin L. Vanzant, MD
Assistant Professor
Department of Surgery
University of Florida College of Medicine
Gainesville, Florida

Roberto J. Vidri, MD, MPH, FACS
Division of Surgical Oncology
Department of Surgery
University of Wisconsin School of Medicine and Public Health
Madison, Wisconsin

Charles M. Vollmer, Jr., MD
Professor of Surgery
Department of Surgery
Perelman School of Medicine at the University of Pennsylvania
Director, Pancreatic Surgery
Department of Surgery
Hospital of the University of Pennsylvania
Philadelphia, Pennsylvania

Sharon M. Weber, MD
Professor
Chief, Division of Surgical Oncology
Medical Director of Surgical Oncology
Department of Surgery
University of Wisconsin Health
Madison, Wisconsin

Ujwal R. Yanala, MBBS
Advanced GI/MIS/Bariatric Surgery Fellow
Department of Surgery
University of Nebraska Medical Center
Omaha, Nebraska

Dennis Yang, MD
Associate Professor of Medicine
Division of Gastroenterology and Hepatology
Department of Internal Medicine
University of Florida College of Medicine
Interventional Endoscopist
University of Florida Health
Gainesville, Florida

Victor M. Zaydfudim, MD, MPH
Associate Professor of Surgery
Department of Surgery
University of Virginia Health System
Charlottesville, Virginia

Herbert J. Zeh, III, MD
Professor and Chair of Surgery
Department of Surgery
UT Southwestern
Dallas, Texas

Ivan R. Zendejas, MD
Transplant and Hepatobiliary Surgeon
Abdominal Transplant Services
Intermountain Medical Center
Salt Lake City, Utah

Amer H. Zureikat, MD
Associate Professor of Surgery
University of Pittsburgh School of Medicine
Chief, Division of Surgical Oncology
Director, Surgical Oncology, UPMC Hillman Cancer Center
Vice Chair of Surgery for Surgical Oncology
Department of Surgery
University of Pittsburgh Medical Center
Pittsburgh, Pennsylvania

Nicholas J. Zyromski, MD
Professor of Surgery
Department of Surgery
Indiana University School of Medicine
Indianapolis, Indiana

PART 4 OPERATIVE TECHNIQUES IN COLON AND RECTAL SURGERY

Matthew Albert, MD, FACS, FASCRS
Medical Director, Surgical Innovation
Digestive Health and Surgical Institute
AdventHealth Orlando
Department of Colorectal Surgery
AdventHealth
Orlando, Florida

Daniel Albo, MD, PhD, FACS
Chair, Department of Surgery
Director, Cancer Center Service Line
The University of Texas Rio Grande Valley (UTRGV) School of Medicine
Harlingen Texas

Daniel A. Anaya, MD
Chief, Division of GI Surgery
Head, Hepatobiliary Section
Department of GI Oncology
Moffitt Cancer Center
Tampa, Florida

Avo Artinyan, MD, MS
CEO
Academic Surgical Associates
Los Angeles, California

Erik Paul Askenasy, MD
Assistant Professor of Surgery
Department of Surgery
McGovern Medical School
University of Texas Health Science Center at Houston
Houston, Texas

Valerie P. Bauer, MD, FACS, FASCRS
Director Colorectal Surgery
Department of Surgery
Cape Regional Medical Center
Cape May Court House, New Jersey

Jaime L. Bohl, MD
Associate Professor of Surgery
Chief, Division of Colon and Rectal Surgery
Department of Surgery
Virginia Commonwealth University
VCU Health
Richmond, Virginia

George J. Chang, MD, MS
Chair and Professor
Department of Colon and Rectal Surgery
The University of Texas MD Anderson Cancer Center
Houston, Texas

Navin Rajindra Changoor, MD
Colon and Rectal Surgeon
Department of Colon and Rectal Surgery
AdventHealth Medical Group
Orlando, Florida

William C. Chapman, Jr., MD
Department of Surgery
Washington University School of Medicine
Saint Louis, Missouri

Angel M. Charles, MD
Department of General Surgery
University of Florida College of Medicine
Gainesville, Florida

Robert R. Cima, MD, MA
Professor of Surgery
Division of Colon and Rectal Surgery
Mayo Clinic College of Medicine and Science
Rochester, Minnesota

Bidhan Das, MD
Clinical Associate Professor
Colon and Rectal Surgery
Department of Surgery
University of Texas Health Science Center at Houston
Houston, Texas

Vijian Dhevan, MD, MBA
Vice Chair for Clinical Affairs
Department of Surgery
The University of Texas Rio Grande Valley (UTRGV) School of Medicine
Harlingen, Texas

Kristen D. Donohue, MD
Assistant Professor
Department of Surgery
Rutgers New Jersey Medical School
New Brunswick, New Jersey

Antonio D'Urso, MD, PhD
Senior Consultant
IRCAD
Department of Digestive and Visceral Surgery
Nouvel Hospital Civil
University Hospital of Strasbourg
Strasbourg, France

Roosevelt Fajardo, MD, MBA, FACS
Associate Professor
Los Andes University School of Medicine
Department of Surgery
Director of Education
Fundación Santa Fe de Bogota University Hospital
Bogotá, Colombia

Barry W. Feig, MD
Professor of Surgical Oncology
Department of Surgical Oncology
The University of Texas MD Anderson Cancer Center
Houston, Texas

Daniel L. Feingold, MD, FACS, FASCRS
Professor of Surgery
Department of Surgery
Rutgers New Jersey Medical School
New Brunswick, New Jersey

Wayne A. I. Frederick, MD, MBA
Professor
Department of Surgery
Howard University
Washington, D.C.

Roger M. Galindo, MD
Assistant Professor of Surgery
Department of Surgery
The University of Texas Rio Grande Valley (UTRGV) School of Medicine
Trauma Medical Director
Department of Surgery
Valley Baptist Medical Center Harlingen
Harlingen, Texas

Julio Garcia-Aguilar, MD, PhD
Benno C. Schmidt Chair in Surgical Oncology
Chief, Colorectal Service
Department of Surgery
Director, Colorectal Cancer Research Center
Memorial Sloan Kettering Cancer Center
Professor of Surgery
Weill Cornell Medical College
New York, New York

Kelly A. Garrett, MD
Associate Professor of Surgery
Department of General Surgery
New York Presbyterian Hospital
Weill Cornell Medicine
New York, New York

Eric Mitchell Haas, MD
Chief, Division of Colon and Rectal Surgery
Houston Methodist Hospital
Houston, Texas

Karin M. Hardiman, MD, PhD
Associate Professor
Department of Surgery
University of Alabama at Birmingham School of Medicine
Surgeon
University of Alabama at Birmingham Health System
Birmingham Veterans Affairs Medical System
Birmingham, Alabama

Andrew G. Hill, MBChB, MD, FRACS, FACS
Professor of Surgery
Department of Surgery
University of Auckland
Middlemore Hospital
Auckland, New Zealand

Joshua S. Hill, MD
Assistant Professor
Division of Surgical Oncology
Department of Surgery
Levine Cancer Institute, Atrium Health
Charlotte, North Carolina

Mehraneh Dorna Jafari, MD, FACS, FASCRS
Associate Professor
Department of Surgery
Weill Cornell Medicine
New York, New York

Anish Jay Jain, MD
Department of Surgery
Howard University College of Medicine
Howard University Hospital
Washington, D.C.

Lillian S. Kao, MD, MS
Professor
Department of Surgery
McGovern Medical School at University of Texas
Houston, Texas

Hasan T. Kirat, MD
Associate Professor of Surgery
Department of Surgery
New York University
Colorectal Surgeon
Department of Surgery
New York University Langone Health
New York, New York

Cherry E. Koh, MBBS(Hons), MS, PhD, FRACS
Associate Professor
Department of Colorectal Surgery
Royal Prince Alfred Hospital
Director of Surgical Outcomes Research Centre
Sydney, New South Wales, Australia

Sang W. Lee, MD
Professor and Chief, Colon and Rectal Surgery
Department of Colon and Rectal Surgery
Keck School of Medicine of the University of Southern California
Los Angeles, California

Edward A. Levine, MD
Professor of Surgery
Department of Surgery
Wake Forest University School of Medicine
Winston-Salem, North Carolina

Luis Jorge Lombana, MD
Colo-Rectal Surgeon
Department of Surgery
Hospital San Ignacio Universidad Javeriana
Bogotá, Columbia

Lillias Holmes Maguire, MD
Assistant Professor
Department of Surgery
Perelman School of Medicine at the University of Pennsylvania
Hospital of the University of Pennsylvania
Philadelphia, Pennsylvania

Michael R. Marco, MD
Postdoctoral Clinical Fellow
Department of Colon and Rectal Surgery
Weill Cornell Medicine
Colorectal Surgery Clinical Fellow
Department of Colon and Rectal Surgery
New York Presbyterian Hospital
New York, New York

Jacques Marescaux, MD, FACS, Hon. FRCS, Hon. FASA, Hon. FJSES, Hon. FJSS
Professor of Surgery
President and Founder of IRCAD, Research Institute against Cancers of the Digestive System
University Hospital of Strasbourg
Strasbourg, France

John H. Marks, MD, FACS, FASCRS
Professor
Lankenau Institute for Medical Research
Chief of Colorectal Surgery
Lankenau Medical Center
Wynnewood, Pennsylvania

Craig A. Messick, MD
Associate Professor of Surgery
Department of Colon and Rectal Surgery
The University of Texas MD Anderson Cancer Center
Houston, Texas

Stefanos G. Millas, MD
Associate Professor
Department of Surgery
McGovern Medical School at University of Texas
LBJ General Hospital
Houston, Texas

Somala Mohammed, MD, MPH
Assistant Professor of Surgery
Harvard Medical School
Pediatric Surgeon
Department of General Surgery
Boston Children's Hospital
Boston, Massachusetts

Jayson Moloney, MBBS
Senior Lecturer
University of Queensland
Staff Surgeon
Department of Colorectal Surgery
Royal Brisbane and Women's Hospital
Brisbane, Australia

Arden M. Morris, MD, MPH
Professor
Department of Surgery
Stanford University School of Medicine
Stanford, California

Matthew G. Mutch, MD
Solan and Bettie Gershman Professor of Surgery
Chief, Section of Colon and Rectal Surgery
Department of Surgery
Washington University School of Medicine
Saint Louis, Missouri

Didier Mutter, MD, PhD, FACS, FRSM
Professor of Surgery
IRCAD
Chair, Digestive and Endocrine Surgery Department
Department of Digestive and Endocrine Surgery
University Hospital of Strasbourg
Strasbourg, France

Govind Nandakumar, MD, FACS, FASCRS
Chief, GI Surgery
Department of Surgery
Mawipal Hospitals
Bangalore, India

Dana M. Omer, MD
Research Scholar
Department of Surgery, Colorectal Service
Memorial Sloan Kettering Cancer Center
New York, New York

Tolulope A. Oyetunji, MD, MPH, FACS
Associate Professor of Surgery
Department of Surgery
University of Missouri-Kansas City School of Medicine
Director, Health Outcomes Research
Department of Surgery
Children's Mercy Hospital
Kansas City, Missouri

Rodrigo Pedraza, MD
Colon and Rectal Surgeon
Center for Advanced Surgery
The Oregon Clinic
Portland, Oregon

Alessio Pigazzi, MD, PhD
Chief, Colorectal Surgery
Department of Surgery
Weill Cornell Medicine
New York, New York

Harsha Polavarapu, MD, FACS, FASCRS
Attending Surgeon
Department of Surgery
Blessing Hospital
Quincy, Illinois

Dhruvesh M. Ramson, MBBS (Hons)
Adjunct Research Associate
Department of Surgery
Monash University
Melbourne, Australia
Surgical Registrar
Department of Surgery
Counties Manakau Health
Auckland, New Zealand

Scott E. Regenbogen, MD, MPH
Associate Professor
Department of Surgery
University of Michigan Medical School
Ann Arbor, Michigan

Henry A. Reinhart, MD
Assistant Professor
Department of Surgery
The University of Texas Rio Grande Valley (UTRGV) School of Medicine
Harlingen, Texas

Feza H. Remzi, MD
Professor of Surgery
Department of Surgery
New York University
Colorectal Surgeon
Department of Surgery
New York University Langone Health
New York, New York

Saul J. Rugeles, MD
Professor of Surgery
Department of Surgery
Pontificia Universidad Javeriana
Colon and Rectal Surgeon
Department of Colon and Rectal Surgery
Hospital Universitario San Ignacio
Bogotá, Colombia

Perisa Ruhi-Williams, MD
Department of Surgery
University of California, Irvine Medical Center
Orange, California

Tarik Sammour, BHB, MBChB, FRACS, CSSANZ, PhD
Associate Professor
Faculty of Medical and Health Sciences
University of Adelaide
Colorectal Unit
Department of Surgery
Royal Adelaide Hospital
Adelaide, Australia

William M. Sánchez, MD, FACS
Chair, Department of Surgery
Universidad Militar Nueva Granada
Hospital Militar Central
Bogotá, Colombia

Brendan F. Scully, MD
Fellow
Department of Colon and Rectal Surgery
Rutgers New Jersey Medical School
New Brunswick, New Jersey

Shiva Seetahal, MD, FACS
Medical Director, Bariatric and Weight Loss Surgery
AdventHealth Heart of Florida
Davenport, Florida

Perry Shen, MD, FACS, FSSO
Professor of Surgery
Department of Surgery
Wake Forest University Medical Center
Winston-Salem, North Carolina

Eric J. Silberfein, MD, FACS
Associate Professor of Surgery
Associate Program Director, General Surgery
Division of Surgical Oncology
Michael E. DeBakey Department of Surgery
Baylor College of Medicine
Chief, Surgical Oncology
Chief, General Surgery
Ben Taub Hospital
Huston, Texas

Mark Soliman, MD, FACS, FASCRS
Chair, Department of Colon and Rectal Surgery
AdventHealth Medical Group
Orlando, Florida

Michael J. Solomon, MB BCH (Hons), BAO, MSc, DMedSc (USYD), DMed (NUI)
Professor of Surgical Research
Faculty of Medicine and Health
University of Sydney
Academic Head & VMO, Department of Colorectal Surgery
Royal Prince Alfred Hospital
Sydney Local Health District
New South Wales, Australia

Andrew RL Stevenson, MB, BS, FRACS, FASCRS (Hon)
Clinical Professor
Department of Surgery
University of Queensland
Senior Colorectal Surgeon
Department of Colorectal Surgery
Royal Brisbane and Women's Hospital
Brisbane, Australia

Zhifei Sun, MD
Assistant Professor
Section of Colorectal Surgery
Department of Surgery
Georgetown University Medical Center
Washington, D.C.

David Graham Taylor, MBBS, FRACS
Colorectal Surgeon
Department of Surgery
Royal Brisbane and Women's Hospital
Herston, Queensland, Australia

James P. Taylor, MBBChir, MPH
Colorectal Fellow
Department of Colon and Rectal Surgery
New York Presbyterian Hospital
Weill Cornell Medicine
New York, New York

Ryan M. Thomas, MD
Associate Professor
Department of Surgery
University of Florida College of Medicine
Section Chief, Department of General Surgery
North Florida/South Georgia Veterans Healthcare System
Gainesville, Florida

Kathrin Mayer Troppmann, MD, FACS
Professor Emeritus
Department of Surgery
University of California Davis School of Medicine
Sacramento, California

Cristian D. Valenzuela, MD
Clinical Fellow, Complex General Surgical Oncology
Department of Surgical Oncology
Wake Forest University School of Medicine
Wake Forest Baptist Atrium Health
Winston-Salem, North Carolina

Elsa B. Valsdóttir, MD
Assistant Professor
University of Iceland
Surgeon
Department of Surgery
Landspítali University Hospital
Reykjavík, Iceland

Oliver Adrian Varban, MD
Associate Professor of Surgery
Chief, Division of Minimally Invasive Surgery
Department of General Surgery
University of Michigan Medical School
Ann Arbor, Michigan

Theodoros Voloyiannis, MD, FACS, FASCRS
Chair, Colon and Rectal Surgery
US Oncology Network
Medical Director, Oncologic Surgery
HCA Houston Healthcare, Gulf Coast Division
Houston, Texas

Konstantinos I. Votanopoulos, MD, PhD, FACS
Professor of Surgery
Department of Surgery
Wake Forest University School of Medicine
Winston-Salem, North Carolina

Rebecca L. Wiatrek, MD, FACS
Surgical Oncologist
Texas Oncology Surgical Specialists
Austin, Texas

Curtis J. Wray, MD, MS
Professor
Department of Surgery
McGovern Medical School at University of Texas
Houston, Texas

Jane Yang, MD
Fellow
Colorectal Surgery
Department of Surgery
Lankenau Medical Center
Wynnewood, Pennsylvania

Y. Nancy You, MD, MHSc
Professor
Department of Colon and Rectal Surgery
The University of Texas MD Anderson Cancer Center
Houston, Texas

Jonathan Benjamin Yuval, MD
Fellow
Department of Surgery
Memorial Sloan Kettering Cancer Center
New York, New York

PART 5 OPERATIVE TECHNIQUES IN BREAST, ENDOCRINE, AND ONCOLOGIC SURGERY

Shoshana Woo Ambani, MD
Medical Director
Department of Plastic & Reconstructive Surgery
Henry Ford Allegiance Health
Jackson, Michigan

Christina V. Angeles, MD
Assistant Professor
Department of Surgery
University of Michigan Medical School
Ann Arbor, Michigan

Peter Angelos, MD, PhD
Professor of Surgery
Chief, Endocrine Surgery
Director MacLean Center for Clinical Medical Ethics
Department of Surgery
University of Chicago
Chicago, Illinois

Adil Ayub, MD
Department of Surgery
University of Texas Medical Branch
Galveston Texas

Haripriya S. Ayyala, MD
Microsurgery Fellow
Division of Plastic and Reconstructive Surgery
Department of Surgery
Memorial Sloan Kettering Cancer Center
New York, New York

Russell S. Berman, MD
Professor of Surgery
Department of Surgery
New York University Grossman School of Medicine
Vice Chair for Education and Faculty Affairs
Chief, Division of Surgical Oncology
Director, Surgical Residency Program
Department of Surgery
NYU Langone Health
New York, New York

Janet Sybil Biermann, MD
Professor
Service Chief, Musculoskeletal Oncology
Department of Orthopedics
University of Michigan Medical School
Ann Arbor, Michigan

Joshua Alex Bloom, MD
Department of Surgery
Tufts University School of Medicine
Tufts Medical Center
Boston, Massachusetts

Judy C. Boughey, MD
W.H. Odell Professor in Individualized Medicine
Chair, Division of Breast & Melanoma Surgical Oncology
Professor of Surgery
Mayo Clinic College of Medicine and Science
Mayo Clinic Hospital, Methodist Campus
Rochester, Minnesota

David L. Brown, MD
William C. Grabb Professor of Plastic Surgery
University of Michigan Medical School
Ann Arbor, Michigan

Michael J. Carr, MD, MS
Research Fellow
Department of Surgical Oncology
Moffitt Cancer Center
Tampa, Florida

Anees B. Chagpar, MD, MSc, MPH, MA, MBA
Professor
Department of Surgery
Yale University
New Haven, Connecticut

Abhishek Chatterjee, MD, MBA, FACS
Associate Professor of Surgery
Tufts University School of Medicine
Chief of Breast Surgery, Chief of Plastic Surgery
Division of Plastic Surgery
Department of Surgery
Tufts Medical Center
Boston, Massachusetts

Betzaira Getzemani Childers, MD
Department of General Surgery
University of Cincinnati
Cincinnati, Ohio

Robin M. Cisco, MD
Clinical Assistant Professor
Department of Surgery
Stanford University School of Medicine
Stanford, California

Amy S. Colwell, MD
Professor of Surgery
Department of Surgery
Massachusetts General Hospital
Boston, Massachusetts

Amy C. Degnim, MD
Professor of Surgery
Department of Surgery
Mayo Clinic College of Medicine and Science
Consultant
Division of Breast & Melanoma Surgical Oncology
Mayo Clinic College of Medicine and Science
Rochester, Minnesota

Danielle K. DePalo, MD
Cutaneous Oncology Research Fellow
Department of Cutaneous Oncology
H. Lee Moffitt Cancer Center and Research Institute
Tampa, Florida

Vasu Divi, MD, FACS
Associate Professor
Department of Otolaryngology – Head and Neck Surgery
Stanford University School of Medicine
Stanford, California

Gerard M. Doherty, MD
Moseley Professor of Surgery
Chair, Department of Surgery
Harvard Medical School
Surgeon-in-Chief
Brigham and Women's Hospital
Boston, Massachusetts

Alison B. Durham, MD
Associate Professor
Department of Dermatology
University of Michigan Medical School
Ann Arbor, Michigan

Michael E. Egger, MD, MPH
Assistant Professor of Surgery
Hiram C Polk, JR MD Department of Surgery
University of Louisville
Louisville, Kentucky

Kelly M. Elleson, MD
Cutaneous Oncology Research Fellow
Department of Cutaneous Oncology
H. Lee Moffitt Cancer Center and Research Institute
Tampa, Florida

Douglas L. Fraker, MD
Jonathan Rhoads Professor of Surgery
Department of Surgery
Perelman School of Medicine at the University of Pennsylvania
Philadelphia, Pennsylvania

Henry Jean François, MD
Professor
Department of General Endocrine and Metabolic Surgery
Aix-Marseille University
Conception Hospital, Assistance Publique Hôpitaux de Marseille
Marseille, France

Paul J. Gagnet, MD
Department of Orthopaedic Surgery
University of Michigan Medical School
Ann Arbor, Michigan

Isaac Gendelman, MD
Department of Surgery
Tufts University School of Medicine
Tufts Medical Center
Boston, Massachusetts

Jeffrey E. Gershenwald, MD
Professor
Department of Surgical Oncology
The University of Texas MD Anderson Cancer Center
Houston, Texas

Joseph S. Giglia, MD
Professor
Interim Chief, Vascular Surgery
Department of Surgery
University of Cincinnati
Cincinnati, Ohio

Raymon H. Grogan, MD, MS, FACS
Associate Professor
Chief of Endocrine Surgery
Michael E. DeBakey Department of Surgery
Baylor College of Medicine
Houston, Texas

Janie G. Grumley, MD FACS
Professor
Saint John's Cancer Institute
Director Comprehensive Breast Program
Margie Petersen Breast Center
Providence Saint John's Health Center
Santa Monica, California

Steven C. Haase, MD, FACS
Professor of Plastic and Orthopedic Surgery
Department of Plastic Surgery and Orthopedic Surgery
University of Michigan Medical School
Ann Arbor, Michigan

Eric G. Halvorson, MD
Adjunct Associate Professor
University of North Carolina
Plastic Surgery Center
Asheville, North Carolina

D. Brock Hewitt, MD, MPH, MS
Fellow
Division of Surgical Oncology
Department of Surgery
The Ohio State University School of Medicine
Columbus, Ohio

Melissa E. Hogg, MD, MS
Clinical Professor
Department of Surgery
University of Chicago
Chicago, Illinois
Director HPB Surgery
Department of Surgery
Northshore University Health System
Evanston, Illinois

Rolfy A. Perez Holguin, MD
Department of Surgery
Penn State Milton S. Hershey Medical Center
Hershey, Pennsylvania

Dennis Ricky Holmes, MD, FACS
Breast Program Director
Department of Surgery
Adventist Health Glendale Medical Center
Glendale, California

Jessica Jen-Tau Hsu, MD, PhD
Assistant Professor
Section of Plastic Surgery
Department of Surgery
Michigan Medicine
Ann Arbor, Michigan

David T. Hughes, MD
Associate Professor of Surgery
Division of Endocrine Surgery
Department of Surgery
University of Michigan Medical School
Ann Arbor, Michigan

Folasade Imeokparia, MD
Assistant Professor
Department of Surgery
Indiana University School of Medicine
Indianapolis, Indiana

Oscar V. Imhof, EKP/ECCP
Clinical Perfusionist
Department of Heartbeat
University Medical Center of Utrecht
Utrecht, The Netherlands

William B. Inabnet, III, MD, MHA, FACS
Johnston-Wright Endowed Professor and Chair
Surgeon-in-Chief
Department of Surgery
University of Kentucky College of Medicine
Lexington, Kentucky

James W. Jakub, MD
Professor of Surgery
Department of Surgery
Mayo Clinic College of Medicine and Science
Jacksonville, Florida

Michael Gwynne Johnston, MD, FACS
Assistant Professor
Department of General Surgery
Uniformed Services University of the Health Sciences
Bethesda, Maryland
Endocrine and General Surgeon
Department of Surgery
Naval Medical Center Portsmouth
Portsmouth, Virginia

Edwin L. Kaplan, MD
Professor
Department of Surgery
University of Chicago
Chicago, Illinois

Cary S. Kaufman, MD, FACS
Clinical Professor
Department of Surgery
School of Medicine, University of Washington
Seattle, Washington

Erika King, MD, MA
Department of General Surgery
Henry Ford Allegiance Health
Jackson, Michigan

Jeffrey H. Kozlow, MD, MS
Associate Professor
Section of Plastic Surgery
Department of Surgery
University of Michigan Medical School
Ann Arbor, Michigan

Bin B.R. Kroon, MD, PhD, FRCS
Emeritus Professor of Surgery
Department of Surgery
The Netherlands Cancer Institute
Amsterdam, The Netherlands

Hidde M. Kroon, MD, PhD
Associate Professor of Surgery
Department of Surgery
Adelaide Medical School
University of Adelaide
Gastro-intestinal and Oncological Surgeon
Department of Surgery
Royal Adelaide Hospital
Adelaide, South Australia, Australia

Anita R. Kulkarni, MD
Private Practice Plastic Surgeon
DC Plastic Surgery Boutique
Washington, D.C.

Nishant Ganesh Kumar, MD
House Officer
Section of Plastic Surgery
Department of Surgery
University of Michigan Medical School
Ann Arbor, Michigan

Anna Kundel, MD, FACS
Clinical Assistant Professor
Department of Surgery
ICAHN School of Medicine at Mount Sinai
New York, New York
Medical Director
Department of Endocrine Surgery
Valley Medical Group
Ridgewood, New Jersey

Theodore A. Kung, MD
Associate Professor of Surgery
Section of Plastic Surgery
Department of Surgery
University of Michigan Medical School
Ann Arbor, Michigan

Eric James Kuo, MD
Fellow
Department of Endocrine Surgery
Columbia University Vagelos College of Physicians and Surgeons
New York, New York

James A. Lee, MD
Edwin K. & Anne C. Weiskopf Professor of Surgery
Chief, Endocrine Surgery
Department of Surgery
Columbia University Medical Center
New York, New York

Dana T. Lin, MD
Clinical Assistant Professor
Department of Surgery
Stanford University School of Medicine
Stanford, California

Erin C. MacKinney, MD
Clinical Assistant Professor
Department of Endocrine Surgery
University of Wisconsin School of Medicine and Public Health
Madison, Wisconsin
Endocrine Surgeon
Department of Surgery
UW Swedish American Hospital
Rockford, Illinois

Kerry M. Madison, MD
Surgical House Officer
Department of Surgery
University of Michigan Medical School
Ann Arbor, Michigan

Gabriele Materazzi, MD
Associate Professor
Department of Surgery
University of Pisa
Chief of Endocrine Surgery
Department of Surgery
Azienda Ospedaliero Universitaria Pisana
Pisa, Italy

Evan Matros, MD, MMSc, MPH
Associate Professor
Division of Plastic and Reconstructive Surgery
Department of Surgery
Memorial Sloan Kettering Cancer Center
New York, New York

Rachel Louise McCaffrey, MD
Assistant Professor
Department of Surgery
Vanderbilt University
Nashville, Tennessee

Christopher R. McHenry, MD, FACS
Professor of Surgery
The Cleveland Clinic Lerner College of Medicine of Case Western University
Vice Chair, Department of Surgery
MetroHealth Medical Center
Cleveland, Ohio

Scott A. Mclean, MD, PhD
Clinical Associate Professor
Department Otolaryngology-Head & Neck Surgery
University of Michigan Medical School
Ann Arbor, Michigan

Kelly M. McMasters, MD, PhD
Ben A Reid, Sr MD Professor and Chair
Hiram C Polk, JR MD Department of Surgery
University of Louisville
Louisville, Kentucky

Roberto D. Lorenzi Mendez, MD, MPH
Department of Surgery
Florida Atlantic University
Boca Raton, Florida
Research Fellow
Department of Plastic and Reconstructive Surgery
Massachusetts General Hospital
Boston, Massachusetts

Paolo Miccoli, MD
Professor Emeritus
Department of Surgical Physiopathology
Università di Pisa
Pisa, Italy

Claire W. Michael, MD
Professor
Department of Pathology
The Cleveland Clinic Lerner College of Medicine of Case Western University
Senior Pathologist
Department of Pathology
University Hospitals Cleveland Medical Center
Cleveland, Ohio

Barbra S. Miller, MD
Professor of Surgery
Division of Surgical Oncology
Department of Surgery
The Ohio State University School of Medicine
Surgeon
Department of Surgery
The James Cancer Hospital and Solove Research Institute
The Ohio State University Wexner Medical Center
Columbus, Ohio

Adeyiza O. Momoh, MD
Professor of Surgery
Section of Plastic Surgery
Department of Surgery
University of Michigan Medical School
Ann Arbor, Michigan

Jeffrey S. Montgomery, MD, MHSA, FACS
Professor
Department of Urology
University of Michigan Medical School
Ann Arbor, Michigan

Paige L. Myers, MD
Assistant Professor
Department of Surgery
University of Michigan Medical School
Ann Arbor, Michigan

Lisa A. Newman, MD, MPH, FACS, FASCO
Chief, Section of Breast Surgery
Chief, Breast Cancer Disease
Department of Surgery
Weill Cornell Medicine
Chief, Breast Surgical Oncology
Department of Surgery
New York Presbyterian Hospital
New York, New York

Omgo E. Nieweg, MD, PhD, FRACS
Clinical Professor of Surgery
Department of Surgery
The University of Sydney
Melanoma Institute Australia
Sydney, New South Wales, Australia

Nunzia Cinzia Paladino, MD, PhD
Department of General Endocrine and Metabolic Surgery
Aix-Marseille University
Conception Hospital, Assistance Publique Hôpitaux de Marseille
Marseille, France

Barnard J. A. Palmer, MD, MEd
Associate Professor
Department of Surgery
University of California, San Francisco – East Bay
Oakland, California

Judy C. Pang, MD
Associate Professor
Department of Pathology
University of Michigan Medical School
Ann Arbor, Michigan

Cindy Eliana Parra, MD
Micrographic Surgery and Dermatologic Oncology Fellow
Department of Dermatology
University of Michigan Medical School
Michigan Medicine
Ann Arbor, Michigan

Robert M. Pride, MD
Department of Surgery
Mayo Clinic College of Medicine and Science
Rochester, Minnesota

Richard A. Prinz, MD
Clinical Professor of Surgery
Department of Surgery
The University of Chicago Pritzker School of Medicine
Chicago, Illinois
Senior Attending Surgeon
Department of Surgery
NorthShore University HealthSystem
Evanston, Illinois

Merrick I. Ross, MD, MSHCT
Charles McBride Professor of Surgery
Section Chief, Melanoma
Department of Surgical Oncology
The University of Texas MD Anderson Cancer Center
Houston, Texas

Michael S. Sabel, MD, FACS, FSSO
Professor
Department of Surgery
University of Michigan Medical School
Ann Arbor, Michigan

Amod A. Sarnaik, MD
Associate Professor
Department of Cutaneous Oncology
Moffitt Cancer Center
Tampa, Florida

Brian D. Saunders, MD, FACS
Professor and Vice Chair
Department of Surgery
Penn State College of Medicine
Section Chief, Endocrine Surgery
Department of Surgery
Penn State Health Milton S. Hershey Medical Center
Hershey, Pennsylvania

Anneke T. Schroen, MD, MPH
Professor
Department of Surgery
University of Virginia
Charlottesville, Virginia

Frédéric Sebag, MD
Professor
Department of General Endocrine and Metabolic Surgery
Aix-Marseille University
Conception Hospital, Assistance Publique Hôpitaux de Marseille
Marseille, France

Ashok R. Shaha, MD, FACS
Jatin P. Shah Chair, Head and Neck Surgery and Oncology
Department of Surgery, Head and Neck Service
Memorial Sloan Kettering Cancer Center
New York, New York

Andrew G. Shuman, MD, FACS
Associate Professor
Division of Head and Neck Oncology
University of Michigan Medical School
Ann Arbor, Michigan

Geoffrey W. Siegel, MD
Assistant Professor
Division of Musculoskeletal Oncology
Department of Orthopaedic Surgery
University of Michigan Medical School
Ann Arbor, Michigan

Vernon K. Sondak, MD
Richard M. Schulze Family Foundation Distinguished Endowed Chair
Department of Cutaneous Oncology
Moffitt Cancer Center
Tampa, Florida

Jeffrey J. Sussman, MD
Professor of Surgery
Department of Surgery
University of Cincinnati College of Medicine
Cincinnati, Ohio

Mark S. Talamonti, MD
Clinical Professor
Department of Surgery
The University of Chicago Pritzker School of Medicine
Chicago, Illinois
Chair, Department of Surgery
NorthShore University HealthSystem
Evanston, Illinois

Geoffrey B. Thompson, MD
Professor Emeritus
Department of Surgery
Mayo Clinic College of Medicine and Science
Rochester, Minnesota

Tiffany A. Torstenson, DO
Breast Surgical Oncologist
Department of Surgery
Mercy One Medical Center
Des Moines, Iowa

Eleni Anastasia Tousimis, MD, MBA, FACS
Professor
Department of Surgery
Director, Cancer Center
Department of Oncology
Cleveland Clinic Indian River Hospital
Vero Beach, Florida

Douglas Tyler, MD, MSHCT
Johns Woods Harris Distinguished Chair in Surgery
Professor and Chair, Department of Surgery
University of Texas Medical Branch
Adjunct Professor
Department of Surgical Oncology
The University of Texas MD Anderson Cancer Center
Galveston, Texas

Hunter J. Underwood, MD
Clinical Lecturer
Department of Surgery
University of Michigan Medical School
Ann Arbor, Michigan

Charles C. Vining, MD
Assistant Professor of Surgery
Division of Surgical Oncology
Department of Surgery
Penn State Health Milton S. Hershey Medical Center
Hershey, Pennsylvania

Roi Weiser, MD
Fellow
Department of Surgical Oncology
The University of Texas MD Anderson Cancer Center
Houston, Texas

Jonathan S. Zager, MD
Chair and Professor
Department of Oncologic Sciences
University of South Florida Morsani College of Medicine
Chief Academic Officer and Senior Member
Department of Cutaneous Oncology
H. Lee Moffitt Cancer Center and Research Institute
Tampa, Florida

PART 6 OPERATIVE TECHNIQUES IN VASCULAR SURGERY

Steven D. Abramowitz, MD, RPVI
Assistant Professor of Surgery
Chair, Department of Vascular Surgery
Georgetown University School of Medicine
Washington, D.C

Georges E. Al-Khoury, MD
Assistant Professor of Surgery
Division of Vascular Surgery
University of Pittsburgh Medical Center
Pittsburgh, Pennsylvania

Olamide Alabi, MD, FACS
Assistant Professor of Surgery
Division of Vascular Surgery and Endovascular Therapy
Department of Surgery
Emory University School of Medicine
Atlanta, Georgia

Adham N. Abou Ali, MD
Division of Vascular Surgery
Department of Surgery
University of Pittsburgh Medical Center
Pittsburgh, Pennsylvania

Shipra Arya, MD, SM
Associate Professor of Surgery
Division of Vascular Surgery
Department of Surgery
Stanford University School of Medicine
Stanford, California
Section Chief, Vascular Surgery
VA Palo Alto Health Care System
Palo Alto, California

Bernadette Aulivola, MD, MS, RVT, RPVI
Professor
Department of Surgery
Loyola University Stritch School of Medicine
Director, Division of Vascular Surgery and Endovascular Therapy
Department of Surgery
Loyola University Medical Center
Maywood, Illinois

Kellie R. Brown, MD
Professor of Surgery, with Tenure
Division of Vascular and Endovascular Surgery
The Medical College of Wisconsin
Milwaukee, Wisconsin

Christopher Burke, MD
Assistant Professor of Cardiac Surgery
Department of Cardiac Surgery
University of Washington
Seattle, Washington

Ruth L. Bush, MD, JD, MPH, FACS
Associate Dean for Medical Education
Professor
University of Houston College of Medicine
Houston, Texas
Vascular Surgeon
Department of Surgery
Central Texas VA Healthcare System
Temple, Texas

Rabih A. Chaer, MD, MSc
Professor of Surgery
Department of Surgery
University of Pittsburgh Medical Center
Pittsburgh, Pennsylvania

Venita Chandra, MD, FACS
Clinical Associate Professor of Surgery
Division of Vascular Surgery
Department of Surgery
Stanford University School of Medicine
Stanford, California

Mark F. Conrad, MD, MMsc
Associate Professor of Surgery
Department of Surgery
Harvard Medical School
Boston, Massachusetts
Chief, Vascular and Endovascular Surgery
Department of Surgery
St. Elizabeth's Hospital
Brighton, Massachusetts

Esmaeel Reza Dadashzadeh, MD, MS
Vascular Surgery Fellow
Department of Vascular Surgery
Washington University School of Medicine
Saint Louis, Missouri

Ronald L. Dalman, MD
Walter Clifford Chidester and Elsa Rooney Chidester Professor of Surgery
Department of Surgery
Stanford University School of Medicine
Stanford Healthcare
Stanford, California

Brian G. DeRubertis, MD
Assistant Professor
Chief, Division of Vascular and Endovascular Surgery
Department of Surgery
Weill Cornell Medicine
New York, New York

Peter DeVito, Jr., MD
Division of Vascular Surgery and Endovascular Surgery
Department of Surgery
University of Arizona Health Sciences
Tucson, Arizona

Kathryn Lambeth DiLosa, MD, MPH
Division of Vascular Surgery
Department of Surgery
University of California Davis School of Medicine
Sacramento, California

Shernaz S. Dossabhoy, MD, MBA
Division of Vascular Surgery
Department of Surgery
Stanford University School of Medicine
Stanford, California

Anahita Dua, MD, MSc, MBA
Assistant Professor
Division of Vascular Surgery
Department of Surgery
Harvard Medical School
Vascular Surgeon
Massachusetts General Hospital
Boston, Massachusetts

Audra A. Duncan, MD, FACS, FRCSC
Professor
Department of Surgery
Western University
Chair/Chief, Division of Vascular Surgery
London Health Sciences Centre
London, Ontario, Canada

Javairiah Fatima, MD, FACS, RPVI, DFSVS
Associate Professor of Surgery
Georgetown University School of Medicine
Co-Director of Complex Aortic Center
Department of Vascular Surgery
MedStar Heart and Vascular Institute
Washington Hospital Center
Washington, D.C.

Arash Fereydooni, MD, MS, MHS
Department of Vascular Surgery
Stanford University School of Medicine
Stanford, California

Julie Ann Freischlag, MD
CEO, Atrium Health Wake Forest Baptist
Dean, Wake Forest University School of Medicine
CAO, Atrium Enterprise
Department of Vascular and Endovascular Surgery
Wake Forest University School of Medicine
Winston-Salem, North Carolina

Elizabeth Leigh George, MD, MSc
Division of Vascular Surgery
Department of Surgery
Stanford University School of Medicine
Stanford, California

Ashley R. Gutwein, MD
Assistant Professor of Surgery
Department of Vascular Surgery
Indiana University School of Medicine
Indianapolis, Indiana

E. John Harris, Jr., MD
Professor
Division of Vascular Surgery
Department of Surgery
Stanford University School of Medicine
Stanford Healthcare
Stanford, California

Joseph Patrick Hart, MD, MHL, FACS
Associate Professor of Surgery and Radiology
Division of Vascular and Endovascular Surgery
Department of Surgery
The Medical College of Wisconsin
Froedtert Hospital
Milwaukee, Wisconsin

Stephen Heisler, DPM, MHSA
Podiatrist
Department of Surgery
University of North Carolina School of Medicine
Chapel Hill, North Carolina

Thomas S. Huber, MD, PhD
Edward R. Woodward Professor and Chief
Division of Vascular Surgery
Department of Surgery
University of Florida College of Medicine
Gainesville, Florida

Misty D. Humphries, MD, MAS, RPVI, FSVS, FACS
Associate Professor of Surgery
Department of Surgery
University of California Davis School of Medicine
Sacramento, California

Jeffrey Jim, MD, MPHS
Chair, Vascular and Endovascular Surgery
Minneapolis Heart Institute
Abbott Northwestern Hospital
Minneapolis, Minnesota

Erika R. Ketteler, MD, MA
Associate Professor
Department of Surgery
University of New Mexico School of Medicine
Chief, Vascular Surgery
Albuquerque VA Medical Center
Albuquerque, New Mexico

Sharon C. Kiang, MD
Chief, Vascular and Endovascular Surgery
Chair, Institutional Review Board
Medical Director, Non-Invasive Vascular Laboratory
Associate Professor of Surgery
Department of General Surgery
Division of Vascular and Endovascular Surgery
Loma Linda Veterans Healthcare System
Loma Linda, California

Young Kim, MD, MS
Vascular Surgery Clinical Fellow
Division of Vascular and Endovascular Surgery
Massachusetts General Hospital
Harvard Medical School
Boston, Massachusetts

Dean Edward Klinger, MD, FACS
Professor of Surgery
Department of Surgery
The Medical College of Wisconsin
Milwaukee, Wisconsin

Lindsey Marie Korepta, MD, RPVI
Assistant Professor of Surgery
Division of Vascular and Endovascular Surgery
Department of Surgery
Loyola University Stritch School of Medicine
Loyola University Medical Center
Maywood, Illinois

Ashley Nicole Krepline, MD
Department of Surgery
The Medical College of Wisconsin
Milwaukee, Wisconsin

Nathan W. Kugler, MD
Assistant Professor
Division of Vascular Surgery
Department of Surgery
The Medical College of Wisconsin
Froedtert Memorial Lutheran Hospital
Milwaukee, Wisconsin

Gregory J. Landry, MD
Professor and Chief, Vascular Surgery
Department of Surgery
Oregon Health & Science University
Portland, Oregon

Cheong Jun Lee, MD
Associate Professor
Department of Surgery
University of Chicago
Chicago, Illinois
Division Chief, Vascular Surgery
Department of Surgery
NorthShore University HealthSystem
Evanston, Illinois

Jason T. Lee, MD
Professor
Department of Surgery
Stanford University School of Medicine
Chief, Division of Vascular Surgery
Department of Surgery
Stanford Healthcare
Stanford, California

Meryl Simon Logan, MD
Adjunct Assistant Professor
Department of Surgery
Texas A&M University College of Medicine
Vascular Surgeon
Department of Surgery
Central Texas Veterans Health Care System
Temple, Texas

Diletta Loschi, MD
Contract Lecturer
Medical Assistant
Department of Cardiothoracic Surgery
Vita-Salute University, San Raffaele Scientific Institute
Milan, Italy

Gregory A. Magee, MD, MSc, FACS, FSVS
Assistant Professor of Surgery
Division of Vascular Surgery and Endovascular Therapy
Department of Surgery
Keck School of Medicine of the University of Southern California
Los Angeles, California

Robyn A. Macsata, MD†

Germano Melissano, MD
Professor, Chair of Vascular Surgery
Department of Vascular Surgery
Vita-Salute San Raffaele University
Milan, Italy

Matthew W. Mell, MD, MS
Professor and Chief
Division of Vascular Surgery
Department of Surgery
University of California Davis School of Medicine
Sacramento, California

Erica L. Mitchell, MD, MEd
Professor and Interim Chief, Vascular and Endovascular Surgery
Department of Surgery
University of Tennessee Health & Science Center
Medical Director, Vascular & Endovascular Surgery
Elvis Presley Trauma Center
Regional One Health
Memphis, Tennessee

Mark D. Morasch, MD, FACS, RPVI
Chief, Vascular and Endovascular Surgery
Vascular Specialists at St. Mark's
St. Mark's Hospital
Salt Lake City, Utah

Courtney M. Morgan, MD
Assistant Professor of Surgery
Department of Vascular Surgery
University of Wisconsin School of Medicine and Public Health
University of Wisconsin Hospital Clinics
Madison, Wisconsin

†deceased

Raghu L. Motaganahalli, MD, FRCS, FACS
Professor
Division of Vascular Surgery
Department of Surgery
Indiana University School of Medicine
Indianapolis, Indiana

Robin B. Osofsky, MD
Department of Surgery
University of New Mexico School of Medicine
University of New Mexico Health Sciences Center
Albuquerque, New Mexico

Laura B. Pride, MMSc, PA-C
Medical College of Georgia
Athens, Georgia

Benjamin Pomy, MD
Department of Surgery
George Washington University Hospital
Washington, D.C.

Alyssa Jaesun Pyun, MD
Department of Surgery
Keck School of Medicine of the University of Southern California
Los Angeles, California

John E. Rectenwald, MD, MS
Professor of Surgery
Division of Vascular Surgery
Department of Surgery
University of Wisconsin School of Medicine and Public Health
Madison, Wisconsin

Kyle B. Reynolds, MD, RPVI
Assistant Professor of Surgery
Site Chief, MedStar Montgomery Medical Center
Department of Vascular Surgery
Georgetown University School of Medicine
Washington, D.C.

Enrico Rinaldi, MD
Chair, Department of Vascular Surgery
Vita-Salute San Raffaele University
San Raffaele Scientific Institute
Milan, Italy

Matthew John Rossi, MD
Department of Vascular Surgery
MedStar Washington Hospital Center
Washington, D.C.

Peter J. Rossi, MD
Professor and Chief, Division of Vascular and Endovascular Surgery
Department of Surgery
The Medical College of Wisconsin
Milwaukee, Wisconsin

Vincent Lopez Rowe, MD
Professor of Surgery
Department of Surgery
Keck School of Medicine of the University of Southern California
Los Angeles, California

Salvatore T. Scali, MD
Professor of Surgery
Division of Vascular and Endovascular Surgery
Department of Surgery
University of Florida College of Medicine
Staff Surgeon
Division of Vascular and Endovascular Surgery
Department of Surgery
University of Florida Health Shands Hospital
Gainesville, Florida

Oonagh H. Scallan, MD
Western University
London, Ontario, Canada

Malachi G. Sheahan, MD
Claude C. Craighead, Jr. Professor and Chair
Division of Vascular and Endovascular Surgery
Louisiana State University Health Sciences Center
New Orleans, Louisiana

Benjamin W. Starnes, MD, FACS, DFVS
Professor and Chief, Division of Vascular Surgery
Department of Surgery
University of Washington
Harborview Medical Center
Seattle, Washington

Kathryn Marie Swanson, MD
Department of Surgery
Louisiana State University Health Sciences Center
New Orleans, Louisiana

Matthew P. Sweet, MD, MS
Associate Professor
Division of Vascular Surgery
Department of Surgery
University of Washington
University of Washington Medical Center
Seattle, Washington

Robert W. Thompson, MD
Professor of Surgery
Director, Center for Thoracic Outlet Syndrome
Section of Vascular Surgery
Department of Surgery
Washington University School of Medicine
Attending Surgeon
Department of Surgery
Barnes-Jewish Hospital
Saint Louis, Missouri

Gabriela Velazquez-Ramirez, MD, FACS
Associate Professor
Department of Vascular and Endovascular Surgery
Wake Forest University School of Medicine
Winston-Salem, North Carolina

Harold Davis Waller, MD
Department of Surgery
Massachusetts General Hospital
Boston, Massachusetts

Fred Arthur Weaver, MD, MMM
Professor
Department of Surgery
Keck School of Medicine of the University of Southern California
Chief, Division of Vascular Surgery and Endovascular Therapy
Department of Surgery
Keck Hospital of USC
Los Angeles, California

Lauren N. West-Livingston, MD, PhD, MSL
Division of Vascular and Endovascular Surgery
Duke University School of Medicine
Department of Surgery
Durham, North Carolina

Edward Y. Woo, MD
Professor of Surgery
Georgetown University School of Medicine
President
MedStar Medical Group
Washington, D.C

Jacob C. Wood, MD
Assistant Professor
Department of Surgery
University of North Carolina School of Medicine
Chapel Hill, North Carolina

Mohamed A. Zayed, MD, PhD
Associate Professor with Tenure
Department of Surgery, Radiology, Molecular Cell
Department of Biology & Biomedical Engineering
Department of Surgery, Section of Vascular Surgery
Washington University School of Medicine
Department of Surgery
Barnes-Jewish Hospital
Saint Louis, Missouri

Wei Zhou, MD
Professor and Chief, Vascular Surgery
Department of Surgery
University of Arizona
Banner-University Medical Center
Tucson, Arizona

PART 7 OPERATIVE TECHNIQUES IN TRAUMA AND CRITICAL CARE

Christofer B. Anderson, MD
Department of Surgery
Tulane University School of Medicine
New Orleans, Louisiana

Jeffery H. Anderson, MD
Assistant Professor of Clinical Surgery
Department of Surgery
Lewis Katz School of Medicine at Temple University
Philadelphia, Pennsylvania

Jessica H. Beard, MD, MPH, FACS
Assistant Professor
Division of Trauma Surgery and Surgical Critical Care
Department of Surgery
Lewis Katz School of Medicine at Temple University
Philadelphia, Pennsylvania

Bennett J. Berning, MD
Assistant Professor
Department of Surgery
University of Nebraska
Trauma and Acute Care Surgeon
Department of Surgery
University of Nebraska Medical Center
Omaha, Nebraska

Walter L. Biffl, MD
Division Head, Trauma/Acute Care Surgery
Vice-Chair Department of Surgery
Scripps Clinic Medical Group
Trauma Medical Director
Department of Surgery
Scripps Memorial Hospital La Jolla
La Jolla, California

Kevin M. Bradley, MD, MBA, FACS, FCCM
Section Chief of Trauma
Department of Surgery
ChristianaCare
Newark, Delaware

Tejal Sudhirkumar Brahmbhatt, MD
Assistant Professor
Department of Surgery
Boston University School of Medicine
Chief of Surgical Critical Care
Boston Medical Center
Boston, Massachusetts

Karen J. Brasel, MD, MPH
Professor
Department of Surgery
Oregon Health & Science University
Portland, Oregon

Clay Cothren Burlew, MD
Professor of Surgery
University of Colorado School of Medicine
Director, Surgical Intensive Care Unit
Program Director, Surgical Critical Care Fellowship
Program Director, Trauma & Acute Care Surgery Fellowship
Denver Health Medical Center
Denver, Colorado

James P. Byrne, MD, PhD
Assistant Professor of Surgery
Division of Trauma and Acute Care Surgery
Department of Surgery
Johns Hopkins Hospital
Baltimore, Maryland

S. Ariane Christie, MD
Trauma, Acute and Critical Care Surgery Fellow
Department of Trauma and Acute Care Surgery
University of Pittsburgh Medical Center
Pittsburgh, Pennsylvania

John J. Como, MD, MPH
Professor of Surgery
Department of Surgery
The Cleveland Clinic Lerner College of Medicine of Case Western University
MetroHealth Medical Center
Cleveland, Ohio

Jennifer T. Cone, MD, MHS
Assistant Professor
Department of Surgery
University of Chicago
Chicago, Illinois

Martin A. Croce, MD, FACS
Professor of Surgery
Department of Surgery
University of Tennessee Health Science Center
Sr. Vice President and Chief Medical Officer
Regional One Health
Memphis, Tennessee

Elizabeth Dauer, MD
Associate Professor of Surgery
Department of Surgery
Lewis Katz School of Medicine at Temple University
Temple University Hospital
Philadelphia, Pennsylvania

Kimberly A. Davis, MD, MBA
Professor of Surgery
Chief, Division of General Surgery, Trauma and Surgical Critical Care
Department of Surgery
Yale School of Medicine
New Haven, Connecticut

Marc Anthony de Moya, MD
Professor
Department of Surgery
The Medical College of Wisconsin
Chief of Trauma and Acute Care Surgery
Froedtert Trauma Center
Milwaukee, Wisconsin

Tracey A. Dechert, MD
Associate Professor of Surgery
Department of Surgery
Boston University School of Medicine
Director, Surgical Intensive Care
Department of Trauma and Acute Care Surgery
Boston Medical Center
Boston, Massachusetts

Christopher J. Dente, MD
Professor of Surgery
Department of Surgery
Emory University
Senior Surgeon
Department of Surgery
Grady Memorial Hospital
Atlanta, Georgia

Rushabh Prakash Dev, MD
Trauma Fellow
Division of Acute Care Surgery
Department of Surgery
McGovern Medical School at University of Texas
Red Duke Trauma Institute
Houston, Texas

Sharmila Dissanaike, MD, FACS, FCCM
Peter C. Canizaro Chair and Professor
Department of Surgery
Texas Tech University Health Sciences Center
Lubbock, Texas

John Donkersloot, MD
Surgical Critical Care Fellow
Department of Surgery
University of Michigan Medical School
Michigan Medicine
Ann Arbor, Michigan

Adam Joseph Doyle, MD
Associate Professor of Surgery
Associate Program Director Vascular Surgery Integrated Residency Program
Medical Director Noninvasive Vascular Laboratory
Department of Surgery
University of Rochester School of Medicine and Dentistry
Vascular Surgeon
Department of Surgery
University of Rochester Medical Center
Rochester, New York

David T. Efron, MD
Professor of Surgery
Department of Surgery
University of Maryland School of Medicine
Medical Director and Chief of Trauma
R. Adams Cowley Shock Trauma Center
Baltimore, Maryland

Paula Ferrada, MD, FACS, FCCM, MASE
Professor of Medical Education
University of Virginia
Division and System Chief, Trauma and Acute Care Surgery
Inova Healthcare System
Falls Church, Virginia

Joseph M. Galante, MD, MBA, FACS
Professor of Surgery
Department of Surgery
University of California Davis School of Medicine
Sacramento California

Arvin C. Gee, MD, PhD
Assistant Professor
Department of Surgery
Oregon Health & Science University
Portland, Oregon

Mitchell D. Gorman, DO
Trauma and Surgical Critical Care Fellow
Department of Surgery
Sidney Kimmel Medical College at Thomas Jefferson University
Philadelphia, Pennsylvania

Melike N. Harfouche, MD
Assistant Professor
Department of Surgery
University of Maryland School of Medicine
Attending Surgeon
R. Adams Cowley Shock Trauma Center
University of Maryland Medical Center
Baltimore, Maryland

John Andrew Harvin, MD, MS
Associate Professor of Surgery
Department of Surgery
McGovern Medical School at University of Texas
Memorial Hermann Texas Medical Center
Houston, Texas

Alex Helkin, MD
Assistant Professor
Department of Surgery
The Ohio State University Wexner Medical Center
Columbus, Ohio

David I. Hindin, MD, MS
Surgical Critical Care Fellow
Department of Surgery
Stanford University Hospital
Stanford, California

Natalie J. Hodges, MD, MPH
Department of Surgery
School of Medicine
Texas Tech University Health Services Center
Lubbock, Texas

Kenji Inaba, MD, FACS
Professor of Surgery
Department of Surgery
Vice Chair, Program Director Department of Surgery
Chief of Trauma and Critical Care
LAC+USC Medical Center
University of Southern California
Los Angeles, California

Christina L. Jacovides, MD
Fellow
Division of Traumatology, Surgical Critical Care and Emergency Surgery
Department of Surgery
Perelman School of Medicine at the University of Pennsylvania
Philadelphia, Pennsylvania

Sagar S. Kadakia, MD
Assistant Professor of Surgery
Division of Acute Care Surgery
Thomas Jefferson University Hospital
Philadelphia, Pennsylvania

Matthew P. Kochuba, MD
Assistant Professor of Surgery
Department of Surgery
University of Florida College of Medicine
Jacksonville, Florida

Rosemary A. Kozar, MD, PhD
Professor of Surgery
Department of Surgery
University of Maryland School of Medicine
Co-Director, Shock Trauma Anesthesia Research (STAR) Center
Shock Trauma Department
Baltimore, Maryland

Claire Lauer, MD
Department of General Surgery
Geisinger Medical Center
Danville, Pennsylvania

Irma J. Lengu, MD
Assistant Professor
Department of Urology
The Cleveland Clinic Lerner College of Medicine of Case Western University
Department of Surgery
MetroHealth Medical Center
Cleveland, Ohio

Louis Jude Magnotti, MD, MS
Professor
Department of Surgery
University of Tennessee Health Science Center
Memphis, Tennessee

Zoë Maher, MD
Associate Professor of Surgery
Department of Surgery
Lewis Katz School of Medicine at Temple University
Temple University Hospital
Philadelphia, Pennsylvania

Joshua A. Marks, MD, FACS
Associate Professor of Surgery
Division of Acute Care Surgery
Program Director, Surgical Critical Care Fellowship
Associate Program Director, General Surgery Residency
Sidney Kimmel Medical College at Thomas Jefferson University
Philadelphia, Pennsylvania

Joseph P. Minei, MD, MBA
Professor and Executive Vice Chair
Department of Surgery
UT Southwestern Medical Center
Surgeon-in-Chief
Parkland Health and Hospital System
Dallas, Texas

Michael J. Nabozny, MD
Assistant Professor
Department of Surgery
University of Rochester School of Medicine and Dentistry
Rochester, New York

Caroline Park, MD, MPH, FACS
Assistant Professor
Department of Surgery
University of Texas Southwestern Medical Center
Dallas, Texas

Pauline K. Park, MD
Professor
Department of Surgery
University of Michigan Medical School
Attending Physician
Co-Director, Surgical Intensive Care Unit
Department of Surgery
Michigan Medicine
Ann Arbor, Michigan

Devanshi D. Patel, MD
Department of Surgery
University of Tennessee Health Science Center
Memphis, Tennessee

Abhijit S. Pathak, MD, FACS, FCCM
Professor of Surgery
Department of Surgery
Lewis Katz School of Medicine at Temple University
Philadelphia, Pennsylvania

Andrew B. Peitzman, MD
Mark M. Ravitch Professor of Surgery
Department of Surgery
University of Pittsburgh School of Medicine
Chief, University of Pittsburgh Medical Center Trauma System
University of Pittsburgh Medical Center, Presbyterian
Pittsburgh, Pennsylvania

Craig J. Profant, MD
Department of Surgery
Temple University Hospital
Philadelphia, Pennsylvania

Lisa Rae, MD, FACS
Associate Professor of Surgery
Department of Surgery
Lewis Katz School of Medicine at Temple University
Medical Director, Temple Burn Center
Temple University Hospital
Philadelphia, Pennsylvania

Lisbi del Valle Rivas Ramirez, MD
Assistant Professor
Department of Surgery
Johns Hopkins University
Baltimore, Maryland
Trauma and Acute Care Surgeon
Department of Surgery
Suburban Hospital
Bethesda, Maryland

Jennifer E. Reid, MD, MS
Fellow
Department of Surgery
University of California, San Francisco
San Francisco, California

Patrick M. Reilly, MD, FACS
C. William Schwab Professor of Surgery
Perelman School of Medicine at the University of Pennsylvania
Philadelphia, Pennsylvania

Aaron Powel Richman, MD
Assistant Professor
Department of Surgery
Boston University School of Medicine
Trauma & Critical Care Surgeon
Department of Surgery
Boston Medical Center
Boston, Massachusetts

Kaitlin A. Ritter, MD
Trauma/Critical Care Fellow
Department of General Surgery
University of Colorado School of Medicine
Denver Health Medical Center
Denver, Colorado

Selwyn O. Rogers, Jr., MD, MPH
Professor
Department of Surgery
University of Chicago Medicine
Chicago, Illinois

Lucy Ruangvoravat, MD, FACS
Assistant Professor
Division of General Surgery, Trauma, and Surgical Critical Care
Department of Surgery
Yale School of Medicine
New Haven, Connecticut

Noelle N. Saillant, MD, FACS
Assistant Professor of Surgery
Division of Trauma, Emergency Surgery and Surgical Critical Care
Department of Surgery
Harvard Medical School
Massachusetts General Hospital
Boston, Massachusetts

Thomas A. Santora, MD, MBA
Professor of Surgery
Lewis Katz School of Medicine at Temple University
Interim Chair, Department of Surgery
Temple University Hospital
Philadelphia, Pennsylvania

Morgan Schellenberg, MD, MPH, FRCSC, FACS
Assistant Professor
Division of Acute Care Surgery
LAC+USC Medical Center
University of Southern California
Los Angeles, California

Mark J. Seamon, MD, FACS
Director of Research, Director of Education
Professor of Surgery
Division of Traumatology, Surgical Critical Care and Emergency Surgery
Department of Surgery
Perelman School of Medicine at the University of Pennsylvania
Philadelphia, Pennsylvania

Carrie Sims, MD, PhD
Professor
Division Chair, Trauma, Critical Care and Burns
Department of Surgery
The Ohio State University Wexner Medical Center
Columbus, Ohio

Lars Ola Sjoholm, MD
Associate Professor
Department of Surgery
Temple University Hospital
Philadelphia, Pennsylvania

Randi N. Smith, MD, MPH
Assistant Professor
Department of Surgery
Emory University
Trauma Surgeon
Department of Acute Care Surgery
Grady Memorial Hospital
Atlanta, Georgia

David A. Spain, MD
Professor and Chief, Acute Care Surgery
Department of Surgery
Stanford University School of Medicine
Stanford, California

Nicole A. Stassen, MD, FACS, FCCM
Professor of Surgery
Department of Surgery
University of Rochester School of Medicine and Dentistry
Rochester, New York

Deborah M. Stein, MD, MPH
Professor
Department of Surgery
University of Maryland School of Medicine
Director of Critical Care Services
R. Adams Cowley Shock Trauma Center
University of Maryland Medical Center
Baltimore, Maryland

Kelly M. Sutter, MD
Fellow
Department of Trauma & Surgical Critical Care
MedStar Washington Hospital Center
Washington, D.C.

Sharven Taghavi, MD, MPH, MS, FACS
Assistant Professor of Surgery
Department of Surgery
Tulane University School of Medicine
New Orleans, Louisiana

Christopher Thacker, MD
Department of Surgery
Geisinger Medical Center
Danville, Pennsylvania

Christine T. Trankiem, MD, FACS
Associate Professor
Georgetown University School of Medicine
Chief, Trauma and Acute Care Surgery
Department of Surgery
MedStar Washington Hospital Center
Washington, D.C.

Denise Torres, MD, FACS
Division Chief
Acute Care Surgery
Geisinger Health System
Danville, Pennsylvania

Esther S. Tseng, MD, FACS
Assistant Professor
The Cleveland Clinic Lerner College of Medicine of Case Western University
Division of Trauma, Critical Care, Burns, and Emergency General Surgery
Department of Surgery
MetroHealth Medical Center
Cleveland, Ohio

Michael A. Vella, MD, MBA
Assistant Professor
Department of Surgery
University of Rochester School of Medicine and Dentistry
Rochester, New York

George C. Velmahos, MD, PhD, MSEd
John F. Burke Professor of Surgery
Harvard Medical School
Division of Trauma, Emergency Surgery and Surgical Critical Care
Department of Surgery
Massachusetts General Hospital
Boston, Massachusetts

Natalie M. Wall, MD
Department of General Surgery
Virginia Commonwealth University
Richmond, Virginia

Kojo Wallace, MD
Surgical Critical Care Fellow
Department of Surgery
Emory University School of Medicine
Grady Memorial Hospital
Atlanta, Georgia

Anne H. Warner, MD, FACS
Trauma, Acute Care, Surgical Critical Care Attending
Associate Medical Director, Surgical Critical Care
Department of Surgery
ChristianaCare
Newark, Delaware

Brian K. Yorkgitis, DO, FACS
Associate Professor of Surgery
Department of Surgery
University of Florida College of Medicine
Jacksonville, Florida

Valeda Yong, MD
Department of Surgery
Temple University Hospital
Philadelphia, Pennsylvania

Scott A. Zakaluzny, MD, FACS
Assistant Professor
Department of Surgery
Uniformed Services University
Bethesda, Maryland
Volunteer Assistance Clinical Professor
Department of Surgery
University of California Davis School of Medicine
Sacramento, California

Jeanette Zhang, MD
Assistant Professor of Surgery
Department of Surgery
University of Florida College of Medicine
Jacksonville, Florida

Preface

Operative interventions are complex, technically demanding, and rapidly evolving. *Operative Techniques in Surgery* seeks to provide highly visual step-by-step instructions to perform these complex tasks. This comprehensive text covers the multitude of approaches for the procedures including open and minimally invasive, endoscopic, endovascular, and percutaneous techniques.

The text is organized anatomically in sections covering esophageal and upper gastrointestinal surgery, hepatopancreaticobiliary surgery, colorectal surgery, breast surgery, endocrine surgery, trauma and critical care, and topics related to surgical oncology and modern approaches to vascular surgery. In this second edition, many chapters are augmented by video clips dynamically demonstrating the critical steps of the procedure.

The editors are renowned surgeons with expertise in their respective fields. Each is a leader in the discipline of surgery, each recognized for superb surgical judgment and outstanding operative skill. Breast surgery, endocrine procedures, and surgical oncology topics were edited by Dr. Michael S. Sabel of the University of Michigan. Esophageal, foregut, and upper gastrointestinal surgery topics were edited by Dr. Aurora D. Pryor of Stony University, with Dr. Steven J. Hughes of the University of Florida directing the section on hepatopancreaticobiliary surgery. Dr. Daniel Albo of University of Texas Rio Grande directed the section dedicated to colorectal surgery. Dr. Kellie R. Brown of Medical College of Wisconsin edited topics related to vascular surgery, including both open and endovascular approaches. New this year, we have added a section on Trauma and Critical Surgery, led by Dr. Amy J. Goldberg of Temple University.

In turn, the editors have recruited contributors that are world-renowned; the resulting volumes have a distinctly international flavor. Surgery is a visual discipline. *Operative Techniques in Surgery* is lavishly illustrated with a compelling combination of line art and intraoperative photography. The illustrated material provides a uniform style emphasizing clarity and strong, clean lines. Intraoperative photographs are taken from the perspective of the operating surgeon so that operations might be visualized as they would be performed. The accompanying text is intentionally sparse, with a focus on crucial operative details and important aspects of postoperative management and potential complications. The text is designed for surgeons at all levels of practice, from surgical residents to advanced practice fellows to surgeons of wide experience. *Operative Techniques in Surgery* would be possible only at Wolters Kluwer, an organization of unique vision, organization, and the talent of Brian Brown, executive editor, Keith Donnellan, senior acquisition editor, and Ashley Fischer, senior development editor.

I am deeply indebted to Dr. Michael W. Mulholland, a master surgeon and leader and the editor in chief of the first edition of *Operative Techniques in Surgery*. Without his leadership, this project would not have been successful. I am grateful to our new and returning section editors for their vison on how to make the second edition even more impactful. Curating and editing a major surgical techniques textbook during a worldwide pandemic has not been seamless, yet the outcome is masterful.

Mary T. Hawn, MD, MPH

Contents

Section III Surgery of the Pancreas

Section IV Surgery of the Spleen

Part 4 Operative Techniques in Colon and Rectal Surgery

Section I Surgery of the Small Intestine

Section II Surgery of the Colon, Appendix, Rectum, and Anus

Volume Two

Part 5 Operative Techniques in Breast, Endocrine, and Oncologic Surgery

Section I Breast Surgery

Video Contents List

Volume One

Part 3 Operative Techniques in Hepato-Pancreato-Biliary Surgery

Section I Surgery of the Biliary System

Section II Surgery of the Liver

Section III Surgery of the Pancreas

Part 5 Operative Techniques in Breast, Endocrine, and Oncologic Surgery

SECTION I: BREAST SURGERY

SECTION I: Breast Surgery

Chapter 1 Breast Cyst Aspiration

Rachel Louise McCaffrey

DEFINITION

- Cyst aspiration is a technique used to drain large or symptomatic breast cysts. If a cyst has complex architecture (eg, internal septations, cyst wall nodularity, or internal debris), there is benefit in aspiration to rule out malignancy; however, complex cysts are often accompanied by core needle biopsy (CNB) of nodular or solid portions. For the purpose of this chapter, simple cyst aspiration will be described.
- Breast cysts typically form due to involution or aging of ducts within the breast. Cysts are a common cause of palpable breast masses in premenopausal women in the fourth and fifth decade of life. In women under 40, additional benign pathology must be considered when a palpable breast mass is found. Cysts are well circumscribed, mobile, and can be tender to palpation.
- Historically and in remote-access areas, breast aspiration is used as a primary method of diagnosis for a new breast mass to determine solid vs cystic and malignant vs benign pathology. With modern imaging methods including mammogram and ultrasound, cysts are often identified prior to intervention (**FIGURE 1**).

DIFFERENTIAL DIAGNOSIS

- Benign (fibroadenoma, fibrocystic change, benign appearing calcifications, cysts)
- Malignant (cystic adenocarcinoma)

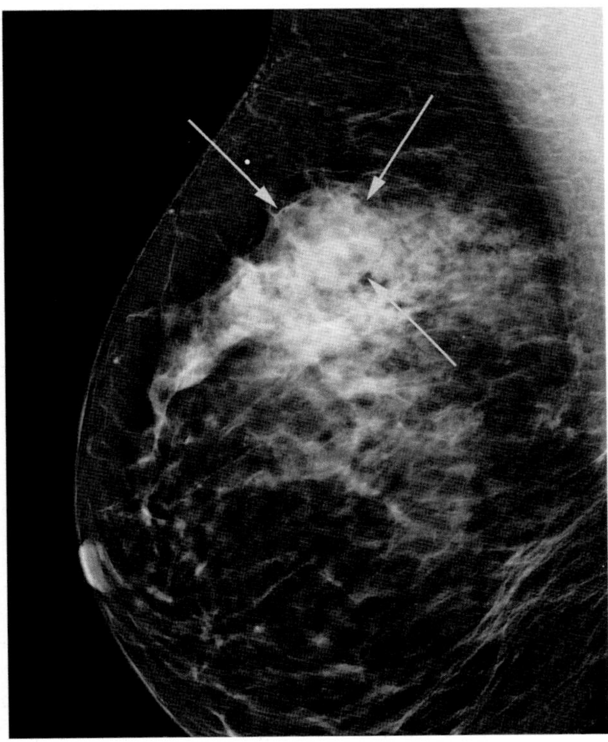

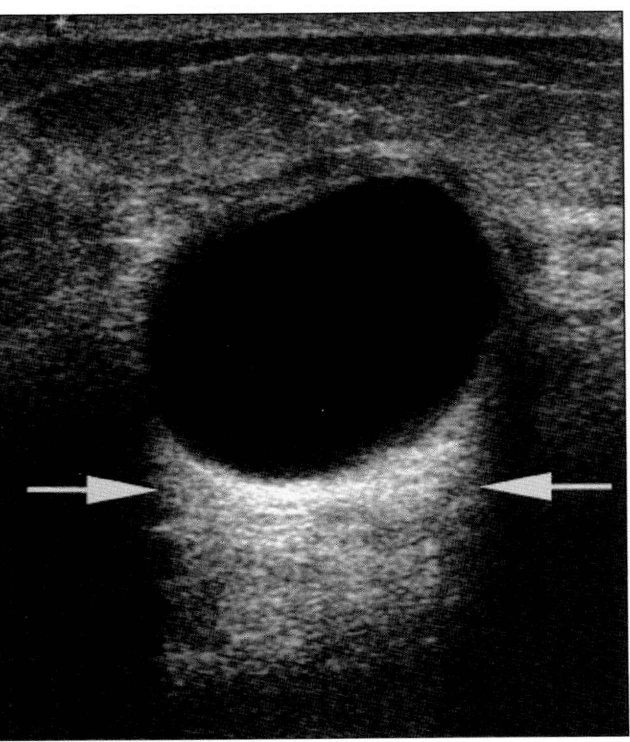

FIGURE 1 ● Simple cyst. **A,** Right breast mediolateral oblique (MLO) digital mammogram. A simple cyst. The isodense cyst (*arrows*) has sharp borders and no calcifications. **B,** Right breast ultrasound of the lesion **(A)**. This is the classic appearance of a benign simple cyst. The cyst is a round well-circumscribed anechoic mass with very thin cyst–parenchymal transition. Posterior acoustic enhancement (*arrows*) is commonly found immediately posterior to a cyst. (Reprinted with permission from Smith WL. *Radiology 101*. 4th ed. Wolters Kluwer; 2014. Figure 11.4.)

PATIENT HISTORY AND PHYSICAL FINDINGS

- A focused history and physical exam should be obtained from the patient including how the mass was first discovered (ie, on self-examination or via routine screening), associated symptoms such as nipple discharge or pain, palpable mass, changes in mass size, or fluctuations with menstrual cycle. Any prior history of breast trauma or malignancies should be evaluated. The physical examination should include palpation of the mass/cyst, both breasts and both axillary lymph node basins. The exam should also include a skin evaluation for changes in color, warmth, thickening or edema, as well as changes to the nipple-areola complex.
- There are no absolute contraindications to cyst aspiration; however, patients on anticoagulants or antiplatelet agents may be asked to hold these medications prior to the procedure to reduce the risk of hematoma.

IMAGING AND OTHER DIAGNOSTIC STUDIES

- On review of imaging, note should be taken of the cyst size, cyst depth, as well as any complex cystic features (septations, wall nodularity, heterogeneous cyst contents).
- Noncomplex cysts are benign in 99% of cases. The risk of malignancy increases with more complex features found on imaging; approach to complex cysts is discussed later in this chapter.
- For this review, we will focus on techniques for nonimage guided aspiration of cysts in the breast. Although aspiration can be performed on palpable cysts, using preprocedural imaging, if available, is useful to determine the best needle trajectory and insertion depth. The imaging can offer guidance on depth of needle insertion depending on the mass size, location relative to the chest wall or skin, and the overall quadrant location in the breast.
- If preprocedural imaging has not been performed or is not available, point-of-care ultrasound to confirm the presence of a cystic lesion and its resolution after aspiration can be very helpful. If imaging is not available, as in rural or underserved settings, proceeding with an aspiration attempt is reasonable given the low risk and higher benefit of diagnostic value.

NONOPERATIVE MANAGEMENT

- For patients who are asymptomatic and/or decline cyst aspiration, interval imaging and examination should be obtained at 6 months to document stability. Of note, <5% of breast cysts, both complex and noncomplex, harbor malignancy and <1% of simple cysts harbor malignancy. Increased concern for malignancy includes rapid growth of cysts, multiple cyst septations on imaging, internal echoes on ultrasound, wall nodularity on imaging, both solid and cystic components on imaging, and any posterior shadowing on ultrasound (**FIGURE 2**).[1,2] Patients with these findings should be encouraged to undergo aspiration for cytologic analysis and possibly CNB of solid components of the cyst.

SURGICAL MANAGEMENT

Beyond Aspiration

- Alternatives to cyst aspiration include cyst excision with care to remove the entire cyst wall.
- Proceeding to excisional biopsy is appropriate if the cyst has reaccumulated in a 4 to 6 week period after initial aspiration attempts, the cyst is complex, or if there is concern for malignancy after cyst aspiration.
- If during the aspiration the fluid is bloody, particularly tenacious, or no fluid can be evacuated due to solid components, all these are indications for excisional breast biopsy.
- If the fluid is bloody or thickened, cytologic analysis of the aspirate may be of benefit.
- If aspirate cytology demonstrates atypical or malignant cells—this is also cause for excisional biopsy to provide tissue architecture for definitive pathological diagnosis and immunohistochemical analysis. A general algorithm for management is included in **FIGURE 3**.[3,4]
- If the cyst has complex features such as wall nodularity, multiple septations, or solid components within or adjacent to the cyst, consider CNB in addition to cyst aspiration. The core biopsy and cyst fluid should be sent for pathology and cytology, respectively, to rule out malignancy. A biopsy clip should be placed at the time of CNB to facilitate excisional biopsy if atypia or malignancy is present on pathology.

PREOPERATIVE PLANNING

- Discuss risks, benefits, and reasoning behind cyst aspiration. Aspiration of large, tender cysts can provide immediate symptomatic relief to patients, but this is not guaranteed if underlying mastodynia is present.
- Use any preprocedural imaging coupled with physical exam findings to determine needle insertion trajectory and depth. Often if imaging is present prior to procedure, a rough volumetric assessment can be determined for larger cysts. This thought process can aid in the selection of larger syringes for compete cyst evacuation.
- If preprocedural imaging demonstrates complex cystic components, a determination must be made if the patient would benefit more from image-guided simultaneous cyst aspiration and CNB for definitive diagnosis.
- Ensure the patient has stopped NSAID and anticoagulants accordingly to reduce hematoma risk.

POSITIONING

- For in-office cyst aspiration, the patient should be positioned supine on the procedure table, with arms at the patient's side if the cyst is easily isolated with the surgeon's nondominant hand.
- If the cyst is very large or deeper within the breast, having the patient raise their ipsilateral arm overhead may provide tension to the breast to help stabilize the cyst to be aspirated.

Approaches

- Cyst aspiration is approached with a needle and syringe technique with fluid sent for cytologic analysis as needed, it is best to plan to have all equipment available for cytologic preparation at the time of aspiration.
- Of note, the techniques used for cyst aspiration also translate well to in-office seroma or abscess aspiration.
- The aspiration needle should be guided tangential to patient's chest wall whenever feasible to avoid pectoral muscle injury and (rarely) pneumothorax.

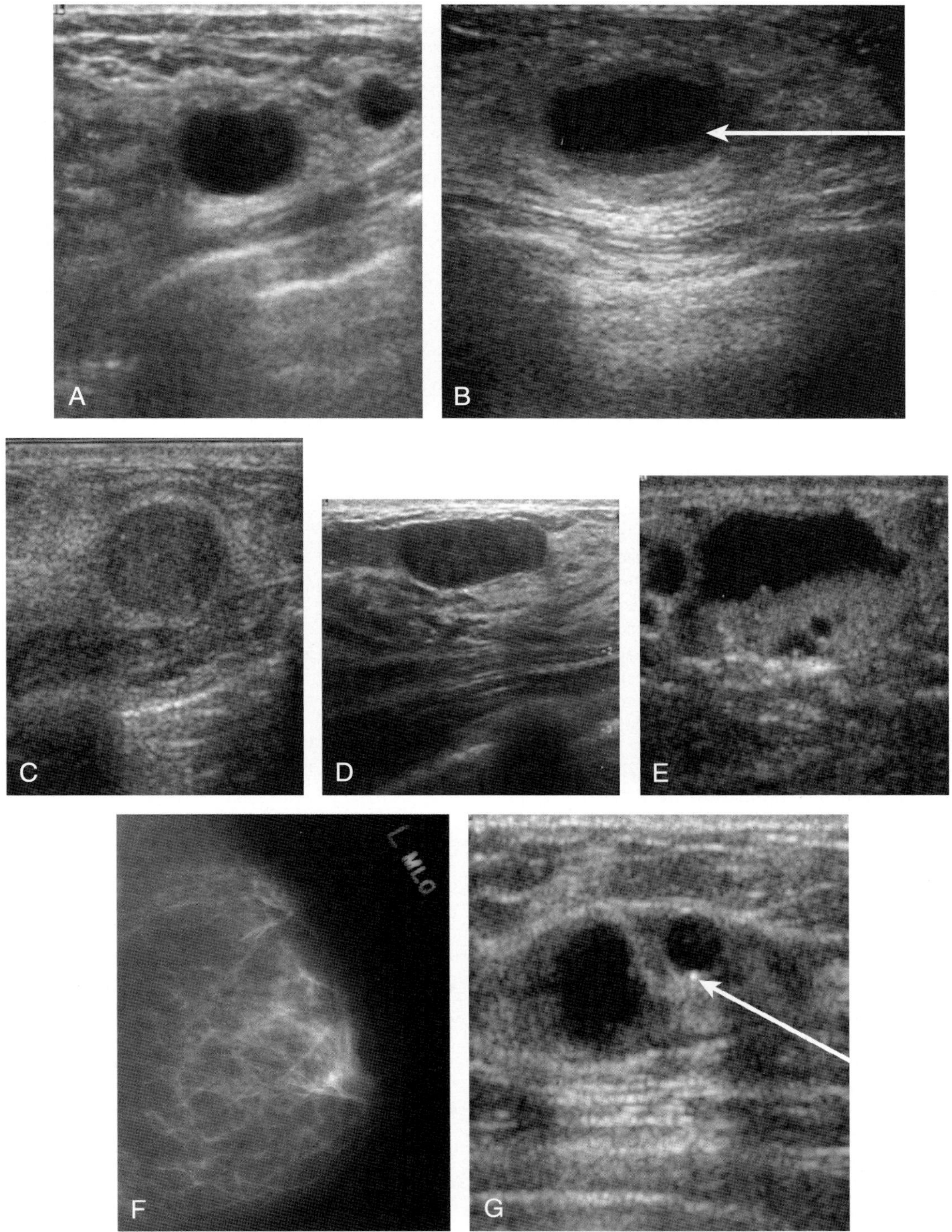

FIGURE 2 ● Complex cyst image findings. Cysts: simple, complicated, and complex. **A,** Simple cysts. Anechoic, circumscribed, oval or macrolobulated masses with acoustic enhancement satisfy the requirements for simple cysts. No action is necessary unless the patient is symptomatic. Management: routine follow-up for the age of the patient. **B,** Complicated cysts may have fluid-debris levels (arrow) that shift slowly as the patient changes her position, as in this case. Aspiration may not be necessary. **C** and **D,** Complicated cysts may have low-level internal echoes throughout, and these masses may be difficult to distinguish from benign solid masses, such as fibroadenomas. The mass on the left **(C)** is a complicated cyst; on the right **(D)**, similar in appearance, is a fibroadenoma. **E** and **F,** Complex cystic mass: hematomas. Complex cystic masses have echogenic and anechoic components. They may have thick septa and mural nodules. This palpable posttraumatic hematoma **(E)** is an example. The abnormality is inapparent on the mammogram **(F)**, where a small metallic marker has been placed on the skin to denote the palpable area. **G,** Complex cystic mass. This mass has benign-appearing shape, margins, and parallel orientation. Its heterogeneity led to ultrasonography-guided core biopsy with histopathologic diagnosis of fibrocystic disease. The echogenic focus (*arrow*) is a calcification. (Reprinted with permission from Harris JR, Lippman ME, Morrow M, et al. *Diseases of the Breast*. 3rd ed. Wolters Kluwer; 2005. Figure 12.3.)

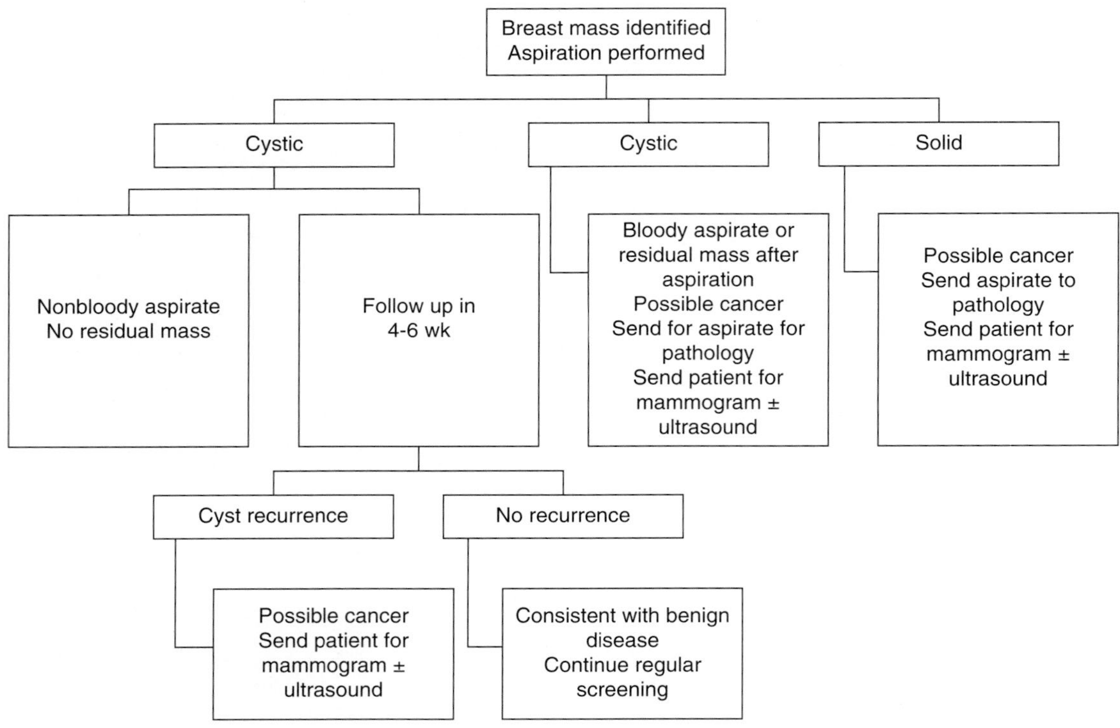

FIGURE 3 ● Algorithm for non–image-guided breast mass aspiration. Assumes no preprocedural imaging.[5]

Equipment for Cyst Aspiration

- Cleaning solution (chlorhexidine or povidone iodine)
- 1% lidocaine without epinephrine
- Optional: 8.4% bicarbonate solution
- 3-mL syringe for anesthetic
- 23- and 25-gauge needle for anesthetic infiltration
- 10 to 20 mL syringe for aspiration
- 1.5-in, 21- or 22-gauge needle for aspiration
- Cytologic fixative fluid
- Slides and slide slip cover

TECHNIQUES

- Palpate the breast to relocalize the cyst. Mark the needle insertion site on the skin.
- Clean the site appropriately and drape.
- With aseptic technique, infiltrate the skin with lidocaine/bicarbonate solution with a 25-gauge needle to create a skin wheel. If the cyst is deeper, transition to a 1.5-in 23-gauge needle to introduce more local anesthetic.
- Prep the aspiration needle with a 1.5-in 21-gauge needle by pulling back the plunger to allow some air into the syringe. This will allow for expulsion of any residual fluid in the needle for cytology analysis if needed.
- Stabilize the breast with the nondominant hand using thumb and index finger.
- Insert the aspiration needle and syringe by holding the syringe as if for injection in the palm and use the thumb or fourth finger to pull back on the plunger and generate negative pressure (**FIGURE 4**).
- Insert the aspiration needle along the trajectory of injected anesthetic into the cyst.
- During aspiration, move the nondominant hand to palpate the aspirated area to assess for resolution of the palpable cyst.
- If nonbloody straw or green colored serous fluid is obtained, this is likely benign. If confirmation of complete cyst collapse can be obtained by palpation, point-of-care ultrasound or postprocedural imaging, this fluid does not require cytological analysis.
- If the fluid is bloody, particularly thick, the residual cyst is palpable on exam, or there is clinical concern for malignancy, send the fluid for cytological analysis (**FIGURE 5**).
- For cytology, all fluid from the aspiration syringe and needle should be injected into a specimen cup containing an alcohol-based preservative as PreservCyt or SurePath fluid. This method is comparable to more historic approaches of slide smears prepped during the procedure.
- For solid lesions, a CNB or fine needle aspiration biopsy can be performed, please refer to Part 5, Chapter 3 for reference.
- Hold pressure over the site of aspiration for 5 minutes and place a bandage over the needle insertion site.
- Document the site of aspiration (clock position on the breast as well as distance in centimeters from the nipple).

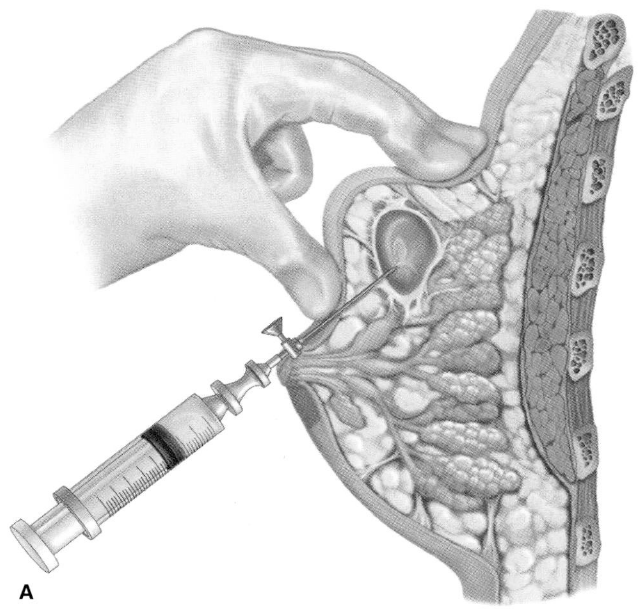

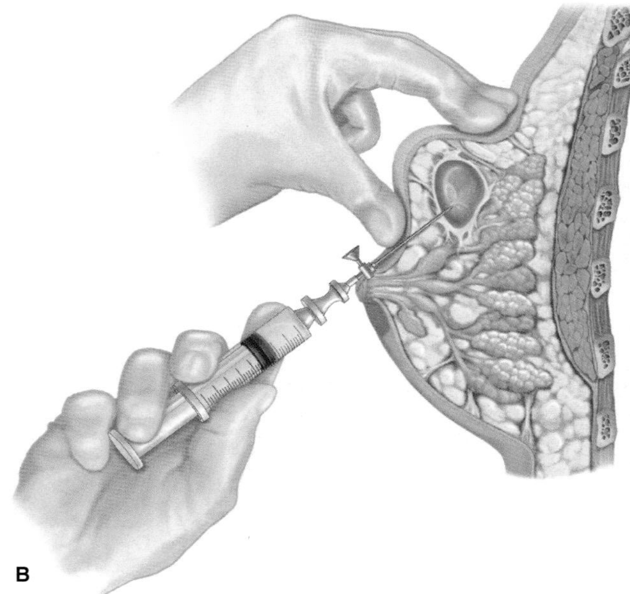

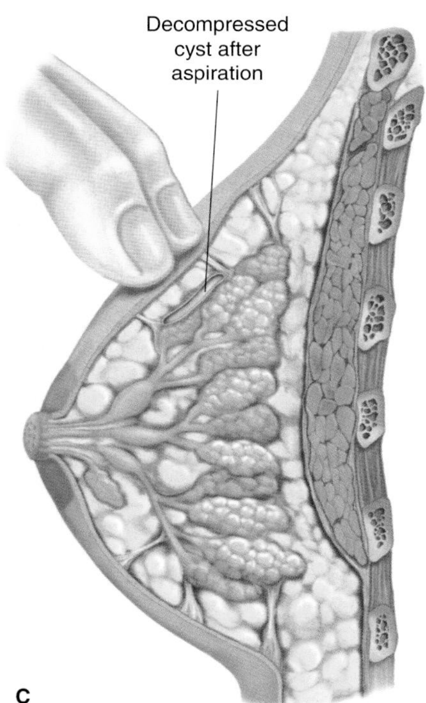

FIGURE 4 ● Free-hand aspiration of palpable cyst. **A,** Stabilize palpable cyst between the thumb and the forefinger of non-dominant hand. **B,** Hold needle and syringe across palm of the dominant hand, applying traction on plunger with fourth finger. **C,** Collapsed cyst after aspiration. (Reprinted with permission from Bland KI, Klimberg VS. *Master Techniques in Surgery: Breast Surgery*. 2nd ed. Wolters Kluwer; 2019. Figure 3.4.)

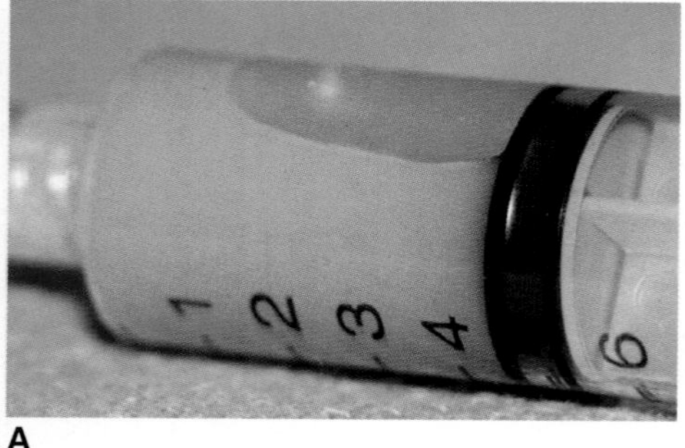

A

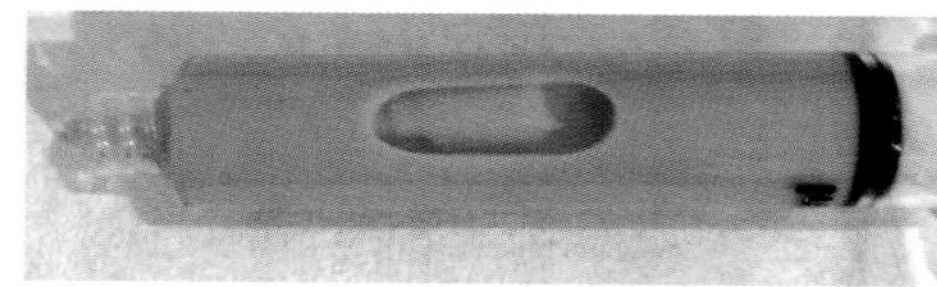

B

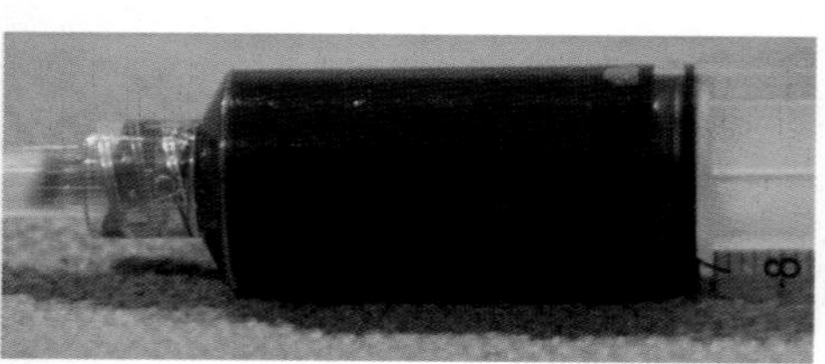

C

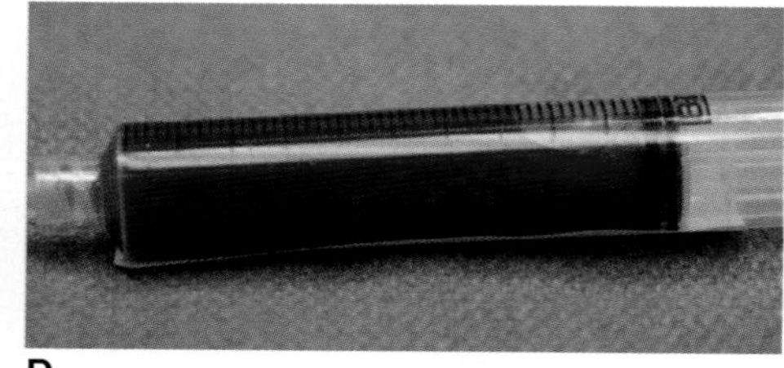

D

FIGURE 5 ● Abnormal breast aspirates. **A,** Aspirated cyst fluid. Free flowing opaque cream-colored fluid. **B,** Aspirated cyst fluid. The fluid is free-flowing, dark brown to green in color. **C,** Aspirated fluid, purulent in appearance. If an abscess is suspected clinically, this type of fluid is submitted for Gram stain, culture, and sensitivity. **D,** Grossly bloody fluid. If bloody fluid is obtained following an atraumatic tap, submit the sample for cytology. As illustrated by these examples, the fluid in cysts is highly variable in appearance. Except for the grossly bloody or purulent aspirates, all other fluid is typically discarded. (Reprinted with permission from Cardenosa G. *Breast Imaging Companion*. 4th ed. Wolters Kluwer; 2018. eFigure 9.8.)

PEARLS AND PITFALLS

Indications	■ Symptomatic breast cysts. ■ Can also be used for postoperative seromas or abscesses. For the latter, consider a larger gauge needle and send the specimen for gram stain, culture, and sensitivities. ■ For complex cysts with concerning features, core biopsy should be considered in addition to aspiration, with a biopsy clip placed at the time.
Imaging	■ Ultrasound can be used to assure cysts are simple vs complicated or complex. ■ Ultrasound can also be used to determine resolution following aspiration.
Placement of needle	■ Avoid needle insertion perpendicular or at a steep angle to avoid muscle hematoma or pneumothorax.
Follow-up	■ Reaccumulating fluid—follow up in 4-6 weeks for repeat aspiration or discussion of surgical excisional biopsy. ■ If atypia or malignant cells are seen on pathology, the patient will require excisional biopsy for definitive pathological analysis and diagnosis.

POSTOPERATIVE CARE

- After aspiration pressure is held over the area for 5 to 10 minutes to reduce the risk of hematoma. The patient is instructed to refrain from anticoagulants or NSAIDs for 2 days after biopsy.
- The patient should be placed in a well-fitting sports bra to help maintain hemostasis, reduce edema, and immobilize the breast to reduce pain. The garment should be worn for 2 days after aspiration.
- Postprocedural follow-up is important. The patient should return 4 to 6 weeks after aspiration for physical exam and follow up mammography or ultrasound to confirm resolution of cyst. Cytology should also be reviewed.

COMPLICATIONS

- Hematoma
- Infection (cellulitis or abscess)
- Inadequate aspiration with residual fluid, may require additional aspiration attempts
- Reaccumulating fluid within a cyst, repeat aspiration, or surgical excision required
- Identification of malignancy

REFERENCES

1. Lucas JH, Cone DL. Breast cyst aspiration. *Am Fam Physician*. 2003;68:1983-1986, 1989.
2. Bhate RD, Chakravorty A, Ebbs SR. Management of breast cysts revisited. *Int J Clin Pract*. 2007;61(2):195-199. doi: 10.1111/j.1742-1241.2006.01192.x
3. Heisey RE, McCready DR. Office Management of a palpable breast lump with aspiration. *CMAJ (Can Med Assoc J)*. 2010;182(7):693-696. doi: 10.1503/cmaj.090416
4. Sanders LM, Lacz NL, Lara J. 16 year experience with aspiration of noncomplex breast cysts: cytology results with focus on positive cases. *Breast J*. 2012;18(5):443-452. doi: 10.1111/j.1524-4741.2012.01277.x
5. Ponka D, Baddar F. Breast cyst aspiration. *Can Fam Physician*. 2012;58(11):1240.

Chapter 2 Fine Needle Aspiration of a Breast Mass

Judy C. Pang and Claire W. Michael

DEFINITION

- Fine needle aspiration (FNA) biopsy is a percutaneous procedure that uses a fine gauge needle with or without a syringe to sample fluid from a cyst or extract cells from a solid palpable mass for cytologic analysis.

PATIENT HISTORY AND PHYSICAL FINDINGS

- A focused history should be obtained from the patient including duration of the mass, changes in size, associated pain, or fluctuations of the mass with menstrual cycle. Prior history of trauma or malignancies should also be ascertained. On physical examination, localizing the mass as within the breast parenchyma, lower axilla, or subcutaneous/cutaneous tissue of the chest wall is important. The differential diagnoses may be different. In addition, noting any skin changes such as redness, warmth, or edema is also helpful. Determining the size and quality of the mass as well as the depth and relation to other structures is essential for an adequate sample while minimizing complications. There are no absolute contraindications to FNA.

IMAGING AND OTHER DIAGNOSTIC STUDIES

- Mammographic and ultrasound findings can be helpful in arriving at an accurate diagnosis. Knowing whether a lesion is solid or cystic can help select the appropriate needle and syringe. For lesions that are nonpalpable or difficult to palpate, image-guided (ie, ultrasound) FNA is recommended to ensure proper sampling of the mass.

DIFFERENTIAL DIAGNOSIS

- Benign (ie, fibroadenoma, cyst)
- Malignant (ie, carcinoma, lymphoma)
- Atypical (core biopsy or surgical excision required for definitive diagnosis)

NONOPERATIVE MANAGEMENT

- For patients who opt not to undergo a biopsy, short-term follow-up (4-6 months) with repeat imaging and clinical examination to document stability or changes is recommended.

SURGICAL MANAGEMENT

- Alternative procedures to FNA biopsy are core needle biopsy and surgical excision of mass.
- For solid masses, FNA biopsy provides cells for cytology, whereas core needle biopsy obtains tissue. In situations where an experienced cytopathologist is not available or tissue architecture is necessary to make a diagnosis (eg, differentiating between in situ and invasive disease), core needle biopsy is preferred.
- Surgical excision should be reserved for cases where FNA or core needle biopsy was inconclusive. It may be considered for small breast masses where the patient is strongly desirous of excision.

Preoperative Planning

- Prior to the FNA, the location of the palpable mass should be confirmed with the patient. The mass should be examined in the upright and supine position to determine the ideal position for the biopsy.

Positioning

- The patient may be upright or supine depending on the location of the mass. The patient should be positioned to optimize palpation and sampling of the mass.

Approach

- FNA can be performed using (1) a needle, syringe, and syringe holder; (2) a needle and syringe; or (3) a needle only.

EQUIPMENT

- Alcohol pads to cleanse the skin and gauze pads to apply pressure after completion of the procedure.
- Local anesthetic is optional.
- Beveled hypodermic needles
  - A 23-gauge needle is preferred and typically the one to start with. If inadequate material is obtained, a 22-gauge needle can be used especially for lesions with minimal stroma (ie, lymphoma, melanoma) or a 25-gauge needle for rubbery or fibrous masses (ie, fibroadenoma).
  - The length of the needle is typically 5/8 in to 11/2 in, which is just long enough to reach the target. Shorter needles are easier to manipulate because they will not bend.
- A slip-tip syringe is best as it is easy to handle and provides a good seal. A Luer lock syringe may also be used, but it can be difficult to remove the needle. A 10-mL syringe is preferred as it allows the hand to be closer to the target and only 2 to 4 mL of suction is needed for aspiration. For larger cystic lesions, a 20-mL syringe may be advantageous.
- A syringe holder allows for one-handed grip and application of suction leaving the other hand free to stabilize the target.
- Glass slides and cover slips.
- Slide holder for air-dried slides.
- Ninety-five percent ethanol (EtOH) in a jar for fixation of slides or spray fixative. If the jar is not slotted for separating slides, using paper clips on alternating slides can achieve the same goal.
- There are different rapid stains that can be used for adequacy checks including toluidine blue, rapid hematoxylin and eosin, rapid Papanicolaou for fixed slides, and Giemsa and Diff-Quik for air-dried slides.
- Needle rinses can be performed in RPMI (cell block or flow cytometry for lymphoma), 10% buffered formalin (cell block), or CytoLyt (thin prep).

FINE NEEDLE ASPIRATION USING NEEDLE, SYRINGE, AND SYRINGE HOLDER[1,2]

- Carefully palpate the mass to estimate the size and depth as well as assess the structures nearby to avoid (ie, major blood vessels, bone, and lung especially with small breasts).
- Fix the mass firmly in place with the fingers.
  - For large lesions, use the thumb and opposing finger (**FIGURE 1**).
  - For smaller lesions, place the forefinger and middle finger on top of the mass and then spread them apart, stretching the skin (**FIGURE 2**).
- Plan the angle of the needle at the entrance point of the skin and determine the depth of penetration.
  - If the needle enters at 90° to the mass, the needle should penetrate the skin on top of the mass (**FIGURE 3A** and **B**).
  - If the needle enters at a 30° to 45° angle, which is oftentimes more comfortable and practical, compensate for the acute angle by penetrating the skin adjacent to the mass and not on top of the mass (**FIGURE 4A** and **B**).
  - When entering at 90°, penetrating too deep with the needle can potentially result in a pneumothorax. If this is a concern (eg, mass near the chest wall), a 30° to 45° angle is preferred.
  - To stabilize the instrument, rest the barrel of the syringe on the forefinger of the palpating hand or use the thumb to stabilize the syringe as you enter the mass. Once the needle is in the mass, the thumb can be removed (**FIGURE 4A**).
- Extracting material
  - For cystic lesions, applying suction without back and forth movement is sufficient.
  - For solid masses, 15 to 20 excursions are made before suction is released and the needle is removed from the mass. If blood is seen at the hub, the number of excursions should be limited and suction should be released before reaching 15 to 20. Always release the suction before pulling the needle out of the patient; otherwise, all the material will flow into the barrel of the syringe, which will be very difficult to extract (**FIGURE 5**).
- Adequate sampling
  - To sample different areas of a well-defined large lesion, it is preferable to make separate passes to sample different areas. This is also preferable in well-defined lesions. In ill-defined targets, especially fibrocystic changes

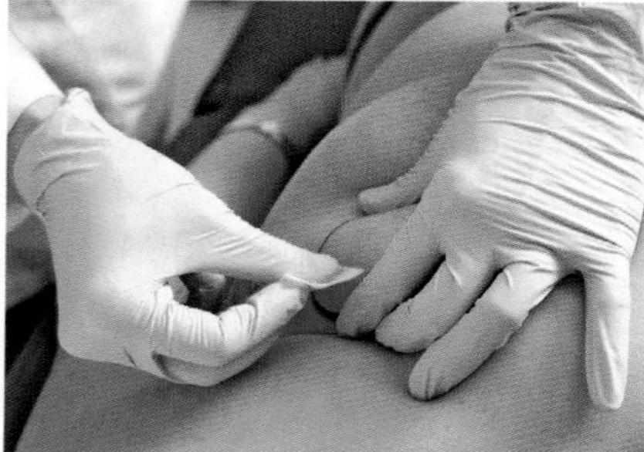

FIGURE 1 ● Fixation of a large mass using the thumb and opposing finger.

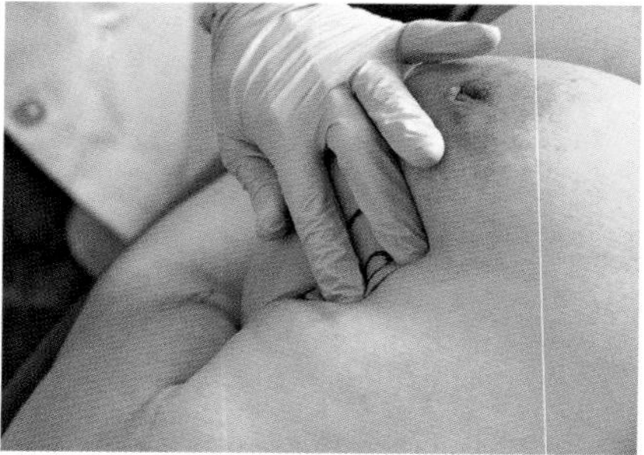

FIGURE 2 ● Fixation of smaller mass using the forefinger and middle finger.

of the breast, it is best to redirect while sampling in a fanlike fashion. To avoid tearing the tissue and causing bleeding, the needle should be retracted to the surface of the target (but still in the patient) before redirecting (**FIGURE 6**).

- Typically, two to three passes are adequate. Additional passes are performed if the target is large or the sample is inadequate. However, typically more than three passes is not recommended as often times the yield of diagnostic material decreases with each subsequent pass due to blood. The first pass is traditionally the best.
- Zajdela's technique uses only the needle without a syringe or syringe holder (**FIGURE 7A**). This technique is ideal for small targets as it increases sensitivity to the difference in

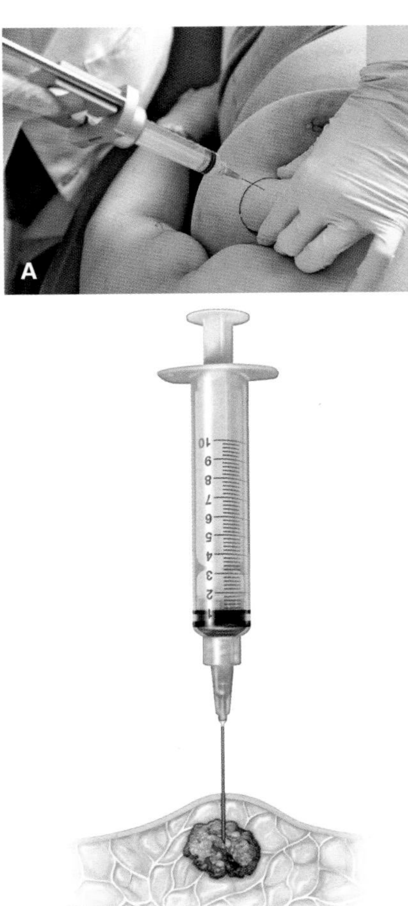

FIGURE 3 ● **A** and **B,** Needle entering 90° to the mass should penetrate the skin on top of the mass.

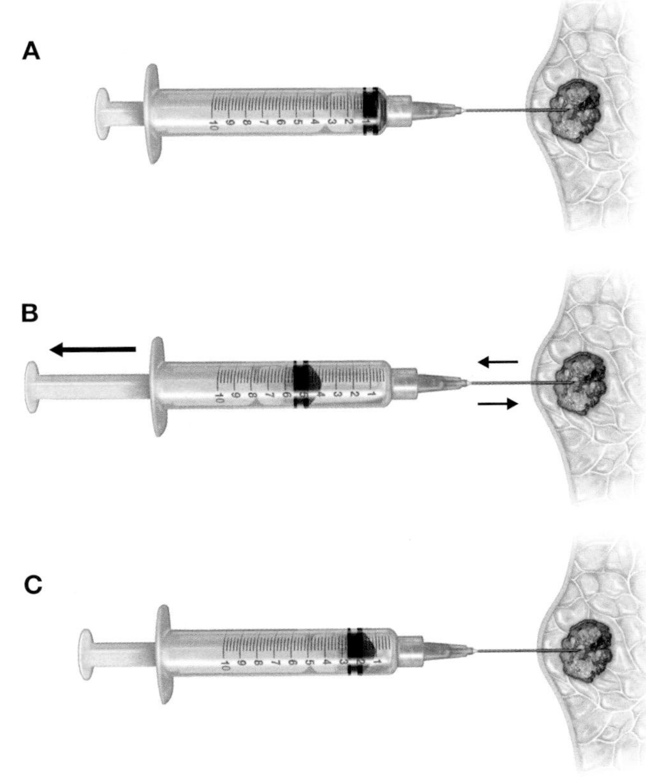

FIGURE 5 ● **A,** Needle placed in mass. **B,** Withdraw plunger creating 2 to 4 mL of vacuum/suction and perform 15 to 20 excursions. **C,** Release the plunger/suction before pulling needle out of the patient.

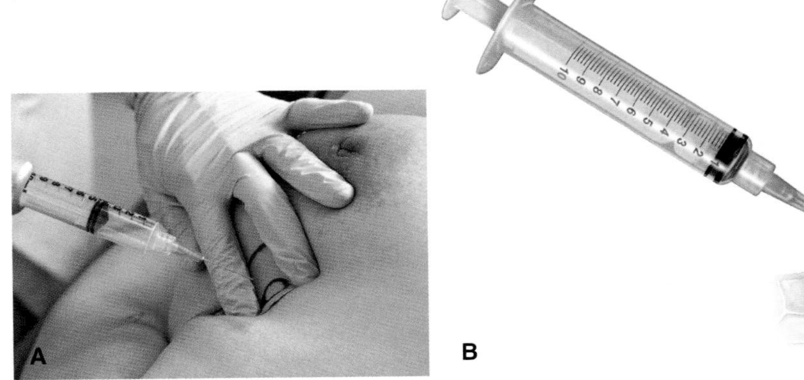

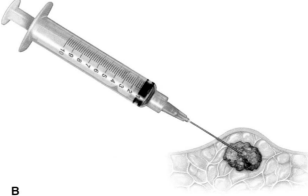

FIGURE 4 ● **A,B,** Needle entering 30° to 45° to the mass should penetrate the skin adjacent to the mass and not on top of the mass.

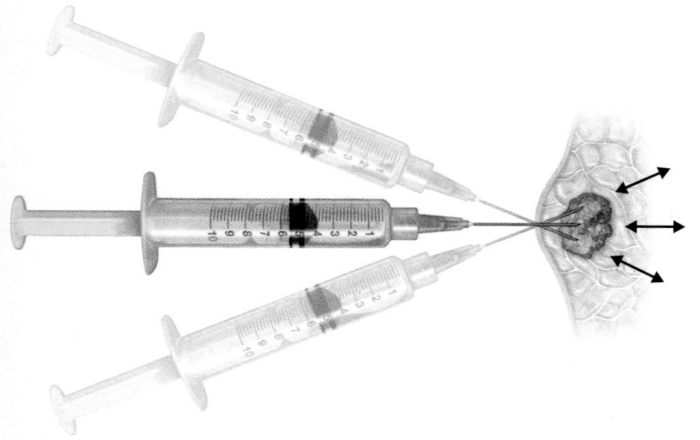

consistencies between normal breast tissue and the lesion that cannot be appreciated as well with a syringe and syringe holder. In addition, it is less bloody. However, this technique often yields less material than when suction is used, and there is a risk of overflow of material if the lesion is cystic. A syringe (without the plunger) can be used if needed (**FIGURE 7B**).

FIGURE 6 ● To sample different areas, redirect the needle in a fanlike fashion.

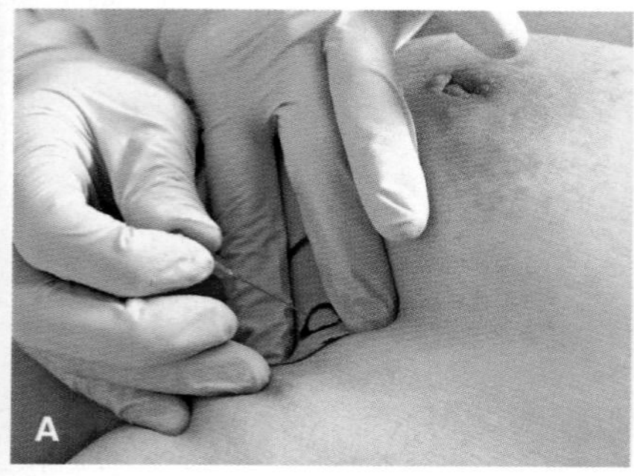

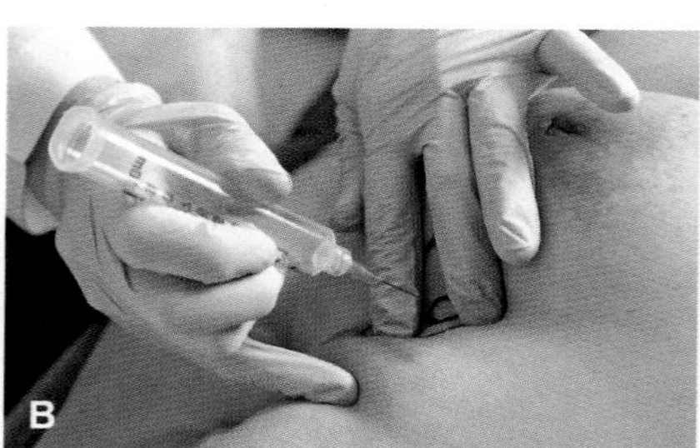

FIGURE 7 ● Zajdela technique using only a needle **(A)** or a needle and a syringe without the plunger **(B)**.

PREPARING SLIDES[1,2]

- Expulsion of material
  - The needle is first disconnected from the syringe (**FIGURE 8**). The plunger is then pulled back all the way before reattaching the needle (**FIGURE 9A** and **B**). If using the Zajdela technique with the needle and syringe, disconnect the needle from the syringe before putting the plunger back into the syringe.

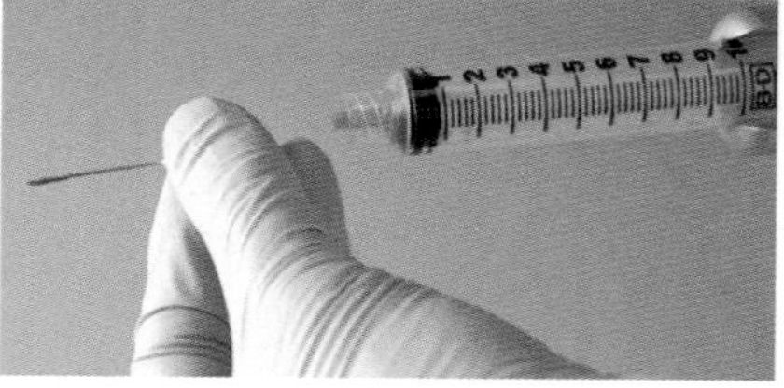

FIGURE 8 ● Disconnect needle from syringe.

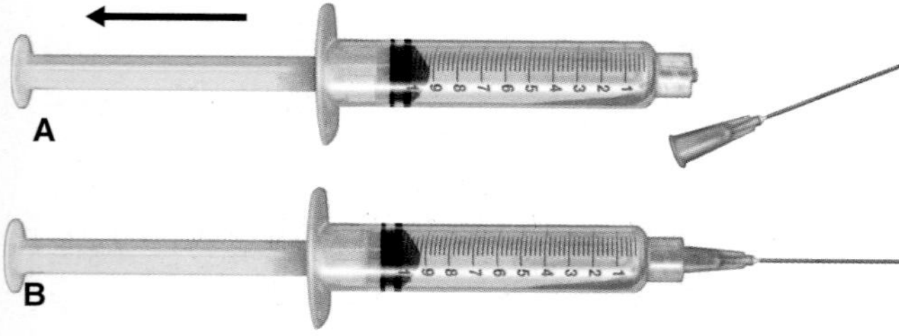

FIGURE 9 ● **A** and **B,** The plunger is pulled back all the way **(A)** before reattaching the needle **(B)**.

- With the tip of the needle on the slide (bevel down), the plunger is forcefully pushed so that all the material is on one slide (**FIGURE 10A** and **B**). If there is abundant

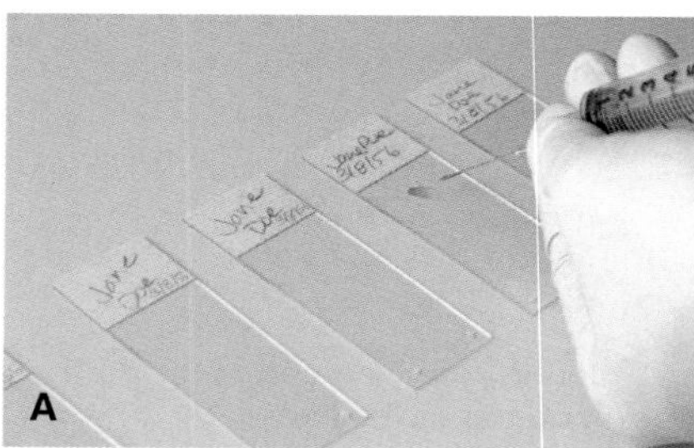

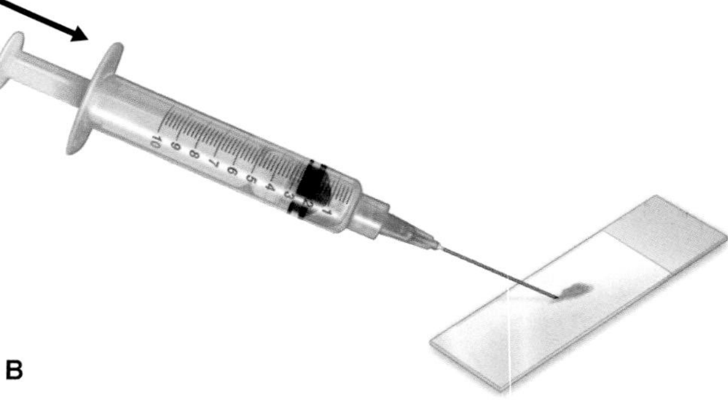

FIGURE 10 ● **A** and **B,** With the tip of the needle on the slide (bevel down), the plunger is forcefully pushed so that all the material is on one slide. If there is abundant material, the plunger can be pushed slowly so that only a small amount of material is placed on each slide.

material, the plunger can be pushed slowly so that only a small amount of material is placed on each slide. The slides should be labeled with patient identifiers (ie, name and birth date) with a pencil.

  - If there is remaining material in the hub, it can be rinsed for cytocentrifugation (in CytoLyt) or cell block (10% buffered formalin or RPMI) (**FIGURE 11**). If additional smears are desired, the flip technique can be used where the needle is secured in the rubber top of a Vacutainer tube, or if available, a needle safety device. The hub is then flicked repeatedly onto a slide. Droplets of the material on the slides can then be smeared (**FIGURE 12**).
- Smearing techniques
  - Rest the edge of a second slide on top of the slide that contains the aspirate material (**FIGURE 13**).
  - Rotate the top slide so that it is level with the bottom slide (**FIGURE 14**).
  - Keeping both slides level, apply light pressure and slide the top slide over the bottom slide (**FIGURE 15**).
  - The end product should be a slide with material in an oval configuration of even thickness (**FIGURE 16**). Virtually, all the material should be on the bottom slides. Microscopically, the cells should be well preserved with intact cytoplasm. If too much pressure is applied, there will be crushed nuclei and few cells with preserved cytoplasm. If the slides are not maintained level to each other, the material will be scraped and lost and distortion will be present.
- Other techniques
  - Place a clean slide exactly parallel to the bottom slide containing the aspirate material and slide apart. The

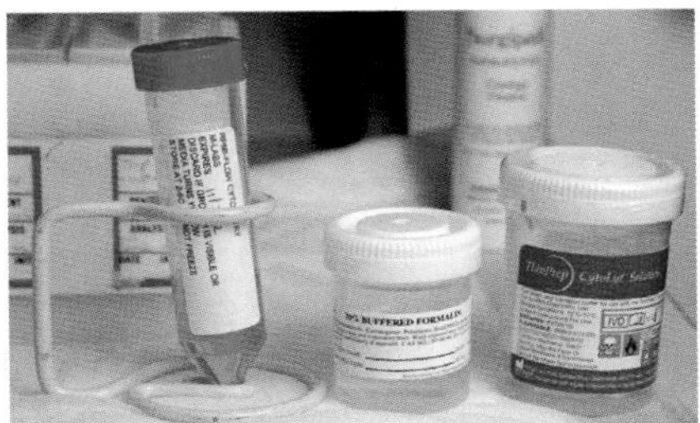

FIGURE 11 ● The needle can be rinsed in RPMI, 10% buffered formalin, or CytoLyt.

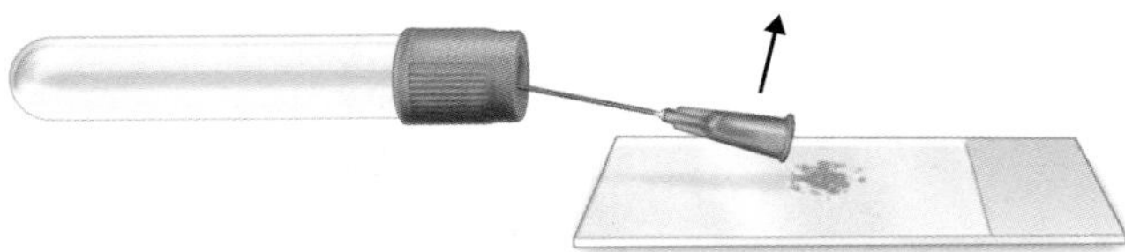

FIGURE 12 ● Secure the needle in the rubber top of a Vacutainer tube. Flick the hub repeatedly onto a slide.

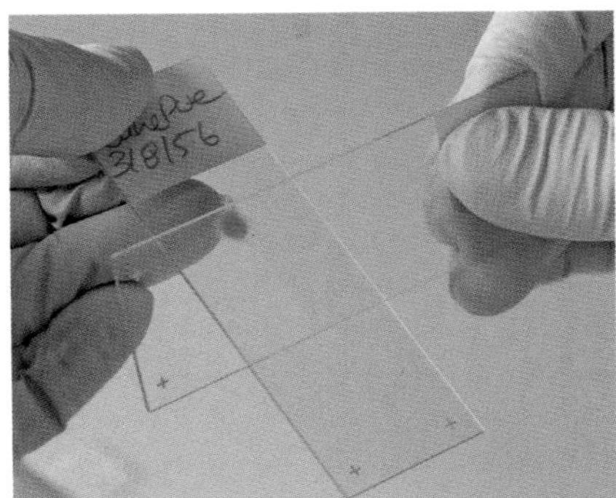

FIGURE 13 ● Rest a slide on top of the slide that contains the aspirate material.

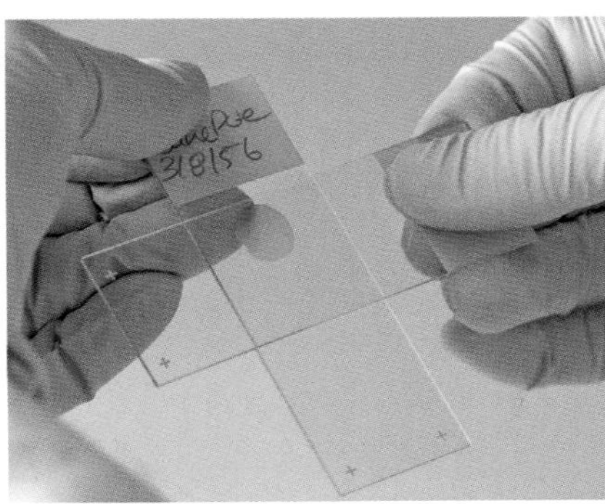

FIGURE 14 ● Rotate the top slide so that it is parallel to the bottom slide.

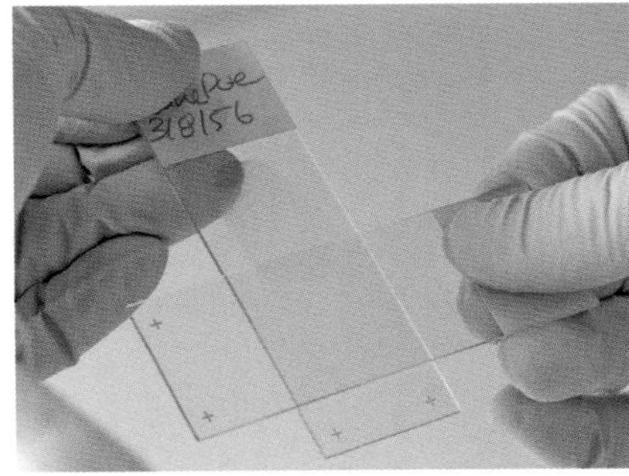

FIGURE 15 ● Apply light pressure and slide the top slide over the bottom slide.

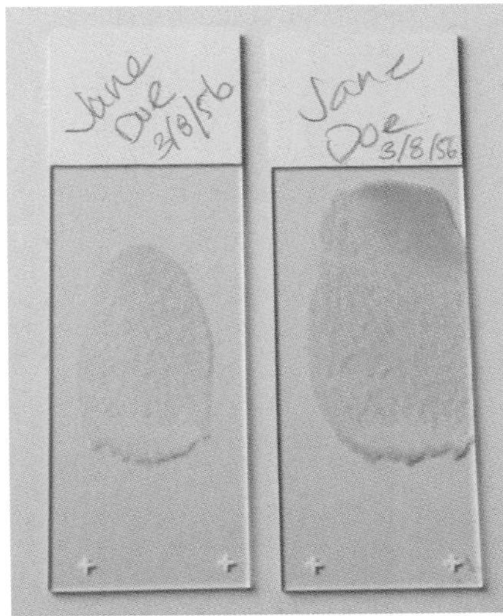

FIGURE 16 ● End product with material in an oval configuration.

material will be present on both slides (also produces good smears) (**FIGURE 17A** and **B**).

- For bloody aspirates, tilt the slide and allow the blood to drain into the collecting media (**FIGURE 18A** and **B**). The particulates remaining on the slide are then scraped with the edge of another slide and then smeared onto a separate slide (**FIGURE 18C** and **D**). Alternatively, the particulates on the original slide can be smeared directly with a separate clean slide (**FIGURE 18E**).

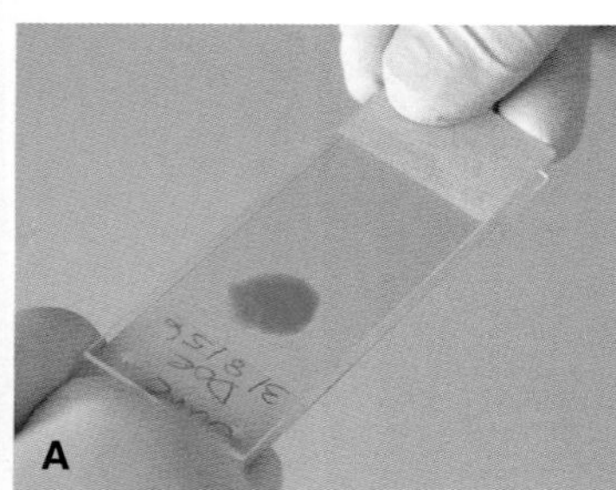

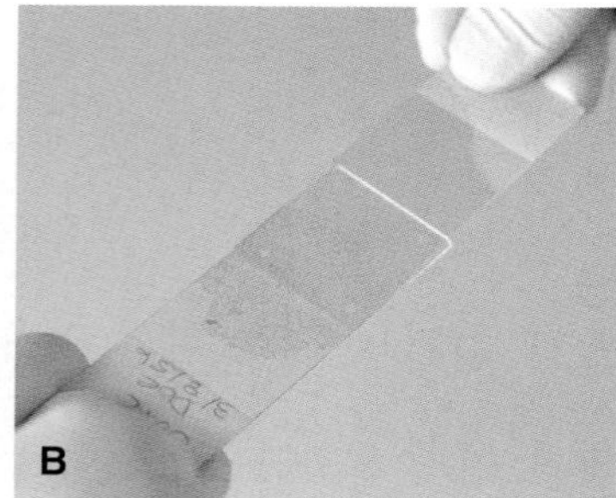

FIGURE 17 ● **A** and **B,** Place a clean slide exactly parallel to the bottom slide containing the aspirate material and slide apart.

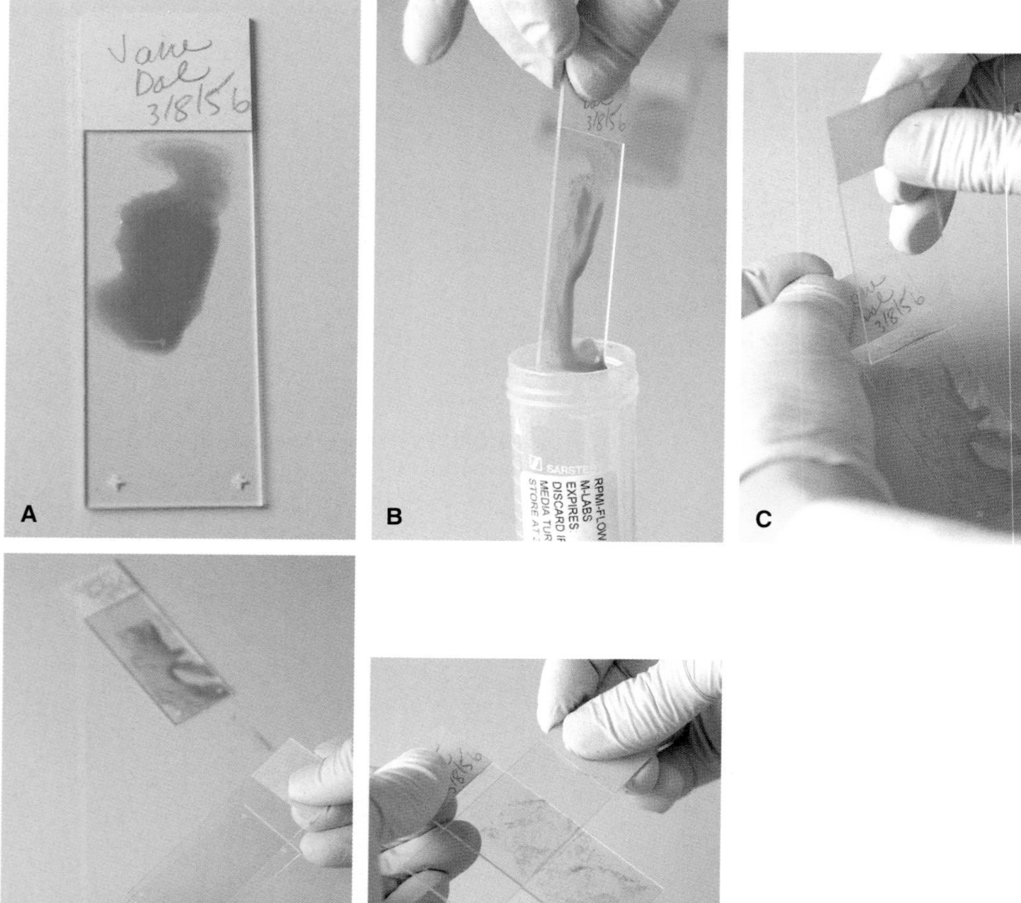

FIGURE 18 ● **A,** Bloody aspirate. **B,** Tilt the slide and allow the blood to drain into the collecting media. **C,** Scrape remaining particulates on the slide with the edge of another slide and then smear onto a separate slide **(D)** or smear the particulates on the original slide directly with a separate clean slide **(E)**.

FIX SLIDES

- The slides should be immersed in 95% EtOH or fixed by spray fixation (**FIGURE 19**). This should be done as quickly as possible after smearing the slides to prevent air-dry artifact. Alternatively, slides may be left to air dry without fixation. Ideally, both air-dried and fixed slides should be made for cytologic evaluation.

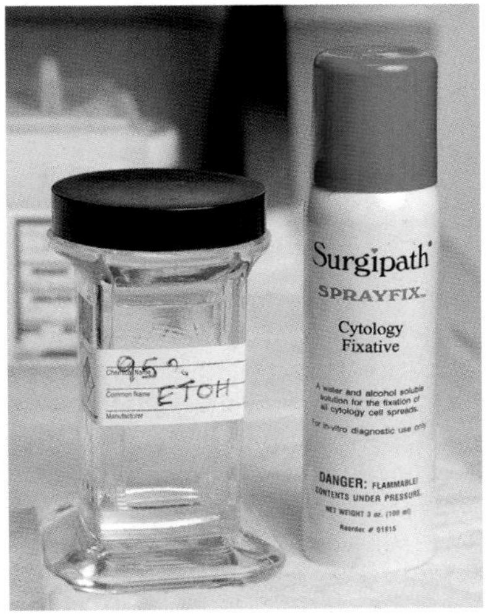

FIGURE 19 ● Fix slides immediately in 95% liquid EtOH or spray fix.

PEARLS AND PITFALLS[3]

Indications	■ Palpable masses: a brief history and focused physical examination should be performed ■ Diagnostic: primary neoplasms (benign vs malignant), tumor recurrence, secondary or metastatic tumors, inflammatory diseases (uncommon), atypical epithelial lesions (require additional studies) ■ Therapeutic: evacuation of simple cysts
Major diagnostic pitfalls	■ False negative: small focus of carcinoma arising in a background of a predominantly benign lesion (ie, fibrocystic change), carcinoma arising in a complex proliferative lesion (ie, papilloma), well-differentiated carcinomas, rare tumor types, extensively necrotic or cystic carcinomas, sampling error, inadequate smears ■ False positive: fibroadenoma, papilloma/papillary lesions, atypical ductal hyperplasia, pregnancy-associated/lactational changes, fat necrosis, collagenous spherulosis, skin adnexal tumors
Major limitations	■ Inability to distinguish between invasive and in situ carcinoma ■ Accuracy is often dependent on the size of the lesion (less sensitive if <0.5 cm) ■ Low accuracy in tumors with a predominant necrotic/cystic component ■ Lack of specific diagnosis for majority of benign lesions ■ Need for biopsy (core or excisional) of all lesions with an "atypical" diagnosis ■ Ability to perform hormone receptor and *HER-2/neu* analysis can only be done with accuracy if an adequate sample is obtained

POSTOPERATIVE CARE

- Pressure should be applied to the site for a few minutes to assure hemostasis, and then a sterile dressing is applied.

OUTCOMES

- 80% to 100% sensitivity, with a specificity of over 99%
- 3% to 5% false-negative and 0.5% to 2% false-positive rate
- Implementing the "triple test" is essential (correlation of clinical, radiologic, and cytologic findings)

COMPLICATIONS

- Low complication rate and most complications are minor
- Pain
- Bleeding/hematoma
- Infection
- Vasovagal reaction
- Pneumothorax
- Epithelial displacement/tumor seeding
- Artifacts occurring after aspiration may interfere with radiographic interpretation and histologic evaluation of surgical resection (epithelial displacement can mimic invasive carcinoma).

REFERENCES

1. Dusenbery D. The technique of fine needle aspiration of palpable mass lesions of the head and neck. *Otolaryngol Head Neck Surg.* 1997;8(2):61-67.
2. Ljung BM. *Fine Needle Aspiration Biopsy (FNA) Techniques video.* USCAP Your Academy. Website. August 2018. https://www.youtube.com/watch?v=mXh9en_nCBU
3. Ali SZ, Parwani AV. *Breast Cytopathology.* Springer; 2007.

Chapter 3 Percutaneous Breast Core Needle Biopsy

Rachel Louise McCaffrey

DEFINITION

- A core needle biopsy (CNB) is a percutaneous procedure that uses a larger bore needle to obtain a tissue sample from a mass. The biopsy is performed both with and without image localization either with ultrasound, mammography, or MRI.
- CNB provides tissue and architecture that can differentiate between benign, in situ, or invasive disease in the breast and is the preferred method for diagnosis of breast malignancy.
- CNB has remained a mainstay of breast mass diagnosis and is typically the subsequent step after a breast abnormality has been discovered on screening imaging or physical exam and confirmed with additional diagnostic imaging.

DIFFERENTIAL DIAGNOSIS

- Benign (fibroadenoma, papilloma, fibrocystic change, cysts)
- Malignant (carcinoma, sarcoma, lymph node containing lymphoma)
- Atypical or high-risk lesions (may require surgical excision for final diagnosis or to rule out associated malignancy)

PATIENT HISTORY AND PHYSICAL FINDINGS

- A focused history and physical exam should be obtained from the patient including how the mass was first discovered (ie, on self-examination or via routine screening), associated symptoms such as nipple discharge or pain, palpable mass, changes in mass size, or fluctuations with menstrual cycle. Any prior history of breast trauma or malignancies should be evaluated. The physical examination should include palpation of the mass, both breasts and both axillary lymph node basins. The differential may be different depending on the location and physical characteristics of the mass. The exam should also include a skin evaluation for changes in color, warmth, thickening, or edema as well as changes to the nipple-areolar complex.
- There are no absolute contraindications to CNB; however, patients on anticoagulants or antiplatelet agents may be asked to hold these medications prior to the procedure to reduce the risk of hematoma.
- CNB is the first step for pathologic diagnosis of any suspicious breast lesion and is sufficient for diagnosis of most benign breast lesions and breast cancers. Diagnostic excisional breast biopsy should be the exception, not the rule. For example, diagnostic excisional breast biopsy can be performed when there is imaging and pathologic discordance from a CNB.

IMAGING AND OTHER DIAGNOSTIC STUDIES

- Here, we will describe techniques for non–image-guided CNB of palpable lesions in the breast. Although CNB can be performed on palpable lesions, using preprocedural imaging is still key to determine the best approach for biopsy. Imaging can offer guidance on depth of needle insertion depending on the mass size, location relative to the chest wall or skin, and the overall quadrant location in the breast in conjunction with findings on physical exam (**FIGURE 1**).
- Mammographic, ultrasound, and MRI findings are key to accurate diagnosis. Often masses or areas of calcifications eligible for CNB are not felt on physical examination and these should be biopsied via image guidance, which is beyond the scope of the chapter. Of note, the imaging modality that demonstrates the suspicious area in question should be used to guide CNB; for example, calcifications are often only seen on mammogram. Therefore, in order to obtain a biopsy, a stereotactic biopsy using mammogram for localization of the calcifications is the best course of action.

NONOPERATIVE MANAGEMENT

- Patients with suspicious masses on physical exam and imaging should be highly encouraged to proceed with CNB. If the patient declines biopsy, short-term interval imaging and physical exam in 3 months should be recommended to document change and encourage diagnosis with CNB.
- For patients who decline initial biopsy for likely benign masses, such as a younger woman with a history and imaging findings consistent with fibroadenoma, these patients should be followed with interval imaging and physical examination in 6-month intervals. This will document stability or changes to the area under evaluation and determine further recommendations for surveillance vs biopsy.

SURGICAL MANAGEMENT

PreProcedural Planning

- The majority of CNB procedures can be performed in the office or procedure room if the breast mass is easily palpable. If the lesion is difficult to palpate or nonpalpable, biopsy should be performed under image guidance.
- Informed consent is obtained.
- Allergies to local anesthetics should be reviewed.
- Mild anxiolysis can be offered, but is often unnecessary with a good bedside manner and use of local anesthetic.
- Ensure the patient has stopped NSAID and anticoagulants accordingly to reduce hematoma risk.
- Discuss with the patient that you will be placing a biopsy marker during the procedure to identify the biopsy site on future imaging or for localization if an excisional biopsy is required.

Positioning

- The patient should be positioned supine on the procedure table, with the ipsilateral arm overhead to provide some tension and stability to breast tissue.
- A bolster or towel behind the patient's ipsilateral shoulder will aid in placing the lesion directly over the chest wall;

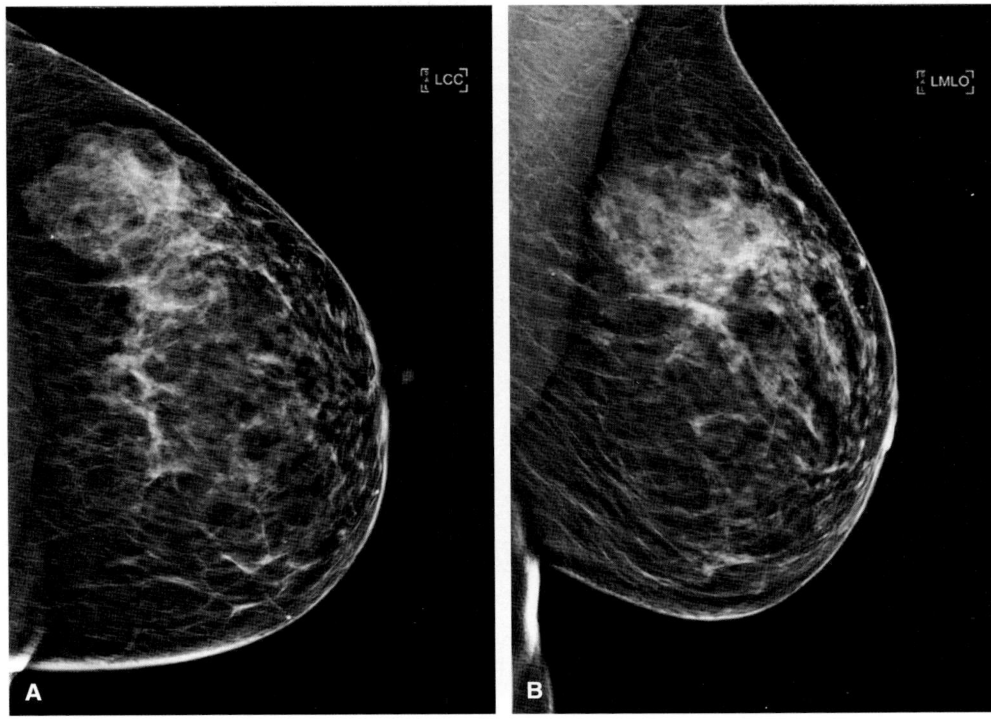

FIGURE 1 ● Craniocaudal **(A)** and mediolateral oblique **(B)** mammograms of a clinically palpable mass amenable to core needle biopsy. Identified proximity to the skin and depth adjacent to pectoralis major.

this aids in optimal stabilization and immobilization of the breast during biopsy.

- Occasionally for very lateral and inferior lesions it is preferable to have the patient positioned laterally to facilitate ergonomic CNB trajectory for the physician; however, with a bolster and table height adjustment, a lateral position is rarely needed. The surgeon may also consider standing on the patient's contralateral side to facilitate a medial to lateral needle trajectory.

ANTICIPATING LESION LOCATION

- On review of imaging, note should be taken of the depth of the mass, as a mass close to the chest wall may influence the planned trajectory for CNB in order to avoid damage to muscle or the underlying lung.
- Although rare, pneumothoraxes with biopsy can occur, making three-dimensional awareness of your biopsy needle trajectory critical.
- The best approach is to plan a needle trajectory parallel to the chest wall with the shortest distance between the skin entry point and the lesions to be biopsied while avoiding the nipple-areolar complex and allowing enough distance for the sample notch (see anatomy and deployment section below) to be fired into the mass accordingly.
- Have imaging displayed in the room at time of biopsy.

APPROACHES

- CNB can be approached with hand-held spring-loaded devices or larger vacuum-assisted devices, for the purposes of percutaneous CNB, a technique involving a spring-loaded device will be described here and is more practical in the use of free-hand, non–image-guided biopsy.
- If CNB is being used for large fungating masses (**FIGURE 2**), it is useful to obtain a deeper sampling of the mass with CNB as opposed to a punch biopsy or incisional biopsy of the fungating mass surface. A CNB is useful as it reduces bleeding risk and can obtain a less confounding sample. Superficial samples of fungating masses are often plagued with environmental contaminants and inflammatory tissue, which make malignancy diagnosis and staining for hormone and growth receptors difficult. In addition, adequate hemostasis from incisional biopsies of fungating masses is quite difficult. It is advisable to approach the mass from an area of intact skin to reduce postprocedural bleeding and to use the introducer needle as described below to minimize tissue trauma.

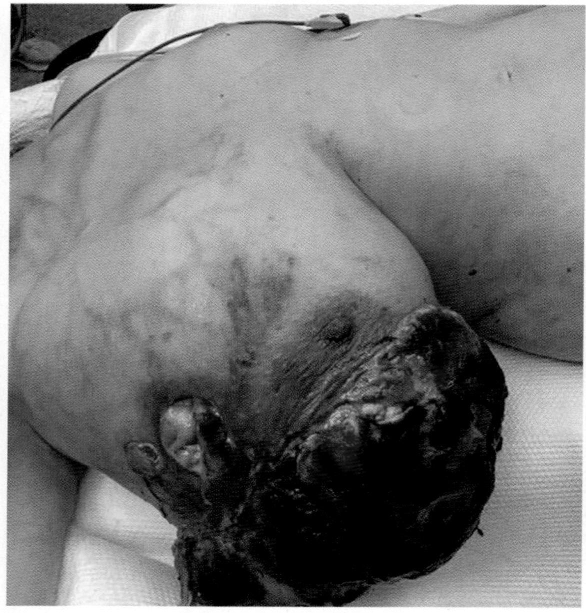

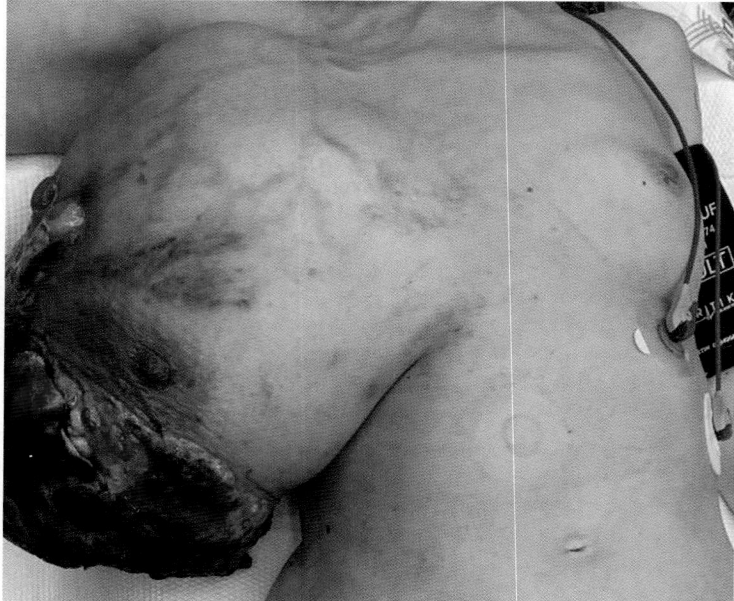

FIGURE 2 ● Fungating breast mass on the lateral breast, best approached with the biopsy needle directed from medial to lateral to avoid the chest wall and through an area of intact skin to improve hemostasis.

- Many patients with fungating masses have reduced or absent sensation; however, local anesthetic with epinephrine should still be used for the intact skin and along the biopsy tract for patient comfort and to aid in hemostasis. In most of these cases, a biopsy marker is not necessary given the patient is likely to progress to systemic therapy with or without mastectomy.

Equipment for Core Needle Biopsy

- Cleaning solution (chlorhexidine or povidone iodine)
- 1% lidocaine with epinephrine
- Optional: 8.4% bicarbonate solution
- 10 mL syringe for anesthetic
- 25-gauge needle for superficial local anesthetic
- 1.5-inch, 21-gauge needle for deep local anesthetic infiltration
- #11 blade
- Spring Loaded Core Needle Biopsy Device with introducer needle and trocar
- Test tube like collection jar
- 3 to 4 mL normal saline into test tube
- Specimen jar with permanent fixative for biopsy submission to pathology
- Surgical glue or Steri-Strips

Preparation of Local Anesthetic

- Take note of patient weight and maximal safe dosing for the anesthetic used.
- Typically, the amount of 1% lidocaine drawn into a 10 mL syringe will be below this dose limit.
- Mix 2 mL 8.4% bicarbonate solution with 8 mL 1% lidocaine with epinephrine.
- A note on bicarbonate—aids in the transit of local anesthetic to nerve endings and reduces the "stinging" effect of lidocaine and marcaine upon injection and is useful for any local anesthetic application.

SPRING-LOADED CORE NEEDLE BIOPSY ANATOMY AND DEPLOYMENT

- There are many types of core biopsy devices that vary in needle gauge and length (**FIGURE 3**). The spring-loaded core biopsy devices are button activated, which deploys a high-speed stylet into a target lesion, rapidly followed by a cutting cannula in swift motion. It is best to fire the device once prior to biopsy, allowing the patient to hear the "click" the device makes so they are not startled during the procedure.
- Often the core biopsy device will have an introducer needle and trocar as separate devices (**FIGURE 4**). The trocar is placed inside the introducer needle and this device is used to create the initial path in the patient's tissue for biopsy sampling after local anesthetic is applied. The trocar is subsequently removed, and the core biopsy device placed through the introducer needle for biopsy collection. This introducer needle remains in place throughout the procedure and can minimize damage to tissue that would otherwise be subjected to multiple passes of the core needle device. Of note, both the introducer needle and the core biopsy needle are marked in 1-cm increments to aid in precision.
- The dimensions of the core biopsy needle are important including the device's throw length, which is the distance the sampling notch protrudes from the end of the biopsy needle. This length varies from 10 to 20 mm and the operator must ensure any sensitive structures including skin, muscle ,and the operator's hand are not in the potential path of the throw length. The notch itself is the area where the core is

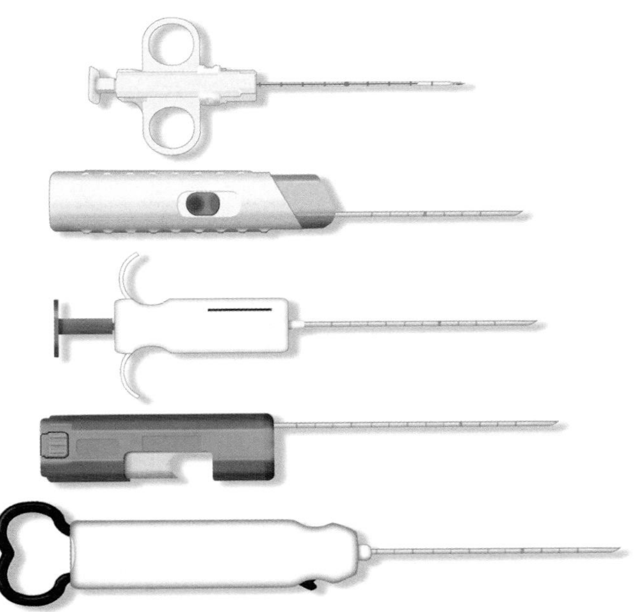

FIGURE 3 ● Examples of various spring-loaded core needle biopsy devices.

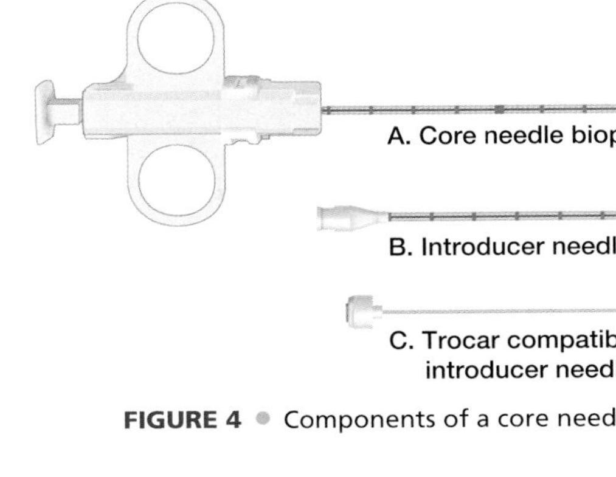

FIGURE 4 ● Components of a core needle biopsy.

collected once the cutting cannula slides over the inner stylet and notch to isolate the specimen.

- Also consider the dead length, which is the distance from the distal notch to the tip of the core biopsy stylet (**FIGURE 5**). If the lesion is large enough, the needle tip can be positioned at its margin before being deployed. If the lesion is small, the tip should be positioned far enough away to ensure the sample notch traverses the lesion after deployment.

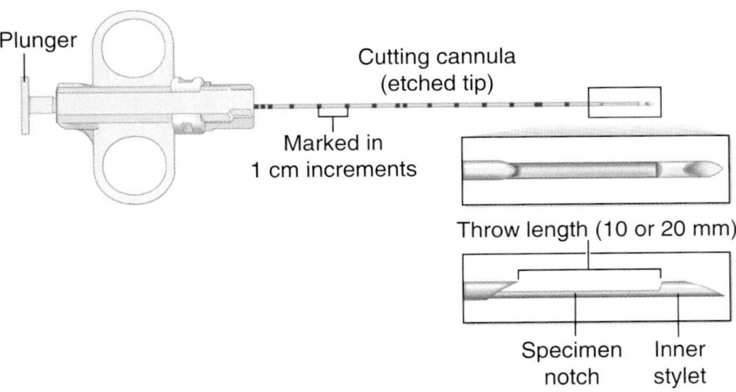

FIGURE 5 ● Terminology of core biopsy needle.

PERFORMANCE OF BIOPSY

Prep and Local Anesthesia

- Sterilize the skin with povidone-iodine or chlorhexidine solution and drape the patient after appropriate prep dry time.
- Assemble the biopsy tray, the surgeon should remain consistent in placement of all biopsy components for efficiency and safety.
- Detach the introducer trocar from the introducer needle to ensure smooth separation and perform a test deployment of the biopsy device to confirm proper function.
- With the aid of imaging displayed in the room, plan the trajectory of the biopsy needle into the mass via a specific site on the skin.
- Create a skin wheel of anesthetic with a 25-gauge needle at the biopsy insertion site.
- Apply local anesthetic with the 1.5-in 21-gauge needle along the planned trajectory path of the biopsy needle. Take care to inject past the planned length of the biopsy needle including the throw distance and dead length (up to 3 cm) as this keeps the patient most comfortable during the procedure.
- Make a small skin incision with a #11 blade to allow passage of the introducer needle and inner trocar (**FIGURE 6**).

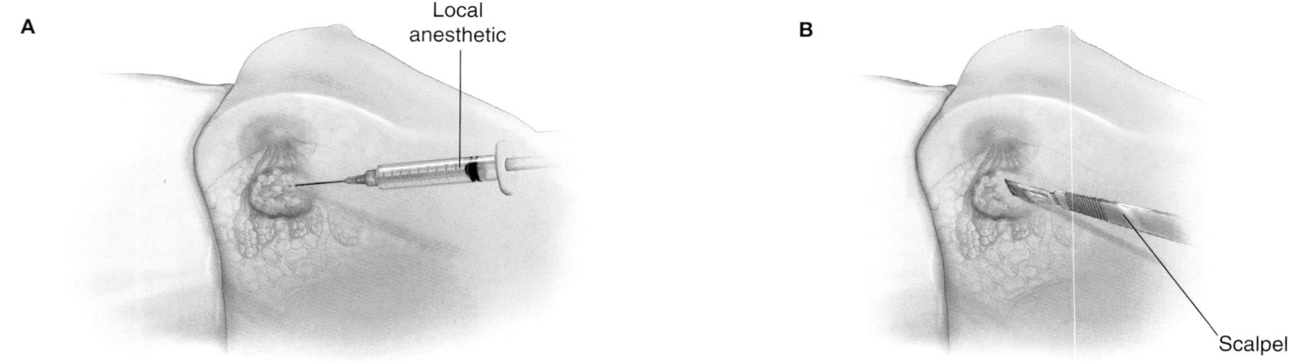

FIGURE 6 ● **A,** Application of local anesthetic along biopsy tract. **B,** Incision of skin.

INTRODUCER NEEDLE AND CORE BIOPSY DEVICE

- The surgeon immobilizes the breast with their nondominant hand. The surgeon ensures that in the planned needle trajectory, the supportive hand will not be in the needle's path.
- The surgeon places the trocar in the introducer needle and advance the introducer through the skin and along the trajectory of the local anesthetic. The surgeon assures here that the patient is not feeling any sharp pain. Ideally, the surgeon should follow the same trajectory as the anesthetic and that the patient remains comfortable (**FIGURE 7**).
- Once the needle is advanced at the edge of or into the mass (usually signaled by an increased resistance and aided by the surgeon's three-dimensional knowledge of the distance required) the surgeon removes the trocar from the introducer needle. It is best to target a central portion of the mass to improve sampling if the mass is large or fungating.

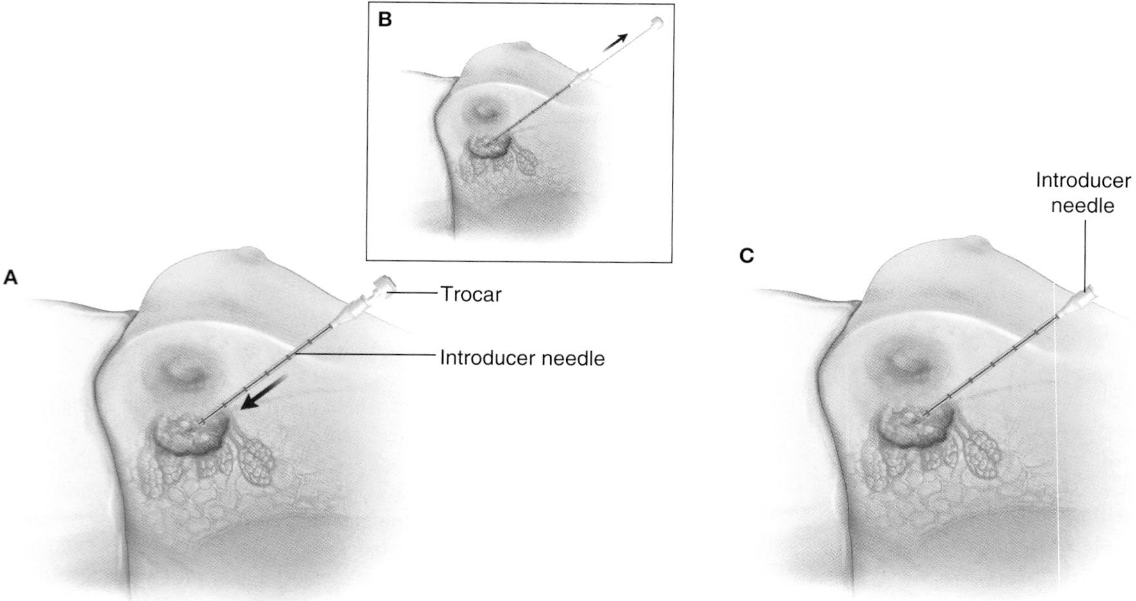

FIGURE 7 ● **A,** Placement of introducer needle along the path of the local anesthesia to the mass. **B,** Removal of trocar. **C,** Introducer needle in place ready for core needle insertion.

OBTAINING SAMPLES AND MARKING BIOPSY SITE

- The surgeon inserts the CNB device through the introducer needle and five core biopsy specimens are obtained, typically in a rotating clockwise fashion where the sampling notch of the biopsy needle is rotated to a different portion of the mass (**FIGURE 8**).
- After each firing of the CNB, the surgeon removes the specimen from the biopsy needle notch by swirling it in a test tube containing 3 to 4 mL of 0.9% saline solution or by using an additional needle to remove the core specimen onto a designated 4 × 4 gauze. The surgeon inspects the cores to ensure at least 1 cm of tissue was obtained, ideally the core should be cylindrical.
- Once all five specimens are collected, the specimens are poured or placed into to a permanent fixative such as a 10% formaldehyde solution. Of note, if the saline technique is used, the diminutive amount of saline applied during transfer does not compromise sample fixation.
- It can sometimes be helpful to deploy a biopsy marker at the same depth of invasion as the CNB device, particularly if neoadjuvant chemotherapy is anticipated for a possible cancer diagnosis. Most biopsy clip devices are a push mechanism on a device and shaft similar to CNB devices. Using the biopsy marker deployment device, the shaft is inserted to the same depth as the CNB device. The 1-cm markings on both the CNB and the biopsy marker deployment device increases accuracy of biopsy marker placement.
- The surgeon removes the introducer needle and applies Steri-Strips or surgical glue to the skin incision.
- To reduce the risk of hematoma, manual pressure is applied to the breast for 10 minutes.

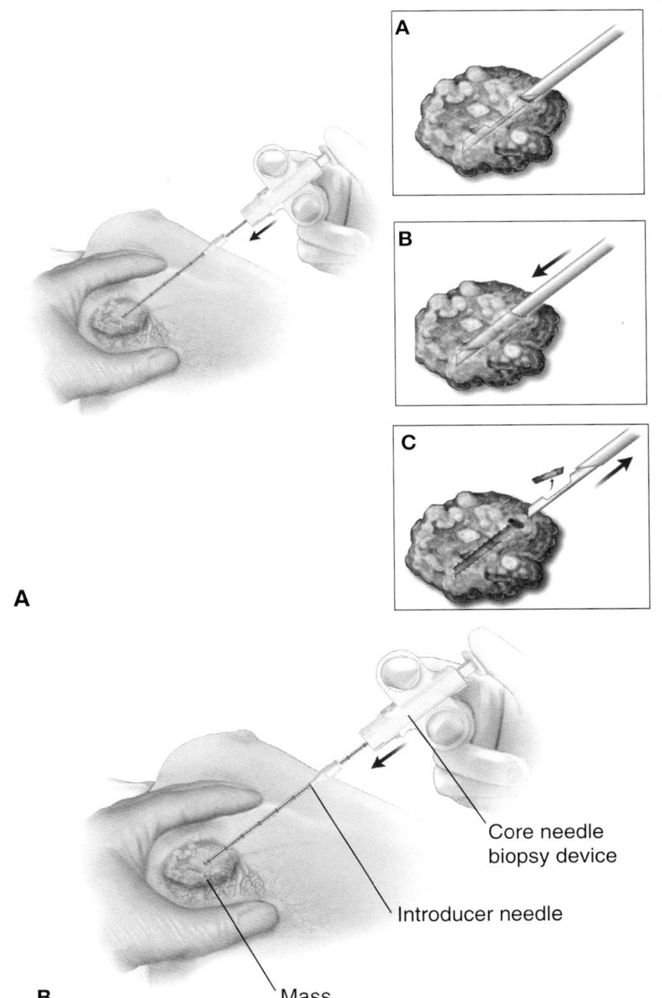

FIGURE 8 ● **A,** Introduction of CNB through introducer needle. **B,** Inset of biopsy needle throw length into the mass and advancement of cutting cannula and retrieval of biopsy specimen, repeated 5 times for adequate sampling.

PEARLS AND PITFALLS

Indications	■ Palpable lesions can be biopsied without image guidance. ■ If there is any ambiguity, image-guided CNB should be pursued.
Position of biopsy needle	■ Always know location and depth of the target. ■ Angle away from the chest wall to avoid pneumothorax. ■ Avoid compromising skin for superficial lesions by knowing the throw length and dead length. ■ Use the most hemostatic pathway for fungating masses.
Diagnostic pitfalls	■ Inadequate sampling—requires repeat CNB or excisional biopsy. ■ Biopsy marker migration—If the biopsy marker is displaced, localization and certainty of biopsy clip removal during excision biopsy can be difficult. ■ Discordance—Prebiopsy imaging and biopsy results must be concordant otherwise an excisional biopsy is indicated.

POSTOPERATIVE CARE

- If a biopsy marker was deployed, a postprocedural mammogram with mediolateral and craniocaudal views of the ipsilateral breast are obtained to document the deployment and location of the biopsy marker. This imaging will also confirm if the lesion sampled correlates with prior mammography findings.
- The patient is instructed to avoid heavy lifting or strenuous activity of the ipsilateral arm for 2 to 3 days.
- The patient is encouraged to wear a breast binder or snug sports bra for 2 to 3 days with only removal for showers.
- Postprocedural pain is typically minimal, but if medication is required, acetaminophen is a good option provided the patient has no contraindications.
- Anticoagulant and NSAID medications can be resumed in 1 to 2 days.
- Once the pathology has resulted, a determination of concordance between mammography findings and the pathology is made. If there is discordance, excisional biopsy is indicated and should be discussed with the patient.

COMPLICATIONS

- Hematoma
- Infection (cellulitis or abscess)
- Biopsy marker migration
- Milk fistula in lactating patients
- Failure to sample the mass requiring repeat biopsy or excisional biopsy
- Potential need for excisional biopsy due to discordant results between imaging and biopsy results

SUGGESTED READING

1. Jain A, Khalid M, Qureshi MM, et al. Stereotactic core needle breast biopsy marker migration: an analysis of factors contributing to immediate marker migration. *Eur Radiol.* 2017;27:4797-4803. doi:10.1007/s00330-017-4851-7
2. Kirshenbaum K, Keppke A, Hou K, et al. Reassessing specimen number and diagnostic yield of ultrasound guided breast core biopsy. *Breast J.* 2012;18:464-469. doi:10.1111/j.1524-4741.2012.01269.x
3. McMahon P, Reichman M, Dodelzon K. Bleeding risk after percutaneous breast needle biopsy in patients on anticoagulation therapy. *Clin Imag.* 2021;70:114-117. doi:10.1016/j.clinimag.2020.09.014
4. Schnitt SJ Problematic issues in breast core needle biopsies. *Mod Pathol.* 2019;32:71-76. doi:10.1038/s41379-018-0137-0
5. Winkler N. Ultrasound guided core breast biopsies. *Tech Vasc Interv Radiol.* 2021;24(3):100776. doi:10.1016/j.tvir.2021.100776

Chapter 4 Wire-Localized Breast Biopsy

Michael S. Sabel

DEFINITION

- The wire-localized excisional biopsy (or needle-localized biopsy) is used to obtain tissue for the diagnosis of a nonpalpable, image-detected abnormality. While several technologies are being used to move away from wires, such as radiocolloid occult lesion localization, infrared/electromagnetic, magnetic seed, and radiofrequency identification localization, wire localization is still the most frequently used method and is described in this chapter.
- It is preferable to use image-guided biopsy as a first step (stereotactic, ultrasound, or magnetic resonance imaging–guided biopsy), as this avoids surgery in patients with benign disease and allows for planning a definitive oncologic operation in patients with malignant disease. Thus, the wire-localized excisional biopsy should be limited to patients who failed image-guided biopsy (or have discordant findings), are not suitable candidates, or require excision secondary to a risk of upstaging.
- Wire-localized lumpectomy is a similar procedure for patients who have already been diagnosed with breast cancer, where the goal is a complete excision of the cancer with an adequate margin of surrounding normal tissue. For wire-localized lumpectomy, often, two wires are needed to "bracket" the cancer in order to assure complete removal.

PATIENT HISTORY AND PHYSICAL FINDINGS

- A bilateral breast examination should be performed in all patients for whom wire-localized breast biopsy is being contemplated for two reasons. First, to assess whether or not the lesion is truly nonpalpable. If the abnormality is palpable, then wire localization will not be necessary. If an abnormality is palpated, it is critical to review with the radiologist to be sure that the palpable abnormality corresponds to the imaging abnormality being recommended for biopsy. The second reason for bilateral breast examination is to make sure there are no other palpable occult abnormalities that may also require biopsy.
- For patients with biopsy-proven cancer who are to undergo wire-localized lumpectomy, a thorough history and physical examination is necessary to make sure they are suitable candidates for breast conservation therapy (BCT). Contraindications to BCT include prior radiation, collagen vascular disease, first or second trimester of pregnancy, multicentric cancer, or widespread calcifications (see Part 5, Chapter 9).

IMAGING AND OTHER DIAGNOSTIC STUDIES

- The preoperative imaging is essential to the procedure. Prior to the decision to perform a wire-localized breast biopsy, the breast imaging should be reviewed to determine whether the patient is a suitable candidate for an image-guided biopsy, as this is the preferable first step. The patient's allergies and medications (specifically aspirin or anticoagulants) or the presence of a bleeding diathesis should be reviewed. Contraindications to stereotactic core needle biopsy include an inability to adequately visualize the target lesion or an inability of the patient to remain in the position required for the procedure. Some patients may exceed the weight limit for the stereotactic table. Other factors that may preclude stereotactic core needle biopsy include higher breast density or faint calcifications, limiting visualization; lesions close to the skin, chest wall, or axilla; or the presence of breast implants.
- Prior to coming to the operating room (OR), the patient undergoes needle localization under image guidance. After local anesthesia, a rigid introducer needle with a hooked wire within it is directed toward the site of the abnormality using biplanar mammography (**FIGURE 1A**) or ultrasound (**FIGURE 1B**). The rigid needle is then removed, leaving the wire secured by the hook so it is not easily withdrawn or redirected (**FIGURE 2A** and **B**).
- Wire-localized excisional biopsy is also used in patients in whom the diagnosis is discordant or in benign lesions at high risk of "upstaging" upon excision. Several prospective studies have led to changes in the recommendations for wire-localized excision of benign, concordant lesions of the breast.[1]

SURGICAL MANAGEMENT

Preoperative Planning

- Performing a breast examination after the localization will be difficult, as the wire will be secured by a variety of methods that will preclude physical examination. These should not be removed until the patient is positioned in the OR to minimize the chance of dislodging the wire during transport.
- Prior to taking the patient back to the OR, the localization films should be reviewed. Specifically, the surgeon should note the proximity of the abnormality to the wire, the direction of the wire from the point of skin entry, and how far the lesion is from the skin, as this may impact the degree of sedation (if any).
- Although the risk of infection after breast surgery is low, it tends to be higher than average for a clean surgical procedure, and several studies have shown that antibiotic prophylaxis significantly reduces the risk of postoperative infection.[2]

Positioning

- The patient should be positioned supine. Often, the localization wire is placed laterally, so the ipsilateral arm may need to be at 90°.
- Once the patient is on the OR table and positioned, the tape and dressings securing the wire should be removed carefully as not to dislodge the wire. A gentle breast examination can be performed at this point to see if the lesion is palpable. In addition, light palpation while watching the external portion

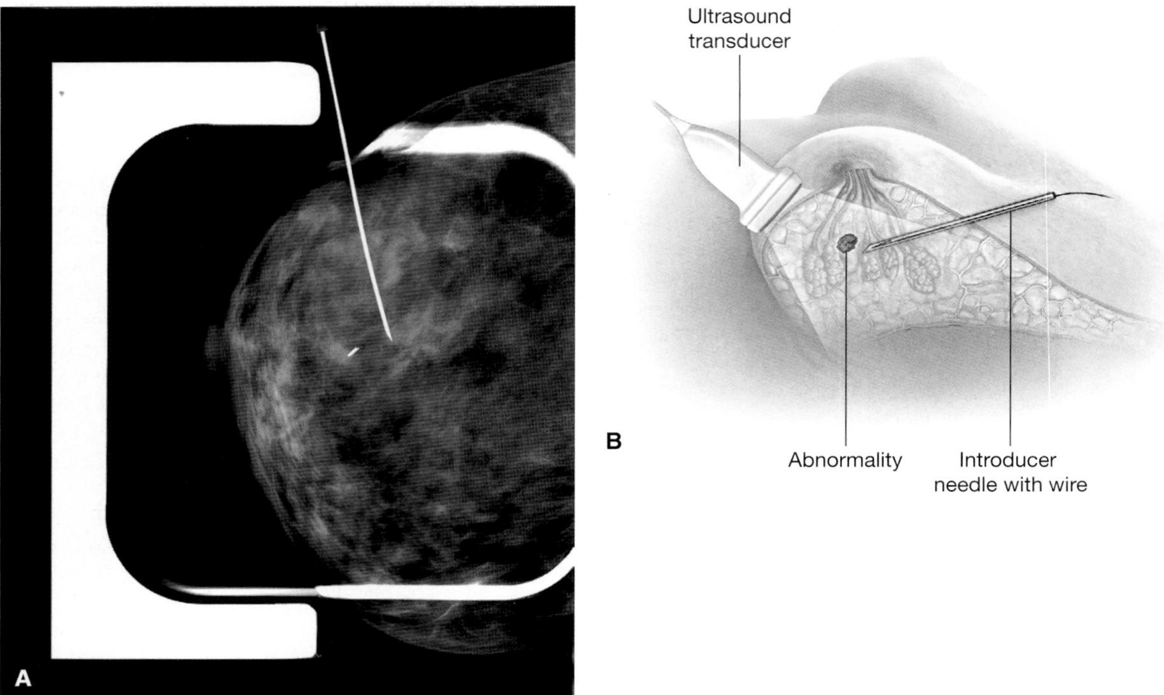

FIGURE 1 ● Placement of the rigid needle using biplanar mammography **(A)** or ultrasound (**B**).

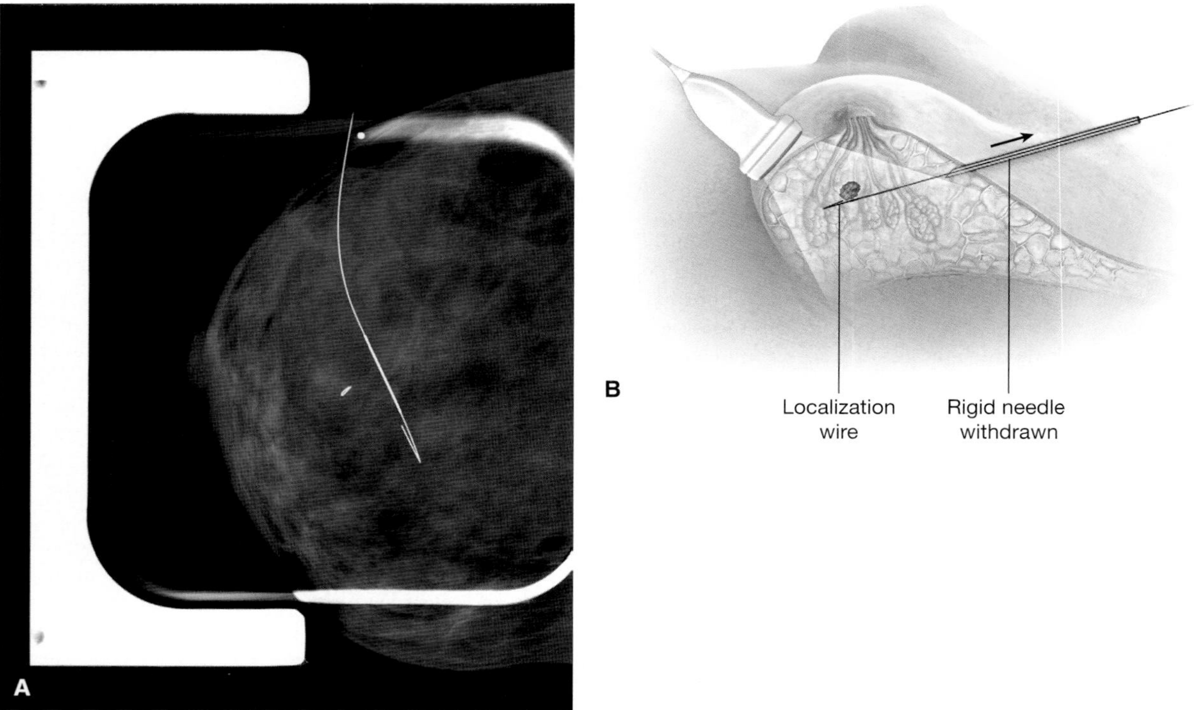

FIGURE 2 ● **A** and **B,** The rigid needle is withdrawn, leaving the wire in the location of the abnormality.

of the wire can give the surgeon an idea of what direction the wire is heading.

- The localization wire is often quite long and with a significant portion outside of the skin. The case will be facilitated by cutting the wire to a more workable length. Care must be taken not to advance the wire or pull the wire back (or out). It is also important not to cut the wire so close to the skin that it disappears. Secure the wire at the level of the skin prior to cutting with a wire cutter (**FIGURE 3**).

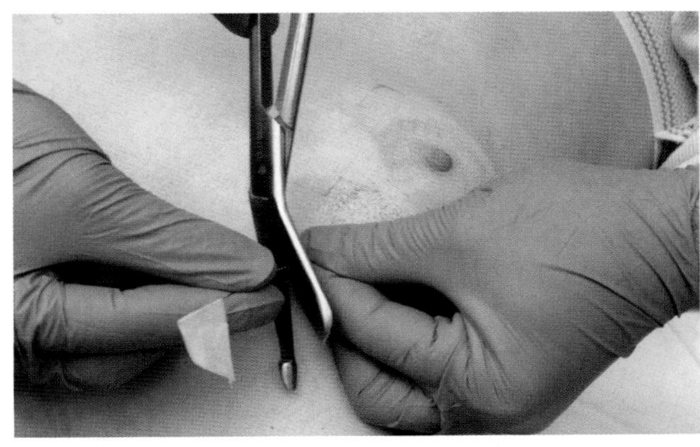

FIGURE 3 ● The wire is secured at the level of the skin while excess wire is cut. It is important not to dislodge the wire as well as to leave an adequate amount.

ANTICIPATING THE LOCATION OF THE ABNORMALITY

- After the dressings have been removed, the surgeon uses the site and direction of the wire along with the craniocaudal (CC) and lateral-medial (LM) views to determine the location of the abnormality in the breast. A small ball bearing is usually placed at the site where the wire enters the skin, so it is possible to estimate how far through the breast tissue the wire extends. Remember, the breast is compressed during the mammography but not on the OR table, so the measurement on the film may not be exact. It is often helpful to identify the nipple on the mammogram as an additional landmark.
- The CC view (**FIGURE 4A**) demonstrates both the anterior-posterior and the lateral-medial location of the abnormality but gives no information regarding the superior-inferior location. With a laterally placed wire, the CC view can be used to estimate how deep the lesion is and how medial (especially when also using the nipple as an additional landmark).
- The LM view (**FIGURE 4B**) demonstrates the anterior-posterior orientation as well as the superior-inferior but gives no information regarding the lateral-medial location. Again, with a laterally placed wire, the deviation from the skin ball bearing to the hook of the wire can be used to assess whether the wire is heading superiorly or inferiorly.
- Using both views, the surgeon should also note where the abnormality is in relation to the wire. Typically, the radiologist attempts to place the reinforced portion of the wire in close proximity to the lesion. It is crucial to know the relative proximity of the wire to the lesion and in what direction the wire sits relative to the lesion.

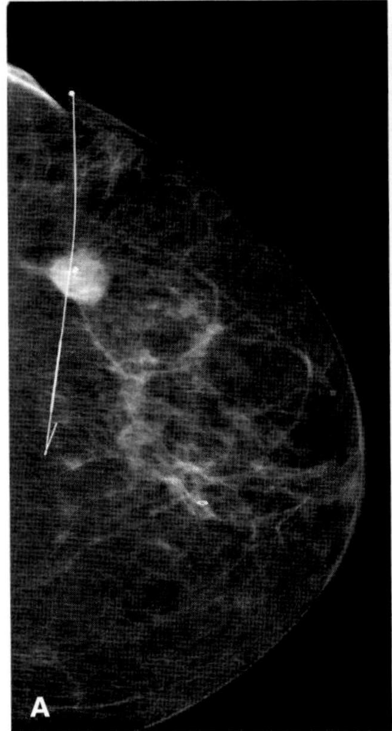

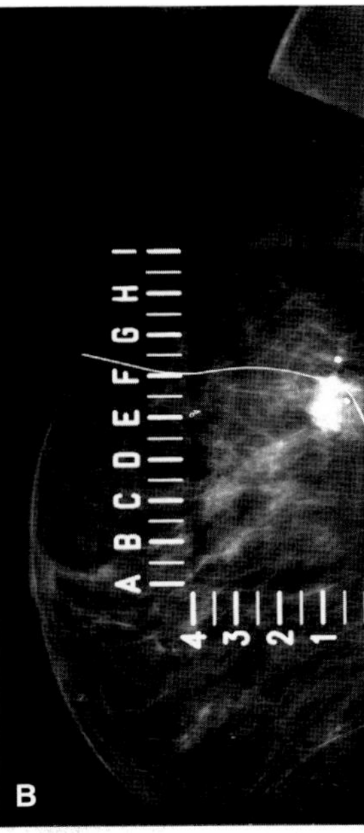

FIGURE 4 ● The localization films show the relationship between the skin, the wire, and the abnormality. In the CC view **(A)**, the *dot* shows the entry point in the skin. The film shows the lesion to be posterior and lateral, but this film does not reveal the anterior-posterior position. The hook and reinforced portion of the wire are distal (medial) to the lesion. In the LM view **(B)**, you can again see the lesion is posterior, but now you can see that it sits superiorly. It may seem like the wire travels through the breast for some distance but most of that is external. The *white dot* shows where it enters the skin.

SKIN INCISION AND IDENTIFICATION OF THE WIRE

- Using both the preoperative imaging and examination of the breast, the surgeon can estimate the direction of the wire and the distance to the reinforced portion of the wire. The incision can be placed directly over the anticipated site of the lesion (**FIGURE 5**) or can be placed laterally, circumareolar or in the inframammary fold, which will improve the cosmetic outcome. The greater the distance between the target and the incision site, the more tunneling will be needed, and this will impact the amount of local anesthetic and sedation that may be needed.
- When marking the incision, it should be kept in mind that if this lesion is malignant, you may be returning for a re-excision lumpectomy or a mastectomy. Therefore, the incision should be placed in a way that does not compromise that.
- The incision should be kept small at first, as it can be lengthened later if need be (**FIGURE 6**). As these are typically performed with just local anesthesia or light sedation, the skin is anesthetized prior to any incision.

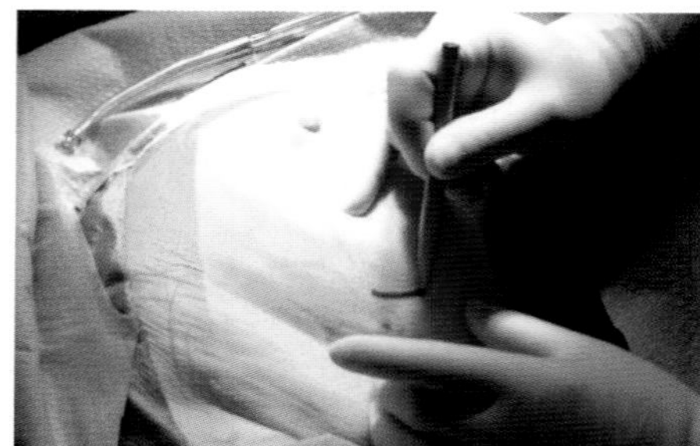

FIGURE 5 ● An incision is marked out over the anticipated site of the abnormality, keeping in mind a re-excision lumpectomy or mastectomy should the pathology return as malignant.

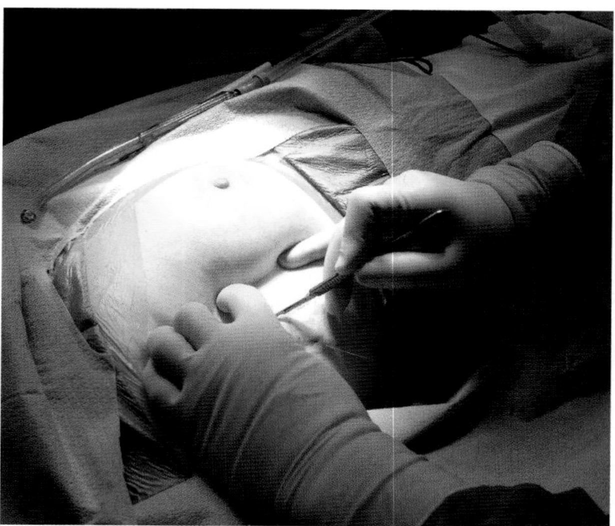

FIGURE 6 ● A small incision is made in the skin after infiltration of local anesthesia.

EXCISION

- The goal of the wire-localized excisional biopsy is to make the diagnosis while removing as little breast tissue as possible. If the CC and LM views suggest that the lesion is deep to the incision, the dissection is continued posteriorly so as to avoid removing excessive tissue anterior to the lesion and wire (**FIGURE 7A**). For more superficial lesions, flaps should be elevated shortly after incision but kept thick enough to avoid concavity at the site (**FIGURE 7B**).
- If the incision does not incorporate the entry site of the wire, the next step is to identify the shaft of the wire proximal to the lesion. Dissection is carried down to the wire, taking care not to land on top of the abnormality but rather on the wire proximal to the abnormality (**FIGURE 8**).
- Once the wire is identified, it is grasped with a hemostat on the specimen side, and the shaft of the wire is retracted into the wound. Take care to secure the wire adequately so it is not dislodged (**FIGURE 9A** and **B**).
- At the point where the wire enters the breast, grasp the tissue with an Allis clamp. Be careful to grasp above or below the wire and not the wire directly, as retraction on the clamp may dislodge the wire (**FIGURE 10**).
- Dissection then continues parallel to the wire, maintaining a circumference of approximately 1 cm of breast tissue around the wire. This is modified based on the size of the

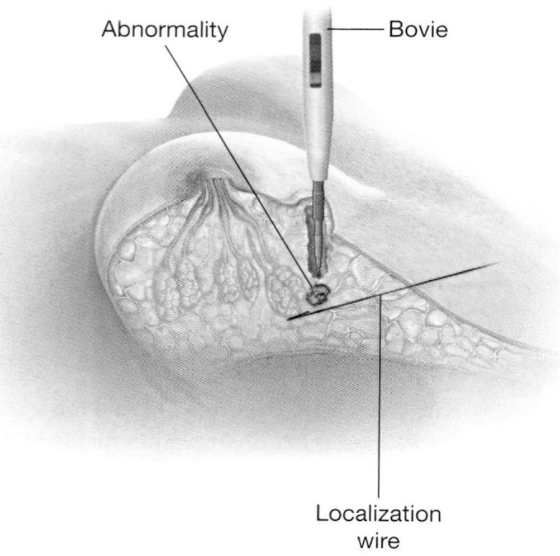

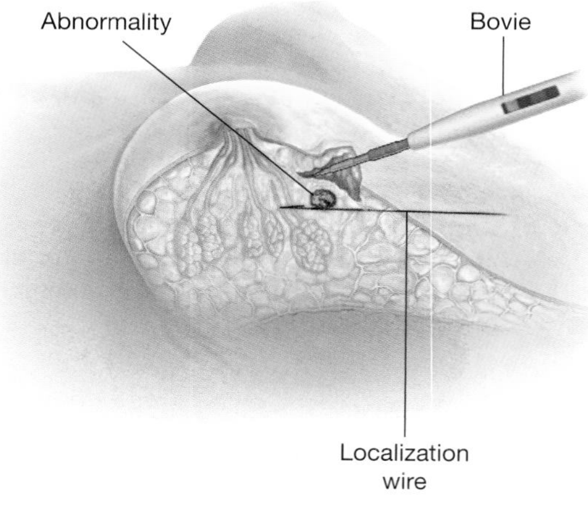

FIGURE 7 ● The subcutaneous fat and breast parenchyma are divided with cautery. For deep lesions **(A)**, dissect a fair distance to avoid taking excessive tissue anterior to the lesion (causing concavity). For superficial lesions **(B)**, thick flaps should be elevated shortly after incision.

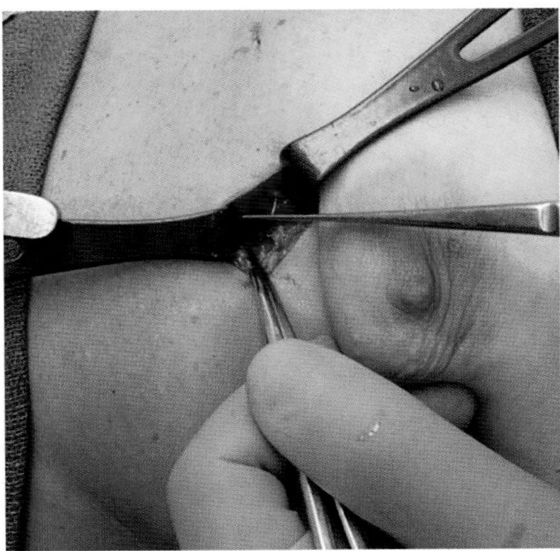

FIGURE 8 ● The wire is identified proximal to the anticipated site of the abnormality.

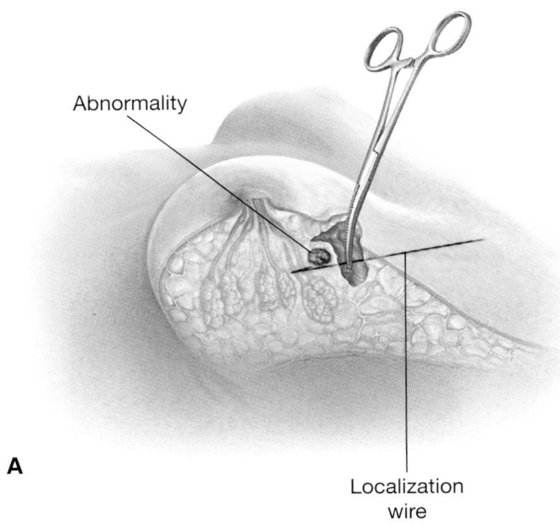

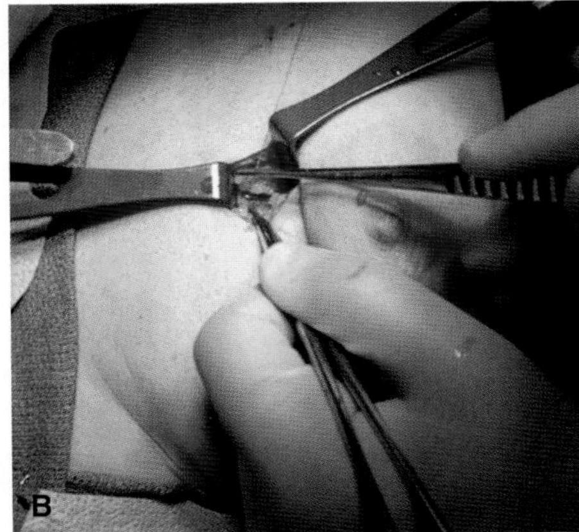

FIGURE 9 ● **A,** The wire is secured at the breast with a hemostat. **B,** Forceps are then used to pull the external portion of the wire through the skin and out of the wound.

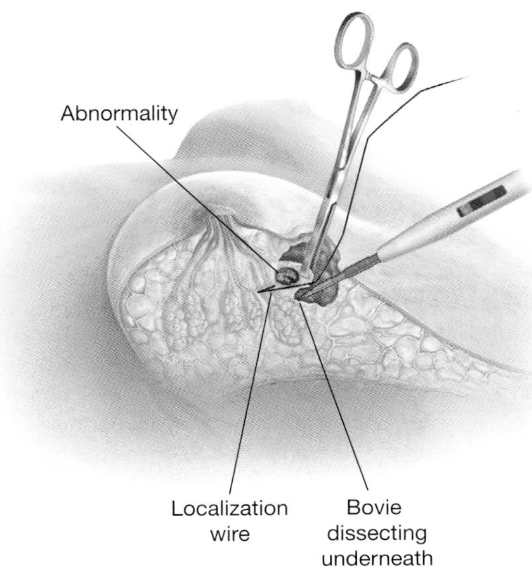

FIGURE 10 ● An Allis clamp is used to grasp the breast tissue (do not grab the wire) and dissection continues parallel to the wire in all directions.

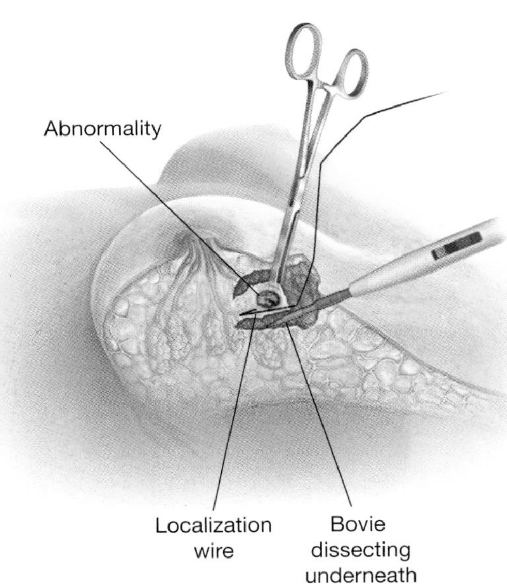

FIGURE 11 ● Once the circumferential dissection is past where you estimate the lesion to be, the specimen is transected, taking care not to divide the wire (and leave the hook).

abnormality and the relationship between the wire and the lesion. For example, for a lesion sitting approximately 1 cm anterior to the wire, a larger margin is taken anteriorly, whereas a smaller margin can be taken deep to the wire.

- For mammographic masses, palpation along the wire may allow the surgeon to identify the abnormality and proceed with excision, simplifying the procedure.
- Dissection continues until you are confident you are past the location of the abnormality and the specimen can be transected (**FIGURE 11**). Often, the wire will be encountered

during this step, so take care not to divide the wire, potentially leaving the hooked end in the patient. If the wire is identified at this point, visualize where on the wire you are. If you are at the hook and the films show the hook is distal to the lesion, you should be fine. If you encountered the reinforced portion of the wire, grasp the remaining tissue in the direction of the wire and continue the dissection until you are past the hook.

ORIENTATION

- Immediately upon removing the lesion, maintain the orientation and place 2-0 silk sutures for the pathologist. If this returns as cancer, this allows for simple re-excision of any involved margin as opposed to a re-excision of the entire cavity. It is often preferable to place one or two orienting sutures before complete removal of the specimen.
- Three sutures are recommended to orient the mass correctly for the pathologist and avoid errors.[3] We recommend placing a short suture superiorly, a long suture laterally, and a double suture deep posteriorly (**FIGURE 12**).
- It may also be beneficial to place radiopaque clips on the specimen to allow for orientation of the lesion on the specimen mammograms. For example, if the wire enters laterally, placing a single clip superiorly and a double clip posteriorly allows you to orient the specimen on the films (**FIGURE 13A** and **B**). In the case of a wire-localized lumpectomy for cancer, this allows for re-excision of a potentially close margin. For a biopsy, if the abnormality is not within the specimen, this may help the surgeon identify in what direction additional tissue should be sampled.

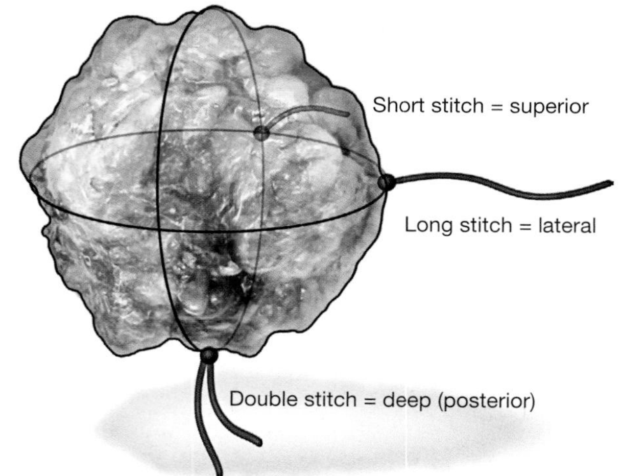

FIGURE 12 ● The lesion is oriented with three marking sutures prior to sending to radiology for specimen mammography.

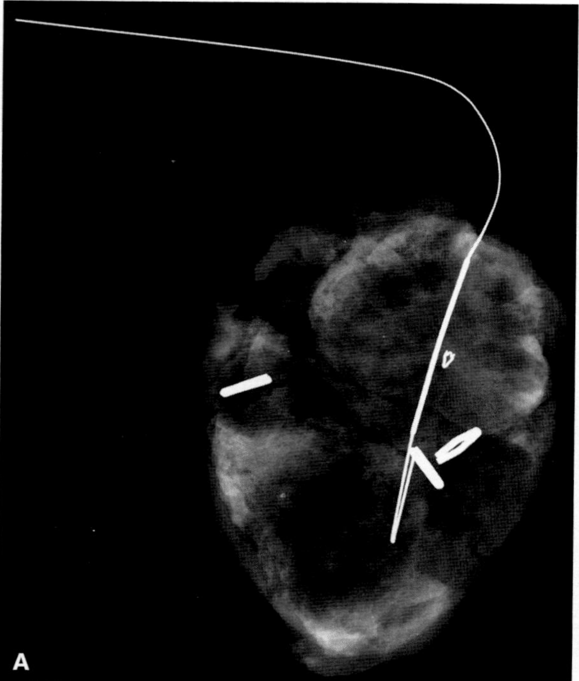

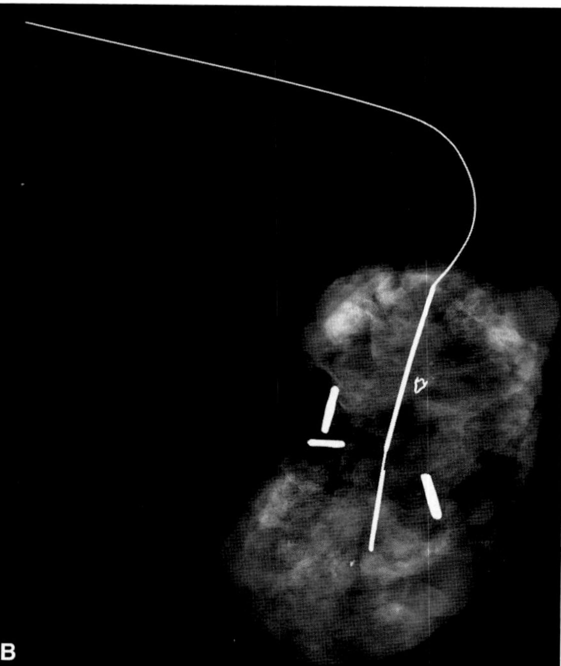

FIGURE 13 ● A and **B**, Specimen mammography shows the clip and wire to be completely removed.

SPECIMEN RADIOGRAPHY AND ADDITIONAL TISSUE

- Specimen radiography is performed to confirm that the area of concern has been removed (**FIGURE 13A** and **B**). The specimen mammogram should demonstrate the presence of the microcalcifications of concern or the presence of a clip placed within the specimen. It should also show that the entire wire has been removed. If the wire becomes separated from the specimen, send both to radiology to document its removal.
- If the lesion is identified on specimen radiography, the wound can be closed. If the lesion is not present, then additional tissue should be excised and sent to radiology. It may be clinically evident what area needs further excision based on exposure of the wire during the dissection. The use of radiopaque clips on the specimen, as well as other landmarks on the original mammograms, may also help identify where to excise additional tissue.
- If a second specimen fails to identify the lesion, it becomes a judgment call whether to continue or abandon the procedure. For ultrasound-visible lesions, intraoperative ultrasound may be able to identify the abnormality. In the case of a clip that should have been in the specimen, sometimes these can get dislodged and suctioned out. Filtering and x-raying the fluid in the suction canister can sometimes reveal a dislodged clip. Otherwise, it may be prudent not to continue and plan on reimaging and, if necessary, returning to the OR rather than taking an excessive amount of breast tissue.

CLOSURE

- Once the biopsy is complete, hemostasis is assured and the wound is irrigated with saline.
- For an excisional biopsy, the surgeon should *not* try to reapproximate the breast tissue. The cavity will fill with seroma and fibrin and, ultimately, fibrous tissue, which will maintain the normal contour.
- The incision is closed with absorbable deep dermal sutures, followed by either a subcuticular stitch or tissue adhesive. Drains should not be used.

PEARLS AND PITFALLS

Indications	■ Image-guided biopsy is the preferred approach to the nonpalpable abnormality. Review the case with the radiologist to confirm whether this is an option.
Placement of incision	■ Keep in mind that, if the lesion is malignant, the patient may need a re-excision lumpectomy or mastectomy. Place your incision with this in mind.
Identifying the wire	■ Take care not to move or dislodge the wire during the positioning, prepping, and draping of the patient. ■ Identify the wire early and secure it while bringing it into the wound so that it does not become dislodged during the procedure.
Excision	■ Grasp the tissue, not the wire, while excising the lesion so as not to accidently pull the wire out. ■ During dissection, palpate the area to identify a mass or if you are too close to the wire.
Specimen mammography	■ Three orientation sutures are necessary to avoid error. ■ Clips can help orient the specimen on the mammography so as to guide a re-excision.
Closure	■ Do not try to reapproximate the breast tissue or place a drain.

POSTOPERATIVE CARE

- After a breast biopsy, the patient should be placed in a breast binder or supportive brassiere. This helps sustain hemostasis and relieves tension on the skin closure imposed by the weight of the breasts. This should remain in place for 48 hours.
- After 48 hours, the patient may remove the binder and shower. We recommend the patient continue to wear a comfortable bra, including while sleeping, for the remainder of a week.

OUTCOMES

- In experienced hands, the failure rate of wire-localized biopsy is low, approximately 2.5%.[4] Factors associated with failure include lesion type and size, distance from the wire, breast shape and size, and volume of excised tissue.[4-6]

COMPLICATIONS

- Seroma
- Hematoma
- Infection (cellulitis or abscess)

- Pneumothoraces (rare)
- Retained wire fragments
- Failure to identify abnormality

REFERENCES

1. American Society of Breast Surgeons. *Consensus Guideline on Concordance Assessment of Image-Guided Breast Biopsies and Management of Borderline or High-Risk Lesions*. Accessed December 30, 2021. https://www.breastsurgeons.org/docs/statements/Consensus-Guideline-on-Concordance-Assessment-of-Image-Guided-Breast-Biopsies.pdf?v2
2. Bunn F, Jones DJ, Bell-Syer S. Prophylactic antibiotics to prevent surgical site infections after breast cancer surgery. *Cochrane Database Syst Rev*. 2012;9(3):CD005360. 10.1002/1465858.CD005360.pub3.
3. Molina MA, Snell S, Franceschi D, et al. Breast specimen orientation. *Ann Surg Oncol*. 2009;16:285-288.
4. Mayo RC, Kalambo JM, Parikh JR. Preoperative localization of breast lesions: current techniques. *Clin Imag*. 2019;56:1-8.
5. Abrahamson PE, Dunlap LA, Amamoo MA, et al. Factors predicting successful needle-localized breast biopsy. *Acad Radiol*. 2003;10(6):601-606.
6. Kouskos E, Gui GP, Mantas D, et al. Wire localization biopsy of non-palpable breast lesions: reasons for unsuccessful excision. *Eur J Gynaecol Oncol*. 2006;27(3):262-366.

Chapter 5 Subareolar Duct Excision

Anneke T. Schroen and Amy C. Degnim

DEFINITION

- Subareolar duct excision is defined as the surgical removal of lactiferous ducts in the immediate subareolar space. The terms "major duct excision" and "central duct excision" refer to excision of the entire bundle of ducts contained within the central nipple stalk; microdochectomy refers to selective excision of a single abnormal duct.

ANATOMY

- The lactiferous ducts drain converging ducts from lobes of the breast gland and serve as a conduit for milk egress via the nipple during lactation (**FIGURE 1**). Most women have approximately 7 to 20 ducts that are distinct and functional sources of milk during lactation. At the base of the nipple, the lactiferous ducts widen centrally in a spindle shape over a short distance. This region is called the lactiferous sinus and can expand in lactation to 8 mm as a reservoir for milk. Surrounding the lactiferous ducts is a system of smooth muscle fibers that contract in response to nipple stimulation and oxytocin release, facilitating milk flow through the nipple.[1]

PATIENT HISTORY AND PHYSICAL FINDINGS

- Subareolar duct excision is undertaken in cases of abnormal nipple discharge for two purposes:
  - To obtain diagnostic biopsy tissue and rule out malignancy
  - To provide resolution of the bothersome discharge
- Abnormal, or "pathologic," nipple discharge is characterized by the following features:
  - Discharge from a single duct
  - Spontaneous discharge
  - Clear or bloody discharge
  - Discharge associated with skin changes or a mass

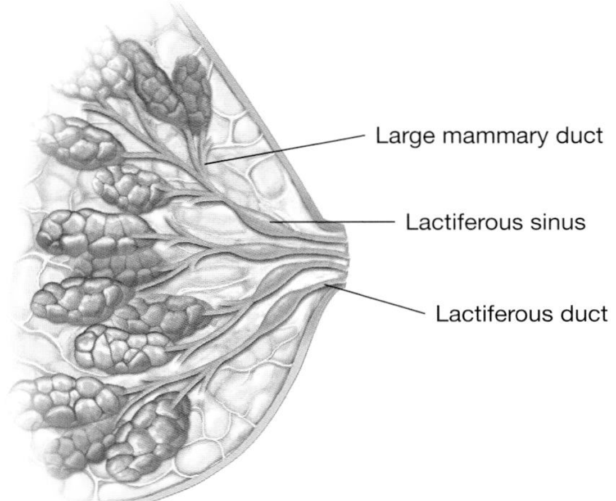

FIGURE 1 ● Normal anatomy of subareolar lactiferous ducts and sinuses.

- The history should be focused on questions to determine the laterality and quality of the discharge as well as whether it is spontaneous or only occurs with manual expression.
- Physical examination should include a thorough examination of both breasts and axillae.
- In addition, a detailed examination is necessary for both nipple-areolar complexes and the subareolar tissues.
- Inspect the nipples for crusting, bloodstained ducts, or any visible protuberances or nodules.
- The deep tissue of the areolae should be palpated carefully for any small nodules and to determine if subareolar pressure or trigger point results in nipple discharge.
- The nipple itself should be palpated by rolling the nipple between the thumb and forefinger in order to best detect any small nodules located centrally within the nipple stalk. This should be performed first for the breast without discharge to set a normal comparison with the breast that is symptomatic.
- Additional maneuvers that may help elicit discharge include clockwise massage of tissue from the periphery toward the nipple or application of a warm compress.
- Throughout the examination, for any nipple discharge observed, its location (o'clock position) and quality of the fluid should be noted.

IMAGING AND OTHER DIAGNOSTIC STUDIES

- Women over age 30 years and all men with abnormal nipple discharge should undergo diagnostic mammogram and ultrasound. The imaging team should be informed about the symptom of nipple discharge and which breast is affected. If initial standard imaging is negative, breast MRI or ductography may be helpful.[2] Ultrasound alone may be reasonable for women who are under 30 years or pregnant.
- The purpose of diagnostic imaging is to look for possible signs of underlying malignancy and to evaluate the subareolar tissues for any findings that would explain the presence of nipple discharge.
- Generally, subareolar ducts are not visible with ultrasound unless they are abnormally dilated. A small nodule visualized within a dilated subareolar duct indicates a likely diagnosis of intraductal papilloma (**FIGURE 2**).
- Breast magnetic resonance imaging (MRI) has been shown to have high sensitivity for invasive cancer detection but relatively low specificity.[2] In addition, breast MRI may detect lesions located more peripherally than included in central duct excision, ductography, or subareolar ultrasound.[3] MRI for nipple discharge is best employed when MRI-directed biopsy is available.
- Ductography is a radiographic procedure that entails cannulation of the duct with abnormal discharge, then injection of contrast dye with immediate mammographic imaging. This procedure can identify and map out abnormal ducts and identify some intraductal filling defects, but it does not

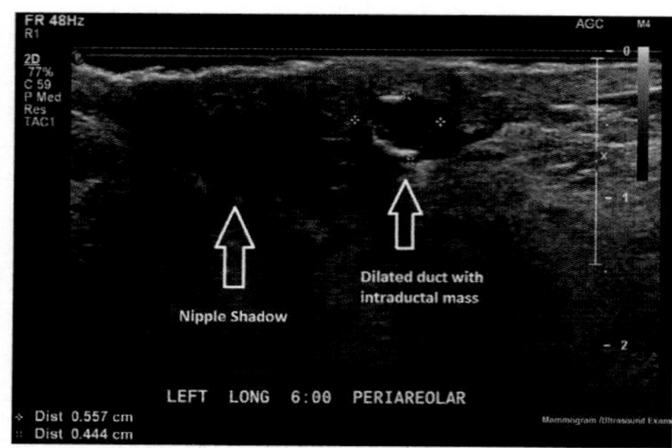

FIGURE 2 ● Ultrasound of a subareolar nodule.

provide diagnostic tissue. Although ductography may help to localize the etiology of the discharge, it cannot reliably exclude malignancy or eliminate the need for duct excision.[3,4]

- Studies have shown that surgery with image-guided localization of a lesion results in higher likelihood of identifying the cause of nipple discharge than duct excision alone.[5]
- Another approach to diagnostic evaluation is via ductoscopy, a microendoscopic procedure to directly visualize the duct(s) with discharge. This requires special equipment and skill, with a learning curve for technical success. Ductoscopy can help to identify lesions and guide excision but has not been proven in large numbers of women to improve diagnosis to the point that duct excision can be avoided.[6,7]

DIFFERENTIAL DIAGNOSIS

- Intraductal papilloma
- Duct ectasia
- Carcinoma, either invasive or ductal carcinoma in situ
- Paget disease

NONOPERATIVE MANAGEMENT

- Nonoperative management can be considered for cases of nipple discharge when
  - The discharge occurred on only one occasion and was not reproducible on examination.
  - Both mammogram and ultrasound show no abnormalities.[8,9] Addition of breast MRI may provide further reassurance that an invasive malignancy is not missed.
  - In this case, 3-month follow-up history and physical examination is recommended.
- If imaging identifies a benign-appearing lesion and percutaneous core biopsy confirms a benign intraductal papilloma with complete or near-complete removal by imaging, then observation is also appropriate with follow-up imaging in 6 months.
- Practice regarding nonsurgical management of radiologic-pathologic concordant papillomas without atypia is evolving.[10]

SURGICAL MANAGEMENT

- Subareolar duct excision removes the lactiferous ducts under the nipple, the primary connection between the nipple and the milk-producing lobules of the breast, so patients must be counseled that lactation from the operated breast should not be possible after surgery.
- Selective and focused excision of the single abnormal duct may be performed in an attempt to preserve other ducts for future lactation, but due to the very close proximity of the remaining ducts, scar tissue from the operation may still impair future lactation.
- In women who are past childbearing age, a plan to remove the entire bundle of subareolar ducts is preferred because future lactation is not needed. This approach reduces the chance of recurrent discharge from another duct and need for repeat operation in a field of scar tissue. If the location of the lesion is not known, the central duct excision should extend at least 2 to 3 cm deep to the nipple in order to maximize the likelihood of including the lesion causing the pathologic discharge.
- The patient should be informed of the possibility of a diagnosis of malignancy yet reassured that benign findings are most likely.
- Localized excision of a lesion remote from the nipple without formal duct excision is reasonable if no pathologic discharge persists. Controversy exists surrounding the need for true duct excision with all discharging ducts if etiology of discharge is identified and no discharge persists.

Preoperative Planning

- For subareolar mass lesions that are nonpalpable and identified only by imaging, preoperative localization with either a wire or a radioactive seed should be performed to ensure intraoperative guidance to the target.
- Before surgery, patients should be counseled that they may experience continued discharge in the first few weeks postoperatively, as postoperative fluid in the subareolar space may discharge via the nipple duct until healing is complete. This should resolve completely by 4 to 6 weeks. Patients should also be counseled on change in nipple sensation, including hyper- or hyposensitivity, that may last for several weeks.

Positioning

- The patient should be positioned supine.
- The ipsilateral arm is generally positioned at approximately 90°, although the arm could also be tucked.

Approach

- The general approach is to dissect under the areola toward the nipple, isolate and excise the central duct bundle, and follow any abnormal ducts to complete removal, along with simultaneous excision of any nonpalpable lesions identified on preoperative imaging.

INCISION PLANNING

- In general, incisions are placed at the areolar edge.
- An incision at the inferior areolar edge is preferred if possible for better cosmesis, especially if the involved duct is located centrally on the nipple surface and the imaging does not demonstrate any abnormalities (**FIGURE 3**).
- Otherwise, incisions can be placed along the areolar border in the o'clock position of the abnormality, either for a peripherally located duct with discharge or if there is an imaging abnormality a few centimeters from the nipple.
- The length of the incision should be large enough that the surgeon has adequate visualization of the subareolar space without requiring excess retraction and ischemia of the areolar edge. Depending on the areolar size, the incision may go up to 50% of the circumference of the areola, but a shorter incision is preferred when possible to help preserve blood supply to the nipple and areolar dermis.

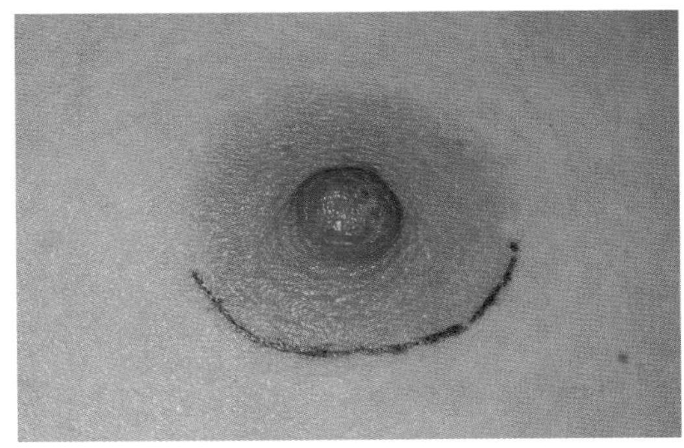

FIGURE 3 ● Incision at inferior areolar border.

- Prior to incision, correct surgical site and plan should be confirmed with the operative team.

DUCT CANNULATION

- Once the field is prepped and draped, attempt should be made to cannulate the involved duct.
- A fine lacrimal duct probe (4-0) should be held ready in the dominant hand for cannulation prior to expressing the nipple discharge.
- The nipple should be grasped between the thumb and forefinger of the nondominant hand at the nipple base and drawn upward gradually (**FIGURE 4**). If no discharge is seen, increasing pressure can be applied to a reasonable degree. The goal is to elicit a single tiny drop of fluid at the skin surface; a smaller drop of fluid will be more helpful in identifying the location of the abnormal duct (**FIGURE 5**).
- The nipple should be pulled away from the breast gently in order to elongate the subareolar lactiferous sinus and improve the chance of cannulation (**FIGURE 6**).
- The lacrimal duct probe should be gently probed along the nipple skin surface at the site of the expressed fluid. The goal is to find the opening rather than make a false passage; the probe will slide easily into the duct once it is in the right location (**FIGURE 7**).
- The probe should be gently advanced as far as it will easily go. If it does not pass greater than 1 cm beyond the nipple skin surface, then the depth of the cannulation should be noted as a sign that there may be a very superficial obstructing mass lesion.
- If no discharge is identified or if the duct cannot be cannulated despite several attempts, the procedure should proceed to incision.

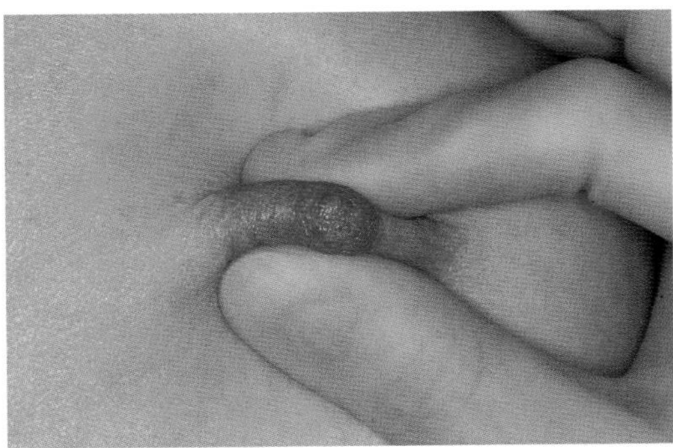

FIGURE 4 ● Manual expression of nipple discharge.

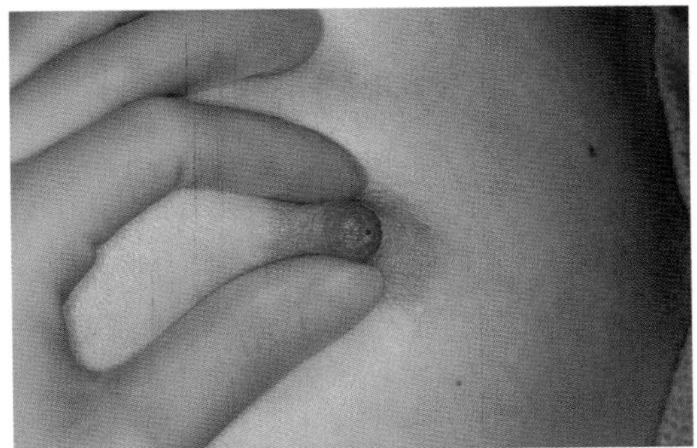

FIGURE 5 ● Visible tiny drop of fluid at nipple surface.

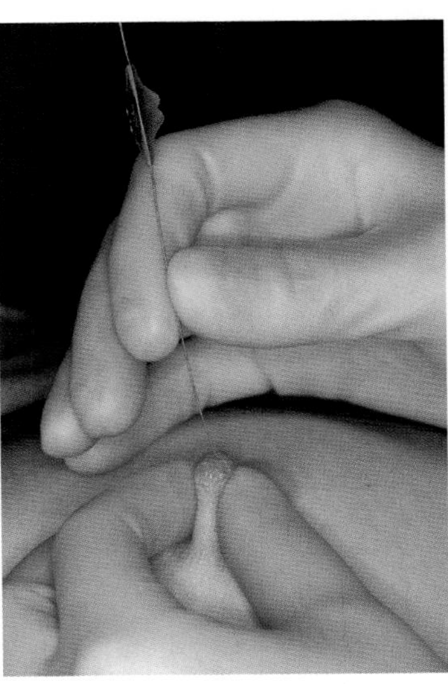

FIGURE 6 ● Cannulation technique.

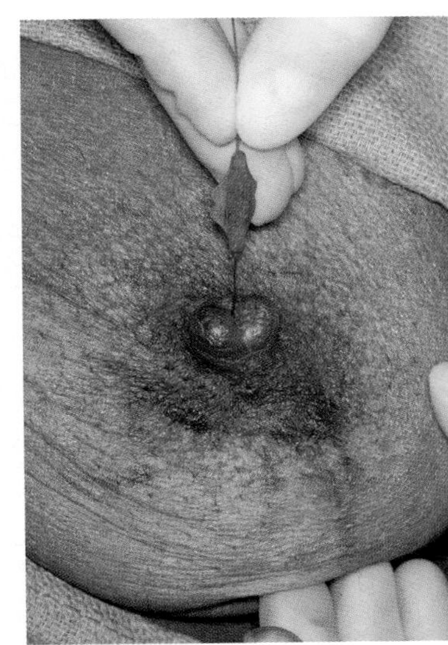

FIGURE 7 ● Cannulated duct with probe advanced.

INCISION

- Prior to incision, local anesthetic can be used but should not be injected directly into the area of the subareolar ducts. If used, it should be injected intradermally directly at the planned incision site (no more than 1 mL) and additionally in a peripheral fashion into the four quadrants of the breast to create a local field block. Local anesthetic can also be injected prior to closure when using general anesthesia.
- The skin should be incised sharply with a scalpel, taking care to maintain a blade angle that is perpendicular to the skin.
- The incision should be deepened a few millimeters into the subcutaneous fatty tissue (**FIGURE 8**).

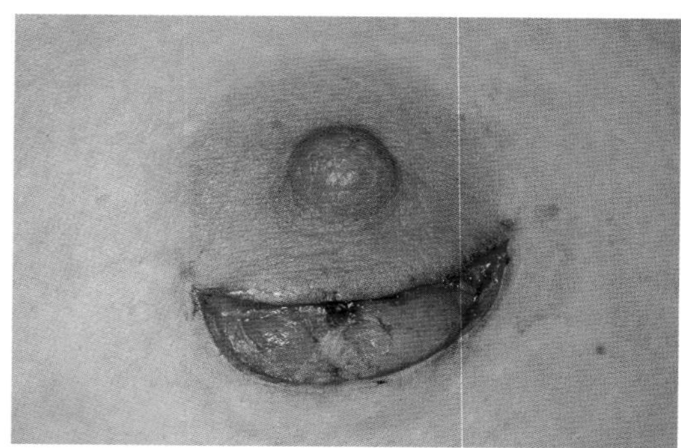

FIGURE 8 ● Incision into subcutaneous tissue.

ELEVATION OF THE AREOLAR SKIN FLAP

- The areolar skin edge is then retracted superiorly (skin hooks or sutures could be used), and dissection proceeds in the direction of the nipple toward the central duct bundle (**FIGURE 9**).
- Care should be taken to perform the dissection at a depth to preserve some subcutaneous fatty tissue under the areolar skin, as this will help to protect the viability of the areolar skin and nipple. Similarly, the lateral edges of the dissection field should narrow as the central duct bundle is approached (**FIGURE 10**).
- Attention should be paid to the location of dissection and its proximity to the nipple, looking closely for the ducts, which appear as narrow vertical tubular or strand-like structures. The ducts may be visibly discolored (**FIGURE 11**).

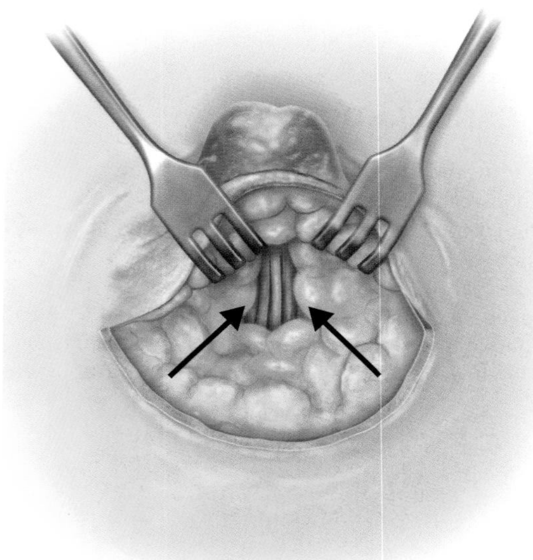

FIGURE 10 ● Narrowing the dissection field toward the nipple.

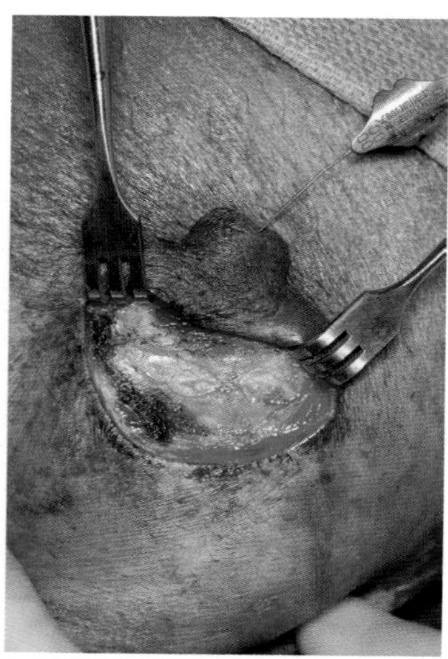

FIGURE 9 ● Retraction of the skin flap.

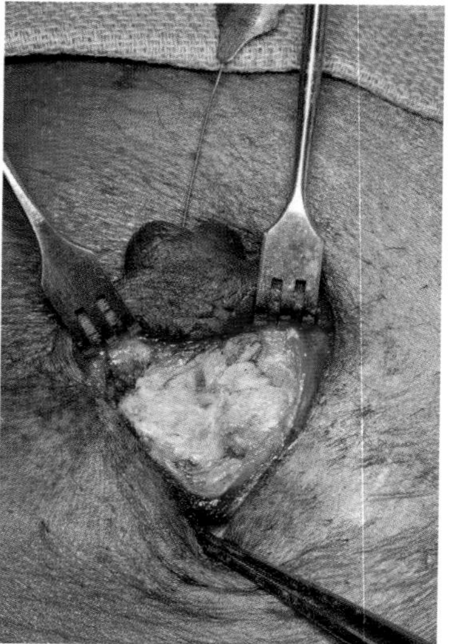

FIGURE 11 ● A visibly abnormal duct with discolored intraluminal fluid.

ISOLATION AND EXCISION OF THE CENTRAL DUCT BUNDLE

- Dissection then proceeds in vertical fashion on the lateral sides of the duct bundle under the nipple. This should proceed to the far side of the nipple (**FIGURE 12**).
- The duct bundle should be palpated between the thumb and finger to confirm the presence of the duct probe and any other small palpable nodules.
- The central duct bundle should then be transected at the deep aspect of the nipple dermis. If using electrocautery, the "cutting" mode should be chosen at a low energy setting to minimize thermal damage to the nipple dermis.
- As the duct bundle is transected, the cannulating probe will be identified. It may be withdrawn if it becomes difficult to maintain its position in the duct (**FIGURE 13**).
- The duct bundle should be retracted away from the breast, dissecting circumferentially around the duct bundle to a depth of approximately 3 to 5 cm or farther along a particular grossly abnormal duct (**FIGURE 14**).
- The tissue specimen should be transected at its base and oriented for the pathologist (**FIGURE 15**).
- The open wound should be palpated for any abnormalities, and the nipple dermis should be palpated between the thumb and finger to ensure that there are not any superficial nodules present that were not excised. In the event of a small nodule within the nipple dermis, a tiny skin incision in the nipple can be made to remove the lesion, or a small spatulation of the transected duct end may facilitate removal of a very superficial intraductal lesion.

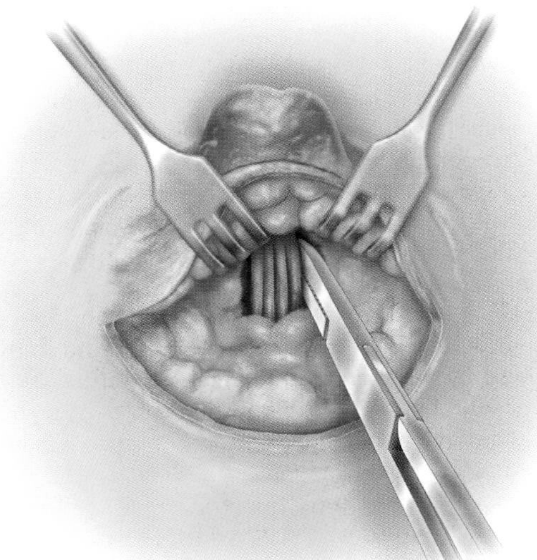

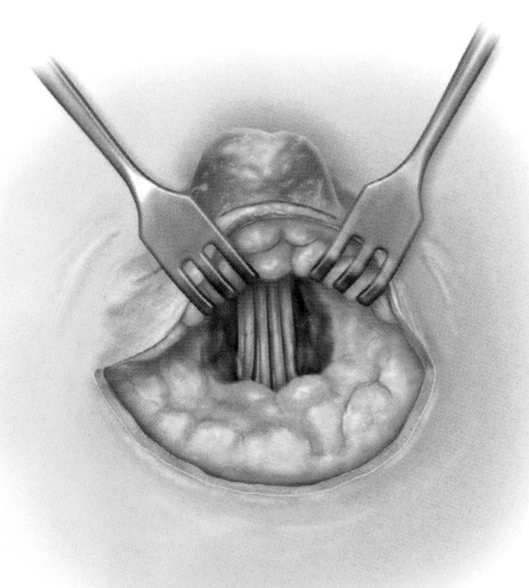

FIGURE 12 ● Vertical dissection along both sides of the duct bundle.

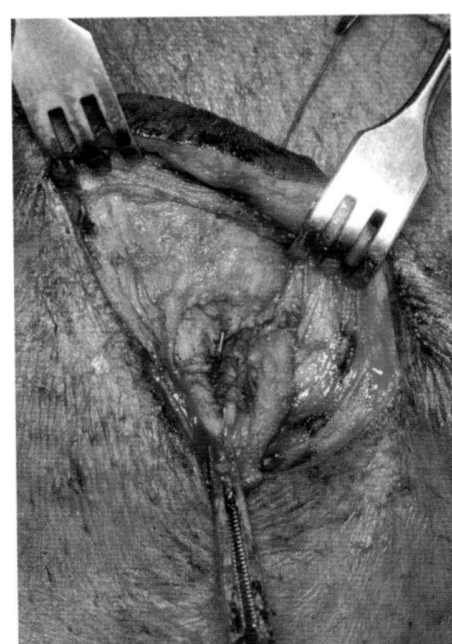

FIGURE 13 ● Transection of the ducts just deep to the nipple dermis.

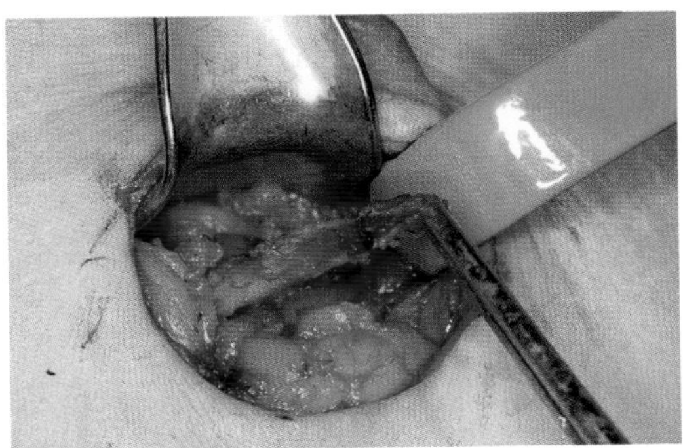

FIGURE 14 ● Dissection of ducts deeper into the breast parenchyma.

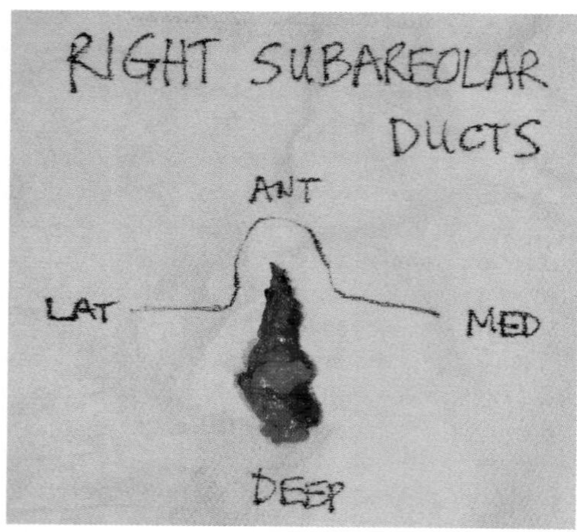

FIGURE 15 ● Orientation of the specimen.

CLOSURE

- After hemostasis, the parenchymal and subcutaneous tissue defect in the subareolar region must be closed in order to avoid nipple retraction in the healing phase. If there is a solid buttress of tissue underlying the nipple-areolar complex, the nipple will be less likely to retract.
- The parenchymal closure may be performed as a simple direct approximation of tissues, in whatever orientation results in least tension and absence of skin dimpling (**FIGURE 16**). If the defect is larger, it may require a small local tissue advancement flap or undermining of the breast gland from the skin. In that case, it is preferable to avoid further dissection under the areolar skin and obtain donor tissue from the other side of the cavity.
- If the nipple is effaced, it may be helpful to place a purse-string stitch in the deep dermis around the nipple base to recreate the normal nipple shape and prevent nipple retraction in the healing phase (**FIGURE 17**).
- The skin should be closed in two layers, with buried interrupted sutures in the deep dermis and subcutaneous tissue, followed by a running intradermal stitch in the skin edge. Care should be taken to place the deep dermal sutures so that the areolar skin edge is at or slightly above the breast skin edge (but not lower) (**FIGURE 18**), or the nipple-areolar complex will have a sunken-in appearance. If the areola is small, resulting in an incision with greater curvature, the final layer of skin closure should use multiple shorter bites (**FIGURE 19**).
- Adhesive dressings on the dermis of the nipple itself should be avoided. If an incision was required in the nipple dermis for an intradermal nodule, the nipple incision should be closed with fine interrupted nonabsorbable sutures.
- Dressings that create excess pressure on the nipple should also be avoided. If a pressure dressing is desired, it should have a "donut" opening for the nipple.

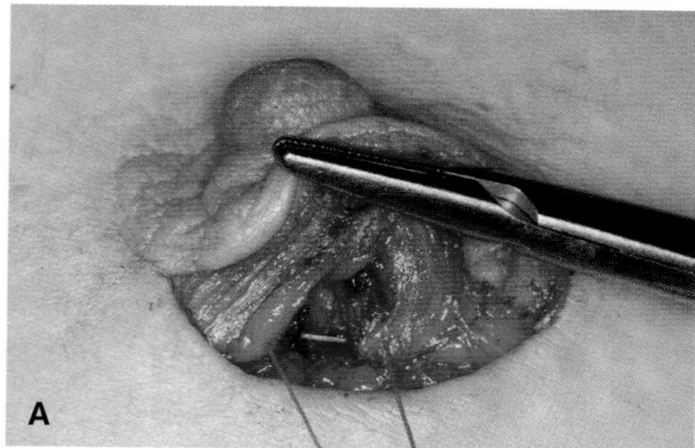

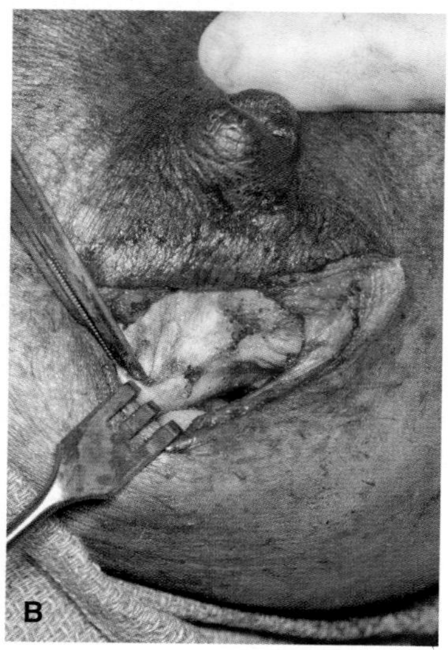

FIGURE 16 ● Closure of the deep tissue. **A,** Medial-to-lateral closure, **B,** Superior-to-inferior closure.

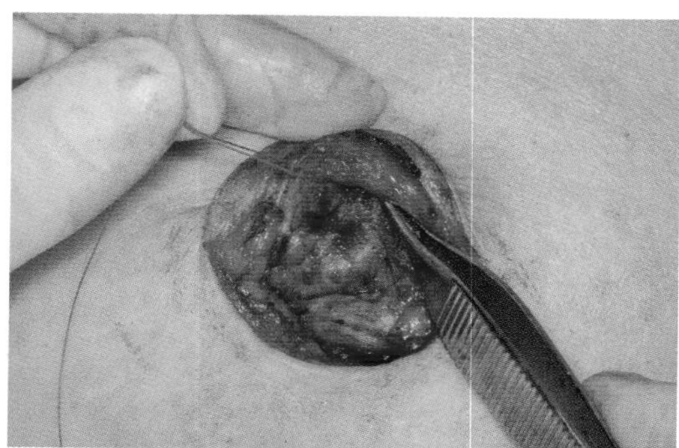

FIGURE 17 ● Purse-string suture in the deep dermis of the nipple.

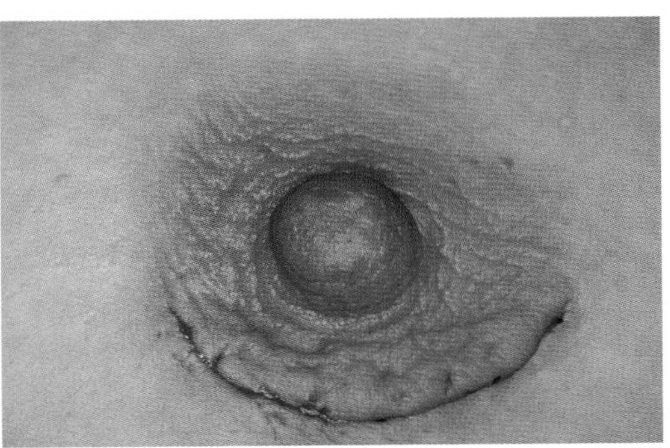

FIGURE 18 ● Appearance after closure of the deep dermal layer of incision, with the areolar edge at or above the breast skin.

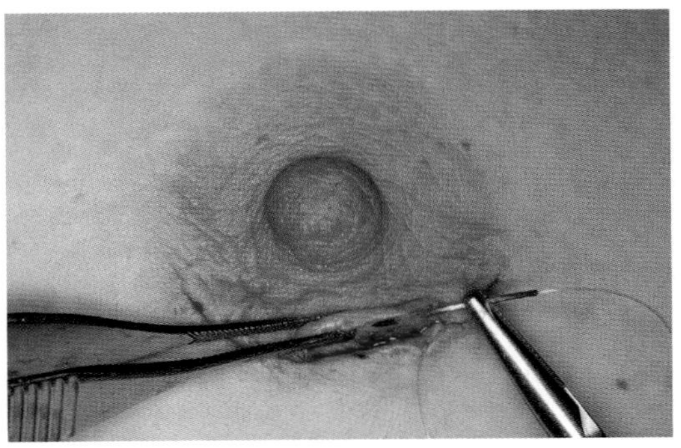

FIGURE 19 ● Intradermal suture for final layer of closure.

PEARLS AND PITFALLS

Preoperative counseling	■ Preoperative counseling should address ■ Focused duct excision vs excision of the entire duct bundle ■ Inability to lactate after surgery from the operated breast ■ Likely pathologic findings ■ Possible nipple discharge in the postoperative healing period ■ Temporary change in nipple sensation
Incision planning	■ Inferior areolar edge is preferred.
Subareolar dissection	■ Be careful to preserve subcutaneous fat under the areolar skin and to limit dissection to as narrow a field as possible to reduce risk of skin necrosis.
Closure	■ Proper closure of the deep and superficial tissues under the nipple-areolar complex is critical to avoid nipple retraction with healing, and consider a purse-string stitch to reestablish normal nipple projection.

POSTOPERATIVE CARE

- The incision should be kept clean and dry.
- Clothing that creates excess pressure on the nipple should be avoided, and patients may choose to use a donut-type foam dressing to relieve any pressure on the nipple.
- Showering is permitted.
- If any nonabsorbable sutures were placed in the nipple skin, they are removed at 1 week.

OUTCOMES

- Subareolar duct excision for abnormal nipple discharge is highly successful, with resolution of discharge in the vast majority. Recurrent discharge is reported in the range of less than 5%.[11]
- Pathology findings are most often benign (papilloma or duct ectasia), but malignancy is found in the range of 0% to 20%.[10-12]
- The likelihood of successful lactation after duct excision is not well characterized.

COMPLICATIONS

- Bleeding and infection are possible complications after every surgical procedure but are rare with this procedure. Avoidance of antiplatelet therapies and anticoagulants per surgical routine will help to minimize risk of bleeding, and a single preoperative dose of intravenous antibiotics is recommended prophylactically.
- Skin necrosis is also rare but devastating if it occurs; for this reason, careful attention should be paid to preserving blood supply to the areolar tissue and limiting the extent of dissection under the areolar skin, with focused excision of the central ductal tissue.

REFERENCES

1. Fritsch H, Kühnel W. *Color Atlas of Human Anatomy: Internal Organs*. Vol. 2. 5th ed. Thieme; 2008:418.
2. Expert Panel on Breast Imaging; Lee SJ, Trikha S, Moy L, et al. ACR Appropriate Criteria evaluation of nipple discharge. *J Am Coll Radiol*. 2017;14:S138-S153.

3. Morrogh M, Morris EA, Liberman L, et al. The predictive value of ductography and magnetic resonance imaging in the management of nipple discharge. *Ann Surg Oncol*. 2007;14(12):3369-3377.
4. Dawes LG, Bowen C, Venta LA, et al. Ductography for nipple discharge: no replacement for ductal excision. *Surgery*. 1998;124:685-691.
5. Van Zee KJ, Ortega Perez G, Minnard E, Cohen MA. Preoperative galactography increases the diagnostic yield of major duct excision for nipple discharge. *Cancer*. 1998;82:1874-1880.
6. Fisher CS, Margenthaler JA. A look into the ductoscope: its role in pathologic nipple discharge. *Ann Surg Oncol*. 2011;18:3187-3191.
7. Khan SA, Mangat A, Rivers A, et al. Office ductoscopy for surgical selection in women with pathologic nipple discharge. *Ann Surg Oncol*. 2011;18:3785-3790.
8. Gray RJ, Pockaj BA, Karstaedt PJ. Navigating murky waters: a modern treatment algorithm for nipple discharge. *Am J Surg*. 2007;194:850-855.
9. Sabel MS, Helvie MA, Breslin T, et al. Is duct excision still necessary for all cases of suspicious nipple discharge? *Breast J*. 2012;18(2):157-162.
10. Racz JM, Carter JM, Degnim AC. Challenging atypical breast lesions including flat epithelial atypia, radial scar, and intraductal papilloma. *Ann Surg Oncol*. 2017;24:2842-2847.
11. Morrogh M, Park A, Elkin EB, et al. Lessons learned from 416 cases of nipple discharge of the breast. *Am J Surg*. 2010;200:73-80.
12. Kooistra BW, Wauters C, van de Ven S, et al. The diagnostic value of nipple discharge cytology in 618 consecutive patients. *Eur J Surg Oncol*. 2009;35:573-577.

Chapter 6 Reflector Localized Breast Biopsy

Folasade Imeokparia

DEFINITION

- A reflector localized breast biopsy can acquire tissue for diagnostic purposes when an abnormality is not palpable. The SCOUT reflector device that is deployed for this method uses radar technology. The device measures smaller than a grain of rice. The detection of the radar pulse emitted from the reflector (up to 50 million pulses per second) allows for identification of the device up to a range of 60 mm. The SCOUT system allows for accurate 1 mm distance measurement in vivo from the reflector in a multidirectional manner.[1]
- Until recently, wire localized breast biopsy was the most frequently used method for localization of breast abnormalities. However, advancements in options such as the SCOUT system have brought about a "wire-free" era.
- As with other localization techniques, image-guided biopsy should be the first step. If image-guided biopsy can obtain a concordant diagnosis, surgery may be avoided. If a malignancy has been diagnosed prior to surgery, reflector localized lumpectomy is identical to reflector localized breast biopsy, with the exception that attention to sufficient margins and/or intraoperative margin assessment should be actively sought for the former.

DIFFERENTIAL DIAGNOSIS

- Given the diagnostic goal of a reflector localized breast biopsy, there are numerous potential lesions that may be observed on final pathologic assessment. These include benign, high-risk and malignant lesions. The most common benign lesions include fibroadenoma, benign phyllodes, benign mucocele-like lesions, pseudoangiomatous stromal hyperplasia (PASH), benign papillary lesions, complex sclerosing lesion or radial scar, intraductal papilloma and others. High-risk lesions may include flat epithelial atypia (FEA), atypical ductal hyperplasia (ADH), atypical lobular hyperplasia (ALH), or lobular carcinoma in situ (LCIS). Malignancies such as ductal carcinoma in situ (DCIS), invasive ductal carcinoma (IDC), invasive lobular carcinoma (ILC), or sarcomas may be diagnosed after excision. Additional surgical management, workup, and treatment are considered for certain lesions.

PATIENT HISTORY AND PHYSICAL FINDINGS

- Prior to any surgery, a bilateral breast exam must be completed. If a reflector localized breast biopsy is planned, the surgeon will verify the same considerations as for a wire localized breast biopsy: that the lesion is not palpable, it is concordant with imaging, and there are no additional lesions (especially any that may be palpable) requiring workup or excision.
- For patients with biopsy-proven cancer who are to undergo reflector localized lumpectomy, a thorough history and physical examination is necessary to make sure they are suitable candidates for breast conservation therapy (BCT). Contraindications to BCT include prior radiation, collagen vascular disease, first or second trimester of pregnancy, multicentric cancer, or widespread calcifications (see Part 5, Chapter 9).

IMAGING AND OTHER DIAGNOSTIC STUDIES

- In the workup prior to a reflector localized breast biopsy, all pertinent imaging should be reviewed. In addition, appropriate assessment of the patient's candidacy for surgical intervention should be completed carefully.
- Patient selection is important. The maximum depth the signal would have validation from the skin for is 6 cm. Thus, patients with very deep lesions may not be ideal candidates for reflector-guided biopsy and may be better suited for wire localization. With more experience, deeper lesions may be candidates for reflector-guided biopsy by making the incision based on the imaging and dissecting closer to the region before using the probe to identify the signal from the reflector.
- The reflector can be inserted well in advance of the procedure. After instillation of local anesthesia, a rigid introducer needle, which contains a preloaded reflector device, is directed toward the site of the abnormality using biplanar mammography or ultrasound (**FIGURE 1**). The needle is advanced until the tip is about 1 cm beyond the center of the target. The radar reflector is then deployed under mammographic guidance to ensure proper placement and the needle is removed.
- As with other excisional breast biopsies, a reflector localization may be recommended following stereotactic or ultrasound-guided biopsy results that necessitate additional tissue for evaluation (ie, FEA, LCIS, ADH, or ALH).[2-5]

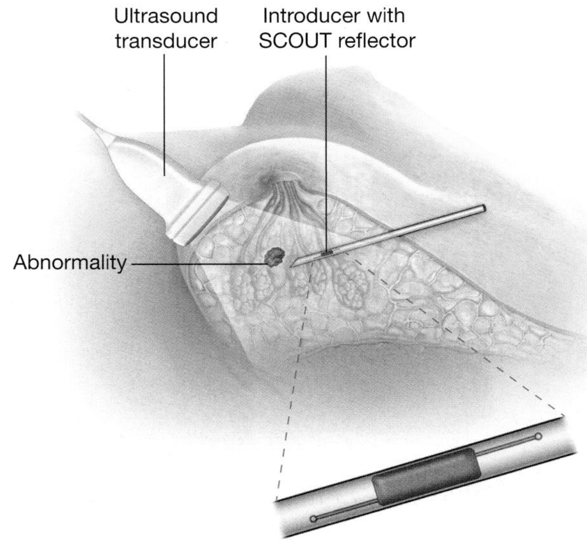

FIGURE 1 • Placement of a rigid needle with SCOUT device using biplanar mammography or ultrasound.

SURGICAL MANAGEMENT

Preoperative Planning

- Reflector localized breast biopsies are diagnostic. The objective is to obtain adequate tissue for further, or initial, pathologic assessment. This will guide further treatment, including surgical intervention, if necessary. Thus, the indications for and optimal localization technique should be carefully reviewed carefully for each patient. After reflector placement, a physical exam will be limited. Verifying that a clinically significant hematoma has not developed is typically sufficient.
- Given that the reflector can be placed well in advance of the operative day, the post-procedure mammograms should be reviewed and discussions with the radiologists should occur before surgery. It is important to review the post-procedure report and mammography with the radiologist directly, to verify successful deployment of the reflector near the target/abnormality of interest. It is also critical to verify that the device was functional with signal confirmation at the time of insertion. The distance of the reflector from the skin, distance of the lesion from the skin, and location of the reflector with respect to the abnormality are important to note.
- Migration of the device is possible, often secondary to a procedural hematoma. Typically, this is evident at the time of placement when radiology cannot verify the signal at the area of interest or the mammogram shows evidence of migration. In this case, it may be necessary to place a second reflector at the area of concern and the malpositioned reflector can be retrieved intraoperatively.
- The Joint Commission on Accreditation of Healthcare Organizations has national patient safety guidelines that include recommendations to limit surgical site infections (SSI). Prophylactic antibiotics that are administered within 1 hour of surgical incision, use of chlorhexidine surgical bath preoperatively, and clipping of hair, when appropriate, all reduce risk of SSI.[6]

Positioning

- The patient is laid supine on the OR table with the ipsilateral arm at 90°. The patient is secured to the table with the use of appropriate seat/table belts. Especially if there may be a need to tilt the table for adequate excision, the secure positioning of the patient is essential.
- When the patient is secured and positioned, the probe can be used to accurately localize the position of the reflector ex vivo (on the skin). The location will be identified by noting the highest audible frequency emitted by the device and observing/noting the shortest distance (in mm) visible on the front face of the SCOUT console screen.

TECHNIQUES

ANTICIPATING THE LOCATION OF THE ABNORMALITY

- By reviewing the craniocaudal (CC) and lateral–medial (LM) views from the pre- and post-procedure mammograms, the surgeon can estimate the approximate position of the lesion of interest prior to employing the SCOUT hand-held probe.
- The CC view (**FIGURE 2A**) demonstrates the anterior–posterior and the lateral–medial location of the abnormality but not the superior–inferior location. The CC view can be used

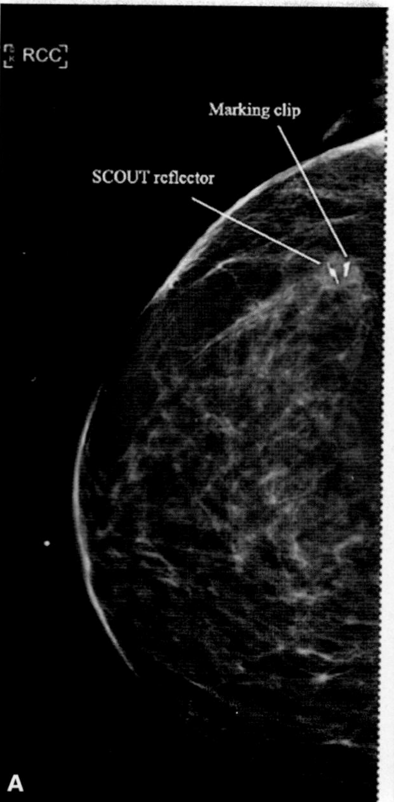

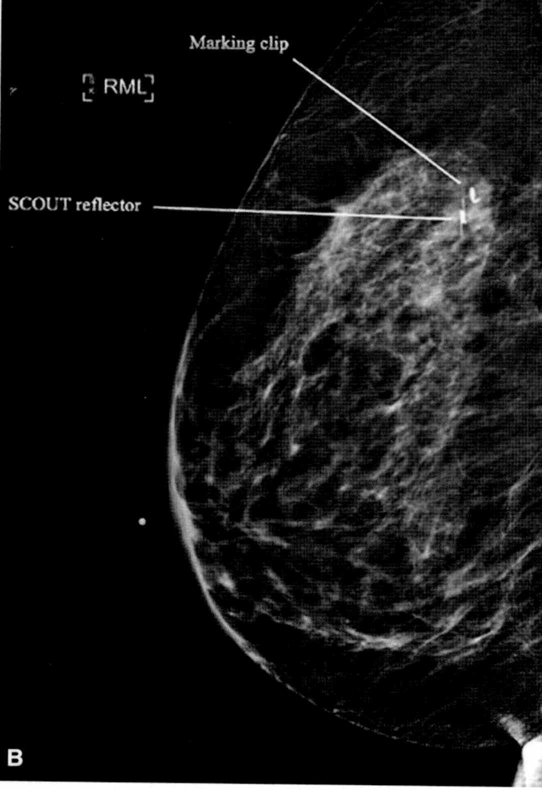

FIGURE 2 ● Localization films show the relationship between the skin, the reflector, and the abnormality. **A,** CC view. The film shows the abnormality is posterior to the reflector, but this film does not reveal the superior–inferior position. **B,** In this LM view, the abnormality is posterior to the reflector, but it also sits slightly superiorly to the reflector.

to estimate how deep the lesion is from the skin along with review of any mention from the radiologist regarding measurements during placement.

- The LM view (**FIGURE 2B**) demonstrates the superior–inferior as well as the anterior–posterior orientation but not the lateral–medial location. The CC view, as mentioned, can be used for this coordination.
- Using the biplanar views, it is important to assess the relationship of the reflector to the abnormality as the goal is to excise both the device and the lesion en bloc.

SKIN INCISION AND IDENTIFICATION OF THE SCOUT REFLECTOR

- Prior to incision, the surgeon can detect the exact location of the reflector with aid/review of preoperative imaging. This is achieved by moving the probe along the skin ex vivo and using the real-time feedback information from the console to confirm the location. This feedback information includes the distance measurement and the auditory frequency emitted. To confirm location of the reflector, the surgeon should use the smallest distance measurement noted (in mm) and the highest auditory signal heard. The skin should be marked using a water-soluble pen to note the location of the reflector (**FIGURE 3A** and **B**).
- The skin should be anesthetized prior to incision. The position of the incision utilized is at the discretion of the surgeon, however, peri-areolar incisions, upper outer quadrant incisions, or other "hidden" scars are valued by patients (**FIGURE 4**).

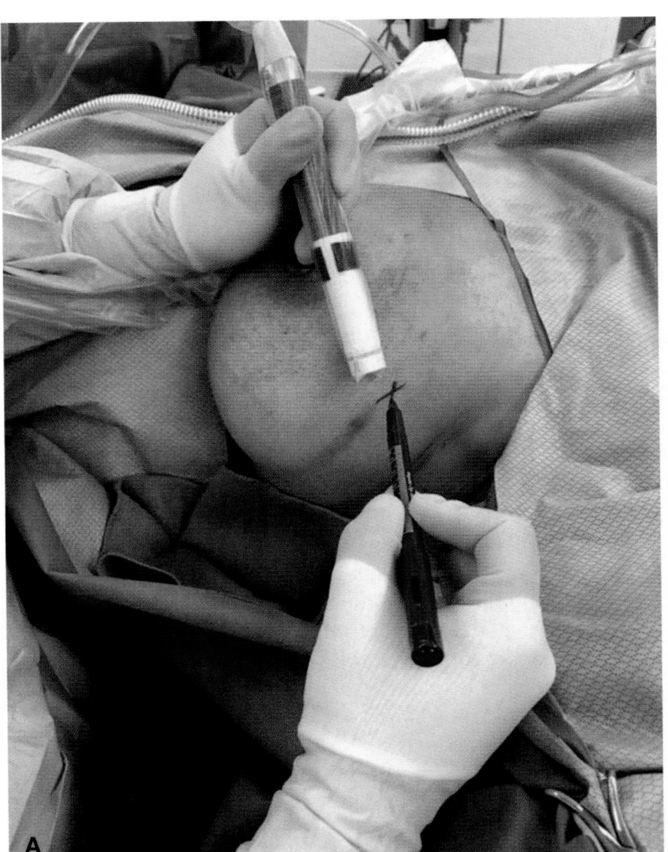

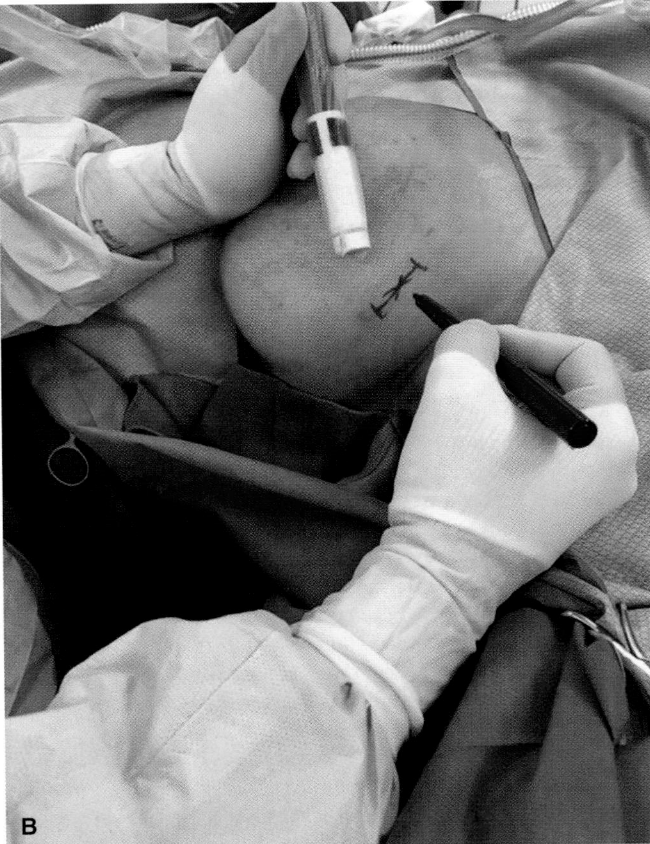

FIGURE 3 ● **A** and **B,** The SCOUT reflector's location is detected ex vivo on the skin using the SCOUT guide and a water-soluble pen is used to mark the location of the reflector and planned incision.

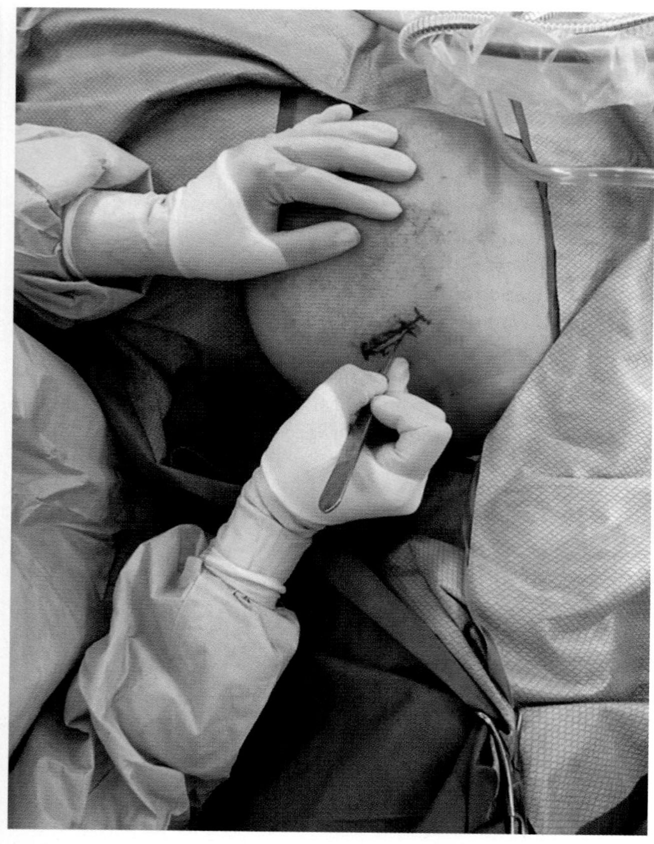

FIGURE 4 ● A small incision is made in the skin after infiltration of local anesthesia.

EXCISION

- A reflector localized breast biopsy is optimized when the surgeon understands the location of the abnormality as previously discussed. In the tissue, the probe is used in a manner such that the frequency, or cadence, of the audio sound emitted from the console increases as an indication that the probe is physically nearing the reflector (an inverse relationship). In real time, the surgeon can also observe the console screen and take note of the estimated distance measurement from the probe to the reflector. While holding the probe, the surgeon's hand is centered, pointing at the target, and moves to act as a fulcrum to accurately detect the best angle of approach to the target (**FIGURE 5A** and **B**).
- If the targeted abnormality is estimated to be superficial, or in the anterior-third of the breast tissue, the surgeon should dissect to the target and reflector such that adequate anterior flaps are maintained to avoid skin necrosis or ischemia. This thoughtful dissection can also prevent contour deflects at the conclusion of the case. If the lesion is suggested to be in the middle or posterior-third of the breast tissue, the dissection can be carried deep to the skin surface and down to an estimated depth that allows for removal of the lesion and reflector without excessive tunneling or large cavities. Regardless of the depth of the lesion within the parenchyma, the incision can be placed in a cosmetically appealing location even if the abnormality and reflector are not in close distance to the incision. It is imperative in these cases to use a multidirectional approach with the probe to determine where to elevate flaps, appropriate depth of those flaps, and in which relative direction the reflector sits. Marking the skin ex vivo assists in this endeavor.
- Knowing the dimensions of the abnormality to be removed, its estimated proximity to the reflector, and using the probe in vivo, the surgeon ensures circumferential dissection prior to complete excision.
- Care should be taken to avoid cauterization too close to the reflector, as this may short circuit the device and make localization using the probe challenging or impossible. The localization is at the center of the device which measures 12 mm. Once the measurement is at about 5 to 6 mm, the probe is so close to the area of dissection that it is likely that cautery could cause signal loss. If this occurs, intraoperative ultrasound can help identify the reflector and/or the biopsy clip relatively well and allow you to complete the biopsy.
- Either just before removal from the breast, or just after, confirm the reflector is present in the excisional tissue using the probe (**FIGURE 6**).

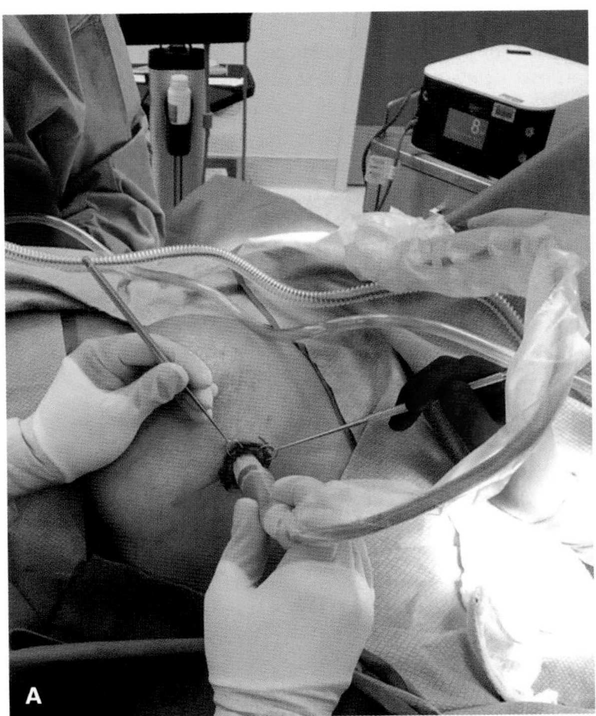

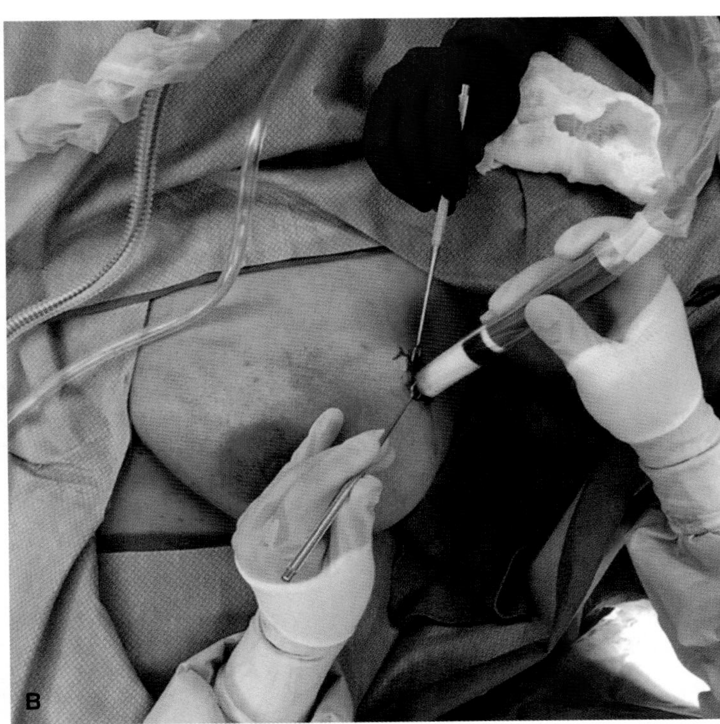

FIGURE 5 ● **A** and **B,** The reflector is identified at the anticipated site of the abnormality in vivo.

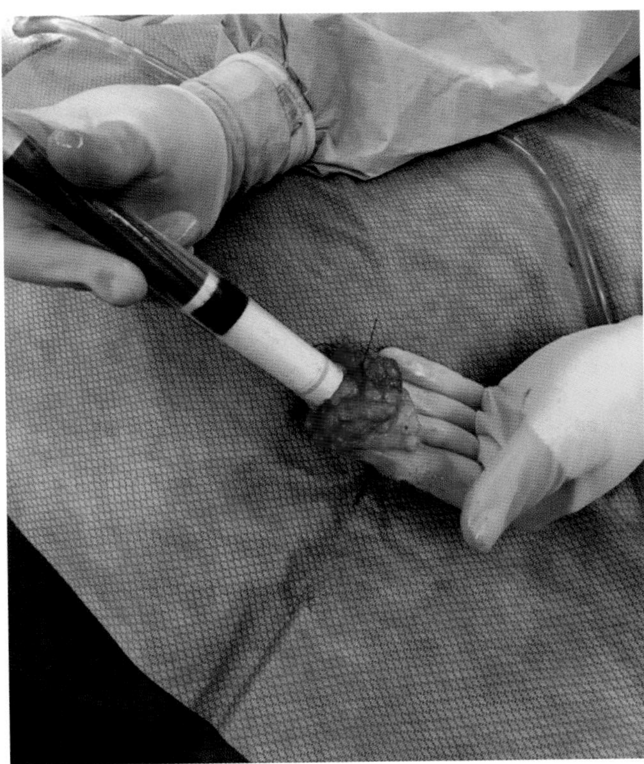

FIGURE 6 ● The reflector is confirmed to have been removed after circumferential dissection and completion of excision.

ORIENTATION

- Once the reflector localized tissue is removed, proper orientation is imperative. This step is identical to that used in a wire-guided biopsy. Silk sutures placed on three adjacent margins are preferred. Frequently, one or more of these sutures can be placed prior to the amputation and removal of the excisional tissue in vivo. Commonly, sutures are placed at the superior, lateral, and deep (or posterior) aspects. In naming the margins for pathology orientation, the surgeon can use a clever alliteration technique, for example, "short" suture for "superior," "long" suture for "lateral," and "double" suture for "deep." Some surgeons may opt to use sutures of a different dye color to distinguish the margins. Whatever the technique, orientation can reduce confusion and inadvertent errors for the pathologists, as well as assist in identification of appropriate margins should re-excision be required[7] (**FIGURE 7A** and **B**).

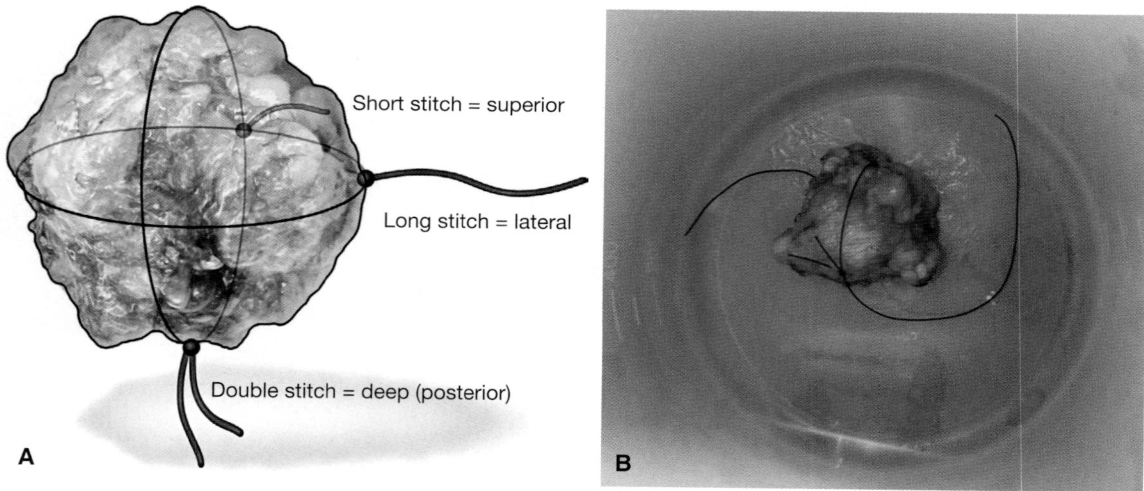

FIGURE 7 ● **A** and **B,** The lesion is oriented with three marking sutures prior to specimen mammography.

SPECIMEN RADIOGRAPHY AND VERIFICATION

- Specimen radiography confirms removal of the lesion of interest as well as removal of the reflector (**FIGURE 8A** and **B**). Typically, this confirmation is done intraoperatively.
- Inadvertent dislodgment of the reflector is possible. If the reflector is not seen on radiograph, it should be assumed that it is still be present in the tissue. Careful observation of the surgical cavity should be done first. It may be present but dislodged. Next, sweeping the probe throughout the surgical cavity may yield a response from the reflector as described above (ie, auditory signal vs observed distance measurement). Given its size, it is uncommon for the reflector to pass through standard suction devices (eg, Yankauer or Frazier suction tips). If a dislodged device should be retrieved, its intact removal must be documented by radiograph as well as sending the device alongside the tissue to pathology.
- If a reflector is not identified on any radiograph despite additional tissue excision, the surgeon may need to postpone the remainder of the procedure and obtain radiology's assistance to identify the device with additional mammography postoperatively. Unfortunately, an abandoned excision may require an additional operative procedure to extract the device once reidentified.
- In a situation where the lesion of interest is not seen on radiograph, additional excision is warranted and the surgeon can utilize palpation and additional exposure to aid in the lesion's retrieval, especially if the reflector is no longer present or active. If the reflector has been inadvertently short-circuited and is no longer active, the use of mammographic orientation may help in additional dissection.

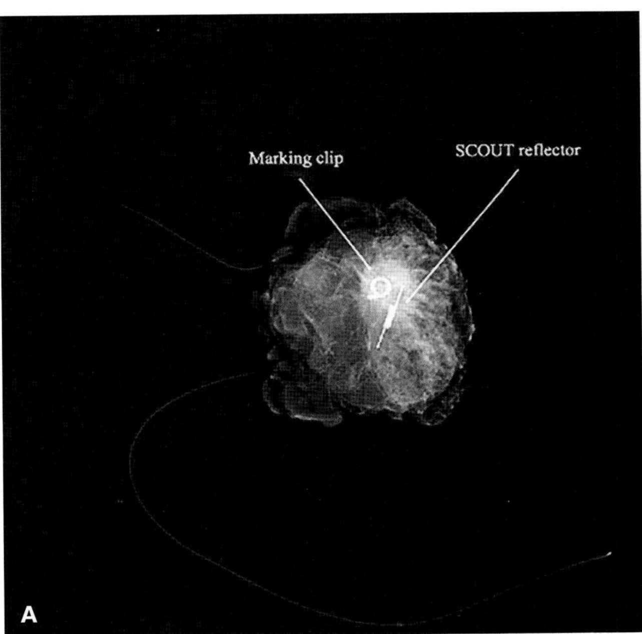

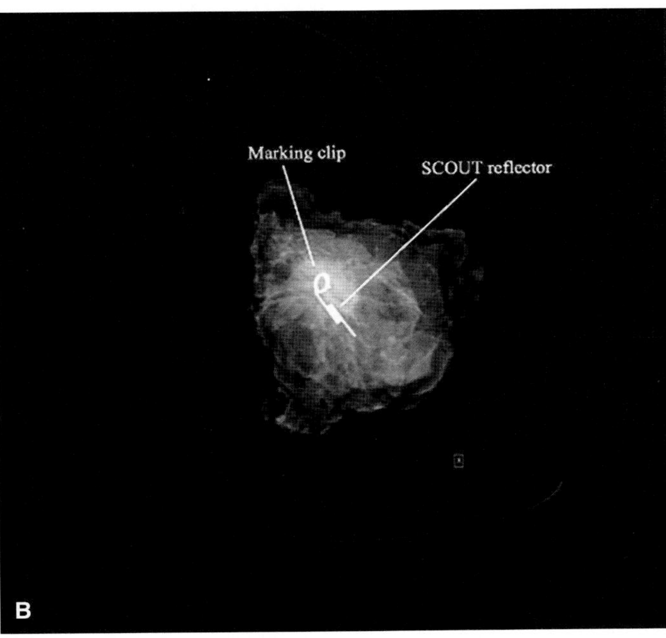

FIGURE 8 ● **A** and **B,** Specimen mammography displays that the SCOUT reflector and clip are completely removed.

CLOSURE

- Closure should take place once the lesion and reflector are identified on specimen radiograph. The surgical bed can be irrigated, and hemostasis should be obtained prior to closure. For most excisions, the resulting surgical cavity will not require tissue rearrangement to prevent deformity and an expected seroma will allow the breast tissue to hold its shape. Appropriate anticipation of flaps at the initiation of the dissection aids in a cosmetically appealing outcome.
- Skin closures are completed in two layers. The skin edges should be healthy and well-vascularized. If, for any reason, the skin edges appear nonviable or compromised, they should be debrided to allow for the most successful closure. The first layer is the deep connective tissue and reticular dermis, which are closed with an interrupted, absorbable suture. Last, a running, absorbable subcuticular stitch is completed followed by skin adhesive glue or adhesive bandage. It is reasonable to forgo the subcuticular stitch and only use adhesive.

PEARLS AND PITFALLS

Indications	■ Image-guided biopsy is the preferred approach to the nonpalpable abnormality. Review the case with the radiologist to confirm whether this is an option.
Placement of incision	■ Keep in mind that if malignant, the patient may need a re-excision lumpectomy or mastectomy.
Patient selection	■ Lesions deeper than 6 cm may not allow for identification of the signal ex vivo and may be better suited for wire localization.
Identifying the reflector	■ Review preoperative imaging and understand the relationship of the device to the abnormality. ■ Mark the skin with a pen ex vivo after the location of the device is approximated.
Excision	■ Utilize the real-time, multidirectional feedback from the SCOUT system to localize the device and abnormality of interest.
Specimen mammography	■ Three orientation sutures are necessary to avoid error. ■ Clips can help orient the specimen on the mammography so as to guide a re-excision.
Closure	■ Review preoperative imaging and understand the relationship of the device to the abnormality.

POSTOPERATIVE CARE

- A chest binder or bra should be applied to the patient or placed on the patient as the final step. Various sizes should be available for optimal patient fit. This outer material serves as external support, to offload tension on the tissue and relieve pain. It also provides compression, to reduce gravitational pull, without crushing the tissue or making it difficult for the patient to breathe deeply. The patient should be encouraged to wear the binder or bra for at least 48 hours.

OUTCOMES

- The success rate of reflector localization breast excisions is typically 100%.[8-10] Reviewing Pearls and Pitfalls (see previous section) can help support successful reflector localizations. A difficult excision or failure to excise the abnormal lesion is typically secondary to reflector mispositioning and/or dislodgement, or a challenging breast shape and/or size.

COMPLICATIONS

- Seroma
- Hematoma
- Infection (cellulitis or abscess)
- Pneumothoraces from placement of reflector (rare)
- Retained reflector device or fragments (if inadvertently transected)
- Failure to identify/excise the abnormality

ACKNOWLEDGMENT

Special thanks to the assistance of Dr. Betty Fan for her media contribution to this content.

REFERENCES

1. Merit Medical. *SCOUT Radar Localization*. 2021. https://www.merit.com/merit-oncology/localization/breast-soft-tissue-localization/scout-radar-localization/
2. American Society of Breast Surgeons. *Consensus on Image-Guided Percutaneous Biopsy of Palpable and Nonpalpable Breast Lesions*. 2018. https://www.breastsurgeons.org/docs/statements/Consensus-Guideline-on-Image-Guided-Percutaneous-Biopsy-of-Palpable-and-Nonpalpable-Breast-Lesions.pdf
3. American Society of Breast Surgeons. *Consensus Guideline on Concordance Assessment of Image-Guided Breast Biopsies and Management of Borderline or High-Risk Lesions*. 2018. https://www.breastsurgeons.org/docs/statements/Consensus-Guideline-on-Concordance-Assessment-of-Image-Guided-Breast-Biopsies.pdf?v2
4. Racz JM, Carter JM, Degnim AC. Challenging atypical breast lesions including flat epithelial atypia, radial scar, and intraductal papilloma. *Ann Surg Oncol*. 2017;24(10):2842-2847.
5. Rudin AV, Hoskin TL, Fahy A, et al. Flat epithelial atypia on core biopsy and upgrade to cancer: a systemic review and meta-analysis. *Ann Surg Oncol*. 2017;24(12):3549-3558.
6. Joint Commission. *Surgical Site Infections*. 2021. https://www.jointcommission.org/resources/patient-safety-topics/infection-prevention-and-control/surgical-site-infections/
7. Molina MA, Snell S, Franceschi D, et al. Breast specimen orientation. *Ann Surg Oncol*. 2009;16:285-288.
8. Cox CE, Russell S, Prowler V, et al. A prospective, single arm, multisite, clinical evaluation of a nonradioactive surgical guidance technology for the location of nonpalpable breast lesions during excision. *Ann Surg Oncol*. 2016;23(10):3168-3174.
9. Mango VL, Wynn RT, Feldman S, et al. Beyond wires and seeds: reflector-guided breast lesion localization and excision. *Radiology*. 2017;284(2):365-371.
10. Taback B, Jadeja P, Ha R. Enhanced axillary evaluation using reflector-guided sentinel lymph node biopsy: a prospective feasibility study and comparison with conventional lymphatic mapping techniques. *Clin Breast Cancer*. 2018;18(5):e869-e874.

Chapter 7

Magnetic Seed Localized Breast Biopsy

Michael S. Sabel

DEFINITION

- There are several methods that may be utilized to excise a nonpalpable, image-detected abnormality, including wire localization, radiocolloid occult lesion localization (ROLL), infrared/electromagnetic, magnetic seed, and radiofrequency identification (RFID) localization. Each of these technologies has advantages and disadvantages compared to each other as well as to wire localization.
- Advantages of seed localization include the ability to place the seed prior to the operative day (facilitating scheduling) and avoiding the risks of dislodging or transecting the wire.
- For magnetic seed localization, a small (5 × 1 mm) stainless steel seed is placed at the site of the target (**FIGURE 1**). The seed can be placed at any time prior to the planned surgical procedure using ultrasound or stereotactic guidance. A probe that senses the magnetic signal is then used to locate the magnetic marker and excise the tissue surrounding it.
- Magnetic seed localization is a highly accurate method for excising nonpalpable lesions.[1-3] A systemic review and pooled analysis of magnetic seed localization demonstrates a high rate of successful placement (94.42%), successful localization (99.86%), and in the case of lumpectomies, no significant difference in re-excision rates.[4]

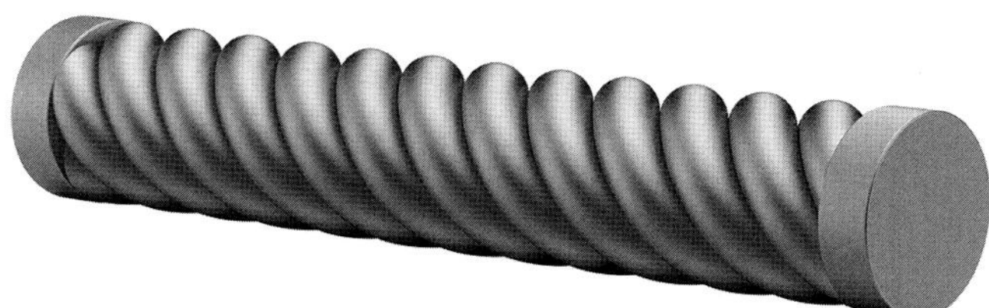

FIGURE 1 ● The Magseed magnetic marker. (Image courtesy of Endomag.)

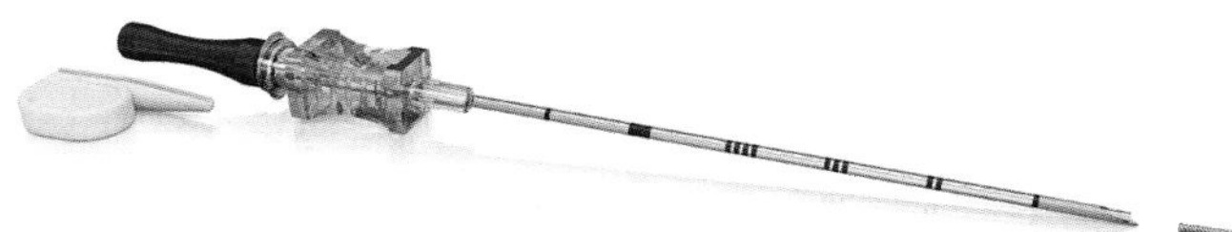

FIGURE 2 ● A preloaded deployment needle is used to place the magnetic marker at the location of the breast abnormality. (Image courtesy of Endomag.)

INDICATIONS

- For newly diagnosed mammographic abnormalities, it is preferable to use image-guided biopsy as a first step (stereotactic biopsy or ultrasound or magnetic resonance imaging [MRI]-guided biopsy). This helps avoid surgery in patients with benign disease and allows for preoperative staging and planning a definitive oncologic operation in patients with malignant disease. Thus, excisional biopsy should be limited to patients who failed image-guided biopsy or are not suitable candidates.
- Magnetic seed localized excisional biopsy is also used in patients in whom the diagnosis is discordant, or in benign lesions at high risk of "upstaging" upon excision.[5]
- The techniques described here can also be utilized for magnetic seed lumpectomy, where the goal is a complete excision of the cancer with an adequate margin of surrounding normal tissue.

EQUIPMENT

- The magnetic seed is stainless steel and measures 5 × 1 mm (**FIGURE 1**). The seed itself is not magnetic, but is induced to become a magnet under the influence of the detector. A preloaded 18-gauge deployment needle is used to insert the seed (**FIGURE 2**).
- The surgeon uses a magnetometer that generates an alternating magnetic field that transiently magnetizes the seed and then measures the magnetic field emitted by the seed. The base unit has a detachable hand-held probe that senses the magnetic signal allowing the surgeon to locate the magnetic marker (**FIGURE 3**). The presence of the seed is indicated

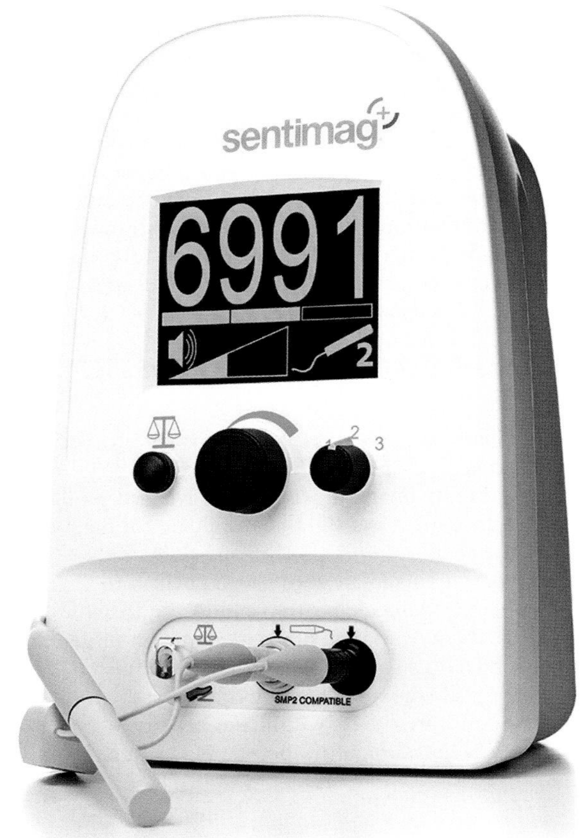

FIGURE 3 ● The Sentimag console. (Image courtesy of Endomag.)

both by a change in pitch (frequency) of an audio output as well as a numerical representation on the base unit.

- The system needs to be balanced at the start of the case, and potentially rebalanced during the case. This is done by stepping on a footswitch connected to the unit.
- The probe is activated by metal instruments. Therefore, it is extremely helpful to have either plastic or titanium (which is not magnetizable) instruments for retraction and to grasp the tissue.

PATIENT HISTORY AND PHYSICAL FINDINGS

- The patient's allergies, medications (specifically aspirin or anticoagulants), or the presence of a bleeding diathesis should be reviewed.
- The use of the magnetic seed marker is not officially indicated for use in patients with nickel allergies. While the steel in the marker has less than 0.23% Ni content, and exposure is less than with stainless-steel guide wires, patients should be asked about nickel allergies and alternative approaches be considered.
- A bilateral breast exam should be performed in all patients for whom magnetic seed localized biopsy is being contemplated for two reasons. First, to assess whether or not the lesion is truly nonpalpable. If the abnormality is palpable, then localization will not be necessary. If an abnormality is palpated, it is critical to review with the radiologist to be sure that the palpable abnormality corresponds to the imaging abnormality being recommended for biopsy. The second reason for bilateral breast examination is to make sure there are no other palpable occult abnormalities that may also require biopsy.
- For patients with biopsy-proven cancer who are to undergo lumpectomy, a thorough history and physical examination is necessary to make sure they are suitable candidates for breast conservation therapy (BCT). Contraindications to BCT include prior radiation, collagen vascular disease, first or second trimester of pregnancy, multicentric cancer, or widespread calcifications (see Part 5, Chapter 9).

IMAGING AND OTHER DIAGNOSTIC STUDIES

- The preoperative imaging is essential to the procedure. Prior to the decision to perform a magnetic seed localized excision, the breast imaging should be reviewed to determine whether the patient is a suitable candidate for magnetic seed placement.
- More than one magnetic seed can be placed to "bracket" a wider area of microcalcifications; however, the seeds should be at least 2 cm from each other to allow the surgeon to distinguish the two signals. This can be technically challenging, and wire-bracketing may be preferred.
- For lesions located deep within the breast, the signal may be quite low and difficult to detect. When starting out with magnetic seed localization, it may be worth limiting the procedure to more superficial lesions (within 6 cm of the skin). With more experience using the system, deeper lesions can be targeted with magnetic seeds.
- Prior to coming to the operating room (OR), a preloaded deployment needle is used to insert the seed (**FIGURE 4**). The magnetic seed can be placed well in advance of the operative day. The surgeon should confirm successful deployment of the seed prior to the day of the operation.

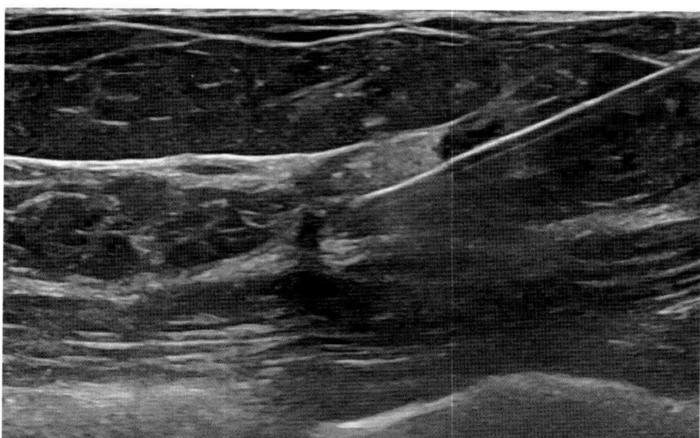

FIGURE 4 ● Ultrasound is used to guide the deployment needle to the site of the abnormality and place the magnetic marker.

SURGICAL MANAGEMENT

Preoperative Planning

- Prior to taking the patient back to the OR, the localization films should be reviewed. Specifically, the surgeon should note the proximity of the seed to the abnormality. As magnetic seed-guided excision is typically utilized following an image-guided biopsy, there is usually a clip at the site, and the magnetic seed should be placed in close proximity to the clip.
- The surgeon should also note the relative location of the lesion within the breast. This will help narrowing the search for the signal. The mammogram should be reviewed to estimate the location of the magnetic seed. The CC view (**FIGURE 5A**) demonstrates both the anterior–posterior and the lateral–medial location of the abnormality but gives no information regarding the superior–inferior location. The LM view (**FIGURE 5B**) demonstrates the anterior–posterior orientation as well as the superior–inferior but gives no information regarding the lateral–medial location.
- The surgeon should also note how far the target is from the skin, as this may impact the degree of sedation.
- Although the risk of infection after breast surgery is low, it tends to be higher than average for a clean surgical procedure, particularly when the patient has had instrumentation prior to surgery. Several studies have shown that antibiotic prophylaxis significantly reduces the risk of postoperative infection.[6]

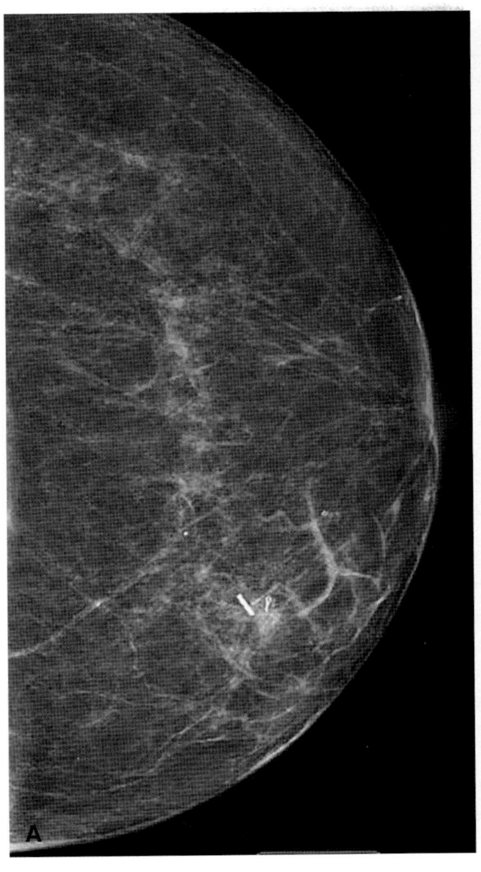

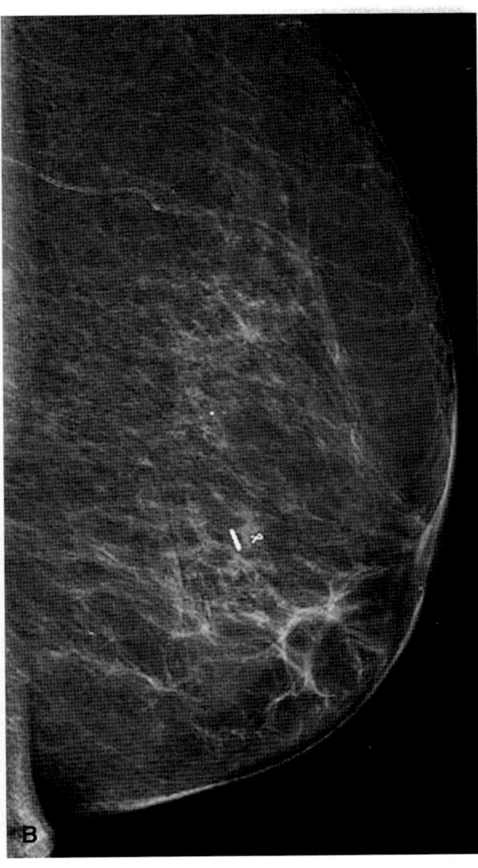

FIGURE 5 ● The magnetic seed is demonstrated in proximity to the clip placed at the initial biopsy on **(A)** cranial–caudal view and **(B)** lateral–medial view.

See **Video 1**.

ANTICIPATING THE LOCATION OF THE ABNORMALITY

- The patient should be positioned supine with the ipsilateral arm at slightly less than 90°. The patient and arms should be appropriately strapped down. Often the table may be tilted for more lateral lesions.
- Prior to prepping and draping, the detector should be used to localize the magnetic signal and confirm that the equipment is functioning properly.
- The breast is then prepped and draped and the probe is sterilely draped.
- In the region you estimate the magnetic seed to be, place the probe on top of the skin and move around until a clear signal is established (**FIGURE 6**). As you get closer to the signal, the numbers on the console will turn from red (negative) to yellow (positive) and increase, as will the intensity and pitch of the sound.
- For deeper lesions, it may be necessary to press the probe down into the breast while scanning, angling it in different directions (**FIGURE 7**). The signal and volume pitch will increase as the probe gets closer to the magnetic seed. Once the highest peak is determined, mark the area.
- It is important to note that the intensity of the signal reflects the depth. This can be used to help estimate the distance to the target; the higher the number, the closer you are.

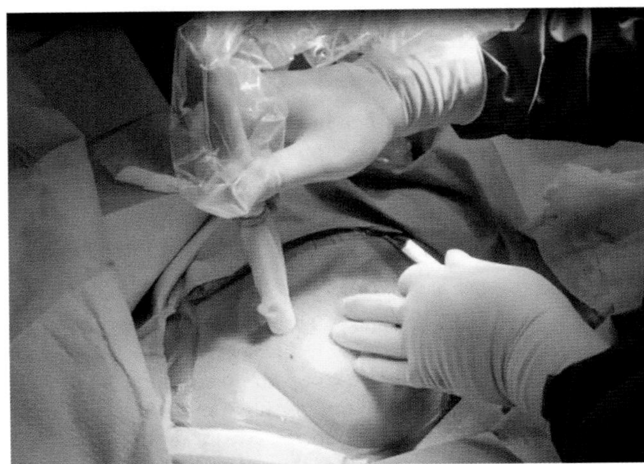

FIGURE 6 ● The probe is used to scan the skin to determine the location of the magnetic marker.

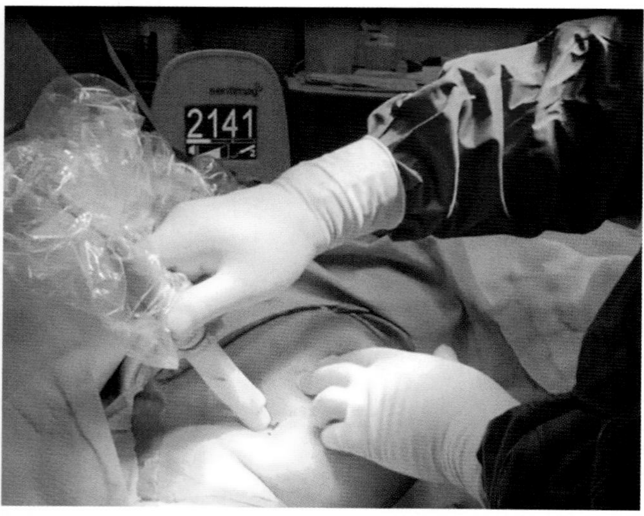

FIGURE 7 ● For deeper lesions, the probe is gently pressed into the breast and the angle of the probe is changed in order to identify the location with the maximum counts.

SKIN INCISION AND FLAP ELEVATION

- Using the preoperative imaging and the site of the "hottest" spot, the incision is planned. The incision can be placed directly over the maximum signal, which will facilitate excision, or can be placed circumareolar, lateral, or in the inframammary fold, which will improve the cosmetic outcome. The greater the distance between the target and the incision site, the more tunneling will be needed and this will impact the amount of local anesthetic and sedation that may be needed. In addition, if the lesion is malignant, you may be returning for a re-excision lumpectomy or mastectomy, so the incision should be placed in a way that does not compromise that.
- Following the skin incision, cautery is used to divide the tissue and then flaps are developed. It will be important to elevate adequate flaps so that the probe can easily be maneuvered around the cavity during the dissection.
- If the imaging and the counts suggest that the lesion is deep to the incision, the dissection is continued posteriorly prior to flap creation so as to avoid removing excessive tissue anterior to the lesion. For more superficial lesions, flaps should be elevated shortly after incision but kept thick enough to avoid concavity at the site.

EXCISION

- After elevating the flaps, the probe is used to identify the highest intensity of the signal. Plastic retractors should be used to retract the skin and soft tissue and allow access to the cavity. The probe can be used to determine the direction of the magnetic seed as well as the distance to the seed (**FIGURE 8**).
- For counts <2500 (on setting 2), you still have 1 to 2 cm between the magnetic seed and the probe. For counts around 5000, you are within 1 cm of the magnetic seed. Counts of >9000 suggest you are right on top of the magnetic seed.
- Once you feel you are close to the seed, but with some tissue between the seed and the probe, you should begin dissecting peripherally around where you anticipate the target. Repeated scanning with the probe will assure you are continuing in the right direction.
- Remember that each time you probe the cavity, you will need to move any metal instruments away as not to interfere with the signal. If you need to grasp the tissue surrounding the lesion while scanning, there are titanium and plastic instruments that can be used. When you are not using the probe, it is advisable to keep it away from metal, but often the probe needs to be reset before you use it. Aim the probe straight up and press the foot pedal to reset the probe.
- With the highest signal centered within the tissue, dissect past the target peripherally. The probe has side-sensing zones, so as the probe tip moves past the seed, the signal will decrease and drop from yellow to red (**FIGURE 9**). This can be used to estimate when you are past the target.

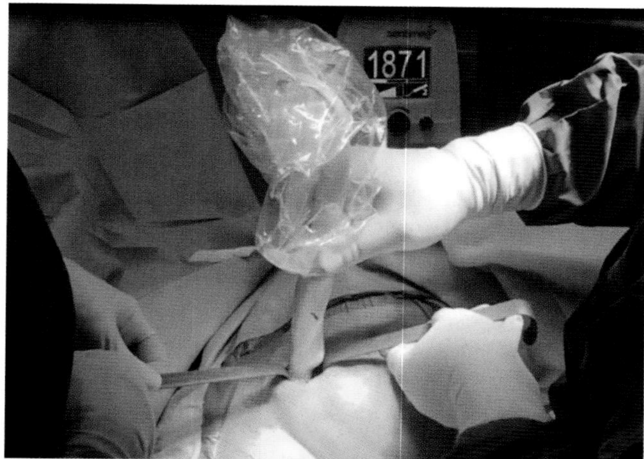

FIGURE 8 ● Using plastic retractors, the probe is used within the developing cavity to guide the dissection and determine proximity to the marker.

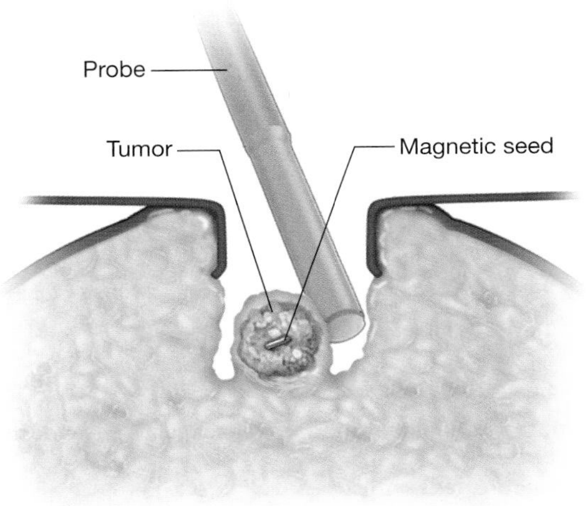

- During the dissection, try to avoid using suction, particularly with a Yankauer suction tip. In some cases, if the clip or seed is at the periphery of the specimen, it can be dislodged and potentially suctioned out.

FIGURE 9 ● As dissection continues, the probe can be placed past the anticipated target to determine when the deep aspect of the dissection is completed.

ORIENTATION

- Immediately upon removing the lesion, maintain the orientation and place three 2-0 silk sutures for the pathologist. If this returns as cancer, this allows for simple re-excision of any involved margin as opposed to a re-excision of the entire cavity. Do this prior to scanning the specimen for the seed to avoid losing the orientation.
- Once the lesion is oriented, use the probe to confirm that the seed has been excised. Be sure that there is no metal beneath the specimen as you scan the specimen to avoid false findings. In the case of cancer, it can also be helpful to note where the strongest signal is within the specimen (where the seed is closest to) as this can help guide any re-excision.
- If the seed is not present in the specimen, scan the cavity again for the signal. While the seed is small, it can be visualized and may be identified loose within the cavity. If so, it should be grasped with pick-ups and included with the specimen for mammography to confirm that it has been removed. If the signal is deeper within the tissue, additional excision should be performed to assure that the tissue surrounding the seed has been excised and all specimens should be sent to radiology.

SPECIMEN RADIOGRAPHY AND ADDITIONAL TISSUE

- Specimen radiography is performed to confirm that the area of concern has been removed (**FIGURE 10**). The specimen mammogram should demonstrate the presence of the lesion (mass or microcalcifications), the seed, and any clips placed at the time of the image-guided biopsy. Once confirmed, the wound can be closed.
- If the seed is present but the lesion or the clip is not present, then additional tissue should be excised and sent to radiology. The potential location may be estimated by using the initial imaging (the relationship between the clip and the seed) and the location of the seed within the specimen. The use of radiopaque clips on the specimen, as well as other landmarks on the original mammograms, may also help identify where to excise additional tissue.
- If a second specimen fails to identify the lesion, it becomes a judgment call whether to continue or abandon the procedure. For ultrasound-visible lesions, intraoperative ultrasound may be able to identify the abnormality. In the case of a clip that should have been in the specimen, sometimes these can get dislodged and suctioned out. Filtering and x-raying the fluid in the suction canister can sometimes reveal a dislodged clip. Otherwise, it may be prudent not to continue and plan on reimaging and, if necessary, returning to the OR rather than taking an excessive amount of breast tissue.

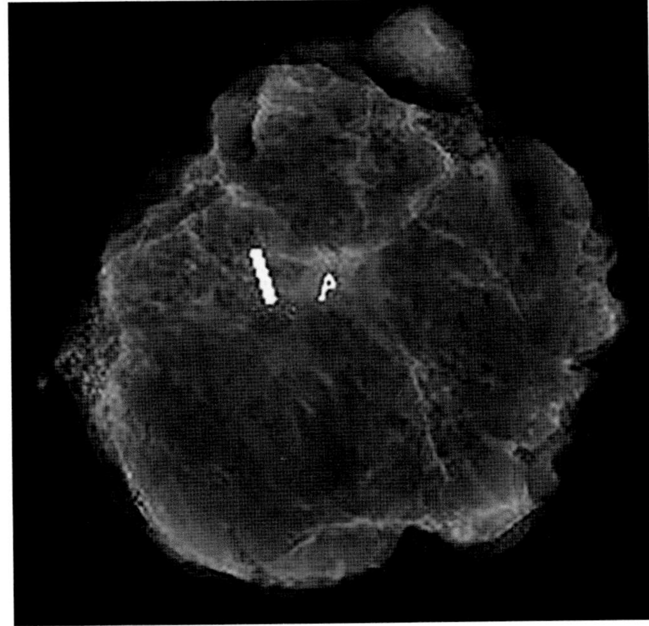

FIGURE 10 ● Specimen mammogram confirms excision of the mass, biopsy clip, and magnetic seed.

CLOSURE

- Once the biopsy is complete, including confirmation that the abnormality, seed, and biopsy clip has been removed, hemostasis is assured and the wound is irrigated with saline.
- For an excisional biopsy, the surgeon should *not* try to reapproximate the breast tissue. The cavity will fill with seroma and fibrin, and ultimately, fibrous tissue, which will maintain the normal contour.

The incision is closed with absorbable deep dermal sutures, followed by either a subcuticular stitch or tissue adhesive. Drains should not be used.

PEARLS AND PITFALLS

Indications	▪ Image-guided biopsy is the preferred approach to the nonpalpable abnormality. Review the case with the radiologist to confirm whether this is an option. ▪ Deep lesions may be more challenging to use magnetic seeds until you have more experience.
Placement of incision	▪ Keep in mind that if malignant, the patient may need a re-excision lumpectomy or mastectomy. Plan your incisions with this in mind.
Identifying the seed	▪ Review preoperative imaging for the relationship between the seed and the clip (or abnormality), location within the breast, and distance to the skin. ▪ Scan the breast prior to prepping and draping to confirm the location of the seed and mark the relative location of the device.
Excision	▪ Use plastic retractors and either plastic or titanium instruments during the incision. ▪ Repeatedly scan during dissection to confirm the correct direction and begin dissecting around the lesion before coming too close to it. ▪ If counts are not consistent, reset the probe by holding it upward and pressing on the foot pedal.
Specimen mammography	▪ Three orientation sutures are necessary to avoid error. ▪ Clips can help orient the specimen on the mammography so as to guide a re-excision.

POSTOPERATIVE CARE

- After a breast biopsy, the patient should be placed in a breast binder or supportive brassiere. This helps sustain hemostasis and relieves tension on the skin closure imposed by the weight of the breasts. This should remain in place for 48 hours.
- After 48 hours, the patient may remove the binder and shower. We recommend the patient continue to wear a comfortable bra, including while sleeping, for the remainder of a week.

COMPLICATIONS

- Seroma
- Hematoma
- Infection (cellulitis or abscess)
- Pneumothoraces (rare)
- Failure to identify abnormality

REFERENCES

1. Miller ME, Patil N, Li P, et al. Hospital system adoption of magnetic seeds for wireless breast and lymph node localization. *Ann Surg Oncol*. 2021;28:3223-3229.
2. Zatceky J, Kubula O, Coufal O, et al. Magnetic seed localization in breast cancer surgery: a multicentre clinical trial. *Breast Care*. 2021;16:383-388.
3. Zacharioudakis K, Down S, Bholah Z, et al. Is the future magnetic? Magseed localization for non palpable breast cancer. A multi-centre non randomized control study. *Eur J Surg Oncol*. 2019;44(11):2016-2021.
4. Gera R, Tayeh S, Al-Reefy S, Mokbel K. Evolving role of Magseed in wireless localization of breast lesions: systematic review and pooled analysis of 1,559 procedures. *Anticancer Res*. 2020;40:1809-1815.
5. American Society of Breast Surgeons. *Consensus Guideline on Concordance Assessment of Image-Guided Breast Biopsies and Management of Borderline or High-Risk Lesions*. Accessed 12/30/2021. https://www.breastsurgeons.org/docs/statements/Consensus-Guideline-on-Concordance-Assessment-of-Image-Guided-Breast-Biopsies.pdf?v2
6. Bunn F, Jones DJ, Bell-Syer S. Prophylactic antibiotics to prevent surgical site infections after breast cancer surgery. *Cochrane Database Syst Rev*. 2012;2012(1):CD005360. doi:10.1002/14658858.CD005360.pub3

Chapter 8 Cryoablation of Breast Fibroadenomas

Cary S. Kaufman

CRYOABLATION TREATMENT FOR BREAST FIBROADENOMAS

- Cryoablation is an innovative treatment that is a minimally invasive, office-based procedure that is administered without the use of general anesthesia, involving minimal patient discomfort and little to no scarring. The treatment is performed in an office setting rather than in an operating room, resulting in a cost-effective and patient-friendly procedure. Published reports demonstrate that cryoablation as primary treatment for breast fibroadenomas is safe and effective and at long-term follow-up demonstrates progressive resolution of the treated area, with excellent patient and physician satisfaction (see **TABLE 1**).
- About 80% of the approximately 1.3 million biopsies performed annually in the United States reveal benign conditions, primarily benign tumors or fibrocystic change. The most common benign breast tumor is a fibroadenoma.[1-3]
- Although not life-threatening, benign breast tumors can cause fear, anxiety, and discomfort in the patient, and definitive treatment is often desired.[3-5]
- Fibroadenomas consist of a proliferation of epithelial and connective tissue elements within the lobular region of the breast. They are usually sharply demarcated from the adjacent breast tissue and give the clinical and imaged appearance of being encapsulated.[5]
- They often grow to a size of 2 to 3 cm and are multiple in 20% of women.[4,6-9]
- Approximately 10% of women will experience a fibroadenoma in their lifetime. Although most common in young women, fibroadenoma occurs in every age group, from adolescents to octogenarians.[1,2,7,10,11]
- Not all fibroadenomas are symptomatic and not all have progressive growth.

Table 1: Reasons to Consider Ablation Technologies

Reasons to consider ablation techniques:
Small incision
A procedure not surgery
Less scarring
Mild discomfort
Shorter recovery time
Less invasive
Newer technology
Less expensive

DIFFERENTIAL DIAGNOSIS

- These benign breast tumors have a classic physical examination: rubbery texture, smooth and well defined, circular to oval, most often painless and freely moveable within the breast.
- Other breast lesions that may have similar clinical presentations include benign phyllodes tumors, juvenile fibroadenomas, medullary carcinomas, or even breast cysts. Diagnosis is resolved by imaging and core needle biopsy.
- Cryoablation has been proven therapeutically effective for biopsy-proven fibroadenomas[12-16] (see **TABLE 2**).

PATIENT HISTORY AND PHYSICAL FINDINGS

- Patients with the appropriate size and location of fibroadenomas may be treated with cryoablation. Candidates for cryoablation treatment should have small to medium-sized, single tumors that are not too close to the skin or nipple (see **TABLE 3**). Other requirements include:
  - The target lesion must be clearly visible with ultrasound.
  - Target lesion location within the breast must not be within 1 cm of the skin and not immediately deep to the nipple.
  - A histologic diagnosis using a core biopsy should demonstrate a classic fibroadenoma without atypia. Other histologic lesions are not appropriate for cryoablation at the time of writing.

Table 2: Published Reports of Cryoablation for Fibroadenomas

Author	Fibroadenomas (n)	Mean size (cm)	Freeze time (min)	Skin injury (%)	Any growth @ 1 y	Still palpable @ 1 y (%)	Volume decrease @ 1 y (%)	Cosmesis by patient @ 1 y (%)	Satisfied patient @ 1 y (%)
Edwards[a]	310	1.8	N/A	0	None	33	97	92	100
Nurko[b]	444	1.8	22	0	None	35	71	82	88
Hahn[c]	23	<3.0	10	4	None	22	76	96	96
Kaufman[d]	70	2.1	15	6	None	25	89	100	97
Total/Average	847	1.9	16	3	None	29	83	93	95

[a] *Edwards MJ, et al. Am J. Surg. 2004;188:221-224.*
[b] *Nurko J, et al. Am J Surg. 2005;190:647-652.*
[c] *Hahn M, et al. Ultraschall in Der Medizin. 2013;34:64-68.*
[d] *Kaufman CS, et al. J Am Coll Surg. 2004;198:914-923.*

Table 3: Indications and Contraindications for Cryoablation for Fibroadenomas

Inclusion criteria for fibroadenoma cryoablation:

1. Lesion must be sonographically visible.
2. Diagnosis of fibroadenoma must have histologic confirmation.
3. Lesion size must be less than 3 cm in largest diameter.

Contraindications for cryoablation:

1. Pathology suggestive of phyllodes tumor or malignancy.
2. Poor ultrasound visualization.
3. Pathologic diagnosis of fibroadenoma nonconcordant with imaging or physical examination.

Note: After cryoablation, patients should be followed with ultrasound assessment and physical examination at 6, 12, 18, and 24 months post procedure.

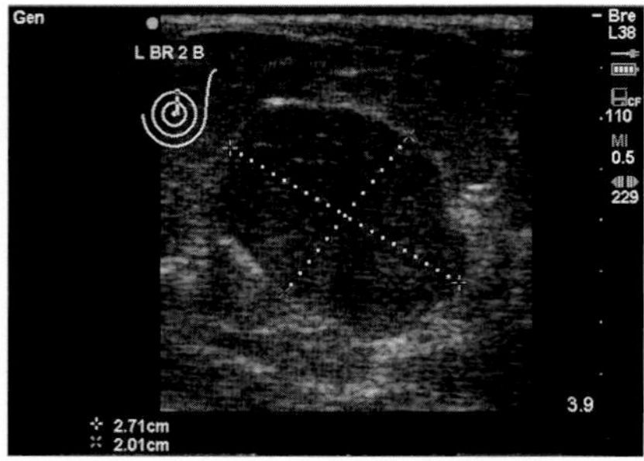

FIGURE 1 ● Ultrasound of fibroadenoma prior to treatment. Size, position, and two orthogonal views are taken.

- Fibroadenomas should be measured in three dimensions and the longest dimension used to calculate freezing time. Larger tumors require longer freezing times (see **FIGURE 1**)
- The patient should understand the process of cryoablation and the eventual progressive resorption of the residual necrotic debris over time (see **FIGURE 2**).
- The patient should not currently have breast cancer in the ipsilateral breast and be otherwise healthy.
- If the patient is in the mammography screening age group, a pretreatment screening mammogram should be obtained and be without suspicion except for the fibroadenoma (see **FIGURE 3**).
- Patients should not be pregnant or breast feeding. The patient should not have breast implants.

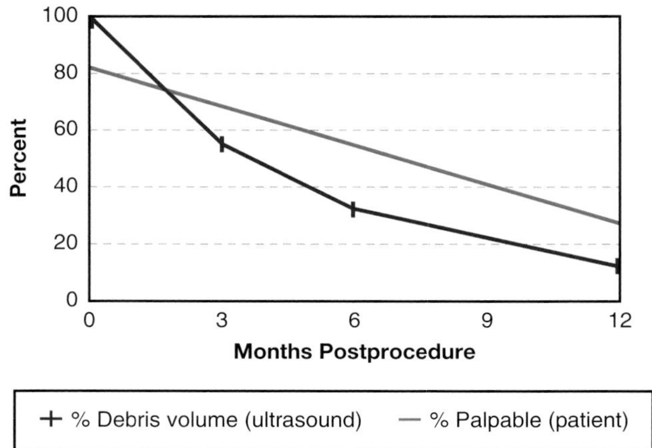

FIGURE 2 ● Postcryoablation resolution of palpable and ultrasound-visible cryolesion over the first year. In most patients tumors fully dissolve over the year, but tumors larger than 2 cm will take a longer to resorb.

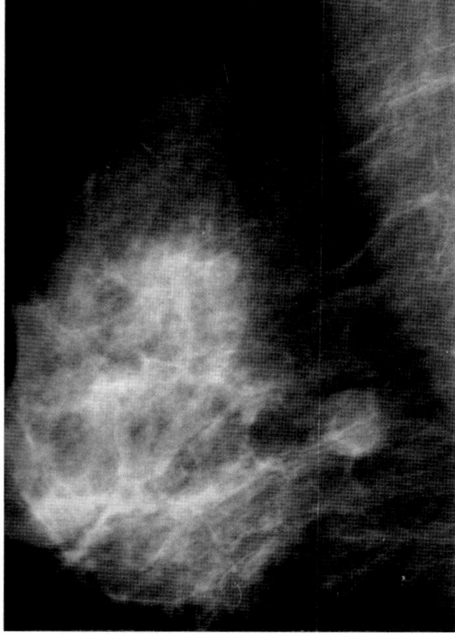

FIGURE 3 ● Mammogram demonstrating oval fibroadenoma.

IMAGING AND OTHER DIAGNOSTIC STUDIES

- There are classic imaging findings of fibroadenoma on both ultrasound and mammography, but histology is needed for an accurate diagnosis[1,3,9,17] (**FIGURES 3, 4A** and **B**, ultrasound and mammogram of a fibroadenoma).
- The differential diagnosis includes the larger and faster-growing juvenile fibroadenomas and phyllodes tumors, although these are less common.[1,6,9]
- Large-core needle biopsy is the diagnostic method of choice because of the high degree of differentiation between benign and malignant tumors in general and fibroadenoma from phyllodes tumor in particular.[1,9]

SURGICAL MANAGEMENT

- There are three treatment options for a confirmed fibroadenoma: (1) serial observation ("watchful waiting"), (2) surgical removal, and (3) cryoablation. Surgery for fibroadenoma provides a definitive treatment while confirming the diagnosis and eliminating patient anxiety and future monitoring. Drawbacks to surgical excision include patient discomfort, anesthetic and surgical recovery, skin incision and potential scarring, as well as operating room costs.[18]
- Many women choose serial observation since many lesions will not grow over time. The advantages include absence of

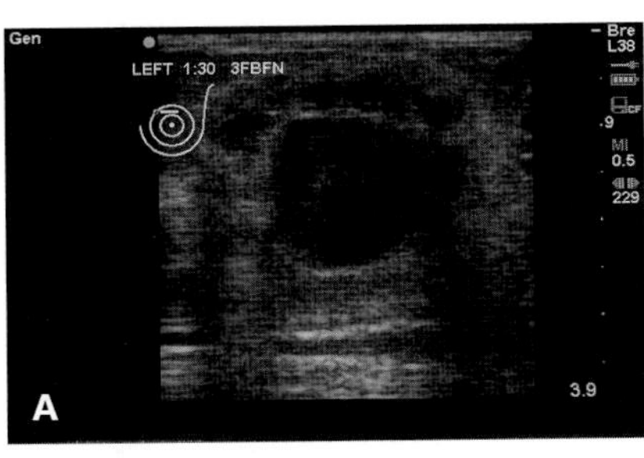

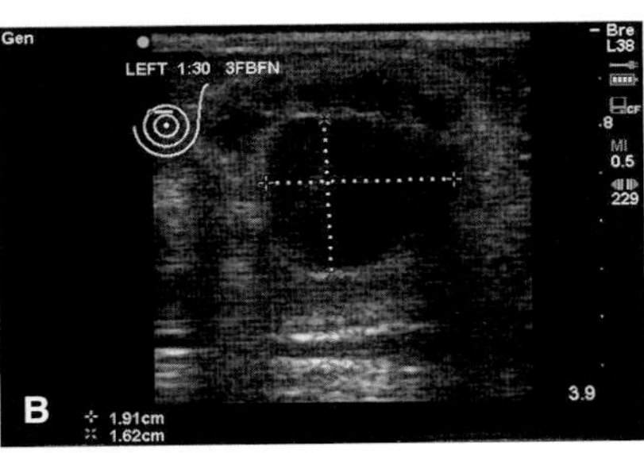

FIGURE 4 ● A and B, Classic ultrasound image of fibroadenoma demonstrating well-defined borders, homogeneous solid mass with edge shadowing.

surgical pain, avoidance of the operating room and anesthesia, less cost compared with surgical excision, and only a minimal scar from the large-core needle biopsy. Drawbacks to conservative management include ongoing patient anxiety, potential growth of a lump, the inconvenience of serial office visits, and the potential new lesion developing midst the confusion of a mass on physical examination and on mammography.[7,19]

- Cryoablation for fibroadenoma has the advantage of being an office-based procedure with no need for systemic anesthesia, minimal discomfort, skin puncture similar to the core biopsy site, and the expectation of lower overall costs of treatment compared with surgical excision.
- Multiple reports in the United States and Europe of favorable outcomes make cryoablation for fibroadenoma an attractive alternative for patients.[12-16,20]
- As a result of these reports, the American Society of Breast Surgeons has produced a statement in support of cryoablation as an acceptable alternative method of treatment of fibroadenoma.[21]

POSITIONING AND PROCEDURE DESCRIPTION

- Most cryoablation devices have an automated treatment program that uses the longest tumor dimension to calculate treatment times. The cryoablation machine should be programmed for treatment using the longest axis of the fibroadenoma.
- Specifics of the cryoablation machine preparation should be completed, which may include obtaining a supply of liquid nitrogen and filling the dewars with liquid nitrogen. Care must be taken when using liquid nitrogen to avoid burns while filling dewar flasks.
- Cryoablation is an office-based sterile procedure with preparation like that of an ultrasound-guided core needle biopsy. Have a sterile cryoprobe available and a sterile field setup with equipment similar to that needed for core needle biopsy. In addition to the sterile instruments, several syringes of sterile saline should be available for injections to distance the skin away from the cryoprobe during the procedure.
- The cryoprobe should be tested just prior to use. A backup probe should be available in case the probe tests defective. During the test, the probe is placed in sterile saline to observe a practice iceball formation. No air bubbles should be discharged from the tip of the probe.
- To initiate the automated treatment protocol on the cryoablation device, enter the fibroadenoma size measurement into the cryomachine. Each machine will have its unique process and calculations.
- Note the distance beyond the fibroadenoma that the probe must extend for the symmetric distribution of the freezing.
- Identify the ideal skin entry site to create a cryoprobe pathway along the long axis of the fibroadenoma with adequate circumferential distance for the cryoprobe iceball to be entirely within the breast and away from the skin.
- Inject local anesthetic in the skin and along the path toward the fibroadenoma. Infiltrate some local anesthetic deep to and around the periphery of the target lesion. Some local is valuable beyond the target for the "past pointing" of the cryoprobe beyond the tumor.
- Use a #11 scalpel blade to make a 3-mm entry site for the cryoprobe.
- Using ultrasound visualization, carefully place the tested cryoprobe along the desired track into and through the fibroadenoma. This may take some time to be sure the cryoprobe lies within the center of the fibroadenoma. Before a final pathway is accepted, be sure that the cryoprobe lies in the mid center of the target lesion. Move your targeting ultrasound in all directions to confirm the cryoprobe's central placement both longitudinally and transversely (see **FIGURE 5A-C**, two orthogonal ultrasound views of position of cryoprobe within fibroadenoma, showing examination of transverse evaluation).
- Some fibroadenomas are very dense, causing the cryoprobe to deviate off the desired central pathway. It may take repeated efforts to place the probe in the very rubbery tumor.
- **"TIP"** One method to facilitate central probe position is to obtain a core needle biopsy just prior to placing the probe. If the core needle biopsy is obtained from the desired central pathway, it will be easier to place the treatment cryoprobe in the same path.
- Once the cryoprobe has adequately been placed and the distal "past pointing" has been measured, you are ready to initiate the cryoablation sequence.
- Press the start button and use the ultrasound unit to document the development of the iceball. Obtain multiple measurements especially iceball size at the end of each of the three phases of treatment: first freeze, thaw, and second freeze (see **FIGURE 6A** and **B**)

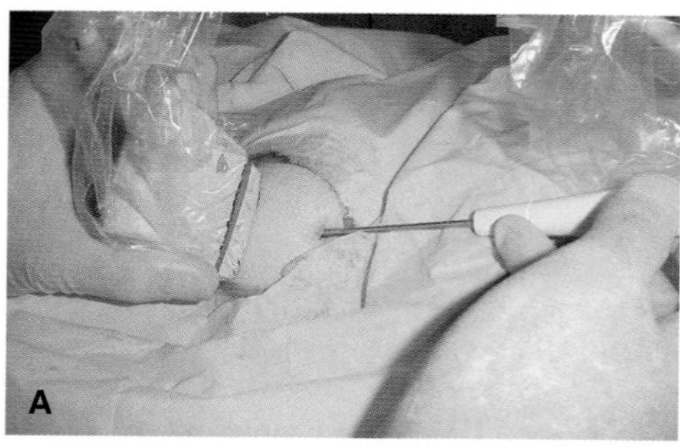

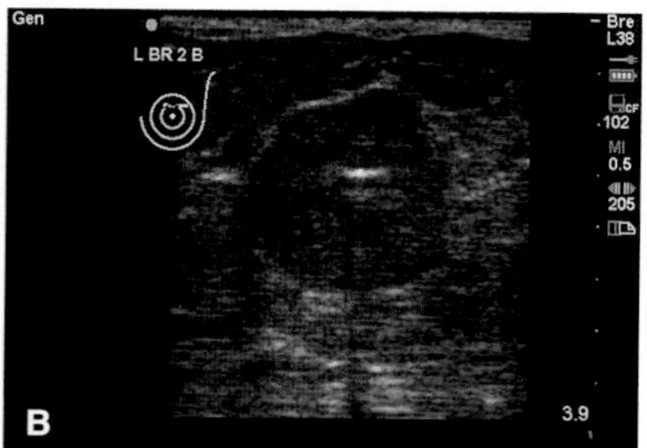

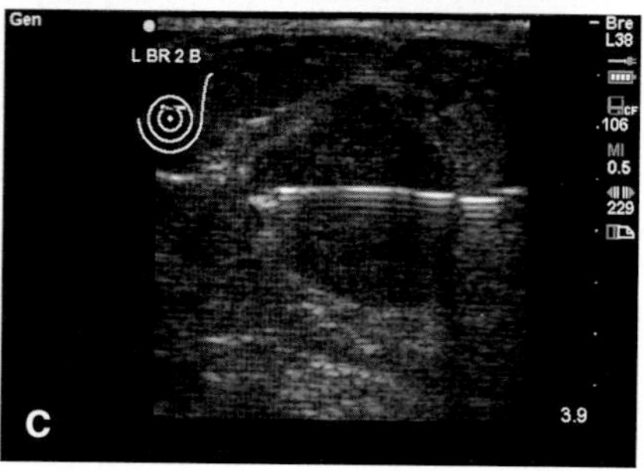

FIGURE 5 ● **A,** Ultrasound examination of probe placement to confirm central location within fibroadenoma. **B,** Ultrasound view of probe in tumor via transverse image. **C,** Ultrasound view of probe in tumor via longitudinal image.

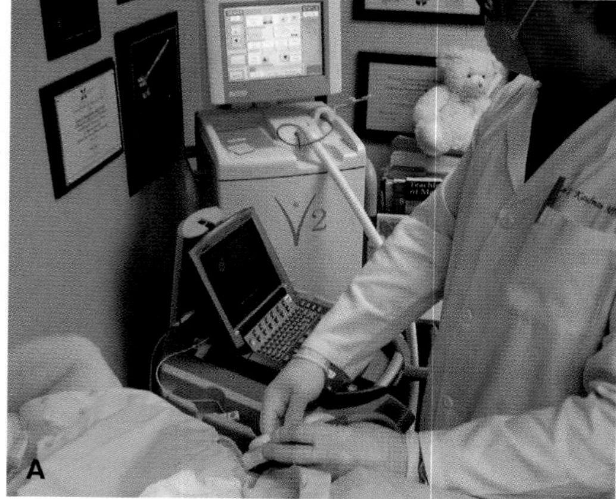

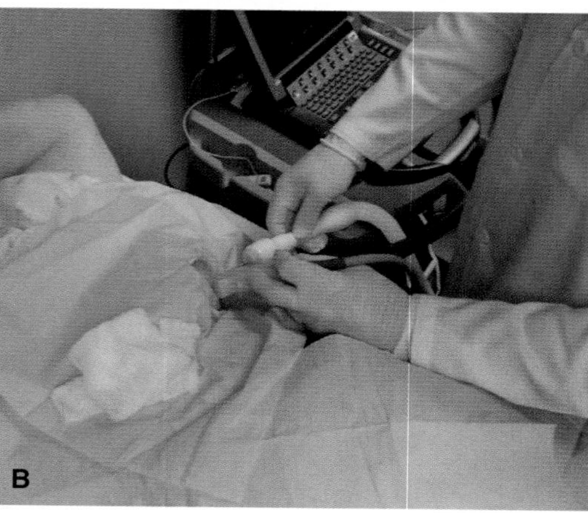

FIGURE 6 ● **A,** During procedure, surgeon holds both cryoprobe and ultrasound transducer. Continuous visualization of both cryoablation machine and ultrasound image is required. **B,** Ongoing ultrasound monitoring of skin bridge is necessary. Avoid pressing skin too close to iceball formation with ultrasound transducer.

- During the procedure, continuously monitor the skin bridge (distance between the skin and the developing iceball) to be sure the skin does not get frozen and attached to the iceball. Freely inject saline between the iceball and the skin to "lift" the skin away from the developing iceball. Skin that becomes attached to the iceball may be injured and result in scar.
- **"Tips"** to avoid skin injury during cryoablation include: (1) Palpate the skin and move the skin horizontally overlying the iceball formation to confirm there is a large subcutaneous portion of mobile fat separating the iceball from the skin. Repeated movement of the skin overlying the iceball confirms it is not becoming attached. If the skin does not freely move, inject more saline to lift the skin away from the freezing iceball (see **FIGURE 7A** and **B**). (2) Avoid continuous downward pressure of the monitoring ultrasound transducer pushing the skin down onto the developing iceball narrowing the distance between the iceball and the skin. (3) Holding the cryoprobe, angle the distal end of the cryoprobe toward the posterior (chest wall) direction so that the distance from the developing iceball to the skin is maximized. (4) Continuously monitor the distance from the iceball to the skin and inject saline between the skin and iceball to "lift" the skin away from the iceball development. This can be done repeatedly as needed. Avoid adherence of the skin to the iceball at all times.
- The treatment consists of two high-freeze cycles separated by a thaw cycle. Each cycle is usually the same length of time, that is, 8 minutes each for a total treatment time of 24 minutes. A single freeze cycle may only injure the tumor but two freeze cycles creates necrosis of the tumor.
- The cryoablation device will freeze high for the first and second freeze cycles. During the freezing continuous ultrasound monitoring will visualize an iceball growing as it envelopes the target lesion. At the end of the first freeze, the iceball will be much larger than the targeted tumor. That is normal since the edge of the iceball is injured but may not be necrotic (see **FIGURE 8A-D**).
- When the automated cryoablation machine reaches the end of the second freeze, it will automatically go into a warming mode. The cryoprobe cannot be removed while it is frozen. The tip of the probe will warm after about 30 seconds of warming so that it may be gently removed.
- At the end of the procedure, the patient will still be able to feel a firm frozen area, which is the iceball (see **FIGURE 9**).

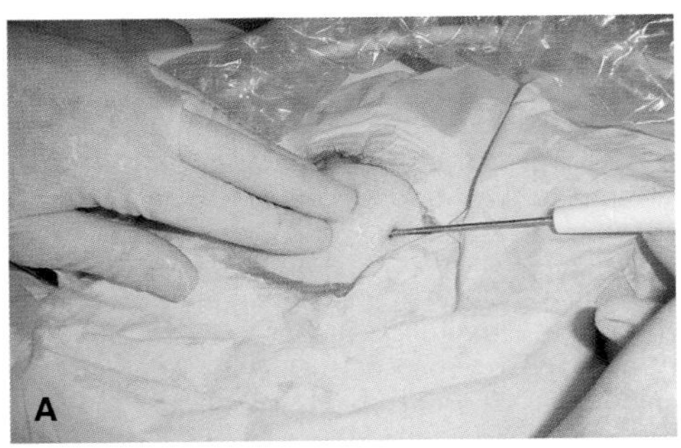

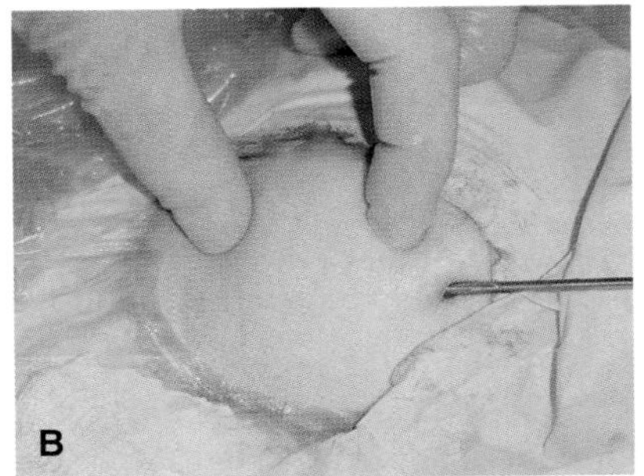

FIGURE 7 ● **A,** Use of palpation over iceball to confirm skin is moveable and not frozen to iceball, which can cause skin damage. **B,** Palpation of iceball during cryoablation confirming skin not attached to iceball.

That will thaw within an hour, but there will still remain a palpable mass, which is the residual necrotic debris. It will take several months for the debris to be resorbed. This normal fact must be communicated adequately to the patient and her primary care provider.

- A Steri-Strip is placed on the entry wound similar to a core needle biopsy dressing. Careful not to place a tight adhesive bandage on the area since it will swell significantly over the next 2 days and blisters can develop (see "Postoperative Care").

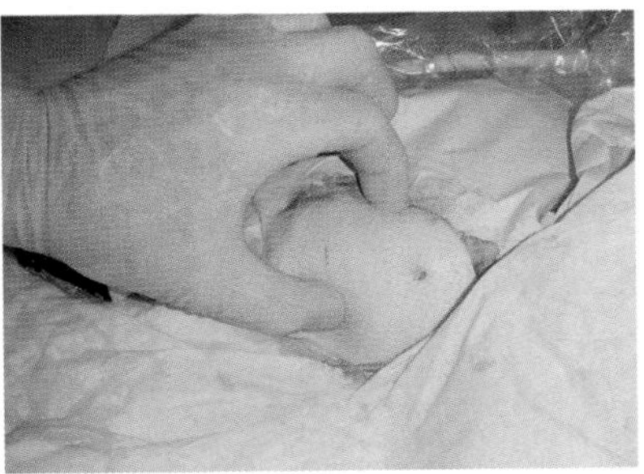

FIGURE 9 ● Immediate posttreatment palpation of iceball.

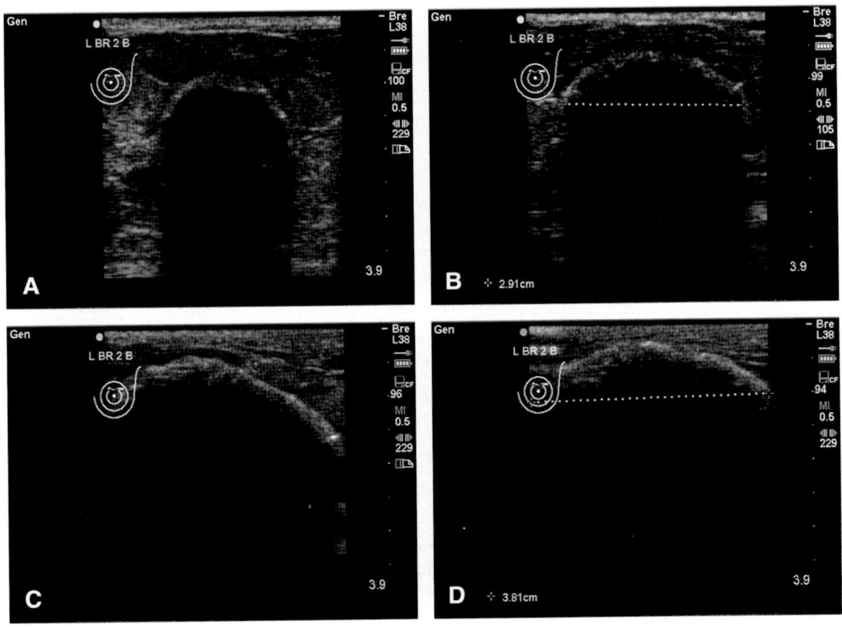

FIGURE 8 ● Serial ultrasound images of cryoablation. **A,** During initial iceball development. **B,** Transverse view of iceball at the end of first freeze cycle. **C,** Longitudinal view of iceball at end of second freeze cycle. **D,** Transverse view of iceball after cryoprobe removal.

PEARLS AND PITFALLS

Lesion Location	
Very close to the chest wall	After placement of the probe, during the initial icing phase, lift directly up off the chest wall with the probe in the tumor. This will allow the iceball to form without attachment to the pectoralis major muscle. After the iceball is adequately formed, about 2 min into the freezing, you can release the traction away from the chest wall.
Close to the skin but away from nipple	After placing the probe into the tumor and confirming satisfactory position, inject lidocaine in the space between the skin and the tumor. Try to spread your fluid within the remaining space between the skin and the tumor. After you have over 1 cm of fluid in the ultrasound "window" proceed with freezing. Be ready to inject further saline/lidocaine during the freezing period for the first 4 min. Thereafter, the iceball will unlikely get too much bigger until the second freeze. The main problem is that there is a progressive iceball enlargement, and frequent skin reassessment must be made to avoid freeze injury. An easy way to tell if the iceball is getting too close to the skin is to examine the mobility of the skin over the iceball. If the skin has much movement, (similar to the skin of your hand over your knuckles) then the iceball is not too close. If there is limited horizontal movement of the skin, inject more fluid. If there is no skin movement, stop the procedure until you can inject more fluid and create a better bridge.
Immediately deep to areolar, close to true nipple	One is concerned if the tumor is immediately below the nipple, especially if the patient is a young woman who wishes to breast feed in the future. During the cryoablation, the immediate surrounding tissues may be injured or destroyed. This usually is not a problem within the body of the breast, since a small surrounding margin of normal breast tissue is often removed with fibroadenoma excision. But when the immediate surrounding tissue includes major milk ducts, one must be cautious in treating that patient. There is no literature of treating these patients and later determining the ability of these women to breast feed. My habit is to refrain from treating those fibroadenomas that lie immediately below the nipple and immediately adjacent to the true nipple.
Candidates for Treatment	
Benign tumors other than fibroadenoma	There are anecdotal data on cryoablation of nonfibroadenomas. Although early in our experience other lesions were treated with success, the current published acceptable indications for cryoablation are for treatment of fibroadenomas. In the small series of patients with nonfibroadenoma, they acted similar to the fibroadenoma cryoablated patients. However, a clinician would have little literature support if there were complications on a nonfibroadenoma patient. We would refrain from treating those patients.
Pregnant patients	There are little data on cryoablation during pregnancy. Surgery should be considered for rapidly growing or painful lesions during pregnancy while others may wait. Be sure to rule out malignancy in this clinical situation.
More than one fibroadenoma	For two tumors close together in the same quadrant, both less than 2 cm, it is possible to place the probe through both lesions at one time and treat both simultaneously. If they cannot be treated simultaneously, then using the same probe in the same quadrant would be reasonable if the entry site were unchanged. If there are two separate punctures to be made, or if the lesions are in different quadrants of the same breast, then two separate probes would be optimal. When treating fibroadenomas of both breasts, two separate probes should be used.
Technical Challenges	
Difficulty placing probe in a firm fibroadenoma	Some fibroadenomas are very dense and seem to forbid entry of the cryoprobe. The best approach is to reevaluate your entry site and your options to "hold" the tumor in place while you advance the probe into it. One must be cautious to avoid "past pointing" and pushing through the tumor once the probe enters it fully. One technique is to start the probe into the lesion and then use your opposite hand to manually brace the tumor while you advance slowly the probe with your dominant hand. A slow twisting of the probe may allow the cryoprobe to enter the lesion. Use plenty of lidocaine. If it seems impossible to enter the lesion, consider temporarily removing the cryoprobe and using a spring-loaded core needle to take a few "bites" of the tumor at the planned trajectory of the cryoprobe. By creating a small bore-hole with the needle biopsy device, the cryoprobe may be able to enter the tumor more easily. Care should be taken to keep the cryoprobe sterile while you use the core biopsy tool. If the patient did not have an adequate pretreatment core biopsy, these extra cores can be submitted.
Patient desires sedation	Most patients tolerate this very well under local anesthesia alone, as with core needle biopsy. Adequate infiltration of the entry pathway of the cryoprobe and some anesthetic immediately in and around the fibroadenoma facilitates this process. Moving the procedure from the office to an outpatient treatment facility in order to administer sedation complicates the process by moving equipment and requiring recovery time and nurses. This increases the overall cost and minimizes the financial benefit. We have not had to perform this procedure under sedation or general anesthesia due to the inherent anesthetic properties of extreme cold. Use enough local anesthetic but do not inject much volume directly in the ultrasound "window" between the skin and the tumor for fear of obstructing your ultrasound "view." The only objection has been the time it takes to treat. Some patients want to listen to their music during the procedure.
Choice of treatment device	There are several cryoablation devices on the market. Although early versions used super-cooled argon gas, currently the majority of devices use liquid nitrogen as coolant. This is easier to obtain and simple to use, but the liquid nitrogen does not store well, so it requires replacement on a regular basis.

Postoperative pitfalls

- **The patient has much more pain in the first few days than I expected.** Sometimes, surrounding tissue is damaged and swells more than expected. If the lesion was on the chest wall, cryoablation of pectoralis muscle will be more painful than breast tissue ablation. Supportive pain medicine will allow this to resolve as with any surgical procedure. In other patients, there is significant swelling in and around the cryoablated tissue. This is more likely with longer ablations or larger areas of normal breast tissue ablated. This occurs with cancer ablations due to longer treatment times. With tissue swelling, one must be cautious of skin taping or Steri-Strips during these first few days. Owing to the swelling, there may be a sheering force on the skin by the tape, and skin blisters may occur. This is strictly due to tape applied too tight for the amount of tissue swelling that may occur. Avoid tape close to the cryoablation area. Pain may be due to blisters forming under the tape. Finally, since this is essentially a tissue burn, icepacks after the cryoablation may be helpful for the first few days.
- **The ecchymosis after the treatment is more than I expected.** All blood cells within the cryoablated area will be lysed during the treatment. The free hemoglobin will come to the surface over the first few days and make a noticeable bruise. This will all resorb within the first 2 weeks. Since there is a relatively small area of treatment, the distribution of the lysed products may be larger than expected but normal (see **FIGURE 10A-C**).

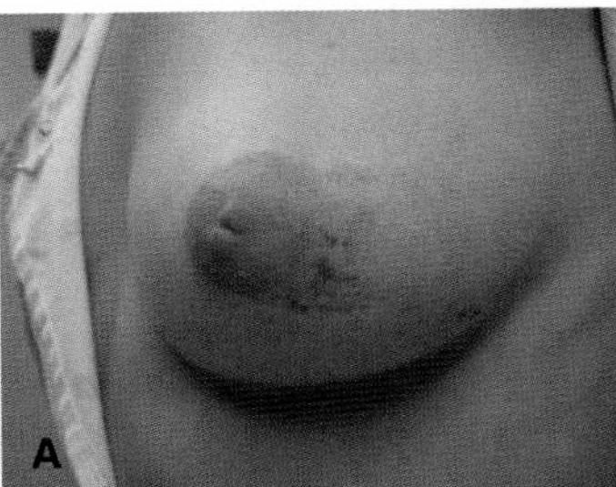

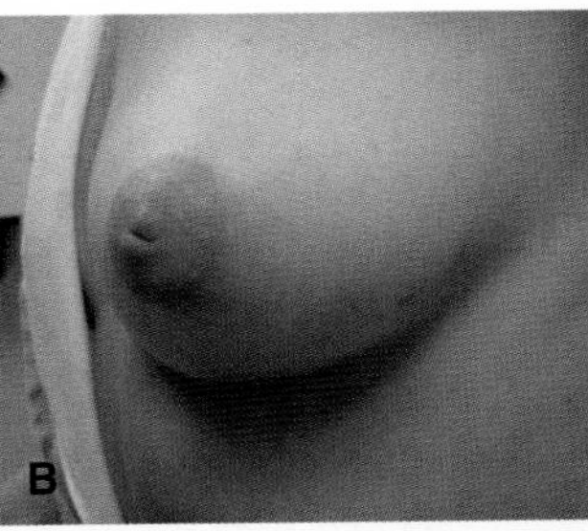

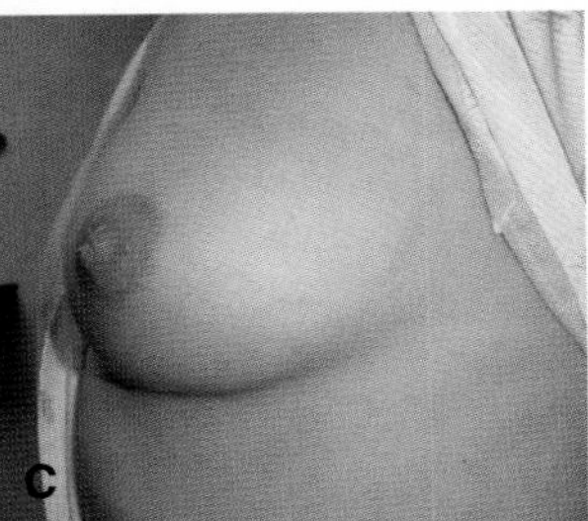

FIGURE 10 ● **A-C,** Clinical images of patient postcryoablation at 1 week, 1 month, and 6 months. Note, the ecchymosis extends in a larger area than the fibroadenoma due to the lysis of blood cells in the area but resolves promptly.

- **The patient has a large palpable mass in an area where nothing was palpable before.** The iceball is usually at least 30% larger than the treated lesion. The tissue within the iceball becomes firm and much more noticeable than the prior tumor. Nonpalpable tumors become palpable "cryolesions" immediately. Over the first 1 to 2 months, these areas will start to decrease in firmness. It would not be until about 6 months before they dissolve. Continue to reassure the patient that the firmness they feel is normal and expected. Anxiety of finding a new mass (although temporary) when none was present previously can readily undo the expected benefits of the procedure.
- **The patient has a persistent firm mass for 6 to 9 months, and she and the physician are worried that something is wrong.** The findings at the late stage of these patients are primarily related to the adequacy of the initial treatment. If the cryoprobe was placed accurately, and the treatment given properly, these patients will need to wait for the expected resolution of the palpable mass. For lesions over 2 cm, it will take over 6 months before their lesions start to noticeably decrease in size. Signs of a successful cryoablation include no growth in the palpable mass after the first month and that after 6 months there seems to be a slight softening of the mass, although it is difficult to notice. There should be no progressive measurable growth in the "mass." Reassurance is necessary for both the doctor and the patient during this time. By 9 months, it is clear that the cryolesion is getting smaller and the firmness is decreasing. By 12 months, there is noticeable change, even if the lesion is not gone. Progressive decrease in size is noticeable on ultrasound and palpation. The answer is patience.
- **Follow-up ultrasound after cryoablation shows a suspicious hypoechoic shadowing lesion, suspicious for breast cancer.** The ultrasound picture of cryoablated tissue is similar to surgical scar. There is typically an irregular hypoechoic shadowing mass, noticeably more suspicious on ultrasound that prior to cryoablation. The clues of normalcy are that there is no progressive growth but slow and progressive decrease in overall size. These lesions are followed but not biopsied unless there is growth. A well-informed experienced imager will steer clear of anxiety and simply follow over time. (See **FIGURE 11A** and **B,** shows the ultrasound 4 years post cryoablation of a fibroadenoma.)

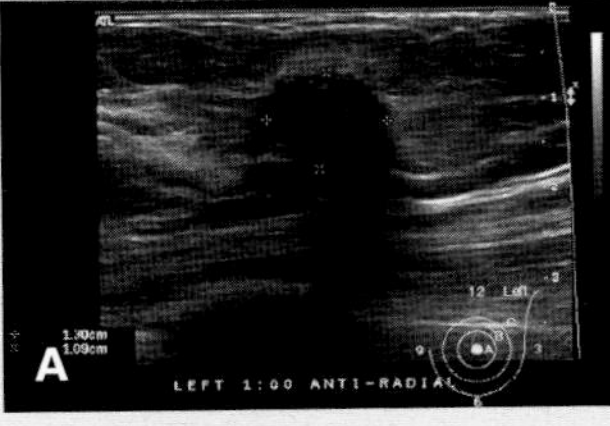

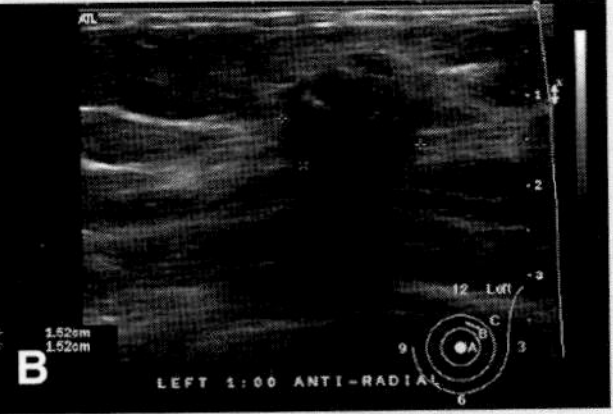

FIGURE 11 ● **A** and **B,** Ultrasound images of cryoablation site 4 years after treatment. Site is smaller and has residual scar of necrotic debris where lesion had previously been.

Key pearls	▪ Choose your target wisely, biopsy proven benign fibroadenoma away from the skin and nipple typically less than 2.5 cm in a willing patient who is informed of the long-term gradual resolution of the cryolesion. ▪ Confirm technical accuracy of probe placement and adherence to cryoablation treatment protocol. ▪ At each postprocedure appointment, examine the regressing cryolesion, check for clinical changes, and restate the long-term expected clinical outcomes. ▪ Maintain routine age-specific breast health monitoring, which may include screening mammogram and clinical breast examinations.

POSTOPERATIVE CARE

- Bandage dressing over the entry site is very important to absorb some fluid that may drain out of the entry site. The treatment is essentially a burn of the interior of the breast. As with other burns, the area will swell over the next 2 to 3 days. A dressing over the area must accommodate the skin stretching and tissue swelling; otherwise, there will be blistering of the skin where tape or other adhesive dressings are placed.
- The entry site is closed with a Steri-Strip. Over the Steri-Strip can be placed a couple 2 × 2 gauze pads and then all covered with a Tegaderm-like adhesive waterproof dressing. Be careful NOT to stretch the adhesive dressing over the gauze since the tissue will swell. Stretch the skin and lay the unstretched dressing over the gauze so that the swelling of the skin over the next couple days would not create blistering at the corners of the dressing from a sheer effect that occurs with tissue swelling under a tight Tegaderm-like plastic. Do not stretch the Tegaderm-like plastic dressing on the skin but rather stretch the skin as you place the unstrectched Tegaderm-like dressing over the gauze. Instruct the patient to peel back the edges if it starts to irritate at the edges as the tissue swells.
- Immediately after the procedure, patients have a cold firm spot on their breast that is numb. They typically are able to drive themselves home after a few minutes of relaxation while getting dressed.
- Inform the patient that her tissue will swell significantly over the next few days, which may also be tender. Local treatments of ice packs and ibuprofen will aid in decreasing the swelling. Patients who are warned of the swelling and local tenderness will less likely be alarmed when and if it occurs.
- Owing to the complete destruction of all cells within the cryoablation target, all blood cells will lyse and exude their hemoglobin into the tissues. The entire treated area will turn a deep shade of red-purple merging to yellow-green over the next week to 10 days. The person is not bleeding but the blood within the cryotreated area has lysed. An informed patient will not be alarmed when these color changes occur. By 2 weeks all the color is gone.
- The patient is advised to call the office as needed for the first 5 days to let us know of the changes that have been described. It is not likely at all to have a significant posttreatment hemorrhage or infection. However, patients will think both of these events might be happening due to the typical changes post cryoablation.
- After these initial changes, the patient will be able to feel a firm oval mass at the site of the cryoablation zone. It will not be very tender but will be larger than the patient's original lesion, or if it was nonpalpable prior to cryoablation, it is now palpable to the patient. Knowing this change in physical examination will occur is helpful to prevent the patient's concern when they first palpate the area after the initial swelling is gone.

Long-Term Postprocedure Management

- See **FIGURE 2**.
- After the initial healing period, the patient enters a long-term resolution phase. During this time the patient will have very slow resolution of the residual mass left by the necrotic central cryoablative zone. The length of time is directly related to the size of the cryoablated tissue. Typically, there is little pain in the area. Properly informed patients express little concern when feeling the persistent cryonecrotic mass over several months as it resolves.
- Follow-up office visits. Some clinicians treat the patients and simply advise the patients of expected local changes in the breast and do not follow their patients in the office. This is not the advised method of follow-up, but some clinicians just wait for patients to call or return as needed. This method creates unnecessary anxiety in the patient and likely decreases patient satisfaction. We recommend regular follow-up examinations for 1 year after cryoablation. This avoids the frantic call from the primary care provider who finds a new mass in the breast, not previously seen.
- As time goes on, the patient is seen less frequently to confirm the residual mass is decreasing as well as to reassure the patient that all is well. The first posttreatment visit is about 2 to 4 weeks after the cryoablation. The next visit is 2 months later. The next visit is 3 to 4 months after that. Thereafter, every 3 to 6 months till the lesion has disappeared. This ranges from 9 months to 2 years.
- With each visit the area is examined with or without focal ultrasound measurements. With each examination note the size of the residual cryonecrosis and reassure the patient of slow and progressive absorption.
- Most patients are under 40 years and not candidates for routine mammographic screening. If they are over 40 years, preferably their most recent mammogram was just prior to their cryoablation. Routine screening may follow. The first mammogram post cryoablation will have imaging changes from the procedure. If the imager is unaware of the treatment, they will note increased density and mass effect with indistinct margins in the area of the previously benign-appearing lesion. The unaware imager may consider the image BIRADS 4 and suggest a biopsy. However, clarifying the treatment events will modify the reading to either BIRADS 3 or 2 suggesting serial follow-up imaging.[22,23]

- The speed of resorption of the residual cryoablation debris relates to the original size of the target lesion. For tumors less than 2 cm, the area normally disappears within 1 year post treatment. For those larger than 2 cm, it may take longer than a year. Almost all lesions over 2 cm are not palpable by 2 years. Ultrasound visualization of the residual cryoablated tissue remains visible for longer periods, but that is similar to scar after surgical excision seen by ultrasound. Ultrasound identification of the treated area is difficult to find by 3 years.
- Long-term (over 3 years) imaging changes vary from no evidence of treatment to residual scar similar to surgical biopsy changes. Mammograms may occasionally show focal calcifications in the area or radiating fibrosis, but the most common mammographic image is fatty replacement of the treatment area.[22] Ultrasound imaging most often demonstrates nonspecific breast tissue with some areas of hypoechoic scar over time.

OUTCOMES

- Many reports have demonstrated the effectiveness of cryoablation of fibroadenomas. These reports are consistent in their results in properly chosen patients. After treatment, clinical and imaging evidence of the lesion slowly resorbs until the area disappears. Imaging evidence of the targets also disappears.
- After initial positive reports of this technique, a CPT code was assigned to this process. Many payers reimbursed for this procedure. However, owing to limited use of this method of treatment, many payers reversed their acceptance of payment and reclassified this procedure as investigational. However, the data supporting this method of treatment as acceptable have been repeated in the peer-reviewed literature in many sites. The few negative comments are mostly reports of slow resorption of the treated lesion.
- As this procedure is the marriage of imaging by ultrasound and surgical percutaneous procedure, many surgeons have become less interested in performing this procedure while radiologists have become more interested. This trend seems to be steady over time.[24]

COMPLICATIONS

- Most complications can be prevented, or said another way, most complications are iatrogenic. These include choosing a patient who has too narrow a window between the skin and the lesion, making skin injury more likely.
- Other complications include blistering on the skin due to swelling of the skin under adhesive from Steri-Strips or the Tegaderm-like dressing.
- Although ecchymosis and swelling is expected, significant hemorrhage and infection is quite rare.
- Although infections can occur, proper sterile technique is associated with a very minimal risk of infection.

REFERENCES

1. Smith BL. Fibroadenomas. In: Harris JR et al, ed. *Breast Diseases*. JB Lippincott; 1991: 34-37.
2. Haagensen CD. *Diesases of the Breast*. WB Saunders; 1986.
3. Greenberg R, Skornick Y, Kaplan O. Management of breast fibroadenomas. *J Gen Intern Med*. 1998;13(9):640-645.
4. Dixon JM, Dobie V, Lamb J, Walsh JS, Chetty U. Assessment of the acceptability of conservative management of fibroadenoma of the breast. *Br J Surg*. 1996;83(2):264-265.
5. Houssami N, Cheung MN, Dixon JM. Fibroadenoma of the breast. *Med J Aust*. 2001;174(4):185-188.
6. Yilmaz E, Sal S, Lebe B. Differentiation of phyllodes tumors versus fibroadenomas. *Acta Radiol*. 2002;43(1):34-39.
7. Isaacs JH. Benign neoplasms. In: Marchant DJ, ed. *Breast Disease*. WB Saunders;1997: 66-67.
8. Rosen PP. Fibroepithelial neoplasms. In: Rosen PP, ed. *Rosen's Breast Pathology*. Lippincott-Raven Press; 1996:143-155.
9. Hughes LE, Mansel RE, Webster DJT. *Fibroadenoma and Related Tumors. Benign Disorders and Diseases of the Breast: Concepts and Clinical Management*. WB Saunders; 1999:73-94.
10. Kaufman CS, Bachman B, Littrup PJ, et al. Office-based ultrasound-guided cryoablation of breast fibroadenomas. *Am J Surg*. 2002;184(5):394-400.
11. Hindle WH. Fibroadenoma. In: Hindle WH, ed. *Breast Care: A Clinical Guidebook for Women's Primary Health Care Providers*. Springer-Verlag; 1999:191-193.
12. Kaufman CS, Littrup PJ, Freman-Gibb LA, et al. Office-based cryoablation of breast fibroadenomas: 12-month followup. *J Am Coll Surg*. 2004;198:914-923.
13. Kaufman CS, Littrup PJ, Freeman-Gibb LA, et al. Office-based cryoablation of breast fibroadenomas with long-term follow up. *Breast J*. 2005;11:344-350.
14. Kaufman CS, Bachman B, Littrup PJ, et al. Cryoablation treatment of benign breast lesions with 12 month follow up. *Am J Surg*. 2004;188:340-348.
15. Edwards MJ, Broadwater R, Tafra L, et al. Progressive adoption of cryoablative therapy for breast fibroadenoma in community practice. *Am J Surg*. 2004;188:221-224.
16. Nurko J, Mabry CD, Whitworth P, et al. Interim results from the FibroAdenoma cryoablation treatment registry. *Am J Surg*. 2005;190(4):647-651.
17. Stavros AT, Rapp CL, Parker SH. *Breast Ultrasound*. Lippincott Williams & Wilkins; 2003.
18. Sperber F, Blank A, Metser U, et al. Diagnosis and treatment of breast fibroadenomas by ultrasound-guided vacuum-assisted biopsy. *Arch Surg*. 2003;138(7):796-800.
19. Foxcroft L, Evans E, Hirst C. Newly arising fibroadenomas in women aged 35 and over. *Aust N Z J Surg*. 1998;68(6):419-422.
20. Hahn M, Pavlista D, Danes J, et al. Ultrasound guided cryoablation of fibroadenomas. *Ultraschall der Med*. 2013;34(1):64-68.
21. *Statement on Use of Ablative Techniques for Benign Tumors*. ASBS website. Accessed June 26, 2022. https://www.breastsurgeons.org/docs/statements/Management-of-Fibroadenomas.pdf
22. Kaufman CS. Mammographic appearance of fibroadenoma disappears after cryoablation. *Scientific paper*. 2002 RSNA annual meeting, December, 4, 2002, Chicago, Illinois.
23. Brenner RJ, Pfaff JM. Mammographic changes after excisional breast biopsy for benign disease. *AJR Am J Roentgenol*. 1996;167(4):1047-1052.
24. Sheth M, Lodhi U, Chen B, Park Y, McElligott S. Initial institutional experience with cryoablation therapy for breast fibroadenomas: technique, molecular science, and post-therapy imaging follow-up. *J Ultrasound Med*. 2019;38(10):2769-2776.

Chapter 9 Lumpectomy for Breast Cancer

Michael S. Sabel

DEFINITION

- Lumpectomy is defined as the complete excision of a breast tumor with an adequate margin of surrounding normal tissue. Lumpectomy plus breast irradiation are the essential components of successful breast conservation therapy (BCT).
- Lumpectomies for nonpalpable cancers require some form of localization, such as wire localization, infrared/electromagnetic, or magnetic seed localization (see Part 5, Chapters 4-6). This chapter focuses on a lumpectomy for a palpable breast mass.

PATIENT HISTORY AND PHYSICAL FINDINGS

- For BCT to be successful, it must be possible to (1) obtain negative surgical margins around the tumor while still maintaining a cosmetically acceptable result and (2) safely deliver radiation therapy. A thorough history and physical examination is necessary to carefully select patients for BCT. Absolute contraindications to BCT are listed in **TABLE 1**.
- A thorough history should be performed prior to treatment, including a detailed past medical history, present medications and allergies, and a personal and family history of cancer.
- Prior radiation to the breast is a contraindication to BCT. For patients who may have had chest wall radiation for indications other than a prior breast cancer (such as mantle radiation for Hodgkin disease), it may be helpful to obtain the prior records and review the fields treated. These patients may be eligible for a partial breast irradiation technique.
- Patients with a history of autoimmune or collagen-vascular diseases, such as scleroderma, lupus, or dermatomyositis, may have abnormal reaction to radiation therapy, which significantly compromises the cosmetic outcome. For some types of collagen-vascular diseases, such as Raynaud phenomenon, rheumatoid arthritis, or Sjögren syndrome, the response to radiation is not as severe and these patients may be considered for BCT.
- A detailed family history is critical to assess the risk of a future breast cancer, and consider genetic counseling and testing. High-risk patients may want to consider bilateral mastectomy as they are at considerable risk of a second primary cancer. A systematic review demonstrates that BCT in BRCA mutation carriers have a higher rate of ipsilateral breast cancer recurrence (which likely includes some new primary cancers), but this was not associated with adverse short- or long-term survival outcomes.[1] The decision to pursue BCT in known BRCA1/2 carriers should be made following extensive discussion with a genetic counselor.
- Patient age, nodal status, histologic tumor type, tumor grade, and extensive intraductal component (EIC) are not contraindications to BCT as long as negative margins can be obtained.
- If an adequate lumpectomy can be performed, prior breast augmentation with breast implants are not an absolute contraindication, and radiation can be delivered to the augmented breast using standard techniques and doses. However, capsular contraction is a risk. If the tumor is close to the implant the capsule surrounding the implant may need to be included in the specimen, or the implant may need to be removed, to obtain negative margins (cancers sometimes invade the fibrous capsule around the implant).
- A complete, bilateral breast examination should focus on both assessing the cosmetic implications of lumpectomy and identifying additional areas of concern to rule out multicentric disease. Any additional suspicious masses should be biopsied, and cancer ruled out, prior to proceeding with BCT.
- The size of the mass relative to the size of the breast, location of the mass, proximity to the skin and amount of skin needed to be resected, and symmetry of the breasts should be noted. For some patients with a large tumor relative to the size of the breast, neoadjuvant chemotherapy may be considered to downstage the primary tumor. For other patients in whom a poor cosmetic outcome with standard lumpectomy is predicted, an oncoplastic approach should be considered (Part 5, Chapters 10, 11, 12, and 13).
- A detailed examination of the bilateral axillary, supraclavicular, and cervical lymph nodes should be undertaken, and any suspicious lymphadenopathy worked up prior to surgery.

Table 1: Absolute Contraindications to Breast-Conserving Surgery

Unable to receive radiation therapy
Previous chest wall irradiation
Need to deliver radiation during pregnancy
Scleroderma or active systemic lupus erythematosus
Multicentric disease
Diffuse suspicious calcifications on mammography
Inability to achieve adequately negative margins

IMAGING AND OTHER DIAGNOSTIC STUDIES

- All patients require bilateral mammographic evaluation, with appropriate magnification views, within 3 months of surgery (**FIGURE 1**). Patients who received neoadjuvant chemotherapy will need updated imaging following the completion of therapy. The tumor size, the presence of microcalcifications, and the extent of calcifications outside of the mass should be noted. Some patients with palpable cancers may still require wire localization of the calcifications to assure complete removal at the time of lumpectomy.
- Any additional areas of abnormality should be worked up and biopsied to rule out multicentric cancer. Multicentric disease is typically a contraindication to BCT; however, patients

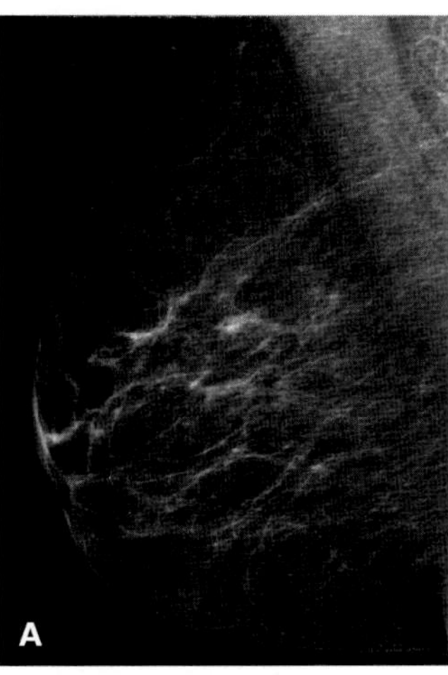
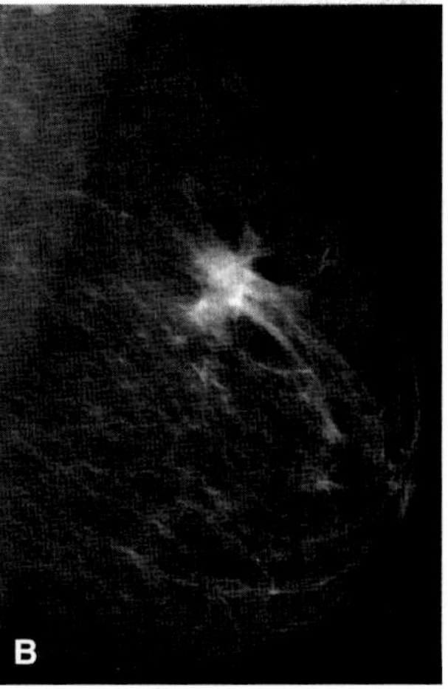
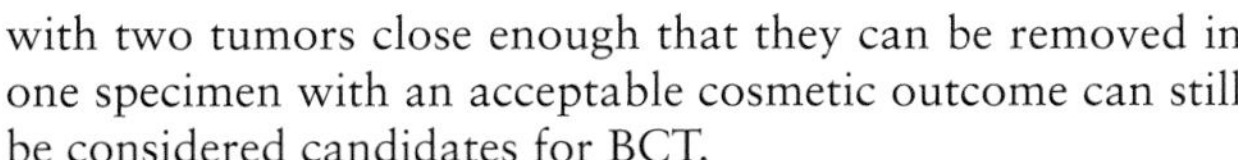

FIGURE 1 ● Bilateral mammogram demonstrating a left breast cancer. **A,** Right breast. **B,** Left breast.

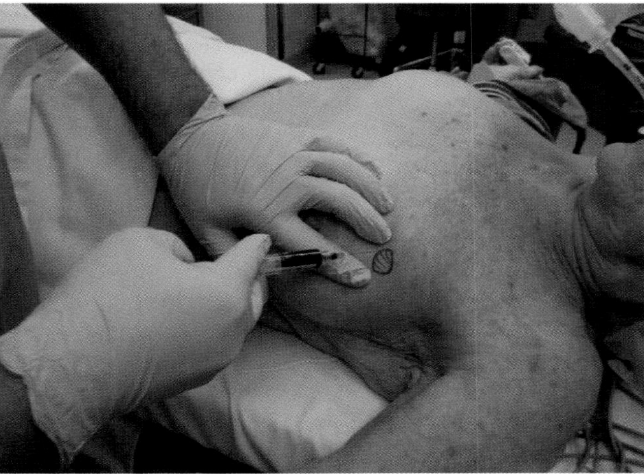

FIGURE 2 ● Peritumoral injection of blue dye prior to lumpectomy for performance of sentinel lymph node (SLN) biopsy.

with two tumors close enough that they can be removed in one specimen with an acceptable cosmetic outcome can still be considered candidates for BCT.

- The use of magnetic resonance imaging (MRI) to determine eligibility for BCT has been increasing. Although MRI may more accurately determine the extent of the tumor or identify multicentricity, particularly in women with dense breast tissue (for whom mammography is less sensitive), its use is controversial. MRI is highly sensitive but has limited specificity and is limited in its ability to visualize ductal carcinoma in situ (DCIS). A meta-analysis of preoperative MRI showed no evidence of an effect on rates of re-excision, reoperation, or positive margins, but was associated with an increased likelihood of ipsilateral mastectomy and contralateral prophylactic mastectomy.[2] Preoperative MRI also does not reduce the risk of breast cancer recurrence.[3] The need for MRI should be evaluated on a case-by-case basis.
- Accurate histologic assessment of the primary tumor, including histologic subtype, grade, hormone receptor status, and Her-2/neu overexpression, is necessary in evaluating the breast cancer patient. This is best accomplished through a core needle biopsy rather than fine needle aspiration biopsy or excisional biopsy.
- In addition to down-staging larger tumors, neoadjuvant chemotherapy is also often utilized in patients with triple-negative or Her-2 over-expressing tumors. In many cases, a palpable tumor prior to systemic therapy is no longer palpable at the time of surgery. For patients presenting for lumpectomy following neoadjuvant treatment, be sure to repeat your examination and update the imaging prior to planning surgery, as localization may be necessary.

SURGICAL MANAGEMENT

Preoperative Planning

- Prior to taking the patient back to the operating room (OR), the presence of the palpable cancer should be confirmed with the patient. In the preoperative area, the mass should be examined in both the upright and supine positions.
- With the patient in the supine position with the arm extended, the mass should be carefully marked.
- Although the risk of infection after breast cancer surgery is low, it tends to be higher than average for a clean surgical procedure, and several studies have shown that antibiotic prophylaxis significantly reduces the risk of postoperative infection.[4]

Positioning

- Lumpectomy is often performed in conjunction with a sentinel lymph node biopsy. Therefore, the patient should be positioned supine with the ipsilateral arm at 90°. Unless intraoperative analysis of the sentinel lymph node with intraoperative analysis and possible axillary lymph node dissection is planned, the ipsilateral arm can be secured.
- If a sentinel lymph node biopsy is to be performed in conjunction with lumpectomy, then the blue dye should be injected at this point. The skin is prepped with alcohol and either isosulfan or methylene blue dye is injected peritumoral (see Part 5, Chapter 16) (**FIGURE 2**).

- See **Video 1**.

PLACEMENT OF INCISION

- Skin incisions can be placed directly over the tumor, or placed in more cosmetically appealing locations such as circumareolar, lateral, or within the inframammary fold. The decision should be made based on the estimated distance between the tumor and the skin, the size of the tumor (and subsequent size of the incision), and the distance between the planned incision and the tumor so that excessive tunneling is not needed.
- Often, the skin incision is placed directly over the palpable mass (**FIGURE 3**) as this helps avoid excessive tunneling, which may compromise the margins and make a re-excision for close or positive margins unnecessarily difficult.

- When there is adequate distance between the skin and the tumor, skin does not need to be removed. However, when the tumor is close to the skin, an ellipse of skin over the tumor should be removed with the lumpectomy specimen.
- In the upper hemisphere of the breast, curvilinear incisions following the Langer lines (the normal lines of tension in the skin) are ideal. In the lower hemisphere, the incisions can either be curvilinear or radial (**FIGURE 4**). For smaller tumors in relatively larger breasts, where there is adequate breast parenchyma, curvilinear incisions are acceptable. However, when skin or a fair amount of tissue is to be removed, curvilinear incisions will collapse the breast inferiorly so that the nipple points downward. In this situation, radial incisions will result in less distortion of the nipple–areolar complex.
- Incisions should be planned with an eventual mastectomy in mind should attempts at breast conservation fail (**FIGURE 5**). The incision size needs to be adequate to remove the mass and surrounding margin. Using a small incision for cosmetic benefit may result in excessive manipulation of the tumor and involved margins that prompt subsequent re-excision.

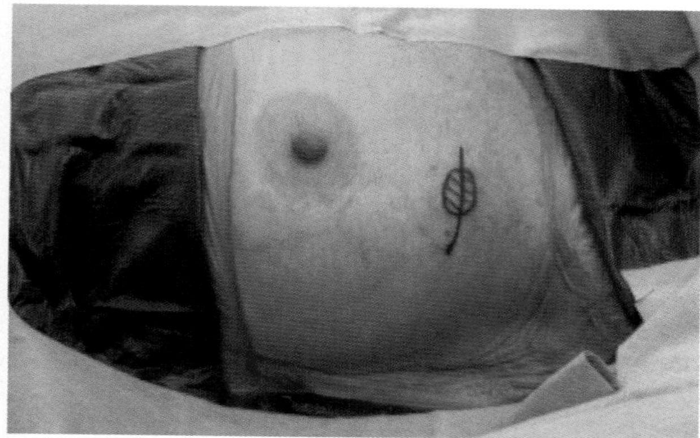

FIGURE 3 • Placement of incision within the Langer lines of the breast directly over the palpable cancer. The incision is planned large enough to remove the cancer without excess manipulation.

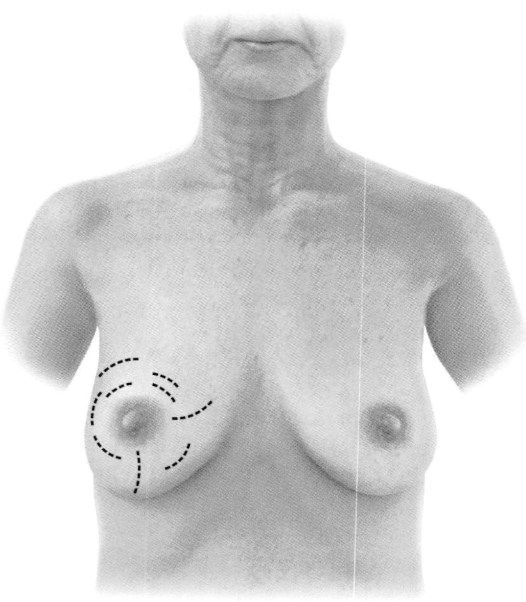

FIGURE 4 • Potential lines of excision for breast lumpectomy. In the upper hemisphere of the breast, curvilinear incisions are best, keeping within the Langer lines of the skin. In the lower hemisphere, either curvilinear or radial incisions are acceptable.

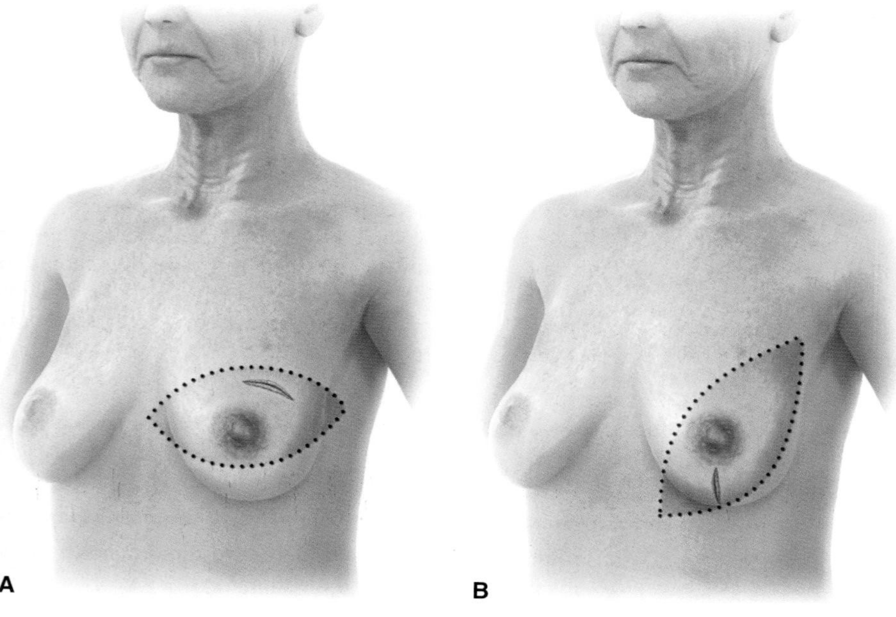

FIGURE 5 • Potential mastectomy incisions if breast conservation fails. Lumpectomy incisions should be planned with a possible mastectomy in mind should negative margins not be attainable.

SKIN INCISION AND RAISING OF FLAPS

- An incision is made in the skin going just deep to the dermis. For lesions closer to the skin, skin flaps should be immediately elevated in all directions over the mass (**FIGURE 6**). Adequate subcutaneous fat should be left on the flaps, which should get progressively thicker as the flaps are elevated. Excessively thin flaps lead to excessive retraction and concavity with radiation and should be avoided by excising the skin over the mass.
- For deep-seated tumors, after dividing the skin, the breast tissue may be divided straight down to approximately 1 cm over the mass before beginning the dissection around the tumor (**FIGURE 7**).

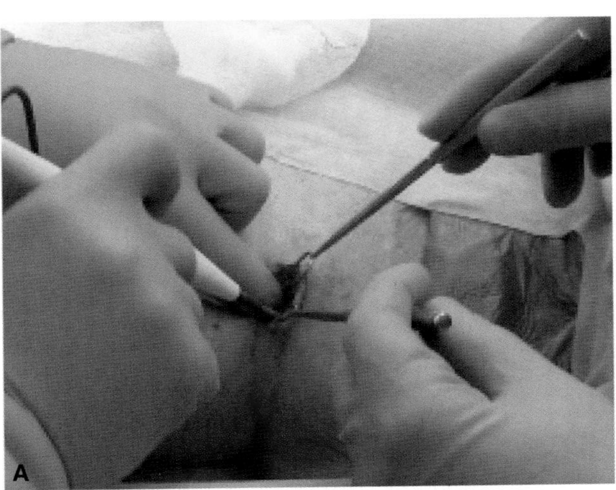

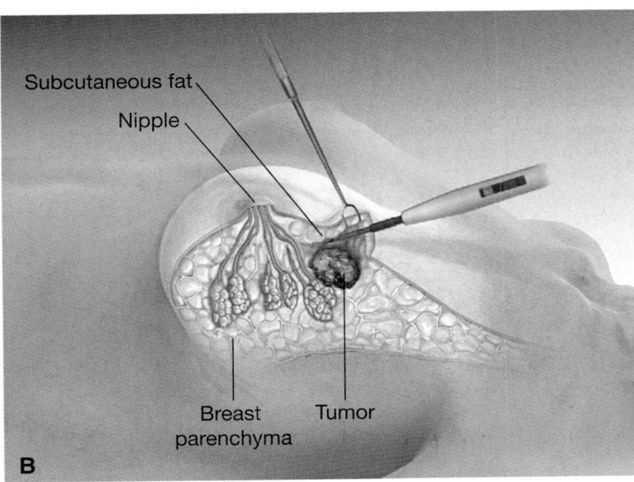

FIGURE 6 ● Raising of flaps over the tumor. Excessively thin flaps should be avoided. The flaps should get thicker as they are elevated.

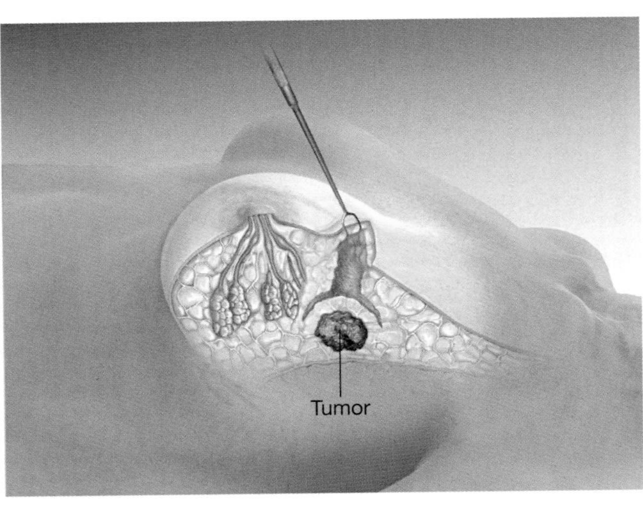

FIGURE 7 ● The breast parenchyma is divided until approximately 1 cm above the tumor before dissecting around the tumor for a deep-seated tumor.

EXCISION

- The excision is then carried out with the goal of maintaining 1-cm grossly free margins around the mass. This is best accomplished by retracting the mass with the index finger of the nonoperative hand to be constantly aware of the margin and maintaining a 1-cm rim of normal breast tissue or fat as dissection continues toward the chest wall (**FIGURE 8A** and **B**).
- The tissue is divided circumferentially around the mass. Once it is free, it can usually be elevated out of the wound (**FIGURE 9**). The skin incision must be large enough so that the resected portion can be easily brought out; struggling to deliver a mass through a small incision may lead to excessive manipulation and positive margins on final pathology.
- Before the lesion is completely removed from the body, the specimen should be oriented with 2-0 silk sutures. Orientation is critical so that if re-excision for close or positive margins are needed, this can be limited to just the involved margin (as opposed to re-excising the entire cavity). Three sutures are necessary to orient the mass correctly for the pathologist and avoid errors (**FIGURE 10**).[5] At this juncture, we recommend placing a short 2-0 silk suture at the superior margin and a long silk suture at the lateral margin (**FIGURE 11**).

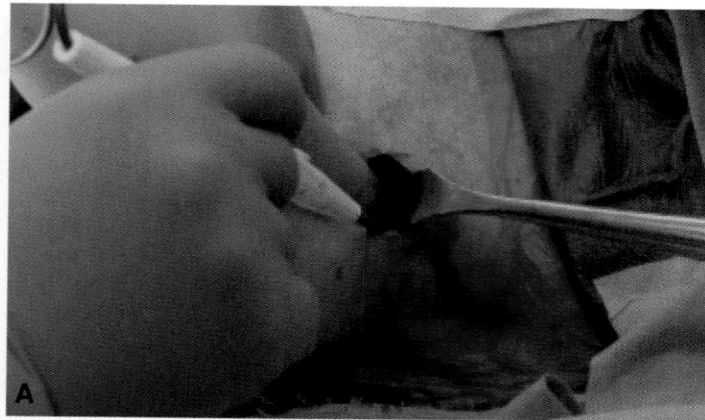

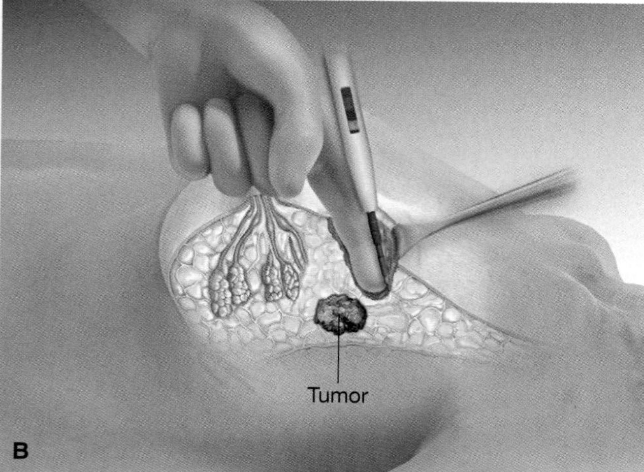

FIGURE 8 ● With the tumor retracted with the index finger, the surgeon dissects around it, maintaining 1 cm of normal breast tissue around the tumor.

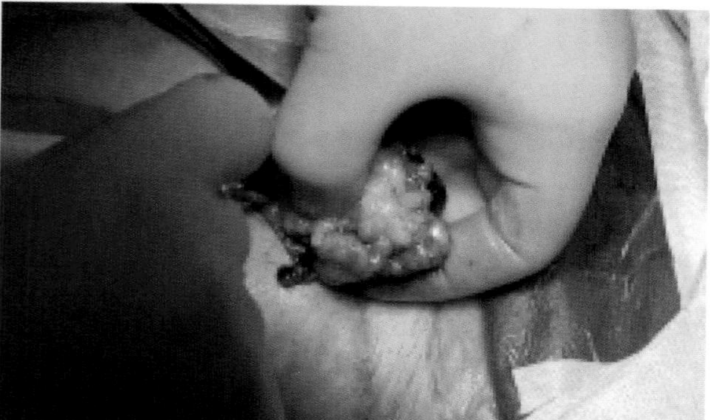

FIGURE 9 ● The entire tumor is excised circumferentially and delivered from the wound.

- The specimen is now completely removed by dividing the deep margin (**FIGURE 12**). For lesions close to the chest wall, the deep margin should include the fascia of the pectoralis major muscle. In rare cases, excision of some of the pectoralis is necessary to assure a negative deep margin. Once excised, a third double-stranded orientation suture is placed at the deep margin (**FIGURE 13**).

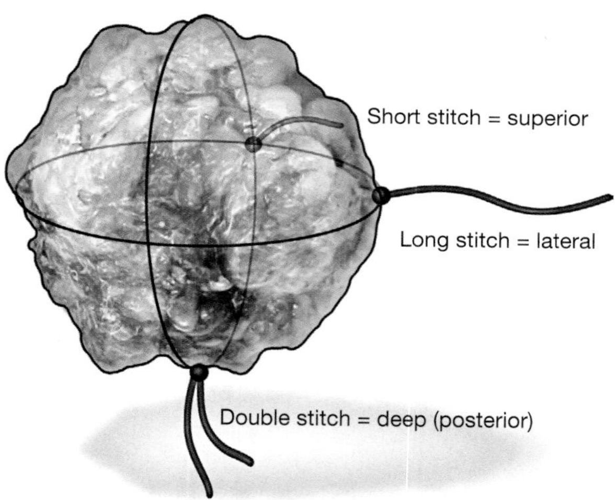

FIGURE 10 ● Three suture marking system for lumpectomy specimens. A 3-0 silk short stitch is placed superiorly, a long stitch is placed laterally, and a double stitch is placed deep (posteriorly).

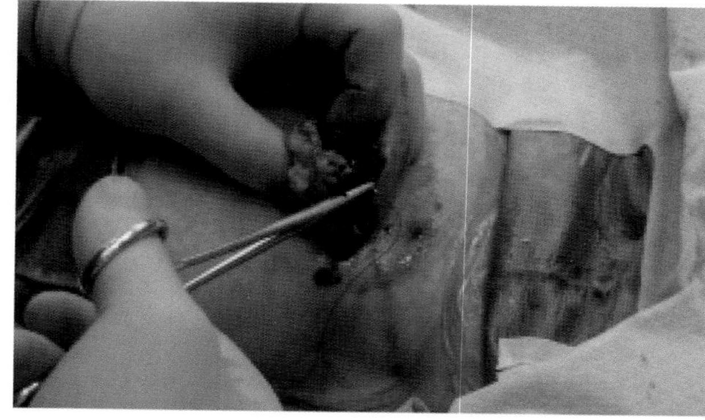

FIGURE 11 ● Marking sutures are placed prior to complete excision of the specimen so as not to lose the orientation.

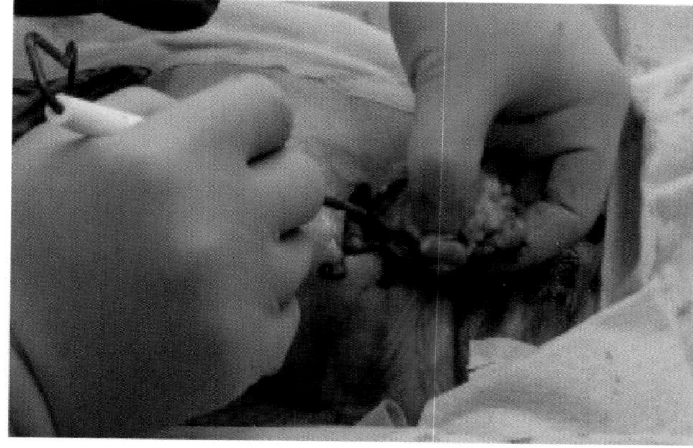

FIGURE 12 ● The posterior tissue is divided last, completing the lumpectomy.

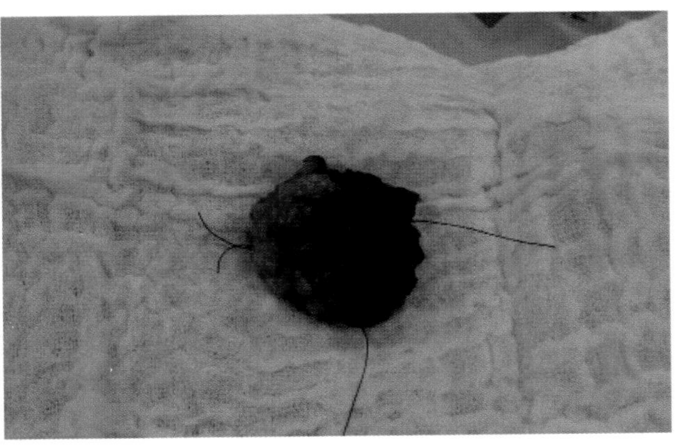

FIGURE 13 ● Lumpectomy specimen with marking sutures.

INTRAOPERATIVE MARGIN ANALYSIS

- Without intraoperative margin analysis, re-excision rates to obtain negative margins can be as high as 30% to 50%. Intraoperative margin analysis is highly recommended to minimize re-excision rates to well below 5%.[6] After orientation, the margins of the specimen are inked using six colors and then sectioned at 2- to 3-mm intervals (**FIGURE 14**).
- After gross examination of the margin status, sections are taken for each suspicious margin (**FIGURE 15**). Sections 6- to 7-μm thick are cut on a −20 °C cryostat and stained with a rapid hematoxylin and eosin technique (with two levels of each tissue block examined). Any margins in which invasive or in situ carcinoma extend to within 2-mm are reported to the surgeon (**FIGURE 16**).
- In cases where intraoperative margin analysis is not available, gross examination of the specimen may help identify margins close to the tumor so that an additional margin may be obtained. In some cases, obtaining six cavity shave margins at the time of lumpectomy may be performed to minimize the chance of negative margins, but this may increase the volume of resected tissue and the impact on local recurrence data is unknown.[7]
- A re-excision of the close margin can then be performed by grasping the top of the margin with an Allis clamp and excising back another 0.5 to 1 cm around the hemisphere in need of re-excision (**FIGURE 17A** and **B**). The new margin should be appropriately marked for the pathologist (**FIGURE 18**).

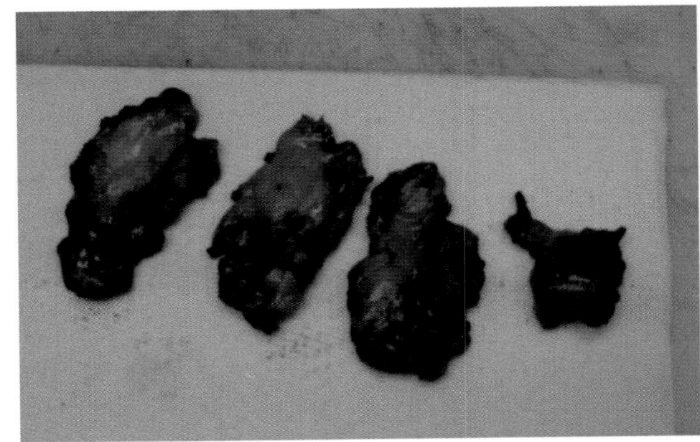

FIGURE 15 ● The sections are grossly examined for involved margins.

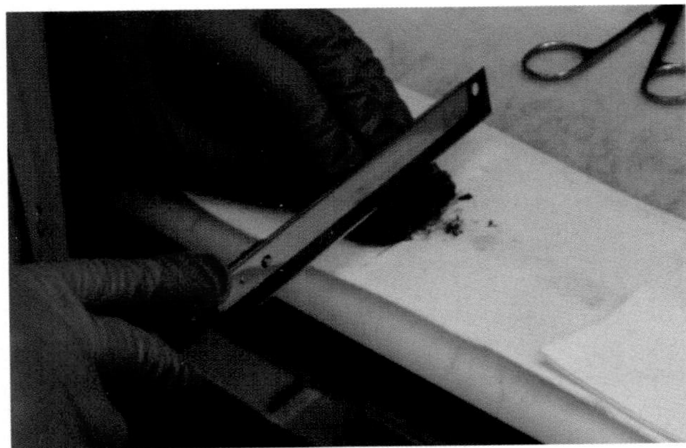

FIGURE 14 ● The specimen is inked with six colors and sectioned for intraoperative margin analysis.

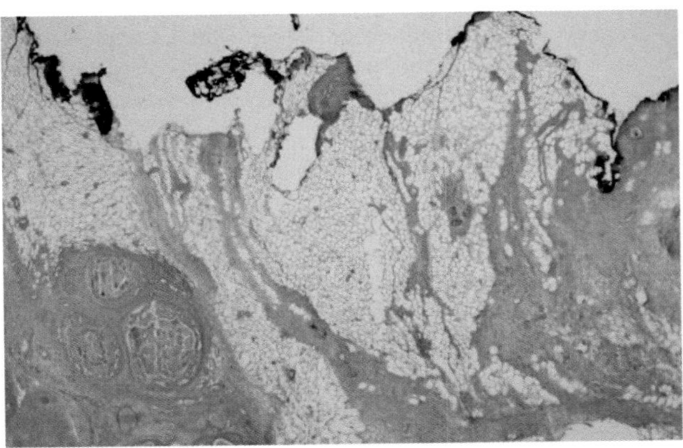

FIGURE 16 ● DCIS is identified close to the margin. This information is relayed to the surgeon so a re-excision of that margin can be performed.

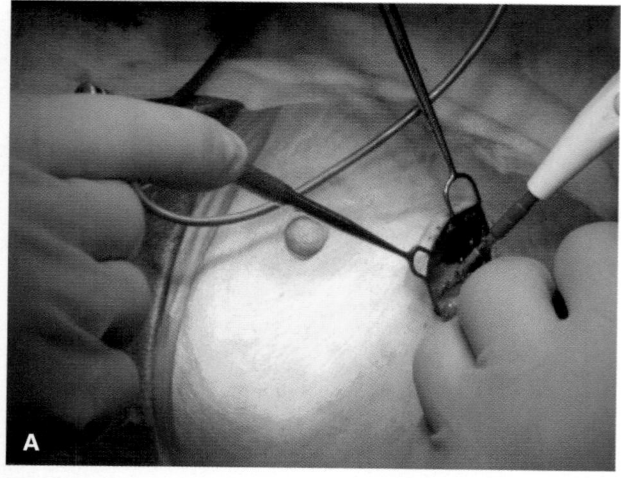

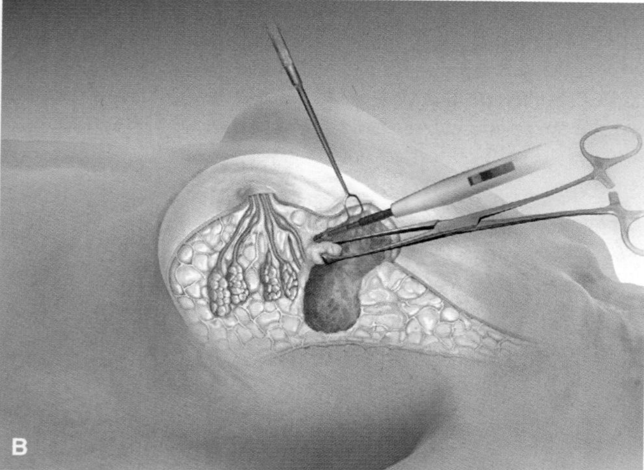

FIGURE 17 ● **A,** An additional inferior margin is obtained based on the intraoperative margin analysis. **B,** The top of the cavity is grasped with an Allis and the entire hemisphere is excised approximately 1 cm back from the cavity.

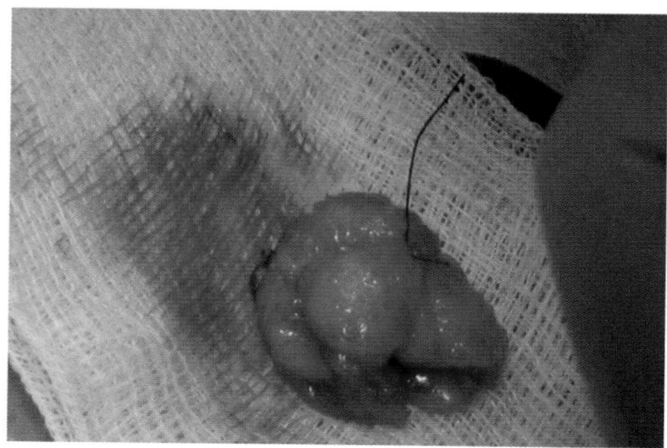

FIGURE 18 ● A marking stitch designating the new, true margin after re-excision.

CLOSURE

- Once the lumpectomy is complete, hemostasis is assured and then surgical clips are placed within the cavity at the six anatomic locations (anterior, posterior, medial, lateral, superior, and inferior) (**FIGURE 19**). This helps in the planning of radiation therapy, particularly for a boost or for partial breast irradiation.
- For the standard lumpectomy, the surgeon should *not* try to re-approximate the breast tissue. The cavity will fill with seroma and fibrin, and ultimately fibrous tissue, which will maintain the normal contour. For large defects, oncoplastic techniques can be considered, which are discussed in Part 5, Chapter 15.
- The incision is closed with absorbable deep dermal sutures, followed by either a subcuticular stitch or tissue adhesive (**FIGURE 20**). Drains should not be used.

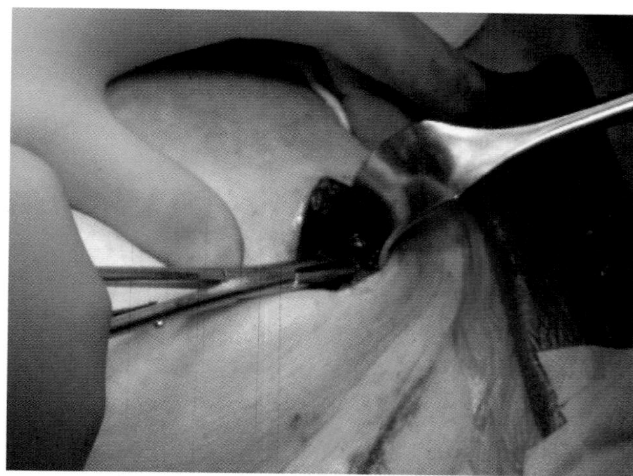

FIGURE 19 ● Clips are placed around the lumpectomy cavity to aid in the delivery of radiation.

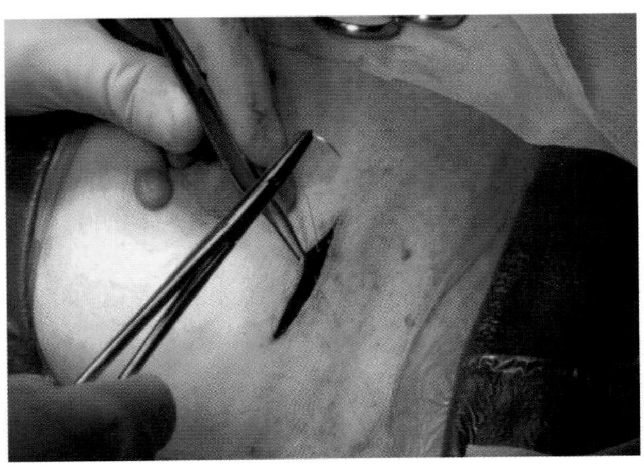

FIGURE 20 ● The skin is reapproximated with absorbable deep dermal sutures.

PEARLS AND PITFALLS

Indications	■ A complete history and physical and review of the breast imaging should take place to assure the patient is a suitable candidate for BCT. ■ Suspicious lesions on exam or imaging should be biopsied prior to proceeding with BCT.
Placement of incision	■ Incisions should be planned keeping in mind a possible re-excision or a mastectomy should BCT fail. ■ In the inferior portion of the breast, radial incisions can give superior cosmetic outcomes compared to curvilinear incisions. ■ Make the incision large enough to remove the tumor without excessive manipulation. This decreases the close/positive margin rate and the need for re-excision.
Raising of flaps	■ Thin flaps will lead to excessive retraction and concavity after radiation. Avoid them by excising the skin over the tumor with the lumpectomy. ■ Flaps should get progressively thicker as they are raised.
Excision	■ Maintain at least 1 cm of grossly normal margins around the mass throughout the excision. ■ Intraoperative margin analysis can greatly reduce re-excision rates, leading to lower mastectomy rates and improved cosmetic outcome.
Orientation	■ Three orientation sutures are necessary to avoid error. ■ Place two sutures before complete excision of the tumor to avoid losing the orientation.
Closure	■ Do not try to reapproximate the breast tissue or place a drain.

POSTOPERATIVE CARE

- After a lumpectomy, the patient should be placed in a breast binder or supportive brassiere. This helps sustain hemostasis and relieves tension on the skin closure imposed by the weight of the breasts. The patient should be encouraged to wear a supportive bra day and night for 1 week after surgery.
- Patients who had microcalcifications on preoperative mammography extending outside of the mammographic mass should undergo postlumpectomy mammogram to assure complete clearance of the microcalcifications.

OUTCOMES

- Margins should be histologically negative (no tumor on ink) following lumpectomy. Patients with a positive margin should return to the operating room for re-excision lumpectomy. Obtaining wider histologic margins between tumor and ink (eg, 2 mm) are no longer recommended with the use of no ink on tumor as the standard for an adequate margin.[8]
- In a meta-analysis of 33 eligible studies between 1965 and 2013, the median prevalence of in-breast tumor recurrence following lumpectomy and radiation was 5.3% (interquartile range, 2.3%-7.6%).[9] Survival rates are equivalent.[10]

COMPLICATIONS

- Seroma
- Hematoma
- Infection (cellulitis or abscess)
- Altered sensation to the nipple
- Close or positive margins
- Poor cosmetic outcome

REFERENCES

1. Co M, Liu T, Leung J, et al. Breast conserving surgery for BRCA mutation carriers—a systematic review. *Clin Breast Cancer.* 2020;20(3):e244-e250.
2. Houssami N, Turner RM, Morrow M. Meta-analysis of pre-operative magnetic resonance imaging (MRI) and surgical treatment for breast cancer. *Breast Cancer Res Treat.* 2017;165:273-283.
3. Houssami N, Turner R, Macaskill P, et al. An individual person data meta-analysis of preoperative magnetic resonance imaging and breast cancer recurrence. *J Clin Oncol.* 2014;32:392-401.
4. Bunn F, Jones DJ, Bell-Syer S. Prophylactic antibiotics to prevent surgical site infection after breast cancer surgery. *Cochrane Database Syst Rev.* 2012;3:CD005360. doi: 10.1002/1465858.CD005360.pub3
5. Molina MA, Snell S, Franceschi D, et al. Breast specimen orientation. *Ann Surg Oncol.* 2009;16:285-288.
6. Sabel MS, Jorns JM, Wu A, et al. Development of an intraoperative pathology consultation service at a free-standing ambulatory surgical center: clinical and economic impact for patients undergoing breast cancer surgery. *Am J Surg.* 2012;204(1):66-77. doi:10.1016/j.amjsurg.2011.07.016
7. Chagpar AB, Killelia BK, Tsangaris TN, et al. A raondomized, controlled trial of cavity shave margins in breast cancer. *NEJM.* 2015;373:503-510.
8. Moran MS, Schnitt SJ, Giuliano AE, et al. Society of surgical oncology-American society for radiation oncology consensus guideline on margins for breast-conserving surgery with whole-breast irradiation in stages I and II invasive breast cancer. *Int J Radiat Oncol Biol Phys.* 2014;88:553-564.
9. Houssami N, Macaskill P, Marinovich ML, et al. The association of surgical margins and local recurrence in women with early stage invasive breast cancer treated with breast conserving therapy: a meta-analysis. *Ann Surg Oncol.* 2014;21:717-730.
10. Clarke M, Collins R, Darby S; Early Breast Cancer Trialists' Collaborative Group (EBCTCG). Effects of radiotherapy and of differences in the extent of surgery for early breast cancer on local recurrence and 15-year survival: an overview of the randomized trials. *Lancet.* 2005;366(9503):2087-2106.

Chapter 10

Oncoplastic Breast Surgery: Parallelogram Mastopexy Lumpectomy

Cary S. Kaufman

DEFINITION

- For most patients, adequate margins and excellent cosmetic outcomes can be achieved with a simple lumpectomy without specific attempts to eliminate the residual seroma defects (Part 5, Chapter 9).
- For patients with larger defects, seroma absorption and the effects of radiation may lead to excessive retraction, depression, and deviation of the nipple. Oncoplastic resections allow for resection of the tumor and reapproximating the dead space to avoid this.
- One of the simpler oncoplastic approaches for tumors of the upper breast is the ***parallelogram mastopexy lumpectomy***, named for its rounded parallelogram skin incision.[1] This procedure is based on Veronesi's "quadrantectomy" with its radially oriented, full-thickness glandular excision.[2]
- The parallelogram mastopexy lumpectomy allows resection of wide margins around a cancer with concurrent mastopexy lift for small to moderate ptosis (**FIGURE 1**).
- Subsequent undermining of the breast gland with reapproximation of the tissues at the chest wall (mastopexy closure) reduces the extent of postoperative skin retraction and cavitation, but may lead to asymmetry. That asymmetry may be desired in a patient such as this who has ptosis that can be corrected with this simple procedure. On the other hand, without ptosis, a patient may have a high nipple or may require a contralateral breast lift and/or reduction for symmetry restoration.

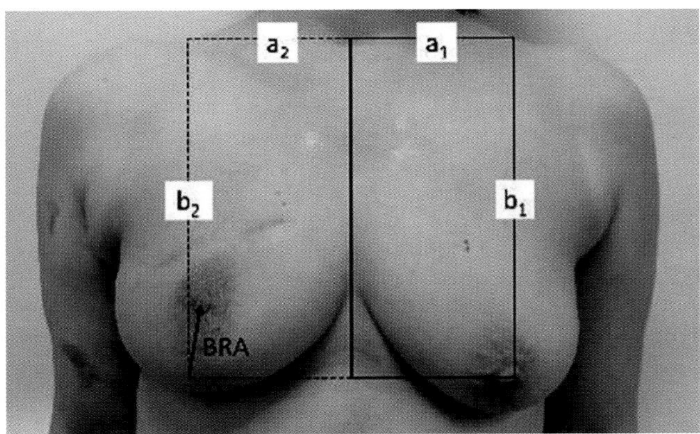

FIGURE 1 ● The untreated left breast has mild to moderate ptosis while the right breast, after a parallelogram mastopexy, has the benefit of a breast/nipple lift as well as wide excision of the cancer. (From Chen CY, Wang PJ, Huang CS, et al. Increased asymmetry with larger breast size following the oncoplastic parallelogram mastopexy lumpectomy for cancer. *Breast J*. 2021;27:409-411. Copyright © 2021 The Authors. Reprinted by permission of John Wiley & Sons, Inc.)

PATIENT HISTORY AND PHYSICAL EXAMINATION

- All breast cancer patients undergoing donut mastopexy lumpectomy should undergo a thorough history and physical examination as described in Chapter 9.
- Beyond the oncologic concerns, the physical exam should include an assessment of the size of the breasts, the size and locations of their tumors, estimated volume of tissue to be excised (including margins), the degree of ptosis, as well as their degree of satisfaction with their current breast appearance.
- Attention should be paid to contraindications to standard or oncoplastic breast conservation surgery, including widespread microcalcifications and multicentric disease. Any other suspicious lesions on imaging should be biopsied to rule out multicentric disease and for definitive surgical planning.

IMAGING AND OTHER DIAGNOSTIC STUDIES

- Evaluation of the extent of disease is facilitated by full-field digital mammography, selective use of breast and axillary ultrasound (US), and in some cases, contrast-enhanced breast magnetic resonance imaging (MRI).
- Breast MRI may be particularly helpful for evaluation of extent of disease for mammographically occult cancers and infiltrating lobular carcinoma. When planning an oncoplastic resection, it may give additional information on the proximity of the malignancy to the adjacent skin or chest wall. Breast MRI may also be helpful following neoadjuvant chemotherapy.
- Wire or wireless localization procedures are required to guide resection of nonpalpable lesions. Larger nonpalpable lesions may benefit from bracketing using multiple localization devices. Techniques for localization are reviewed in Part 5, Chapters 4, 6, and 7.
- For patients with locally advanced disease (T4 or N2 disease or higher), staging with CT scan of the chest, abdomen, and pelvis and bone scan should be considered.
- Preoperative lymphoscintigraphy by nuclear medicine may be considered if this is a malignant lesion and sentinel lymph node biopsy is anticipated, although this is not always necessary for SLN biopsy (Part 5, Chapters 16 and 17).

PATIENT SELECTION

- The parallelogram mastopexy lumpectomy involves removal of the skin island located directly superficial to the known disease and is most commonly used for superior pole or lateral cancers.[3]
- For upper inner quadrant lesions, the skin island excisions should be small or performed using a simple reapproximation of breast tissue and skin without removal of any skin island.[4]
- Removal of the overlying parallelogram of skin avoids excessive, redundant skin from being left behind after excision and helps prevent declivity.

PLANNING THE ELLIPSE

- Care must be taken when designing the skin ellipse as removal of too broad of an island can cause substantial shifting of the nipple-areolar complex (NAC).
- A rounded parallelogram with two equal length lines is drawn, thus marking the skin island to be excised in conjunction with the underlying target lesion and surrounding tissues (**FIGURE 2**).
- For lesions in the upper breast, incisions should be curvilinear, whereas lesions located within the lower breast, including the 3- and 9-o'clock positions, should have a radially placed parallelogram.
- The proposed skin incision is incised down to the breast parenchyma (**FIGURE 3**).
- After excision of the skin island, short-distance mastectomy-type skin flaps are raised along both sides of the wound.
- Dissection is carried down to the chest wall, the breast gland is lifted off the pectoralis muscle (**FIGURE 4**), and a standard tumor resection is performed.
- Four to six marking clips are typically placed at the base of the defect within the surrounding fibroglandular tissue. A three-dimensional tissue marker is an alternative method of marking the lumpectomy bed for the radiation oncologist.
- Once resection is complete and hemostasis obtained, the fibroglandular tissue at the level of the pectoralis fascia is undermined so that full thickness breast tissue advancement can be performed over the muscle (**FIGURE 5**).
- The margins of the residual cavity are then shifted together by the advancement of breast tissue over muscle and the defect is sutured at the deepest edges using 3-0 absorbable suture. The direction of tissue advancement can be adjusted depending on the location of the fibroglandular defect and the excess tissue that can be shifted to close it. The goal of the mastopexy is to perform as complete of a closure over the pectoralis muscle as possible to discourage communication between the anterior skin and the deeper tissues (**FIGURE 6**).
- The superficial tissue layer is closed with interrupted subdermal absorbable sutures (we use 3-0 sutures), whereas the skin is closed by absorbable subcuticular sutures (we use 4-0 sutures) in routine fashion (**FIGURE 7**).

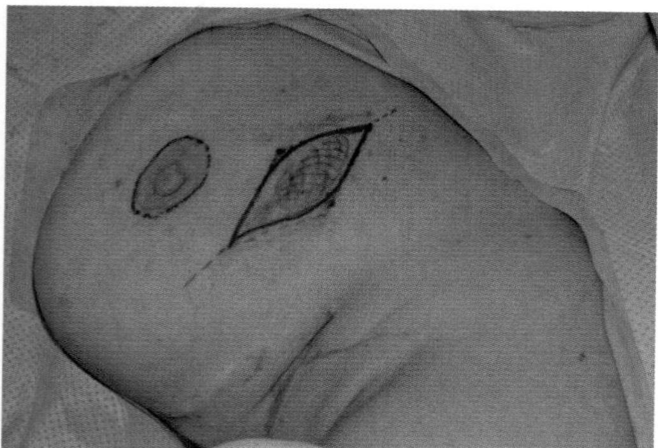

FIGURE 2 ● The rounded parallelogram, with two equal line lengths, to excise a skin island en bloc with the tumor.

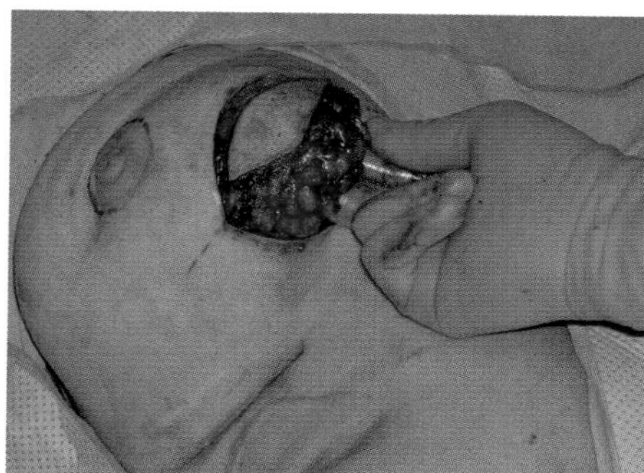

FIGURE 4 ● Full thickness resection down to the pectoralis muscle is performed.

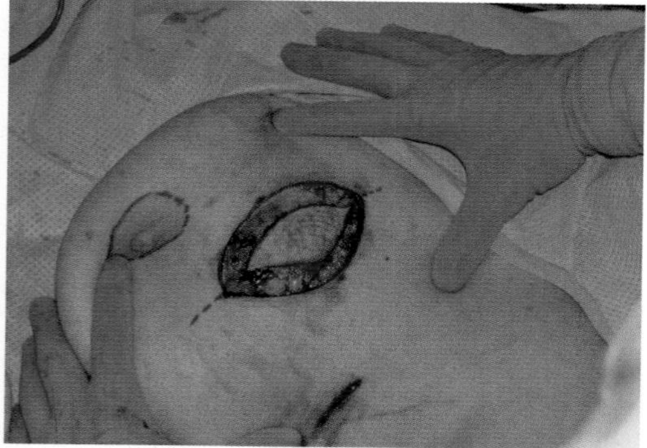

FIGURE 3 ● The skin of the rounded parallelogram is divided with a scalpel down to the breast parenchyma.

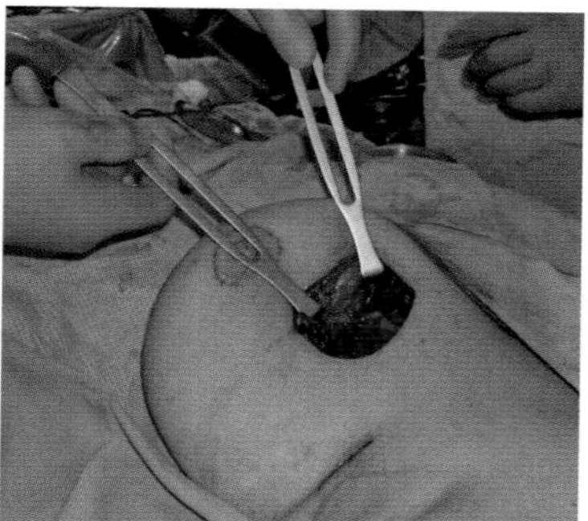

FIGURE 5 ● The remaining fibroglandular tissue is elevated off of the pectoralis fascia to allow advancement over the muscle.

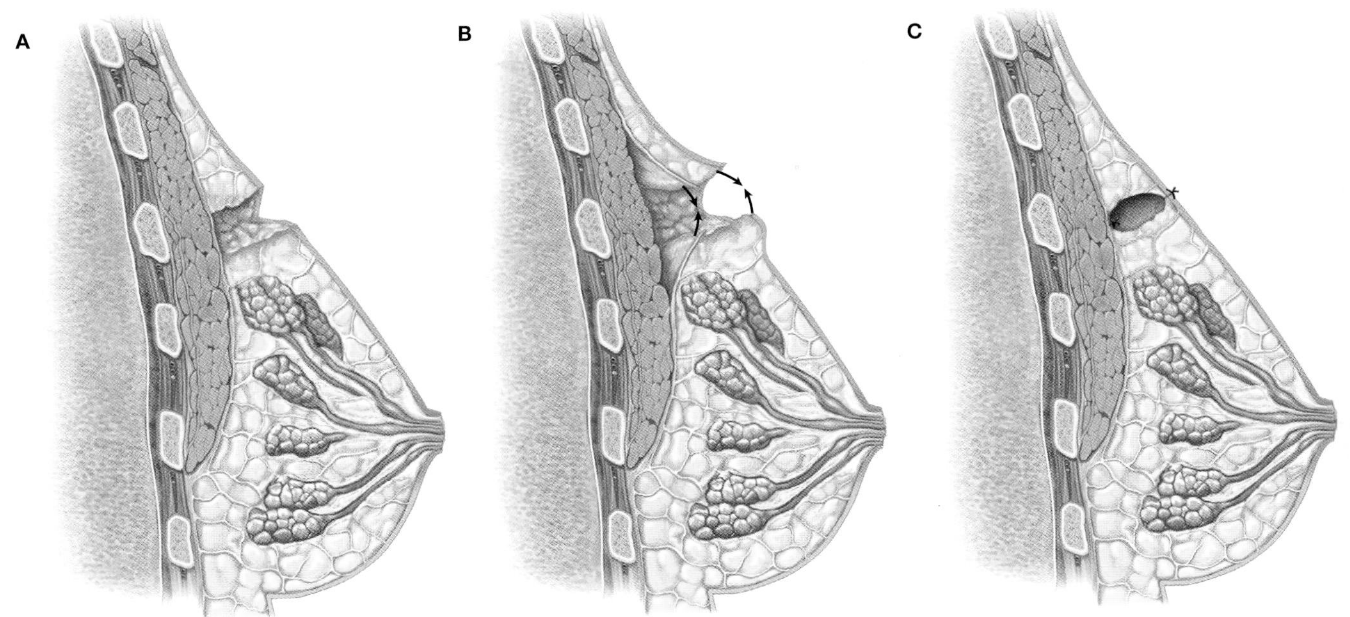

FIGURE 6 ● The fibroglandular tissue is advanced over the pectoralis muscle to separate the deeper tissues from the overlying skin. **A,** Excision of breast tissue from skin to pectoralis fascia. **B,** Mobilization of adjacent tissue off fascia to achieve approximation. **C,** Closure of all layers of wound to minimize residual space.

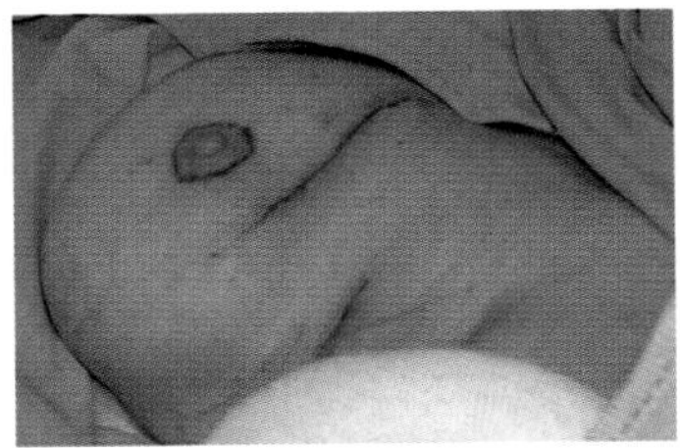

FIGURE 7 ● Two-layer skin closure with interrupted subdermal absorbable sutures followed by absorbable subcuticular sutures.

PEARLS AND PITFALLS OF PARALLELOGRAM MASTOPEXY LUMPECTOMY

Indications	■ Indications include an upper pole cancer location and the presence of mild to moderate ptosis:
	  ■ Patient should desire ptosis correction.
	■ The same contraindications exist as with traditional lumpectomy:
	  ■ Multicentric disease
	  ■ Radiation contraindication
	  ■ Inability to obtain negative surgical margins

Nipple areolar uplifting and asymmetry	■ May occur with this technique. Ensure the patient is informed. ■ Contralateral reduction and/or lift may be necessary.
Seroma formation	■ Less common with parallelogram mastopexy since the open space is completely closed. ■ Drains rarely used.
Inadequate margins	■ Wide excision promotes negative margins including deep and anterior margins. ■ Multiple involved margins may require mastectomy to clear.
Long-term outcomes	■ Appear to have superior cosmetic results with similar local recurrence rates.

POSTOPERATIVE CARE

- Drains are rarely required in standard partial mastectomy cases, as any seroma is avoided by closure of the lumpectomy cavity.

OUTCOMES

- As with traditional lumpectomy, the main goal of all the oncoplastic approaches remains negative surgical margin resection.
- Excision of calcified lesions, masses, and the intended targeted lesion should be confirmed with specimen radiography during surgery.
- Some centers use intraoperative analysis with frozen section or cytology to aid in decisions regarding the resection of additional segments of tissue. This can be particularly helpful for oncoplastic resections where re-excisions can be challenging.
- Additional oriented margins can be resected prior to mastopexy closure when intraoperative analysis or the specimen radiograph suggests inadequate resection may have occurred, hopefully eliminating the need for a delayed re-excision. Tomosynthesis 3D specimen mammograms may also be helpful to assess margins intraoperatively.
- If subsequent re-excision is needed for inadequate surgical margins following the initial resection, use of the same incision is preferred.
- The parallelogram specimen is easy to orient and multiple sutures or colored ink should be applied for the occurrence of a positive margin.
- When the positive margin involves a minority of the specimen, the entire biopsy cavity does not need to be re-excised with only the involved margins of the previous biopsy cavity taken.
- When all the margins of resection are involved, mastectomy may be needed to attain satisfactory surgical clearance. In this instance, it may be technically challenging to include both the initial oncoplastic incision and the NAC in a subsequent total mastectomy and consultation with the plastic surgeon in the event that immediate postmastectomy reconstruction is mandatory.
- Several studies have demonstrated that oncoplastic approaches are sound options for breast conservation therapy.[5-7] As these techniques often result in wider margins of resection than traditional lumpectomy, one would expect future studies should continue to confirm the oncologic benefits of oncoplastic breast surgery.

COMPLICATIONS

- When using oncoplastic approaches, surgeons without formal training must determine which procedures they are comfortable performing without plastic surgery consultation or intraoperative collaboration.
- Using the parallelogram mastopexy lumpectomy is a variant of standard lumpectomy and thus has a very low complication rate. No devascularization of the nipple occurs, no necrotic flaps should occur. The most significant challenge specific to the parallelogram mastopexy is the inadequate planning of the incision anticipating the final result. Gradual progressive experience will attend to that problem.

ACKNOWLEDGMENTS

The authors would like to thank Benjamin O. Anderson and Kristin Calhoun for their prior contributions to Operative Techniques in Surgery.

REFERENCES

1. Anderson BO, Masetti R, Silverstein MJ. Oncoplastic approaches to partial mastectomy: an overview of volume-displacement techniques. *Lancet Oncol*. 2005;6(3):145-157.
2. Veronesi U, Cascinelli N, Mariani L, et al. Twenty-year follow-up of a randomized study comparing breast- conserving surgery with radical mastectomy for early breast cancer. *N Engl J Med*. 2002;347(16):1227-1232.
3. Kraissl CJ. The selection of appropriate lines for elective surgical incisions. *Plast Reconstr Surg*. 1951;8:1-28.
4. Grisotti A. Conservation treatment of breast cancer: reconstructive problems. In: Spear SL, ed. *Surgery of the Breast: Principles and Art*. Lippincott-Raven Publishers; 1998:137-153.
5. Carter SA, Lyons GR, Kuerer HM, et al. Operative and oncologic outcomes in 9861 patients with operable breast cancer: single institution analysis of breast conservation with oncoplastic reconstruction. *Ann Surg Oncol*. 2016;23:3190-3198.
6. De La Cruz L, Blankenship SA, Chatterjee A, et al. Outcomes after oncoplastic breast-conserving surgery in breast cancer patients: a systematic literature review. *Ann Surg Oncol*. 2016;23:3247-3258.
7. Kaufman CS. Increasing role of oncoplastic surgery for breast cancer. *Curr Oncol Rep*. 2019;21:111.

Chapter 11

Batwing Mastopexy Lumpectomy

Joshua Alex Bloom, Isaac Gendelman, and Abhishek Chatterjee

DEFINITION

- Oncoplastic breast surgery (OPS), a form of breast-conservation surgery (BCS), is a safe oncologic and reconstructive technique that allows for a large partial mastectomy followed by volume displacement or volume replacement surgery.[1-3] Not only does this allow for the surgeon to restore symmetry and overall cosmesis, but it also decreases the positive margin rate (5%-10%) compared to standard partial mastectomy (20%-30%).[4] Furthermore, this technique consistently scores above other forms of breast reconstruction on patient-reported outcome measures (PROMs) such as the BREAST-Q.[5]
- OPS is subdivided into volume displacement and volume replacement techniques by the percentage of tissue excised.[2] Volume displacement is further subdivided into level 1 (<20% breast tissue removed) and level 2 (20%-50% breast tissue removed) techniques. Batwing mastopexy lumpectomy is one such level 1 volume displacement technique that is designed for central upper pole tumors.[6,7]

PATIENT HISTORY AND PHYSICAL FINDINGS

- Given that the batwing mastopexy lumpectomy is a form of BCS, it is imperative to first perform a thorough history and physical examination to ensure that the patient is a proper candidate.
  - Specifically, the patient should be asked about family history of cancers, any known genetic syndromes, and prior radiation treatment as absolute contraindications for BCS include widespread disease, multicentric disease, diffuse microcalcifications, BRCA 1 or 2 mutations, and prior chest wall radiation.[8] Past surgical history, medical history, allergies, and medications (eg, aspirin or anticoagulants) should also be reviewed.
- A bilateral breast exam, including evaluation of the axillae, should be performed on all patients.
  - In addition to palpating for masses and lymphadenopathy, the size of the breasts and degree of ptosis should be noted.
- As the batwing mastopexy allows for preservation of the breast shape in addition to elevation of the lower half of the breast and nipple-areolar complex (NAC), it provides the best outcome with ptotic breasts.[9]
- With regard to patient expectations, it is imperative that the patient understands that scars will be visually placed on the breast skin and that, especially if unilateral surgery is performed without a contralateral symmetry lift, the breasts would appear different not only by volume measurements but also nipple positioning.
- While the batwing mastopexy is relatively quicker and simpler to perform than a circumvertical or wise pattern mastopexy (with associated pedicles), skin incisions are better hidden with the latter option.
- The batwing mastopexy does allow direct skin excision in the upper and upper outer quadrants; thus, for a superficial or ulcerating lesion in these areas, it does allow for a clear anterior margin.
- Fundamentally, the surgeon should also discuss these options with the patient and under shared patient-surgeon discussion decide which oncoplastic option is most appropriate.

IMAGING AND OTHER DIAGNOSTIC STUDIES

- Proper planning is an essential step prior to any surgical intervention, especially when dealing with suspected or confirmed malignancy. The patient should first undergo a complete workup including a bilateral screening mammogram, targeted diagnostic mammogram, ultrasound of the area, and core-needle biopsy for complete workup of the breast mass.
- Once the pathology results have been analyzed, the case and proposed surgical plan should be discussed in a multidisciplinary tumor board that includes a breast surgeon, plastic surgeon, radiation oncologist, and medical oncologist.
- If the lesion is palpable, then it is permissible to proceed to the operating room (OR) directly. However, if it is not palpable, then it should be wire localized preoperatively. Other considerations include preoperative lymphoscintigraphy by nuclear medicine if this is a malignant lesion and sentinel lymph node biopsy is anticipated.

SURGICAL MANAGEMENT

Preoperative Planning

- The patient should be marked standing up in the preoperative area. The batwing mastopexy lumpectomy involves a crescent-shaped central area around the NAC with two triangle-shaped areas extending from both sides of the areola. The lower half of the marking should include the upper half of the NAC (**FIGURE 1**). This allows for a large resection extending medial and lateral to the NAC.[7,10]
- It is important to understand that the nipple will be elevated with a batwing mastopexy, and any nipple elevation of greater than 1 cm on the breast with cancer should

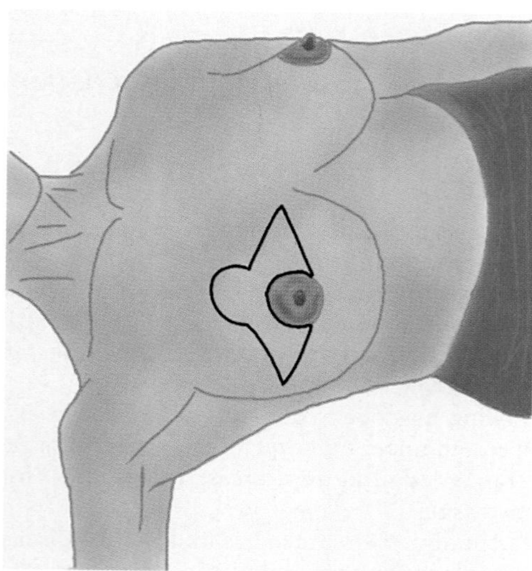

FIGURE 1 ● Batwing mastopexy incision markings. (Courtesy of Issac Gendelman.)

necessitate a contralateral symmetry mastopexy discussion with the patient.

- In order to reduce opioid consumption, preoperative pain medication and/or regional blocks should be considered in oncoplastic surgery.[11] Antibiotic prophylaxis should be administered prior to the incision (preferably a first-generation cephalosporin if no history of an anaphylactic reaction) and sequential compression devices are applied and consideration for deep vein thrombosis anticoagulation prophylaxis prior to induction of anesthesia is considered based on the Caprini Score.[12]

Positioning

- The patient is positioned supine with arms out at 90°. The skin is widely prepped and draped. The contralateral breast should be included in the field in order to compare throughout the procedure to arrive at a reasonably symmetrical result, especially if a contralateral procedure is not performed at the index operation.

SKIN INCISION AND EXCISION OF THE LESION

- After a timeout is performed, the markings are again reviewed to ensure that the breast is positioned centrally over the pectoralis muscle.[7] If necessary, tailor tacking the batwing mastopexy markings and sitting the patient up after intubation will give a reasonable estimation on breast shape and nipple positioning before making the incisions.
- Subsequently, a full-thickness incision is made along the marked batwing incision (**FIGURE 1**). The dissection is carried down through the skin and glandular tissue with electrocautery until deep to the lesion, or to the pectoralis fascia if dealing with a breast malignancy. The specimen is removed in one piece as it is peeled off of the chest wall (**FIGURE 2**).

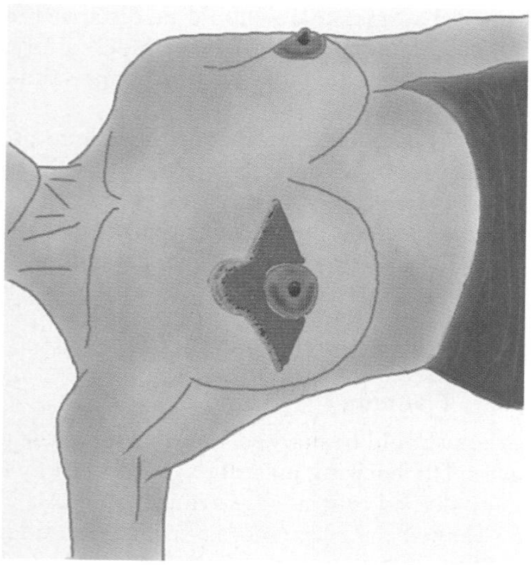

FIGURE 2 ● Resection cavity of Batwing resection following removal of specimen. (Courtesy of Issac Gendelman.)

ORIENTATION OF THE SPECIMEN AND MARKING OF THE TUMOR BED

- The specimen is marked using a nonabsorbable suture with a short suture tail superiorly and a long suture tail laterally.
- Clips are placed onto the tissue of the borders of the resection cavity in case pathology returns with positive margins and to aid with targeting of postoperative radiotherapy if required.[13]

CLOSURE

- Once the specimen is removed and the resection cavity is marked, glandular flaps are elevated both cranially and caudally and advanced to achieve a tension-free closure.
- Drains are not typically necessary unless the patient is on therapeutic anticoagulation.
- Glandular tissue is reapproximated with absorbable suture in multiple layers (**FIGURE 3**).
- Skin is closed with a running subcuticular absorbable suture and reinforced with skin glue and Steri-Strips.

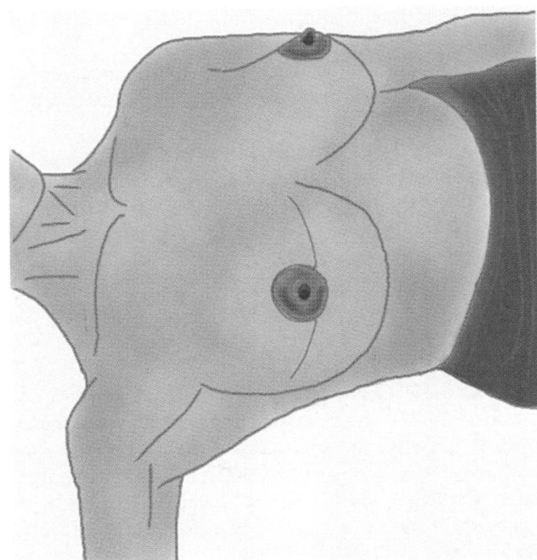

FIGURE 3 ● Closure of Batwing mastopexy. (Courtesy of Issac Gendelman.)

PEARLS AND PITFALLS

Indication	■ Batwing mastopexy lumpectomy is an option in patients with central upper pole tumors who are eligible for breast-conservation therapy, but who are not able to or do not wish to undergo more complicated volume displacement oncoplastic designs such as circumvertical or wise patterns (with their associated pedicles). ■ The batwing mastopexy lumpectomy is ideal in older and/or sicker patients who would benefit from less operative time compared to more complex oncoplastic techniques for patients who do not mind scars in the central regions of the breast skin. ■ It is also indicated for patients who have superficial or ulcerating cancers in the region where the batwing design will remove the skin (ensuring a negative anterior margin).
Incision	■ Center markings around NAC and ensure that breast mass is centered over pectoralis muscle.
Excision	■ The posterior margin should include the pectoralis fascia if dealing with confirmed or suspected malignant lesion. This increases the likelihood of a negative margin especially in the setting of extensive ductal carcinoma in situ.
Specimen orientation	■ Mark the specimen with short stitch superior and long stitch lateral. The resection bed should be marked with surgical clips.
Closure	■ Close the glandular tissue in multiple layers to eliminate dead space and elevate the lower half of the breast/NAC.

POSTOPERATIVE CARE

- Steri-Strips remain in place until they fall off.
- The patient should wear a surgical bra for 1 week postoperatively. However, the patient may remove the bra when showering and may shower on postoperative day 1.

OUTCOMES

- Cosmesis may be superior compared to standard partial mastectomy, but the batwing mastopexy does leave a central scar on the breast. Furthermore, if there is no contralateral symmetry procedure, there will be some degree of asymmetry.
- While the batwing mastopexy design does have reasonable cosmetic outcomes, when compared to the level 2 volume displacement-wise skin incision pattern, it has comparably inferior cosmetic outcomes.[14]
- Lastly, from an oncologic perspective, the positive margin rate is reported between 5% and 10%, and a return to the OR may be required for clean margins.[4]

COMPLICATIONS

- Infection
- Seroma
- Hematoma
- Asymmetry/poor cosmesis
- Positive margin

REFERENCES

1. Losken A, Chatterjee A. Improving results in oncoplastic surgery. *Plast Reconstr Surg*. 2021;147(1):123e-134e.
2. Chatterjee A, Gass J, Patel K, et al. A consensus definition and classification system of oncoplastic surgery developed by the American Society of Breast Surgeons. *Ann Surg Oncol*. 2019;26(11):3436-3444.
3. Margenthaler JA, Dietz JR, Chatterjee A. The landmark series: breast conservation trials (including oncoplastic breast surgery). *Ann Surg Oncol*. 2021;28(4):2120-2127.
4. Campbell EJ, Romics L. Oncological safety and cosmetic outcomes in oncoplastic breast conservation surgery, a review of the best level of evidence literature. *Breast Cancer*. 2017;9:521-530.
5. Char S, Bloom JA, Erlichman Z, Jonczyk MM, Chatterjee A. A comprehensive literature review of patient reported outcome measures (proms) among common breast reconstruction options: what types of breast reconstruction score well? *Breast J*. 2021;27(4):322-329.
6. Patel K, Bloom J, Nardello S, Cohen S, Reiland J, Chatterjee A. An oncoplastic surgery primer: common indications, techniques, and complications in level 1 and 2 volume displacement oncoplastic surgery. *Ann Surg Oncol*. 2019;26:3063-3070.
7. Holmes DR, Schooler W, Smith R. Oncoplastic approaches to breast conservation. *Int J Breast Cancer*. 2011;2011:303879. doi:10.4061/2011/303879
8. Fajdic J, Djurovic D, Gotovac N, Hrgovic Z. Criteria and procedures for breast conserving surgery. *Acta Inform Med*. 2013;21(1):16-19.
9. Anderson BO, Masetti R, Silverstein MJ. Oncoplastic approaches to partial mastectomy: an overview of volume replacement techniques. *Lancet Oncol*. 2005;6(3):145-157.
10. Manie TM, Youssef MMG, Taha SN, Rabea A, Farahat AM. Batwing mammoplasty: a safe oncoplastic technique for breast conservation in breast cancer patients with gigantomastia. *Ann R Coll Surg Engl*. 2020;102:115-119.
11. Buzney CD, Lin LZ, Chatterjee A, Gallagher SW, Quraishi SA, Drzymalski DM. Association between Paravertebral block and pain score at the time of hospital discharge in oncoplastic breast surgery: a Retrospective Cohort Study. *Plast Reconstr Surg*. 2021;147(6):928e-935e.
12. Pannucci CJ, Bailey SH, Dreszer G, et al. Validation of the Caprini risk assessment model in plastic and reconstructive surgery patients. *J Am Coll Surg*. 2011;212(1):105-112.
13. Riina MD, Rashad R, Cohen S, et al. The effectiveness of intra-operative clip placement in improving radiotherapy boost targeting following oncoplastic surgery. *Pract Radiat Oncol*. 2020;10(5):e348-e356.
14. Hashem T, Farahat A. Batwing versus wise pattern mammoplasty for upper pole breast tumours: a detailed comparison of cosmetic outcome. *World J Surg Onc*. 2017;15:60.

Chapter 12 Donut Mastopexy Lumpectomy

Dennis Ricky Holmes and Michael S. Sabel

DEFINITION

- The donut mastopexy lumpectomy level is a level I oncoplastic volume displacement procedure that is variably described in the literature as modified Benelli mammaplasty, round block technique, periareolar mastopexy, and circumareolar mastopexy.
- The procedure was developed by Louis Benelli with the goal of limiting the mammoplasty scar to the areolar margin. More recently, the procedure has been modified to permit resection of benign or malignancy breast abnormalities, and as such is appropriately considered a therapeutic mammaplasty procedure.
- Donut mastopexy lumpectomy utilizes a pair of concentric or eccentric circumareolar skin incisions, one placed at or near the areolar margin and the second whose diameter is at least 1 cm larger. The intervening ring of skin or "donut" is de-epithelialized and then incised to provide access for resection of a lesion in the central or peripheral breast.
- A distinguishing feature of the round block approach compared to the donut mastopexy lumpectomy is the use of cerclage, nonabsorbable suture to encircle and secure the outer areolar margin (ie, outer donut). This cerclage prevents the areola from being dilated and stretched in response to centrifugal forces exerted by surrounding breast skin.

DIFFERENTIAL DIAGNOSIS

- Donut mastopexy was originally developed as a cosmetic procedure that has been modified to facilitate resection of malignant or benign lesions.

PATIENT HISTORY AND PHYSICAL FINDINGS

- All breast cancer patients undergoing donut mastopexy lumpectomy should undergo a thorough history and physical examination as described in Part 5, Chapter 9.
- Beyond the oncologic concerns, the physical exam should include an assessment of the size of the breasts, the size and locations of the tumors, estimated volume of tissue to be excised (including margins), the degree of ptosis, as well as the degree of patient satisfaction with their current breast appearance.
- Attention should be paid to contraindications to standard or oncoplastic breast conservation surgery, including widespread malignant microcalcifications and multicentric disease. Any other suspicious lesions on imaging should be biopsied to rule out multicentric disease for definitive surgical planning.
- Donut mastopexy lumpectomy may be used for resection of a lesion in any quadrant of the breast that does not involve the nipple-areolar complex (NAC) position.
- The procedure is particularly useful for patients with small to medium sized ptotic breasts who would benefit from a modest mastopexy.
- As a mastopexy procedure, the donut may be used to maintain, elevate, or recentralize the NAC.

IMAGING AND OTHER DIAGNOSTIC STUDIES

- Evaluation of the extent of disease is facilitated by full-field digital mammography, selective use of breast and axillary ultrasound, and contrast-enhanced breast MRI, as needed.
- Breast MRI may be particularly helpful for evaluation of extent of disease for mammographically occult cancer, infiltrating lobular carcinoma, assessment of proximity of the malignancy to the adjacent skin or chest wall, and evaluation of response to neoadjuvant systemic therapy.
- Wire or wireless localization procedures are required to guide resection of nonpalpable lesions. Larger nonpalpable lesions may benefit from bracketing using multiple localization devices. Techniques for localization are reviewed in Part 5, Chapters 10, 11, and 13.
- Intraoperative ultrasound can also be used in place of or as an adjunct to localization devices to aid surgical resection and assessment of macroscopic surgical margins.
- For patients with locally advanced disease (T4 or N2 disease or higher), staging with CT scan of the chest, abdomen, and pelvis and bone scan should be considered.
- Other considerations include preoperative lymphoscintigraphy by nuclear medicine if this is a malignant lesion and sentinel lymph node biopsy is anticipated.

SURGICAL MANAGEMENT

Preoperative Planning

- Initial skin markings are performed in the preoperative holding area using an indelible marker. Skin markings are best performed with the patient in a standing position with arms at her side and the surgeon seated. In this position, the surgeon should mark the final position of superior areolar margin, which is generally 16 to 19 cm from suprasternal notch depending on the indication (eg, mastopexy, recentralization, or skin resection). The surgeon should also determine the desired areolar diameter (usually 42-50 mm or smaller), depending on patient preference and symmetry.
- Photographic documentation of the preoperative appearance and postoperative results will help the surgeon evaluate and improve their results over time. In addition, the confidential sharing of these photos with prospective patients will provide a clearer understanding of expected surgical results.
- Donut mastopexy lumpectomy patients should be forewarned that they should expect to see pleating or creased skin along the outer areolar margin, a feature that will gradually resolve over 2 to 3 months in patients with thin skin and over 6 months in patients with thick skin.

Positioning

- Upon arriving in the operating room, patients are maintained in the supine position following induction of anesthesia. Securement of both arms to the arm board allows the patient's torso to be elevated to the upright seated position for evaluation of nipple position, breast shape, symmetry, and skin tethering prior to wound closure.

- The contralateral breast should be included in the field in order to compare throughout the procedure in order to arrive at a reasonably symmetrical result, especially if a contralateral procedure is not performed at the index operation.

TECHNIQUES

DETERMINING POSITION OF NIPPLE-AREOLAR COMPLEX

- As a mastopexy procedure, the donut may be used to maintain or reposition the NAC. Maintenance of the nipple position can be accomplished with a concentric donut where an equal distance is maintained between the inner and outer rings of the donut, permitting the outer ring to be conformed around the stationary areola. This approach is most appropriate when there is no significant ptosis, when the surgeon aims to minimize the need for a contralateral symmetrization procedure, or when a patient simply does not desire ptosis correction.[1]
- For small to moderate size breasts, ptosis correction can be accomplished with an eccentric donut where the outer margin of the donut is shifted cephalad along the breast meridian (**FIGURE 1A**). By increasing the distance between the top edges of the inner and outer donuts and decreasing the distance between the bottom edges of the two donuts, the final nipple position is shifted cephalad when the inner and outer donuts are approximated (**FIGURE 1B**).
- It is best to limit the degree of nipple elevation (eg, the distance between the top edges of the inner and outer donuts) to <3 cm to avoid excessive skin pleating and undesirable flattening of the central breast when the two margins of the donuts are sutured together. If the degree of ptosis warrants >3 cm nipple elevation, a level II mammoplasty procedure (eg, Wise-pattern reduction) should be employed that is capable of correcting a greater degree of ptosis while also improving breast projection. However, despite its limitations, donut mastopexy lumpectomy is sometimes favored by patients wishing to avoid long breast incisions and also by surgeons aiming to avoid extensive tissue mobilization and reduce operative time for patients at higher risk of complications.

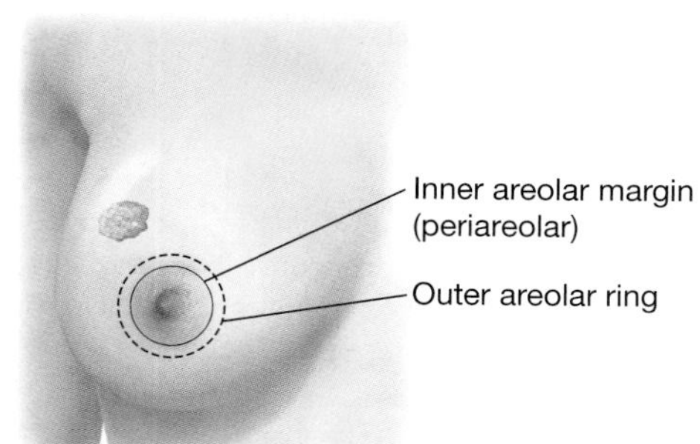

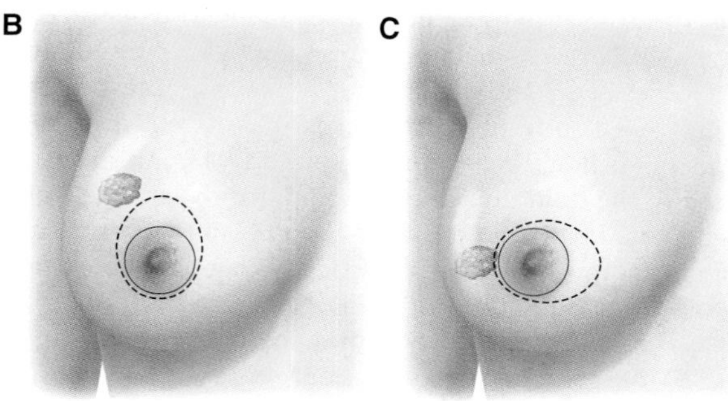

FIGURE 1 ● **A,** Inner and outer areolar margin. **B,** Eccentric outer areolar margin helps correct a slight ptosis. **C,** Oval ring directed medially to correct anticipated lateral displacement of the NAC following resection of the tumor.

- A third application of the donut mastectomy is nipple recentralization, which may be required when the resection of skin at the medial or lateral areolar margin would produce medial or lateral displacement of the NAC (**FIGURE 1C**). Less commonly, donut mastectomy may be utilized to reduce the areolar diameter in a patient with a large, asymmetric, or irregular areola for whom resizing of the areola is desired.

SKIN INCISION

- If the native areolar diameter is to be maintained, the surgeon may mark the existing areolar margin with an indelible marker. On the other hand, if a smaller areola is desired, the surgeon may use an areolatome (ie, cookie cutter) or areolar marker to score the areola surface, which is then traced with an indelible marker. This outlines the circumference of the neoareola. The outer areolar margin is drawn on the skin, the diameter and position of which depends on the surgical indication.
- For periareolar tumors in proximity to the overlying skin, the anterior skin margin can be incorporated within the donut to permit a dermoglandular resection. Alternatively, for a more peripheral tumor approximating the skin, the anterior skin margin may be excised using a radial extension from the outer edges of the donut.
- With the assistant holding uniform circumferential retraction of the skin away around the areola, the surgeon may use a scalpel to incise the superficial skin of the outer and inner areolar margins to the level of the superficial deep dermis (**FIGURE 2**). The pigmented dermis between both incisions is then de-epithelialized in the usual manner. Depending on the lesion location, the adjacent deep dermis is widely incised to provide easy access to the tumor site.
- Intraoperative ultrasound may be helpful to avoid excessive breast tissue removal and positive margins.

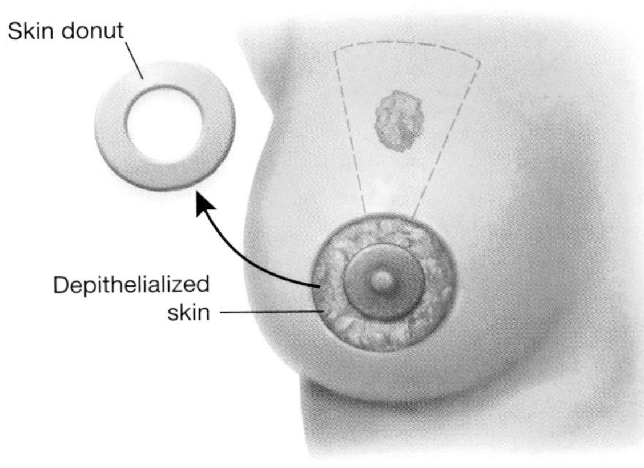

FIGURE 2 ● The "donut" of skin surrounding the areola is de-epithelialized, leaving the underlying vascularized dermis intact.

SKIN FLAP DISSECTION

- Generally, up to half of the areolar circumference is incised to gain access to the tumor, leaving the remaining dermis intact as a vascular pedicle for the NAC. In some cases, multiple incisions are made in the de-epithelialized dermis to provide access to lesions in the upper and lower poles of the breast. Infrequently, a fully circumferential incision is made in the de-epithelialized skin to permit complete redraping of the skin over the breast mound.
- Using skin hooks and/or skin retractors, the surgeon may utilize electrocautery or sharp dissection to widely elevate a thick or thin subcutaneous tissue flap (depending on tumor depth) over the tumor. The width of flap elevation is directly proportional to the size of the planned resection. Whenever possible, the thickness of the flap should increase as dissection extends peripherally to optimize perfusion to the central skin (**FIGURE 3**).
- The incision in the de-epithelialized dermis should be placed a few millimeters away from the adjacent epithelialized skin to protect the epithelialized skin edges from instrument trauma.
- For tumors close to the NAC, a subareolar flap can be raised. It is important to preserve adequate perfusion of the undermined NAC.

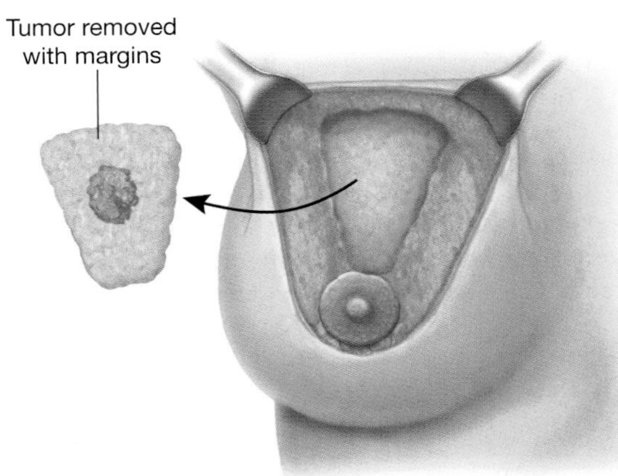

FIGURE 3 ● The breast parenchyma is excised from the subcutaneous tissue to and including the underlying pectoralis fascia. Image also shows tumor location and planned resection volume.

TUMOR RESECTION

- Through the periareolar skin opening, the surgeon may perform a lumpectomy (partial mastectomy) or excisional biopsy.
- Resection of malignant lesions generally involves full-thickness glandular resection extending from the subcutaneous plane to the underlying muscular fascia, which is included as the posterior margin (**FIGURE 3**). For periareolar tumors in proximity to the overlying skin, the anterior surgical margin can be incorporated within the donut to permit a neuroglandular resection. Alternatively, for more peripheral tumor approximating the skin, the anterior skin margin may be excised using a radial extension from the outer edge of the donut.
- In patients with benign tumors, donut mastopexy lumpectomy provides access for excisional biopsy of masses in multiple quadrants (eg, multicentric fibroadenomas).[2] Donut mastopexy lumpectomy also permits imbrication of stretched or redundant skin remaining after resection of a large benign mass (eg, juvenile fibroadenoma, phyllodes tumors, gynecomastia, and pseudogynecomastia).[3,4]
- Intraoperative ultrasound and specimen radiography may be used to evaluate intraoperative margins, with resection of additional margins as needed. Specimen orientation is performed using sutures, clips, or paint. Intraoperative pathology consultation (eg, gross section, frozen section, and touch prep) may also be utilized to evaluate uncertain margins.

PARENCHYMAL CLOSURE

- Fiducial markers may be applied to the surgical margins if postoperative radiotherapy is planned.
- Dual plane undermining of the subcutaneous tissue and glandular tissue may be performed to facilitate approximation of the surgical margins and full-thickness parenchymal closure without tension. Interrupted simple or figure-of-8 absorbable sutures may be placed in one or more layers for tissue approximation without tissue strangulation to prevent fat necrosis. On the other hand, dual planing must be performed judiciously in fatty breasts due to an increased risk of fat necrosis.
- At this point in the operation, it should be apparent if additional dissection is required in the subcutaneous plane to release tethered or dimpled skin.
- Temporary skin closure with staples (ie, tailor tacking) and sitting the patients upright permits assessment and adjustment of the skin flaps and breast contour prior to definitive wound closure.

SKIN CLOSURE

- Skin closure may be initiated with placement of a purse string suture in the deep dermis along the outer areolar margin using a nonabsorbable translucent (ideally) monofilament suture or white suture (eg, Gore-Tex) to minimize visibility through the skin, especially in thin-skinned or pale patients (**FIGURE 4A**). A 4-0 or larger-gauge suture will reduce risk of suture breakage from pressure.
- With the assistant holding the cookie cutter over the nipple, the purse string may be cinched down to reduce the diameter of the outer areolar margin down to the diameter of the cookie cutter to achieve the desired areolar diameter (**FIGURE 4B**). The purse string is then tied with multiple throws to prevent slippage. The resulting knot is then buried deep to prevent erosion through the incision.
- Skin staples or absorbable deep dermis sutures are then used to inset the nipple-areolar complex in the outer areolar margin by tacking the inner areolar margin to the outer areolar margin at the 12:00, 3:00, 6:00, and 9:00 positions. Multiple interrupted absorbable sutures may then be used to approximate the inner and outer donuts along the entire perimeter of the areola at the level of the deep dermis. Another strategy for reducing the outer areolar margin and insetting the NAC is the "wagon wheel" closure (**FIGURE 5**).
- Finally, an absorbable suture should be placed in a subcuticular manner to approximate the epidermis, taking smaller bites on the inner donut and larger bites of the outer donut to make up for the length discrepancy between the two donuts.

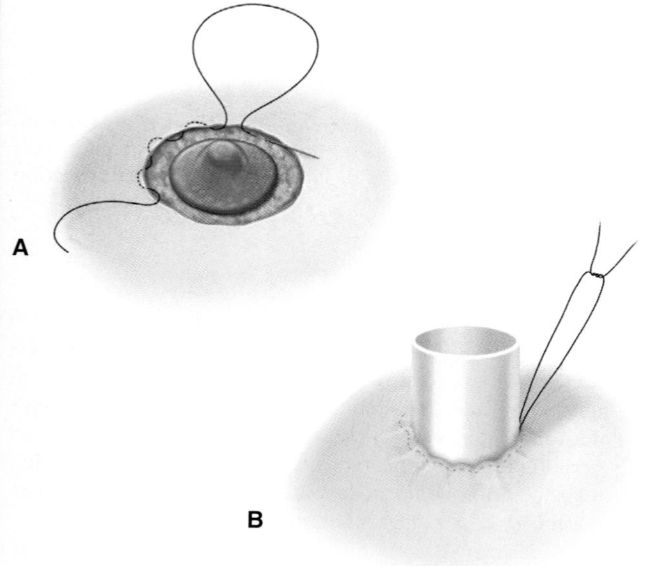

FIGURE 4 ● **A,** Purse string placement along outer areolar margin; **B,** Tying down or closure of purse string suture around areolatome and NAC.

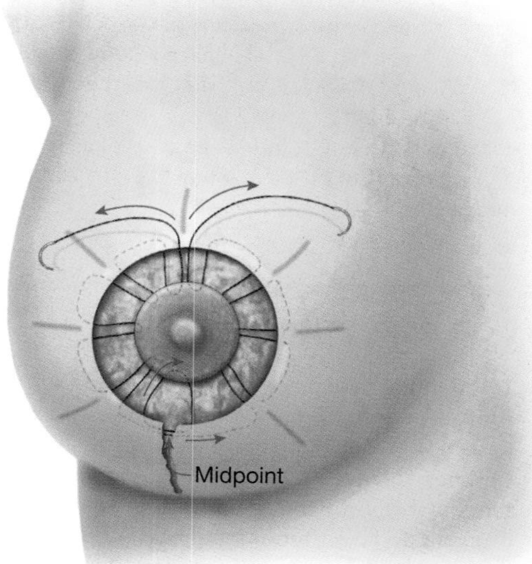

FIGURE 5 ● Wagon Wheel closure of NAC.

MANAGEMENT OF THE CONTRALATERAL BREAST

- Mastopexy, breast reduction, or a contralateral donut mastopexy lumpectomy with or without mirror resection may be performed to reduce or correct breast asymmetry resulting from oncoplastic breast conserving surgery.
- Symmetrization surgery can be performed at the time of the oncoplastic resection, at a second operation after assessment of surgical margins, or at a later time depending on the clinical setting, patient's wishes, surgeon's skill set, and/or availability of plastic surgery expertise.
- The key steps of a bilateral donut mastopexy procedure with resection are displayed in **FIGURE 6**.

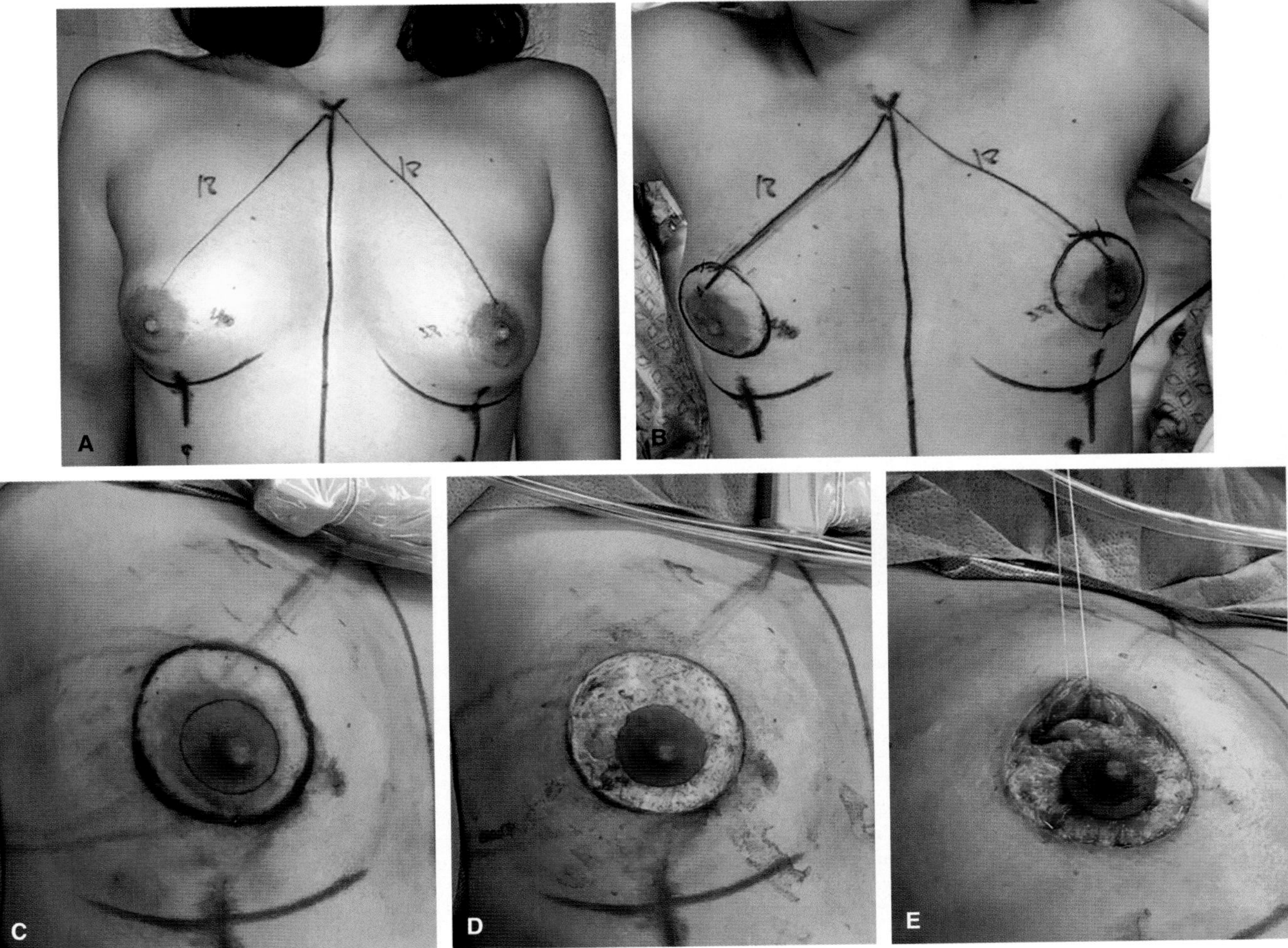

FIGURE 6 ● Donut mastopexy with bilateral excisional biopsies in a 34-year-old woman with A-cup breasts and history of bilateral breast autologous fat injections resulting in symptomatic palpable masses in the right (5.1 × 3.2 cm) and left (5.3 × 4.4 cm) breasts. **A** and **B,** preoperative skin markings, **C,** outer and inner ("neoareola") areolar skin margins, **D,** de-epithelialized skin between outer and inner areolar margins, **E,** placement of purse string suture using Gore-Tex suture following resection of breast mass and approximation of glandular margins after tissue resection, **F,** areolatome used to resize outer areolar margin of right breast, **G,** resized outer areolar margin before insetting nipple areolar complex, **H,** areolatome used to resize outer areolar margin of left breast after tissue resection, **I,** closure of bilateral areolas with periareolar skin pleating, **J,** breast appearance 1 week after surgery, and **K,** breast appearance 4 months after surgery.

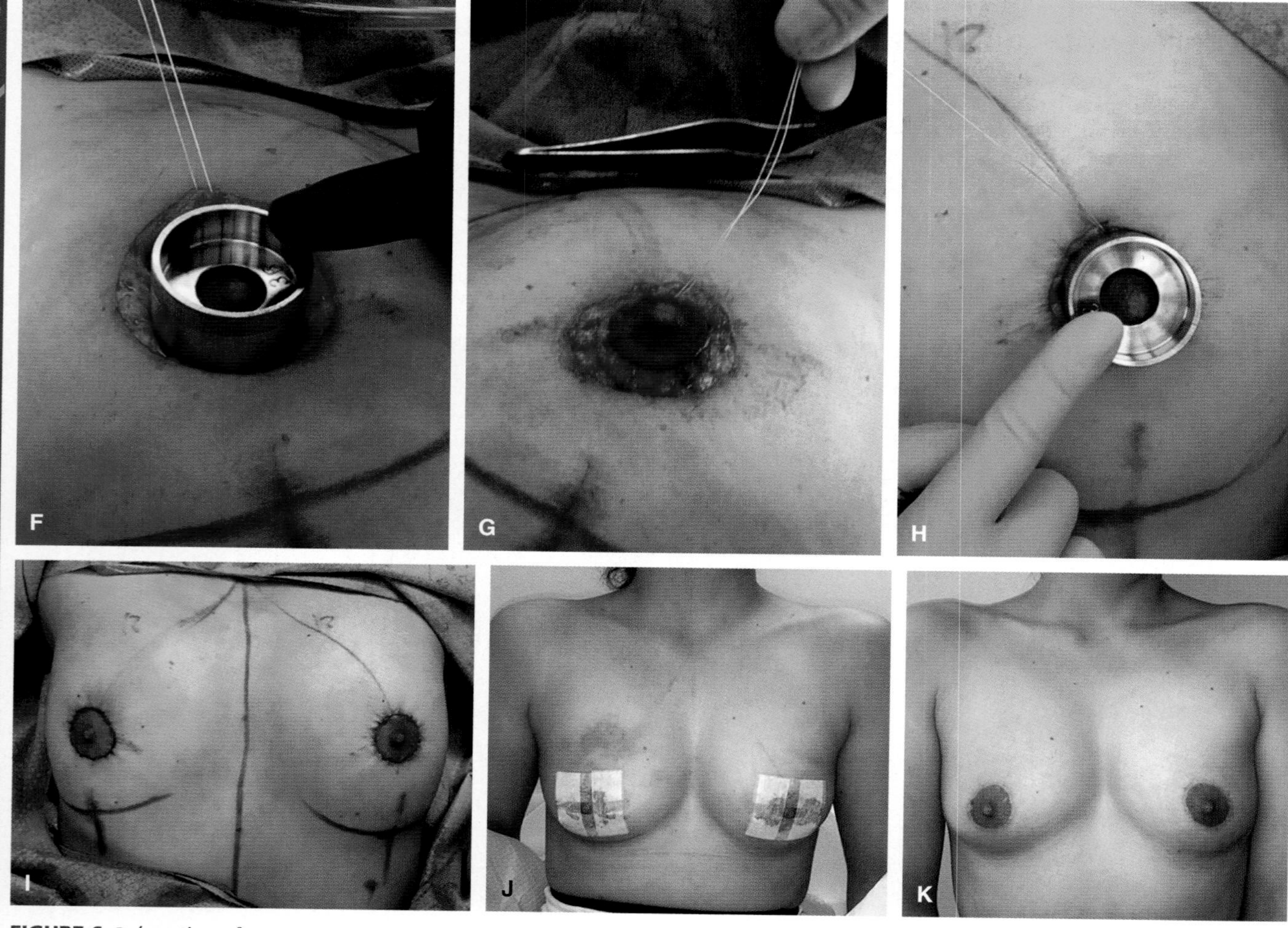

FIGURE 6 • (*continued*)

PEARLS AND PITFALLS

Indications	▪ Oncoplastic resection of lesion in any quadrant of the breast, including subareolar location. ▪ May include radial skin excision for tumors close to the skin. ▪ Other oncoplastic resections should be considered for tumors close to or involving the NAC. ▪ May be used to correct ptosis <3 cm.
Skin incision	▪ The shape and distance of the outer ring should be determined by several factors, including tumor location and degree of ptosis. ▪ Take great care to only de-epithelialize the "donut" and to limit full thickness incisions around the areola.
Tumor resection	▪ Undermine the skin widely over the involved quadrant(s). ▪ Full thickness resection of a wedge or segment of tissue around the tumor. ▪ Intraoperative margin analysis is strongly recommended.
Filling the defect	▪ Place clips to assist with radiation planning. ▪ Raise flaps above the pectoralis fascia to facilitate tissue flap rotation. ▪ Advance the breast parenchyma and close in multiple layers. ▪ Closure of outer ring with nonabsorbable purse string suture prevents delayed dilatation of NAC.
Postoperative management	▪ Assure negative pathologic margins and resection of all microcalcifications. Patients may require re-excision or mastectomy. ▪ Many patients will require contralateral lift or reduction to achieve symmetry. This is best performed in a delayed fashion.

POSTOPERATIVE CARE

- Donut mastopexy lumpectomy is performed as an outpatient procedure.
- Use of a surgical drain is optional depending on the extent of dissection.
- Use of a surgical bra or sports bra reduces postoperative pain, swelling, and bruising.
- Activity level is restricted during the first month of recovery.

COMPLICATIONS

- With any breast-conserving procedure, infection, seroma, hematoma, asymmetry, and retraction are possible, as are positive margins.
- Smoking, diabetes, obesity, chronic obstructive pulmonary disease (COPD), longer operative time, and bleeding disorder have been reported as independent predictors of 30-day morbidity following oncoplastic surgery.[5]
- Although the donut mastopexy lumpectomy requires considerably less dissection than the typical level II mammoplasty procedure, the requirement for greater tissue dissection necessitates careful tissue handling.
- Extensive undermining of the fatty breast may increase the risk of fat necrosis or seroma formation. Excessive undermining of the NAC may increase the risk of NAC ischemia, necrosis, and nipple sensation loss.
- Areolar widening and nipple retraction are more likely to occur if a cerclage is omitted.[6]

REFERENCES

1. Holmes DR, Schooler W, Smith R. Oncoplastic approaches to breast conservation. *Int J Breast Cancer*. 2011;2011:303879.
2. Lai HW, Kuo YL, Su CC, et al. Round block technique is a useful oncoplastic procedure for multicentric fibroadenomas. *Surgeon*. 2016;14(1):33-37.
3. Lai HW, Chih-Wei L, Yu-Hsein L, et al. Juvenile giant fibroadenomas with apparent breast asymmetry successfully managed by round-block technique. *JPRAS Open*. 2015;6:40-43.
4. Wyrick DL, Roberts M, Young ZT, Mancino AT. Changing practices: the addition of a novel surgical approach to gynecomastia. *Am J Surg*. 2018;216(3):547-550.
5. Cil TD, Cordeiro E. Complications of oncoplastic breast surgery involving soft tissue transfer versus breast-conserving surgery: an analysis of the NSQIP database. *Ann Surg Oncol*. 2016;23:3266-3271.
6. Kim MK, Kim JK, Jung SP, et al. Round block technique without cerclage in breast-conserving surgery. *Ann Surg Oncol*. 2013;20:3341-3347.

Chapter 13

Reduction Mammoplasty Lumpectomy

Janie G. Grumley

DEFINITION

- Oncoplastic surgery has become a common term used in breast cancer surgery, which is broadly defined as the use of an aesthetic approach to breast cancer surgery. In this broad definition, oncoplastic surgery may refer both to approaches to mastectomy or breast-conserving surgery (BCS). Oncoplastic BCS is a specific term that refers to the combination of partial mastectomy (lumpectomy or quadrantectomy) using plastic surgery techniques to improve aesthetic outcomes.
- Chatterjee et al[1] have divided oncoplastic BCS into two main categories:
  1. Volume displacement: defined reapproximation of the lumpectomy defect with redistribution of breast tissue to preserved breast appearance. Displacement techniques are further subdivided into level 1 (resection of <20% of breast tissue volume) and level 2 (resection of 20%-50% of breast tissue volume).
  2. Volume replacement: oncoplastic techniques where volume is added using tissue flaps or implants to correct the partial mastectomy defect.
- The reduction mammoplasty lumpectomy uses traditional reduction mammoplasty incisions to perform an oncologic partial mastectomy and is typically considered a level 2 oncoplastic breast-conserving operation.

PATIENT HISTORY AND PHYSICAL FINDINGS

- Careful evaluation of the patient with thorough history and physical exam should be completed to ensure that BCS is the appropriate surgical approach. A detailed approach to the breast cancer patient considering breast conservation is described in Part 5, Chapter 9.
- A detailed family history of cancer, particularly breast, ovarian, colon, pancreatic, prostate, and thyroid cancer, will help to determine if the patient is a candidate for hereditary risk assessment and genetic testing. Patient with a genetic predisposition for breast cancer may choose an alternative surgical approach in treatment of their breast cancer.
- Personal history of prior breast surgery may limit the ability to use this approach as blood supply to the breast may be unpredictable. Likewise, a prior history of radiation therapy may preclude breast conservation.
- Physical exam focused on location of the cancer, span of disease, size of breast, and grade of ptosis will impact the ability to use this technique.

IMAGING AND OTHER DIAGNOSTIC STUDIES

- Standard breast imaging should be performed prior to surgery:
  - Mammogram of both breasts to ensure number of lesions and location disease.
  - Ultrasound if architectural distortion or spiculated mass is shown on mammogram.
- Percutaneous biopsy to confirm diagnosis and obtain prognostic markers.
- MRI of the breast should be considered, especially in patient with heterogeneously dense breasts to ensure no other areas of concerns are identified.

MULTIDISCIPLINARY APPROACH

- Breast cancer care requires a multidisciplinary approach to provide the patient with the best possible outcome. Consultations with medical, surgical, and radiation oncology are needed to formulate the best possible approach to an individual's treatment plan.
- Patient goals of treatment must also be considered as the oncology team formulates the treatment plans. In some patients, radiation therapy may not be acceptable therefore breast conservation may not be the ideal approach. On the other hand, patients who are motivated for breast conservation despite large span disease may consider neoadjuvant systemic therapy or alternatively consider extreme oncoplastic breast-conserving surgical techniques.
- Oncoplastic BCS requires an additional skill set beyond general surgery training. While some surgeons have been trained to perform advanced oncoplastic surgery techniques in surgical breast oncology fellowship, most have limited exposure to these techniques. For surgeons wanting to add oncoplastic surgery techniques to their skill set, additional graduate medical education courses have been set up through many national societies to help those interested in learning.
- Surgeons without specialty training in oncoplastic surgery may seek to collaborate with plastic surgery to provide their patients with oncoplastic BCS.

SURGICAL MANAGEMENT

Preoperative Planning

- Preoperative planning for oncoplastic resection starts with the physical exam and breast imaging. Understanding of breast anatomy and blood supply is critical for optimal outcome. Location, span of disease, size of breast, and degree of ptosis (**FIGURE 1**) need to be considered when planning an oncoplastic partial mastectomy.
- Selecting an incision:
  - There are a number of incisions that may be used in planning an oncoplastic mammoplasty (**FIGURE 2**).
  - *Wise pattern* is the most common incision used. This approach results in the commonly seen inverted T-incision.
    - Pro: This versatile incision may be used for cancers in every quadrant.
    - Con: Long inframammary incision with T-junction that may have compromised blood supply.

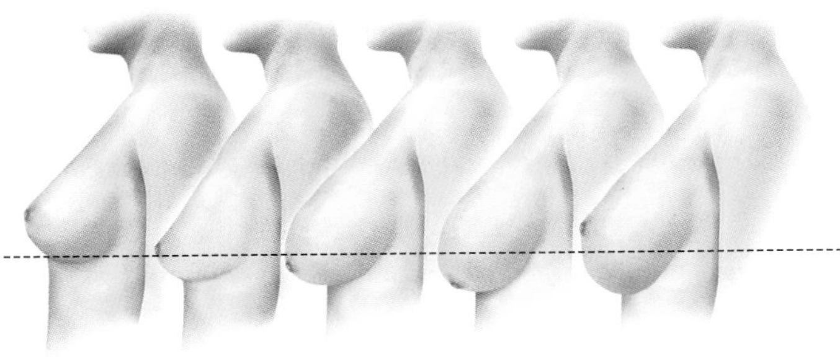

FIGURE 1 ● Grade of breast ptosis.

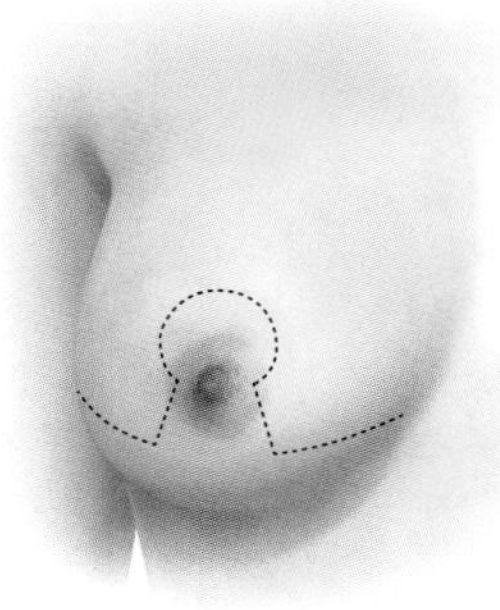

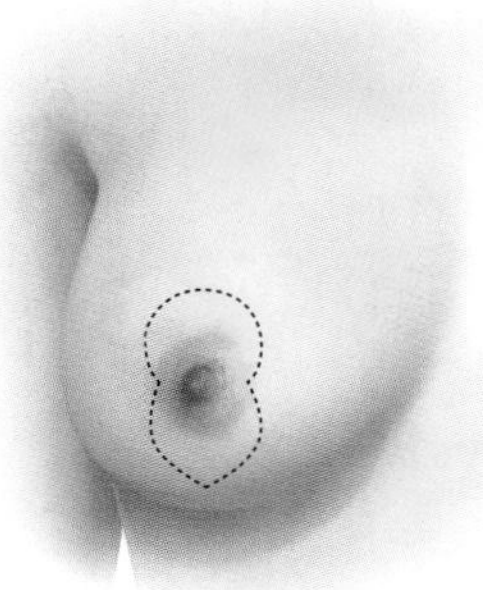

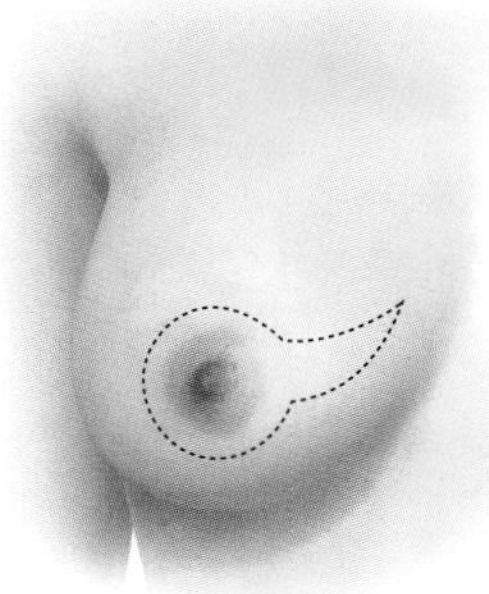

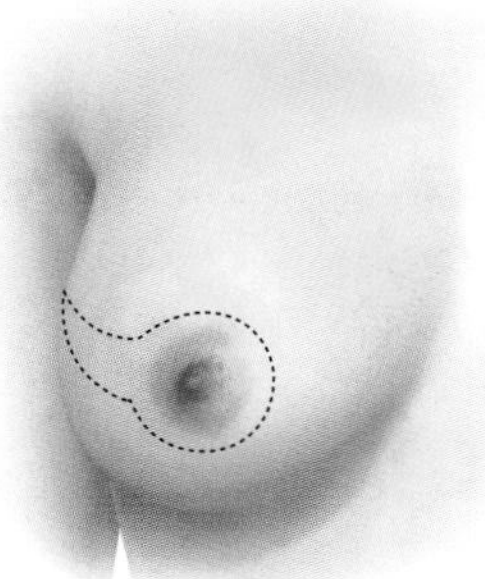

FIGURE 2 ● Commonly used incision.

- ***Vertical mammoplasty*** incision allows for resection of cancers in most quadrants and may be especially useful in patients with lesions at 6:00.
  - Pro: avoidance of the inframammary incision and T-junction, minimizing risk of ischemia
  - Con: Limited use in patients with upper pole breast cancers. This approach may leave redundant skin along the inferior aspect of the vertical incision and may require revision.
- ***Medial mammoplasty*** incision allows for resection of superficial medial lesions.
  - Pro: resection of skin overlying lesions in the medial aspect of the breast.
  - Con: incision that extends to the medial aspect of the breast. Limited to lesions in the medial aspect of the breast.
- ***Lateral mammoplasty*** incision allows for resection of lesions in the lateral aspect of the breast.
  - Pro: resection of skin overlying lesions in the lateral aspect of the breast and avoids the inframammary incision and high risk T-junctions.
  - Con: incision that extends laterally with small risk of lateral displacement of the nipple-areolar complex (NAC). Limited to lesions in the lateral aspect of the breast.

Selecting a Pedicle

- Oncoplastic reduction mammoplasty may be used for cancers in any quadrant; however, understanding of pedicles used for reduction mammoplasty is critical for optimal outcome.

- Blood supply to the nipple is abundant and therefore pedicles may be designed to accommodate site of cancer. In patients with prior breast surgery, it is important to understand where prior surgery may have compromised blood supply to the nipple and avoid pedicles based in that area.
- Major blood supply of the breast comes from (**FIGURE 3**).
  - Branches of the internal mammary artery
  - Branches of the axillary artery
  - Lateral thoracic
  - Intercostal perforators
- ***Inferior pedicle*** is one of the most commonly used pedicles (**FIGURE 4A**).
  - Pro:
    - Predictable blood supply and nervous supply to the nipple.
    - Allows for resection of tumor in all quadrants with the exception of lesions in located at 6:00.
  - Con:
    - May result in less upper breast fullness.
    - Well-defined pedicle may result in indentation along the medial and lateral aspect of the pedicle after radiation therapy.
- ***Superior medial pedicle*** is another commonly used pedicles (**FIGURE 4B**).
  - Pro:
    - Sustained cosmetic results over time.

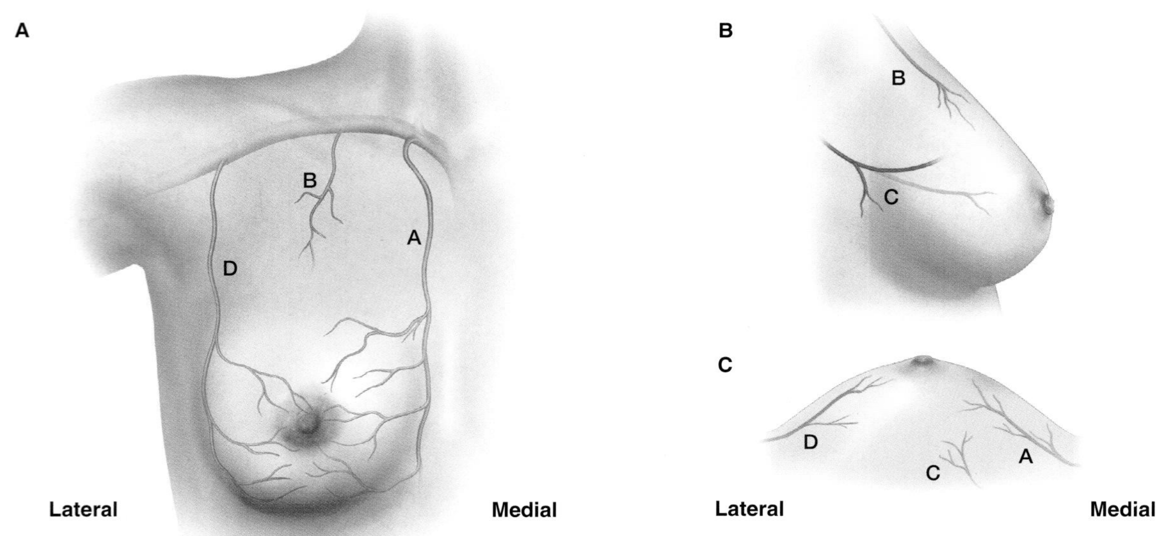

FIGURE 3 ● Blood supply to the breast. **A,** Branches from internal mammary (thoracic) artery. **B,** Supraclavicular branches. **C,** Perforator from intercostal system. **D,** Lateral thoracic system.

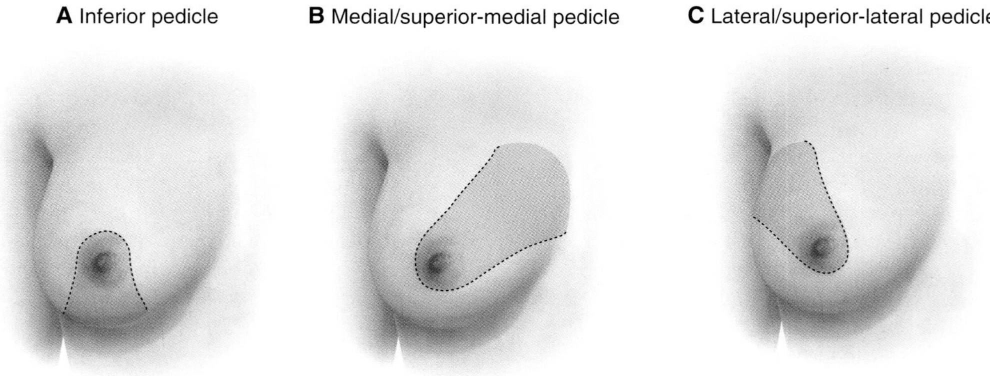

FIGURE 4 ● Glandular Pedicles options. **A,** Inferior pedicle. **B,** Medial/superior-medial pedicle. **C,** Lateral/superior-lateral pedicle.

- Allows for resection of tumors in all quadrants with the exception of lesions in the upper inner quadrant.
- Very useful pedicle in patients with a lesion at 6:00.
- Con:
  - Significant void at 6:00 may result in scaring and indentation that may give a bird beak appearance.
  - May be a challenging approach if a there is significant ptosis or significant macromastia.
- *Superior lateral pedicle* is a less commonly used pedicle (**FIGURE 4C**).
  - Pro:
    - Allows for resection of lesion in any quadrant except lesions in the upper outer quadrant of the breast.
  - Con:
    - Less predictable blood supply.
    - Resection may result in lateral fullness.
- Other pedicles: any combination of the above pedicles may be designed to provide patients with wide excision and optimal cosmetic outcome.

Preoperative Marking

- Preoperative marking of the patient in a standing or sitting position is critical (**FIGURE 5**). Important landmarks for all mammoplasty incisions:
  - Sternal notch
  - Midline
  - Meridian
  - Site of desired location for areola or nipple
  - The remaining mammoplasty incisions are then marked depending on the incision chosen.

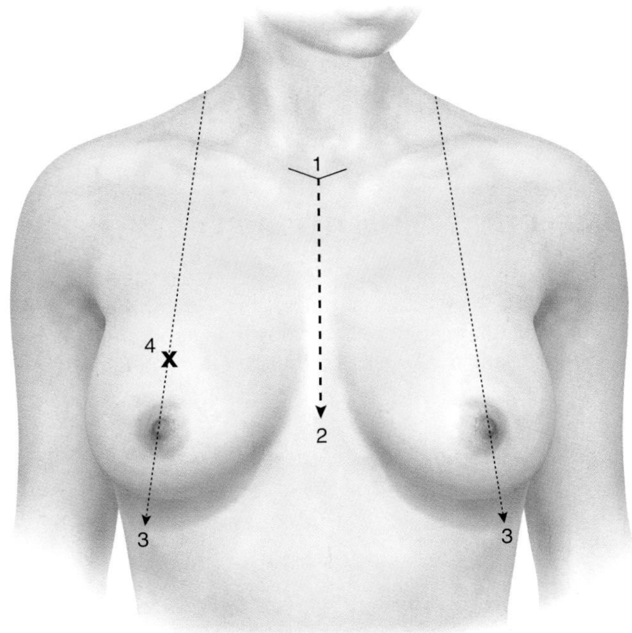

FIGURE 5 ● Preoperative marking. 1) Sternal notch, 2) Midline, 3) Meridian, 4) Site of desired location for areola or nipple.

- There are a number of tools commercially available to help with the remaining mammoplasty incision. Simple protractor and premade molds or stencils may be used to mark the incision lines.

- Localization is an important part of BCS. Any available method may be used when performing oncoplastic BCS. Reliable localization is especially important in patients with macromastia as lesion may move with positioning of the patients.

POSITIONING

- The patient should be placed in a supine position with arms secured on arm boards out toward the side. Taking care to cushion the elbow to avoid undue pressure on nerves. Arms should be well secured since reverse Trendelenburg or sitting position may be needed intraoperatively to assess for symmetry.

DEFINING THE PEDICLE

- Once the patient is anesthetized, prepped and draped, the patient's areola is marked with nipple sizers. The typical nipple sizer used for marking the areola is 34 to 50 mm. Choose the size that will suit the ultimate size of the breast. Local anesthesia or a mixture of tumescent may be injected into the breast to minimize pain.
- After marking the areola, the predetermined breast pedicle should be marked and de-epithelialized. The pedicle is then defined using electrocautery.

PERFORMING THE PARTIAL MASTECTOMY

- Once the pedicle has been defined, it should be well protected as the partial mastectomy is performed.
- Using the desired localization technique, identify the area of resection. Always keep in mind the shape of resection and ability to reapproximate the area after resection.

- Partial mastectomy is then performed, specimen marked for orientation, and specimen radiograph performed to confirm resection of the desired area and margins. If additional margins are deemed necessary, they should be resected and oriented.
- In most patients, if axillary staging is indicated, the procedure may be performed through the mammoplasty incision by tunneling along the plane between the breast parenchyma and anterior fascia of the pectoralis major muscle up toward the axilla.

COMPLETING THE MAMMOPLASTY

- If a wise-pattern mammoplasty is planned (**FIGURE 6**); additional areas of tissue may need to be removed from the superior triangle above the nipple, medial triangle, and or lateral triangle in order to complete the mammoplasty.

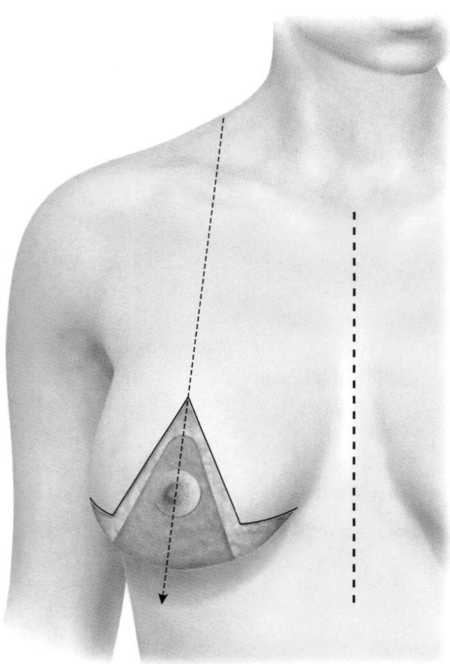

FIGURE 6 ● Additional tissue removal for closure for wise-pattern reduction mammoplasty.

- For the vertical mammoplasty (**FIGURE 7**); Once the partial mastectomy and axillary staging has been done, additional tissue may need to be removed from the superior aspect of the mammoplasty pattern to accommodate for the rotation of the areolar pedicle into position.

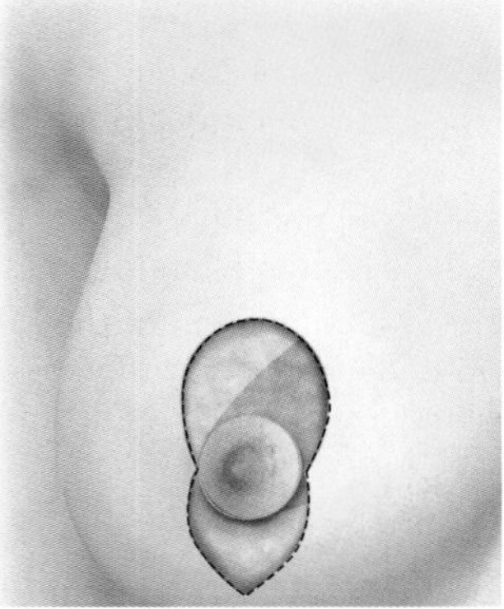

FIGURE 7 ● Additional tissue removal for closure for vertical mammoplasty.

- Regardless of the incision used, it is important to note the location, relationship, and orientation of all additional tissue removed in relation to the site of partial mastectomy to fully assess margins. In cases where a contralateral symmetry procedure it planned, specimen weights need to be documented to aid resection on the contralateral side.

CLOSURE OF THE MAMMOPLASTY

- Prior to closure of the mammoplasty, it is critical to mark the site of partial mastectomy in order to aid adjuvant radiation therapy. Simple surgical clips may be used to mark the perimeter of the partial mastectomy site.
- Reapproximation of the partial mastectomy should be done when possible. In some cases, elevation of the breast parenchyma off the pectoralis major muscle may need to be performed to allow for advancement of the parenchyma and closure of the defect.
- In order to close the wise pattern mammoplasty, skin flaps may be elevated superior laterally and superior medially to close the inverted T-incision at the inframammary fold (**FIGURE 8**).
- If preoperative markings were made with a simple protractor, the inverted T-incision is closed and the final site of the areola is marked with the same size nipple sizer used to mark the areola at start of the operation. This circular patch of skin is then excised and the NAC elevated and secured to skin.
- If a stencil with premarked areolar site was used to mark the patient, then the areola will be secured in the premarked areolar site (**FIGURE 9**).
- Closure of the vertical, lateral, or medial mammoplasty is done with reapproximation of tissue and in some cases rotation of the NAC into the final areolar position (**FIGURE 10**).

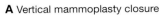

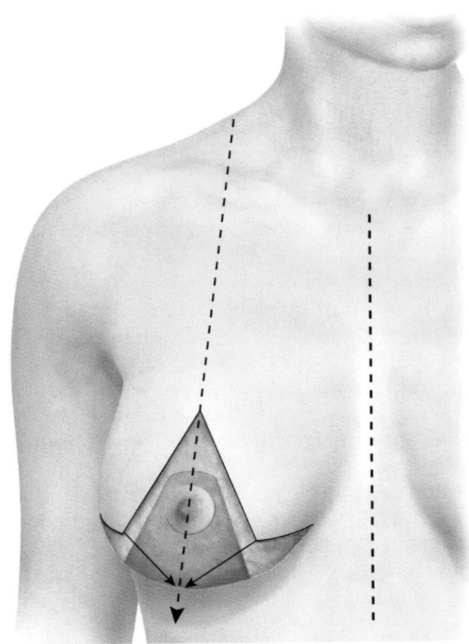

FIGURE 8 ● Wise-pattern mammoplasty skin closure.

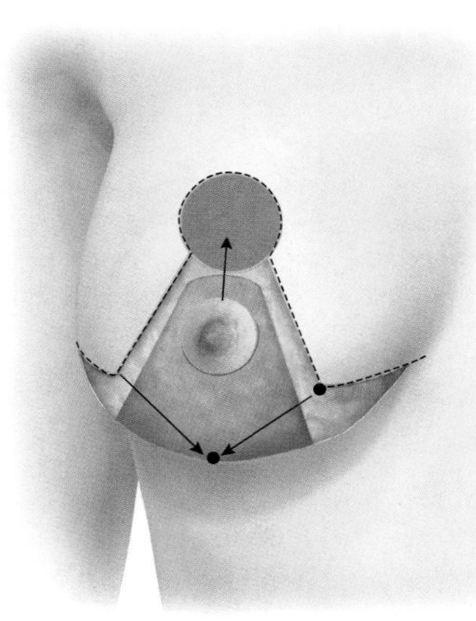

FIGURE 9 ● Placement of the NAC in the final position.

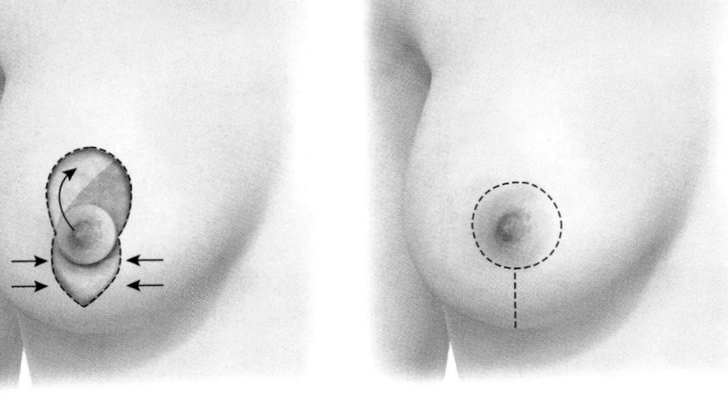

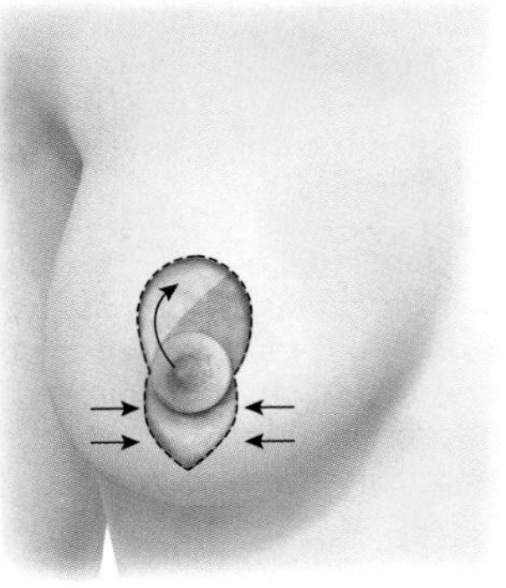

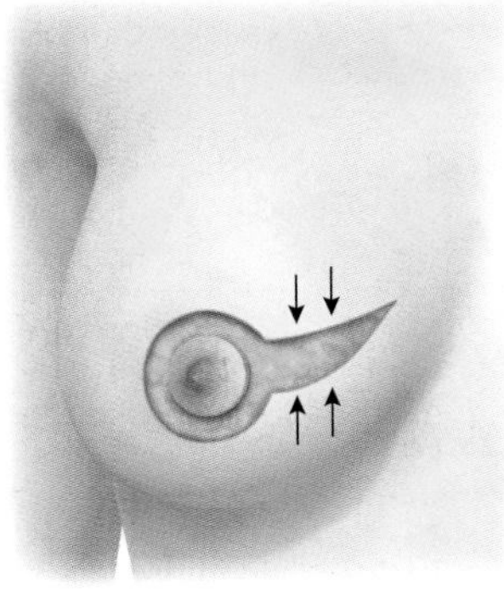

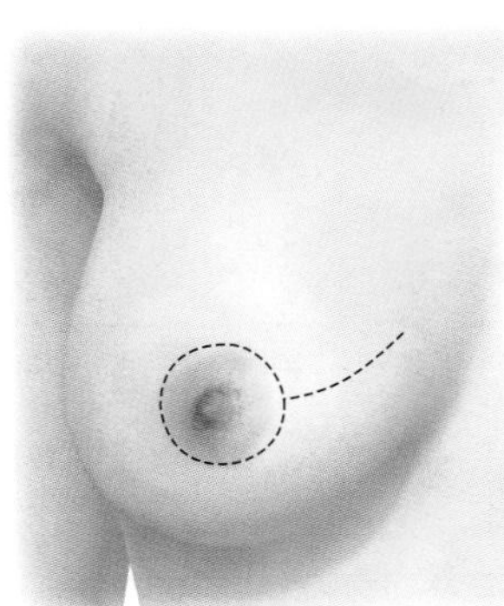

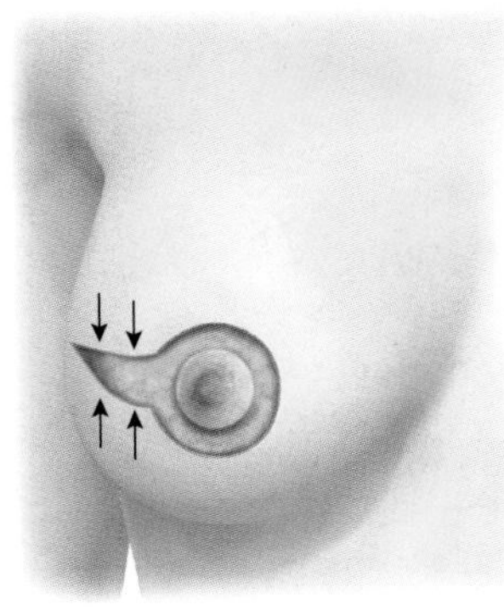

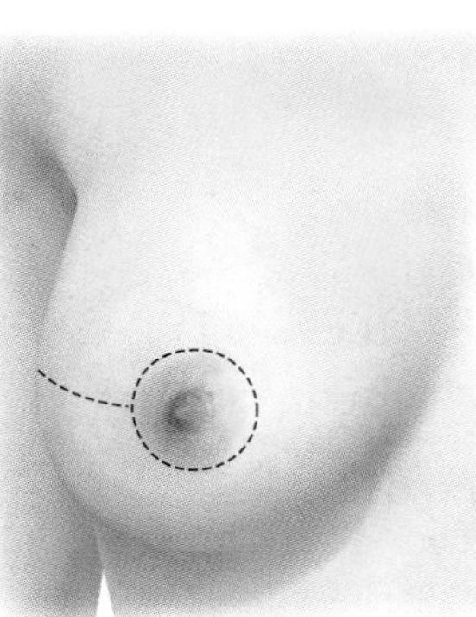

FIGURE 10 ● Skin closure for vertical, lateral, and medical mammoplasty. **A,** Vertical mammoplasty closure. **B,** Medial mammoplasty closure. **C,** Lateral mammoplasty closure.

PEARLS AND PITFALLS

Surgeon experience	■ The reduction mammoplasty lumpectomy is a complex oncoplastic surgery. Surgeon experience is critical. ■ Working with a mentor, taking oncoplastic courses, or working collaboratively with a plastic surgeon is strongly recommended.
Patient selection	■ Since a reduction mammoplasty allows for resection of large volumes of breast tissue from multiple sites, patients with large span disease or multiple areas disease may consider using this approach if they are motivated for breast conservation. ■ In appropriate patients, neoadjuvant chemotherapy may be used to reduce volume of disease to allow for breast conservation. However, neoadjuvant chemotherapy may have suboptimal results for patients with hormone positive, lower grade disease. Therefore, an oncoplastic reduction mammoplasty may allow patient the option of BCS without the need for neoadjuvant systemic therapy.[2,3] ■ In patients with prior mammoplasty or breast implants, make note of prior incisions and if possible, obtain prior detailed operative reports to better assess blood supply to the NAC. In these more complicated cases, it may be best to work with their prior plastic surgeon to provide patients with the best results. ■ Patients with obesity, diabetes, or history of prior radiation therapy may be at higher risk of wound complications and therefore proper patient counseling is needed when discussing these approached in these patients.[4-6] ■ This approach will often leave patients with potential asymmetry. Patient should be advised of this asymmetry and offered a symmetry procedure if so desired, either simultaneously or in a delayed fashion.
Tumor resection	■ Plan the areas of tissue resection carefully, both for removal of the cancer and for closure of the mammoplasty. ■ Limit the number of specimens and orient the specimens accurately as to not complicate margin assessment. ■ Intraoperative margin analysis may be beneficial in reducing the need for re-excision.
Pedicle formation	■ Wide-based pedicles can improve cosmetic outcomes, preserve blood supply, and nervous innervation of the NAC. ■ For patients undergoing radiation, a narrow inferior pedicle can result in significant scarring and indentation at the medial and lateral edge of the pedicle. This can be minimized using a wide-based pedicle along the entire inframammary fold.

POSTOPERATIVE CARE

- Oncoplastic surgery does not require unique postoperative care compared to a patient who undergoes standard partial mastectomy. In most cases, surgical drains are not required.
- Wounds are dressed using wound closure glue or surgical adhesive bandages.
- A surgical bra is usually placed to support the breast post operatively. Patients are advised to keep the supportive garments on for 2 to 4 weeks.
- Postoperative pain control should maximize the use of NSAID and other non-narcotic pain medications.

COMPLICATIONS

- Complications associated with this approach is uncommon. Most widely reported complications:
  - Wound dehiscence (4.6%)
  - Fat necrosis (4.3%)
  - Infection (2.8%)
  - Partial or total nipple loss (0.9%)
  - Hematomas (0.9%)
  - Seromas (0.6%)
- Overall, rate of complications is low and similar to reported complication associated with traditional BCS. Crown et al[7] compared perioperative complication in standard vs oncoplastic surgery. Their series reported lower overall complication with oncoplastic surgery. Most complication may be avoided with careful attention to blood supply and careful tissue handling.
- Management of complications:
  - Wound dehiscence, skin ischemia, and nipple necrosis can all be managed with local wound care. For larger area of dehiscence or necrosis, it may take many weeks of local wound care before the wound granulates and heals. In very rare incidences, skin grafting may be needed in order expedite wound healing.
  - Fat necrosis does not require intervention. With time, area of fat necrosis may become a palpable solid mass. At times, imaging may appear suspicious, and biopsy may be done to rule out disease recurrence. In rare cases, symptomatic patients may consider resection.
  - Hematomas are rare. Early recognition of large hematomas should be evacuated. Smaller hematomas will resolve with time.
  - Seroma may develop postoperatively. Small seromas will resolve with time. Larger seromas may require aspiration.

REFERENCES

1. Chatterjee A, Gass J, Patel K, et al. A consensus definition and classification system of oncoplastic surgery developed by the American Society of Breast Surgeons. *Ann Surg Oncol*. 2019;26(11):3436-3444. doi:10.1245/s10434-019-07345-4
2. Crown A, Handy N, Weed C, et al. Oncoplastic breast-conserving surgery: can we reduce rates of mastectomy and chemotherapy use in patients with traditional indications for mastectomy? *Ann Surg Oncol*. 2021;28:2199-2209.
3. Crown A, Laskin R, Rocha FG, Grumley J. Extreme oncoplasty: expanding indications for breast conservation. *Am J Surg*. 2019;217(5):851-856. doi:10.1016/j.amjsurg.2019.01.004
4. Piper ML, Esserman LJ, Sbitany H, Peled AW. Outcomes following oncoplastic reduction mammoplasty. *Ann Plast Surg*. 2016;76:S222-S226. doi:10.1097/SAP.0000000000000720
5. Myung Y, Heo CY. Relationship between obesity and surgical complications after reduction mammaplasty: a systematic literature review and meta-analysis. *Aesthetic Surg J*. 2017;37(3):308-315.
6. Gust MJ, Smetona JT, Persing JS, Hanwright PJ, Fine NA, Kim JYS. The impact of body mass index on reduction mammaplasty: a multicenter analysis of 2492 patients. *Aesthetic Surg J*. 2013;33(8):1140-1147.
7. Crown A, Scovel LG, Rocha FG, Scott EJ, Wechter DG, Grumley JW. Oncoplastic breast conserving surgery is associated with a lower rate of surgical site complications compared to standard breast conserving surgery. *Am J Surg*. 2019;217(1):138-141. doi:10.1016/j.amjsurg.2018.06.014

Chapter 14

Techniques for Correcting Lumpectomy Defects

Jessica Jen-Tau Hsu and Paige L. Myers

DEFINITION

- Most women with breast cancer are candidates for breast conservation therapy (BCT); the combination of lumpectomy or partial mastectomy with radiation. This allows women to avoid mastectomy without compromising survival. For many women, simple lumpectomy (Part 5, Chapter 9) can achieve negative margins and excellent cosmesis.
- For some women, with larger tumors relative to the size of their breasts, there are several simple oncoplastic resection techniques that can allow for tissue rearrangement to maintain the contour of the breast while performing wider resections. Several of these are described in prior chapters (Parallelogram, Batwing, Donut, and Reduction Mastopexy).
- Other patients may require more complex tissue rearrangement and replacement techniques for correcting lumpectomy defects to minimize the risk for asymmetry from volume loss and radiation changes.
- There will also be a portion of women who will present following radiation therapy with concavity, volume loss or significant asymmetry that may require surgery to correct lumpectomy defects.

PATIENT HISTORY AND PHYSICAL FINDINGS

- For patients with larger tumor-to-breast size ratios, where a significant defect is anticipated, preoperative assessment by both the breast surgeon and the plastic surgeon is recommended to plan potential immediate or staged reconstruction.
- Patients may also be referred to the plastic surgeon following completion of breast conservation therapy to address contour deformities, volume deficit, and/or nipple-areolar complex (NAC) malposition.
- A comprehensive breast and oncologic history with previous and/or anticipated surgical and nonsurgical interventions should be obtained. One should note the size of the primary tumor, location within the breast, and proximity to skin (and the NAC) and muscle. The stage, including regional metastases, and the potential need for lymph node dissection, adjuvant chemotherapy, and radiation therapy (or if these treatments have already occurred). The history should also include previous elective breast surgeries such as benign excisional biopsies, breast augmentation, reduction, or mastopexy.
- Patient factors that could affect surgical planning and outcome should be considered including current use of nicotine, vasospastic drugs, immunosuppressants, and comorbidities such as diabetes. These factors can impact nipple perfusion, tissue viability, and wound healing.
- A thorough breast exam should document breast size, breast footprint, overall contour, nipple position, degree of ptosis, inframammary fold (IMF) position, and scars on or around the breast. The plastic surgeon should measure and compare the sternal notch to nipple and nipple to IMF distances bilaterally. Any asymmetries compared to the contralateral breast should be noted.
- For patients seen prior to planned breast conservation surgery, it is important to discuss with the patient their expectations regarding ideal breast shape and size in the face of anticipated surgery and radiation therapy. If the patient has a large breast with ptosis, she may be a candidate for oncoplastic breast reduction or require symmetrizing a procedure for the contralateral breast.
- A multidisciplinary approach is essential for patients who are likely to have substantial volume loss or contour deformity following BCT. For these individuals, it is best to work with the breast surgeon, and perhaps the radiation oncologist, prior to lumpectomy to determine the optimal approach, understand the expected location and volume of resection, discuss potential reconstructive options, and the ideal timing for reconstructive procedures. It is also important to discuss the potential of mastectomy with immediate or delayed reconstruction as an alternative to large volume resections with tissue rearrangement.

IMAGING AND OTHER DIAGNOSTIC STUDIES

- Oncologist workup for patients with anticipated or previous BCT include bilateral mammography (**FIGURE 1A**), and in some cases, magnetic resonance imaging (MRI) (**FIGURE 1B**).
- Standard clinical photographs of the breasts and potential donor sites should be obtained.

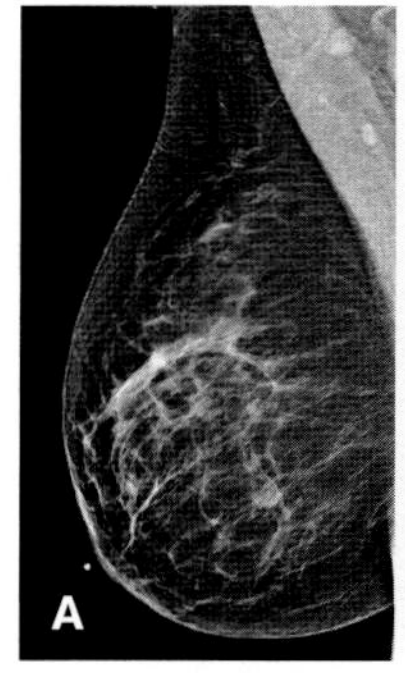

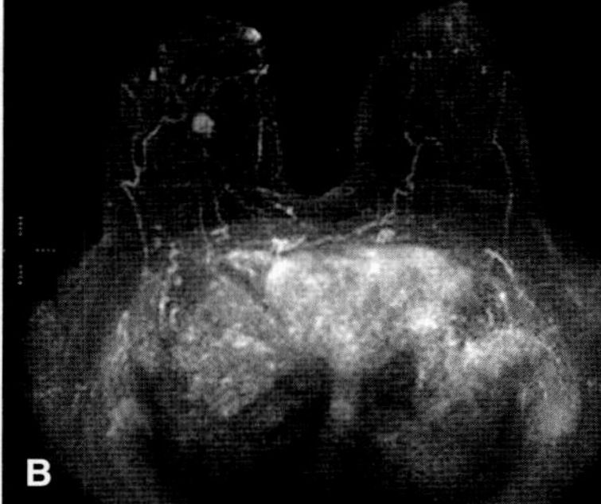

FIGURE 1 • Mammogram **(A)** and MRI **(B)** of patient with 1.1 × 1.0 × 0.8 cm right-sided breast cancer at 5-o-clock position.

- Additional imaging, such as computed tomography angiography, may be necessary to further delineate vascular anatomy depending on the reconstructive plan.

GOALS AND EXPECTATIONS

- Timing: For patients who are planning breast conservation, it is important to have discussions with the patient, the breast surgeon, and occasionally, the radiation oncologist. The timing of oncoplastic reconstruction may be dictated by the clinical scenario. In some cases, reconstruction needs to be staged to ensure negative margins or complete removal of calcifications prior to rearrangement of breast tissue. In this setting, the plastic surgeon and surgical oncologist should plan the resection approach together and with consideration for the eventual reconstruction.
- A staged approach has the advantage of reducing the risk for completion mastectomy if there is residual disease whereas an immediate oncoplastic reconstruction at the time of the lumpectomy reduces the number of operations.
- Procedures on the contralateral breast for symmetry can also be done in an immediate or delayed fashion. Some surgeons prefer to reduce and/or lift the contralateral breast at the same time as the breast-conserving surgery. This requires an estimation of the appearance of the ipsilateral breast following radiation therapy, and may require leaving the involved breast slightly larger in anticipation of contraction, which is common following radiation. Another drawback to immediate contralateral procedures is that some patients may need to return for re-excisions and greater volume loss should they have involved margins or residual calcifications. For these reasons, many surgeons prefer to delay any contralateral procedures until after completion of radiation therapy.
- Goals: The goal of oncoplastic reconstruction is to achieve the best possible aesthetic outcome in the setting of oncologically sound breast preservation after lumpectomy. This will require obliteration of parenchymal dead space, maintenance of NAC perfusion, optimization of NAC position, and management of the soft tissue envelope.
- Surgical Approach: There are two principles for oncoplastic reconstruction:
  - ***Volume displacement*** techniques use residual parenchyma to recreate the aesthetic breast shape.
  - ***Volume replacement*** techniques use local, regional, and distant tissue to restore volume. In addition to tissue flaps, fat grafting is a replacement technique for correcting focal or diffuse volume deficiencies and contour/shape irregularities. It can be used as an adjunct procedure for tethered scar release following BCT.
- Tumor size and location are important considerations. If there will be enough residual parenchyma with nipple-areolar complex perfusion, then volume displacement (ie, intrinsic tissue rearrangement, reduction techniques, mastopexy) can be used (**FIGURE 2**). If there is insufficient tissue, then volume replacement techniques will need to be employed.

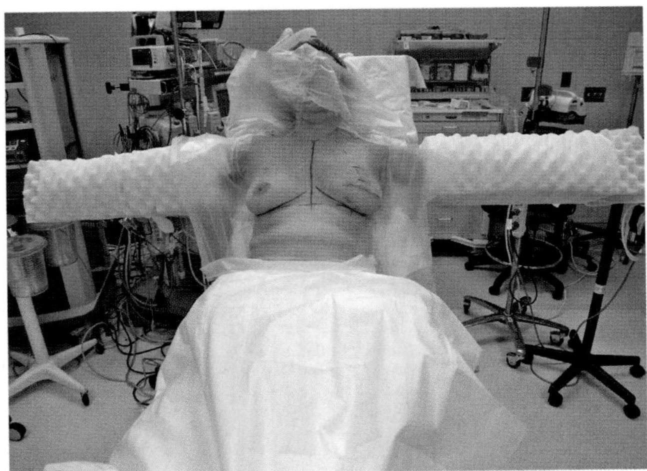

FIGURE 2 ● Positioning of a patient with both arms abducted, padded, and secured, enabling seating the patient during surgery to assess for symmetry of reconstruction.

SURGICAL MANAGEMENT

Preoperative Assessment

- In the preop area, the patient should be examined and the surgeon should note the breast size, overall contour, nipple position, degree of ptosis, and position of the inframammary fold.
- The plastic surgeon should mark the distances from the sternal notch to the nipples and between the nipples and IMF.

Positioning

- The patient is positioned supine with arms secured to padded, adjustable arm boards (**FIGURE 3**). Ensure the anterior superior iliac crest is placed at the break of the bed if the patient is to be placed in a sitting position for oncoplastic surgery. The shoulders should be straight.

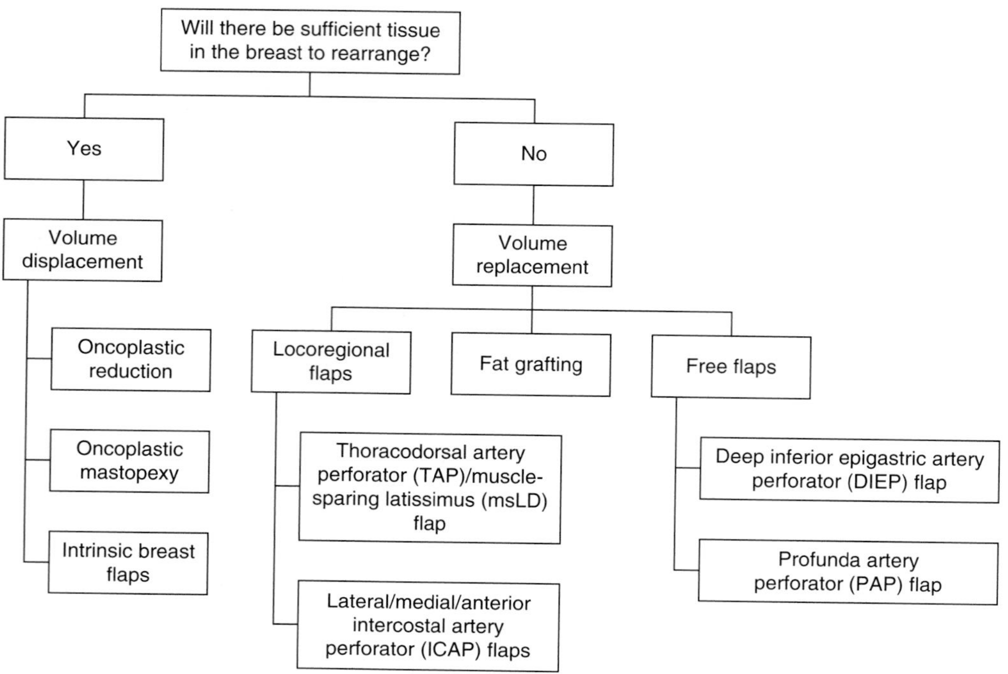

FIGURE 3 ● Algorithm for oncoplastic surgery.

TECHNIQUES

ASSESSING THE DEFECT

- In the operating room (OR), either at the time of the BCT or in a delayed fashion, the lumpectomy cavity is examined, and any seroma evacuated. Initially, the seroma will mask the defect, so this is an important step to appreciate the extent of necessary reconstruction.
- Evaluate the perfusion and soft tissue support to the NAC. Confirm perfusion via clinical exam (bleeding edges, capillary refill) or through indocyanine green fluorescent angiography. If during surgery, the NAC is dangerously undermined NAC, a free nipple graft (FNG) can be performed: the NAC is excised as a full-thickness skin graft, defatted, secured to a de-epithelialized bed in the appropriate position on the breast mound, and secured in place with a bolster dressing.

VOLUME DISPLACEMENT PROCEDURES:

Freestyle Intrinsic Breast Flaps

- Dermoglandular flaps maintain support to the NAC, obliterate dead space, and minimize lumpectomy deformity after radiation, it is particularly helpful if there is minimal parenchyma between the skin and underlying muscle.
- After either the breast surgeon has completed the lumpectomy or the prior lumpectomy cavity has been opened and the seroma released, the size of the defect is measured, and the remaining breast parenchyma is evaluated for availability of tissue for intrinsic flap creation.
- Flap design should incorporate the principles of random pattern flaps (**FIGURE 4A**). The breast parenchyma is then dissected free from the skin superficially and pectoralis muscle deep (**FIGURE 4B**).
- Flaps should be designed as random pattern flaps (though they can have a perforator-based blood supply, this pedicle is not identified during the dissection), ensuring a broad base to maximize perfusion to the distal end of the flap. The flap

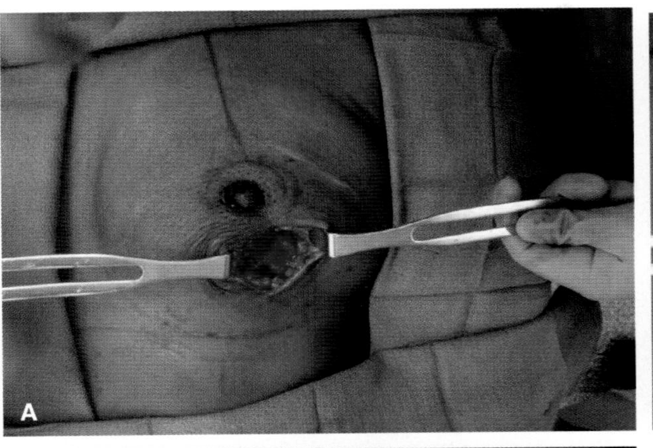

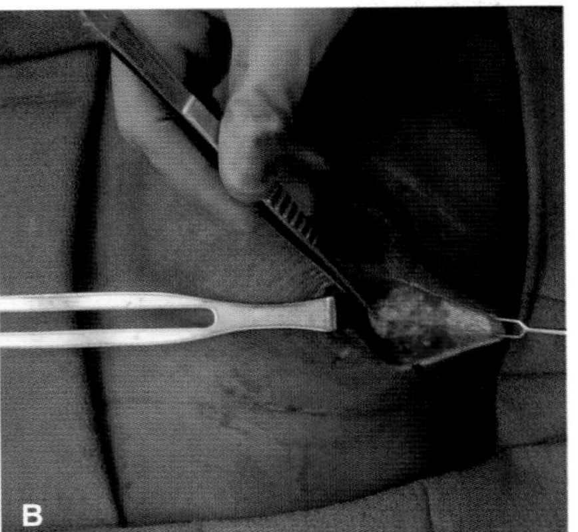

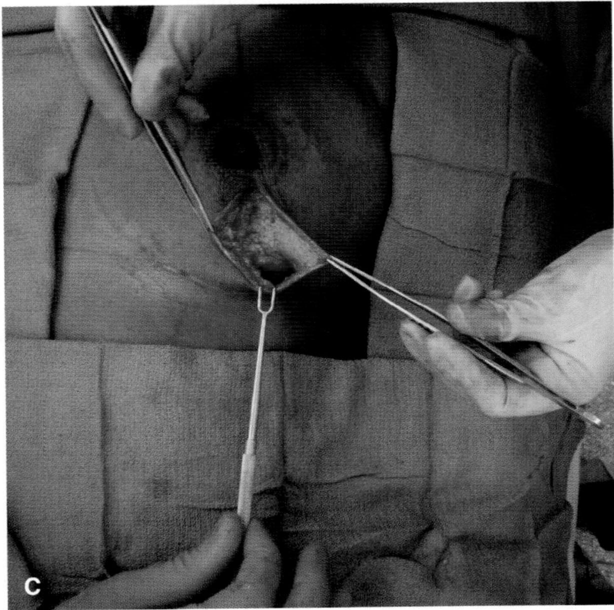

FIGURE 4 ● **A,** The lumpectomy cavity and surrounding breast tissue is examined. **B,** An intrinsic flap is raised by elevating the skin from the breast parenchyma and the breast tissue off the underlying pectoralis. **C,** The flap is advanced into the defect and secured, obliterating the dead space.

is then advanced or rotated to fill the lumpectomy cavity and to maintain support to NAC (**FIGURE 4C**).

- Excess skin is resected, and the wound is closed. This should not be too tight to compress the flap perfusion. Tailor tack the incisions frequently to confirm there is no inadvertent misshaping the of the breast.

VERTICAL MAMMAPLASTY TECHNIQUE FOR INFERIOR POLE DEFECTS

Preoperative Marking

- This approach is an option for patients with larger breasts, moderate ptosis, and lumpectomy defects in the inferior pole of the breast.
- With the patient in the upright position, landmarks are drawn—sternal notch, midline, and breast meridian—a line from the midclavicular point to the midbreast. The new position of NAC is marked out at Pitanguy point—a point transposed from the IMF to the anterior breast along the meridian.
- The breast is mobilized laterally and a vertical line is drawn medially. Then the breast is mobilized medially and a vertical line is drawn laterally. The vertical components are then connected with a curved line approximately 2 to 4 cm above the IMF. A mosque-shaped marking is drawn for inset of the NAC (**FIGURE 5**). These markings may need to be slightly modified based on any asymmetries of the breast.

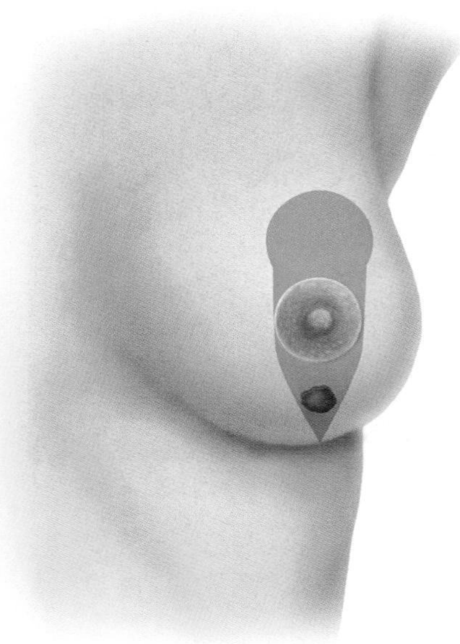

FIGURE 5 ● A vertical reduction pattern.

Conversion to a Vertical Reduction

- Additional breast tissue can be resected as needed to allow for an acceptable final shape. The breast tissue is undermined inferiorly only. Tissue is resected around the vertical incision creating medial and lateral "pillars" that are then approximated centrally.
- Skin closure in a standard fashion. A small horizontal excision is made along the IMF if needed to further reduce the skin.
- Though initially this approach may result in a conical-shaped breast with a protuberant and flat lower pole, it is important that the patient and staff appreciate that this will become ptotic over the course of the next several weeks to settle into an aesthetic breast shape.
- Because this approach often results in volume loss, a contralateral reduction will often be needed. This can be done at the same setting or in a delayed fashion. For patients who are yet to have radiation, it may be preferable to return to the OR for the contralateral reduction approximately 6 months following radiation to allow for a better assessment of the final appearance of the ipsilateral breast.

WISE PATTERN REDUCTION WITH INFERIOR PEDICLE FOR SUPERIOR POLE DEFECTS

Preoperative Marking

- With the patient in the upright position, the landmarks are drawn, including the sternal notch, midline, and the breast meridian. The breast meridian is a line from the midclavicular point to the midbreast. The new position for the NAC is marked out at Pitanguy point—a point transposed from the IMF to the anterior breast along the meridian.
- To mark the skin excision, the breast is mobilized laterally and a vertical line is drawn medially. Next, the breast is mobilized medially and a vertical line drawn laterally. These generally measure 8 to 10 cm based on the size and shape of the breast. The vertical components connect to the IMF with a curved line (**FIGURE 6**). It is important to note any asymmetries at this time that may impact these markings.

Creation of the Inferior Pedicle

- An 8-cm inferior pedicle is marked and the pedicle de-epithelialized after marking the NAC with a 42-mm areolar sizer. The pedicle is freed from the surrounding tissue down to the chest wall along its medial, lateral, and superior margins.

Perform a Wise Pattern Reduction

- Along the superior Wise pattern incision, skin flaps are raised that are approximately 1 to 2 cm thick, based on the patient's

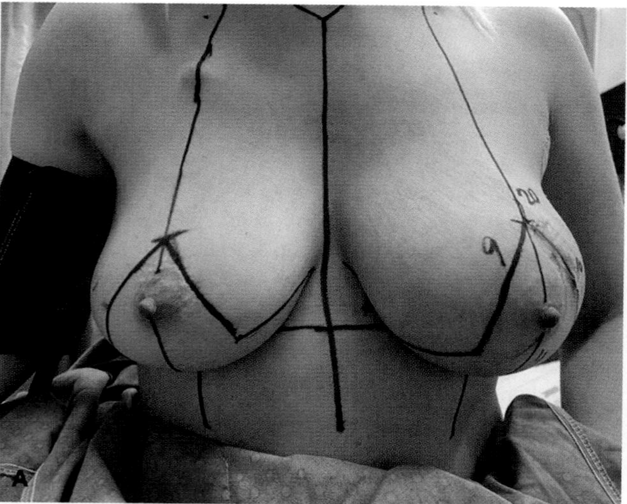

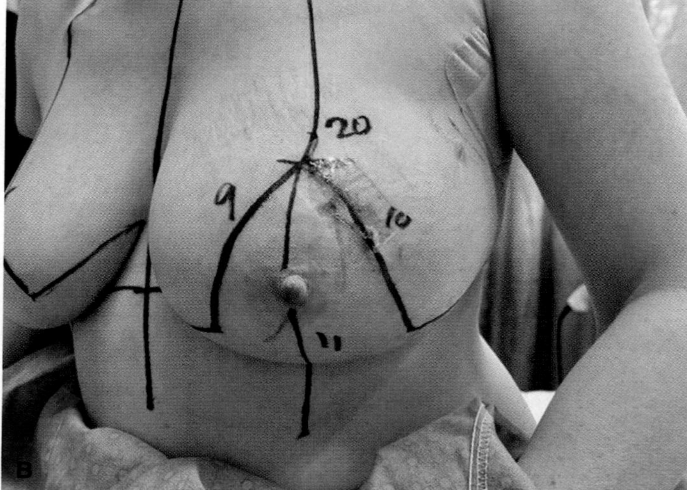

FIGURE 6 ● A Wise pattern reduction mastopexy with inferior pedicle, photographs postlumpectomy. Note previous lumpectomy incision hidden within Wise pattern.

natural parenchymal anatomy. The intervening soft tissue is excised, often including the lumpectomy cavity.

- If the inferior pedicle is long and ptotic, the pedicle can be imbricated in a horizontal fashion and then secured medially to the chest wall.
- The ends of the vertical limb are secured to their correct position along the IMF incision, just medial to the breast meridian. The breast is then tailor tacked into place.
- In the sitting position, the breast is examined for overall size and shape. If a contralateral reduction is being performed, symmetry is also assessed.
- The new NAC position is marked and closing proceeds in the standard fashion.

VOLUME REPLACEMENT TECHNIQUES

Pedicled Flaps

- For patients with larger defects for which displacement techniques are insufficient, replacement techniques may be necessary. In general, pedicled flaps are recommended. In some cases, free tissue transfer may be considered; however, one must consider future reconstructive challenges should the patient develop a recurrence or a new primary tumor that requires a mastectomy.
- While there are several locoregional perforator flaps, the most commonly used is the *thoracodorsal artery perforator (TAP) flap*, which is based on the perforators from the descending or the horizontal branches of the thoracodorsal vessels for superolateral defects (**FIGURE 7**). Other locoregional perforator flaps such as the Lateral Intercostal Artery Perforator (LICAP) flap, the anterior intercostal artery perforator (AICAP) flap, or the superior epigastric artery perforator (SEAP) flap are used less commonly and beyond the scope of this chapter.

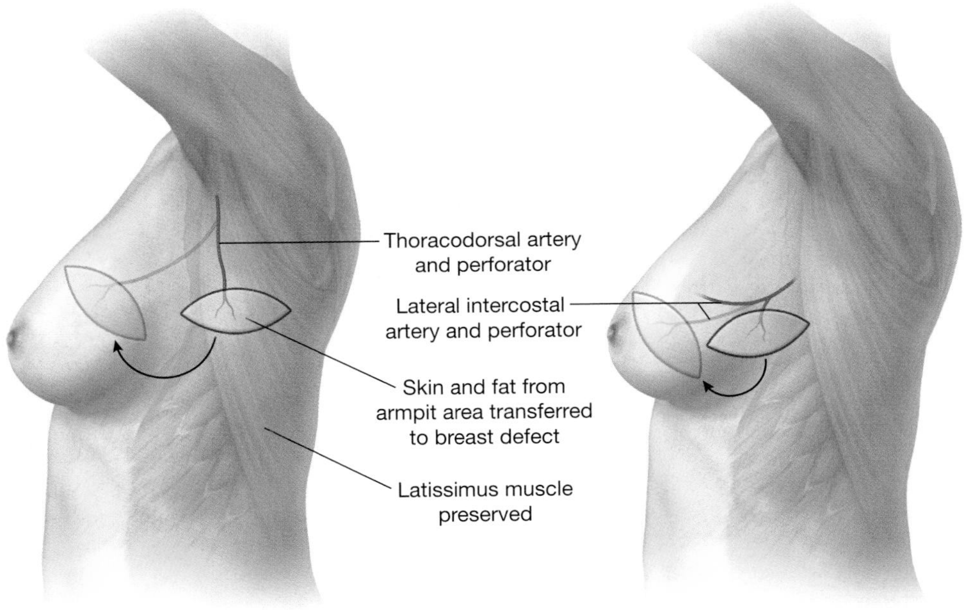

FIGURE 7 • The TAP and MSLD flap.

THORACODORSAL ARTERY PERFORATOR FLAP OR MUSCLE-SPARING LATISSIMUS DORSI FLAP

Preoperative Marking

- With the patient in the upright position, landmarks are marked out, including the sternal notch, midline, and the breast meridian—a line from the midclavicular point to the midbreast.
- Mark the new NAC position if required based on its location on the contralateral breast. This may need to be adjusted accordingly if there is a plan for a symmetrizing procedure.
- Identify and mark the tip of scapula and the anterior edge of the latissimus dorsi muscle.
- A pinch test should then be performed to determine the amount of redundant skin to determine the size of flap.
- The perforator location is marked with a Doppler ultrasound device. It emerges approximately 8 to 10 cm from the posterior axillary crease and 2 cm posterior to anterior border of the latissimus (**FIGURE 8**).
- Based on the perforator location, the amount of excess soft tissue and the size of the defect, the surgeon can design the flap with different skin paddle orientations:
    - The ***Horizontal*** (or "bra line") orientation has a better cosmetic outcome as it is often hidden within clothes.

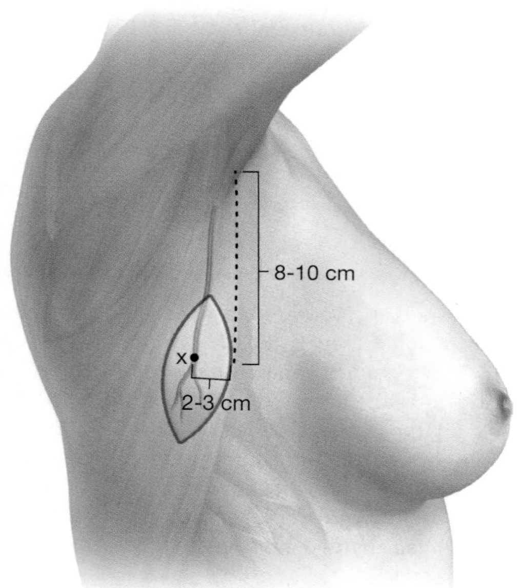

FIGURE 8 ● The patient is placed in the lateral decubitus position to locate the perforators and design the flap. The *dotted line* is the anterior border of the latissimus dorsi muscle. "X" marks the main perforator artery for the flap, located 2 to 3 cm from the anterior margin of latissimus and 8 to 10 cm from the posterior axillary crease.

- The ***Oblique*** orientation is oriented along relaxed skin tension lines, which allows for greater volume harvest and less tension upon closure.
- The ***Vertical*** orientation along the anterior edge of the latissimus is more likely to capture the perforator with dissection.

Creation of Lateral Tunnel From the Breast Pocket

- The patient should be placed on a beanbag. Initially, the patient will be supine. The chest and upper abdomen are sterilely prepped into the field.
- After the lumpectomy cavity is assessed, a tunnel is then created from the lumpectomy cavity to the anterior edge of the latissimus muscle.
- Once the latissimus muscle is identified, the skin edges are temporarily reapproximated with skin staples and the wound is covered.

Flap Harvest

- The patient is repositioned in the lateral decubitus position.
- The perforating vessels are confirmed by a handheld pencil Doppler as they may have adjusted with position. Once the perforators have been identified, the flap orientation is adjusted as necessary.
- The skin of the flap is incised with a scalpel, beveling to capture as much sub-Scarpa fat as needed. Dissection is then carried down to the muscle.
- Dissect in a subfascial plane anteriorly from the midline until the perforators are identified (**FIGURE 9**). The latissimus dorsi fascia should be included with the flap. Complete dissection to isolate perforators.

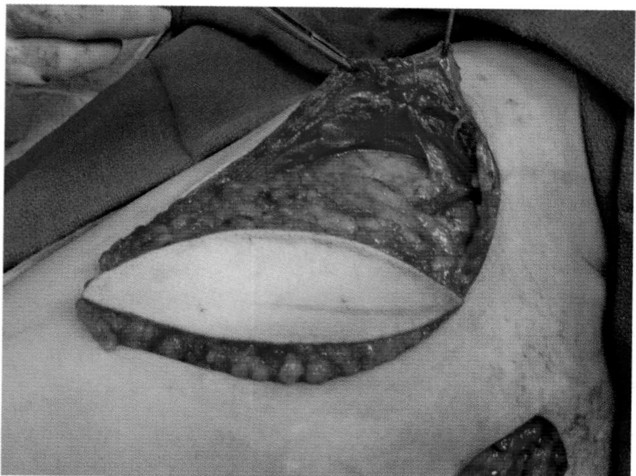

FIGURE 9 ● The latissimus dorsi muscle is completely dissected from anterior to midline to identify the perforators.

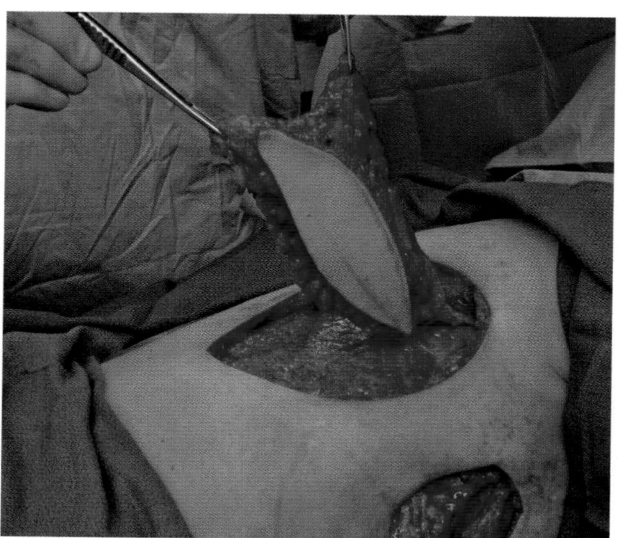

FIGURE 10 ● Once the flap has been elevated, a drain is placed, and the skin is reapproximated. The patient is then repositioned supine.

- At this point, it becomes necessary to decide between a TAP flap or an MSLD flap based on the perfusion of the tissues, especially the venous drainage.
  - For a TAP flap, just one perforator is isolated. The muscle is then split, and the descending branch of the thoracodorsal artery is dissected to the takeoff point of the transverse branch of the thoracodorsal vessels.
  - For an MSLD flap, multiple perforators within 1 to 3 cm of the anterior edge of the latissimus need to be captured within the substance of the muscle. Harvest the descending branch of the thoracodorsal artery at the takeoff point of the transverse branch.
- Following flap harvest, it is mobilized into the breast cavity through the tunnel (**FIGURE 10**); the skin is closed in a standard fashion over a closed-suction drain.

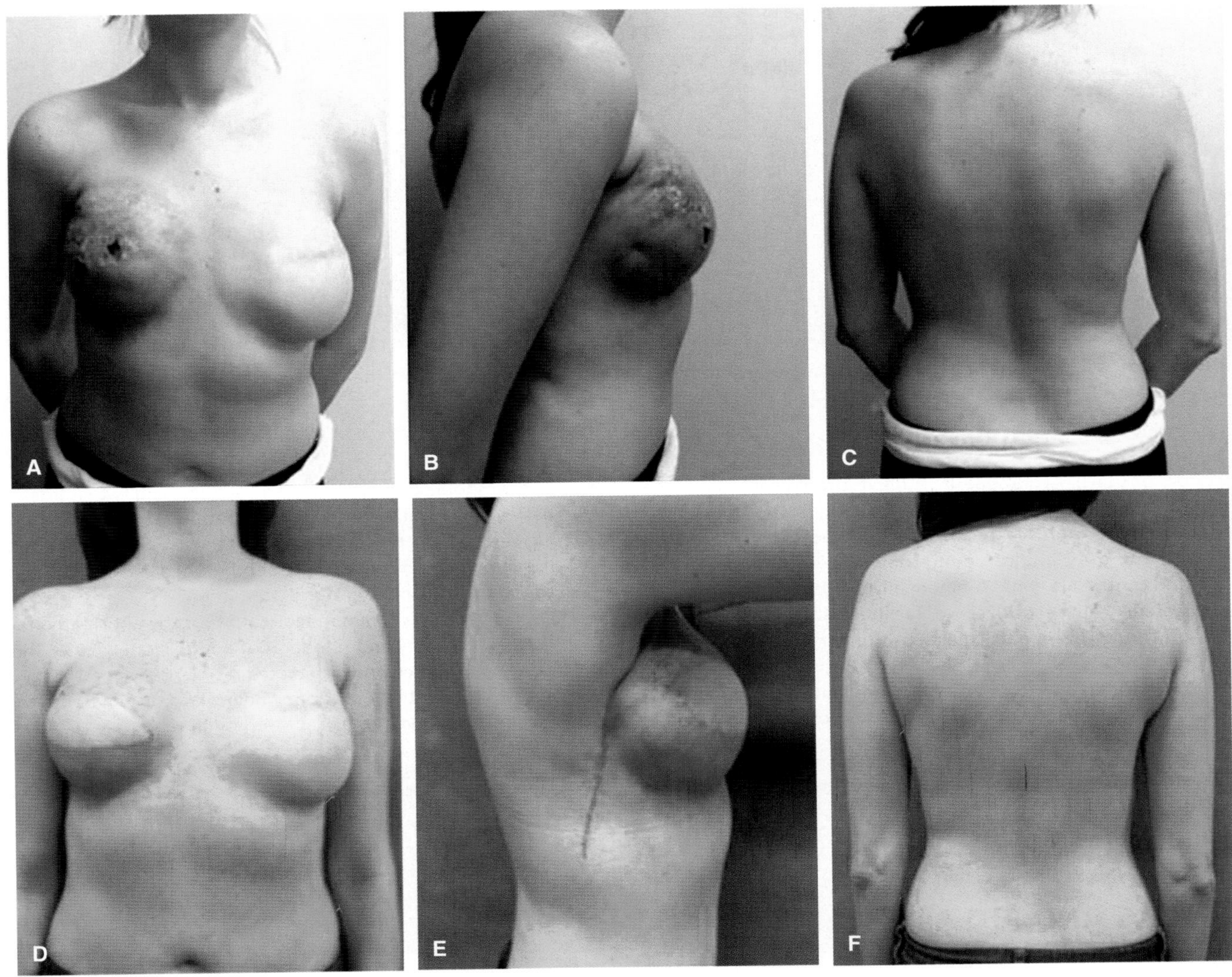

FIGURE 11 ● After a poor outcome with a superior lateral lumpectomy **(A-C)**, the defect was corrected using a TAP **(D-F)**.

Flap Inset

- The patient is repositioned supine and the two breasts are compared with the patient in the upright position. The flap is inset to fill the volume defect and support the NAC.
- It is often necessary to de-epithelialize the skin, but a small skin island should be maintained for monitoring of the flap. The patient should be monitored in the hospital for 1 to 2 days postoperatively (**FIGURE 11**).

FAT GRAFTING

Preoperative Evaluation and Marking

- It is generally recommended to wait a minimum of 4 to 6 months following radiation treatment or most recent surgery before performing fat grafting.
- Physical examination is needed to determine volume deficit, location of deficit, and to identify any areas of contour deformity.
- In addition, the patient is examined to identify potential donor sites. Most common donor sites include abdomen, flank, thigh, and buttock.
- In the preoperative area, mark breast anatomic landmarks bilaterally along with topographic contour lines based on volume deficit and excess for both recipient and donor sites, respectively (**FIGURE 12A**).

Technique

- Tumescent solution comprising a dilute solution of lidocaine and epinephrine is typically infiltrated into the donor site for both hemostatic effect and postoperative pain control. This can be performed either before or after harvest.
- Hand-assisted or vacuum-assisted liposuction with a large diameter, blunt cannula is performed for fat harvest from

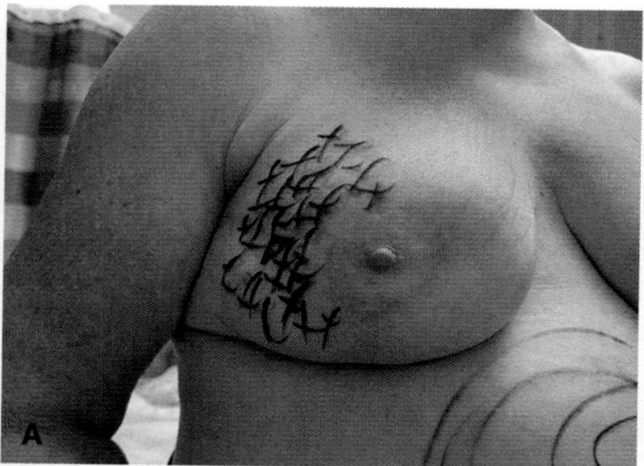

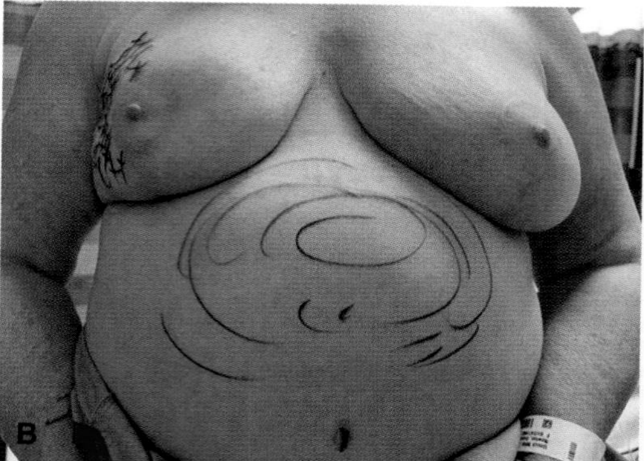

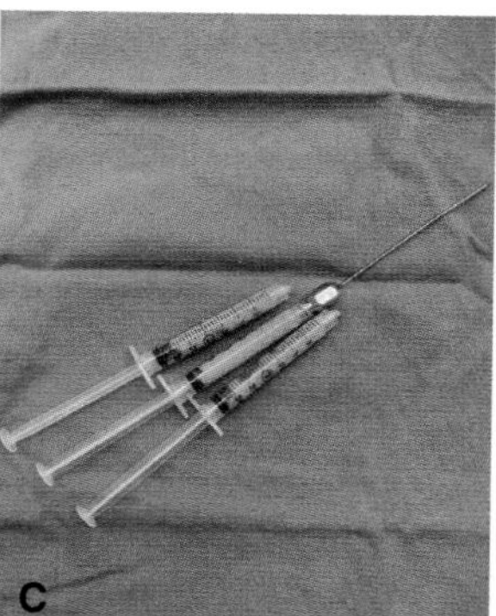

FIGURE 12 ● **A** and **B,** Tethered scar of a breast lumpectomy defect following radiation with markings for fat grafting and liposuction. **C,** Fat harvested ready to be grafted in small aliquots.

donor site(s). Avoid superficial harvest to prevent donor site contour irregularities.

- There are multiple techniques to process the harvested fat for grafting including rolling, decanting, washing, and centrifugation. Commercially available fat processing systems can be utilized to facilitate fat preparation for grafting. This is particularly useful for larger-volume fat grafting.
- Fat grafting is performed to the recipient site through small stab incisions and using a blunt infiltration cannula.
- The fat should be grafted in small aliquots and with multiple passes to maximize contact of the grafted fat with surrounding vascularized tissue (**FIGURE 12 C**).
- It is important to consider the depth of harvest and grafting to avoid additional contour deformities.
- Overcorrection is common to account for the anticipated fat graft survivability and retention of approximately 50%. This can be less in previously irradiated recipient sites.
- It may be helpful to fat graft under areas of released tethered scar to prevent recurrent tethering.

PEARLS AND PITFALLS

Timing—Immediate oncoplastic reconstruction	■ Patient must be seen prior to lumpectomy. ■ Resection and reconstruction approach should be planned and marked together. ■ Risk is possible need for completion mastectomy.
Timing—delayed oncoplastic reconstruction	■ Wait at least 6 months after radiation. ■ Assess tissues for adequate recovery before procedures on radiated breast.
Patient factors	■ Consider risks for delayed wound healing and tissue viability. ■ Avoid procedures that may delay radiation treatment.
Preoperative counseling	■ Managing expectations is key: patients should be prepared that multiple procedures may be required for definitive reconstruction. ■ Engage patients in shared decision making. ■ Asymmetries are expected and will worsen over time; radiated and nonradiated tissue behave differently.
Adjuvant therapy	■ Can place clips in lumpectomy defect prior to reconstruction as needed to guide radiation therapy. ■ Implant-based reconstruction has a relatively high complication rate in the setting of radiation, so autologous techniques are generally recommended.
Intrinsic flaps	■ Ideal if sufficient tissue is available. ■ Avoids additional donor sites.
Oncoplastic reduction	■ Communication with surgical oncologist is key to ensure lumpectomy markings are in planned incision for reduction.

Flap reconstruction	▪ Evaluate the lumpectomy defect during first surgery to plan flap type/design. ▪ Intraoperative perfusion assessment with indocyanine green dye fluorescent angiography is a useful tool if concern for flap perfusion, nipple viability or pending skin necrosis. ▪ For perforator flaps, identifying and monitoring the perforator with a handheld Doppler ultrasound is key.
Fat grafting	▪ Gentle processing and grafting in small, dispersed aliquots increase survivability. ▪ Often requires multiple episodes of grafting due to variable graft survivability, especially in radiated bed. ▪ Place fat below tethered scar in radiated areas to prevent recurrence.

POSTOPERATIVE CARE

- Patients undergoing oncoplastic reduction or fat grafting may be outpatient. Patients receiving flap reconstruction likely observed for 1 to 2 days.
- Surgical support bra but avoid excessive compression to flap or areas of fat grafting. Compression garments to fat grafting harvest sites will limit postoperative ecchymosis and edema.
- Any postoperative wounds or infection must be addressed immediately to avoid delays to radiation therapy.
- Drains can be used to minimize risk of postoperative seroma and edema.
- Counsel patients that fat grafting can often result in changes to mammography and other breast imaging, which can result in patient anxiety and additional need for biopsy.

COMPLICATIONS AND CONSIDERATIONS

- Fat necrosis and oil cysts can occur and are more common with larger volume fat grafting and if excessive fat is injected with each pass.
- Full/partial flap loss may result in fat necrosis and the need for revision.
- Wound healing complications or infection can delay radiation therapy.
- Need for future revisions, persistent asymmetry. Recommend 3+ month intervals between repeat episodes of fat grafting to the same location.
- Injection of fat into large vessels can result in fat embolism, which is rare when blunt and appropriately sized injection cannulas are used.
- Loss of NAC—may require reconstruction or FNG if this occurs.

ACKNOWLEDGMENTS

We gratefully acknowledge the contributions of Julie E. Park, Jonathan Bank, and David H. Song as portions of their chapter were retained in this revision.

SUGGESTED READINGS

1. Hamdi M, Van Landuyt K, de Frene B, et al. The versatility of the inter-costal artery perforator (ICAP) flaps. *J Plast Reconstr Aesthet Surg*. 2006;59(6):644-652.
2. Hamdi M, Van Landuyt K, Hijjawi JB, et al. Surgical technique in pedicled thoracodorsal artery perforator flaps: a clinical experience with 99 patients. *Plast Reconstr Surg*. 2008;121(5):1632-1641.
3. Losken A, Styblo TM, Carlson GW, et al. Management algorithm and outcome evaluation of partial mastectomy defects treated using reduction or mastopexy techniques. *Ann Plast Surg*. 2007;59(3):235-242.
4. Roughton MC, Shenaq D, Jaskowiak N, et al. Optimizing delivery of breast conservation therapy: a multidisciplinary approach to oncoplastic surgery. *Ann Plast Surg*. 2012;69(3):250-255.

Chapter 15 Cryoablation of Breast Cancer

Michael S. Sabel

DEFINITION

- Cryoablation is a percutaneous procedure that uses freezing temperatures to destroy tumors. It has been used successfully to treat a variety of tumors, including breast cancer (**FIGURE 1**).
- Cryoablation as a cancer treatment is based on the immediate and delayed impact of freezing temperatures on cellular structure. When tissues are frozen to temperatures less than −40°C, extracellular water freezes, intracellular osmolarity increases, and water is drawn out of cells leading to cellular dehydration. During thawing, this reverses, the cells swell and rupture. In addition, ice crystals damage organelles and plasma membranes. Cryoablation also causes endothelial dysfunction, thrombus formation, ischemia, and platelet aggregation.
- Once injured by freezing, tissues conduct cold temperature even more efficiently. A second freeze enhances those lethal effects and expands the area of tumor necrosis. Thus, cryoablation of breast cancer utilizes two freeze-thaw cycles.
- There is emerging, promising data from phase II clinical trials examining cryoablation as an alternative to lumpectomy for early-stage breast cancer.[1,2] However, lumpectomy (or mastectomy) should still be considered the standard of care. Cryoablation may be considered in patients who are not candidates for surgery, or who refuse surgery.

PATIENT HISTORY AND PHYSICAL FINDINGS

- The initial workup to the patient should be the same as with any patient with early-stage breast cancer.
- Cryoablation is typically considered in older patients with hormone receptor positive, Her-2/neu negative disease, and as such many patients being considered for cryoablation may not need radiation therapy (RT). However, if postablation radiation therapy is planned as a component of local therapy, contraindications to radiation should be ruled out. This includes patients with prior radiation to the breast or chest wall, or a history of collagen-vascular diseases such as scleroderma, lupus, or dermatomyositis.
- A detailed family history is important to determine whether genetic counseling and testing is indicated. High-risk patients may want to consider bilateral mastectomy for both treatment of the known cancer and risk reduction.
- A complete, bilateral breast exam should be performed to characterize the mass and potentially identify additional areas of concern that may represent multicentric disease. Lesions involving or extremely close to the skin or nipple may be poor candidates for cryoablation.
- Physical exam of the axillary, supraclavicular, and cervical should be performed to rule out clinical node involvement. Suspicious adenopathy should prompt appropriate imaging and biopsy.
- For clinically node-negative patients, it should be determined whether the patient will need a sentinel lymph node (SLN) biopsy. Cryoablation does not require intravenous (IV) sedation or general anesthesia. If SLN biopsy is indicated and cryoablation is desired, the procedure can be performed in the operating room (OR) at the same time as the SLN biopsy. Alternatively, SLN biopsy can be performed prior to cryoablation if the information will guide local therapy decisions.

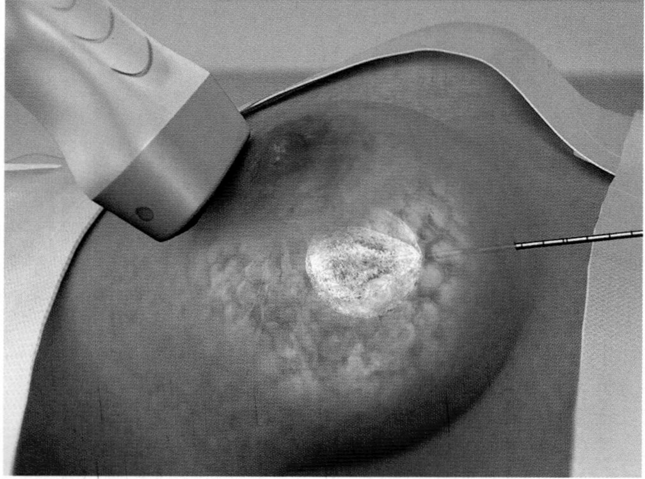

FIGURE 1 ● Cryoablation involves the percutaneous placement of a probe in the center of a tumor under ultrasound guidance and freezing the tumor and a margin of normal breast tissue surrounding the tumor. (Figure courtesy of IceCure Medical, LTD.)

IMAGING AND OTHER DIAGNOSTIC STUDIES

- To determine whether a patient is a candidate for cryoablation, a mammogram and ultrasound is essential. Magnetic resonance imaging (MRI) may also be useful, and some clinicians consider MRI an essential component of the preoperative workup.
- The tumor must be visualized under ultrasound to be a candidate for cryoablation. The best clinical results are achieved when the primary tumor is <15 mm in size.[3-5]
- In addition to the size of the lesion, attention should be paid to how close the lesion is to the skin and to the chest wall. While rarely reported, thermal injury (frostbite and possible skin necrosis) is the most concerning complication of cryoablation. Lesions too close to the skin may be poor candidates for cryoablation. Likewise, lesions close to the pectoralis major muscle may be less suitable candidates, although some freezing of the muscle can be tolerated.
- Core needle biopsy is critical in determining whether a patient is suitable for cryoablation. Cryoablation is dependent upon imaging, and certain histologies may be associated with underestimation of size on imaging. Initial trials of cryoablation have shown that cryoablation is less effective in patients with lobular carcinoma or patients with an extensive intraductal component (EIC).[3,4]

- In addition to histology, grade, ER, PR, and Her-2/neu status should be considered when selecting patients for cryoablation. Most of the data regarding the efficacy of cryoablation has been in women with grade 1 or 2, hormone sensitive, Her-2/neu negative tumors. While cryoablation may be considered in patients with other subtypes, there is less data regarding outcomes.

- See **Video 1**.

ROOM SETUP AND PRETREATMENT CALCULATIONS

- Cryoablation is an office-based procedure that requires the user to use ultrasound for both probe placement and monitoring the development of the ice ball. The room should be set up so that the physician has access to both the ultrasound and cryoprobe and visualization of both monitors (**FIGURE 2**).
- Before prepping and draping assure that the cryoablation machine is working and that there is an adequate supply of liquid nitrogen. The cryoablation system typically has a diagnostic run-through that includes holding the cryoprobe in sterile water to observe the development of ice at the tip of the probe.
- Prior to prepping and draping, an ultrasound should be performed to confirm that the lesion is (1) still visible on ultrasound and (2) has not increased in the size beyond the maximum dimensions. It should be assured that the probe can be easily placed and the saline can be injected; otherwise, the patient can be repositioned.
- Measurements are taken and should include the tumor length and width, the distance from the skin to the top of the tumor, and the distance from the bottom of the tumor to the chest wall.
- Based on the size of the tumor, calculate the necessary distance from the tip of the probe to the far end of the tumor. The probe has a defined segment that freezes (**FIGURE 3**).
  - The ice ball that develops will typically be an oval along the length of the probe and the center of the tumor should be the center of the freezing segment. The formula is the width of the tumor subtracted from the freezing segment length, divided by 2.
  - As an example, if there is a 4-cm freezing segment and a 1.8-cm wide tumor, the tip of the probe should be (40-18)/2 or 11 mm past the far edge of the tumor.
- As the best candidates for cryoablation at this time are usually older women, calculate the maximum volume of xylocaine that can be used during the case. For plain lidocaine, the maximum dose is 4.5 mg/kg. The volume then depends on the concentration. One percent lidocaine is recommended, which is 10 mg per 1 mL, so divide the maximum dose by 10 to calculate the maximum volume.
  - As an example, a 150 lb patient is 68 kg. Therefore the maximum dose is 68 × 4.5 or 306, which translates to a maximum volume for 1% lidocaine of 30 mL.

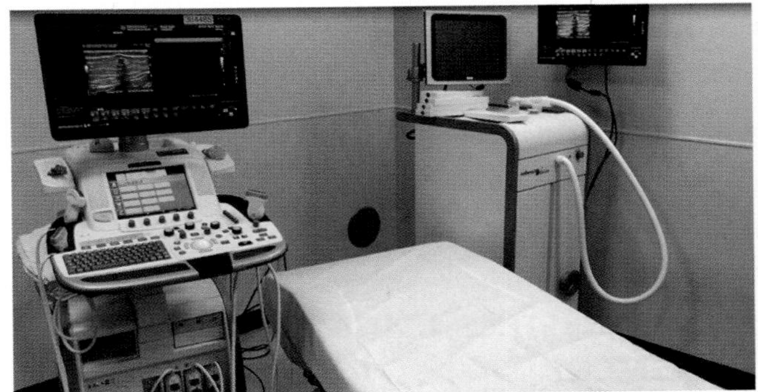

FIGURE 2 ● Room setup for breast cancer cryoablation. The physician has access to the probes and visualization of both monitors.

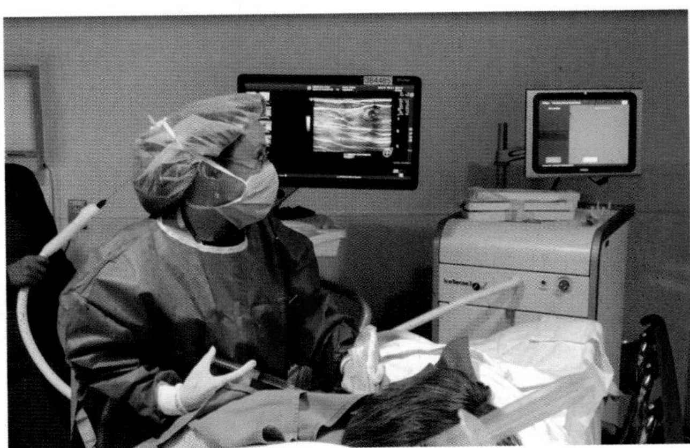

FIGURE 3 ● Xylocaine is used to anesthetize between the insertion site and the tumor. It should also be injected above and below the tumor both for anesthesia and to increase the distance between the tumor and the skin and/or chest wall.

POSITIONING

- The patient is positioned in a way that allows for the following:
  - Insertion of the cryoprobe parallel to the chest wall so it can be easily advanced through the center of the tumor. Often, the scar from the core biopsy incision is the best insertion site for the cryoprobe.
  - Injection of xylocaine or saline between the tumor and the skin or between the tumor and the chest wall.
- The patient may either be supine, or slightly angled with a wedge placed beneath the shoulder. In rare cases, the patient may be in the lateral decubitus position.
- The arm is positioned so it does not interfere with probe placement. This may be above the head. It is important to keep in mind that the patient will need to maintain this position for 30 to 40 minutes, so ensure the patient is comfortable before beginning. This may require support for the arm.

PREPPING AND DRAPING

- The sterile setup should include sterile gel, syringes, and needles for injection of xylocaine. Syringes, needles, and extension tubing for injection of saline, and an 11-blade scalpel.
- The entire breast is prepped and draped in aseptic fashion, allowing adequate access. The ultrasound transducer is placed in a sterile drape.

LOCAL ANESTHESIA AND PROBE PLACEMENT

- The entire procedure is performed under ultrasound visualization. Using a 25-gauge needle, xylocaine is used to raise a wheal at the site of insertion, which is often the scar from the prior core biopsy. An 11-blade is then used to make a small nick in the skin. A slightly larger needle (21 g) can then be used to anesthetize the breast tissue leading to the mass (**FIGURE 3**).
- Lidocaine should then be injected above and below the lesion. In addition to local anesthesia, this can be used to increase the distance between the ice ball and the skin and/or chest wall.
- For lesions close to the chest wall, injection beneath the tumor can move the tumor away from the chest wall. However, there may be some freezing of the muscle, and so the muscle beneath the tumor should also be anesthetized.
- Once adequately anesthetized, the cryoprobe is placed through the skin nick and advanced toward the tumor under ultrasound visualization. The safest approach is to keep the probe parallel to the chest wall, which is facilitated by proper patient positioning.
- The probe is then placed through the center of the tumor. This should be visualized in both the sagittal and transverse orientations to assure the probe is centrally placed and that the distal end of the probe is the appropriate distance from the far margin of the tumor (**FIGURE 4**).

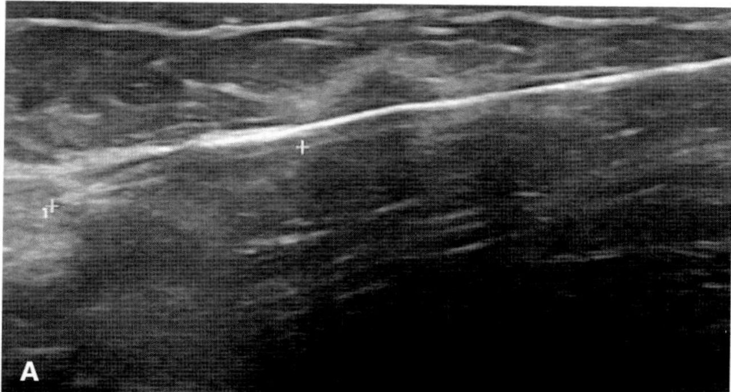

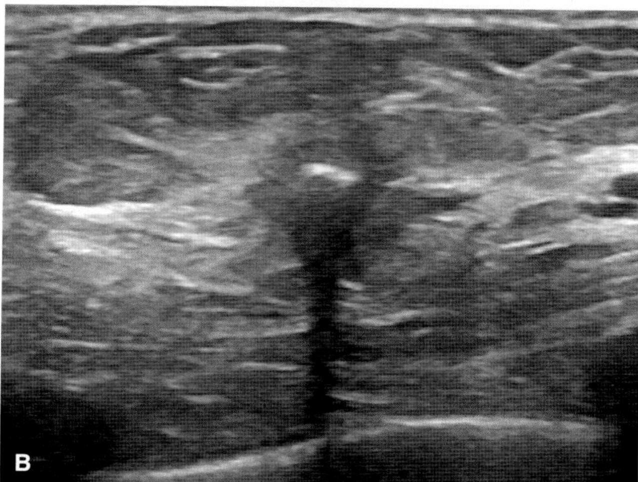

FIGURE 4 ● The probe is confirmed to be in the center of the tumor in both sagittal **(A)** and transverse orientations **(B)**. The distance the tip of the probe needs to go past the tumor is calculated as one-half the difference between the freezing segment of the probe and the tumor size.

CRYOABLATION

- Once proper position of the cryoprobe is assured, the freezing is initiated. Cryoablation involves two freeze-thaw cycles. The length of time for the cycles is determined by the size of the tumor and the necessary margins.
- During the first freeze cycle, the generation of the ice ball around the tumor is easily visualized with US (**FIGURE 5**).
- The most concerning complication of cryoablation is thermal injury to the skin and this is prevented by using hydrodissection to "push" the skin away from the enlarging ice ball. Under US guidance, a needle connected to an extension tube and then a large syringe of saline is advanced between the ice ball and the skin (**FIGURE 6**). Alternatively, a three-way stopcock and a larger bag of saline can be used to avoid having to consistently change syringes. As the saline is slowly injected, the distance between the ice ball and the skin enlarging can be observed. This may need to be done repeatedly as the ice ball enlarges.
- For lesions close to the chest wall, saline can be injected beneath the tumor. Alternatively, once there is an ice ball, the probe can be torqued to move the ice ball away from the chest wall.
- The ice ball should be monitored in both sagittal and transverse orientation. Near the end of the first freeze cycle, measurements of the size of the ice ball should be recorded (**FIGURE 7**).
- At the conclusion of the first freeze cycle, a passive thaw cycle is initiated. During this time, change or refill the dewar containing the liquid nitrogen so as not to run out during the second freeze cycle.
- During the second freeze cycle, saline will still be needed to inject between the skin and ice ball to prevent thermal injury. The second ice ball will develop slightly faster and larger than the first.
- Following the second freeze cycle, the probe cannot be removed until it is actively warmed. Gently twist the probe to assure it is loose, and then the probe can be withdrawn. Hold pressure for several minutes to assure hemostasis.

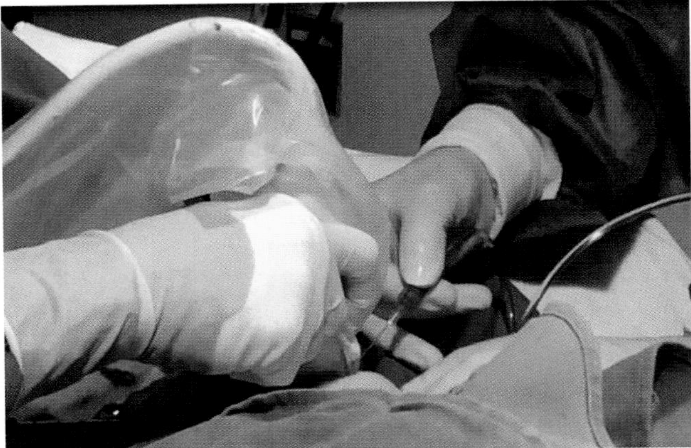

FIGURE 5 ● During the procedure, saline is injected between the tumor and the skin to avoid frostbite of the overlying skin.

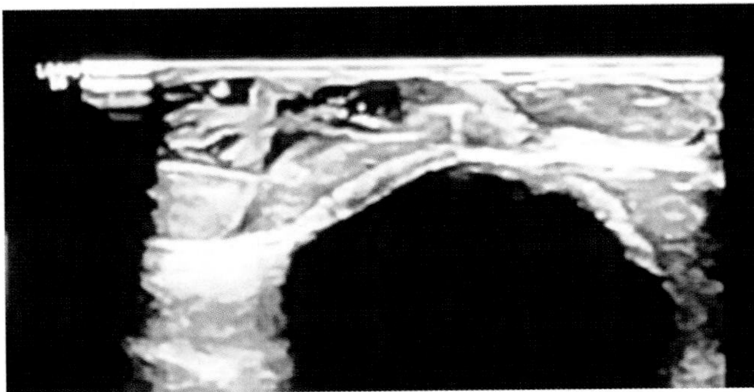

FIGURE 6 ● Ultrasound shows the infiltration of saline in the subcutaneous tissues above the tumor and the increasing distance between the skin and the expanding ice ball.

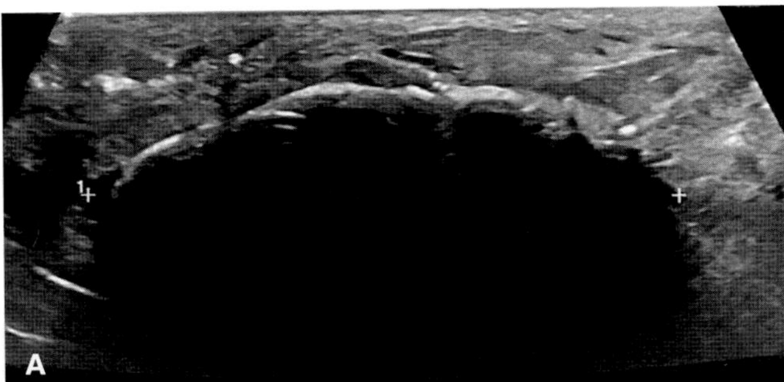

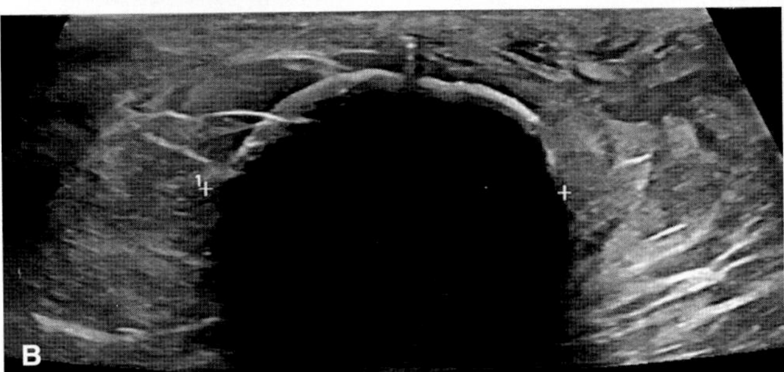

FIGURE 7 ● The ice ball is easily visualized encompassing the tumor with ultrasound. At the completion of the first freeze, measurements are obtained in the **(A)** transverse and **(B)** sagittal views.

PEARLS AND PITFALLS

Patient selection	▪ While the initial data is encouraging, lumpectomy and mastectomy remain the standard of care for breast cancer. Cryoablation may be considered in patients who are high-risk surgical candidates or who refuse surgery. ▪ Studies of cryoablation have shown high success rates with invasive ductal carcinomas ≤1.5 cm. Lobular cancers, DCIS, and cancers with extensive ductal carcinoma may extend beyond what is visualized on imaging and may not undergo complete ablation. ▪ To date, the majority of data detailing the success of cryoablation has been in older patients with hormone sensitive, Her-2 negative, clinically node-negative cancers.
Tumor location	▪ Tumors close to the skin risk frostbite with cryoablation. Injecting saline between the tumor and the skin can avoid this, but tumors too close to the skin, particularly the nipple-areolar complex, are poor candidates for cryoablation. ▪ Tumors close to the chest wall can also be successfully treated by lifting the tumor off the chest wall, and the pectoralis muscle can tolerate some freezing, but tumors abutting or involving the chest wall are poor candidates for cryoablation.
Imaging	▪ With single-probe cryoablation, tumors must be confirmed to be less than 1.5 cm on mammography and ultrasound. Ultrasound is used to guide the procedure so it is essential that the lesion be clearly visible on ultrasonography. MRI can be useful in confirming whether the patient is an appropriate candidate for cryoablation.
Preprocedure	▪ Prior to prepping and draping, confirm that the lesion is ultrasound visible and repeat measurements as these can sometimes differ from prebiopsy measurements. ▪ Calculate how much xylocaine can be used and the distance that the tip of the probe needs to go past the edge of the tumor to assure complete ablation of the tumor with adequate margins. ▪ Make sure the patient is in a comfortable position that allows adequate access.
Procedure	▪ Have plenty of saline available to inject between the skin and the tumor as the ice ball enlarges in order to protect the skin (or beneath the tumor to protect the muscle). ▪ Deep tumors can be moved away from the muscle by angling the probe after the ice ball has started. ▪ Two freeze-thaw cycles are performed. The first thaw is passive, and the second is active in order to remove the probe. ▪ During the second freeze, the ice ball will expand more quickly, and will be larger, so before beginning, make sure you have adequate saline for subcutaneous injection.
Follow-up	▪ Following the procedure, have the patient follow-up in 1 wk to assess for complications and then set up short-term surveillance with imaging. As cryoablation does not allow for margin analysis, close follow-up is critical. ▪ Patients should be referred for adjuvant therapy as the clinical situation warrants. ▪ Follow-up imaging will show classic signs of fat necrosis in the area of the ablation. Any unusual findings or concerns on follow-up imaging should undergo image-guided biopsy.

Postoperative Care

- Following direct pressure, steri-strips can be used to re-approximate the skin incision. Sterile gauze should be secured over this, as there may be some drainage of fluid from the site.
- Over the next few days, patients will experience some swelling, erythema, and tenderness at the site. This is typically well-controlled with acetaminophen or ibuprofen. If some of the pectoralis major is frozen, this can increase post-operative pain, although narcotics are rarely needed.
- Patients should be informed of the swelling and that there may be some color changes in the skin following cryoablation.
- The patient should return to the office in 1 week for a post-treatment visit. Quite often the patient had a nonpalpable tumor at diagnosis, but now there will be a palpable mass at the site of the ablation, and the patient should be made aware that this will likely remain palpable for at least 6 months, and potentially >1 year.
- At this postoperative visit, the patient should be schedule for close surveillance, and set up with referrals to radiation oncology or medical oncology as indicated by the clinical case, no different than if the patient had a lumpectomy.

REFERENCES

1. Simmons RM, Ballman KV, Cox C, et al. A phase II trial exploring the success of cryoablation therapy in the treatment of invasive breast carcinoma: results from ACOSOG (Alliance) Z1072. *Ann Surg Oncol*. 2016;23:2438-2445.
2. Fine RE, Gilmore RC, Dietz JR, et al. Cryoablation without excision for low-risk early-stage breast cancer: 3-year interim analysis of ipsilateral breast tumor recurrence in the ICE3 trial. *Ann Surg Oncol*. 2021;28:5525-5534.
3. Sabel MS, Kaufman CS, Whitworth PW, et al. Cryoablation of early stage breast cancer: work-in-progress report of a multi-institutional trial. *Ann Surg Oncol*. 2004;11:542-549.
4. Poplack SP, Levine GM, Henry L, et al. A pilot study of ultrasound-guided cryoablation of invasive ductal carcinomas up to 15 mm with MRI follow-up and subsequent surgical resection. *AJR Am J Roentgenol*. 2015;204:1100-1108.
5. Pfleiderer SO, Freesmeyer MG, Marx C, et al. Cryotherapy of breast cancer under ultrasound guidance: initial results and limitations. *Eur Radiol*. 2002;12:3009-3014.

Chapter 16 Sentinel Lymph Node Biopsy for Breast Cancer

Anees B. Chagpar

DEFINITION

- Sentinel lymph node biopsy (SLNB) is a minimally invasive means to accurately stage the axilla in patients with breast cancer.

PATIENT HISTORY AND PHYSICAL FINDINGS

- As always, a complete history and physical examination is warranted. If the patient has obvious clinically enlarged axillary lymph nodes on physical examination, ultrasound and/or fine needle aspiration or core needle biopsy may provide diagnostic information. If the biopsied node is positive, one could proceed to neoadjuvant chemotherapy. Although historically a positive node on needle biopsy would mandate an axillary lymph node dissection (ALND) if primary surgery is planned, trials such as the American College of Surgeons Oncology Group (ACOSOG) Z-11 trial have now found that such patients should still undergo SLNB as patients with one to two positive nodes may be able to avoid ALND. If the needle biopsied node is negative, sentinel node biopsy is still indicated for definitive evaluation.[1]

IMAGING AND OTHER DIAGNOSTIC STUDIES

- Lymphoscintigraphy is commonly obtained prior to SLNB in breast cancer following the injection of the radioactive tracer; however, it is not truly required in the majority of patients with breast cancer.[2] Many surgeons opt to forgo lymphoscintigraphy and inject the radioactive tracer themselves in the operating room. For patients who have had previous sentinel node biopsy and/or axillary node dissection, repeat sentinel node biopsy may be considered for staging ipsilateral recurrent or new primary disease. In this circumstance, alternative drainage patterns are possible, and therefore, preoperative lymphoscintigraphy may be useful.[3]

SURGICAL MANAGEMENT

- Sentinel node biopsy is indicated for staging of patients with invasive breast cancer or those with ductal carcinoma in situ undergoing mastectomy.

Preoperative Planning

- It has now been well established that, in clinically node negative patients undergoing neoadjuvant chemotherapy, SLNB after neoadjuvant chemotherapy can accurately stage the axilla, particularly if a dual tracer technique is used and several sentinel nodes are harvested.[4,5] This will allow patients who have had a pathologic complete response to be spared the morbidity of a complete axillary dissection. For patients who were clinically node positive prior to neoadjuvant chemotherapy, a targeted dissection should be planned.

Positioning

- Patients are positioned supine. A roll may be placed under the ipsilateral shoulder so as to elevate the latissimus dorsi muscle. Care should be exercised to ensure that the arm is supported on folded sheets so as to avoid a brachial plexus stretch injury (**FIGURE 1**).
- Intravenous lines, pulse oximeter devices, and blood pressure cuffs should be placed on other extremities if possible.

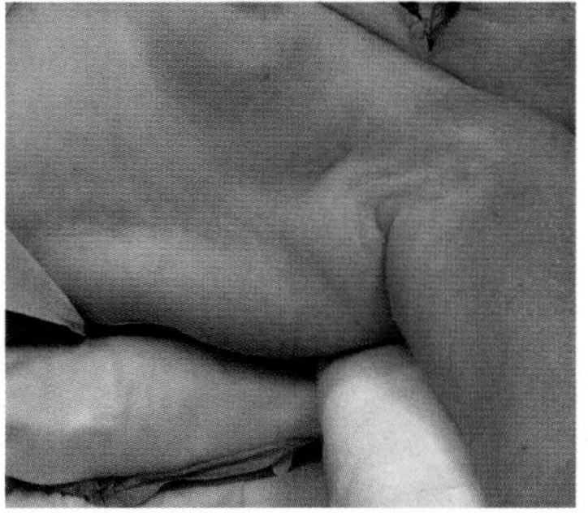

FIGURE 1 ● Patient positioned with roll under ipsilateral latissimus and folded sheets to support arm.

INJECTION OF RADIOACTIVE TRACER AND/OR BLUE DYE

- Use of dual tracer has been shown to be associated with higher identification and lower false-negative rates[6]; however, particularly in patients undergoing skin-sparing mastectomy, surgeons may wish to forgo blue dye, as the dye may discolor the skin and make it more difficult to evaluate for skin ischemia or necrosis.
  - In general, the radioactive tracer used is technetium-99m, sulfur colloid. This is often injected in nuclear medicine in a periareolar fashion prior to lymphoscintigraphy. However, lymphoscintigraphy is not absolutely necessary, so this can be injected in the operating room, after induction. This may be beneficial to the patient, as the injection can be quite painful. Generally a dose of 0.5 mCi is used.
  - Both isosulfan and methylene blue dye have been used for SLNB; they vary in their color, complication profile, and cost. Isosulfan blue is a more azure blue (which is easier to distinguish from venous structures) but is associated with less than 1% risk of anaphylaxis[7] and is significantly more costly than methylene blue. Methylene blue is darker, associated with a higher rate of skin necrosis, but is far less expensive.[8] In general, 5 mL of these tracers is used.
- Blue dye may be injected peritumoral, or using a subareolar approach, which allows for lymphatic mapping of multiple tumors and those that are not palpable[9] (**FIGURE 2**).

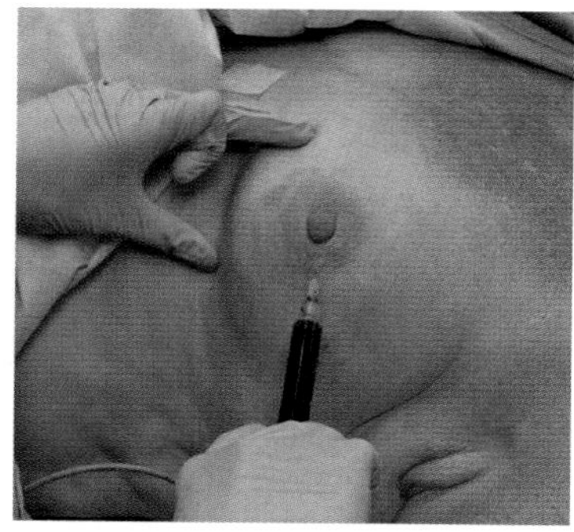

FIGURE 2 ● Subareolar injection of blue dye.

PREPPING AND DRAPING

- The arm is prepped circumferentially along with the breast. The arm is draped into the field and kept free such that the surgeon may move the arm in a sterile fashion during the case (**FIGURE 3**).

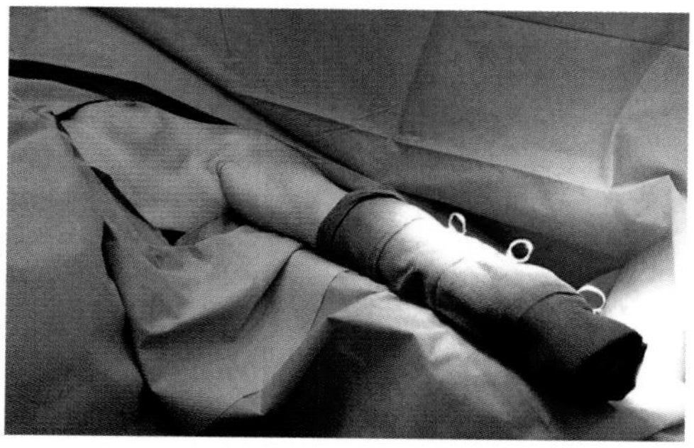

FIGURE 3 ● Patient draped with breast and axilla in the field; the ipsilateral arm is draped in the sterile field.

INCISION

- Identification of the area of maximal radioactivity in the axilla using a handheld gamma probe allows one to position the incision over the sentinel node.
- Landmarks of the pectoralis and latissimus dorsi muscle are used to fashion an incision for an axillary dissection of which the sentinel node incision would be a segment (**FIGURE 4**). A lazy S incision will allow for optimal cosmesis and will allow for extension superiorly and inferiorly if needed for maximal visualization. Alternatively, if a conventional mastectomy is planned, the sentinel node biopsy can often be performed through the lateral aspect of the same incision.
- Local anesthetic may be used for preemptive analgesia. The incision is taken down through skin, subcutaneous tissue, and clavipectoral fascia.

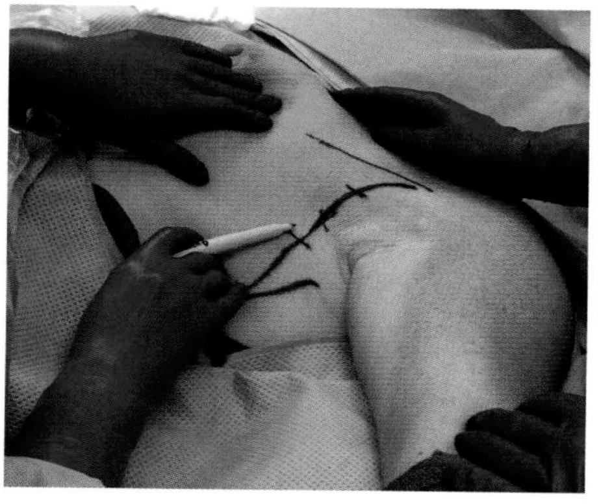

FIGURE 4 ● Incision planning. The pectoralis and latissimus dorsi muscle borders are identified. An "X" marks the area of maximal radioactivity. A lazy S incision is fashioned for a potential axillary dissection going through the X. A smaller segment (marked by the crosshatch lines) delineates the incision for the sentinel node biopsy.

IDENTIFICATION OF SENTINEL NODES

- Care is taken to remove the hottest node and any node with radioactive counts greater than 10% of the ex vivo counts of the hottest node. In addition, all blue nodes and those at the end of a blue lymphatic channel are also removed (**FIGURE 5**).
- Palpation is critical to identify any clinically suspicious lymph nodes; these should also be removed regardless of whether they are blue or hot, as tracers may not have traveled to positive lymph nodes if lymphatics are obstructed with tumor.
- Although some have argued that the procedure can be terminated after three sentinel lymph nodes (SLNs) have been removed,[10] others have argued that all nodes that fit the earlier mentioned criteria be removed.[11] On average, however, two sentinel nodes are identified.

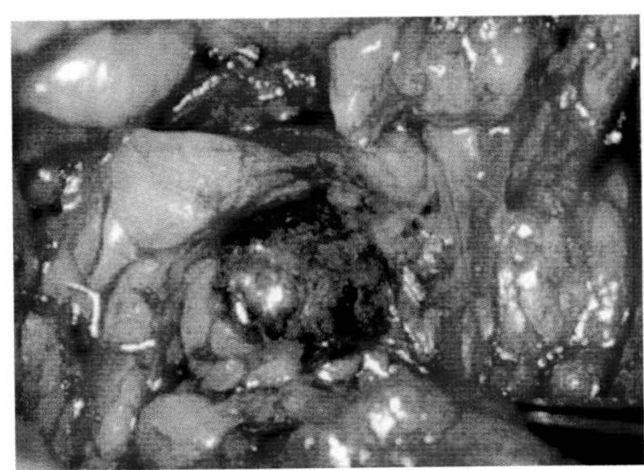

FIGURE 5 ● Blue SLN at the end of a blue lymphatic channel.

INTRAOPERATIVE EVALUATION

- Intraoperative evaluation with either touch preparation cytology or frozen section has been found to have a high specificity and fairly high sensitivity (**FIGURE 6**).
- Some surgeons may opt to forgo intraoperative evaluation if they do not intend to complete the axillary node dissection at the same operative setting given the findings of the sentinel node biopsy. For patients who fit the American College of Surgeons Oncology Group Z0011 criteria, completion axillary node dissection may be avoided if only one to two sentinel nodes are positive and whole breast irradiation after partial mastectomy is planned.[1]

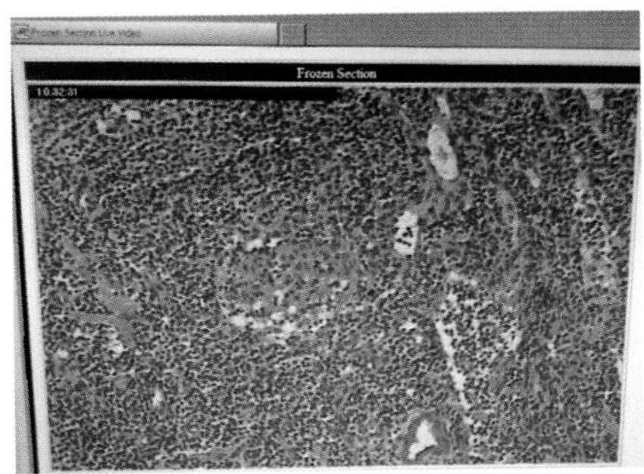

FIGURE 6 ● Intraoperative frozen section results.

CLOSURE

- In general, if axillary node dissection is not performed, no drains are required. The incision is closed in standard fashion with subdermal and subcuticular sutures followed by Steri-Strips. If, however, an axillary dissection is indicated, the incision can be extended (as planned in the earlier discussion).

POSTOPERATIVE CARE

- After sentinel node biopsy alone (ie, without axillary dissection), patients can go back to usual activities. No special exercises are required nor is there any need for lymphedema compression garments.

OUTCOMES

- Outcomes after sentinel node biopsy alone are outstanding, with no detriment in survival or local recurrence. Morbidity is low, especially compared with axillary dissection.

COMPLICATIONS

- Bleeding/hematoma
- Infection
- Seroma
- Numbness/paresthesia
- Lymphedema
- Allergic reaction to isosulfan blue dye
- "Blue breast" from blue dye injection
- Skin or fat necrosis from methylene blue dye

REFERENCES

1. Giuliano AE, Ballman KV, McCall L, et al. Effect of axillary dissection vs no axillary dissection on 10-year overall survival among women with invasive breast cancer and sentinel node metastasis: the ACOSOG Z0011 (Alliance) randomized clinical trial. *JAMA*. 2017;318(10):918-926.
2. McMasters KM, Wong SL, Tuttle TM, et al. Preoperative lymphoscintigraphy for breast cancer does not improve the ability to identify axillary sentinel lymph nodes. *Ann Surg*. 2000;231:724-731.
3. Port ER, Fey J, Gemignani ML, et al. Reoperative sentinel lymph node biopsy: a new option for patients with primary or locally recurrent breast carcinoma. *J Am Coll Surg*. 2002;195:167-172.

4. Kuehn T, Bauerfeind I, Fehm T, et al. Sentinel-lymph-node biopsy in patients with breast cancer before and after neoadjuvant chemotherapy (SENTINA): a prospective, multicentre cohort study. *Lancet Oncol*. 2013;14(7):609-618.
5. Boughey JC, Suman VJ, Mittendorf EA, et al. Sentinel lymph node surgery after neoadjuvant chemotherapy in patients with node-positive breast cancer: the ACOSOG Z1071 (Alliance) clinical trial. *JAMA*. 2013;310(14):1455-1461.
6. Chagpar AB, Martin RC, Scoggins CR, et al. Factors predicting failure to identify a sentinel lymph node in breast cancer. *Surgery*. 2005;138:56-63.
7. Albo D, Wayne JD, Hunt KK, et al. Anaphylactic reactions to isosulfan blue dye during sentinel lymph node biopsy for breast cancer. *Am J Surg*. 2001;182:393-398.
8. Simmons RM, Smith SM, Osborne MP. Methylene blue dye as an alternative to isosulfan blue dye for sentinel lymph node localization. *Breast J*. 2001;7:181-183.
9. Chagpar A, Martin RCIII, Chao C, et al. Validation of subareolar and periareolar injection techniques for breast sentinel lymph node biopsy. *Arch Surg*. 2004;139:614-618.
10. Zakaria S, Degnim AC, Kleer CG, et al. Sentinel lymph node biopsy for breast cancer: how many nodes are enough? *J Surg Onc*. 2007;96:554-559.
11. Chagpar AB, Scoggins CR, Martin RC, et al. Are 3 sentinel nodes sufficient? *Arch Surg*. 2007;142:456-459.

Chapter 17

Sentinel Lymph Node Surgery With Resection of the Index Biopsy-Proven Positive Node (Targeted Axillary Dissection)

Robert M. Pride and Judy C. Boughey

DEFINITION

- Neoadjuvant chemotherapy has become a more common component of treatment plans for breast cancer patients, particularly for patients with more aggressive tumor biology (triple-negative and HER2-positive breast cancer) and those with advanced disease.[1-4]
- Axillary pathologic complete response (pCR) following neoadjuvant chemotherapy is achieved in approximately 40% of node-positive breast cancer patients.[5,6] Rates of pCR vary by biologic subtype with rates as high as 70% in HER2-positive disease treated with neoadjuvant chemotherapy and targeted anti-HER2 therapy.
- Growing evidence suggests that axillary lymph node dissection may be omitted for patients presenting with biopsy-proven node-positive disease that converts to sentinel node-negative disease following neoadjuvant chemotherapy.[5-9]
- Recent focus has centered around decreasing the false-negative rate of axillary sentinel lymph node surgery following neoadjuvant therapy. Sentinel lymph node surgery plus ensuring resection of the index biopsy-proven positive lymph node with the use of preoperative localization (called targeted axillary dissection [TAD]) has been identified as a reliable technique to minimize the false-negative rate of sentinel lymph node surgery after neoadjuvant chemotherapy.[5,10-15]
- TAD is utilized to assess response after neoadjuvant therapy to identify the subset of patients with eradication of nodal disease, also known as a nodal pCR. These patients can thus avoid completion axillary dissection, greatly reducing the risk of long-term associated morbidities.
- This technique has become an acceptable alternative to axillary dissection in select breast cancer patients with confirmed nodal disease at initial diagnosis who have a good clinical and imaging response to neoadjuvant therapy.

PATIENT SELECTION

- Sentinel lymph node surgery/targeted axillary dissection should be considered in patients presenting with invasive breast cancer and biopsy-proven nodal disease who are treated with neoadjuvant chemotherapy. Eligible patients include those with cN1 nodal disease; however, this has also been extrapolated to selected patients with cN2 and cN3 disease such as those whose axillary disease burden is low and extra-axillary disease will be treated with radiation.
- For patients who present with clinically positive nodal disease by imaging and are treated with neoadjuvant hormone therapy alone without chemotherapy, sentinel lymph node surgery/targeted axillary dissection is an option. However, nodal pCR rates with hormone therapy are low and thus likelihood of negative sentinel lymph nodes is low.[16,17]
- Currently, TAD is not recommended in patients with inflammatory breast cancer.
- Data are lacking in patients with recurrent breast cancer, although the concept can be extrapolated to this group on a case-by-case basis.
- Upfront knowledge of which patients are most likely to respond well to neoadjuvant chemotherapy is also important for patient selection and pretreatment counseling. Factors associated with nodal pCR include[2,18-21]:
  - Lower clinical N category at presentation (cN1 vs cN2-3)
  - HER2-positive status
  - Triple-negative status

PATIENT HISTORY AND PHYSICAL FINDINGS AT INITIAL BREAST CANCER DIAGNOSIS

- A comprehensive history and physical examination are performed as part of the initial consultation at the time of diagnosis with breast cancer. The history should be detailed, including questions pertaining to medical conditions, medications, prior surgeries, and allergies. It is important to query any musculoskeletal issues that could impact operative positioning. It is also important to evaluate for any family history of breast or ovarian cancer.
- Genetic testing should be offered and available to all patients with a current breast cancer diagnosis, as outlined by the American Society of Breast Surgeon guidelines.[22] If a strong family history of breast or ovarian cancer exists, genetic counseling and genetic testing should be strongly recommended as this can not only impact surgical recommendations but also systemic therapy options.
- Physical examination starts with an inspection of bilateral breasts. The patient should be examined first with the arms at the patients' side followed by having the arms elevated. Assessment should focus on any asymmetry, nipple retraction, prior scars, or skin changes.
- Palpation of the breasts should be performed both in a sitting and supine position and can be in a circular or vertical pattern. Palpable masses should have bidimensional measurements and should be assessed for chest wall adherence and skin proximity. Document distance from the nipple and "o'clock" position. Photographs of any visible abnormalities should be taken. These characteristics should be well-documented, as it will be important for comparison to assess response to therapy.
- A thorough examination of the lymph node basins should be performed, including the axillary, cervical, supraclavicular, and infraclavicular nodes.

IMAGING AND OTHER DIAGNOSTIC STUDIES PRIOR TO NEOADJUVANT THERAPY

Preoperative Imaging

- Comprehensive breast imaging should be performed prior to initiation of any neoadjuvant therapy. The goals of pretherapy imaging are to determine the extent of disease for local-regional staging and screening of the contralateral breast.
- Diagnostic mammography should be obtained and should include full-field craniocaudal, mediolateral oblique, and mediolateral views, with spot compression or magnification at the site of interest. Full-field craniocaudal and mediolateral oblique views of the contralateral breast should also be obtained. Digital breast tomosynthesis may be utilized as part of the diagnostic evaluation.
- A targeted breast ultrasound should be performed to help characterize any mass(es).
- Core needle biopsy of the breast mass(es) can subsequently be performed under ultrasound, stereotactic, or magnetic resonance imaging (MRI) guidance. The biopsy tissue should be assessed for pathology including in situ carcinoma or invasive disease. Immunohistochemistry assays should also be performed to assess for receptor status, specifically estrogen receptor, progesterone receptor, and human epidermal growth factor receptor 2 (HER2), and consider Ki67 testing in hormone receptor–positive, HER2-negative disease.
- All patients with biopsy-proven invasive breast cancer should undergo ultrasound of the ipsilateral regional axillary nodal basin. Some centers also routinely image the infraclavicular and internal mammary nodes. Abnormal nodes are defined as having eccentric cortical thickening to >3 mm, having irregular margins, or having hilar fat displacement.
- Biopsy of the most abnormal node should be performed for pathologic evaluation. If metastasis is demonstrated, this lymph node should be marked (using a clip, or tattoo or marking device). The most common practice is to place a titanium clip into the sampled lymph node. Use of a large, sonographically visible clip is recommended to assist with identification after neoadjuvant therapy. Appropriate placement of the clip can then be confirmed with postprocedural X-ray (**FIGURE 1**).
- If disease is identified within any lymph node(s) during the workup, a multidisciplinary team should be assembled to consider neoadjuvant therapy options for node-positive breast cancer.
- For patients who will receive neoadjuvant therapy, bilateral breast MRI should be obtained to further characterize extent of disease prior to therapy. Breast MRI also captures axillary disease burden and can be used later as reference to assess response.
- If there are any signs and/or symptoms of metastatic disease, further workup including labs and more extensive imaging (PET-CT or CT chest/abdomen/pelvis and bone scan) is recommended.[23] Staging for distant disease is recommended in the setting Stage III disease and considered in cases with extensive nodal disease and high-risk tumor biology.

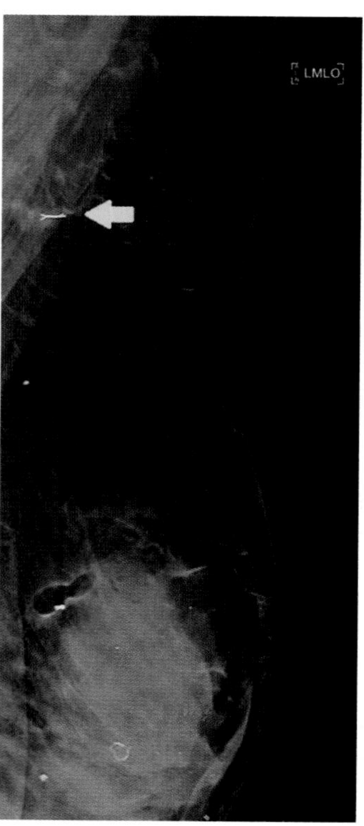

FIGURE 1 • Postprocedural X-ray confirming appropriate position of clip within abnormal axillary lymph node. *Yellow arrow* points to the node containing an X-shaped titanium clip.

POST-NEOADJUVANT THERAPY EVALUATION AND IMAGING

- At present, no test is reliable enough to determine pCR without surgery. However, physical examination together with imaging do yield insight into the likelihood of pCR following neoadjuvant therapy. This information can be used to guide surgical decision-making, particularly with regards to use of sentinel lymph node surgery/targeted axillary dissection.
- After completion of neoadjuvant therapy, patients should be reexamined to assess for response both in the breast and in the axilla. A thorough physical examination, as described earlier, should be performed and compared to the examination findings from the initial consultation visit. The overall accuracy of clinical breast examination for determining pCR in patients with locally advanced breast cancer after neoadjuvant hormonal or chemotherapy is roughly 50% with a negative predictive value (ability to correctly predict pCR) of only about 30%.[24]
- Mammography and ultrasound should also be repeated. Both offer better overall accuracy than physical examination, at 74% and 79% as well as higher negative predictive values at 41% and 44%, respectively.[24]
- Many physicians will utilize MRI in the post-neoadjuvant setting. It has a reported accuracy of 84% and a negative predictive value of 65%.[24] In general, the imaging modality that best demonstrated extent of disease at presentation is usually the best modality to use to assess response in an individual.

- Importantly, preoperative axillary ultrasound following neoadjuvant therapy should be performed to assess response in the axillary lymph nodes and to confirm whether the marked node is visible. Post-neoadjuvant chemotherapy axillary ultrasound has been reported to decrease the false-negative rates at the time of sentinel lymph node surgery to below 10% for patients with normal axillary ultrasound findings.[25]
- Response in the breast and response in the axilla are often similar; therefore, when considering sentinel lymph node surgery, surgeons should consider both the breast and axillary response by physical examination and imaging. If there is progression of disease in the breast or significant residual tumor in the breast, it is unlikely that there is a nodal pCR.
- The benefit of sentinel lymph node surgery is for those patients who have converted to pathologic negative nodes (ie, nodal pCR). Thus, the benefit of sentinel lymph node surgery is likely low when the post-therapy examination or imaging is consistent with residual disease. Therefore, many surgeons would not offer sentinel lymph node surgery in these scenarios, although it is not an absolute contraindication.

Preoperative Localization of Clipped Node

- Prior to surgery, the clipped axillary lymph node needs to be identified and localized. There are several methods to localize this node for retrieval in the operating room which are outlined below:
  - Iodine-125 seed
    - A radioactive I-125 titanium seed can be placed into the node under imaging guidance. Location is then confirmed by postprocedural X-ray (**FIGURE 2**).

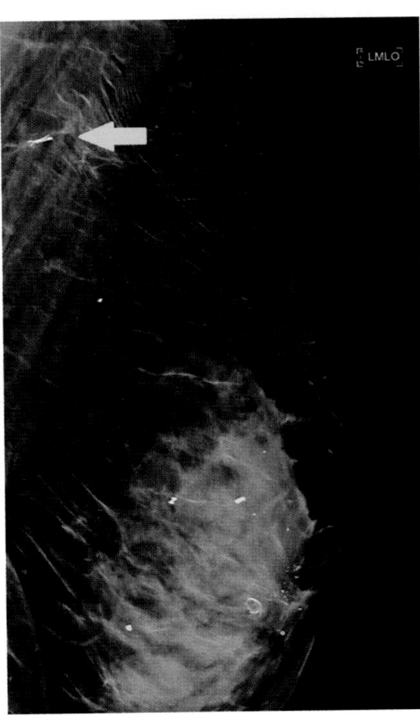

FIGURE 2 ● Postprocedural X-ray confirming appropriate position of seed within previously clipped axillary lymph node following neoadjuvant therapy. *Yellow arrow* points to the node containing both the radioactive seed and an X-shaped clip.

    - These seeds have a half-life of 60 days but are typically placed within 5 days of the planned surgery depending on licensing limitations.
    - In most circumstances, the seed is placed under ultrasound guidance. However, cases where the clip is not sonographically visible can be technically challenging. CT-guided placement of the seed is an alternative method for these challenging cases.
  - Wire localization of the clipped node can be utilized, rather than a seed.
  - Multiple additional methods are now available on the market including SAVI SCOUT and Magseed among other methods, some of which can be placed in the lymph node at time of diagnosis and not require an additional localization procedure prior to surgery.[11-13,26]
  - Tattooing
    - Carbon or charcoal tattooing of the node at the time of initial biopsy has been successfully utilized.[10,27] This method obviates the need for an additional localization procedure prior to surgery and relies on the surgeon being able to visualize the tattooed node.

Preoperative Radioisotope Injection

- Multiple studies have shown that sentinel lymph node identification rates following neoadjuvant chemotherapy are improved with dual-tracer nodal mapping and that dual-tracer mapping decreased the false-negative rate of sentinel lymph node surgery in this setting.[5,7-9,14,28] Thus, dual-tracer mapping should be the standard approach for patients who present with node-positive breast cancer, are treated with neoadjuvant therapy, and subsequently undergo sentinel node surgery.
- Dual-tracer mapping refers to the use of both a radioactive isotope injected preoperatively and an injection of a blue dye at the time of the operation with the goal that the sentinel lymph nodes take up at least one of the agents. This increases the chance that a sentinel node is identified.
- The standard radioisotope utilized for sentinel lymph node surgery is technetium-99 sulfur colloid. It has a half-life of approximately 6 hours and thus is generally injected intradermally at the edge of the areola or subareola on the morning of surgery or the afternoon prior.
- Lymphoscintigraphy can be performed after administration of the tracer to confirm uptake by nodes within the axilla and track any drainage to extra-axillary lymph node basins, although this is not generally necessary in cases without prior breast or axillary surgery.

SURGICAL MANAGEMENT

Preoperative Planning

- All imaging (both from the time of diagnosis and post-neoadjuvant chemotherapy) should be thoroughly reviewed, and preoperative seed localization of the clipped node scheduled, prior to proceeding to the operating room.
- Localization imaging should be reviewed to confirm location of clip(s) and seed(s) in the breast and lymph nodes.
- Appropriate informed consent should be obtained preoperatively, which should include the risks, benefits, and alternatives to the planned operation. It should be clearly discussed that even if preoperative examination and imaging suggest

good response to neoadjuvant therapy, there is still a possibility that residual cancer resides within the lymph nodes and that a completion axillary dissection is recommended if a positive lymph node is identified at sentinel lymph node surgery/targeted axillary dissection.

Positioning

- Patients should be in a supine position with the side of the planned axillary surgery close to the edge of the operating table. The endotracheal tube should be positioned toward the contralateral side of the mouth. Arms should not be abducted greater than 90° to prevent injury to the brachial plexus. Arms should be placed on padded arm boards and positioned in a way that pressure points are alleviated. The arms should be secured to the arm board.
- Blood pressure cuffs and intravenous access lines should be placed on the contralateral upper extremity.
- Sequential compression devices should be placed.
- If the duration of the operation is anticipated to exceed 4 hours, then a Foley catheter should be placed. Otherwise, the patient should void on call to the operating room.

There should be enough space between the operating table and anesthesiologist cart to allow an assistant to stand above the arm.

Blue Dye Injection

- If using methylene blue dye, mix 0.5 cc dye with 3.5 cc dextrose in a 5 cc syringe (1:8 dilution).
  - Alternatively, 1% isosulfan blue is an alternative blue dye that can be used instead of methylene blue. It does not cause nipple necrosis but has been associated with anaphylactic reactions.
- After a preprocedural pause, prior to prepping and draping, the blue dye is injected. If the planned operation includes sparing of the nipple-areolar complex, the dye should be injected in the subareolar space to minimize the risk of nipple necrosis (**FIGURE 3A** and **B**). If the planned operation

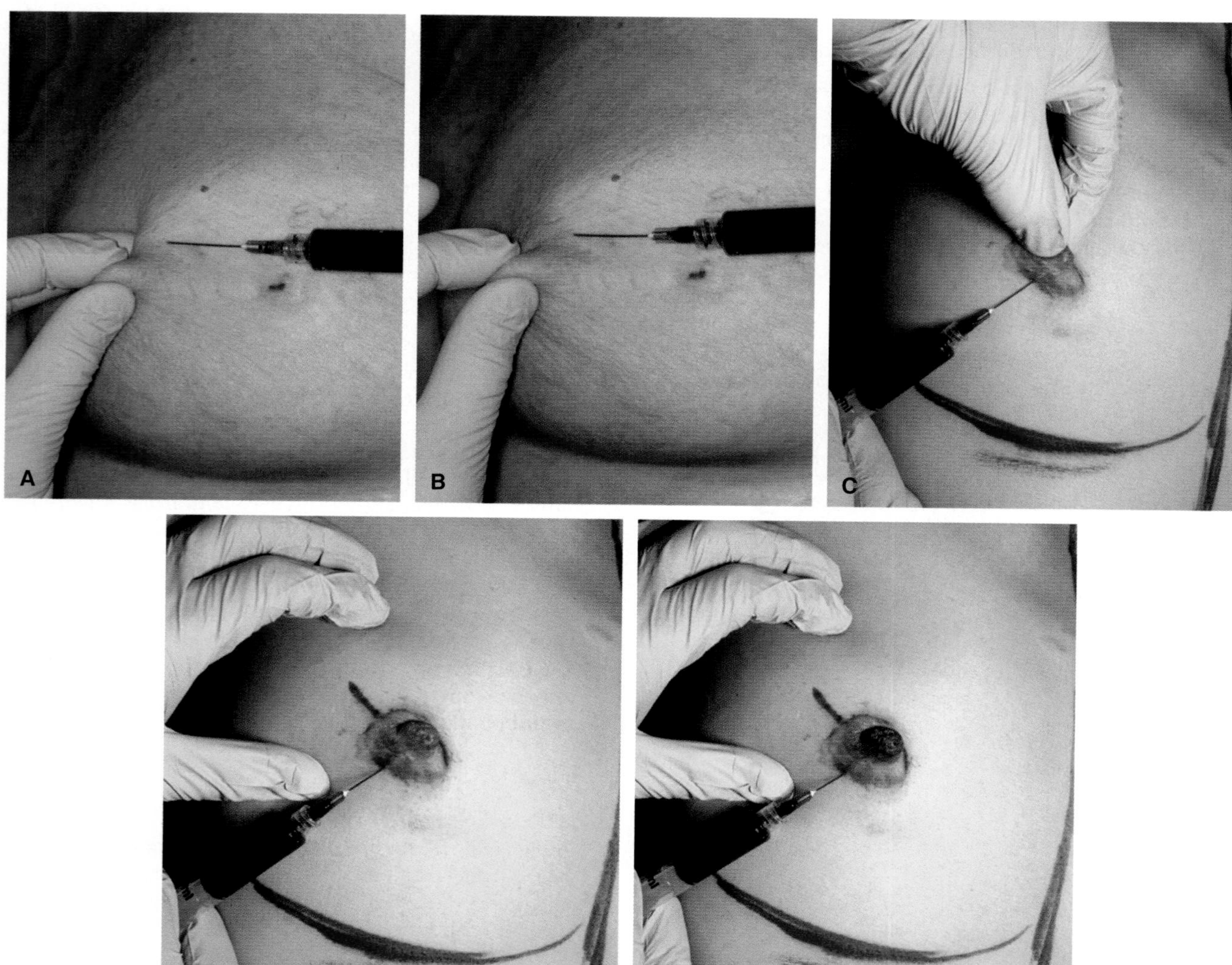

FIGURE 3 ● **A**, In the case of nipple sparing procedures, blue dye is injected in the subareolar space to minimize the risk of nipple necrosis. **B**, A faint blue hue can be seen in the subareolar space, indicating appropriate depth of dye injection. **C**, If the nipple-areolar complex is to be resected as part of the procedure, the blue dye can be injected directly within the nipple. **D**, The nipple begins to turn blue, indicating appropriate location of dye injection. **E**, The nipple becomes entirely blue as more dye is injected.

includes resection of the nipple-areolar complex, the blue dye can be injected directly in the nipple (**FIGURE 3C-E**).

- A 22-gauge needle is typically used, although smaller needles are also acceptable.

Surgical Prep and Incision

- Surgical prep should include the breast and axilla and extend across the midline, inferiorly onto the abdomen, superiorly to the neck and the upper arm, and laterally to the level of the operating table. Draping should ensure preservation of a sterile field with exposure of the entire breast and axilla.
- Prior to marking out an axillary incision, the gamma probe (on the I-125 setting) should be maneuvered over the axilla to ensure the seed is present in the expected location. This can also give an approximate idea for the incision and direction of dissection within the axilla.
- Similarly, the gamma probe (on the technetium-99 setting) can then be utilized to assess whether there was uptake of technetium in the sentinel nodes of the axilla.
- Incision and approach for targeted axillary dissection depends on the planned operation. If a lumpectomy is planned, a 3 to 4 cm axillary incision can be drawn, most commonly just inferior to the hair-bearing line of the axilla. This incision is the same incision as would typically be made for sentinel lymph node biopsy. This incision can be extended in the event that a complete axillary dissection is warranted.
- If a mastectomy is planned, the sentinel lymph node surgery/targeted axillary dissection can often be approached through the mastectomy incision without a separate counter incision in the axilla.

TECHNIQUES

IDENTIFICATION OF TARGETED NODE

- If axillary approach through a separate skin incision is planned, dissection is carried down through the subcutaneous tissue, through the clavipectoral fascia, and into the axilla. Utilizing the handheld gamma probe on the I-125 setting to guide the direction of dissection, the targeted node is identified. It may or may not contain blue dye and may or may not be Tc^{99} radioactive, as nearly 25% of targeted nodes are not sentinel nodes.[15,28] Fine instruments are used to tease out the surrounding fat to isolate the node containing the seed. Small titanium clips or suture ties can be used to ligate visible capillaries and lymphatic channels. Ideally, both the efferent and afferent nodal lymphatics are identified and ligated.
- The same techniques described earlier are used to identify and resect the targeted node via a mastectomy incision (**FIGURE 4**).
- It is good to evaluate and document whether the seed localized lymph node with the clip is blue or not and whether it is technetium-99 radioactive.
- Once the targeted node is resected, intraoperative specimen X-ray is utilized to confirm and document that the excised node contains both the preoperatively placed clip and the radioactive seed (**FIGURE 5**).
- The seed localized lymph node is then sent to pathology labeled as "sentinel lymph node #1 containing seed" or "targeted axillary node containing seed." It is of the utmost importance to communicate with the pathology team that the specimen contains a radioactive seed so that the seed is not accidently cut or lost during processing. Appropriate handling and disposal of the radioactive seed are crucial.

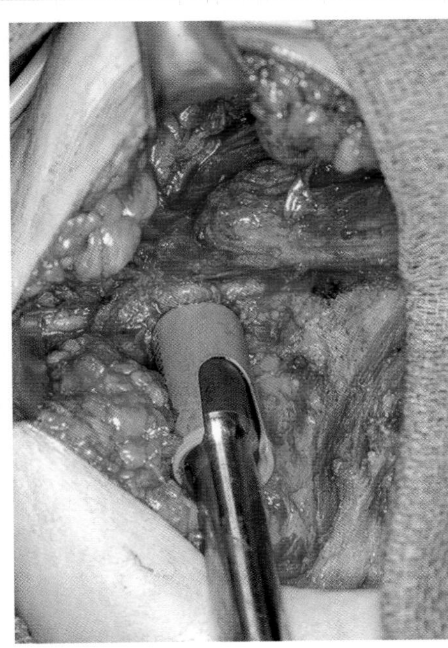

FIGURE 4 ● Utilization of the gamma probe to direct dissection within the axilla.

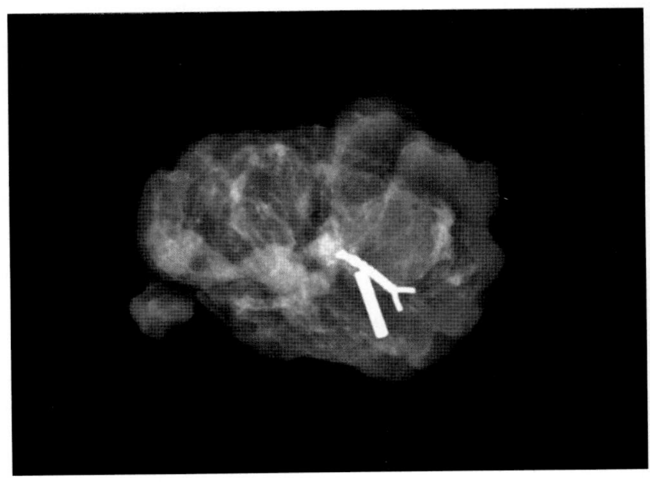

FIGURE 5 ● Intraoperative X-ray confirming the resected node contains both radioactive seed and clip.

TECHNIQUES

SENTINEL LYMPH NODE RESECTION

- Dual-tracer nodal mapping has been shown to improve sentinel lymph node identification and decrease the false-negative rate of a targeted axillary dissection.[5,7-9,14,28]
- Following removal of the targeted node, the gamma probe setting should be switched to technetium-99.
- With the gamma probe on technetium-99 setting, proceed with resection of all additional sentinel lymph nodes.
- Blue lymphatic channels are often encountered. These channels can be very useful to guide dissection toward a sentinel node (**FIGURE 6A-C**).
- All nodes that are dyed blue should be removed and sent to pathology as a sentinel lymph node for review (**FIGURE 6D**). Additionally, all nodes present at the end of a blue dye filled lymphatic channel should be removed and submitted as a sentinel lymph node, even if the node itself is not stained blue.
- All nodes that have uptake of radioisotope (>10% of the hottest node) should be removed and sent to pathology as sentinel lymph nodes.
- All nodes that are palpably suspicious (large or firm) should also be removed and sent to pathology as sentinel lymph nodes.

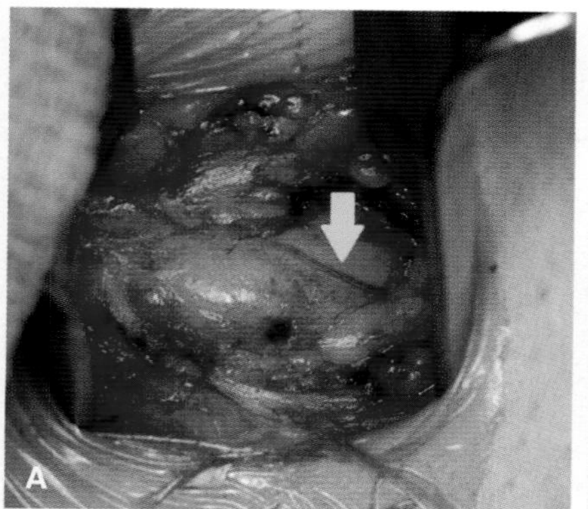
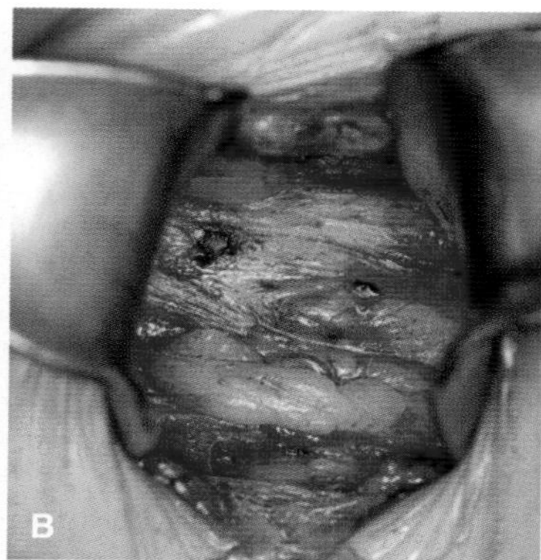
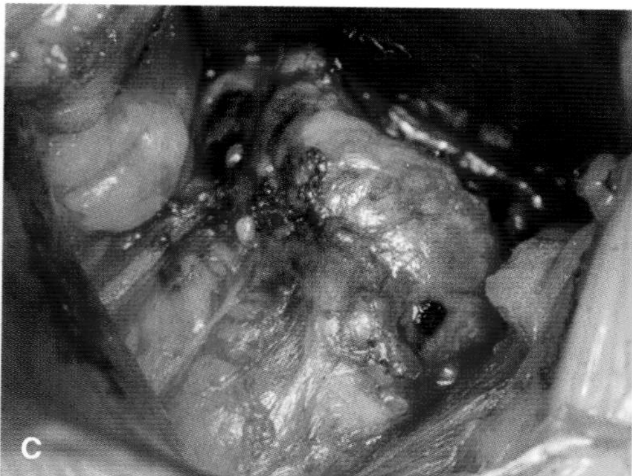
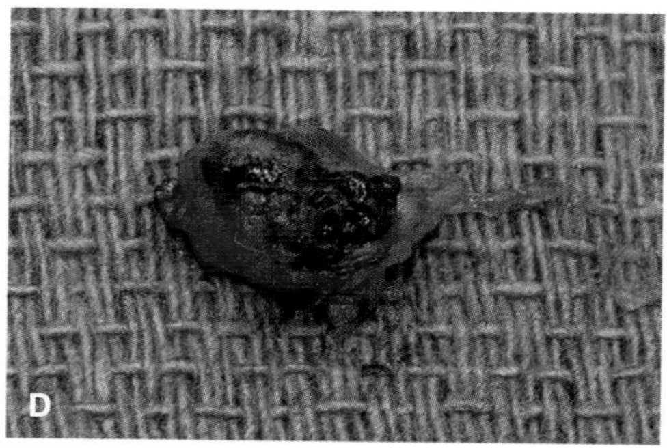

FIGURE 6 ● **A**, Lymphatic channel containing blue dye within the axilla. **B**, Axillary sentinel lymph node containing blue dye can be seen through overlying tissue. **C**, Further dissection reveals the blue node. **D**, Following resection, the blue node is sent for pathologic review.

INDICATIONS TO PROCEED TO COMPLETION AXILLARY LYMPH NODE DISSECTION

- Currently, it is recommended to proceed with completion axillary lymph node dissection if residual disease is identified in any of the lymph nodes resected during sentinel lymph node surgery/targeted axillary dissection following neoadjuvant therapy.
- In cases with failed lymphatic mapping and no sentinel lymph node identified, axillary lymph node dissection is recommended.
- In cases where a single sentinel lymph node is identified and does not contain the clip or biopsy site changes or treatment effect, axillary lymph node dissection is recommended.
- If a single negative node containing the clip or biopsy site changes is identified, complete axillary dissection is not necessarily required, as false-negative rates in this situation are still sufficiently low.[15]

PEARLS AND PITFALLS

- Multiple trials have evaluated and demonstrated the feasibility of sentinel lymph node surgery following neoadjuvant therapy for breast cancer patients with clinically node-positive disease at presentation.
- A key principle identified in these trials for successful de-escalation of axillary lymph node surgery is the reduction of the false-negative rate of the evaluated nodes.
- Targeted axillary dissection which refers to sentinel lymph node surgery along with ensuring resection of the initially biopsied positive node (targeted axillary dissection) is one technique that has been shown to decrease the false-negative rate.[5,10-15]
- Other factors that have been identified that decrease false-negative rate of sentinel lymph node surgery in this setting include:
  - Use of dual tracer to identify the sentinel lymph nodes[5,7-9,14,28]
  - Resection of at least two sentinel lymph nodes[5,10-15]
  - Ultrasound imaging of the axilla following neoadjuvant therapy, for patient selection, prior to surgery[25]
  - Performing immunohistochemistry on the removed sentinel lymph nodes to detect low volume disease[8,9]

POSTOPERATIVE CARE

- If all the lymph nodes removed during sentinel lymph node surgery/targeted axillary dissection are negative, the patient can avoid an axillary dissection, and thus the risk of lymphedema is drastically lower. Potential complications are the same as those associated with sentinel lymph node biopsy.
- It is important to counsel patients preoperatively that urine can be a blue-green color for up to 48 hours postoperatively secondary to methylene blue or isosulfan blue injection.
- Although uncommon, occasionally the clipped node is unable to be targeted with radioactive seed or by the other methods discussed earlier. In such cases, intraoperative palpation and ultrasound can be utilized to try to identify the clipped node. Additionally, the clipped node is one of the sentinel nodes in 75% of cases. Additionally if 3 or more nodes are resected the clipped node is identified in 88% of cases.

REFERENCES

1. Fisher B, Brown A, Mamounas E, et al. Effect of preoperative chemotherapy on local-regional disease in women with operable breast cancer: findings from National Surgical Adjuvant Breast and Bowel Project B-18. *J Clin Oncol*. 1997;15(7):2483-2493.
2. Murphy BL, Day CN, Hoskin TL, Habermann EB, Boughey JC. Neoadjuvant chemotherapy use in breast cancer is greatest in excellent responders: triple-negative and HER2+ subtypes. *Ann Surg Oncol*. 2018;25:2241-2248.
3. Untch M, Konecny GE, Paepke S, von Minckwitz G. Current and future role of neoadjuvant therapy for breast cancer. *Breast*. 2014;23(5):526-537.
4. Haddad TC, Goetz MP. Landscape of neoadjuvant therapy for breast cancer. *Ann Surg Oncol*. 2015;22(5):1408-1415.
5. Boughey JC, Suman VJ, Mittendorf EA, et al. Sentinel lymph node surgery after neoadjuvant chemotherapy in patients with node-positive breast cancer: the ACOSOG Z1071 (Alliance) clinical trial. *JAMA*. 2013;310:1455-1461.
6. Mamtani A, Barrio AV, King TA, et al. How often does neoadjuvant chemotherapy avoid axillary dissection in patients with histologically confirmed nodal metastases? Results of a prospective study. *Ann Surg Oncol*. 2016;23(11):3467-3474.
7. Kuehn T, Bauerfeind I, Fehm T, et al. Sentinel lymph node biopsy in patients with breast cancer before and after neoadjuvant chemotherapy (SENTINA): a prospective, multicentre cohort study. *Lancet Oncol*. 2013;14:609-618.
8. Boileau JF, Poirier B, Basik M, et al. Sentinel node biopsy after neoadjuvant chemotherapy in biopsy-proven node-positive breast cancer: the SN FNAC study. *J Clin Oncol*. 2015;33:258-264.
9. Classe JM, Loaec C, Gimbergues P, et al. Sentinel lymph node biopsy without axillary lymphadenectomy after neoadjuvant chemotherapy is accurate and safe for selected patients: the GANEA 2 study. *Breast Cancer Res Treat*. 2019;173:343-352.
10. Park S, Koo JS, Kim GM, et al. Feasibility of charcoal tattooing of cytology-proven metastatic axillary lymph node at diagnosis and sentinel lymph node biopsy after neoadjuvant chemotherapy in breast cancer patients. *Cancer Res Treat*. 2018;50(3):801-812.
11. Plecha D, Bai S, Patterson H, Thompson C, Shenk R. Improving the accuracy of axillary lymph node surgery in breast cancer with ultrasound-guided wire localization of biopsy proven metastatic lymph nodes. *Ann Surg Oncol*. 2015;22(13):4241-4246.
12. Trinh L, Miyake KK, Dirbas FM, et al. CT-guided wire localization for involved axillary lymph nodes after neo-adjuvant chemotherapy in patients with initially node-positive breast cancer. *Breast J*. 2016;22:390-396.
13. Lim GH, Teo SY, Gudi M, et al. Initial results of a novel technique of clipped node localization in breast cancer patients postneoadjuvant chemotherapy: skin mark clipped axillary nodes removal technique (SMART trial). *Cancer Med*. 2020;9:1978-1985.
14. Boughey JC, Ballman KV, Le-Petross HT, et al. Identification and resection of clipped node decreases the false-negative rate of sentinel lymph node surgery in patients presenting with node-positive breast cancer (T0-T4, N1-N2) who receive neoadjuvant chemotherapy: results from ACOSOG Z1071 (Alliance). *Ann Surg*. 2016;263:802-807.
15. Caudle AS, Yang WT, Krishnamurthy S, et al. Improved axillary evaluation following neoadjuvant therapy for patients with node-positive breast cancer using selective evaluation of clipped nodes: implementation of targeted axillary dissection. *J Clin Oncol*. 2016;34(10):1072-1078.
16. Montagna G, Sevilimedu V, Fornier M, Jhaveri K, Morrow M, Pilewskie ML. How effective is neoadjuvant endocrine therapy (NET) in downstaging the axilla and achieving breast-conserving surgery? *Ann Surg Oncol*. 2020;27(12):4702-4710.
17. Schipper RJ, de Bruijn A, Voogd AC, et al. Rate and predictors of nodal pathological complete response following neoadjuvant endocrine treatment in clinically biopsy-proven node-positive breast cancer patients. *Eur J Surg Oncol*. 2021;47(8):1928-1933.
18. Vila J, Mittendorf EA, Farante G, et al. Nomograms for predicting axillary response to neoadjuvant chemotherapy in clinically node-positive patients with breast cancer. *Ann Surg Oncol*. 2016;23:3501-3509.
19. Piltin MA, Hoskin TL, Day CN, et al. Oncologic outcomes of sentinel lymph node surgery after neoadjuvant chemotherapy for node-positive breast cancer. *Ann Surg Oncol*. 2020;27:4795-4801.
20. Cortazar P, Zhang L, Untch M, et al. Pathologic complete response and long-term clinical benefit in breast cancer: the CTNeoBC pooled analysis. *Lancet*. 2014;384(9938):164-172.

21. Leon-Ferre RA, Hieken TJ, Boughey JC. The landmark series: neoadjuvant chemotherapy for triple-negative and HER2-positive breast cancer. *Ann Surg Oncol*. 2021;28(4):2111-2119.
22. Plichta JK, Sebastian ML, Smith LA, et al. Germline genetic testing: what the breast surgeon needs to know. *Ann Surg Oncol*. 2019;26:2184-2190.
23. National Comprehensive Cancer Network. Breast Cancer (Version 8.2021). Accessed September 22, 2021, http://www.nccn.org/professionals/physician_gls/pdf/bone.pdf.
24. Croshaw R, Shapiro-Wright H, Svensson E, Erb K, Julian T. Accuracy of clinical examination, digital mammogram, ultrasound, and MRI in determining postneoadjuvant pathologic tumor response in operable breast cancer patients. *Ann Surg Oncol*. 2011;18(11):3160-3163.
25. Boughey JC, Ballman KV, Hunt KK, et al. Axillary ultrasound after neoadjuvant chemotherapy and its impact on sentinel lymph node surgery: results from the American College of Surgeons Oncology Group Z1071 trial (Alliance). *J Clin Oncol*. 2015;33(30):3386-3393.
26. Hartmann S, Kühn T, de Boniface J, et al. Carbon tattooing for targeted lymph node biopsy after primary systemic therapy in breast cancer: prospective multicentre TATTOO trial. *Br J Surg*. 2021;108(3):302-307.
27. Laws A, Dillon K, Kelly BN, et al. Node-positive patients treated with neoadjuvant chemotherapy can be spared axillary lymph node dissection with wireless non-radioactive localizers. *Ann Surg Oncol*. 2020;27(12):4819-4827.
28. Boughey JC, Alvarado MD, Lancaster RB, et al; I-SPY 2 Investigators. Surgical standards for management of the axilla in breast cancer clinical trials with pathological complete response endpoint. *NPJ Breast Cancer*. 2018;4:26.

Chapter 18 Simple Mastectomy

Michael S. Sabel and Lisa A. Newman

DEFINITION

- A simple mastectomy, also commonly referred to as a total mastectomy, is the surgical removal of all breast tissue, including the nipple-areolar complex and enough overlying skin to allow a flat closure. This can be performed in conjunction with a sentinel lymph node biopsy, but a simple mastectomy does not include removal of the axillary contents. When the breast tissue and axillary lymph nodes are removed en bloc, this is referred to as a modified radical mastectomy (MRM) (see Part 5, Chapter 20). Variations of the simple mastectomy, typically performed in concert with immediate reconstruction include the "skin-sparing mastectomy," where the nipple–areolar complex is removed but the overlying skin is preserved; and the "nipple-areolar sparing mastectomy," where the native skin and nipple-areolar complex are preserved. These are described in Part 5, Chapter 19.

PATIENT HISTORY AND PHYSICAL FINDINGS

- In clinically early-stage breast cancer, survival is largely driven by risk of distant organ micrometastatic disease and ability to control/eliminate this aspect of the cancer with adjuvant systemic therapy. Locoregional manifestations of disease in the breast and axilla can usually be controlled with surgery and radiation. Multiple prospective, randomized clinical trials have therefore documented survival equivalence between breast-conserving and mastectomy surgery for invasive breast cancer as well as for ductal carcinoma in situ (DCIS). Lumpectomy for a diagnosis of breast cancer is usually followed by breast radiation to sterilize microscopic/occult foci of disease in the remaining breast tissue, thereby reducing the incidence of ipsilateral breast tumor recurrence. Many women will nonetheless undergo total mastectomy as the primary breast surgical option either because of personal preference, medical contraindication to breast radiation, or because of disease features suggesting inability to achieve a margin-negative lumpectomy with a cosmetically acceptable result (eg, diffuse suspicious-appearing microcalcifications on mammogram, multiple breast tumors not amenable to resection within a single lumpectomy, unfavorable tumor-to-breast size ratio). It is important for the clinician to remember that esthetic acceptability must be defined by the patient. Total mastectomy is also the conventionally accepted surgical approach for breast cancer prophylaxis in high-risk women such as those with hereditary susceptibility.
- A detailed history and physical examination is imperative on the first consultation with these patients. In addition to the details of their breast cancer diagnosis, the history should cover medical comorbidities, medications, surgeries, allergies, and any musculoskeletal issues that could affect operative positioning and/or radiation treatment planning. Prior chest wall irradiation (such as for Hodgkin lymphoma or as part of breast-conserving treatment for a past ipsilateral breast cancer) is a contraindication to reirradiation and breast conservation for a new or recurrent breast cancer. Connective tissue disorders such as Sjögren syndrome or scleroderma can result in severe radiation-related toxicity and patients with these medical conditions will typically require mastectomy for management of breast cancer, even if the tumor is detected at a small size that would otherwise have been amenable to breast-conserving surgery. Patients who are unable to raise the arm above shoulder level may have difficulty tolerating the breast radiation tangents.
- All breast cancer patients should have a detailed family cancer history, focusing on both the maternal and paternal sides of the family. Patients with a strong family history, particularly of breast and ovarian cancer, should receive genetic counseling. These patients may want to consider bilateral mastectomies for prevention of second cancers.
- A bilateral breast and lymph node examination, including the axillary, cervical, and supraclavicular lymph nodes, is critical. Any patient with clinically evident lymph nodes should undergo further evaluation, including axillary ultrasound and fine needle aspiration (FNA) biopsy.
- Breast examination should focus on the size and location of the tumor, fixation to the underlying musculature or overlying skin, and skin changes, particularly those consistent with inflammatory breast cancer (erythema, swelling, peau d'orange) or locally advanced disease (bulky tumors, tumors with secondary inflammatory changes, or cancers associated with matted nodal disease). These patients may require neoadjuvant chemotherapy in order to downstage the cancer and to improve resectability. A coordinated multidisciplinary approach, including input from medical and radiation oncology specialists promptly following the breast cancer diagnosis, is important for efficient management planning and is vital to the successful treatment of these patients.
- Early-stage breast cancer patients with a clinically negative axillary exam undergoing total mastectomy require axillary staging, which can usually be performed as lymphatic mapping and sentinel lymph node (SLN) biopsy. Mastectomy patients with axillary metastases documented by either needle biopsy or SLN dissection require standard levels 1 and 2 axillary lymph node dissection (ALND) or MRM, and postmastectomy locoregional radiation needs are then determined by the full pathologic extent of disease identified in the breast and axillary contents.
- All patients planning mastectomy should be presented the option of immediate reconstruction and a consultation with a plastic surgeon. Patients who opt for immediate reconstruction may be candidates for a skin-sparing or nipple-areolar–sparing mastectomy. If postmastectomy radiation is being considered, this might impact both short-term and long-term outcomes with immediate breast reconstruction.

IMAGING AND OTHER DIAGNOSTIC STUDIES

- Breast imaging plays a vital role in the screening and diagnostic workup for breast cancer. Imaging can define the extent of the disease and help assess for any abnormalities in the contralateral breast. Bilateral mammography is essential for any patient with breast cancer. Any suspicious contralateral lesions should be worked up before making the final surgical decision.
- Axillary ultrasound can be performed in many patients with a biopsy-proven invasive cancer to identify suspicious nodes suggestive of regional involvement. Suspicious nodes on axillary ultrasound should undergo an FNA biopsy with ultrasound guidance.
- It should not be assumed that any axillary node that is palpable or suspicious on ultrasound is malignant, as often they may be reactive. They should always be interrogated with FNA biopsy; and if the FNA is negative, then definitive axillary staging should be performed by SLN biopsy. At the time of lymphatic mapping and sentinel node dissection, it is important to excise any palpable/suspicious node, regardless of whether the node has any appreciable radiocolloid or blue dye uptake. If local resources permit, intraoperative evaluation of the sentinel node(s) with frozen section analysis can also be useful so that the patient can proceed onto immediate completion of the ALND if metastatic nodal disease is confirmed. When frozen section analyses are available and planned, the patient must be consented preoperatively for possible conversion from total mastectomy to MRM.
- The use of magnetic resonance imaging (MRI) is controversial. For patients undergoing mastectomy, MRI may detect contralateral cancers that were not visualized on mammography. For patients who hope to pursue breast-conserving surgery, a preoperative breast MRI may detect suspicious foci of disease in the breast such that mastectomy may be recommended. MRI usage has therefore been associated with increased rates of bilateral mastectomies. However, MRIs are sensitive but not specific and may lead to false-positive findings that necessitate additional biopsies. Furthermore, the natural history of MRI-detected multifocal/multicentric lesions in the cancerous breast is unclear, as these areas of otherwise occult disease would typically be radiated following lumpectomy for the known cancer. Retrospective and prospective studies of the outcome following breast-conserving surgery in patients whose breast-conserving surgery eligibility was planned with vs without breast MRI have failed to demonstrate any significant differences in cancer-related outcomes.[1-3] We do not recommend routine MRI but rather its use should be on a patient-by-patient basis.
- In the absence of locally advanced disease (skin or muscle involvement, multiple matted nodes, and inflammatory breast cancer), routine staging tests, such as computed tomography (CT) scan of the chest, abdomen, and pelvis, bone scan, or positron emission tomography (PET) scan, are not indicated.

SURGICAL MANAGEMENT

Preoperative Planning

- In the preoperative area, the breast to be removed should be clearly marked and confirmed with the patient.
- Prophylactic antibiotics have been shown to reduce postoperative infections and are indicated.[4] Sequential compression devices should be placed prior to initiation of general anesthesia for venous thromboembolism (VTE) prevention.

Positioning

- The patient should be positioned supine with the arm out laterally, taking care not to abduct the arm greater than 90° as this may cause an injury to the brachial plexus. For a simple mastectomy, it is not necessary to prep and drape the ipsilateral arm into the field. However, if an SLN biopsy with frozen section and possible ALND is planned, it may be reasonable to include the arm using a sterile stockinette and Kerlix wrap. The endotracheal tube should be positioned toward the contralateral side of the mouth from the side of the mastectomy.
- Position the table and lights to allow enough room above the arm for an assistant to stand.
- If an SLN biopsy is to be performed and blue dye is to be injected, this can be done at this time. Either isosulfan blue dye or methylene blue dye can be injected subareolar, periareolar, or peritumoral, according to surgeon preference. Given the risk of allergic reaction with isosulfan blue dye, we prefer methylene blue dye. One risk of methylene blue dye is skin necrosis, so we prefer a subareolar or periareolar injection to avoid any retained blue dye within the skin flap.
- The chest wall, axilla, and upper arm are prepped into the field. Be sure to prep widely, extending across the midline and onto the abdomen and neck.

TECHNIQUES

- See **Video 1**.

CHOICE OF INCISION

- The standard incision for a simple mastectomy is the classic Stewart incision, an ellipse oriented medial to lateral, encompassing the nipple-areolar complex and any prior biopsy scar (**FIGURE 1**). Alternatively, the modified Stewart incision is angled toward the axilla. It has been suggested that the modified Stewart incision, by excising more of the dermal lymphatics running toward the axilla, may provide better local control.
- In addition to the Stewart and modified Stewart, there are alternate options for a simple mastectomy. The placement and orientation of the incision must be based on the location of the biopsy scar and/or the location of the tumor. For a palpable tumor, particularly one close to the skin, the skin over the tumor should be included in the excised skin. Planning of the skin incision in conjunction with the plastic surgeon can be quite helpful in patients undergoing skin-sparing mastectomy and immediate reconstruction. If the patient has a surgical cancer biopsy incision, this scar

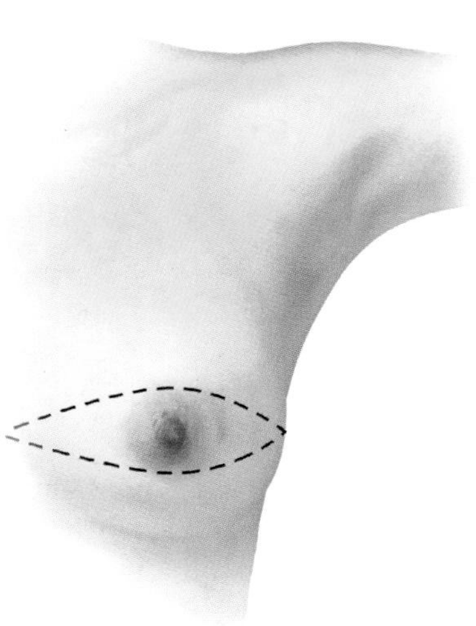

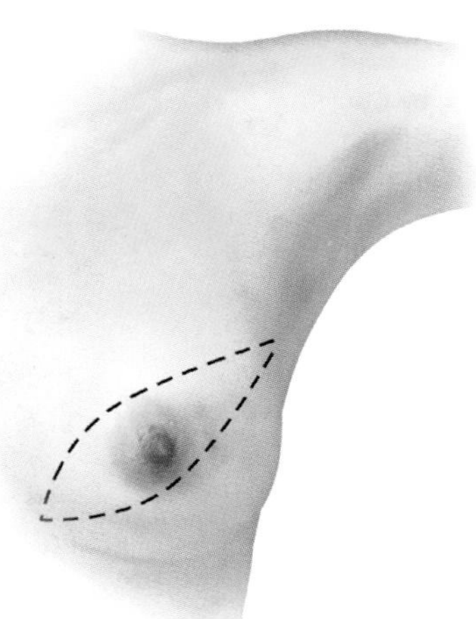

FIGURE 1 ● Standard incisions for a simple mastectomy. The Stewart incision **(left)** involves a horizontal ellipse that encompasses the nipple-areolar complex and adequate skin to allow a flat closure. The modified Stewart incision is angled toward the ipsilateral axilla.

should be resected with the underlying mastectomy specimen. Incisions located in proximity to the nipple-areolar complex can be resected within the central skin ellipse that is being sacrificed. Incisions that are located remote from the central nipple-areolar skin can sometimes be resected as a separate ellipse of sacrificed skin, as long as the remaining skin bridge is wide enough to remain viable. The original surgical cancer biopsy scars should not be left intact in the mastectomy skin flaps because of the oncologic concern that this skin may potentially harbor cancer cells (and the mastectomy skin is usually not being radiated, as is the case following lumpectomy); and from a wound healing perspective, the subcutaneous fat deep to the traumatized incisional skin will be less healthy and more likely to necrose. Old surgical biopsy scars that are unrelated to the cancer diagnosis can be left in place. Also, percutaneous needle biopsy scars can be left intact on the skin flaps, as these have not been shown to contribute to risk of local recurrence.

- It is important to remove enough skin so that there is no redundancy but not so much that there is undue tension on the incision. A useful method to determine the placement of the superior and inferior incisions is to hold a marking pen in the air over the nipple and retract the breast inferiorly. Mark this site on the skin and then retract the breast superiorly to mark the inferior extent (**FIGURE 2A** and **B**).
- When designing the ellipse, closure will be facilitated by making sure the superior and inferior incisions are of equal length (**FIGURE 3**). This can easily be assessed using a 3-0 silk suture.
- Before making the incision, mark the boundaries of the breast tissue. Although the breast is an obvious external feature of the human anatomy, its boundaries deep to the skin are less well defined. Lacking any clear-cut capsule to delineate breast tissue from surrounding fat and subcutaneous tissue, the surgeon must identify anatomic landmarks that serve as reasonable and relatively constant

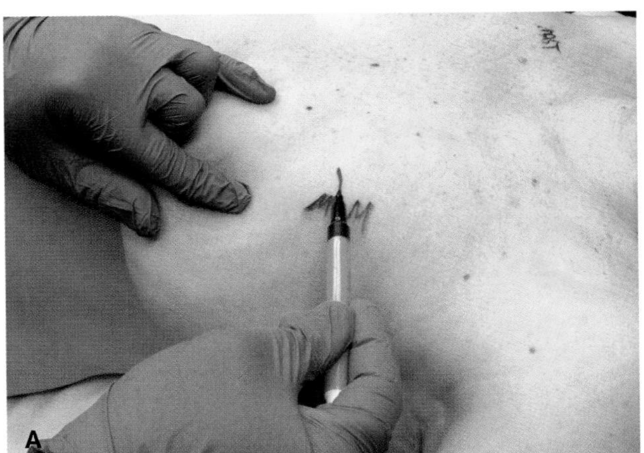

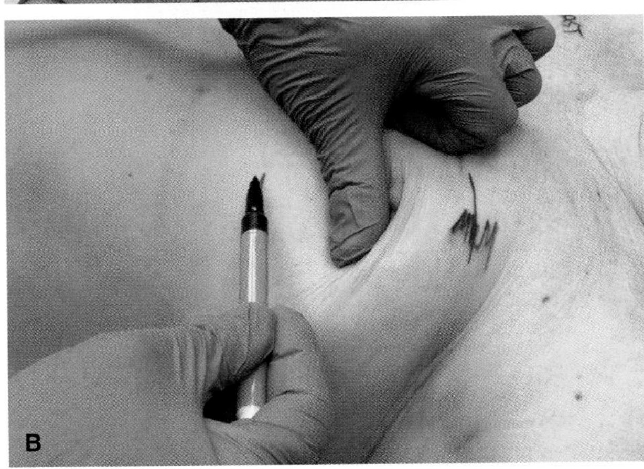

FIGURE 2 ● With a marking pen held over the nipple, the breast is retracted inferiorly **(A)** and the extent of the superior flap is marked. The breast is then retracted superiorly **(B)** and the inferior extent is marked. This allows the surgeon to estimate how much skin should be excised to eliminate redundancy without undue tension.

structures, beyond which it is unlikely to find significant amounts of breast tissue. These radial boundaries for the skin flaps essentially serve as a picture frame; and once these flaps are completed, the breast is dissected off the pectoralis major muscle en bloc with the pectoralis fascia. The conventionally accepted peripheral mastectomy flap boundaries are as follows: superior margin—clavicle or second rib (identified by palpation); inferior margin—inframammary fold (IMF); medial margin—lateral border of the sternum (identified by palpation); lateral margin—the lateral extent of the breast tissue can be marked externally on the skin surface and the edge of the latissimus dorsi muscle is a useful vertical boundary that can be visually identified from within the mastectomy surgical field (**FIGURE 4**).

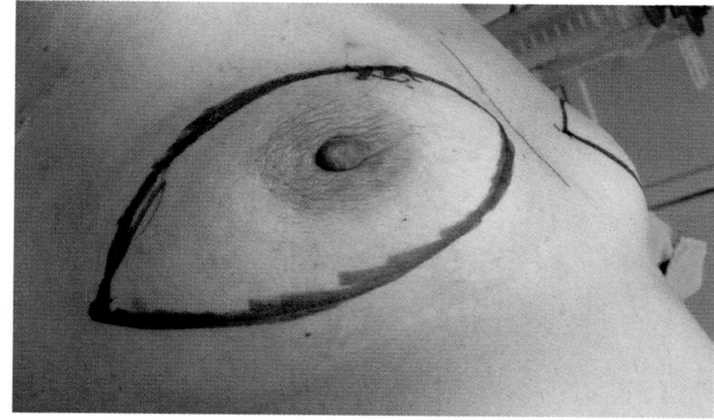

FIGURE 3 ● Confirming the superior and inferior incisions are of equal length will facilitate closure.

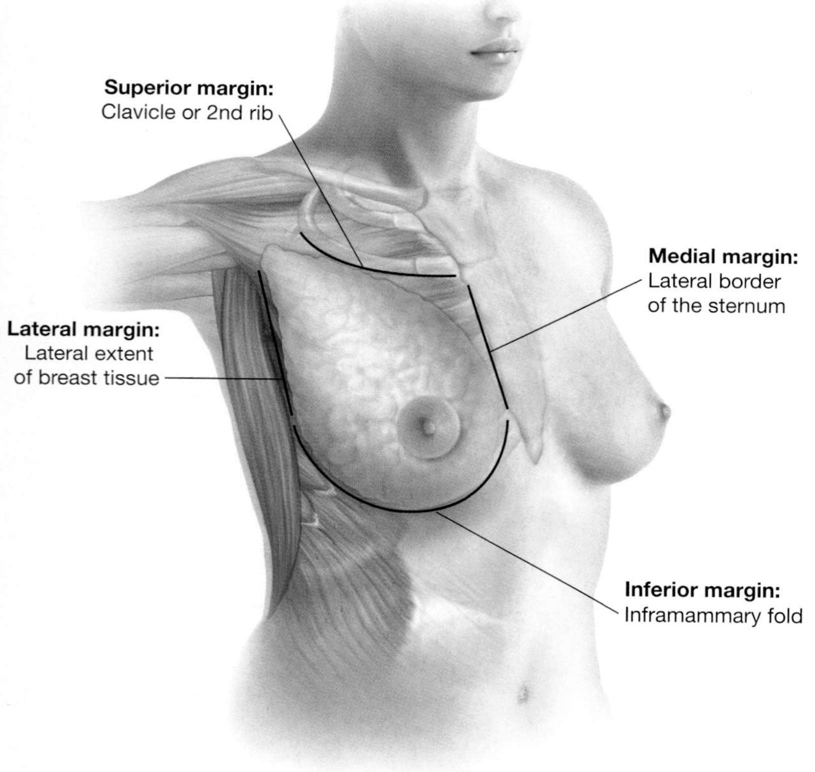

FIGURE 4 ● To assure removal of all breast tissue, the dissection is performed to the clavicle or second rib superiorly, the IMF inferiorly, the lateral border of the sternum medially, and the lateral extent of the breast tissue or edge of the latissimus dorsi muscle laterally.

SKIN INCISION AND CREATION OF FLAPS

- Once the skin incision has been mapped out on the breast, a scalpel is used to cut through the skin and dermis. Cautery is used to then obtain hemostasis. It is important to get into the right plane to raise flaps at the start. The initial incision should extend through full-thickness skin, just barely exposing the subcutaneous fat, and no further. Incising through deeper layers of subcutaneous fat will result in a splaying out of those fatty planes, and these deeper tissues will spuriously appear as anterior margin surfaces when analyzed and inked in the pathology laboratory. The actual anterior margin of the mastectomy specimen (beyond the central ellipse of sacrificed nipple-areolar skin) should be defined by the surgeon via dissection of the appropriate-thickness skin flaps. Failing to leave a small amount of tissue beneath the dermis can lead to ischemia and wound complications, and this can be particularly concerning in cases involving immediate reconstruction. Conversely, an excessively thick skin flap leaves the patient at risk for residual breast tissue on the chest wall, thereby increasing risk of local recurrence.

- Starting with the superior flap, skin hooks are used to elevate the skin and provide appropriate tension for elevation of the flap (**FIGURE 5**). The key to elevating an appropriate flap is the tension on the breast tissue. Initially, a forceps can be used to get into the right plane; but once that plane is identified, traction with the contralateral hand of the surgeon using a laparotomy pad on the breast tissue will be critical. As the flap elevation proceeds, it is important to reposition the contralateral hand accordingly.
- It is imperative that the assistant holding the skin hooks maintain retraction straight up (**FIGURE 6**). Often, an assistant, such as a resident or medical student, will retract toward themselves so they have a better view of the dissection. However, this can lead to exposing the dermis and possibly a buttonhole injury to the skin.
- The correct plane will leave a small amount of subcutaneous fat beneath the dermis so that the blood supply is preserved while not leaving any breast tissue. This plane is often avascular (**FIGURE 7**). Intermittently inspecting and palpating the flap will assure the correct thickness. Older women (where much of the breast is fatty-replaced) and heavier patients often have a thicker flap of subcutaneous fat separating the skin from the underlying breast parenchyma. In contrast, younger and thin patients may have breast tissue closely abutting the dermis, allowing for a very narrow margin of error while raising the flap.
- Flaps can be elevated using cautery, scissors, or a scalpel. Cautery will help provide hemostasis during the procedure. If sharp dissection is used, pressure on the breast with a laparotomy sponge will help maintain hemostasis.
- The superior flap is complete when you reach the level of the clavicle. At this point, the pectoralis muscle should be identified and the pectoralis fascia is divided (scored) along the length of the flap (**FIGURE 8**).
- In patients for whom SLN biopsy with intraoperative analysis and possible conversion to MRM is being considered, it may be prudent to perform the SLN biopsy at this time to allow adequate time for pathologic assessment. The lateral edge of the pectoralis muscle is identified and the clavipectoral fascia is identified and divided. This allows access to the fibrofatty tissue of the axilla. The sentinel nodes can now be identified by using the gamma probe or by following any blue-stained lymphatics. Alternatively, the SLN biopsy can be performed following removal of the breast tissue.
- The medial extent of the dissection should extend to the lateral edge of the sternum. Going too far medially can lead to excessive dog-earing, which will need excision and thus lengthen the incision. In the case of bilateral mastectomies, going too far medially can accidently connect the two incisions, potentially contaminating the prophylactic side and complicating reconstruction.

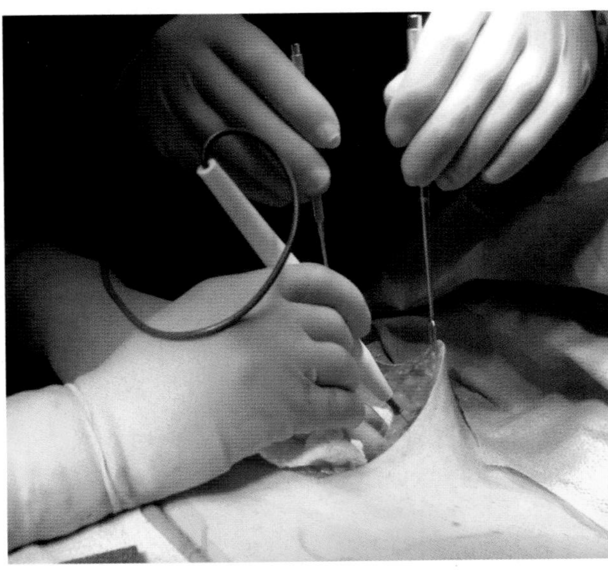

FIGURE 6 ● It is important that the assistant retracts straight up while the flap is raised; otherwise, exposure of the dermis or injury of the flap is more likely.

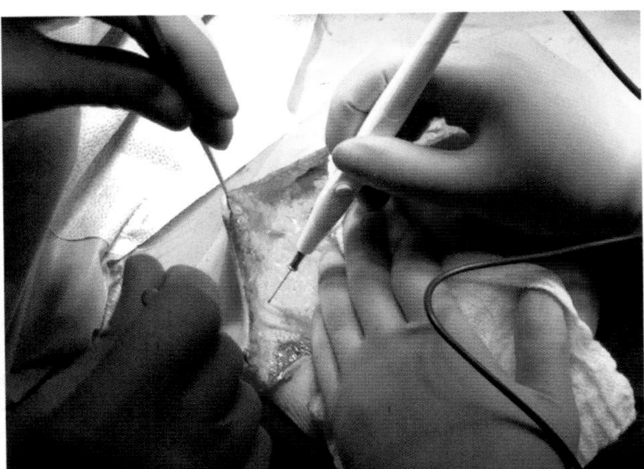

FIGURE 5 ● The surgeon's opposite hand is used to provide adequate tension on the breast tissue to allow elevation of the superior flap in the correct plane.

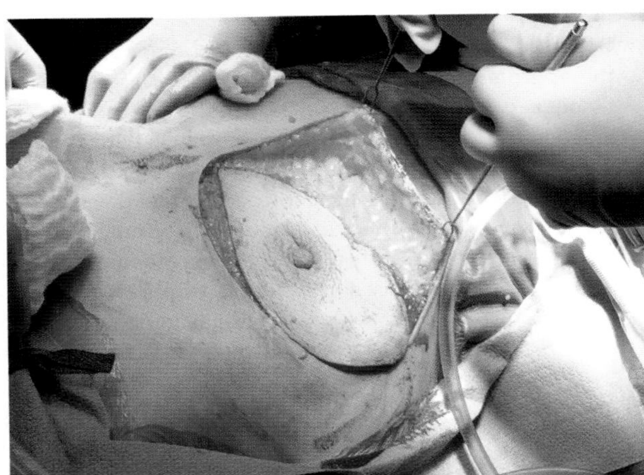

FIGURE 7 ● If done correctly, there will be a small amount of subcutaneous fat beneath the dermis so that the blood supply is preserved.

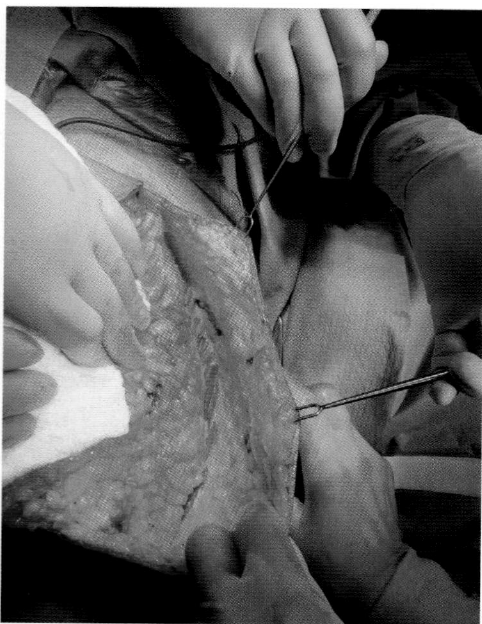

FIGURE 8 ● At the superior extent (clavicle or second rib), the pectoralis fascia is divided along its length.

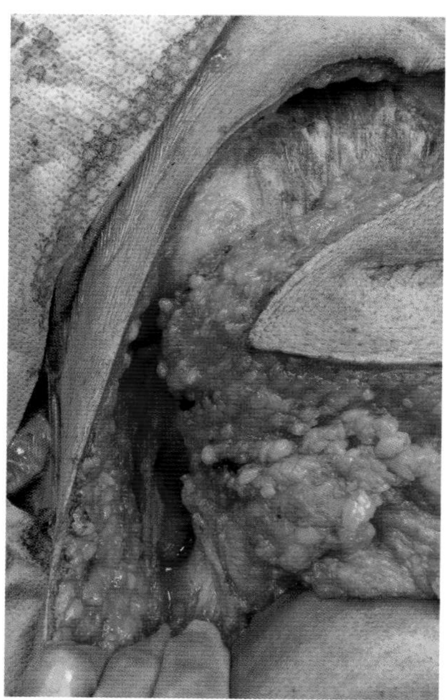

FIGURE 9 ● Visualization of the edge of the latissimus dorsi muscle assures the completeness of the lateral flap.

- The inferior flap is then elevated in an identical manner to the level of the IMF. It is important to mark this, as it can easily be lost while elevating the flap. The assistant can provide feedback to the surgeon as the IMF is approached. Elevating past the IMF is not only unnecessary but can also complicate reconstruction, necessitating the plastic surgeon to recreate it to assure symmetry.
- Finally, the lateral margin is developed. As this is not an MRM, it is not necessary to thoroughly mobilize the latissimus dorsi muscle but identifying the edge of these fibers can enhance the completeness of the lateral flap (**FIGURE 9**). Avoiding an unnecessary mobilization of the latissimus dorsi muscle in total mastectomy patients undergoing immediate reconstruction is especially important, as creating extra dissection flaps in this lateral tissue can compromise the plastic surgery esthetics.
- It is important that the lateral extent of the breast tissue is removed. This includes the axillary tail of Spence, which extends around the superior aspect of the pectoralis muscle to the clavipectoral fascia. Identification of the clavipectoral fascia can help assure that the lateral extent of the breast tissue is removed without removing the node-bearing axillary fat.

REMOVAL OF THE BREAST TISSUE

- Once the flaps have been completed circumferentially to the appropriate landmarks, it is time to excise the breast tissue and the pectoralis fascia off the pectoralis major muscle. It is important to remove the fascia with the specimen to assure negative margins. Failure to excise the fascia with the specimen may lead to a positive deep margin, which may prompt the use of postmastectomy radiation or increase chest wall recurrence.[5] Deep to the tumor, it can be useful to resect a tiny sample of pectoralis muscle fibers (labeled as sample of additional posterior margin) to serve as pathologic documentation that the mastectomy specimen included the pectoralis fascia. Some patients may have diffuse DCIS extending throughout the breast to its posterior surface, but by definition, the noninvasive nature of this disease is such that documenting resection of the pectoralis fascia is consistent with an adequate resection and further local therapy in the form of postmastectomy radiation is unnecessary. Patients with palpable breast tumors abutting the chest wall surface should have a wedge of underlying pectoralis muscle at the site of the tumor resected en bloc with the mastectomy specimen.
- The breast tissue is retracted inferiorly. This is typically done with the contralateral hand but grasping the fascia with a right-angle clamp can facilitate this. The fascia is elevated off the muscle using cautery, moving the cautery back and forth in the direction of the fibers of the muscle (**FIGURE 10**). This technique minimizes the damage to the pectoralis muscle.
- Small perforators extending from the pectoralis to the breast should be grasped with a hemostat or forceps and cauterized. There are slightly larger perforators medially. It is best to preserve these if possible. If not, these should be grasped and cauterized or suture ligated (**FIGURE 11**). If these are accidentally divided, they often retract into the muscle and can be difficult to control.

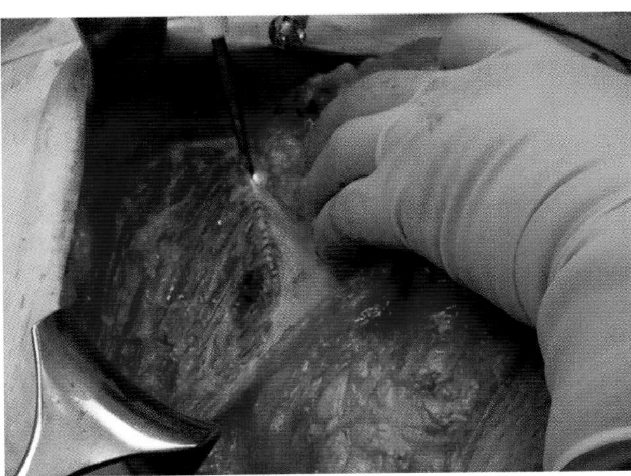

FIGURE 10 ● Retracting the breast inferiorly, the breast tissue and pectoralis fascia are taken off the pectoralis major. The cautery is moved back and forth in the direction of the fibers of the muscle.

- Some patients (especially older and/or less fit patients) will have a weakened, attenuated, and fatty-replaced pectoralis musculature. Caution should be exercised during the lateral retraction of the breast in these cases, as overly aggressive tugging on the breast can result in the muscle being inadvertently avulsed from its costochondral and sternal attachments.

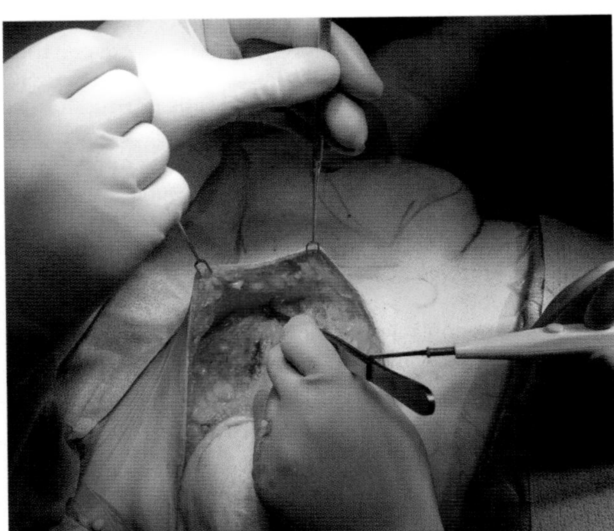

FIGURE 11 ● Medial perforators are grasped and cauterized.

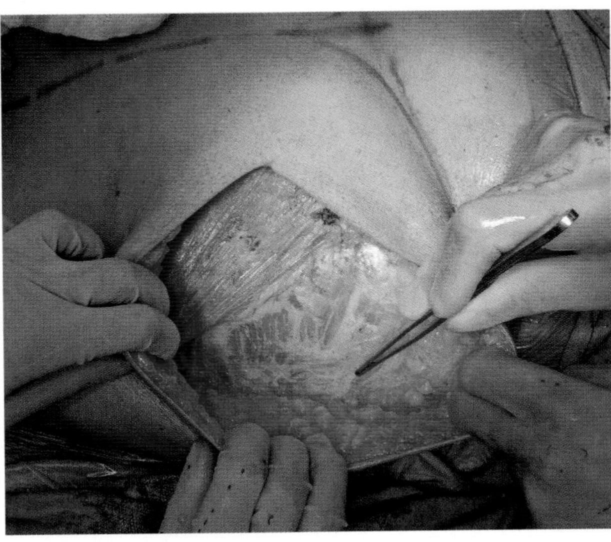

FIGURE 12 ● As opposed to the pectoralis fascia, which is taken with the breast tissue, the fascia over the serratus anterior is left intact.

- Dissection of the breast off the pectoralis muscle continues inferiorly toward the IMF and then out laterally. Resecting the pectoralis fascia has oncologic significance; however, fascia overlying the serratus anterior muscle can be left intact (**FIGURE 12**). Dissecting deep to this fascia and exposing the serratus muscle bed results in unnecessary bleeding and can place the long thoracic nerve at risk for injury, because this important motor nerve is not routinely identified through visual exposure unless the patient is undergoing an ALND.
- Intercostal nerve block: Many mastectomy patients will benefit from intraoperative injection of approximately 5 mL of 0.5% ropivacaine into 2 or 3 intercostal spaces along the surgical field lateral to the pectoralis muscle. The surgeon should notify the anesthesia staff who will then give the patient a few extra deep breaths. At maximal end expiration, the patient is taken off the ventilator while the surgeon injects the long-acting anesthetic just at the inferior edge of the selected rib to block the associated intercostal nerves. Ventilator-assisted respirations then resume. If intercostal nerve blocks as well as incisional long-acting anesthetic injection are planned, then the maximum volume of safe anesthetic delivery (based on body weight of the patient) should be calculated.

DRAIN PLACEMENT

- A closed suction drain is placed over the pectoralis major muscle through a separate stab incision and sutured in place with a monofilament suture (**FIGURE 13**). When inserting the drain through the skin flap, it is useful to be mindful of the location of the latissimus dorsi muscle. Inadvertent insertion of the drain through this muscle can result in excessive bleeding from the tract. In cases where the drain tract does bleed excessively, the best remedy is to simply remove the drain, apply pressure, and replace the drain through a different tract.

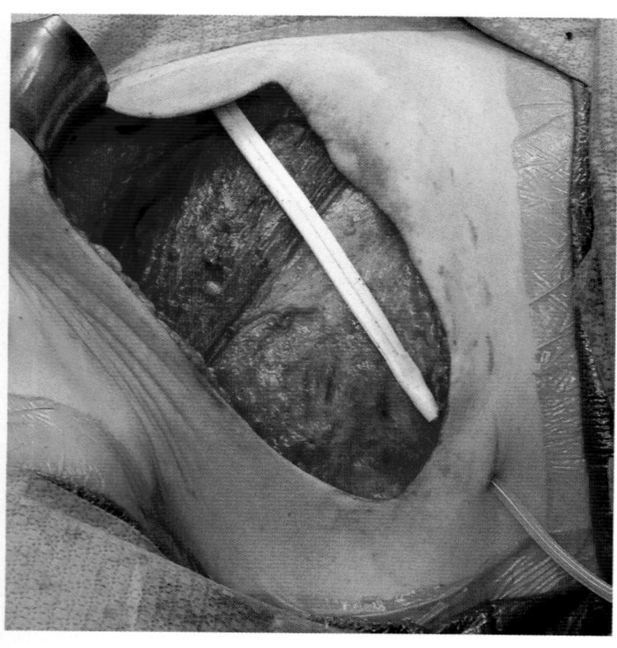

FIGURE 13 ● A flat channel drain is placed over the pectoralis major muscle through a separate stab incision prior to closing.

CLOSURE

- Although excess tension on the incision can lead to wound complications, excess skin will lead to redundant flaps, which can be uncomfortable for the patient; they can be difficult to monitor for recurrence and can interfere with wearing a prosthesis. In cases where postmastectomy radiation and delayed reconstruction is planned, it may be helpful to leave the skin flaps a little looser, but a floppy anterior skin flap will be unsightly and serves as a site for recurrent seroma accumulation. Excess skin can be excised, so that the incision approximates flat on the chest wall. Remember that the patient is lying flat back, but once awake will slouch forward slightly, so a small amount of tension will be released.
- Commonly, the medial and lateral aspects of the incision will "dog ear." Often, these can be easily excised as an ellipse. There are times, particularly in older, heavier women, where excising the lateral dog ear simply moves the dog ear more posteriorly. In these cases, a fish-tail plasty (**FIGURE 14A-C**) can be useful.[6]
- The dermal layer should be closed with interrupted deep dermal absorbable sutures. Because the Jackson-Pratt (JP) drain will evacuate the postoperative seroma formation, the mastectomy skin flap closure should be subject to minimal tension. A reasonable closure alternative can therefore rely on a few interrupted sutures to line up the appropriate skin closure, followed by a running, continuous absorbable deep dermal suture. The skin can be approximated with an absorbable 4-0 monofilament suture in a running subcuticular closure or a surgical adhesive.

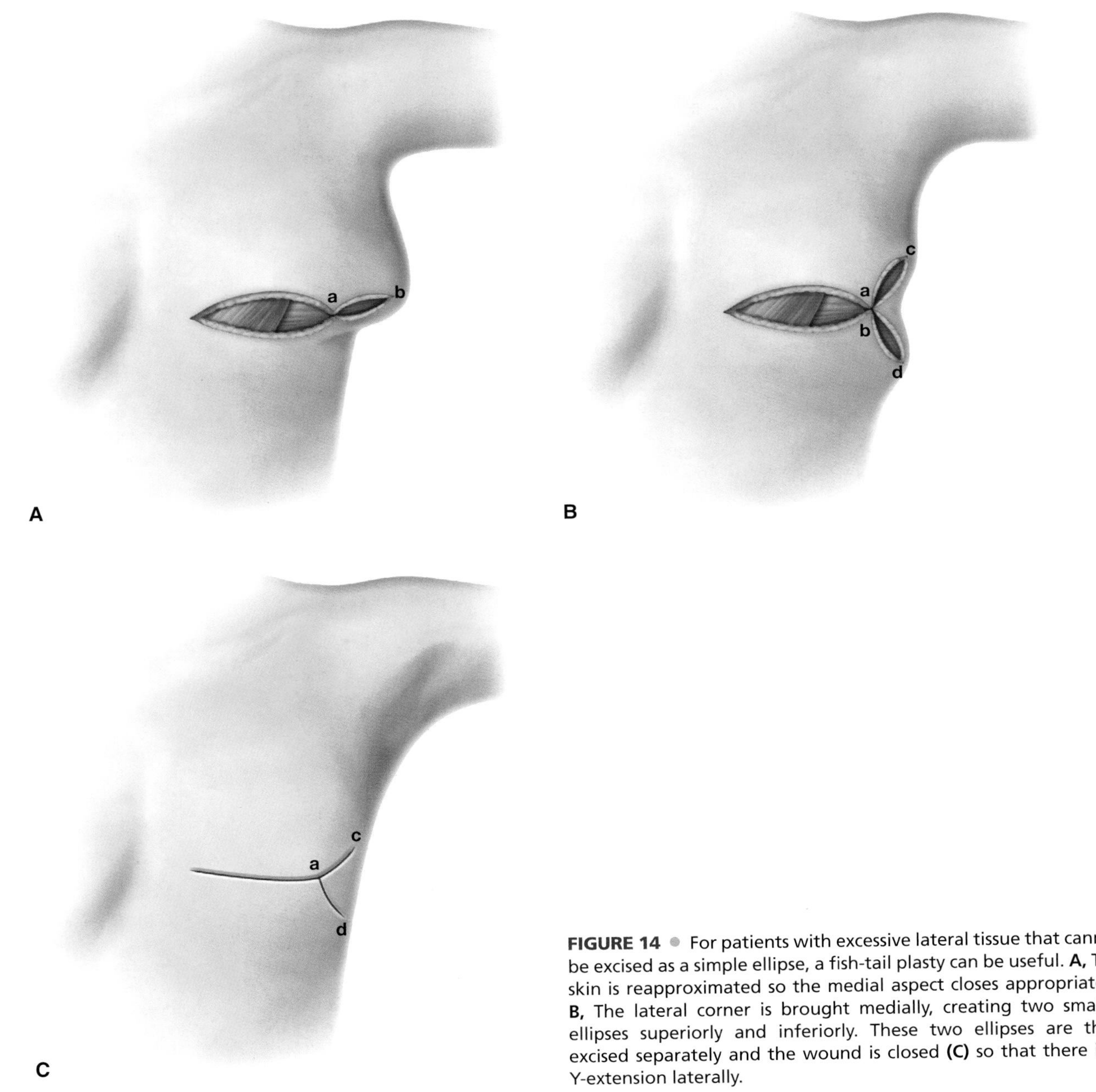

FIGURE 14 ● For patients with excessive lateral tissue that cannot be excised as a simple ellipse, a fish-tail plasty can be useful. **A,** The skin is reapproximated so the medial aspect closes appropriately. **B,** The lateral corner is brought medially, creating two smaller ellipses superiorly and inferiorly. These two ellipses are then excised separately and the wound is closed **(C)** so that there is a Y-extension laterally.

PEARLS AND PITFALLS

Patient expectations	■ Patients who are candidates for breast conservation therapy (BCT) should understand there is no improvement in survival with a mastectomy. ■ All patients undergoing mastectomy should be offered consultation with a plastic surgeon to discuss reconstruction options. ■ Patients may have concerns regarding cosmesis and sexual identity after mastectomy that should be addressed preoperatively. ■ Patients should also understand the potential for redundancy or dog ears after mastectomy and how these can be addressed.

Planning the incision	■ Include the excisional biopsy scar in the ellipse. For palpable tumors, include an adequate amount of skin over the tumor. ■ Plan the ellipse so that it will lie flat, without excess laxity, yet not too tight. ■ Measure the superior and inferior incisions to confirm they are roughly the same length.
Raising the flaps	■ Make sure to start in the right plane with the initial incision and not go too far into the subcutaneous fat. ■ The assistant should hold the skin hooks straight up. Bending the skin backward can inadvertently lead to exposing dermis or "buttonholing." ■ Countertension with the opposite hand is the key to being in the right plane. As you progress, reposition the hand accordingly. ■ Be careful not to pass the IMF while raising the inferior flap.
Removing the breast	■ Retract the breast inferiorly and move the cautery medial to lateral, parallel to the pectoralis major muscle fibers. ■ Remove the fascia of the pectoralis with the specimen. ■ Grasp perforators with a forceps or clamp and coagulate rather than try to directly cauterize. ■ Do not retract the breast laterally with excess force, this will avulse the muscle from the sternum.
Closure	■ Excise excess skin so that the flaps close flat against the chest wall. ■ Medial and lateral dog ears should be excised, but do not keep repositioning a lateral dog ear more posteriorly. A plasty can eradicate a dog ear but can make reconstruction more difficult. A dog ear can always be corrected at a later date under local anesthetic.

POSTOPERATIVE CARE

- A nonadherent dressing can be placed over the incision. Patients can be placed in a breast binder with Kerlix fluffs in order to apply even compression. This will help prevent hematoma but should not be excessively tight.
- Patients do not need to be admitted to the hospital overnight, they may be safely discharged to home. Arranging for a visiting nurse can be helpful for drain management and wound checks.
- The drain can be removed when the output is less than 30 mL/24 hours for 2 days in a row.

OUTCOMES

- Overall, local (chest wall) recurrence after mastectomy is low, ranging from 0.6% to 9.5%, increasing with increasing stage, the presence of nodal metastases, and positive margins after mastectomy. However, local recurrence rates also appear to be decreasing as systemic therapies improve.[7] Local recurrence is also related to the histologic subtype, with luminal subtype tumors (ER/PR positive) less likely to recur than *HER2/neu* overexpressing or triple negative tumors after mastectomy.[8]
- Because local recurrence rates remain higher among patients with node-positive disease or positive margins, postmastectomy radiation therapy (PMRT) should be considered in these situations. PMRT is strongly indicated for patients with positive margins or positive lymph nodes.

COMPLICATIONS

- Seroma
- Wound infection
- Hematoma
- Wound dehiscence
- Flap necrosis
- Positive margins

REFERENCES

1. Turnbull L, Brown S, Harvey I, et al. Comparative effectiveness of MRI in breast cancer (COMICE) trial: a randomized controlled trial. *Lancet*. 2010;376(9714):563-571.
2. Peters NH, van Esser S, van den Bosch MA, et al. Preoperative MRI and surgical management in patients with nonpalpable breast cancer: the MONET-randomised controlled trial. *Eur J Cancer*. 2011;47:879-886.
3. Solin LJ, Orel SG, Hwang WT, et al. Relationship of breast magnetic resonance imaging to outcome after breast-conservation treatment with radiation for women with early-stage invasive breast carcinoma or ductal carcinoma in situ. *J Clin Oncol*. 2008;26:386-391.
4. Tejirian T, DiFronzo LA, Haigh PI. Antibiotic prophylaxis for preventing wound infection after breast surgery: a systematic review and metaanalysis. *J Am Coll Surg*. 2006;203(5):729-734.
5. Dalberg K, Krawiec K, Sandelin K. Eleven-year follow-up of a randomized study of pectoral fascia preservation after mastectomy for early breast cancer. *World J Surg*. 2010;34(11):2539-2544.
6. Hussien M, Daltrey IR, Dutta S, et al. Fish-tail plasty: a safe technique to improve cosmesis at the lateral end of mastectomy scars. *Breast*. 2004;13(3):206-209.
7. Yi M, Kronowitz SJ, Meric-Bernstam F, et al. Local, regional, and systemic recurrence rates in patients undergoing skin-sparing mastectomy compared with conventional mastectomy. *Cancer*. 2011;117:916-924.
8. Lowery AJ, Kell MR, Glynn RW, et al. Locoregional recurrence after breast cancer surgery: a systematic review by receptor phenotype. *Breast Cancer Res Treat*. 2012;133:831-841.

Chapter 19 Skin-Sparing and Nipple/Areolar-Sparing Mastectomy

Eleni Anastasia Tousimis

DEFINITION

- Skin-sparing mastectomy is defined as removal of the breast tissue while preserving the natural skin envelope for immediate breast reconstruction. This is an effective treatment option for patients with operable breast cancer without skin involvement. By preserving the patient's skin envelope with a smaller incision, it markedly improves the aesthetics of the breast reconstruction.
- To further enhance cosmesis, the nipple and areola can be preserved at the time of mastectomy in select patients, which is called nipple/areola or nipple-sparing mastectomy. The selection criteria for nipple-sparing mastectomy have widened extensively to include any patient who does not have nipple areolar involvement with tumor. The nipple-areolar complex (NAC) is considered like any other margins and as long as free of tumor then oncologically safe to preserve.

ANATOMY

- As with all types of mastectomy, a thorough understanding of the anatomy of the breast, chest wall, and axilla is necessary. The goal of mastectomy is to remove the breast tissue while maintaining the viability of the skin envelope.
- The breast tissue is encapsulated by the superficial fascia that adheres to the subcutaneous tissue in a lobulated fashion (**FIGURE 1**). This makes it difficult to remove all of the breast tissue during mastectomy and maintain skin viability.
- The boundaries of the breast (**FIGURE 2**) are defined by the clavicle superiorly, the sternum medially, the sixth rib inferiorly, and the latissimus dorsi muscle laterally.
- The axillary tail of the breast extends from the upper outer quadrant of the breast superior and laterally toward the low axilla. Posteriorly, the breast adheres to the pectoralis major muscle and is separated from the chest wall by the deep fascia of the breast (see **FIGURE 1**).
- A skin-sparing mastectomy involves preserving the skin envelope while removing the NAC and underlying breast via a small incision (**FIGURE 3**). Nipple-sparing mastectomy is a total skin-sparing mastectomy with preservation of the NAC. Several approaches are feasible, including inframammary, circumareolar, or lateral. The choice of incision is usually a joint decision between the breast surgeon and the plastic surgeon. The nipple-sparing mastectomy is often performed through an inframammary skin incision when possible.
- When performing a skin-sparing mastectomy, it is important to remove as much breast tissue as possible while maintaining the viability of the skin. From the oncologic standpoint, this is a balance between removing the majority of the breast tissue but not making the skin flaps so thin that it results in skin necrosis and flap loss. The anatomic plane that separates the subcutaneous tissue and the underlying breast parenchyma is formed by the superficial fascia of the breast. This is an ill-defined thin layer visualized by a faint white fascial line (see **FIGURE 1**). The dissection is carefully performed in this plane. The remaining tissue on the skin envelope usually ranges in thickness between 2 and 5 mm depending on the patient's body mass index and anatomy.
- It is crucial to flap viability to preserve both the subcutaneous venous plexus under the skin as well as the branches of the second intercostal perforator in the upper medial flap as it exits the ribs. This is the largest blood supply to the skin flap (**FIGURE 4A** and **B**).
- Once the flaps are created to the clavicle superiorly including the axillary tail of Spence, medially to the lateral edge of the sternum, laterally to the latissimus dorsi muscle, and inferiorly to the sixth rib, the breast is then removed posteriorly from the pectoralis major muscle including the underlying deep fascia overlying the muscle. It is important when creating the flap medially not to extend across the sternum to the contralateral breast.

PATIENT HISTORY AND PHYSICAL FINDINGS

- Patients with operable breast cancer are candidates for either breast conservation therapy (BCT) or skin-sparing mastectomy with or without reconstruction. It is important

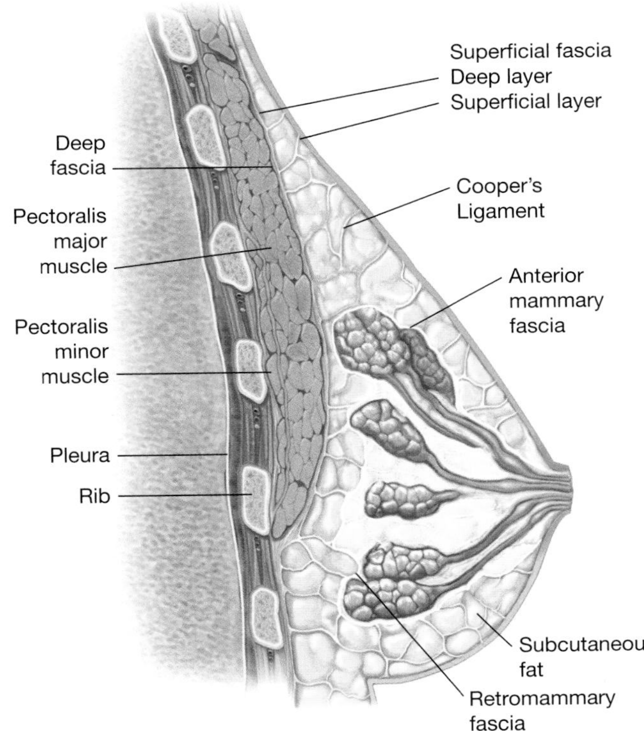

FIGURE 1 • Cross section of the breast demonstrating the superficial fascia, including both the superficial and deep layers.

for patients to understand that the survival between BCT and mastectomy is equal. However, mastectomy does carry a slightly lower locoregional recurrence rate of about 2% vs 5% in 10 years after BCT.[1]

- Another important difference between the two surgical treatment options is that mastectomy usually does not require postoperative radiation therapy. Postmastectomy radiation is recommended for patients with tumors greater than 5 cm in size, patients with positive margins after mastectomy, or select patients with axillary lymph node involvement for locoregional control and to improve survival.[2]
- Prior to determining whether a patient will be a candidate for mastectomy or BCT, a thorough history and physical examination should be performed.
- The medical history should focus on the patient's family history of breast cancer in first-degree relatives and ovarian cancer in the family. Patients with a strong family history of breast or ovarian cancer, patients with premenopausal breast cancer, patients with bilateral breast cancer, male family members with breast cancer, those of Ashkenazi Jewish descent, or those with a personal history of breast cancer should be recommended for genetic counseling and testing for the BRCA 1 and 2 gene mutations. Also included in the medical history, the surgeon should ask about personal risk factors for developing breast cancer such as early menses, late menopause, a personal history of an atypical breast biopsy, lobular carcinoma in situ, a history of previous chest wall radiation for Hodgkin lymphoma, or use of hormone replacement therapy. Many of these high-risk patients who decide to undergo mastectomy also opt for contralateral mastectomy at the time of mastectomy to decrease their risk of a future breast cancer. Another reason for the recent increased incidence of contralateral prophylactic mastectomy is because of patient's anxiety, fear, and desire to reduce future risk of recurrence and cosmetic symmetry.[3]
- After obtaining a thorough medical history, a detailed physical examination would include examination of the patient in both the upright and supine positions (**TABLE 1**). While placing the patient's hands on her hips in the upright position, the patient is visually examined for symmetry, evidence of skin changes, or dimpling. The cervical and axillary areas are palpated for adenopathy, and the breasts are examined. The patient is then placed supine with both arms over her head. The breasts are examined again for palpable masses and nipple discharge, and the axillae are palpated again while lowering the arms to the side. The abdomen is then examined for hepatosplenomegaly.

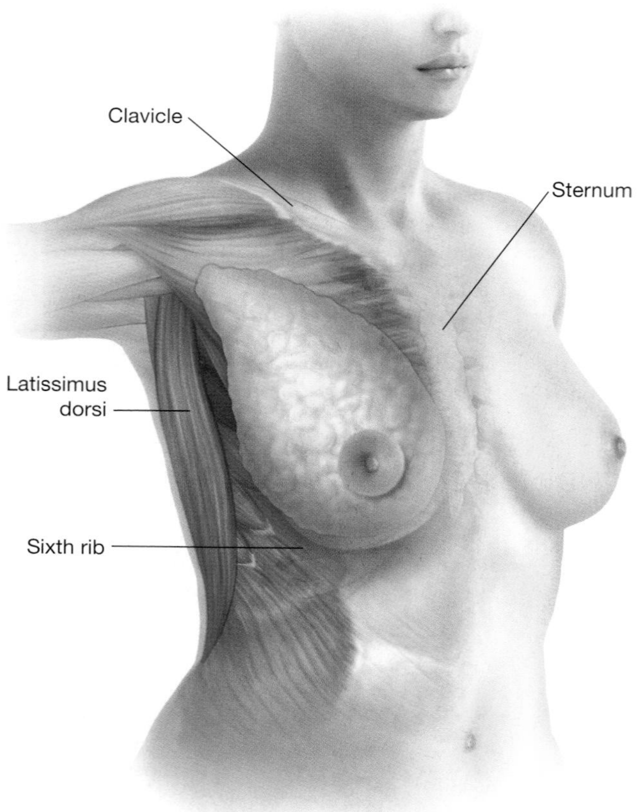

FIGURE 2 ● Anatomic boundaries of the breast.

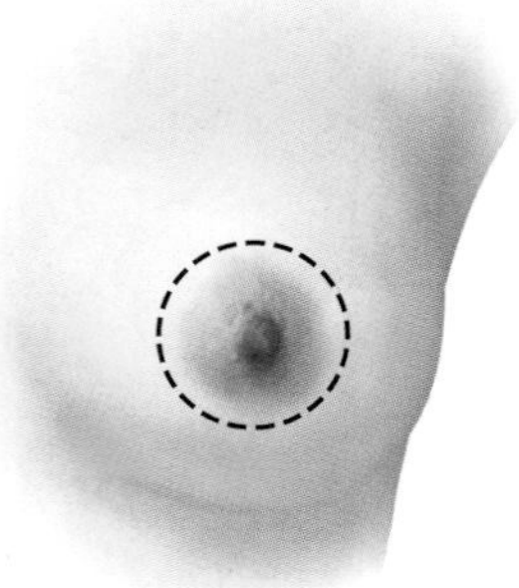

A. Round periareolar

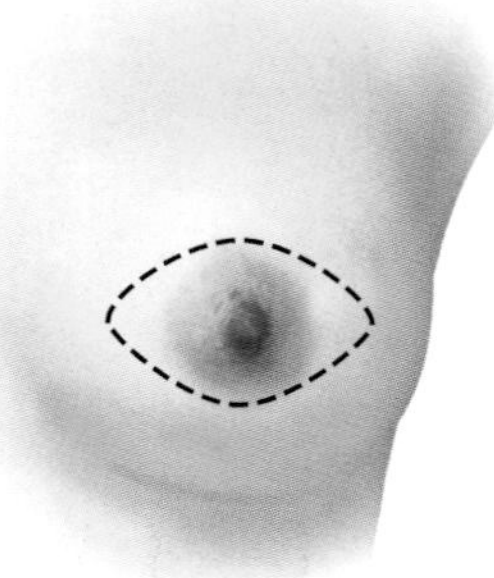

B. Small eliptical periareolar

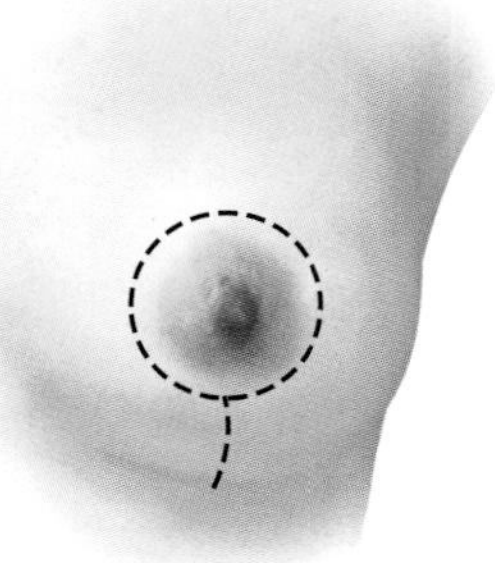

C. Periareolar with inferior extension

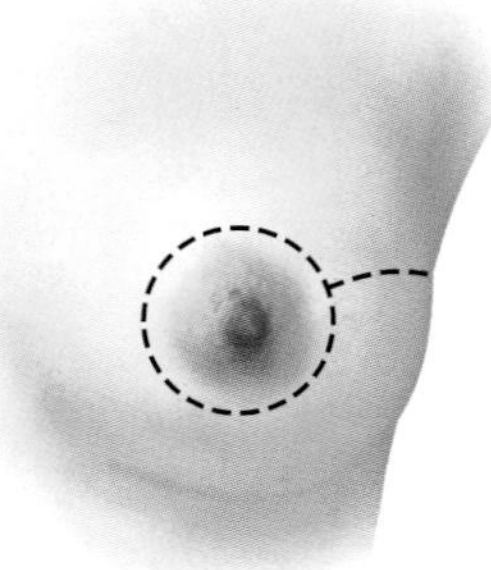

D. Periareolar with lateral extension

FIGURE 3 ● **A-D,** Surgical incisions used for a skin-sparing mastectomy.

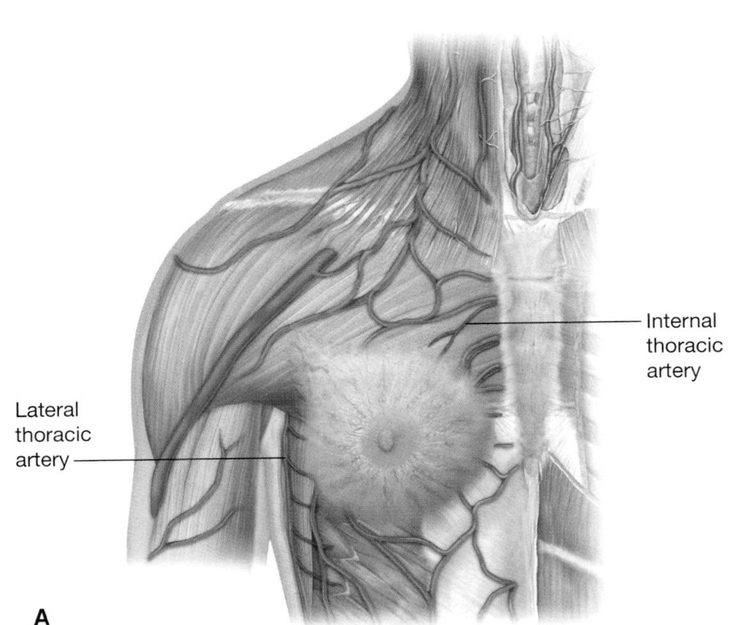

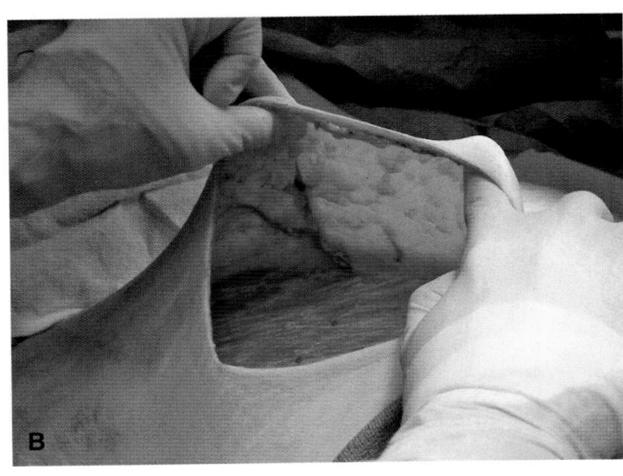

FIGURE 4 ● **A,** The blood supply to the breast comes primarily from the lateral (mammary) thoracic artery, the internal (mammary) thoracic artery, and the intercostal arteries. It is crucial to preserve the branches of the second intercostal artery in the upper medial flap to ensure viability. **B,** The subcutaneous venous plexus and branch off the second intercostal artery are seen preserved with the flap.

Table 1: Methods for Examining the Breast and Pathognomonic Signs

Examination	Technique	Grading	Significance
Breast examination	Upright Supine	Symmetry	Cancer causing enlargement
		Skin changes	Peau d'orange, associated with inflammatory breast cancer, or an underlying tumor pulling on Cooper ligaments
		Palpable masses	Cancer, benign mass, or cysts
		Adenopathy	Lymph node metastasis or reactive lymph nodes
		Nipple discharge	Bloody or clear spontaneous unilateral discharge associated with carcinoma risk

PREOPERATIVE IMAGING AND OTHER DIAGNOSTIC STUDIES FOR OPERABLE BREAST CANCER

- The purpose of preoperative imaging is to clinically stage the patient, determine operability, assist with surgical decision making, and assess the need for preoperative chemotherapy for downstaging. All patients prior to mastectomy require a recent bilateral mammogram including craniocaudal and medial lateral views. On mammogram, one should look for spiculated masses, tumor size and location to skin and nipple, additional tumors, involvement of the skin and/or NAC, and associated calcifications (**FIGURE 5**).
- For patients with dense breast tissue or young age, a breast sonogram may be a helpful addition to assess the presence of additional lesions in dense breast tissue and the extent and depth of the tumor.
- Ultrasonography is also helpful to assess the axilla radiographically. Suspicious nodes have a very characteristic appearance with an obliterated hilum and nondistinct borders. An ultrasound-guided fine needle aspiration (FNA) can be performed preoperatively for suspicious nodes (**FIGURE 6**).

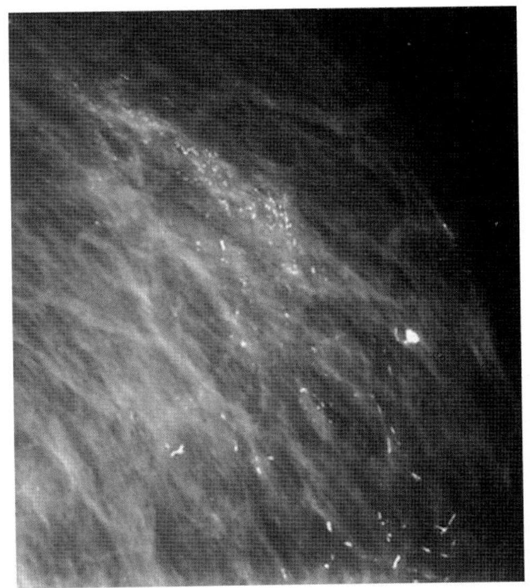

FIGURE 5 ● Magnification mammogram showing pleomorphic calcifications suspicious for carcinoma.

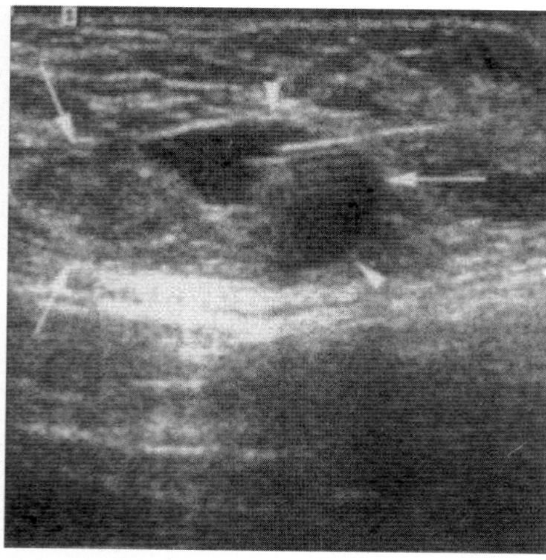

FIGURE 6 ● Ultrasound-guided FNA biopsy of axillary lymph node metastases. The arrows are pointing to the axillary lymph node.

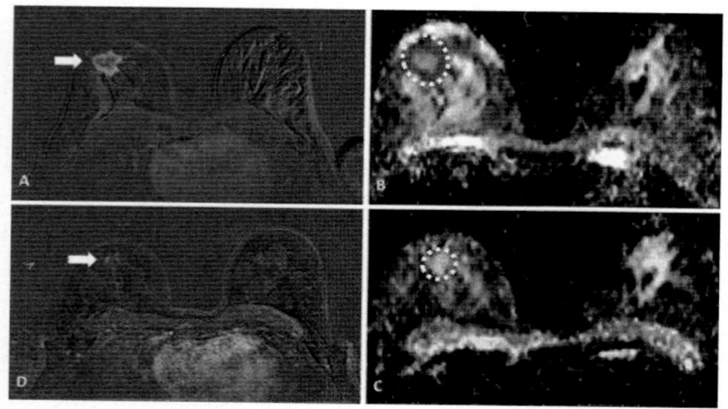

FIGURE 7 ● MRI showing response to chemotherapy before treatment **(A)** and after treatment **(B)**.

- Magnetic resonance imaging (MRI) of the breast is used selectively for patients who are having mastectomy. One indication is for patients with invasive lobular cancer because of a higher incidence of contralateral disease.[4]
- MRI may also be used preoperatively for high-risk patients such as those with the BRCA 1 or 2 mutation, a strong family history, dense breast tissue, difficult breast examinations, large tumors with questionable skin involvement, or those undergoing neoadjuvant chemotherapy. In patients undergoing preoperative chemotherapy, MRI helps to monitor the response to treatment. An MRI is performed before treatment begins and then repeated again during systemic treatment or after is completed for comparison. The MRI shows a nice relationship of the tumor location to the overlying skin or NAC for treatment planning and choice of surgical incision for mastectomy (**FIGURE 7**).
- Staging tests to rule out metastatic disease, such as positron emission tomography–computed tomography (PET/CT) or alternatively a computed tomography (CT) scan of the chest, abdomen, and pelvis and bone scan should be considered in patients with lymph node involvement or large tumors or those patients with signs or symptoms suggestive of metastases (**TABLE 2**).

Table 2: Indications for Preoperative Positron Emission Tomography–Computed Tomography (PET/CT)

Examination	Indications Preoperatively
PET/CT	Large tumor size Evidence of lymph node metastasis Symptomatic disease (ie, bone pain) Locally advanced breast cancer

SURGICAL MANAGEMENT

- Indications for skin-sparing mastectomy include patients with macromastia or ptosis who choose mastectomy to reduce their risk of a future local recurrence and patients with the *BRCA* gene mutation, other high-risk patients who have a strong family history of breast cancer, or patients with young age at diagnosis. The patient must have operable breast cancer and not have extensive skin involvement or fungating, ulcerating lesions.
- Indications for nipple-sparing mastectomy include patients who are undergoing prophylactic surgery, *BRCA* gene mutation carriers, and patients who have operable cancers not located close to the nipple.[5] Patients who should not undergo nipple-sparing mastectomy are those patients with cancers located directly under the nipple, patients with radiographic evidence of nipple involvement, or those with suspicious nipple discharge or nipple retraction. Patients must be informed that it is not possible to remove all the tissue under the nipple and that there is a reported risk of recurrence in the nipple and nipple necrosis of less than 5%.[6]
- Patients with macromastia or ptosis who wish to undergo nipple-sparing mastectomy may be candidates especially if they are able to undergo a lumpectomy with oncoplasty to raise the nipple above the inframammary fold followed by nipple-sparing mastectomy after 10 to 12 weeks from the first surgery. It is important that the breast and reconstructive surgeon work closely together to determine whether the patient is a good candidate for a two-stage nipple-sparing mastectomy.

Preoperative Planning

- All preoperative radiographic studies should be performed prior to surgery to determine tumor location, size, and depth.
- The breast cancer surgeon and patient discuss the optimal type of skin-sparing mastectomy preoperatively and determine whether they are candidates for skin-sparing simple mastectomy or nipple-sparing mastectomy.
- All patients undergoing immediate reconstruction consult with a reconstructive surgeon prior to surgery for preoperative planning. After the reconstructive surgeon examines the patient and determines the optimal reconstruction depending on the patient's body habitus, breast size, and clinical stage, the reconstructive surgeon collaborates with the breast surgeon for the optimal oncologic approach with the best cosmesis.
- Patients with palpable tumors close to skin or those considering nipple-sparing mastectomy with tumors close to the areola may benefit from a preoperative breast MRI to

address distance of tumor to the skin or disease below the NAC. This may alter treatment planning such as the use of neoadjuvant chemotherapy to achieve negative margins as well as surgical decision making.

Positioning

- The optimal operative position for all patients undergoing skin-sparing mastectomy is supine with the arms abducted approximately 45°. Care is taken not to hyperextend the arms in anticipation for a long surgery. The arm boards are padded in order to protect the elbows from pressure compression causing a median nerve palsy.
- Compression boots are placed preoperatively, and there is no need for additional anticoagulation unless the patient is at high risk for deep vein thrombosis (DVT), including obesity, a personal history of DVT, or cardiac valves requiring prophylaxis.
- Upon induction, if the patient is undergoing immediate breast reconstruction, they should receive a dose of intravenous (IV) antibiotics to cover gram-positive bacteria, usually a first-generation cephalosporin such as cephazolin.

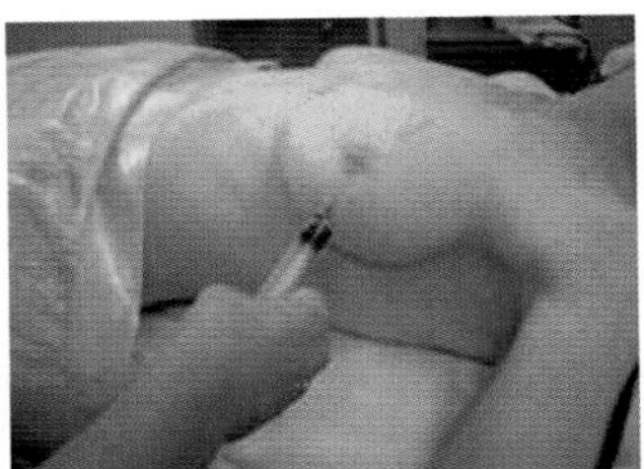

FIGURE 8 ● Patient positioning and preoperative injection of blue dye in a subareolar fashion.

- For flap reconstruction with a prolonged anesthetic time, a Foley catheter is inserted after induction.
- Prior to prepping the patient, methylene blue dye is injected subareolar for those surgeons who use dual tracer to identify the sentinel lymph node (**FIGURE 8**).
- Once prepped, the patient's arm is wrapped with a free arm dressing in anticipation of an axillary node dissection if axillary metastasis is known; otherwise, the arm is draped outside the field.

SKIN-SPARING MASTECTOMY

- Prior to surgery, the patient is skin marked by both the reconstructive and breast cancer surgeons. The NAC is removed by a small elliptical skin incision. There are many options of excision depending on breast size and tumor location as well as type of reconstruction (see **FIGURE 3**).
- The NAC is incised in an elliptical fashion with a no. 15 blade scalpel into the dermis. Skin hooks are placed on the flap and pulled upward by the first assistant. Care is taken to ensure the first assistant pulls directly perpendicular to the chest wall to avoid an inadvertent buttonhole in the flap (**FIGURE 9**).
- By retracting the breast downward against the upward traction of the skin, the superficial fascial plane is identified.

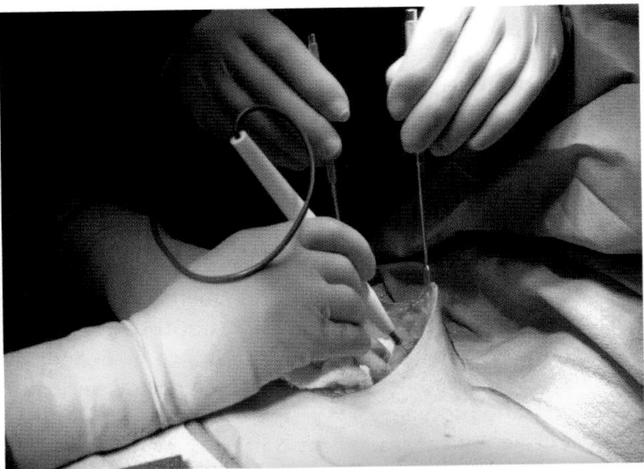

FIGURE 9 ● Skin hooks are placed on the flap and pulled upward by the first assistant. Care is taken to ensure the first assistant pulls directly perpendicular to the chest wall to avoid an inadvertent button hole in the flap.

The surgeon uses cautery to create the flaps by dissecting just above the superficial fascia in order to remove as much of the breast tissue as possible. Alternatively, some surgeons may use either the knife or scissors to create the mastectomy flaps. As long as the surgeon is in the correct anatomic plane, it should be relatively avascular.

- As the surgeon progresses further posteriorly, medium-sized Richardson retractors or lighted retractors are used to assist with retraction (see **FIGURE 15**). Because the skin ellipse opening may be quite small, the flaps are created in a spiral fashion until the pectoralis muscle is identified.
- The surgeon's hand is then used to examine the flaps. If the surgeon is in the proper plane, the flaps will only be a couple of millimeters thick and even throughout. Care is taken to ensure that the axillary tail of the breast has been adequately dissected and removed en bloc with the specimen.
- Next, the breast is removed from the pectoralis muscle. Medium-sized or large Richardson retractors are used to retract the skin superiorly, and Kelly clamps may be placed on the superior aspect of the breast to assist with downward traction.
- Electrocautery is then used to separate the breast from the pectoralis muscle by dissecting parallel to the muscle fibers from medial to lateral (**FIGURE 10**). All perforating vessels are carefully cauterized prior to cutting to prevent retraction into the muscle and subsequent bleeding.
- Once the breast is removed from the chest wall, a silk stitch is used to mark the axillary tail for orientation for the pathologist. The breast is passed off the field for permanent section, and attention is paid to the axilla to perform either a sentinel lymph node biopsy or axillary lymph node dissection, depending on the stage of the cancer. This may be performed via the mastectomy incision if there is no tension on the wound. If the axilla is too far away, a separate axillary incision is made.

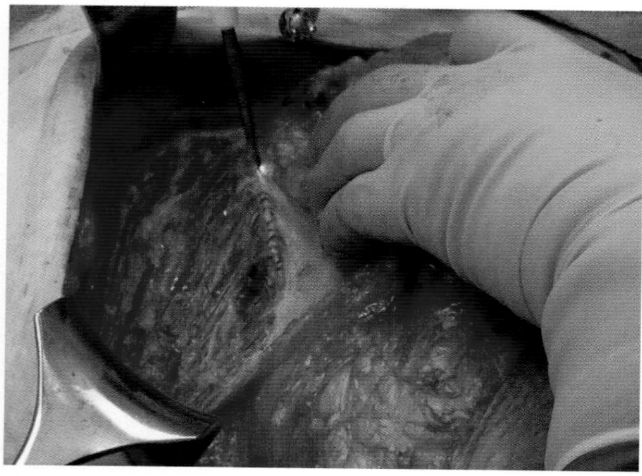

FIGURE 10 ● Electrocautery is used to dissect the breast and pectoralis fascia off the underlying muscle. Cautery is moved parallel to the muscle fibers from medial to lateral.

NIPPLE-SPARING MASTECTOMY

- Nipple-sparing mastectomy is performed similar to skin-sparing mastectomy (**FIGURE 11**); however, the NAC is spared. This can be done through various approaches (**FIGURE 12**).
- The inframammary incision is the most cosmetically appealing and may be associated with less nipple areolar ischemia by not disrupting the blood flow around the NAC (**FIGURE 13A** and **B**).[7] The entire flap is created from the inframammary fold inferiorly to the clavicle superiorly. This is a long flap and is therefore best used on women with small to medium-sized breasts. A generous inframammary fold incision can be made to allow adequate exposure. The most challenging technical aspect of this approach is getting sufficient upward traction of the skin in order to create the flap in the appropriate plane.

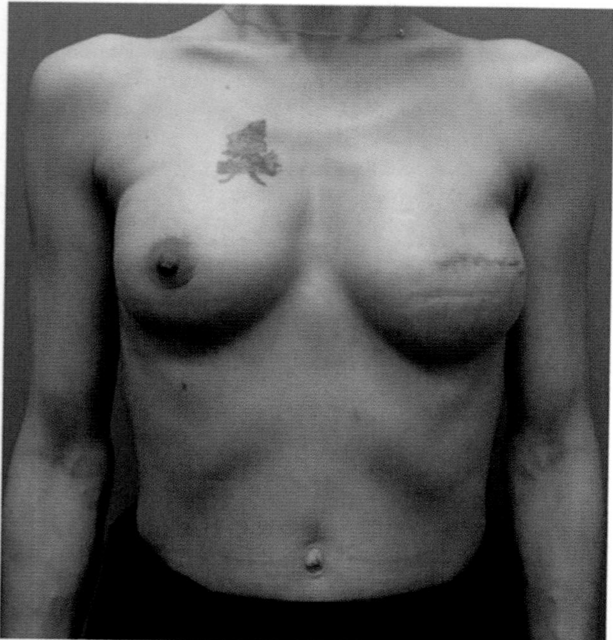

FIGURE 11 ● Nipple-sparing mastectomy via inframammary skin incision vs skin-sparing mastectomy on patient with left centrally located tumor. (Photo courtesy of Sherman J, MD.)

- Skin hooks are used for upward traction, as in the traditional skin-sparing mastectomy. However, when approaching the NAC, it is best to have the first assistant retract the nipple upward with a lighted retractor under the NAC in order to visualize the area adequately (**FIGURES 14** and **15**).
- The ductal tissue posterior to the nipple is usually more dense and lighter in color (**FIGURE 16**). Once through this area, the lighted retractors are advanced in order to complete the superior aspect of the flaps to the clavicle. The first assistant can apply gentle traction of the skin flap by placing the palm of their hand on the superior aspect of the flap and pushing away superiorly toward the patient's head. This upward traction takes a curve and makes a straight plane, which is easier for dissection.
- To create even flaps, it is important that both the first assistant and surgeon apply steady, even traction and avoid readjusting multiple times.
- After the breast is removed from the chest wall, attention is paid to the nipple to take an additional nipple margin.
- The surgeon's finger is placed on the outside of the nipple and the nipple is everted. An Allis clamp is then placed on the tissue inside the nipple and a no. 15 blade scalpel is used to perform a shave biopsy of any residual ductal tissue within the nipple. The tissue is then sent to pathology for permanent section. Frozen section of this additional nipple margin is discouraged since it is difficult to freeze such a small specimen and can be inaccurate.
- If there is disease on permanent section of the additional nipple margin, the standard treatment is to take the patient back for excision of the NAC (**FIGURE 17**).
- For patients with ptotic breasts who are not ideal candidates for nipple-sparing mastectomy, we recommend performing a two-stage procedure suggested by Spear and colleagues[8] where the patient undergoes a primary mammoplasty followed by nipple-sparing mastectomy 10 to 12 weeks later (**FIGURE 18**).

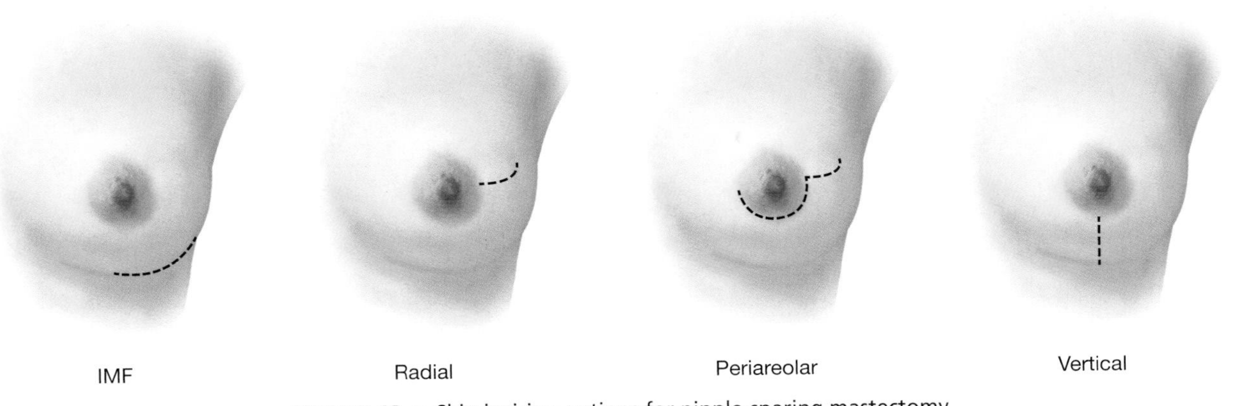

FIGURE 12 ● Skin incision options for nipple-sparing mastectomy.

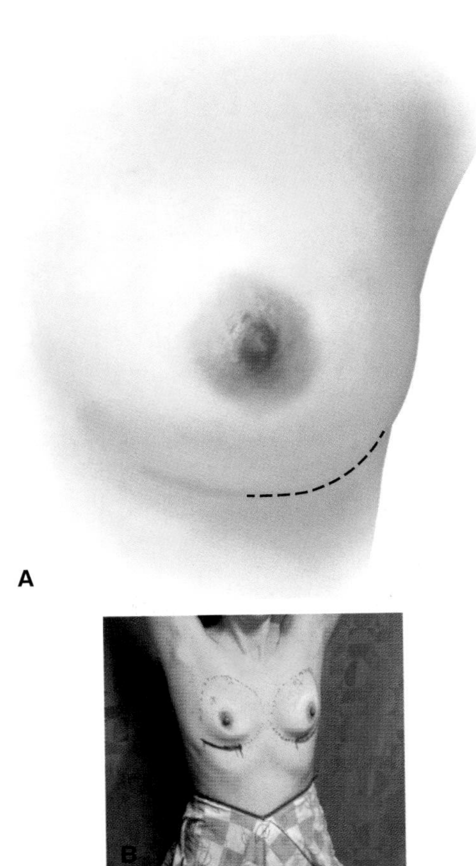

FIGURE 13 ● **A,** Nipple-sparing mastectomy via inframammary fold skin incision. **B,** Preoperative skin marking for inframammary skin incision.

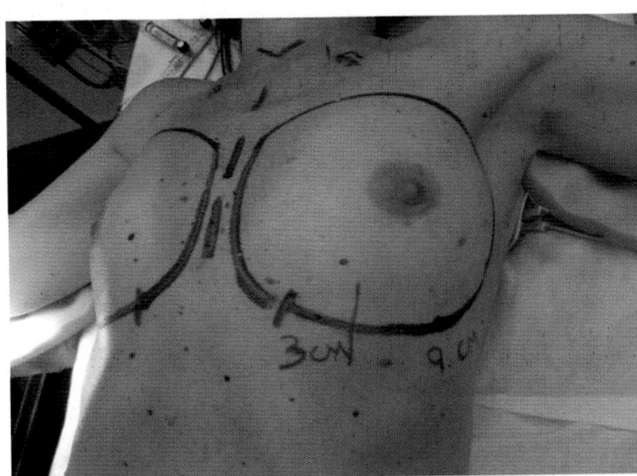

FIGURE 14 ● Extended incision for more exposure if necessary.

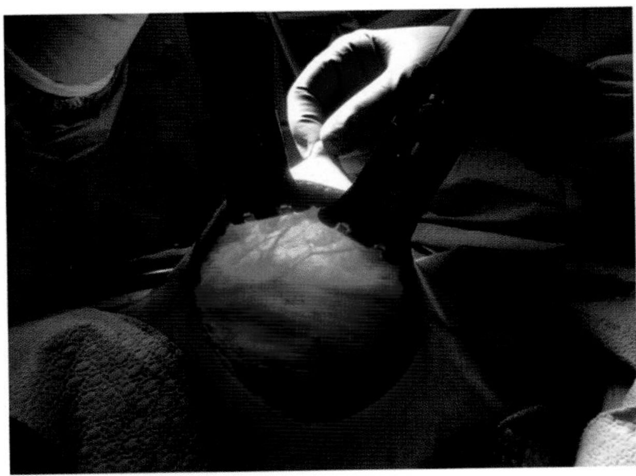

FIGURE 15 ● Gentle upward traction of the nipple by the first assistant to create plane behind the nipple.

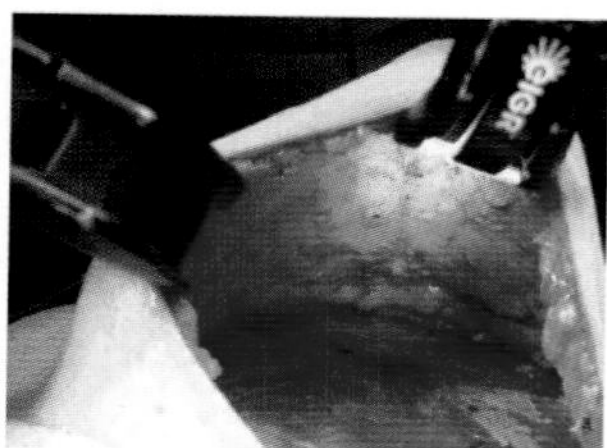

FIGURE 16 ● Inside of nipple area appears lighter compared with the surrounding tissue.

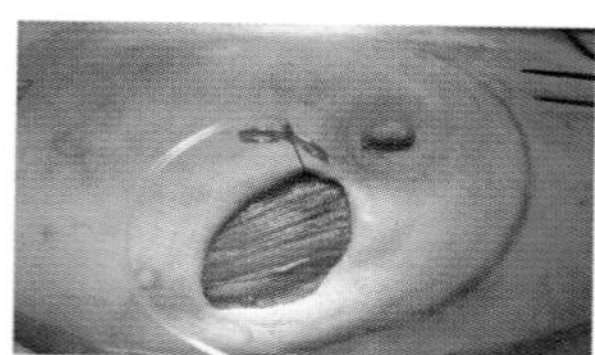

FIGURE 17 ● Expansion of the tissue expander after a nipple-sparing mastectomy with immediate reconstruction.

Analgesia after Mastectomy

- Mastectomy is performed under general anesthesia with an enhanced recovery after surgery (ERAS) protocol to decrease the use of narcotics. Intraoperatively, a long-acting local anesthetic may be injected into the borders of the mastectomy wound just below the cut edge of the fascia. Postoperatively, patients are given anti-inflammatories and an oral narcotic as needed for pain. Valium may be used to relax the muscle and prevent muscle spasm and tightness after retropectoral reconstruction. For patients with prepectoral reconstruction and the ERAS protocol with a local injectable anesthetic, same day discharge is possible if they meet postanesthesia care unit (PACU) criteria for discharge. We have found preoperative counseling and drain teaching help facilitate same day discharge after prepectoral breast reconstruction.

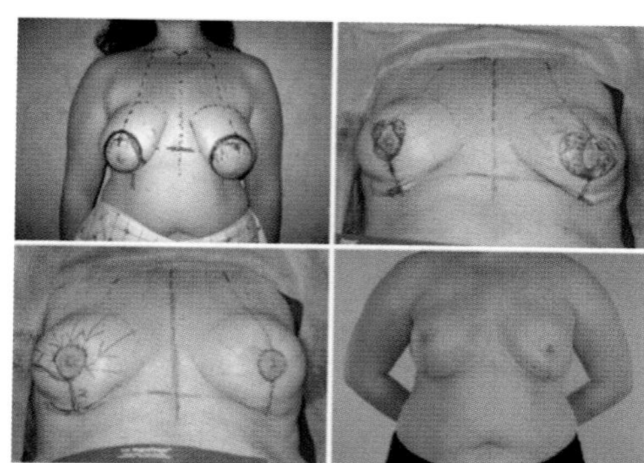

FIGURE 18 ● Staged nipple-sparing mastectomy following reduction for macromastia or ptotic breasts. (Photo courtesy of Spear S, Rottman S, Seiboth L, et al. Breast reconstruction using a staged nipple-sparing mastectomy following mastopexy or reduction. *Plast Reconstr Surg*. 2012;129(3):572-581.)

PEARLS AND PITFALLS

Possible Pitfalls of Skin-Sparing Mastectomy	Pearls
Flap necrosis	■ Identify fascial plane below subcutaneous tissue; stay just above this line to create flap. ■ Maintain even traction/countertraction in order to create even flaps. ■ Preserve the subcutaneous venous plexus and the second intercostal perforator to prevent flap necrosis. ■ Avoid denuding the skin.
Nipple necrosis	■ Do not denude the nipple. ■ Avoid too much traction on the nipple for prolonged periods of time. ■ Avoid cautery under the nipple.
Infection	■ Treat reconstructive patients with preoperative IV antibiotics and postoperative oral antibiotics until the drains are removed. ■ Irrigate thoroughly with normal saline after the mastectomy is performed. ■ Obtain careful hemostasis.

POSTOPERATIVE CARE

- Patients who undergo prepectoral implant reconstruction have the possibility of same day discharge if they meet PACU criteria postop.
- Patients who undergo flap reconstruction are admitted longer depending on the type of flap reconstruction.
- They are maintained on oral first-generation cephalosporin until the Jackson-Pratt (JP) drains are removed.
- The patients are discharged with a surgical bra and the JP drains attached to the bra.
- They may resume showering after 48 hours and are taught how to empty and record the drain output.

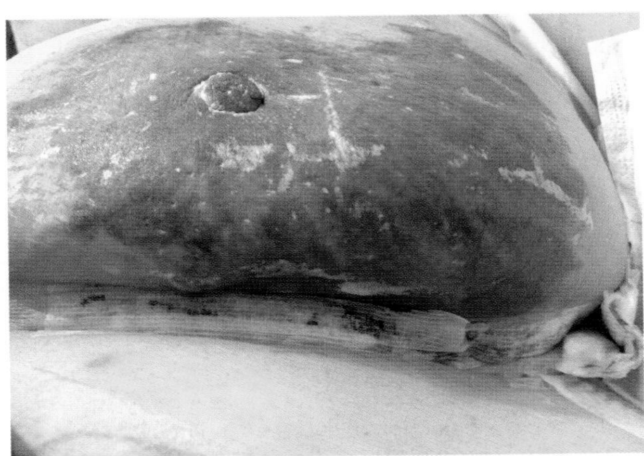

FIGURE 19 ● Nipple and flap necrosis after nipple-sparing mastectomy via inframammary skin incision.

- The patient returns in 1 week to have the drains removed if she is draining less than 30 mL/d from each drain and to discuss the pathology report.
- Patients are then referred to medical oncology for adjuvant treatment and a radiation oncologist if indicated.
- When the breast is removed, the sensory innervations to the skin are also removed, resulting in loss of sensation. This resulting band of numbness gets narrower over time but never completely resolves.
- Following mastectomy, patients are seen in follow-up by the breast surgeon or advanced practice provider every 6 months for 5 years to examine the skin for recurrent disease, then yearly thereafter.
- An instruction book of postmastectomy stretching exercises is given to the patient after the drains are removed to increase mobility and prevent frozen shoulder. For patients who develop decreased mobility after surgery, they are referred to a specially trained physical therapist.

OUTCOMES

- Include functional and prosthetic survivorship data, as applicable.

COMPLICATIONS

- Skin flap necrosis (**FIGURES 19** and **20**)
- Nipple necrosis
- Infection
- Seroma
- Hematoma

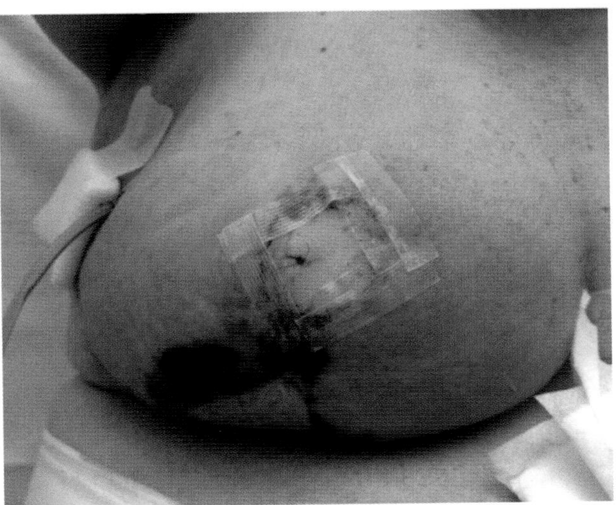

FIGURE 20 ● Inferior flap necrosis after skin-sparing mastectomy with deep inferior epigastric perforator (DIEP) flap reconstruction.

REFERENCES

1. Veronesi U, Cascinelli N, Mariani L, et al. Twenty-year follow-up of a randomized study comparing breast-conserving surgery with radical mastectomy for early breast cancer. *N Engl J Med.* 2002;347(16):1227-1232.
2. Vilarino-Varela M, Chin YS, Makris A. Current indications for post-mastectomy radiation. *Int Semin Surg Oncol.* 2009;6:5.
3. Howard-McNatt M, Schroll RW, Hurt GJ, et al. Contralateral prophylactic mastectomy in breast cancer patients who test negative for BRCA mutations. *Am J Surg.* 2011;202(3):298-302.
4. Heil J, Buehler A, Golatta M, et al. Do patients with invasive lobular breast cancer benefit in terms of adequate change in surgical therapy from a supplementary preoperative breast MRI? *Ann Oncol.* 2012;23(1):98-104.
5. Smith BL, Tang R, Rai U, et al. Oncologic saftey of nipple sparing mastectomy in women with breast cancer. *J Am Coll Surg.* 2017;225(3):361-365. doi: 10.1016/j.jamcollsurg.2017.06.013.
6. Petit JY, Veronesi U, Orecchia R, et al. Risk factors associated with recurrence after nipple-sparing mastectomy for invasive and intraepithelial neoplasia. *Ann Oncol.* 2012;23(8):2053-2058.
7. Frey JD, Salibian AA, Levine JP, Karp NS, Choi M. Incision choices in nipple-sparing mastectomy: a comparative analysis of outcomes and evolution of a clinical algorithm. *Plast Reconstr Surg.* 2018;142(6):826e-835e.
8. Spear S, Rottman S, Seiboth L, et al. Breast reconstruction using a staged nipple-sparing mastectomy following mastopexy or reduction. *Plast Reconstr Surg.* 2012;129:572-581.

Chapter 20 Modified Radical Mastectomy

Tiffany A. Torstenson and Judy C. Boughey

DEFINITION

- Modified radical mastectomy (MRM) is a surgical procedure that removes the breast tissue from the chest wall and the lymphatic-bearing tissue from the axilla. This operation removes the nipple-areolar complex, the majority of the excess skin, and level I and II axillary nodes but spares the pectoralis major muscle. It can also be termed as a total mastectomy with an axillary lymph node dissection.

PATIENT HISTORY AND PHYSICAL FINDINGS

- There has been a huge evolution in types of the mastectomy over the years. We have moved away from the radical mastectomy to more cosmetic procedures such as simple/total mastectomy, skin-sparing mastectomy, and nipple-sparing mastectomy. In patients undergoing mastectomy who have node-positive disease, axillary lymph node dissection is often (but not always) recommended.
- Patients undergoing an MRM usually have documented axillary lymph node metastases diagnosed on percutaneous biopsy preoperatively or on sentinel lymph node surgery intraoperatively and either elect to have a total mastectomy or require a mastectomy (ie, are not candidates for breast-conserving therapy) and are not interested or are not candidates for immediate reconstruction. Patients diagnosed with inflammatory breast cancer should also undergo an MRM after neoadjuvant chemotherapy according to National Comprehensive Cancer Network (NCCN) guidelines.[1]
- For patients with large tumors and tumors involving the skin, it is crucial to decide from the beginning if these patients are operable candidates and whether neoadjuvant systemic therapy (with chemotherapy or endocrine therapy) should be considered to decrease the extent of disease prior to surgery. A multidisciplinary approach is vital in the treatment success of these patients. Involvement of a medical oncologist and radiation oncologist early in the management of these patients helps treatment planning and to streamline patient care. All patients with inflammatory breast cancer should receive neoadjuvant chemotherapy.
- A comprehensive history and physical examination is imperative on the first consultation with these patients. The history should be very detailed and include questions pertaining to medical conditions, medications, surgeries, allergies, and also about any musculoskeletal issues, which could affect operative positioning. It is important to evaluate for any family history of breast or ovarian cancer.
- If there is a strong family history of breast or ovarian cancer, it is essential to offer genetic counseling and possibility of genetic testing. However, given the broad availability and decreased cost of genetic testing, and potential implications to both medical and surgical recommendations, genetic testing should be offered to all patients with breast cancer.
- Physical examination starts with an inspection of bilateral breasts both with arms at the patient's side and with the arms elevated, noting any asymmetry, nipple retraction, prior scars, or skin changes.
- Palpation of the breasts should always be done both in a sitting and supine position in a circular or vertical pattern. Palpable masses should have bidimensional measurements and should be assessed for chest wall adherence and proximity to the skin and to the nipple. Any palpable masses that do not correspond to radiologic findings require further testing and tissue biopsy.
- A thorough examination of the lymph node basins should be performed, including the axillary, cervical, supraclavicular, and infraclavicular nodes. If there is adenopathy on palpation, patients should undergo an in-office or radiologic ultrasound. Any suspicious nodes on imaging should undergo a fine needle aspiration or core needle biopsy. Placement of a clip in a positive node (or at time of biopsy of a very abnormal node that most likely will be positive) should be performed for patients to ensure this node is resected at surgery. (This is not critical for inflammatory breast cancer but should be performed in patients being considered for neoadjuvant therapy where systemic therapy may lead to axillary downstaging and the potential to avoid axillary lymph node dissection [and thus MRM (see Part 5, Chapter 16)]).
- Imaging and pathology diagnoses should be shared and explained to the patient. It is helpful to map out the incisions for the patients to see preoperatively. Explain to patients the need for either neoadjuvant or adjuvant chemotherapy as well as likely need for postmastectomy radiation in patients with node-positive disease.
- Neoadjuvant chemotherapy can increase rates of breast-conserving therapy as well as potentially avoid axillary lymph node dissection.
- Postmastectomy radiation in node-positive disease decreases rates of locoregional recurrence and increases disease-free and breast cancer–specific survival.
- Inquire if patients are seeking immediate reconstruction or desire to go flat chested. Patients with inflammatory breast cancer are not candidates for immediate reconstruction.
- Allocate enough time to spend with these patients in order to answer all their questions and be empathetic to their needs during this emotional time. Keep interruptions with pagers and cell phones to a minimum.

IMAGING AND OTHER DIAGNOSTIC STUDIES

- Breast imaging plays a vital role in the screening and diagnostic workup for breast cancer. Imaging can define the extent of the disease and help assess for any abnormalities in the contralateral breast. It is also used as a monitor for local recurrence in patients postoperatively.
- Mammography is the initial imaging test in the breast cancer workup. Mammograms are very sensitive in detecting abnormalities and have been shown to decrease breast cancer mortality approximately by 30%. Screening mammograms should begin yearly in women who are 40 years of age and asymptomatic.[2]

- Diagnostic mammograms should be obtained in any patient being considered for an MRM (**FIGURE 1**). Spot and magnification views can help to focus and distinguish abnormalities. Implant displacement views (Eklund views) should be obtained in women with implants.[2,3] Request films so you can review them if they were done at an outside institution. An ultrasound should also be performed to further assess the size of the tumor and the proximity of it to the skin and chest wall. Lesions that are suspicious on ultrasound and/or mammogram should undergo a percutaneous core needle biopsy.
- Axillary ultrasound should be performed in patients with a biopsy-proven invasive cancer. Lymph nodes should be evaluated for their size, shape, and morphology. Suspicious nodes on imaging or clinically palpable nodes should undergo a fine needle aspiration biopsy or core needle biopsy with ultrasound guidance (**FIGURE 2**).
- Magnetic resonance imaging (MRI) usage is controversial but can be used as an additional imaging tool for screening patients at high risk of breast cancer development, staging of known breast cancers, and evaluating the contralateral breast. MRIs are highly sensitive tests but lack specificity leading to an increased false-positive rate. Studies have also demonstrated an increased rate of mastectomies in patients undergoing MRIs. The decision to order an MRI should be based on the recommended indications and individualized.
- According to NCCN guidelines, positron emission tomography (PET) scans can be used to evaluate for distant metastasis in patients with stage IIIA breast cancer, but this is a category 2B recommendation. Systemic staging is not recommended for patients with early-stage breast cancer in the absence of symptoms.[1]
- When a suspicious lesion is identified on imaging, a tissue biopsy is needed to differentiate between a benign and malignant process. Percutaneous biopsy is preferred over an excisional biopsy, which can lead to unnecessary surgeries for benign entities. Core needle biopsy is preferred to evaluate histology and differentiate in situ from invasive disease and to have enough tissue for receptor evaluation (estrogen receptor [ER], progesterone receptor [PR], and Her2 expression). Most breast lesions will undergo a core needle biopsy using ultrasound or stereotactic guidance. MRI-guided core needle biopsy can also be performed for lesions not visible on ultrasound or mammography, but these are more technically challenging. If cancer is identified, there should be a detailed pathologic assessment, including subtype and hormone receptor status (ER, PR, and Her2 status). In cases with morphologically abnormal lymph nodes on ultrasound, fine needle aspiration biopsy or core biopsy of the most abnormal lymph node should be performed.
- After any percutaneous breast biopsy, a marking clip should always be placed. This is extremely important in patients receiving neoadjuvant chemotherapy.

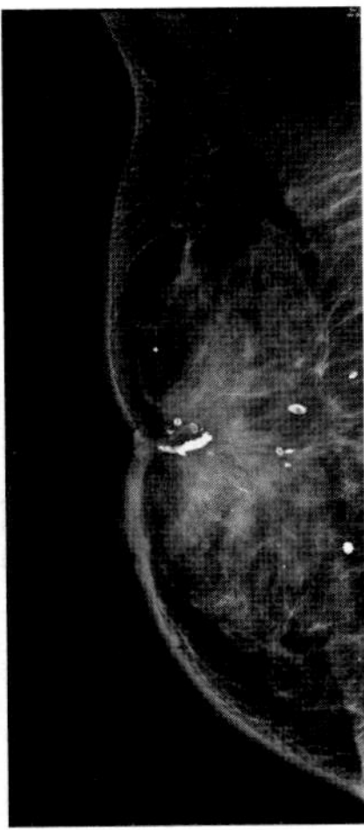

FIGURE 1 ● Mammogram showing a right invasive ductal carcinoma invading the skin and causing skin retraction.

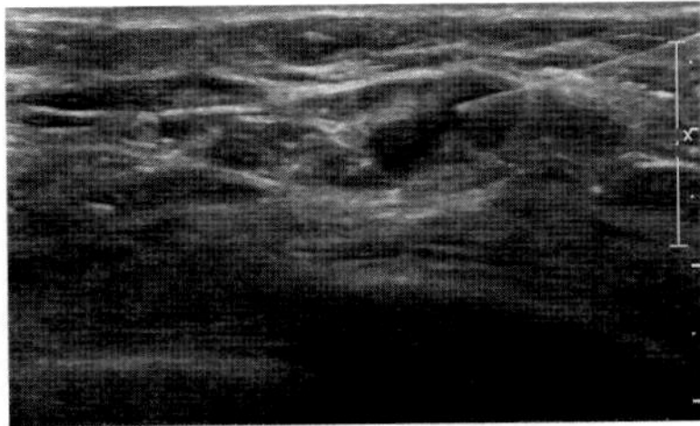

FIGURE 2 ● Ultrasound-guided fine needle aspiration of an axillary lymph node that revealed metastatic carcinoma in a male patient with breast cancer who underwent an MRM.

SURGICAL MANAGEMENT

Preoperative Planning

- Preoperatively, patients can be considered for regional anesthesia at the surgeon's and anesthesiologist's discretion. Paravertebral blocks (PVBs) are sometimes used for breast surgery and are more commonly favored over epidural blocks. They can be performed as single- or multiple-level injections or as a continuous catheter infusion. PVBs have been shown to shorten recovery times and length of hospital stays, decrease opiate usage, and decrease the incidence of vomiting. It is also hypothesized this type of regional anesthesia may protect the immune system and decrease metastasis.[4]
- PVBs are preferred over epidural blocks because they induce less hypotension and less urinary retention, are technically easy to learn, and have less severe side effects. Patients who are coagulopathic or who have musculoskeletal deformities such as kyphosis or scoliosis should not be considered for a PVB.[5,6]
- Potential complications associated with a PVB are pneumothorax, vascular penetrance, sepsis, and hematoma. Pneumothoraces are more common with multiple-level injections in comparison with single-level injections. Patients can either be seated with the spine in a kyphotic curve or be placed in a lateral decubitus position (**FIGURE 3**). The local anesthetic is injected in the paravertebral space where the thoracic spinal nerves emerge.
- Ultrasound can also help guide the correct placement of the local anesthetic. Patient comfort improves when an ultrasound is used, and the pneumothorax rate decreases due to the direct visualization of the pleura.
- Pectoralis nerve blocks (PECS) are increasingly used over PVB.
- Before patients enter the operating theater, they should be site marked in the preoperative area to ensure the correct side is being operated on. Radiologic imaging should be thoroughly reviewed prior to the procedure to ensure the location of the tumor and the proximity of it to the skin.

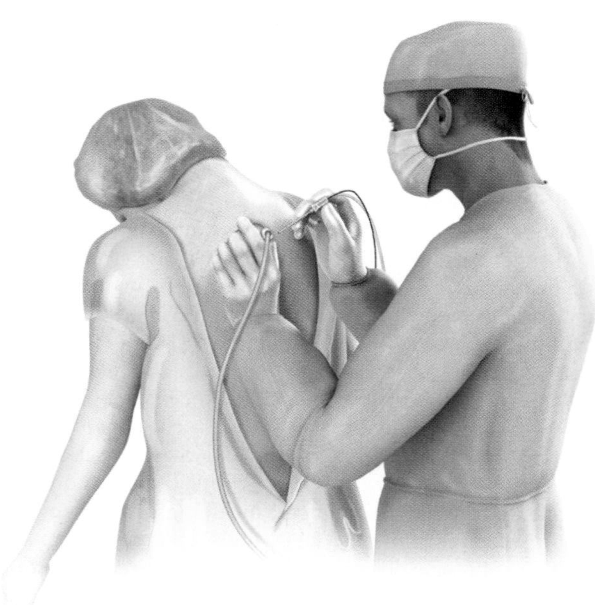

FIGURE 3 ● When performing a PVB, the patient can be seated with the spine positioned in a kyphotic curve. (Redrawn and modified from Kopp SL, Smith HM. ParaVertebral block. In: Hebl JR, Lennon RL, eds. *Mayo Clinic Atlas of Regional Anesthesia and Ultrasound-Guided Nerve Blockade*. Mayo Clinic Scientific Press and Oxford University Press; 2010:323-330.)

- Prophylactic antibiotics have been shown to reduce postoperative infections and should be administered prior to incision.[7] Most surgeons prefer to avoid the use of paralytics during an MRM in order to aid identification of important motor nerves, but excessive handling of these nerves is discouraged to prevent axonal injury.
- Prophylactic anticoagulants for prevention of venous thromboembolism (VTE), such as subcutaneous heparin, should be considered. Sequential compression devices should be placed prior to initiation of general anesthesia for VTE prevention.

Positioning

- Correct positioning of patients undergoing an MRM is vitally important. Patients should be in a supine position with the side of the MRM close to the edge of the operating table. The endotracheal tube should be positioned toward the contralateral side of the mouth from the side of the MRM. Arms should not be abducted greater than 90° to prevent injury to the brachial plexus. Arms should be placed on padded arm boards and positioned in a way that pressure points are alleviated. It is often helpful, particularly with bulky adenopathy, to prepare the ipsilateral arm into the field and wrap it with a sterile stockinette and Kerlix wrap (**FIGURE 4**). This allows for movement of the arm intraoperatively to relax the pectoral muscles and provide easier access to the axilla.
- The arm should be secured to the arm board. Blood pressure cuffs and intravenous (IV) lines should be placed in the contralateral upper extremity (**FIGURE 5**). Allow enough room between the operating table and anesthesiologist cart to allow an assistant to stand above the arm.
- Surgical preparation should include the breast and axilla and extend across the midline, inferiorly onto the abdomen, superiorly to the neck and the upper arm, and laterally to the level of the operating table. Draping should ensure preservation of a sterile field with exposure of the whole breast and axilla (**FIGURE 6**).

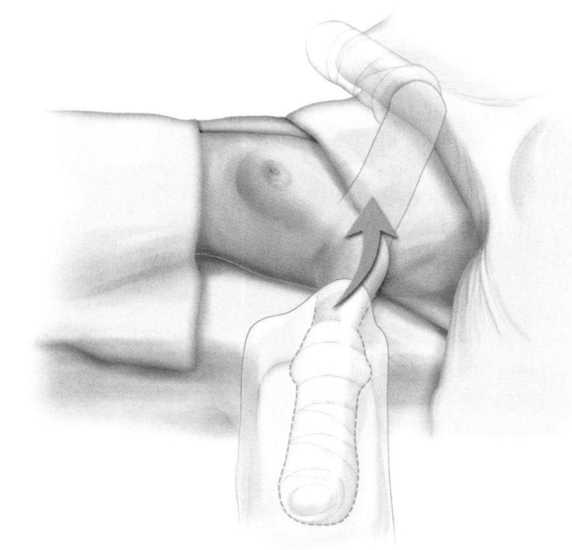

FIGURE 4 ● Positioning and draping of a patient for an MRM. (Redrawn and modified from Donohue JH, Van Heerden J, Monson JRT, eds. *Atlas of Surgical Oncology*. Cambridge, MA: Blackwell Science; 1995.)

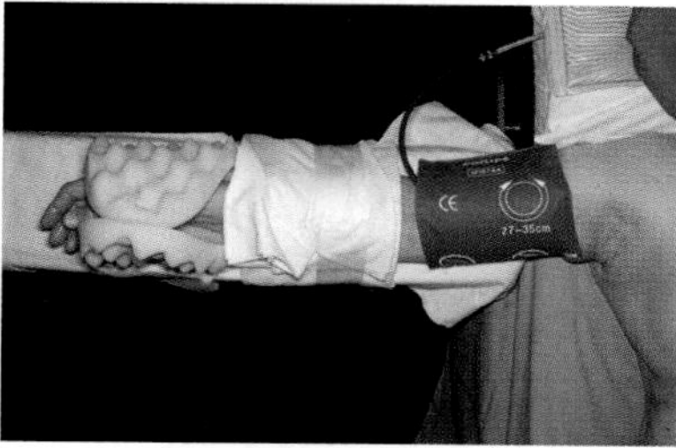

FIGURE 5 ● The contralateral arm should contain the IV and blood pressure cuff.

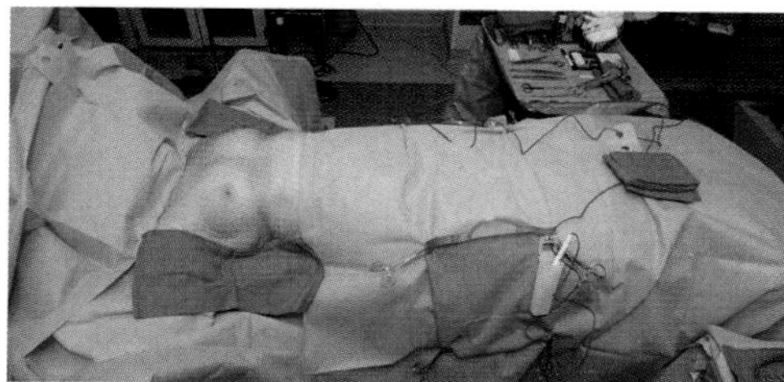

FIGURE 6 ● Draping should ensure preservation of a sterile field with exposure of the whole breast and axilla.

INCISION PLACEMENT

- There are many options for incisions for a total mastectomy that are based on the tumor location. In an MRM, it is important to have an incision that provides good exposure to the axilla and reduces skin redundancy. The incision should include the skin overlying the tumor in cases where the tumor is close to the skin and a 1- to 2-cm margin around the tumor and ideally include the previous biopsy site.
- The classic Stewart incision is a transverse elliptical incision, provides access to the axilla, and is the preferred incision of many plastic surgeons for patients seeking delayed reconstruction (**FIGURE 7**).
- When mapping the incision, it is important to make sure there will be adequate skin for a tension-free closure without excess skin for redundancy (**FIGURE 8A** and **B**). Most of these patients will be receiving postmastectomy radiation, which can lead to incision breakdown, and this is increased when incisions are under tension. The boundaries of the breast (clavicle superiorly, inframammary fold inferiorly, sternum medially, and midaxillary line laterally) define the extent of the flap dissection.

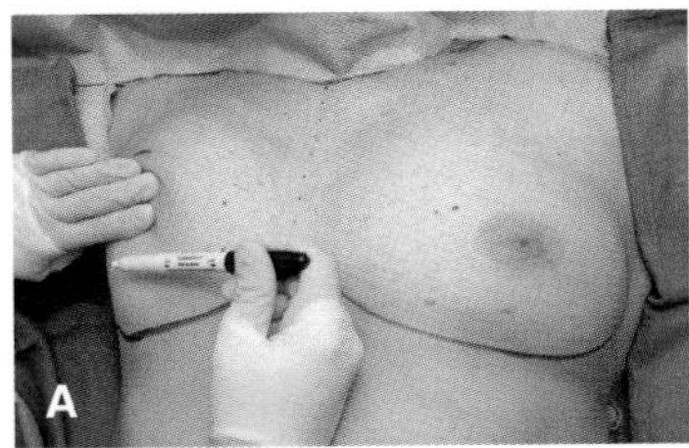

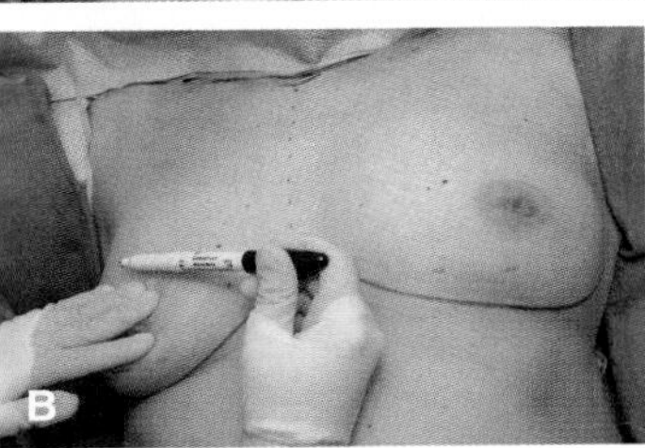

FIGURE 8 ● **A** and **B,** Measuring the distance from the superior to the inferior incision with a marking pen will help provide a tension-free closure and reduce skin redundancy.

- Measuring the length of the planned superior incision and inferior incision to ensure that these are equal in length can help guide adjustments to allow equal-length skin flaps.

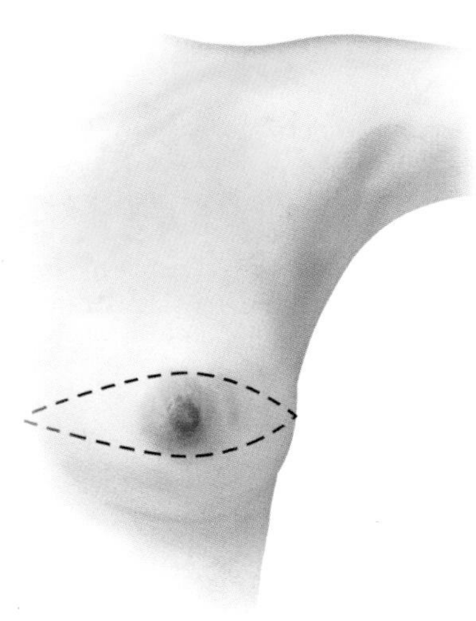

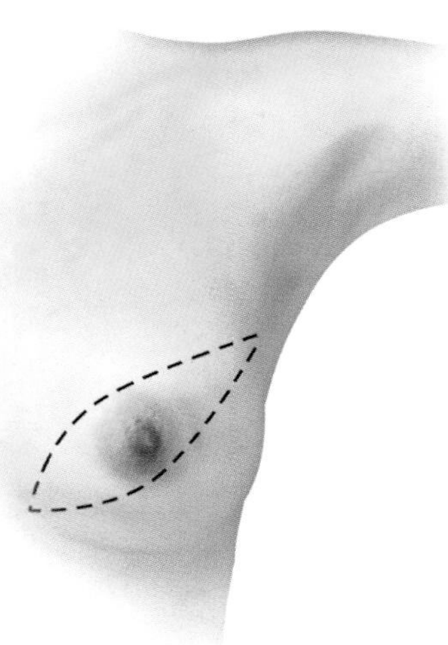

FIGURE 7 ● The two most common and preferred incisions for an MRM, which provide good axillary exposure. **Left:** Stewart incision. **Right:** Modified Stewart incision. (Redrawn and modified from Donohue JH, Van Heerden J, Monson JRT, eds. *Atlas of Surgical Oncology*. Cambridge, MA: Blackwell Science; 1995.)

SKIN INCISION AND CREATION OF FLAPS

- Once the skin incision has been mapped out on the breast, a scalpel is used to cut through the skin and dermis. A small edge of tissue is raised below the dermal layer to develop the flap (**FIGURE 9**). Skin hooks are used to provide traction for flap elevation, and these should be replaced with deeper retractors or lighted retractors when the dissection flaps are extended (**FIGURE 10**). Traction of the contralateral hand of the surgeon with a sponge also provides necessary tension for appropriate plane dissection. Flap dissection can be done sharply or with electrocautery, but electrocautery will provide better hemostasis during the dissection.
- The goal of flap elevation is to remove all the breast tissue while maintaining vascular supply to the flaps. The dissection plane should be developed between the breast tissue and subcutaneous fat. Frequently, there will be an avascular plane that can help guide in the dissection. It is important to keep traction on the breast to assist in finding the correct plane, and intermittent flap palpation should be performed to determine the correct thickness of the flaps. Flap thickness will vary among patients and is dependent on the patient's body habitus.
- The superior flap should be extended up to the inferior border of the clavicle, and the medial flap should be dissected to the sternal border (**FIGURE 11**). When creating the medial

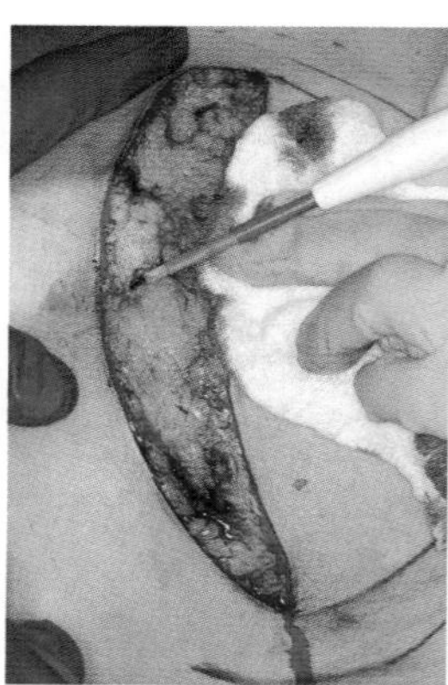

FIGURE 9 ● Raise an area of tissue under the dermis to begin the flap dissection. Using a sponge in the opposite hand can help provide traction, which will help in the flap creation.

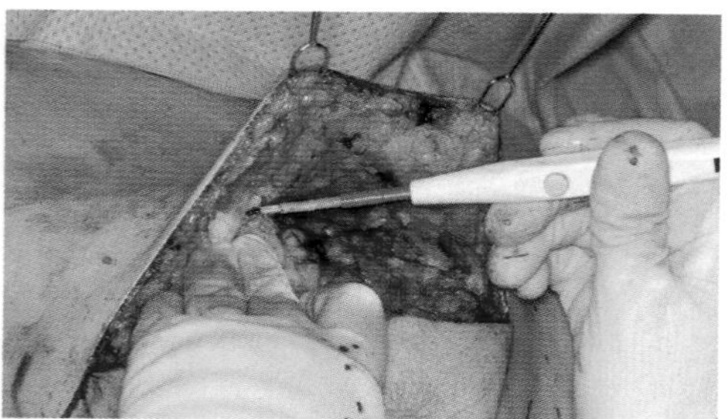

FIGURE 10 ● Joseph retractors or skin hooks are used at the beginning of the flap dissection. These should be switched out for deeper retractors as the dissection is extended.

flap, careful attention should be directed to the medial perforators. These perforators should be preserved where feasible to maintain vascular supply to the flap. When these need to be sacrificed, clips or suture ligation should be used to assure hemostasis. The lateral flap should be extended to the latissimus dorsi, and the inferior flap should be dissected to the inframammary fold (**FIGURE 12**). It is important to avoid excess traction as the dissection is extended to avoid flap ischemia. The inferior aspect of the dissection is the inframammary fold, and there should not be any ridge of tissue left in this area. Marking the inframammary fold preoperatively is helpful to guide this extent.

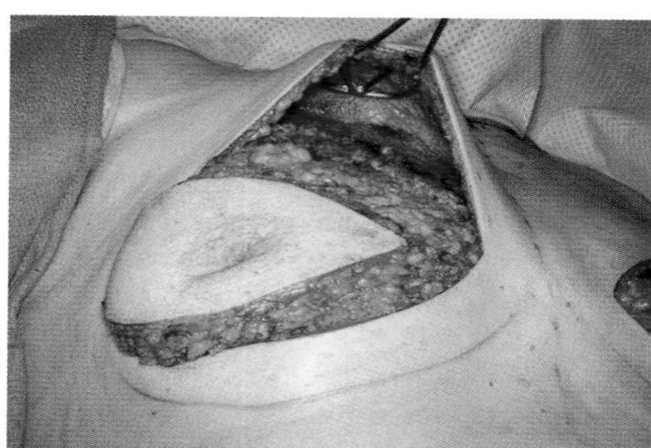

FIGURE 11 ● The superior flap dissection is extended up to the clavicle where the underlying muscle can then be exposed.

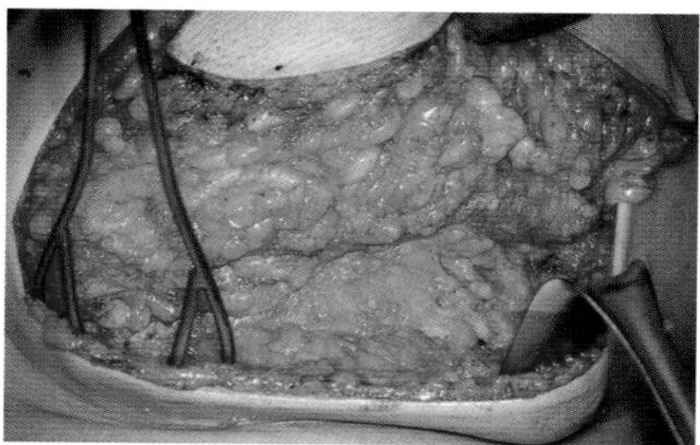

FIGURE 12 ● The inferior flap dissection is carried to the inframammary fold.

DISSECTION FROM THE PECTORAL MUSCLES

- When the flaps are completed to the appropriate landmarks, the breast tissue is dissected off the pectoralis muscle taking the pectoral fascia with the breast tissue using the electrocautery. The dissection should be started superiorly at the level of the clavicle. Traction should be applied with the contralateral hand to visualize the dissection plane (**FIGURE 13**).
- The dissection should continue inferiorly and in a medial-to-lateral fashion to follow the muscle fibers. The fascia surrounding the muscle should be dissected off with the breast in order to prevent local recurrence.[8,9] Careful attention should be provided to preserve the serratus anterior muscle fascia laterally and inferiorly and the rectus sheath fascia inferiorly. The axillary tail of the breast should remain attached in order to keep the breast and axillary contents as one pathologic specimen and also to guide the axillary dissection.

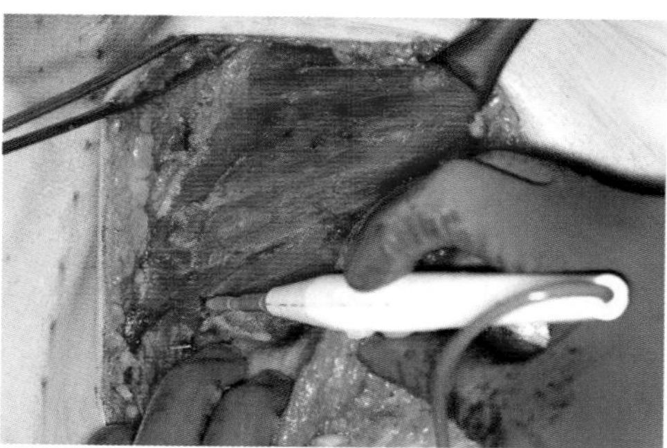

FIGURE 13 ● Dissection of the breast tissue off the pectoralis major muscle should be done with electrocautery in a medial-to-lateral fashion taking the pectoralis major muscle fascia with the specimen.

AXILLARY DISSECTION

- The axilla has a pyramidal shape and is located between the upper arm and thoracic chest wall. It is bounded superiorly by the axillary vein, anteriorly by the pectoralis muscle, medially by the serratus anterior muscle, and posterolaterally by the latissimus dorsi.
- The axilla can be reached when the breast tissue is positioned laterally and the dissection is continued under the pectoralis major muscle (**FIGURE 14**). The clavipectoral fascia should be incised along the edge of the pectoralis major muscle, which will free up the pectoralis major and minor muscle from the nodal tissue (**FIGURE 15**). Close attention should be paid to identify the medial pectoral neurovascular bundle. It sweeps laterally along the pectoralis minor, and care should be taken to preserve the bundle. The inferior border of the dissection should extend to the fourth or fifth rib to ensure that all level I nodes are included in the specimen.[10]
- Once the axillary fat pad is encountered, the subcutaneous fat appears darker and is glistening. Once the axillary space is entered, it is vitally important to identify landmarks to guide your dissection and to prevent neurovascular injury. This axillary lymph node dissection describes a lateral-to-medial approach to the axillary lymph node dissection. A medial-to-lateral approach is described in Part 5, Chapter 34.
- The first vital structure to identify is the thoracodorsal bundle, and this is facilitated by visualizing the latissimus dorsi laterally (**FIGURE 16**). The thoracodorsal nerve inserts approximately 4 cm inferior to the axillary vein, and the bundle can be followed superiorly to its posterior insertion on the axillary vein (**FIGURE 17**).
- The next step is to identify the axillary vein. Richardson retractors should be used at this time to provide exposure to the vein by retracting the pectoral muscles (**FIGURE 18**). The

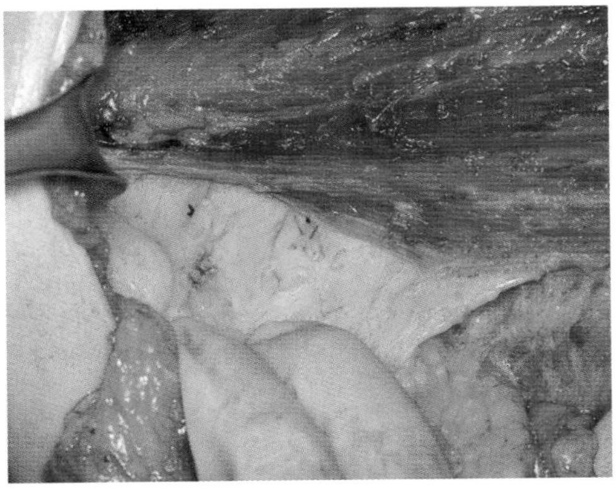

FIGURE 14 ● The axilla can be reached when the breast tissue is positioned laterally and the dissection is *continued* under the pectoralis major muscle, where the clavipectoral fascia is exposed.

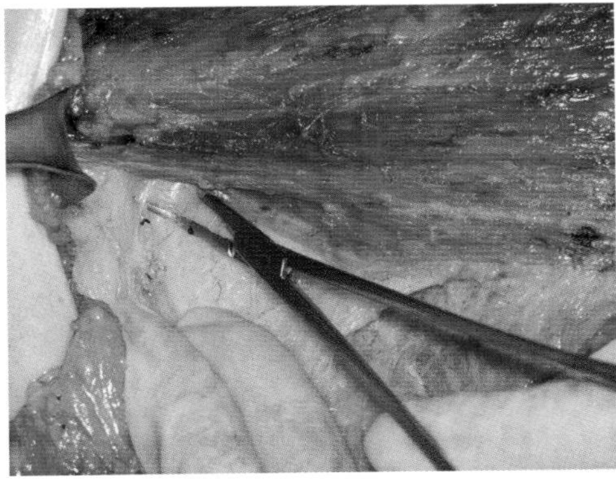

FIGURE 15 ● The axillary fat pad is entered when the clavipectoral fascia is incised.

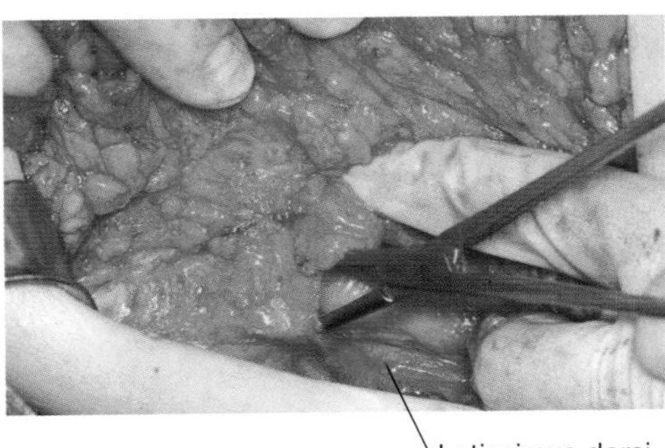

FIGURE 16 ● Dissect laterally to identify the latissimus dorsi muscle and enter axilla just anterior to latissimus dorsi to find the thoracodorsal bundle.

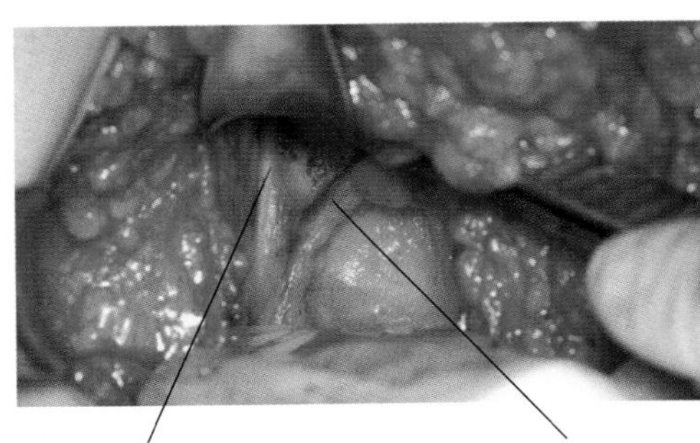

FIGURE 17 ● The thoracodorsal bundle.

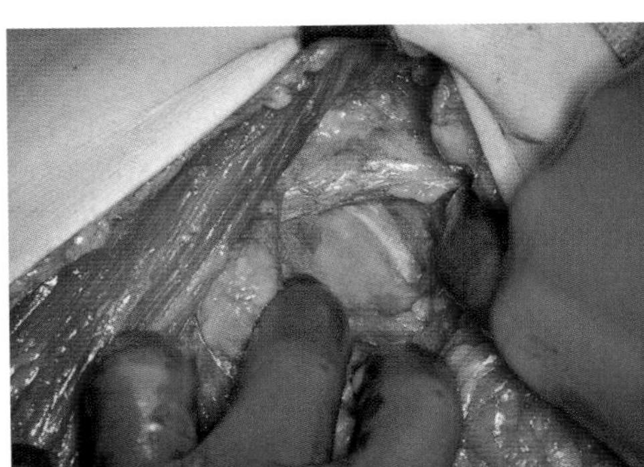

FIGURE 18 ● The Richardson retractor is used to expose the axillary vein by retracting the pectoral muscles. The thoracodorsal bundle is seen posterior to the axillary vein.

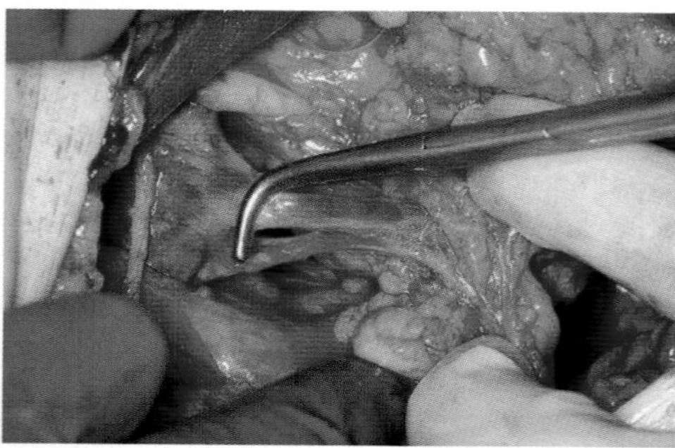

FIGURE 19 ● The thoracoepigastric vein is the only superficial tributary of the axillary vein and should be ligated with clips or ties.

axillary vein can be easily identified using blunt dissection of the axillary fat once the clavipectoral fascia has been divided. Once the vein is identified, the dissection should continue inferiorly to it. The nodal tissue superior to the axillary vein should be preserved to reduce lymphedema and brachial plexus injury. The thoracoepigastric vein is the only superficial tributary of the axillary vein and should be ligated with clips or ties (**FIGURE 19**). Before any ligation of this branch is performed, care must be taken to not mistake this vein for the thoracodorsal vein, which lies deep to it. All other lymphatic channels should be clipped and divided using scissors, and superficial branches of the axillary vein should be divided sharply between clips or sutures.

- Level II nodes are located underneath the pectoralis muscle, and level III nodes are located medial to the muscle. Level III nodes are rarely involved in most breast cancer metastasis and are not included in the traditional axillary lymph node dissection.[11] To gain access to the level II nodes, the Richardson retractor should retract the pectoral muscles medially. When placing the retractor deep under the muscles, pay careful attention to the medial pectoral bundle to prevent damage to these structures (**FIGURE 20A** and **B**). The dissection should continue to extend medially along the axillary vein, and the lymphatic tissue on the chest wall should be retracted inferolaterally. This tissue should be dissected off the chest wall with ties or clips to prevent lymphatic leaks.
- The long thoracic nerve lies along the chest wall and is superficial to the investing fascia of the serratus anterior muscle (**FIGURE 21**). This nerve can be difficult to identify, and palpation of this nerve can help to recognize it. The nerve feels like a string of spaghetti when running a finger along the serratus anterior muscle. Care should be taken to not retract the nerve off the chest wall with the specimen. If this nerve is inadvertently injured, it will cause patients to have a winged scapula. Dissection of the lymphatic tissue close to the nerve should be done with sharp dissection and not electrocautery.
- The thoracodorsal bundle is found lateral to the long thoracic nerve. The lymphatic tissue between the two nerves should be dissected and removed. The thoracodorsal bundle should be skeletonized. Any lymphatic channels or superficial branches should be clipped or suture ligated. The branches of the thoracodorsal vein and artery entering the chest medially should be preserved where possible (**FIGURE 22**).

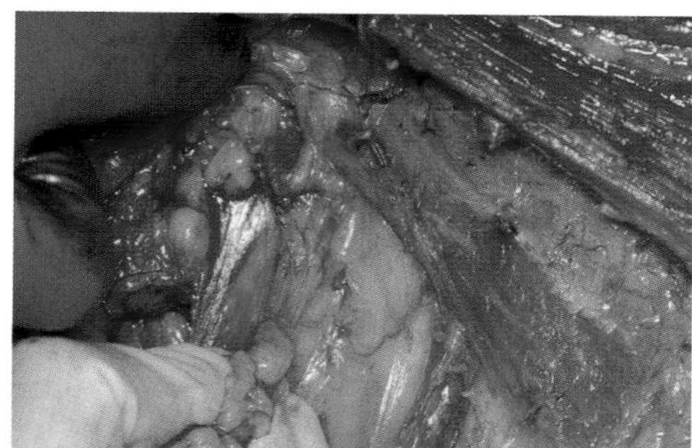

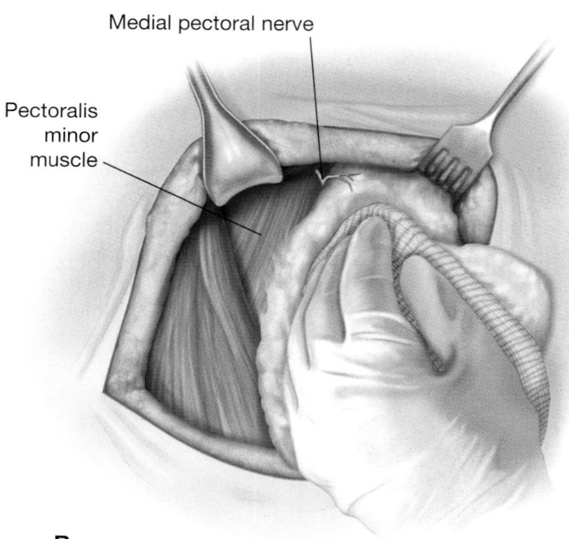

FIGURE 20 ● **A** and **B,** When placing the retractor deep under the muscles, pay careful attention to the medial pectoral bundle to prevent damage to these structures. The medial pectoral nerve wraps around the underside of the pectoralis minor muscle. (Redrawn and modified from Donohue JH, Van Heerden J, Monson JRT, eds. *Atlas of Surgical Oncology*. Blackwell Science; 1995.)

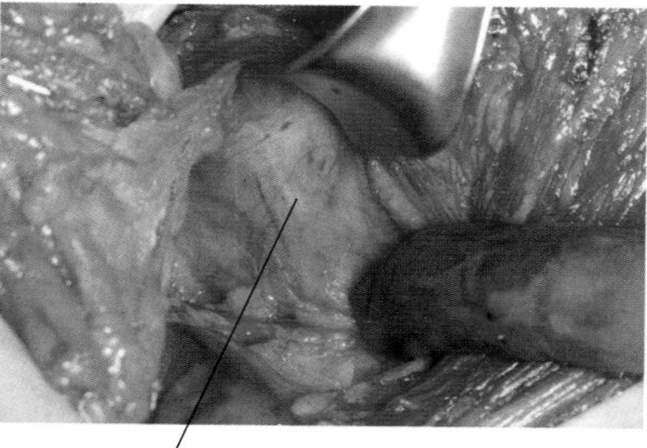

FIGURE 21 ● The long thoracic nerve lies along the chest wall and is superficial to the investing fascia of the serratus anterior muscle. Care should be taken to not pull the nerve laterally during the axillary dissection. The nerve can be difficult to identify and sometimes will only be felt on palpation. Running a finger along the lateral chest wall can aid in identifying the nerve.

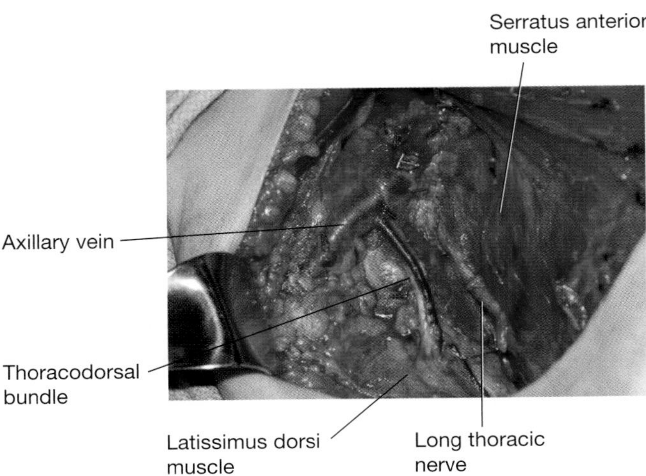

FIGURE 22 ● The axilla after removal of level I and II lymph nodes, with thoracodorsal bundle and long thoracic nerve and axillary vein intact.

- Attempts should also be made to try to preserve the intercostobrachial nerves, but if the path of the nerve is directly through the specimen, it can be ligated with clips and scissors (**FIGURE 23**). Patients should know that the intercostobrachial nerves may need to be sacrificed preoperatively, and explain to them that ligating the nerve will cause loss of sensation to their upper inner arm.
- The breast and attached nodal tissue should be excised en bloc by dividing the remaining lateral pedicle. The specimen should be sent to pathology with sutures placed for orientation (**FIGURE 24**).

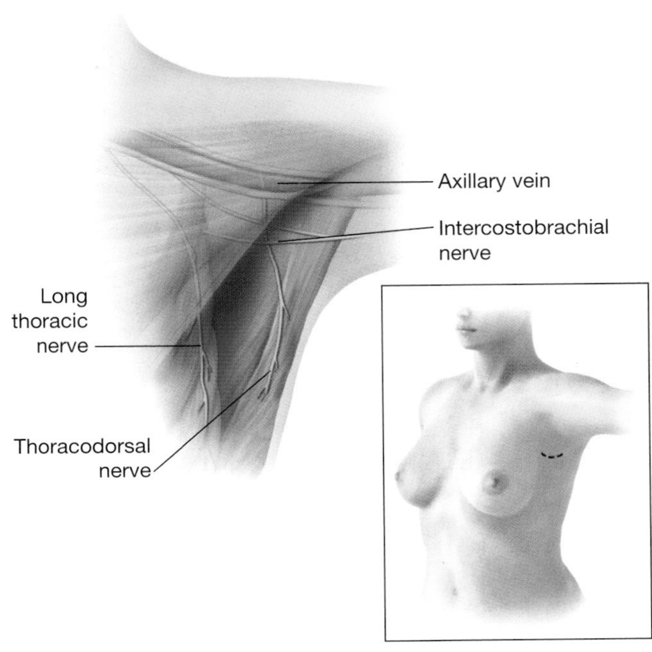

FIGURE 23 ● Schematic drawing of the relationship of the axillary nerves to each other. The intercostobrachial nerves should be preserved if possible. (Used with permission of Mayo Foundation for Medical Education and Research. All rights reserved.)

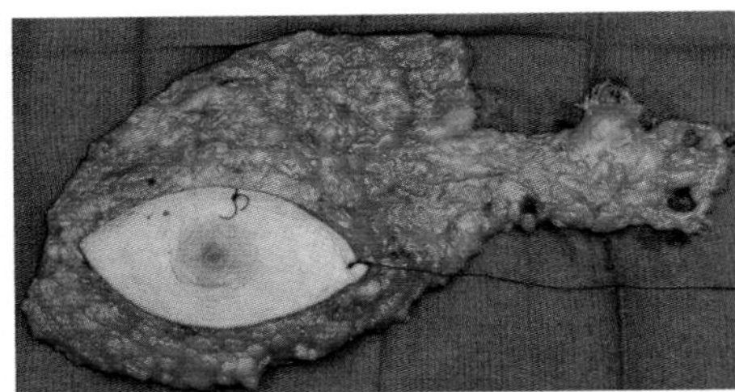

FIGURE 24 ● Suture orientation should be done before the specimen is passed off to pathology. A short stitch should be placed superiorly and a long stitch laterally.

DRAIN PLACEMENT

- Two closed suction drains should be placed to prevent seroma formation. Studies have shown two drains are superior in comparison with one drain placed.[12] One drain should be placed over the pectoralis major muscle, and the other drain should be placed in the axillary space (**FIGURE 25A** and **B**). The drains should be sutured in place with a monofilament suture and dressed appropriately based on surgical preference.
- Local anesthetic is important for postoperative pain control. There are many different options for local anesthetic administration:
  - For patients with a PVB placed, additional local anesthetic is not needed.
  - When a PVB is not used, local anesthetic can be infiltrated into the skin incision prior to incision and in the base of the mastectomy flaps prior to closure like a field block to aid immediate postoperative pain.
  - Another option shown to provide excellent postoperative pain control is the use of long-acting liposomal bupivacaine. This provides anesthesia for 72 hours after the procedure. For unilateral case 30 cc of liposomal bupivacaine mixed with 20 cc of bupivacaine for a total volume of 50 cc can be used and infiltrated into the base of the skin flap, the low axilla (avoiding placing the solution near the brachial plexus), the muscle and also ensuring to infiltrate into the drain site.
- Quilting sutures to tack the mastectomy flaps down to the underlying muscle have been shown to decrease risk of postoperative seroma. These improve healing of the mastectomy flaps to the underlying muscle and change the dead space from one large cavity to multiple smaller cavities for healing. These can be used per surgeon preferences on all total mastectomy cases or selectively in patients who are at higher risk of postmastectomy seroma, namely, those patients on steroids and patients with high body mass index, diabetes, etc.

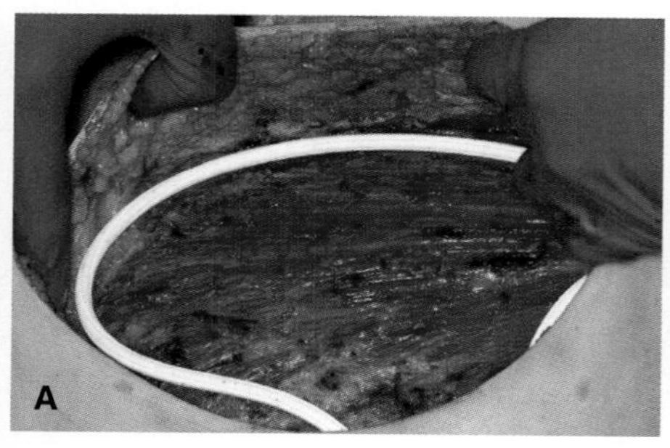

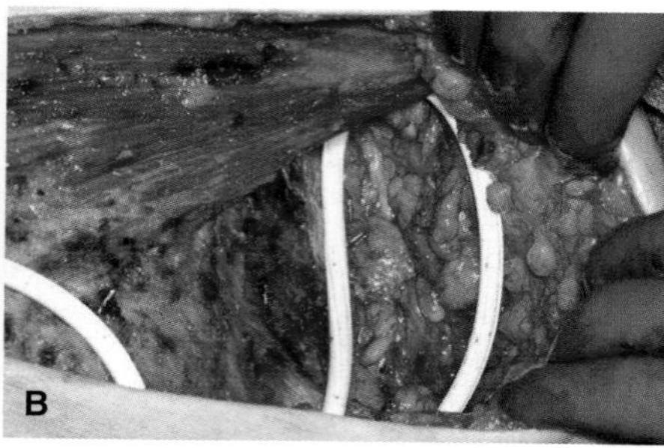

FIGURE 25 ● **A,** One drain should be placed over the pectoralis major muscle, **(B)** and the other should be placed in the axillary space. The drains should be secured to the skin.

CLOSURE

- A cosmetically pleasing closure is important for psychologic reasons. The goal is to provide a closure that will cause the chest to have a very flat appearance without excess skin redundancy.
- If the skin edges are traumatized, they should be excised with scissors or scalpel. Many times, dog ears appear at the medial and lateral edges of the incision. These should be excised to make the incision have a smoother and flatter appearance. The dermal layer should be closed with an inverted interrupted closure using absorbable suture. The skin should be approximated with an absorbable 4-0 monofilament suture in a running subcuticular closure (**FIGURE 26**). Staples should not be used for mastectomy closure.

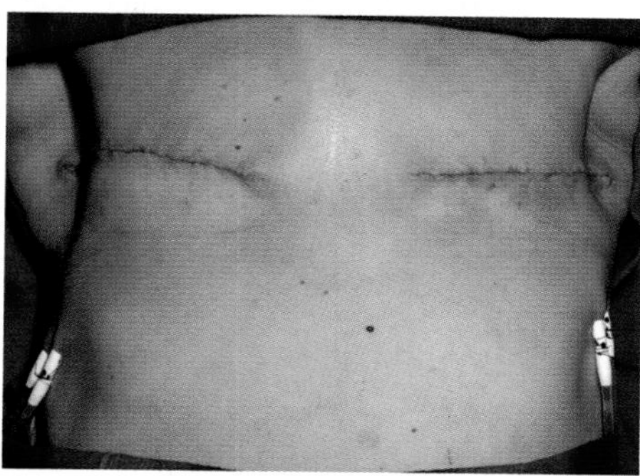

FIGURE 26 ● A cosmetic closure with a flat-appearing chest wall without skin redundancy is the goal.

PEARLS AND PITFALLS

Indications	▪ A comprehensive history and physical examination should be undertaken, as well as review of the radiographic images of the breast and axilla and pathology from all biopsies. Patients with node-positive disease either not amenable to breast conservation or electing mastectomy are candidates for modified radical mastectomy, which encompasses a simple/total mastectomy together with an axillary lymph node dissection. ▪ Once a cancer diagnosis is made, multidisciplinary coordination is essential for successful treatment planning.
Incision placement	▪ When choosing an incision for a modified radical mastectomy, the goal is to provide great exposure to the axilla and a good cosmetic outcome. ▪ The incision should include a 1- to 2-cm margin around the tumor (if close to the skin) and include the previous biopsy site. ▪ The classic Stewart incision is the preferred incision for a modified radical mastectomy providing the necessary exposure and cosmetic outcome.
Flap dissection	▪ Flaps should be extended to the borders of the breast tissue. Careful attention needs to be paid to ensure all the breast tissue is resected and the vascular supply to the remaining skin flaps is preserved to avoid flap ischemia.
Axillary lymph node dissection	▪ Careful identification of vital structures and the axillary borders will define the dissection. ▪ Close attention needs to be paid to the preservation of the axillary vein, thoracodorsal bundle, and long thoracic nerve during the dissection.
Closure	▪ The goal is to reduce skin redundancy and create a smooth flat incision. Avoid medial and lateral dog ears. Two closed suction drains should be placed to avoid seroma.
Rehabilitation	▪ Patients should have access to counseling or therapy to help in coping with issues of body image. Patients who do not desire reconstruction should also be set up to be fitted for a breast prosthesis. ▪ All patients should meet with a lymphedema specialist to coordinate an exercise plan and be provided with compression garments if needed. Initial consultation ideally should be prior to surgery.

POSTOPERATIVE CARE

- Patients after an MRM should be placed in an Ace wrap following their surgery (**FIGURE 27**). This will provide good compression to decrease risk of hematoma. Steri-Strips or Xeroform dressing can be placed directly over the incisions. Fluffs or Kerlix gauze can be placed over the incision to act as a barrier between the incision and ACE wrap.
- Patients who have undergone an MRM will face a variety of rehabilitation issues pertaining to lymphedema, body image, and sexual dysfunction. It is important to have all these concerns addressed preoperatively, during their hospital stay, or at follow-up appointments. The most dreaded complication of having an axillary lymph node dissection is lymphedema. All patients should be scheduled to meet with a lymphedema therapist preoperatively and again approximately 2 weeks from their surgery or after drain removal. The therapists can help educate patients on lymphedema and how to prevent the complication and provide them with exercises to avoid restricted shoulder range of motion.
- Patients who have undergone MRM without reconstruction should be referred to be fitted for a breast prosthesis after the drains are removed and the swelling has gone down.

OUTCOMES

- Patients who undergo an MRM are at risk for developing secondary lymphedema. This is one of the most dreaded fears of many breast cancer survivors, and many women are not educated on this complication preoperatively.
- Many patients undergoing an MRM will require postmastectomy radiation. The addition of radiation after a nodal dissection can substantially increase the risk of development of lymphedema to over 40%. Successful diagnosis and treatment of patients suffering from lymphedema should focus on risk-reducing therapies and lifelong self-directed care.[13,14]
- Survival outcomes in patients undergoing MRM are not based solely on the operative procedure but dependent on the tumor stage, nodal stage, and tumor biology. Studies have shown in node-positive patients that the number of positive lymph nodes, patient age, tumor grade, and race are significant variables to affect survival.[15]

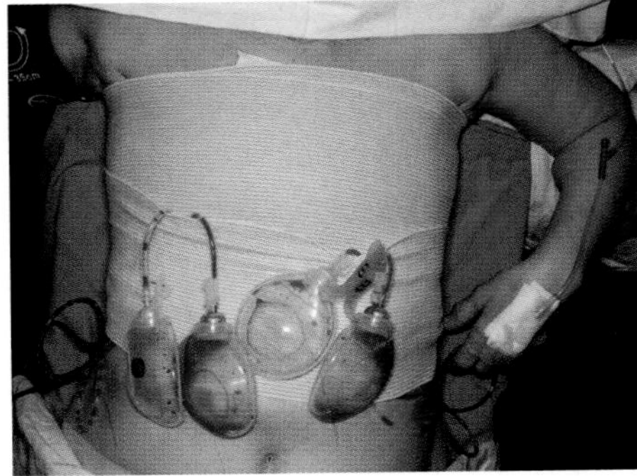

FIGURE 27 ● Patients should be wrapped in an Ace binder to provide compression. The drains should be in view to monitor output and consistency.

COMPLICATIONS

- Seroma
- Wound infection
- Hematoma
- Wound dehiscence
- Flap necrosis
- Positive margins
- Brachial plexus injury
- Nerve injury
- Winged scapula
- Axillary vein thrombosis
- Lymphedema

REFERENCES

1. *NCCN Clinical Practice Guidelines in Oncology: Inflammatory Breast Cancer*. National Comprehensive Cancer Network. Published March 2022. Accessed May 21, 2022. http://www.nccn.org
2. Kopans DB. The positive predictive value of mammography. *AJR Am J Roentgenol*. 1992;158(3):521-526.
3. Handel N, Silverstein MJ, Gamagami P, et al. Factors affecting mammographic visualization of the breast after augmentation mammaplasty. *JAMA*. 1992;268(14):1913-1917.
4. Exadaktylos AK, Buggy DJ, Moriarty DC, et al. Can anesthetic technique for primary breast cancer surgery affect recurrence or metastasis? *Anesthesiology*. 2006;105(4):660-664.
5. Coveney E, Weltz CR, Greengrass R, et al. Use of paravertebral block anesthesia in the surgical management of breast cancer: experience in 156 cases. *Ann Surg*. 1998;227(4):496-501.
6. Kairaluoma PM, Bachmann MS, Rosenberg PH, et al. Preincisional paravertebral block reduces the prevalence of chronic pain after breast surgery. *Anesth Analg*. 2006;103(3):703-708.
7. Tejirian T, DiFronzo LA, Haigh PI. Antibiotic prophylaxis for preventing wound infection after breast surgery: a systematic review and metaanalysis. *J Am Coll Surg*. 2006;203(5):729-734.
8. Dalberg K, Johansson H, Signomklao T, et al. A randomized study of axillary drainage and pectoral fascia preservation after mastectomy for breast cancer. *Eur J Surg Oncol*. 2004;30(6):602-609.
9. Dalberg K, Krawiec K, Sandelin K. Eleven-year follow-up of a randomized study of pectoral fascia preservation after mastectomy for early breast cancer. *World J Surg*. 2010;34(11):2539-2544.
10. Ung O, Tan M, Chua B, et al. Complete axillary dissection: a technique that still has relevance in contemporary management of breast cancer. *ANZ J Surg*. 2006;76(6):518-521.
11. Rosen PP, Lesser ML, Kinne DW, et al. Discontinuous or "skip" metastases in breast carcinoma. Analysis of 1228 axillary dissections. *Ann Surg*. 1983;197(3):276-283.
12. Terrell GS, Singer JA. Axillary versus combined axillary and pectoral drainage after modified radical mastectomy. *Surg Gynecol Obstet*. 1992;175(5):437-440.
13. Herd-Smith A, Russo A, Muraca MG, et al. Prognostic factors for lymphedema after primary treatment of breast carcinoma. *Cancer*. 2001;92(7):1783-1787.
14. Aitken RJ, Gaze MN, Rodger A, et al. Arm morbidity within a trial of mastectomy and either nodal sample with selective radiotherapy or axillary clearance. *Br J Surg*. 1989;76(6):568-571.
15. Fisher ER, Anderson S, Redmond C, et al. Pathologic findings from the National Surgical Adjuvant Breast Project protocol B-06. 10-year pathologic and clinical prognostic discriminants. *Cancer*. 1993;71(8):2507-2514.

Chapter 21 Direct-to-Implant Breast Reconstruction

Amy S. Colwell and Roberto D. Lorenzi Mendez

DEFINITION

- Mastectomy is increasingly performed for breast cancer treatment or risk reduction in high-risk patients. The goal of breast reconstruction is to rebuild the breast and restore a sense of normalcy.

ANATOMY

- The breast glandular tissue extends to the clavicle superiorly, the inframammary fold (IMF) inferiorly, sternum medially, and latissimus dorsi laterally (**FIGURE 1**). With a skin-sparing or nipple-sparing mastectomy, the glandular tissue is removed and the skin is spared, thus making direct-to-implant breast reconstruction possible. In implant-based subpectoral breast reconstruction, a space is created underneath the pectoralis muscle with release of the inferior attachment, and the serratus anterior is sometimes used to help define the lateral border of the reconstructed breast (**FIGURE 2**). In prepectoral breast reconstruction, the implant is placed above the muscle.

NATURAL HISTORY

- Mastectomy offers potential cure in breast cancer patients and prevention for those at high risk for cancer. Immediate breast reconstruction offers an improvement in health-related quality of life and patient satisfaction for women choosing mastectomy as part of their treatment plan.[1-3]

PATIENT HISTORY AND PHYSICAL FINDINGS

- Patient selection in immediate direct-to-implant breast reconstruction is one of the keys to success. A history is obtained to check for comorbidities that are known risk factors for increased complications including smoking, diabetes, body mass index (BMI), and previous breast radiation. On physical exam, the breast is assessed for skin quality, size, scars from previous procedures, symmetry, position of the IMF, and nipple position if a nipple-sparing mastectomy is being considered.

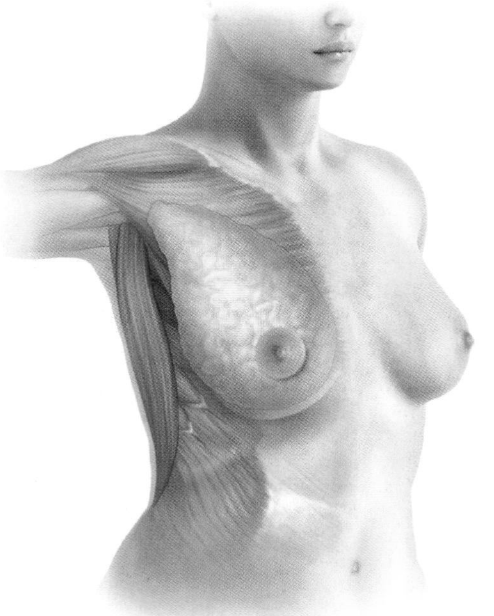

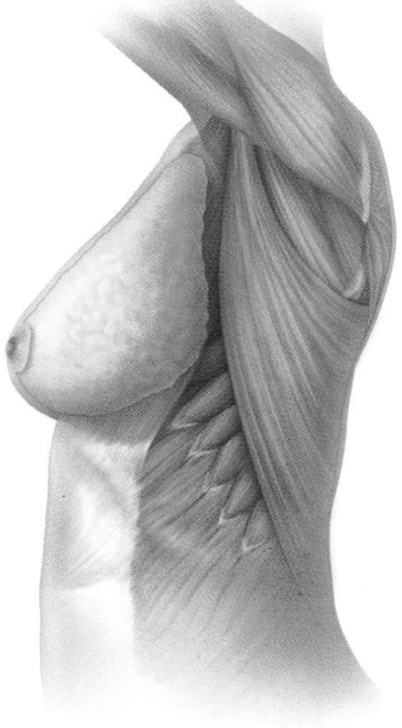

FIGURE 1 ● The anatomic boundaries of the breast are the clavicle, sternum, inframammary fold, and latissimus dorsi.

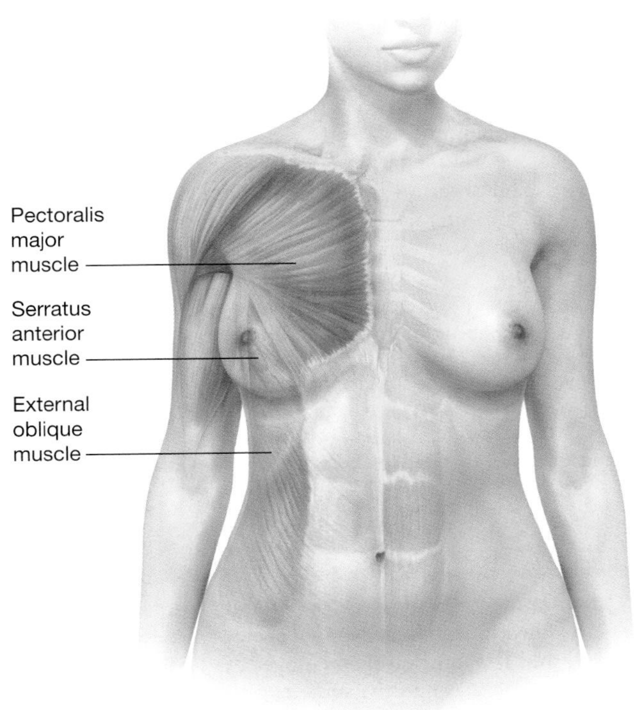

FIGURE 2 ● A plane is created under the pectoralis muscle for implant placement. The pectoralis thus covers the implant superior and medially. The serratus muscle is sometimes elevated for lateral coverage or support.

DIFFERENTIAL SURGICAL TREATMENT OPTIONS

- Two-stage tissue expander–implant reconstruction
- Autologous reconstruction using tissue from the body including the abdomen (TRAM, transverse rectus abdominis myocutaneous; DIEP, deep inferior epigastric perforator; SIEA [superficial inferior epigastric artery] flaps), buttocks (SGAP, superior gluteal artery perforator; IGAP [inferior gluteal artery perforator] flaps), thighs (TUG [transverse upper gracilis] flap), and back (latissimus dorsi)
- Fat transfer
- No, or delayed, reconstruction

NONOPERATIVE MANAGEMENT

- Breast reconstruction is a choice, and patients undergoing mastectomy may not elect to pursue reconstruction. If no reconstruction is planned, the breast skin is closed and the chest remains flat in contour. If desired, external breast prostheses are available for women to wear in their clothing to give the appearance of a breast.

SURGICAL MANAGEMENT

- The goals of reconstruction are considered in determining if the reconstruction is designed to augment, reduce, or maintain the current breast size. In general, if a woman wants a significant increase in breast size, this is more safely done in two stages using a tissue expander followed by exchange to implant in a second surgery (see Part 5, Chapter 22). For single-stage implant reconstruction, the implant may be placed directly in a partial subpectoral pocket in order to allow superior soft tissue coverage with muscle in the cleavage area of the breast and to help prevent contracture around the implant.[4] The implant is subcutaneous inferiorly, which allows a more natural teardrop shape, and is typically supported by a surgical acellular dermal matrix (ADM) or mesh. Currently, the most common ADM is AlloDerm (human dermis, LifeCell, Branchburg, NJ), but a variety of ADM or mesh material derived from human dermis, porcine dermis, bovine pericardium, fetal bovine dermis, silk, titanium, poly-4-hydroxybutyrate (P4HB), and Vicryl exist. Direct-to-implant reconstruction with partial muscle coverage offers excellent long-term results. However, a potential drawback includes temporary movement of the implant with pectoralis flexion (animation deformity). Alternatively, the implant may be placed on top of the muscle (prepectoral) and is most commonly supported by ADM or mesh. Prepectoral DTI mostly avoids animation; however, the implant has less soft tissue coverage and is therefore more visible with a higher incidence of rippling deformity.

Preoperative Planning

- With immediate implant reconstruction, a foreign body (implant) is placed into a skin envelope that has been partially devascularized with the mastectomy. Therefore, sterility is an important component of preoperative planning and operative management. The patient sits upright and is marked prior to the procedure. Important landmarks include the IMF position, its relation to the IMF on the contralateral breast, and the lateral border of the breast. The mastectomy portion of the procedure is performed first followed by the reconstruction.

Positioning

- The patient is positioned supine with the arms secured on arm boards at the side, angled approximately 80° to 85° from the operating table (**FIGURE 3**). This allows access to

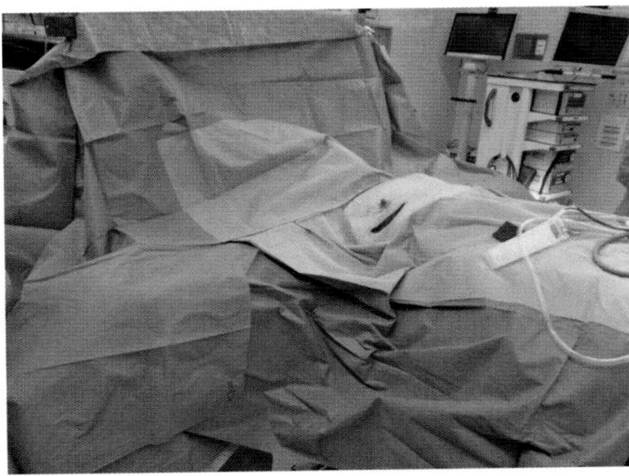

FIGURE 3 ● The patient is positioned supine with arms out on arm boards at approximately 80° to 85° from the operating room table. Care is taken to secure the arms firmly as the back of the operating room table will be raised to a sitting position to check implant placement in the breast pocket while the patient is under anesthesia.

the axillary lymph nodes for sampling during the mastectomy. Both breasts are prepped and draped into the field.

Approach

- The mastectomy and reconstruction may be performed using various incisions. If a nipple-sparing approach is chosen, the safest option is to use a radial lateral incision extending from the areola toward the axilla without a full-thickness incision around the nipple. The incision that maximizes cosmesis is an inferolateral or standard IMF incision under the breast.[5] For skin-sparing mastectomies, the incision is made around the areola and extended laterally if needed for access. For larger breasts, a skin-reducing pattern is designed to remove excess skin in a vertical or horizontal direction. The inverted T/Wise/anchor skin pattern is typically avoided (secondary to higher risk of skin necrosis and complications). The pectoralis muscle is partially released inferiorly to accommodate the implant size and allow more natural breast shape if a subpectoral approach is planned. The challenge of direct-to-implant breast reconstruction is in replacement of the breast volume with an implant that closely matches the breast base diameter and centralizes nipple position, but does not place undue stress on the breast skin envelope. If this cannot be achieved in one stage, a two-stage approach is used with a tissue expander intermediary step.

TECHNIQUES

- See **Video 1**.

SUBPECTORAL DIRECT-TO-IMPLANT BREAST RECONSTRUCTION WITH PARTIAL PECTORALIS MUSCLE COVERAGE AND ACELLULAR DERMAL MATRIX

- Following mastectomy, the patient is paralyzed in order to allow easier dissection and pocket creation under the pectoralis muscle. The color of the skin and thickness of the skin flaps are observed to determine if the patient is a candidate for direct-to-implant reconstruction. If there are ischemic changes to the skin marked by pink or blue discoloration, or if the skin flaps are very thin with areas of dermis exposed on the undersurface, it is unlikely that the skin will be able to support the additional stress and weight of a full-size implant at the time of mastectomy. If the skin color is good and the skin flaps have a uniform marbling of subcutaneous fat on the undersurface, then the patient is a candidate for direct-to-implant reconstruction. A sizer is placed into the subcutaneous pocket and inflated to determine implant volume and to confirm candidacy for direct-to-implant reconstruction. The implant size and profile are determined by the volume and breast base diameter.

Pectoralis Muscle Release

- Using the same access incision used for the mastectomy, the pectoralis muscle is raised from lateral to medial in the loose areolar tissue plane underneath the muscle until the medial origin on the sternum is reached. The pectoralis muscle is then detached from its origin on the external oblique aponeurosis and rectus sheath inferiorly. Dissection continues to the medial muscle origin on the sternum at approximately the 4-o'clock or 8-o'clock position on the chest wall (**FIGURE 4**) using electrocautery. Inadequate medial release will lead to lateral malposition of the implant. The remaining pectoralis attachment to the sternum is preserved. If necessary, the muscle may be released further to the 3-o'clock or 9-o'clock position on the chest wall to facilitate medial positioning, but this also results in greater pectoralis muscle retraction and thus less muscle coverage over the implant. The pectoralis muscle becomes the superior and medial border of the implant pocket.

Pocket Creation

- Although the pectoralis muscle serves as the superior and medial pocket borders, the inferior and lateral pocket borders are formed by the ADM. The ADM is washed and rehydrated according to the manufacturer. The ADM is then first stitched to the medial border of the released pectoralis muscle (**FIGURE 5**). If the IMF is intact inferiorly, the ADM may be sewn to the IMF using simple buried interrupted sutures;

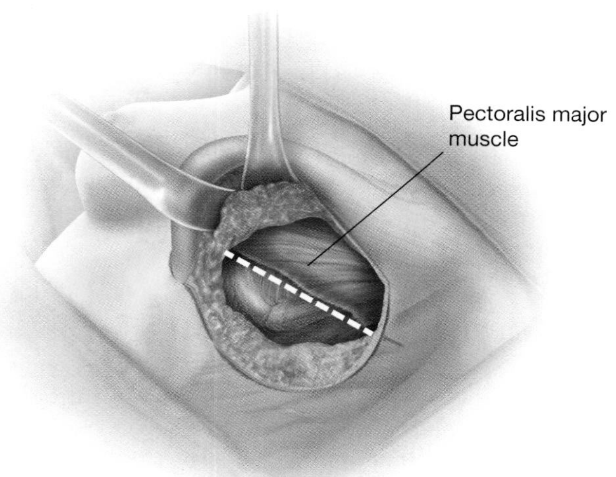

FIGURE 4 ● The pectoralis muscle is released from its insertion inferiorly to the 4-o'clock or 8-o'clock position on the chest wall to allow medial placement of the implant.

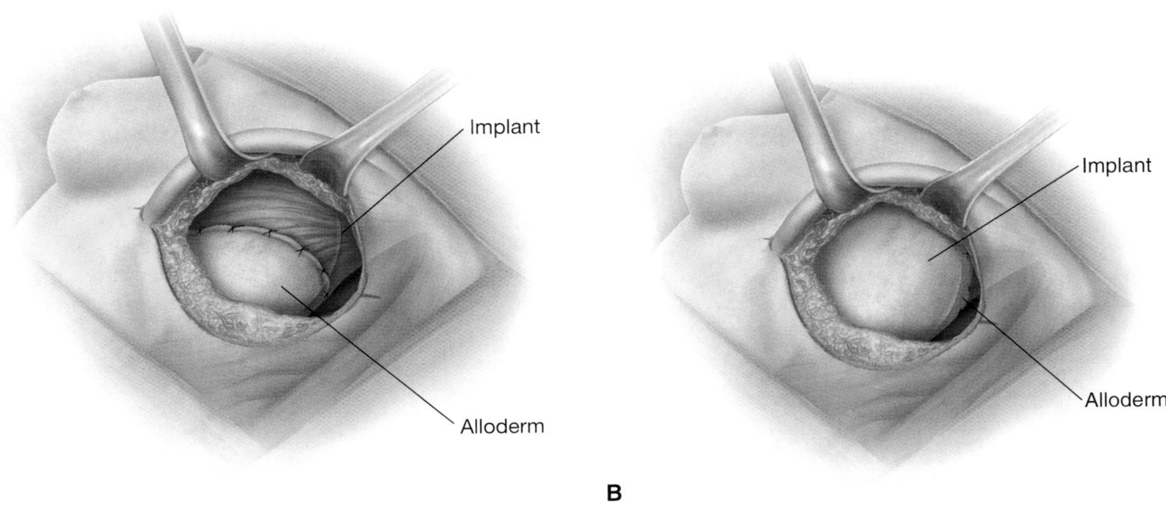

FIGURE 5 ● **A,** To create the inferior and lateral portions of the implant pocket, an ADM or scaffold is sewn to the IMF or chest wall inferiorly and laterally. The implant is placed inside the pocket and then the pectoralis-ADM pocket is closed using absorbable sutures. **B,** Alternatively, ADM covers the entire anterior surface of the implant for long term support using either one large sheet or 2 smaller contour sheets of ADM.

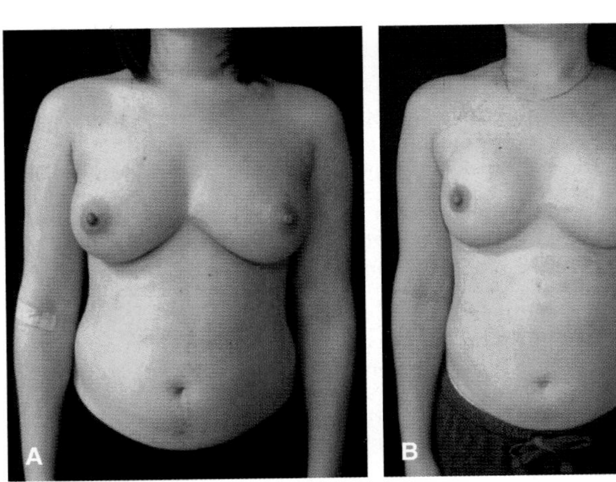

FIGURE 6 ● This 34-year-old female developed breast cancer and had bilateral nipple-sparing mastectomy procedures through inferolateral IMF incisions with single-stage direct-to-implant reconstructions. **A,** Preoperative photo. **B,** Postoperative photo.

however, the implant will drop 2 to 3 cm 4 to 6 weeks after surgery. Instead, the ADM can be sewn to the chest wall at the desired location for the IMF using a permanent suture (0 Ethibond) with more predictable postoperative position. Care is taken to leave the ADM loose medially in preparation for accommodating an implant. Laterally, the ADM is sewn to the chest wall at the lateral border of the breast as marked preoperatively at a position 1 cm more narrow than the permanent implant, or to a raised edge of serratus muscle if the ADM is insufficient in horizontal length. A sizer is then replaced into the subpectoral, sub-ADM pocket and one or two sutures are placed from the pectoralis muscle to the ADM to keep the sizer in place in the pocket. The skin is stapled shut and the patient is sat upright on the operating room table. The breast reconstruction is observed for shape and symmetry.

- The pocket is copiously irrigated with a triple-antibiotic solution of cefazolin, gentamicin, and bacitracin. The surgeon's gloves are changed and the implant is inserted into the newly created pectoralis-ADM pocket. The pocket is closed using figure-of-eight or horizontal mattress absorbable sutures (2-0 Vicryl) from lateral to medial (**FIGURE 6A** and **B**). Two closed suction drains are placed with one inside the ADM pocket along the IMF and the other outside the pocket in the axilla. The skin edges are trimmed and closed in two layers. Incisions are sealed with surgical glue (Dermabond) and covered with a clear semipermeable dressing (Tegaderm). A chlorhexidine-impregnated sponge (Biopatch) can be used around the drains. If desired, Microfoam tape can be placed laterally and inferiorly to help support the implant position.

TECHNIQUES

PREPECTORAL DIRECT-TO-IMPLANT BREAST RECONSTRUCTION

Following mastectomy, the skin is assessed for viability and eligibility for direct-to-implant reconstruction similar to partial muscle coverage. A sizer is placed to confirm candidacy for DTI and to choose a permanent implant.

To help hold the implant and offer a smoother transition from the chest wall to the implant, a small slip of superior pectoralis muscle is raised for inset of the ADM or mesh. The surgeon may choose one large piece of ADM to tailor to the implant's dimensions, or it is the authors' preference to use two contour pieces of ADM inset to precisely conform to the implant and allow adjustment of the tension for a hand-in-glove fit.

The pocket dimensions are set 1 cm more narrow than the implant diameter. The inferior contour ADM is sewn to the chest wall with 0-Ethibond sutures and medially to the skin flap to allow medial positioning of the implant. The superior contour ADM is sewn medially to the skin flap, superior to the slip of superior pectoralis muscle, and laterally to the chest wall.

The reconstruction proceeds with drain placement and antibiotic irrigation. Once the implant is placed, the tension is set by sewing the two pieces of ADM together from lateral to medial using 2-0 Vicryl or PDS sutures. The skin edges are de-epithelialized and closed.

PEARLS AND PITFALLS

Lateral malposition of implant	■ Check placement of lateral sutures and determine if lateral border should be medialized to shift implant position. If appropriate, check base diameter of implant to ensure proper fit into pocket. Make sure pectoralis muscle is appropriately released to sternal origin medially and to the 4-o'clock or 8-o'clock position on the chest wall.
Asymmetry of IMF positions	■ Preoperative marks should determine whether the IMF position is similar on the breasts. If asymmetric, a decision is typically made to change the IMF position on one breast to match the other breast. Inferior suture placement is checked on both sides for bilateral reconstruction to make sure both are sewn to similar positions on the chest wall or IMF.
Lateralization of nipples on nipple-sparing mastectomy	■ For large breasts, medial positioning of implants may result in lateralization of the nipples. A preoperative discussion with the patient sets expectations and determines whether it would be better to pursue a skin-sparing mastectomy as an alternative. A radial inferior incision yields better nipple position in these breasts but places greater tension on the skin, thus making single-stage reconstruction less likely.
Implant choice	■ For skin-sparing mastectomies, a moderate-plus or full profile implant best matches goals for projection and breast base diameter in most patients. For nipple-sparing mastectomies, a low-plus or moderate profile implant is used more often to help centralize the nipple for small to medium sized breasts.
Learning curve	■ There is a learning curve for surgeons using this technique ie primarily related to the ability to assess the perfusion of the breast skin flap. If the limits of perfusion are surpassed, the result is skin necrosis. Experience with the technique, experience with the breast surgeon, and novel devices to assess skin perfusion decrease the complication rate for this technique.
Fat transfer	■ Fat transfer is increasingly used in implant-based breast reconstruction to fill in defects around the implant. This is not recommended at the time of immediate breast reconstruction with implants, but may be safely done in a second procedure.

POSTOPERATIVE CARE

- The patient may be discharged on the same day of surgery if pain and nausea are controlled. Prior to discharge, a loose-fitting surgical bra is placed. Care is taken to avoid a tight or constricting dressing or bra that may compromise the blood flow of the mastectomy skin flaps. Patients are seen weekly until drains are removed. Criteria for drain removal is less than 30 mL/d. If skin necrosis develops, it is treated aggressively with sharp debridement and closure. For smooth round implants, gentle medial massage of the implants is started 4 weeks postoperatively to help prevent implant contracture.

OUTCOMES

- Immediate breast reconstruction following mastectomy leads to improved psychosocial outcomes and patient satisfaction compared to patients who decide not to have reconstruction.

COMPLICATIONS

- Total complications following direct-to-implant reconstruction are 3% to 15%.[6-9] The explant rate ranges from 1% to 4%. The most common complication is skin necrosis. Other complications include infection, seroma, hematoma, nipple necrosis, implant malposition, and deep venous thrombosis. The most common late complication is capsular contracture.

REFERENCES

1. Alderman AK, Wilkins EG, Lowery JC, et al. Determinants of patient satisfaction in post-mastectomy breast reconstruction. *Plast Reconstr Surg*. 2000;106:769-776.
2. Alderman AK, Kuhn LE, Lowery JC, et al. Does patient satisfaction with breast reconstruction change over time? Two-year results of the Michigan Breast Reconstruction Outcomes Study. *J Am Coll Surg*. 2007;204:7-12.
3. Christensen BO, Overgaard J, Kettner LO, et al. Long-term evaluation of postmastectomy breast reconstruction. *Acta Oncol*. 2011;50(7):1053-1061.
4. Breuing KH, Colwell AS. Inferolateral AlloDerm hammock for implant coverage in breast reconstruction. *Ann Plast Surg*. 2007;59(3):250-255.
5. Colwell AS, Gadd M, Smith BL, et al. An inferolateral approach to nipple-sparing mastectomy: optimizing mastectomy and reconstruction. *Ann Plast Surg*. 2010;65(2):140-143.
6. Colwell AS, Tessler O, Lin AM, et al. Breast reconstruction following nipple-sparing mastectomy: predictors of complications, reconstruction outcomes, and 5-year trends. *Plast Reconstr Surg*. 2014;133(3):496-506.
7. Colwell AS, Christensen JM. Nipple-sparing mastectomy and direct-to-implant breast reconstruction. *Plast Reconstr Surg*. 2017;140:44S-50S.
8. Colwell AS, Damjanovic B, Zahedi B, et al. Retrospective review of 331 consecutive immediate single-stage implant reconstructions: indications, complications, trends, and costs. *Plast Reconstr Surg*. 2011;128:1170-1178.
9. Salzberg CA, Ashikari AY, Koch RM, et al. An 8 year experience of direct-to-implant immediate breast reconstruction using human acellular dermal matrix (AlloDerm). *Plast Reconstr Surg*. 2011;127(2):514-524.

Chapter 22 Two-Stage Implant Breast Reconstruction

Eric G. Halvorson

DEFINITION

- Two-stage implant breast reconstruction is performed in either the immediate or delayed setting following mastectomy.
- The advantages of two-stage implant reconstruction (compared with autologous reconstruction) include shorter operation, lack of donor site, shorter hospital stay, shorter recovery, patient control over final volume, and a rounder and perkier result.
- The disadvantages of two-stage implant reconstruction include multiple postoperative office visits for expansions, discomfort associated with the expansion process, a second (albeit outpatient) surgery, and the permanent risks of implants (capsular contracture, rupture, rippling, infection, malposition, exposure, breast implant illness [BII], and breast implant–associated anaplastic large cell lymphoma [BIA-ALCL]).

PATIENT HISTORY AND PHYSICAL FINDINGS

- It may be beneficial for the initial consultation to occur separate from multidisciplinary clinic visits focused on cancer care. Patients presenting to the plastic surgeon after such visits are often overloaded with information and overwhelmed by all the options and information related to reconstruction. It is critical to determine the patient's goals for reconstruction and to ascertain their preferences with respect to breast size, breast shape, willingness to accept surgical risk, willingness to accept donor site morbidity, operative length, hospital stay, recovery process, postoperative follow-up protocol, secondary surgeries, and long-term complications.
- Having a physician extender well versed in reconstructive options to meet with patients and show them patient photographs is an incredibly helpful prelude to the physician-patient consultation.
- Patients are screened for the **six well-established risk factors** for surgical complications following mastectomy with expander placement: **BMI >30, smoking, history of radiation, recent chemotherapy, diabetes, and autoimmune disease.**
- Physical examination of the breasts is performed to evaluate any masses and whether or not skin involvement or peau d'orange is present. The overall size and degree of ptosis is noted. Patients with significant ptosis will typically require skin excision. If performed as an inverted "T" or Wise pattern, there is increased risk for mastectomy flap necrosis. Alternatively, one can perform a generous horizontal, vertical, or oblique ellipse, or a two-stage Wise pattern excision with the vertical closure first and a horizontal excision at the inframammary fold (IMF) 3 to 6 months later.
- The breast width, height, and projection are measured in centimeters. These measurements are used for selecting a tissue expander (as described in the following text).

SURGICAL MANAGEMENT

- Ideal candidates for two-stage implant reconstruction are thin nonsmokers undergoing bilateral mastectomy who have not, and will not, receive radiotherapy. Smokers are prone to mastectomy flap necrosis and infection. Radiotherapy increases the risk of infection, implant exposure, and capsular contracture. Previously radiated skin will not expand well.
- Patients without ptosis who wish to be larger often require expansion. Most patients having nipple-sparing mastectomy end up having direct-to-implant reconstruction, although those who wish to be larger may require expansion. Patients having skin-sparing mastectomy who wish to be bigger need expansion. Patients who have minimal ptosis and want their breasts to be similar in size are candidates for single-stage implant reconstruction. Large-breasted women with ptosis often require two-stage implant reconstruction to allow staged management of the skin envelope.
- Although obesity increases the risk of complication for any type of reconstruction, heavier patients tend to have better cosmetic results with autologous reconstruction than with implants, as it can be difficult to match the opposite breast after a unilateral mastectomy or give adequate volume/ptosis after a bilateral mastectomy.
- Prepectoral implant reconstruction has gained popularity and is currently the most common approach in some centers. It usually involves at least complete anterior coverage of the expander with an acellular dermal matrix (ADM), and therefore it should be approached with caution in patients who are at increased risk for ADM-related complications (obesity, smoking, history of radiation). Early outcome studies show similar rates of complications, although there can be a higher risk of seroma with prepectoral reconstruction.[1,2] The author's approach is to consider prepectoral reconstruction when the mastectomy flaps are at least 1 cm thick in nonsmokers with no history of radiation. When mastectomy flaps are <1 cm, prepectoral reconstruction can result in a very obvious implant border at the upper pole and an increased need for fat grafting compared with submuscular reconstruction. Some patients who are very concerned about pectoral function may request prepectoral reconstruction.

Preoperative Planning and Implant Selection

- Good communication with the breast surgeon is important to ensure oncologic goals are maintained and that reconstruction is appropriately staged. Patients with advanced disease, requirement for immediate postoperative adjuvant therapy, multiple risk factors, unstable social environment, and/or uncertainty regarding goals for reconstruction may be better served by delayed reconstruction.
- Surgeons will have different risk tolerances when it comes to patient selection; however, the author's approach is to offer **immediate reconstruction for patients with 0 to 1 risk**

factors, consider delayed reconstruction for patients with 2 risk factors, and offer delayed reconstruction only for patients with 3 or more risk factors.

- Prior to mastectomy, the patient must be marked in the standing position. The IMF is marked on each side, and the midline is drawn between the sternal notch and xiphoid process. The overall outline of the breasts is marked. Although a transverse ellipse around the nipple-areolar complex (NAC) is commonly used for the mastectomy incision, the author's preference is an oblique ellipse parallel to the pectoralis major fibers (**FIGURE 1**). This renders the medial scar less visible in clothing, allows for better subincisional muscular coverage, and facilitates a stair-step approach during the exchange procedure (as described in the following text). Once a good relationship with the breast surgeon/s is established, they will learn to mark the patients as this will save time and allow the plastic surgeon to schedule other procedures during the mastectomy portion of the case.
- Tissue expanders are selected preoperatively based on the width of the patient's breast. There are many different tissue expanders to choose from, but most are anatomic, providing lower pole projection. Although smooth expanders with multiple suture tabs to prevent rotation have become more popular due to concerns for BIA-ALCL, no cases have been reported following temporary placement of textured expanders followed by smooth implant placement, and therefore it is the author's practice to use textured anatomic expanders. Some expanders are taller than they are wide, some are wider than they are tall (author's preference), and some are semicircular or crescentic and focus on lower pole expansion. Most have integrated metal ports that are located with magnets, although a remote port is useful when placing the expander under a thick flap (such as a latissimus dorsi flap in an obese patient). In such patients, finding the port with a magnet can be difficult and a long needle is required, placing the expander at risk for rupture. There is currently a dual-port expander that has an integrated drain that can be accessed to aspirate or flush fluid, which may allow salvage of the device in the setting of seromas or infections.[3]

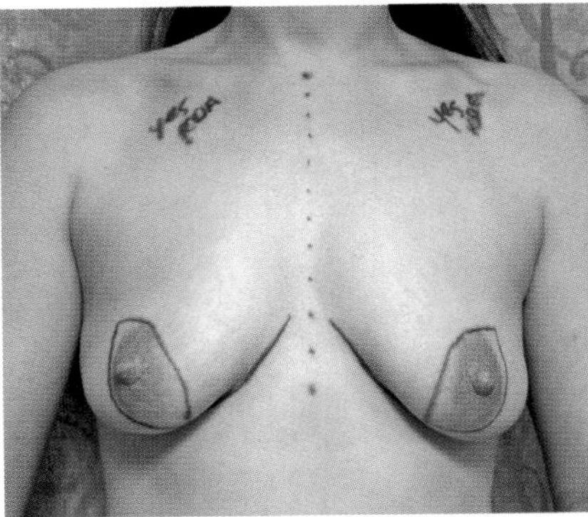

FIGURE 1 ● This patient will be used for the majority of photographs in this chapter. She is a woman in her late 20s with genetic predisposition (*BRCA* gene mutation) undergoing bilateral prophylactic mastectomy and two-stage implant reconstruction. Preoperative markings for the mastectomy are shown, demonstrating the oblique ellipses for incision preferred by the author.

- Intraoperatively, a ruler is used to measure the width of the surgically created implant pocket, which ultimately determines the expander to be used. Alternatively, one can create a pocket wide enough to accommodate the desired expander. The medial implant edge should be approximately 1 cm lateral to the medial breast border, and the lateral implant edge should be approximately 1 cm medial to the lateral breast border. If the lateral breast border has been obscured, as is often the case, then the anterior axillary line can be used or one can select a width that corresponds to that of the final implant that is expected to be placed.
- Prior to the exchange procedure, the patient is again marked in the standing position. The midline is marked, and asymmetries in implant position are noted. The ideal contour for the final implants is marked.
- The US Food and Drug Administration (FDA) now requires that surgeons review a "patient decision checklist" with patients undergoing implant placement, reviewing the risks of implants including BII and BIA-ALCL. Implant manufacturers are only allowed to sell implants to surgeons who comply with this mandate.
- Final implants are selected primarily based on volume, although width should be taken into consideration. A full discussion of implant types is beyond the scope of this chapter. The majority of surgeons use smooth, round, high-profile cohesive silicone implants for reconstructive purposes. Although textured anatomic implants can offer a more natural look, they typically feel firmer and are more fixed in position. There is also a small risk of rotation and an extremely low risk for BIA-ALCL, which has made them much less popular. Patients with very wide chests may require a moderate-profile implant that will have a larger base diameter for a given volume (although less projection). Most smooth implants today have a similar rate of capsular contracture. Traditional single-lumen saline implants usually have a higher risk of rupture, whereas newer dual-lumen "structural" saline implants have a similar risk of rupture (compared with silicone implants).[4] The author's preference is to offer all types of implants to patients and let them decide, understanding the following:
    - Saline
        - Advantages: Implant rupture is immediately detected; removal of a ruptured implant is simpler.
        - Disadvantages: Reexpansion may be required if implant ruptures and is not replaced expeditiously; less natural feel than silicone; higher potential for rippling if underfilled; higher risk of rupture.
    - Silicone
        - Advantages: Softer, more "natural" feel.
        - Disadvantages: Rupture is often clinically silent until capsular contracture or extracapsular rupture is present, removal of a ruptured implant can be challenging (especially with older implants and extracapsular rupture), monitoring for implant rupture with MRI/US as recommended by the FDA can be associated with false-positive results.

Positioning

- Patients are placed in supine position under general anesthetic with arms padded circumferentially and abducted at <90°. Following mastectomy, the patient is positioned such that the sternum is parallel to the floor.

TISSUE EXPANDER PLACEMENT

First Step—Wound Assessment

- Following mastectomy, the wounds are irrigated and hemostasis is obtained. The mastectomy flaps are evaluated by examining their thickness and assessing color and capillary refill. Areas where dermis is exposed internally should be carefully evaluated externally. Areas where the external skin is pale without capillary refill should be considered for debridement. Laser-assisted indocyanine-green fluoroscopy has been promoted to assess mastectomy flap perfusion; however, guidelines for its use and interpretation have not been firmly established.[5]
- Use of tumescent solution by the extirpative surgeon makes assessment of mastectomy flaps difficult and has been shown in some studies to be associated with a higher rate of mastectomy flap necrosis.[6-8]
- When there is significant concern for mastectomy flap necrosis, or if debridement of questionable tissue will lead to closure under tension or an open wound, then aborting reconstruction is strongly advised.
- If necessary, the IMF can be recreated with interrupted suture; however, the position of the inferior edge of the expander will ultimately determine the IMF, which can be adjusted further during an exchange procedure if desired. Some surgeons try to establish the native IMF during this initial procedure (which may make the exchange procedure simpler), whereas others intentionally place the expander lower than the IMF to increase lower pole expansion and projection (which requires recreation of the IMF with suture during the exchange procedure). The author's preference is to preserve the native IMF when performing single-stage implant reconstruction, when placing a significant initial fill volume in the expander, or when the IMF is already low. When performing delayed two-stage implant reconstruction or when placing minimal initial fill volume in the expander, placing the implant below the IMF will preferentially expand the lower pole and permit the surgeon to create minimal ptosis at the exchange procedure (as described in the following text).

Second Step—Creation of Implant Pocket

- The tissue expander cannot be covered by the mastectomy flaps alone, which are thin and offer poor soft tissue coverage. Ideally, the surgeon should provide complete musculofascial coverage with the pectoralis major and serratus anterior muscles (**FIGURE 2**), use an ADM (or other product) in addition to the pectoralis major muscle, or cover the entire expander with ADM in prepectoral reconstruction.
- Submuscular placement:
  - The lateral edge of the pectoralis major muscle is pinched between the surgeon's index finger and thumb and pulled away from the chest, revealing a loose areolar plane between the pectoralis major and minor muscles. Dissection in this plane commences with Bovie cautery, but once the subpectoral space is entered, much of the superior and medial implant pocket can be created via blunt digital dissection before using lighted retractors for direct visualization. A lighted retractor is quite helpful to finish medial dissection, as great care must be taken to ligate or cauterize intercostal perforators (**FIGURE 3**).
  - The medial boundary is defined externally by the preoperative markings that define the patient's native breast form. Internally, it is quite common to release the medial and inferomedial origins of the pectoralis major muscle. It is important not to release this area excessively, as symmastia can result and is difficult to correct.
  - After the subpectoral plane is developed, the inferior insertion of the pectoralis major muscle is examined (**FIGURE 4**). If the patient's muscle reaches the IMF, then a submuscular pocket can be created down to the IMF with supple and adequate soft tissue coverage that will respond well to expansion (**FIGURE 5**). More commonly, however, the pectoralis major inserts above the IMF. In

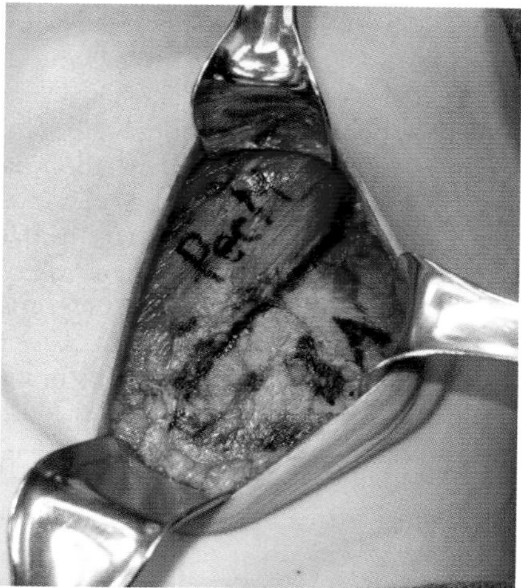

FIGURE 2 ● Following mastectomy, the pectoralis major and serratus anterior muscles are visualized as these are the muscles used for expander coverage in a total submuscular approach. If these muscles have been affected by mastectomy, if the pectoralis major does not extend to the IMF, if an increased initial fill volume is desired, or if a prepectoral approach is planned, use of an ADM is considered.

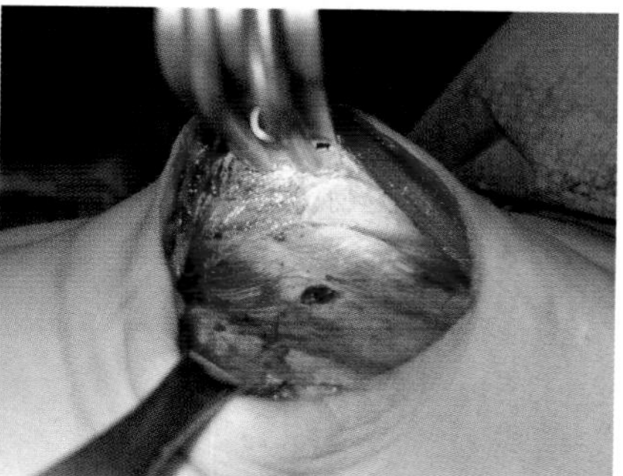

FIGURE 3 ● A lighted retractor is very helpful for both expander placement and the implant exchange procedure. Here, the lighted retractor is shown during creation of the subpectoral pocket superomedially, where dissection proceeds carefully so intercostal perforators can be visualized and carefully ligated if necessary.

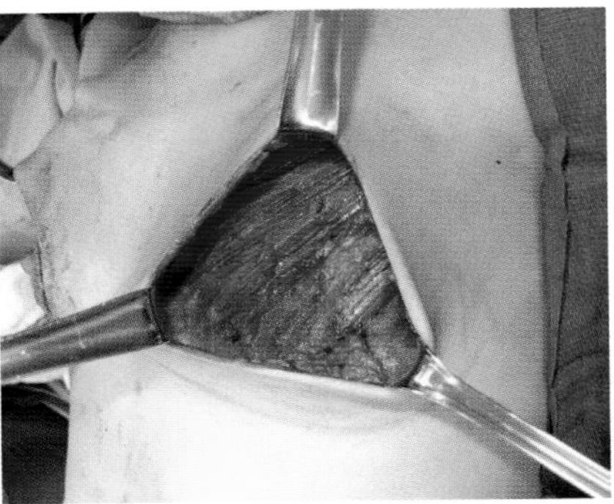

FIGURE 4 ● The relationship between the most caudal extent of the pectoralis major muscle and the IMF determines whether or not the anterior rectus sheath will be necessary to provide complete submusculofascial coverage of the expander. If the muscle originates at or below the IMF, as shown in this figure, then there is no need to elevate the anterior rectus sheath.

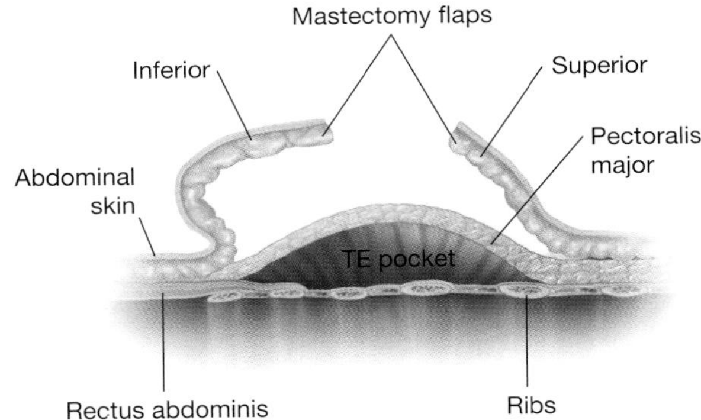

FIGURE 5 ● Schematic diagram of patient anatomy when the pectoralis major originates at or below the IMF. In this case, a submuscular pocket can be created down to the IMF that will be supple and respond well to expansion. TE, tissue expander.

this scenario, to provide autologous implant coverage inferiorly, one must continue dissection past the pectoralis major insertion and under the anterior rectus sheath until just below the IMF. Transitioning from the subpectoral plane to underneath the anterior rectus sheath is sometimes technically difficult and may result in a few gaps in coverage that can be closed after the pocket is fully created. A lighted retractor is necessary for this portion of the procedure. The anterior rectus sheath is quite stiff and will not expand well unless an incision is made transversely across the sheath just below the IMF, entering the subcutaneous plane (**FIGURES 6** and **7**). If the anterior rectus sheath is released above the IMF, one would obviously enter the implant pocket. The goal is to provide complete and supple submusculofascial coverage without gap between the pectoralis major and the IMF.

- This approach is beneficial in patients with multiple risk factors for ADM-related complications.
- Following creation of a subpectoral pocket with or without elevation of the anterior rectus sheath, inferolateral coverage must be provided. Autologous coverage is provided by elevating the serratus anterior fascia if robust, or a partial thickness muscle flap if the fascia is thin or traumatized from the mastectomy. An incision in the serratus anterior is made at the level of, and parallel to, the inferolateral edge of the pectoralis major muscle and a fascial or musculofascial flap is elevated to the anterior axillary line (**FIGURE 8**). Alternatively, one can determine the width of the implant pocket based on the width of the desired tissue expander and stop lateral dissection when a sufficient pocket width is achieved (usually 1 cm wider than the tissue expander). At this point, the inferior and lateral dissections will be complete, but the inferior serratus and superolateral external oblique muscles will still be attached to the chest wall. By retracting inferiorly and laterally, this plane is exposed and the

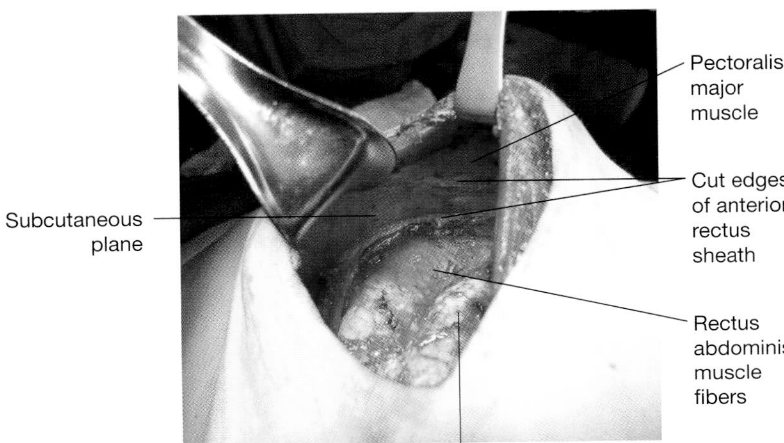

FIGURE 6 ● At or just below the IMF, the anterior rectus sheath is divided horizontally to enter the subcutaneous plane. If this is not performed, lower pole expansion will be limited by the stiff anterior rectus sheath.

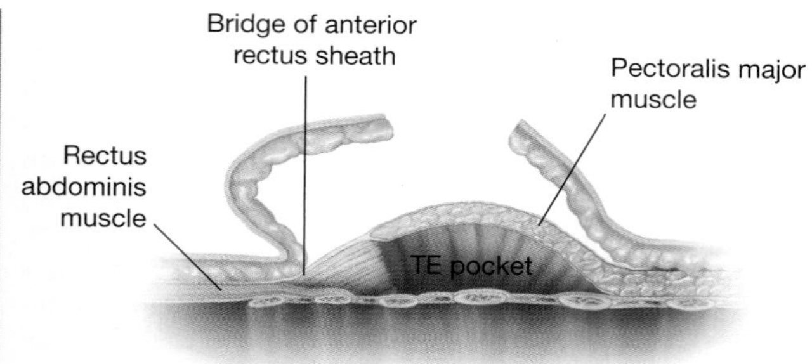

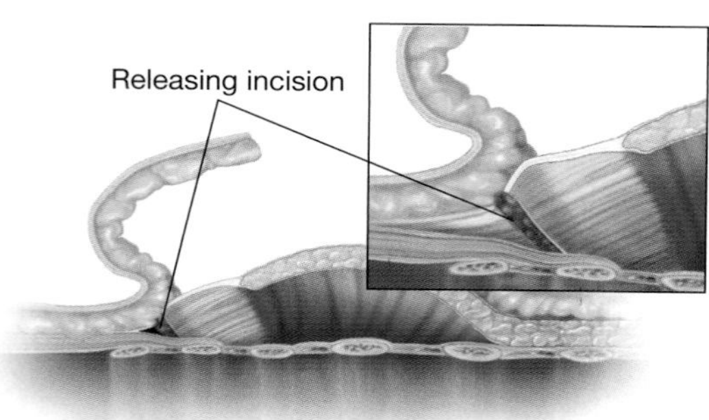

FIGURE 7 • Schematic diagram of patient anatomy when the pectoralis major muscle originates above the IMF. In this case, the gap between the caudal border of the pectoralis and IMF must be bridged by elevating the anterior rectus sheath. At or just below the IMF, the sheath must be incised horizontally to enter the subcutaneous space; otherwise, the inferior pocket will not expand well. Alternatively, an ADM can be used to bridge this gap. TE, tissue expander.

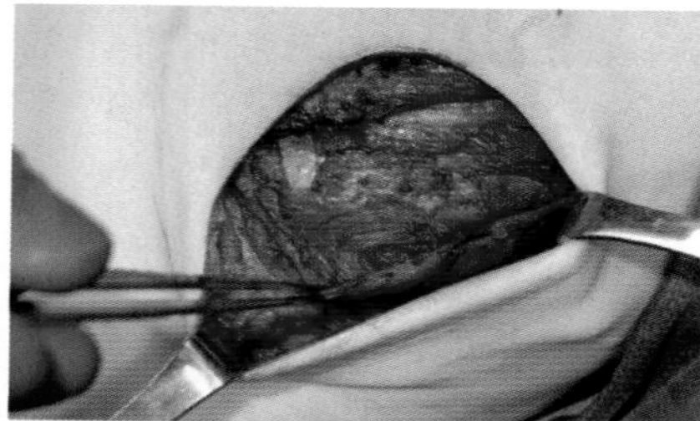

FIGURE 8 • For lateral and inferolateral coverage in a submuscular approach, a partial-thickness serratus anterior muscle flap is elevated and shown in this photograph. If the fascia is robust and intact, that can be used alone; however, this is seldom the case. An incision in the muscle parallel to the inferolateral edge of the pectoralis major muscle is made, and the flap is elevated laterally until the anterior axillary line or sufficiently to create the desired pocket width for the chosen expander.

muscles can be elevated off the chest wall to open the inferolateral pocket (**FIGURE 9**).

- Submuscular placement with ADM:
  - The inferior and inferomedial origins of the pectoralis major are divided, releasing the muscle from the chest wall. A piece of ADM (or other product) can be sewn to the IMF inferiorly and the cut edge of the muscle superiorly.

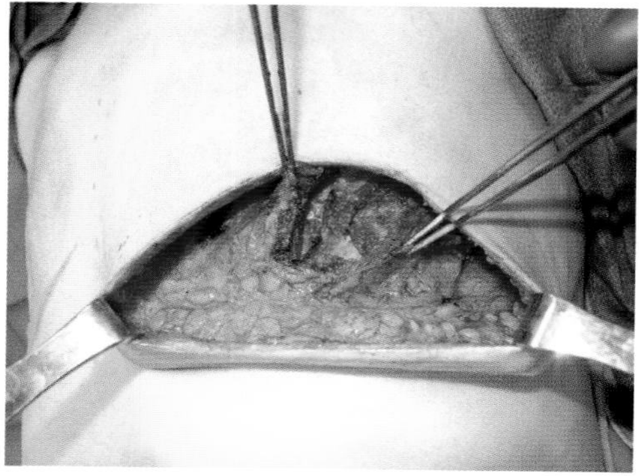

FIGURE 9 • Following elevation of the serratus anterior muscle, the inferolateral aspect of the implant pocket will still be adherent to the chest wall. If retractors are placed under the pectoralis major and serratus anterior muscles, this area of adhesion will be exposed and inferolateral dissection will elevate the serratus anterior and external oblique muscles off the chest wall to complete implant pocket dissection.

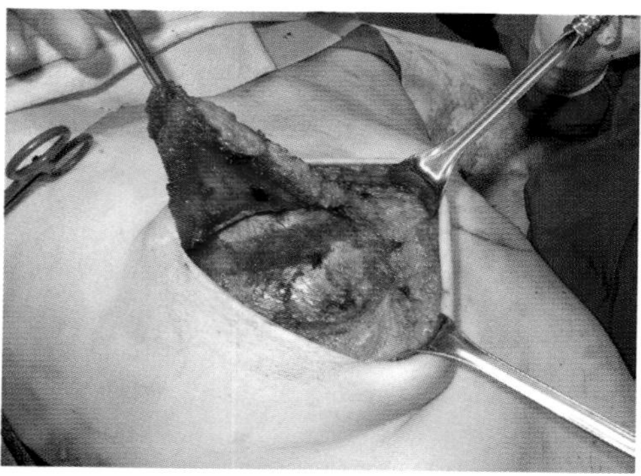

FIGURE 10 • If an ADM is used, the pectoralis major muscle is elevated from the chest wall by dividing its inferior and inferomedial origin.

  - This approach allows for an increased initial fill volume and is therefore often employed in women with larger breasts who have extra skin.
  - If an ADM is used, the origin of the pectoralis major is taken down starting inferolaterally and extending medially and then superiorly along the sternal origin to approximately the third or fourth rib (**FIGURE 10**). The ADM will provide inferolateral implant coverage and there is no need to elevate the serratus anterior. In this case, the IMF and anterior axillary line are marked internally and the ADM is sutured along a line that transitions in an arc from the IMF to the anterior axillary line (**FIGURE 11**). Alternatively, one can mark the lateral mammary fold based on the width of the desired tissue expander and suture the ADM to this line (**FIGURE 12**). One can tailor the surgically created IMF to match the contralateral native IMF during unilateral reconstruction. If performing bilateral reconstruction, then it is imperative to create symmetric IMFs.
  - The advantages of using an ADM are that it avoids any morbidity associated with elevation of the rectus sheath and serratus anterior, it allows for a greater initial fill volume (and potentially fewer postoperative

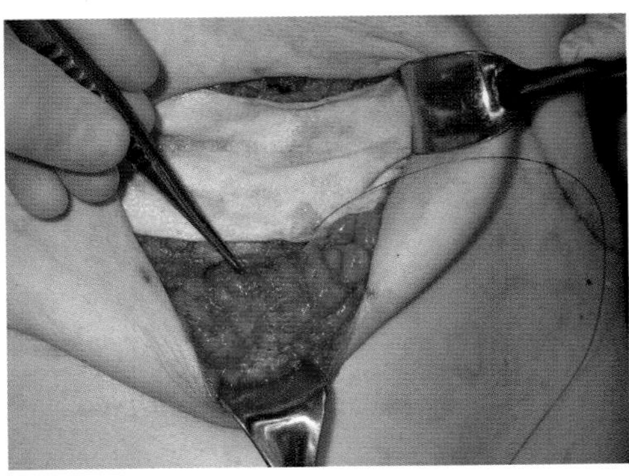

FIGURE 11 ● A piece of ADM is prepared appropriately, according to the manufacturer's recommendations, and is sewn in with the epidermis side facing the expander. The inferomedial and inferolateral corners of the ADM are trimmed to create a curved inferior border (unless a contoured product is used) and it is secured to the IMF and lateral pocket using interrupted 2-0 braided absorbable suture. The transition from the IMF to the lateral pocket must be a gentle arc that mimics the opposite side.

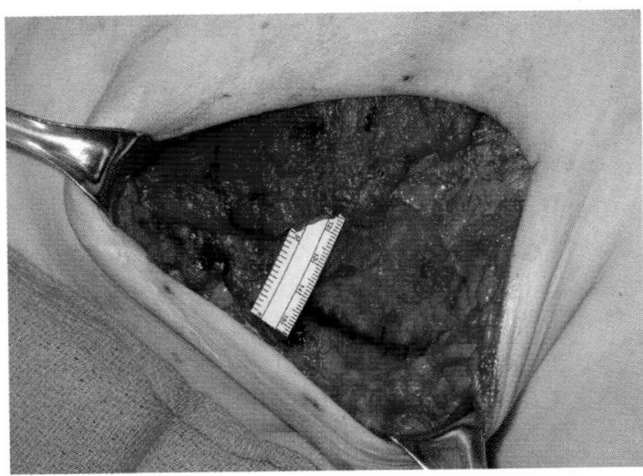

FIGURE 12 ● A ruler is used to measure the width of the surgically created pocket. The proper pocket width can be determined either by patient anatomy (eg, the anterior axillary line) or the dimensions of the expander desired.

expansions), it allows precise control of the IMF, it may reduce operative time, and it may preserve lower pole fullness. Disadvantages include cost and an increased incidence of seroma, infection, and reconstructive failure in patients with risk factors such as obesity, smoking, and/or radiation.[9] Although some surgeons use an ADM routinely and others do not, the author's preference is to use ADM selectively (**FIGURE 13**). It is used for every prepectoral reconstruction (indications discussed above). If the anterior rectus sheath or serratus anterior has been affected by the mastectomy and will not provide adequate coverage, ADM is an option, provided the patient does not have risk factors such as prior radiation, obesity, or smoking. In patients who have excess skin, it is advantageous to take advantage of this by placing a higher initial fill volume, and an ADM will allow the surgeon to do this (again, provided the patient does not have the risk factors mentioned earlier). When the pectoralis major does not extend down to the IMF in a patient with some excess skin and no risk factors, ADM is a good option. However, in a

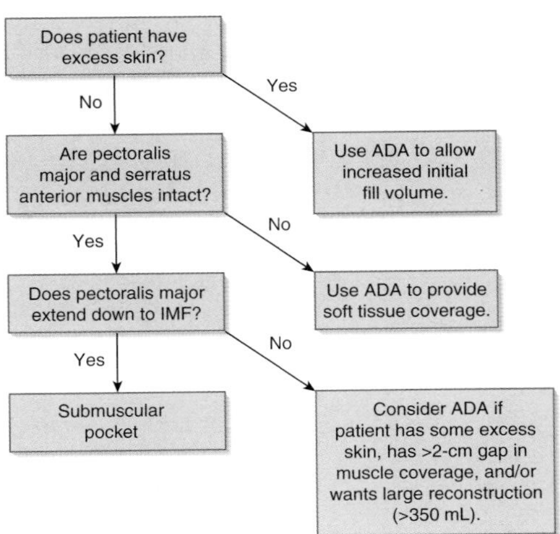

FIGURE 13 ● Algorithm to determine when to use ADM. IMF, inframammary fold.

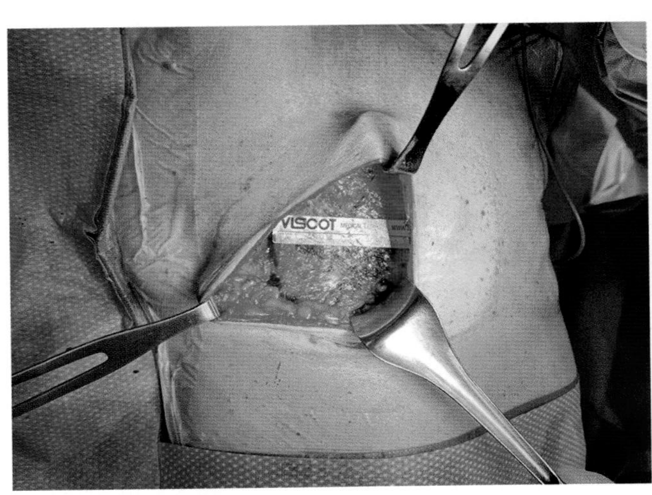

FIGURE 14 ● A ruler is placed in the prepectoral pocket and the lateral border of the pocket is marked according to the desired expander width.

patient without skin excess, who desires small breasts, and in whom very little initial fill volume will be placed, submusculofascial coverage can be provided without ADM.

- Prepectoral placement with ADM:
  - Surgeons may cover the expander with ADM (or other product) prior to implantation or after. It is the author's belief that only anterior coverage is required; therefore, the ADM is typically placed first and then the expander is placed under it. Some surgeons like to wrap the expander with ADM ex vivo while the mastectomy is performed. The author's preference is to have other cases scheduled simultaneously in another operating room during the mastectomy (see **FIGURES 14** and **15**).
  - The implant is positioned on the chest wall in the desired location. Integrated tabs and/or the ADM can be sutured to the chest wall to stabilize the expander and prevent rotation.

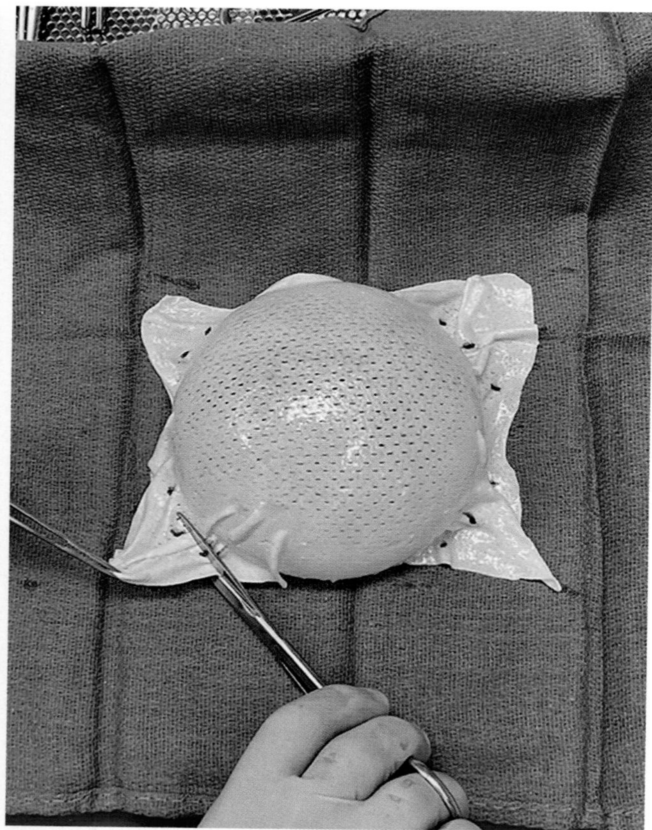

FIGURE 15 ● A large piece of meshed ADM is draped over the expander and trimmed accordingly to remove excess ADM.

Third Step—Preparation of Tissue Expander

- Tissue expanders come with air in them to prevent the inner shell from sticking to itself. There are usually markings for orientation, but it is helpful to draw a vertical line on the expander with a marking pen to assist with positioning the expander in the pocket. A needle (usually 23 gauge) is inserted into the port and all air is removed. The most commonly used tissue expanders are anatomic (creating lower pole expansion) and thus they are textured (to prevent rotation). Alternatively, they can be smooth with integrated tabs to secure the expander to the chest wall to prevent rotation. There is typically more shell inferiorly, and while deflating the expander, it is important to fold excess shell inward as opposed to folding it upward and on to itself, where it might cover the port and get punctured (**FIGURE 16**).
- The author's preference is to place 60 to 180 mL of sterile saline in the tissue expander prior to placement, which allows the anterior shell to move away from the rigid backing. It is important to control positioning of this backing as it is what determines final expander position.
- It can be helpful to put 1 mL of methylene blue in 1 L of injectable saline and use this for the initial expander fluid. If the expander is punctured during closure, it will be evident due to the dye. In addition, during expansions in clinic, the blue dye will confirm when the port is accessed.

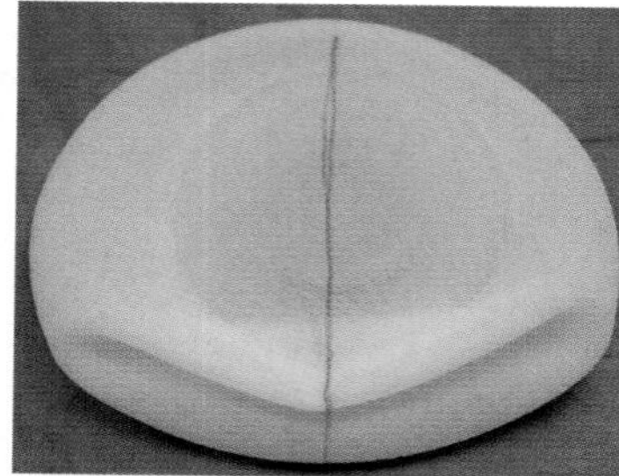

FIGURE 16 ● The tissue expander is marked with a vertical line for orientation. All air is removed with the excess inferior implant folded inward as shown to avoid puncturing the inferior implant while placing needles for expansion in clinic postoperatively. A minimum of 60 mL of saline is instilled, dyed with methylene blue. This allows for quick identification of inadvertent implant rupture during wound closure and also allows the clinic staff to confirm placement of the filling needle during subsequent expansions.

Fourth Step—Placement of Tissue Expander and Closure

- The pectoralis and/or ADM is retracted away from the chest wall, and the expander is placed into the pocket taking great care to orient it correctly. It is important to note the rigid backing of the expander and place the caudal edge at the IMF or below if desired. Be sure to unfold all edges of the expander. If performing bilateral reconstruction, symmetry in expander placement should be confirmed by palpating the expander ports on each side and ensuring symmetric horizontal and vertical positioning. If an expander requires adjustment in positioning, it is critical to grasp the rigid backing of the implant and then adjust the position. If only the ports or anterior shell are adjusted, this usually has no effect on the position of the backing, which determines implant position once fully inflated.
- The inferolateral edge of the pectoralis major muscle is sutured to the anteromedial edge of the serratus anterior muscle with running absorbable 2-0 braided suture, closing the pocket. A small opening is left superolaterally to allow egress of fluid. Alternatively, if an ADM is used, the pectoralis major muscle is sewn to the ADM with interrupted figure-of-8 braided absorbable 2-0 suture (**FIGURE 17**). If prepectoral placement is performed and ADM coverage was performed prior to implantation, then the expander is simply placed in position and secured to the chest wall. Alternatively, the expander is placed, ADM coverage is provided, and then the tabs and/or ADM are secured to the chest wall (see **FIGURES 18** and **19**).
- The author's preference is to inflate the tissue expander with sterile saline as much as the soft tissue (muscle/skin) will allow without undue tension. This is typically 180 to 240 mL but depends on the patient's anatomy. It is important to do this prior to skin closure, as placing the needle through the muscle will occasionally cause bleeding, which can be controlled directly. Otherwise, a hematoma could expand in the subcutaneous space without notice until the patient is out of surgery. In cases where there is significant concern regarding the cutaneous circulation, then only 0 to 60 mL of inflation is advisable.
- Two closed suction drains are placed in the subcutaneous space. One is oriented superiorly and the other inferiorly. The

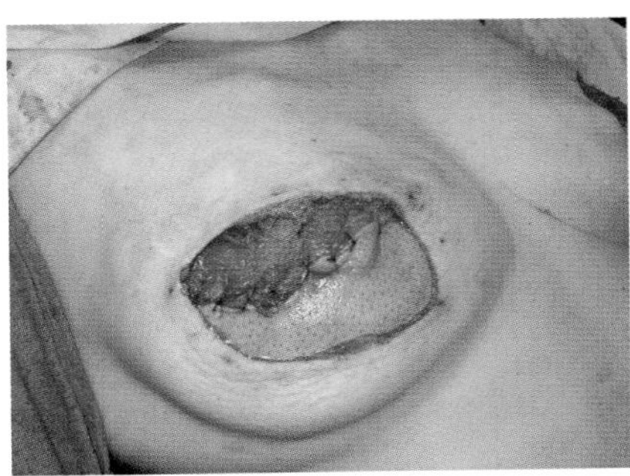

FIGURE 17 ● The inferolateral edge of the pectoralis major is sewn to the superomedial edge of the serratus anterior with interrupted horizontal mattress (inferiorly) and figure-of-8 (laterally) 2-0 absorbable braided suture to cover the implant. If an ADM is used, the pectoralis major is sewn to the edge of the ADM with interrupted horizontal mattress (inferiorly) and figure-of-8 (laterally) 2-0 absorbable braided suture, as shown. Use of horizontal mattress sutures inferiorly and figure-of-8 sutures laterally is due to the orientation of the pectoralis fibers, so the sutures do not pull through.

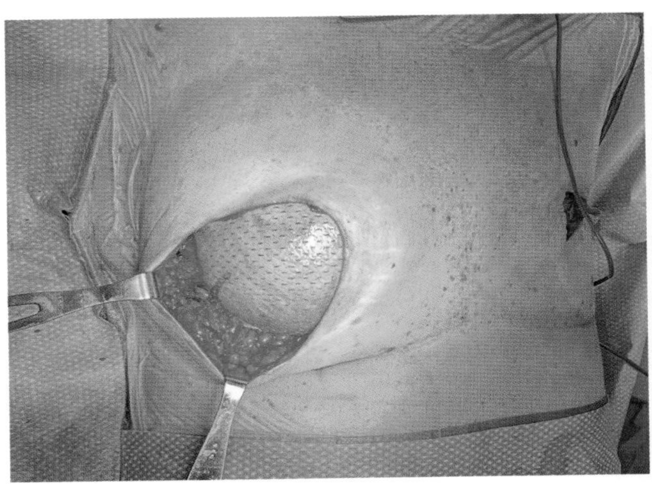

FIGURE 19 ● The expander is shown in position with ADM coverage prior to drain placement and skin closure.

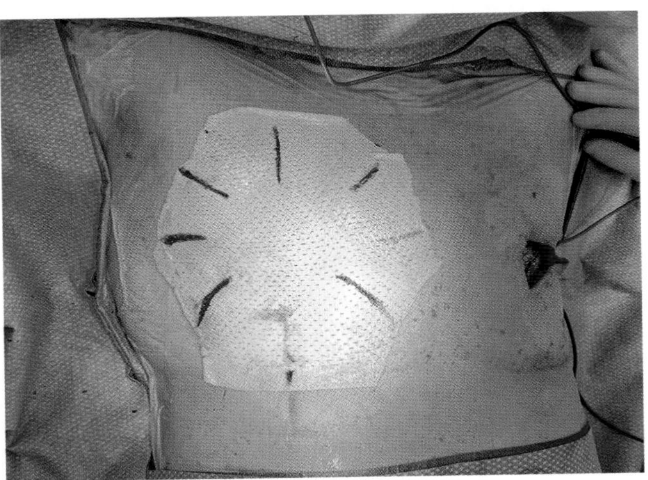

FIGURE 18 ● The ADM is marked for orientation and placed in the implant pocket with the epidermis side facing the expander. The ADM is secured to the inframammary fold and chest wall at the markings with interrupted braided absorbable 2-0 suture.

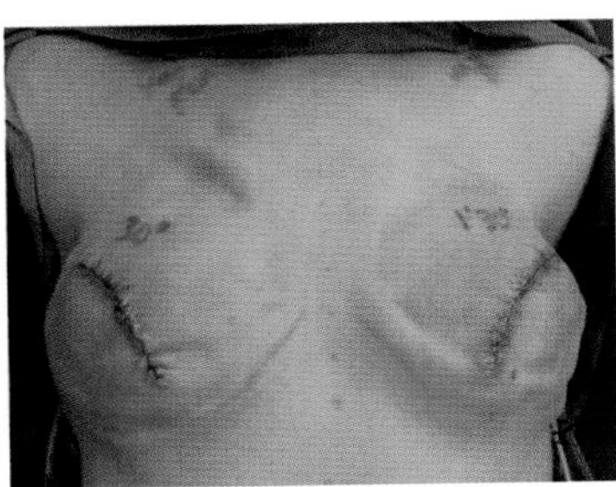

FIGURE 20 ● The patient is shown following placement of tissue expanders and closure over two closed suction drains on each side. Internal absorbable sutures are used, with skin glue as the only dressing. One packet of nitroglycerin ointment is applied on each side and covered with occlusive dressings (removed in 48 h prior to showering). No bra is applied, which might apply pressure to tenuous mastectomy flaps.

skin is closed with interrupted deep dermal and running subcuticular absorbable monofilament suture (**FIGURE 20**). The author's preference is to use skin glue alone as a dressing, without placement of a surgical bra, which applies pressure to the tenuous mastectomy flaps and is an impediment to physical examination. One packet of nitroglycerin is applied to the skin around the incisions on each side and covered with occlusive dressings that are removed after 48 hours.

- Antibiotics are continued parenterally for 24 hours postoperatively. Prolonged postoperative antibiotics do not seem to prevent infections, yet a single preoperative dose is not adequate either.[10] The ideal duration of postoperative antibiotic prophylaxis has yet to be determined and may be different according to patient risk factors. Drains are removed when output is less than 30 mL/d for 2 days in a row, and expansion is begun typically 4 weeks postoperatively unless there is a rush to expand prior to radiation. Expansion can continue on a weekly or biweekly basis, adding as much fluid as the patient will tolerate without discomfort (usually 60-120 mL). Some surgeons expand until the patient's desired volume is reached (keeping in mind that the final implant volume should be slightly larger to account for the volume of the integrated expander port), whereas others will overexpand to create some excess skin to allow minimal ptosis (described later).

IMPLANT EXCHANGE

First Step—Removal of Tissue Expander

- As noted earlier, the patient is marked in the standing position. Asymmetries are noted and the ideal position for the final implants is marked.
- The mastectomy scars have often widened during expansion and these can be excised. If the expander is submuscular, a stair-step approach to the implant pocket should be performed, so any wound breakdown in one layer does not expose the suture line of the other layer. If the scar is oriented obliquely (**FIGURE 21**), 2 to 4 cm of superomedial skin elevation will expose the pectoralis major, which can be incised parallel to the muscle fibers (**FIGURES 22** and **23**). If a transverse approach was used, then superolateral and inferomedial skin elevation is required to expose the pectoralis major and allow for an incision parallel to the muscle fibers. Incisions that go through the skin and immediately down to the implant through muscle can result in indented scars due to contracture.
- For prepectoral reconstructions, a stair-step approach can also be utilized; however, with sufficient flap thickness it is probably safe to go straight down through the allograft to the implant pocket in low-risk patients.
- The implant pocket is entered and the capsule is bluntly separated from the expander, which is removed. If the expander is too large, it can be ruptured with a needle or scalpel to assist in removal. If there was any doubt about the final expander volume, it can be measured at this point.

Second Step—Creation of Implant Pocket

- Ideally, the expanders can be removed and the permanent implants placed without further intervention; however, this is almost never the case. Superior capsulotomy is often required to soften the transition from the chest wall to the implant or to elevate the pocket (**FIGURE 24**). With prepectoral reconstruction, one may choose not to perform this capsulotomy so fat grafts can be placed in the subcutaneous

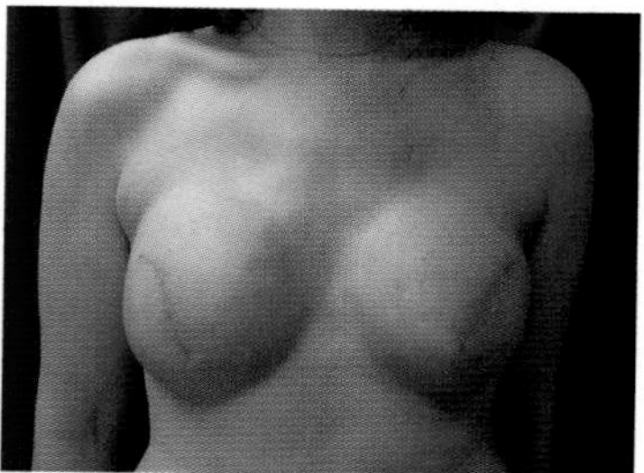

FIGURE 21 ● The patient is shown prior to the exchange procedure, 1 month following the last expansion in clinic. She has been expanded to 600 mL and desires 550-mL implants.

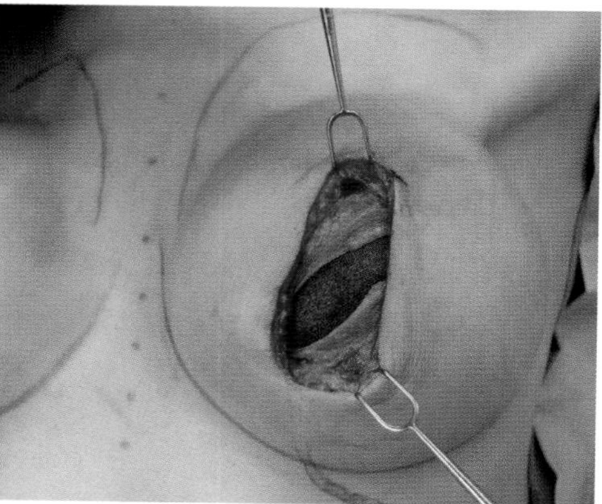

FIGURE 23 ● A muscular incision is made parallel to the pectoralis major muscle fibers to access the implant pocket. The capsule is also incised with cautery and the expander is bluntly separated from the capsule.

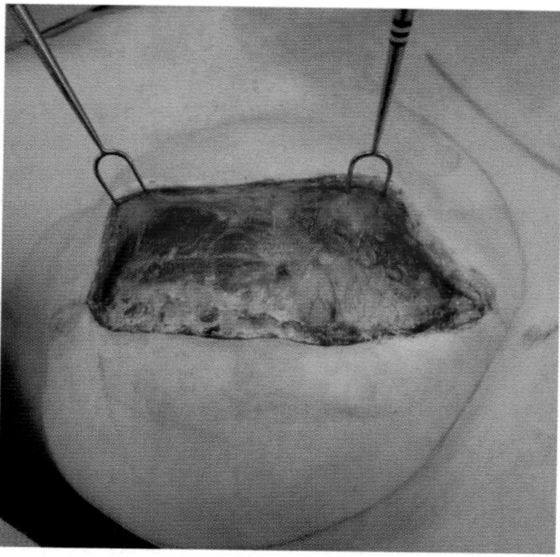

FIGURE 22 ● If the oblique incision is used for mastectomy, it is easy at the exchange procedure to elevate a superomedial flap exposing the pectoralis major muscle where it tends to be thicker. This will allow a "stair-step" approach to the implant pocket. Any wound healing issue at one level will not expose the suture line at the other level.

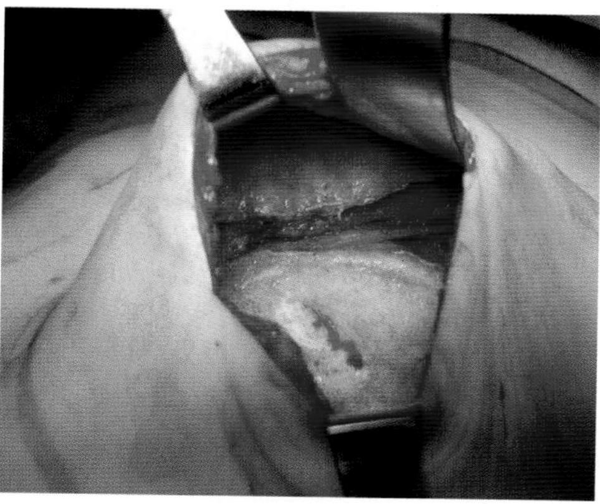

FIGURE 24 ● A superomedial and superior capsulotomy is made just above the chest wall using a lighted retractor. This will soften the transition from chest wall to implant and allow for more implant mobility within the pocket. Some surgeons will not perform capsulectomy superiorly if planning fat grafting in this location.

space at the superior border of the implant without injecting fat into the implant pocket.

- The pocket may need to be medialized, lateralized, elevated, or displaced inferiorly. These can all be accomplished through capsulotomy with or without capsulorrhaphy. If the final implant is roughly the same width as the expander, then a corresponding capsulorrhaphy at the opposite side of the pocket is necessary. Minimal tightening of the pocket can be performed using thermal (aka "popcorn") capsulorrhaphy by grasping the capsule with an insulated forceps and applying cautery set on 50. This causes a full-thickness burn of the capsule, resulting in contracture of the capsule and tightening of the implant pocket. The durability of thermal capsulorrhaphy has not been formally evaluated. If more tightening is required, then a combination of thermal and suture capsulorrhaphy is performed. If the implant is wider than the expander, this may not be necessary as the capsulotomy will increase pocket diameter.
- If the expander was placed below the IMF, or if the IMF needs to be elevated, this is accomplished with figure-of-8 interrupted 0 braided absorbable suture following thermal capsulorrhaphy. The patient is sat upright (**FIGURE 25**) and the inferior mastectomy flap is lifted away from the chest wall. Usually, the old IMF can be visualized and marked (**FIGURE 26**); otherwise, the desired IMF can be marked. The needle is passed through the capsule and the IMF marking externally is visualized. The needle tip should just catch the deep dermis, resulting in a small indentation when tied. These indentations will resolve in several weeks. After passing the needle through the capsule/dermis, tension can be adjusted by examining the fold externally (**FIGURE 27**) and elevating it as desired. Internal inspection with the suture still under tension will indicate where the corresponding suture throw in the chest wall must be made. Suturing into the rib should be avoided, as this results in pain. The first suture is placed at the center of the IMF, and then one to two sutures are placed medially and laterally until an adequate fold is created (**FIGURES 28** and **29**).

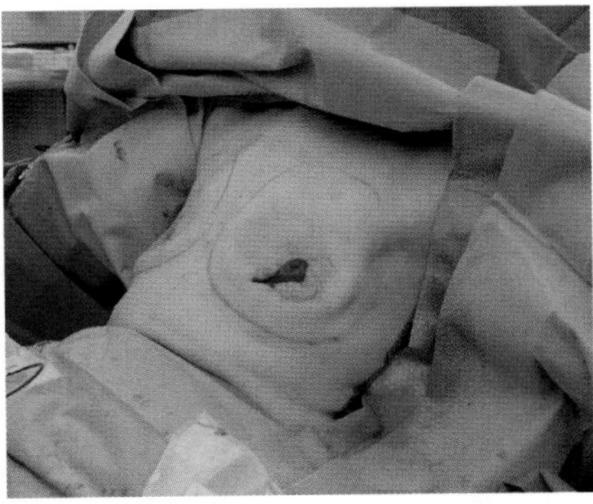

FIGURE 25 ● The patient is positioned upright with both upper extremities well padded and secured to arm boards abducted less than 90°.

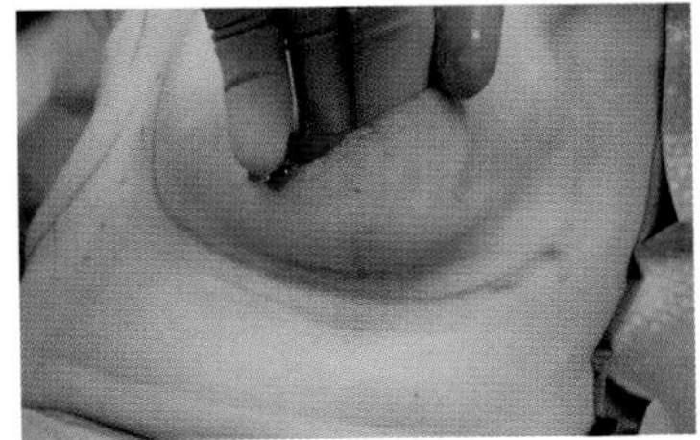

FIGURE 26 ● When the inferior mastectomy flap is elevated gently from the chest wall, the patient's original IMF is usually still visible and can be marked for recreation of the native IMF. A higher or lower IMF can also be created.

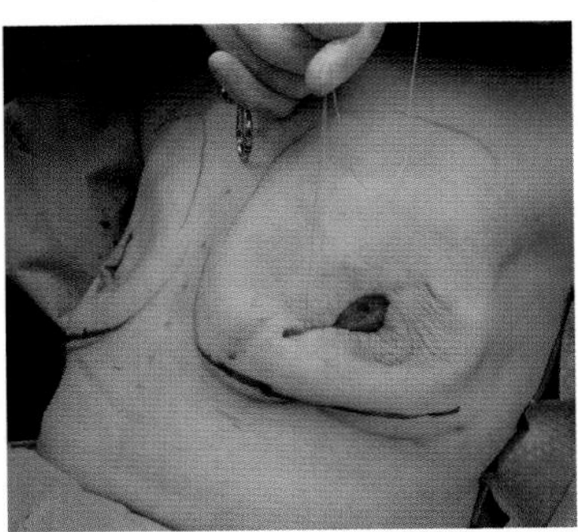

FIGURE 27 ● A suture is placed in the center of the IMF, through the capsule and just catching the deep dermis. The suture is pulled upward and the level of the IMF adjusted as desired to recreate a sharp and well-defined IMF. Once held in appropriate position, internal inspection will reveal where a suture should be placed on the chest wall. To minimize pain, suturing to the ribs should be avoided if possible. If the lower portion of the expander was placed at the IMF and good lower pole expansion and a crisp IMF in good position has resulted, then this maneuver is unnecessary.

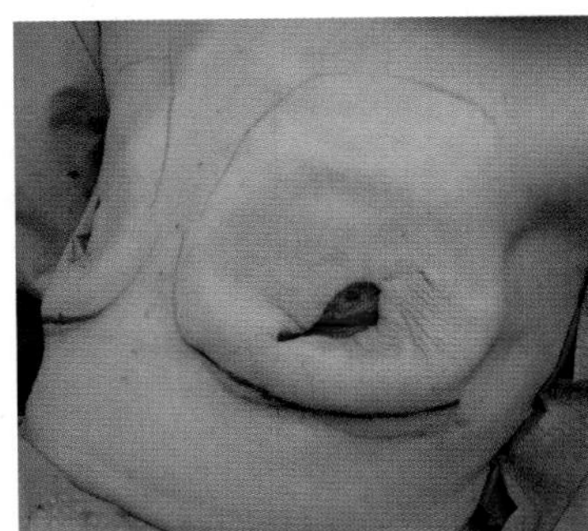

FIGURE 28 ● The IMF has been reestablished with multiple figure-of-8 capsulorrhaphy sutures, starting in the center of the IMF and proceeding medially and laterally until an adequate IMF is recreated. A temporary implant sizer is helpful to assess the reconstructed IMF during this process.

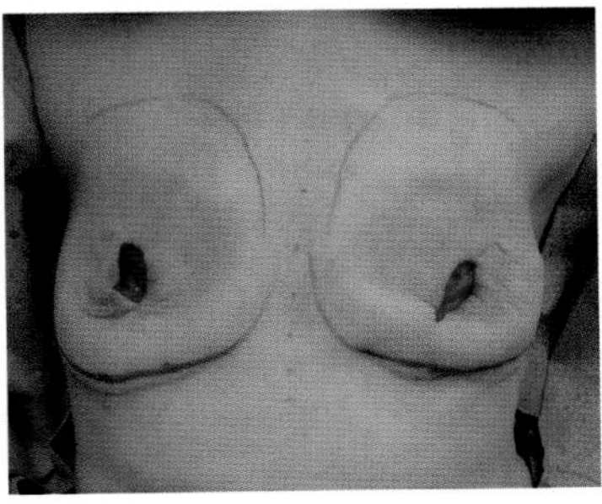

FIGURE 29 ● Comparison of the left side, where the IMF has been recreated, and the right side, where it has not.

- Some surgeons prefer to establish the IMF at the initial operation, potentially with an ADM, which has the added benefit of permitting a higher initial fill volume. A higher initial fill volume has the potential to better preserve lower pole fullness. No time is spent reconstructing the IMF at the exchange procedure. Although this may be a simpler approach, it may result in a blunted IMF. The author's preference is to treat each case individually and surgically create a crisp IMF at the exchange procedure if necessary. For example, patients undergoing delayed reconstruction will benefit from significant lower pole expansion and thus the expander is placed inferior to the desired IMF and the IMF is reconstructed at the exchange procedure. A patient with ptosis undergoing immediate reconstruction will benefit from an ADM to maximize the initial fill volume (preserve lower pole fullness), establish the IMF, and avoid inferior capsulorrhaphy at the exchange procedure.
- To further expand the lower pole and create minimal ptosis, capsulotomy of the inferior pocket is then performed. A horizontal capsulotomy half way up the inferior mastectomy flap, at least 4 cm off the chest wall, will expand the lower pole of the pocket (**FIGURE 30**). Additional radial capsulotomies can be added for further lower pole expansion or elsewhere to create symmetric pockets.
- During pocket creation, it is helpful to have a temporary sizer placed into the implant pocket to assess position, shape, and volume.

Third Step—Implant Selection and Closure

- When ordering implants for the exchange procedure, it is the author's preference to order implants that are slightly larger than the fill volume at which the patient was happy, as the expander includes the additional volume of the fill apparatus.
- When placing conventional saline implants, choose an implant that has the desired volume as the upper end of its volume range. For example, if 380 mL is the desired implant volume, use an implant with a volume range of 360 to 390 mL. This avoids rippling at the expense of making the implant slightly firmer. Some surgeons will in fact overfill the implant by 10% to avoid rippling. Newer dual-lumen saline implants are usually not overfilled, as they inherently have less rippling.
- If fat grafting is to be performed, it is performed prior to closure through the existing incision or via additional stab incisions. Following fat grafting, the implants should be removed to confirm their integrity and the pocket should be irrigated to remove any free-floating fat grafts. Alternatively, one can perform fat grafting with sizers in place or even without any implants in place.
- The pockets are irrigated, hemostasis is obtained, and the final implants are opened. Although many surgeons will reprep the patient, place new drapes, dip retractors in prep solution, and handle the implants with fresh gloves, there are no data to support these practices. The author does not take any special precautions, as the procedure is a clean, sterile procedure. The implants are placed, and the muscular (or dermal allograft) closure is performed with a running 2-0 braided absorbable suture. No drains are placed. The skin is closed with interrupted deep dermal and running subcuticular 3-0 monofilament absorbable suture (**FIGURE 31**). Skin glue is applied, and a bra is only used if supporting the implant in a particular position is desired.

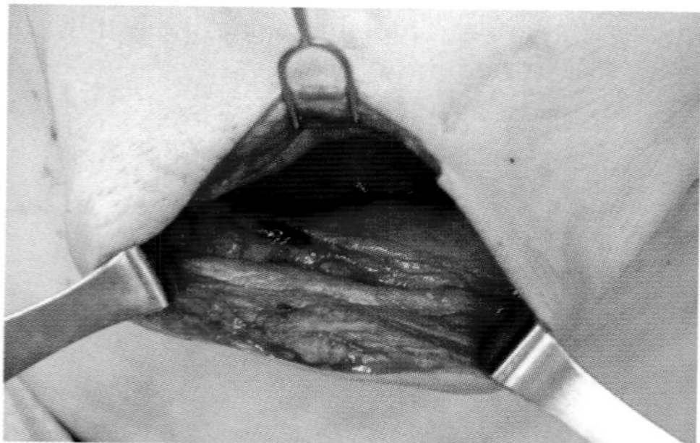

FIGURE 30 ● A horizontal capsulotomy approximately half way up the inferior mastectomy flap is performed to further expand the lower pole and create minimal ptosis. Multiple radial capsulotomies (perpendicular to the horizontal capsulotomy) will further expand the lower pole.

Additional Procedure—Nipple Reconstruction and Revisions

- When examined with a critical eye, almost all patients have some degree of asymmetry or contour deformity following reconstruction (**FIGURE 32**). Approximately 30% or more

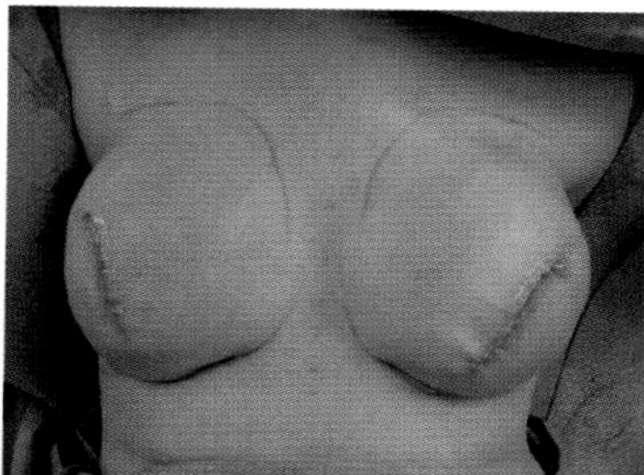

FIGURE 31 ● The implants have been placed and the wounds closed without drains. Skin glue has been applied. The dimpling observed at the IMFs will resolve in several weeks.

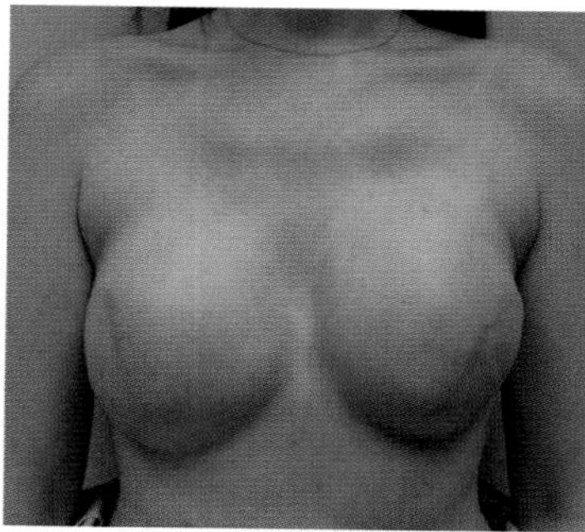

FIGURE 32 ● Three months following the exchange procedure, the patient is very happy and interested in nipple reconstruction. The right IMF is 2 cm lower than the left IMF, but the patient does not desire correction. It is important to establish the final implant position prior to nipple reconstruction; otherwise, later implant repositioning will affect how the nipple is positioned on the breast mound. There is minimal step-off from the chest wall to the implants, which is the result of mastectomy and commonly seen in implant reconstruction. This can be corrected with fat grafting, which this patient declined.

will request a third revision procedure. Correcting the unfavorable result in implant breast reconstruction is a complex subject, involving techniques to alter implant position, breast shape, implant type, and soft tissue characteristics. Many patients ultimately opt for NAC reconstruction (**FIGURE 33**) (see Part 5, Chapter 26). In many cases, minor revisions can be performed at the time of NAC reconstruction; however, the nipple should only be created once the breast mound is in its final position, and thus it is not advisable to adjust the implant pocket and create the nipple during the same operation.

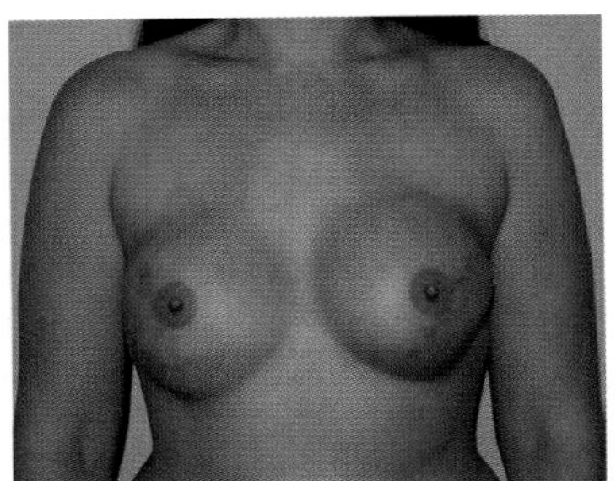

FIGURE 33 ● Options for nipple-areolar complex (NAC) reconstruction include tattoo only, nipple reconstruction with areola tattoo, and nipple reconstruction with areola graft. This patient opted for a "3-D" tattoo performed by a professional tattoo artist, which is becoming standard of care. She is very happy with the aesthetic result, although she has some chronic discomfort lateral to the right breast, has asymmetry of implant position, and very obvious implant borders superiorly. The implants have dropped slightly, resulting in a more obvious step-off from the chest wall to the implants, and could be corrected with elevation of the implants (which would affect NAC position on the breast mound) or fat grafting.

PEARLS AND PITFALLS

Indications	■ Patients with a history of radiation are poor candidates for implant reconstruction. ■ Risk factors for infection and wound healing complications include smoking, radiation, and obesity.
Incision placement	■ An oblique incision parallel to the pectoralis muscle fibers provides the best cosmesis and easiest approach for the exchange procedure. ■ Excess skin can be excised through a linear incision, as additional incisions will compromise circulation and risk mastectomy flap necrosis. Secondary procedures are frequently necessary in patients with excess skin.
Expander selection	■ Expanders are selected based on breast width, not volume.
Expander placement	■ Marking the expander assists in correct orientation. ■ Remove all air and place saline dyed with methylene blue to allow detection of implant rupture as well as confirmation of port access for staff performing expansions. ■ Provide at least 24 h of postoperative antibiotics.
Implant selection	■ Implants are selected based on volume primarily, taking breast width into consideration. High-profile implants are typically used, except in patients with wide chests who benefit from wider profile implants.
Patient expectation	■ Two-stage implant breast reconstruction is typically a year-long process. ■ Symmetry in the nude is always the goal but is seldom achieved. Symmetry in clothing is the most reasonable expectation.

POSTOPERATIVE CARE

- Following the mastectomy and tissue expander placement, the patient is maintained on intravenous antibiotics for 24 hours (unless they are discharged in which case a short course of oral antibiotics is prescribed). Drains remain in place at least 5 to 7 days and then are removed when output is less than 30 mL/d for 2 days in a row. Only one drain from each side should be removed at a time, as sometimes the output of the second drain will increase after the first drain is removed. The author's preference is to allow patients to shower after 48 hours with drains in place, although there are data to suggest showering the next day is acceptable. Many plastic surgeons still prohibit their patients from showering while drains are in place, which is a practice that makes no sense when considering the basic tenets of asepsis established over a century ago. The patient should be seen within 1 to 2 weeks to evaluate for postoperative infection and/or mastectomy flap necrosis and to remove drains if appropriate. Expansion is begun 4 weeks after surgery and continued on a biweekly basis thereafter until the patient and surgeon are happy with the final volume. If radiation is required soon after mastectomy, then the expansion schedule can be rushed, starting approximately 2 weeks after surgery and continued on a weekly basis. The exchange procedure is scheduled at least 3 months after the initial surgery and 3 weeks after the last expansion to allow the tissues to heal and soften.

- Following the exchange procedure, patients may shower after 48 hours. Although the author feels very strongly about giving patients postoperative prophylactic antibiotics after mastectomy and expander placement, the exchange procedure is a clean procedure and the mastectomy flaps have been delayed and have robust perfusion. Thus, no postoperative antibiotics are usually given. There are little data to support practices such as repreping the patient, changing drapes, changing gloves, or dipping retractors in prep solution, although this is commonly performed by surgeons placing implants.

OUTCOMES

- Patient satisfaction with implant breast reconstruction is high, provided the preoperative consultation appropriately identified the patient's priorities, goals, and preferences with respect to reconstructive options, and realistic expectations were discussed (**FIGURES 34-36**). Although some studies have indicated that patients undergoing prosthetic reconstruction are less satisfied than those undergoing autologous tissue reconstruction,[11,12] other studies have shown significant improvements in psychosocial outcomes regardless of the type of reconstruction.[13]
- It is common to tell patients undergoing implant reconstruction that, on average, they will require some form of surgery every 10 to 15 years. These could be procedures for symmetry, infection, rupture, or capsular contracture. Although surgeons used to exchange silicone implants every 10 years due to a much higher risk of extracapsular rupture with older-generation implants, most surgeons currently only offer surgery if a problem is identified. One study evaluated long-term outcomes of autologous vs implant reconstruction and noted stable survival of 90% of autologous reconstructions vs a gradual decline to 70% survival of implant reconstructions.[14] In general, autologous reconstructions improve or remain stable with time, whereas implant reconstructions tend to worsen over time.
- There is no increased risk of breast cancer recurrence in patients undergoing therapeutic mastectomy and implant reconstruction. Detection of recurrence and outcome when recurrence is detected are not affected by the presence of an implant reconstruction.[15]

COMPLICATIONS

- Bleeding
- Infection
- Injury to surrounding structures (eg, cutaneous nerves)
- Mastectomy flap necrosis
- Long-term risks of implants: capsular contracture, rupture, rippling, infection, malposition, exposure, BII, BIA-ALCL
- Asymmetry, less than desired cosmetic result

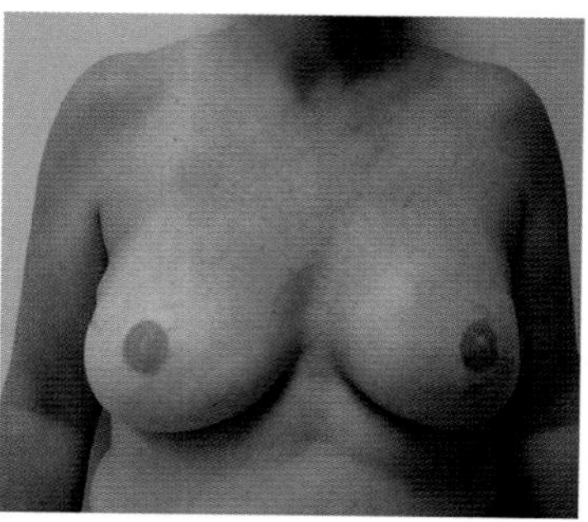

FIGURE 34 ● This patient is 1 year out from the exchange procedure and 6 months out from NAC reconstruction with local flaps to reconstruct the nipple and areola tattoo. She has a higher body mass index (BMI) and more subcutaneous fat, and the mastectomy did not extend very far superiorly. Thus, she has a smooth transition from the chest wall to the implants.

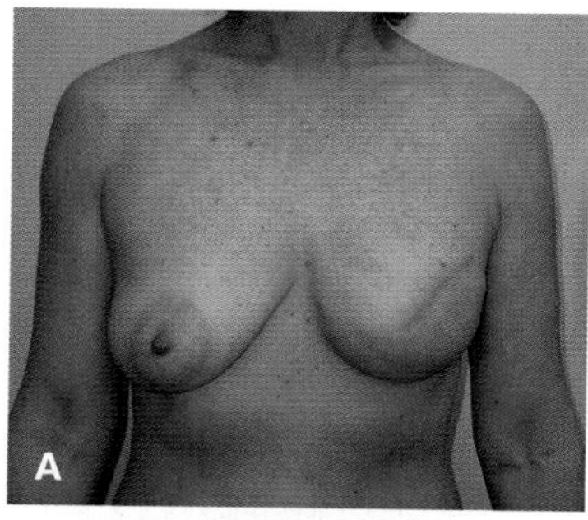

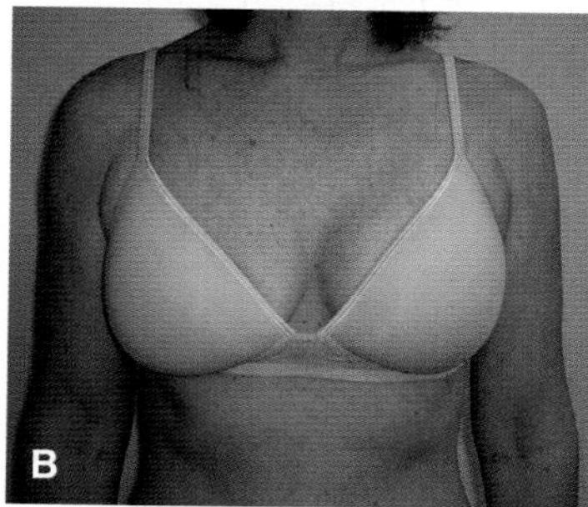

FIGURE 35 ● **A** and **B,** This patient is 6 months out from unilateral reconstruction. She did not desire NAC reconstruction or a contralateral mastopexy for symmetry. She has a very acceptable appearance in a bra.

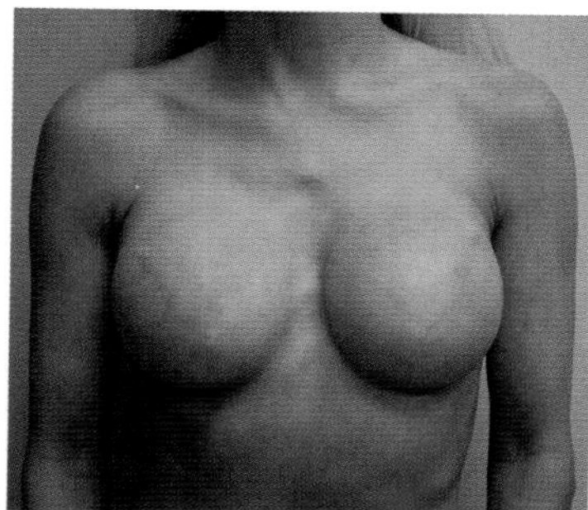

FIGURE 36 ● This patient is 9 months out from her exchange procedure. She had prior augmentation mammaplasty and thin soft tissue coverage inferiorly; therefore, an ADM was used to augment soft tissue coverage of the expanders.

REFERENCES

1. Nelson JA, Shamsunder MG, Vorstenbosch J, et al. Prepectoral and subpectoral tissue expander–based breast reconstruction: a Propensity-Matched analysis of 90-day clinical and Health-related quality-of-life outcomes. *Plast Reconstr Surg*. 2022;149(4):607e-616e.
2. Campbell CA, Losken A. Understanding the evidence and improving outcomes with implant-based prepectoral breast reconstruction. *Plast Reconstr Surg*. 2021;148(3):437e-450e.
3. Momeni A, Li AY, Tsai J, et al. The impact of device innovation on clinical outcomes in expander-based breast reconstruction. *Plast Reconstr Surg Glob Open*. 2019;7(12):e2524.
4. Nichter LS, Hardesty RA, Anigian GM. Ideal implant structured breast implants: core study results at 6 years. *Plast Reconstr Surg*. 2018;142(1):66-75.
5. Moyer HR, Losken A. Predicting mastectomy skin flap necrosis with indocyanine green angiography: the gray area defined. *Plast Reconstr Surg*. 2012;129(5):1043-1048.
6. Abbott AM, Miller BT, Tuttle TM. Outcomes after tumescence technique versus electrocautery mastectomy. *Ann Surg Oncol*. 2012;19(8):2607-2611.
7. Seth AK, Hirsch EM, Fine NA, et al. Additive risk of tumescent technique in patients undergoing mastectomy with immediate reconstruction. *Ann Surg Oncol*. 2011;18(11):3041-3046.
8. Chun YS, Verma K, Rosen H, et al. Use of tumescent mastectomy technique as a risk factor for native breast skin flap necrosis following immediate breast reconstruction. *Am J Surg*. 2011;201(2):160-165.
9. Ho G, Nguyen TJ, Shahabi A, et al. A systematic review and meta-analysis of complications associated with acellular dermal matrix-assisted breast reconstruction. *Ann Plast Surg*. 2012;68(4):346-356.
10. Clayton JL, Bazakas A, Lee CN, et al. Once is not enough: withholding postoperative prophylactic antibiotics in prosthetic breast reconstruction is associated with an increased risk of infection. *Plast Reconstr Surg*. 2012;130(3):495-502.
11. Alderman AK, Wilkins EG, Lowery JC, et al. Determinants of patient satisfaction in postmastectomy breast reconstruction. *Plast Reconstr Surg*. 2000;106:769-776.
12. Christensen BO, Overgaard J, Kettner LO, et al. Long-term evaluation of postmastectomy breast reconstruction. *Acta Oncol*. 2011;50(7):1053-1061.
13. Wilkins EG, Cederna PS, Lowery JC, et al. Prospective analysis of psychosocial outcomes in breast reconstruction: one-year postoperative results from the Michigan Breast Reconstruction Outcome Study. *Plast Reconstr Surg*. 2000;106(5):1014-1025; discussion 1026-1027.
14. Rusby JE, Waters RA, Nightingale PG, et al. Immediate breast reconstruction after mastectomy: what are the long-term prospects?. *Ann R Coll Surg Engl*. 2010;92(3):193-197.
15. McCarthy CM, Pusic AL, Sclafani L, et al. Breast cancer recurrence following prosthetic, postmastectomy reconstruction: incidence, detection, and treatment. *Plast Reconstr Surg*. 2008;121(2):381-388.

Chapter 23

Pedicled Latissimus Dorsi Flap for Breast Reconstruction After Mastectomy

Nishant Ganesh Kumar and Adeyiza O. Momoh

DEFINITION

- The latissimus dorsi myocutaneous flap was originally performed for chest wall reconstruction after radical mastectomy by Iginio Tansini in 1906 but fell out of favor when mastectomies were primarily closed or skin grafted.[1] Although the latissimus flap remained a dependable option for anterior chest wall reconstruction,[2-4] it was not until 1977 when it was first described to reconstruct a true breast mound in combination with a prosthetic implant.[5]
- The latissimus dorsi myocutaneous flap currently remains a viable and frequently used option for breast reconstruction. Typically, patients who have undergone chest wall irradiation or either unwilling or unable (lack of donor site tissue volume) to undergo other autologous flap options for breast reconstruction will proceed with this option. Furthermore, this flap has found use in the reconstruction of congenital breast mound defects such as in Poland syndrome.[6]
- For the purpose of breast reconstruction, this technique usually requires flap transfer combined with an initial tissue expansion process followed by a subsequent saline- or silicone-filled prosthetic permanent implant. Breast reconstruction with a latissimus dorsi myocutaneous flap without an implant is also possible but less commonly used due to flap volume limitations.[7] Recently, the latissimus dorsi flap has been used in conjunction with immediate fat transfer into the flap for complete autologous breast reconstruction.[8,9] This option can be considered in carefully selected patients as a viable alternative to other autologous means of breast reconstruction with satisfactory long-term outcomes.
- Relative indications and contraindications for latissimus dorsi flap reconstruction exist. Relative indications include implant-based reconstruction in the setting of prior radiation therapy, for candidates who desire autologous reconstruction where other options (eg, deep inferior epigastric perforator [DIEP] flap, profunda artery perforator [PAP] flap, transverse upper gracilis [TUG] flap) may not be possible, and to reconstruct small volume lumpectomy or mastectomy defects. Relative contraindications can include prior axillary node dissection resulting in trauma to the pedicle or neurovascular bundle, imaging findings suggesting pedicle damage or affected blood flow to the flap, attenuated latissimus dorsi muscle, active smoking, and prior surgical incisions at the site of flap harvest (eg, from lateral thoracotomy) that might result in damage to the muscle or pedicle.[10]

ANATOMY

- The latissimus dorsi is a large, flat, triangle-shaped muscle on the back measuring approximately 25 × 35 cm; it mirrors the pectoralis major posteriorly.
- The muscle origin is a broad aponeurosis that spans the lower six thoracic vertebrae (superomedially), supraspinous ligament (central medial region), thoracolumbar fascia (inferomedially), and posterior iliac crest (inferiorly).
- The lateral border of the muscle separates from the serratus anterior as a free potential space until one encounters the small slips of origin from the 10th to 12th ribs, where the latissimus interdigitates with the slips of origin of the external oblique and serratus anterior muscles.
- The superior border of the muscle has an area of adhesion to the region of the inferior angle of the scapula but otherwise contains free potential space with the underlying layer.
- The muscle converges in the axilla to insert on the crest of the lesser tuberosity of the humerus.
- The latissimus dorsi adducts, extends, and rotates the humerus medially ("pull-up," rowing, or free-style swimming motions).
- The latissimus dorsi flap is a Nahai-Mathes type V myocutaneous flap, meaning that it may survive based solely on either the thoracodorsal artery or the segmental perforators from the intercostal and lumbar arteries.
- The thoracodorsal artery (arising from the subscapular branch off the axillary artery) enters the deep surface of the latissimus dorsi muscle in the posterior axilla approximately 10 cm inferior to the muscle insertion into the humerus and 2.6 cm medial to the lateral border of the muscle (**FIGURE 1**).
- The artery then divides into the medial (also known as transverse) and the lateral (also known as vertical or descending) branches. The medial branch is located approximately 3.5 cm below and parallel to the superior border. The lateral branch is located approximately 2.6 cm medial and parallel to the lateral border. The serratus branch (artery to the serratus anterior), which joins the thoracodorsal artery just before its entrance to the latissimus muscle, is a useful landmark as it guides one directly to the thoracodorsal pedicle. There is usually a single vena comitans of the thoracodorsal artery.[11,12]
- Knowledge of the vascular branching pattern of the thoracodorsal artery has supported the use of muscle-sparing latissimus dorsi flaps for breast reconstruction that relies on the descending branch of the artery. Advocates have cited minimal functional deficits and acceptable aesthetic scar outcomes to support the use of the muscle sparing latissimus dorsi for breast reconstruction.[13]
- The thoracodorsal motor nerve enters the muscle with the vascular pedicle. Cutaneous sensory nerves arise from the intercostal nerves at the midaxillary line and also in the paraspinal region.

PATIENT HISTORY AND PHYSICAL FINDINGS

- A thorough history and physical examination are critical in preparing for reconstruction. Appropriate coordination with physicians involved in the patient's care should be carried out prior to surgery.

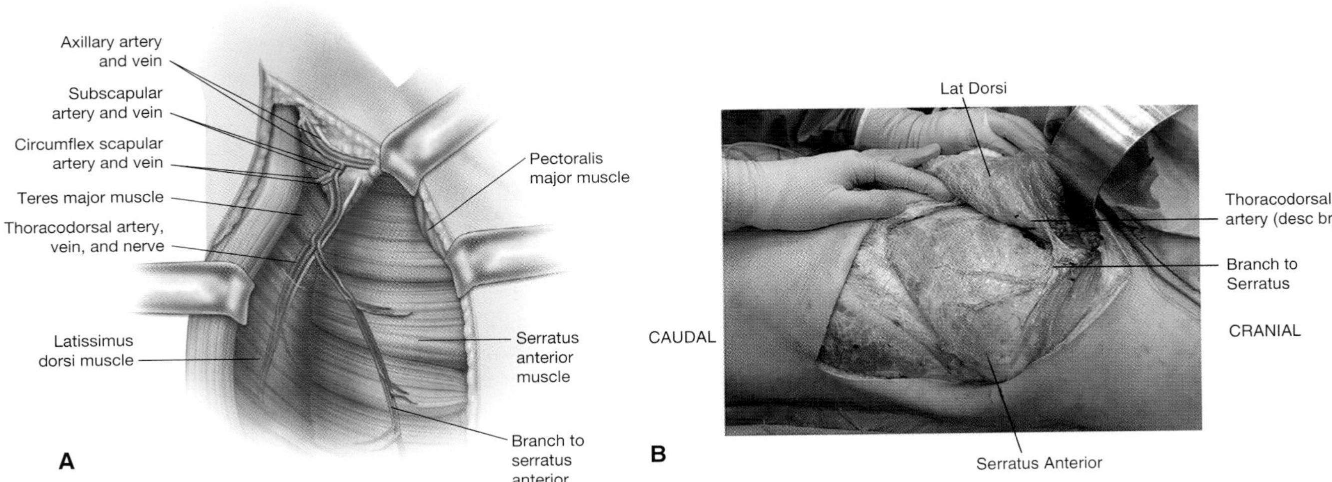

FIGURE 1 ● **A,** Illustration and **(B)** intraoperative representation of the vascular anatomy of the latissimus dorsi muscle and thoracodorsal neurovascular bundle.

- Pertinent aspects of the history include previous axillary or thoracic operations (eg, lymph node dissections or biopsies, lateral thoracotomy) and medical conditions that would preclude patients from an operation of moderate length under general anesthesia.
- Certain patients (eg, paraplegic or wheelchair-dependent individuals) who cannot afford even a minimal weakening of shoulder strength, probably should not undergo latissimus dorsi breast reconstruction as some individuals may experience functional deficits with shoulder function after surgery (see outcomes below).
- A focused examination of the axilla and back for scars that may preclude use of the muscle flap or affect placement of the skin paddle is necessary.
- The presence of a viable and innervated muscle may be confirmed by having the patient activate the muscle by placing the hands on the hips and pushing firmly. However, a vigorous muscle contraction does not necessarily indicate an intact thoracodorsal arterial pedicle, as the nerve is quite separated from the thoracodorsal artery proximal to the branch point from the subscapular artery and could be potentially preserved despite ligation of the artery.

IMAGING AND OTHER DIAGNOSTIC STUDIES

- Imaging is not absolutely necessary preoperatively in patients who have not undergone prior surgeries; however, it can help in preoperative planning.
- Preoperative computed tomography (CT) angiography of the donor site (**FIGURE 2**) is recommended in patients with previous surgical procedures during which the thoracodorsal arterial pedicle may have been sacrificed (eg, axillary lymph node dissection or modified radical mastectomy).

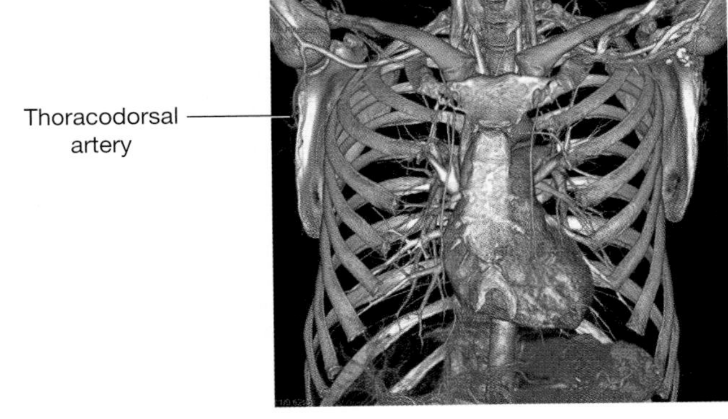

FIGURE 2 ● Preoperative CT angiography of the thoracodorsal vessels.

SURGICAL MANAGEMENT

- In consulting with patients, decisions about the timing of reconstruction (immediately after mastectomy or delayed) and the type of reconstruction (eg, implant based or complete autologous and, prepectoral or subpectoral implant placement) are made taking patient factors and tumor characteristics into consideration.
  - Patient factors of significance include the following:
    - Patient preference
    - Smoking history
    - History of previous axillary operations that compromise the vascular pedicle of the donor site
    - Medical comorbidities that would preclude patients from undergoing an operation of moderate length
  - Tumor characteristics as they relate to the following:
    - The need for postmastectomy radiation therapy

- The need for close postmastectomy surveillance prior to reconstruction
- In general, patients known to require postmastectomy radiation therapy are reconstructed in a delayed fashion to avoid the detrimental effects of radiation on flaps. A history of radiation therapy also serves as a relative indication for use of an autologous form of reconstruction, as implant-only reconstructions in the setting of radiation are prone to higher rates of complications and failure.

- Reconstruction goals in planning latissimus dorsi flap:
  - A clear understanding of the patient's goals for breast reconstruction and final breast mound size, shape, and projection is necessary. Furthermore, patient preferences regarding complete autologous or use of implants should be clearly understood taking into consideration risk profile, long-term surveillance, and reconstruction goals.
  - The patient should understand limitations in the size and shape possible for breast reconstruction using the latissimus dorsi with or without an implant. These include limitations in breast base width and implant size, the need for tissue expansions, and ultimately the type of permanent implant being used.
  - Recent advances in latissimus dorsi and implant-based reconstruction have also led to placement of the implant in the prepectoral plane with complete latissimus dorsi coverage. Advocates for prepectoral implant position in latissimus dorsi reconstruction include avoiding the need to expand the irradiated pectoralis muscle that occurs in subpectoral placement and limiting the functional implications of latissimus dorsi and subpectoral placement that has been associated with reduced shoulder strength and shoulder stiffness.[14-16]
  - Therefore, surgeons and patients should have a thorough discussion regarding possible reconstructive options before proceeding with latissimus dorsi breast reconstruction surgery.

Preoperative Planning

- Preoperative labs and appropriate clearance from the patient's medical providers should be obtained.
- Preferably, all anticoagulant and antiplatelet medications should be stopped prior to the operation in discussion with the patient's primary care physician and specialist providers. In instances where continuing anticoagulation is necessary, bridging should be considered or preadmission to the hospital for anticoagulation drip.
- Smokers are required to quit for a minimum of 4 weeks prior. It is useful to obtain a urine cotinine to confirm absence of nicotine prior to surgery.
- Patients receive preoperative antibiotics with intraoperative redosing. If the patient is admitted after surgery, our practice is to administer 24 hours of perioperative intravenous (IV) antibiotics. If an expander or permanent implant is also placed, a short course of postoperative oral antibiotics may or may not be prescribed on discharge depending on surgeon practice. Ongoing clinical investigations are trying to determine the efficacy of postoperative oral antibiotics in the setting of implant-based breast reconstruction.
- Patients receive deep vein thrombosis (DVT) prophylaxis with use of a pneumatic compression device at the beginning of the case; preoperative subcutaneous heparin can be used; however, this is not typically performed in our practice.
- A Foley catheter will be needed, given the length of the case.
- A headlight may be helpful in the harvest of the latissimus dorsi muscle.
- A deflatable beanbag is needed for lateral decubitus positioning.
- A sterile Doppler probe is helpful to have available in case there is any concern for the location or integrity of the thoracodorsal pedicle during the case.

Marking and Positioning

Preoperative Marking

- The inframammary fold (IMF), medial limit, and lateral limit of the breast should be marked with the patient upright.
- With the patient in the sitting position, have the patient activate the latissimus muscle (by placing hands on the hips and coughing or pushing against the hips) and mark the anterolateral margin of the muscle.
- Other key landmarks for the limits of the latissimus muscle are the tip of scapula, vertebral column, and posterior iliac crest. They should be marked for additional orientation.
- The pivot point for the flap is the approximate pedicle location: It should be marked 2 to 3 cm medial to lateral border and 9 cm below the apex of the axilla.
- The size of the skin paddle required should be assessed preoperatively based on the anticipated skin defect after mastectomy. In instances of delayed reconstruction, consideration should be given to excision of contracted scars or focal areas of skin compromise secondary to radiation that may hinder the final reconstructive outcome.
- About 8- to 10-cm-wide skin paddles can generally be closed primarily (verify adequate skin laxity by pinching). The skin paddle must be placed over the muscular portion of the latissimus, as the vascularity of the skin over the thoracolumbar fascia is notoriously poor. In most patients, it is necessary to stay at least 8 cm superior to the posterior iliac crest to avoid the thoracolumbar fascia (**FIGURE 3**).
- Verify that the skin paddle has been designed correctly for rotating to the planned anterior position by measuring from the estimated pedicle pivot point to the inferolateral tip of the skin paddle. This distance must equal the distance from the pivot point to the medial limit of your planned mastectomy incision.

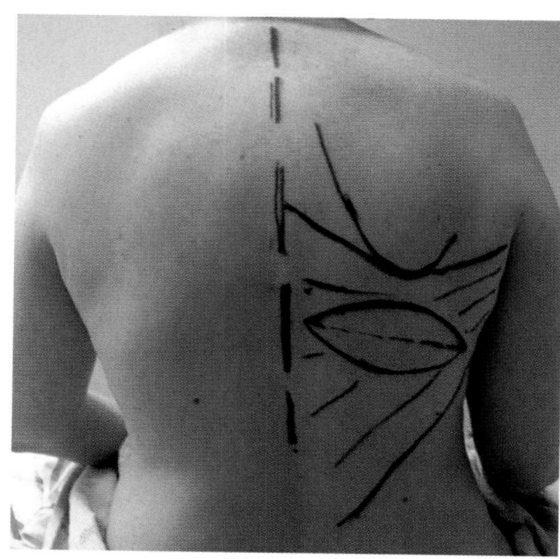

FIGURE 3 • Flap markings.

- The orientation of the axis of the skin paddle can be varied and can commonly include horizontal or obliquely oriented skin paddles (**FIGURE 4**). A horizontally oriented skin paddle allows the scar to be hidden by a bra strap but may limit the size of the paddle harvested. Obliquely oriented paddles can allow for wider skin paddles at the cost of scar visibility.
- If an expander or permanent implant is being used, measure the breast base width to guide choice of tissue expander size.

Positioning

- Patient positioning varies by surgeon. Harvesting a full latissimus dorsi flap requires a lateral decubitus position with a special arm support for the ipsilateral arm and an axillary roll under the contralateral axilla to prevent brachial plexopathy. The lower extremities will also require adequate padding.
- Placing patients in the supine position during the earlier or latter parts of the case is based on surgeon preference and laterality of reconstruction (unilateral vs bilateral). Bilateral procedures absolutely require position changes.
- In bilateral latissimus dorsi cases, the prone position will be required to adequately access both flaps. In unilateral cases, the lateral decubitus position is preferred.
- Adequate padding and positioning is critical and generally requires a combination of a beanbag, foam padding, and pillows or rolled sheets.
- The description in the following text will include multiple position changes to make clear the sequence of events for the procedure. In addition, it will describe reconstruction with a tissue expander in the prepectoral and subpectoral pocket. This sequence as well as pocket for expander placement can be modified.

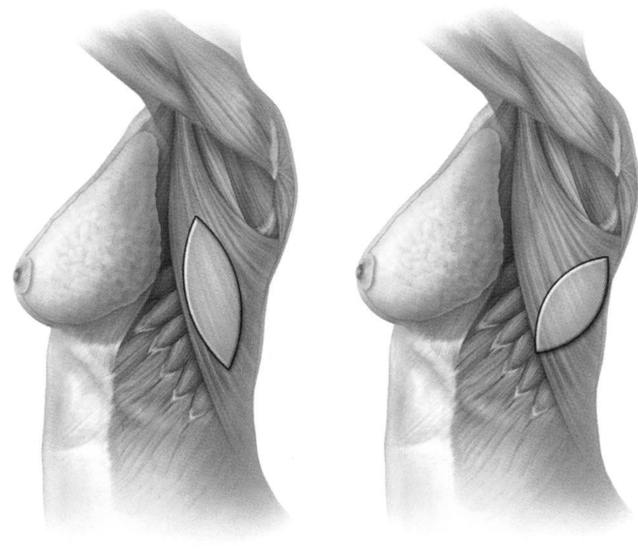

FIGURE 4 ● Possible orientations of the latissimus dorsi flap skin paddles.

RECIPIENT SITE PREPARATION (IN EITHER SUPINE OR LATERAL POSITION)

- Develop the recipient site with the patient in supine position: Elevate the skin and subcutaneous flaps off the pectoralis major to recreate the mastectomy defect in cases of delayed reconstruction; for immediate reconstruction, the mastectomy skin flaps are already developed by the breast surgeon. Any skin that appears nonviable or tenuous should be excised. The anticipated skin defect should be measured to confirm the skin paddle is of appropriate size.
- Natural borders of the breast should be preserved, including the IMF and skin adherence to the sternum along the midline. A possible exception would be in delayed reconstruction where the inferior dissection can extend approximately 0.5 to 1.0 cm inferior to the IMF to allow the expander to sit at the IMF after the latissimus is inset.
- Limit the lateral dissection, when possible, to the anterior axillary line with the exception of a three- to four-fingerbreadth tunnel created to allow for transfer of the flap. This tunnel should not violate the IMF. It is important to make the tunnel large enough to avoid compression or kinking of the pedicle.
- The lateral dissection is performed in a suprafascial plane within the tunnel and extends to the lateral border of the latissimus.
- Dissect 2 to 3 cm past the border of the latissimus, on its deep surface, to facilitate flap elevation when the patient is repositioned (**FIGURE 5**).
- Elevation of the pectoralis major muscle is then performed, disinserting the muscle from its attachments to ribs at the IMF. This disinsertion is terminated at the lateral border of the sternum.
- The anterior chest surgical site is then packed with moist laparotomy sponges, tucking a sponge laterally under the lateral border of the latissimus. This also helps identify this border of the flap during harvest in the lateral decubitus position. An Ioban sheet is then used to seal the mastectomy defects.

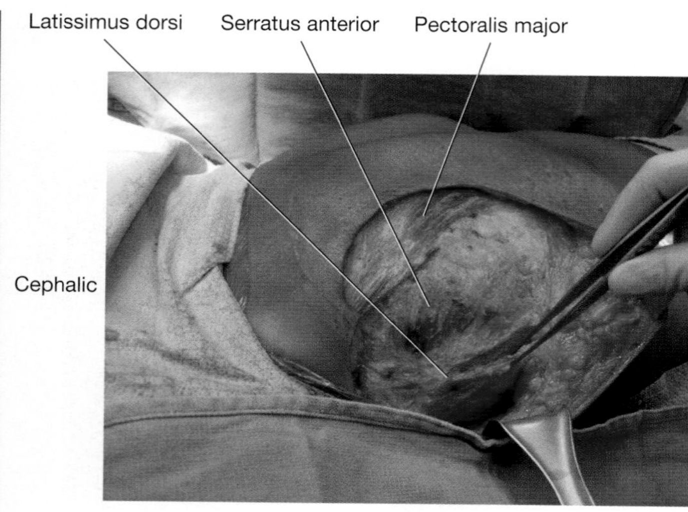

FIGURE 5 ● View of the chest wall with exposure of the pectoralis major, serratus anterior, and lateral border of the latissimus dorsi muscle.

FLAP HARVEST

- The patient is placed either in a lateral decubitus position (**FIGURE 6**) for a unilateral flap harvest or in a prone position for bilateral flap harvests.
- All position changes require reprepping and redraping of the operative fields.
- The incision is made on the lines of the designed skin paddle. As soon as subcutaneous fat is visualized, the plane of dissection should be beveled outward in a fashion to preserve as many vascular perforators as possible. In some instances, it may be helpful to use temporary tacking sutures to secure the skin paddle to the muscle to prevent shear or inadvertent avulsion of the skin paddle off the muscle.
- The skin and subcutaneous tissue are elevated off the latissimus muscle until the superior, medial, and inferior limits of the muscle are visualized. Careful dissection in the correct plane and observation of the orientation of the muscle fibers can be helpful to avoid inadvertent elevation of the trapezius medially and serratus muscle deep and lateral to the latissimus.
- Retraction can be a challenging aspect of this step. A Deaver or Harrington retractor and Bovie electrocautery extension are helpful (**FIGURE 7**).
- Dissection under the lateral edge of the latissimus is now initiated, starting in the area inferolaterally. Note that the anterior edge of the muscle often approaches the midaxillary line.
- Identification of the lateral border of the muscle is easy if elevation is begun while the patient is supine, with placement of a laparotomy sponge under the muscle edge as outlined previously.
- Dissection deep to the latissimus near the pedicle should be done cautiously with electrocautery to minimize the chance for pedicle damage. It is important to recognize that the pedicle and neurovascular bundle lie in a plane deep to the muscle surrounded by fatty tissue.
- Visualization of the pedicle is not necessary for most pedicled flaps with the exception of flaps requiring a division of the muscle insertion or flaps requiring denervation.
- Note that the serratus branch artery (**FIGURE 1**) can guide you from the serratus anterior muscle to the superiorly located thoracodorsal vessels. It is good practice to preserve

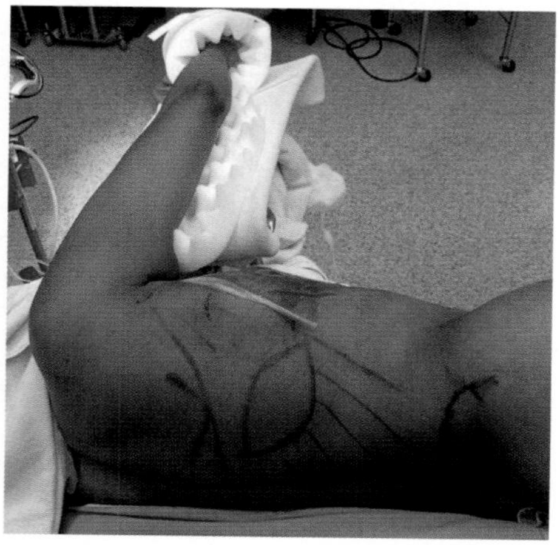

FIGURE 6 ● Patient positioning (lateral decubitus) for flap harvest.

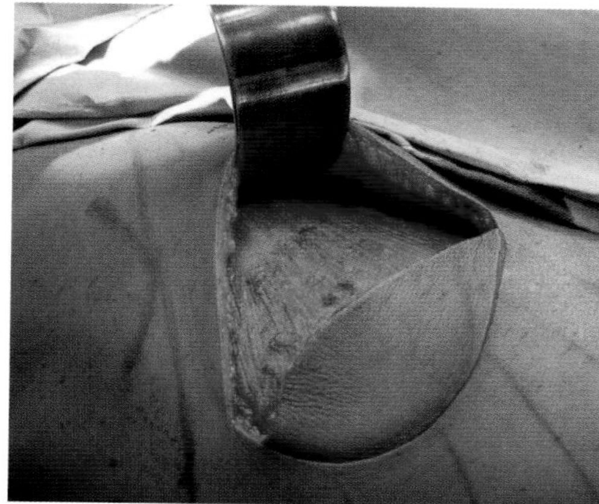

FIGURE 7 ● Exposure of superficial surface of the muscle during flap harvest.

the serratus branch given that it may be possible to sustain the flap on the serratus branch in the event of proximal injury to the thoracodorsal vessels.

- Lateral and medial row segmental pattern perforators to the skin will be encountered in the paraspinal region and should be meticulously cauterized.
- The latissimus muscle is divided medially and inferiorly at the point where the muscle fibers transition into the thoracolumbar fascia.
- Deep to the latissimus muscle, the dissection should be limited to muscle only, leaving behind adipose tissue, as this contains many lymphatic channels; preserving this lymphatic circulation is thought to reduce the risk for seroma.
- The fully elevated flap (**FIGURE 8**) is then rotated into the previously created lateral chest wall tunnel for passage to the mastectomy defect.
- Placing a large silk stitch on the medial edge of the flap skin paddle is helpful for locating the flap within the tunnel and subsequently for traction to slide the flap through the subcutaneous tunnel.
- It is important to avoid inadvertent kinking, twisting, or compression of the pedicle during flap inset and transfer into the tunnel.
- One or two drain tubes are placed in the back donor site.
- The back donor site is then closed in layers after adequate irrigation and hemostasis is obtained.

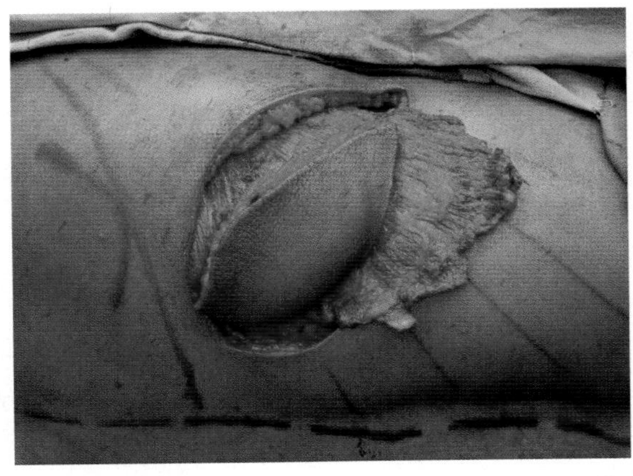

FIGURE 8 ● Elevated latissimus dorsi myocutaneous flap.

- Some surgeons advocate for the use of progressive tension sutures or quilting sutures during the back closure to aid in minimizing seroma formation.
- Prior to closure, fibrin sealant such as Tisseel or Evicel can be instilled into the donor site. Although not absolutely necessary, this maneuver is thought to reduce the risk for seroma.
- Dressings in the form of a skin glue product, Steri-Strips, or an ointment are then applied to the suture line.

INSETTING OF THE FLAP

- The patient is repositioned to the supine position. If necessary, appropriate reprepping and redraping is performed.
- The latissimus muscle is advanced into the recipient site. Any restricting bands of tissue near the pedicle pivot point can be carefully lysed to yield better flap rotation and an ideal position of the pedicle.
- Complete skeletonization of the pedicle is not necessary. Disinsertion of the muscle attachments to the humerus can be performed to gain a few additional centimeters of reach. If additional arc of rotation is required, and there are no concerns about the thoracodorsal pedicle, consideration can be given to sacrificing the serratus branch to increase arc of rotation.
- Ligation of the thoracodorsal nerve eliminates contraction of the muscle, which can be bothersome to some patients. Most patients, however, do not complain about persistent muscle contractions after transposition of this muscle without sacrificing the motor nerve.
- The latissimus muscle is then inset to the IMF with interrupted absorbable sutures.
- In the subpectoral approach, a tissue expander is selected based on the patient's chest wall dimensions (primarily breast base width) that is then placed in the pocket flanked superiorly by the pectoralis major muscle flap and inferiorly by the latissimus dorsi myocutaneous flap (**FIGURE 9**). The pectoralis major muscle is then approximated to the latissimus muscle with interrupted or running absorbable sutures.
- In the prepectoral approach, no elevation of the pectoralis major muscle is required. A tissue expander is selected based on the patient's chest wall dimensions (primarily base width), and the expander is secured and covered exclusively by the latissimus dorsi muscle (**FIGURE 10**).
- Tissue expanders with suture tabs can be used, as they allow the expander to be secured to the chest wall temporarily, preventing migration and optimizing expansion of desired areas of the breast mound.
- If there are concerns for tension on the flap, filling of the tissue expander (**FIGURE 11**) should be delayed.

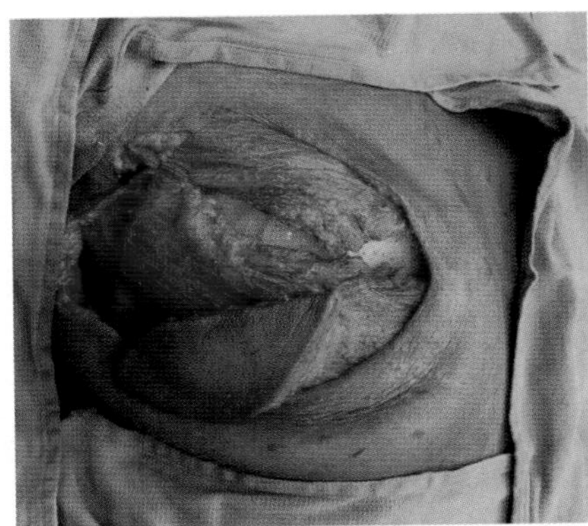

FIGURE 9 ● Tissue expander placed behind the pectoralis major (superior) and latissimus dorsi (inferior) muscle flaps within the mastectomy defect.

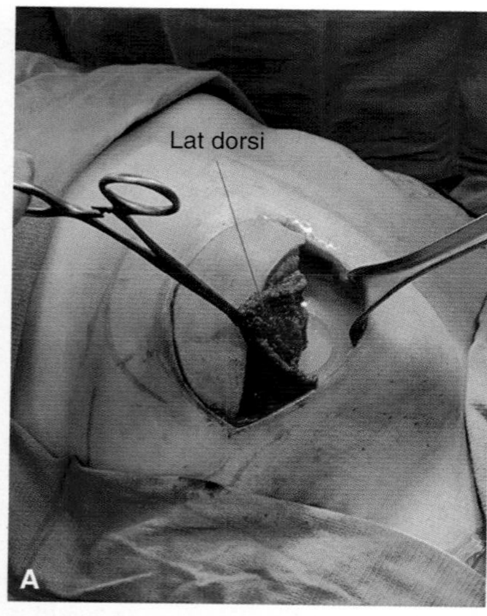

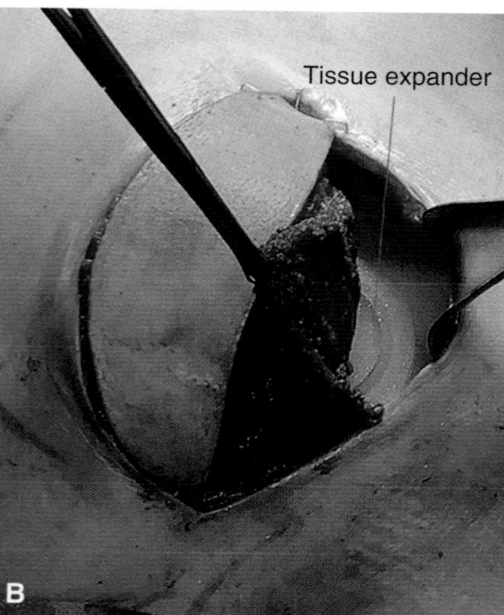

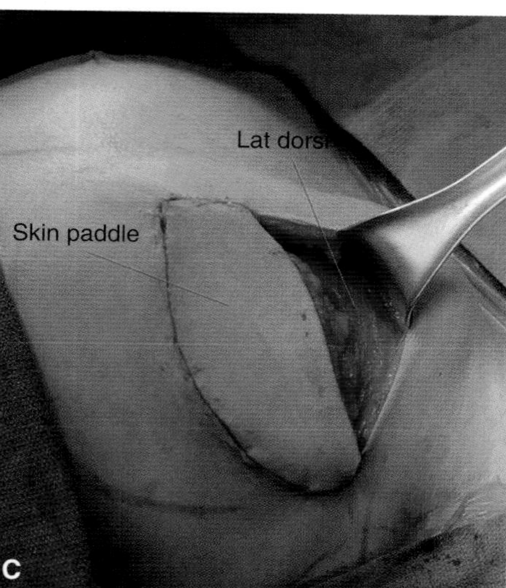

FIGURE 10 ● Intraoperative photo of prepectoral coverage of tissue expander for breast reconstruction using myocutaneous latissimus dorsi flap. **A,** Inset of the latissimus dorsi flap in breast defect with underlying tissue expander, **B,** Zoomed-in image of latissimus dorsi muscle covering the tissue expander **(C)**. Complete inset of the latissimus dorsi over the expander (not visible) with skin paddle secured in a tension-free manner with good capillary refill.

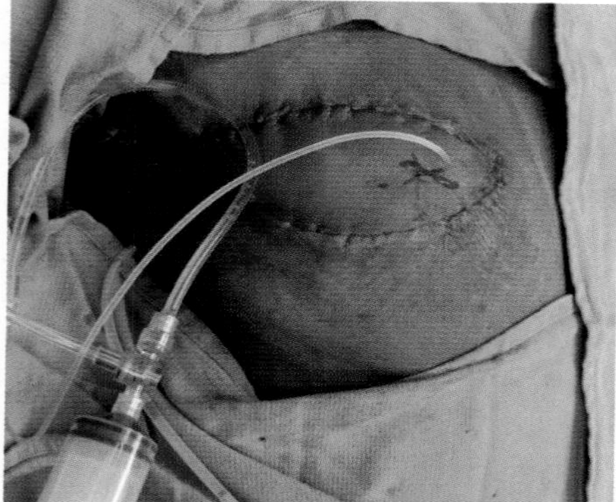

FIGURE 11 ● Intraoperative fill of the tissue expander.

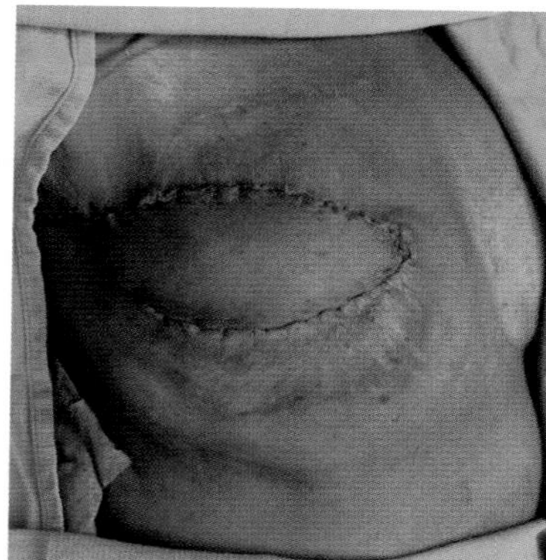

FIGURE 12 ● Inset flap skin paddle.

- The subcutaneous tunnel opening to the lateral tissue expander pocket can be closed to prevent lateral migration of the implant.
- The use of sterile techniques (eg, no touch technique, Betadine and antibiotic irrigation) are recommended for expander or implant insertion.
- A drain tube is placed deep to the skin flaps but superficial to the muscle flaps at the inferior pole of the breast, exiting at the lateral chest wall.
- Skin closure is performed in layers with absorbable interrupted deep dermal sutures and a running subcuticular suture (**FIGURE 12**).
- Dressings in the form of a skin glue product, Steri-Strips, or an ointment are then applied to the suture line.

PEARLS AND PITFALLS

Preoperative planning	■ Preoperative CT angiography is worthwhile when axillary lymph node dissection or preoperative radiation has been performed previously. The thoracodorsal vessels are occasionally ligated during axillary dissections or their caliber affected by preoperative radiation. ■ It is important to appropriately position and orient the skin paddle to ensure it covers the anticipated skin defect based on the expected arc of rotation.
Positioning	■ Minimizing the position changes will reduce surgical duration. For instance, a lateral position for both recipient site preparation and donor site harvest followed by supine positioning for the inset and expander placement takes advantage of a single position change. ■ If adjustments to markings are made after repositioning, this should be done with extreme caution as the muscle orientation and overlying skin position can change compared with standing preoperative markings.
Freeing the latissimus dorsi	■ Identifying and beginning the dissection underneath the lateral border of the latissimus while the patient is supine allows for an easier flap elevation once the patient is in a lateral position. ■ When elevating the flap from the medial to lateral, ensure that adipose tissue deep to the flap is left on the chest wall to avoid inadvertent elevation of the serratus. ■ The serratus branch should not be ligated without confirmation of the patency of the thoracodorsal vessels. ■ Disinserting the muscle attachments to the humerus improves the reach of the muscle. ■ Ensure a tunnel of adequate size to accommodate the flap and avoid inadvertent flap pedicle compression.
Donor site management	■ Avoid taking out donor site drains too early as seromas are common with this flap elevation. ■ Consider the use of adjuncts such as progressive tension sutures, or procoagulant products to minimize chances of seroma and hematoma.

POSTOPERATIVE CARE

- Patients can be transferred from the operating room to a postanesthesia care unit or directly to a unit with nursing capabilities for flap monitoring.
- Flaps are monitored by physical examinations (color, temperature, capillary refill) performed every hour for the first 4 hours, and then checks can be spaced out to every 2 and 4 hours over subsequent hospital days.
- DVT prophylaxis is the only form of anticoagulation used routinely. In our practice, weight-based Lovenox (or heparin if Lovenox is contraindicated) is administered approximately 6 to 8 hours after the operation.
- Diet is advanced from clear liquids to regular on postoperative day 1; there are no restrictions on caffeine.
- Patients are assisted to ambulate beginning on postoperative day 1.
- Foley catheters and IV fluids are discontinued; IV medications/patient-controlled analgesias are converted to orals on postoperative day 1.
- Patients are typically ready for discharge home from postoperative days 2 to 4.
- With recent advances in multimodal pain control and careful patient selection, some surgeons have also advocated for latissimus dorsi–based breast reconstruction to be performed in an outpatient ambulatory setting.[17]
- Surgical drains are discontinued once the output is less than 30 mL for 2 consecutive days.
- Activities are limited and weight-lifting restrictions are in place for 6 weeks postoperative.
- The first postoperative visit is at 1 week following discharge.
- Postoperative results for a left delayed breast reconstruction in an irradiated patient (**FIGURE 13**).

OUTCOMES

- In general, excellent outcomes can be achieved using the latissimus dorsi flap with high patient levels of satisfaction and without adverse functional impacts on the back and shoulder.[18]
- An evaluation of patient satisfaction showed that latissimus dorsi breast reconstruction patients are generally satisfied with their decision, with 80% of surveyed patients indicating that they would both recommend the surgery to another person and undergo the surgery again if given the choice. Over 70% of surveyed patients found the size, shape, and scars associated with their reconstructions to be "good" or "excellent." However, contrary to what is previously believed, over one-third of patients questioned reported moderate to severe loss of shoulder force and function. By strict physiometric measurements, there is comparable shoulder range of motion and slight decrease in shoulder strength when compared with preoperative measurements at 1 year postoperatively. This amount of change does not substantially affect the ability to perform daily activities for most patients.[19] Also, reoperation rate was 50% for prosthesis-related problems at a mean follow-up time of 14.9 years.[20]
- Several studies have elucidated the functional consequences of latissimus dorsi for breast reconstruction. A review by Blackburn et al[21] found functional recovery varies between studies with conflicting results on long-term functional outcomes. In a prospective study using validated patient reported outcomes, Yang et al[22] found that, in women undergoing latissimus dorsi breast reconstruction at 1 year postoperatively, although shoulder strength and range of motion returned to baseline, there was some functional disability that persisted as measured by the Disabilities of the

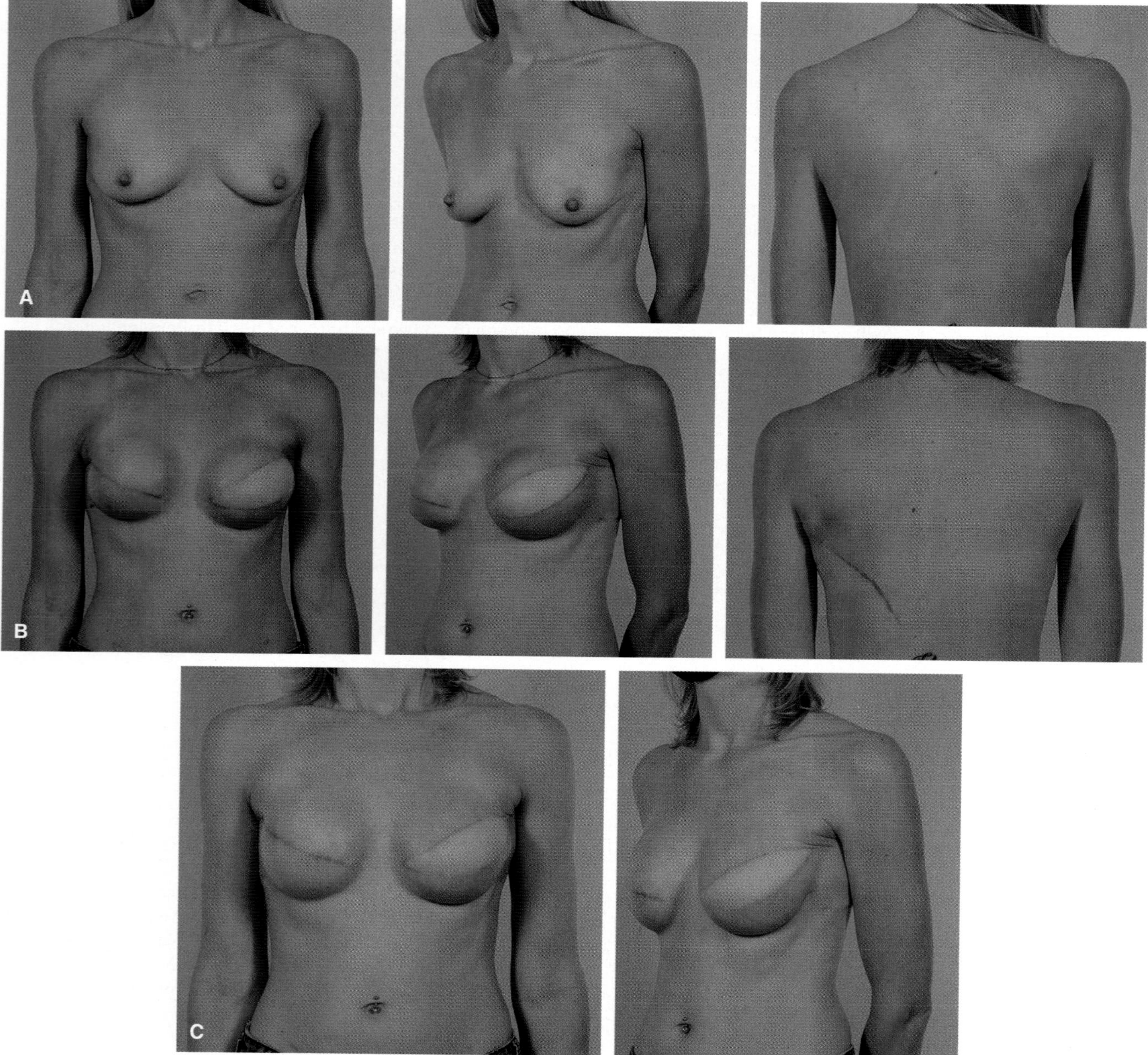

FIGURE 13 ● A patient with left breast invasive ductal carcinoma who underwent bilateral mastectomies and left chest wall radiation. **A,** Preoperative photos; **B,** Approximately 4 months postoperative, after completion of tissue expansion **(C)**. Approximately 9 months postoperative after exchange of expanders for implants.

arm, shoulder, and hand instrument. Using robot-assisted measures of shoulder strength and stiffness, and multiple patient-reported outcomes surveys, Leonardis et al[16] found that latissimus dorsi and subpectoral implant placement significantly reduced shoulder strength and stiffness when compared with subpectoral only and deep inferior epigastric artery perforator flap patients. Furthermore, Leonardis et al found that it was the disinsertion of the latissimus, and not the disinsertion of the pectoralis major or radiotherapy, that contributed to the strength deficits in latissimus-based reconstructions.[23]

- Therefore, shoulder function should be an important part of the patient-provider discussion and decision-making process when considering latissimus-based reconstructions.
- Breast reconstruction patients are typically satisfied in the short term (<5 years) with their choice of reconstruction across implant-based to autologous forms of reconstruction.[24]
- Over the long term (>8 years), satisfaction with abdominal-based flap reconstruction is maintained, whereas satisfaction with implant-based techniques tends to depreciate.[24]
- Studies have also shown greater satisfaction with autologous reconstruction in patients requiring unilateral reconstructions.

This is likely the result of better symmetry with the natural contralateral breast.[24]

- Patient satisfaction in bilateral reconstructions has been found to be similar across all techniques provided that the same technique is used on both sides,[24] highlighting again the importance of symmetry.

COMPLICATIONS

Flap-Related Complications

- Infections/implant extrusions—risks for these complications are elevated for implant-only reconstruction of irradiated sites. Autologous tissue transferred to the chest over a prosthesis offers greater resistance to infection or implant extrusion than do prostheses alone on irradiated sites.[25,26]
- Delayed wound healing—this complication typically occurs at the interface between the mastectomy flap and latissimus flap skin paddle. It often is a result of marginal mastectomy flap necrosis from poor skin perfusion, which is more likely in smokers and in the previously radiated breast skin.
- Partial flap loss—an uncommon complication (~3% or less) that is also related to poor perfusion.[27,28] It can be the result of poor skin paddle design, exacerbated in reconstruction of obese or higher-BMI patients or in patients with significantly attenuated latissimus dorsi muscles. An excision of the necrotic segment is usually required.
- Total flap loss—this is one of the most devastating complications encountered and occurs in less than 1% of reconstructions.[27,28]
- Capsular contracture—recent studies based on the newest-generation implants report approximately 16%.[29]

Donor Site Complications

- Seroma—approximately 9% of latissimus dorsi flap donor sites encounter a seroma.[27,28] Some studies report as high as 34%.[29]
- Delayed wound healing—wound healing problems are encountered often in morbidly obese patients, diabetic patients, and smokers. These wounds are managed by debridement and dressing changes with healing by secondary intention.

REFERENCES

1. Maxwell GP. Iginio Tansini and the origin of the latissimus dorsi musculocutaneous flap. *Plast Reconstr Surg*. 1980;65(5):686-692.
2. Davis HH, Tollman JP, Brush JH. Huge chondrosarcoma of rib. *Surgery*. 1949;26:699.
3. Campbell D. Reconstruction of the anterior thoracic wall. *J Thorac Surg*. 1950;19(3):456.
4. Olivari N. The latissimus flap. *Br J Plast Surg*. 1976;29(2):126-128.
5. Schneider WJ, Hill HL Jr, Brown RG. Latissimus dorsi myocutaneous flap for breast reconstruction. *Br J Plastic Surg*. 1977;30(4):277-281.
6. Hester TR Jr, Bostwick JIII. Poland's syndrome: correction with latissimus muscle transposition. *Plast Reconstr Surg*. 1982;69(2):226-233.
7. Chang DW, Youssef A, Cha S, et al. Autologous breast reconstruction with the extended latissimus dorsi flap. *Plast Reconstr Surg*. 2002;110(3):751-759.
8. Economides JM, Song DH. Latissimus dorsi and immediate fat transfer (LIFT) for complete autologous breast reconstruction. *Plast Reconstr Surg Glob Open*. 2018;6(1):e1656.
9. Brondi RS, de Oliveira VM, Bagnoli F, et al. Autologous breast reconstruction with the latissimus dorsi muscle with immediate fat grafting: long-term results and patient satisfaction. *Ann Plast Surg*. 2019;82(2):152-157.
10. Sood R, Easow JM, Konopka G, Panthaki ZJ. Latissimus dorsi flap in breast reconstruction: recent innovations in the workhorse flap. *Cancer Control*. 2018;25(1):1073274817744638.
11. Zenn MR, Jones GE. *Reconstructive Surgery: Anatomy, Technique, and Clinical Applications*. Quality Medical; 2012.
12. Strauch B, Yu H-L. *Atlas of Microvascular Surgery: Anatomy and Operative Techniques*. 2nd ed. Thieme; 2006.
13. Saint-Cyr M, Nagarkar P, Schaverien M, et al. The pedicled descending branch muscle-sparing latissimus dorsi flap for breast reconstruction. *Plast Reconstr Surg*. 2009;123(1):13-24.
14. Akyurek M, Dowlatshahi S, Quinlan RM. Two-stage prosthetic breast reconstruction with latissimus flap: prepectoral versus subpectoral approach. *J Plast Reconstr Aesthetic Surg*:2020;73(3):501-506.
15. Pacella SJ, Vogel JE, Locke MB, Codner MA. Aesthetic and technical refinements in latissimus dorsi implant breast reconstruction: a 15-year experience. *Aesthetic Surg J*. 2011;31(2):190-199.
16. Leonardis JM, Lyons DA, Kidwell KM, et al. The influence of functional shoulder biomechanics as a mediator of patient-reported outcomes following mastectomy and breast reconstruction. *Plast Reconstr Surg*. 2021;147(1):181-192.
17. Ayyala HS, Atamian EK, Le TT, Cohen S. Autologous can be ambulatory: the outpatient latissimus dorsi myocutaneous flap for breast reconstruction. *Plast Reconstr Surg*. 2021;147(2):361e-362e.
18. Koh E, Watson DI, Dean NR. Quality of life and shoulder function after latissimus dorsi breast reconstruction. *J Plast Reconstr Aesthetic Surg*. 2018;71(9):1317-1323.
19. Glassey N, Perks GB, McCulley SJ. A prospective assessment of shoulder morbidity and recovery time scales following latissimus dorsi breast reconstruction. *Plast Reconstr Surg*. 2008;122(5):1334-1340.
20. Tarantino I, Banic A, Fischer T. Evaluation of late results in breast reconstruction by latissimus dorsi flap and prosthesis implantation. *Plast Reconstr Surg*. 2006;117(5):1387-1394.
21. Blackburn NE, Mc Veigh JG, Mc Caughan E, Wilson IM. The musculoskeletal consequences of breast reconstruction using the latissimus dorsi muscle for women following mastectomy for breast cancer: a critical review. *Eur J Cancer Care*. 2018;27(2):e12664.
22. Yang JD, Huh JS, Min YS, et al. Physical and functional ability recovery patterns and quality of life after immediate autologous latissimus dorsi breast reconstruction: a 1-year prospective observational study. *Plast Reconstr Surg*. 2015;136(6):1146-1154.
23. Leonardis JM, Diefenbach BJ, Lyons DA, et al. The influence of reconstruction choice and inclusion of radiation therapy on functional shoulder biomechanics in women undergoing mastectomy for breast cancer. *Breast Cancer Res Treat*. 2019;173(2):447-453.
24. Hu ES, Pusic AL, Waljee JF, et al. Patient-reported aesthetic satisfaction with breast reconstruction during the long-term survivorship period. *Plast Reconstr Surg*. 2009;124(1):1-8.
25. Kroll SS, Schusterman MA, Reece GP, et al. Breast reconstruction with myocutaneous flaps in previously irradiated patients. *Plast Reconstr Surg*. 1994;93(3):460-469.
26. Spear SL, Boehmler JH, Taylor NS, et al. The role of the latissimus dorsi flap in reconstruction of the irradiated breast. *Plast Reconstr Surg*. 2007;119(1):1-9.
27. De Mey A, Lejour M, Declety A, et al. Late results and current indications of latissimus dorsi breast reconstructions. *Br J Plast Surg*. 1991;44(1):1-4.
28. Moore TS, Farrell LD. Latissimus dorsi myocutaneous flap for breast reconstruction: long-term results. *Plast Reconstr Surg*. 1992;89(4):666-672.
29. Sternberg EG, Perdikis G, McLaughlin SA, et al. Latissimus dorsi flap remains an excellent choice for breast reconstruction. *Ann Plast Surg*. 2006;56(1):31-35.

Chapter 24

Pedicled Transverse Rectus Abdominis Myocutaneous Flap Breast Reconstruction

Shoshana Woo Ambani and Erika King

DEFINITION

All patients undergoing mastectomy, or those who have undergone a prior mastectomy, are potential candidates for breast reconstruction. The choice whether or not to pursue breast reconstruction is a personal one. The options available for breast reconstruction are impacted by an individual's anatomic limitations, surgical history, radiation history, and personal preferences. Consideration must also be made of the patient's current breast size and goal breast size, along with the surgeon's technical preferences and perioperative resources.

The pedicled transverse rectus abdominis myocutaneous (pTRAM) flap was first described by Hartrampf in 1982 and was considered the "work horse" of autologous breast reconstruction for many decades. However, with the advent of microsurgery, that is, free tissue transfer or free flaps, the pTRAM has fallen out of favor. Currently, the deep inferior epigastric perforator (DIEP) flap, superficial inferior epigastric artery (SIEA) flap, and the muscle-sparing TRAM flap (ms-TRAM) are preferred when microsurgical resources are available, as they are associated with decreased donor site morbidity and high patient satisfaction. They are also preferred in cases of bilateral autologous tissue breast reconstruction in order to minimize postoperative abdominal wall weakness and risk of bulge or hernia. Still, pTRAMs are associated with lower costs, decreased resource utilization, and fewer postoperative complications as compared with free flaps and continue to be performed in many hospital systems.

The pTRAM remains a viable option for breast reconstruction in a variety of scenarios: (1) when microsurgical resources are not available, such as in developing countries and resource-constrained areas within Ghana and India; (2) when patients have comorbid conditions and are unable to tolerate the long operative times associated with free flaps, (3) if the patient prefers using their own tissue instead of having implants, and/or (3) if a patient has had a prior history of radiation. Generally, autologous tissue options, both pedicled and free, are preferred in cases of radiation, which is associated with a high risk of capsular contracture around implants.

PATIENT HISTORY AND PHYSICAL FINDINGS

- A complete medical and surgical history is essential. Prior comorbidities should be identified, and the decision for preoperative anesthesia evaluation should be made.
- Related history should also include cancer stage; *BRCA* status; other genetic testing, if any; and prior breast treatments including lumpectomy, breast or lymph node biopsy, neoadjuvant chemotherapy, and radiation.
- Accurate documentation of any prior abdominal, pelvic, groin, and cardiac surgery that would cause vascular disruption of the rectus abdominus muscle is necessary to evaluate the candidacy for a pTRAM flap.
- Diabetic patients, smokers, and patients with an elevated body mass index (BMI) or a pendulous pannus have a higher risk of flap failure.
- A history of pregnancy or plans for pregnancy should also be considered. Pregnancy after pTRAM leads to a slightly higher risk of abdominal bulge than after a DIEP flap. Young patients without any gestational history were shown to have a lower incidence of postoperative abdominal bulge.
- Current breast size, the patient's goal for breast size, and the amount of infraumbilical abdominal soft tissue present on examination will also guide surgical planning.
- The need for a contralateral breast surgery for symmetry should also be considered.
- Preoperative imaging including computed tomography (CT) or CT angiography can be a beneficial adjunct to surgical planning, particularly if there is a history of prior abdominal surgery. This allows the surgeon to evaluate the thickness of the abdominal wall muscular, along with a surgical roadmap of the vascular blood supply to the flap. Ultrasonography can also be used as a cost-effective alternative to CT for cross-sectional area analysis of muscle thickness and has been used in developing countries.
- Risks, benefits, and alternate therapies must be reviewed with the patient, including other autologous flaps (free and pedicled) and implant-based reconstruction, prior to obtaining surgical consent.

Anatomy

- As with any surgical technique, a thorough working knowledge of the anatomy of the chest and abdominal wall and its variations is essential. The primary blood supply of the breast originates from internal mammary perforating branches. Secondary blood supply is received via perforating arteries from the lateral thoracic, pectoral, thoracic, and lateral intercostal arteries. Many of these vessels are injured during mastectomy, compromising mastectomy flap blood supply. Mastectomy flap perfusion often relies on dermal-subdermal and subcutaneous vessels running just deep to the dermis.
- The abdominal wall is made of skin, varying thickness of subcutaneous adipose tissue, and the anterior rectus fascia overlying the paired rectus abdominis muscles (**FIGURE 1**).
- Deep to the muscles is the posterior rectus fascia, which is made up of the transversus fascia and internal oblique muscle fascia above the arcuate line and the transversus fascia below the arcuate line.
- The paired rectus muscles originate from the pubic bone and extend to the cartilage of the sixth, seventh, and eighth ribs. The rectus muscle has two pedicles: the dominant deep inferior epigastric vessels and the deep superior epigastric vessels (**FIGURE 2**). Additional blood supply comes from the posterior perforating vessels accompanying the 8th through 12th intercostal neurovascular bundles.

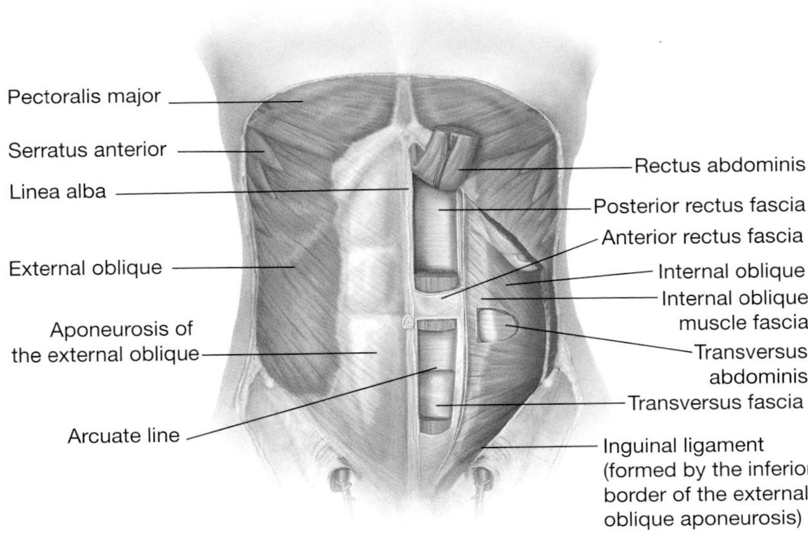

FIGURE 1 ● Abdominal wall musculature.

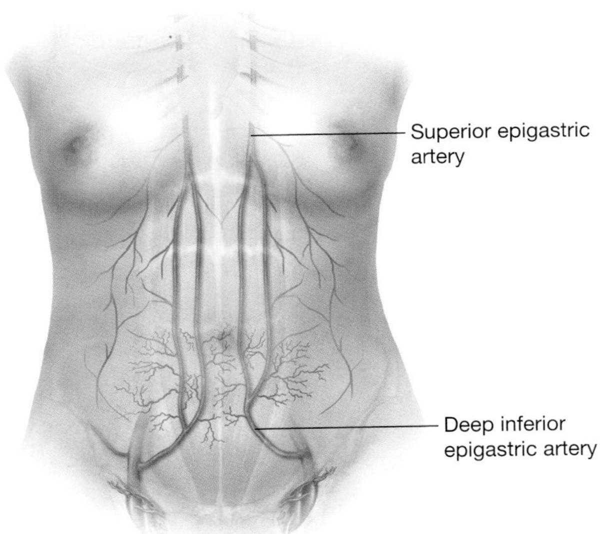

FIGURE 2 ● Abdominal wall blood supply.

- The pTRAM flap is based on the superior epigastric vessels, and the deep inferior epigastric vessels are ligated with release of the inferior muscular attachments to allow for flap transfer to the breast.
- The patterns of anastomosis between the deep superior epigastric artery and the deep inferior epigastric artery with the rectus abdominal muscle have been described: type I involves a single deep superior epigastric artery and deep inferior epigastric artery (29%); type II involves a double-branched system (57%); and type III involves a system of three or more major branches (14%) (**FIGURE 3**). These connections are made or increased with the surgical delay technique, in which the deep inferior epigastric artery is ligated several weeks prior to flap transfer.
- Musculocutaneous perforators pass through the muscle and anterior rectus fascia to supply the overlying skin (**FIGURE 4**). They are often gathered in the periumbilical area. There is often a medial row and a lateral row of perforators, separated by approximately 1.5 to 2 cm.
- Hartrampf's conventional perfusion zones of the lower abdominal flap were described to help with selection of the flap tissue: the vascularity decreases as the zone number increases (**FIGURE 5**). With the advent of the DIEP and SIEA flaps and their variations, newer classification systems have been developed.

SURGICAL MANAGEMENT

Preoperative Planning

- For patients at high risk for flap necrosis, surgical delay (ie, ligation of the deep inferior epigastric artery and vein) should be considered. This is performed at least 10 to 14 days prior to the mastectomy. This is often performed at the time of sentinel lymph node biopsy in order to limit events requiring anesthesia.
- On the day of reconstruction, the patient is marked first in the standing position.
- At the breast, the inframammary fold (IMF), midline with a line 1 cm off the midline on either side, the lateral breast extensions, and proposed or prior mastectomy skin incisions are marked. The based width of the proposed breast reconstruction is measured, as this will guide the ideal width of the abdominal flap, which is particularly important in delayed breast reconstruction where there is often a paucity of breast skin (**FIGURE 6**).
- On the abdomen, the midline is marked and an ellipse of skin including the umbilicus is marked. A pinch test is performed to estimate the maximum height of the ellipse that would still allow primary closure of the donor site, usually around 13 cm (**FIGURE 6**).
- The patient is then seated, and further extensions of the incisions are marked laterally to remove any standing cutaneous deformities. The soft tissues and markings are also assessed in the supine position as this best represents the intraoperative surgical field, and any adjustments to the markings can be made at this time.

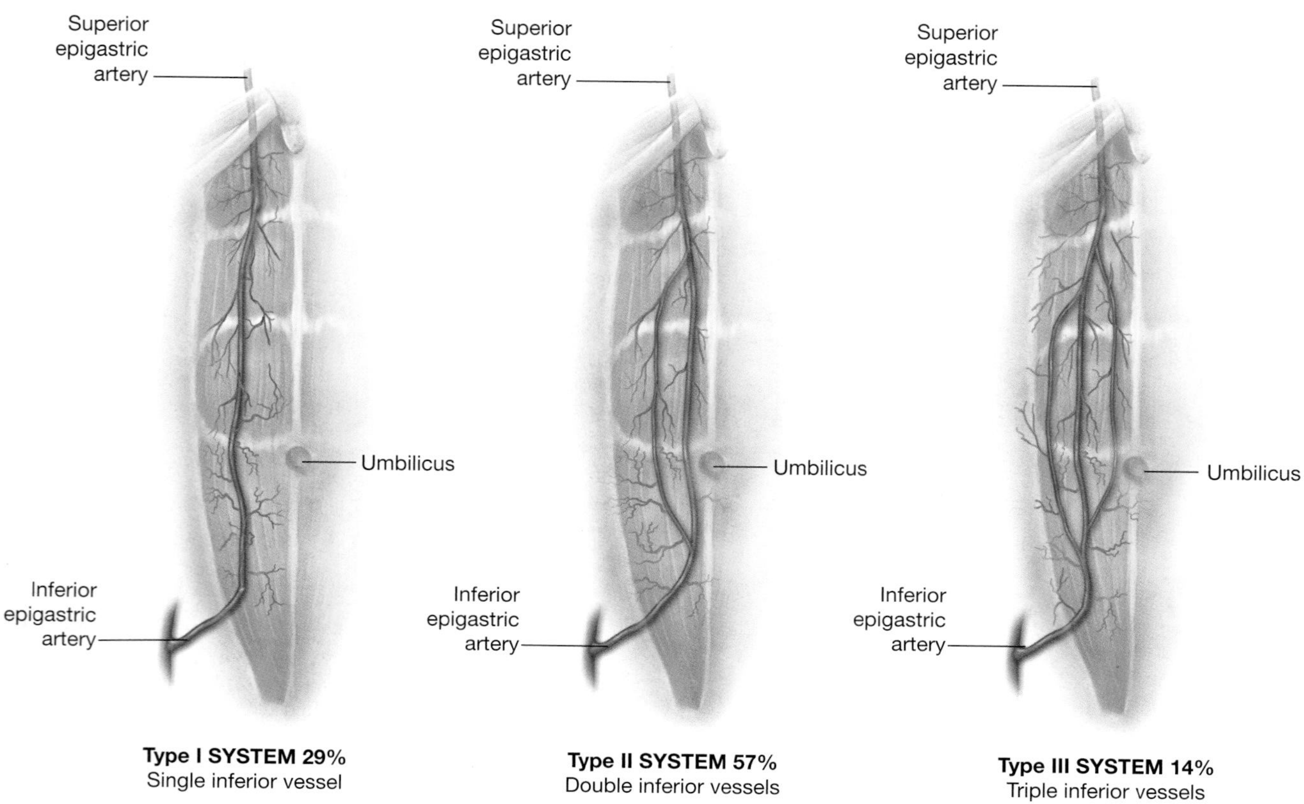

FIGURE 3 ● Moon: There are three patterns of blood supply to the rectus muscle, types I-III. (Redrawn from Moon HK, Taylor GI. The vascular anatomy of rectus abdominis musculocutaneous flaps based on the deep superior epigastric system. *Plast Reconstr Surg*. 1988;82(5):815-832. doi:10.1097/00006534-198811000-00014)

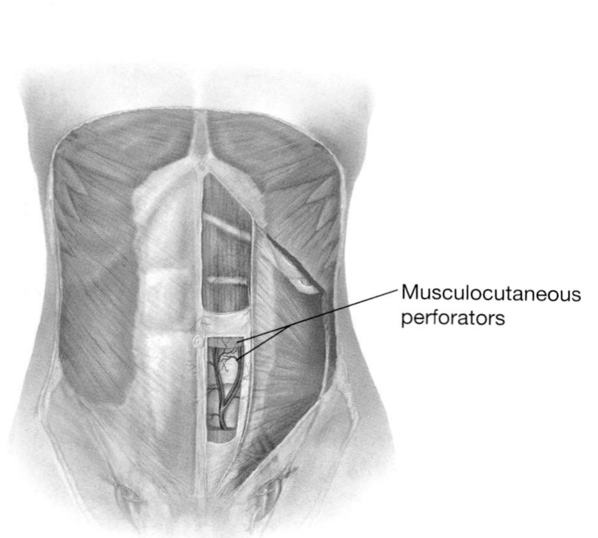

FIGURE 4 ● Surgical delay is performed to ligate the deep inferior epigastric artery and vein at least 10 to 14 days prior pTRAM transfer, in order to improve flap vascularity.

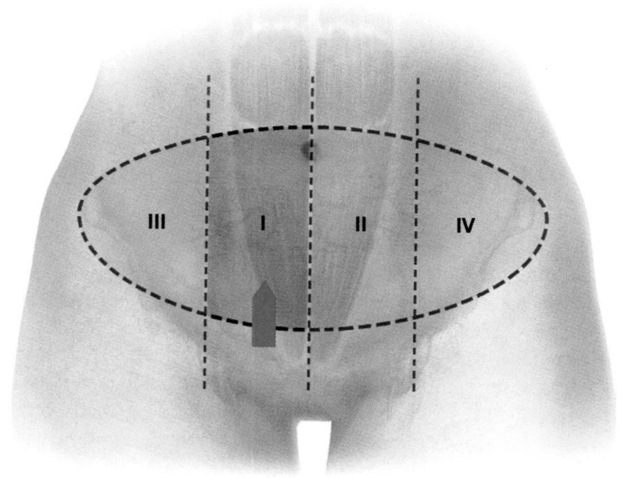

FIGURE 5 ● Hartrampf zones of perfusion from I-IV for pTRAM indicates vascularity of the soft tissue with zone I (overlying the pedicle) having the most robust blood supply, and zone IV having the weakest blood supply. Red block arrow indicates location of pedicle. (Redrawn Holm C, Mayr M, Höfter E, Ninkovic M. Perfusion zones of the DIEP flap revisited: a clinical study. *Plast Reconstr Surg*. 2006;117(1):37-43.)

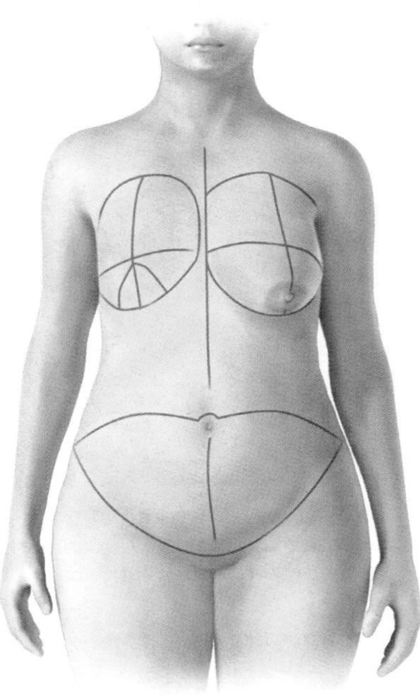

FIGURE 6 ● Preoperative marking of chest and abdomen in the standing position. Note the lateral dimension of the planned breast should correlate to the height of the planned pTRAM flap. The pTRAM flap is centered on the site of the largest perforators at the periumbilical region.

- Perioperative antibiotics are provided. A Foley catheter and sequential compression device (SCD) boots are placed. Warming devices must be employed to maintain normothermia.
- The flap can be raised while the mastectomy is being performed. The umbilicus is released with an 11 blade and Metzenbaum scissors down to fascia. Next the superior incision is made, and the upper abdominal skin flap is raised off the anterior fascia to the level of the costochondral cartilages. On the side of the planned reconstruction, a tunnel is made through the IMF into the mastectomy pocket wide enough for the planned flap.
- The inferior incision is then made. The flap is then elevated with electrocautery above the level of the fascia from lateral to medial until the lateral border of the rectus abdominis muscle is identified. At this point, low cautery is used to further identify both the medial and lateral rows of perforators (**FIGURE 7**). If a bilateral reconstruction is planned, the midline incision is made to facilitate the dissection (**FIGURE 8**). No perforators should be sacrificed at this time.
- Once all perforators have been identified, flap vascularity is clinically assessed. Intraoperative indocyanine green (ICG) angiography, which is often used to assess mastectomy flap perfusion (Munabi 2014), can also be used to assess flap viability at this time. Partial debridement of ischemic areas can then be performed accordingly. Of note, in unilateral reconstruction cases, the flap with the heartier blood supply is chosen, whether ipsilateral or contralateral. Studies have shown that the ipsilateral pTRAM flap tends to have better blood supply and less risk of necrosis.
- The planned fascial incisions are then marked to include each row of perforators and only the intervening fascia. A no. 10 blade and tenotomies are used to incise the fascia and sharply dissect around the outside of each medial and lateral perforator under loupe magnification (**FIGURES 9** and **10**). The width of this fascia (approximately 2 cm) is also included in the flap superiorly to the level of the costochondral cartilage

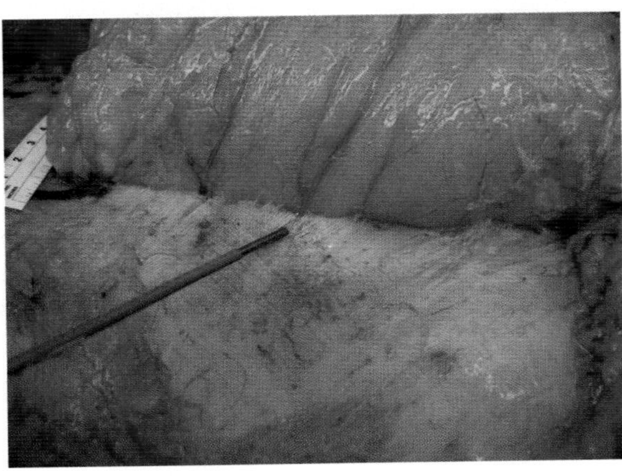

FIGURE 7 ● Lateral flap elevation: From lateral to medial, the flap is elevated with electrocautery above the level of the fascia to the lateral border of the rectus abdominis muscle. At this point, low cautery is used to complete the identification of both the medial and lateral rows of perforators.

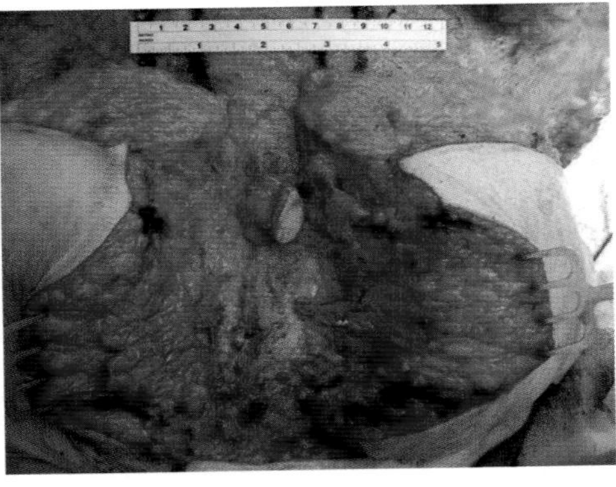

FIGURE 8 ● If a bilateral reconstruction is planned, the midline incision may also be made to help in exposure for dissection.

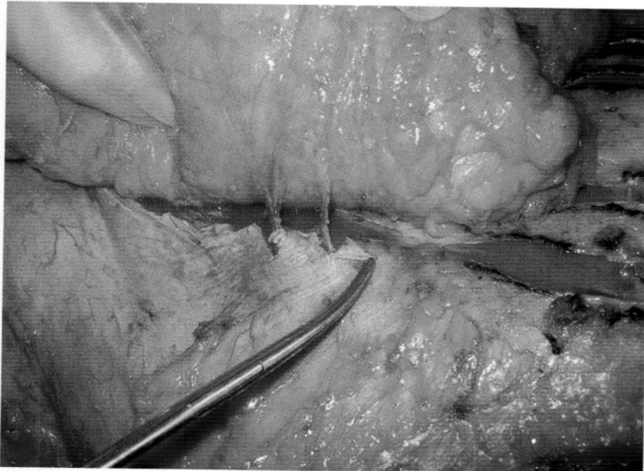

FIGURE 9 ● Methylene blue is used to mark the planned fascia incisions to include each row of perforators and only the intervening fascia.

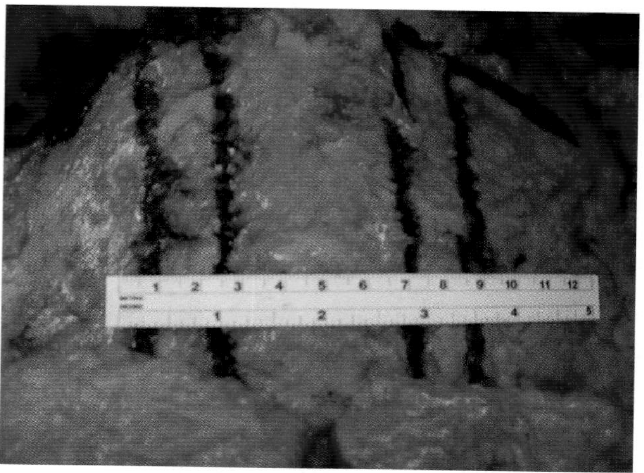

FIGURE 11 ● Flap elevation: The width of the fascia within the pTRAM (approximately 2 cm) is also included in the flap superiorly to the level of the costochondral cartilage.

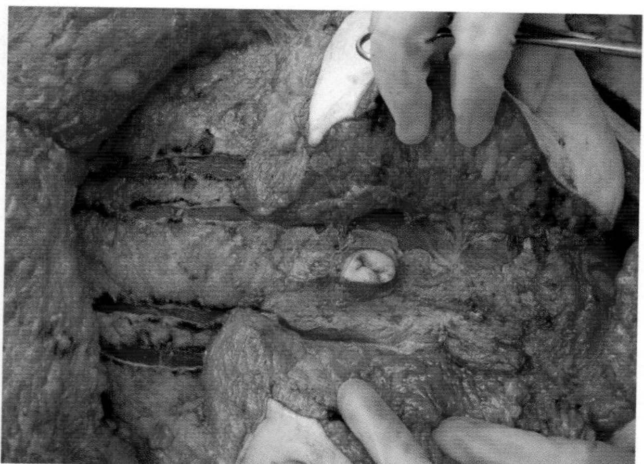

FIGURE 10 ● Perforator dissection. A no. 10 blade and tenotomy scissors are used to incise the fascia and perform a sharp dissection around the outside of each medial and lateral perforator under loupe magnification.

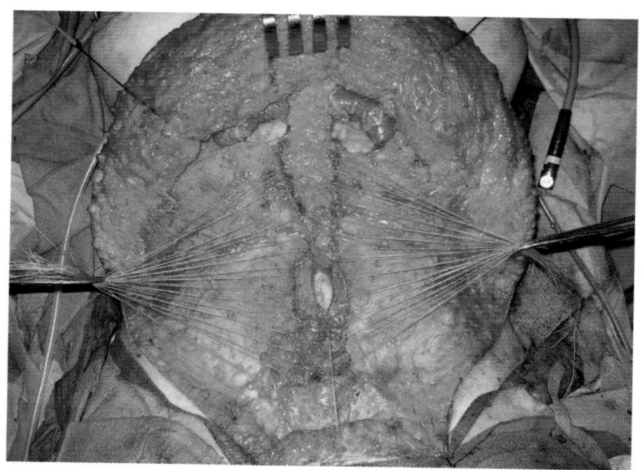

FIGURE 12 ● Fascia closure: The anterior rectus fascia is closed with interrupted 0-Vicryl and a running 0-PDS suture. The posterior sheath has not been violated.

(**FIGURE 10**). The underlying rectus muscle is then secured to the anterior rectus fascia and overlying Scarpa fascia with a 3-0 Vicryl to prevent the skin paddle from being avulsed from the muscle.

- Circumferential muscle dissection is then performed. The deep inferior epigastric artery is identified and ligated. The inferior portion of the muscle is then released with electrocautery. The flap is elevated from inferior to superior, taking care to ligate any posterior perforators or intercostal nerves along the way (**FIGURE 11**). At the superior border of the fascial dissection, a back cut is made to allow the flap to rotate superiorly without tension or kinking of the blood supply. The flap is then delivered through the tunnel into the mastectomy pocket.
- The donor site is verified for hemostasis, particularly at the site of the deep inferior epigastric vessel ligation. The gap in the anterior rectus fascia is closed with 0-Vicryl and 0-polydioxanone (PDS) sutures (**FIGURE 12**). In unilateral cases, a plication may be performed on the contralateral side to restore the umbilicus to the midline. This plication and closure should extend from the costochondral margin to the pubic bone to create a smooth desirable abdominal contour. Mesh can be considered to bolster the fascial repair. The bed is then flexed at the hip, and two drains are placed exiting through inferolateral stab incisions. Scarpa fascia is approximated with 0-Vicryl sutures. The deep dermis is closed with buried 3-0 Vicryl. A subcuticular running 4-0 Monocryl is then performed, followed by dermal glue application.
- A small oval or inverted U-shaped hole is made in the abdominal skin to deliver the umbilicus. The umbilicus is inset with 3-0 Vicryl deep dermal and 5-0 Monocryl subcuticular sutures.
- By this time, the mastectomy flaps are clinically assessed for viability; ICG angiography can be employed at the surgeon's discretion. In cases of questionable pTRAM or mastectomy flap viability, inset may be delayed, and any further debridement can be performed 3 to 5 days later. If skin-sparing mastectomy is performed through an incision around the nipple-areolar complex (NAC), the pTRAM flap is mostly de-epithelialized except for the spot resurfacing the NAC area. If a nipple-sparing mastectomy is performed, the flap is completely de-epithelialized and buried (**FIGURE 13**). Inset

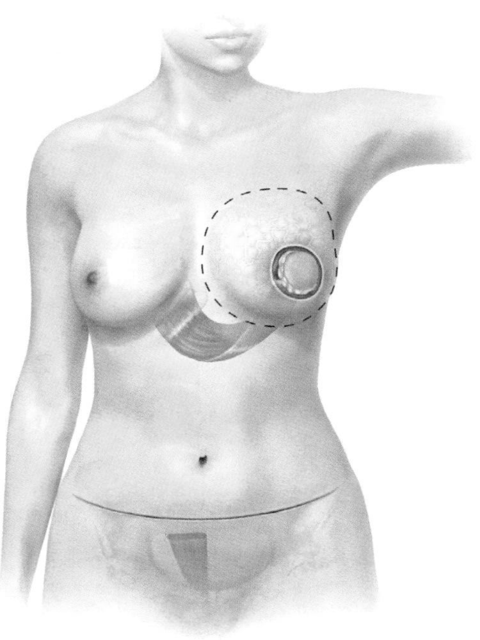

FIGURE 13 ● Flap placement: The flap is then rotated into the ipsilateral or contralateral mastectomy defect via the prepared tunnel.

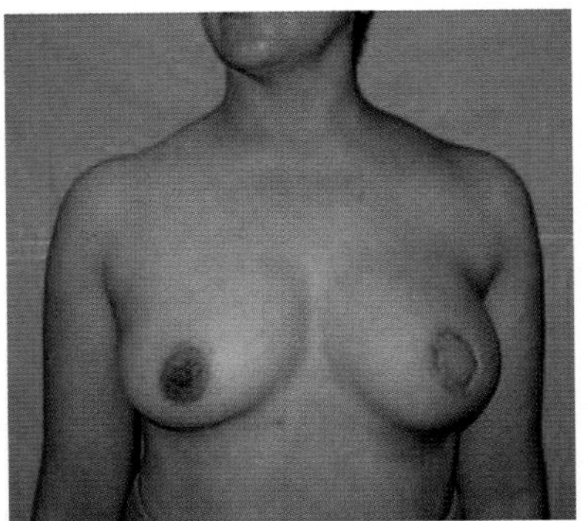

FIGURE 14 ● Immediate pTRAM reconstruction for left skin sparing mastectomy.

involves securing the flap medially and superiorly with Vicryl sutures to the pectoralis fascia. A drain is placed along the IMF, exiting through a lateral stab incision. A second drain is placed if an axillary lymph node dissection has been performed. The remaining skin is closed with deep dermal 3-0 Vicryl sutures and a 4-0 Monocryl subcuticular suture followed by dermal glue (**FIGURE 14**).

PEARLS AND PITFALLS

Preoperative planning	■ A thorough discussion regarding goals and reasonable expectations is essential. ■ A surgical delay procedure can be considered prior to pTRAM transfer in order to optimize flap vascularity in high-risk patients. ■ Smoking cessation should be strongly encouraged. ■ Preoperative imaging can be used to evaluate blood flow to the rectus abdominus muscles if there is a history of prior abdominopelvic or cardiac surgeries.
Patient marking	■ Careful markings are performed in both the standing and seated positions.
Intraoperative technique	■ Use either bipolar or very low cautery to avoid injury to the medial and lateral rows of perforators. ■ Carefully assess mastectomy flap viability. Excise any questionable areas or consider delaying flap inset. Use nitroglycerine paste to support blood flow.

POSTOPERATIVE CARE

- When transferring from the operating table to the inpatient bed, keep the patient in the flexed position to avoid tension on the abdominal closure.
- No bra is initially placed to prevent compression of the pedicle. A surgical bra without underwire is placed in clinic on the first visit once the mastectomy flap has matured.
- An abdominal binder is placed when patient is ambulating but not while in the seated position to avoid compression of the pedicle. The abdominal binder is recommended for up to 6 to 8 weeks for support and to minimize swelling.
- Routine inpatient postoperative care includes removal of the Foley catheter, SCD boots, early postoperative ambulation including the evening of surgery, and chemoprophylaxis for venous thromboembolism beginning 6 to 8 hours after the procedure is completed, per the Caprini scale. Incentive spirometry is encouraged hourly.
- Patients are discharged between 1 and 3 days after the procedure or on the day of inset if inset has been delayed.

COMPLICATIONS

- Patients with age >60 years and smokers have an increased risk for immediate complications. Patients with BMI >30 have an increased risk for late complications. Frequently, evaluations and early recognition of postoperative complications is paramount.
- Mastectomy flap necrosis is a common complication related to breast reconstruction. Keeping the mastectomy flaps as thick as possible while still performing an oncologically sound operation is critical in the ability to achieve a successful reconstruction. Use of nitroglycerine paste to ischemic mastectomy skin can help decrease the risk of necrosis when breast reconstruction is immediately performed.
- Partial flap loss or fat necrosis can be limited by preoperative smoking cessation for at least 2 to 4 weeks and/or performing a surgical delay procedure in preparation for pTRAM transfer. Complete flap loss is unusual.
- Abdominal bulge, hernia, and back pain are also reported complications of pTRAM patients. The rate of abdominal bulge and hernia can be decreased by almost half (from about 8% to 4.5%) with use of mesh to support the rectus sheath when closing the pTRAM donor site and has been shown to be a cost-effective technique. The authors would caution against bilateral pedicled TRAM reconstructions, as rates of bulge or hernia up to 48% have been reported. In these cases, muscle-sparing free tissue transfer techniques would be preferred.
- Deep venous thrombosis and pulmonary embolism are life-threatening complications associated with long operative times in patients diagnosed with cancer. Following the most current VTE guidelines with proper Caprini risk assessment is important for patient safety.

OUTCOMES

- Patients are generally satisfied with pTRAM breast reconstruction.
- Common secondary procedures include NAC reconstruction, scar revision to address standing cutaneous deformities, fat grafting to improve contours or increase breast volume, and contralateral symmetrizing procedures such as breast reduction, mastopexy, and/or augmentation (**FIGURE 15**).

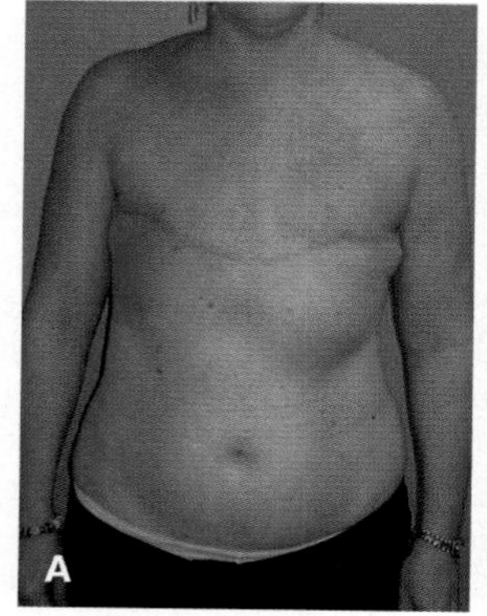

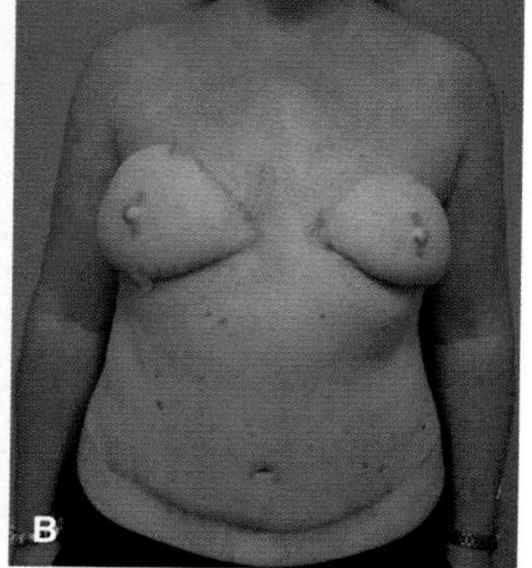

FIGURE 15 ● **A** and **B**, Pre- and postoperative images of delayed TRAM flap breast reconstruction.

SUGGESTED READINGS

1. Anuar NAA, Awang RR, Khoo ET, Anthonysamy D, Darail NAH, Emran NA. Pedicled transverse rectus abdominis myocutaneous flap breast reconstruction: hospital Kuala Lumpur's early experience. *Int Surg J*. 2021;8(10):2872-2875.
2. Atisha DM, Comizio RC, Telischak KM, et al. Interval inset of TRAM flaps in immediate breast reconstruction: a technical refinement. *Ann Plast Surg*. 2010;65(6):524-527.
3. Bharti G, Groves L, Sanger C, Thompson J, David L, Marks M, Minimizing donor-site morbidity following bilateral pedicled TRAM breast reconstruction with the double mesh fold over technique, *Ann Plast Surg*. 2013;70(5):484-487. doi:10.1097/SAP.0b013e31828569c0
4. Chatterjee A, Ramkumar DB, Dawli TB, Nigriny JF, Stotland MA, Ridgway EB. The use of mesh versus primary fascial closure of the abdominal donor site when using a transverse rectus abdominis myocutaneous flap for breast reconstruction: a cost-utility analysis. *Plast Reconstr Surg*. 2015;135(3):682-689. doi:10.1097/PRS.0000000000000957
5. Fu A, Liu C. Is pregnancy following a TRAM or DIEP flap safe? A critical systematic review and meta-analysis. *Aesthetic Plast Surg*. 2021;45:2618-2630.
6. Gdalevitch P, Van Laeken N, Bahng S, et al. Effects of nitroglycerin ointment on mastectomy flap necrosis in immediate breast reconstruction: a randomized controlled trial. *Plast Reconstr Surg*. 2015;135(6):1530-1539. doi:10.1097/PRS.0000000000001237
7. Golpanian S, Gerth DJ, Tashiro J, et al. Free versus pedicled TRAM flaps: cost utilization and complications. *Aesth Plast Surg*. 2016;40:869-876. doi:10.1007/s00266-016-0704-z
8. Hartrampf CR, Scheflan M, Black PW. Breast reconstruction with a transverse abdominal island flap. *Plast Reconstr Surg*. 1982;69(2):216-225.
9. Holm C, Mayr M, Höfter E, Ninkovic M. Perfusion zones of the DIEP flap revisited: a clinical Study. *Plast Reconstr Surg*. 2006;117(1):37-43. doi:10.1097/01.prs.0000185867.84172.c0
10. Ireton JE, Kluft JA, Ascherman JA. Unilateral and bilateral breast reconstruction with pedicled TRAM flaps: an outcomes analysis of 188 consecutive patients. *Plast Reconstr Surg Glob Open*. 2013;1(2):1-7. doi:10.1097/GOX.0b013e3182944595
11. Jankau J, Kolacz S, Moderhak M. IPSI vs CONTRA TRAM—old doubts new answers: evaluation TRAM flap survival with static and active dynamic thermography in pedicled flap breast reconstruction. *Indian J Surg*. 2021;83:306-310.
12. Kanchwala SK, Bucky LP. Optimizing pedicled transverse rectus abdominis muscle flap breast reconstruction. *Cancer J*. 2008;14(4):236-240.
13. Kerrigan CL, Collins ED. Are perforator flaps truly more cost-effective than TRAM flaps? How good is the evidence. *Plast Reconstr Surg*. 2001;107(3):881-883.
14. Knox ADC, Ho AL, Leung L, et al. Comparison of outcomes following autologous breast reconstruction using the DIEP and pedicled TRAM flaps: a 12-year clinical retrospective study and literature review. *Plast Reconstr Surg*. 2016;138(1):16-28. doi:10.1097/PRS.0000000000001747
15. Mata Ribeiro L, Meireles RP, Brito IM, et al. Risk factors for delayed autologous breast reconstruction using pedicled TRAM and latissimus dorsi flaps. *Eur J Plast Surg*. 2021;44:333-344.
16. Mizgala CL, Hartrampf CR Jr, Bennett GK. Assessment of the abdominal wall after pedicled TRAM flap surgery: 5- to 7-year follow-up of 150 consecutive patients. *Plast Reconstr Surg*. 1994;93(5):988-1002.
17. Moon HK, Taylor GI. The vascular anatomy of rectus abdominis musculocutaneous flaps based on the deep superior epigastric system. *Plast Reconstr Surg*. 1988;82(5):815-832. doi:10.1097/00006534-198811000-00014. PMID: 2971981.
18. Munabi NC, Olorunnipa OB, Goltsman D, Rohde CH, Ascherman JA. The ability of intra-operative perfusion mapping with laser-assisted indocyanine green angiography to predict mastectomy flap necrosis in breast reconstruction: a prospective trial. *J Plast Reconstr Aesthetic Surg*. 2014;67(4):449-455. doi:10.1016/j.bjps.2013.12.040

19. Nair N, Atisha DM, Streu R, et al. An innovative approach to the primary surgical delay procedure for pedicle TRAM flap breast reconstruction. *Plast Reconstr Surg*. 2010;125(4):173e-174e.
20. Serletti JM. Breast reconstruction with the TRAM flap: pedicled and free. *J Surg Oncol*. 2006;94(6):532-537.
21. Shestak KC. Breast reconstruction with a pedicled TRAM flap. *Clin Plast Surg*. 1998;25(2):167-182.
22. Teyhen DS, Gill NW, Whittaker JL, Henry SM, Hides JA, Hodges P. Rehabilitative ultrasound imaging of the abdominal muscles. *J Orthop Sports Phys Ther*. 2007;37(8):450-466.
23. Thoma A, Veltri K, Khuthaila D, Rockwell G, Duku E. Comparison of the deep inferior epigastric perforator flap and free transverse rectus abdominis myocutaneous flap in postmastectomy reconstruction: a cost-effectiveness analysis. *Plast Reconstr Surg*. 2004;113(6):1650-1661.
24. Tieman JT, Nourian MM, Agbenorku P, Hoyte-Williams PE, Farhat B, Goodwin IA, Swistun L, Foreman KB, Rockwell WB. Developing a breast reconstruction program in a resource-constrained Ghanaian teaching hospital. *Ann Plast Surg*. 2021;86(2):129-131.
25. Tokumoto H, Akita S, Kubota Y, Mitsukawa N. Relationship between preoperative abdominal wall strength and bulging at the abdominal free flap donor site for breast reconstruction. *Plast Reconstr Surg*. 2022;149(2):279e-286e.

Chapter 25

Deep Inferior Epigastric Perforator Flap Breast Reconstruction After Mastectomy

Theodore A. Kung and Adeyiza O. Momoh

DEFINITION

- The deep inferior epigastric perforator (DIEP) flap remains the most common choice for autologous breast reconstruction. While many other autologous flaps have been described for free flap breast reconstruction, the DIEP flap continues to be the best option for a majority of mastectomy patients due to its vascular reliability, sufficient soft tissue volume, and well-tolerated donor site. Compared with implant-based reconstruction, abdominal flaps such as the DIEP flap provide distinct advantages, including more natural contour, superior symmetry and appearance of the reconstructed breast mound, and higher patient satisfaction.[1,2] In addition, a secondary benefit of DIEP flap reconstruction is improvement of the abdominal contour.
- Hartrampf et al[3] first described the use of a pedicled transverse rectus abdominis myocutaneous (TRAM) flap for breast reconstruction in 1982, with its benefits of providing a soft, ptotic, aesthetically pleasing reconstruction that closely approximates the natural breast. Subsequently, continued advancements in the field of microsurgery and efforts to limit donor site morbidity led to the description of the deep inferior epigastric perforator (DIEP) flap by Koshima and Soeda[4] in 1989 with later popularization by Allen and Treece[5] in 1994. Further technical refinements have resulted in less abdominal wall weakness, bulging, and hernias.[6-8] Currently, the DIEP flap is considered the primary choice for autologous breast reconstruction in mastectomy patients with a suitable abdominal donor site.

ANATOMY

- The DIEP flap is an adipocutaneous flap based on intramuscular perforators from the deep inferior epigastric artery (DIEA) and deep inferior epigastric vein (DIEV).
- The DIEA and DIEV originate from the external iliac vessels within the groin and course superomedially toward the lateral border of the rectus abdominis muscle.
- The vascular pattern of the deep interior epigastric system is classified by the number of dominant branches: Type I vessels have a single dominant branch, type II vessels bifurcate in the vicinity of the arcuate line, and type III vessels demonstrate a trifurcating pattern (**FIGURE 1**). Superior to the umbilicus, these vessels coalesce with the terminal branches of the superior epigastric vessels.
- The most common branching pattern is type II. Perforators supplying the lower abdominal skin and adipose tissue come off branches of the pedicle at various levels and are referred as medial or lateral rows of perforators, indicating their relative position within the rectus abdominis muscle and their points of entry point into the DIEP flap. The most reliable perforators are found within a 10-cm radius from the umbilicus. Zones of perfusion based on fluorescent perfusion studies[9] are illustrated in **FIGURE 2**. Zone I is the area of the DIEP flap over each rectus abdominis muscle and pedicle (left or right); the other zones are relative to zone I.
- In general, perfusion of the hemiabdominal flap ipsilateral to its perforators (zones I and II) is more robust than it is to the contralateral abdominal flap across the midline (zones III and IV).

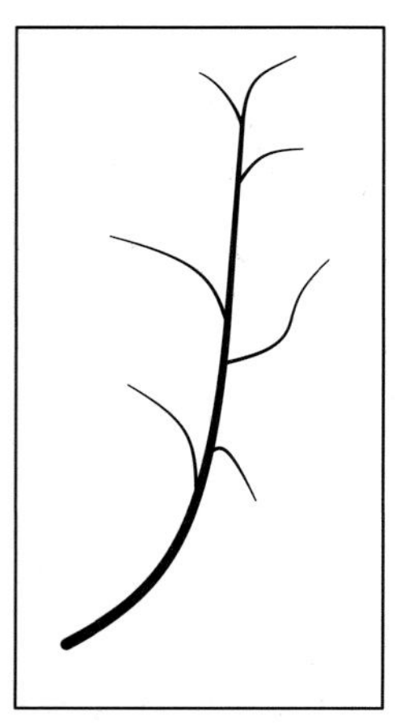

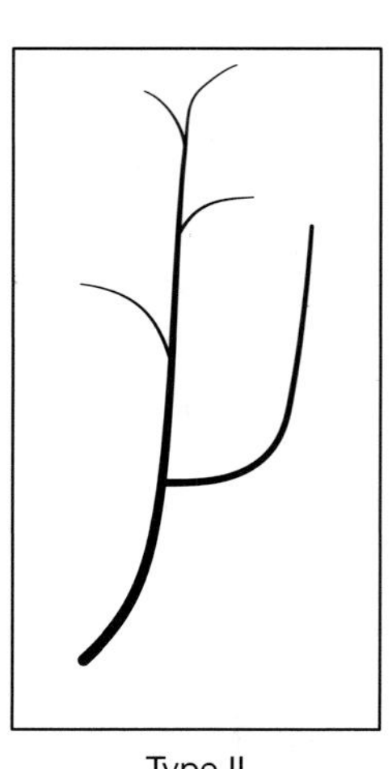

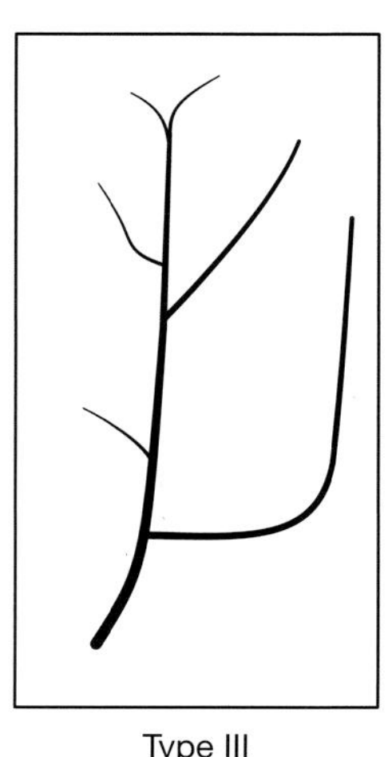

FIGURE 1 • Type I, type II, and type III vascular branching patterns.

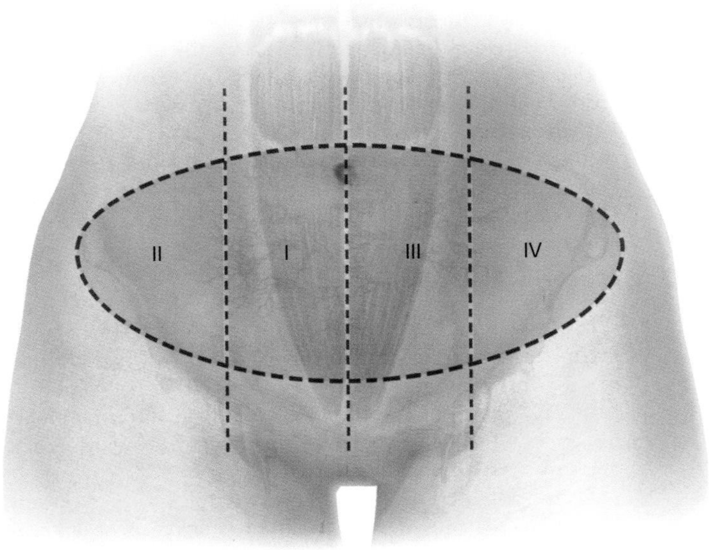

FIGURE 2 • Zones of perfusion of the lower abdomen based on fluorescent perfusion studies. In this figure, the zones are depicted relative to the perfusion of the right-sided pedicle.

- However, medial row perforators have a greater likelihood of perfusing tissue across the midline than do lateral row perforators. For extended DIEP flaps that cross midline (into zone III) to maximize tissue volume, inclusion of one or more medial perforators will optimize viability of the flap.
- In contrast, lateral row perforators have a greater likelihood of perfusing the most lateral extent of the ipsilateral hemiabdominal flap (zone II) compared with medial row perforators.
- Medial and lateral rows of perforators communicate via the subdermal plexus.
- There is also communication between the deep inferior epigastric system and the superficial inferior epigastric system.
- In some patients, the superficial inferior epigastric vein (SIEV) is the dominant outflow vessel for the DIEP flap. Preoperative imaging studies can help identify patients where the SIEV may be needed to during flap transfer to ensure adequate venous outflow.

PATIENT HISTORY AND PHYSICAL FINDINGS

- Pertinent aspects of the history include previous abdominal or chest wall operations and medical conditions that would preclude patients from a lengthy operation under general anesthesia.
- A focused abdominal examination is performed to evaluate the amount of lower abdominal adipose tissue and skin available for breast reconstruction. Any existing surgical scars over the abdomen should be noted. In general, small scars from laparoscopic procedures are not problematic. Other incisions such as a Kocher incision or a McBurney incision may have a detrimental effect on perfusion to either the DIEP flap or the abdominal donor site.
- A history of radiation therapy to the chest wall is a relative indication for autologous breast reconstruction.
- In our practice, DIEP flap reconstruction is not offered to active smokers due to the increased risk of wound healing problems and known exacerbation of abdominal donor site morbidity.
- Morbid obesity (body mass index > 40) is not necessarily a contraindication to DIEP flap reconstruction. However, the patient should be counseled about additional risks to the surgery due to the morbid obesity, and the surgeon should consider including more perforators during flap harvest to optimize flap perfusion.
- Risks factors for thrombosis should be ascertained and mitigated if possible. DIEP flap surgery in patients with known thrombogenicity (eg, heterozygous factor V Leiden) is controversial but may be performed without incident in consultation with a hematologist.

IMAGING AND OTHER DIAGNOSTIC STUDIES

- Preoperative computed tomography (CT) angiography of the donor site has been advocated in recent years. The preoperative scans provide a road map for flap perforators, with information on perforator location, size, and distribution (**FIGURE 3**).
- In patients with previous abdominal surgery, preoperative imaging permits confirmation of the integrity of the deep inferior epigastric vessels.
- Information gathered from scans has been shown to decrease operative times.[10] CT scans, however, are not an absolute requirement for preoperative planning.
- Alternatively, some authors have used magnetic resonance angiography for preoperative planning before DIEP flap reconstruction.[11]

SURGICAL MANAGEMENT

- In consulting with patients, decisions are made regarding the timing of reconstruction (immediately after mastectomy or in a delayed fashion) and the patient's preferences and unique factors are considered to create an individualized surgical plan.
- Several aspects of breast cancer treatment will affect breast reconstruction:

- In patients who have previously received radiation therapy to the chest wall, implant-based reconstructions are associated with higher rates or complications and failure; therefore, a history of radiation is a relative indication for autologous reconstruction.
- The need for postmastectomy radiation should be carefully considered. Patients undergoing prophylactic mastectomy for genetic mutations and patients with in situ breast cancer have a low risk of needing radiation therapy after mastectomy. In contrast, patients with aggressive invasive cancer or known nodal spread have a high likelihood of needing radiation therapy.
- Nipple-sparing mastectomy is increasingly more common. From a plastic surgery standpoint, the best nipple-sparing mastectomy candidates are women with minimal ptosis, good nipple symmetry, and healthy skin flaps after mastectomy.

Preoperative Planning

- In addition to obtaining basic laboratory tests, patients should be typed and screened, particularly in cases of bilateral reconstructions.
- All anticoagulant and antiplatelet medications should be stopped a week prior to the operation. Warfarin can be bridged with enoxaparin also a week prior.
- Smokers are required to quit for a minimum of 4 weeks prior.
- Patients receive preoperative antibiotics with intraoperative redosing if necessary.
- Patients receive deep vein thrombosis (DVT) prophylaxis through the use of a pneumatic compression device and subcutaneous heparin at the beginning of the case.
- Unless cardiovascular indications are present, arterial lines are not necessary for DIEP flap surgery.

Positioning

Marking/Positioning

- Preoperative markings of the breast are performed with the patient in the upright position.
- Key landmarks include the chest midline, inframammary fold, and anterior axillary line. The breast base width is also measured (**FIGURE 4A**).
- A variety of incisions can be drawn for the mastectomy. For many patients, a periareolar incision with or without an extension is appropriate when the mastectomy does not

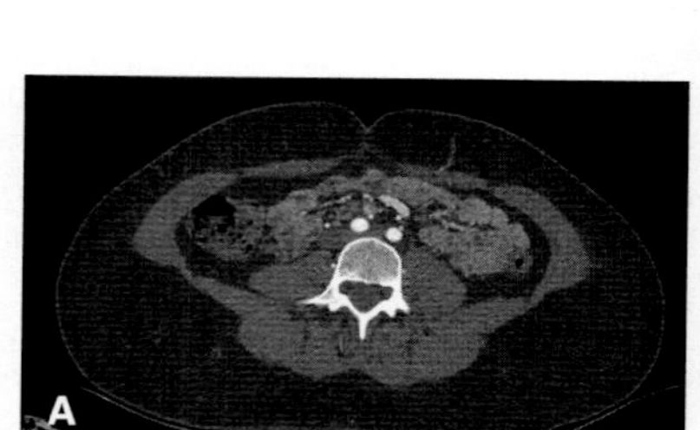

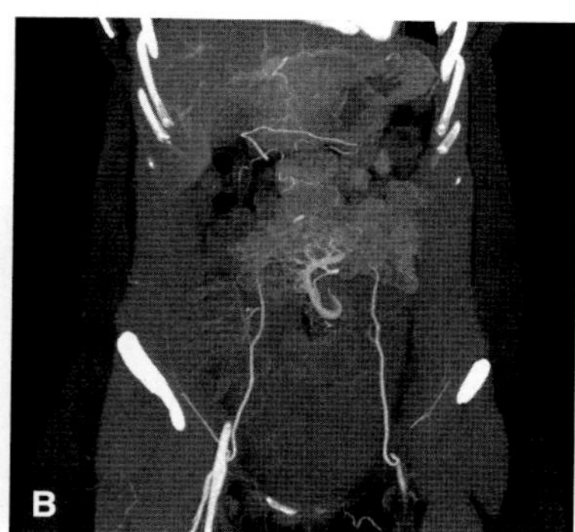

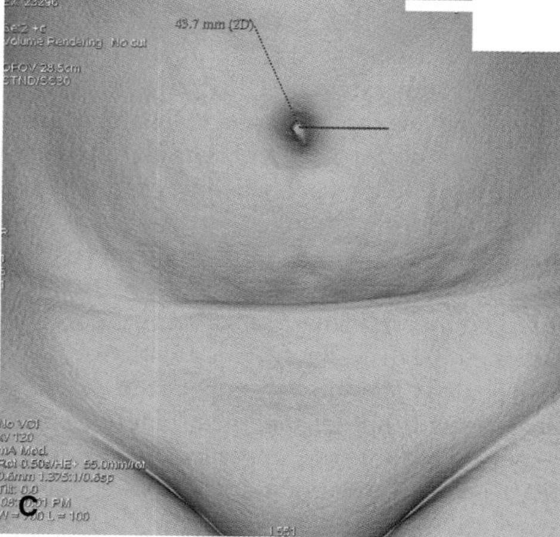

FIGURE 3 ● **A** and **B,** Preoperative CT angiography of the lower abdomen. **C,** A 3-D rendering of the abdominal soft tissue. Perforator locations based on axial cuts are transposed to the skin surface to enhance preoperative planning.

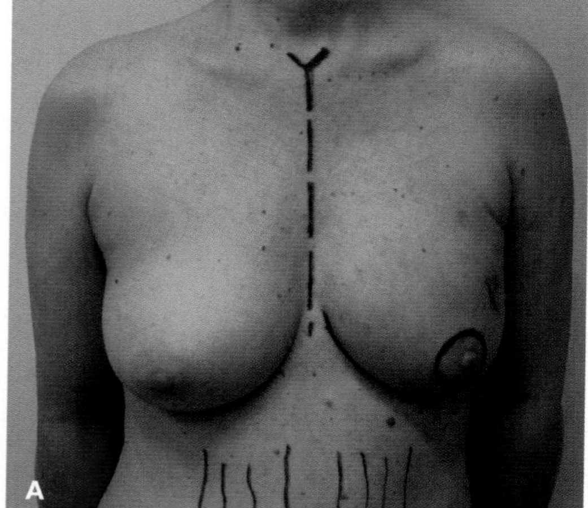

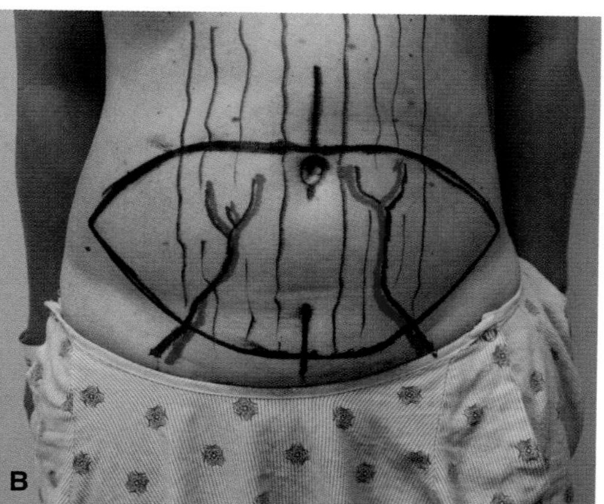

FIGURE 4 ● **A,** Breast preoperative marking. **B,** Abdominal preoperative marking.

spare the nipple. A lateral extension is selected when there is minimal breast ptosis. Alternatively, vertical extension can be used when there is a larger degree of ptosis; this vertical scan can be incorporated into a Wise-pattern mastopexy procedure later.

- For nipple-sparing mastectomies, an inferior periareolar incision can be made with or without an extension. Alternatively, an inframammary or lateral inframammary incision can be used for patients with smaller breasts (B cup or smaller).
- The upper marking for the abdominal flap is made at or just above the umbilicus. Preoperative imaging is used to ensure capture of the periumbilical perforators. The breast base width is used to mark the possible vertical distance from the upper marking to the lower marking. The lower marking is then made to complete the elliptical pattern (**FIGURE 4B**).
- Patient positioning in the operating room (OR) is supine and the table is turned 180° from the anesthesiologist, which provides better access for two surgical teams (**FIGURE 5**).

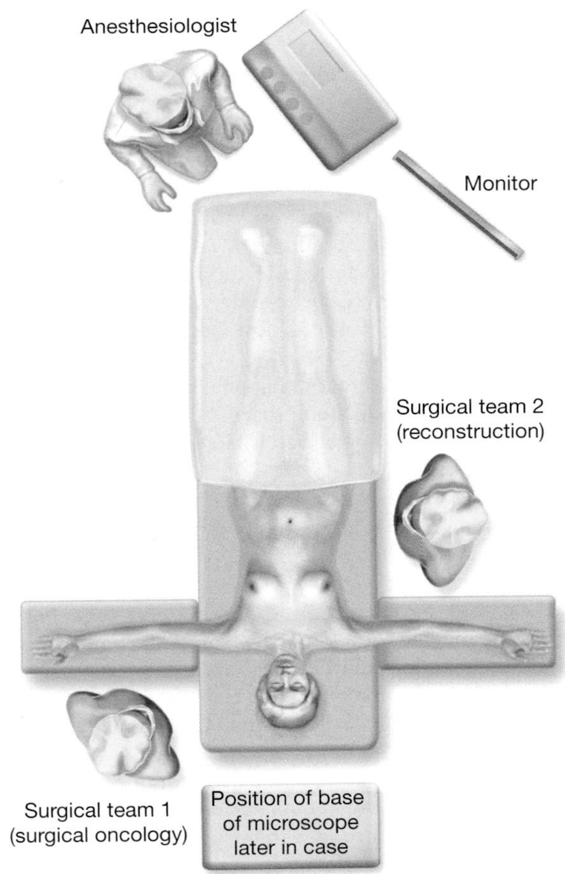

FIGURE 5 ● Patient positioning in the OR.

FLAP HARVEST

- The breasts and abdomen are prepped and draped in a sterile fashion.
- The upper abdominal incision is made with a scalpel, and dissection through the adipose tissue down to anterior abdominal wall fascia is performed with electrocautery. If necessary, the dissection can be beveled out to maximize flap volume by including additional sub-Scarpa fat.
- The adipocutaneous abdominal flap is elevated cranially with electrocautery, ending at the xiphoid centrally and at the costal margins laterally. Less elevation may be needed in patients with ample skin laxity.
- The OR table is reflexed, and the elevated upper abdominal flap is transposed inferiorly to assess the ability of this skin edge to meet the planned lower abdominal markings for closure. The lower abdominal markings are at this time adjusted as needed, and the table is returned to its original position.
- The lower abdominal incision is made superficially with a scalpel, and careful dissection through the adipose tissue is performed to identify the SIEV, typically above Scarpa fascia (**FIGURE 6**). If the SIEA is present and of sufficient caliber, it may be dissected proximally and a SIEA flap may be considered.

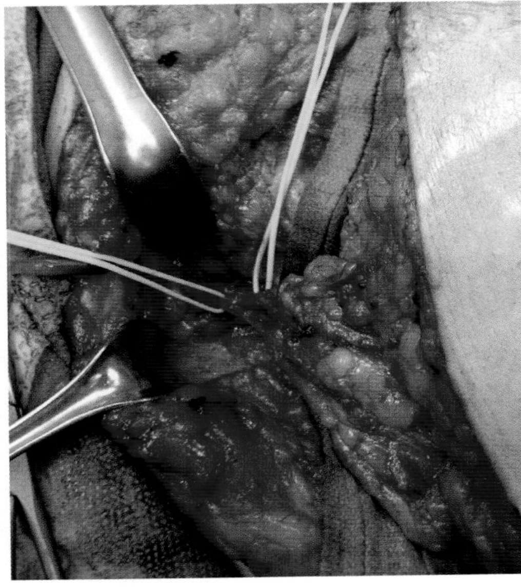

FIGURE 6 ● Dissection of the SIEV within the lower abdominal incision.

- Once the superficial epigastric vessels are visualized, a Weitlaner retractor may be introduced to provide further exposure. The vessels are dissected out toward the external iliac vessels with use of tenotomy scissors and bipolar electrocautery. In patients who are not good candidates for the SIEA flap, a length of the SIEV is still preserved whenever possible in case it is needed to augment venous drainage.
- Dissection down to the anterior abdominal wall fascia is then completed with electrocautery.
- Flap elevation is performed in the suprafascial plane from lateral to medial with electrocautery until the lateral row of perforators are encountered just medial to the edge of the rectus fascia (**FIGURE 7**).
- An incision is made around the umbilicus and along the midline of the flap in bilateral reconstruction cases or in cases where a hemiabdominal flap is large enough for unilateral reconstruction.
- The umbilical stalk is dissected out with blunt-tipped scissors, and division of the flap down the midline is completed with electrocautery. A ring of fat is preserved around the umbilical stalk to improve its vascularity.
- In unilateral reconstructions that require use of a flap that cross the midline for additional volume, the umbilicus is dissected out without splitting the flap.
- Suprafascial elevation of the flap from its medial edge is then performed with electrocautery until the medial row of perforators are encountered.
- Complete dissection around all perforators is achieved with a low-energy electrocautery. All perforators are then assessed for their size and location within the flap.
- Small perforators (<1.5 mm in diameter) are ligated with hemoclips, and one or more perforators within either the medial or lateral row are selected for use.
- Laser angiography with indocyanine green fluorescent dye can be employed at this point to assist with perforator selection. Acland clamps are placed on all perforators excluding the few selected, and the dye is administered intravenously. Within a few minutes of the dye administration, a real-time perfusion map of the flap is visualized (**FIGURE 8**).

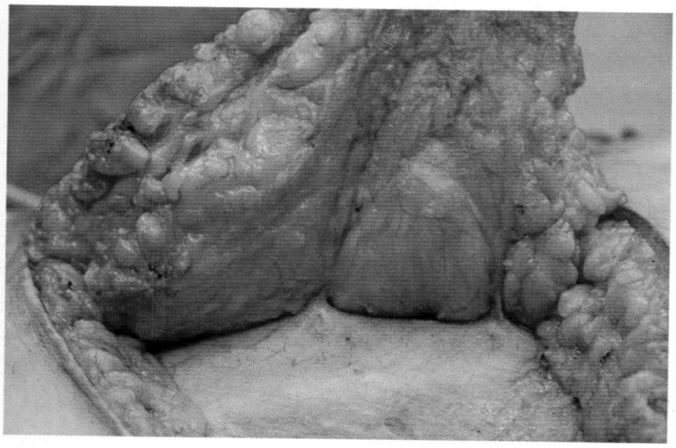

FIGURE 7 ● The lateral row of perforators visualized with suprafascial flap elevation.

- Alternatively, capillary refill can be assessed with the Acland clamps in place for a few minutes to determine adequacy of flap perfusion based on the few selected perforators.
- The anterior rectus fascia adjacent to the selected row of perforators is incised with electrocautery in a craniocaudal orientation (**FIGURE 9**).
- A small cuff of fascia is cut with tenotomy scissors around the perforator, freeing it from the surrounding anterior rectus fascia.
- Heparinized saline, 2 to 3 mL, is then injected into the rectus muscle adjacent to the individual perforators with an olive-tipped cannula. The heparinized saline used in this fashion hydrodissects the surrounding soft tissue away from the perforator and aids with visualization of the perforator's course. This technique is repeated as needed throughout the course of the intramuscular dissection (**FIGURE 10**).
- The perforators are dissected through the rectus muscle with the aid of a bipolar electrocautery down to the larger deep inferior epigastric vessels that run along the undersurface of the muscle.
- The continuation of the deep epigastric vessels to the superior epigastric vessels is encountered above the most cephalad perforator, and these vessels are ligated with hemoclips 1 to 2 cm cephalad to the perforator.
- The submuscular dissection then proceeds toward the external iliac vessels in the pelvis. The deep inferior epigastric vessels are dissected to a point where their length and size are of an appropriate size match for the recipient vessels in the chest (**FIGURE 11**).

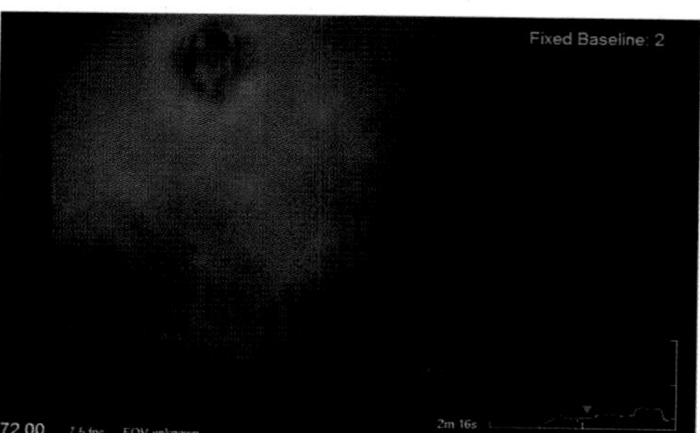

FIGURE 8 ● Perfusion map with laser-assisted indocyanine green fluorescent dye with dark areas (lateral aspects of the left hemiabdomen) indicating poor perfusion.

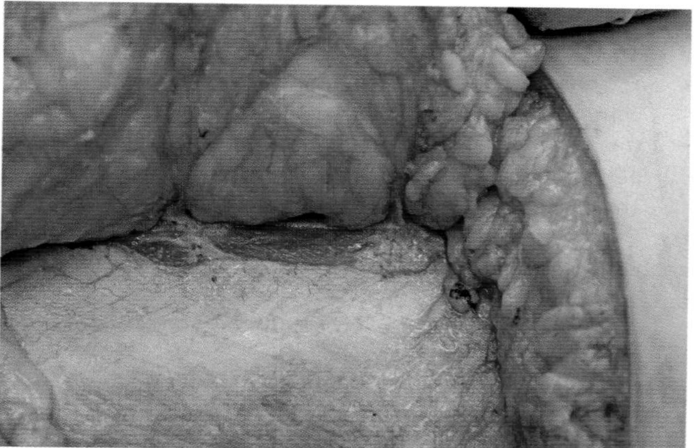

FIGURE 9 ● Subfascial exposure of flap perforators.

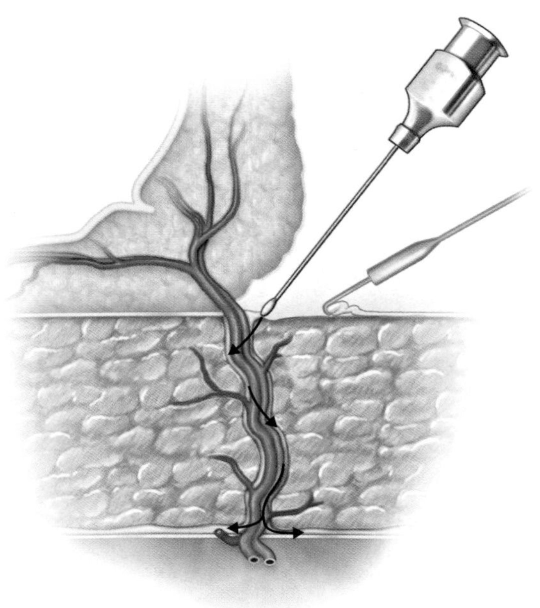

FIGURE 10 ● Hydrodissection technique for intramuscular perforator dissection illustrated. Heparinized saline is injected adjacent to the perforator and creates a dissection plane between the perforators and muscle. The *arrows* illustrate the course of the heparinized saline, which tracks along the perforator with each injection.

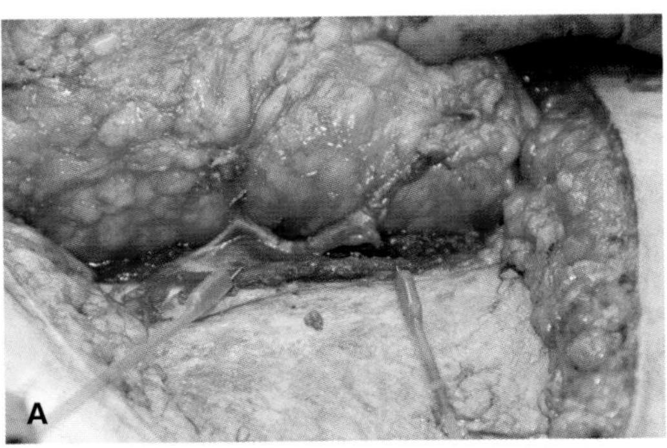

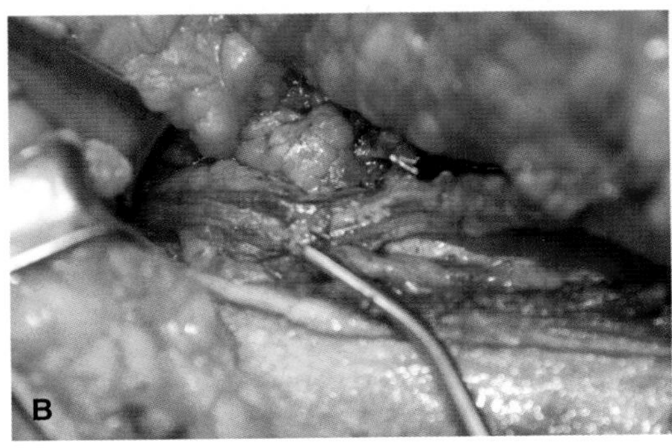

FIGURE 11 ● **A,** Intramuscular and submuscular dissection of perforators and vascular pedicle. **B,** DIEP flap pedicle prior to ligation.

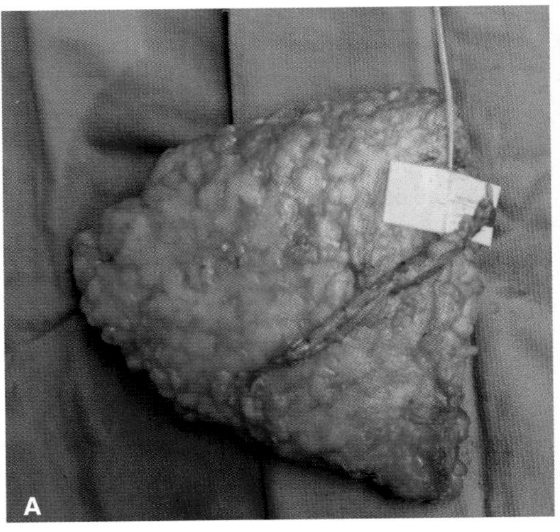

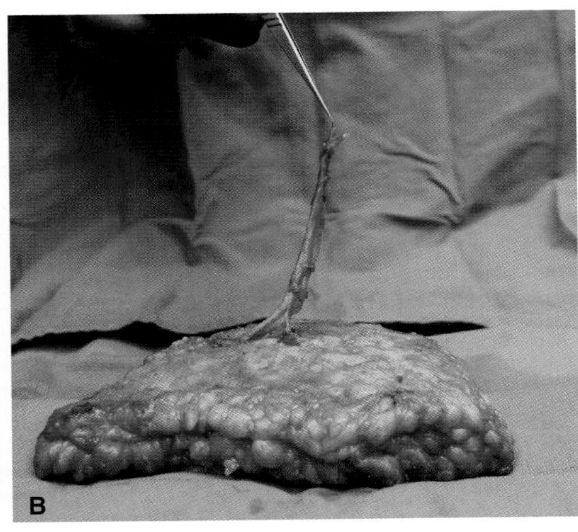

FIGURE 12 ● **A** and **B,** Flap harvested and prepped on a back table.

- Once ready for transfer to the chest, the artery is first ligated distally with hemoclips followed by the vein(s).
- A tenotomy scissors is used to divide the vessels proximal to the clips.
- The harvested flap (**FIGURE 12**) is prepared on a back table by flushing the flap from its arterial end with heparinized saline until the venous outflow runs clear.

RECIPIENT VESSEL EXPOSURE (INTERNAL MAMMARY)

- A common choice and the authors' preference for recipient vessels are the internal mammary artery and vein. Alternatively, the thoracodorsal artery and vein can be used.
- Once the mastectomy is complete, the defect is irrigated and hemostasis with electrocautery is performed as needed.
- The medial cartilaginous aspect of the third rib is palpated through the pectoralis major muscle. The muscle fibers over this medial aspect of the rib are split (ideally along the fibers) with electrocautery and a Weitlaner retractor is introduced

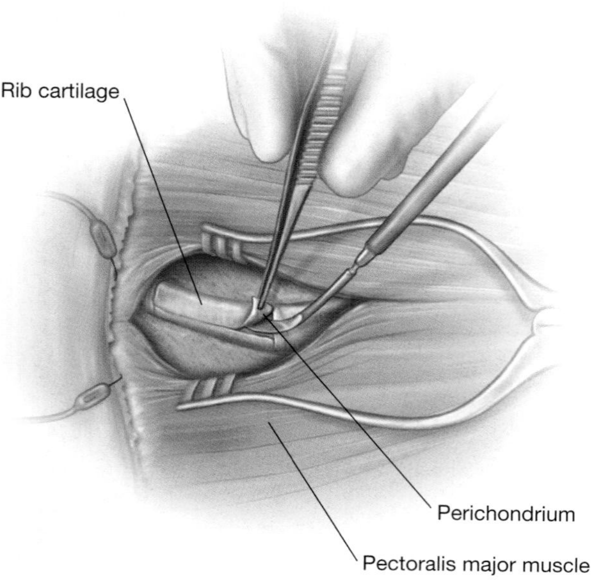

FIGURE 13 ● Elevation of the rib perichondrium.

between the muscle fibers to provide exposure. The muscle split is performed from the lateral edge of the sternum to a point approximately 6 cm laterally.

- The anterior costal perichondrium is scored along its length with the electrocautery and also perpendicular to the lengthwise incision at the medial and lateral extents of the exposed cartilage.
- A freer or narrow periosteal elevator is then used to elevate the perichondrium off the underlying cartilage circumferentially (**FIGURE 13**).
- The cartilage is then excised with a rongeur from lateral to medial, exposing the posterior perichondrium. The internal mammary artery and vein are sometimes visible through the posterior perichondrium at this point.
- A second Weitlaner is introduced perpendicular to the first using the lateral cut end of the rib as an anchor for one end of the retractor while the opposite end retracts the medial mastectomy flap out of the field.

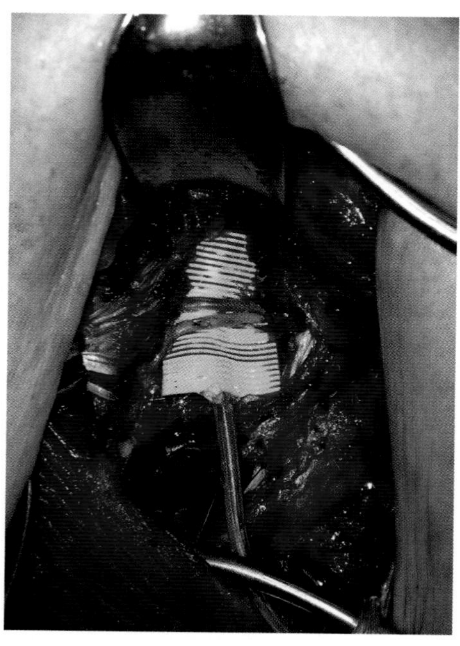

FIGURE 14 ● Exposed IMA and IMV with placement of a background mat with suction.

- An incision is made laterally through the posterior perichondrium with a scalpel, and a freer is then introduced underneath the perichondrium and used to push all soft tissue and recipient vessels downward.
- The posterior perichondrium is then split from lateral to medial, exposing the underlying internal mammary artery (IMA) and internal mammary vein (IMV).
- The posterior perichondrium is bluntly dissected off the underlying vessels with a freer and excised completely to provide optimal exposure of the recipient vessels. Intercostal muscle can be excised en bloc as needed along with the posterior perichondrium to maximize exposure of the internal mammary vessels between the second and fourth ribs.
- The IMA and IMV are dissected circumferentially, and a background mat with attached suction is placed beneath both vessels (**FIGURE 14**).

MICROVASCULAR ANASTOMOSIS

- The harvested DIEP flap is transferred to the chest and secured to the chest wall with sutures.
- Through the use of an operative microscope, the flap vessel ends are prepared, sharply cutting away irregular vessel ends and loose adventitia.
- Achland clamps are placed on the IMA and IMV proximally, and the distal ends are clipped and divided. The cut vessel ends are flushed with heparinized saline.
- Anastomosis of the arteries and veins can be performed in any order based on the surgeon's preference. The authors preferentially perform venous coupling prior to the arterial anastomosis.
- A vessel sizer is used to determine the approximate vein diameter for both the flap vein and the IMV. The smaller of the two vessels determines the coupler size to be used.
- The flap vein is first placed in one end of the coupler followed by the IMV and the coupler is closed without placing tension on either vessel. The previously placed Achland clamp is then taken off the IMV. Heparinized saline can be flushed through the flap artery to confirm flow through the venous coupler.
- For the arterial anastomosis, a double-opposing Acland clamp may be used to algin the arterial ends.
- An end-to-end anastomosis of the arterial ends is performed with 8-0 or 9-0 nylon sutures in an interrupted or running fashion (**FIGURE 15**).
- Once the anastomosis is complete, the double-opposing Achland clamp is taken off prior to taking off the clamp on the IMA.

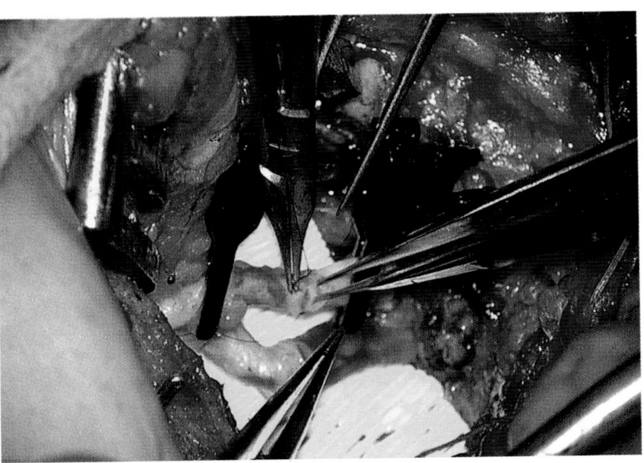

FIGURE 15 ● Microvascular anastomosis under an operating microscope. A double opposing Acland clamp holds the arterial ends in place, and an end-to-end anastomosis is being performed with interrupted 8-0 nylon sutures. The DIEV has been coupled to the IMV in the background.

- With flow reestablished, papaverine is infiltrated into the adventitia of the arteries to prevent spasm.
- The flap and anastomosed vessels are warmed with warm saline and allowed to reperfuse for a few minutes.
- Doppler signals are identified on the flap skin and may be marked with sutures.
- If a flow coupler is used, the Doppler probe is secured into its housing on the venous coupler and audible signal used to confirm flow through the coupler.
- Fat grafts obtained from either the abdominal donor site or flap edge are placed around the anastomosis to help ensure the desired position of the vessels and reduce malposition.

FLAP INSET/DONOR SITE CLOSURE

- Peripheral zones of the flap that may be less optimally perfused are excised.
- The flap is then placed within the mastectomy defect, and interrupted absorbable sutures are used to secure the flap to the medial aspect of the chest wall (ie, medialization).
- The pattern of the skin paddle is marked, and all skin (epidermis and dermis) outside of the paddle is excised with electrocautery (**FIGURE 16**). De-epithelialization is also an option.
- A drain is placed along the inferior aspect of the mastectomy defect and exits the skin along the anterior axillary line.
- Skin closure for the flap inset is performed in layers with absorbable interrupted deep dermal sutures and a running subcuticular suture.
- The abdominal fascial incisions are closed with 2-0 Vicryl figure-of-eight sutures. This is then oversewn with a 1 PDS suture.
- In some patients, closure of the infraumbilical fascial incisions create a relative supraumbilical bulge. For these situations, supraumbilical rectus plication can be performed to avoid undesirable epigastric fullness after surgery.
- The OR table is reflexed to allow for closure of the abdominal. Two drains are placed in the abdominal donor site, and closure of the defect is performed with approximation of Scarpa fascia, the deep dermis, and subsequently the a subcuticular stitch is run. The umbilicus is delivered through the skin flap above the horizontal abdominal closure along the midline by creating an appropriate-sized oval with a full-thickness excision. The umbilicus is then inset with a layered closure.
- Minimal dressings in the form of a skin glue product, Steri-Strips, or an ointment are then applied to all suture lines.

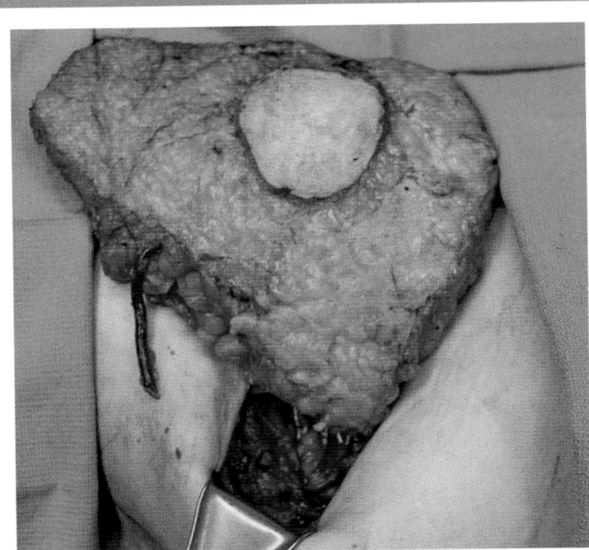

FIGURE 16 ● Flap with all skin outside of the skin paddle excised; preserved SIEV can be seen on the medial aspect of the flap.

PEARLS AND PITFALLS

Preoperative evaluation	■ Preoperative CT angiography is a useful tool to assist with perforator selection—it provides information on perforator location and size but does not give information on perfusion. ■ Flap perfusion based on a few perforators is better assessed by laser-assisted indocyanine green fluorescent dye or by physical examination with occlusion of all perforators with the exception of the few selected perforators.
Patient positioning	■ With the patient in supine position, the table can be turned 180° from the anesthesiologist, providing better access for two surgical teams.
Dissection of the vessels	■ Preserve as long a length of the SIEV (≥5 cm) as possible for use as an additional outflow vessel in flaps with venous congestion after elevation or transfer to the chest. ■ The hydrodissection technique used for the intramuscular perforator dissection simplifies this portion of the operation, creating dissection planes and allowing for better visualization of the perforators and small vascular branches.

POSTOPERATIVE CARE

- Patients can be transferred from the OR to a postanesthesia care unit or directly to a unit with nursing staff trained in flap monitoring.
- Flaps are monitored by physical examinations (color, temperature, capillary refill, and handheld Doppler signals) performed every hour for the first 24 hours, and then checks can be spaced out to every 2 and 4 hours over subsequent hospital days.
- Additional flap monitoring with continuous near-infrared spectroscopy tissue oximetry or audible flow coupler signal is employed for 72 hours postoperatively.
- DVT prophylaxis is the only form of anticoagulation used routinely.
- The patient's bed is kept in the semi-Fowler position at all times.
- Diet is advanced from clear liquids to regular on postoperative day (POD) 1 with restrictions to caffeine intake.
- Patients are assisted out of bed to a chair on POD 1, and they ambulate beginning on POD 2.
- Foley catheters and intravenous (IV) fluids are discontinued, and IV medications/patient-controlled analgesias are converted to orals on POD 2.
- Patients are typically ready for discharge home from POD 3 to POD 5.
- Surgical drains are discontinued once the output is less than 30 mL for two consecutive days.
- Activities are limited and weight-lifting restrictions are in place for 6 weeks postoperatively.
- The first postoperative visit is at 1 week following discharge.
- Preoperative photographs of a patient with a left breast invasive cancer who opted for DIEP flap reconstructions are presented in **FIGURE 17A** and **B**.
- The same patient's postoperative results after immediate bilateral DIEP flap breast reconstruction and subsequent revisions are presented in **FIGURE 17C** and **D**.

OUTCOMES

- The goals of breast reconstruction are to create breast mounds that are aesthetically pleasing, symmetric, and similar to the natural breast in appearance and feel.
- Patient satisfaction is of great importance in assessing outcomes of reconstruction.
- Breast reconstruction patients are typically satisfied in the short term (<5 years) with their choice of reconstruction across implant-based to autologous forms of reconstruction.[12]
- Over the long term (>8 years), satisfaction with abdominal-based flap reconstruction is maintained, whereas satisfaction with implant-based techniques tends to depreciate.[12]
- Studies have also shown greater satisfaction with autologous reconstruction in patients requiring unilateral reconstructions.[13] This is likely the result of autologous flaps achieving better symmetry and feel compared with the natural contralateral breast.
- Patient satisfaction in bilateral reconstructions has been found to be similar across all techniques provided that the same technique is used on both sides,[13] highlighting again the importance of symmetry.

COMPLICATIONS

Flap-Related Complications

- Infections—Surgical site infections are rare as these are clean cases and the autologous tissue transferred to the chest offer greater resistance to infection than do implants.
- Delayed wound healing—This complication typically occurs at the interface between the mastectomy flap and DIEP flap skin paddle. It often is a result of marginal mastectomy flap necrosis from poor skin perfusion, which is more likely in smokers and in previously radiated breast skin.
- Fat necrosis—Varying degrees of fat necrosis are encountered in 10% to 15% of autologous reconstructions; it occurs in relatively small peripheral segments of flap adipose tissue with poor perfusion. This complication is apparent within a few weeks of the operation and presents as a firm palpable nodule, which occasionally causes some discomfort. These areas of necrosis can be directly excised or managed with liposuction (ultrasound assisted or suction assisted) during revision procedures.
- Partial flap loss—an uncommon complication that is also related to poor perfusion. Here, a segment of the flap is lost. It can be the result of poor perforator selection or thrombosis of one or more of the selected perforators. An excision of the necrotic segment is usually required.
- Total flap loss—This is one of the most devastating complications encountered and occurs in less than 2% of

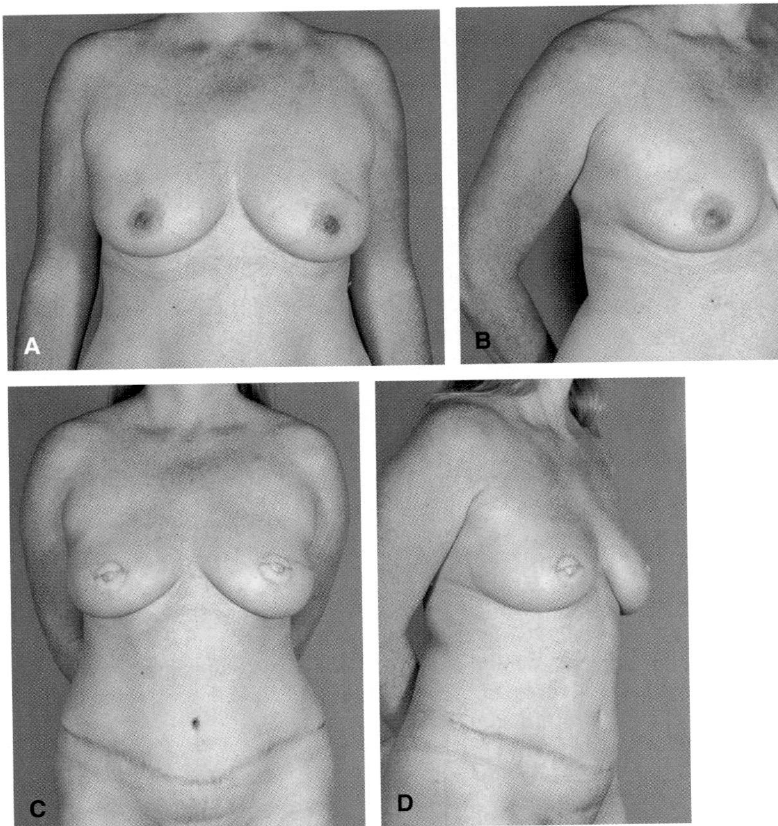

FIGURE 17 ● **A** and **B,** Preoperative photographs of a patient with a left breast invasive cancer. **C** and **D,** Postoperative photographs of the breasts and abdominal donor site after immediate bilateral DIEP flap reconstruction with subsequent revisions including bilateral nipple reconstructions. The patient will undergo nipple tattooing as a final procedure.

reconstructions. The cause of flap loss is a thrombosis of the vascular pedicle (either artery or vein), which could be brought about by a variety of factors ranging from technical problems to hypercoagulable conditions. Early detection of thrombosis with a return to the OR and correction of the inciting problem leads to flap salvage in most cases.

Donor Site Complications

- Hernias/bulges—This complication results from weakening of the abdominal wall after DIEP flap harvest. It is seen much less commonly compared with the TRAM flap, which by definition takes muscle and fascia as part of the flap harvest. The incidence of this complication has been shown to decrease with use of mesh reinforcement in TRAM flap harvests.
- Delayed wound healing—Wound healing problems are encountered often in morbidly obese patients, diabetic patients, and smokers. Perfusion to the infraumbilical portion of the abdominal donor site is marginal in some patients; fat necrosis occurs in this area and ultimately results in a wound dehiscence. These wounds are managed by debridement and dressing changes with healing by secondary intention.

REFERENCES

1. Santosa KB, Qi J, Kim HM, Hamill JB, Wilkins EG, Pusic AL. Long-term patient-reported outcomes in postmastectomy breast reconstruction. *JAMA Surg*. 2018;153(10):891-899.
2. Toyserkani NM, Jørgensen MG, Tabatabaeifar S, Damsgaard T, Sørensen JA. Autologous versus implant-based breast reconstruction: a systematic review and meta-analysis of Breast-Q patient-reported outcomes. *J Plast Reconstr Aesthet Surg*. 2020;73(2):278-285.
3. Hartrampf CR, Scheflan M, Black PW. Breast reconstruction with a transverse abdominal island flap. *Plast Reconstr Surg*. 1982;69:216-225.
4. Koshima I, Soeda S. Inferior epigastric artery skin flaps without recuts abdominis muscle. *Br J Plast Surg*. 1989;42:645-648.
5. Allen RJ, Treece P. Deep inferior epigastric perforator flap for breast reconstruction. *Ann Plast Surg*. 1994;32:32-38.
6. Blondeel N, Vanderstraeten GG, Monstrey SJ, et al. The donor site morbidity of free DIEP flaps and free TRAM flaps for breast reconstruction. *Br J Plast Surg*. 1997;50:322-330.
7. Nahabedian MY, Dooley W, Singh N, et al. Contour abnormalities of the abdomen after breast reconstruction with abdominal flaps: the role of muscle preservation. *Plast Reconstr Surg*. 2002;109:91-101.
8. Momoh AO, Colakoglu S, Westvik TS, et al. Analysis of complications and patient satisfaction in pedicled transverse rectus abdominis myocutaneous and deep inferior epigastric perforator flap breast reconstruction. *Ann Plast Surg*. 2012;69(1):19-23.
9. Holm C, Mayr M, Hofter E, et al. Perfusion zones of the DIEP flap revisited: a clinical study. *Plast Reconstr Surg*. 2006;117:37-43.
10. Smit JM, Dimopoulou A, Liss AG, et al. Preoperative CT angiography reduces surgery time in perforator flap reconstruction. *J Plast Reconstr Aesthet Surg*. 2009;62:1112-1117.
11. Vasile JV, Levine JL. Magnetic resonance angiography in perforator flap breast reconstruction. *Gland Surg*. 2016;5(2):197-211.
12. Hu ES, Pusic AL, Waljee JF, et al. Patient-reported aesthetic satisfaction with breast reconstruction during the long-term survivorship period. *Plast Reconstr Surg*. 2009;124:1-8.
13. Craft RO, Colakoglu S, Curtis MS, et al. Patient satisfaction in unilateral and bilateral breast reconstruction. *Plast Reconstr Surg*. 2011;127:1417-1424.

Chapter 26 Nipple-Areolar Complex Reconstruction

Haripriya S. Ayyala, Anita R. Kulkarni, and Evan Matros

DEFINITION

- Nipple-areolar complex (NAC) reconstruction is often the final stage of breast reconstruction after mastectomy and is a critical consideration for the creation of an aesthetically pleasing breast.

PATIENT HISTORY AND PHYSICAL FINDINGS

- The ideal reconstructed NAC recreates both the projected nipple and surrounding areola and should achieve symmetry with the contralateral NAC.[1]
- Nipple-areolar reconstruction is performed approximately 3 months after the final stage of breast mound reconstruction, including both autologous and implant-based methods. This allows the final breast shape and position to be obtained prior to placement of the NAC, as the NAC position may not be easily moved postoperatively. Reconstruction can also be performed in a delayed fashion at any time a patient desires, including months or years after breast mound reconstruction.
- The presence of an NAC increases patient satisfaction and provides a sense of symmetry, completeness, and closure.[2]

SURGICAL MANAGEMENT

- There are many described techniques for nipple reconstruction, including nipple sharing, local flaps, cartilage grafts, dermal grafts, and prostheses.[3] Local flaps are the most popular option and are described in detail in this chapter.
- Reconstructed nipples lack the rigid ductal and smooth muscle elements of a natural nipple; therefore, the long-term maintenance of nipple projection continues to be the most challenging aspect of NAC reconstruction.[4]
- Multiple autologous and prosthetic materials (auricular cartilage, rib cartilage, toe pulp, acellular dermal matrix, calcium hydroxylapatite, polytetrafluoroethylene implants, etc.) have been attempted to give permanent rigidity to the nipple; however, no single technique has demonstrated definitive superiority.[3]
- Areolar reconstruction is primarily done by skin grafting, tattoo, or both.
- The first described technique in this chapter is a skate flap for nipple reconstruction with a full-thickness skin graft for areolar reconstruction. This procedure is typically done in the operating room under sedation or general anesthesia.
- The second described technique is a CV flap for nipple reconstruction, which can be used in combination with a tattoo for areolar reconstruction. This procedure can be done in the office under local anesthesia.
- An alternative, nonsurgical technique for NAC restoration includes 3D tattooing. While this does not restore anatomic projection of the papilla, this requires no surgical intervention and can be done without anesthesia.

Preoperative Planning

- In unilateral NAC reconstruction, the position, size, and shape of the opposite nipple are taken into consideration to design the reconstruction in addition to anatomic landmarks. In bilateral reconstruction, anatomic landmarks and standard measurements are utilized to position and design the NAC.
- Anatomically, the NAC is located at the anterior-most projecting part of the breast mound at the level of the inframammary fold, centered on the reconstructed breast mound.
- The nipple has an average projection of 5 mm, and the areola has an average diameter of 35 to 45 mm.

Positioning

- In the operating room, patients are positioned supine with arms at 90° secured to armboards. Both breasts are prepped into the field to allow for evaluation of symmetry. Patients are secured to the operating table to allow upright evaluation intraoperatively.
- In the clinic, patients are positioned supine with arms at sides.

Skate Flap (Nipple) + Full-Thickness Skin Graft (Areola)

- The patient is placed in supine position with arms abducted at 90°. Arms are secured on armboards.
- The NAC position is selected at the anterior-most projecting part of the reconstructed breast with the patient in an upright position. In unilateral nipple reconstruction, the NAC is placed symmetrically to the opposite side (**FIGURE 1**).
- A donor site is chosen for the full-thickness skin graft, which will be used to reconstruct the areola. Commonly used sites include the lower abdomen and the groin crease. In addition, the areolar graft can be taken adjacent to any of the patient's existing scars.
- A 38- or 42-mm nipple sizer is used to mark the areolar skin graft. An ellipse is drawn tangent to the areolar graft to allow linear closure of the donor site.

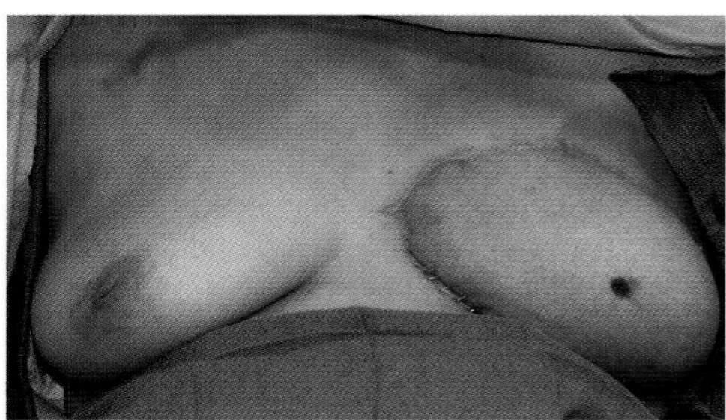

FIGURE 1 • Nipple position is selected symmetrically to the native nipple.

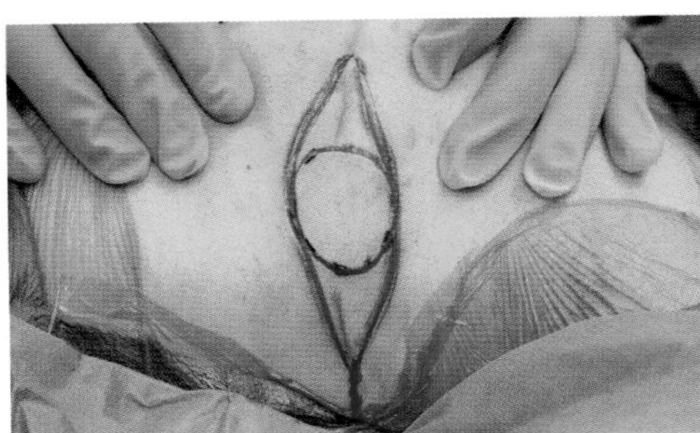

FIGURE 2 ● Areolar skin graft is marked with a 38-mm nipple sizer. An ellipse is drawn tangentially to facilitate linear closure.

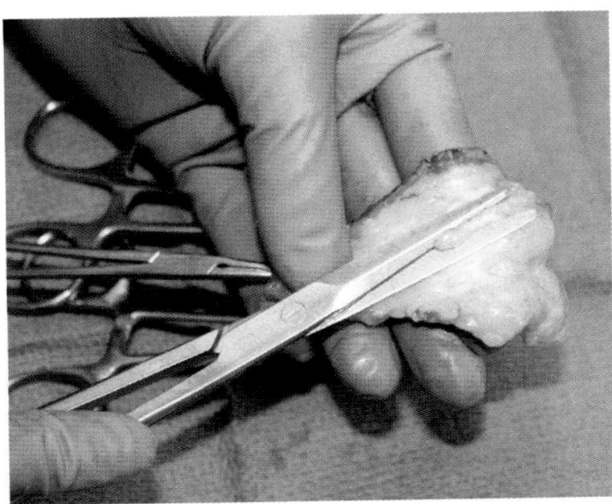

FIGURE 3 ● Areolar skin graft is aggressively defatted.

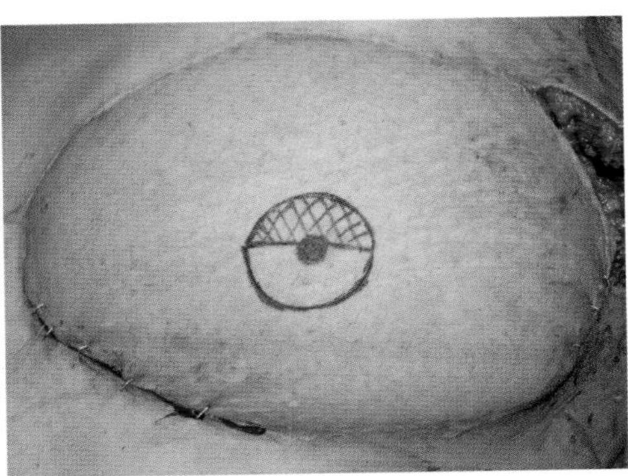

FIGURE 4 ● Skate flap design.

- The areolar skin graft is scored with a knife prior to harvest. The ellipse is then excised as a full-thickness skin graft (**FIGURE 2**).
- The areolar graft is aggressively defatted with a small sharp scissor, leaving only full-thickness skin behind (**FIGURE 3**).
- The skate flap is designed at the previously marked site (**FIGURE 4**).
  - A 1- to 1.5-cm circle is drawn at the planned location of the nipple.
  - A 38- or 42-mm nipple sizer is used to mark the areola centered on the nipple.
  - A horizontal line is drawn across the circle at the superior edge of the marked nipple.

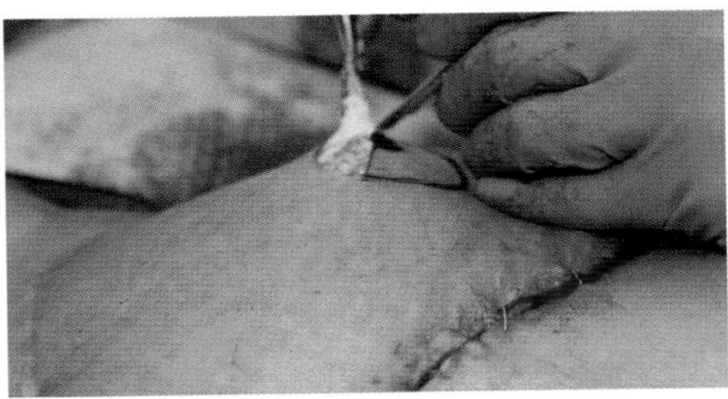

FIGURE 5 ● Crosshatched area is de-epithelialized.

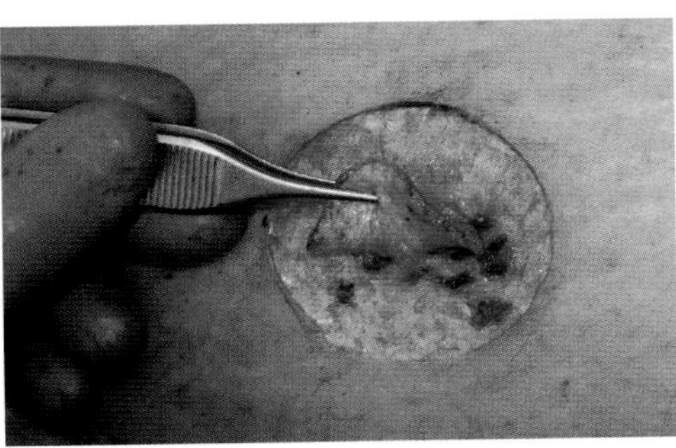

FIGURE 6 ● Skate flap is raised in the mid-dermal plane, leaving central pedicle attached.

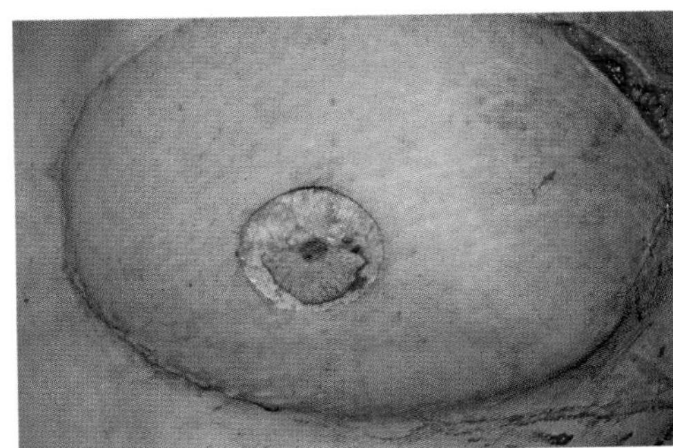

FIGURE 7 ● Skate flap is shown raised.

  - The upper portion of the circle is crosshatched to mark the area that will be de-epithelialized.
  - The lower portion of the circle will be raised as the "skate flap" to create the new nipple.
- The epidermis is scored along all incisions.
- The crosshatched semicircle is de-epithelialized (**FIGURE 5**).
- The flap is then raised from the edges at the level of the mid-dermis. The deepest layer of dermis is left down in order to provide a vascularized bed for the areolar skin graft (**FIGURE 6**).
- The flap remains attached to the deep dermis at the marked nipple. The flap is raised in a slightly deeper plane at the center in order to include some fat with the flap to provide bulk (**FIGURE 7**).
- The corners of the flap are centralized and sutured to the underlying dermis using 5.0 rapide (**FIGURE 8**).
- The edges of the flap are sutured together using interrupted 5.0 rapide (**FIGURE 9**).

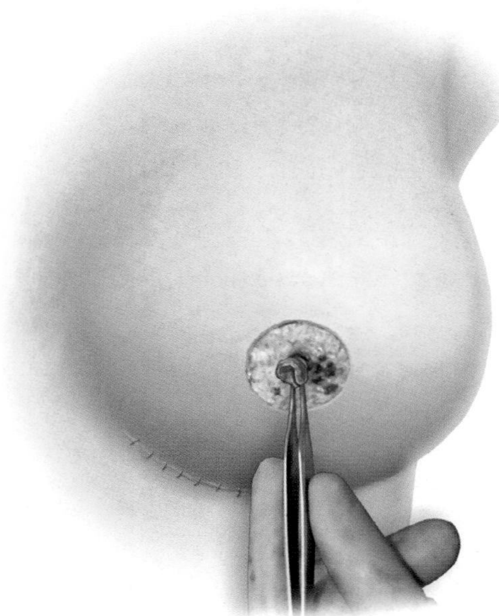

FIGURE 8 ● Edges of skate flap are brought together centrally to recreate nipple.

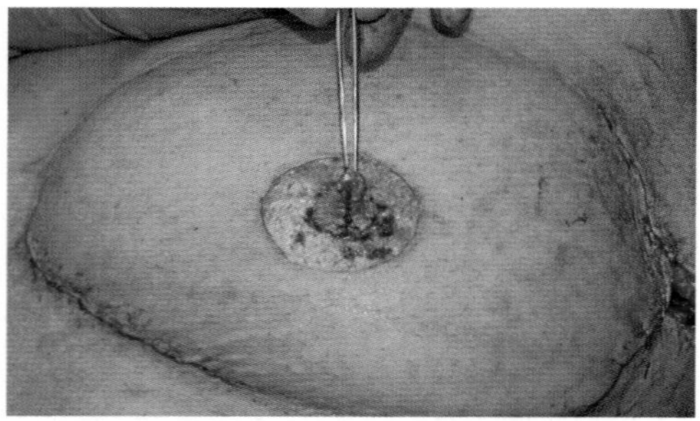

FIGURE 9 ● Edges are sutured together in midline.

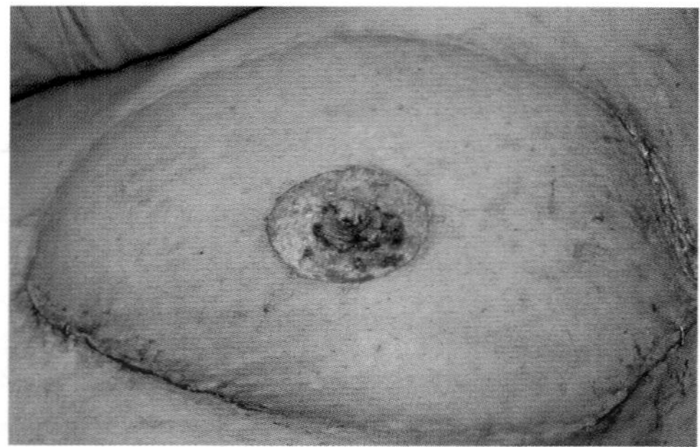

FIGURE 10 ● Open end of nipple is sutured down as a cap.

- The cap is sutured down to close off the nipple (**FIGURE 10**).
- The full-thickness skin areolar skin graft is sutured to the bed using 4.0 chromic half-buried horizontal mattress sutures. The buried portion of suture is placed along the native breast skin to avoid scarring on the breast (**FIGURE 11**).
- A 1-cm hole is cut in the center of the areolar graft to expose the nipple (**FIGURE 12**).

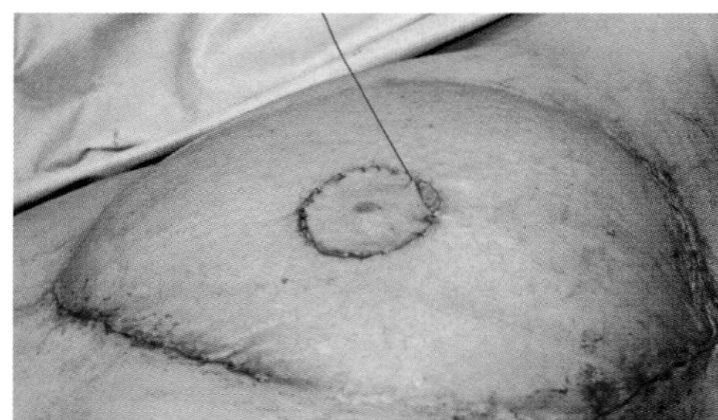

FIGURE 11 ● Areolar skin graft is sutured to skin edges.

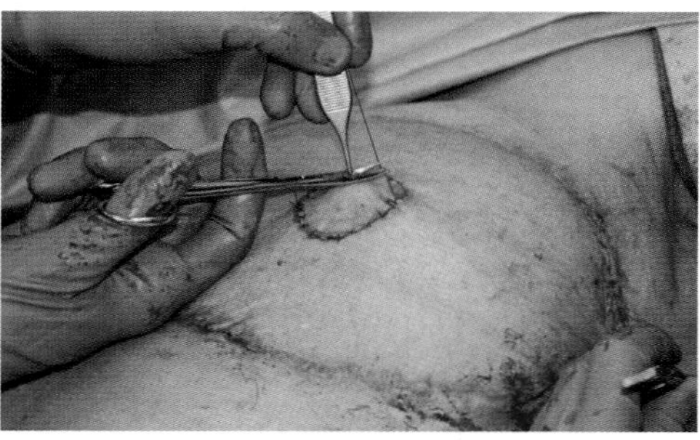

FIGURE 12 ● Central hole is cut in areolar skin graft to allow nipple to protrude.

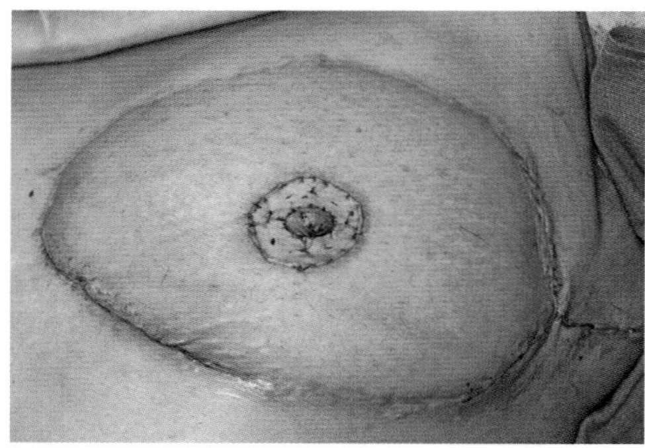

FIGURE 13 ● Tacking sutures and pie-crust incisions are placed in areolar skin graft.

- The graft is secured to the nipple using interrupted 5.0 chromic sutures.
- 4.0 Chromic tacking sutures and pie crust incisions are placed in the areolar graft (**FIGURE 13**).
- A protective dressing is applied using Mastisol liquid adhesive (Eloquest Healthcare, Ferndale, MI, USA) on the native breast, crisscrossed Steri-Strips (3M, Two Harbors, MN, USA), 2 × 2 fluffed gauze, and foam tape (**FIGURE 14A-D**). The goal of the dressing is to protect the nipple-areolar reconstruction without putting any pressure on the skate flap.
- The dressing is kept in place for 5 to 7 days after surgery, at which time it is removed in clinic.

CV Flap

- This procedure can be performed under local anesthesia with the patient awake.

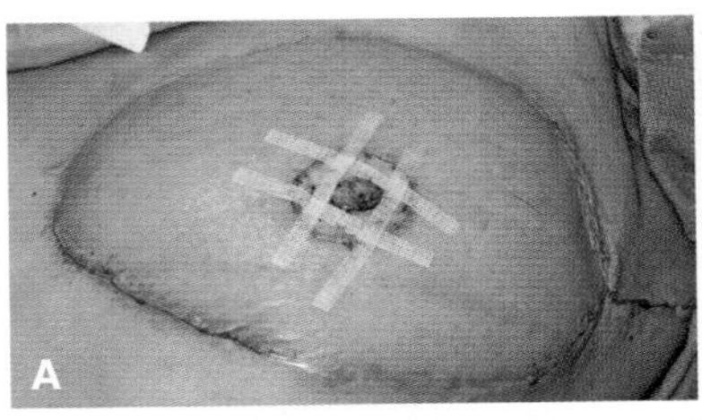

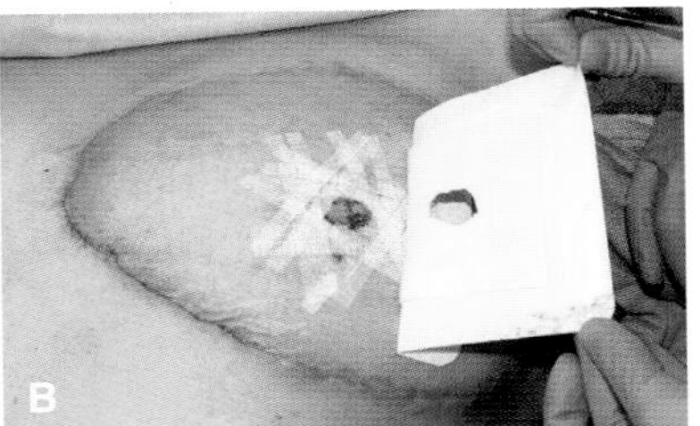

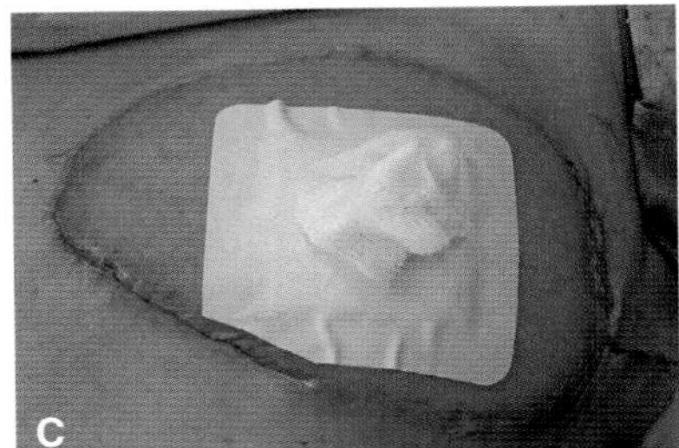

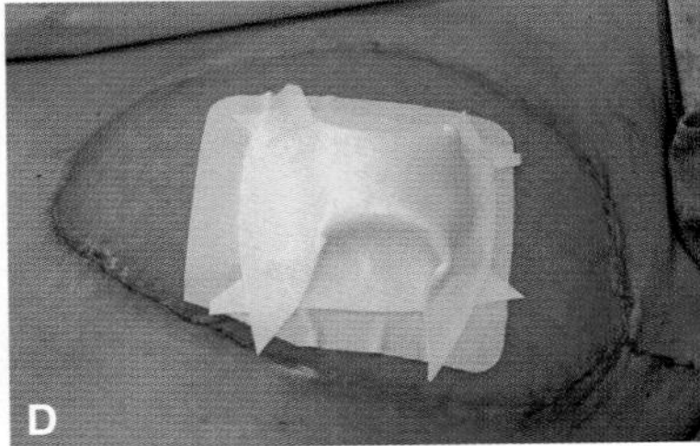

FIGURE 14 ● Bolster dressing. **A,** Mastisol is applied to the surrounding breast skin, followed by tightly adherent Steri-Strips placed in a crosswise fashion to apply pressure to the graft. **B,** Foam tape dressing with a central hole for nipple is placed over crosswise Steri-Strips. **C,** A 2 × 2 fluffed gauze is placed over the nipple. **D,** Additional foam tape is tented over the fluffed gauze without putting any pressure on nipple reconstruction.

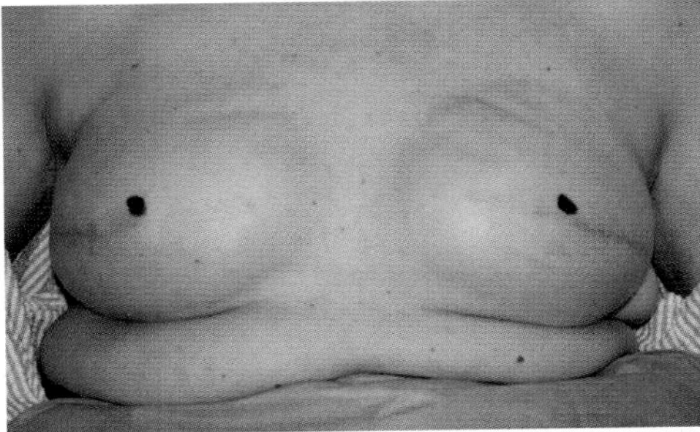

FIGURE 15 ● Bilateral nipple position marked at the anterior-most projecting part of breast mounds adjacent to mastectomy scars.

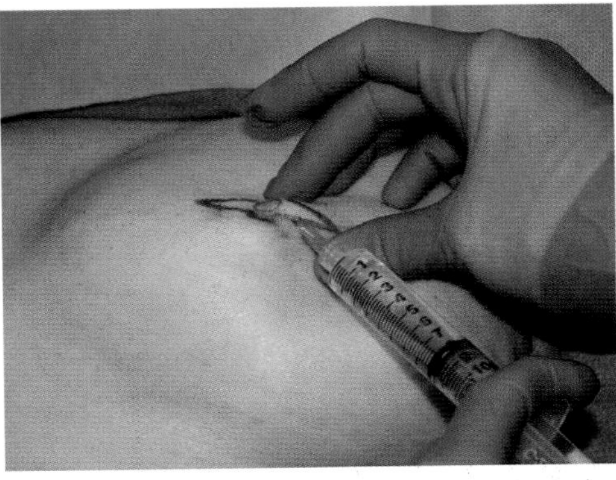

FIGURE 17 ● Lidocaine, 1%, with 1:100,000 epinephrine is injected subcutaneously.

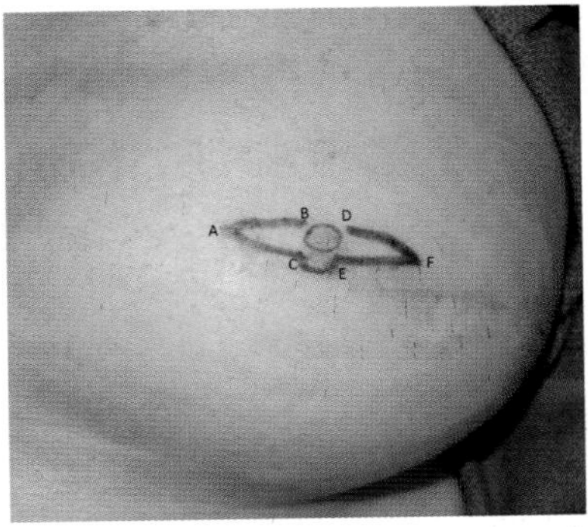

FIGURE 16 ● Markings for CV flap. Length from *A* to *F* is approximately 5 cm, width from *BD* to *CE* is approximately 1.5 cm.

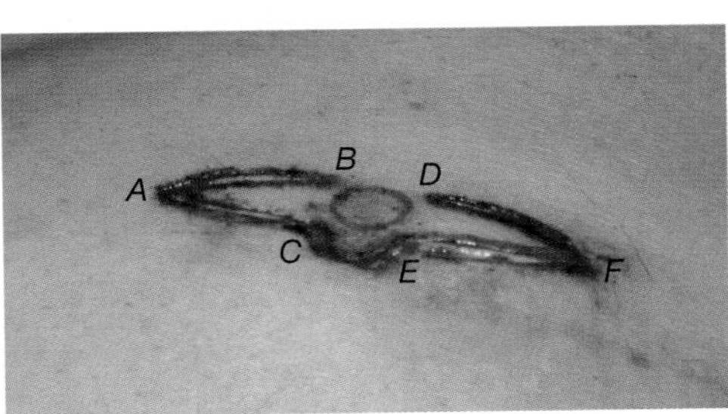

FIGURE 18 ● The CV flap is incised through to mid-fat level along all incisions except *B* to *D*.

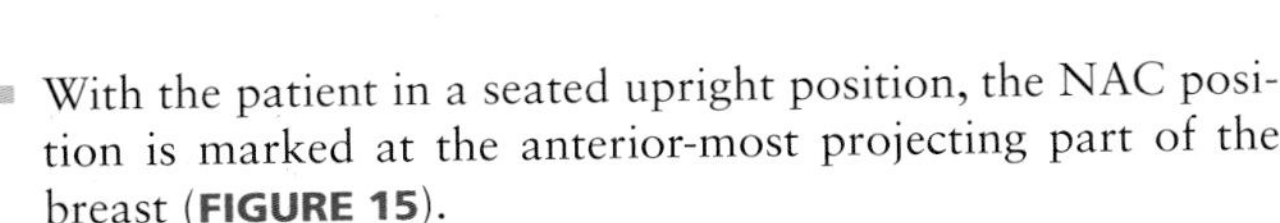

- With the patient in a seated upright position, the NAC position is marked at the anterior-most projecting part of the breast (**FIGURE 15**).
- The CV flap is drawn as shown. The length of the flap is approximately 5 cm (A to F), and the width is approximately 1.5 cm. The width of the flap (BD to CE) determines the projection of the nipple (**FIGURE 16**).
- The subcutaneous tissue is infiltrated with 1% lidocaine with 1:100,000 epinephrine (**FIGURE 17**).
- Incisions are made along all edges **except** points B to D at the base of the nipple. This area is left attached and serves as the blood supply to the flap (**FIGURE 18**).
- The flap is raised from both sides in the mid-subcutaneous fat plane (**FIGURE 19A** and **B**).
- The incision is closed from point B to C and D to E (**FIGURE 20**).
- One flap edge (point A) is brought to the center and sutured in place with 5.0 rapide (**FIGURE 21**).

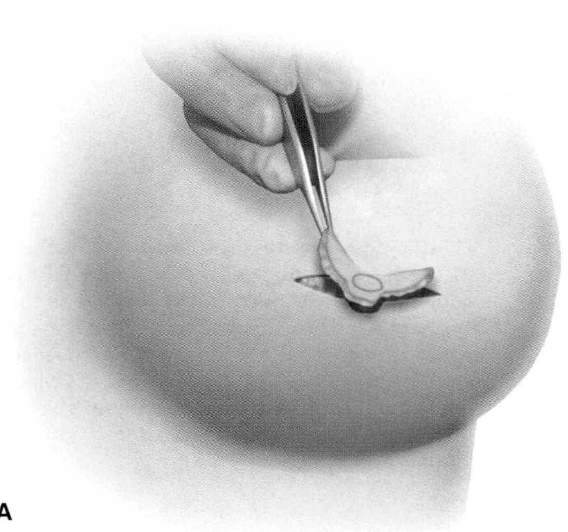

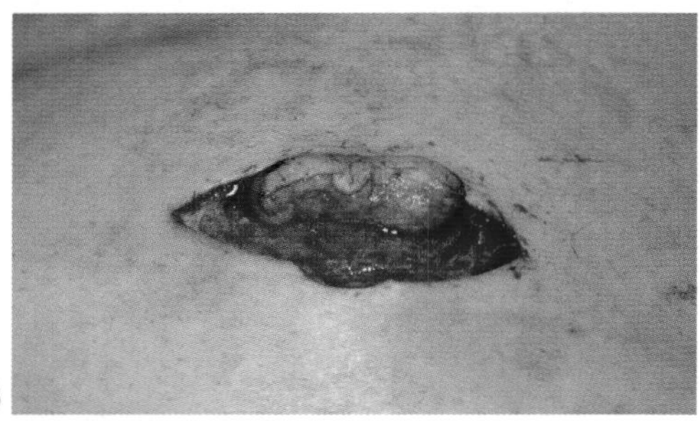

FIGURE 19 ● **A,** The CV flap is raised in the mid-fat plane. **B,** The CV flap is shown raised.

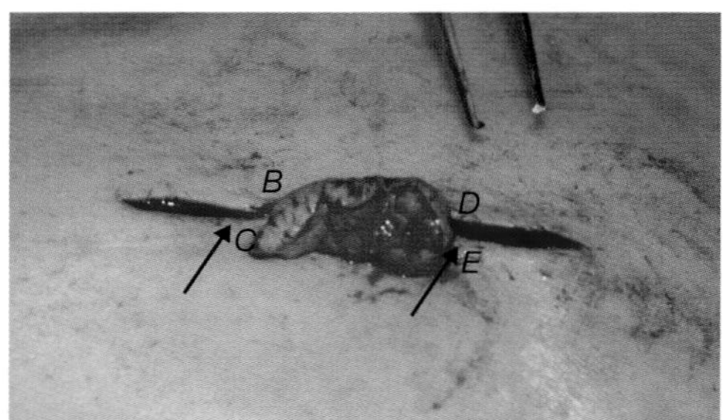

FIGURE 20 ● Incision is closed (point *B* to *C* and *D* to *E*).

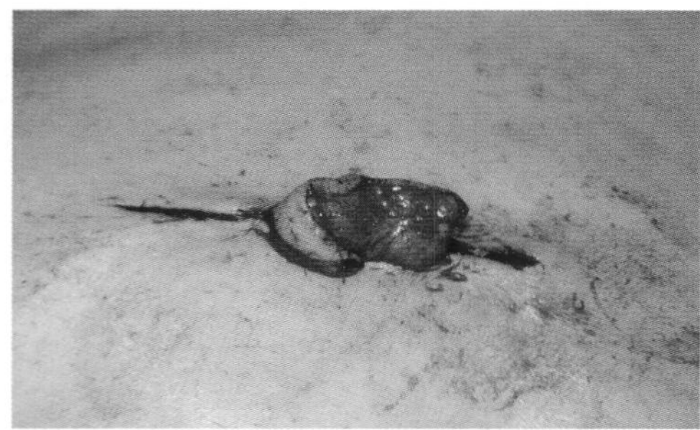

FIGURE 21 ● One flap edge (point *A*) is centralized and sutured to the deep surface.

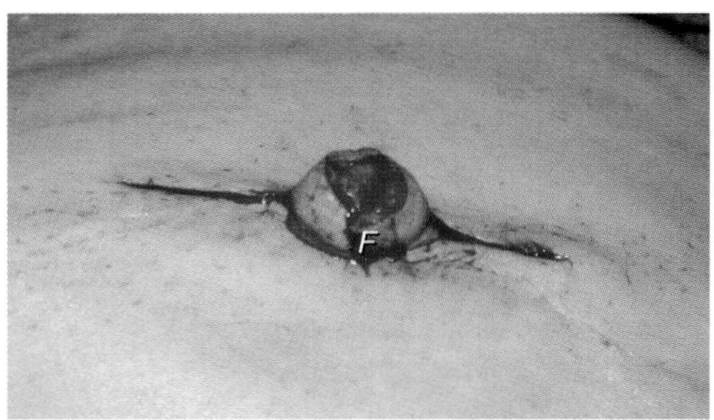

FIGURE 22 ● Opposite flap edge (point *F*) is centralized and sutured to point *A*.

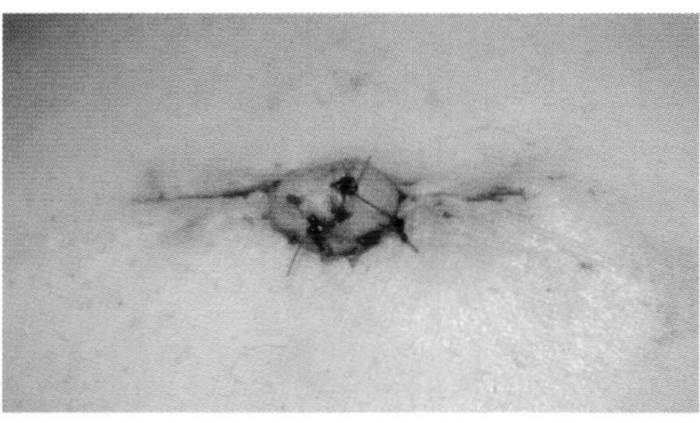

FIGURE 23 ● Cap is sutured down to close off nipple, and all incisions are closed with interrupted sutures.

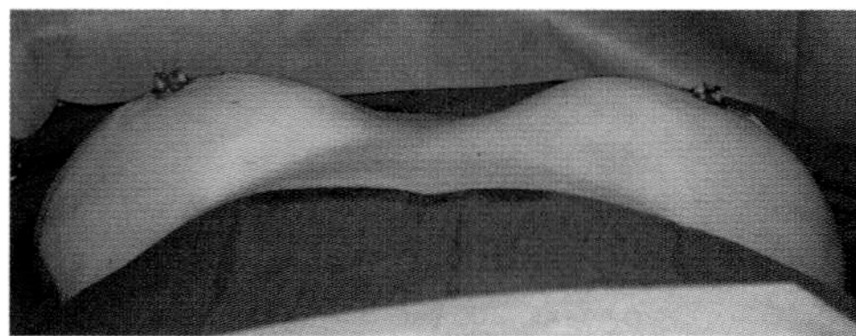

FIGURE 24 ● Final result showing projection of bilateral CV flaps.

- The opposite flap edge (Point F) is brought to the center and sutured to the first flap edge (**FIGURE 22**).
- The cap is sutured down to close the top of the nipple and the remainder of the incision is closed with 4.0 vicryl deep and 4.0 monocryl running subcuticular (**FIGURE 23**).
- Nipple projection is shown after complete reconstruction (**FIGURE 24**).

3D Tattoo

- This procedure can be performed without anesthesia by an experienced nipple tattoo artist. This technique avoids additional incisions and surgical scarring.
- Consideration is given to the patient's skin tone when selecting pigment for bilateral cases or matched to the contralateral nipple in unilateral cases.
- Pigment is applied using needles with shading techniques to create the appearance of a 3D NAC, completing the visual aesthetic unit of the NAC (**FIGURE 25**).

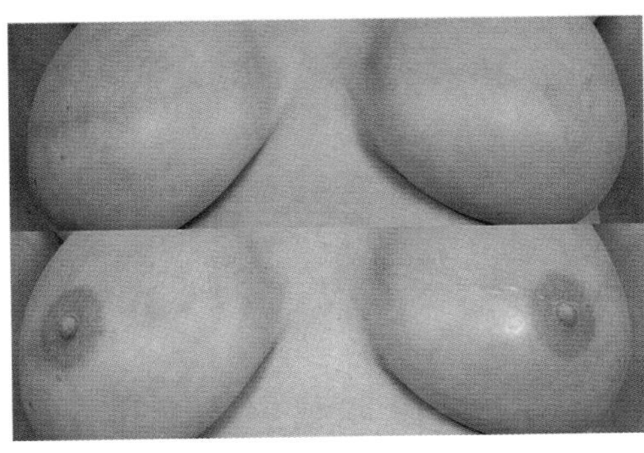

FIGURE 25 ● Final result of a 3D tattooed nipple areolar complex.

PEARLS AND PITFALLS

Indications	▪ Nipple areolar reconstruction should be deferred until the final breast mound shape is obtained for best cosmesis.
Placement of incision	▪ Flaps should be based adjacent to the mastectomy scar whenever possible to avoid additional scarring and ensure viability of the reconstructed complex.
Projection	▪ Nipple projection will decrease by 50% in the first year; therefore, projection should be overestimated at the time of reconstruction. ▪ Projection can be increased later with dermal fillers such as collagen or hyaluronic acid.
Areola	▪ Areolar tattoo is often used in addition to skin grafting or as a primary modality for areolar reconstruction. ▪ Tattoos often need more than one application spaced over several months in order to achieve the final desired color.

POSTOPERATIVE CARE

- After nipple reconstruction, a protective dressing should be applied and maintained in place for 1 week postoperatively. Brassieres should be avoided for the first 6 weeks to prevent pressure on the nipple flap.
- If no skin graft is used, patients may shower after the dressing is removed 1 week postoperatively.
- If a skin graft is used for areolar reconstruction, the bolster is removed 1 week postoperatively in the clinic, and daily petroleum gauze dressing changes are performed for 1 week. After 2 weeks, patients may shower and apply moisturizer to the graft.

OUTCOMES

- All modes of nipple reconstruction result in some degree of loss of projection over time, up to 50%.[5] Most loss of projection occurs within the first 3 months, and final nipple shape and size is typically achieved by 1 year.[6] CV flaps tend to lose more projection than skate flaps over time.
- Dermal fillers such as collagen and hyaluronic acid can be injected into the nipple to increase projection.

COMPLICATIONS

- Loss of nipple projection
- Partial or complete flap necrosis
- Partial or complete loss of areolar skin graft
- Infection

REFERENCES

1. Lewin R, Amoroso M, Plate N, et al. The aesthetically ideal position of the nipple-areola complex on the breast. *Aesthetic Plast Surg.* 2016;40(5):724-732. doi:10.1007/s00266-016-0684-z
2. Momoh AO, Colakoglu S, de Blacam C, et al. The impact of nipple reconstruction on patient satisfaction in breast reconstruction. *Ann Plast Surg.* 2012;69(4):389-393. doi:10.1097/SAP.0b013e318246e572
3. Boccola MA, Savage J, Rozen WM, et al. Surgical correction and reconstruction of the nipple-areola complex: current review of techniques. *J Reconstr Microsurg.* 2010;26(9):589-600. doi:10.1055/s-0030-1263290
4. Farhadi J, Maksvytyte GK, Schaefer DJ, et al. Reconstruction of the nipple-areola complex: an update. *J Plast Reconstr Aesthetic Surg.* 2006;59(1):40-53. doi:10.1016/j.bjps.2005.08.006
5. Shestak KC, Gabriel A, Landecker A, et al. Assessment of long-term nipple projection: a comparison of three techniques. *Plast Reconstr Surg.* 2002;110(3):780-786. doi:10.1097/00006534-200209010-00010
6. Few JW, Marcus JR, Casas LA, et al. Long-term predictable nipple projection following reconstruction. *Plast Reconstr Surg.* 1999;104(5):1321-1324. doi:10.1097/00006534-199910000-00012

Chapter 27 Excisional and Incisional Biopsies of Skin and Soft Tissue Lesions

Cindy Eliana Parra and Alison B. Durham

DEFINITION

- The elliptical excision is a versatile and straightforward procedure that can be performed in the outpatient office setting.[1] Proper planning and technique yield excellent cosmetic outcomes with minimal risk to the patient, as it may be performed with local anesthesia. The elliptical excision is more properly termed the fusiform excision, as the ends are pointed rather than rounded.[2] This shape maximizes cosmetic outcomes by minimizing incision length while removing the redundant tissue along the length of either end of the extirpated lesion, or "dog ears," with one incision.
- The traditional fusiform shape can be designed by creating a 3:1 ratio between the diameter of the lesion (plus appropriate margins, if needed) to be excised and the long axis of the ellipse.
- The ideal tip angle is typically 30°, though this may vary in actual practice.[3] The excision can easily be designed to hide the final sutured line and subsequent scar within skin tension lines and results in excellent cosmesis with well executed side-to-side closure.
- The technique may be used for both the diagnosis and management of benign and malignant lesions of the skin and subcutaneous tissues. An excisional biopsy refers to the technique where the entire lesion is removed from the skin. In contrast, an incisional biopsy is a technique that removes only a portion of the lesion for the purpose of diagnosis or may be used to remove a benign lesion and minimize the appearance of the final scar.

DIFFERENTIAL DIAGNOSIS

- Optimal planning and execution of an excision requires an understanding of the type of lesion (ie, benign vs malignant) and the location of the lesion (ie, within the skin or within the subcutaneous tissue).
- Benign lesions can include epidermal inclusion cysts, pilar cysts, keloids, and others.
- Malignant lesions may include melanoma and nonmelanoma skin cancers, dermatofibrosarcoma protruberans, and others. Additionally, an understanding of the purpose of the excision is required prior to design and execution, as excisions being performed for the diagnosis of a lesion will differ from an excision being performed for definitive treatment.
- For example, if an elliptical excision is to be performed for diagnosis of a lesion suspected to be melanoma, an excisional biopsy of the entire clinical lesion with a narrow (0.2 cm) margin is the preferred method. This technique allows the histopathologist to evaluate the entirety of the lesion and provide accurate prognostic information in order to determine optimal final treatment.
- For large lesions where complete excision is not possible, an incisional biopsy through the area clinically suspected to be deepest is recommended in the case of suspected melanoma. If an incisional biopsy is performed and the pathology result does not show the suspected malignancy, rebiopsy should be considered to rule out sampling error.
- In general, excisional biopsies should not include standard treatment margins prior to obtaining a definitive diagnosis of a lesion suspected to be a malignancy. If a narrow margin excisional biopsy is performed for diagnosis of a lesion on an extremity, which is suspected to be malignant, the orientation should optimally be along the longitudinal axis to facilitate closure of the skin if a definitive wide local excision is indicated and to minimize disruption of the dermal lymphatics if sentinel lymph node biopsy were to be recommended as part of treatment.

PATIENT HISTORY AND PHYSICAL FINDINGS

- The elements involved in planning an excision should include the physical exam or adequate description of the lesion, the precise location, and size of the lesion.
- Knowledge of cutaneous surgical anatomy and anatomic danger zones are essential prior to planning an excision. For instance, removal of a lesion located along the temple could compromise the temporal branch of the facial nerve or removal of lesions along the lateral jawline could affect the marginal mandibular branch of the facial nerve.
- The location of a lesion along a free margin should also be taken into account, as primary closure of the skin after removal of the lesion could distort local anatomy if not properly planned and executed. Excisions along the cheek near the eye could lead to ectropion if not appropriately designed.
- Care should thus be taken to orient the tension vectors of the ellipse perpendicular to the free margin. Orienting the length of the excision along relaxed skin tension lines allows for the final scars to fall parallel to natural motion lines.
- Ensuring that the final scar falls at the border of cosmetic subunits, rather than crossing them, also facilitates improved cosmesis.
- A clinical lymph node exam should be performed to assess for regional lymph node involvement in cases

involving melanoma, Merkel cell carcinoma, squamous cell carcinomas, or other cancers with potential to metastasize to regional lymph nodes. Palpable lymph nodes on clinical exam warrant evaluation with an ultrasound and fine needle aspiration (FNA) if malignancy is suspected.

IMAGING AND OTHER DIAGNOSTIC STUDIES

- Imaging may be considered prior to the elliptical excision in certain cases and may better delineate the clinical extent of the lesion or help determine extension or adherence to surrounding structures such as tendons or even bony extension. Magnetic resonance imaging (MRI) may be used to assess soft tissue involvement whereas computed tomography (CT) can help determine bony involvement. Imaging may also help identify whether a lesion such as a lipoma is above or below the muscle and thus assist in preoperative planning. The use of other imaging modalities, such as tetrahertz pulsed imaging and reflectance confocal microscopy, have been proposed to delineate margins of nonmelanoma skin cancers.[4,5] Reflectance confocal microscopy could also be considered to better evaluate the margins of melanomas prior to cutaneous surgery but is not used routinely at this time.[6]

SURGICAL MANAGEMENT

Preoperative Planning

- Preoperative planning (**TABLE 1**) should include a thorough patient history examination that includes current medications, allergies, cardiac history, and history of joint replacements or joint infections. Patient factors such as uncontrolled hypertension should be optimized prior to proceeding with the elliptical excision. The patient's functional status, ability to understand and follow basic instructions, and ability to tolerate the procedure should also be considered. Pregnancy is not a contraindication to outpatient dermatologic surgery; however, procedures should be performed in the second trimester or the postpartum period if possible to avoid impact during organogenesis in the first trimester or triggering preterm labor in the third trimester.[7] Few absolute contraindications to the elliptical excision exist; however, relative contraindications include an infected surgical site.

Table 1: Pertinent Health History and Preoperative Checklist

Preoperative health history checklist
Allergy or sensitivity to local anesthesia?
Allergy to antibiotics?
Latex allergy/sensitivity?
Adhesive sensitivity?
HIV/Hepatitis?
Bleeding disorder, thrombocytopenia, or uncontrolled hypertension?
Taking blood thinner?
Taking Bruton tyrosine kinase inhibitor?
Pacemaker/defibrillator?
Other implanted electrical device?
Heart valve replacement?
Joint replacement?
Currently pregnant?

- Patients on oral anticoagulants, such as aspirin, warfarin, or direct-acting oral anticoagulants, may safely undergo elliptical excision. Patients may safely discontinue nonclinically indicated supplements that may increase bleeding risk (ie, fish oil, garlic, ginger, gingko, danshen).[8] Suspension of clinically indicated oral anticoagulation is generally not recommended, as the risk of holding these medications is typically higher than the risk of intraoperative bleeding.
- Bruton tyrosine kinase (BTK) inhibitors are new drugs used to treat chronic lymphocytic leukemia and mature B cell malignancies and have been associated with serious bleeding events.[9] BTK and TEC (tyrosine kinase expressed in hepatocellular carcinoma) are expressed in platelets and act downstream in glycoprotein (GP)VI signaling involved in collagen-mediated platelet aggregation. Holding medications in this class (ibrutinib, acalabrutinib, tirabrutinib, and zanubrutinib) should be strongly considered prior to cutaneous surgery to avoid adverse patient outcomes.[10,11] Consultation with the primary prescribing provider should occur prior to withholding any medication, as timing may vary depending on the type of drug being held.
- Patients with thrombocytopenia should be evaluated on a case-by-case basis in order to determine the safety of proceeding with cutaneous surgery.[12] Thrombocytopenia is defined as a platelet count below 150×10^9 L^{-1} and is a common issue that arises in the perioperative setting. Thrombocytopenia has been subcategorized for surgical purposes into mild (100×10^9 L^{-1}, moderate (50×10^9 L^{-1}), and severe ($<50 \times 10^9$ L^{-1}). The clinical utility of this categorization is limited, as the relationship between platelet count and bleeding risk is nonlinear and depends on platelet function and other patient-related variables. The risk of spontaneous bleeding is difficult to predict until platelet count decreases to values below 10×10^9 L^{-1}. There are also limited data to inform perioperative management of patients with thrombocytopenia, and threshold recommendations are based on low quality evidence, expert opinion, or practice review. In dermatologic surgery, a threshold of 20×10^9 L^{-1} is typically used. A hematologist is typically consulted in patients with lower platelet levels who require cutaneous surgery in order to optimize platelet counts prior to the procedure.[13]
- Presurgical planning should include review of allergies to local anesthetics, antiseptics, latex, oral antibiotics, and adhesives. True IgE-mediated anaphylaxis to local anesthesia is very rare, and most reports of true local anesthetic immediate hypersensitivity result from the amide class of anesthetics (articaine, bupivacaine, levobupivacaine, dibucaine, etidocaine, lidocaine, mepivacaine, prilocaine, and ropivacaine).[14] This predominance is postulated to be due to the preferential use of amides over esters in current clinical practice rather than enhanced allergenicity of amides over esters.
- Other adverse non–IgE-mediated reactions attributed to local anesthetics are often reported, including delayed type hypersensitivity, epinephrine reactions, vasovagal response, local reaction from needle trauma, or rarely anesthetic toxicity. It is important to clarify whether reported allergies are true allergies during the presurgical planning phase. If deemed necessary, allergy testing for adverse reactions can either be performed through skin prick or intradermal testing (immediate hypersensitivity testing) or patch testing (delayed hypersensitivity testing).

Table 2: Possible High-Risk Factors for Infective Endocarditis and Prosthetic Joint Infection

High-risk factors for infective endocarditis	Possible high-risk factors for prosthetic joint infection
Prosthetic cardiac valve Previous infective endocarditis Unrepaired cyanotic congenital heart disease Fully repaired congenital heart defects with a prosthetic material, <6 mo after procedure Repaired congenital heart disease with residual defects at or adjacent to the site of prosthetic device Cardiac transplant recipients with cardiac valvulopathy	First 2 y following joint replacement Previous prosthetic joint infections Immunocompromised status (ie, solid organ and bone marrow transplant, receiving chemotherapy, and chronic steroid use)

Adapted with permission from Bae-Harboe YSC, Liang CA. Perioperative antibiotic use of dermatologic surgeons in 2012. Dermatol Surg. 2013;39(11):1592-1601.

- Use of an alternate class of topical anesthetic is a suitable option (amide vs ester) in cases of a true documented immediate hypersensitivity. In a case series involving 2978 patients, only 29 (0.97%) of patients were found to have a true IgE-mediated allergy to local anesthetic.[15] Immediate hypersensitivity to latex among the general population is estimated at 1% to 5% in the general population, and is thus far more common than allergies to local anesthetics.[16]
- The need for antibiotic prophylaxis (**TABLE 2**) perioperatively may be considered for higher risk populations to prevent infectious endocarditis or prosthetic joint infection in cases where the surgery breaches the oral mucosa or if excision is planned within an infected surgical site.[15] Though no evidence-based guidelines exist specific to dermatologic surgery, consensus recommendations to guide prophylactic antibiotics in high-risk patients receiving dental work have been made by the American Heart Association (AHA), American Dental Association (ADA), and American Academy of Orthopedic Surgery (AAOS).[17] These recommendations have been extrapolated for use in dermatologic surgery.
- Presence of pacemaker, defibrillator, or other implantable devices (ie, cochlear implant, implantable medication pumps, etc) should be discussed. While modern pacemakers typically have override systems that prevent the disruption of their transmission during electrocautery, care should still be taken. It is not advisable to use prolonged electrosurgery directly over the pacemaker or lead wires, or in an area within 15 cm of the implanted device.[18]
- Electrocautery may be used in lieu of typical electrosurgery in such patients. Electrocautery seals small blood vessels using a heated wire and does not produce electrical currents or high-frequency electromagnetic interference. Bipolar electrocoagulation is another option for patients with implantable defibrillators, as the current is concentrated across the two terminal tips. This minimizes the distal dispersion of electricity and interference with implanted devices.[13] Electrocautery should also be considered in patients with other types of implantable devices to avoid interference or damage of the device.

Positioning

- Once the history has been completed, the ellipse should be marked and the site is verified with the patient. The ellipse should be designed such that the length of the ellipse runs parallel to skin tension lines, to minimize the amount of tension placed on the skin edges during closure (**FIGURE 1**). When designing the ellipse, the patient should be positioned in a way that allows the surgeon to examine the patient and properly evaluate the lines of skin tension (ie, if the lesion is on the back, the patient should be sitting upright or standing with their arms by their sides). Care should be taken to avoid design of an ellipse that crosses multiple cosmetic subunits, when possible, to improve final cosmesis (**FIGURE 2**).

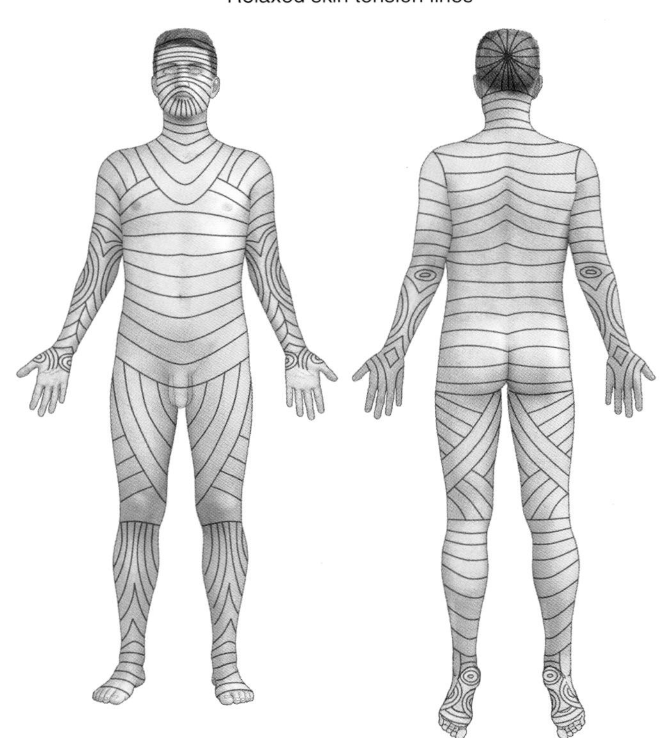

FIGURE 1 ● Relaxed skin tension lines. Langer's lines, or the relaxed skin tension lines of the skin should be kept in mind when orienting the direction of the fusiform ellipse.

- For the procedure, the patient should be placed in a position that allows the surgeon optimal access to the excision site. Ergonomics for the surgeon should be kept in mind during patient positioning to reduce the risk of work-related injury.[19] In a 2010 survey of 354 dermatologic surgeons by Liang and colleagues, 90% of surgeons reported musculoskeletal injury most commonly involving the neck, shoulder, and back, and over 50% of surgeons reported they worked through pain so as to not hinder work quality.[20] Chan et al proposed optimizing ergonomics of dermatologic surgery through modifications

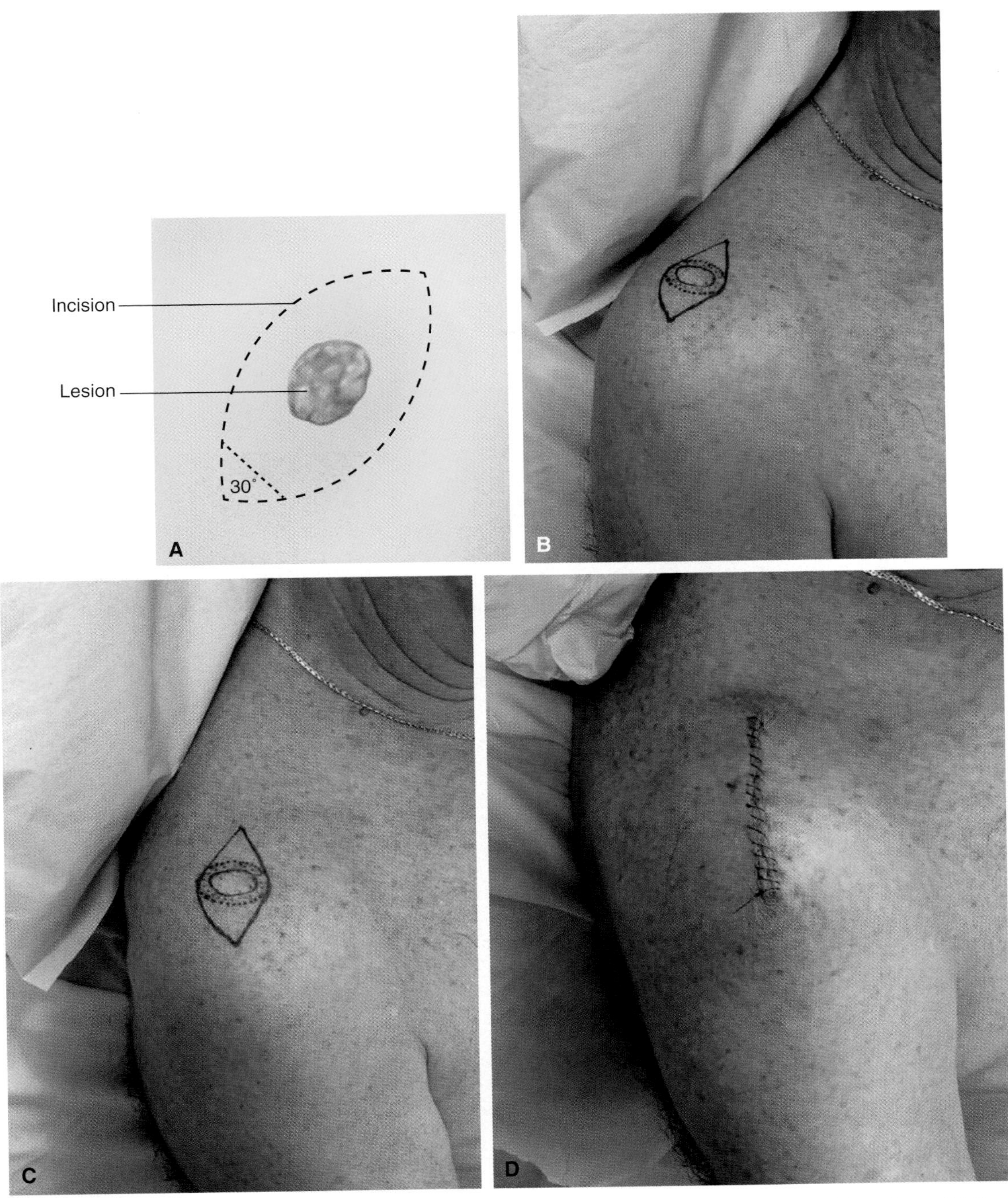

FIGURE 2 ● The fusiform or elliptical excision design. **A,** The fusiform design with a 3:1 length to width ratio and 30° angles at the apex. **B,** Intraoperative design of the elliptical excision, front view. **C,** Intraoperative design of the elliptical excision, lateral view. **D,** Postoperative, final epidermal running suture placement.

in treatment room layout and organization, instrumentation and work flow, patient positioning, and surgeon mechanics and posture.[21] Specifically, the patient should be positioned in a chair that allows the surgeon to maintain an upright posture with the spine and arms at a 90° angle between the spine and forearm, and with elbows close to the body throughout the procedure. Patients should be positioned as flat as tolerated in order to achieve a surgical plane that is parallel, rather than perpendicular, to the floor to optimize freedom of motion and neutral body position. Lights should be centered over the surgical table so they can be easily reached and repositioned to illuminate the desired surgical site with minimal shadow to optimize visualization. The use of compression socks and antifatigue mats can also help to reduce surgeon fatigue and musculoskeletal injury.

SKIN INCISION

- The skin should be incised with the scalpel blade placed at a 90° angle to the skin surface, in order to promote even skin approximation during suturing (**FIGURE 3**). Three-point counter tension should be applied to the surrounding skin as the scalpel breaches the skin. The incision should begin at the apex and extend to the opposite apex, and extend to the desired anatomic depth of excision.[22] Incising the skin with the scalpel blade at less or more than a 90° angle to the skin surface will create a beveled edge, which makes it more challenging to approximate the wound edges and which may lead to less-than-ideal cosmetic results (**Video 1**).
- Once the incision has been made to the desired depth, skin hooks or forceps can then be used to gently grasp the apex of the ellipse and lift the excision specimen to maintain counter tension. A consistent and even plane of dissection across the deep margin should be maintained as the ellipse is removed, either with a scalpel or scissors (**FIGURE 4**) (**Videos 1** and **2**). Once the excision specimen has been removed, hemostasis should be achieved by meticulously cauterizing any actively bleeding vessels. To facilitate tissue orientation, placement of marking sutures may be considered to allow the pathologist to describe the location of any positive margin.[23]

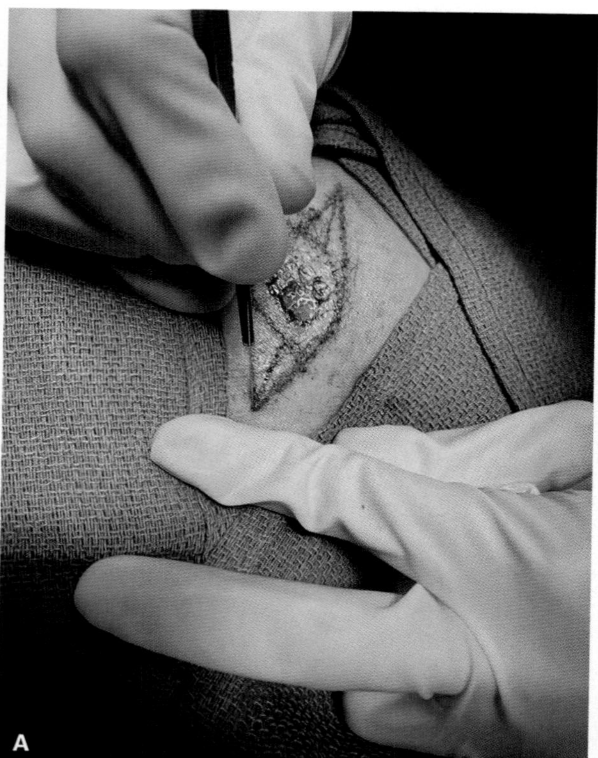

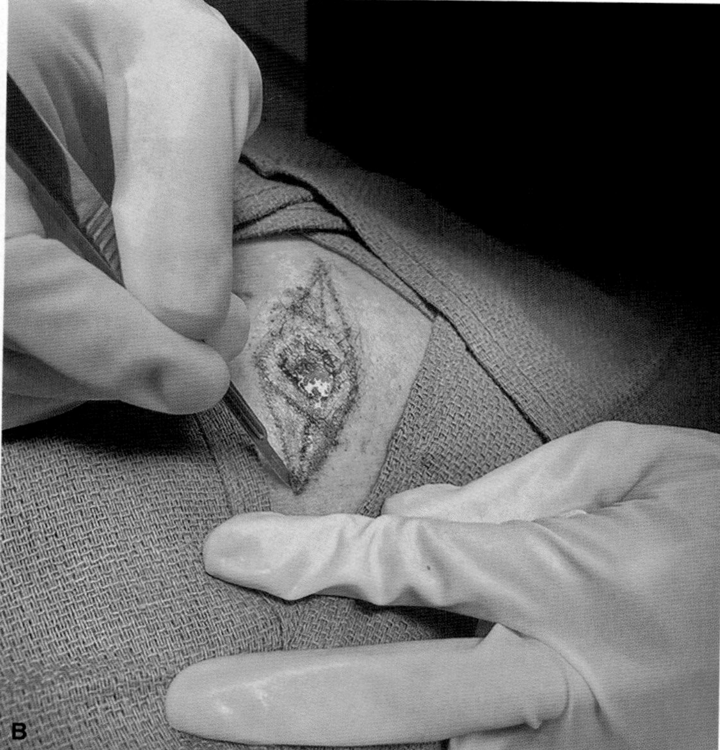

FIGURE 3 ● **A,** 90° approach to the skin incision vs **(B)** beveled skin incision.

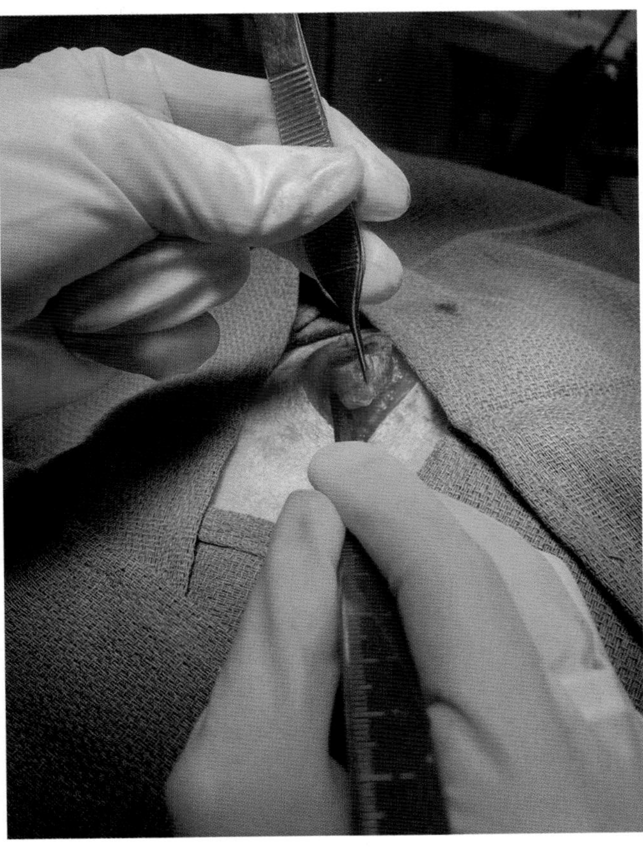

FIGURE 4 ● Removing the excision specimen.

CLOSURE

- The goal of side-to-side closure is precise wound edge approximation with eversion. Sharp or blunt undermining should be performed to facilitate sliding of the surrounding skin over the excision defect. The depth of undermining usually corresponds to the depth of tissue excised, and may vary by anatomic site.[22] For instance, the optimal undermining plane on the trunk or extremities for small or superficial defects is the mid-deep fat. The optimal undermining planes on the head and neck differ by cosmetic subunit. The mid subcutaneous plane should be used when on the cheek, temple, and forehead to avoid transecting branches of the facial nerve whereas excisions on the scalp should be undermined along the avascular subgaleal plane, which has the advantage of minimizing bleeding.
- Precise execution of skin cutting and undermining prepares the wound for placement of buried and superficial sutures.[24] The use of the buried vertical mattress suture decreases dead space, minimizes wound tension on the dermal and epidermal edges, and provides wound edge eversion if executed correctly.[25] The needle path should start at the bottom of the undermined edge of the wound, and peak at the mid dermis or papillary dermis a few millimeters from the wound edge (**FIGURE 5**). The needle should then be rotated downward slightly to exit at a slightly deeper depth in the reticular dermis. The arc of the needle should resemble the shape of a half heart loop. The mirror image loop should be completed on the opposing side by starting the needle's path in

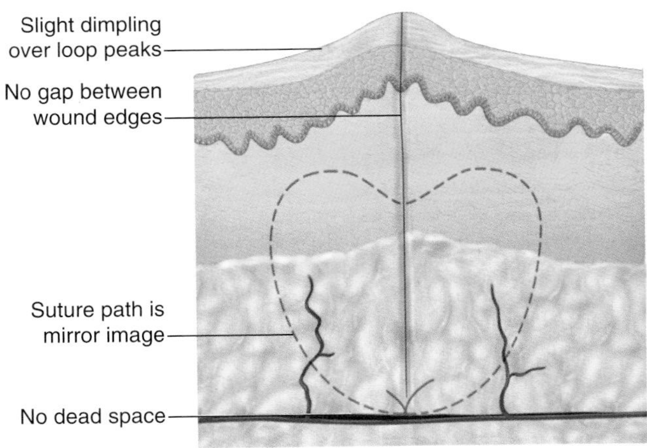

FIGURE 5 ● Placement of the vertical buried suture.

the reticular dermis with a slightly upwards angle allowing the path to peak a few millimeters from the cut edge. The needle should then be rotated to allow for exit at the base of the undermined skin edge. The final shape of the needle trajectory should be a heart-shaped loop, with the knot of the suture buried in the deep margin. Atraumatic handling of the skin during suture placement is imperative to achieve optimal cosmetic outcomes. This can be achieved by avoiding pinching the epidermal edges when guiding the needle into the skin if using tissue forceps. Retracting the skin edge

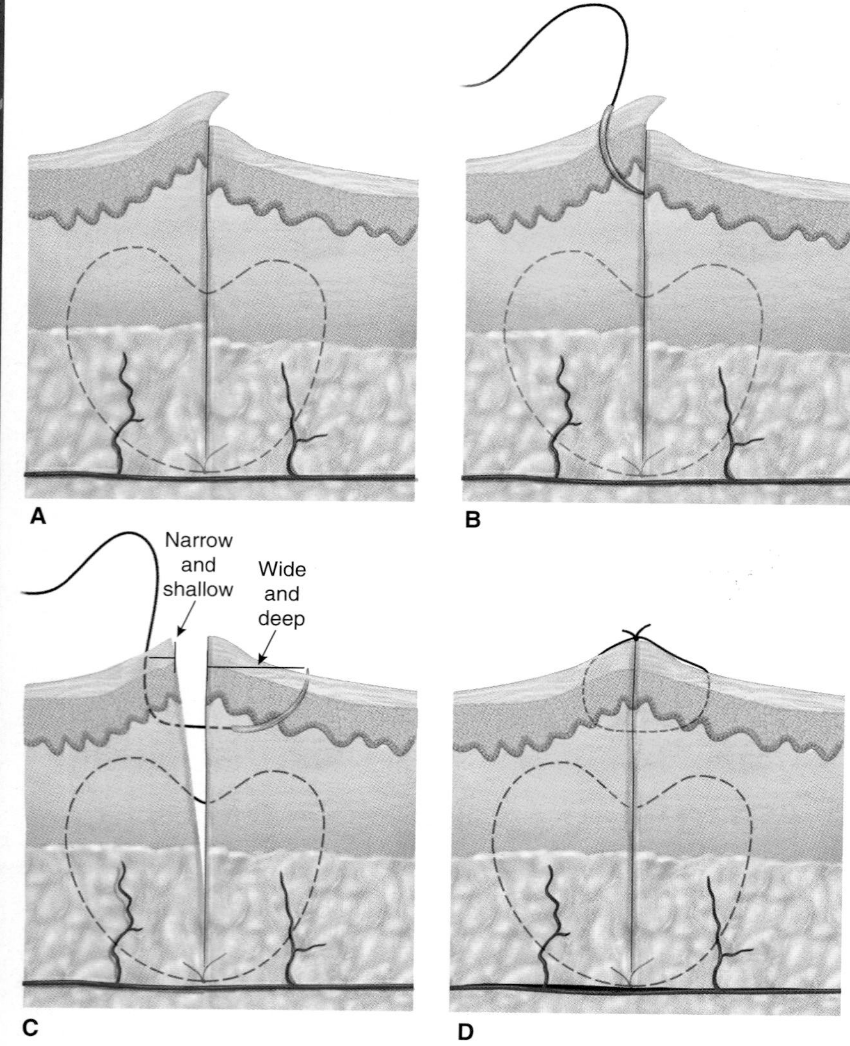

FIGURE 6 ● Placement of the epidermal suture to fix height discrepancy.

with one tooth of the forceps or a skin hook can also be used to avoid trauma at the epidermal edge that could impede wound healing[24] (**Videos 3** and **4**).

- Finally, the placement of epidermal sutures helps to precisely approximate the wound edges.[24] If a height discrepancy has been created by imperfect placement of the deep sutures, this may be corrected with well-placed epidermal sutures (**FIGURE 6**). The general rule is to "bite high on the high side and bite low on the low side."[24] The higher side of the wound should be approached with a shallow bite of the needle in the papillary dermis, closer to the wound edge. This wound edge should then be depressed to match the lower height of the opposite side of the wound. The needle should then enter the opposing lower side deeper and wider to achieve precise epidermal approximation and correct the height discrepancy.[24]

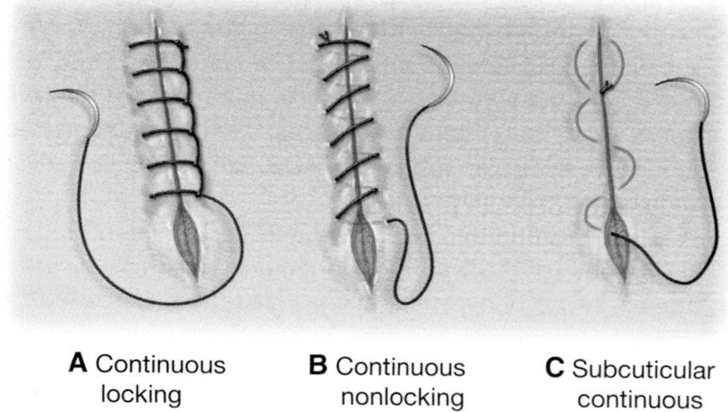

FIGURE 7 ● Epidermal suture types.

- Different epidermal suturing techniques may be used, though the simple running standard suture is most commonly used due to its ease of use and efficiency (**FIGURE 7**). Other techniques may be utilized for specific indications. For instance, a running interlocking suture may be used if additional hemostasis is needed. Horizontal mattress sutures may be used if additional wound eversion or hemostasis is desired. Running subcuticular sutures may also be used if there is additional concern about cosmesis. Though the width of the final scar does not vary significantly when compared to the simple running suture technique when used in dermatologic surgery, the running subcuticular suture eliminates the creation of track marks from exit and entry of the top suture through the surface of the skin.[26]
- Choice of suture type and needle size depends on the anatomical site of the excision. The most commonly used needle in dermatologic surgery is 3/8 circle reverse cutting needle (**TABLE 3**).

Table 3: Sutures Used by Site and Removal Time Frames

Site	Deep suture	Superficial suture	Removal
Face	4-0 or 5-0 polyglactin 910 or poliglecaprone 25	5-0 or 6-0 nylon, polypropylene, or fast gut	7-10 d
Neck	4-0 or 5-0 polyglactin 910 or poliglecaprone 25	5-0 or 6-0 nylon, polypropylene, or fast gut	7-10 d
Trunk and proximal extremities	3-0 or 4-0 polyglactin 910 or poliglecaprone 25	3-0 or 4-0 nylon or polypropylene	2-3 wk
Mucosa	None	5-0 silk or polyglactin 910	

Adapted from Bolognia J, Jorizzo JL, Schaffer JV, eds. Wound Closure Materials and Instruments. *4th ed.*

PEARLS AND PITFALLS

Indications	Excisional and incisional ellipse biopsies are techniques used for the diagnosis and management of benign and malignant lesions of the skin and subcutaneous tissues.
Orientation of ellipse	Consider placing the excision along relaxed skin tensions line or within cosmetic subunits. Keep in mind the orientation if a re-excision is required.
Excision technique	Use three-point counter tension when incising the skin at the apex. Incise the skin with the blade at a 90° angle to the skin surface to avoid beveling the edges. Use forceps to retract the specimen while excising at the desired anatomic plane.
Closure	Precise side-to-side closure with eversion can be achieved through placement of buried vertical mattress sutures. Ensure atraumatic handling of the skin. Placement of epidermal sutures can be used to approximate epidermal wound edges or correct height discrepancies.

POSTOPERATIVE CARE

- Pressure dressings (nonadherent dressing, dry gauze, and adhesive tape) are commonly used after skin surgery to prevent seroma or hematoma formation.[27] We apply Vaseline to the sutured area, then cover it with a nonadherent dressing and cotton balls, and adhere the aforementioned to the adjacent skin with several layers of stretchable adhesive tape. For extremities, we also apply a pressure wrap. We typically instruct patients to maintain the pressure bandage in place for 24 hours after surgery and to maintain the dressing dry during this time frame. Once the bandage is removed, patients are instructed to gently wash the sutured area with soap and water, taking care not to scrub the area vigorously or soak the site for prolonged periods of time. Vaseline should be applied to the wound daily to aid with wound healing and may be covered with a bandage until suture removal.
- We instruct patients to take care not to shave over the sutured site if located on hair-bearing skin.[28] We also discuss activity restrictions with patients to prevent wound dehiscence or hematoma formation. The restrictions include minimizing lifting objects heavier than 5 lb, refraining from cardiovascular exercise, and activities that would otherwise place excessive tension on the sutured excision site. The timing of suture removal depends on the location of the surgical site. Sutures on the face are generally removed 7 to 10 days after excision, while those on the trunk and extremities are typically removed 14 to 21 days after surgery.

COMPLICATIONS

- Complications may arise during the postoperative period. These include bleeding and hematoma formation, allergic reactions, and infection. Bleeding after the procedure can first be managed by applying direct pressure to the area for 20 to 30 minutes at a time, which usually stops minor bleeding. Formation of a hematoma or persistent subcutaneous bleeding that does not improve with manual pressure may require evacuation. Though this is a relatively rare scenario, cases where a hematoma is rapidly expanding may require removal of sutures, identification of active bleeding source, and meticulous hemostasis. Stable and nonexpanding hematomas may be decompressed by inserting an 18-gauge needle along the wound edge and draining the subcutaneous fluid. If the

Table 4: Proposed Risk Factors for Dermatologic Surgical Site Infection

Wound characteristics	Host factors	Body site	Complex surgery
Bacterial contamination	Immunosuppression Diabetes Smoking	Below the knee Nose and ear Mucosal site Groin	Prolonged procedure Flap on the nose Graft repair Wedge excision on the nose and ear

Adapted from: Harlan C, Nguyen N, Hirshburg J, Hirshburg JM. Updates on recommendations for prophylactic antibiotics in dermatologic surgery.[15]

hematoma is stable, nonexpanding, and does not cause excessive tension on the wound, it may be left to resorb on its own.

- Allergic contact dermatitis should be suspected in cases where pruritus, pseudo or frank vesiculation starts within 24 hours of the procedure, or sooner if the patient has been previously sensitized to the allergen. Typically, these early reactions are due to allergens from cleansers (ie, chlorhexidine, iodine) or other materials used intraoperatively. Erythema or vesiculation in a geometric configuration may also occur at later time points from a bandage or topical antibiotic used postoperatively. Management includes the prompt identification of the intraoperative or postoperative allergen, prompt removal if possible, and its future avoidance.
- Infections should be suspected with increasing warmth, tenderness, purulence, or wound induration that starts around 4 to 8 days postoperatively (**TABLE 4**). For cutaneous elliptical excisions, the risk of postoperative wound infection has consistently been found to be quite low at 1% to 3%. The most common organisms isolated from surgical wound infections include methicillin-susceptible *Staphylococcus aureus*.[29] If a surgical site infection develops, an empiric oral antibiotic course that covers methicillin-susceptible *S. aureus* or a first-generation cephalosporin, such as Cephalexin, is indicated. Wound cultures can be obtained to help guide further oral antibiotic management or in nonresponders to empiric therapy.[30] Intravenous antibiotics may be considered in patients with worsening systemic symptoms, in whom bacteremia is suspected, or in patients with an inability to tolerate oral antimicrobial therapies.

REFERENCES

1. Dunlavey E, Leshin B. The simple excision. *Dermatol Clin.* 1998;16(1):49-64.
2. Goldberg LH, Alam M. Elliptical excisions: variations and the eccentric parallelogram. *Arch Dermatol.* 2004;140(2):176-180.
3. Moody BR, McCarthy JE, Sengelmann RD. The apical angle: a mathematical analysis of the ellipse. *Dermatol Surg.* 2001;27(1):61-63.
4. Fan B, Neel VA, Yaroslavsky AN. Multimodal imaging for nonmelanoma skin cancer margin delineation. *Lasers Surg Med.* 2017;49(3):319-326.
5. Flores E, Yélamos O, Cordova M, et al. Peri-operative delineation of non-melanoma skin cancer margins in vivo with handheld reflectance confocal microscopy and video-mosaicking. *J Eur Acad Dermatol* Venereol. 2019;33(6):1084-1091.
6. Cinotti E, Belgrano V, Labeille B, et al. In vivo and ex vivo confocal microscopy for the evaluation of surgical margins of melanoma. *J Biophotonics.* 2020;13(11). doi:10.1002/jbio.202000179
7. Sweeney SM, Maloney ME. Pregnancy and dermatologic surgery. *Dermatol Clin.* 2006;24(2):205-214.
8. Strickler AG, Shah P, Bajaj S, et al. Preventing complications in dermatologic surgery: presurgical concerns. *J Am Acad Dermatol.* 2021;84(4):883-892.
9. Mock J, Kunk PR, Palkimas S, et al. Risk of major bleeding with ibrutinib. *Clin Lymphoma Myeloma Leuk.* 2018;18(11):755-761.
10. Parra CE, Newsom E, Lee EH, Allan JN, Minkis K. Association of ibrutinib treatment with bleeding complications in cutaneous surgery. *JAMA Dermatol.* 2017;153(10):1069-1070.
11. Lebas D, Preta LH, Leguern A, Modiano P, Wiart T. Haemorrhagic complications following ibrutinib intake after dermatological surgery. *Annales de Dermatologie et de Venereologie.* 2020;147(11):775-779.
12. Nagrebetsky A, Al-Samkari H, Davis NM, Kuter DJ, Wiener-Kronish JP. Perioperative thrombocytopenia: evidence, evaluation, and emerging therapies. *Br J Anaesth.* 2019;122(1):19-31.
13. Kaur RR, Glick J, Siegel D. Achieving hemostasis in dermatology - Part 1: preoperative, intraoperative, and postoperative management. *Indian Dermatol Online J.* 2013;4(2):77-81.
14. Fathi R, Serota M, Brown M. Identifying and managing local anesthetic allergy in dermatologic surgery. *Dermatol Surg.* 2016;42(2):147-156.
15. Harlan CA, Nguyen N, Hirshburg J, Hirshburg JM. Updates on recommendations for prophylactic antibiotics in dermatologic surgery. *Dermatol Surg.* 2021;47(2):298-300.
16. Bousquet J, Flahault A, Vandenplas O, et al. Natural rubber latex allergy among health care workers: a systematic review of the evidence. *J Allergy Clin Immunol.* 2006;118(2):447-454.
17. Surgeons AAoO. Recommendations for the Use of Intravenous Antibiotic Prophylaxis in Primary Total Joint Arthroplasty. https://aaos.org/globalassets/about/bylaws-library/information-statements/1027-recommendations-for-the-use-of-intravenous-antibiotic-prophylaxis-in-primary-total-joint-arthroplasy.pdf
18. Porres JM, Laviñeta E, Reviejo C, Brugada J. Application of a clinical magnet over implantable cardioverter defibrillators: is it safe and useful? *PACE.* 2008;31(12):1641-1645.
19. Bhatia AC, Xu S, Robinson JK. The need for ergonomics education in dermatology and dermatologic surgery: sit up straight, stand up tall, and carry a sharp scalpel. *JAMA Dermatol.* 2017;153(1):13-14.
20. Liang CA, Levine V, Dusza S, Hale E, Nehal KS. Musculoskeletal disorders and ergonomics in dermatologic surgery: a survey of Mohs surgeons in 2010. *Dermatol Surg.* 2012;38(2):240-248.
21. Chan J, Kim DJ, Kassira-Carley S, Rotunda AM, Lee PK. Ergonomics in dermatologic surgery: lessons learned across related specialties and opportunities for improvement. *Dermatol Surg.* 2020;46(6):763-772.
22. Miller CJ, Antunes MB, Sobanko JF. Surgical technique for optimal outcomes: part I. Cutting tissue: incising, excising, and undermining. *JAAD.* 2015;72(3):377-387.
23. Nantel-Battista M, Murray C. Dermatologic surgical pearls: enhancing the efficacy of the traditional elliptical excision. *J Cutan Med Surg.* 2015;19(3):287-290.
24. Miller CJ, Antunes MB, Sobanko JF. Surgical technique for optimal outcomes: part II. Repairing tissue: suturing. *JAAD.* 2015;72(3):389-402.
25. Kantor J. The set-back buried dermal suture: an alternative to the buried vertical mattress for layered wound closure. *JAAD.* 2010;62(2):351-353.
26. Alam M, Posten W, Martini MC, Wrone D, Rademaker AW. Aesthetic and functional efficacy of subcuticular running epidermal closures of the trunk and extremity: a rater-blinded randomized control trial. *JAMA Dermatol.* 2006;142(10):1272-1278.
27. Kontos M, Petrou A, Prassas E, et al. Pressure dressing in breast surgery: is this the solution for seroma formation? *J BUON.* 2008;13(1):65-67.
28. Elsaie M, Nouri K, Choudhary S. Side-to-side closure. In: Nouri K, ed. *Dermatologic Surgery: Step by Step.* Blackwell Publishing Ltd; 2013:Chapter 14.
29. National nosocomial infections surveillance (NNIS) system report, data summary from january 1992 through june 2004, issued october 2004. *Am J Infect Control.* 2004;32(8):470-485.
30. Stevens DL, Bisno AL, Chambers HF, et al. Practice guidelines for the diagnosis and management of skin and soft tissue infections: 2014 update by the infectious diseases society of America. *Clin Infect Dis.* 2014;59(2):e10-e52.

Chapter 28 Wide Excision of Primary Cutaneous Melanoma

Roi Weiser, Russell S. Berman, and Jeffrey E. Gershenwald

DEFINITION

- Wide excision (WE) of a primary cutaneous melanoma is the term used to describe the definitive surgical management of the primary melanoma site. It is defined as the surgical removal of the primary tumor and/or the biopsy site that includes a defined radial margin of normal-appearing skin and underlying subcutaneous tissue. The appropriate margin of resection is determined by the Breslow thickness of the primary tumor as discussed in this chapter.
- Depending on primary tumor characteristics and clinical nodal status, WE may be performed concomitantly with either intraoperative lymphatic mapping and sentinel lymph node biopsy (SNB) (for patients with clinically negative nodes and a primary tumor suggesting sufficient risk of occult regional node metastasis) or regional lymphadenectomy (for patients with clinically involved regional lymph nodes without distant metastasis)[1] (refer to Part 5, Chapters 33-38, 39 and 40).
- The main goal of the WE is to remove the primary tumor along with any nearby microscopic melanoma cells, thereby minimizing the risk of local recurrence. In addition to following oncologic principles, the surgeon should also aim to simultaneously minimize dysfunction or disfigurement. This procedure is also known as a wide local excision.

DIFFERENTIAL DIAGNOSIS

- A WE should not be performed unless a definitive pathological diagnosis of melanoma has been obtained.

PATIENT HISTORY AND PHYSICAL FINDINGS

- A patient with newly diagnosed melanoma should undergo a comprehensive history that includes assessment of age, gender, personal or family history of melanoma, or other malignancy as well as history of any nevus syndromes. The patient should also be assessed for any other significant medical and surgical history or issues, medications used, and allergies.
- History of sun exposure and use of tanning beds, if any, should also be obtained. A thorough history may also provide clinical clues as to the extent of disease present at diagnosis. Symptoms such as worsening headaches or abdominal cramps may suggest distant metastatic disease and warrant additional workup.
- A physical examination is extremely important in the newly diagnosed melanoma patient. If a biopsy has been performed, the anatomic site and orientation of the biopsy should be documented along with the presence or absence of any residual pigmented lesion.
- It is imperative to confirm the specific site(s) of any primary melanoma to be treated. Although this may seem obvious, many patients have had concomitant and/or prior skin biopsies, and further clarification with source information, including prebiopsy photographs and/or direct consultation with the referring clinician, may be necessary. Because biopsy sites may heal prior to treatment, photographic images are ideally obtained to document location(s) of all biopsy sites for which treatment is/may be planned. This will facilitate future identification by the surgeon prior to excision, as well as by nuclear medicine personnel to facilitate proper radiotracer injection during lymphoscintigraphy. This documentation is particularly relevant in the emerging era of neoadjuvant therapy. This strategy is currently focused largely on patients with clinically positive regional disease, some of whom may have been diagnosed in the setting of concomitant primary tumor. Neoadjuvant therapy can result in complete tumor regression; as such, in addition to photographic documentation, some clinicians may choose to tattoo the location of the primary tumor.
- Skin and soft tissue between the primary site and draining regional nodal basin(s) should be examined for any signs of satellite or in-transit metastases. Melanoma most commonly metastasizes via regional lymphatics to regional lymph nodes. Nonetheless, because melanoma may metastasize to both regional and distant nodes, all accessible lymph node basins should be carefully examined in the new melanoma patient, including cervical, supraclavicular, axillary, epitrochlear, inguinal, and popliteal nodes. For patients with a melanoma in a region of ambiguous drainage (typically considered to be the head and neck and trunk regions), drainage to multiple nodal basins is possible. Given the importance of the lymphatics in melanoma, meticulous attention to the lymphatic examination is essential. Evidence of lymphedema in the melanoma-bearing extremity should also be noted, as it may also suggest regional nodal disease and/or a vascular issue.
- The clinician should document the presence of any lymphadenopathy along with details such as firm, fixed, or matted nodes. Clinically suspicious lymph nodes should be evaluated by fine needle aspiration and/or core needle biopsy (often performed with ultrasound guidance) and cytological and/or pathological analysis. In patients where the ability to palpate lymph nodes is limited due to body habitus, as well as patients with clinically negative lymph nodes but whose primary tumors have high-risk features, an ultrasound of the potential lymphatic basins can be performed, with biopsy of any suspicious nodes. Biopsy-proven regional metastasis renders a SNB procedure unnecessary to diagnose stage III disease in the involved basin.
- Importantly, palpable "reactive" lymphadenopathy may sometimes develop following biopsy of the primary melanoma, thus highlighting the importance of pathological confirmation of metastatic melanoma before definitive treatment of the basin with lymphadenectomy or neoadjuvant systemic treatment is considered.

- Newly diagnosed melanoma patients should also undergo a head-to-toe skin examination to identify the presence of other suspicious skin lesions. Although it is beyond the scope of this section to review biopsy techniques in detail, an appropriate biopsy should include the epidermis, dermis, and at least a cuff of subdermal fat. This allows the dermatopathologist to accurately report the essential components of primary melanoma tumor histopathological microstaging, discussed later in the chapter.
- When signs and/or symptoms are suggestive of additional disease, a well-performed physical examination may raise suspicion for distant metastasis. Particular attention should be paid to the neurologic examination, assessing for any localizing symptoms or mental status changes. The finding of hepatomegaly, abdominal mass, or a rectal examination significant for mass or occult blood should prompt further workup. Finally, distant dermal or subcutaneous nodules or distant adenopathy also warrant further investigation.

IMAGING AND OTHER DIAGNOSTIC STUDIES

- Treatment planning for patients with primary melanoma is based largely on primary tumor histologic microstaging.
- In the absence of symptoms, the use of imaging studies as part of a staging workup has not been shown to significantly impact survival or the treatment algorithm of the newly diagnosed, clinically node-negative, melanoma patient. For asymptomatic preoperative stages I and II melanoma patients, preoperative cross-sectional imaging has a very low yield.[2] In one study, out of 515 preoperative imaging studies conducted on stage IA-IIC patients, 132 of which were advanced imaging studies, only seven studies had suspicious findings. Notably, none of these findings were eventually proven to be melanoma, and there was no change to clinical management based on the preoperative imaging.[3] Nonetheless, some clinicians do chose to obtain preoperative cross-sectional imaging for patients with high-risk primary cutaneous melanomas.
- Among asymptomatic occult stage III patients (ie, sentinel node positive), cross-sectional imaging studies infrequently identify distant metastatic melanoma.[4] However, as more effective adjuvant systemic therapy has recently been approved for use in patients with stages II and III melanoma, and clinical trials are ongoing, use of cross-sectional imaging to exclude systemic metastases prior to initiation of adjuvant therapy is indicated; additional details regarding the utility of such imaging studies represent an area of ongoing study.
- Although positron emission tomography (PET)/computed tomography (CT) generally includes images of the extremities, regions not typically imaged during standard CT or magnetic resonance imaging (MRI), a benefit for routine use of PET/CT has yet to be demonstrated in this patient population.
- In the otherwise asymptomatic patient with clinically palpable adenopathy, the detection rate of asymptomatic distant metastasis is higher, approximating 4% to 16%, warranting baseline imaging for staging. Several studies have demonstrated a higher sensitivity and specificity for PET/CT, but current guidelines support the use of either PET/CT or CT chest/abdomen/pelvis, with the addition of a brain MRI for preoperative staging.[5,6]
- There is no specific tumor marker or biochemical parameter that has been validated and employed for melanoma screening or recurrence. Elevated serum lactate dehydrogenase (LDH) level is an adverse prognostic factor in patients with distant metastatic melanoma and is included in the American Joint Committee on Cancer (AJCC) eighth edition staging system for stage IV disease. Patients with or without elevated LDH levels are designated as (1) or (0) in the M category; for example, a patient with distant metastases to non-CNS visceral sites and an elevated LDH is categorized as M1c(1).[7,8]

SURGICAL MANAGEMENT

Preoperative Planning

Biopsies

- Most cutaneous lesions suspicious for melanoma have been biopsied by a dermatologist or other health care provider prior to treatment referral.
- If the biopsy of a lesion suspicious for melanoma has not yet been performed, the surgeon should plan and perform a biopsy to establish a definitive histologic diagnosis with appropriate microstaging of the lesion (if melanoma is confirmed), while optimizing the potential for primary closure of the subsequent WE (see Part 5, Chapter 27).
- An excisional biopsy should include a narrow 1 to 3 mm margin of normal-appearing skin around the suspicious lesion along with a cuff of underlying subcutaneous fat to provide the dermatopathologist with sufficient material to fully diagnose and, if melanoma, to histologically microstage the primary tumor.
- An excisional biopsy of the extremities is typically oriented parallel to the long axis of the extremity (**FIGURE 1**). On the trunk and head and neck, the orientation of the biopsy should ideally follow the lymphatic drainage of the involved skin while also being mindful of the lines of tension for optimal closure.
- Incisional biopsies are sometimes preferred for large lesions, especially in cosmetically sensitive areas. Such a biopsy approach does not always reflect the full microstaging of the lesion, including margin assessment, and such limitations need to be considered during definitive treatment planning.
- Superficial shave biopsies are not generally recommended when a cutaneous lesion is suspicious for melanoma, as the full extent of the lesion (especially Breslow thickness) may not be included in the biopsy, resulting in underestimation in microstaging. The American Academy of Dermatology distinguishes such superficial shave biopsies from deep shave biopsies or saucerization. The latter are the most common diagnostic technique used by dermatologists and usually extend to the deep reticular dermis, below the plane of the lesion.[9]
- In cases with a suboptimal biopsy (eg, shave with a positive deep biopsy margin), we do not recommend

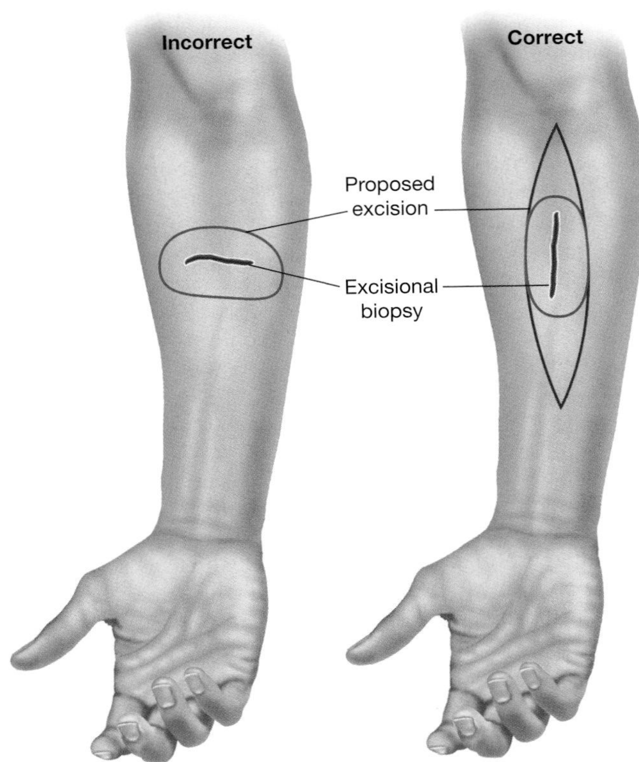

FIGURE 1 ● Importance of orientation of excisional biopsy. An excisional biopsy of the extremity is typically oriented parallel to the long axis of the extremity (right panel). In this example, incorrect orientation (left panel) would likely result in the need for skin graft closure, while primary closure could likely be achieved if the biopsy had been correctly orientated (right panel). Note that in the right panel example, the overall excision has been extended to accommodate primary closure. It is always important to consider next steps when performing a biopsy.

additional biopsy of the shave biopsy site solely based on the positive deep biopsy margin prior to surgical WE. If, however, there is significant intact residual pigmented component, an additional biopsy(ies) is/are generally reserved for infrequent clinical scenarios in which additional histopathological information of clinically suspicious findings would alter treatment planning, with a wider margin of excision, expanded appreciation of the extent of the primary tumor process, and/or recommendation for SNB.

- Confirmation of the melanoma biopsy site(s) must be performed prior to any planned definitive treatment.

Histopathological Microstaging of Primary Melanoma

- In order to determine the appropriate extent of surgery for a patient with a primary melanoma—including extent of WE margins and whether to recommend intraoperative lymphatic mapping and SNB—assessment of several of the primary tumor's histopathological features is essential.
- Breslow thickness (in millimeters), presence or absence of primary tumor ulceration, and the biopsy margin status (peripheral and deep margins) are all essential to define T category and to guide appropriate surgical therapy and should be assessed by a dermatopathologist. Additional primary tumor information that may be useful for the operating surgeon's treatment planning include the mitotic rate (expressed in mitoses/mm^2), the presence or absence of lymphovascular invasion, perineural invasion, microscopic satellitosis, regression, the extent of tumor-infiltrating lymphocytes, and histologic subtype.

Margins of Excision

- WE includes a radial margin of the skin and underlying subcutaneous tissue, with margins appropriate for tumor thickness.
- The radial margin chosen for the excision is based on the primary tumor (Breslow) thickness. At least six prospective randomized trials conducted over the past 3 decades informed an evidence-based approach. Although detailed discussion is beyond the scope of this section, the recommendations from the National Comprehensive Cancer Network (NCCN) for the radial margin are as follows, with recommended margins referring to margins measured by the surgeon from the edge of the biopsy and/or intact residual component at the time of surgery and not those measured on the specimen by the histopathologist[5]:
  - Melanoma in situ: 0.5 to 1 cm margin
    - Note: For large or poorly defined melanoma in situ, lentigo maligna or acral lentiginous subtypes, margins >0.5 cm may be considered to adequately treat occult early invasive disease.
  - Less than or equal to 1.0 mm tumor thickness (T1): 1.0 cm margin
  - Greater than 1.0 to 2.0 mm (T2): 1 to 2 cm margin
  - Greater than 2.0 to 4.0 mm (T3): 2 cm margin
  - Greater than 4.0 mm thickness (T4): 2 cm margin

Positioning

General Positioning Strategies

- Depending on primary tumor characteristics and other considerations, lymphatic mapping and SNB may be indicated. In such cases, every effort should be made to perform these procedures in conjunction with the WE of the primary tumor.[10] For this reason, proper patient positioning should account for both the location of the primary melanoma and the location(s) of draining regional nodal basins. This may become challenging when the primary melanoma drains to multiple nodal basins and/or to interval, ectopic, and/or in-transit sites. In addition, potential "shine through" from the primary tumor radiotracer injection site during SNB should be taken into account when considering the optimal operative positioning strategy for an individual patient.
- For patients with de novo stage III disease with clinically positive nodes, both regional node dissection and primary tumor WE are usually indicated, either initially or following neoadjuvant systemic therapy (the latter preferably in the context of a clinical trial). The surgeon should optimize positioning to accommodate concomitant operative procedures. Less frequent but similar situations include planned

synchronous resection of local and/or in-transit and/or regional node metastases.

- Intraoperative repositioning of the patient should be considered whenever concomitant excisions are not feasible without repositioning, or whenever operative quality would be compromised by attempting to excise multiple sites in a single position.
- Skin graft donor sites or other reconstructive issues must also be considered when positioning the patient.

Proximal Extremity

- For proximal upper extremity lesions, a supine position is generally appropriate for WE and SNB. For more posterior lesions near the shoulder, a modified supine position using a shoulder roll or a lateral decubitus position provides easy access for WE and closure, as well as to the axillary and cervical/supraclavicular nodal basins. The arm, prepped circumferentially, should be supported to prevent injury to the brachial plexus and/or shoulder.
- For proximal lower extremity lesions, the supine position provides excellent exposure of anterior or lateral sites, allowing both WE and SNB, and even groin dissection, when indicated. When the melanoma is on the posterior proximal leg or the buttock, the WE may be performed with the patient in the lateral or prone position. Pressure points need to be padded and axillary and chest rolls need to be appropriately positioned. Some surgeons are comfortable performing both WE and inguinal SNB in the lateral position; a potential advantage is that repositioning is not required. Alternately, SNB can be performed in the supine position, and the patient repositioned for the WE.

Distal Extremity

- In general, a supine position is appropriate for most distal extremity lesions. If SNB or lymph node dissection is also to be performed, access to the axillary, epitrochlear, and inguinal nodal basins is readily achieved. If a patient's melanoma drains to the popliteal nodal basin, then an alternative position other than the supine approach should be considered. Options include frog leg, lateral decubitus, and the prone position, with the position selected based on surgeon preference and patient characteristics. When a popliteal dissection is indicated, the prone position is most often used.
- Heel melanomas not only have the potential to drain to the popliteal basin but may also require specialized reconstructive approaches (eg, wound VAC device, rotational flaps, and/or vascularized free flaps). In this situation, use of a beanbag on the operating room table allows for repositioning as needed.

Truncal Sites

- When an SNB is performed with WE of a truncal melanoma, the possibility of multiple nodal basin drainage patterns must be considered when devising an operating room positioning strategy. A preoperative lymphoscintigraphy will demonstrate afferent lymphatic drainage patterns to major and/or unusually situated (eg, ectopic, interval) nodal basins. The preoperative lymphoscintigraphy should always be reviewed prior to the operation to inform operative positioning and overall operative strategy.
- For most anterior truncal melanomas (eg, chest and abdomen), the supine position allows for access to the primary lesion and draining regional nodal basins. For lateral truncal melanomas, ideal positioning for the WE may include placing the patient in a partial or formal lateral position (with appropriate padding and brachial plexus protection). This position also facilitates concomitant access to draining regional lymphatic basins.
- When performing a WE only (eg, for a thin melanoma without adverse risk features), back melanomas may be excised in the prone or lateral positions at the discretion of the surgeon. Appropriate padding and brachial plexus protection must be employed and airway protection is essential. If SNB is being performed in the same operative setting, the patient must be positioned to facilitate access to draining nodal basins, including multiple and/or unusually situated nodal basins. This can occasionally be achieved with a lateral decubitus position, but repositioning the patient after the SNB and before the WE might be necessary (**FIGURES 2** and **3**).

Head and Neck Sites

- Head and neck melanoma patients must also be carefully positioned with consideration of the WE, reconstructive requirements, and access to draining regional nodal basins if SNB is to be performed. Whether in a supine, prone, or lateral position, the head and neck must be appropriately supported and padded. Additionally, the airway, eyes, and ears must be protected.

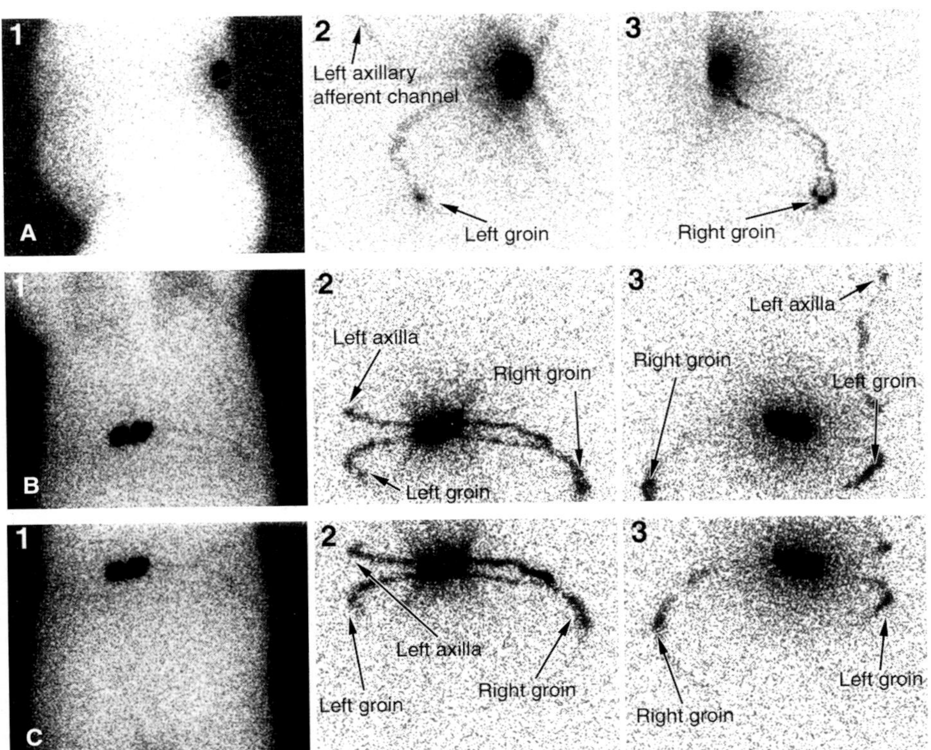

FIGURE 2 ● Lymphoscintigraphic images of a patient with a primary cutaneous melanoma of the midline mid back demonstrate radiotracer uptake activity in the bilateral groins and the left axilla. **(A)** Lateral views, **(B)** AP and PA views, superior aspect, **(C)** AP and PA views, inferior aspect.

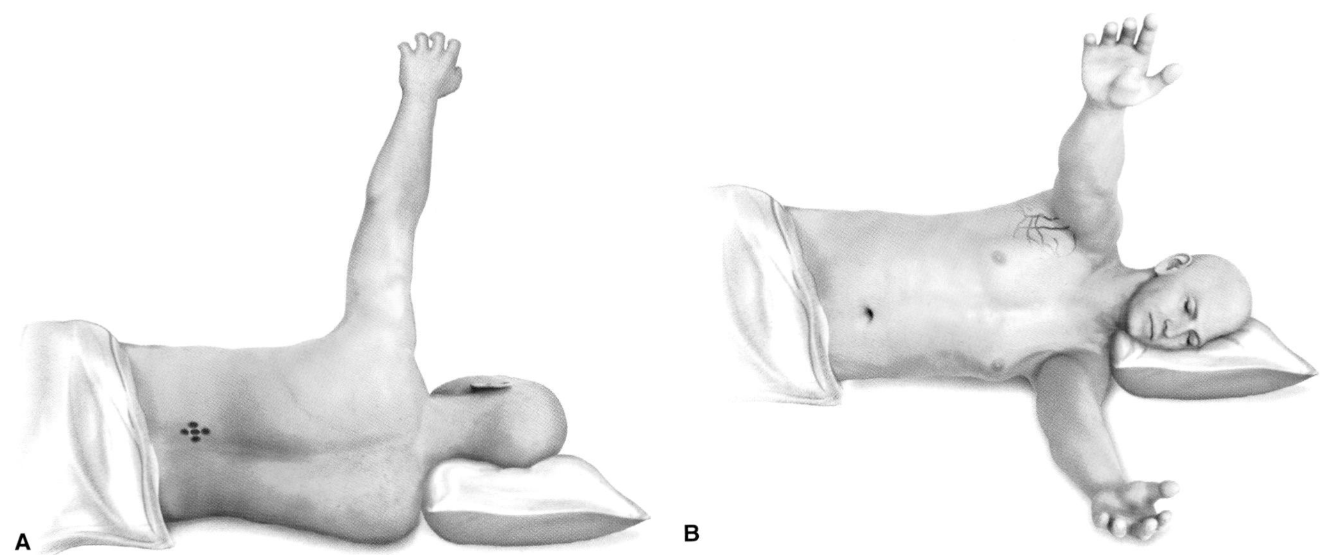

FIGURE 3 ● Example of an operative positioning strategy for patient with the midline melanoma of the mid back undergoing wide excision and lymphatic mapping and sentinel node biopsy in the same operative procedure. (Note lymphoscintigraphic drainage to the bilateral groin regions and left axilla as shown in **FIGURE 2**.) Due to radiotracer "shine through" from the primary injection site in the midline back, the patient was placed in the lateral decubitus position to address both the left axillary drainage and primary tumor site (midline back) **(A** and **B)**. The patient was then repositioned to supine to perform bilateral inguinal sentinel node biopsies **(C)**. Note that if radiotracer shine through was not a problem, then the patient could have been initially positioned in the supine position (after intradermal injection of both isosulfan blue dye and radiocolloid around the mid back lesion) to address the bilateral inguinal nodal basins as well as left axillary nodal basin and then repositioned into the lateral decubitus position to perform the wide excision of the back melanoma. Regardless of the approach, it is important to scan regions between primary tumor and draining nodal basin(s) with the gamma probe.

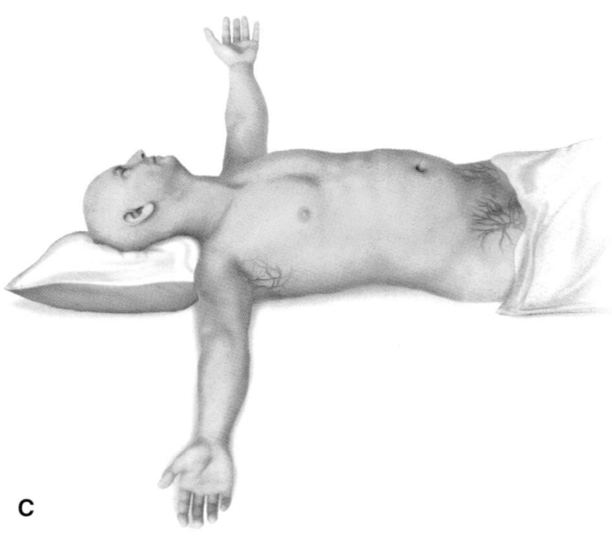

FIGURE 3 ● Continued

WIDE EXCISION MARGIN

- The planned margin of excision of the primary melanoma is based on the Breslow tumor thickness as described earlier and refers to the radial margin of normal-appearing skin to be resected. If the primary melanoma is entirely or partially intact, the margin should be measured from the periphery of the visible lesion. When the entire pigmented lesion has been excised by the previous biopsy, the margin should be measured from the periphery of the biopsy scar.

PLACEMENT AND ORIENTATION OF INCISION

- Proper planning of the incision is critical. The surgeon must consider the required radial margin (ie, margin of excision), the specific anatomic primary site involved, and the quality and quantity of local soft tissue.
- Because the resulting final incision may be significantly longer than what the patient might have otherwise anticipated, based on the usually "small" biopsy site, we strongly recommend that this theme be integrated into the surgical consultation and preoperative visits: a "scale" drawing presented to the patient at the time of initial and/or preoperative visit is often very instructive.
- The recommended margins of excision generally produce a circular or oval defect that is marked on the skin (**FIGURE 4A** and **B**). When a primary closure is planned, the circle or oval can be modified into an ellipse prior to WE to improve cosmetic outcome and facilitate primary closure (**FIGURE 5**).

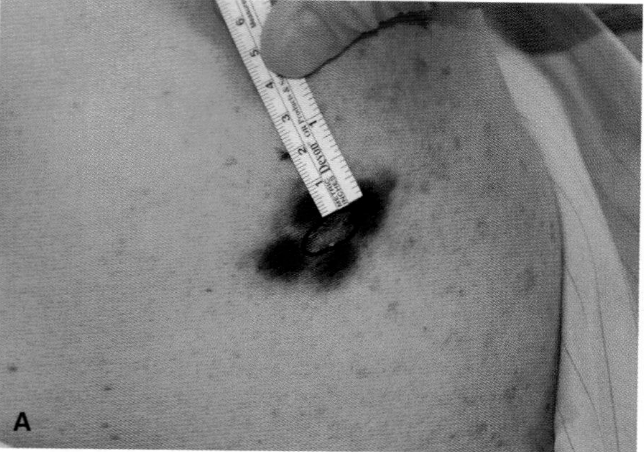

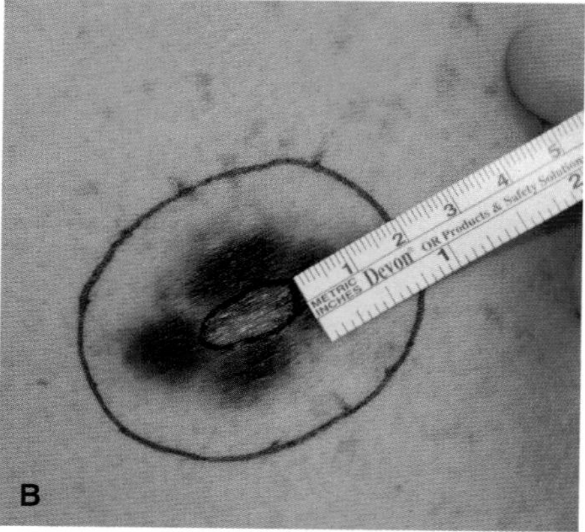

FIGURE 4 ● **A** and **B**, In this example, the patient has already been injected with both Tc-99 sulfur colloid and isosulfan blue intradermally around the biopsy site for a lymphatic mapping and sentinel biopsy procedure at the time of wide excision in the same operative setting. The recommended margin of excision is based on primary tumor thickness and is measured from either the edge of the intact melanoma or biopsy scar, generally resulting in the proposed circular or oval defect marked on the skin.

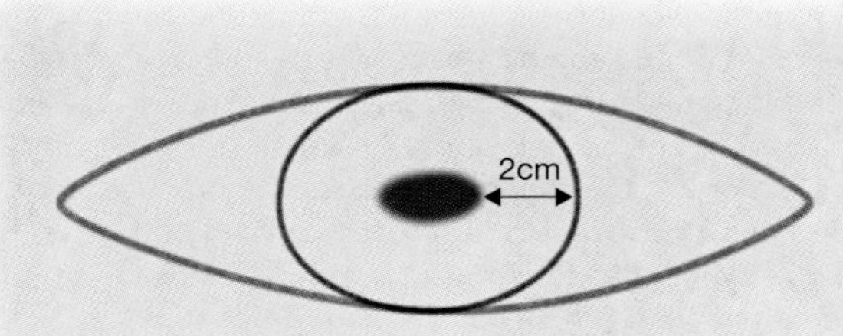

FIGURE 5 ● When a primary closure is planned, the circle or oval is generally fashioned into an ellipse prior to wide excision to improve cosmetic outcome and facilitate primary closure.

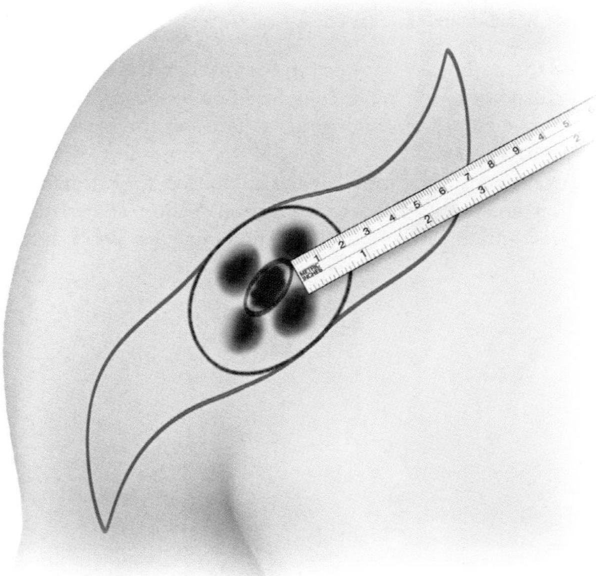

FIGURE 6 ● Depending on the lines of tension of the skin, a modified ellipse such as lazy S or hurricane-type incision may facilitate closure.

Excision of an ellipse of tissue results in a more gradual transition in wound contour and minimizes "dog ears" at the poles of the incision.

- Creation of an ellipse approximately three times as long as it is wide has often been recommended in textbooks; cosmetically acceptable closure can often be achieved with a smaller ratio and should be individualized.
- Alternatively, tissue that may contribute to dog ears can be resected after the oncologic portion of the WE. Depending on the lines of tension of the skin, a modified ellipse such as lazy S or hurricane-type incision (**FIGURE 6**) may facilitate closure, generally as triangular-shaped segments of the skin and underlying subcutaneous tissue are excised.
- When feasible, the incision should be oriented to facilitate primary closure. On the extremities, for example, the WE incision is usually oriented parallel to the long axis of the limb. This facilitates primary closure, results in greater excision of lymphatics that are at risk for melanoma tumor cell emboli, and may decrease subsequent lymphedema.
- Specific considerations by primary site:
  - Breast: Primary cutaneous melanoma of the skin of the breast should be managed with similar principles as cutaneous melanoma elsewhere. A mastectomy is not required to achieve oncologic control.
  - Hand, foot, and digits: General margin guidelines for cutaneous melanoma should be followed and consideration for preservation of function should be maximized. As a general principle, it is not usually necessary to remove bone to obtain oncologic control of the primary melanoma. However, amputation is usually necessary if standard WE for subungual or distal digit invasive cutaneous melanoma leaves insufficient soft tissue to maintain a functional digit without partial phalanx bony resection (see Part 5, Chapter 31). Phalanx-preserving approaches can sometimes be employed for distal digit/subungual melanoma in situ. For webspace lesions, phalanx preservation can also often be achieved.
- Perianal skin melanomas should be treated as cutaneous melanomas.

SKIN INCISION

- The skin incision is typically made with a no. 10 or 15 blade scalpel, initially to the level of the deep dermis. The remainder of the dermis can be divided either using the electrocautery on cutting mode or by using a scalpel. Care is required to avoid cautery to the skin edges, as this may result in wound healing issues.
- The excision continues by deepening the initial incision into the subcutaneous tissue to the level of the muscular fascia; care must be taken to maintain an angle of attack through the subcutaneous tissue that is perpendicular to the skin surface. The actual depth of excision will vary according to the anatomic location of the primary melanoma. It is rarely necessary to include fascia with WE, as it does not decrease the rate of local recurrence[5,11]; an exception is when prior surgery at the site included or abutted the fascia such that clear margin cannot be achieved or in the uncommon clinical scenario of obvious tumor involvement at the fascia.
- The surgeon should be aware of superficial (subcutaneous) motor nerves (eg, superficial peroneal or spinal accessory nerves). This is especially true for head and neck cases, particularly when a neck dissection is required. In such cases, a minimal use of paralytic agents should be discussed with the anesthesia team to ensure preservation of nerve function and facilitate detection in the operative field.

EXCISION OF SPECIMEN

- Once the depth of the resection has reached the underlying muscular fascia, the WE is completed by dissecting skin and soft tissue from the underlying fascia using the electrocautery (**FIGURE 7**).
- WE specimens are almost always submitted for permanent section analysis; intraoperative frozen section analysis is a rare exception. When reconstruction may be significantly impacted by an involved margin, "rush" permanent pathology (turnaround about 24-48 h) may be coordinated with the pathology team (see also "Delayed Wound Closure" in this chapter).
- It is important to properly document the orientation of the specimen prior to submitting for pathological assessment in the event that final margins are involved and an additional resection (usually as a separate operative procedure) is required (**FIGURE 8**).

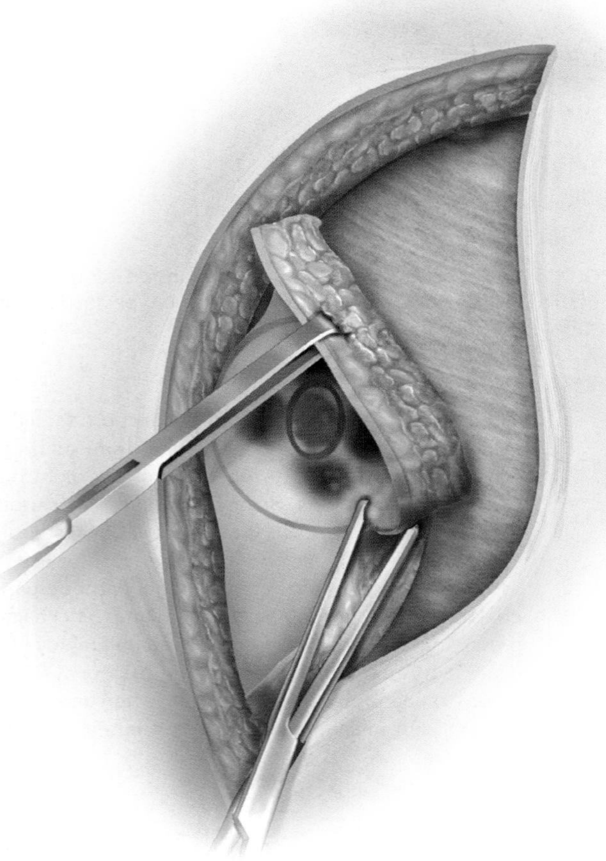

FIGURE 7 ● The depth of wide excision down to the muscular fascia is demonstrated. Once this depth is reached, the skin and soft tissue are dissected off the underlying fascia, completing the wide excision.

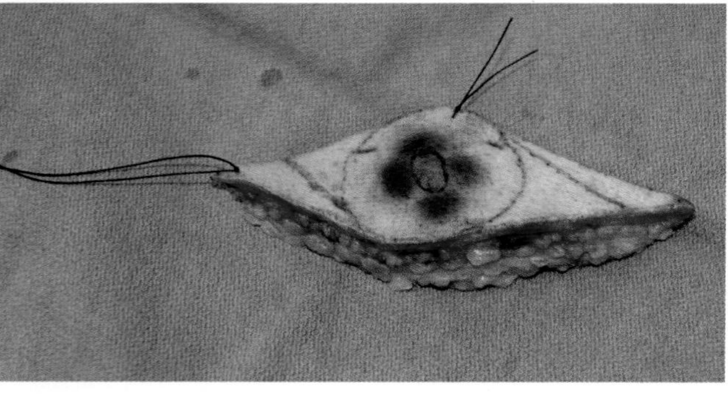

FIGURE 8 ● The resected specimen is carefully oriented to ensure accurate margin assessment by the pathologist. It is also important to orient in such a fashion that reexcision of involved margins can be accurately mapped back to the patient.

CLOSURE

- The majority of 1-cm margin defects and many 2-cm margin defects can be closed primarily. Recruitment of adjacent tissue by fashioning local flaps often facilitates primary closure and is dependent on the primary tumor location, margin, and the laxity of adjacent skin. Surgical defects may often be closed by mobilizing tissue flaps that have been created by undermining in a suprafascial plane and include full-thickness skin and underlying subcutaneous fat (**FIGURE 9A** and **B**).
- Complex closure of a WE defect involves placement of one or two layers of deep absorbable sutures (**FIGURE 10**), followed by placement of an intradermal layer of a buried absorbable suture. Skin closure can be carried out using a number of techniques, depending on the tissue tension, anatomic location, mobility, and surgeon preference. A subcuticular skin closure may be performed using an absorbable monofilament suture or a nonabsorbable pull-through suture that requires removal. Interrupted or running nonabsorbable sutures or skin staples may also be used as per surgeon preference (**FIGURE 11**). Dermal adhesives or adhesive bands may be used to directly cover the skin.

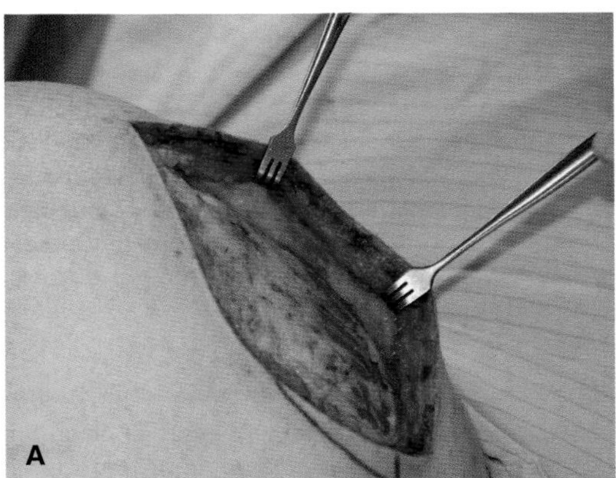

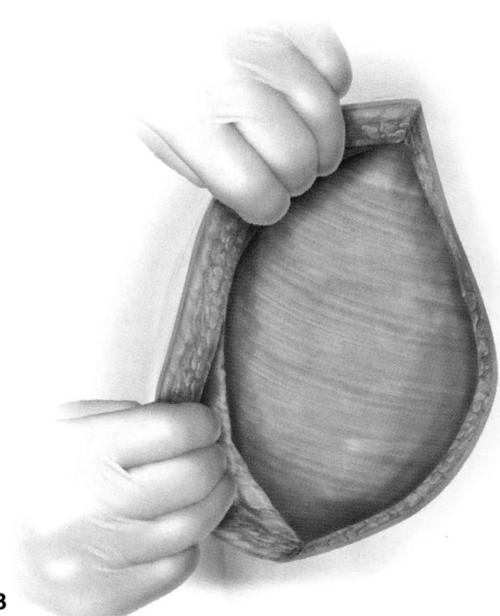

FIGURE 9 ● Photo **(A)** and illustration **(B)** demonstrating the mobilization of tissue flaps by undermining the full thickness of skin and subcutaneous fat at a level just superficial to the muscular fascia.

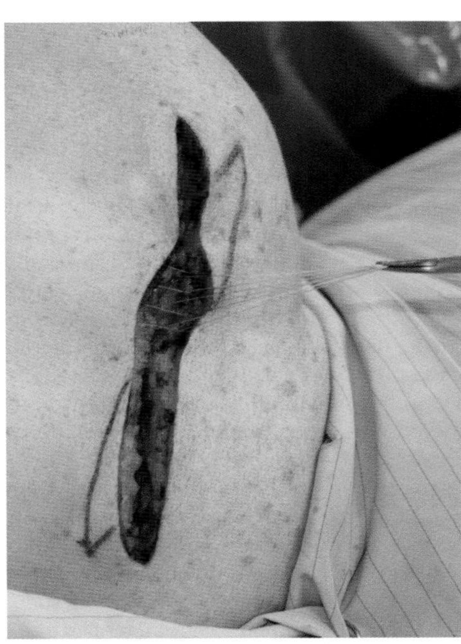

FIGURE 10 ● Photo demonstrating placement of deep absorbable sutures to facilitate complex primary closure of a wide excision. Typically one or two layers of deep absorbable sutures are used.

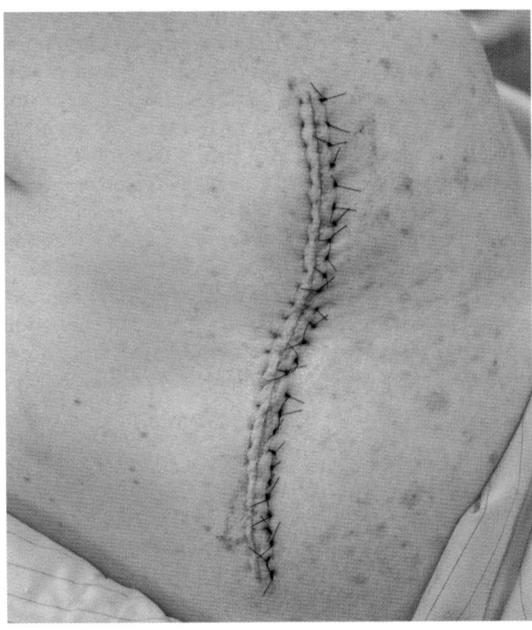

FIGURE 11 ● After reapproximation of deep layer(s), the skin may be closed using a number of different techniques and sutures depending on location, tension, and surgeon preference. In this photograph, interrupted vertical mattress sutures were used.

- At the discretion of the surgeon, closed suction drainage may be used when extensive undermining or large flaps is necessary or when considerable dead space persists after layered closure. If a drain is used, the exit site should generally be placed in line with the incision so that any potential recurrence can be reexcised without jeopardizing subsequent wound closure. Alternatively, suture plication of the more superficial tissue to the underlying fascia may sometimes be used and obviate the need for drainage, even when larger flaps are used.

RECONSTRUCTION

- When primary closure is not feasible, consideration should be given to skin grafts or local tissue flaps. The advantage of a skin graft is that it is a relatively straightforward procedure that minimizes adjacent tissue manipulation, allows for easy long-term monitoring of the primary melanoma site, and does not disrupt lymphatic drainage pathways. Skin grafts, however, are insensate, provide little protection to underlying tissue, and may result in a more pronounced contour defect. Furthermore, compared to local tissue flaps, skin grafts may result in more disfigurement and prolonged healing, as well as a longer need for distal extremity immobilization in a splint to prevent premature movement (eg, supination or pronation) that can otherwise result in suboptimal graft take due to shearing of the graft. Skin grafts are discussed in detail in Part 5, Chapter 30.
- Typically, split-thickness skin grafts are harvested from the posterior or proximal lateral thigh. Of note, when a lower extremity melanoma requires a skin graft closure, the graft should be harvested from the contralateral extremity.
- Full-thickness skin grafts can be harvested from multiple locations, allowing for better skin color and texture matching to skin adjacent to the melanoma excision. Full-thickness skin grafts may be harvested from the inguinal groin crease, the lower neck region overlying the clavicle, or behind the ear. After an appropriately sized ellipse of skin is excised down into the subcutaneous fat, the donor site is primarily closed, resulting in less morbidity than the typical split-thickness skin graft donor site. The full-thickness harvested skin is defatted and secured in place as a skin graft.
- The decision to proceed with a local tissue or rotational flap should be made after careful consideration of the features of the local tumor, including risk of satellite or in-transit metastases, the potential benefit to the patient from the functional and cosmetic perspective, the comorbidities of the patient, and the local tissue options available. The advantages of local flaps include durable, sensate, similar thickness, and textured skin. Disadvantages include rearrangement of regional soft tissue at risk for in-transit/satellite metastatic disease. Advancement and rotational flaps are discussed in detail in Part 5, Chapter 29.

DELAYED WOUND CLOSURE

- The majority of WE defects are closed or reconstructed during the same operation as the WE. There are circumstances, however, when delayed reconstruction is the most appropriate course of action. These situations include cases where accurate margin assessment is needed prior to reconstruction, either due to the complexity of the reconstruction and the potential adverse impact on cosmesis or functionality of a reexcision, or due to the large diameter or poorly defined nature of the melanoma, where margins are clinically equivocal at time of WE. Unlike its common use for assessment of margins for nonmelanoma skin cancer, intraoperative frozen section margin assessment for melanoma has been shown to be inaccurate compared to standard paraffin-embedded sections, and therefore it is infrequently employed for intraoperative margin assessment of primary melanoma WE.[12]
- Delayed reconstruction may also be beneficial when time is needed for a granulation bed to form in order to facilitate grafting, such as after excision of a heel melanoma where skin grafting onto a granulating bed is often performed in such a fashion (**FIGURE 12**).
- When wound closure is delayed, options for wound coverage include temporary wound dressings with routine dressing changes or a vacuum-assisted sponge dressing device (eg, vacuum-assisted closure [VAC] device). VAC devices are sometimes not available until negative margins are confirmed.
- In these situations, a request for rush permanent pathology of the WE specimen may be coordinated in advance with the pathology team, thus facilitating advance surgical planning (often at 48 h postoperative) both in terms of operating room space and collaboration with the reconstructive team. In such cases, a temporary occlusive dressing is often used to protect the WE site until final margins are available.

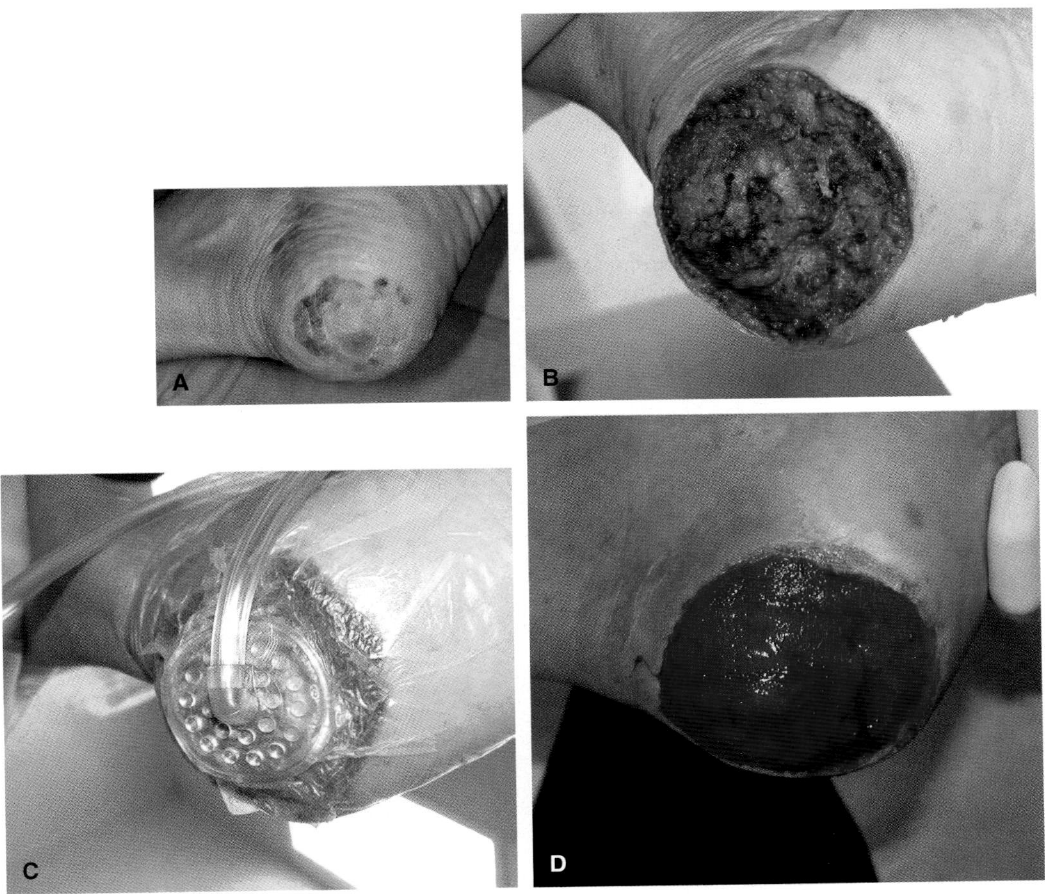

FIGURE 12 ● Photographs demonstrating use of delayed reconstruction for a large heel melanoma **(A)**. Upon completion of the wide excision **(B)**, a vacuum-assisted sponge dressing device is placed intraoperatively **(C)**. The recipient granulation bed, shown here after use of a vacuum-assisted device for approximately 3 weeks, is now optimized for skin grafting **(D)**.

PEARLS AND PITFALLS

Preoperative strategies	■ Orientation of biopsy is important whenever performed. ■ Photo documentation of the biopsy site is critical for subsequent site confirmation by the surgical team, and if lymphoscintigraphy is performed, by nuclear medicine personnel, to ensure that the correct site is addressed. ■ Complete history and physical examination is essential to identify additional suspicious primary lesions as well as potential sites of in-transit metastasis, satellites, and clinical nodal disease.
Operative positioning	■ Pad all pressure points. ■ Include potential interval and/or in-transit drainage sites within operative field, if SNB is to be performed. ■ Do not harvest skin grafts from in-transit region (ie, between primary tumor and draining nodal basin); as a practical approach, it is generally not prudent to harvest skin grafts from ipsilateral extremity.
Placement of incision	■ Extremities: Incision is generally oriented parallel to the long axis of extremity. ■ Always consider reconstructive options when placing and planning incision for WE. ■ Use radial margins appropriate for tumor thickness. ■ Be aware of superficial (subcutaneous) motor nerves (eg, superficial peroneal and portion of spinal accessory).
Intraoperative considerations	■ Excision should be performed up to, but not including, the underlying muscular fascia, unless the fascia itself is involved with tumor or the prior biopsy procedure. ■ Maintain perpendicular orientation through subcutaneous tissue. ■ Frozen section margin analysis is unreliable and rarely employed for primary melanoma WE. ■ Proper orientation of WE specimen is essential to facilitate reexcision of involved margins when necessary.
Closure	■ Consider overall risks of locoregional and other metastases with any extensive reconstruction option employed. ■ Consider closing dead space where appropriate to reduce likelihood of seroma formation.

POSTOPERATIVE CARE

- Specific postoperative care is dependent on the type of closure, the use of absorbable or permanent suture material, the extent of tension on the wound, and the presence or absence of a drain.
- In general, the patient can shower in 24 to 48 h unless skin grafts are used.
- Drains (if used) usually stay in place until collected volumes remain 30 mL or less for two consecutive days.
- Specific restrictions may apply depending on anatomic location (eg, restrictions on weight bearing for melanomas on the plantar surface of foot) and type of closure (eg, skin graft).
- Progressive increase in activity, weight bearing, and lifting over a 4- to 6-week period is recommended.

OUTCOMES

- After an appropriate WE based on tumor thickness, true local melanoma recurrences are uncommon and likely represent lymphatic tumor emboli. Some "local recurrences" are a result of an incompletely or inadequately excised primary melanoma.
- Functional outcome is critical and early use of physical therapy is encouraged when appropriate.

COMPLICATIONS

- Infection (cellulitis or abscess)
- Seroma
- Hematoma/bleeding
- Wound dehiscence or separation
- Failure of take of skin graft or flap
- Poor functional or cosmetic outcome
- Numbness and/or hyperesthesia and/or pain
- Edema/lymphedema

REFERENCES

1. Gershenwald JE, Ross MI. Sentinel-lymph-node biopsy for cutaneous melanoma. *N Engl J Med*. 2011;364(18):1738-1745. doi:10.1056/NEJMct1002967
2. Sabel MS, Wong SL. Review of evidence-based support for pretreatment imaging in melanoma. *J Natl Compr Canc Netw*. 2009;7(3):281-289. doi:10.6004/jnccn.2009.0021.
3. Haddad D, Garvey EM, Mihalik L, Pockaj BA, Gray RJ, Wasif N. Preoperative imaging for early-stage cutaneous melanoma: predictors, usage, and utility at a single institution. *Am J Surg*. 2013;206(6):979-985; discussion 985-986. doi:10.1016/j.amjsurg.2013.08.017
4. Aloia TA, Gershenwald JE, Andtbacka RH, et al. Utility of computed tomography and magnetic resonance imaging staging before completion lymphadenectomy in patients with sentinel lymph node-positive melanoma. *J Clin Oncol*. 2006;24(18):2858-2865. doi:10.1200/JCO.2006.05.6176
5. National Comprehensive Cancer Network. NCCN Guidelines Version 3.2022. Cutaneous Melanoma. Accessed May 26, 2022. https://www.nccn.org/professionals/physician_gls/pdf/cutaneous_melanoma.pdf
6. Xing Y, Bronstein Y, Ross MI, et al. Contemporary diagnostic imaging modalities for the staging and surveillance of melanoma patients: a meta-analysis. *J Natl Cancer Inst*. 2011;103(2):129-142. doi:10.1093/jnci/djq455
7. Gershenwald JE, Scolyer RA, Hess KR, et al. Melanoma staging: evidence-based changes in the American Joint Committee on Cancer eighth edition cancer staging manual. *CA Cancer J Clin*. 2017;67(6):472-492. doi:10.3322/caac.21409
8. Gershenwald JE, Scolyer RA, Hess KR, et al. Melanoma of the skin. In: Amin A, Edge SB, Greene FL, et al., eds. *AJCC Cancer Staging Manual*. 8th ed. Springer; 2017:563-585.
9. Swetter SM, Tsao H, Bichakjian CK, et al. Guidelines of care for the management of primary cutaneous melanoma. *J Am Acad Dermatol*. 2019;80(1):208-250. doi:10.1016/j.jaad.2018.08.055
10. Gannon CJ, Rousseau DL, Ross MI, et al. Accuracy of lymphatic mapping and sentinel lymph node biopsy after previous wide local excision in patients with primary melanoma. *Cancer*. 2006;107(11):2647-2652. doi:10.1002/cncr.22320
11. Grotz TE, Glorioso JM, Pockaj BA, Harmsen WS, Jakub JW. Preservation of the deep muscular fascia and locoregional control in melanoma. *Surgery*. 2013;153(4):535-541. doi:10.1016/j.surg.2012.09.009
12. Prieto VG, Argenyi ZB, Barnhill RL, et al. Are en face frozen sections accurate for diagnosing margin status in melanocytic lesions? *Am J Clin Pathol*. 2003;120(2):203-208. doi:10.1309/J1Q0-V35E-UTMV-R193

Chapter 29 Advancement and Rotational Flaps

Jeffrey H. Kozlow

DEFINITION

- Advancement and rotational flaps are tissue transfer techniques used in reconstructive surgery for the closure of acquired defects.
- A flap is an area of tissue designed for movement to another area while remaining vascularized. This is in contrast to a graft, which is transferred in a nonvascularized fashion and becomes revascularized only with local incorporation and vascular neogenesis.
- Advancement and rotation flaps are both considered local flaps because they borrow from the tissue adjacent to the defect. Distant flaps use tissue from areas away from the defect, and free flaps involve the transfer of tissue from a distant site by means of a microsurgical anastomosis.
- Local flaps can be defined by their vascularity. Random flaps are based on blood flow through the subdermal plexus to provide vascularity to the distal end of the flap (**FIGURE 1**). Axial flaps are based on a longitudinal blood vessel incorporated into the flap design that can extend the effective length of a flap (**FIGURE 2**). Perforator flaps are based on underlying septocutaneous or musculocutaneous perforators into the central area of the flap (**FIGURE 3**).
- Local flaps can also be defined by the geometry of the incisions used with example of common designs shown in the following text.
- Flap design includes evaluation of tissue laxity, optimization of scar position, and management of standing cutaneous deformities.

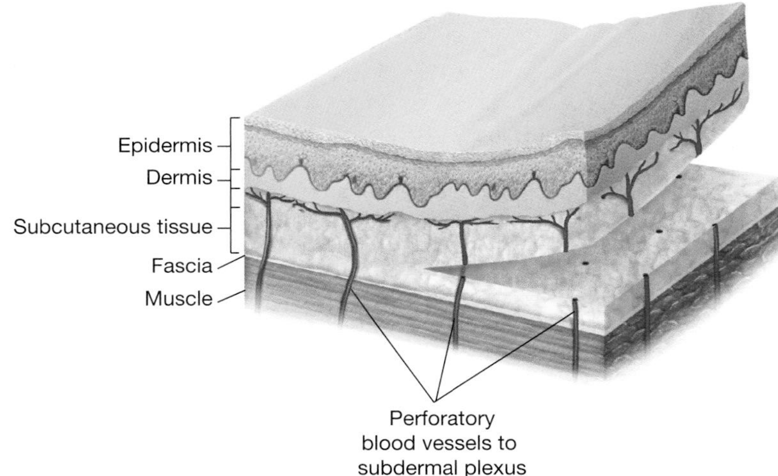

FIGURE 1 • Demonstration of a "random" pattern flap based on the subdermal plexus—the distal aspect of the flap remains vascularized through the small vessels running underneath the dermis only. As the length of the flap increases, the blood flow through the subdermal plexus decreases.

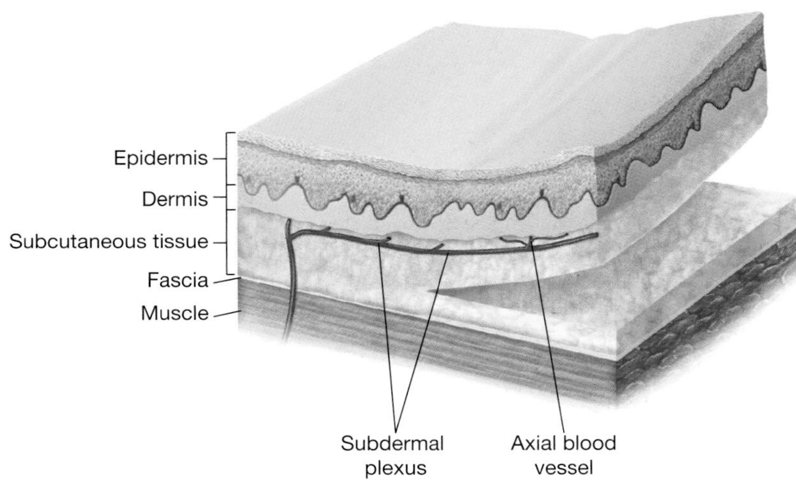

FIGURE 2 • Demonstration of an axial pattern flap—the flap design incorporates a named arterial supply along the length of the flap, which increases perfusion to the distal aspect of the flap compared with a random pattern flap.

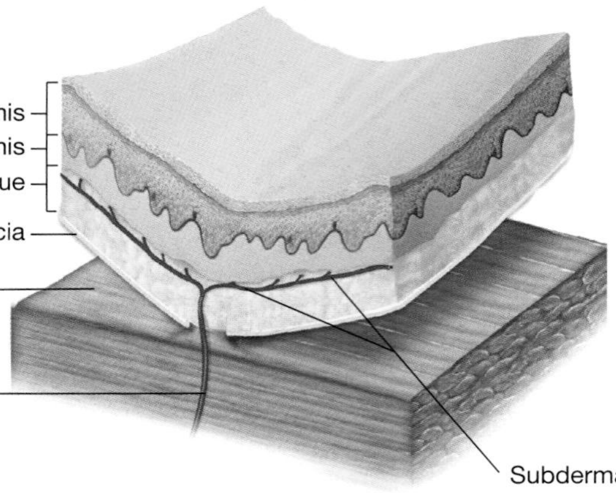

FIGURE 3 ● Demonstration of a perforator-based flap—the flap is centered on a single blood vessel, which perforates through the fascial layer from the underlying muscle or muscular septa to then supply the subdermal plexus.

PATIENT HISTORY AND PHYSICAL FINDINGS

- The choice and design of local flaps is dependent on multiple factors including the region on the body for reconstruction, local and regional soft tissue laxity, relationships with underlying critical anatomy, relaxed lines of skin tension for scarring, and underlying flap vascularity.
- Poor quality of tissue adjacent to the defect may preclude the use of local flaps.
- Local radiation damage will often limit the pliability of tissues for transfer and inhibit the healing potential of tissue.
- Each patient is different, and flap choice must be tailored to the individual, the size of the defect, and the location of the defect.
- There are often multiple different flaps that will adequately reconstruct a defect; there is no "one right answer" for any given case.
- Flap design should also consider potential oncologic implications including the need for recurrence monitoring, secondary reconstruction techniques, and margin management when reconstruction is done immediately after resection and margin status cannot be confirmed.
- For patients with lower extremity defects, an evaluation of arterial status and venous insufficiency should be considered.

IMAGING AND OTHER DIAGNOSTIC STUDIES

- In general, local flaps do not require preoperative imaging or diagnostic studies.
- Doppler can be used to identify either axial or perforating blood vessels if clinically indicated.

SURGICAL MANAGEMENT

Preoperative Planning

- A reconstructive plan can only be made after the resection is designed. In cases that may require a plastic and reconstructive surgeon for advanced reconstructive techniques, it is always best to plan accordingly ahead of time and not consult intraoperatively.
- Preoperative markings may include important regional anatomic landmarks (such as facial rhytids) that may be obscured with the injection of local anesthetic intraoperatively.

Positioning

- Patients should be positioned to optimize not only surgical access for tumor resection but also for access to any local areas potentially usable for the subsequent reconstruction.
- All areas should be prepped widely to allow for access to all local and regional flap options. All extremities should be prepped and draped circumferentially. For areas where symmetry is important (such as the face or breasts), it is important to have the contralateral side in the operative field as well.

TECHNIQUES

- There are multiple local flaps that are available for use in reconstruction. Not all of them can be highlighted in this text; however, the most common flaps for general reconstruction are described in the following text. In some cases, multiple local flaps are required and techniques can be combined to achieve closure of the defect.
- In most flaps, the area is often infiltrated with local anesthesia including 1:100,000 to 1:200,000 parts epinephrine to help with hemostasis and minimize electrocautery injury to dermal edges. However, overinjection of local anesthesia can result in tissue edema that decreases flap mobility.
- Skin hooks are used on the margins of a flap for handling; the use of forceps is discouraged due to injury to the flap edges from overzealous pressure.
- Drains are typically not used unless flaps are large.
- Flaps designed around joints should be inset under the greatest tension of the joint to avoid postoperative dehiscence.

SIMPLE ADVANCEMENT FLAPS

Flap Design

- Flap design is either based on the subdermal plexus as a vascular supply from the base of the flap to the distal end or can include an axial vessel for additional length and degrees of freedom.
- Incisions are designed in a parallel fashion equal to the dimensions of the defect (**FIGURES 4** and **5A**); choice of direction is based on local tissue laxity.
- Classic teaching is that a maximum 3:1 ratio of length to width can be used when the flap is based on the subdermal plexus.

Flap Elevation

- Incisions are made extending from the defect in a parallel fashion toward base of flap.
- Dissection is carried down to the depth of defect or deeper in order to match volumetric dimensions of reconstruction.
- The central portion of the flap is undermined either in the deep subcutaneous level or below the fascia, depending on flap design and reliance on subdermal only vs axial-based blood supply (**FIGURES 4** and **5B**).

Defect Closure

- Careful hemostasis is assured after flap elevation; hematomas under the flap can compromise vascularity and overall outcome.
- Once the flap has adequate advancement to fill the defect, closure often occurs from the base of the flap to help "push" the flap into the defect, which can help alleviate tension over the distal closure (**FIGURE 4C**).
- Standing cutaneous deformities can occur as the base is advanced. These areas can be resected with a scar perpendicular to the direction of the flap.
- Dermal closure is performed using an absorbable suture followed by either a subcuticular or simple external suture (**FIGURE 5C**).

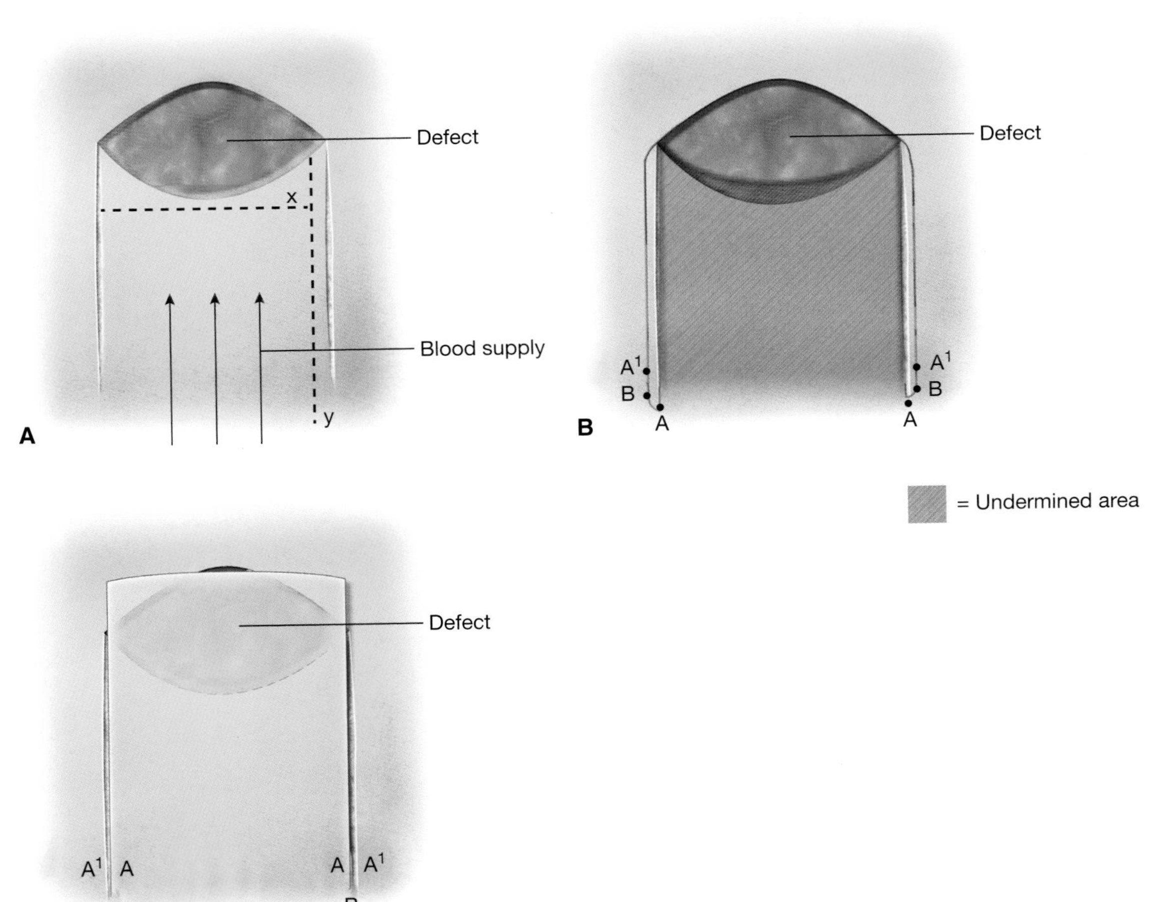

FIGURE 4 ● The design of an advancement flap is based on subdermal blood supply from the base of the flap. The initial parallel incisions are drawn from the wound edges **(A)**. The advancement flap is undermined toward the base, leaving only the subdermal blood supply to vascularize the distal tip **(B)**. The flap is then advanced forward and pushed into the defect. The previous base corner of the flap (point *A*) has been pushed forward and is approximated to point *A*¹ **(C)**.

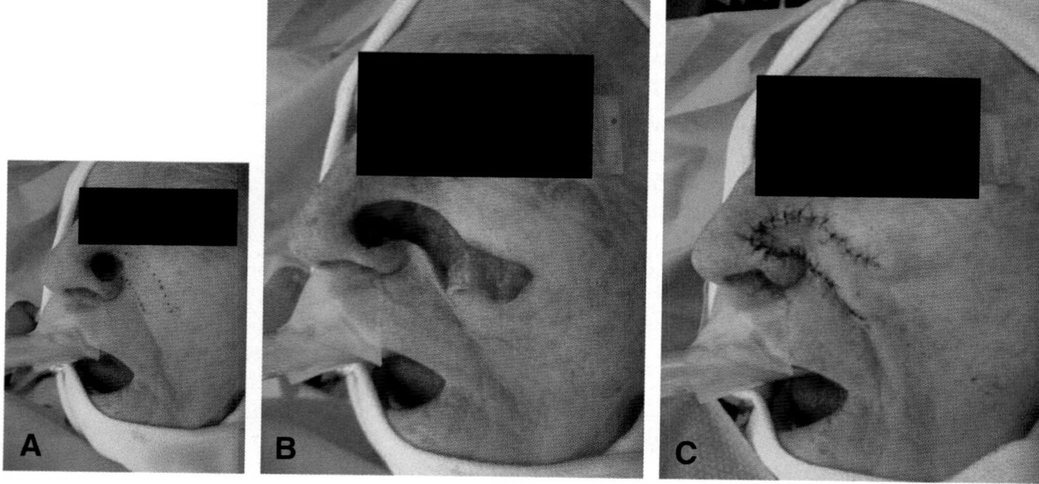

FIGURE 5 ● **A,** In this case, an axial-based advancement flap for nasal reconstruction is designed to incorporate the angular artery for additional length. This undermining is seen in **(B)** as the flap is fold back toward its base prior to advancement. The final advancement and closure of the advancement flap is demonstrated in **(C)**.

ROTATIONAL/TRANSPOSITION FLAPS

Flap Design

- Designed as a semicircle extending from one corner of the defect (**FIGURES 6** and **7A**).
- The direction and orientation of the flap is based on local areas of laxity.
- Based on a pivot point at the "base" of the flap that determines the amount of rotation available.

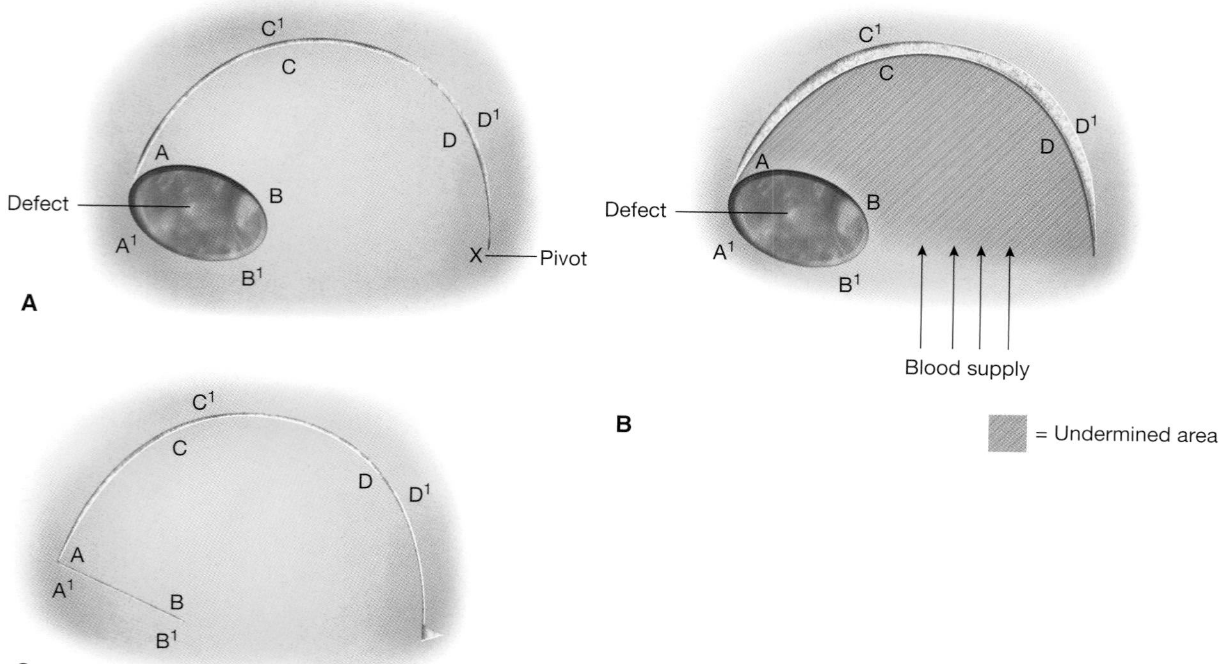

FIGURE 6 ● The semicircular markings for a rotation flap are demonstrated. The subsequent advancement of the flap is demonstrated by the movement of points *A*, *B*, *C*, and *D* to *A*¹, *B*¹, *C*¹, and *D*¹, respectively **(A)**. The rotation flap is undermined back toward the base leaving the distal portion of the tissue perfused through the subdermal plexus. Additional back-cuts across the base should be done judicious to not compromise vascularity of the flap **(B)**. The rotation flap is rotated into the defect for closure. The movement of the flap relative to the adjacent skin is noted by the changed alignment of the *C* and *D* marks to the *C*¹ and *D*¹ marks, respectively. **C,** A small standing cutaneous deformity at the base of the flap may require excision.

Flap Elevation

- Incision is made through the skin and subcutaneous tissues to the depth of the defect or greater.
- The flap is undermined in the same or deeper plane up to the base (**FIGURE 6B**).
- Careful hemostasis is assured in the undermined area to avoid a hematoma that may compromise the flap.

Defect Closure

- The flap is advanced and rotated into the defect with closure often starting at the base of the defect to help push and rotate the flap into the defect (**FIGURE 6C**).
- Dermal closure is performed using an absorbable suture followed by either a subcuticular or simple external suture (**FIGURE 7B**).
- Excision of standing cutaneous deformities should be away from the base of the flap to avoid decreasing flap vascularity.

Additional Designs

- Multiple variations in flap design are commonly used but based on the same principle as earlier. For example,
  - A bilobed flap uses two adjacent rotation/transposition flaps. The flap directly adjacent to the defect is used to close the primary defect and the other flap is then used to close the donor site for the first flap (**FIGURE 8A-C**).
  - A rhomboid flap is designed along the longer edge of a defect and transposes skin from an area of laxity to the defect, allowing for primary closure of the donor site (**FIGURE 9A-C**).

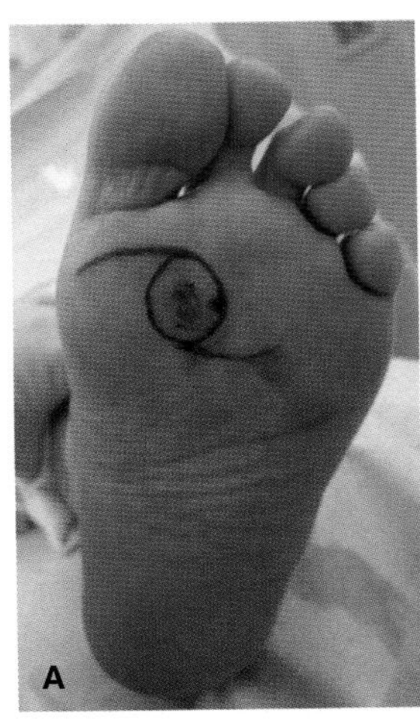

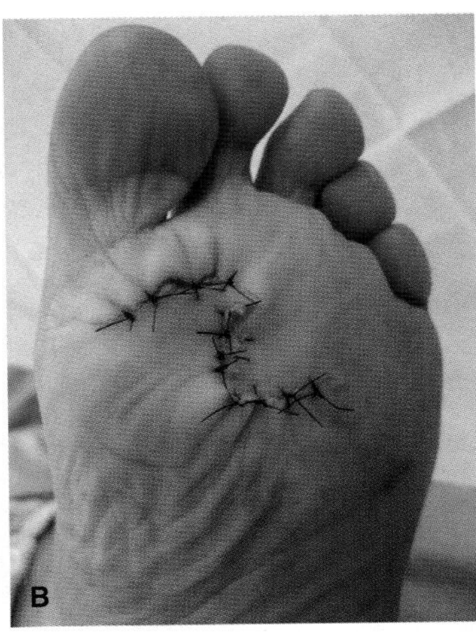

FIGURE 7 ● **A,** In this clinical case, opposing advancement flaps have been designed for reconstruction of a plantar foot wound. **B,** In this case, the opposing flaps have both been advanced to reconstruct the defect.

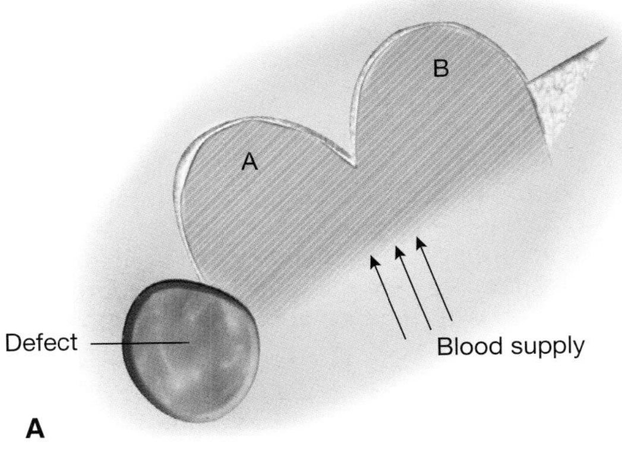

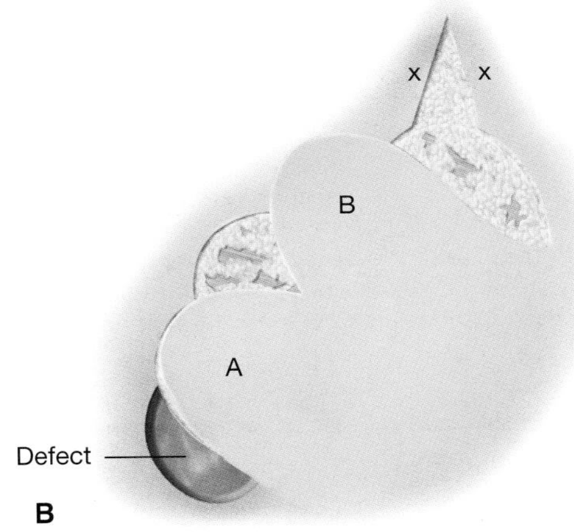

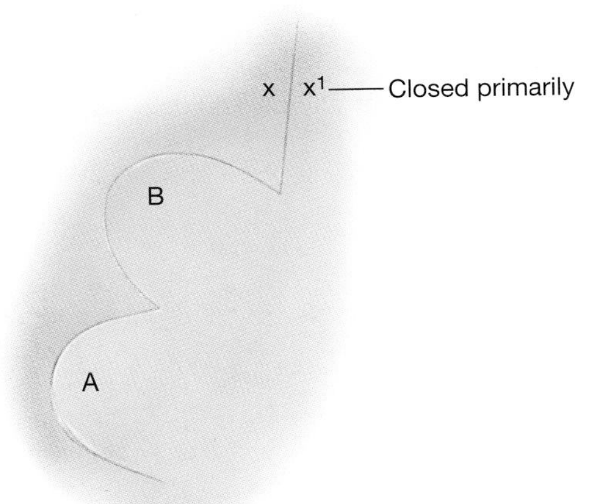

FIGURE 8 ● The bilobed flap uses two rotation-transposition flaps for closure of a defect. **A,** *Flap A* is used to close the primary defect and *flap B* is used to close the donor site from *flap A*. **B,** The flap is elevated in the subcutaneous tissues leaving blood supply from the subdermal plexus at the base of both "lobes" of the flap. **C,** The flaps are then transposed with primary closure of the donor site for *flap B* by reapproximation of *x* to x^1.

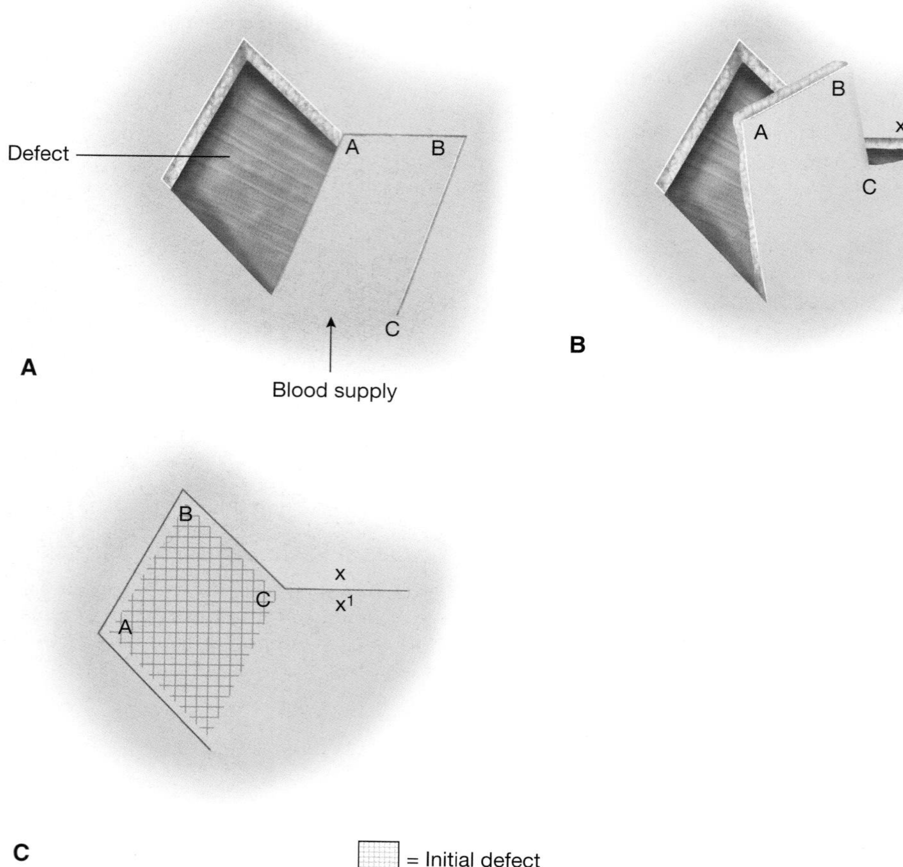

FIGURE 9 ● The rhomboid flap is another variation on the rotation-transposition flap and works well with elliptical or rhomboid-shaped defects. The flap is designed off the "oblique" angle of the defect directly perpendicular to the defect. An additional incision designed parallel to the side of the defect is used to create a mirror image of the defect through the shared border of the flap and the defect **(A)**. The flap is then elevated in the subcutaneous tissues leaving blood supply from the subdermal plexus **(B)**. The flap is then rotated and transposed to fill the defect with the flap donor site closed primarily with approximation of x to x^1 **(C)**.

V-Y ADVANCEMENT FLAP

Flap Design

- The vascularity of the V-Y advancement flap is based on the central perforating vessels.
- Orientation is designed on areas of local laxity and mobility.
- Incisions are designed from the wide part of the defect and then gently tapered into a triangle perpendicular to the wound edge (**FIGURES 10A** and **11A**).
- Care is taken to design a large enough flap to allow for some undermining at the base of the flap for additional advancement while still leaving enough central contact with deeper tissues for vascularity.

Flap Elevation

- Incisions are made through the skin and subcutaneous tissues. Dissection through the subcutaneous tissues should be beveled away from the flap in order to increase the area for capture of underlying perforators into the central flap.
- The fascia can also be divided to allow for additional flap mobility.
- Can undermine the distal and proximal one-fourth of flap to allow for additional advancement but must *not* undermine centrally because this area is key to vascularity (**FIGURE 10B**). This is often done by spreading with a scissors vertically to preserve any potential blood vessels entering the flap.

Defect Closure

- Careful hemostasis is assured after flap elevation; hematomas under the flap can compromise vascularity and overall outcome.
- Closure starts at the "point" of the triangle where the donor site is closed primarily to form the vertical limb of the "Y." This also helps push the flap forward into the defect (**FIGURE 10C**).
- The flap is then pushed forward into the defect by closure of the sides of the triangle (**FIGURE 11B**).

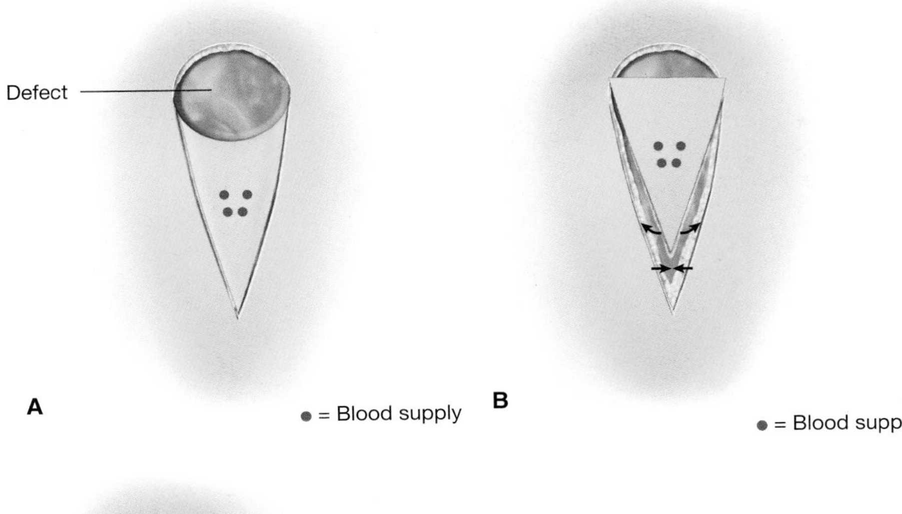

FIGURE 10 ● The V-Y flap is designed as a triangle with the base along the width of the defect and then gently tapered back. The blood supply for this flap is through the central connections with the underlying fascia/muscle **(A)**. The V-Y flap is elevated with gently tapering away from the central portion of the flap to increase the underlying perfusion. Some undermining can be performed at the base of the triangle or at the tip of the triangle if needed, but no undermining can be performed centrally. As the flap is advanced into the defect, the donor site will be closed primarily **(B)**. The V-Y flap is advanced into the defect after the donor site is closed primarily. The closure of the defect leads to the vertical limb of the Y and acts like a zipper to push the flap forward into the defect **(C)**.

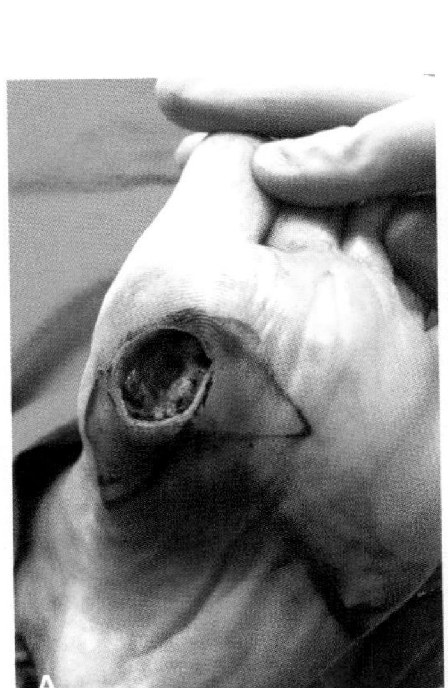

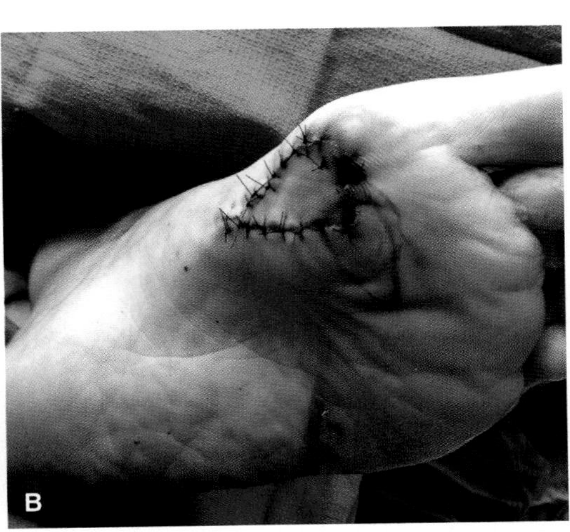

FIGURE 11 ● **A,** In this clinical case, two potential options for a V-Y flap have been designed with the decision to use the flap designed back toward the heel selected due to the relative laxity of that donor site compared with the flap running transversely across the plantar foot. **B,** In this case, the flap has been nicely advanced into the defect with the resultant Y closure demonstrated.

KEYSTONE FLAP

Flap Design

- Flap design is based on central perforators and use of "V-Y" closures to gain local tissue for advancement into the defect.
- A handheld Doppler can be used to identify specific large central perforators for preservation if additional mobilization is expected.
- The flap is most often designed from the longer border of a defect by first marking out the lateral borders of the flap at a 90° angle to the defect (**FIGURE 12A**).
- The flap width is then determined to be at least the width of the defect if not large. The flap is designed to remain this width along the entire length to each of the lateral borders (**FIGURES 12B** and **13A**).

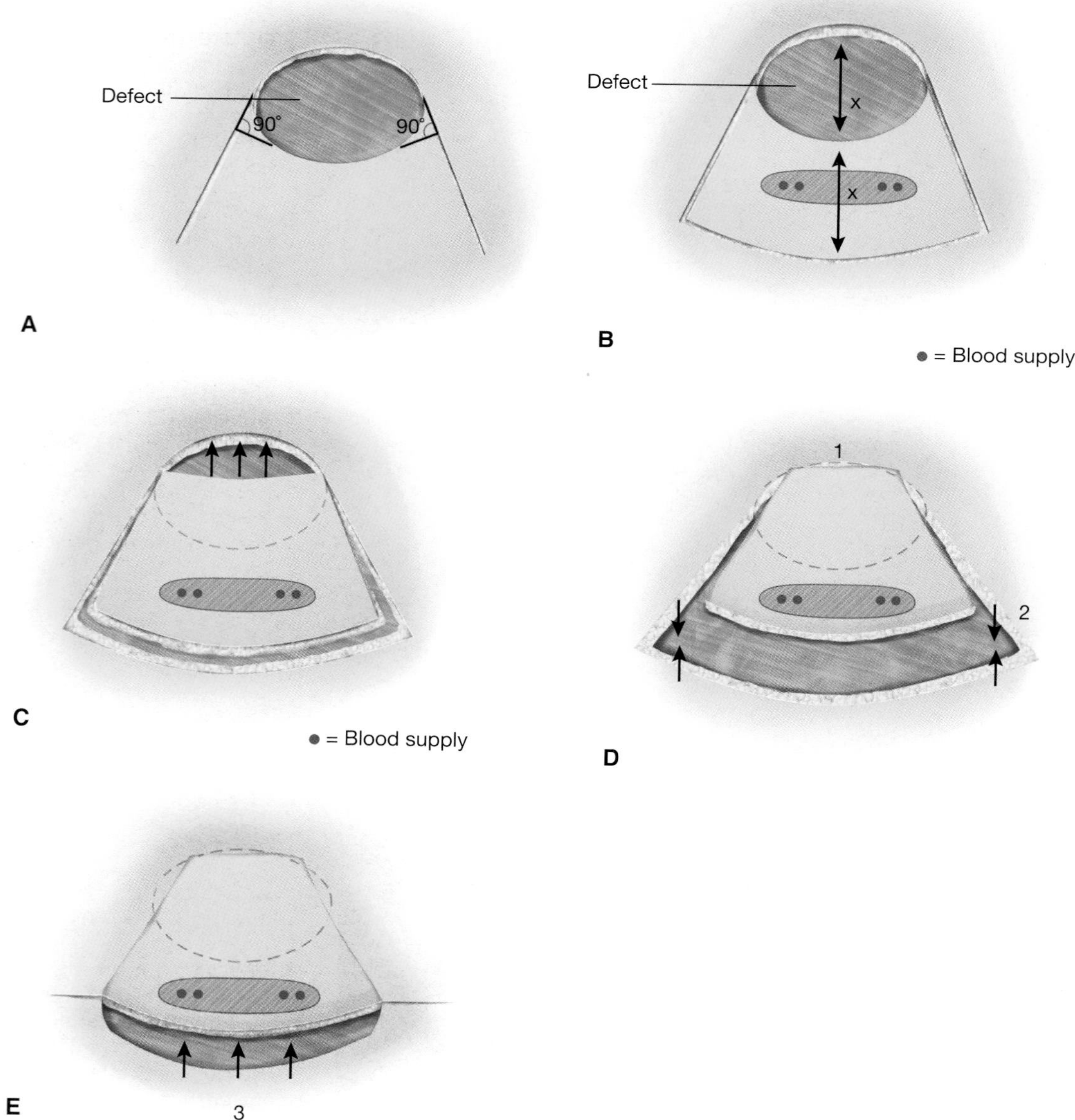

FIGURE 12 ● The first step in designing a keystone flap is to plan incisions from the corners of the defect perpendicular to the defect **(A)**. Next, the flap is designed to be at least the width of the defect with the central blood supply from the underlying tissue providing the vascularity to the flap **(B)**. The flap is elevated by incising through the skin, subcutaneous tissues, and fascia. The flap is then advanced into the defect, and closure occurs first in this area of maximal tension **(C)**. After the flap has been advanced into the defect, the corners of the donor site are closed in a V-Y fashion, which also helps push the flap into the defect and transitions the flap into a rounder shape **(D)**. The incision along the flap border opposite the initial defect is then closed by advancing the adjacent skin flap, which is often undermined **(E)**.

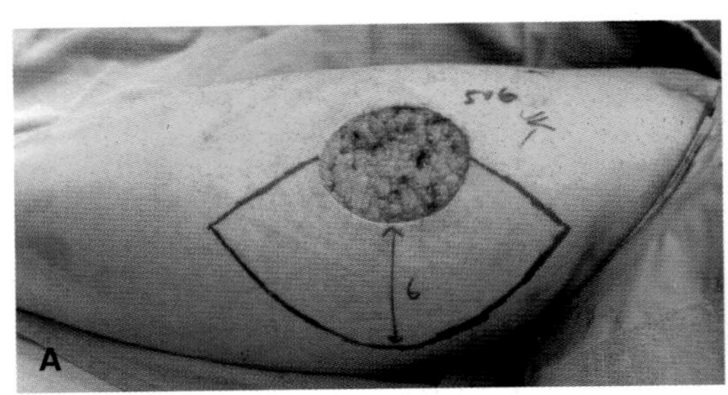

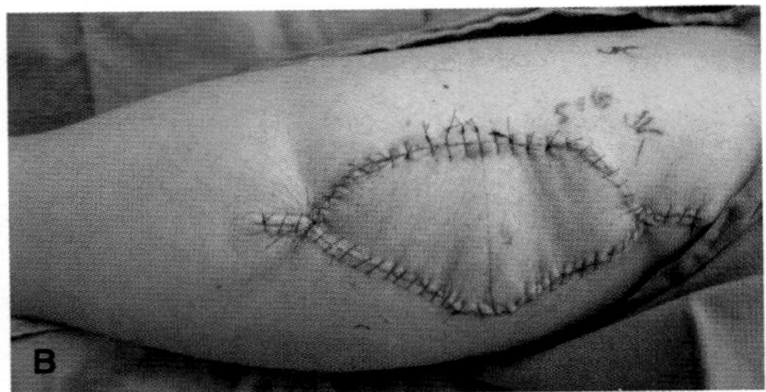

FIGURE 13 ● In this case, a 6-cm wide flap has been designed to match the 6-cm width of the defect **(A)**. In this case, the flap has been advanced and reconstructed the defect. The corners of the flap donor site have been closed in a V-Y fashion, and the flap shape has changed from a "keystone" or semi-arc shape to a rounder shape **(B)**.

Flap Elevation

- Incisions are made through the skin and subcutaneous tissues. This dissection is carried perpendicular to the skin with minimal beveling.
- The underlying fascia may also be divided for additional mobility and can be especially helpful in larger flaps.
- A small amount of subcutaneous or subfascial undermining can be performed, but this must be done judiciously unless large perforators have been knowingly included in the flap design.

Defect Closure

- The leading edge of the flap is advanced into the defect with deep dermal sutures. In situations where this may be initially under significant tension, one can start away from this area and work from peripheral to central, helping push the flap toward the defect (**FIGURE 12C**).
- The defect tissue margin opposite the flap can also be undermined to provide some advancement. Alternatively, an opposing keystone flap may also be designed along this border to provide additional tissue laxity.
- The lateral ends of the flap donor site are then closed in a V-Y fashion to help recruit additional tissue centrally as the flap transitions from a hemi-arc shape to an ellipse (**FIGURE 12D**).
- Finally, the trailing edge of the flap opposite the defect is sutured back to the edge of the donor site. This may require undermining of adjacent skin flaps to ease the overall tension on the closure (**FIGURES 12E** and **13B**).

PEARLS AND PITFALLS

Flap selection	■ Flaps that are not undermined (eg, keystone flaps) should be considered when margin status is unknown.
Flap design	■ Flaps should be large enough for readvancement if necessary.
Flap elevation	■ Care must be taken with perforator-based flaps to avoid central undermining because the subdermal plexus is transected circumferentially around the flap.
Defect closure	■ Care must be taken to avoid hematomas or infections, which can compromise a flap. ■ Postoperative immobilization should be considered for flaps around movable areas. ■ Excision of residual standing cutaneous deformities should be done judiciously to avoid compromise of flap vascularity and can be done at a later operative date if necessary.

POSTOPERATIVE CARE

- Flaps near joints should be immobilized with splinting to prevent mechanical dehiscence.
- Elevation for flaps on the extremities is critical for postoperative edema control.

COMPLICATIONS

- Marginal flap ischemia
- Delayed wound healing
- Infection (cellulitis or abscess)
- Hematoma
- Poor cosmetic outcome
- Flap failure/loss

OUTCOMES

- Outcome data for cutaneous reconstruction are quite heterogeneous due to the multiple body areas, flap techniques, and individual surgeon preferences.
- In general, the average incidence of a major complication is low but increases with the size of the defect and

reconstruction. Minor complications include delayed wound healing, nonoperative infections, and need for secondary revision surgery.[1-3]

- The incidence of total flap failure is low when appropriate reconstructive principles are followed.

REFERENCES

1. Griffin GR, Weber S, Baker SR. Outcomes following V-Y advancement flap reconstruction of large upper lip defects. *Arch Facial Plast Surg*. 2012;14(3):193-197.
2. Coombs CJ, Ng S, Stewart DA. The use of V-Y advancement flaps for closure of pretibial skin defects after excision of cutaneous lesions. *Ann Plast Surg*. 2013;71(4):402-405.
3. Khouri JS, Egeland BM, Daily SD, et al. The keystone island flap: use in large defects of the trunk and extremities in soft-tissue reconstruction. *Plast Reconstr Surg*. 2011;127(3):1212-1221.

Chapter 30 Skin Grafts

David L. Brown and Paige L. Myers

DEFINITIONS

- A graft is different than a flap as it does not bring an independent blood supply with it to the recipient site but rather relies on vascularity from the local wound bed.
- A skin graft is the transfer of cutaneous tissue from one site of the body to another, often to cover large defects. Skin grafts are versatile adjuncts to wound closure in burns, trauma, reconstruction, and other large wounds. After incorporation, skin grafts provide wounds with protection from the environment, pathogens, and heat and water loss similar to normal skin. Skin grafts represent a rung on the proverbial reconstructive ladder above those of primary closure and healing by secondary intention and below local flaps (**FIGURE 1**). With proper defect assessment, reconstructive planning, and attention to detail pre-, intra-, and postoperatively, optimal cosmetic and functional results using skin grafting techniques can be achieved.
- Split-thickness skin graft: contains epidermis and a variable amount of superficial to papillary dermis. Dermal appendages in the papillary dermis contribute to donor site re-epithelialization in 2 to 3 weeks.
- Full-thickness skin graft: includes all of the dermis as well as the epidermis, donor site must be closed primarily or with a skin graft.

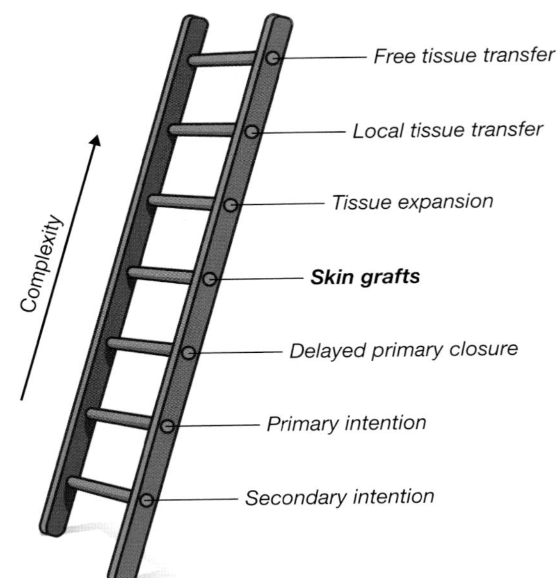

FIGURE 1 ● The reconstructive ladder. Skin grafts occupy an intermediate position in the hierarchy of complexity of closure technique.

- Autograft: one part of an individual's body that is transferred to a different part of the body of that same individual.
- Isograft: genetically identical donor and recipient individuals, such as identical twins in humans.
- Xenograft (heterograft): taken from an individual of one species that is grafted onto an individual of a different species.

PATIENT HISTORY/INDICATIONS

- Primary indications for skin grafting include an inability to perform primary closure, insufficient tissues for local skin flap coverage, and/or comorbid condition precluding a more extensive reconstruction, such as autologous free tissue transfer. This follows the principle of the reconstructive ladder: choose the best option that is simple, fast, and aesthetic.
- Skin grafts are extremely versatile and can essentially be placed on any vascular wound bed: deep partial thickness, full thickness, muscle, tendon (with intact paratenon), cartilage (with intact perichondrium), bone (with intact periosteum), vascularized biologic dressings. Skin grafting boasts applicability in the setting of acute skin loss (burns, trauma, infection), chronic skin loss (venous stasis ulcers), and a planned adjunct reconstruction (covering a muscle flap).
- Absolute contraindications are any situation where a suboptimal environment precludes successful healing. These include active infection (bacterial counts 10^5 CFU/g via quantitative culture), poor vascularity of recipient bed (ie, history of radiation to the area, exposed bone/tendon/nerve without the requisite vascular layer), and anticipation of further underlying reconstruction (ie, nerve or tendon grafting).
- Relative contraindications may pose a risk to successful healing, but skin grafts still may be necessary. Historically, skin grafts were used as wound coverage if there was a possibility of remaining cancer in the wound bed, as a bridge to definitive reconstruction while awaiting pathologic margin control. With the advent of newer wound dressing technology, such as Integra Dermal Regeneration Template (Integra LifeSciences, Princeton, NJ), this is less common. As well, skin grafting can provide for better monitoring of recurrence following resection of high-risk tumors.

IMAGING/OTHER STUDIES

- Adjunct studies are not generally needed for skin grafting.

SURGICAL MANAGEMENT

Preoperative Planning

- Patient counseling
  - Patients should be informed that the donor site is likely to cause more pain than the wound site in the immediate postoperative period. Postoperative care, including the healing stages of the graft and the donor site are discussed.

Some graft loss is to be expected, especially over large areas of grafting and/or uneven surfaces.

- Choice of graft thickness
  - Split-thickness skin grafts (STSGs): 12/1000 in is standard, with 6 to 16/1000 in used for special situations. Thinner grafts exhibit more reliable "take" at the recipient site (imbibition is more successful) and more dermis is left behind for subsequent harvest as necessary. STSGs exhibit less primary contraction and greater secondary contraction. Thicker grafts are more durable, due to increased dermis.
  - Full-thickness skin grafts: Primary contraction is greater, but secondary contraction is less, making them a good choice for joints, neck, eyelids, etc.
- Choice of meshing
  - "Sheet" (unmeshed) grafts have the advantage of better cosmesis but are more likely to develop seroma or hematoma formation underneath them, which can lead to failure.
  - Meshing increases the surface area, advantageous for large wounds. Epithelialization occurs from the skin bridges. If meshing is required, measure the size of the defect, then consider the options for meshing, ranging from 1:1, 1:1.5, 1:2, to 1:4. Meshing of grafts has two primary advantages:
    - Greater recipient surface area with less donor graft. The ratios of 1:1.5 and 1:2 are more commonly used. Larger expansion renders the coverage more tenuous and results in greater secondary contraction.
    - Wound bed drainage and prevention of seroma or hematoma formation minimizing risk of graft failure.

Equipment

- Skin grafts can be harvested with a surgical blade (generally for full-thickness skin grafts), an oscillating Goulian knife, or an air- or electric-powered dermatome (**FIGURE 2**). Dermatome benefits include consistency and the ability to choose specific graft thickness and width (ranging from 1 to 4 in guards).
- Once harvested, the skin graft can be meshed (**FIGURE 3**), allowing for the graft to be expanded.
- Mineral oil is useful to lubricate the donor site (**FIGURE 4**).
- The skin graft should be handled with smooth instruments, such as Adson tissue forceps.

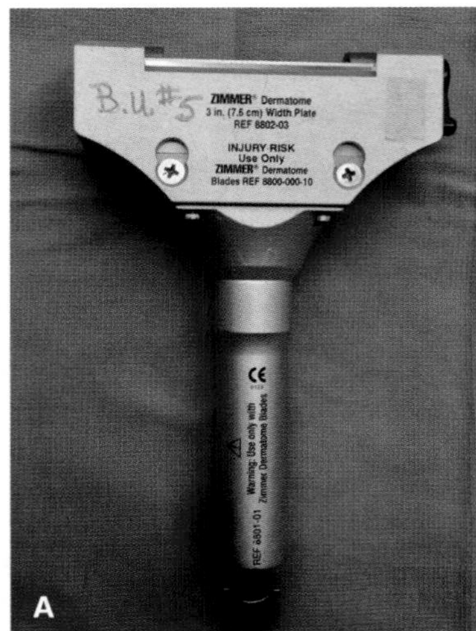

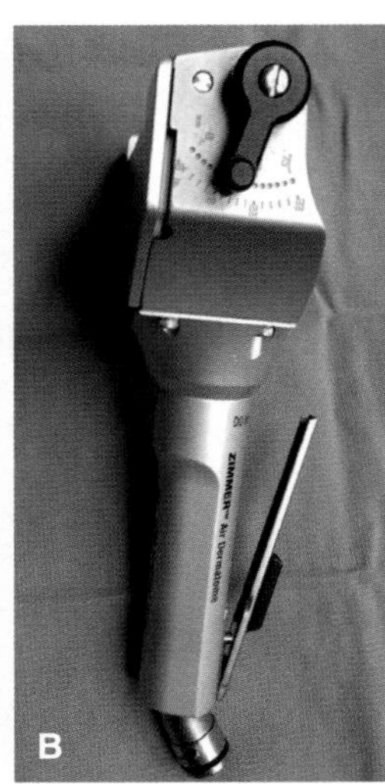

FIGURE 2 ● **A,** Underside of dermatome, with blade and 3-in guard attached. Blade and guard are flush against machine, as assembled. **B,** Dermatome set to 12/1000 in thickness.

Positioning

- Place the patient based in a position to maximize access to the wound as well as the donor site. The anterolateral thigh is generally preferred as it is commonly a flat, wide area. More lateral placement of a single graft harvest site keeps the donor scar off of the patient's lap. The approximate donor site is marked out below the trochanter to above the knee (smaller if less surface area is needed) ensuring enough distance to avoid bony prominences. If the wound is posterior, the back and buttock skin are also acceptable donor sites. The medial thighs are avoided due to friction while walking.
- The donor site is injected with local anesthetic in the subdermal space, using a 22-gauge spinal needle. A mixture of 0.5% lidocaine with a 1:200,000 concentration of epinephrine and 0.25% bupivacaine is the authors' preference for providing both hemostasis and postoperative pain relief (**FIGURE 4**). Mineral oil is spread over the area to allow for smooth gliding of the dermatome over the skin (**FIGURE 4**). Donor sites can be used multiple times after re-epithelialization.

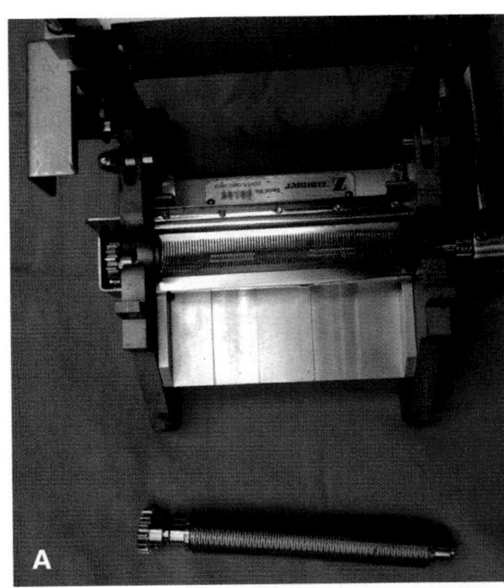
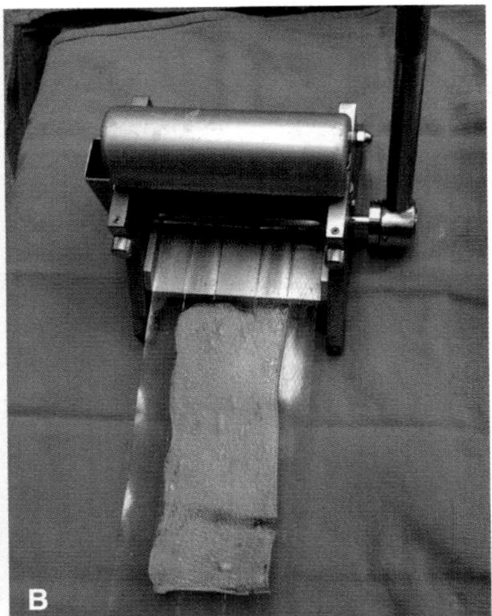
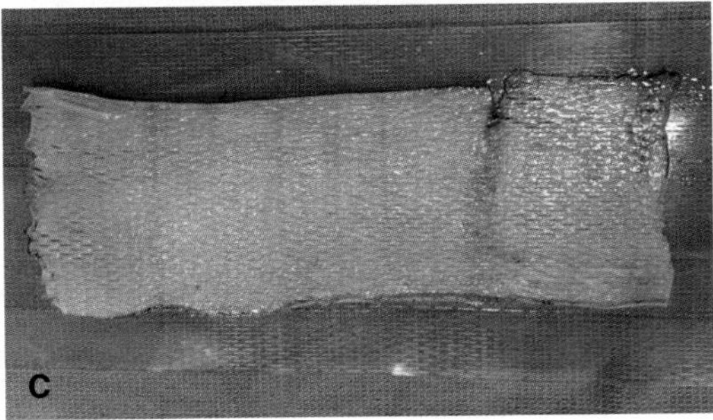

FIGURE 3 ● **A,** View of an opened mesher with space to place the chosen cutting wheel (in this case 1:1.5 ratio). **B,** Graft placed dermal side up on the carrier, which is positioned within the mesher entrance. **C,** Graft, postmeshing.

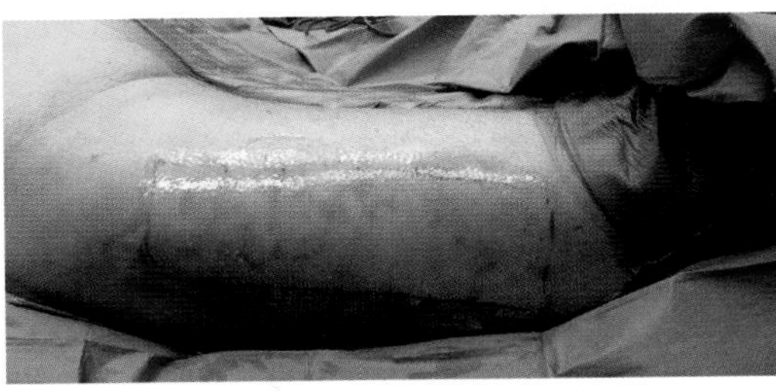

FIGURE 4 ● Prone patient, with the lateral thigh showing from buttock crease (left) to knee (right). Note blanching of skin from epinephrine injection and glossiness of mineral oil application.

- Many consider the most important aspect is the adequate wound bed preparation to accept the graft. The wound must be clean and mechanically debrided (scalpel, dermatome, hydrosurgery device) until the wound bed exhibits brisk, punctate bleeding at the base. Wound edges must be free of nonviable tissues, purulence, biofilm, and exudate.
- The dermatome is assembled, and the appropriate width guard is attached (**FIGURE 2A**). Generally, a 3- or 4-in guard is be used depending on the defect size and size of the patient's donor site. Proper seating of the blade in the machine and underneath the guard is assured; uneven seating can cause an excessively thin graft at one edge and overly thick at the other. The desired thickness of skin harvest is selected via the dial on the side (12/1000 in is shown here, **FIGURE 2B**).
- To harvest the graft, either the surgeon (using their nondominant hand) and/or an assistant will hold manual countertension on the skin (**FIGURE 5A**). The dermatome is pressed against the skin at a 45° angle and with moderate downforce is slowly and evenly advanced along the length of graft harvest (**FIGURE 5B** and **C**). To complete the harvest and separate the end of the graft from the patient, the surgeon lowers the handle of the dermatome toward the patient (decreasing the angle) and slowly lifts off the skin surface (**FIGURE 5D**).
- If meshing is required, the mesher is assembled, and an appropriate cutting wheel is chosen; 1:1.5 shown here (**FIGURE 3A**) is a standard ratio but can be varied up to 1:4 depending on the amount of donor sites available compared

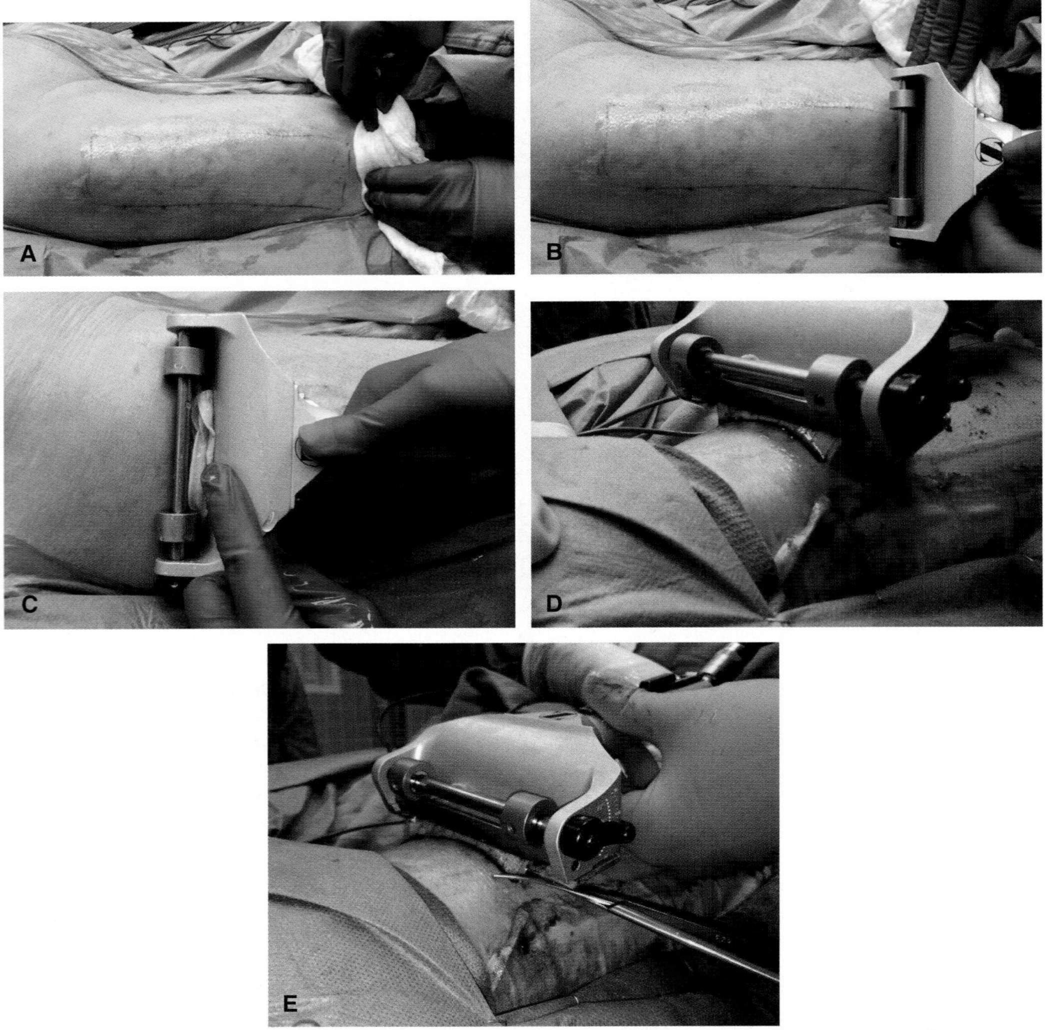

FIGURE 5 ● **A,** Assistant holding countertraction on skin with the use of laparotomy sponge. **B,** Dermatome is placed on skin, running at a 45° angle. **C,** Firm, consistent pressure is applied as the dermatome is moved along the donor site. **D,** At the end of the harvest strip, the surgeon should evaluate the transection of the graft from the donor site. Note the persistent attachment that often requires sharp transection **(E)**.

with the area needing coverage. The graft is placed superficial side down on the carrier and run through the mesher (**FIGURE 3B** and **C**).

- The graft is placed on the wound bed, trimmed appropriately, and secured to the wound edges with surgical staples or dissolvable sutures (ie, 4-0 chromic) (**FIGURE 6A** and **B**). A nonstick dressing is applied. The surgeon may place a tie-over bolster, consisting of cotton soaked with mineral oil, wrapped with petroleum gauze, and tied to the wound edges with nonabsorbable suture (**FIGURE 6C** and **D**). This provides consistent pressure on the graft to the wound bed and keeps the graft moist during the imbibition phase while angio- and vasculogenesis have time to occur. (Pie-crusting of nonmeshed [sheet] grafts has not been found to be successful in avoiding seroma/hematoma formation, and is nonaesthetic, even compared with meshing. A good bolster dressing should suffice.) Alternatively, negative pressure wound therapy atop petroleum gauze is also successful.

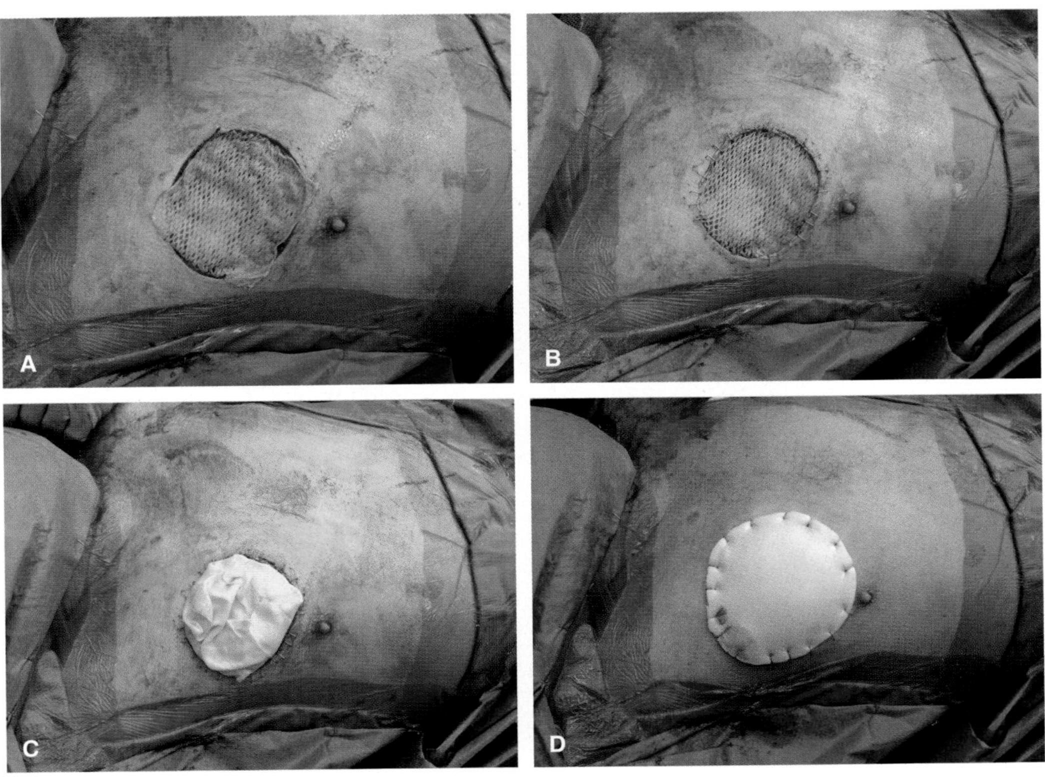

FIGURE 6 ● **A,** Patient with right superior chest wound. Meshed graft placed within wound, dermal side down, and minimally expanded. **B,** The graft is trimmed appropriately and secured with stainless steel clips. **C,** Mineral oil– and saline-soaked cotton batting, wrapped in Xeroform, is shaped to the size of the wound. **D,** A foam bolster is used to secure the dressing over the graft.

PEARLS AND PITFALLS

Recipient site preparation	■ Without adequate wound debridement, the graft will not succeed.
Harvesting the graft	■ Donor site optimization is key. Choose the part of the thigh that can be the flattest, void of bony prominences with tension placed by assistance in all four directions. Lubrication with mineral oil is recommended, both on the skin as well as between the blade and dermatome to ensure minimal friction on the skin. ■ Proper seating of the blade in the machine underneath the guard should be assured; uneven seating can cause an excessively thin graft at one edge and an overly thick one at the other. ■ If the graft is not immediately separated from the donor site at the end of the run with the dermatome, the surgeon should release power to the dermatome and hold it over the skin for an assistant to cut it free with a Metzenbaum scissor. Otherwise, the graft can be pulled back out through the blade entrance, mangling the graft. ■ Rinsing the graft washes away vital procoagulant factors and should be avoided, if possible.
Graft inset	■ To assure consistent application of the graft to the wound bed dermis-side down and to transfer it without bunching, it should be placed on the carrier dermis side up. ■ If the graft is not immediately needed for wound coverage, it can be stored on the back table (appropriately marked to avoid disposal), wrapped in moistened gauze, or left on the carrier and covered with the same. ■ Care should be taken to avoid "tenting" a graft over an uneven wound bed. Extra graft should be placed to allow for complete contour touchdown. ■ Placement of a meshed graft does not need to involve full expansion of the graft; leaving it relatively unexpanded will allow for egress of wound fluids while speeding healing.
Postoperative care	■ Although skin grafting may seem like a relatively straightforward procedure, appropriate patient counseling regarding postoperative course and wound care can help mitigate complications once the patient leaves the hospital.

POSTOPERATIVE CARE

- To cover the donor site of split-thickness grafts, options include petroleum-based gauze versus an occlusive dressing. Patients report more pain with petroleum gauze; however, an occlusive dressing may leak or become a nidus for an infection.
- Bolster dressings on the grafts are usually taken down in 4 to 6 days, unless infection is suspected, and then earlier.
- After bolster removal, the graft is protected with qd or bid daily dressing changes with petrolatum gauze until it is more fully healed (usually another 7-10 days). After this point, the patient should moisturize the graft (and donor site) twice daily for a few months to prevent desiccation, as oil and sweat glands are not transferred with the graft.
- Judgment is exercised to determine the degree of immobilization prescribed, depending on graft location. It is not necessary to splint the foot for grafts on the lower leg, but patients should keep the extremity elevated to prevent swelling and edema and thus graft loss.

COMPLICATIONS

- The most common complication contributing to skin graft failure is hematoma or seroma. The fluid isolates the undersurface of the graft, inhibiting imbibition, and from the endothelial buds of the recipient site so that revascularization cannot take place. If left untreated, they will lead to graft loss.
- Atraumatic tissue handling, cauterization of lymphatic vessels, limited use of electrocautery in the graft bed, and a light pressure dressing minimize the risk of fluid accumulation under the graft.
- Infection can destroy a graft, particularly in the early postoperative period, prior to revascularization. This may be mitigated by carefully preparing the wound bed, using quilting sutures, meshing, or pie-crusting the graft surface to allow egress of subjacent fluids. In the case of unexplained postoperative fevers, the dressings should be removed early and the wound inspected for infection, which can be potentially treated, with graft salvage.
- Secondary contraction of skin grafts is increased with thinner grafts and with greater expansion of meshed grafts. This can affect underlying joint mobility and aesthetics.
- Incompletely debrided or poorly vascularized wound beds can lead to nonadherence and ultimate loss of the graft.

Chapter 31 Digit Amputations

Steven C. Haase

DEFINITION

- Digital amputation refers to the removal of a finger or thumb, most commonly at the level of the phalanges or interphalangeal joints (**FIGURE 1**). More proximal amputations that include a significant portion of the metacarpal are referred to as ray amputations. The techniques found in this chapter have been described chiefly for the hand, although similar procedures can be used on the foot in many cases.
- Digital or ray amputation may be indicated for a variety of diagnoses: malignancy, infection, trauma, burn, frostbite, vascular insufficiency, and other chronic painful conditions, to name a handful. In the case of melanoma, digit amputation is typically used for subungual melanoma or other large invasive melanomas of the finger or thumb.

PATIENT HISTORY AND PHYSICAL FINDINGS

- A patient's age, handedness, occupation, and hobbies should be considered carefully in planning an operation that might significantly affect their function. In some cases, preoperative consultation with a physiatrist and/or occupational therapist may help a patient mentally prepare for what is sometimes an emotionally difficult operation.
- In tumor cases, it is important to assess how long the lesion has been present; how fast it has grown; and whether there has been any history of ulceration, bleeding, or pain. Lesions exhibiting rapid growth in addition to these other findings may require more aggressive treatment.
- Physical examination should include assessment of both the epitrochlear and axillary lymph nodes. For lesions on the toes, examination should include the popliteal and inguinal basins. Clinically node-negative patients with melanoma greater than or equal to 1 mm in thickness, or thin lesions with other worrisome histologic features, may be candidates for sentinel lymph node biopsy at the time of amputation (see Part 5, Chapter 33). Patients with clinically involved nodes should undergo fine needle aspiration biopsy and staging for distant metastases. These patients may require lymph node dissection at the time of amputation.

IMAGING AND OTHER DIAGNOSTIC STUDIES

- Suspicious lesions require biopsy to establish diagnosis. This should include a full-thickness sampling of the skin and/or nail matrix for accurate assessment of depth of the lesion. Increased depth of invasion is consistently associated with worse prognosis.[1]
- For large or fixed lesions, radiographs of the digit should be obtained to assess for the presence of bone involvement. If radiographs demonstrate significant bone destruction, additional imaging with magnetic resonance imaging may be required to assess the full extent of tumor spread in the hand.

SURGICAL MANAGEMENT

Positioning

- For hand operations, patients are positioned supine, with the affected extremity extended on a hand table attached to the operating room table.

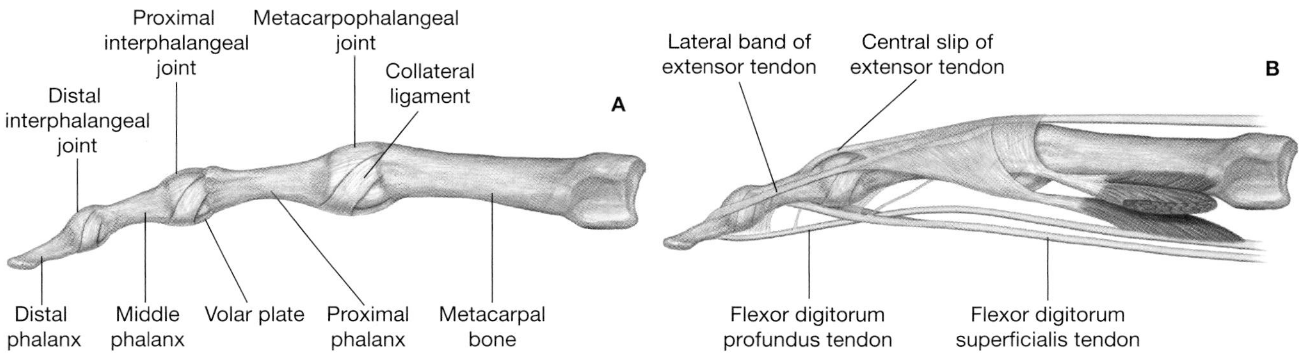

FIGURE 1 ● **A** and **B**, Anatomy of the digit.

DIGITAL AMPUTATION

Skin Incision

- The skin incision should be designed as a "fish mouth," such that dorsal and volar flaps are created that close in a more or less transverse line of closure that gives a smooth, rounded contour to the amputation stump.
- The skin flaps should be designed with enough laxity to close over the underlying skeleton to be preserved. Typically, the level of disarticulation or osteotomy should be a few millimeters proximal to the level of the skin incision.
- Ideally, the volar flap can be designed a bit longer than the dorsal flap (**FIGURE 2A**) to allow resurfacing of the entire opposition surface (contact surface) of the fingertip with the thicker, more densely innervated palmar skin.

Soft Tissue Dissection

- The soft tissue should be divided in a way that minimizes devascularization of the tissues or skin flaps. Sharp scalpel dissection directly to the bone can be performed both dorsally and volarly, dividing the neurovascular bundles, tendons, and periosteum.

Bone Dissection and Osteotomy

- The periosteum should then be sharply elevated proximally using an elevator or scalpel, circumferentially around the digit. This will allow the bone cut to be positioned slightly proximal to the soft tissue dissection.
- Bone division is most efficiently accomplished with a small oscillating power saw. Instruments such as bone cutters or rongeurs tend to crush and fracture the proximal bone stock and are not recommended.
- If disarticulation is planned, the collateral ligaments should be detached from the proximal aspect of the joint, so this bulky, poorly vascularized tissue is discarded with the amputated part.

Traction Neurectomy

- The neurovascular bundle should be identified with delicate dissection. The artery may be cauterized; the nerve should be dissected away from the artery and followed proximally several millimeters. The nerve should be placed on traction, divided proximally, and allowed to retract (**FIGURE 2B**). This will ensure that the neuromas that inevitably form at the end of each digital nerve will be located well proximal to the contact surface of the fingertip.

Closure

- Closure is usually performed with a single layer of nonabsorbable sutures (**FIGURE 2C**), which are removed about 2 weeks later. Do *not* suture the extensor tendon to the flexor tendon over the end of the exposed bone; this will functionally shorten the flexor tendon to that digit, resulting in weakened grip strength due to the quadrigia effect.

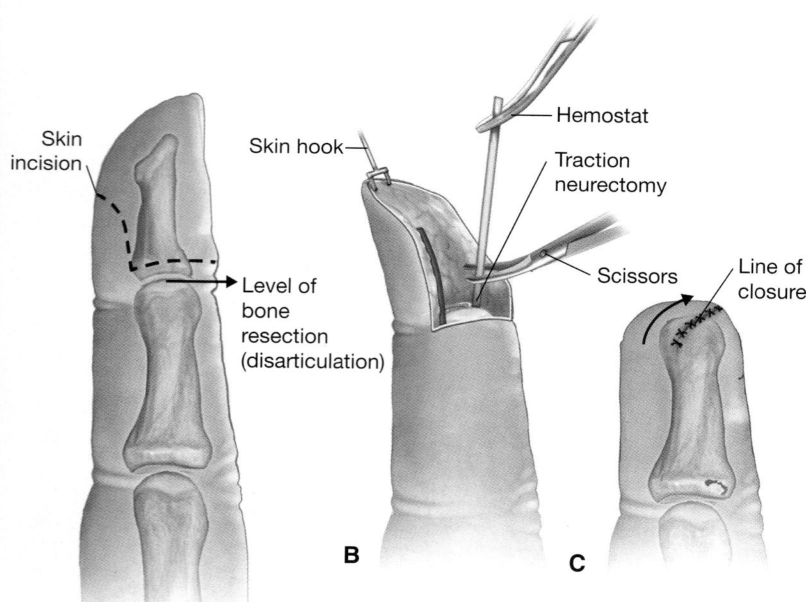

FIGURE 2 ● Digital amputation technique. **A,** The skin incision is designed just distal to the level of planned bone resection or disarticulation. The volar flap is designed longer than the dorsal flap to allow for coverage of the fingertip with more durable, well-innervated volar skin. **B,** After removal of the skeletal elements and nail complex, the neurovascular bundle is identified on the volar flap, and the nerve is gently dissected proximally, ultimately dividing the nerve while on traction, and allowing the stump to retract proximally. **C,** The volar skin is advanced to cover the wound, and a smooth, rounded closure is performed.

RAY AMPUTATION

Skin Incision

- Incisions are designed to avoid a scar in the webspace. Conceptually, the goal is to preserve one webspace and resect the other, rather than having a webspace at the operative site with a contracted scar in its midline (**FIGURE 3A-E**).
- Usually the dissection is performed mostly through a dorsal incision, which extends longitudinally from the base of the finger. Palmar incisions are limited to avoid the possibility of sensitive scarring in that location.

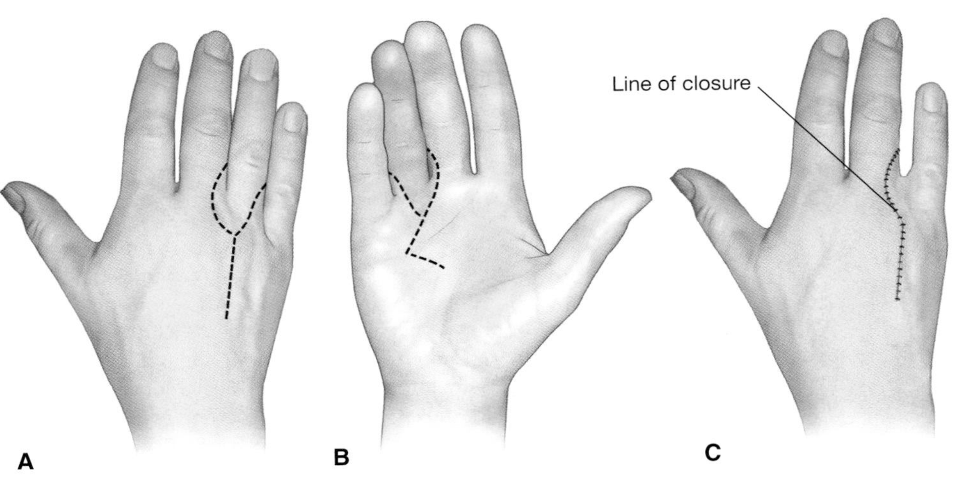

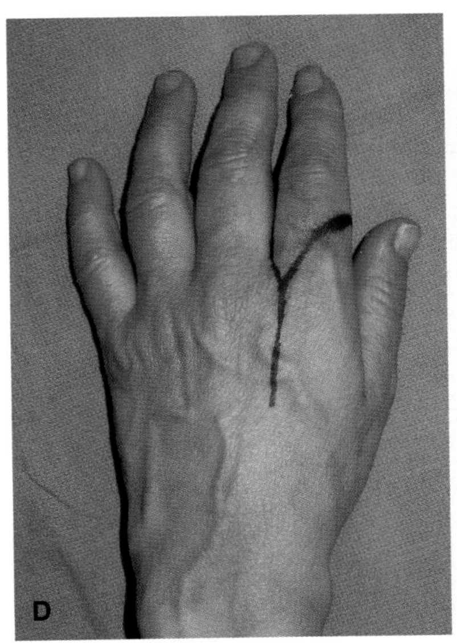

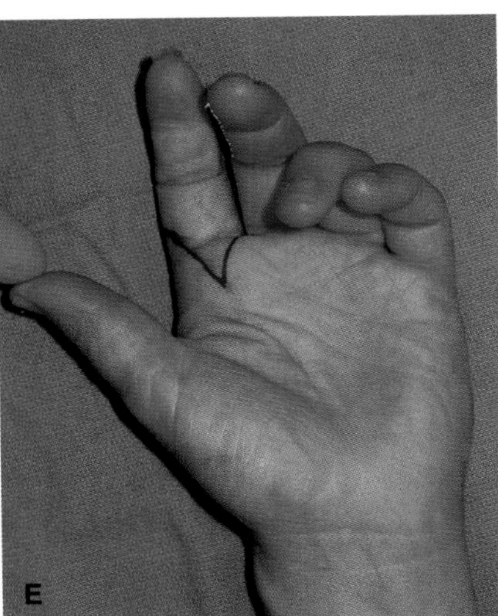

FIGURE 3 ● Skin incision for ray amputation. **A,** Dorsal incision can be designed proximally as a straight line, or as a zigzag, extending distally to encircle the base of the finger to be removed. Note the preservation of an intact webspace for closure, rather than dividing the web with the incision. **B,** Volar incision must be a zigzag or chevron-style incision to avoid longitudinal scars crossing the flexion creases of the palm. **C,** Closure is shown, with preservation of the delicate webspace skin. **D,** Dorsal and **(E)** volar skin markings for index finger ray amputation.

Dorsal Dissection

- Major sensory nerves in the subcutaneous tissue are preserved when possible. The extensor tendon is divided proximally and the metacarpal exposed.
- The periosteum of the metacarpal is incised longitudinally and subperiosteal dissection carried out circumferentially along the shaft of the bone. The attachments of the intrinsic muscles are disrupted with this dissection; most of these do not require transfer or repair, with the exception of the origin of adductor pollicis (**FIGURE 4**). When removed from the middle metacarpal during ray amputation, this muscle origin should be reattached to the index metacarpal with bone anchors or transosseous sutures.

Bone Dissection

- For index, middle, and small finger ray amputations, the osteotomy should be performed distal to the insertion of the wrist extensors: extensor carpi radialis longus, extensor carpi radialis brevis, and extensor carpi ulnaris, respectively (refer to **FIGURE 5**).
- For the ring finger metacarpal, which has no extrinsic tendon attachments, the entire metacarpal can be disarticulated at the base and removed (if no transposition is planned).

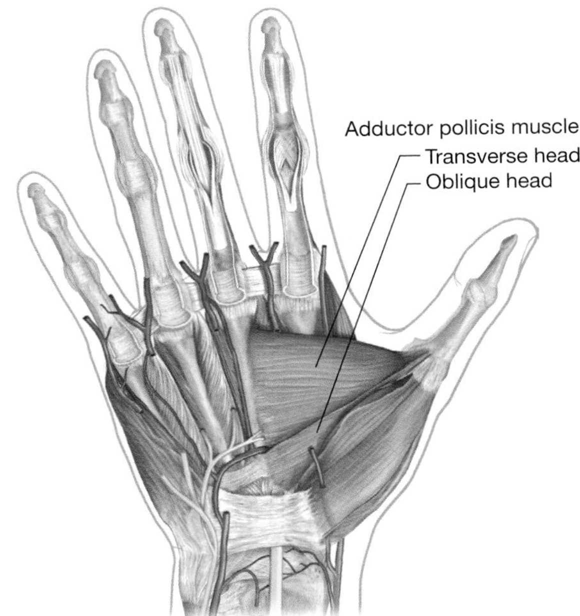

FIGURE 4 ● Anatomy of the adductor pollicis.

- For middle or ring finger ray amputations, some effort should be made in eliminating the troublesome gap between digits that can result.[2,3] This can be accomplished by two principle methods:
  - Meticulous soft tissue repair, including permanent sutures in the intermetacarpal ligaments and careful postoperative splinting (**FIGURE 6**)
  - Transposition of the adjacent border digit, requiring bony fixation of the metacarpal, and often longer postoperative immobilization (**FIGURE 7**)
- Once the bone has been transected, dissection proceeds around the side(s) of the metacarpal head to divide the intermetacarpal ligaments.

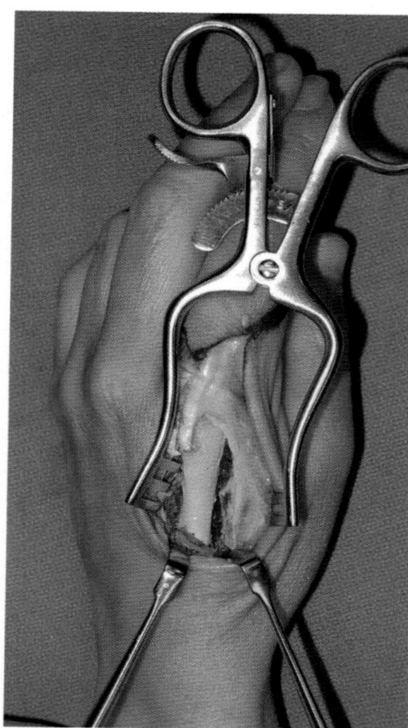

FIGURE 5 ● Dorsal dissection completed, with division of the metacarpal at the proximal shaft, preserving the base with its tendon attachments.

Volar Dissection

- The volar dissection is usually done last. The digital neurovascular bundles are identified and transected distally, keeping them rather long, in contrast to the shortening that is done for phalangeal-level amputations (**FIGURE 8A** and **B**).
- Once the ray amputation is complete, the digital nerves are folded dorsally into the periosteal sleeve left behind after metacarpal removal (**FIGURE 9**). The nerves are secured in this deep, padded area, surrounded by healthy interosseous muscle, where they are protected from trauma during routine hand function.

Closure

- Skin closure should be meticulous, addressing excess laxity and/or standing cutaneous deformities ("dog ears") if encountered (**FIGURE 10A** and **B**). The relative tightness or looseness of the dorsal skin closure, in particular, can help maintain proper orientation of the adjacent digits and help avoid malalignment or "scissoring."

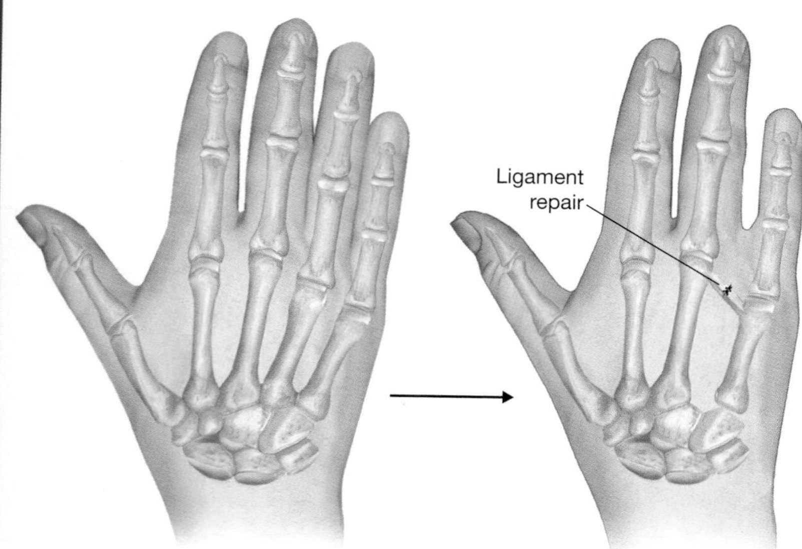

FIGURE 6 ● Ray resection without transposition. Using permanent sutures to reapproximate the intermetacarpal ligament, as well as meticulous skin closure, the finger "gap" can be closed with soft tissue repair alone.

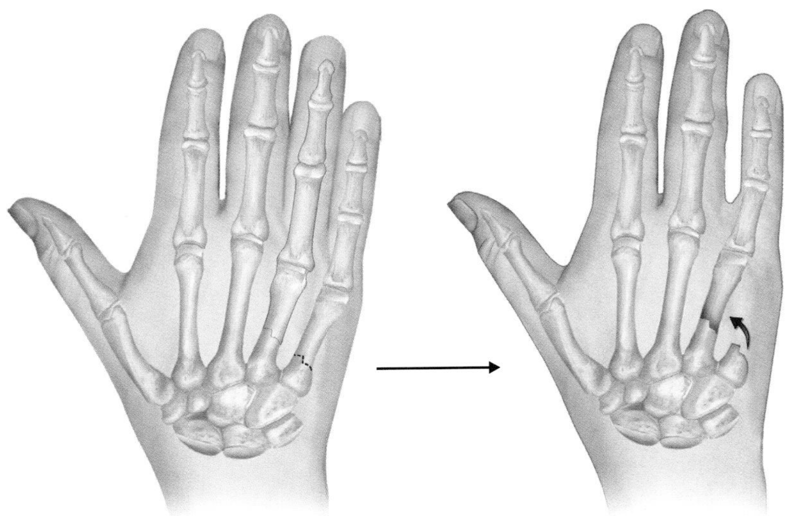

FIGURE 7 ● Ray resection with transposition. Transposition requires osteosynthesis of the involved metacarpals with wires, pins, or plate and screws. One advantage is the potential to minimize length discrepancy of the small finger by preserving added length at the base of the ring metacarpal, as illustrated here.

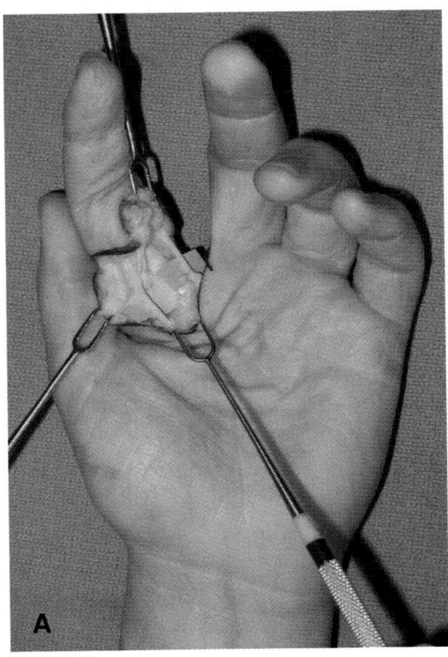

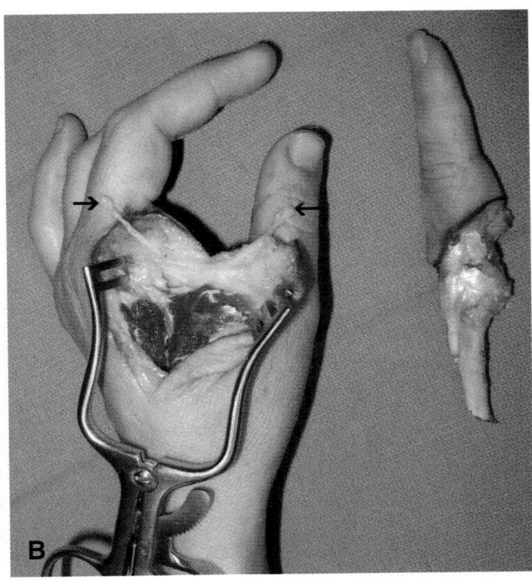

FIGURE 8 ● **A,** Volar dissection with identification of the digital nerves, which are preserved with some length, so they can be relocated in the deeper dorsal tissues at the time of closure. **B,** Ray resection completed, with digital nerves transected (*black arrows*).

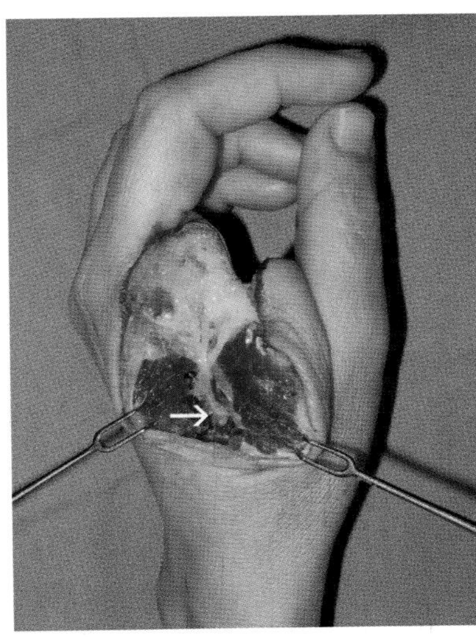

FIGURE 9 ● Digital nerves (*white arrow*) transposed deep into the periosteal sleeve between the interosseous muscles.

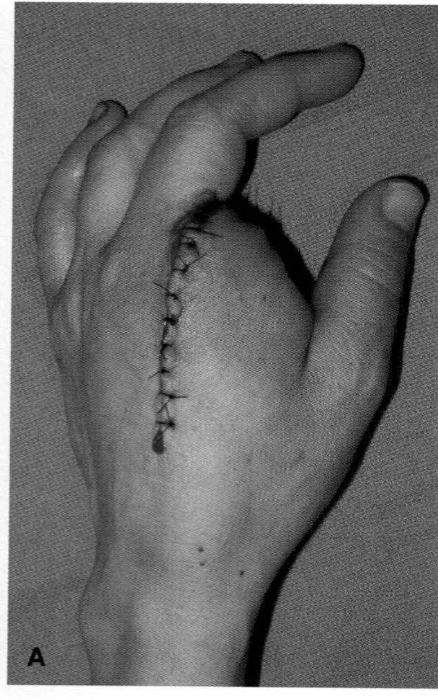

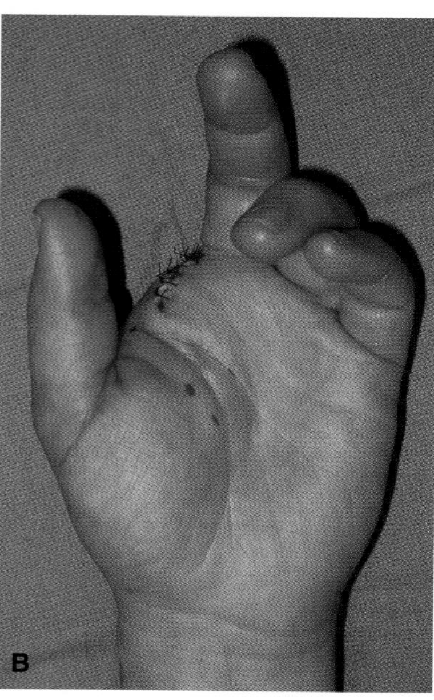

FIGURE 10 ● **A** and **B**, Final wound closure, which avoids extensive incisions on the sensitive palmar skin.

PEARLS AND PITFALLS

Digital amputations	■ When required, retract the skin edges with skin hooks only. This avoids tissue damage that can occur from repeated grasping of the tissues with forceps.
Quadrigia effect	■ Because the flexor digitorum profundus tendons share a common muscular origin, effectively shortening any one of the tendons can lead to an overall decrease in grip strength. During force generation, the foreshortened tendon becomes tight early, preventing transmission of force to the adjacent digits.
Neuroma detection	■ It can be difficult to differentiate symptomatic neuroma from ordinary hypersensitivity after finger amputation. A diagnostic injection of local anesthetic into the specific area of the neuroma, to anesthetize the nerve in isolation, can confirm the diagnosis of neuroma.

POSTOPERATIVE CARE

- For digital amputations, the postoperative dressing should be amply padded to allow for postoperative swelling. A hand-based splint for a short time (1 or 2 weeks) can be used if desired. Prolonged immobilization should be avoided so that the remaining finger joints (including the adjacent digits) do not become stiff.
- For ray amputations, the hand should be splinted for the first 2 weeks, taking care to maintain proper alignment of the digits in the splint, to avoid divergence or convergence of the fingers on either side of the amputation site. Sometimes, temporary pinning of the fingers is warranted to maintain good alignment in this early postoperative period, as the soft tissues are healing. Splinting beyond 2 weeks may still be required for comfort and protection, but the orthosis use should not interfere with early mobilization of the interphalangeal and metacarpophalangeal joints, which may become permanently stiff if immobilized for too long.
- In all cases, consultation with a certified hand therapist may be of benefit to the patient, for help with orthosis fabrication, edema control, joint mobilization, scar massage, desensitization, and molding of the finger stump for prosthesis wear, if desired.

OUTCOMES

- Compared to the contralateral hand, patients with single-ray amputations have on average 13% less key pinch strength, 26% less oppositional strength, and 28% less grip strength at long-term follow-up.[4,5]

COMPLICATIONS

- Acute complications such as bleeding, infection, and delayed healing should be uncommon.

- Chronic complications include phantom pain and painful neuromas:
  - Persistent sensation in an amputated part is common (over 80% in one prospective study) but is not always painful.[6]
  - Neuromas will form at the stump of divided nerves but are not usually symptomatic if the nerve endings are properly padded and located away from contact surfaces.

REFERENCES

1. Warso M, Gray T, Gonzalez M. Melanoma of the hand. *J Hand Surg Am*. 1997;22(2):354-360.
2. Colen L, Bunkis J, Gordon L, et al. Functional assessment of ray transfer for central digital loss. *J Hand Surg Am*. 1985;10(2):232-237.
3. Steichen JB, Idler RS. Results of central ray resection without bony transposition. *J Hand Surg Am*. 1986;11(4):466-474.
4. Peimer CA, Wheeler DR, Barrett A, et al. Hand function following single ray amputation. *J Hand Surg Am*. 1999;24(6):1245-1248.
5. Melikyan EY, Beg MS, Woodbridge S, et al. The functional results of ray amputation. *Hand Surg*. 2003;8(1):47-51.
6. Jensen TS, Krebs B, Nielsen J, et al. Phantom limb, phantom pain and stump pain in amputees during the first 6 months following limb amputation. *Pain*. 1983;17(3):243-256.

Chapter 32 Resection of Head and Neck Melanoma

Scott A. McLean

DEFINITION

- Resection of head and neck cutaneous melanoma is performed with wide surgical margins intended to achieve histologically negative margins. Current guidelines for wide excision of the primary lesion, with an adequate margin of surrounding normal skin and deep soft tissue necessary to achieve clear surgical margins, are based on depth of invasion of the primary lesion (**TABLE 1**).[1] However, given the complex anatomic and functional nature of the head and neck, resection margins are sometimes modified to preserve normal function. Reconstruction of complex head and neck defects is often delayed until final histopathologic evaluation of margins is deemed negative. Reconstruction can be accomplished with primary closure, split or full-thickness skin grafts, local or regional adjacent tissue transfer, or free tissue transfer.
- Patients with invasive melanoma and no clinical evidence or regional metastatic disease may warrant assessment of regional lymph nodes via sentinel lymph node biopsy (SLNB). SLNB has been shown to be both accurate and prognostic in head and neck melanoma.[2,3] Current recommendations on use of SLNB are based on depth of invasion of the primary lesion as well as the presence of adverse histologic features such as ulceration and mitotic rate (**TABLE 2**).[1-5]
- Patients who are found to have micrometastatic disease on SLNB are typically offered close clinical observation with ultrasound of the regional nodal basin every 4 months, with completion lymph node dissection if they have a regional recurrence in the absence of distant metastases. Select patients with a positive sentinel lymph node may be considered for immediate selective neck dissection (see Part 5, Chapter 37; Selective Neck Dissection).
- Patients who present with clinical evidence of regional metastatic disease are offered regional lymph node dissection (LND). Based on the site of the primary lesion, the nodal basins included in the LND may include the postauricular and suboccipital lymph nodes, the parotid gland and its associated lymph nodes, and the cervical lymph nodes levels I-V (**TABLE 3**).[6]

Table 1: Surgical Margin Recommendations for Cutaneous Melanoma

Primary tumor thickness	Clinically measured surgical margin
In situ	0.5-1.0 cm
≤1 mm	1 cm
1.01-2.0 mm	1-2 cm
>2.0 mm	2 cm

Table 2: Recommendations for Sentinel Lymph Node Biopsy

Status of SLN is the most important prognostic indicator for disease-specific survival, recurrence-free survival, and overall survival in patients with primary cutaneous melanoma.
SLNB is not recommended for patients with melanoma in situ or lesions ≤ 1 mm without ulceration and <1 mitosis/mm^2 (T1a lesions).
SLNB should be discussed with patients who have primary lesions 0.8-0.9 mm in thickness with ulceration or ≥1 mitosis/mm^2 (T1b lesions).
SLNB can also be considered in patients with primary lesions ≤0.8 mm with ulceration or increased mitotic rate with other adverse parameters such as angiolymphatic invasion, positive deep margin, or young age.
SLNB should be discussed with patients who have primary lesions >1.0 mm in tumor thickness (T2 or greater).

DIFFERENTIAL DIAGNOSIS

- Cutaneous melanoma of the head and neck usually presents as a pigmented lesion of varying size, shape, and color. Other benign and malignant cutaneous lesions can present in a similar fashion and include:
  - Seborrheic keratosis
  - Junctional nevi
  - Compound nevi
  - Dermal nevi
  - Hemangioma
  - Blue nevus
  - Pyogenic granuloma
  - Spitz nevus
  - Pigmented actinic keratosis
  - Pigmented or nonpigmented basal cell carcinoma
  - Squamous cell carcinoma

PATIENT HISTORY AND PHYSICAL FINDINGS

- A thorough history of the lesion of concern should include the duration of clinical symptoms, the presence of pruritus, and presence of bleeding, and note any changes in the size, shape, or color of the lesion.
- Most cutaneous melanomas will present as either a new pigmented lesion or changes in an existing lesion that exhibit the ABCDE's of melanoma: A—Asymmetry, B—irregular Border, C—varied Color, D—Diameter >6 mm, and E—Evolving changes.

Table 3: Nodal Basins Included in Therapeutic Lymph Node Dissection (TLND)

Primary cutaneous lesion location	Nodal basins included in TLND
Anterolateral scalp, temple, lateral forehead, lateral cheek, ear: all arising anterior to coronal plane through the external auditory canal	Parotid and cervical lymphatic levels I-V
Chin and neck	Cervical lymphatic levels I-V
Scalp and occiput posterior to coronal plane through the external auditory canal	Postauricular, suboccipital, and cervical lymphatics levels II-V

- A thorough past medical history should be performed and include information regarding any previous malignancies, past surgical procedures, current medications and allergies, family history of cancer, problems with anesthesia, and social history, including smoking history, occupation, sun exposure, and history of blistering sunburns.
- A focused review of systems should also be completed and include review of any constitutional, musculoskeletal, neurologic, respiratory, gastrointestinal, hepatic, dermal, and lymphatic signs or symptoms.
- All newly diagnosed patients with melanoma should undergo full body skin evaluation.
- A complete head and neck examination should be performed on every patient and include a thorough skin examination and palpation of the suboccipital, postauricular, parotid, and cervical nodal basins to rule out the presence of clinically palpable regional metastatic disease.
- A detailed cranial nerve examination should be performed to document preoperative cranial nerve function.

IMAGING AND OTHER DIAGNOSTIC STUDIES

- Newly diagnosed patients with localized cutaneous melanoma are not recommended to undergo distant metastatic workup. In the absence of clinical signs or symptoms of distant metastatic disease no imaging modality has been shown to be useful in detecting occult metastatic disease and in fact more often leads to false-positive findings requiring further unnecessary invasive procedures.[1]
- Chest x-ray and serum lactate dehydrogenase are also both insensitive for the detection of occult metastatic disease.
- Most patients will require preoperative chest x-ray, complete blood count, and electrocardiogram depending on age, health status, and need for general anesthesia.

SURGICAL MANAGEMENT

Preoperative Planning

- Prior to proceeding to the operating room, the primary cutaneous lesion should be reexamined and confirmed with the patient. The surrounding skin should also be reexamined to make sure no new lesions have developed. In addition, the plan regarding surgical margins and primary closure vs delayed reconstruction should be confirmed with the patient. All cranial nerve functions in the operative field should also be retested prior to surgery.
- Patients who are scheduled for SLNB in conjunction with excision of their primary cutaneous lesion will undergo lymphoscintigraphy prior to their definitive excision. This procedure is done in the nuclear medicine department and is enhanced by the use of single-photon emission computed tomography–computed tomography (SPECT-CT) imaging.[7] Prior to proceeding to the operating room the SPECT-CT/lymphoscintigraphy should be reviewed to determine the likely location of the sentinel lymph node or nodes (**FIGURES 1** and **2**). These locations should then be discussed with the patient and marked appropriately. If the location of a likely sentinel lymph node is in close proximity to a cranial nerve, this should be discussed with the patient, and the cranial nerve function should be well documented.
- Appropriate use of antibiotics and DVT prophylaxis should also be discussed prior to proceeding to the operating room.
- In addition, it is crucial to have a thorough discussion with the anesthesia team regarding the use of long-acting paralytics. If cranial nerves are likely to be in the operative field, as is almost always the case in the resection of head and neck melanoma, the anesthesia team must be aware to avoid the use of long-acting paralytics.

Positioning

- Patients who are scheduled for wide local excision alone (melanoma in situ or T1a lesions) often can tolerate surgery under

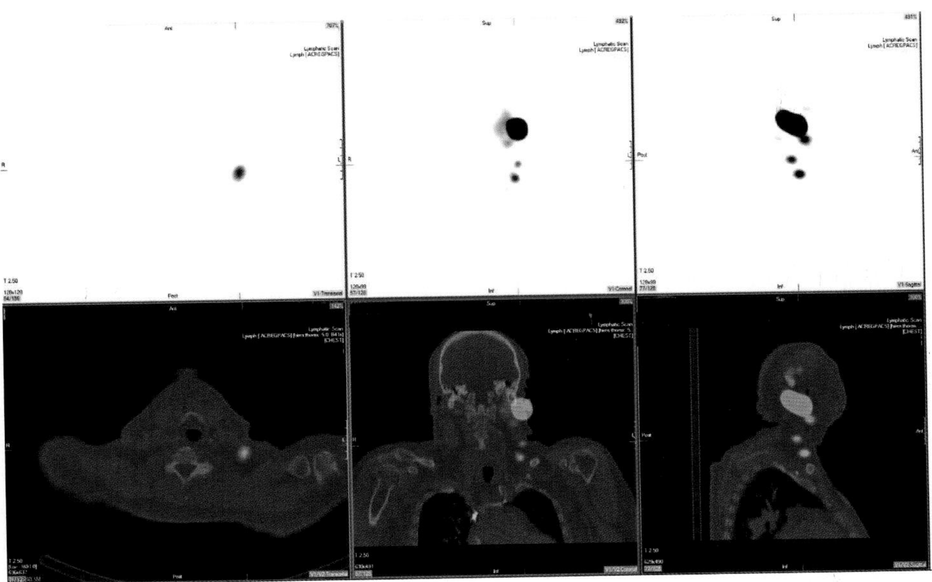

FIGURE 1 ● Lymphoscintigraphy with SPECT-CT imaging after injection of left postauricular primary melanoma site. Imaging reveals a left level II lymph node as well as secondary drainage to left levels Va and Vb.

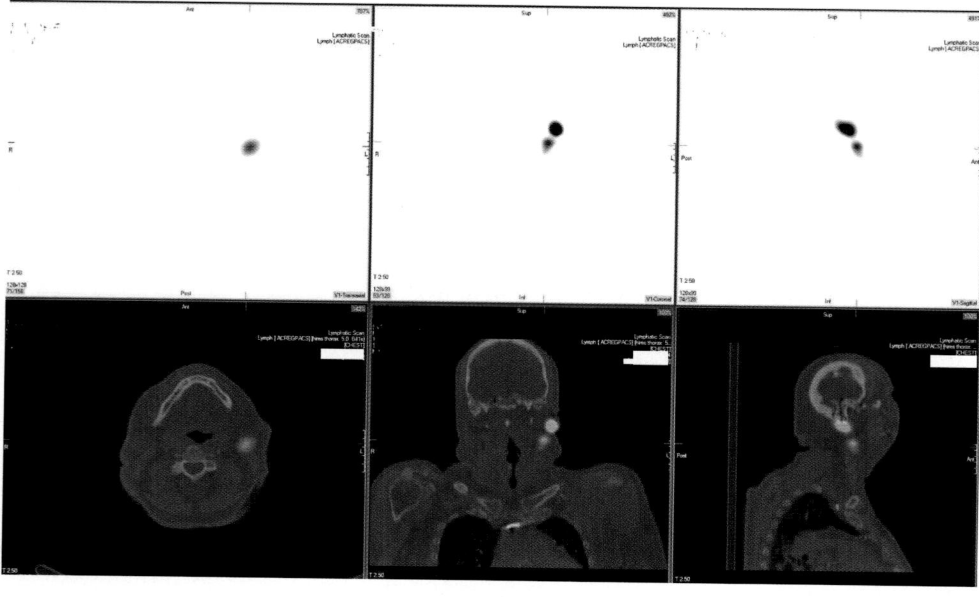

FIGURE 2 ● Lymphoscintigraphy with SPECT-CT imaging after injection of left postauricular primary melanoma site. Careful observation reveals the level II lymph node to be located just inferior to the tail of the parotid and just anterior to the sternocleidomastoid muscle. Likely this represents an external jugular lymph node.

sedation with monitored anesthesia. In these cases the head of the bed is often rotated 90° away from the anesthesia cart to allow for easy access to the surgical field. Oxygen delivery methods can be designed to avoid crossing the surgical field and may include either nasal cannula or mask. In these cases with free flowing oxygen it is very important to discuss the risk of fire with the entire operating room team. The entire face and neck can be prepped into the operative field. Wide draping can then be used with attention to avoid any tenting of drapes, which could lead to pooling of oxygen in the operative field (**FIGURE 3**).

- Patients who are scheduled to undergo sentinel lymph node biopsy in conjunction with the primary excision are almost always placed under general anesthesia. Again, the use of long-acting paralytics must be avoided. The head of the bed can be rotated 180° away from the anesthesia cart to allow for easy surgical access to the operative field. Most primary lesions can be excised with the patient in the supine position. Rarely, the patient may need to be turned prone to allow access to the posterior scalp or suboccipital nodal basin. With the patient intubated either half of the face and neck or the entire face and neck can be prepped and draped depending on the need for surgical access.

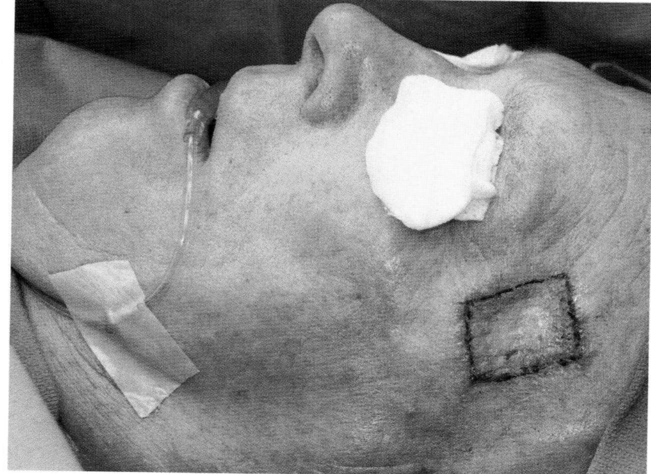

FIGURE 3 ● Patient is under sedation with the entire face prepped to allow for wide draping and to avoid pooling of oxygen within the surgical field.

TECHNIQUES

Placement of Planned Incisions

Primary Lesion Excision Site

- The primary lesion is carefully inspected and cleaned with a moist sponge. The lesion should be marked out with careful attention to include any evidence of dermal extension. This may include any pale, erythematous, or lightly pigmented extension from the primary lesion (**FIGURE 4**).
- With the primary lesion now marked, the appropriate margin is then marked circumferentially around the visible lesion. The excision margin is most often 1 to 2 cm depending on the depth of invasion of the primary lesion.
- In certain functional situations, the excision margin may be left a little short of standard margins. For example, if a lower eyelid lesion requires 2-cm margins, but at 1 cm the excision would cross the lid margin, it may be acceptable to use 1 cm. In this case the surgeon must be willing to re-excise this margin should it return positive on final histopathologic review (**FIGURE 5**).

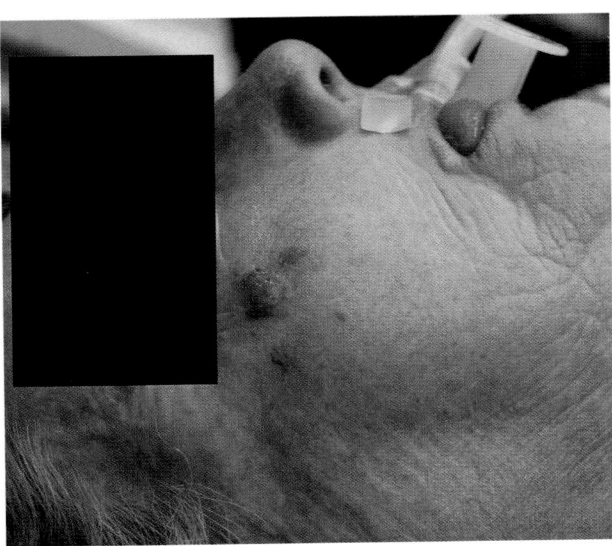

FIGURE 4 ● The main lesion is pink and raised. Notice the pigmented extension into the surrounding skin. The entire pigmented area must be marked out prior to marking out circumferential margins.

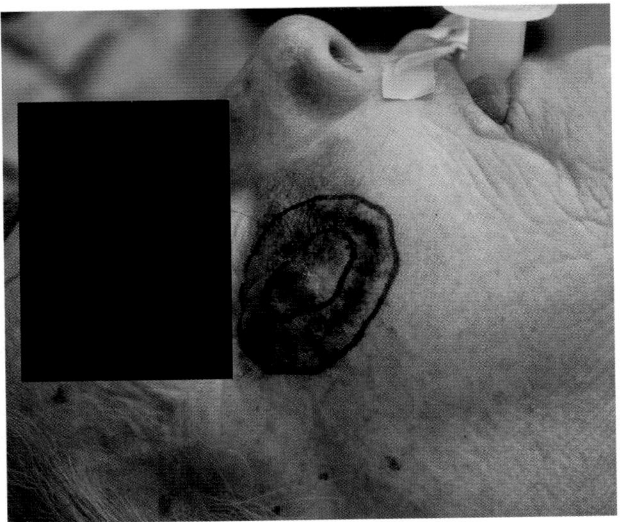

FIGURE 5 ● In this planned resection, the lower eyelid margin is left a little narrow in the hopes of avoiding postoperative ectropion. The margins must be carefully examined by pathology and re-excised should they return positive.

Injection of Methylene Blue Dye

- To assist with sentinel lymph node identification the dermis surrounding the primary lesion is injected with methylene blue dye. Usually only 1 or 2 mL of dye is injected (**FIGURE 6**).
- The injection is made with a 30-gauge needle with the bevel of the needle facing up. There should be slight pressure as the dye is injected and visually the dermis should begin to turn blue. If the dermis is not turning blue or the injection is passing with no resistance the needle is likely too deep. This will cause the subcutaneous tissue to turn blue and can make recognition of tissue planes more difficult.

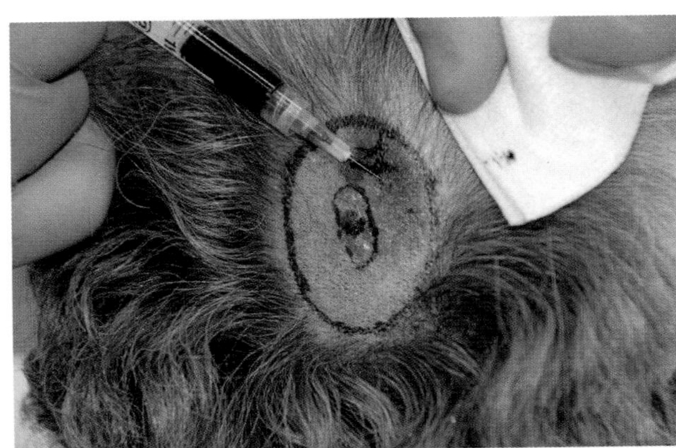

FIGURE 6 ● Methylene blue dye injected circumferentially into the dermis surrounding the lesion. A 30-gauge needle is used, and effort is made to inject directly into the dermis only.

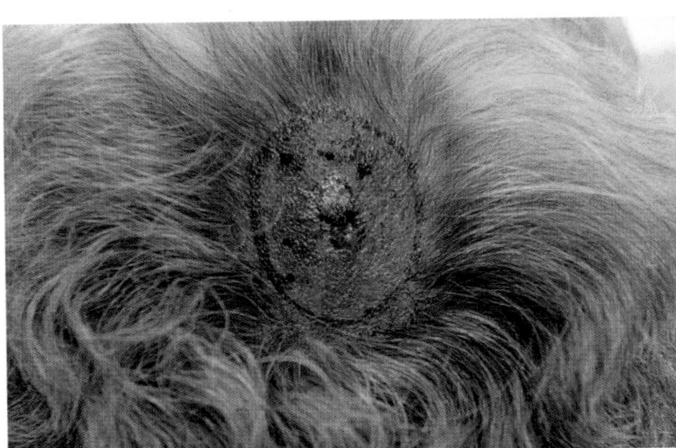

FIGURE 7 ● Methylene blue dye injected into the dermis circumferentially around the lesion.

- Several injections should be made into the dermis surrounding the primary lesion until the lesion is surrounded by blue dye (**FIGURE 7**).

Placement of Incisions for SLNB

- The preoperative lymphoscintigraphy/SPECT-CT is again reviewed to help determine the approximate location of the sentinel lymph nodes in relation to visible or palpable anatomic structures. The intraoperative gamma probe can then be used to confirm the site of the sentinel nodes. Once the location is confirmed incisions are marked to allow access to remove the sentinel nodes (**FIGURE 8**).
- Marking the planned incisions should take into account placement along relaxed skin tension lines. In addition, consideration should be given to any future potential procedures such as rotation flap reconstruction sites or the need for parotidectomy and cervical lymphadenectomy (**FIGURE 9**).
- At this point all planned incisions are usually injected with local anesthesia. Typically, 1% lidocaine with 1:100,000 epinephrine solution is used. A small volume should be used to help avoid inadvertent paralysis of cranial nerves close to the operative sites.

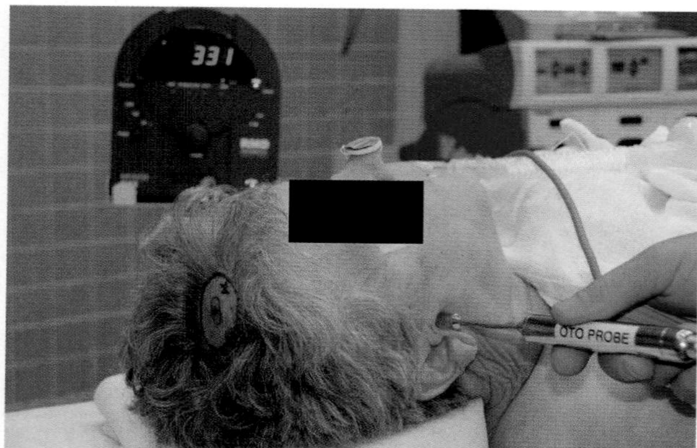

FIGURE 8 ● The intraoperative gamma probe is used to confirm the sites of the potential SLNs.

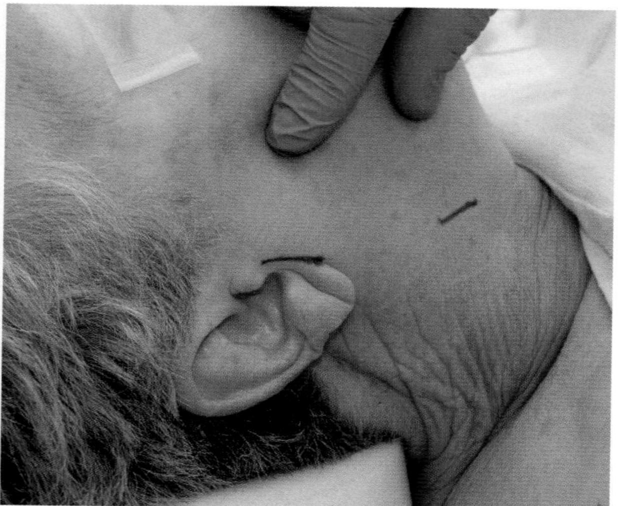

FIGURE 9 ● Small incisions are planned along relaxed skin tension lines.

Excision of the Primary Lesion

Skin Incision

- The skin surrounding the primary lesion is now sharply incised being careful to follow the exact marking. The incision is carried through the subcutaneous tissue now being careful to avoid beveling the cut toward the primary lesion.

Determining the Depth of the Excision

- Once the peripheral incisions are made around the primary lesion the depth of the excision must be determined. In general, the depth of the excision is carried to the fascial plane deep to the subcutaneous tissue. The depth of the excision is highly dependent on the location of the primary lesion, the size and depth of the lesion, and the amount of subcutaneous tissue deep to the lesion.
- For facial lesions the excision is most often carried to a plane just above the facial musculature (**FIGURE 10**).

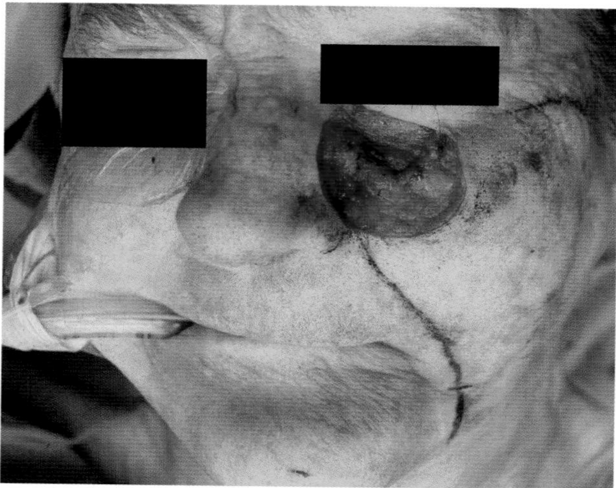

FIGURE 10 ● The facial lesion has been excised to a depth just above the facial musculature.

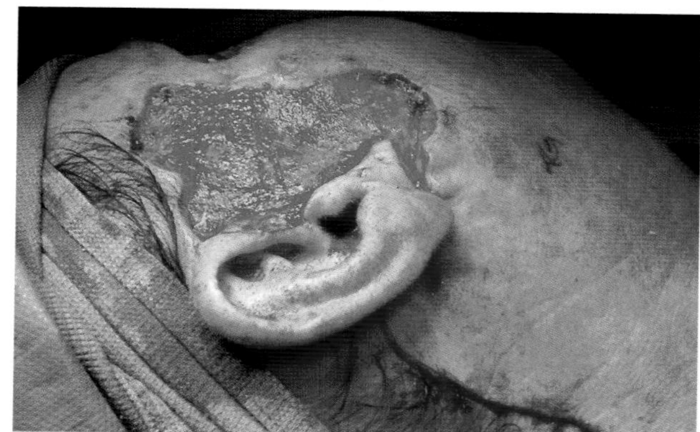

FIGURE 11 ● Preauricular lesions are excised to a depth just above the parotid fascia.

- Preauricular lesions are excised to a depth of the parotid fascia (**FIGURE 11**).
- Nasal lesions are excised above the level of the nasal cartilages.
- Auricular lesions are removed either with or without the underlying cartilage depending on the size of the primary lesion. In many cases the underlying cartilage should be removed to ensure adequate negative margins.
- Scalp lesions are usually excised in a subgaleal plane with the underlying pericranium left intact. In large bulky lesions the underlying pericranium can also be removed to allow for wider clear margins (**FIGURE 12**).
- Neck skin can be excised either with or without the underlying platysma muscle depending on the size of the lesion. If there is any concern about deep invasion it is easy to remove platysma.
- With all excisions attention must be paid to avoiding injury to any underlying cranial nerves.

Orientation

- Once the primary lesion is completely excised it must be carefully oriented and marked for permanent pathology.

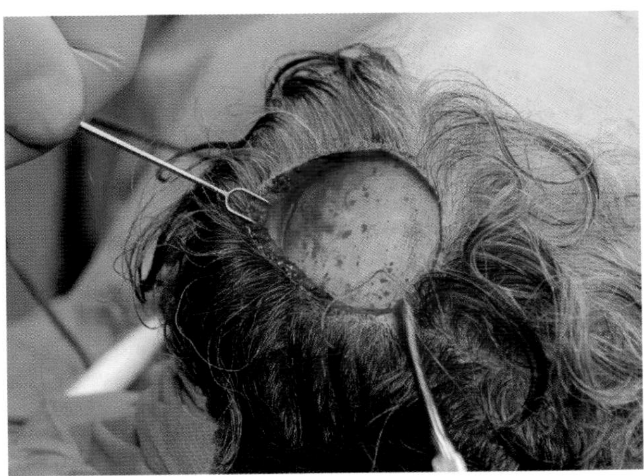

FIGURE 12 ● Scalp lesions are usually excised in a subgaleal plane with the underlying pericranium left intact.

Marking stitches should be easily understood and allow for easy communication between surgeon and pathologist. Any areas of special concern should also be noted on the pathology request, such as when margins are less than ideal due to functional considerations.

Sentinel Lymph Node Biopsy

Intraoperative Gamma Probe

- The intraoperative gamma probe is now used to confirm the site of the sentinel lymph node. In some cases, the primary excision site should be surveyed to look for potential sentinel lymph nodes that may be deep to the primary excision site. These nodes may not appear on the SPECT-CT due to the shadowing caused by the high intensity of the primary lesion injection site. Sometimes a blue lymphatic channel can be seen at the edge of the excision site and can be followed to a sentinel lymph node (**FIGURE 13**).

Incision and Node Dissection

- Before proceeding with lymph node dissection it is important to confirm that the patient has not been given any paralytic agents.
- After confirming the previously marked sentinel lymph node sites with the gamma probe the incision is made and carried to the deep soft tissue. Usually a 2- to 3-cm incision is long enough to allow for easy dissection and visualization.
- With the incision made skin hooks are used to retract the skin edges. Blunt dissection is then used to enter the deeper soft tissue. In the neck, dissection will go deep to the platysma muscle. In the preauricular region the dissection will often proceed deep to the parotid fascia into the parotid parenchyma.
- The intraoperative gamma probe is used frequently to help determine the direction of further dissection. As the tip of the probe gets closer to the sentinel node the gamma counts will increase.
- Often times a blue lymphatic channel can be identified and can then be followed to the sentinel lymph node (**FIGURES 14** and **15**).
- Once the node is identified it is carefully removed with blunt dissection and judicious use of bipolar electrocautery.
- The node is then examined away from the patient to document the gamma count and the presence of blue dye. The node is labeled with the anatomic location, gamma count, and presence of blue dye and sent for histopathology.

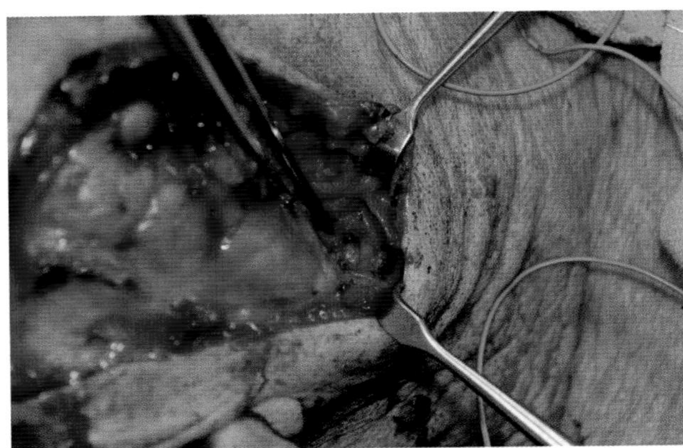

FIGURE 13 ● The SLN is identified deep to the primary excision site.

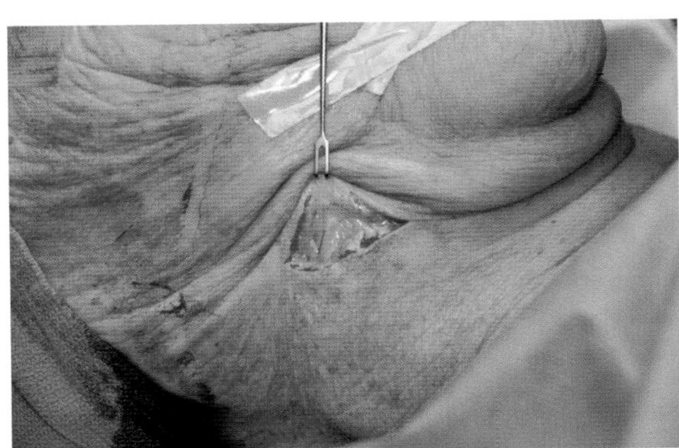

FIGURE 14 ● Oftentimes, a blue lymphatic channel can be identified.

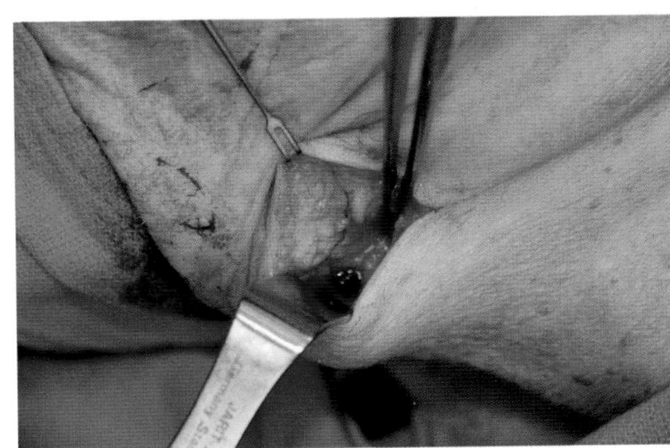

FIGURE 15 ● Lymphatic channels can then be followed to the SLN.

Confirmation and Closure

- After removing the sentinel lymph node the gamma probe is then used to reexamine the surgical bed. The area where the node was removed should now have a very low count compared with the count prior to node removal. As a general rule the count should drop to less than 10% of the count prior to node removal. If the count remains elevated further dissection is warranted to remove any other potential sentinel lymph nodes identified.

- Once all potential sentinel lymph nodes are removed the surgical bed is irrigated with saline. A Valsalva maneuver should be performed to confirm there is no ongoing bleeding. The incision can be closed in standard fashion and a small pressure dressing applied.

Primary Closure vs Delayed Reconstruction of the Primary Site

Primary Closure

- After the primary lesion has been resected and the sentinel lymph node biopsy completed it is time to determine the best method of closing the primary site. If the primary site can be closed without distorting the surgical margins and without the use of rotation flaps or grafts this can be done immediately. Should a margin return positive on permanent pathology it would still be easy to return for wider excision.
- This is usually the case for small lesions or for lesions on the neck where excess skin can easily be advanced.
- In these cases, bilateral Burrow triangle excisions can be performed along the direction of relaxed skin tension lines. The skin is then undermined, advanced, and closed with deep absorbable suture and superficial suture at the skin edge.
- The wound is then dressed with a small pressure dressing, which can be removed after 24 hours.

Delayed Reconstruction

- In many cases reconstruction of the primary resection site will require significant tissue rearrangement, skin grafting, or even free tissue transfer. In these situations, it is preferable to wait for final histopathologic confirmation of negative surgical margins prior to proceeding with definitive reconstruction.
- The size of the wound can often be decreased with use of a circumferential purse-string suture (**FIGURE 16**).
- The wound can then be dressed with a moist bolster dressing using Vaseline or Xeroform gauze, bacitracin, cotton balls, or any foam-type dressing. The bolster dressing can be secured with either silk suture or surgical staples (**FIGURES 17** and **18**).

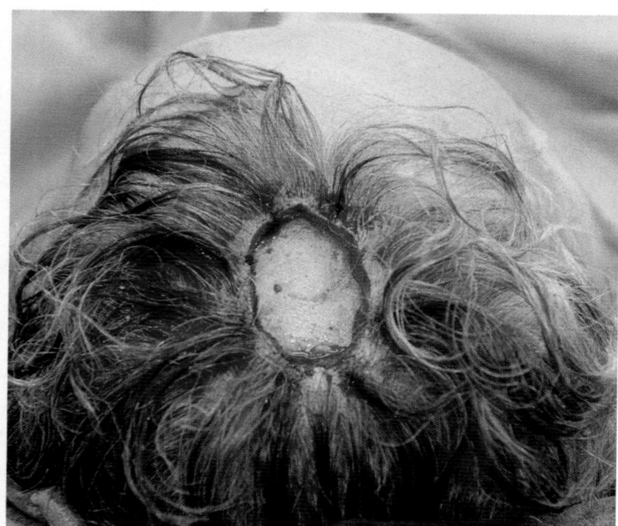

FIGURE 16 ● Circumferential purse-string suture is used to decrease the size of the wound.

- Wound infections are very rare in the head and neck, and therefore, postoperative antibiotics are not routinely used even in the setting of an open wound with a bolster applied. In some cases, such as immune suppression or previous infection, antibiotics may be indicated.

Skin Graft and Rotation Flap Reconstruction

- Once the final surgical margins have returned clear definitive reconstruction can be completed. The method of reconstruction is dependent on the site of the defect and the goals of the patient. Complex facial defects should be addressed by colleagues with experience in facial plastic and reconstructive surgery.
- Facial skin and preauricular skin defects are most often closed with the use of cervicofacial rotation flaps and transposition flaps. Incisions are planned along relaxed skin tension lines when possible and are carried to postauricular and posterior cervical skin. These flaps create standing cutaneous deformities along the arc of rotation, which will need to be excised. Very large defects can be closed and excellent cosmetic outcomes achieved (**FIGURES 19-21**).

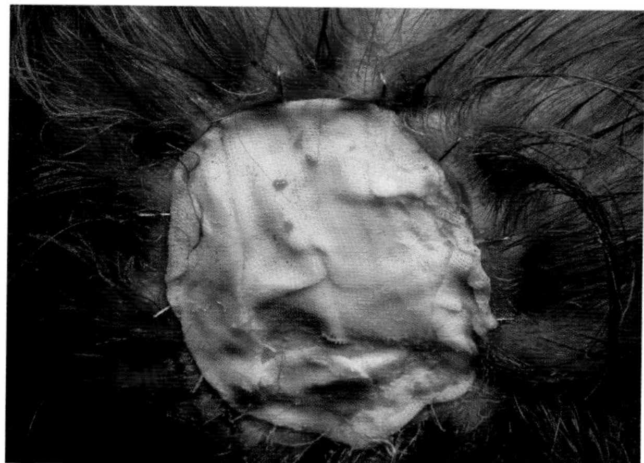

FIGURE 17 ● A Xeroform gauze dressing is placed over the resection site.

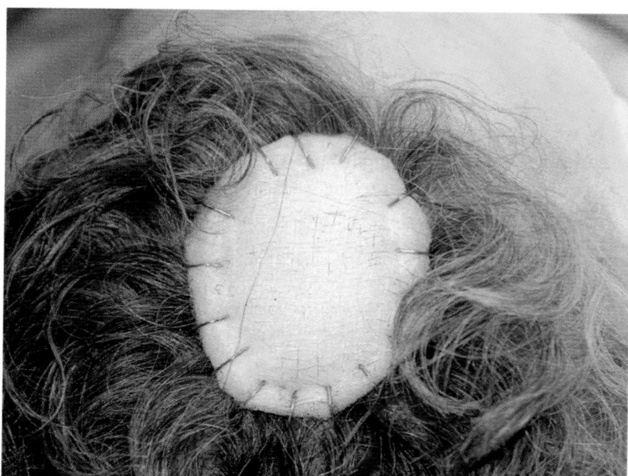

FIGURE 18 ● A Reston foam bolster is secured to the scalp to apply pressure after either resection or skin graft reconstruction.

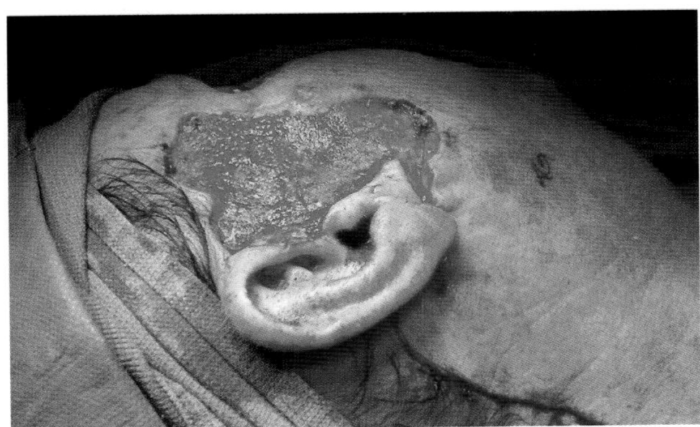

FIGURE 19 ● Large facial defect with posterior cervical incision made to allow for cervicofacial rotation flap reconstruction.

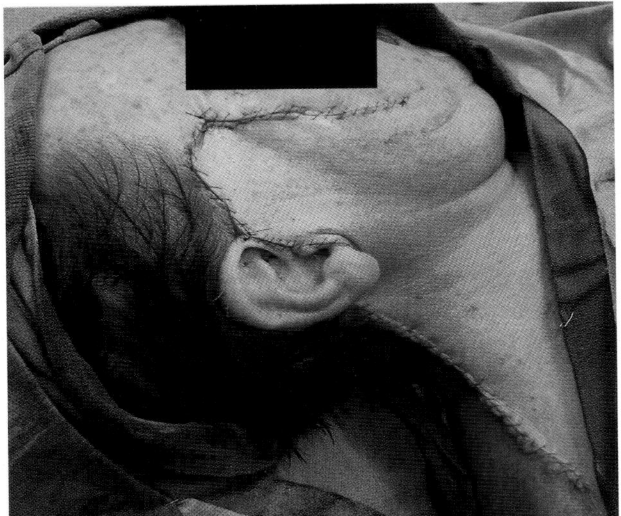

FIGURE 20 ● Cervicofacial rotation flap brought into position.

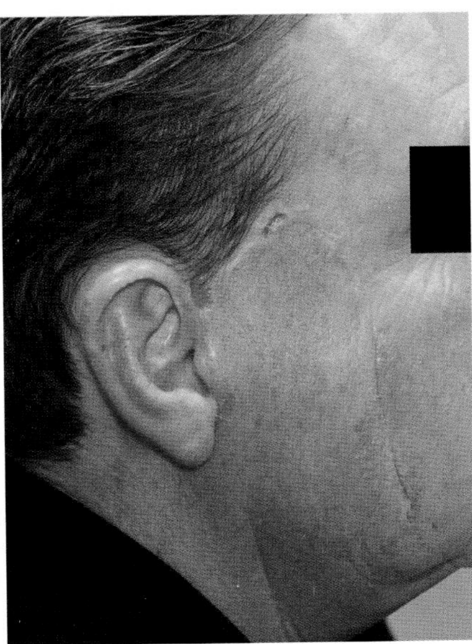

FIGURE 21 ● Excellent cosmetic result several weeks after cervicofacial reconstruction of large facial defect.

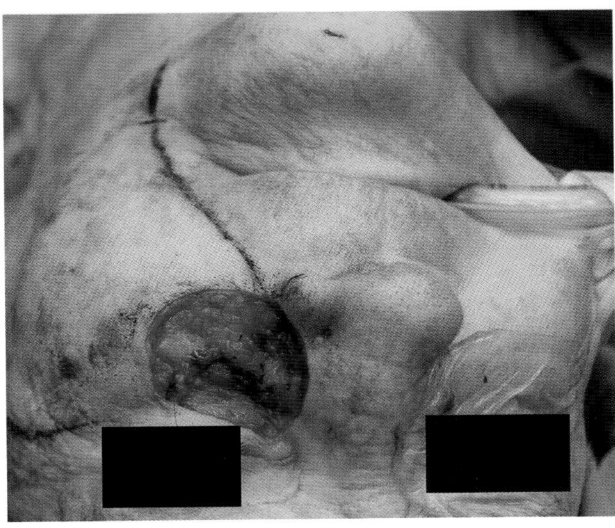

FIGURE 22 ● Large rotation flap designed for reconstruction of lower eyelid defect.

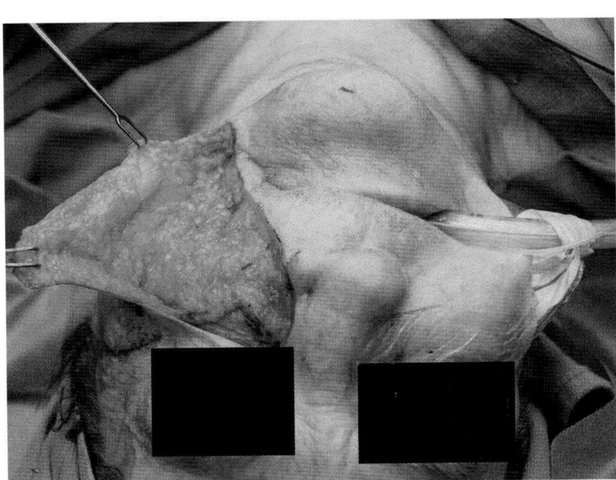

FIGURE 23 ● The flap is raised far enough to allow for tension-free closure.

- Eyelid defects can be very difficult to repair without causing significant ectropion. Lid-tightening procedures can be done in conjunction with skin grafts, transposition flaps, and rotation flaps. Occuloplastic surgeons should be involved if there is concern about postoperative eyelid function (**FIGURES 22-24**).
- Nasal defects can be closed with skin grafts, composite grafts, transposition flaps, advancement flaps, and the interpolated paramedian forehead flap. Each technique can yield excellent results when used in the proper clinical setting (**FIGURES 25-27**).
- Auricular defects are most easily closed with wedge excision and advancement flap closure. Transposition flaps can be used to reconstruct large defects and achieve acceptable cosmetic results (**FIGURES 28** and **29**).
- Scalp defects are most easily closed with the use of full-thickness or split-thickness skin grafts. In older patients large amounts of supraclavicular skin can be harvested and used

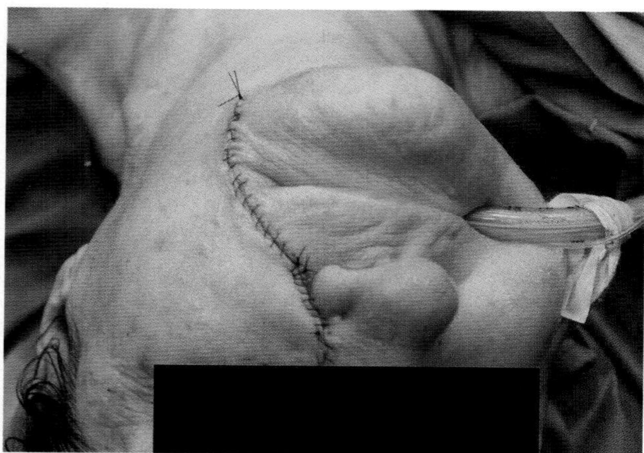

FIGURE 24 ● The rotation flap is sewn into place with no tension inferiorly, thus avoiding postoperative ectropion.

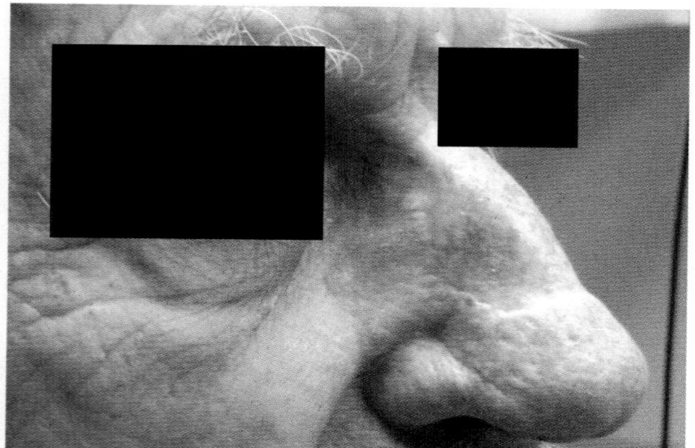

FIGURE 25 ● Postoperative result after full-thickness skin graft reconstruction of the nasal dorsum.

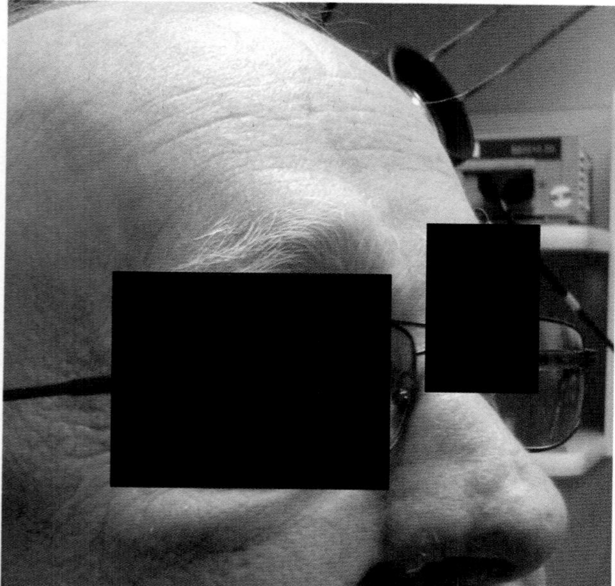

FIGURE 26 ● Postoperative result after paramedian forehead flap reconstruction of right lateral nasal wall and alar rim with use of ear cartilage grafting to alar rim (lateral view).

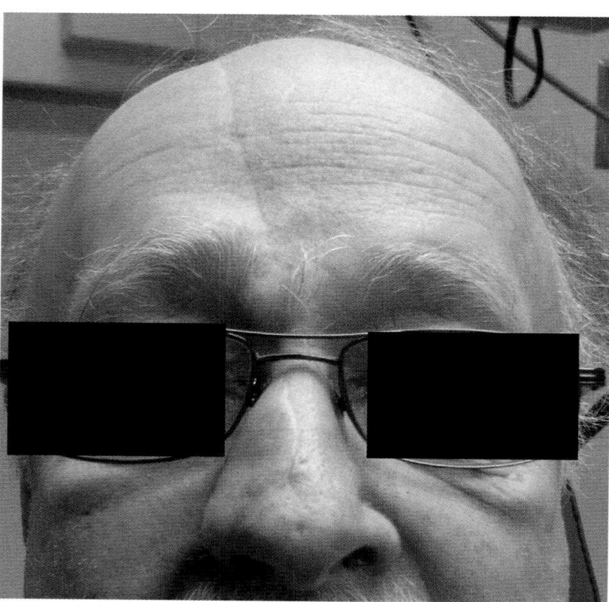

FIGURE 27 ● Postoperative result after paramedian forehead flap reconstruction of right lateral nasal wall and alar rim with use of ear cartilage grafting to alar rim (frontal view).

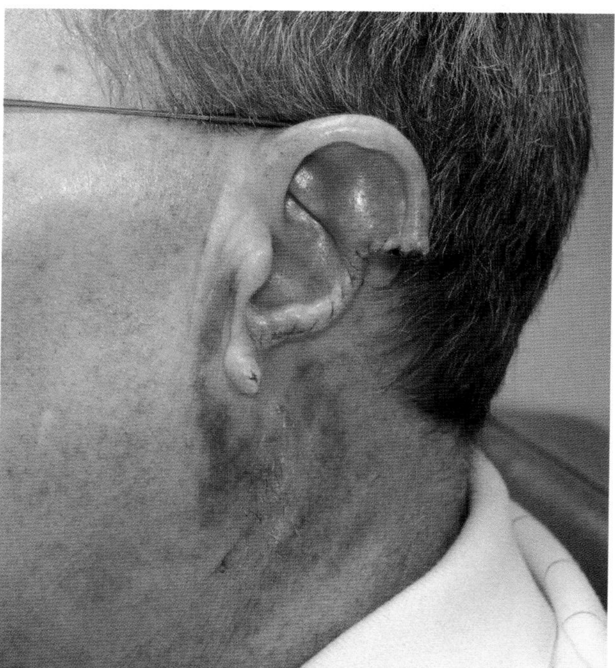

FIGURE 28 ● Resection of left lower ear and helical rim.

to graft large scalp defects. The skin is thinned to the dermal layer making sure to remove all subcutaneous tissue. The skin graft can be placed over intact periosteum or can be grafted directly to exposed bone. In this case a burr can be used to burr down the bone until punctate vessels are seen. The graft is then secured with a bolster dressing and left intact for 7 to 10 days.

- Neck skin defects can almost always be closed with adjacent tissue transfer reconstruction as described earlier.

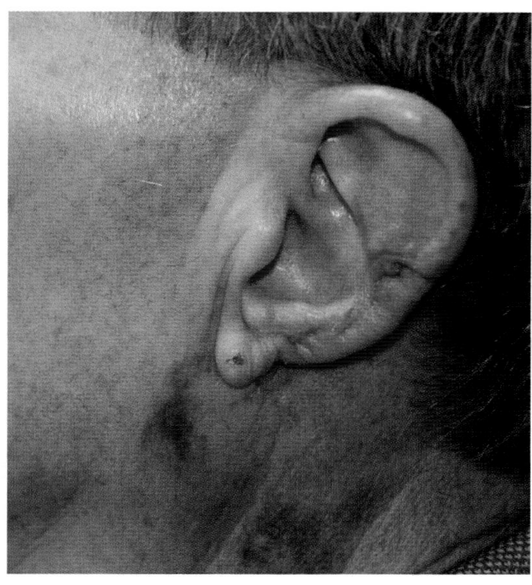

FIGURE 29 ● Reconstruction of left ear with postauricular transposition flaps.

PEARLS AND PITFALLS

Indications and preoperative workup	A complete history and physical examination should be performed including full-body skin check. If SLNB is indicated lymphoscintigraphy with SPECT-CT imaging should be reviewed prior to surgery. A detailed cranial nerve examination should be completed prior to proceeding with surgery.
Excision of primary lesion	The primary lesion should be marked to include any pale, erythematous, or pigmented adjacent skin. Circumferential margins, 1-2 cm, are marked depending on the depth of invasion of the primary lesion and proximity to surrounding structures. The depth of excision needs to include enough normal tissue to ensure complete surgical excision. Mark the specimen with clear orientation sutures to allow for definitive margin analysis.
Sentinel lymph node biopsy	Review preoperative lymphoscintigraphy/SPECT-CT to identify likely sites of sentinel lymph nodes. Inject methylene blue dye circumferentially into the dermis surrounding the primary lesion. Ensure anesthesia has not paralyzed the patient prior to lymph node dissection. Make incisions along relaxed skin tension lines and keeping in mind the possible need for rotation advancement flap reconstruction or future parotid/neck dissection incisions. Utilize intraoperative gamma probe to localize sentinel lymph node and make sure that all potential sentinel lymph nodes are removed.
Closure vs delayed reconstruction	If wound can be closed by simple advancement flap without reorienting margins then wound can be closed primarily. If rotation/transposition flap or skin graft is needed it may be wise to delay reconstruction until final surgical margins are clear. Facial plastic and occuloplastic colleagues should be consulted for closure of complex wounds.

POSTOPERATIVE CARE

- Small pressure dressings are usually applied to small advancement flap reconstruction sites as well as sentinel lymph node biopsy sites and are left intact for 24 hours. Larger cervicofacial advancement flap reconstruction sites are dressed with Jobst pressure dressings and are left intact for 2 to 3 days. When the dressings are removed the incisions should be kept clean with half-strength peroxide and moist with Vaseline. Topical antibiotic ointment may be used for 2 to 3 days but can cause skin irritation with longer use. When skin grafts are used the bolster dressing is left intact for 7 to 10 days. After the bolster is removed the graft is kept moist with Vaseline for 1 to 2 weeks or until the wound has completely healed.

OUTCOMES

- In the hands of experienced head and neck surgeons a sentinel lymph node can be identified in nearly all patients. In patients with cutaneous melanoma of the head and neck with Breslow depth ≥ 1 mm or with Breslow depth between 0.75 and 0.99 mm with other adverse features approximately 20% are found to have a positive sentinel lymph node.
- Among patients with a positive SLN undergoing close clinical observation with serial ultrasounds, approximately 25% of patients will develop regional recurrence.[8] Similarly, approximately 25% of patients with a positive sentinel lymph node undergoing immediate CLND will be found to have at least one more positive nonsentinel lymph node. Approximately 4% of patients with negative sentinel lymph nodes will fail regionally within the sentinel node basin.[2]
- Positive sentinel lymph node status is the factor most strongly associated with decreased recurrence-free survival and decreased overall survival (hazard ratio of 4.23 and 3.33, respectively). The estimated 4-year overall survival approaches 84% in patients with negative sentinel lymph node biopsy and decreases to an estimated 58% in patients with a positive sentinel lymph node.[2]

COMPLICATIONS

- Seroma or hematoma at the sentinel lymph node biopsy site.
- Infection at either the SLNB or primary resection site.
- Wound dehiscence or epidermolysis of the rotation flap reconstruction site.
- Decrease in sensation at either surgical site.
- Theoretical risk of cranial nerve injury.
- Poor cosmetic outcome.

REFERENCES

1. Bichakjian CK, Halpern AC, Johnson TM, et al. Guidelines of care for the management of primary cutaneous melanoma. *J Am Acad Dermatol.* 2011;65:1032-1047.
2. Erman AM, Collar RM, Griffith KA, et al. Sentinel lymph node biopsy is accurate and prognostic in head and neck melanoma. *Cancer.* 2012;118:1040-1047.
3. Gershenwald JE, Thompson W, Mansfield PF, et al. Multi-institutional melanoma lymphatic mapping experience: the prognostic value of sentinel lymph node status in 612 stage I or II melanoma patients. *J Clin Oncol.* 1999;17(3):976-983.
4. Kupferman ME, Kubik MW, Bradford CR, et al. The role of sentinel lymph node biopsy for thin cutaneous melanomas of the head and neck. *Am J Oto.* 2014;35:226-232.
5. Morton DL, Thompson JF, Cochran AJ, et al. Sentinel-node biopsy or nodal observation in melanoma. *N Engl J Med.* 2006;355(13):1307-1317.
6. Schmalbach CE, Johnson TM, Bradford CR. The management of head and neck melanoma. *Curr Probl Surg.* 2006;43:781-835.
7. Zender C, Guo T, Weng C, Faulhaber P, Rezaee R. Utility of SPECT/CT for periparotid sentinel lymoh node mapping in the surgical management of head and neck melanoma. *Am J Oto.* 2014;35:12-18.
8. Faries MB, Thompson JF, Cochran AJ, et al. Completion dissection or observation for sentinel-node metastasis in melanoma. *N Engl J Med.* 2017;376:2211-2222.

Chapter 33 Sentinel Lymph Node Biopsy for Melanoma

Merrick I. Ross

DEFINITIONS

- The sentinel lymph node(s) are defined as the first nodes to receive direct (afferent) lymphatic drainage from the cutaneous site of a primary melanoma and also the most likely lymph node(s) to harbor microscopic metastases. The technique of lymphatic mapping and sentinel lymph node (SLN) biopsy is used to determine the histologic status of the regional lymph node basin(s) in patients with early-stage (American Joint Committee on Cancer [AJCC] clinical stages I and II) melanoma without performing a formal lymph node dissection. The SLN concept as well as the minimally invasive technique, which initially used intradermal injections of vital blue dye only[1] (**FIGURE 1**) and later modified with the addition of radiolabeled colloid injections[2,3] at the site of the primary melanoma, was first studied and reported in detail by Morton and colleagues, demonstrating proof of concept in a large group of patients with primary melanoma and clinically negative regional lymph nodes.[1] This and several subsequent studies have confirmed that the lymphatic drainage patterns from specific regions of the skin can be accurately determined, the SLN is the most likely first site of regional lymph node metastasis, and if the SLNs are histologically negative, the remaining lymph nodes in the mapped basin are unlikely to contain disease. The reported accuracy (sensitivity) of SLN biopsy is 95%.[1,3-5] The term "biopsy" is perhaps a misnomer (particularly to patients) because the biopsy procedure is excisional in nature in that the entire SLN is removed and subjected to rigorous histologic analysis. Alternatively, the term "sentinel lymphadenectomy" can be used to more accurately describe the extent of the surgery.

CLINICAL IMPORTANCE

- Improving outcomes and reducing morbidity: The sobering reality is that when patients with melanoma develop clinically apparent (palpable) regional nodal disease (advanced AJCC stage III), the risk of subsequent distant stage IV disease and recurrent lymph node basin disease, despite treatment with a formal therapeutic lymphadenectomy, is at least 50%[6] and 15% to 50%,[7] respectively. Therefore, the original motivation to study SLN biopsy was to establish an effective method of identifying and then treating lymph node disease early (when microscopic) with a completion lymph node

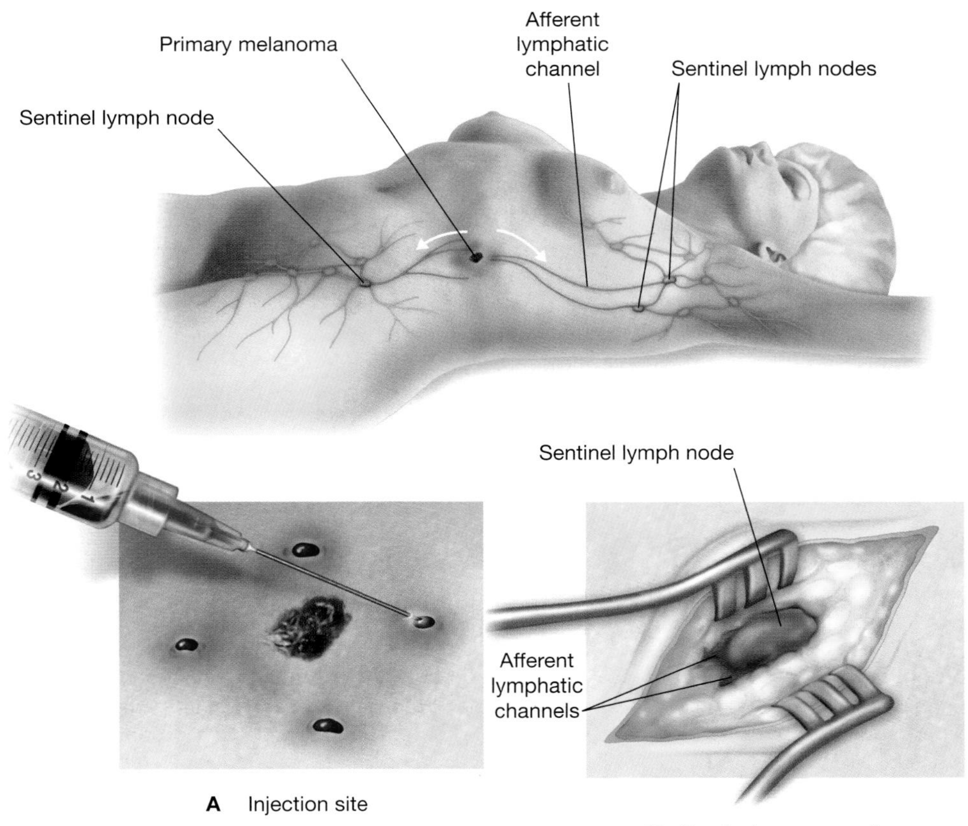

FIGURE 1 ● Sentinel node localization using blue dye injections. An artistic rendition of the sentinel node concept and afferent lymphatic drainage patterns is depicted. After the intradermal injection of blue dye around a primary cutaneous melanoma (left abdominal wall, **Panel A**), afferent lymphatic drainage to a left inguinal sentinel lymph node and two left axillary sentinel lymph nodes is shown. **Panel B** shows surgical exposure, using a self-retaining retractor, of the first of two sentinel nodes in the left axilla. Note the two afferent lymphatic vessels entering the sentinel node. Both nodes in the axilla would be defined as "sentinel" because they each receive first (primary) echelon drainage from a specific afferent lymphatic vessel. Both nodes need to be removed from the axilla as well as the SLN in the groin to complete the surgical procedure of SLN biopsy.

dissection (CLND), an approach termed "selective lymphadenectomy," not to be confused with the aforementioned "sentinel lymphadenectomy," the latter of which refers specifically to the SLN biopsy procedure. Such an approach would prevent the development of clinically palpable nodal disease in most patients and in turn potentially improve the outcomes for the node-positive patients in terms of both regional disease control and survival. The Multi-Center Selective Lymphadenectomy Trial (MSLT)-1, which randomized patients with primary melanoma >1 mm in thickness to wide local excision (WLE) plus SLN biopsy vs WLE alone, was designed to directly test the hypothesis that early surgical treatment of nodal metastases could improve outcomes compared with patients who develop clinically involved nodal disease. The final results of this trial and the collective experience with SLN biopsy demonstrated that proof of concept was established and the two goals of improved regional disease control and melanoma-specific survival in the node-positive subgroups have been achieved.[8,9]

- Additional valuable data derived from MSLT-1 as well as from real world experience with CLND after a positive SLN biopsy demonstrated that, overall, only 10% to 20%[9,10] of patients were found to have additional microscopically involved nodes, referred to as non-SLNs, and that the accepted practice of routine CLND subjected a significant majority of patients the unnecessary morbidity of a CLND. Increasingly, questions were raised about the impact of CLND on melanoma-specific survival,[11] leading to the design and completion of two randomized clinical trials.[12,13] The recently published results of these two trials comparing the outcomes of patients with positive SLNs treated with CLND or nodal basin observation with ultrasound surveillance demonstrated improved regional disease control but no apparent improvement in overall survival with CLND. One of these trials, MSLT-2, also provided compelling data from a multivariable analysis that the presence of non-SLN involvement was the strongest negative prognostic factor even after adjusting for the number of lymph nodes involved,[12] partially explaining why the removal of these additional positive nodes with CLND had little if any impact on long-term melanoma-specific survival. These results confirmed that previously reported findings concerning the prognostic relevance of non-SLN metastases[14,15] were responsible for a global change in practice, which has almost completely replaced routine CLND with either nodal basin observation including nodal basin ultrasound surveillance or a very selective approach to CLND. Subsequent to the publishing of the results of the two aforementioned randomized trials, adjuvant targeted (BRAF-positive patients) and immunotherapy were approved for all node-positive patients, further supporting the clinical management practice away from routine CLND. Overall, these recent evidence-based changes have led to reduced surgery-related morbidity without compromising long-term melanoma-specific survival.[12,15]
- Staging and prognosis: The melanoma patient population with clinical stages I and II (clinically node negative) represent at least 85% of the newly diagnosed patients. The prognosis of this group is very heterogeneous and dependent on a variety of primary tumor factors, specifically tumor thickness, ulceration, and mitotic rate, and probably most importantly, the presence of occult lymph node involvement.[16] The role of SLN biopsy as a staging tool has been well established, as several published multivariable analyses demonstrate that the histologic status of the SLN is the strongest independent predictor of survival for stages I and II and therefore offers another motivation for SLN biopsy.[16,17] The procedure is also intended to identify patients with pathologically node-negative disease for whom additional surgery is not indicated, sparing these patients the morbidity of unnecessary surgery. The patients with melanoma with pathological stages 1b-2a have an excellent prognosis and therefore are not offered any additional treatment but are eligible for long-term surveillance. However, the patients with pathological stages 2b-2c overall have a more guarded prognosis, because of thick and ulcerated primary tumor histological features, and therefore may be offered adjuvant immunotherapy based on the recent results of a completed phase III randomized trial.
- Given the strength of the data derived from the combination of the above-described randomized trials and the real-world experience, the following conclusions can be made about the goals achieved for sentinel lymphadenectomy in the surgical management of patients with melanoma presenting with clinically negative regional lymph node basins:
  - Sentinel lymphadenectomy provides accurate and critical regional lymph node staging information.
  - Removal of all microscopically involved SLNs is therapeutic in terms of melanoma-specific survival.
  - CLND for patients with a positive SLN provides improved regional disease control compared with nodal basin observation but no additional survival benefit above what is achieved with sentinel lymphadenectomy alone.
  - Reduced of surgery, and therefore less overall surgical morbidity is accomplished without compromising long-term survival outcomes.
- SLN biopsy continues to be accepted as a standard of care[19,20] in the surgical management of appropriately selected patients with melanoma. Central to the success of this minimally invasive approach, and in turn achieving the earlier described staging and treatment goals, is the consistent and accurate identification and complete removal of all SLN(s).
- Although in simplest terms SLN biopsy is a straightforward surgical procedure, in reality, the overall approach integrates several necessary components: identification of the appropriate candidates, careful physical examination of the potential nodal basins at risk, preoperative assessment of the lymphatic drainage patterns, intraoperative localization and removal of all the SLN(s), and careful histologic assessment of the SLN(s).

IDENTIFYING THE APPROPRIATE CANDIDATES

- **Histologic evaluation of the primary melanoma:** An experienced dermatopathologist should review all pathology slides related to the melanocytic lesion in question to confirm the diagnosis of melanoma and the histological subtype, as well as to provide the microstaging (tumor thickness and ulceration status) information and the presence of other relevant adverse histologic features (see discussion below). In some situations, however, the primary lesion is essentially intact, and the diagnostic biopsy represents only a small sampling of the entire lesion and/or is very superficial in depth and therefore not reflective of the true biology of the tumor. This type of biopsy may accurately render a definitive diagnosis of melanoma but may lack the histologic features needed to recommend an SLN biopsy. In this situation, the entire lesion should be narrowly removed as an excisional biopsy for complete histologic evaluation.

- Primary invasive cutaneous melanoma: The selection criteria for identifying the appropriate candidates for SLN biopsy is based on the predicted risk for the presence of microscopic lymph node involvement for those patients with newly diagnosed primary melanoma and clinically negative nodes. This is best determined by various primary tumor factors inclusive of tumor thickness and ulceration,[18] which define the five AJCC version 8 stages I and II substages of primary melanoma,[19] mitotic rate, lymphovascular invasion, and microsatellite disease. The consensus recommendations are to offer SLN biopsy to any patient with a primary T-stage tumor of T1b and higher defined as a thickness of ≥0.8 mm and for a thickness <0.8 mm with ulceration (T1b designation) as long as they are safe operative candidates. SLN biopsy should also be considered in patients with a primary melanoma thickness of <0.8 mm if at least one of the following adverse prognostic features are present: two or more mitotic figures per square millimeter in the vertical growth phase, lymphovascular invasion, or microsatellites.[19-23] For these patients with a thickness of <0.8 mm, associated with one of the aforementioned adverse risk factors, a risk of 8% to 12% of SLN involvement is anticipated, similar to patients with T1b primary lesions with tumor thickness between 0.8 and 1.0 mm.[16]
- While these patients overall represent the vast majority of who will be offered an SLN biopsy, a variety of other clinical scenarios are encountered with some frequency, where SLN biopsy may also be considered. These scenarios are described in the six bulleted points that follow directly.
- Primary dermal melanoma: Nodular melanoma lesions have been described where histologically the cells are confined to the dermis without an obvious epidermal junctional component, raising the possibility of a single site of metastases from an unknown primary. Alternatively, such a clinical scenario might represent a primary nodular melanoma that has lost its primary junctional component, or an entity referred to as a "primary dermal" melanoma. Despite the ambiguity of diagnosis, the natural history of these patients is most consistent with a primary lesion rather than a metastasis. Therefore, surgeons have reached a consensus to treat these patients surgically with curative intent, similar to how we treat a primary nodular melanoma with WLE and SLN biopsy when there is no regional lymphadenopathy and no disease identified on imaging studies.[24]
- Desmoplastic melanoma: Approximately 5% to 10% of primary melanomas have some histological desmoplastic component. While the truly mixed histological variant (coexistence of major epithelial and spindle/desmoplastic components) portends a similar prognosis to that of the common primary histological subtypes, and are therefore good candidates for SLN biopsy the "pure" desmoplastic lesions (>90% desmoplasia) seem to have an overall low incidence of associated microscopically involved SLNs and an overall more favorable prognosis. These latter tumors frequently present with a high T-stage, based on tumor thickness, but other adverse primary tumor factors, such as ulceration and lymphovascular invasion, are usually absent. As a result, many surgeons have elected to not routinely offer SLN to patients with **pure** desmoplastic melanoma.[25,26]
- Primary melanoma in an ambiguous (unpredictable) lymphatic drainage site (ie, head and neck or trunk location) and proven synchronous nodal involvement in at least one, but not all, of the potential regional lymph node basins at risk: These patients may be candidates for SLN biopsy to stage the other regional nodal basin(s) proven to receive direct lymphatic drainage from the primary site but without clinical nodal involvement. Generally speaking, these patients will undergo treatment of the primary melanoma and the involved nodal basin with a wide excision and formal therapeutic lymphadenectomy in the same operative setting. In the event that preoperative lymphoscintigraphy (**FIGURE 2**) demonstrates lymphatic drainage to an additional but clinically negative regional nodal basin, SLN biopsy can be performed at the same time in an attempt to be inclusive in the treatment of all nodal disease, both macro- and microscopic.
- Mucosal melanoma: Patients with primary mucosal melanomas that are in locations with easy access for direct injection with the SLN localizing agents, conjunctival and anorectal in particular, can be candidates for SLN biopsy as part of their initial surgical management strategy. Although specific primary tumor criteria for these lesions are not well established for predicting the presence of occult regional node involvement, these tumors are most often diagnosed late and likely to have a high enough inherent risk to consider SLN biopsy.
- True locally recurrent melanoma: Some patients develop recurrent melanoma at the edge of a previous wide excision

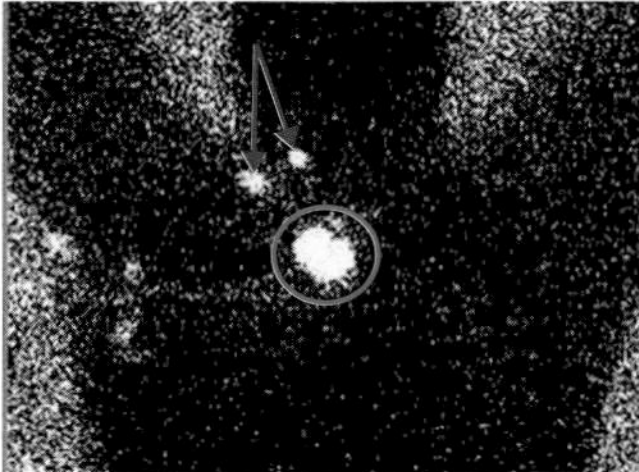

FIGURE 2 ● Lymphoscintigraphy showing lymphatic drainage to more than one nodal basin. An anterior-posterior view of a lymphoscintigraphy is shown, demonstrating lymphatic drainage from a primary melanoma site (*blue circle*) in an ambiguous (unpredictable) drainage location. Afferent drainage is seen to the right axilla and right neck (*red arrows*). This patient presented with a newly diagnosed melanoma in the right midback. Palpable nodes were appreciated on physical examination in the right axilla; an ultrasound-guided fine needle aspiration confirmed metastatic disease. The neck was clinically uninvolved by palpation and ultrasound. The patient underwent surgery with curative intent, which included a right axillary dissection, wide excision of the primary site, and an SLN biopsy in the right neck. Final pathology showed micrometastatic disease in both SLNs removed.

site and may have one of the following three histologic features: in situ disease alone, in situ disease plus an invasive component, or invasive (dermal) component only. All three of these events are likely the result of an inadequate wide excision and an undetected positive margin and therefore represent a "true" local recurrence and have a good chance for long-term survival with surgical treatment. Most of these patients have clinically negative nodes, and in the context of a recurrent invasive component with the appropriate tumor characteristics (see earlier discussion), it is rational to offer these patients an SLN biopsy as a part of the definitive surgical therapy.

- Limited satellite/in-transit metastases: In contrast to the patients with "true" locally recurrent disease, these patients represent manifestations of the biologic disease continuum of regional cutaneous metastases (stage III). Not infrequently, these patients will present with clinically negative regional lymph nodes, stage IIIb. If the extent of the regionally metastatic disease is limited (one or two lesions), a surgical approach to the recurrence is rational. The presence of synchronous microscopic nodal disease not only impacts disease stage, advancing to IIIc and therefore the prognosis, but also the treatment strategies. Therefore, SLN biopsy could also be used in this clinical scenario in conjunction with the resection of the recurrence(s).
- After a wide excision: It is typical and preferable that the SLN biopsy be performed together in a single operative setting in conjunction with the definitive wide excision of the primary melanoma following a diagnostic incisional or excisional biopsy. Occasionally, a patient will have undergone a formal wide excision of the primary melanoma site and then be referred for consideration of an SLN biopsy. A theoretical concern is that the lymphatic drainage pattern of the skin brought together to close the surgical defect or surrounding a skin graft reconstruction has either been altered by the surgery or is far enough away from the original primary lesion that it may not accurately reflect that of the removed skin that was directly adjacent to the primary melanoma, resulting in the identification and removal of the wrong SLN(s). A few publications have put most of these concerns to rest. The data show that, although more afferent lymphatic vessels are likely to be accessed because of the broadened area injected, leading to more SLNs being removed and even the possibility of additional nodal basins explored in sites of ambiguous drainage (trunk and head and neck), the correct SLNs will likely be among the specimens removed, providing accurate nodal staging information.[27] As long as complex rotational flaps were not used for the reconstruction, SLN can be recommended to patients when this clinical setting is encountered.
- Prior surgery in a nodal basin: Occasionally, a primary melanoma will be diagnosed in a location with predicted or possible lymphatic drainage to a regional nodal basin in which surgical intervention has previously been performed, such as an SLN biopsy or lymph node dissection, as treatment for a previous melanoma or other malignancies. An SLN biopsy may still be possible, but a preoperative lymphoscintigraphy is mandated to determine how the lymphatic drainage has been affected or altered by the previous nodal surgery. Lymphatic drainage patterns may be demonstrated in one or more of the remaining nodes (if any exist) in the previously treated basin or diverted to another basin. This information is critical for appropriate surgical planning and operative positioning.

PATIENT HISTORY AND PHYSICAL FINDINGS

- Pertinent information such as a prior personal history of melanoma or other malignancies and current or recent symptoms referable to the presence of metastatic disease should be elicited from the patient during the history.
- Questions about allergic reactions to antibiotics, sulfa in particular, and intravenous (IV) contrast agents should be documented as this information may suggest an increased risk of an allergic reaction to the isosulfan blue dye and therefore may influence the decision to use a different blue dye such as methylene blue or not use any blue dye at all for the SLN procedure (see more details in the following text).
- A thorough head-to-toe skin examination should be performed with the intent of identifying additional suspicious lesions that could represent another primary melanoma or other skin cancers. Diagnostic full-thickness punch or excisional biopsies should be performed on selected lesions.
- Special attention should be paid to the region of the index melanoma. Visual inspection as well as palpation of the biopsy site and surrounding skin and soft tissues should be performed to determine the presence of any residual primary disease and/or satellite and in-transit metastases.
- Skin and soft tissues between the primary lesion and draining lymph node basins should be palpated and closely examined for in-transit disease. All suspicious cutaneous and subcutaneous lesions may undergo fine needle aspiration for pathologic diagnosis.
- All potential regional lymph node basins should be palpated for the presence of clinically apparent disease. This examination should include the epitrochlear and popliteal minor nodal basins when the primary melanoma is located distal to the elbow and knee, respectively.
- Palpable lymph nodes suspicious for metastatic disease should be assessed by either direct fine needle aspiration or further examined with ultrasound and biopsied with ultrasound guidance if confirmed to be radiographically suspicious. Such data may obviate the need for SLN biopsy in that basin and instead invoke a formal radiographic staging evaluation prior to carrying out a therapeutic lymph node dissection of the affected lymph node basin(s).

PREOPERATIVE RADIOGRAPHIC STUDIES

- Although *symptom-directed* preoperative radiographic imaging is a good practice in patients with newly diagnosed melanomas, generally speaking, most newly diagnosed early-stage patients are asymptomatic; therefore, no

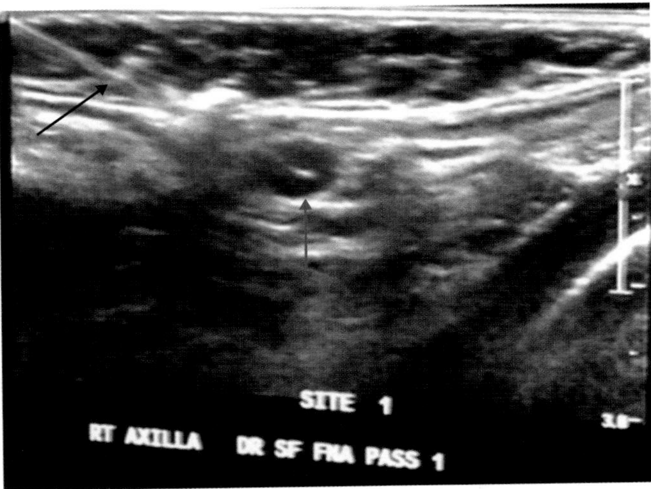

FIGURE 3 ● Ultrasound-guided fine needle aspiration of a suspicious nonpalpable lymph node. A static ultrasound image of biopsy needle (*black arrow*) within the node (*red arrow*) is shown.

special radiographic imaging is required or recommended prior to performing an SLN biopsy for most patients with primary melanoma.[28] In the asymptomatic patient, extensive radiographic staging is more likely to result in false-positive rather than true-positive findings. One possible exception would be the patients with both very thick (>4 mm) and ulcerated primary lesions. Many surgeons would obtain complete radiographic staging inclusive of computed tomography (CT) of chest/abdomen/pelvis or positron emission tomography (PET) scan and magnetic resonance imaging (MRI) of the brain routinely for this high-risk group.[28]

- In contrast, in patients with a locally metastatic lesion or a limited number of in-transit metastases for whom an SLN biopsy is being considered as part of the definitive surgical management, a thorough preoperative radiographic staging evaluation should be performed.[28]
- As mentioned earlier, ultrasound examination should be performed in patients with suspicious palpable nodes. Furthermore, ultrasound evaluation of the regional nodal basins should also be used as an adjunct to physical examination particularly of the axilla, in obese patients, with thick and ulcerated melanomas to evaluate for the presence of macroscopically involved nodes. In these situations, the sensitivity of physical examination is low and the risk of harboring synchronous macroscopically involved nodes is relatively high. Ultrasound examination suspicious for nodal involvement can be confirmed with an ultrasound-guided fine needle aspiration (**FIGURE 3**).
- The success of any SLN program is dependent on the preoperative determination of the lymphatic drainage patterns from the primary melanoma site. Although the nodal basins at risk in extremity melanomas are relatively predictable, such is not the case for head and neck and trunk melanomas where lymphatic drainage patterns are considered ambiguous or unpredictable. Preoperative identification of lymphatic drainage patterns is accomplished with *lymphoscintigraphy*.[28,29]

PREOPERATIVE LYMPHOSCINTIGRAPHY

- Once the decision is made to perform an SLN biopsy, the most important preoperative decision is whether or not to perform a lymphoscintigraphy.
- The technique of cutaneous lymphoscintigraphy provides an objective description of the lymphatic drainage pattern from a primary cutaneous lesion to the nodal basin(s) that receive direct afferent lymphatic drainage. Through the use of external gamma camera images, the migration of the radioactive tracer that is injected intradermally (where the invasive melanoma cells are located) at the site of the primary tumor can be visualized to determine the following: (1) the major lymph node basin(s) receiving direct lymphatic drainage, (2) number and relative location of sentinel nodes within the basin, and (3) the existence and location of SLN(s) located outside of a formal lymph node basin, referred to as either "interval" or "in-transit" SLNs that are located in the subcutaneous tissues between the primary tumor and the formal nodal basin or *ectopic* in completely unpredicted anatomic locations.[29] The lymphatic drainage patterns mimic how melanoma cells metastasize within the lymphatic compartment. Approximately 5% to 10% of the time, an interval or in-transit SLN pattern will be identified during lymphoscintigraphy on the trunk; these nodes are just as likely to be involved with metastatic disease as the SLNs in the formal nodal basins.[30] **FIGURE 4** provides a simplified schematic of potential lymphatic drainage patterns.
- Two radiopharmaceutical agents are now available in the United States to be used for lymphoscintigraphy and for intraoperative SLN localization, both using a dose of 0.5 to 1.0 mCi of the radiotracer technetium-99m. Radiolabeled sulfur colloid has been the historical standard and is still used commonly, to date, but not specifically approved for this use. Recently, the US Food and Drug Administration (FDA) has approved the use of Tilmanocept,[31] which is a formulation of a dextran framework with several attached mannose residues and a technetium-99m binding site.
- In theory, the sulfur colloid particles migrate from the injection site through the afferent lymphatic vessels and are actively taken up by the macrophages in the first draining nodes (the sentinel nodes). Similarly, Tilmanocept migrates to the sentinel nodes from the injection site but is then covalently bound to the macrophages in the sentinel node as a result of the mannose residues, limiting significant pass through to secondary echelon nodes.
- Two types of images can be created. The routine examination is termed "planar" or "biplanar" and delivers images in two perpendicular planes: posterior-anterior (P-A) and/or anterior-posterior (A-P), or both, and perpendicular lateral views[20] (**FIGURE 5**). These images visualize the injection site, the afferent lymphatic channels, and the accumulation of the radiotracer in the SLNs. The A-P and P-A views give

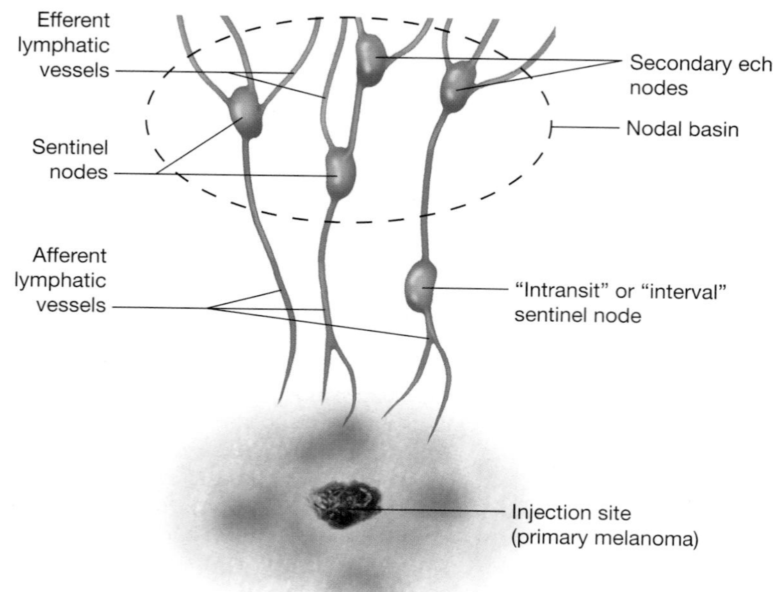

FIGURE 4 ● Lymphatic drainage patterns. A schematic of potential lymphatic drainage patterns from the primary site to the regional nodal basin is shown. The first (primary echelon) node of drainage from a specific afferent lymphatic vessel is defined as an SLN. Up- or downstream drainage from the SLN to another node via efferent lymphatic vessels are considered secondary echelon nodes. Occasionally, primary lymphatic drainage is to a lymph node proximal to the formal basin in the subcutaneous tissue and termed as either an "interval" or "in-transit" SLN.

the clinician medial and lateral as well as superior-inferior orientations, whereas the lateral views provide anterior and posterior localizations and also superior-inferior localizations. A transmission scan adds the contour of the body to the image and provides additional anatomic localizing information. When the radioactive tracer injection site (primary melanoma site) overlies or is in close proximity to a draining lymph node basin in at least one visual plane, the radioactivity in the sentinel node will not be visualized in that plane. Perpendicular images are necessary in order to visualize the sentinel activity separate from the injection site activity.

- More recently, single-photon emission computed tomography–computed tomography (SPECT-CT) lymphoscintigraphy[32,33] has been developed, providing more exact anatomic localizations. With this method, serial cross-sectional, axial, coronal, and sagittal images are obtained and fused with the nuclear images. Relatively precise locations of the SLN and injection sites can be accomplished and is therefore particularly helpful in primary tumor locations such as in the head and neck regions where multiple SLNs may be present or in locations where the potential nodal basins, and therefore the SLNs, may be in close proximity to the injection's site and lie within one of the same visual planes as the injection's site. In this latter situation, the SLN radioactivity will be obscured by activity within the injection site in one or more planes and therefore possibly go undetected on a "planar" study. Although obtaining a perpendicular image may visualize the SLN activity in a different line of sight, as described earlier, the SPECT-CT provides consistent three-dimensional imaging. The SPECT-CT images are also better at determining the presence of and delineating the anatomic location of interval, in-transit, or ectopic SLNs in uncommon and unexpected

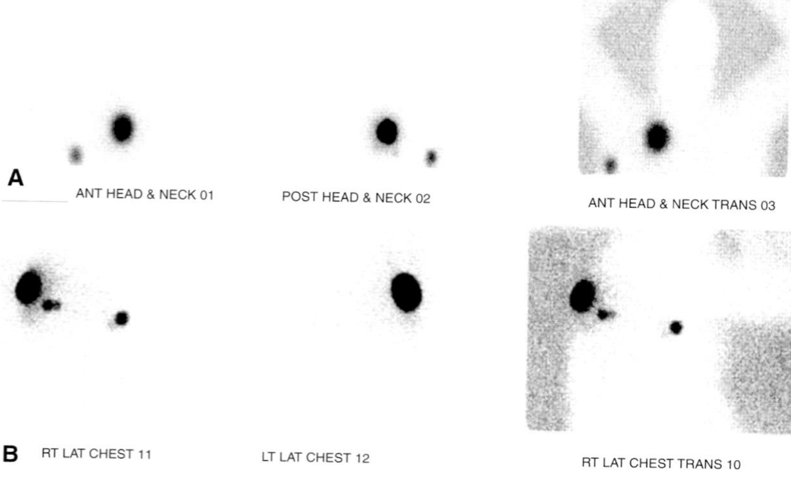

FIGURE 5 ● Planar lymphoscintigraphy. Typical example of a cutaneous lymphatic drainage scan, obtained by injecting the technetium-99m–labeled tracer in the intradermal location at the primary melanoma site, is shown. The injection site, the afferent lymphatic vessels, and the SLNs in the regional nodal basin are visualized. A-P and P-A **(A)** as well as right and left lateral images **(B)** are taken to visualize the drainage pattern in perpendicular visual planes. The last image in both rows is the transmission scan that outlines the contour of the body to facilitate anatomic localization.

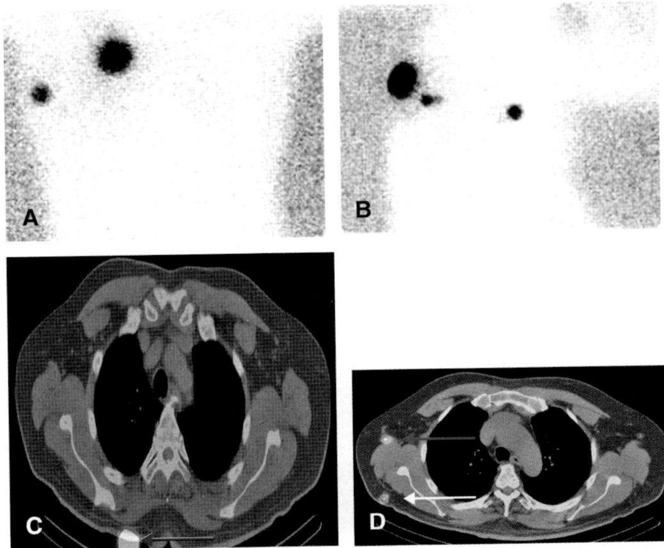

FIGURE 6 • SPECT-CT lymphoscintigraphy. Planar lymphoscintigraphy of primary melanoma is shown in the top row, with anterior view in **(A)** and lateral view in **(B)**. Selected SPECT-CT images of the same patient are seen in the bottom row. Only the axillary SLN is seen in **(A)** and an additional SLN is seen in **(B)**, which was obscured by the overlying activity transmitted to the axilla from the injection site. The additional SLN in **(B)** is likely an in-transit node, the exact anatomic location of which is better visualized in the transaxial view of the SPECT-CT image in **(D)**. In **(C)**, the *blue arrow* indicates the injection site, and in **(D)**, several cross-sectional images inferior to **(C)**, the *white arrow* identifies the in-transit SLN and the *red arrow* identifies the axillary SLN.

locations (**FIGURES 6** and **7**). These studies are critical in helping surgeons locate and remove all of the SLNs at surgery. Complete sentinel lymphadenectomy has become more important since the practice of performing CLND routinely after a positive SLN biopsy has changed to a much more selective approach, so as not to miss the opportunity for a therapeutic benefit achieved in those patients who have disease limited to the SLNs.

- In the management of primary tumors located in cutaneous regions predicted to have ambiguous lymphatic drainage, such as in the head and neck and trunk, a preoperative lymphoscintigraphy is mandated. The extent of ambiguous cutaneous lymphatic drainage includes a very large area of the trunk and head and neck regions and is underestimated by the original classic descriptions of lymphatic drainage patterns. **FIGURE 8** illustrates the actual regions of ambiguous drainage. **FIGURE 9** demonstrates an example of ambiguous drainage.
- For extremity lesions, a formal lymphoscintigraphy is not essential as the basins at risk are predictable and intraoperative scanning can be performed with the handheld gamma probe. Some clinicians, however, will obtain a preoperative study for extremity lesions as well, particularly if the primary tumor is located distal to the knee or elbow to have a preoperative assessment for the presence of popliteal (**FIGURE 10**) or epitrochlear drainage patterns. Even in the proximal extremity locations, a preoperative lymphoscintigraphy can provide useful information in determining whether any upstream drainage from the thigh to the pelvis or the upper arm to the neck is primary (sentinel) or secondary echelon.
- Some clinicians will schedule the lymphoscintigraphy on a day prior to the surgical procedure, whereas others will obtain the study on the day of the surgery. In the latter scenario, the injection of the technetium-99m–labeled radiotracer that is used for the scan can be used for the gamma probe–directed intraoperative localization of the SLN. Because the half-life of technetium-99m is only 6 hours, when the lymphoscintigraphy is performed on a day remote from the surgery, another injection is required on the day of surgery unless a larger (3 times) dose of the radiotracer is given the evening before the surgery.
- The lymphoscintigraphic images should be viewed by the surgeon and displayed in the operating room (OR) at the time of the SLN biopsy surgery to facilitate operative positioning, the intraoperative identification of the SLNs, and subsequent removal of all of the SLNs.

SURGICAL MANAGEMENT

Preoperative Planning

- Except in situations when the patient has already undergone a wide excision of the primary melanoma and then is referred for SLN biopsy, the SLN biopsy is carried out in the same operative setting as the definitive wide excision of the primary site.
- The surgery is performed as a day surgery, most conveniently in an ambulatory OR setting, under general anesthesia or with local anesthesia supported with IV sedation. Therefore, the patient should be nil per os (NPO) after midnight.
- Because frequently the entire index clinical lesion has been removed with either the shave or excisional diagnostic biopsy, identifying the correct site at the time of lymphoscintigraphy or surgical procedure may be difficult. This is further complicated by the fact that these patients frequently have undergone other biopsies of skin lesions either prior to or at the time of the melanoma diagnosis. Because the accuracy of the SLN biopsy is dependent on injecting the correct site, careful documentation of the primary melanoma biopsy location to be injected should be carried out during the first clinic visit when the decision to perform the SLN biopsy is made. Digital images of this site can be obtained and downloaded in the patient's electronic medical record.
- Once the index lesion has been identified and clearly marked in the preoperative holding area and confirmed by the patient and/or family member, the patient can go to nuclear medicine for the radiotracer injection followed by the lymphoscintigraphy if not already completed on a day remote from the actual surgical procedure. The radiotracer is injected intradermally in the normal skin, just adjacent and as close as possible to

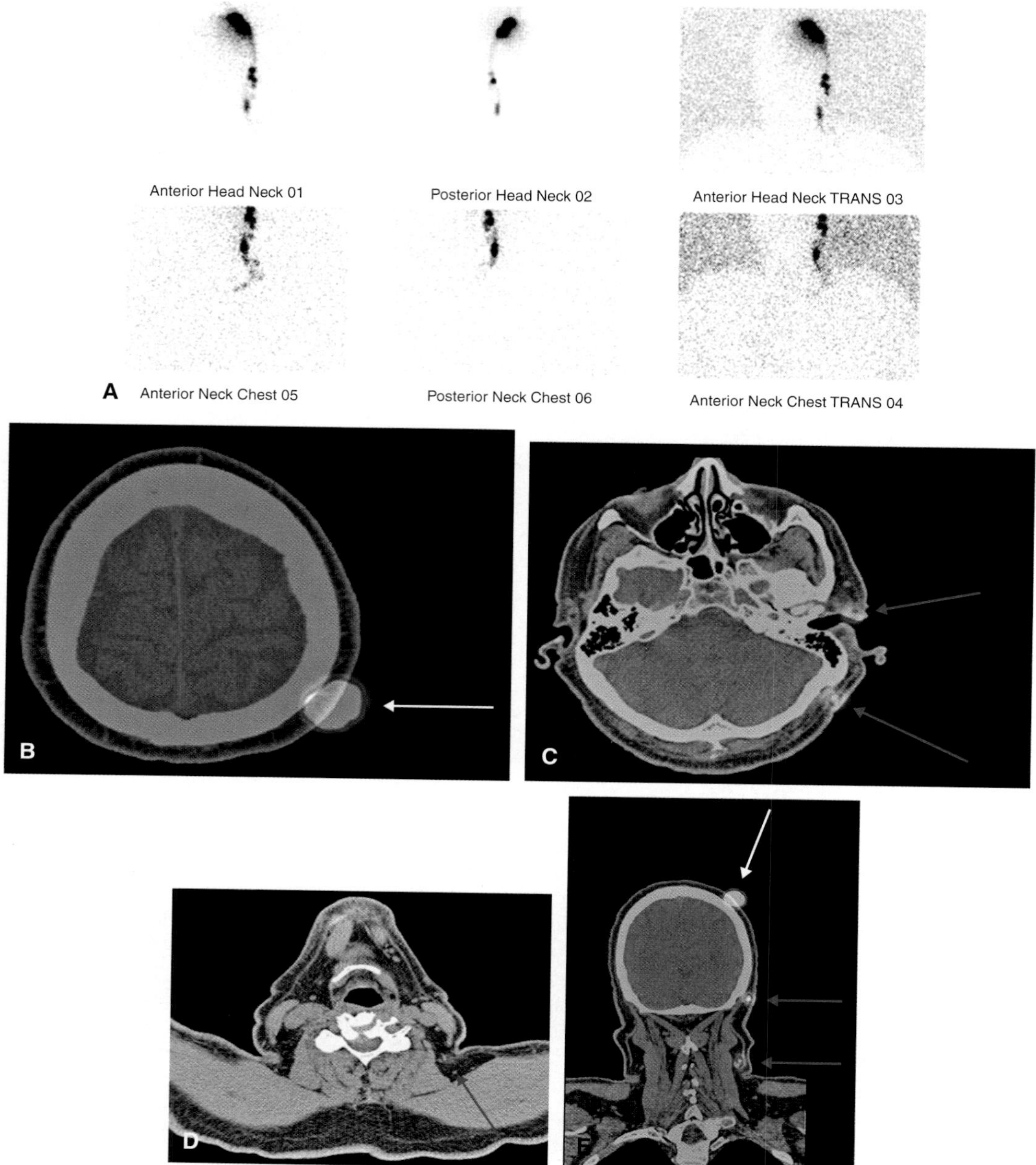

FIGURE 7 ● SPECT-CT lymphoscintigraphy. Planar lymphoscintigraphy of a primary melanoma on the left scalp is shown in **(A)**, demonstrating multiple SLNs, the anatomic locations of which are difficult to define. In **(B-D)**, the SPECT-CT images are shown, with the *white arrows* indicating the injection site and the *red arrows* the SLNs, providing more exact localization with the use of cross-sectional **(B and C)** and coronal views in **(E)**.

the intact residual lesion (if present) or the biopsy site by the radiologist or technician. A four-point injection technique surrounding the lesion is employed with a 30-gauge needle attached to a 1-mL syringe (**FIGURE 11**). The usual dose of the radiotracer is 0.5 to 1 mCi of technetium-99m. For extremity lesions, the surgeon may choose not to obtain a lymphoscintigraphy (see earlier discussion) and have the patient return to the preoperative holding area directly after the injection. Also for extremity primaries, if permissible by the nuclear medicine department and if a lymphoscintigraphy is not going to be obtained, the surgeon can perform the injection of the radiotracer in the OR just prior to injecting the blue dye.

- Generally speaking, scheduling the injection that will be performed by the nuclear medicine staff approximately 1 hour prior to the surgery start time is adequate, but 2 or 3 hours may be required if a SPECT-CT lymphoscintigraphy is planned.
- Open communication with anesthesia personnel should take place prior to arrival in the OR to make sure the IV is placed thoughtfully at a site removed from the planned sites of the surgical procedures.
- The patient should be administered appropriate broad-spectrum antibiotic prophylaxis to reduce the risk of surgical site infection.
- The handheld gamma probe should already be in the OR.

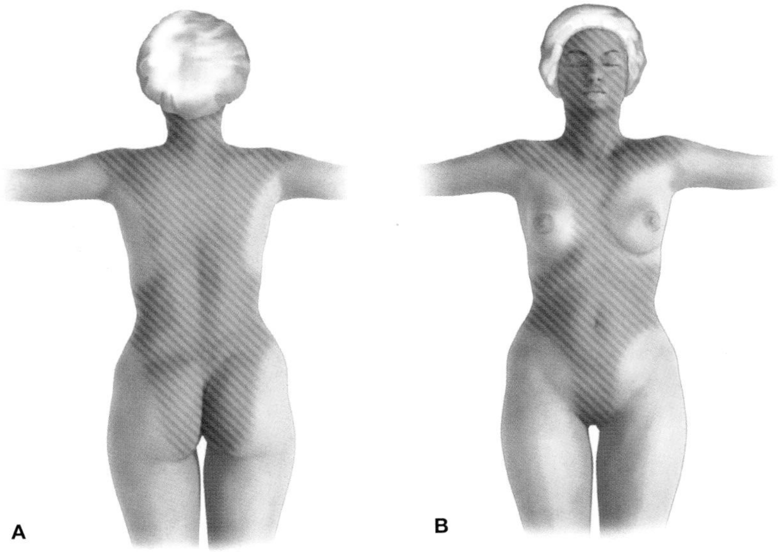

FIGURE 8 ● Areas of ambiguous lymphatic drainage. The regions of ambiguous (unpredictable) cutaneous lymphatic drainage include broad areas of the posterior **(A)** and anterior **(B)** trunk and the entire surface area of the head and neck.

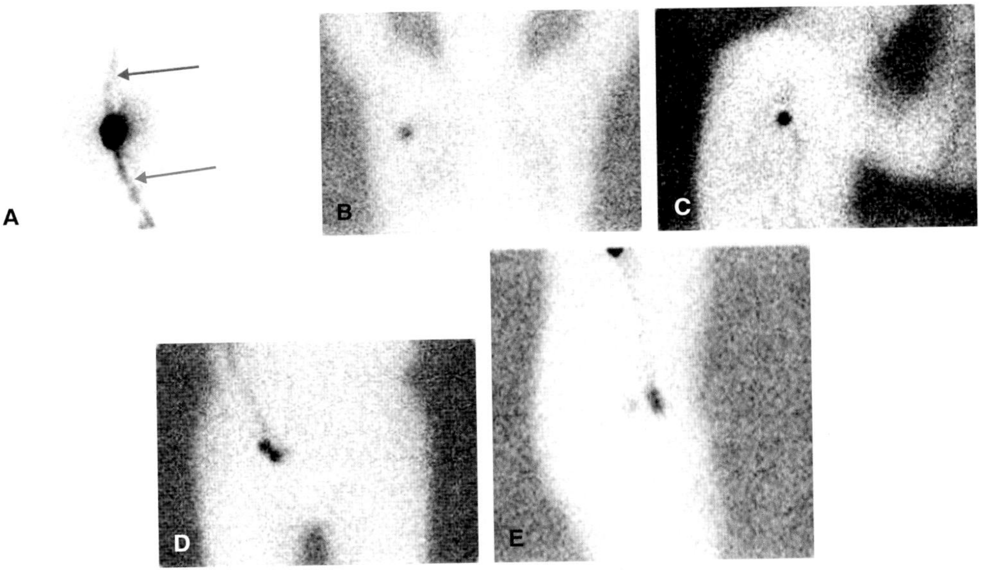

FIGURE 9 ● Ambiguous lymphatic drainage. Lymphoscintigraphy of melanoma on the right flank is displayed. The primary injection site is shown in **(A)**, demonstrating afferent lymphatic vessels draining in a bidirectional fashion to the ipsilateral axilla (*red arrow*) and groin (*blue arrow*). In **(B)** and **(C)**, the axillary SLN is visualized in two perpendicular planes. In **(D)** and **(E)**, the inguinal SLN is visualized in two perpendicular planes.

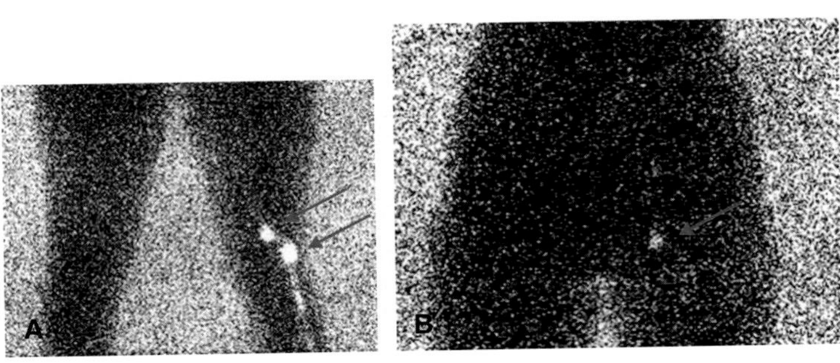

FIGURE 10 ● Visualization of popliteal SLN. Lymphoscintigraphy of melanoma on the plantar surface of the calcaneus demonstrating both popliteal **(A)** and inguinal **(B)** SLNs (*arrows*) is shown.

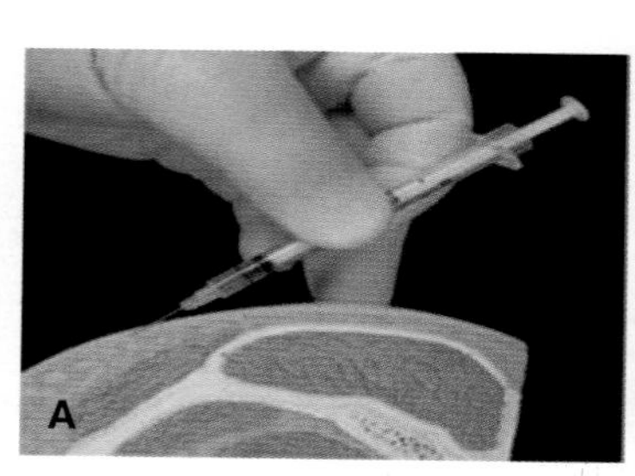

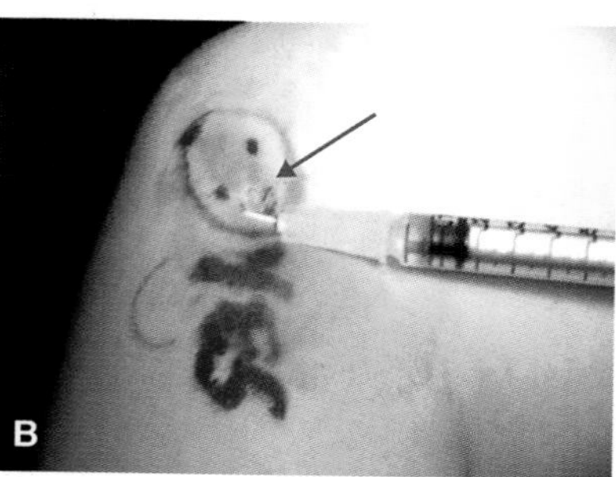

FIGURE 11 • Radiotracer injection technique. The correct technique and needle location for an intradermal injection is shown using a soft tissue model in **(A)**. An actual intradermal injection of the radiotracer at the primary melanoma site using a 1-mL syringe and a 30-gauge needle is shown in **(B)**. Note the wheal formation (*arrow*) confirming the intradermal location.

- If the plan is to use the vital blue dye as another SLN localizing agent, this should be drawn up in 1-mL aliquots in the OR prior to the arrival of the patient.

Operative Positioning

- Thoughtful operative positioning is more of an art than a science but is an important step that will reduce operative times, limit the number of position changes, facilitate intraoperative scanning with the handheld gamma probe, and, more importantly, optimize the complete identification and removal of all SLNs.
- The lymphoscintigraphic images should be displayed in the OR.
- Once in the OR, the gamma probe is used to transcutaneously scan all the planned nodal basins and SLN locations to be explored to make sure that the radiotracer has migrated. Alternatively, the patient can be scanned with the handheld gamma probe in the holding area prior to entering the OR to make sure the radiotracer has migrated in the event that a lymphoscintigraphy was not performed on the day of the surgery or not needed (ie, for extremity primary).
- The gamma probe should also be used to scan potential additional sites that may not have been specifically identified on the lymphoscintigraphy, such as in the epitrochlear and popliteal regions for primary lesions distal to the elbow and knee, respectively; all of the major regional nodal basins in the neck for head and neck and upper trunk primaries close to the midline; contralateral axilla for mid and upper back and chest lesions close to the midline; contralateral inguinal basin for lower abdomen and lower back primaries close to the midline; and ipsilateral axilla and inguinal regions for lateralized flank primaries. Additional SLN sites may be identified, and these findings may influence operative positioning and the regions to be prepped and draped. The arm(s) and leg(s) when performing SLN biopsies in the axillae and groins, respectively, should be circumferentially prepped and draped so position changes can be performed sterilely to facilitate adequate exposure of the lymph node basins intended for biopsy. Moreover, primary lesion(s) intended to undergo WLE should also be clearly visible and accessible.
- Whenever possible, patients should be positioned in a way to expose both the SLN and wide excision sites in one supine or lateral position. This will allow one session of prepping and draping and avoid the time it takes to change positions. This can usually be accomplished when the primary lesion is on one of the extremities, anywhere on the trunk or head and neck locations when all of the SLN sites are on the ipsilateral side of the primary, and anywhere on the anterior trunk and anterior head and neck regions even when the draining nodal basins are bilateral. In contrast, the most problematic locations are posterior neck and trunk lesions close to the midline when bilateral nodal basin (ie, both axillae, both cervical, or both inguinal) drainage is identified or two or more different basins on opposite sides of the body (ie, left axilla and right neck) contain SLNs. In these latter scenarios, at least one position change will be required.
- When foot/lower leg cutaneous lesions localize SLN(s) to the popliteal fossae, prone positioning is best suited for such patients for adequate visualization and access to the SLN(s). The patient may then be subsequently repositioned in the supine or lateral decubitus position for excision of corresponding primary lesions if that site is not accessible in the prone position. Another option for this scenario would be to place the patient in the lateral decubitus position, avoiding a position change.
- The patient should also be positioned to facilitate the surgeon in scanning the nodal basin and the intervening tissues with the handheld gamma probe positioned perpendicular to or in a direction pointed away from the injection site to limit the "shine-through" radioactivity emanating from the injection site that may obscure the radioactivity in the SLN and in turn hamper one's ability to discriminate SLN radioactivity from the injection site activity.
- After the patient is positioned, multiple steps are carried out to accomplish a complete and accurate sentinel lymphadenectomy.[34]

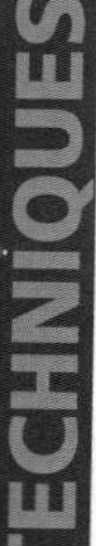

INJECTION OF BLUE DYE

- Once the patient is positioned, the vital blue dye is injected at the primary site using a similar four-point intradermal injection technique that was used for injecting the radiotracer. Approximately 2 to 3 mL of blue dye is injected using 1-mL tuberculin syringes and a 25-gauge needle (**FIGURE 12**).
- Although it is not mandatory that the blue dye be used, most surgeons feel that the two localizing agents complement each other in successfully identifying and removing the SLNs.
- The blue dyes most commonly used are isosulfan blue and methylene blue in the United States and patent Blue V in Europe and Australia. The isosulfan seems to concentrate in the SLNs in a more uniform manner compared with methylene blue, making it easier to visualize. Some surgeons prefer to use methylene blue because of the potential, albeit very low risk, of an allergic reaction to isosulfan blue.[35] However,

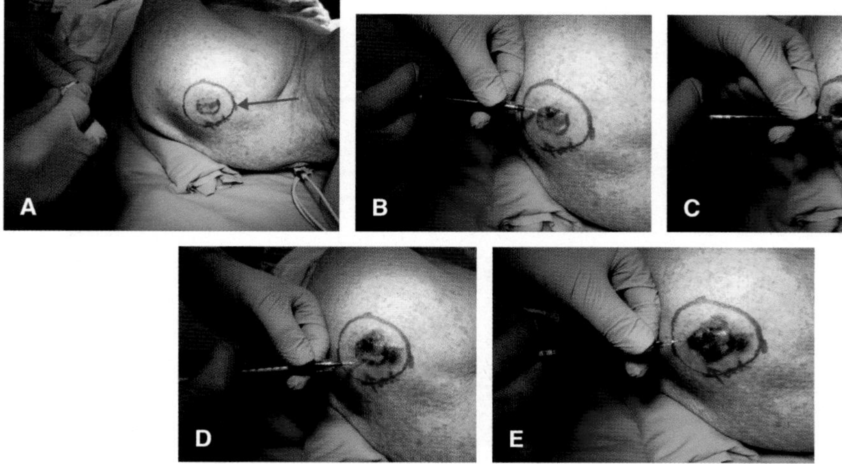

FIGURE 12 • Blue dye injection technique. The primary melanoma is shown **(A)** with planned margins measured and drawn (*arrow*). The four-point intradermal injection of the blue dye is shown in images **(B–E)**.

at least one report documents increased postoperative complications with the use of methylene blue.[36]

- After the blue dye is injected, the patient is then appropriately prepped and draped. The time that transpires during the prepping and draping is long enough for the blue dye to travel through the lymphatic vessels to the SLNs.

INTRAOPERATIVE LOCALIZATION AND SURGICAL EXCISION OF THE SENTINEL NODES

- Most commonly, both the SLN biopsy and the wide excision of the primary site will be performed in the same operative setting. Generally, if the blue dye is used, the nodal basin exploration and removal of the SLN are approached first in order to take advantage of the visualization of the SLN afforded by the blue dye. If the wide excision is performed first, the blue dye will be removed as well, limiting the continued flow of dye to the SLN and in turn the visualization of the SLN.
- The use of the handheld gamma probe is central to this procedure. The probe is placed within a sterile ultrasound cover after the patient is prepped and draped.
- If the planned wide excision site (injection site) is in close proximity to the nodal basin, the shine-through activity may be greater than the sentinel activity. The following maneuvers are used to discriminate SLN activity from the shine-through activity: As the gamma probe is transcutaneously passed from the injection site to the nodal basin, the counts will diminish in proportion to the distance from the injection site. A sentinel node area is identified when the radioactive counts increase as the probe is moved further away from the injection site compared with a location that is closer to the injection site (**FIGURE 13**). The radioactive counts should again decrease as the gamma probe is passed further beyond the sentinel node. The use of a removable collimator can be helpful in reducing shine-through activity. Make sure that, when passing the probe from the injection site to the nodal basin, the probe is positioned perpendicular to or directed away from the injection site. If none of these maneuvers are successful, the wide excision can then be performed first, which very effectively removes the background shine-through counts. This maneuver will also remove the blue dye and stop the continued flow of dye to the nodal basin and in turn significantly reduce the ability to use the blue dye as an aid in identifying the SLN.
- If the patient is positioned correctly, the surgeon will be able to transcutaneously localize the epicenter of the SLN activity with the handheld gamma (which represents a small percentage of the radioactivity at the injection site) within the nodal basin without too much difficulty especially if the injection site is at some distance from the nodal basin (**FIGURE 14**).
- The epicenter of SLN activity is marked with a sterile marking pen and used for surgical incision planning.
- The nodal basin is approached with a small biopsy incision directed by the handheld gamma probe over the epicenter of radioactivity. We make sure that this biopsy incision can be easily incorporated and excised en bloc as part of a formal lymphadenectomy incision if that is required at a later date should the sentinel node reveal metastases (**FIGURE 15**).
- The dermis and subcutaneous tissue are divided with cautery, advancing deeper for approximately 1 to 2 cm at a time between pauses during which time the trajectory of the line of dissection toward the radioactive signal may be confirmed with the gamma probe. Using this technique, the surgeon is able to localize and directly advance to the targeted SLN(s) with minimal tissue disruption (**FIGURE 16**).
- In most situations, the SLNs are deep to the subcutaneous investing fascial layer (ie, Scarpa fascia in the groin and platysma in the neck), which needs to be incised in order to enter the nodal basin proper (**FIGURE 16C**).
- Skin hooks, handheld Richardson-type retractors, or blunt self-retaining retractors can be used for exposure (**FIGURE 16D**).

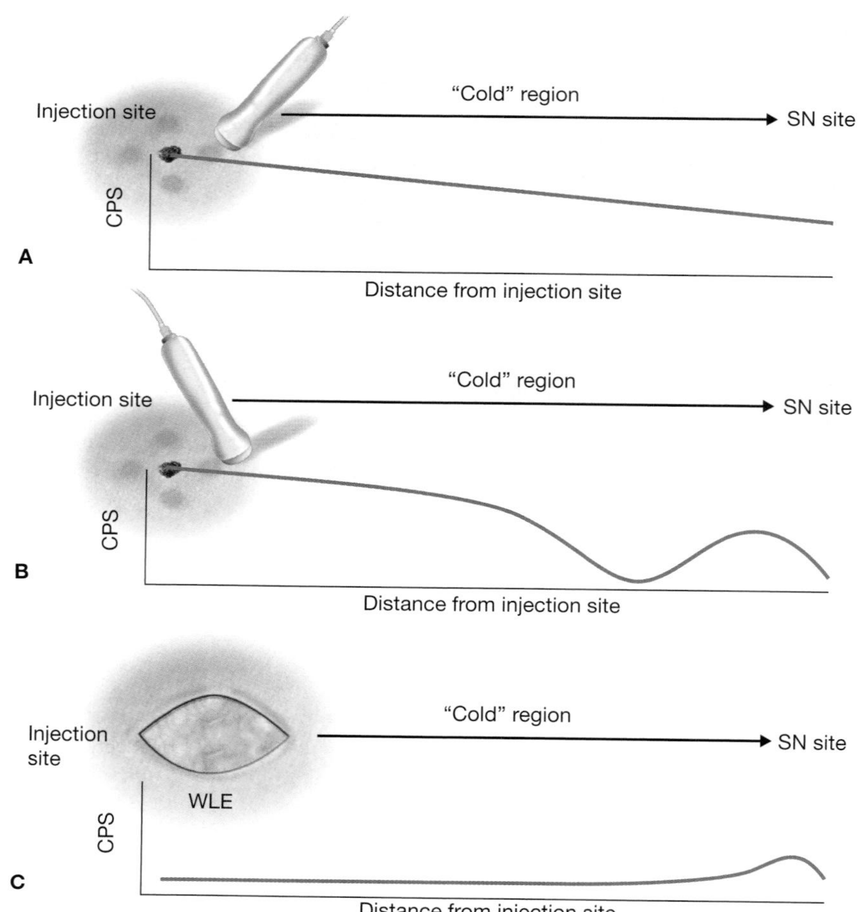

FIGURE 13 ● Conceptualization of intraoperative SLN scanning. Three conceptual graphs are shown, with the x-axis representing radioactive count per second (CPS) and the y-axis distance of the SLN from the injection site. The amount of radioactivity that travels to the SLN is a small percentage of the radioactivity injected. Shine-through radioactivity from the injection site may obscure the ability to detect to the radioactivity in the SLN, particularly if the injection is close to the nodal basin and/or SLNs. Although placing a collimator on the end of the probe may block out much of the shine-through activity and allow the detection of the SLN, it also narrows the exposed area of radioactivity detection crystal on the probe and in turn reduces the counts detected from the node. In **(A)**, scanning for the SLN is performed with the probe pointed at the injection site. Even though the probe is moving away from the site, shine-through counts detected may be greater than the counts in the SLN, limiting the ability to discriminate SLN activity vs shine-through injection activity. In **(B)**, the same maneuver is performed, now with the probe pointed away from the injection site, allowing the detection of a step-up in activity as one reaches the SLN. In **(C)**, the wide excision has been performed, essentially removing any shine-through activity and in turn facilitating the detection of the SLN activity. This latter maneuver is often used when trying to find the remaining SLNs with less radioactivity after the first, most radioactive SLN has been identified and removed.

- Once the nodal basin is entered, the localization of the SLN may be further facilitated by either following a blue-stained lymphatic channel toward the blue node or by direct visualization of the blue-stained lymph node (**FIGURE 16E**).
- The visualization of the blue dye is helpful in rapidly identifying which lymph node has accumulated the radiotracer, discriminating the SLN from the other nonstained surrounding nodes that are usually in close proximity.
- The SLN is then dissected free from the surrounding tissues. This is facilitated by gently grasping the node with a pickup and then delivering the node to a more superficial location in the basin. We prefer to use a pickup with broad and blunt jaws such as Hayes-Martin, rather than a DeBakey or Adson, to avoid tearing the node. Some surgeons place a figure-of-eight stitch in the node for this maneuver, but this can also carry the risk of tearing the node. Once mobilized and delivered, the intervening lymphatic channels can be identified because of the blue dye and are clipped or tied to limit the development of a postoperative seroma. The vascular pedicle is then clamped, cut, and then tied.
- Ex vivo counts of the node are then documented with the handheld gamma probe and recorded (**FIGURE 16F**). After removing the initial SLN, the nodal basin is then scanned for residual radioactive counts with the gamma probe pointed away from the injection site. If the background activity in the nodal basin is still high because of close proximity to the injection site, WLE of the primary site may be performed. This removes any significant background activity (shine through) and allows for a more complete evaluation of residual SLN counts within the nodal basin.
- Additional nodes identified by the presence of high residual radioactivity and/or blue dye staining are then removed and labeled as sentinel nodes, with numbers assigned sequentially in the order of identification. Nodes are defined as sentinel if they are blue and/or contain radioactivity significantly

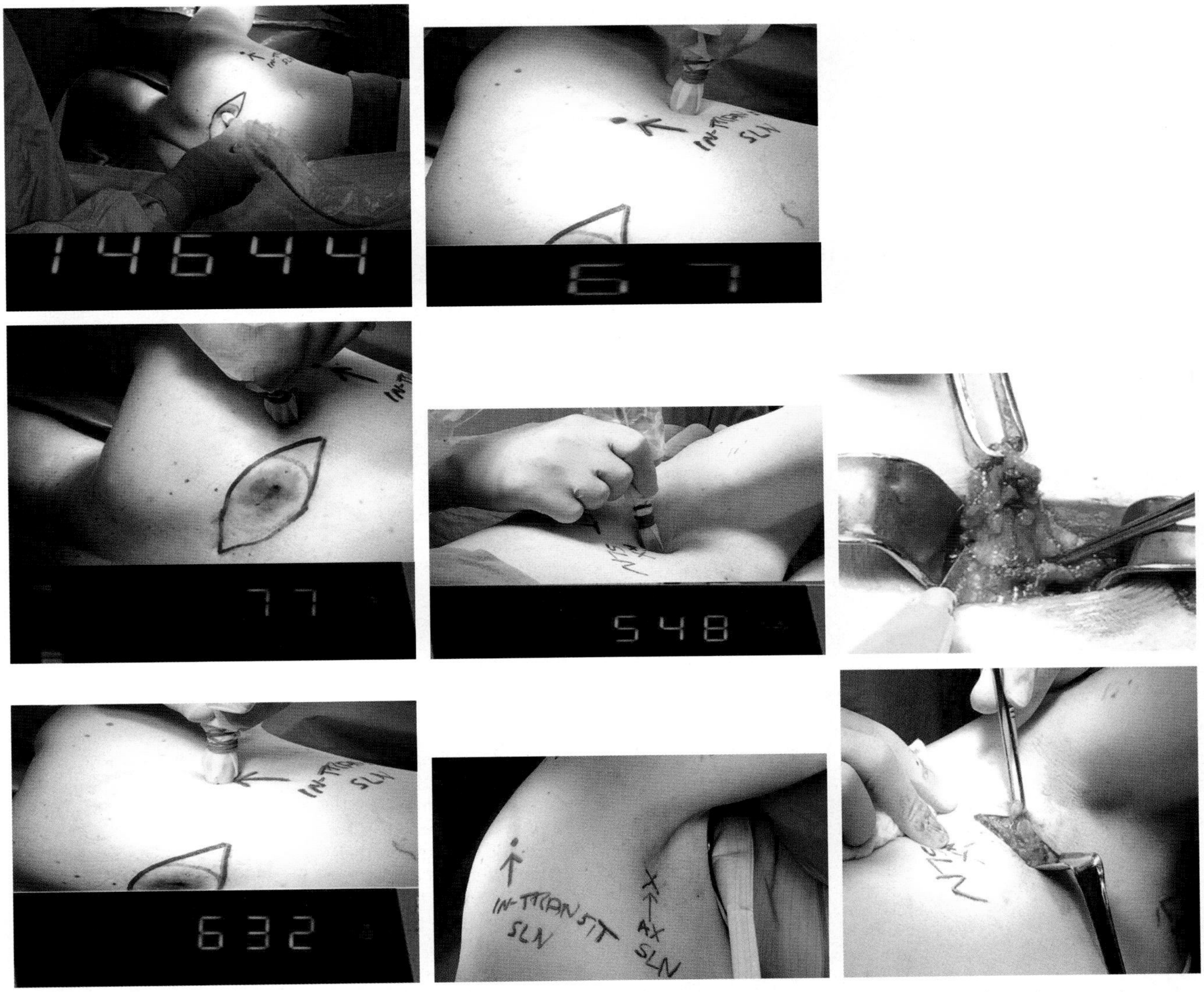

FIGURE 14 ● Thoughtful positioning in the OR. The left lateral position is correctly chosen in this patient with a primary melanoma on the right midback with a lymphoscintigraphy showing drainage to the right axilla and a probable in-transit node over the scapula. This position facilitates not only performing the SLN biopsies and the wide excision without a position change but also scanning for the SLN nodes perpendicular to and directed away from the injection site. Under each frame, the numbers represent the counts per second of radioactivity where the gamma probe is placed. Note that the highest count is over the injection site, then counts decrease moving away from the injection until they increase to identify the in-transit node, then decrease again as the in-transit node is passed, then increase again in the axilla. The last frame in the second column shows the SLN sites marked, and in the last column on the right the two frames show the in-transit SLN and the axillary SLN.

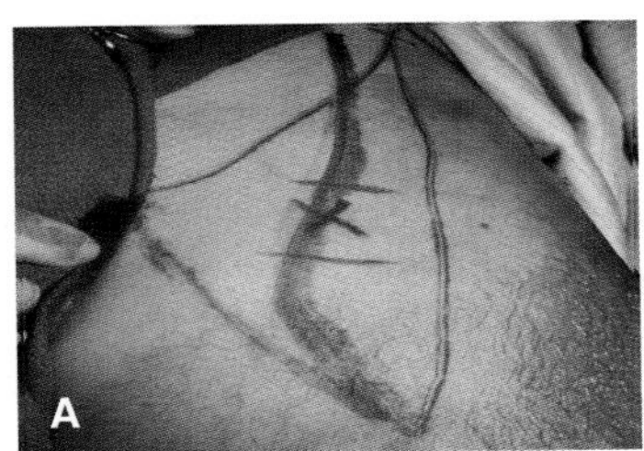

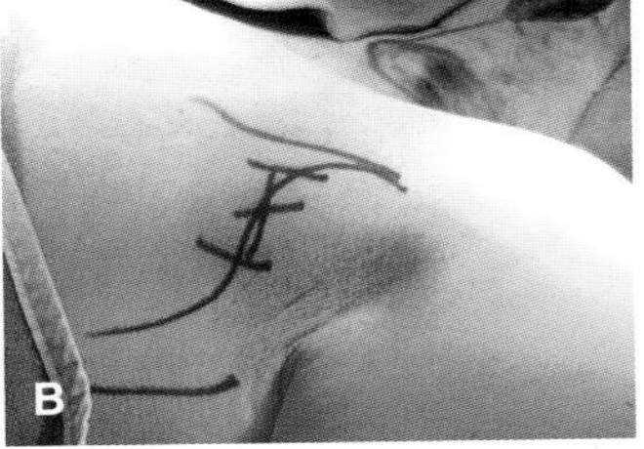

FIGURE 15 ● Skin marking and planned SLN biopsy incision. Examples of transcutaneous SLN localization with the gamma probe in two nodal basins: **(A)** inguinal and **(B)** axillary. In each frame, the SLN biopsy incision is drawn to incorporate the location of the SLN, marked with an "X" as well as a future formal lymphadenectomy should that be required.

above background. Nodes are removed and labeled as "sentinel" until no focal basin radioactivity is >10% of the "hottest" sentinel node removed.

- The skin and soft tissue between the injection site and nodal basin(s) should also be scanned to identify and subsequently remove any "in-transit" or "interval" SLNs. Similarly, if the background counts are too high because of proximity to the injection site, the wide excision can be performed to decrease the shine through and facilitate the exploration for the in-transit SLNs.

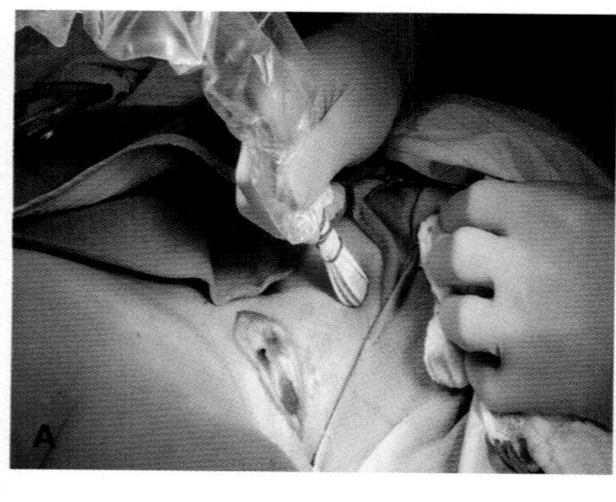

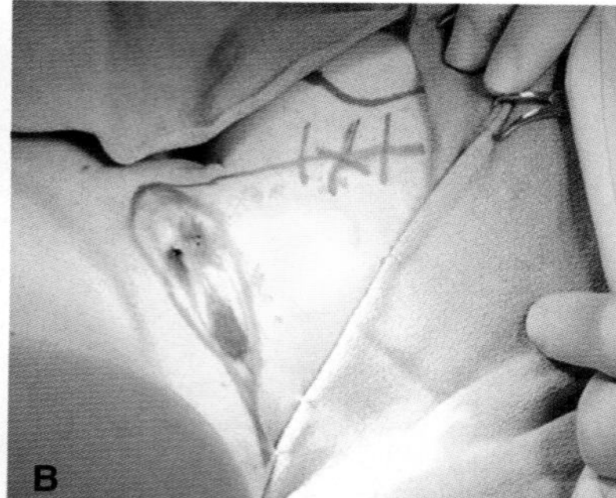

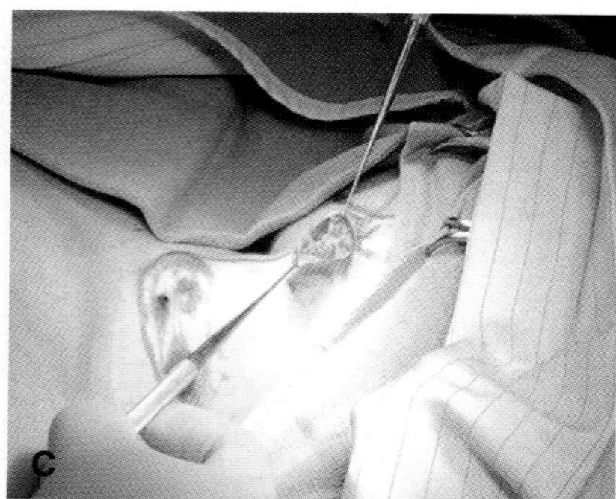

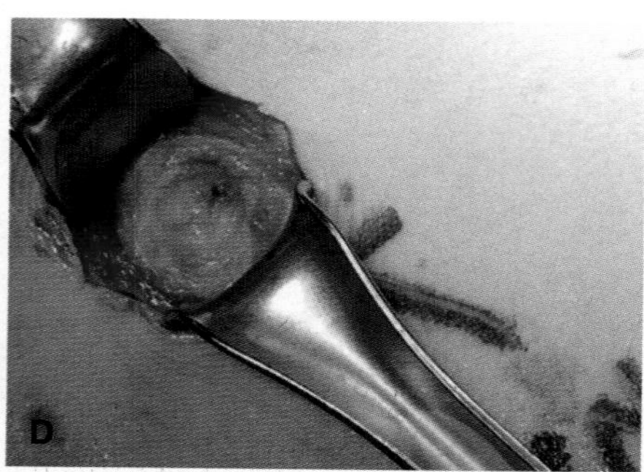

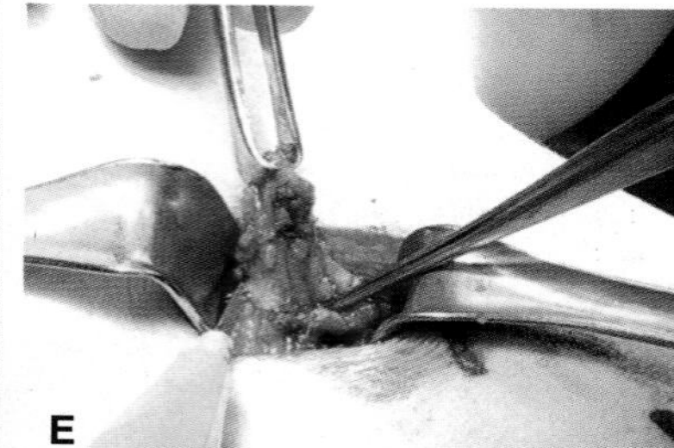

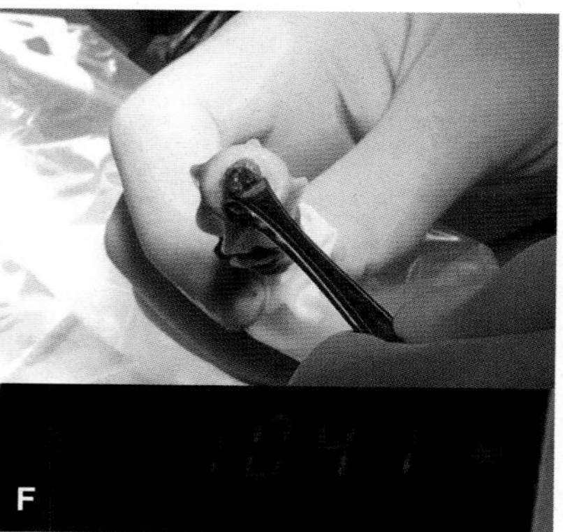

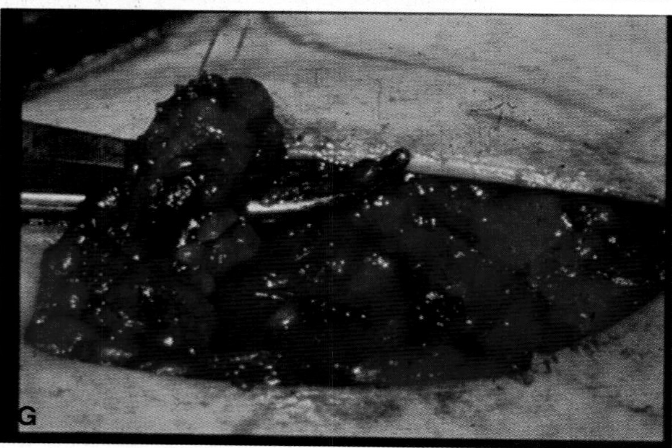

FIGURE 16 • Steps in excising the SLNs. The surgical steps used in the actual removal of the SLNs. **(A)** Transcutaneous localization, **(B)** marking the epicenter of radioactivity and planning the incision, **(C)** making the incision, incising the dermis and the subcutaneous tissue to expose the fascia, **(D)** incising the fascia to enter the nodal basin proper, **(E)** dissecting the SLN from the surrounding tissue, delivering the node into the wound, then removing the node after clipping or clamping then cutting the afferent vessels and vascular pedicle to remove the node, **(F)** ex vivo counting of the SLN, **(G)** rechecking the nodal basin for significant residual radioactivity, and removing additional SLNs.

CLOSURE

- Hemostasis should be ensured and divided fascial layers closed with interrupted 3-0 absorbable sutures. Drains are usually not needed.
- Skin may then be approximated using interrupted, buried absorbable sutures in the dermis followed by a running subcuticular stitch with a 4-0 absorbable monofilament suture. Steri-Strips or a skin adhesive may then be applied.

PATHOLOGIC EVALUATION OF THE SENTINEL NODES

- A dedicated dermatopathologist should process the node and read the pathology slides.
- The SLNs are serially sectioned using either along the long axis of the node or a bread-loafing technique across the short axis of the node (**FIGURE 17**). The width of the serially sliced sections is partly dependent on the size of the node, but usually the sections are made at 2-mm intervals.
- Frozen section evaluation of the SLNs is not recommended out of concern of leaving behind nodal tissue with small-volume diseases in the cryostat, and therefore will go undetected. Such events could reduce the accuracy of the pathologic evaluation of the SLN.[37]
- The tissue slices are embedded in paraffin blocks for permanent section evaluation. All the blocks are stained with hematoxylin and eosin. If these are negative, additional sections are taken for immunostaining.

A

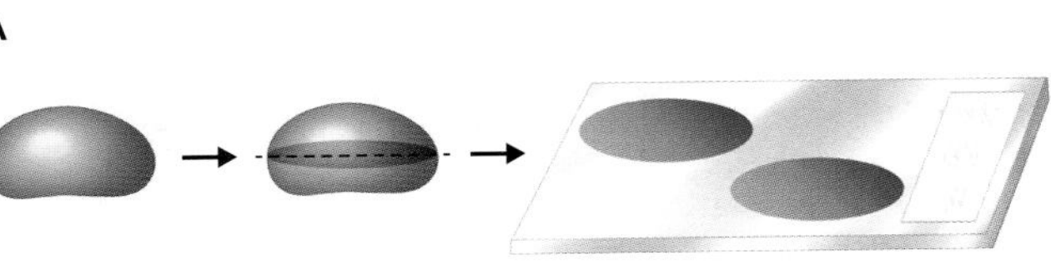

Bisection

B

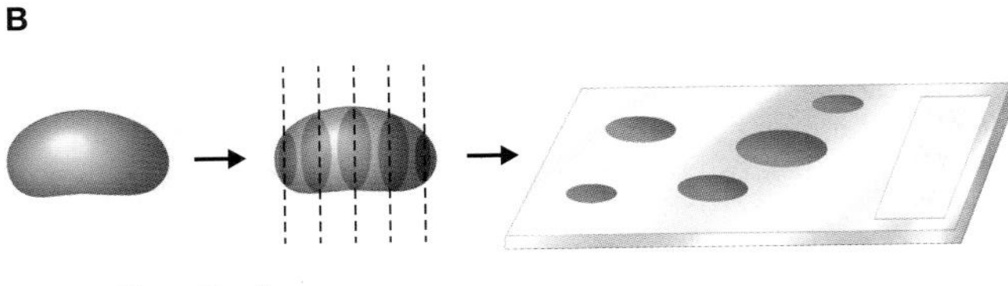

Breadloafing

FIGURE 17 ● Histologic examination of the SLN. Schematic representation of sectioning of lymph nodes, with routine bisection in **(A)** creating two samples to be stained and serial sectioning in **(B)**, resulting in multiple sections for staining.

COMPLICATIONS

- No identifiable drainage to SLN(s)
- Allergic reactions (anaphylaxis and anaphylactoid) to the blue dye (isosulfan blue)
- Removing the "wrong" node and leaving behind the true SLN
- Hematoma
- Seroma
- Infection (cellulitis or infected seroma)
- Paresthesias
- Lymphedema

POSTOPERATIVE CARE

- Always examine the patient before discharge to make sure a hematoma has not developed.
- Instruct the patient what to look for in terms of seroma and surgical site infection.
- Remind them about the blue dye in the urine.
- Keep the SLN site dry for 48 hours.

OUTCOMES

- Using the dual localizing technique of radiotracer and blue dye injections, the SLN identification rate approaches 100%.[3]
- The frequency of a false-negative event defined as the development of clinical nodal disease in the same nodal basin subsequent to the removal of a negative SLN is 3% to 5%.[38] A false-negative event is most commonly a result of very small volume disease undetected by the original pathologic evaluation of the SLN removed, and therefore, a formal lymphadenectomy was not performed. For such an event to occur, another lymph node with subclinical disease was likely present in the same nodal basin at the time of the SLN procedure as the source of the subsequent clinical nodal recurrence. Another reason for a false-negative event leading to a nodal recurrence is the inaccurate identification of the SLN and removing a node that was not sentinel and leaving behind the true SLN that harbored microscopic disease.[38]
- Lymphedema, although rare, can occur and is most common following an SLN biopsy in the groin in conjunction with a wide excision on the thigh or lower leg.

PEARLS AND PITFALLS

Head and neck primaries	■ The lymphatic drainage from these primary lesions is the most ambiguous and least predictable. Therefore, a SPECT-CT lymphoscintigraphy is strongly encouraged. ■ Due to the close proximity to important structures when treating melanomas of the face, the excision margins for the primary lesion may have to be selectively narrowed to avoid injury to these structures and any associated functional or cosmetic impairments (see Part 5, Chapter 32). It is important to note that injected blue dye at the primary site left behind in the remaining skin after the wide excision can tattoo the skin for long periods of time. Therefore, excision margins are clearly delineated with a marking pen prior to the injection of the blue dye. In this way, the volume of dye injected can be adjusted to ensure that the blue staining is limited to the skin to be excised. ■ The SLNs in the neck are surprisingly small; the use of blue dye is particularly helpful. ■ The lymphatic drainage in the head and neck region is very rapid, and the flow of blue dye can be diluted out if too much time transpires between the injection and the exploration of the nodal basin for the SLN. Therefore, in contrast to other primary sites, the blue dye is injected under sterile conditions after the patient is prepped and draped. ■ The SLNs in the neck region are often adjacent to important nerves, such as the spinal accessory, great auricular, and branches of the facial nerve.
Injection of blue dye	■ An injection performed in the intradermal location creates some resistance and can result in the needle becoming separated from the syringe, splattering blue dye on oneself, the patient, and OR staff. Therefore, the use of 1-mL Luer lock–type syringes is recommended. ■ Remember to tell the patient that their urine will be blue/green colored for 24 hours. ■ Any blue dye staining of the skin not removed by the wide excision may take several months to completely fade away. ■ If the patient has already had a wide excision, a preoperative discussion should take place about whether or not to use the blue dye for the planned SLN biopsy. Another excision should not be performed just to remove the blue dye to avoid a tattooing effect. The only time that another excision should take place is when it is necessary to remove the injection site radioactivity that is obscuring your ability to adequately scan the nodal basin for the SLN.
Complications	■ **No drainage observed from the injection site** to an SLN is almost always a result of an error in injection technique. The appropriate technique involves an intradermal injection that raises a wheel and causes some discomfort to the patient. The most common error is injecting the radiotracer too deep into the subcutaneous tissues where the concentration of lymphatic vessels is low or directly into the excisional biopsy site. Hallmarks of a subcutaneous injection include lack of pain during the injection, radiotracer activity seen in the liver on the lymphoscintigraphic images, and no drainage to a nodal basin. ■ **Recurrent seromas** at the SLN biopsy site are conveniently handled by using a "seroma cath" system, composed of a percutaneously placed angiocatheter, a clear tubing, and a small suction bulb. This technique can also be used to treat infected seromas along with antibiotics rather than opening up the wound. ■ **Incorrect identification of the SLN** can lead to pathological understaging and in turn leave behind microscopic nodal disease as a potential source of subsequent clinical lymph node recurrence. One important maneuver to minimize the frequency of such events is to always view the lymphoscintigraphic images prior to the surgery and display the images in the OR rather than depending on the reading by the radiologist. In situations when the primary tumor is on the upper or lower extremity and the surgeon elects to not obtain a lymphoscintigraphy and therefore injects the radiolabeled agent in the OR, it is imperative to scan the intervening skin and soft tissues between the WLE the major nodal basin SLN surgical sites to identify and remove any ectopic/in-transit SLNs.

REFERENCES

1. Morton DL, Wen DR, Wong JH, et al. Technical details of intraoperative lymphatic mapping for early stage melanoma. *Arch Surg*. 1992;127:392-399.
2. Alex J, Krag D. Gamma-probe-guided localization of lymph nodes. *Surg Oncol*. 1993;2:137-144.
3. Gershenwald JE, Tseng CH, Thompson W, et al. Improved sentinel lymph node localization in patients with primary melanoma with the use of radiolabeled colloid. *Surgery*. 1998;124:203-210.
4. Thompson JF, McCarthy WH, Bosch CM, et al. Sentinel lymph node status as an indicator of the presence of metastatic melanoma in regional lymph nodes. *Melanoma Res*. 1995;5:255-260.
5. Cascinelli N, Belli F, Santinami M, et al. Sentinel lymph node biopsy in cutaneous melanoma: the WHO Melanoma Program experience. *Ann Surg Oncol*. 2000;7:469-474.
6. Balch CM, Gershenwald JE, Soong SJ, et al. Multivariate analysis of prognostic factors among 2,313 patients with stage III melanoma: comparison of nodal micrometastases versus macrometastases. *J Clin Oncol*. 2010;28:2452-2459.
7. Lee RJ, Gibbs JF, Proulx GM, et al. Nodal basin recurrence following lymph node dissection for melanoma: implications for adjuvant radiotherapy. *Int J Radiat Oncol Biol Phys*. 2000;46:464-474.
8. Gershenwald JE, Ross MI. Sentinel-lymph-node biopsy for cutaneous melanoma. *N Engl J Med*. 2011;364:1738-1745.

9. Morton DL, Thompson JF, Cochran AJ, et al. Final trial report of sentinel-node biopsy versus nodal observation in melanoma. *N Engl J Med*. 2014;370:599-609.
10. Gershenwald JE, Andtbacka RH, Prieto VG, et al. Microscopic tumor burden in sentinel lymph nodes predicts synchronous nonsentinel lymph node involvement in patients with melanoma. *J Clin Oncol*. 2008;26:4296-4303.
11. Bilimoria KY, Balch CM, Bentrem DJ, et al. Complete lymph node dissection for sentinel node-positive melanoma: assessment of practice patterns in the United States. *Ann Surg Oncol*. 2008;15:1566-1576.
12. Faries MB, Thompson AJ, Cochan RH, et al. Completion dissection or observation for sentinel-node metastases in melanoma. *N Engl J Med*. 2017;376:2211-2222.
13. Leiter U, Stadler R, Mauch C, et al. Final analysis of DeCOG-SLT Trial: no survival benefit for complete lymph node dissection in patients with positive sentinel node. *J Clin Oncol*. 2019;37:3000-3008.
14. Brown RE, Ross MI, Edwards MJ, et al. The prognostic significance of nonsentinel lymph node metastasis in melanoma. *Ann Surg Oncol*. 2010;17:3330-3335.
15. Ross MI. COUNTERPOINT: surgical management of lymph node basin in sentinel lymph node–positive melanoma. At the end of the day, bad biology trumps surgery. *Oncology (Williston Park)*. 2016; 30(10):891. 893-895.
16. Gershenwald JE, Scolyer RA, Hess KR. Melanoma staging: evidence-based changes in the American Joint Committee on Cancer eighth edition cancer staging manual. *CA Cancer J Clin*. 2017;67:472-497.
17. Gershenwald JE, Thompson W, Mansfield PF, et al. Multi-institutional melanoma lymphatic mapping experience: the prognostic value of sentinel lymph node status in 612 stage I or II melanoma patients. *J Clin Oncol*. 1999;17:976-983.
18. Rousseau DL Jr, Ross MI, Johnson MM, et al. Revised American Joint Committee on Cancer staging criteria accurately predict sentinel lymph node positivity in clinically node-negative melanoma patients. *Ann Surg Oncol*. 2003;10:569-574.
19. Balch CM, Morton DL, Gershenwald JE, et al. Sentinel node and standard of care for melanoma. *J Am Acad Dermatol*. 2009;60(5):872-875.
20. *NCCN Clinical Practice Guidelines: Melanoma*. National Comprehensive Cancer Network. Accessed August 14, 2014. http://www.nccn.org/professionals/physician_gls/pdf/melanoma.pdf
21. Wong SL, Faries MB, Kennedy EB, et al. Sentinel lymph biopsy and management of regional lymph nodes in melanoma: American Society of Clinical Oncology and Society of Surgical Oncology clinical practice guideline update. *J Clin Oncol*. 2017;36:399-413.
22. Paek SC, Griffith KA, Johnson TM, et al. The impact of factors beyond Breslow depth on predicting sentinel lymph node positivity in melanoma. *Cancer*. 2007;109:100-108.
23. Doeden K, Ma Z, Narasimhan B, et al. Lymphatic invasion in cutaneous melanoma is associated with sentinel lymph node metastasis. *J Cutan Pathol*. 2009;36:772-780.
24. Doepker MP, Thompson ZJ, Harb JN, et al. Dermal melanoma: a report on prognosis, outcomes, and the utility of sentinel lymph node biopsy. *J Surg Oncol*. 2016;113:98-102.
25. Laeijendecker AE, El Sharouni MA, Sigurdsson V. Desmoplastic melanoma: the role of pure and mixed subtype in sentinel lymph node biopsy and survival. *Cancer Med*. 2020;9:671-677.
26. Pawlik TM, Ross MI, Prieto VG, et al. Assessment of the role of sentinel lymph node biopsy for primary cutaneous desmoplastic melanoma. *Cancer*. 2006;106(4):900-906.
27. Gannon CJ, Rousseau DL Jr, Ross MI, et al. Accuracy of lymphatic mapping and sentinel lymph node biopsy after previous wide local excision in patients with primary melanoma. *Cancer*. 2006;107:2647-2652.
28. Choi EA, Gershenwald JE. Imaging studies in patients with melanoma. *Surg Oncol Clin N Am*. 2007;16:403-430.
29. Uren RF, Howman-Giles R, Thompson JF. Patterns of lymphatic drainage from the skin in patients with melanoma. *J Nucl Med*. 2003;44:570-582.
30. Sumner W, Mansfield P, Ross MI, et al. Implications of lymphatic drainage to unusual sentinel lymph node sites in patients with primary cutaneous melanoma. *Cancer*. 2002;95:354-360.
31. Sondak VK, King DW, Zager JS, et al. Combined analysis of phase III trials evaluating [^{99m}Tc] Tilmanocept and vital blue dye for identification of sentinel lymph nodes in clinically node-negative cutaneous melanoma. *Ann Surg Oncol*. 2013;20:680-688.
32. Uren RF. SPECT/CT lymphoscintigraphy to locate the sentinel lymph node in patients with melanoma. *Ann Surg Oncol*. 2009;16:1459-1460.
33. Quarttuccio N, Garau LM, Arnone A, et al. Comparison of ^{99m}Tc-labeled colloid SPECT/CT and planar lymphoscintigraphy in sentinel lymph node detection in patients with melanoma: a meta-analysis. *J Clin Med*. 2020;9:1680.
34. Ross MI. Lymphatic mapping and sentinel node biopsy for early stage melanoma: how we do it at the MD Anderson Cancer Center. *J Surg Oncol*. 1997;66:273-276.
35. Leong SP, Donegan E, Heffernon W, et al. Adverse reactions to isosulfan blue during selective sentinel lymph node dissection in melanoma. *Ann Surg Oncol*. 2000;7:361-366.
36. Neves RI, Reynolds BQ, Hazard SW, et al. Increased post-operative complications with methylene blue versus lymphazurin in sentinel lymph node biopsies for skin cancers. *J Surg Oncol*. 2011;103:421-425.
37. Scolyer RA, Thompson JF, McCarthy SW, et al. Intraoperative frozen-section evaluation can reduce accuracy of pathologic assessment of sentinel nodes in melanoma patients. *J Am Coll Surg*. 2005;201:821-823.
38. Gershenwald JE, Colome MI, Lee JE, et al. Patterns of recurrence following a negative sentinel lymph node biopsy in 243 patients with stage I or II melanoma. *J Clin Oncol*. 1998;16:2253-2260.

Chapter 34 Axillary Lymph Node Dissection for Melanoma

Michael S. Sabel

DEFINITION

- Axillary lymph node dissection (ALND) involves the surgical excision of the lymph node–bearing tissue from the axilla. The procedure is commonly utilized in breast cancer and melanoma, as well as other cutaneous malignancies such as squamous cell, and Merkel cell carcinomas.
- The axilla is divided into anatomic levels based on the relationship of the nodes to the pectoralis minor muscle (**FIGURE 1**). Level I nodes are located lateral to the pectoralis minor, level II nodes are seated deep to the pectoralis minor, and level III nodes are medial to the pectoralis minor. For patients with clinically evident axillary disease, a level I-III dissection is typically recommended. For patients with a positive axillary SLN biopsy, a level I-III dissection is often performed, but a level I-II dissection may be adequate,[1,2] although ALND for a positive SLN is less common today. This chapter will describe an ALND encompassing levels I, II, and III.

INDICATIONS

- Today, axillary lymph node dissection is primarily indicated for patients with clinically evident axillary nodal involvement (macrometastatic) without evidence of distant metastatic spread. This may include patients who initially present with clinically evident adenopathy or patients with recurrence in the axilla following wide excision alone, a false-negative SLN biopsy, or on nodal observation following a positive SLN biopsy.
- Until recently, ALND for melanoma was indicated for patients following an SLN biopsy that demonstrated micrometastatic disease. However, nodal observation with serial ultrasounds is now an acceptable alternative to completion lymph node dissection in patients with SLN metastasis. Two prospective, randomized clinical trials, the Multicenter Selective Lymphadenectomy Trial II (MSLT-II) and the DeCOG trial,[3,4] showed equivalent melanoma-specific survival for patients with a positive sentinel lymph node randomized to either completion lymphadenectomy or observation with serial clinical examinations and nodal ultrasonography. CLND is reserved for patients with a subsequent isolated regional nodal recurrence. ALND may still be considered in select patients following a positive axillary SLN biopsy based on factors such as nodal tumor burden, patient age, and suitability for adjuvant therapy.

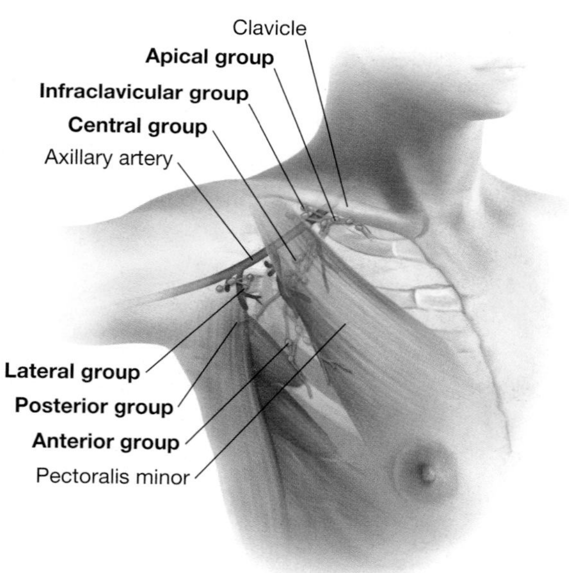

FIGURE 1 ● Levels of axillary lymph nodes. The level I nodes are located lateral to the pectoralis minor muscle, the level II nodes are located deep to the pectoralis minor, whereas the level III nodes are located medial to the pectoralis minor.

PATIENT HISTORY AND PHYSICAL FINDINGS

- The history should focus on the patient's melanoma history, including the histology of the primary tumor, disease-free interval between the primary diagnosis and the diagnosis of regional metastases, and the extent of both locoregional and distant disease. The history should also focus on comorbidities, past medical history, and medications that might impact the patient's surgical candidacy.
- The history should also include a thorough review of systems, specifically looking for symptoms suggestive of distant disease. Patients with symptoms worrisome for stage IV disease should have body imaging before proceeding with surgery.
- A complete physical examination should pay particular attention to signs of local, regional, and distant disease. The site of the primary tumor and the skin between it and the regional basin should be examined for signs of in-transit recurrences. A complete lymph node examination should be performed. This should not just be limited to the axilla of concern but bilateral cervical, supraclavicular, epitrochlear, axillary, and inguinal basins. Suspicious nodes outside of the draining basins may represent stage IV disease.
- For the involved axilla, the examination should focus on the extent of disease, including the size of the involved nodes and fixation. The ipsilateral arm should be examined for lymphedema, weakness, or sensory deficit, as these may be indicative of involvement of the axillary vein or brachial plexus. You should also document any conditions affecting the shoulder or upper extremity, which limits range of motion.
- For patients who had an SLN biopsy or excisional biopsy, it is important to document any sensory or motor deficits that may have occurred at the first surgery as well as any seroma,

hematoma, or infection. It may also be helpful to note the orientation of the incision, as this may impact the orientation of the ALND incision.

- It is important to review with patients the expected postoperative course including drain management and arm exercises, as well as short-term and long-term morbidity, including the risk, prevention, and management of lymphedema.

IMAGING AND OTHER DIAGNOSTIC STUDIES

- As most patients undergoing ALND for melanoma have clinically evident disease or disease recurrence, complete staging is indicated. This should include magnetic resonance imaging (MRI) of the brain and body imaging, either with a computed tomography scan (CT) or positron emission tomography/CT, as there is a large enough chance of detecting metastatic disease that might alter surgical decision making.[5]
  1. For patients with fixed, matted lymph nodes; skin involvement; or neurovascular symptoms of the involved arm (paresthesias, motor and sensory deficits, lymphedema, limited range of motion), MRI of the chest wall can be helpful in determining resectability. Unresectable or borderline resectable patients could be considered for neoadjuvant therapy with BRAF/MEK inhibition (for selected tumors harboring activating mutations in the BRAF V600 codon) or with immune checkpoint blockade immunotherapy (PD-1 blocking antibodies [nivolumab or pembrolizumab] with or without the CTLA-4 blocking antibody ipilimumab).[6]
  2. Patients with large, bulky disease that is technically resectable may also benefit from neoadjuvant therapy. Reducing tumor burden may decrease morbidity, and there may be benefits regarding recurrence and long-term outcomes. Reports from phase II trials suggest that neoadjuvant therapy does not complicate the subsequent node dissection.[7-9] Clinical trials are currently underway examining the safety and efficacy of neoadjuvant immune checkpoint blockade in patients with clinically evident stage III disease, including the possibility of omitting a full nodal dissection in patients with a complete pathologic response.[10-12]

SURGICAL MANAGEMENT

Preoperative Planning

- In the preoperative area, the side of the ALND should be clearly marked and confirmed with the patient before proceeding to the operating room (OR).
- Intravenous (IV) antibiotics are indicated for ALND.[13] Sequential compression devices should be used for deep venous thrombosis (DVT) prophylaxis. Patients with a history of DVT or genetic predisposition toward clotting should receive subcutaneous heparin.

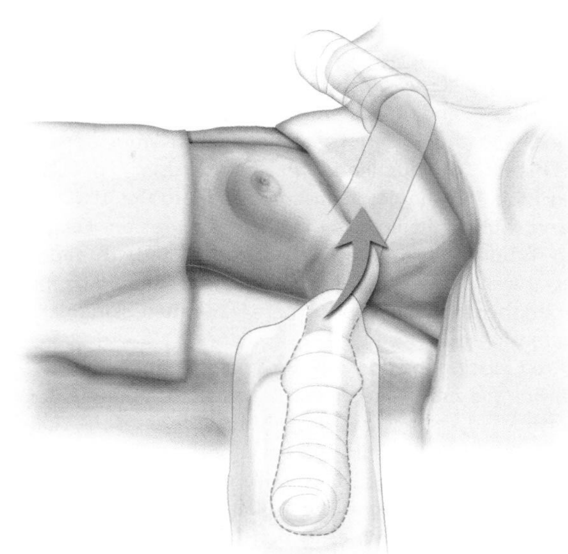

FIGURE 2 ● Preoperative positioning and draping for an ALND. The arm should be prepped into the field with a stockinette and Kerlix wrap so it can be rotated over the chest during the procedure.

- Many surgeons prefer the use of short-acting neuromuscular blocking agents during induction, so that the patients are not paralyzed during the procedure. This allows identification of the thoracodorsal, long thoracic, and medial and lateral pectoral nerves by mechanical stimulation. However, this is not essential and some surgeons prefer paralysis with a long-acting neuromuscular blocking agent to prevent muscular contraction and allow for retraction of the pectoralis major and minor muscles. Either way, this should be discussed with the anesthesiologist prior to the case.

Positioning

- The patient should be positioned supine on the OR table, toward the edge of the side of the ALND so that the posterior axillary line is in line with the edge of the table. The ipsilateral arm is abducted at 90° on a padded arm board. It is important not to extend the arm past 90° to avoid brachial plexus injury.
- The endotracheal tube should be located away from the involved arm, and adequate space should be preserved above the arm for the surgical assistant.
- The chest wall, lower neck, and entire arm should be prepped and draped into the surgical field using a sterile stockinette and Kerlix wrap. This allows the arm to be rotated over the chest, relaxing the pectoralis major and minor (**FIGURE 2**).

INCISION

- Typically, a "lazy S" incision is used along the pectoralis major muscle, extending posteriorly at the level of the axillary hair line, and then inferiorly along the latissimus dorsi muscle (**FIGURE 3**). For patients with a prior excisional or SLN biopsy incision, this should be encompassed into the ALND incision, and thus might impact the choice of incision. For patients with bulky adenopathy, particularly those with nodes close to the skin, the skin overlying the nodes should be included with the specimen. Be sure there is adequate skin to allow for a tension-free closure.
- After incising the skin with a scalpel, electrocautery is used to divide the subcutaneous tissue and elevate skin flaps. Unless mandated by the presence of bulky disease, the skin flaps should not be too thin and get progressively thicker as they are raised. Thin skin flaps will increase the risk of wound complications and give the axilla a sunken-in appearance.
- The skin is elevated using skin hooks or sharp rakes. It is important that the surgical assistant holds the flaps straight up and not retract them back (which residents will sometimes do in order to get a better view). The surgeon retracts the tissue with the opposite hand in order to apply strong countertraction and identify the appropriate tissue plane.
- Surgeons are often hesitant to go too far or too deep while elevating the inferior skin flap at this initial point of the operation for fear of injuring the long thoracic nerve. However, raising an adequate inferior flap allows for greater mobility of the specimen and easier dissection. The inferior flap should be raised to approximately the level of the fifth rib.

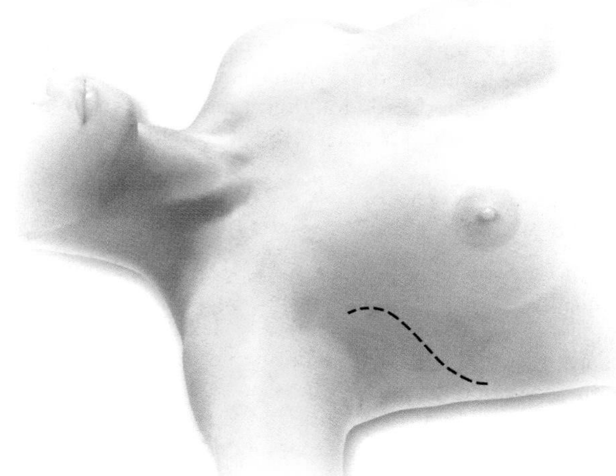

FIGURE 3 ● The "lazy S" incision for an ALND. One can begin with the transverse incision and extend the pectoralis and latissimus arms as needed.

- Once the flaps are elevated, the next step will be to identify some of the borders of the axilla: the pectoralis major and minor muscles, the latissimus dorsi muscle, and the axillary vein. Although individual surgeons have their preferences, there is no correct order, and the presence of large lymph nodes might mandate changing your approach. In this chapter, we will describe a medial-to-lateral approach.

IDENTIFICATION AND RETRACTION OF THE PECTORALIS MAJOR AND MINOR (VIDEO 1)

- The pectoralis major muscle is usually the easiest margin to begin with, as it is often easily palpable upon raising the flaps (and may become apparent while elevating the superior flap). Once the pectoralis major is identified, the length of the lateral border should be exposed (**FIGURE 4**).

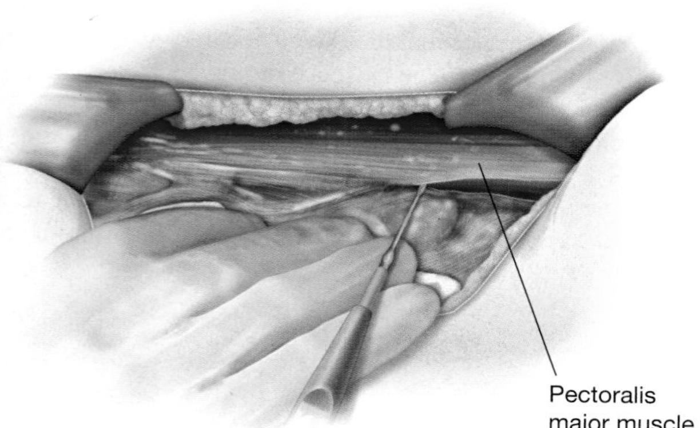

FIGURE 4 ● The pectoralis major muscle is identified and cleaned off along the lateral edge.

- Once the pectoralis major muscle is freed, it is retracted anteriorly and medially to expose the interpectoral nodes and the pectoralis minor muscle. This, and the remainder of the operation, is facilitated by the use of a Thompson retractor (**FIGURE 5**).
- The tissue between the pectoralis major and minor muscle that contains the interpectoral (Rotter) nodes is included with the specimen, dissecting it off the pectoralis minor muscle. As the dissection proceeds onto the pectoralis minor, the medial pectoral bundle can be observed coming either through or lateral to the pectoralis minor (**FIGURE 6**). This should be preserved. There is often an accompanying vein with a branch going into the specimen. This will need to be clipped, taking care not to clip the medial pectoral nerve.
- For patients undergoing an ALND for a positive SLN, the pectoralis minor can be preserved. The lateral edge of the pectoralis minor muscle is freed by dividing the axillary fascia (**FIGURE 7**). The axillary fascia is an extension of the clavipectoral fascia that divides the subcutaneous fat from the axillary fat. Upon dividing the fascia, you will notice the protrusion of a more yellow, globular fat. This is the lymph node–bearing tissue that needs to be excised.
- The axillary contents are now swept laterally and the pectoralis minor muscle exposed along its length. Once this is done, the Thompson retractor can be repositioned so that both the pectoralis major and minor can be retracted anteriorly.
- If there is bulky adenopathy and exposure of the upper axillary lymph nodes is difficult, it may be necessary to divide the pectoralis minor muscle, and this is described subsequently.

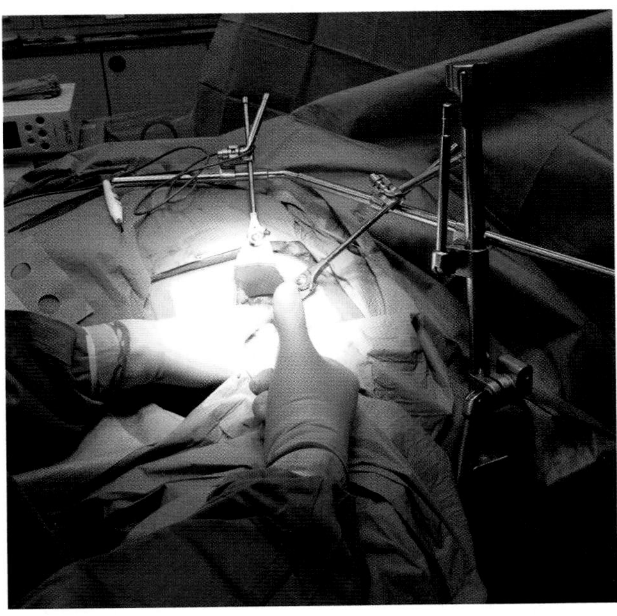

FIGURE 5 ● The Thompson retractor provides excellent exposure for an ALND.

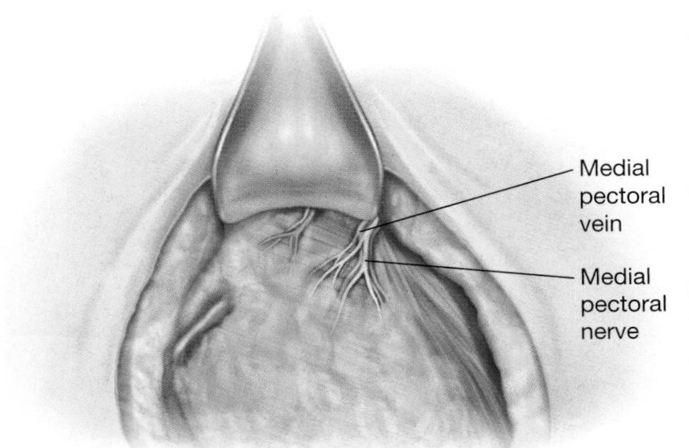

FIGURE 6 ● The medial pectoral nerve.

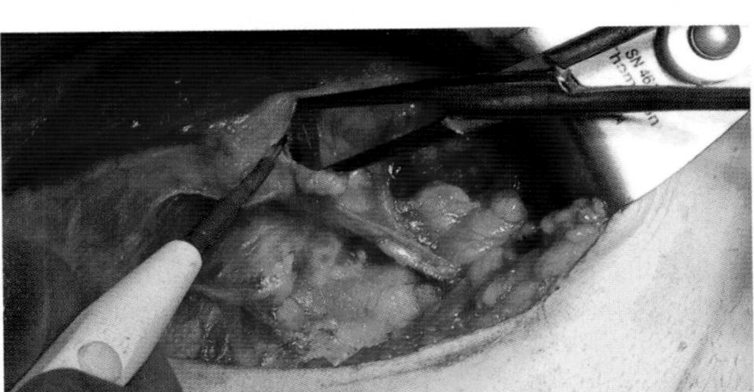

FIGURE 7 ● The axillary (clavipectoral) fascia is divided with cautery, revealing the axillary fat underneath.

IDENTIFICATION OF THE AXILLARY VEIN (VIDEO 1)

- The vein often becomes visible medially during the elevation of the pectoralis musculature. If not, its general location can be anticipated by identifying the underarm dimple at the inferior aspect of the upper arm and tracing it toward the chest wall (**FIGURE 8**). Dissection down to the vein should not be performed directly with cautery to avoid an inadvertent injury, but rather, a careful dissection is recommended (**FIGURE 9**). Small venous branches and lymphatics should be clipped or suture ligated. It is also important not to find yourself superior to the vein, as the axillary artery and brachial plexus can be injured. Once the vein has been identified, the inferior margin should be cleared. It is not necessary to skeletonize the vein.

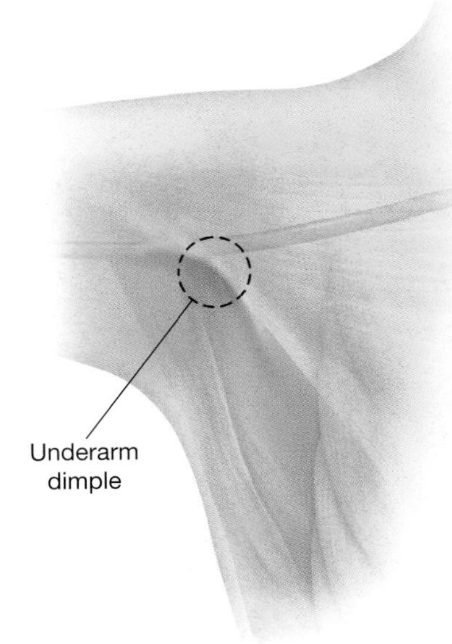

FIGURE 8 ● The position of the axillary vein in the axilla can be estimated by locating the underarm dimple and tracing this back toward the chest wall.

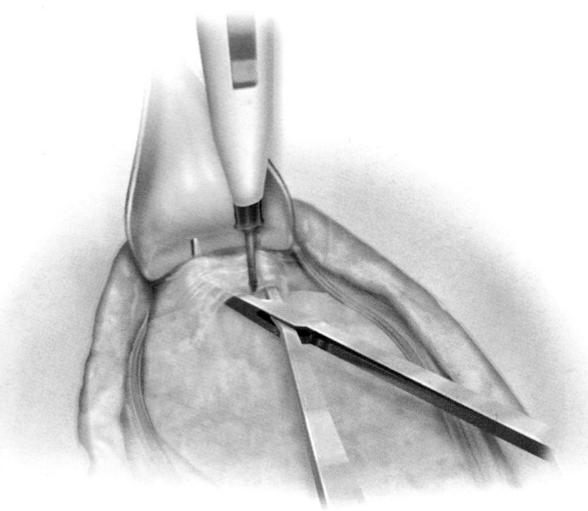

FIGURE 9 ● Exposure of the axillary vein is accomplished by careful dissection with a right angle and cautery.

THE LATISSIMUS DORSI MUSCLE

- The final boundary to identify is the latissimus dorsi muscle. Again, this is often seen during the elevation of the inferior flap. If not, the lateral skin should be retracted laterally using skin hooks or sharp rakes and the axillary contents retracted medially. Dissection down through the subcutaneous fat will identify the muscle (**FIGURE 10**). In obese patients, be careful not to overestimate how lateral the muscle is, as you may dissect past it and raise an unnecessary posterolateral flap. Likewise, being too medial puts the thoracodorsal bundle at risk. Once identified, it should be cleared by staying on the anterior surface of the muscle.
- In a small percentage of cases (approximately 5%–7%), you may identify a more superficial muscle extending from the latissimus dorsi muscle to the pectoralis muscle, over the axillary vein. This is a muscular-tendinous structure known as a Langer arch (**FIGURE 11**). This can often be disorienting, so it is important you be aware of this possibility and continue to dissect laterally to identify the latissimus dorsi. The Langer arch, if present, will need to be divided and excised with the specimen.
- The latissimus muscle should be cleared up to the point where the tendinous insertion is reached beneath the axillary vein.

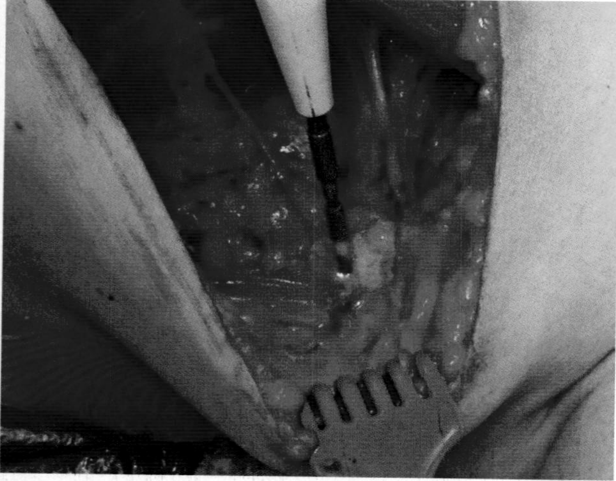

FIGURE 10 ● With lateral traction on the skin, the latissimus dorsi muscle is exposed and cleared on its anterior surface.

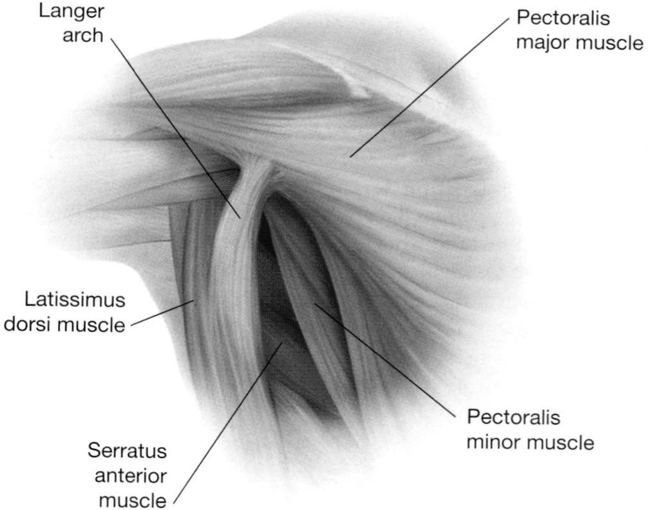

FIGURE 11 ● Anatomy of a Langer arch.

THE THORACODORSAL NEUROVASCULAR BUNDLE (VIDEO 1)

- Once the intersection between the vein and the latissimus is identified, the axillary contents are freed from lateral to medial. Lymphatics should be clipped rather than cauterized. The intercostobrachial nerve will be in this tissue, extending toward the arm, and is commonly sacrificed during this operation. It is important to note that the intercostobrachial nerve does not need to be sacrificed. It can be dissected free by bivalving the specimen and freeing the nerve. However, this is not commonly done when an ALND is being performed for known cancer.

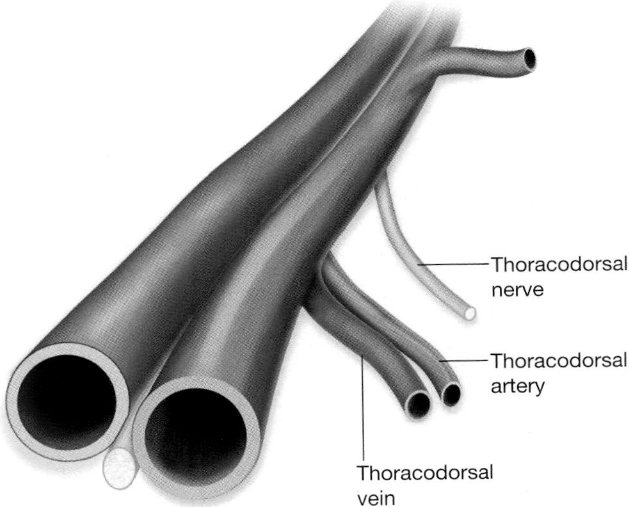

- It is important not to divide the axillary tissue to identify the thoracodorsal vein, but rather, make sure all the tissue between the latissimus dorsi and thoracodorsal bundle is dissected and included with the specimen. Failure to do this, for example, making the thoracodorsal bundle the lateral margin, will leave behind several lymph nodes. As these nodes primarily drain the arm, this is particularly important in melanoma.
- As the axillary vein is cleared medially, the thoracodorsal vein can be identified. The thoracodorsal vein comes off the posterior aspect of the vein. The other large tributary off the axillary vein is the lateral thoracic vein, but this comes off inferiorly, which serves as an important clue that it is not the thoracodorsal vein (**FIGURE 12**). Although the lateral thoracic vein will need to be ligated, this should not be done until the thoracodorsal vein is clearly identified. The thoracodorsal nerve may be directly behind the lateral thoracic vein, so take care when ligating it.
- Once the thoracodorsal vein is visualized, the artery can usually be seen pulsating in close proximity. The nerve, however, at this level, does not run next to the vein but is usually seated more medial, joining the vein and artery 1 to 2 cm inferiorly (**FIGURE 13A** and **B**). The nerve can easily be damaged by assuming it is next to the vein and dividing the more medial tissue. Careful dissection, avoiding the electrocautery, should be used to identify the nerve and trace it inferiorly until it joins the bundle.

FIGURE 12 ● The lateral thoracic nerve enters the axillary vein on the inferior surface, whereas the thoracodorsal vein tends to enter more posteriorly. This can be an important clue as to which vein you are looking at.

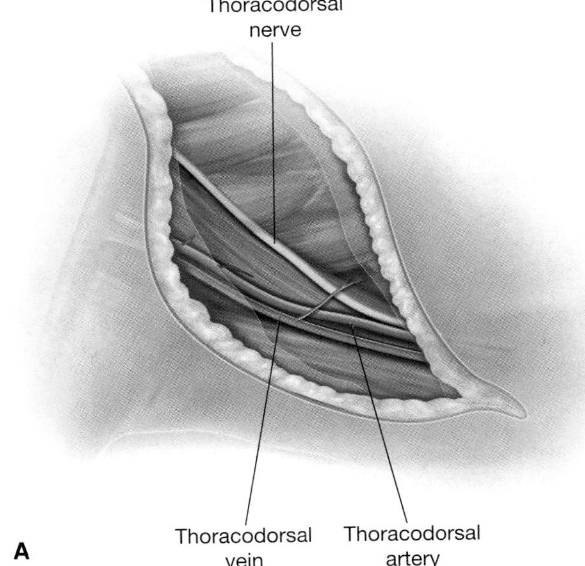

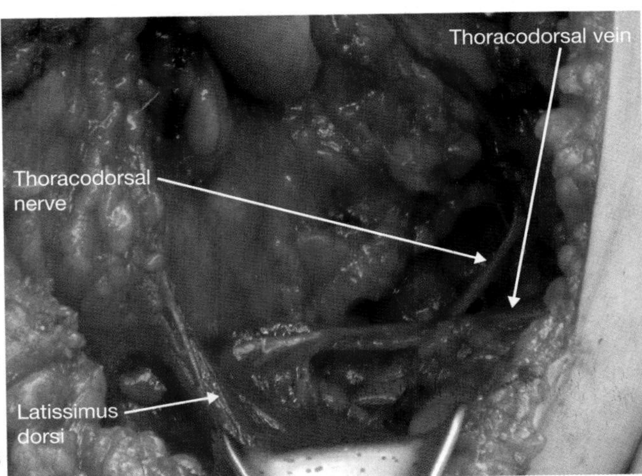

FIGURE 13 ● **A,** Relationship of the thoracodorsal nerve to the artery and vein. **B,** Intraoperative photo showing the nerve medial to the vein and artery and then joining the bundle inferiorly.

- Although these anatomic relationships are generally true, the anatomy can be distorted by both bulky adenopathy and prior surgery. These can distort the relative positions of these structures, and this should be considered when having difficulty identifying them.
- Once the thoracodorsal nerve, artery, and vein are identified, they can be traced and dissected free down to their insertion into the latissimus dorsi. This can be facilitated by retracting the axillary contents anteromedially (which can sometimes be done with the long blade of the Thompson retractor). Although this step can be completed later, we prefer to free the entire bundle now, when visibility is optimized (**FIGURE 14**). There will be branches off of the thoracodorsal toward the specimen that will need to be clipped or ligated.

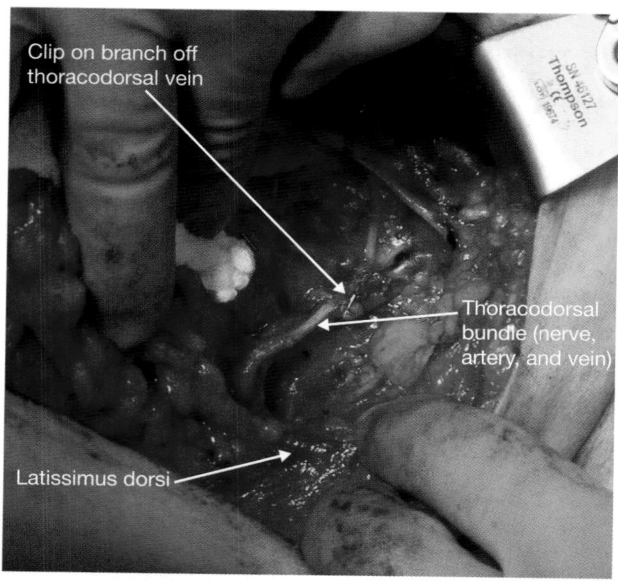

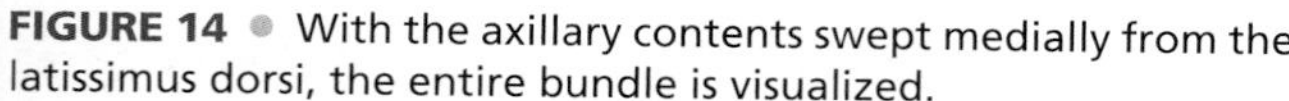

FIGURE 14 ● With the axillary contents swept medially from the latissimus dorsi, the entire bundle is visualized.

DISSECTION OF THE LEVEL II AND LEVEL III NODES (▶ VIDEO 1)

- Once the thoracodorsal is free, the axillary contents are released and the pectoralis major and minor once again retracted medially and anteriorly. The serratus anterior is identified, and you will notice the yellow axillary fat extending up along the serratus, under the pectoralis minor, and along the axillary vein, like the top of a pyramid. This tissue bears the level II and III nodes. The axillary contents are dissected off of the serratus anterior. There is often a large vein that will need to be ligated.
- The intercostobrachial nerve can be seen exiting from the serratus anterior. Although this was likely ligated laterally, it needs to be divided again. The nerve should be cut with scissors flush with the muscle. This minimizes the chance of a neuroma and postoperative neuropathic pain, which is more likely if the nerve is divided with cautery or clips.
- The axillary fat is dissected off of the axillary vein. If you have not already, you will note the axillary fat extending superior to the vein, overlying the brachial plexus. This fat should be included with the specimen. There is a plane of tissue between the fat and the brachial plexus that allows this fat to be retracted inferiorly and can be easily dissected free, dividing only some loose areolar tissue (**FIGURE 15A** and **B**). Excessive cautery near the brachial plexus is strongly discouraged, and care is taken to clip or suture ligate any small vessels.
- Dissection of the upper axillary lymph nodes is facilitated by adducting the arm over the chest and held by an assistant. This allows the surgeon to reposition the Thompson retractor and gain more medial-anterior retraction, opening the axilla. The level II, and in some patients, the level III nodes, can be accessed this way and dissected from the thoracic inlet off the chest wall. It is important to carefully ligate the specimen and any small vessels, as this is a difficult area to return to in the case of bleeding.

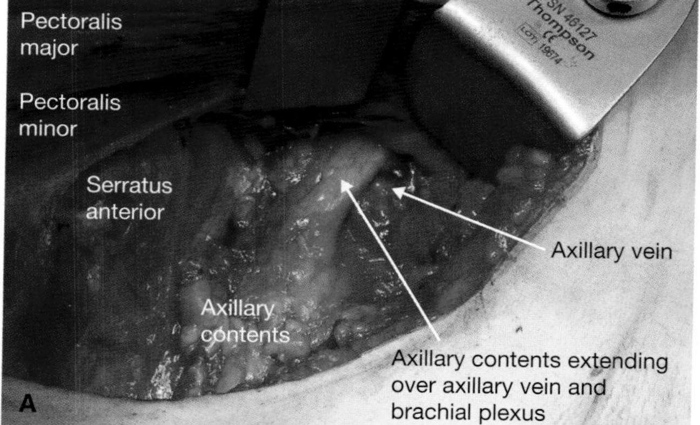

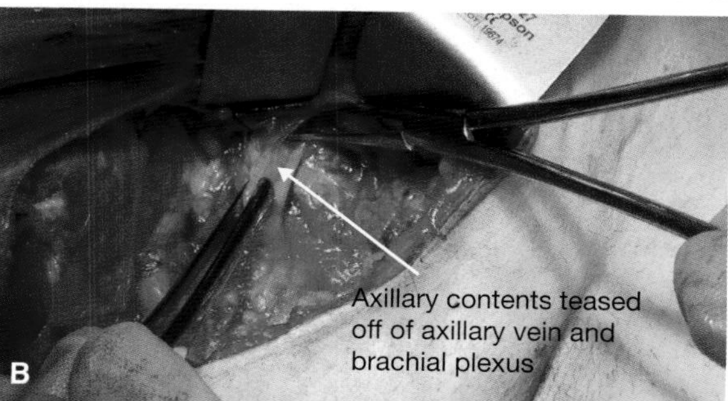

FIGURE 15 ● **A,** Axillary contents extending superiorly over the vein and brachial plexus. **B,** This is teased down with a forceps and included with the specimen.

- In many patients, based on body habitus or in the presence of bulky adenopathy, it is not possible to completely dissect the upper axillary lymph nodes just by adducting the arm over the chest. In this case, there are two options. The pectoralis minor muscle can be divided or an infraclavicular approach can be taken.

DIVISION OF THE PECTORALIS MINOR MUSCLE (PATEY PROCEDURE)

- In some cases, there may be direct involvement of the pectoralis minor muscle by tumor. In this case, the pectoralis minor should be resected en bloc with the axillary contents, dividing the muscle at the insertion point on the coracoid process and dividing it off the chest wall inferiorly (**FIGURE 16**). This greatly facilitates the removal of the level III lymph nodes.

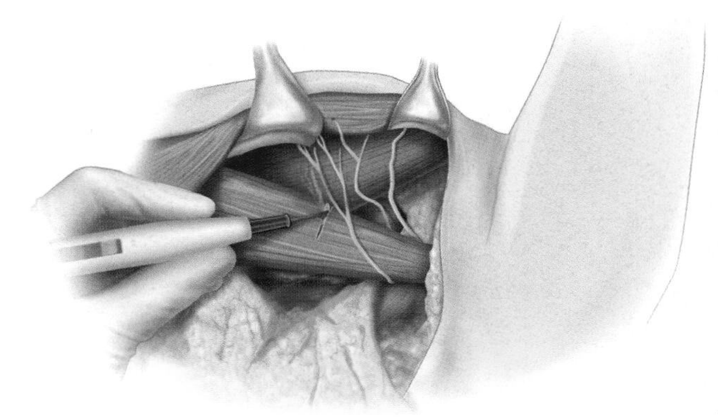

FIGURE 16 ● The pectoralis minor muscle is divided to obtain easier access to the level III lymph nodes, taking care not to injure the pectoral nerves.

INFRACLAVICULAR APPROACH

- An alternate approach is to make a second transverse incision, approximately 2 cm below the clavicle, and then separating the clavicular from the sternal heads of the pectoralis major (**FIGURE 17**). The level III nodes can then be excised, taking care not to injure the neurovascular structures. Division of the pectoralis minor is adequate in the great majority of patients, but the infraclavicular approach can be extremely beneficial in patients with bulky adenopathy at the confluence of the cephalic and axillary veins and in patients who recur in level III after a prior level I and II ALND.

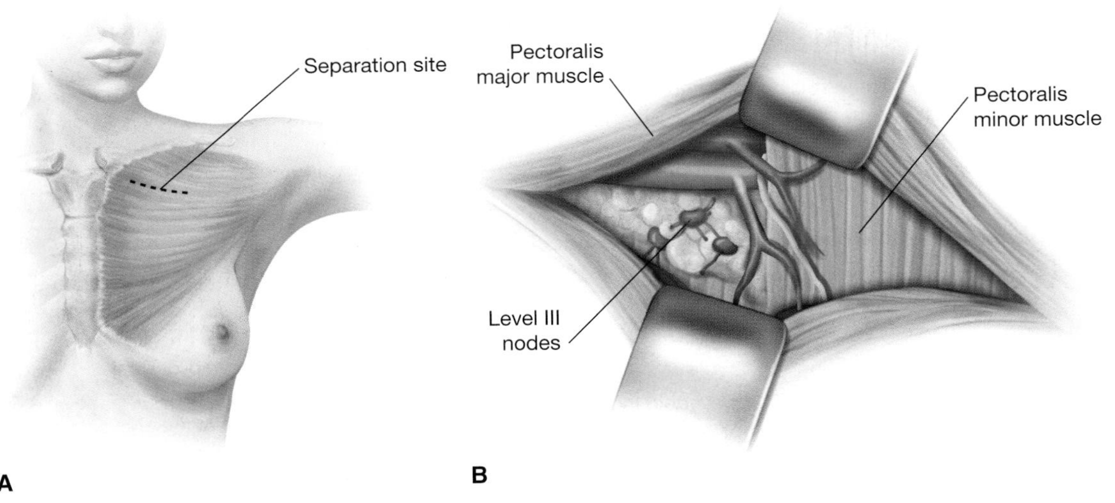

FIGURE 17 ● An alternate approach to the level III axillary nodes is to make an incision 2 cm below the clavicle and separate the clavicular and sternal heads of the pectoralis major.

EXPOSURE OF THE LONG THORACIC NERVE (VIDEO 1)

- Once the level II and III nodes are free, they are brought laterally. The final structure to identify will be the long thoracic nerve. The nerve is commonly described as running along the serratus anterior, but this is incorrect. It is actually outside the fascia of the serratus, and this is exaggerated by the lateral retraction. Therefore, dissection directly on the serratus anterior will not identify the nerve and may lead to inadvertent injury. Dissection should be performed slightly laterally to the chest wall (**FIGURE 18**), and cautery should be used sparingly.
- Two anatomic landmarks can often help identify the nerve or estimate its position. First, the long thoracic and thoracodorsal nerve are roughly in the same anteroposterior (AP) plane. Therefore, by noting the location of the thoracodorsal nerve, you can estimate where you should be looking for the nerve.

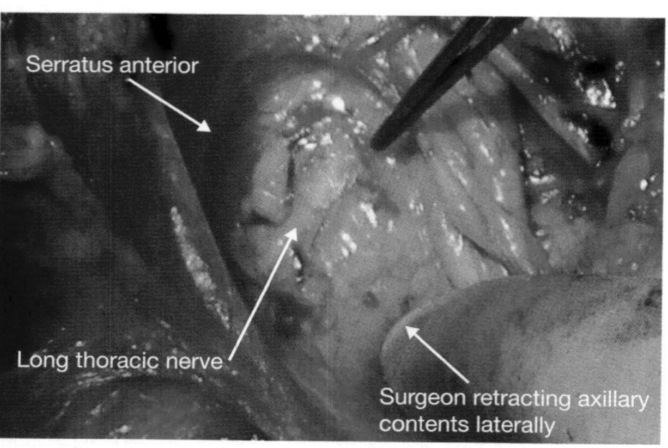

FIGURE 18 ● The long thoracic nerve is identified just lateral to the serratus anterior, which is emphasized by lateral retraction of the specimen.

As before, this relationship can be altered by bulky disease or prior surgery. Second, the thoracodorsal vein often gives off a crossing branch toward the chest wall. This usually enters the chest wall at the level of the nerve.

- Once identified, the specimen is separated from the long thoracic nerve by carefully dissecting laterally to the nerve, allowing the nerve to move medially along the chest wall. This can often be done bluntly, but care should be taken not to stretch the nerve too much, as this can lead to injury and a temporary winged scapula.

REMOVAL OF THE SPECIMEN

- With both nerves free, the next step is to remove the tissue from between the nerves off of the underlying subscapularis muscle. At the level of the axillary vein, the fibrofatty tissue between the nerves should be clamped, taking care to be sure both nerves are free (**FIGURE 19**). The tissue is divided and tied off. This can be done in multiple steps. Once the subscapularis muscle is seen, the tissue can be easily divided off the muscle, constantly visualizing the nerves. Excessive lateral retraction can sometimes pull the serratus and the nerve, leading to accidental injury. This dissection should be carried inferiorly, past the point where both nerves enter their respective muscles. This can be facilitated by repositioning of the Thompson retractor.
- At this point, the specimen may still be attached inferiorly. Other than some veins going to the specimen, which can be suture ligated, this tissue can be divided with cautery, releasing the specimen, which is sent to pathology.

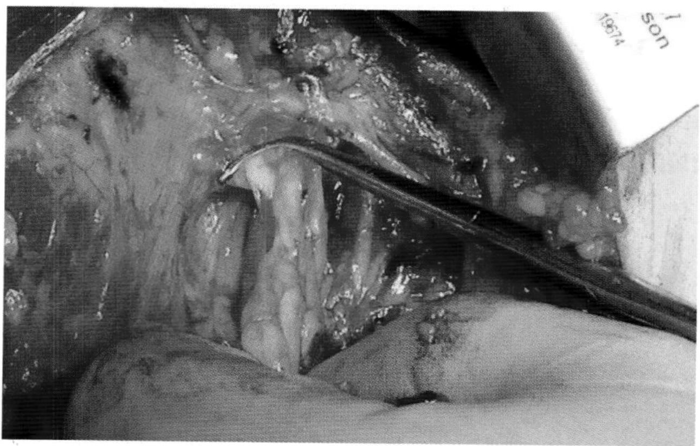

FIGURE 19 ● The axillary tissue below the vein and between the long thoracic and thoracodorsal nerve is clamped, being sure that both nerves are completely free. The tissue is divided and then taken off the subscapularis muscle.

DRAIN PLACEMENT AND INCISION CLOSURE

- The wound should be irrigated with saline or sterile water and thoroughly examined for hemostasis. This should include retraction of the pectoralis major and minor to explore this area. While assuring hemostasis, be careful not to use cautery near the long thoracic or thoracodorsal nerves.
- A single 10-mm flat channel drain is placed through a separate incision inferiorly and sutured to the skin. The drain should be cut so it just lies inferior to the axillary vein. The incision is closed using deep dermal 3-0 absorbable sutures and, for the typical closure, skin adhesive or absorbable monofilament suture. If a large amount of skin is needed to be excised, Nylon sutures may be appropriate.

PEARLS AND PITFALLS

Preoperative planning	■ A thorough neurovascular examination of the involved extremity is critical. Any suggestion of neurovascular involvement should prompt an MRI to assure resectability. ■ For patients who had prior axillary surgery, document any sensory or motor defects, as a nerve injury may have already occurred. ■ Be sure the patient is aware of what to expect postoperatively, including short-term and long-term lymphedema risk reduction and management.

Positioning	■ Having the arm prepped into the field so that it can be retracted over the chest is critical to performing a complete ALND.
Skin flaps	■ Avoid excessively thin flaps as this will lead to wound complications and a "sunken-in" appearance to the axilla. ■ Raise an adequate inferior flap early, as this allows better mobilization of the specimen and better exposure.
Elevating the pectoralis major and minor	■ Every attempt to preserve the medial pectoral nerve should be made. This requires care when mobilizing the pectoralis muscles.
Identifying the latissimus dorsi	■ Careful dissection should land you on the anterior surface of the latissimus dorsi. If you do not see it, slow down and use a right angle rather than continue to cauterize. If you are too medial, you could injure the thoracodorsal bundle. Be careful you are not too lateral (particularly in an obese patient).
Identifying the vein	■ Use the underarm dimple to estimate the location of the axillary vein. Being too far superior risks injury to the brachial plexus.
Thoracodorsal bundle	■ The thoracodorsal vein comes off the axillary vein posteriorly. If you find a vein coming off the inferior aspect of the axillary vein, it is probably the lateral thoracic, but do not ligate it until you have seen the thoracodorsal. ■ The nerve is usually medial to the vein at this level but not always. ■ If you cannot locate the bundle, you can identify it at the level of the latissimus and trace it back toward the axillary vein.
Long thoracic nerve	■ Do not dissect directly on the serratus anterior—you will be medial to the nerve and mobilize it into your specimen. ■ Expect the long thoracic nerve in roughly the same AP plane as the thoracodorsal vein. ■ If you trace the thoracodorsal nerve along its length, a branch will head medially to the chest wall precisely where the long thoracic nerve lies.
Altered anatomy	■ Remember, bulky adenopathy or prior surgery (such as an SLN biopsy) can alter these relationships.

POSTOPERATIVE CARE

- The drain will remain in place until the output falls below 30 mL per 24 hours for 2 days in a row. The patient and their family should be shown how to care for the drain and record the drain output. A visiting nurse can be of assistance.
- Patients should be instructed to avoid repetitive activities with the arm or heavy lifting. Some surgeons also advise avoiding reaching over 90°, particularly if the incision was excessively tight. However, patients should be encouraged to use the arm for normal activities and should be given exercises to maintain normal range of motion. Slings should not be given to patients.
- Once the drains are removed, physical therapy can be extremely helpful with returning to full range of motion.
- Patient should be educated about the signs and symptoms of lymphedema and lymphedema prevention. Early recognition of lymphedema can improve the likelihood of management.
- Patients with stage III melanoma should be referred to medical oncology for a discussion of adjuvant therapies (immunotherapy or targeted therapies) or clinical trial. Patients with disease at high risk for relapse may also be considered for adjuvant radiation.

OUTCOMES

- For prospective trials, the adequacy of an ALND is often based on the number of lymph nodes identified within the axillary specimen. Morton et al[14] in the MSLT-I trial recommended 15 or more nodes for an ALND, and this is a reasonable benchmark. However, this number will vary not only with surgical technique but also body habitus and the pathologist.
- Five-year melanoma-specific survival rates for melanoma metastatic to regional lymph nodes are listed by stage per the eighth edition of the American Joint Committee on Cancer below[15]:
  - Stage IIIA melanoma—93%
  - Stage IIIB melanoma—83%
  - Stage IIIC melanoma—69%
  - Stage IIID melanoma—32%

COMPLICATIONS

- Infection
- Hematoma
- Seroma
- Limited range of motion at the shoulder
- Axillary web syndrome
- Paresthesias of the axilla and upper inner arm
- Axillary vein thrombosis
- Lymphedema
- Winged scapula (injury to the long thoracic nerve)
- Latissimus dorsi paralysis (injury to the thoracodorsal nerve)
- Brachial plexus injury[16]

REFERENCES

1. Namm JP, Chang AE, Cimmino VM, et al. Is a level III dissection necessary for a positive sentinel lymph node in melanoma? *J Surg Oncol*. 2012;105(3):225-258.

2. Nessim C, Law C, McConnell Y, et al. How often do level III nodes bear melanoma metastases and does it affect patient outcomes? *Ann Surg Oncol.* 2013;20(6):2056-2064.
3. Faries MB, Thompson JF, Cochran AJ, et al. Completion dissection or observation for sentinel-node metastasis in melanoma. *N Engl J Med.* 2017;376:2211-2222.
4. Leiter U, Stadler R, Mauch C, et al. Final analysis of DeCOG-SLT trial: no survival benefit for complete lymph node dissection in patients with positive sentinel node. *J Clin Oncol.* 2019;27:3000-3008.
5. Sabel MS, Wong SL. Review of evidence-based support for pretreatment imaging in melanoma. *J Natl Compr Canc Netw.* 2009;7(3):281-289.
6. Amaria RN, Meznies AM, Burton EM, et al. Neoadjuvant systemic therapy in melanoma: recommendations of the international neoadjuvant melanoma consortium. *Lancet Oncol.* 2019;20(7):e378-389.
7. Heiken TJ, Price DL, Piltin MA, Turner JH, Block MS. Surgeon assessment of the technical impact of neoadjuvant systemic therapy on operable stage III melanoma. *Ann Surg Oncol.* 2022;29:780-786.
8. Amaria RN, Reddy SM, Twabi HA, et al. Neoadjuvant immune checkpoint blockade in high-risk resectable melanoma. *Nat Med.* 2018;24(11):1649-1654.
9. Rozeman EA, Menzies AM, van Akkooi AC, et al. Identification of the optimal combination dosing schedule of neoadjuvant ipilimumab plus nivolumab in macroscopic stage III melanoma (OpACIN-neo): a multicentre, phase 2, randomised, controlled trial. *Lancet Oncol.* 2019;20(7):948-960.
10. Neoadjuvant ipilimumab plus nivolumab versus standard adjuvant nivolumab in macroscopic stage III melanoma (NADINA). ClinicalTrials.gov Identifier: NCT04949113.
11. A study to compare the administration of pembrolizumab after surgery versus administration both before and after surgery for high-risk melanoma. ClinicalTrials.gov Identifier: NCT03698019.
12. Blank CU, Reijers IL, Pennington T, et al. First safety and efficacy results of PRADO: a phase II study of personalized response-driven surgery and adjuvant therapy after neoadjuvant ipilimumab and nivolumab in resectable stage III melanoma. *J Clin Oncol.* 2020;38:S10002.
13. Bold RJ, Mansfield PF, Berger DH, et al. Prospective, randomized, double-blind study of prophylactic antibodies in axillary lymph node dissection. *Am J Surg.* 1998;176(3):239-243.
14. Morton DL, Cochran AJ, Thompson JF, et al. Sentinel node biopsy for early-stage melanoma: accuracy and morbidity in MSLT-I, an international multicenter trial. *Ann Surg.* 2005;242:302-313.
15. Gershenwald JE, Scolyer RA, Hess KR, et al. Melanoma staging: evidence-based changes in the American Joint Committee on Cancer eighth edition staging manual. *CA Cancer J Clin.* 2017;67:472-492.
16. Aloia TA, Gershenwald JE, Andtbacka RH, et al. Utility of computed tomography and magnetic resonance staging in patients with stage III melanoma diagnosed by sentinel lymphadenectomy. *J Clin Oncol.* 2006;24:2858-2865.

Chapter **35**

Inguinal Lymph Node Dissection (Inguinofemoral and Ilioinguinal) for Metastatic Melanoma

Amod A. Sarnaik and Vernon K. Sondak

DEFINITION

- Inguinofemoral lymphadenectomy (or superficial inguinal lymph node dissection) is defined as the en bloc removal of all lymphatic tissue contained within the femoral triangle, as well as the node-bearing tissue superior to the inguinal ligament but superficial to the external oblique aponeurosis, up to the level of the anterior superior iliac spine (ASIS).
- The procedure can be combined with a pelvic (also known as deep inguinal) node dissection, in which case it is designated as an ilioinguinal lymphadenectomy, that includes the separate removal of the obturator and external iliac lymph nodes at least up to the level of the iliac bifurcation.
- The procedure has been used for the management of inguinal metastasis from penile, anal, and vulvar carcinomas as well as cutaneous malignancies such as squamous cell, basal cell, adnexal, and Merkel cell carcinomas, but it is most commonly used for metastasis from melanoma, which is the focus of this chapter.

DIFFERENTIAL DIAGNOSIS AND BIOPSY

- Prompt diagnosis of inguinal metastasis by the least invasive means possible is a good start to minimize the morbidity of, and sometimes even the need for, subsequent inguinal node dissection.
- Patients with clinically occult inguinal metastasis from melanoma and other cutaneous malignancies, as well as some anogenital cancers, can be diagnosed with sentinel lymph node biopsy. Inguinofemoral lymphadenectomy for microscopic nodal metastases identified by sentinel lymph node biopsy appears to be associated with less morbidity compared to lymphadenectomy for macroscopic nodal disease; however, completion lymphadenectomy for sentinel node-positive melanoma is much less frequently employed than previously (see below).[1]
- Patients who present with a palpable inguinal mass with a history of melanoma, especially of the ipsilateral lower extremity, trunk, or anogenital region, should be considered to have metastatic melanoma until proven otherwise.
- Patients who present with a palpable inguinal mass without a known history of melanoma should be investigated for a primary malignancy with complete skin/mucosal surface physical examination including the vulva, penis, and perianal skin/anal canal, and a digital rectal examination to evaluate for melanoma, nonmelanoma skin cancer (squamous cell, basal cell, Merkel cell, or adnexal carcinoma), vulvar, penile, and anal cancer.
- For patients presenting with a palpable groin mass but without history or physical evidence of skin/mucosal surface cancers, the differential diagnoses include inguinal/femoral hernias, femoral aneurysm, reactive/infectious lymphadenopathy (cat scratch fever or posttraumatic), lymphoma, and metastatic cancer of unknown primary origin (including melanoma).
- The preferred diagnostic approach for patients with palpable groin masses not consistent with an aneurysm or hernia is needle biopsy—either percutaneous fine needle aspiration or core needle biopsy. If the mass is difficult to palpate or characterize, a diagnostic ultrasound with subsequent ultrasound-guided biopsy could be considered. Open biopsy should be reserved for when needle biopsy is nondiagnostic, as the resulting scar and biopsy cavity from an open biopsy of a palpable mass render subsequent lymphadenectomy technically more difficult and extensive than would otherwise be necessary.[2] In addition, open biopsy can limit the option for neoadjuvant therapy prior to lymphadenectomy, as described below. Concern for a possible diagnosis of lymphoma is no longer an indication for open biopsy, as sufficient tissue to establish the diagnosis and subtype of lymphoma can generally be obtained from core needle biopsies.

INDICATIONS FOR INGUINOFEMORAL AND ILIOINGUINAL LYMPHADENECTOMY

- Nodal observation ("active nodal surveillance") as an alternative to completion lymphadenectomy in melanoma patients with sentinel node metastasis is supported by the results of two multicenter randomized clinical trials involving several thousand patients with sentinel node-positive melanoma: the Multicenter Selective Lymphadenectomy Trial II (MSLT-II) and the DeCOG trial.[3,4] These trials documented equivalent melanoma-specific survival for patients with a positive sentinel lymph node randomized to either completion lymphadenectomy or observation with serial clinical examinations and nodal ultrasonography, with the latter patients undergoing lymphadenectomy only in the event of subsequent isolated regional nodal recurrence. These results have led most practitioners to recommend nodal observation over completion lymphadenectomy for most melanoma patients with positive sentinel nodes.[1] Patients with melanoma in the sentinel node(s) and without prohibitive comorbidities are often offered adjuvant systemic therapy along with nodal observation.[5] The surgeon maintains a role in active nodal surveillance even in patients on adjuvant treatment.
- Ilioinguinal lymphadenectomy is typically reserved for patients with evidence of metastatic disease in both the inguinal and pelvic nodal basins. Although a subset of patients with radiologically normal pelvic nodes will have evidence of occult metastasis if they are removed at the same time as known tumor-containing inguinofemoral lymph nodes, indications for an ilioinguinal lymph node dissection in the face

of radiologically normal pelvic nodes remain controversial. Surprisingly, the long-term morbidity of ilioinguinal lymphadenectomy has not proven to be greater than inguinofemoral lymphadenectomy, despite including the pelvic nodes.[6] Consequently, several indications for ilioinguinal node dissection in the face of radiologically normal pelvic nodes have been proposed. However, the clinical benefit of ilioinguinal lymphadenectomy in patients with biopsy-proven inguinofemoral metastases but radiographically normal pelvic nodes has not been demonstrated in a randomized, prospective trial to date.

- Some surgeons have advocated for the use of intraoperative frozen sections to evaluate the status of the so-called "node of Cloquet," with a positive frozen section result serving as an indication for extending the lymphadenectomy into the pelvis in patients with known inguinal nodal metastasis but radiographically normal pelvic nodes. However, there is a lack of uniform definition of the node of Cloquet, as well as known examples of lymphoscintigraphy performed for sentinel node biopsy showing direct drainage from low or mid-inguinal nodes to pelvic nodes, bypassing that node. Due to these factors, we do not rely on the status of the node of Cloquet in any way.[2]
- Since completion lymphadenectomy is no longer routinely employed after a positive sentinel lymph node biopsy, lymphoscintigraphy evidence of "hot" nodes in the pelvis that were not removed in the sentinel lymph node procedure is no longer considered an indication for ilioinguinal lymphadenectomy.
- Some surgeons have advocated ilioinguinal lymphadenectomy in any patient with palpable inguinofemoral disease.[7] With the widespread use of adjuvant therapy for clinical stage III melanoma, this radical surgical approach is no longer employed at most melanoma centers. During the course of an inguinofemoral lymphadenectomy, if the surgeon can palpate disease deep to the inguinal ligament, extending the dissection into the pelvis would be appropriate.

IMAGING AND OTHER DIAGNOSTIC STUDIES

- Prior to lymphadenectomy, patients who are diagnosed with inguinal metastatic melanoma typically are recommended to undergo whole-body imaging (positron emission tomography–computed tomography [PET/CT] plus brain magnetic resonance imaging [MRI] or equivalent). Systemic therapy is typically pursued if radiologic evaluation shows evidence of distant disease beyond the groin and pelvis.

NEOADJUVANT THERAPY

- Neoadjuvant therapy is defined as an anticancer treatment that is administered prior to surgery to patients with resectable disease. Given the success of systemic therapy for unresectable metastatic melanoma, it is increasingly common for patients with technically resectable nodal metastatic melanoma to undergo neoadjuvant systemic therapy with BRAF/MEK inhibition (for selected tumors harboring activating mutations in the BRAF V600 codon) or with immune checkpoint blockade immunotherapy (PD-1 blocking antibodies [nivolumab or pembrolizumab] with or without the CTLA-4 blocking antibody ipilimumab).[8] Phase III clinical trials are currently underway examining the safety and efficacy of neoadjuvant immune checkpoint blockade, but results of phase II trials indicate that it is relatively rare for neoadjuvant therapy to interfere with the subsequent lymphadenectomy due to either disease progression or toxicity of the treatment. Omission of a full nodal dissection is also being investigated in clinical trials when and if a major pathologic response is achieved by neoadjuvant therapy, as assessed by open excision of an index nodal metastasis whose identification is facilitated by pretreatment fiducial marker placement, with long-term results still pending.[9]

SURGICAL MANAGEMENT

Preoperative Planning

- Preoperative planning for either an inguinofemoral or an ilioinguinal lymphadenectomy starts with careful consideration of the diagnostic procedures required to establish the presence of metastatic disease in the inguinal and/or pelvic nodes. Percutaneous needle biopsy where feasible should be considered for palpable disease as discussed earlier.
- Inguinofemoral and ilioinguinal lymph node dissections are performed under general anesthesia; therefore, the patient should be assessed for perioperative cardiac risk factors and referred for appropriate preoperative testing as clinically warranted.
- Patients should be clinically assessed for any preoperative lymphedema and typically are referred for fitted gradient compression stocking measurements to be used in the postoperative period. Although proof of the value of compression therapy is lacking, it is thought that early institution of compression therapy might minimize the risk of lymphedema in the early postoperative period.[10]
- For clinically node-negative melanoma patients undergoing sentinel node biopsy, orientation of the sentinel node incision should be planned to facilitate any subsequent inguinal lymph node dissection, which should include resection of the sentinel node biopsy scar and cavity.
  - When the sentinel node is located below the inguinal ligament, the sentinel node incision should ideally be vertically oriented and at least 0.5 cm distal to the groin crease (**FIGURE 1A**).
  - When the sentinel node is located above the inguinal ligament (often seen with a flank primary melanoma), the sentinel node incision should ideally be obliquely or transversely oriented and at least 0.5 cm proximal to the groin crease (**FIGURE 1B**).
- As with any surgical procedure, the operative side and site should be identified with the agreement of the patient and/or the representative of the patient in the preoperative holding area.
- Patients with a prior history of deep vein thrombosis (DVT) or known genetic predisposition to thrombosis may be given a prophylactic dose of low molecular weight heparin preoperatively.
- A first-generation cephalosporin such as cefazolin (or another antibiotic with an equivalent spectrum of coverage if allergic to cephalosporins or penicillin) is routinely given

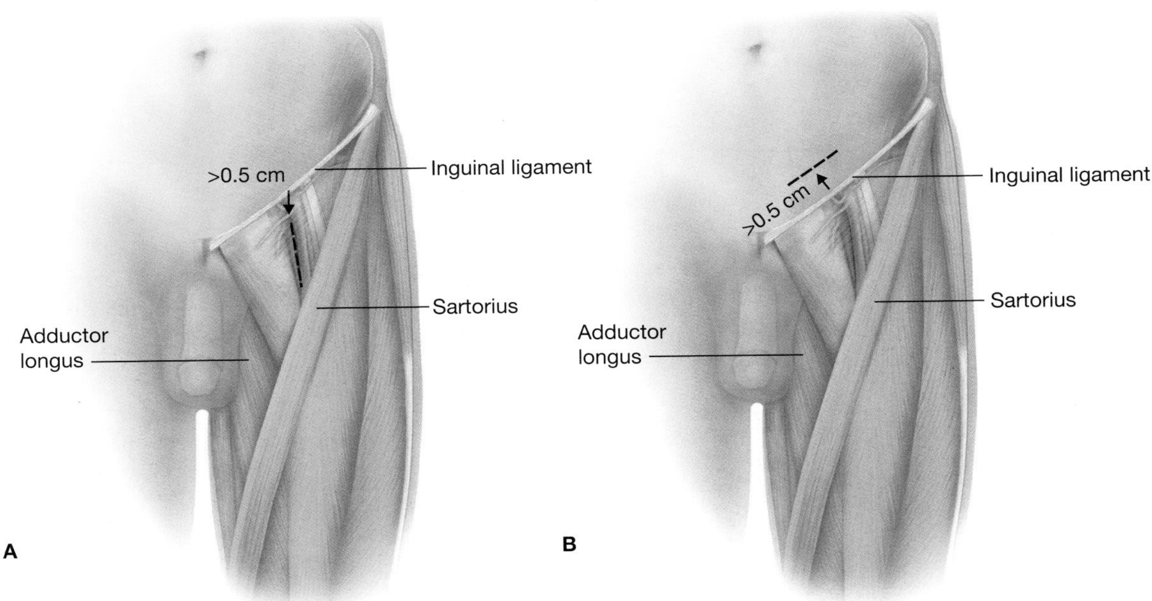

FIGURE 1 ● **A,** The recommended orientation for sentinel node biopsy incision when the draining nodes map to the region inferior (distal) to the groin crease. **B,** The recommended orientation for sentinel node biopsy incision when the draining nodes map to the region superior (proximal) to the groin crease.

intravenously within 30 to 60 minutes of the creation of the skin incision.

- Preoperative stress dose corticosteroids may be entertained for patients with suppression of the hypothalamus–pituitary–adrenal axis, such as for those patients on replacement corticosteroids as a consequence of prior immunotherapy.

Positioning

- The patient is placed in the supine position on a standard operating table. A sequential compression device (SCD) (knee length ipsilateral [omitted if interfering with concomitant wide excision of an ipsilateral leg primary site] and thigh length contralateral) should be placed for DVT prophylaxis prior to induction of anesthesia. General anesthesia is required using either a laryngeal mask or endotracheal tube for inguinofemoral lymphadenectomy, but endotracheal intubation is preferred for ilioinguinal dissections. Long-acting paralytic agents are typically avoided to allow motor nerve stimulation to be evident during the course of the procedure. A urinary catheter is inserted for ilioinguinal dissections but may potentially be omitted for inguinofemoral dissections at the discretion of the surgeon. The patient is placed in a slight frog-leg position with all pressure points padded. The operative field should be prepared from the abdominal wall at the level of the umbilicus or above to the level of the ipsilateral knee. A groin towel secured with a sterile adhesive drape can be used to cover and exclude the genitalia from the field.

INGUINOFEMORAL LYMPHADENECTOMY

Skin Incision and Raising of Flaps

- As stated previously, a well-placed node biopsy incision, or avoiding the creation of a preexisting incision by percutaneous instead of open biopsy of palpable metastasis, is important to minimize the extent of required skin flaps.
- When a preexisting biopsy scar is below the inguinal crease, a curvilinear incision is made in a vertical orientation including the old scar within an ellipse of skin to facilitate excision of the previous cavity of dissection (**FIGURE 2A**). When a preexisting biopsy scar is above the inguinal crease, a transversely or obliquely oriented incision, again including the old scar within an ellipse of skin, is made to excise the previous cavity of dissection. In these cases, a second counterincision can be made below the inguinal crease to reach the lowest femoral nodes (**FIGURE 2B**), although this is rarely necessary as adequate retraction can usually allow for the removal of all the femoral nodes distal to the inguinal crease without the need for the second incision.
- For palpable disease without a preexisting biopsy scar, a skin incision can be configured in a straight line or in a lazy "S" fashion (**FIGURE 2C**). This incision can be extended in a cranial direction if needed for an ilioinguinal lymphadenectomy. If the tumor is close to the skin, an ellipse of skin overlying the palpable tumor should be included.
- Skin flaps are raised in order to clear the anticipated boundaries of the dissection (below) without being so thin as to

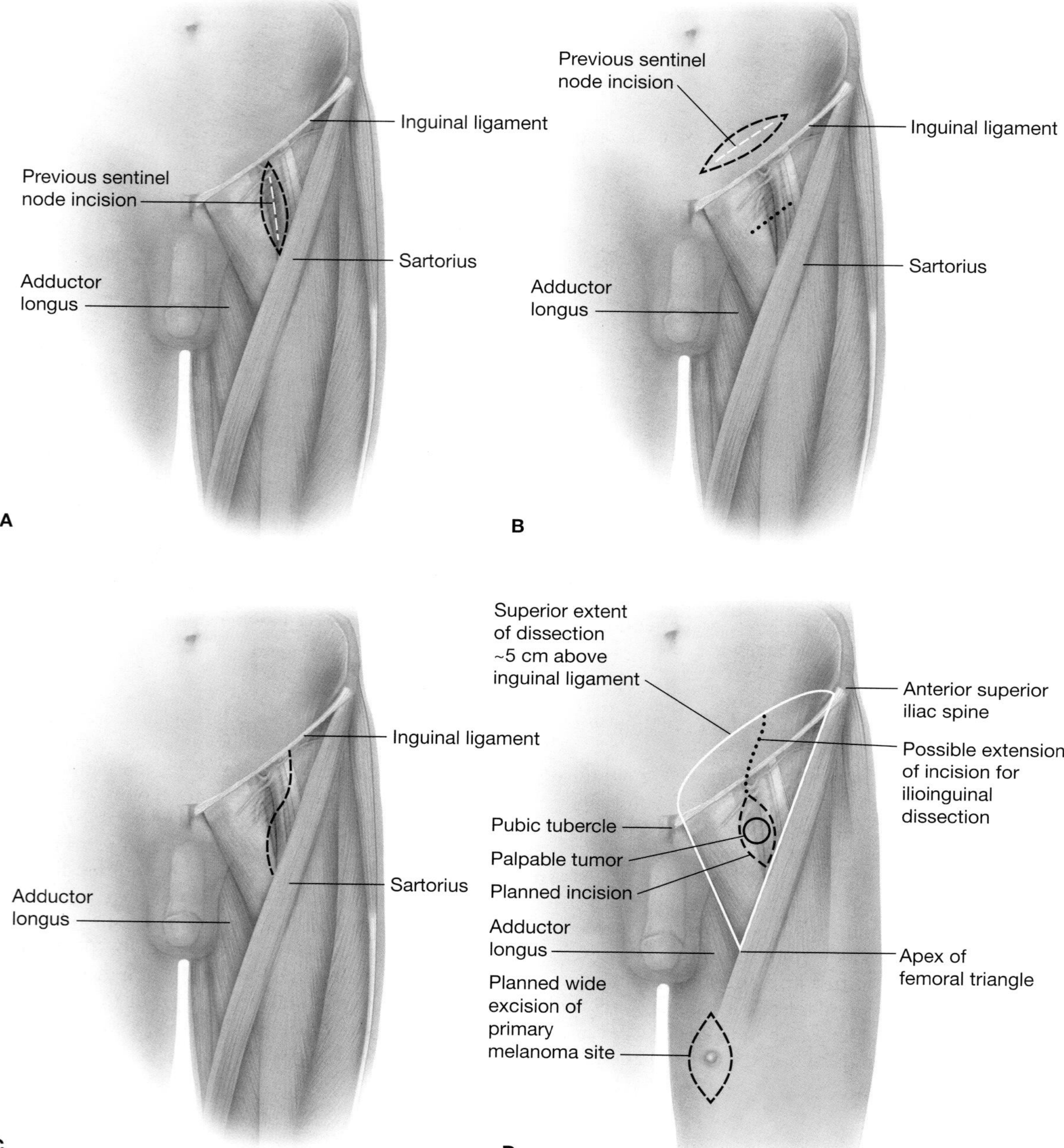

FIGURE 2 ● **A,** The recommended orientation of a curvilinear incision for an inguinal lymphadenectomy with a preexisting biopsy scar inferior to the groin crease. **B,** The recommended orientation of an elliptical incision above the groin crease combined, if necessary, with a linear incision inferior to the groin crease. **C,** The recommended orientation of a lazy S incision that can include an ellipse of skin overlying palpable disease. Of note, to facilitate exposure for an ilioinguinal lymphadenectomy, it may be required for the incision to cross the groin crease. **D,** The operative field with denoted boundaries of the extent of inguinofemoral lymphadenectomy (white line) in a patient with an intact primary melanoma and clinically evident nodal disease. Note that the planned incision includes the palpable metastasis, and that the incision can be optionally extended onto the abdominal wall for an ilioinguinal lymphadenectomy.

increase the risk of postoperative skin necrosis. Limiting the extent of the flaps to the borders of the femoral triangle avoids an unnecessarily wide field of dissection and therefore may be associated with a reduction in morbidity.

- The dissection is continued to the level of the muscular fascia with the following boundaries (**FIGURE 2D**):
  - ASIS superolaterally
  - Pubic tubercle medially
  - The superior extent of dissection should encompass the tissue from the ASIS to the pubic tubercle resulting in approximately 3- to 5-cm clearance above the inguinal ligament while leaving external oblique fascia intact.

- Sartorius muscle laterally, incising the fascia
- Adductor longus medially, incising the fascia
- Junction of the sartorius and adductor longus distally (the so-called apex of the femoral triangle)

- It should be noted that while there have been isolated reports suggesting that incising the fascia of the sartorius and adductor longus may increase lymphedema, this has not been established in large series and most surgeons incise the muscle fasciae as described earlier.
- During the course of the dissection, tissue that potentially contains lymphatic vessels should be clipped, tied, or sealed with harmonic shears.[11]
- A key point of the upper extent of the dissection on the abdominal wall is that the lymphadenectomy clears the node-bearing tissue above the level of the inguinal ligament, specifically removing the subcutaneous node-bearing tissue superficial to the external oblique fascia from the level of the ASIS to the pubic tubercle and down to the shelving edge of the inguinal ligament (**FIGURE 3**). The dissection should typically preserve the spermatic cord in males, but the round ligament can be divided in females, if necessary.

Dissection of the Saphenous Vein Distally

- The distal portion of the saphenous vein is encountered along the medial boundary of the dissection approximately 3 to 5 cm proximal to the apex of the femoral triangle. In most cases, the saphenous vein is tied off distally with 2-0 silk ties and divided. The saphenous vein can potentially be preserved in select cases where the procedure is performed for micrometastatic disease or after an excellent response to neoadjuvant therapy, when and if any existing seroma cavity and scar tissue is separate from the vein.[2,12] Although saphenous vein preservation might theoretically reduce the likelihood of postoperative DVT and lymphedema, this maneuver has never been definitively shown to reduce postoperative complications in any prospective, randomized study. Therefore, saphenous preservation should only be considered in select cases, and the maneuver should never compromise the completeness of the dissection.

Dissection of the Femoral Vessels

- The superficial femoral artery is identified at the distal aspect of the dissection at the apex of the femoral triangle. At this level, the femoral artery lies anterior to the femoral vein. As the dissection proceeds distal to proximal, the femoral artery courses laterally while the femoral vein courses medially. The anterior surfaces of the femoral vessels are skeletonized, and the dissection is extended laterally at the same depth as the surface of the vessels to avoid injury to the femoral nerve, which is generally not directly visualized. The relationship of the femoral vessels to the boundaries of the femoral triangle is shown in **FIGURE 4.** Despite the widely known mnemonic "NAVEL," purporting to describe the relationship of the structures in the femoral triangle at the level of the inguinal ligament from lateral to medial, there is no empty space in the groin and the lymphatics course above the artery and vein and not simply medial to them.

Completion of the Dissection and Ligation of the Saphenofemoral Junction

- The dissection continues in a distal to proximal direction up to the level of the saphenofemoral junction. If the saphenous vein is to be preserved, it is fully freed from the specimen; generally, several small- to medium-sized tributaries draining the specimen need to be divided and ligated individually. Otherwise, the entire portion of the saphenous vein within the femoral triangle is included in the specimen and the remaining soft tissue is circumferentially dissected so that the specimen remains adherent only by the saphenofemoral junction (**FIGURE 5A**).
- The saphenous vein is doubly ligated at the level of the saphenofemoral junction; we typically use a 3-0 silk suture

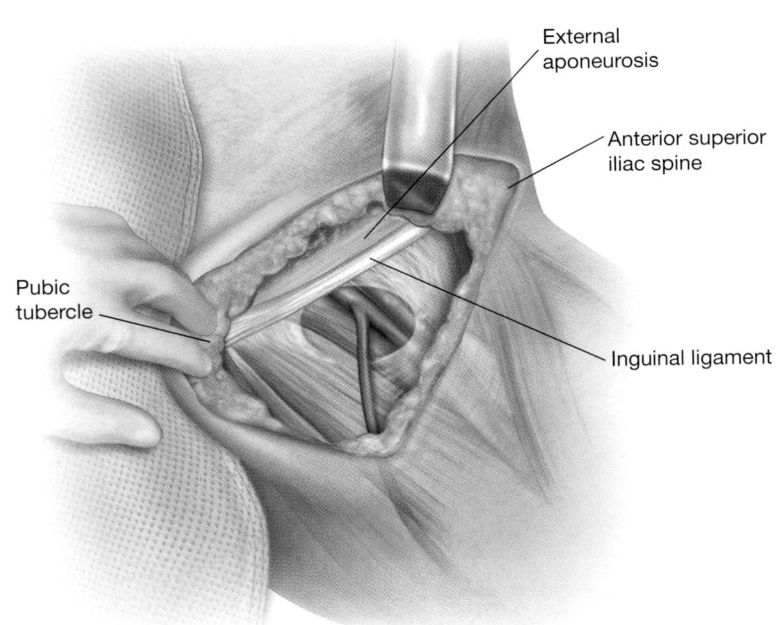

FIGURE 3 ● The superior extent of dissection clears all subcutaneous tissue 3 to 5 cm proximal to the inguinal ligament to a depth bounded by the underlying external oblique aponeurosis.

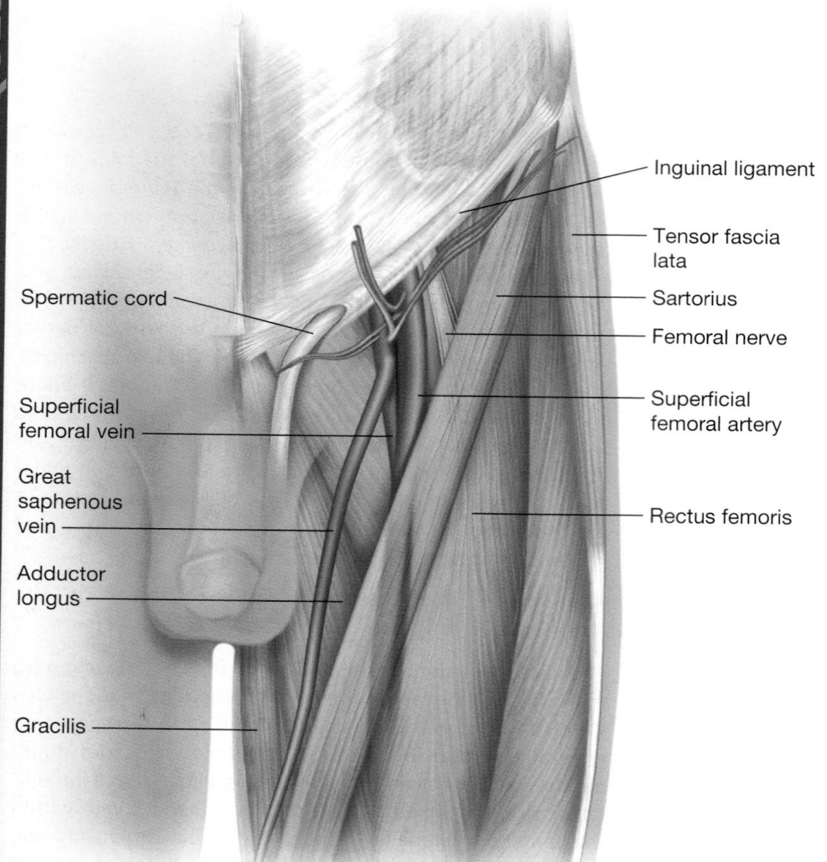

FIGURE 4 ● The relationship of the femoral artery and vein to the boundaries of the femoral triangle. Note at the distal apex of the femoral triangle, the femoral artery lies superficial to the femoral vein.

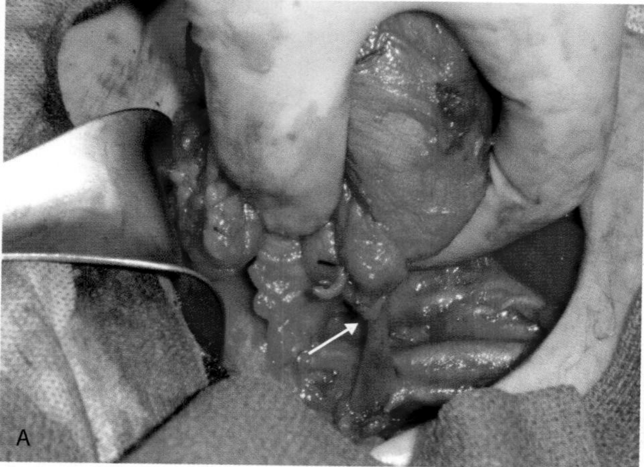

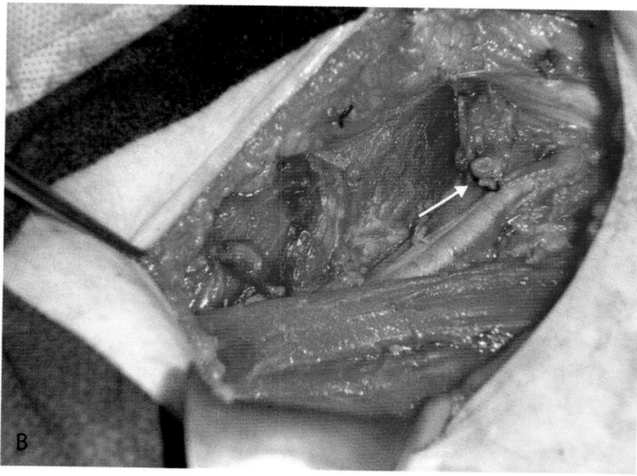

FIGURE 5 ● **A,** The appearance of the completed left inguinofemoral lymphadenectomy dissection with a view of the specimen attached only by the saphenofemoral junction (*arrow*) with the superficial femoral artery immediately lateral. **B,** The appearance of the ligated saphenofemoral junction (*arrow*) after removal of the specimen without any narrowing of the superficial femoral vein, and a view of the superficial femoral artery lateral to the vein as well as the sartorius muscle that forms the lateral boundary of the dissection.

ligature and a 2-0 silk tie, taking care not to narrow the femoral vein (**FIGURE 5B**). A formal closure of the stump with vascular suture is not routinely required but may be necessary if the saphenofemoral junction is very broad or if palpable tumor or dense scar extends in close proximity to the femoral vein itself.

Sartorius Muscle Transposition Flap

- Sartorius muscle transposition is used to cover the exposed femoral vessels in the groin whenever there is concern about the integrity of the overlying skin flap closure. Some surgeons routinely perform this in all cases, whereas others do

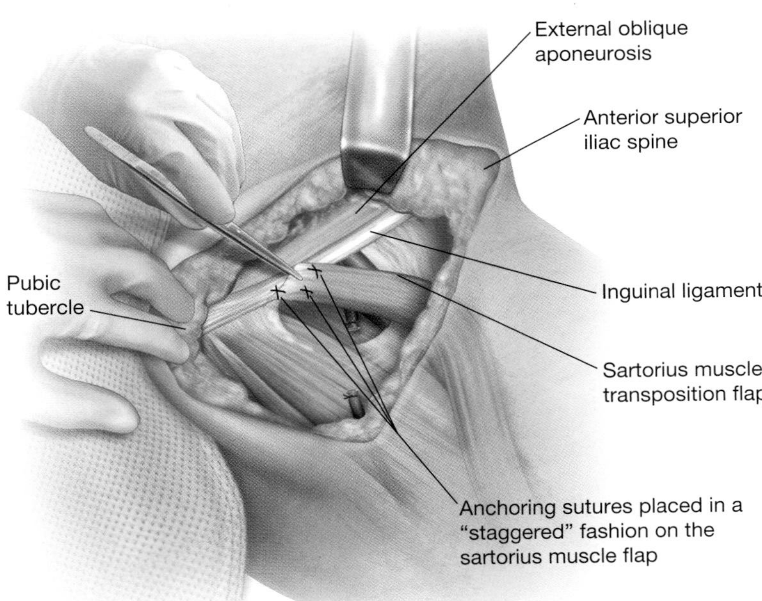

FIGURE 6 ● Sutures that anchor the sartorius muscle transposition flap are placed in the inguinal ligament in a staggered fashion instead of being placed on a single plane in order to avoid weakening the fascia.

it selectively for patients estimated to be at higher risk for wound-related complications due to age or co-morbidities, or not at all.[2,6] We use it in most cases but routinely omit it when the incision is placed high in the groin (ie, not directly overlying the exposed vessels) and in selected younger patients, including children, especially athletes or other very active individuals.

- To perform the transposition, the tendinous portion of the sartorius muscle is divided close to its point of origin at the ASIS with electrocautery, bipolar diathermy, or a stapling device. Dividing the muscle as high as possible will maximize the length of muscle available for the flap. It is critical to obtain meticulous hemostasis at the cut muscle edge, as there is little or no tissue at that level to tamponade bleeding and a small ooze can continue for hours postoperatively. To mobilize the muscle for the transposition flap without tension, a few lateral feeding vessels generally need to be tied off, and the lateral fascia is incised well down the length of the muscle. The muscle is transposed over the femoral vessels and secured in place to the external abdominal oblique aponeurosis/inguinal ligament with three or four interrupted, horizontal mattress 2-0 nonabsorbable, braided polyester sutures oriented so that the knots are pushed down onto the sartorius muscle to minimizing tearing through the muscle fibers. The sutures are placed in a staggered fashion to avoid them all being placed at the same level in the inguinal ligament, which would potentially weaken the fascia (**FIGURE 6**).

Placement of Drain and Closure

- If a concomitant pelvic dissection (ie, superficial and deep lymphadenectomy) is planned, see the following text and muscle transposition and closure is deferred until completion of that portion of the procedure.
- A flat or round closed-suction drain is routinely placed in the bed of dissection and brought out through a separate stab incision relatively close to the wound but away from the thinnest parts of the skin flaps. The incision is closed with interrupted 3-0 absorbable, braided sutures for the subcutaneous tissue and a running suture of 4-0 absorbable, monofilament suture for the subcuticular skin layer. Cyanoacrylate adhesive (or equivalent) is used over the subcuticular closure for extra protection. The leg is wrapped with an elastic bandage (ACE) from the level of the metatarsals to mid-thigh, and a thigh-length SCD is placed over the ACE as well as on the contralateral extremity. The urinary catheter, if used, is generally left in place overnight.

ILIOINGUINAL LYMPHADENECTOMY

Division of the Abdominal Wall and Retroperitoneal Exposure of the Pelvis

- When conducted as a portion of a combined ilioinguinal lymphadenectomy, the pelvic portion of the lymphadenectomy occurs through the same skin incision. The incision may need to be lengthened sufficiently above the inguinal crease to ensure adequate visualization (**FIGURE 2D**).
- The pelvic portion of the ilioinguinal lymphadenectomy involves the removal of the obturator and iliac nodes up to the bifurcation of the iliac vessels through a retroperitoneal approach. The common iliac nodes can be removed if grossly involved by extending the fascial incision cephalad, but paraaortic nodes are considered beyond the scope of the dissection and are rarely accessible through the retroperitoneal approach. Nowadays, radiologic involvement of common iliac nodes would be a strong indication for some form of preoperative therapy prior to any surgical approach.
- Through the same skin incision used for the inguinofemoral dissection, the external and internal oblique aponeuroses are incised parallel to the direction of the fibers of the respective

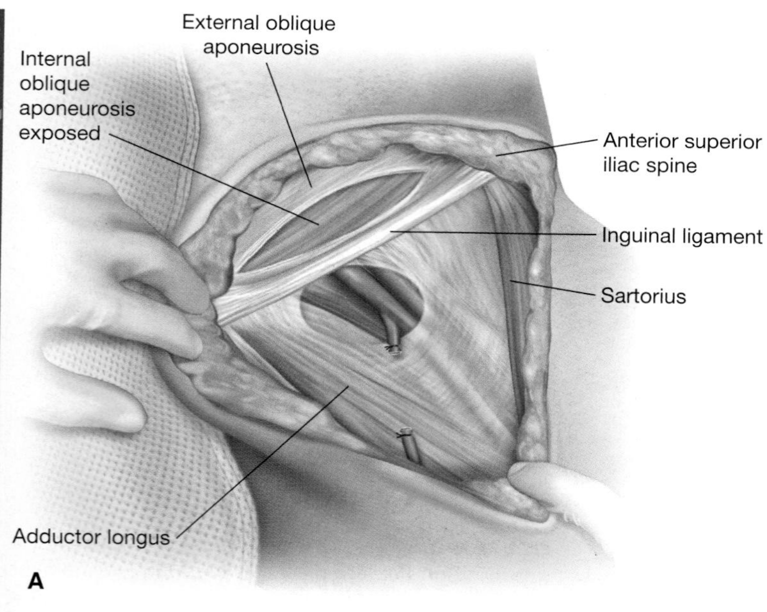

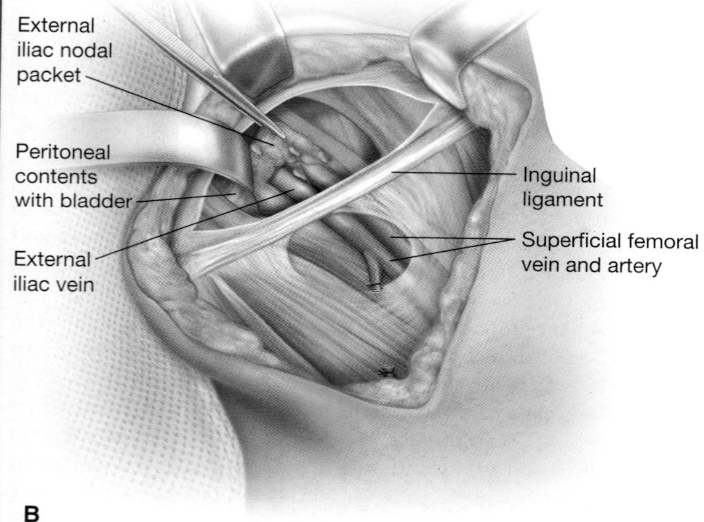

FIGURE 7 ● **A,** The external oblique aponeurosis has been incised in a direction parallel to its fibers, exposing the underlying internal oblique aponeurosis. **B,** Anterior view of the external iliac artery and vein with delivery of the external iliac nodal packet.

muscles (**FIGURE 7A**). A less common approach to the pelvis involves dividing the abdominal wall aponeuroses vertically beginning at the shelving edge of the inguinal ligament and proceeding upward following the course of the iliac vessels. The peritoneum is retracted superiorly and medially, which typically mobilizes the ureter out of the field. Retraction of the peritoneal contents superiorly and medially exposes the external iliac artery and vein with associated node-bearing tissue (**FIGURE 7B**).

Retrieval of Iliac Nodal Tissue

- The external iliac vessels are skeletonized over their anterior aspect. All fibrofatty and lymphatic tissue overlying the iliac vessels is retrieved from the bifurcation proximally to the posterior aspect of the inguinal ligament distally, where the groin and pelvic dissections should essentially meet.

Retrieval of Obturator Nodal Tissue

- The external iliac vein is retracted laterally to expose the obturator space medially. Fibrofatty and lymphatic tissue is removed down to the level of the obturator nerve (**FIGURE 8**). Caution should be taken when dissecting near the nerve as the nearby obturator vessels and their tributaries are difficult to visualize and can be difficult to control if injured.
- The obturator foramen and the pubic rami should be carefully inspected and palpated to ensure that palpable lymph nodes are not left behind in those locations.

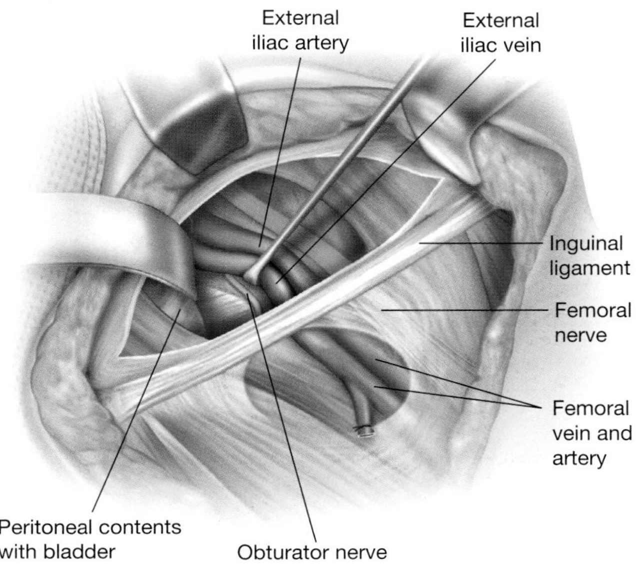

FIGURE 8 ● Appearance of the completed ilioinguinal dissected field with the obturator nerve exposed deep and medial to the external iliac vessels.

Placement of Drain and Closure

- While not absolutely required, a closed-suction drain can be deployed into the bed of the pelvic dissection and brought through the abdominal muscle fibers, exiting the skin through a separate stab incision. The internal and external oblique fasciae are closed with absorbable monofilament or braided sutures. Closure then proceeds as described earlier for the inguinofemoral dissection.

Robotic Approach to Pelvic Lymphadenectomy

The pelvic nodes may be removed via a robotic approach either independently or in conjunction with the inguinal nodes. We advocate the consideration of this minimally invasive approach only for those tumors of sufficiently small size to be extirpated from one of the ports without tumor morcellation or substantial port enlargement. Tumors with significant external iliac vessel involvement—ie, more than a minor abutment—should be removed via the open approach. The operative conduct of this procedure is outside the scope of this chapter but has been described elsewhere.[13]

PEARLS AND PITFALLS

Indications	■ The diagnosis of inguinal metastasis should be made using the least invasive method possible. ■ Palpable disease should be evaluated by percutaneous fine needle aspiration or core needle biopsy rather than open biopsy whenever possible, even in the absence of a known diagnosis of malignancy. ■ Sentinel node biopsy incisions should be fashioned while being mindful of the possibility that inguinal lymphadenectomy may be required in the future. ■ Sentinel node biopsy incisions directly in the inguinal crease are not advised due to difficulty with the subsequent lymphadenectomy incision if necessary. ■ In cases where there is nodal disease without a known primary, a careful physical examination to identify a primary cancer is warranted, including examination of the skin of the lower body, digital rectal examination, and examination of the penis/vulva.
Placement of incision	■ Incisions should be fashioned to avoid crossing the inguinal crease where feasible.
Extent of dissection	■ Saphenous vein preservation may be considered for cases being performed for micrometastatic disease or when neoadjuvant therapy has resulted in an excellent clinical and radiographic response, and when the vein is not involved with tumor, scar, or the seroma/biopsy cavity. ■ Indications for inclusion of pelvic lymphadenectomy in the absence of clear-cut radiographic pelvic involvement have not been definitively established, but this may potentially be considered for macroscopic inguinofemoral disease.
Key postoperative care	■ Patients are typically placed on bedrest overnight with the affected limb elevated. ■ DVT prophylaxis is typically instituted on the evening of the procedure and continued while the patient is in the hospital unless there is clinical concern for hemorrhage. ■ Lymphedema precautions including compression with ACE bandages or fitted compression garments are routinely used, with aggressive institution of lymphedema physical therapy at the first clinical sign of lymphedema. ■ In patients whose hypothalamus–pituitary–adrenal axis may have been altered by neoadjuvant systemic therapy, prompt initiation of steroids may be required if an Addisonian crisis is suspected.

POSTOPERATIVE CARE

- The patient is typically kept on bedrest overnight with the urinary catheter, if used, in place and the affected extremity elevated above the level of the heart. The affected extremity is kept wrapped with an ACE from the metatarsals to midthigh, with thigh-length SCDs in place over the ACE on the ipsilateral extremity as well as on the contralateral extremity.
- If the patient's physical examination and the drain output are not concerning for postoperative bleeding, prophylactic subcutaneous low molecular weight heparin is administered on the evening of the procedure and continued daily while the patient is hospitalized, but generally not longer in the absence of a heightened risk of venous thrombosis.
- On the first postoperative day, the urinary catheter, if present, is removed and the patient is encouraged to ambulate.
- After an inguinofemoral lymphadenectomy, patients are typically discharged after overnight observation, when pain is controlled with oral analgesics.
- After ilioinguinal lymphadenectomy, patients are kept nil per os for the first night. If there is no sign of ileus, the diet can be advanced on postoperative day 1. Patients typically remain in the hospital for 1 to 2 nights and are discharged when pain is controlled with oral analgesics and are tolerating a diet.
- On discharge, patients are encouraged to ambulate to minimize risk of DVT, to wear an ACE or fitted gradient compression stocking on the operated leg during the day, and to elevate the operated leg above the level of the heart at night.
- At the first clinical sign of lymphedema, lymphedema physical therapy is ordered and verification of compliance with the fitted compression stockings is done.

OUTCOMES

- Five-year melanoma-specific survival rates for melanoma metastatic to regional lymph nodes are listed by stage as per the eighth edition of the American Joint Committee on Cancer below[14]:
  - Stage IIIA melanoma—93%
  - Stage IIIB melanoma—83%
  - Stage IIIC melanoma—69%
  - Stage IIID melanoma—32%

COMPLICATIONS AND RELEVANT MANAGEMENT

- Seroma—if symptomatic, can be percutaneously drained; open drainage should be avoided.
- Lymphedema—managed with early compression and lymphedema physical therapy. Severe cases may be considered for postoperative reverse lymphatic mapping and lymphovenous anastomosis.[15]
- Wound dehiscence—risk is minimized by confining area of the flap to the boundaries of the femoral triangle and can be managed with a wound vacuum device as needed.
- Infection/cellulitis—typically managed with oral antibiotics.
- DVT/pulmonary embolism—risk is minimized by the routine use of low molecular weight heparin prophylaxis and high index of suspicion should be maintained for early diagnosis and treatment.
- Sensory deficit is common but typically does not require management unless there is a persistent neuralgia.
- Hypothalamus–pituitary–adrenal axis insufficiency—for patients having received prior immunotherapy, a low threshold for initiation of stress dose corticosteroids should be maintained for postoperative hypotension, severe weakness or confusion, especially for those receiving corticosteroid therapy where postoperative hemorrhage and sepsis have been excluded.
- Recurrence

REFERENCES

1. Bello DM, Faries MB. The landmark series: MSLT-1, MSLT-2 and DeCOG (management of lymph nodes). *Ann Surg Oncol.* 2020;27:15-21.
2. Sarnaik AA, Puleo CA, Zager S, et al. Limiting the morbidity of inguinal lymphadenectomy for metastatic melanoma. *Cancer Control.* 2009;16:240-247.
3. Faries MB, Thompson JF, Cochran AJ, et al. Completion dissection or observation for sentinel-node metastasis in melanoma. *N Engl J Med.* 2017;376:2211-2222.
4. Leiter U, Stadler R, Mauch C, et al. Final analysis of DeCOG-SLT trial: no survival benefit for complete lymph node dissection in patients with positive sentinel node. *J Clin Oncol.* 2019;27:3000-3008.
5. Broman KK, Bettampandi D, Pérez-Morales J, et al. Surveillance of sentinel node-positive melanoma patients who receive adjuvant therapy without undergoing completion lymph node dissection. *Ann Surg Oncol.* 2021;28:6978-6985.
6. Chang SB, Askew RL, Xing Y, et al. Prospective assessment of postoperative complications and associated costs following inguinal lymph node dissection (ILND) in melanoma patients. *Ann Surg Oncol.* 2010;17:2764-2772.
7. Faut M, Kruijff S, Hoekstra HJ, et al. Pelvic lymph node dissection in metastatic melanoma to the groin should not be abandoned yet. *Eur J Surg Oncol.* 2018;44:1779-1785.
8. Amaria RN, Reddy SM, Tawbi HA, et al. Neoadjuvant immune checkpoint blockade in high-risk resectable melanoma. *Nat Med.* 2018;24:1649-1654.
9. Reijers ILM, Menzies AM, van Akkooi ACJ, et al. Personalized response-directed surgery and adjuvant therapy after neoadjuvant ipilimumab and nivolumab in high-risk stage III melanoma: the PRADO trial. *Nat Med.* 2022;26:1178-1188.
10. Paramanandam VS, Dylke E, Clark GM, et al. Prophylactic use of compression sleeves reduces the incidence of arm swelling in women at high risk of breast cancer-related lymphedema: a randomized controlled trial. *J Clin Oncol.* 2022;40:2004-2012.
11. Matthey-Gié M, Deretti S, Demartines N, et al. Prospective randomized study to compare lymphocele and lymphorrhea control following inguinal and axillary therapeutic lymph node dissection with or without the use of an ultrasonic scalpel. *Ann Surg Oncol.* 2016;23:1716-1720.
12. Baur J, Mathe K, Gesierich A, et al. Morbidity and oncologic outcome after saphenous vein-sparing inguinal lymphadenectomy in melanoma patients. *World J Surg Oncol.* 2017;15:99.
13. Dossett LA, Castner NB, Pow-Sang JM, et al. Robotic-assisted transperitoneal pelvic lymphadenectomy for metastatic melanoma: early outcomes compared with open pelvic lymphadenectomy. *J Am Coll Surg.* 2016;222:702-709.
14. Gershenwald JE, Scolyer RA, Hess KR, et al. Melanoma staging: evidence-based changes in the American Joint Committee on Cancer eighth edition staging manual. *CA Cancer J Clin.* 2017;67:472-492.
15. Kong X, DU J, DU X, et al. A meta-analysis of 37 studies on the effectiveness of microsurgical techniques for lymphedema. *Ann Vasc Surg.* 2022 May 16; online ahead of print.

Chapter 36 Minimally Invasive Inguinal Lymph Node Dissection for Melanoma

James W. Jakub

DEFINITION

- Minimally invasive inguinal lymph node dissection (MILND) is defined as an inguinal lymph node dissection performed through trocar ports. Many names have been coined for this videoscopic approach, and unfortunately, minimally invasive has also been used by some to describe an open technique using smaller incisions.[1]
- The terminology surrounding the inguinal node dissection can be confusing. When performing groin dissections, urologists and gynecologic oncologists distinguish the superficial inguinal basin as anterior to the cribriform fascia and the "deep" inguinal nodes as those nodes along the femoral vessels, deep to this fascial layer. Melanoma surgeons have historically referred to both basins as a "superficial inguinal lymph node dissection" or "inguinofemoral" and the pelvic or external iliac/obturator lymph nodes as a "deep inguinal lymph node dissection" or "ilioinguinal." In this chapter, when we describe an inguinal lymph node dissection, it will refer to all the nodes in the groin distal to the inguinal ligament including both superficial and deep to the cribriform fascia. The deep (pelvic) or ilioinguinal dissection is discussed in Part 5, Chapter 39.

ANATOMY

- The anatomy critical to the MILND is identical to that for the conventional open operative approach and is depicted in **FIGURES 1A, B** and **2**. The superficial and deep inguinal lymph nodes are separated by the cribriform fascia, which is violated at the fossa ovalis, where the greater saphenous penetrates to enter the femoral vein. There are approximately 10 lymph nodes in the superficial basin and 5 in the deep.
- The borders of the femoral triangle are graphically depicted in **FIGURE 2**.

NATURAL HISTORY

- Complete inguinal lymph node dissection has historically been advised for any patient with melanoma metastatic to the inguinal lymph nodes in the absence of distant metastases. As a result of the seminal Multicenter Selective Lymphadenectomy Trial II (MSLT II)[2] and effective systemic immunotherapy, the indications for lymph node dissection continue to evolve and are beyond the scope of this chapter.
- Microscopic and macroscopic subclassifications of stage III disease are distinguished as clinical and not pathologic entities.[3] If disease is detected by physical examination, this is considered macroscopic, whereas a positive sentinel lymph node (SLN) represents microscopic disease, regardless of the tumor burden identified pathologically. Stage III melanoma patients represent a very heterogeneous cohort and prognosis varies greatly based on the number of positive lymph nodes, nodal burden in the lymph nodes, and presence or absence of synchronous in-transit metastasis.

PATIENT HISTORY AND PHYSICAL FINDINGS

- An MILND is indicated in most cases that would be considered for traditional inguinal nodal dissection including melanoma, cutaneous squamous cell carcinoma (SCC), and some urologic and gynecologic cancer, as well as select cases of anal or low-lying rectal cancers.
- Physical examination should include inspection for prior scars in the field (SLN) or saphenous vein harvest from prior coronary artery bypass graft. Assessment of the extent of disease, including if the disease is involving the skin and/or fixed suggestive of invasion of deep structures, is critical. Skin thickening and erythema can be signs of cutaneous involvement. Direct extension with overlying cutaneous hyperemia and fixation of disease or nodularity/ulceration is more commonly seen in advanced SCC.
- A comprehensive examination to identify in-transit disease, particularly in the case of melanoma, is critical. These lesions can be subtle and a biopsy in clinic should be performed for any areas of concern, prior to proceeding with groin dissection. Patients with synchronous in-transit disease and clinical nodal disease have a poor prognosis and we would proceed with systemic therapy in this setting.[4]
- Nodal disease can be found cephalad to the inguinal ligament and superficial to the external oblique aponeurosis, especially in cases of a truncal primary.
- For lower extremity disease, the popliteal nodal basin should be evaluated; and for disease of the trunk, consideration for contralateral inguinal or axillary drainage needs to be considered based on the location of the primary.
- If an MILND is being performed for microscopic disease following a positive SLNB, waiting a minimum of 6 weeks from the SLNB to the MILND allows time for the acute operative inflammatory changes to resolve. When performed for macroscopic disease, sound clinical judgment should be used to avoid violating the specimen, assuring an en bloc resection and the disease to be resected will be contained within the contents of dissection.
- MILND is contraindicated in the setting of cutaneous involvement.
- Risk of skin flap necrosis is more of a concern in a radiated field or with active tobacco use.

IMAGING AND OTHER DIAGNOSTIC STUDIES

- Positive SLNB for microscopic disease
  - As noted earlier, based on the results of MSLT-II, patients with a positive SLN most often now undergo active surveillance in our practice. When MILND is performed following a positive SLN biopsy, this is almost always a staged procedure as frozen section analysis is not typically performed on SLNs for melanoma.

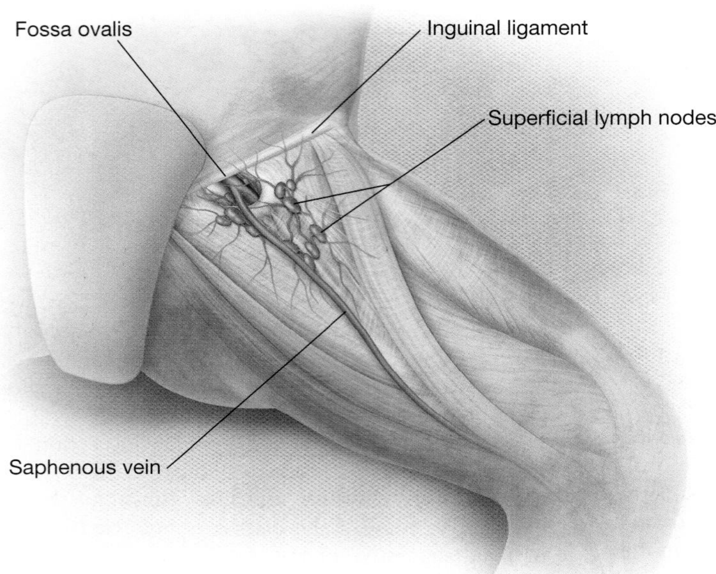

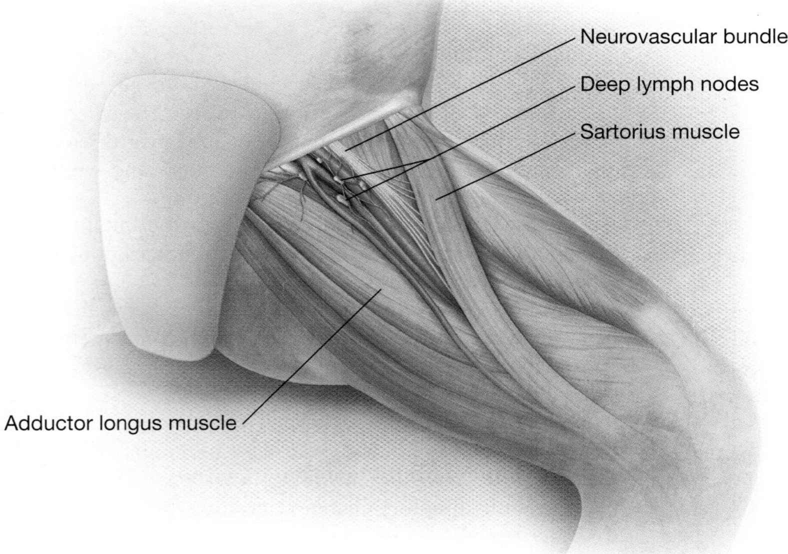

FIGURE 1 ● **A** and **B,** Anatomy of the superficial and deep inguinal basin.

    - The yield of systemic imaging to find clinically occult stage IV disease after a positive SLN is less than 5% and typically not warranted prior to MILND.[5-7]
    - Deep pelvic (external iliac/obturator) node dissection is typically not required.
- Clinical inguinal regional nodal disease
    - In the setting of a palpable inguinal lymph node, a fine needle aspiration to confirm the clinical diagnosis is appropriate prior to embarking on an inguinal node dissection. Excisional diagnostic biopsy is strongly discouraged.
    - A search for systemic disease with whole-body imaging (computed tomography [CT] scan or positron emission tomography [PET]/CT) is reasonable prior to MILND as the true positive rate is above 10%.[8,9]
    - For patients with clinical nodal disease and an unknown primary, a thorough examination is required based on the tumor type and may need to include the skin, genitals, perianal and distal rectal, and/or vaginal mucosa.
    - Historically we performed a combined pelvic dissection for patients with clinical inguinal disease. As a result of contemporary systemic imaging, effective systemic

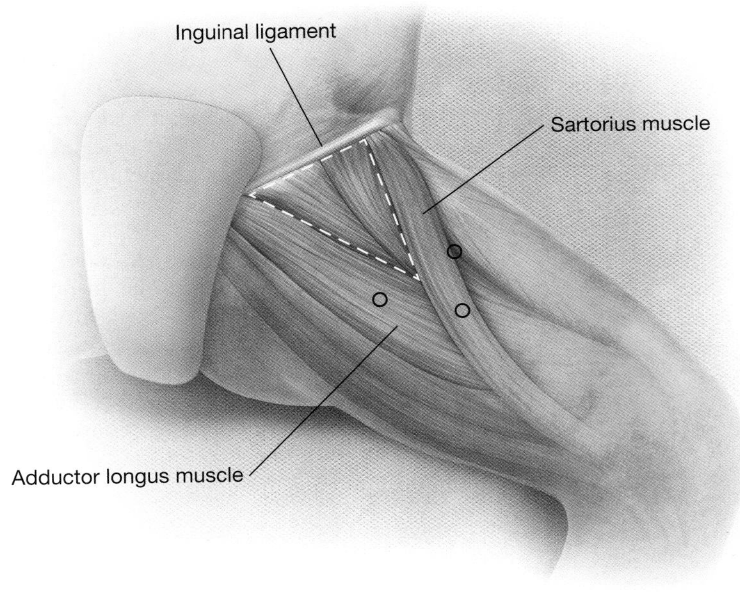

FIGURE 2 ● Borders of the femoral triangle as well as trocar placement for minimally invasive inguinal lymph node dissection.

immunotherapy, and the ability to perform minimally invasive (robotic or laparoscopic) outpatient pelvic dissections, our practice has, for the most part, changed to observation of the pelvis in the setting of inguinal only measurable disease. Unfortunately, an Australian led randomized trial to address this issue closed early secondary to lack of accrual (NCT02166788, personal communication John Thompson).

- The role of neoadjuvant systemic therapy in the setting of clinical measurable stage III disease and the management of patients who have a complete radiographic response are the topics of ongoing clinical trials.

SURGICAL MANAGEMENT

Preoperative Planning

- Preoperative baseline bilateral lower limb volumes are standard at our institution.
- Brief with anesthesia and the operating room (OR) team prior to the start of the procedure:
  - Hypercarbia is to be expected. Unlike laparoscopy performed in an intraperitoneal location, this entire dissection is performed in the subcutaneous plane and much higher levels of carbon dioxide (CO_2) will be systemically absorbed. The anesthesia team needs to be aware and make appropriate ventilatory modifications to avoid the need for conversion.
  - Ensure you have towers in correct position, patient position is rehearsed, and desired equipment, including dissector and laparoscopic supplies, are in the room.
- Prophylactic antibiotics are provided.
- Mechanical venous thromboembolism (VTE) prophylaxis in the form of sequential compression device is placed on the contralateral leg. Chemical VTE prophylaxis in the form of subcutaneous heparin is provided prior to incision and ideally prior to the induction of general anesthesia.
- A Foley catheter is placed sterilely on the prepped field and sealed off from the dissection field with the genitalia by a sterile towel and Ioban.

Positioning

- In the typical setup, the patient is positioned supine with the legs split on a split-leg table (my preference). Yellowfin gel stirrups can be used if it is the only option; however, in my experience this is suboptimal. The operative leg is abducted and slightly flexed at the knee (**FIGURE 3**). If the leg is straight, the surgeon will likely perform the dissection too lateral. The surgeon and the assistant stand so one is between the legs and the other stands lateral to the operative leg. The surgeon and the assistant may change positions during the procedure as desired. The surgical technician stands on the opposite side of the patient's body.
- Video towers are placed at the head of the table, one above each shoulder (**FIGURE 3**). Minimal operative instrumentation is needed on the Mayo stand. If there is a need to emergently convert, appropriate instruments should be immediately available.

Approach

- The standard approach involves en bloc resection of the muscular fascia with the lymphadenectomy specimen. The plane of dissection off the sartorius and adductor muscles may not be as apparent with a minimally invasive approach as during an open procedure, and to be clear that the dissection is in the correct plane, scoring the fascia and visualizing the underlying muscle is routine.
- Resecting the muscular fascia is the approach initially described by Delman et al[10] and the approach we have

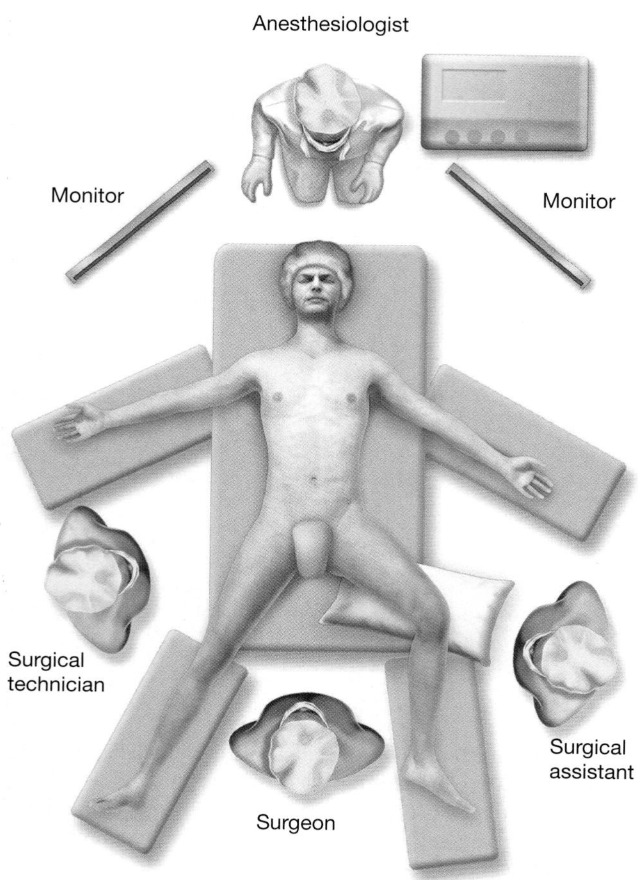

FIGURE 3 ● Operating theater setup and patient position.

followed. Whenever embarking on a new procedure, it is critical that caution is exercised and the procedure is approached with this mindset, assuring that the extent of the oncologic resection is at least as complete as the traditional standard for which it is meant to replace. It is also true that the minimally invasive approach should, as much as possible, exactly mirror the technique of the open approach.

- We initially resected the saphenous vein routinely and now preserve the vein when possible.
- We do not excise the SLNB scar when present. We also do not make an open incision to confirm the adequacy of dissection because the videoscopic view should make this obvious. If there is any question of inadequate resection, a small proximal incision can be made, and the extent of the oncologic operation should not be jeopardized because of a perceived feeling of inadequacy or failure by "converting."

TECHNIQUES

MINIMALLY INVASIVE INGUINAL LYMPH NODE DISSECTION

Operating Room Setup

- In the typical setup, the patient is positioned supine with the legs split on a split-leg table. The operative leg is abducted and slightly flexed at the knee (**FIGURE 3**). The surgeon and the assistant stand so one is between the legs and the other stands lateral to the operative leg. The surgeon and the assistant may change positions as desired. The surgical technician stands on the opposite side of the patient's body.
- Video towers are placed at the head of the table, one above each shoulder (**FIGURE 3**). Minimal operative instrumentation is needed on the Mayo stand. If there is a need to emergently convert, appropriate instruments should be immediately available.
- The anatomy critical to the MILND is identical to that for the conventional open operative approach and is depicted in **FIGURES 1** and **2**.
- External landmarks are identified. Palpation is performed to identify the medial border of dissection, which is the adductor longus muscle. This is marked with a marking pen. Next, similar palpation is performed to identify the sartorius muscle and identify its medial border, which will mark the lateral boundary of the dissection. The convergents of these lines occur at the distal border of dissection, which is the apex of the femoral triangle. Proximal dissection extends 3 to 5 cm cephalad to the inguinal ligament and it includes the soft tissues superficial to the external oblique in this location.
- Next, the three trocar sites are marked. The distal most incision is marked 3 cm from the apex of the femoral triangle. The other two trocars are placed proximal to this, each 5 cm apart, one medial and one lateral (see **FIGURE 5A** and **B**).
- Through one of the trocar sites, blunt dissection is performed with the index finger or fine curved dissector can be used through all the sites, separating along the natural avascular plain deep to the subcutaneous fat. As much of this superficial dissection that can be completed to create an initial working space the better. Three 10/12 mm trocars are next introduced. Short trocars are ideal, and laparoscopic instruments of adequate length should be used to reach the proximal most dissection.
- As a result of the thin subcutaneous tissue, a leak around the trocar can be a challenge early in one's experience. As a result, the incision length should be kept to a minimum and trocars with balloons to minimize the leak are ideal. If finger dissection was performed, this should be limited to one trocar site

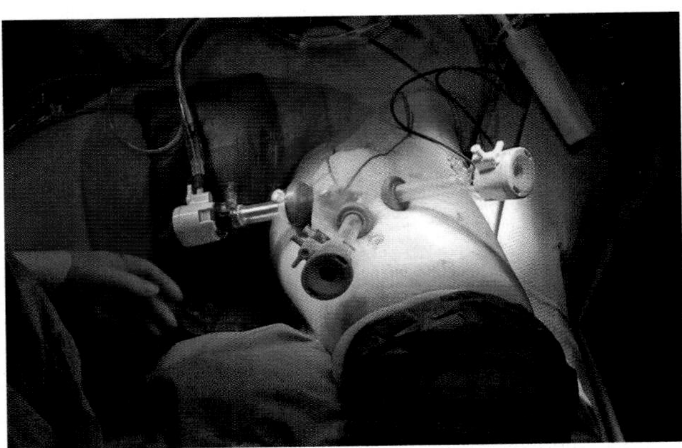

FIGURE 4 ● Photo depicting trocar placement and initial CO_2 insufflation at beginning of case. (Used with permission of Mayo Foundation for Medical Education and Research, all rights reserved.)

and a figure-of-eight suture should be used at this site. The suture is placed prior to trocar placement through the skin and tied snuggly after trocar placement to minimize a leak through this site. This is removed at the end of the case.

- CO_2 insufflation is performed. Initially, 25 mm Hg for 10 minutes and then decreased to 15 mm Hg for the remainder of the procedure (**FIGURE 4**).

Superficial Dissection

- I perform the entire dissection with an ultrasonic dissector (personal preference) except when freeing the tissue from the external oblique aponeurosis where I use a hook cautery.
- Camper fascia is preserved. Dissection is performed superficial to Scarpa fascia.
- Initial dissection starts in a space created by the digital dissection and CO_2 insufflation. The dissection is begun distally and continued proximally. The initial dissection space is limited and dissection to create a functional working space between the subcutaneous tissue and underlying regional contents is undertaken.
- Dissection is performed superficial to Scarpa fascia. This can be appreciated with an external view showing the transillumination of the light source through the skin (**FIGURE 5A** and **B**). The flap will be thin and the transillumination will reveal a red hue of the flap. If it is white, you are on dermis and too thin. If this happens in patchy limited areas, it should not be an issue. Dissection can be assisted by external palpation over the previously marked boundaries of the triangle. Running a finger up and down the previously drawn landmarks while viewing internally assists one in defining the borders and extent of the superficial dissection. As dissection is completed more proximally, the loose areolar tissue overlying the external oblique aponeurosis can be appreciated. The entire anterior dissection within the externally marked triangle should be completed.

Sartorius Exposure

- The next portion of the procedure is the lateral dissection to identify the sartorius muscle. Dissection is performed through the fatty tissue until the sartorius fascia is identified. The fascia is divided, identifying the underlying muscular fibers. This is initiated distally, and once identified, you simply march proximally up this layer. You want to stay medial on the muscle. The fascia is continually scored from distal to proximal as shown in **FIGURE 6**. This is continued up toward the inguinal ligament.

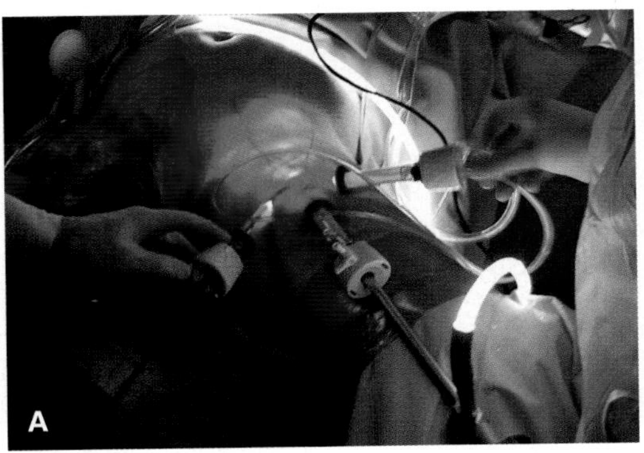

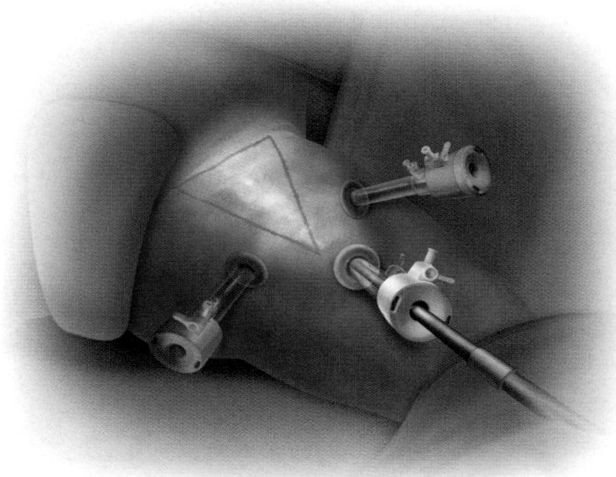

FIGURE 5 ● **A** and **B**, Photo and image demonstrating trocar placement, flap thickness, and drain placement. Dissection is quite superficial and this is demonstrated in these images showing how well the light transilluminates through the skin flaps. (Used with permission of Mayo Foundation for Medical Education and Research, all rights reserved.)

Adductor Longus Exposure

- A similar approach is taken medially to identify the adductor longus muscle (**FIGURE 7**). Because of the crossing saphenous vein, the medial dissection is started more proximal in this location. This dissection is also continued proximally to the inguinal ligament. Again, minimizing the amount of dissection off the muscle by staying on the lateral aspect of the muscle is preferred.
- The specimen is rolled laterally off the adductor. As one progresses proximally, the deep border of dissection becomes the pectineus muscle (**FIGURE 8**).
- It is common for the knee to be "in the way" during portions of the dissection, as a result of the knee bumped and the leg position. For much of the procedure I operate with the handle of the dissection device turned upside down to accommodate.

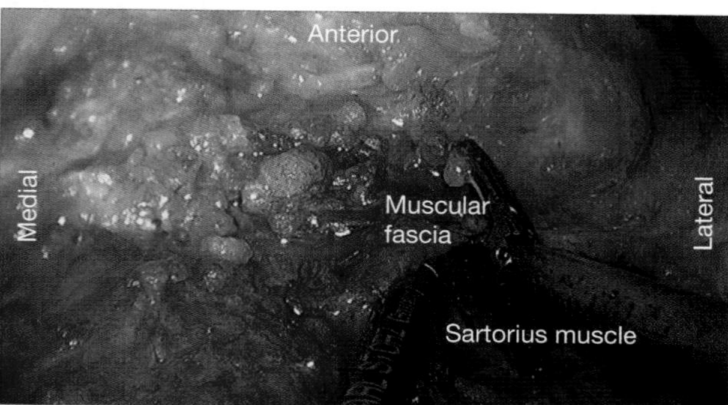

FIGURE 6 ● The lateral border of the deep dissection is shown here. The muscular fascia is scored from distal to proximal exposing the sartorius muscle. (Used with permission of Mayo Foundation for Medical Education and Research, all rights reserved.)

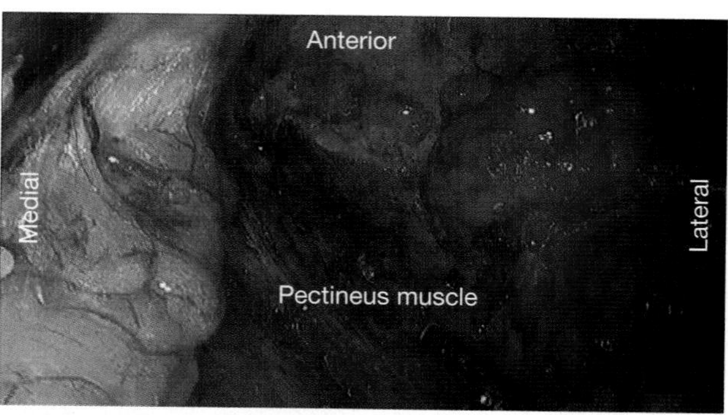

FIGURE 8 ● The pectineus muscle is exposed as the proximal portion of the specimen is rolled from medial to lateral off the adductor. (image © Mayo Clinic, 2014.)

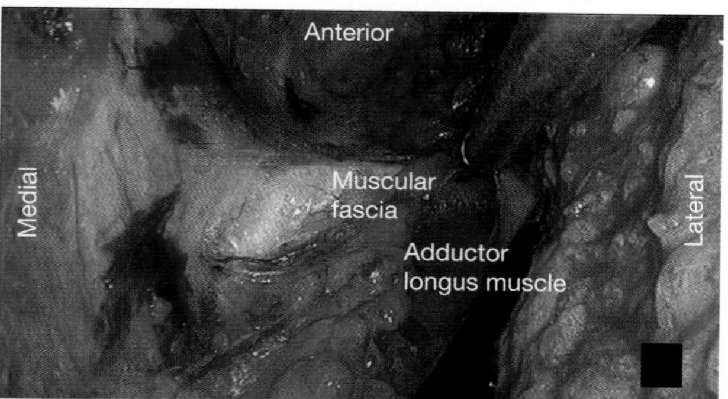

FIGURE 7 ● The medial border of the deep dissection is shown here. The muscular fascia is scored from distal to proximal exposing the adductor longus muscle. (Used with permission of Mayo Foundation for Medical Education and Research, all rights reserved.)

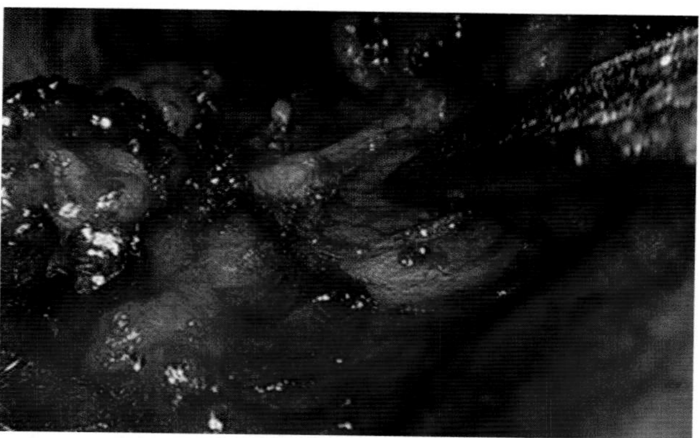

FIGURE 9 ● The distal saphenous vein is being divided as it crosses the adductor longus muscle. (Used with permission of Mayo Foundation for Medical Education and Research, all rights reserved.)

Distal Greater Saphenous Vein

- The saphenous vein is identified and circumferentially dissected out. It is located two-thirds of the distance from the inguinal ligament to the apex of the triangle as the vein crosses the adductor muscle.
- I preserve the greater saphenous vein when possible. If it is to be divided, the vein can be controlled using clips, endovascular stapler, LigaSure or ultrasonic dissector per surgeon preference, and vessel caliber (**FIGURE 9**).

Apex Dissection

- Placing the patient in Trendelenburg position aids in the exposure.
- Next, the apex dissection is completed. This is the remaining soft tissue between the sartorius and the adductor at the distal most aspect of the dissection.
- The contents are grasped and elevated under tension with traction in both the superficial and cephalad directions (**FIGURE 10**). This tissue is controlled with the nondominant hand, as the dissection of the remaining tissue over the apex

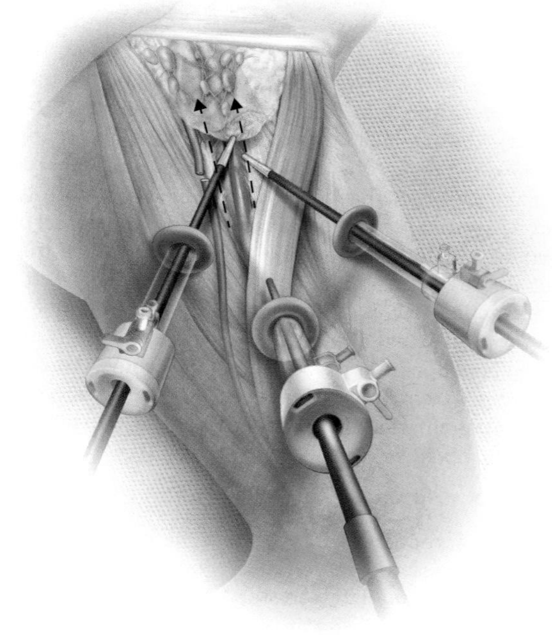

FIGURE 10 ● At the apex of the femoral triangle, the contents are grasped and retracted under tension by pushing the specimen anterior and cephalad.

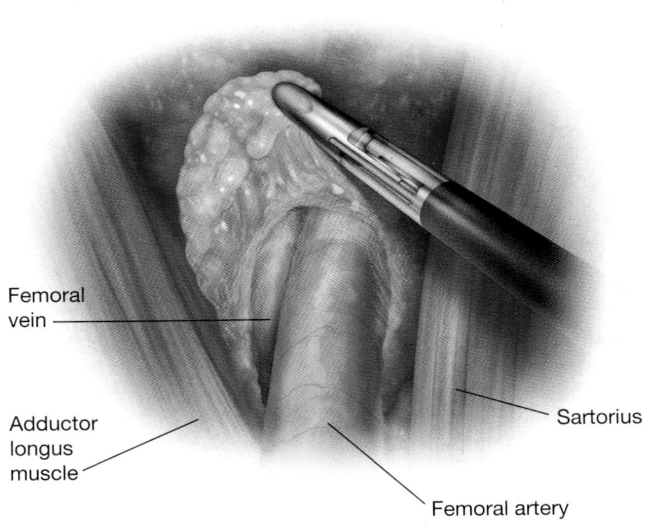

FIGURE 11 ● As the dissection at the apex continues deep from distal to proximal, the femoral vessels will come into view with the artery the first to be encountered.

is completed. I envision my line of dissection is a straight line between the two proximal trocars.

- At this point, the lymphadenectomy is performed by walking up the medial aspect of the sartorius from distal to proximal and rotating the contents medially. Because the femoral nerve lies in this location, a thin rim of fat is left on top of the nerve.
- As this process is repeated and continued, beginning at the apex and dissecting proximally, the femoral vasculature will be identified at this location (**FIGURE 11**).
- As a result of the position of the lower extremity in abduction and flexion, the femoral artery lays anterior to the femoral vein. The femoral vein is deep and medial, and as we dissect proximally, the vessels will spiral, and the two vessels will ultimately become parallel with each other lying in the same plain. Dissection should stay directly on the adventitia of the femoral vessels. A laparoscopic Kittner can aid this dissection. I primarily use the dissection shears. The anterior half of the vessels are completely exposed.
- **FIGURE 12A** and **B** shows the relative position change of vessels in relation to each other as we proceed from distal to proximal; this is accentuated by the leg being in a position of abduction.
- The deep inguinal lymph nodes are resected en bloc with this procedure. Our deep dissection plain is deep to the cribriform fascia. The cribriform fascia is an extension of the fascial lata. It separates the superficial inguinal lymph nodes from the deep inguinal lymph nodes. The cribriform fascia is penetrated by the saphenous vein at the fossa ovalis. The plane of dissection is depicted in **FIGURE 12A** and **B**
- The femoral vein is appreciated deep and medial to the artery, just proximal to the apex. This is dissected out in a similar fashion. The anterior as well as the medial and lateral aspect of the vessels are skeletonized. There is no need to circumferentially dissect out these structures (**FIGURE 13A** and **B**).

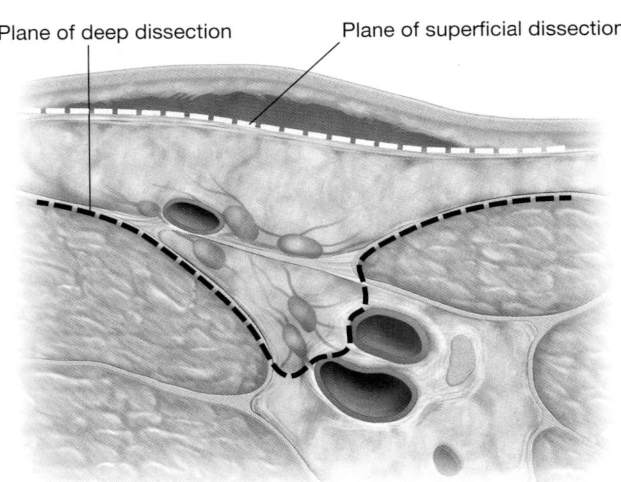

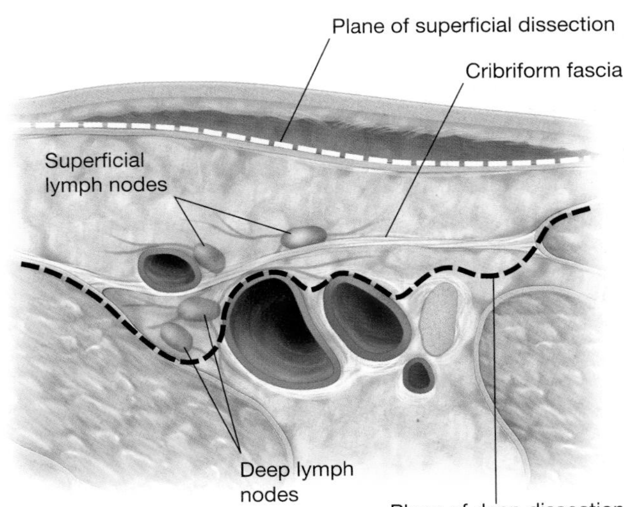

FIGURE 12 ● **A** and **B,** The superficial and deep dissection planes are graphically depicted here. These figures also demonstrate the relative position change of vessels in relation to each other as we proceed from distal to proximal, respectively.

- The femoral vein will be collapsed secondary to the CO_2 insufflation and Trendelenburg position. Its caliber will also be seen to fluctuate with ventilation. If you enter the vein, there will be minimal bleeding until the CO_2 is turned off.
- The medial dissection is completed off the adductor as we progress more proximally. As we continue our dissection, we simply walk up the adductor from distal to proximal. Continued anterior traction is applied to the specimen as we expose the vessels heading toward the inguinal ligament.
- Essentially the lymphadenectomy contents are rotated centrally off their peripheral muscular attachments onto the femoral neurovasculature and the deep dissection off the anterior surface of the femoral vessels proceeds from distal to proximal.
- Note, in very select case, I preserve the cribriform fascia from the apex to the fossa ovalis and do not expose the femoral vessels and deep inguinal lymph nodes until the saphenofemoral junction is reached proximally. This more limited distal

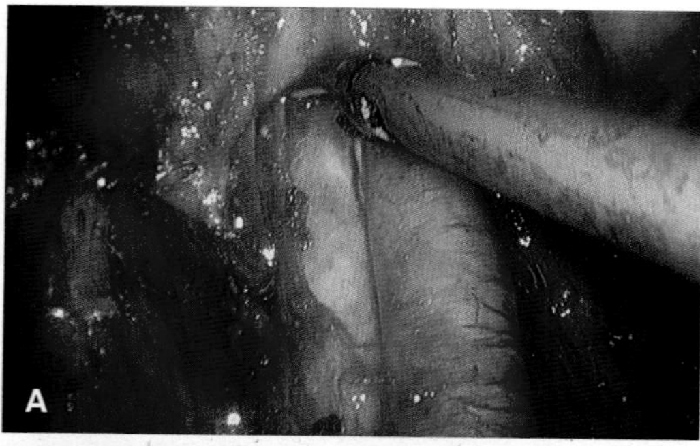

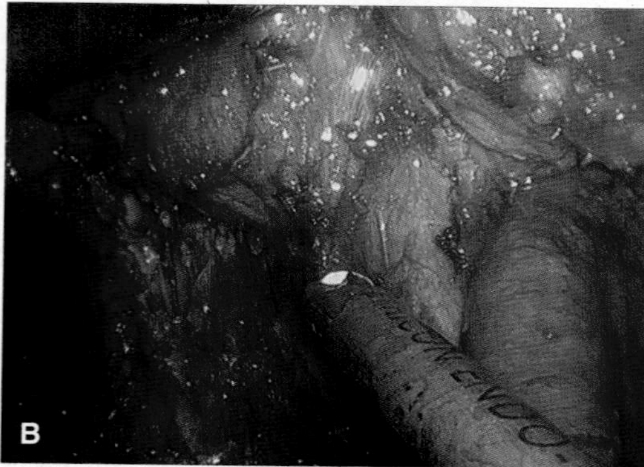

FIGURE 13 ● **A** and **B,** Intraoperative photos of the relationship of the vessels to each other and relative position change from distal to proximal, respectively. (Used with permission of Mayo Foundation for Medical Education and Research, all rights reserved.)

dissection creates a much smaller dead space and makes for a very clear deep plane dissection of the distal contents off the fascia.

Preservation of the Great Saphenous Vein

- Dissection from distal to proximal on the greater saphenous vein should be performed. As the dissection is carried, proximal additional branches entering the vein will need to be divided with clips or energy device. On the posterior aspect of the proximal greater saphenous vein, a small portion of the soft tissue specimen will need to be divided to allow 360° exposure of the vein as it enters the femoral vein and allow the specimen to be completely freed.

Proximal Dissection of Saphenous Vein at the Fossa Ovalis

- The medial and anterior surface of the femoral vein is skeletonized and we continue along medial aspect of this vessel under the inguinal ligament. Based on how far proximal you prefer to dissect here, Cloquet lymph node can be removed en bloc with the specimen. If desired, a suture can be placed to mark Cloquet node.
- The pectineus muscle can be seen here as the deep boundary of dissection. At this point, dissection is deep and proximal to the shelving edge of the inguinal ligament (**FIGURE 14**).
- The tissue is freed from medial to lateral off the previously exposed inguinal ligament.
- At this point, the saphenofemoral junction is identified, coming directly anterior off the femoral vein, approximately 3 cm distal to the inguinal ligament as the saphenous vein penetrates the cribriform fascia at the fossa ovalis. This will be identified as you dissect from distal to proximal along the medial surface of the femoral vein (**FIGURE 15**).
- (Greater saphenous vein resection when required) The saphenofemoral junction is cleared and divided with a linear endovascular stapler (**FIGURE 16**). The proximal/medial tissue must first be freed off the femoral vein before this can be accomplished. It is better to complete this dissection proximal and medial to the saphenofemoral junction and make this window wider than you expect before attempting to introduce the stapler.
- The remaining proximal dissection of the femoral vessels (mostly cephalad and lateral) is then completed, removing the inguinal contents off the remaining attachments with the femoral vessels. Short trocars and long instruments have been necessary in my experience to reach this proximal most dissection.
- If not previously completed, any remaining soft tissue cephalad to the inguinal ligament to be included is dissected off

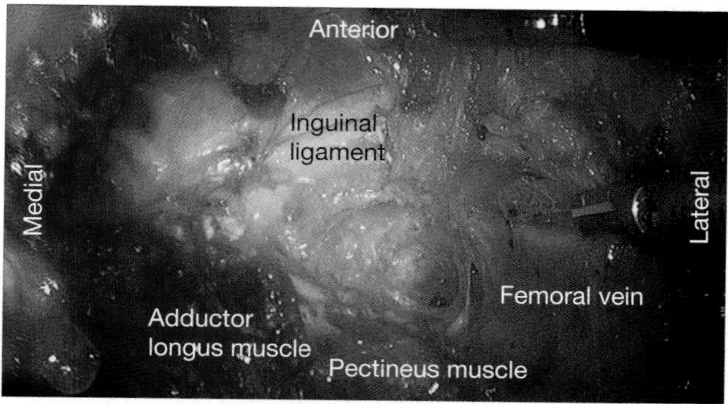

FIGURE 14 ● This image shows the empty space created deep to the inguinal ligament at the proximal/medial aspect of the dissection. The medial aspect of the femoral vein is skeletonized. One can choose to extend proximal to include Cloquet's lymph node with the specimen. (Used with permission of Mayo Foundation for Medical Education and Research, all rights reserved.)

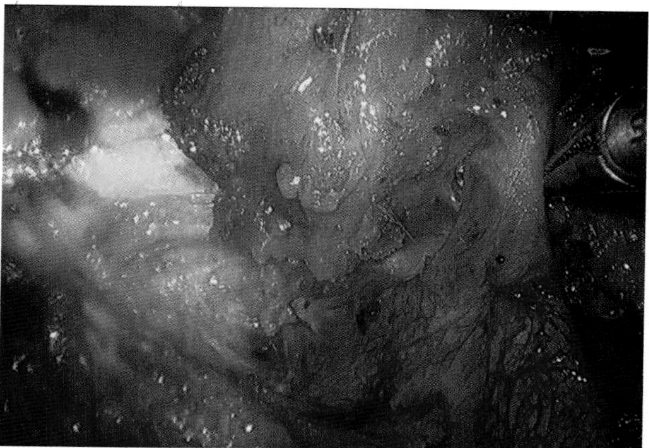

FIGURE 15 ● The saphenofemoral junction is identified as the dissection off the medial and anterior surface of the femoral vein is continued proximally. (Used with permission of Mayo Foundation for Medical Education and Research, all rights reserved.)

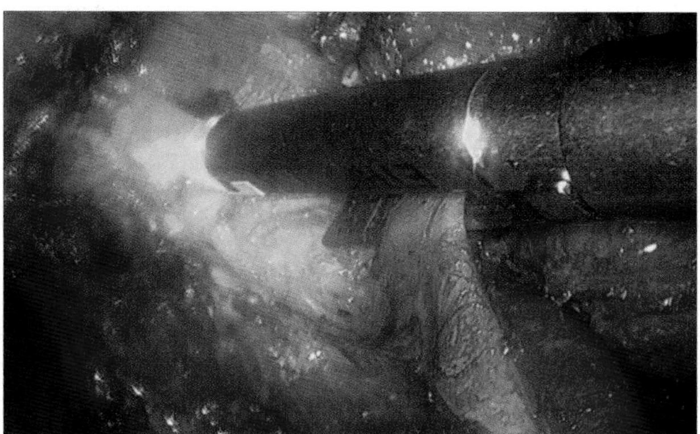

FIGURE 16 ● The intraoperative photo shows the proximal saphenous vein being divided with an endovascular stapler. (Used with permission of Mayo Foundation for Medical Education and Research, all rights reserved.)

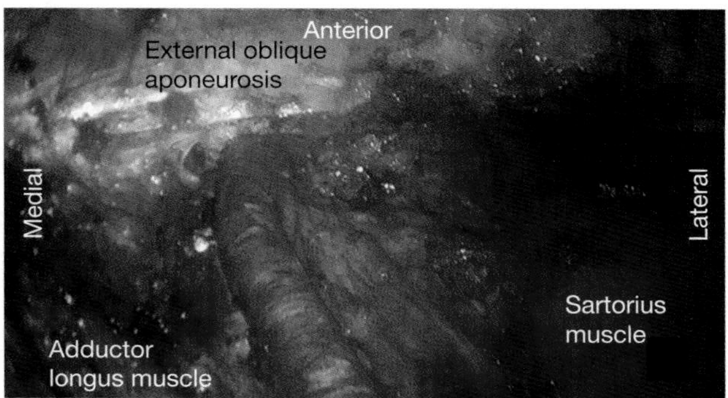

FIGURE 17 ● Intraoperative photo at the completion of the operation showing the musculature of the femoral triangle exposed, including the fascia overlying the external oblique aponeurosis, proximal to the inguinal ligament, and skeletonization of the anterior half of the femoral vessels. (Used with permission of Mayo Foundation for Medical Education and Research, all rights reserved.)

the external oblique aponeurosis. This is easily peeled down using hook cautery and included en bloc with the specimen. The remaining attachments with the inguinal ligament and external oblique aponeurosis are completed.

- In a similar fashion, any remaining lateral attachments are freed off the sartorius followed by the final attachments off the inguinal ligament.

Specimen Removal

- Once the specimen is free, the contents are placed in an endobag.
- The anatomic boundaries are clearly visualized, the adequacy of dissection is inspected and hemostasis confirmed (**FIGURE 17**).
- Once completed, the drain is passed through the lateral trocar site.

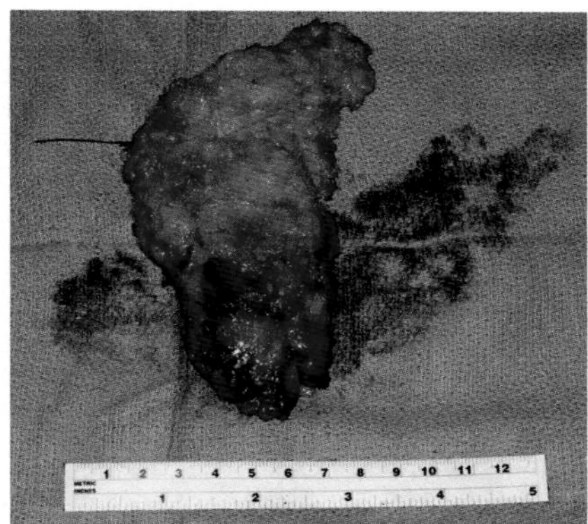

FIGURE 18 ● Photo of the inguinal contents after en bloc resection using the minimally invasive approach. (Used with permission of Mayo Foundation for Medical Education and Research, all rights reserved.)

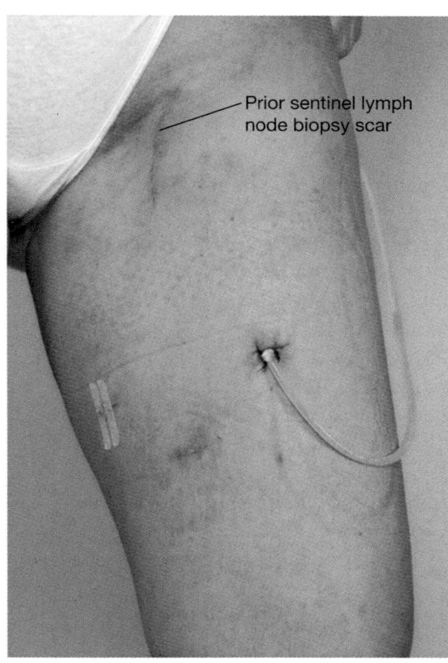

FIGURE 19 ● Photo of operative leg at the first postoperative visit.

- The extracted specimen is depicted in **FIGURE 18**.
- A photo taken 1 week postoperatively is shown (**FIGURE 19**). It should be noted that the proximal longitudinal scar is from the original SLNB and not part of the MILND.
- At the end of the case, the genitals will be edematous from the CO_2 dissection. This is not a concern; the Foley can be removed at the end of the case and this should resolve by morning rounds. Crepitance up to the chest has been reported in some cases but has never been of clinical significance in my experience and to my knowledge. A chest strap during the operation can avoid this.

PEARLS AND PITFALLS

High conversion rate	■ Embarking on this procedure without adequate training ■ Frustration and lack of patience ■ As with any new minimally invasive procedure, this should be scheduled at a date and time when there are limited other external pressures.
Unable to reach proximal dissection	■ Placing trocars too distal or instruments too short.
Dissection too lateral	■ Typically, this is a result of not placing the leg in adequate abduction and external rotation prior to the start of the procedure. You want to have the leg positioned such that the femoral triangle is anterior.
Inadequate lymphadenectomy	■ Not staying within defined anatomic boundaries. ■ Not dissecting anterior to Scarpa fascia. ■ Not dissecting the deep inguinal lymph nodes by staying on the adventitia of the femoral vessels (not dissecting deep to the cribriform fascia). ■ Not dissecting the tissue cephalad to the inguinal ligament.
Conversion secondary to hypercarbia	■ Not briefing with anesthesia team and making appropriate minute ventilation adjustments.
Constant leak during case	■ Finger dissection of more than one port site at the start of case and making incisions too large.
Drain not holding suction	■ Not sealing incision tightly around drain at the end of case. There is no subcutaneous fat between trocar site and cavity, unlike an abdominal procedure or open nodal dissections in which the drain is passed through a subcutaneous tunnel, so this remains very unforgiving.
Seroma/prolonged drain days	■ See section regarding Postoperative Care.

POSTOPERATIVE CARE

- Patients could be outpatient same day discharge as pain is not an issue. We admit as an outpatient overnight stay and discharged within 23 hours. Drain care is reviewed in detail.
- Seromas and prolonged drain days remain an issue in my practice.[11] Patients are encouraged to keep the leg elevated and limit activity until the drain is removed.
- Patients are seen prior to discharge by the physical medicine and rehabilitation lymphedema therapist. Compressive leg wrapping is applied as well as compression to the operative field (compressive biker shorts with a foam insert or sock placed directly over the basin).
- Ensure the drain is holding suction prior to discharge.
- Redness and bruising of the flap noted in the immediate postoperative period is typical and represents mild ischemia. These have all resolved in my experience without any intervention. These findings do not represent cellulitis and antibiotics are not indicated.
- A chlorhexidine disc sealed with Tegaderm is placed around the drain and changed every third day by the patient and the drain site is cleaned with an alcohol wipe with each dressing change.
- I currently remove the drain at 4 weeks regardless of output. Symptomatic seromas are managed with serial aspiration or percutaneous drain placement.
- Patients may shower on postoperative day 1.

OUTCOMES

- The procedure has been established as technically safe and feasible.[12,13] Surgeons who have extensive experience with the open technique, undergoing supervised training on the minimally invasive procedure, attain early competence with a short learning curve.[14] Baseline laparoscopic skills correlate with decreased operative time and operative performance but not complications, conversion rates, or lymph node count.[15]
- The acute morbidity is decreased compared with an open approach.[12,16] Seromas are common and can be prolonged; wound complications requiring more than outpatient oral antibiotics are rare.[11,17] Wound dehiscence has essentially been eliminated.
- The goal of a lymphadenectomy is accurate staging, regional control and ideally cure in patients with regional nodal disease. Surrogate oncologic markers for MILND, such as lymph node count, have been shown to be at least as good as the open approach.[14,17] Two single-institution studies have reported on oncologic outcomes in patients with melanoma.[18,19] A randomized surgical trial (NCT01500304) failed to accrue secondary to patient preference for MILND and many high-volume surgeons no longer have equipoise in randomizing patients.[13]
- A large multi-institutional experience of 14 sites supports the oncologic safety of MILND (228 patients) compared to OILND (299) for melanoma.[20]

- Oncologic principles and the extent of resection should never be jeopardized to accomplish the procedure with the smallest incision possible.

COMPLICATIONS

- Seroma
- Hematoma
- Wound dehiscence (prior scars overlying the flap are most susceptible, such as SLN biopsy incision)
- Flap necrosis
- Major vascular injury
- Femoral nerve injury
- Drain not holding suction
- Recurrence
- Lymphedema
- Infection
- Anesthesia risks
- Hypercarbia
- Inadequate lymphadenectomy

ACKNOWLEDGMENTS

The figures and content were funded in part by the Fraternal Order of Eagles Cancer Research Fund Fellowship Program.

REFERENCES

1. Spillane AJ, Tucker M, Pasquali S. A pilot study reporting outcomes for melanoma patients of a minimal access ilio-inguinal dissection technique based on two incisions. *Ann Surg Oncol.* 2011;18(4):970-976. doi:10.1245/s10434-010-1455-8. Epub 2010 Dec 14.
2. Faries MB, Thompson JF, Cochran AJ, et al. Completion dissection or observation for sentinel-node metastasis in melanoma. *N Engl J Med.* 2017;376(23):2211-2222.
3. Balch CM, Gershenwald JE, Atkins MB, et al. Melanoma of the skin. In: Edge SB, Compton CC, Fritz AG, et al, eds. *AJCC Cancer Staging Manual.* Springer; 2010:325-344.
4. Gonzalez AB, Jakub JW, Harmsen WS, Suman VJ, Markovic SN. Status of the regional nodal basin remains highly prognostic in melanoma patients with in-transit disease. *J Am Coll Surg.* 2016;223(1):77-85.e1. doi:10.1016/j.jamcollsurg.2016.03.025. Epub 2016 Mar 26.
5. Miranda EP, Gertner M, Wall J, et al. Routine imaging of asymptomatic melanoma patients with metastasis to sentinel lymph nodes rarely identifies systemic disease. *Arch Surg.* 2004;139(8):831-836; discussion 836-837.
6. Aloia TA, Gershenwald JE, Andtbacka RH, et al. Utility of computed tomography and magnetic resonance imaging staging before completion lymphadenectomy in patients with sentinel lymph node-positive melanoma. *J Clin Oncol.* 2006;24(18):2858-2865.
7. Gold JS, Jaques DP, Busam KJ, et al. Yield and predictors of radiologic studies for identifying distant metastases in melanoma patients with a positive sentinel lymph node biopsy. *Ann Surg Oncol.* 2007;14(7):2133-2140.
8. Brady MS, Akhurst T, Spanknebel K, et al. Utility of preoperative [(18)]f fluorodeoxyglucose-positron emission tomography scanning in high-risk melanoma patients. *Ann Surg Oncol.* 2006;13(4):525-532.
9. Tyler DS, Onaitis M, Kherani A, et al. Positron emission tomography scanning in malignant melanoma. *Cancer.* 2000;89(5):1019-1025.
10. Delman KA, Kooby DA, Ogan K, et al. Feasibility of a novel approach to inguinal lymphadenectomy: minimally invasive groin dissection for melanoma. *Ann Surg Oncol.* 2010;17(3):731-737.
11. Contreras N, Jakub JW. The achilles heel of minimally invasive inguinal lymph node dissection: Seroma formation. *Am J Surg.* 2020;219(4):696-700. doi:10.1016/j.amjsurg.2019.06.010. Epub 2019 Jun 24.
12. Jakub JW, Terando AM, Sarnaik A, et al. Safety and feasibility of minimally invasive inguinal lymph node dissection in patients with melanoma (SAFE-MILND): Report of a prospective multi-institutional trial. *Ann Surg.* 2017;265(1):192-196.
13. Postlewait LM, Farley CR, Diller ML, et al. A minimally invasive approach for inguinal lymphadenectomy in melanoma and genitourinary malignancy: long-term outcomes in an attempted randomized control trial. *Ann Surg Oncol.* 2017;24(11):3237-3244.
14. Jakub JW, Terando AM, Sarnaik A, et al. Training high-volume melanoma surgeons to perform a novel minimally invasive inguinal lymphadenectomy: Report of a prospective multi-institutional trial. *J Am Coll Surg.* 2016;222(3):253-260.
15. Zendejas B, Jakub JW, Terando AM, et al. Laparoscopic skill assessment of practicing surgeons prior to enrollment in a surgical trial of a new laparoscopic procedure. *Surg Endosc.* 2017;31(8):3313-3319.
16. Abbott AM, Grotz TE, Rueth NM, et al. Minimally invasive inguinal lymph node dissection (MILND) for melanoma: experience from two academic centers. *Ann Surg Oncol.* 2013;20(1):340-355.
17. Sommariva A, Pasquali S, Rossi CR. Video endoscopic inguinal lymphadenectomy for lymph node metastasis from Solid tumors. *Eur J Surg Oncol.* 2015;41:274-281.
18. Sommariva A, Cona C, Tonello M, Pilati P, Riccardo Rossi C. Oncological outcome of videoscopic groin dissection for lymph node metastasis from melanoma. *Surg Endosc.* 2021;35(6):2576-2582.
19. Delman KA, Kooby DA, Rizzo M, et al. Initial experience with videoscopic inguinal lymphadenectomy. *Ann Surg Oncol.* 2011;18(4):977-982.
20. Jakub JW, Lowe M, J. Howard JH, et al. Oncologic outcomes of multi-institutional minimally invasive inguinal lymph node dissection for melanoma compared with open inguinal dissection in the second multicenter selective lymphadenectomy trial (MSLT-II). *Ann Surg Onc.* 2022. doi:10.1245/s10434-022-11758-z

Chapter 37 Selective Neck Dissection for Melanoma

Vasu Divi

DEFINITION

- The goal of a selective neck dissection for melanoma is the complete removal of the lymph nodes and lymphatics that drain a specific region of skin in the head and neck.
- This procedure is indicated for patients presenting with clinically evident regional metastasis in the absence of distant disease. In some cases, neck dissection in patients with documented stage IV disease may provide palliative benefit or prevent morbidity in patients not responding to systemic therapy.
- The indications for a selective neck dissection following a positive sentinel lymph node are evolving. An alternative to complete node dissection is nodal observation with serial ultrasounds, with neck dissection reserved for patients with a subsequent isolated regional nodal recurrence. Two prospective, randomized clinical trials, the Multicenter Selective Lymphadenectomy Trial II (MSLT-II) and the DeCOG trial,[1,2] showed equivalent melanoma-specific survival for patients with a positive sentinel lymph node randomized to either completion lymphadenectomy or observation with serial clinical examinations and nodal ultrasonography. Neck dissection may still be considered in select patients following a positive SLN biopsy based on factors such as nodal tumor burden, patient age, and comorbidities and potential challenges/expected morbidity of a neck dissection in the face of nodal recurrence.

PATIENT HISTORY AND PHYSICAL FINDINGS

- All patients with melanoma of the head and neck should undergo palpation of the regional lymphatics, including the parotid glands and cervical levels 1 to 5.
- Melanomas at the junction of the neck and the chest, back, or shoulder should also include palpation of the axillary lymph nodes.
- All patients with melanoma, particularly those with proven regional metastases, should have a focused review of symptoms, looking for symptoms concerning for metastatic disease.
- All patients with melanoma should also have a complete skin examination, looking for second primary cutaneous malignancies.

IMAGING AND OTHER DIAGNOSTIC STUDIES

- Preoperative imaging of the neck is not necessary in patients without clinically evident neck disease.
- In patients with palpable adenopathy
  - Imaging by contrast-enhanced computed tomography (CT) scan is generally recommended to evaluate the extent of disease.
  - Fine needle aspiration is used to obtain pathologic diagnosis of the enlarged lymph node.
- In cases of distant metastatic disease, new options for treatment using immunotherapy have changed management of melanoma and the treatment paradigm continue to evolve. In very select cases, achievement of regional control in the neck may be necessary.

SURGICAL MANAGEMENT

Preoperative Planning

- Determination of the type of neck dissection to be performed is based on the location of the primary tumor and location of neck disease.
- The relevant lymphatic basins of the head and neck include the parotid lymph nodes, levels 1 to 5, and the postauricular lymph nodes (**FIGURE 1**).
- This serves as a rough guide to when different lymphatic basins should be addressed; ultimately, the clinician should dissect all lymphatic basins that could potentially be harboring clinical disease based on an understanding of lymphatic drainage patterns.
  - The removal of the superficial lobe of the parotid gland is performed for any primary cutaneous tumor anterior to the external auditory canal and above the angle of the mandible.
  - Levels 1 to 4 are dissected with any lesion involving the scalp anterior to the plane of the external auditory canal, facial skin, or anterior neck skin.
  - Levels 2 to 5 are dissected with any lesion involving the scalp posterior to the plane of the external auditory canal or posterior neck skin.
  - If the primary lesion is in the scalp and located very close to the plane of the external auditory canal, dissection should include levels 1 to 5.

Positioning

- Patients are placed supine with the top of the head at the edge of the surgical bed.
- A bump is placed underneath the shoulder blades to allow for extension of the neck, being careful to maintain support of the head on the operating room (OR) table.

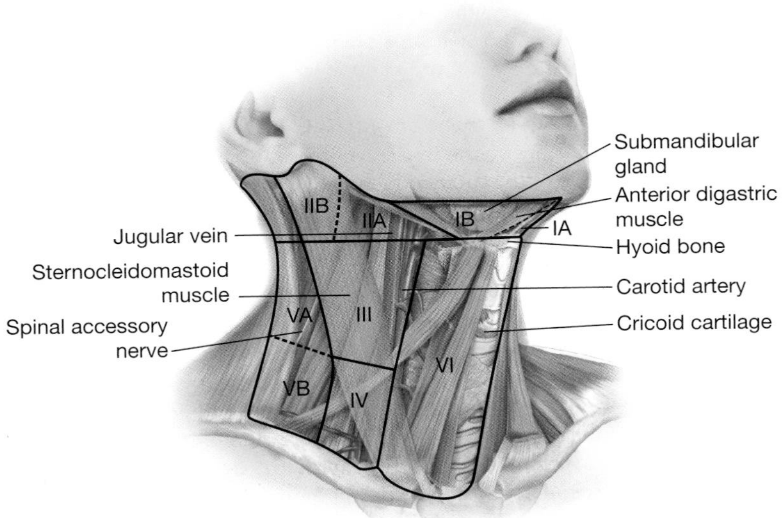

FIGURE 1 ● Levels of the neck. Level 1 includes all nodes between the contralateral anterior belly of the digastric, ipsilateral posterior belly of the digastric, and the inferior edge of the mandible. Level 2 includes the nodes below the skull base between the posterior belly of the digastric, posterior edge of the SCM, and above the level of the hyoid. Level 3 includes all nodes between the hyoid bone and cricoid cartilage arch, between the lateral and the internal carotid artery, and the posterior edge of the SCM. Level 4 includes all nodes between the cricoid cartilage arch and clavicle, between the lateral and the internal carotid artery, and the posterior edge of the SCM. Level 5 includes all nodes from the skull base down to the posterior border of the sternocleidomastoid muscle to the clavicle, anterior to the trapezius muscle.

SELECTIVE NECK DISSECTION LEVELS 1 TO 4

- A curvilinear incision is made midway between the angle of the mandible and the clavicle; the incision travels within a neck crease, extending a few centimeters from the mastoid tip toward the approximate midpoint of the thyroid notch (**FIGURE 2**).
- Skin is incised down through the subcutaneous tissue and platysma.
- Subplatysmal skin flaps are elevated to expose the deeper contents overlying levels 1 to 4 of the neck; this will extend to the mentum, along the strap musculature in the midline, to the posterior border of the sternocleidomastoid muscle (SCM), and down to the level of the clavicle (**FIGURE 3**).
- The marginal mandibular nerve is identified in the superficial layer of the cervical fascia near the angle of the mandible and is identified using nerve stimulation. The nerve is dissected free and elevated over the plane of the mandible (**FIGURE 4**).
- The facial artery and vein are identified and ligated as they cross over the plane of the mandible near the mandibular notch.
- The tissue over the mandible is then incised from the mentum to the angle of the mandible, taking care not to injure the previously dissected marginal mandibular nerve. This tissue is pulled inferiorly, taking care to remove the perifacial lymph nodes located near the facial vessels. During this dissection, the retromandibular vein may be identified and ligated as it travels through the tail of the parotid gland. The periosteum of the mandible should be kept intact—the dissection occurs immediately above this layer.

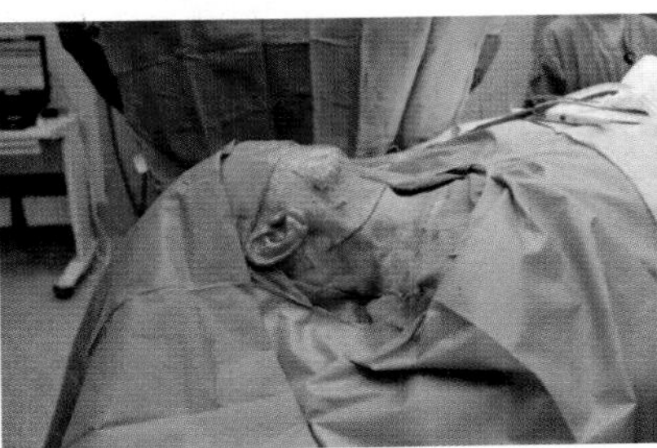

FIGURE 2 ● The neck incision is marked out between the mandible and clavicle.

- Incise soft tissue over contralateral anterior belly of the digastric muscle from mentum down to hyoid bone.
- Begin elevating contents of level 1A by dissecting tissue laterally off the mylohyoid muscle toward the ipsilateral anterior belly of the digastric muscle; this will require division of tissue along the hyoid bone inferiorly.
- Bring packet of tissue over ipsilateral digastric and back onto mylohyoid until the edge of the mylohyoid is reached; see **FIGURE 4**.
- Retract the mylohyoid muscle medially to allow for exposure of the contents deep to the submandibular gland. This may require some blunt dissection in this area. Identify the hypoglossal nerve, lingual nerve, and submandibular duct (**FIGURE 5**).
- Divide the submandibular duct, taking care not to cause excessive bleeding from the nearby veins (**FIGURE 6**).
- Divide the submandibular ganglion and allow the lingual nerve to retract superiorly. The hypoglossal nerve should remain deep in the dissection with a facial plane covering it. There is no need to expose the nerve in this portion of the dissection.

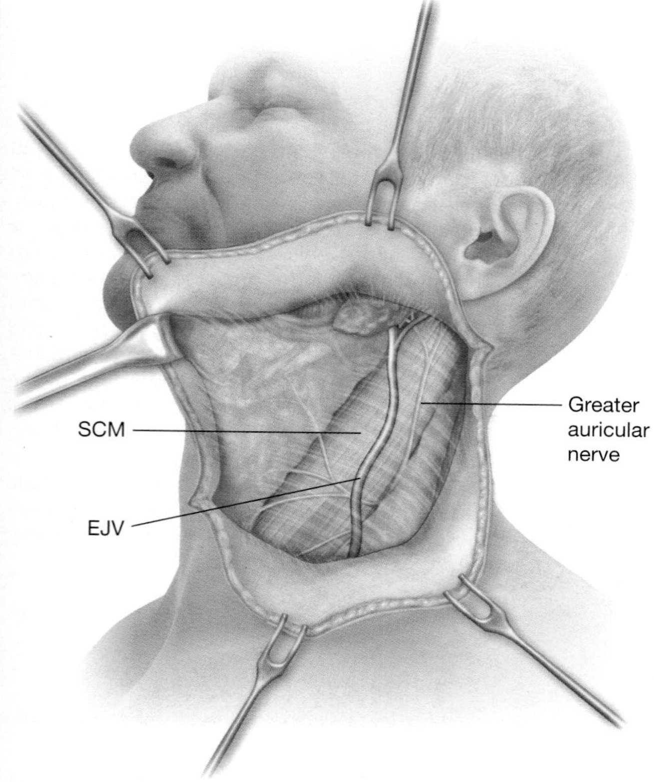

FIGURE 3 ● The neck incision is completed with subplatysmal flaps elevated superiorly and inferiorly.

- Pull the submandibular gland and packet of tissue laterally, carefully dividing the tissue over the posterior belly of the digastric (**FIGURE 7**).
- Approximately halfway up the posterior belly, the facial artery is again seen traveling under the digastric and into the submandibular gland; divide the artery a second time.
- Trace the posterior belly superiorly, dividing the overlying tissue until the SCM is reached. If it has not already been divided, the retromandibular vein is usually encountered as it exits the parotid gland near the angle of the mandible—carefully divide the vein.
- The SCM is then "unwrapped." At the posterior edge of the SCM, incise the fascia over the muscle. This will require division of the cutaneous nerves that course over the muscle; the great auricular branch to the ear as well as the external jugular can sometimes be traced out and saved.
- Pull the fascia medially to unwrap the SCM; be careful to take all tissue over the muscle. Lymph nodes associated with the external jugular vein must be removed due to their potential involvement in cutaneous lesions.
- After the anterior surface of the SCM is wrapped, carefully pull the muscle off the deeper neck and posteriorly to start unwrapping the deep surface; at the junction of the upper one-third and lower two-thirds, the cranial nerve (CN) XI (the spinal accessory nerve) will be encountered as it enters the muscle.
- Continue to unwrap and elevate the muscle of the floor of the neck until the posterior edge is reached, taking care to not stretch or injure CN XI.
- At this point, the posterior belly of the digastric should be traced underneath the SCM and then mobilized so it can be pulled superiorly.
- At the hyoid bone, the omohyoid muscle is identified and traced low into the neck to the posterior edge of the SCM. It is mobilized as well so it can be pulled inferiorly.
- Next, the posterior belly of the digastric is pulled superiorly while CN XI is traced underneath the muscle by dividing the overlying tissue until it courses over the internal jugular (IJ) vein; the nerve usually passes superficial to the vein (80%) but can also pass deep to it (20%) (**FIGURE 8**).
- The spinal accessory nerve is elevated off the deep neck and is circumferentially dissected up to the IJ; the sidewall of the IJ vein is then skeletonized (**FIGURE 9**).

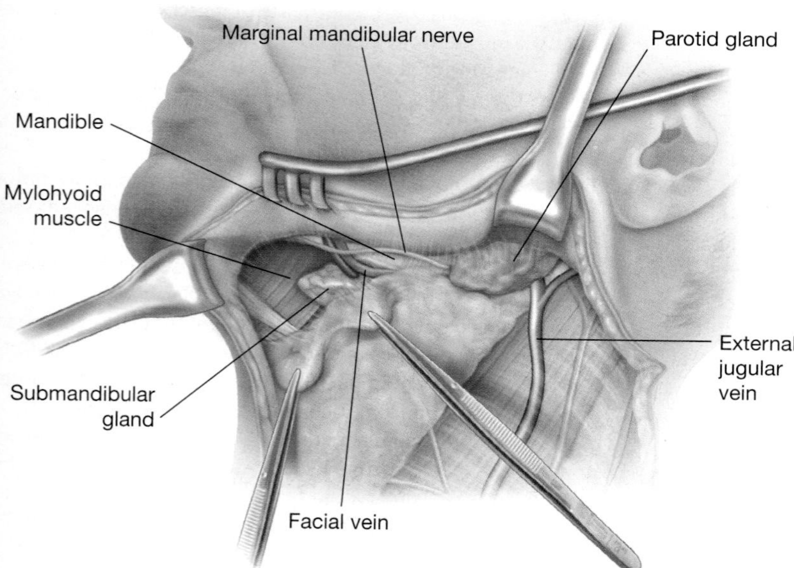

FIGURE 4 ● The marginal mandibular nerve is elevated over the mandible and the contents of level 1A are dissected posteriorly. Division of the facial artery and vein would occur at this point or earlier in the dissection.

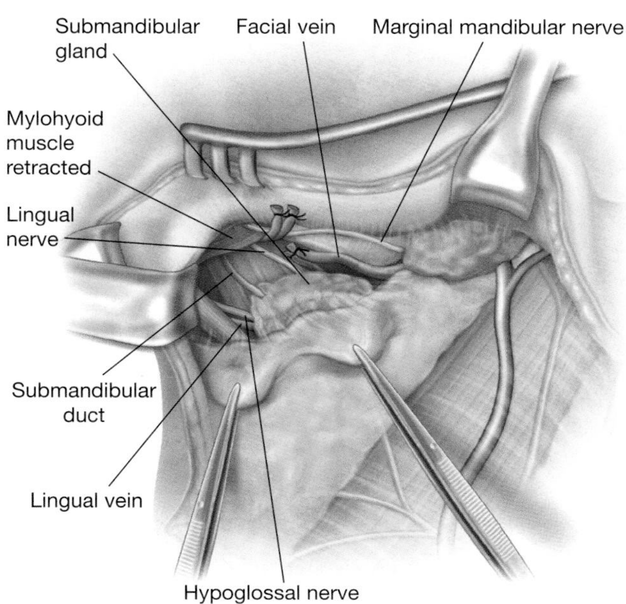

FIGURE 5 ● The mylohyoid muscle is retracted anteriorly exposing the lingual nerve, submandibular duct, and hypoglossal nerve. The hypoglossal nerve is in a deeper plane than the lingual nerve and is only exposed after dividing the overlying fascia.

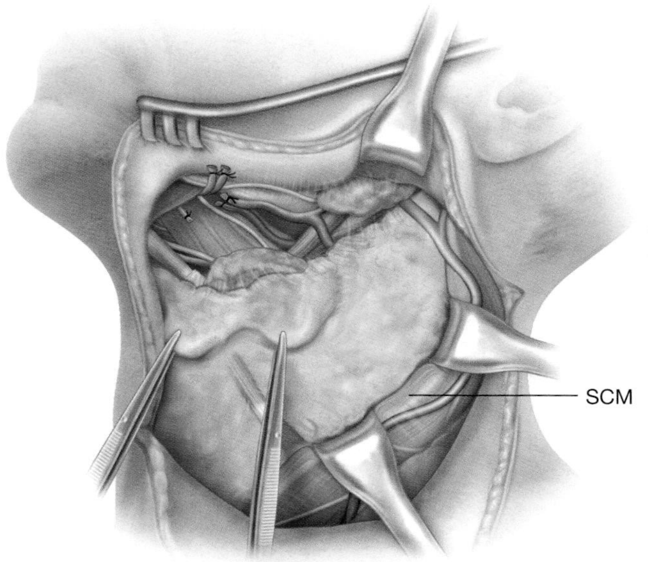

FIGURE 7 ● The contents of level 1B are pulled over the posterior belly of digastric. The facial artery could be dissected free from the gland (as shown) or divided a second time as it crosses under the digastric.

- The transverse process of C1 is palpated on the floor of the neck. This will serve as the superior limit of dissection.
- Lymphatic tissue of level 2B is mobilized by dividing the tissue between the IJ and the posterior edge of the SCM down to the level of the floor of the neck (levator scapulae muscle). Superiorly, the contents of level 2B will need to be pulled underneath the CN XI (**FIGURE 9**).
- The posterior edge of dissection parallels the posterior border of the SCM. This tissue is incised down to the floor of the neck as well, taking care to not divide the cervical rootlets (**FIGURE 10**).
- The inferior margin of dissection is a few centimeters above the clavicle. The omohyoid muscle can be retracted inferiorly or divided to access this area.
- Start by identifying the IJ low in neck and skeletonizing the wall. Next, divide the tissue adjacent to the IJ down to the floor of the neck. This tissue needs to be carefully ligated with sutures or clips due to the presence of the thoracic duct. The tissue is divided between the IJ and the posterior edge of the SCM.
- The tissue is then brought forward off the floor of the neck onto the IJ vein (**FIGURE 11**). Follow the fascia of the floor without violating the fascia covering the deep neck muscles.
- The package of tissue is then brought over the IJ by entering the fascia of the carotid sheath; as the tissue is dissected off the IJ, the branches of the IJ are ligated (**FIGURE 12**). Once the IJ is nearly circumferentially dissected, the carotid artery is in view (**FIGURE 13**).

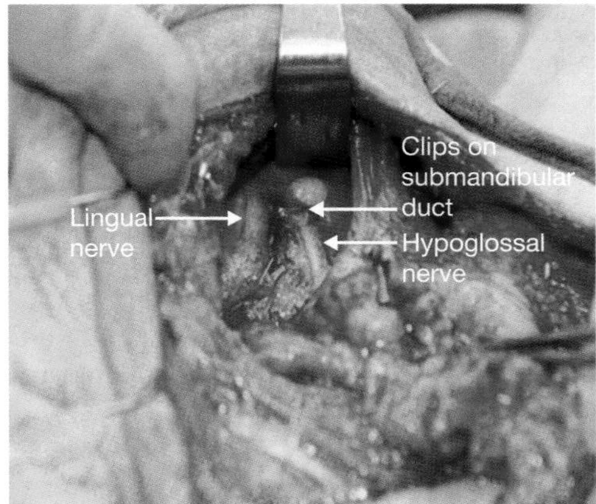

FIGURE 6 ● View of the right neck level 1B with the submandibular gland removed and the mylohyoid muscle retracted anteriorly. Clips are seen on the submandibular duct remnant.

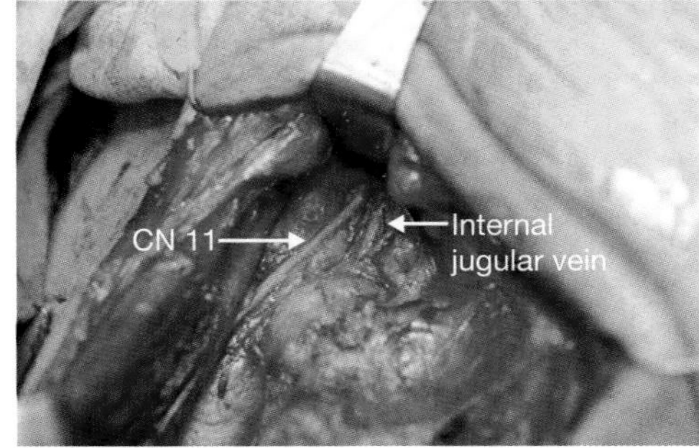

FIGURE 8 ● The contents of the right-sided level 2 are exposed with CN 11 in clear view as it courses over the internal jugular. The posterior belly of digastric is retracted superiorly.

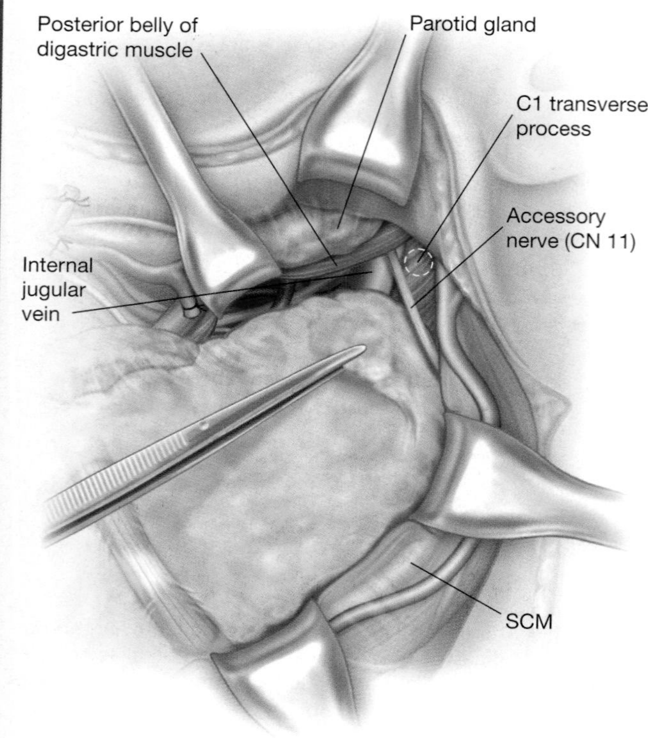

FIGURE 9 ● The contents of level 2B are dissected and passed underneath CN 11. The transverse process of C1 is palpable beneath the muscle.

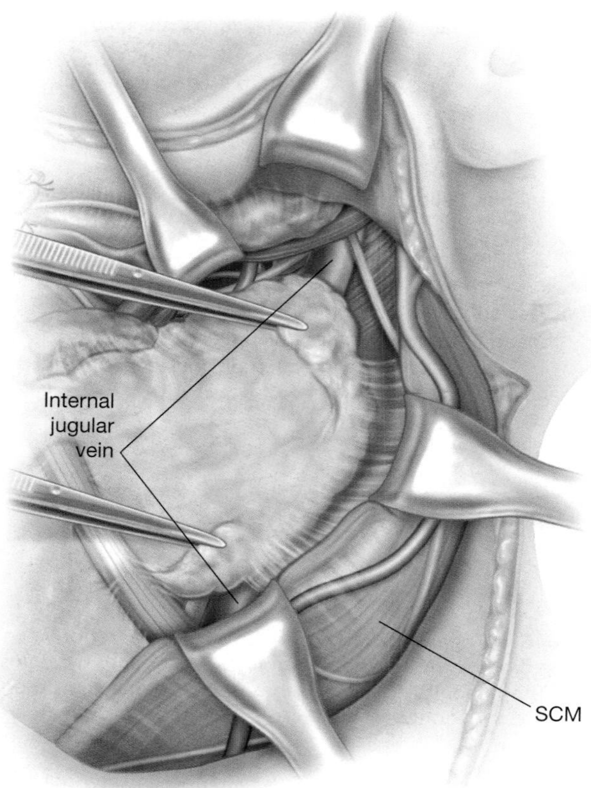

FIGURE 11 ● The inferior dissection at the level of the clavicle is complete, allowing the lymphatic tissue of levels 2, 3, and 4 to be elevated off the floor of the neck.

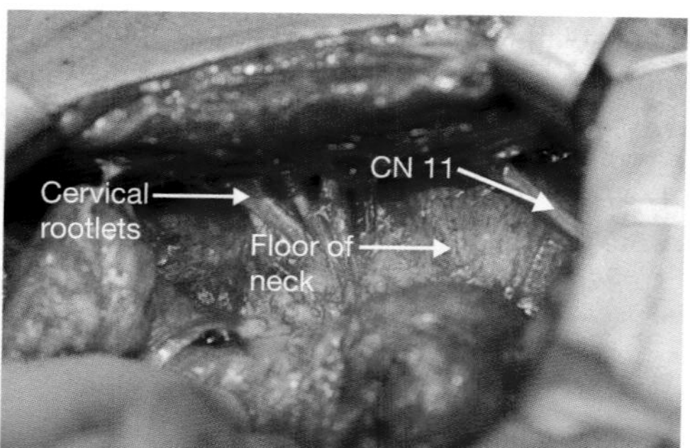

FIGURE 10 ● With the SCM retracted in the right neck, the contents are elevated off the floor of the neck. CN 11 is seen on the right side of the picture, and in the middle of the picture, the cervical rootlets are seen piecing the floor of the neck and wrapped around the posterior SCM.

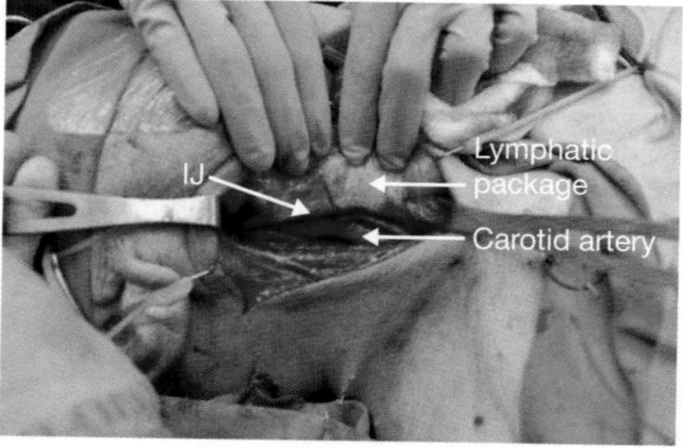

FIGURE 12 ● The lymphatic package is pulled medially in the right neck, still attached to the internal jugular. The package will be taken off of the IJ and onto the visceral space.

- The hypoglossal nerve is identified underneath the digastric. This is traced posteriorly, dividing the overlying tissue and veins until the nerve travels between the carotid and IJ (**FIGURE 14**).
- The package is brought over the carotid until the superior thyroid artery is seen; at this point, transition is made to the fascia of the visceral space (**FIGURE 15**).
- The package of tissue is then truncated at the lateral border of the strap musculature.

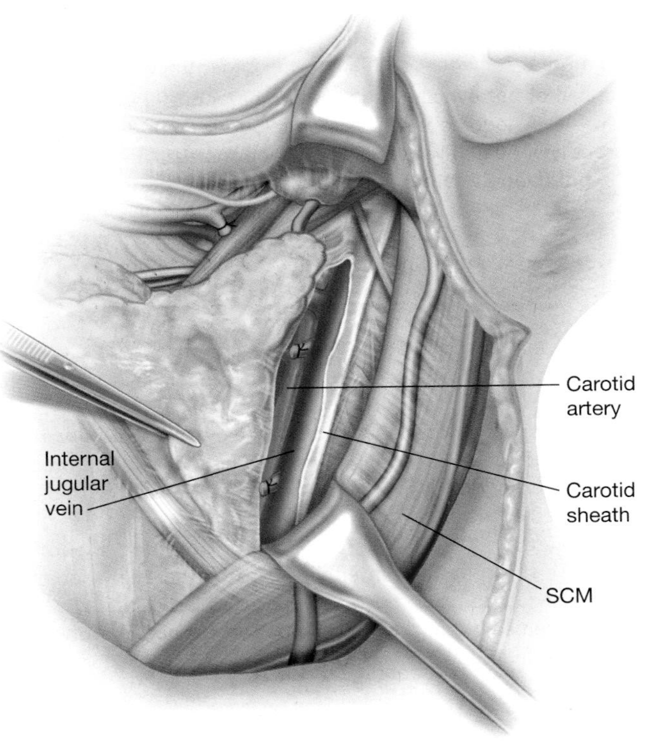

FIGURE 13 ● The carotid sheath is entered and the branches of the IJ are divided allowing the packet to be transitioned onto the carotid artery.

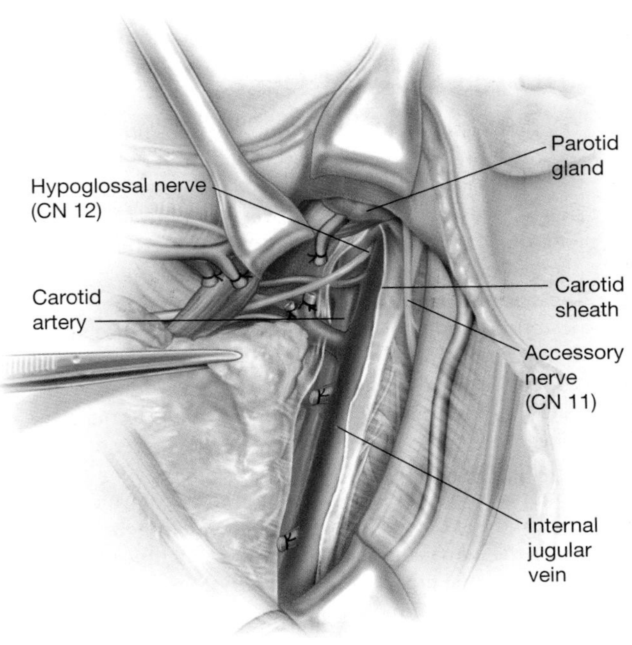

FIGURE 14 ● The hypoglossal nerve is traced out from where it crosses the digastric until it courses between the carotid and the IJ. The overlying veins are delicate and must be divided carefully to avoid significant bleeding, which could obstruct the view of the vein.

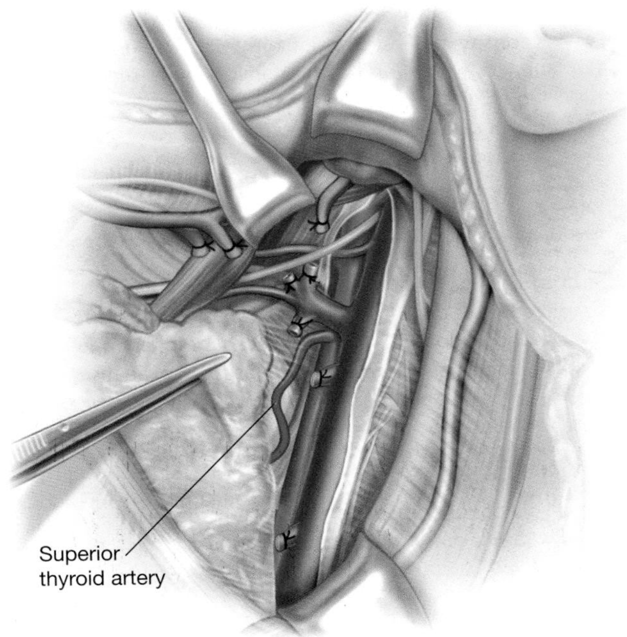

FIGURE 15 ● The packet is transitioned off the carotid space and onto the visceral space carefully preserving the superior thyroid artery.

SELECTIVE NECK DISSECTION LEVELS 2 TO 5 (POSTERIOR-LATERAL NECK DISSECTION)

- The skin incision is modified from the prior procedure being located more posteriorly and traveling lower in the neck.
- Alternatively, a "limb" can be dropped down from the incision to give access to the area over the supraclavicular fossa.
- Posteriorly, the platysma is absent; therefore, the approximate plane of the superficial layer of the cervical fascia is followed.
- The skin flap is raised to the edge of the trapezius muscle posteriorly and inferiorly; the muscle edge is often not seen and therefore must be estimated.
- CN XI is located within the level 5 area. The nerve usually exits the posterior border of the SCM approximately 2 cm above where the great auricular nerve wraps around the muscle. The position is confirmed with nerve stimulation.
- Once the nerve is identified, it is traced from the posterior edge of the SCM until it travels underneath the trapezius muscle; as the nerve approaches the trapezius, it often splits into more than one branch, each of which should be preserved.
- The nerve is then mobilized and elevated from the level 5 contents.
- Next, the posterior superior edge of the SCM is skeletonized.
- This dissection is carried out to the level of the mastoid tip, where the dissection turns posteriorly until the edge of the trapezius is identified.
- In this area, the tissues are cut down to the floor of the neck until the levator scapulae muscle is identified.
- The posterior edge of the SCM and the edge of the trapezius muscle are dissected in their entirety down to the floor of the neck; care is taken to not injure CN XI as it exits and enters these muscles.
- Inferiorly, the tissue at the level of the clavicle is divided heading toward the floor of the neck; careful not to violate the fascia of the floor of the neck to avoid injury to the transverse cervical vessels or the brachial plexus.
- This dissection will connect to both the anterior SCM dissection and the posterior trapezius dissection.
- The omohyoid muscle can be divided near its insertion into the scapula.
- The contents of level 5A and 5B are now brought forward by elevating them off the floor of the neck; during this process, the sensory cervical rootlets can be dissected free and preserved or divided.
- Once the contents are brought to the posterior edge of the SCM, the contents can either be truncated at this point or tucked underneath the SCM.
- The remainder of the levels 2 to 4 neck dissection proceeds as described above; begin by identifying the posterior belly of the digastric muscle and tracing it up to the SCM.

UNIQUE SCENARIOS

- Skin involvement
  - Involvement of the skin can happen from metastatic disease in the neck or from a primary lesion in the neck.
  - Extent of involvement should be determined based on CT scan and palpation with careful attention to the platysma and dermis.
  - Mark at least 1 cm around areas of subcutaneous or dermal involvement; closure is assisted by using elliptical-shaped excisions and paying close attention to resulting skin flaps for rotation or advancement.
  - At the time of skin incision, these areas should be incised down through the level of the platysma.
  - Subplatysmal skin flaps are elevated around the area of involvement, leaving the skin overlying the tumor pedicled on the tumor.
- Involvement of structures
  - Necessity for resection of the SCM, CN XI, IJ, or additional structures is based on involvement seen on imaging studies or at the time of surgery.
  - Tumor should never be violated to preserve any of these structures.

PEARLS AND PITFALLS

Communication with anesthesia	▪ It is essential that the patient is not paralyzed for the operation to allow for monitoring of the marginal mandibular nerve, CN XI, and CN XII. Short-acting paralytics used for induction generally wear off by the time the incision is made.
Placement of incision	▪ The incision should be about two fingerbreadths below the edge of the mandible to avoid injuring the marginal mandibular nerve during skin flap incision and elevation. In level 2-5 dissections, the incision initially parallels the posterior edge of the SCM then curves anteriorly at the level of the cricoid.
Identification of structures	▪ The fascial planes provide excellent boundaries for dissection and should almost always be followed during the neck dissection.
Excision	▪ If grossly positive lymph nodes are encountered, take a cuff of normal tissue to surround the node. This can involve removing a portion of the SCM or sacrificing the IJ or CN XI.

Division of specimen	■ The specimen is typically divided into the corresponding levels of the neck dissection to allow pathology to separately report which levels contained positive lymph nodes.
Prior to closure	■ The level 4 area of the neck is checked for a chyle leak with a sustained Valsalva maneuver. Any evidence of clear or milky fluid should be treated by sewing over or clipping the area.

POSTOPERATIVE CARE

- Following surgery, patients are admitted to the general inpatient unit.
- Postoperative antibiotics are continued for 24 hours.
- Postoperative subcutaneous heparin is used immediately following surgery.
- Closed suction drains are used until output is less than 30 mL/d.
- Patients with extensive CN XI dissection are seen by physical therapy for arm mobilization and strengthening exercises.

OUTCOMES

- The rate of regional recurrence after selective neck dissection for melanoma depends on the extent of cervical disease at the time of resection. Newer approaches with adjuvant immunotherapy have continued to improve recurrence rates and survival.
- Postoperative radiation therapy is considered for patients with extracapsular extension, a single node greater than 4 cm, three or more positive nodes, or for neck dissections following a regional recurrence.
- Recurrent neck disease after neck dissection must be carefully evaluated to determine resectability.

COMPLICATIONS

- Hematoma
- Chyle leak
- CN XI injury
- Hypoglossal injury
- Marginal mandibular weakness
- Stroke

REFERENCES

1. Faries MB, Thompson JF, Cochran AJ, et al. Completion dissection or observation for sentinel-node metastasis in melanoma. *N Engl J Med*. 2017;376:2211-2222.
2. Leiter U, Stadler R, Mauch C, et al. Final analysis of DeCOG-SLT trial: no survival benefit for complete lymph node dissection in patients with positive sentinel node. *J Clin Oncol*. 2019;27:3000-3008.

Chapter 38 Popliteal Dissection

Michael E. Egger and Kelly M. McMasters

DEFINITION

- Popliteal dissection, or popliteal lymphadenectomy, is the removal of all lymph node–bearing tissue from the popliteal fossa. This procedure is most commonly performed for melanoma but may be performed for other malignancies that metastasize to lymph nodes and are best treated with a lymphadenectomy.
- Popliteal dissection, like other lymphadenectomies, is no longer routinely performed for patients with sentinel lymph node positive melanoma. Indications for a popliteal dissection include:
  - Clinically apparent lymph node metastases, in the absence of systemic metastases, in patients unable to undergo systemic therapy
  - Salvage lymphadenectomy after systemic therapy in which nodal disease persists in the popliteal fossa
- Boundaries of the popliteal fossa (**FIGURE 1**):
  - Superomedial: semitendinosus and semimembranosus muscles
  - Superolateral: biceps femoris muscle
  - Inferomedial: medial head of the gastrocnemius muscle
  - Inferolateral: lateral head of the gastrocnemius muscle and plantaris muscle
  - Roof: skin, superficial fascia, deep (popliteal) fascia
  - Floor: popliteal surface of femur, capsule of knee joint, oblique popliteal ligament, fascia overlying popliteus muscle

PATIENT HISTORY AND PHYSICAL FINDINGS

- A thorough history should be elicited prior to treatment, including a detailed past medical and surgical history, present medications and allergies, and a personal and family history of cancer. A complete head-to-toe skin examination should be performed. All lymph node basins (cervical, supraclavicular, axillary, epitrochlear, inguinal, popliteal) should be evaluated for clinically apparent lymph nodes.
- Clinically apparent lymph nodes typically present as a palpable mass. However, enlarged lymph nodes in the popliteal fossa may not be easily palpable because of the thick overlying fascia. Therefore, a careful examination of the popliteal fossa is essential.

IMAGING AND OTHER DIAGNOSTIC STUDIES

- A clinically positive lymph node should be evaluated using fine needle aspiration biopsy. Popliteal dissection is performed for a positive biopsy.
- For patients with clinically negative lymph nodes, preoperative lymphoscintigraphy should be performed at the time of the initial sentinel lymph node biopsy even if the primary melanoma is located on an extremity. Lymphoscintigraphy will demonstrate drainage to popliteal lymph nodes in 1% to 9% of patients with distal lower extremity melanoma (ie, below the knee; **FIGURE 2**).[1-6] By far, the most common locations for primary melanomas that drain to the popliteal fossa are the posterolateral foot and posterior lower leg; however, primary melanomas of the anterior lower leg or anteromedial aspect of the foot will also occasionally drain to the popliteal fossa.[1-4] The overall incidence of a positive popliteal lymph node is 0.3% to 2.8%.[1-3,5]

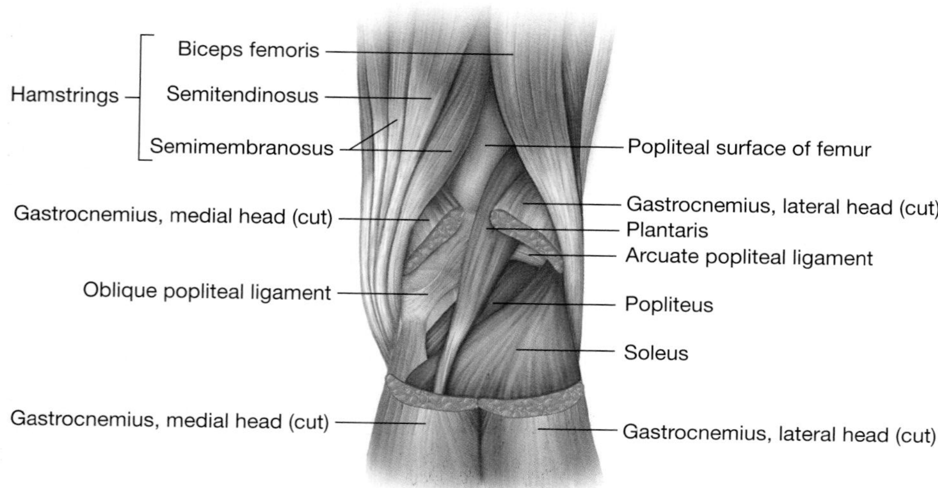

FIGURE 1 ● Boundaries of the popliteal fossa (right leg).

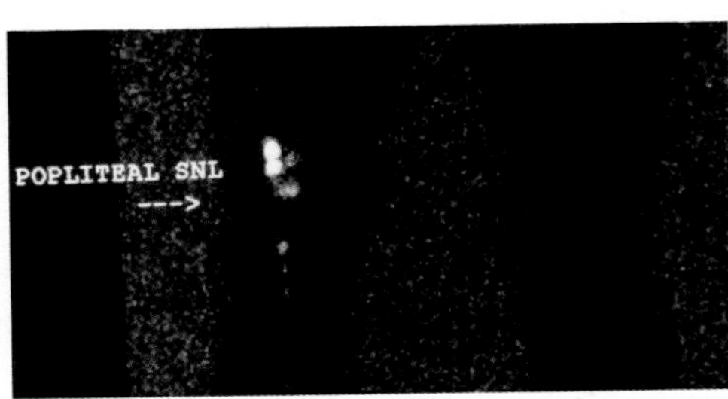

FIGURE 2 ● Lymphoscintigraphy demonstrating lymphatic drainage to the popliteal fossa from a primary melanoma of the distal right foot.

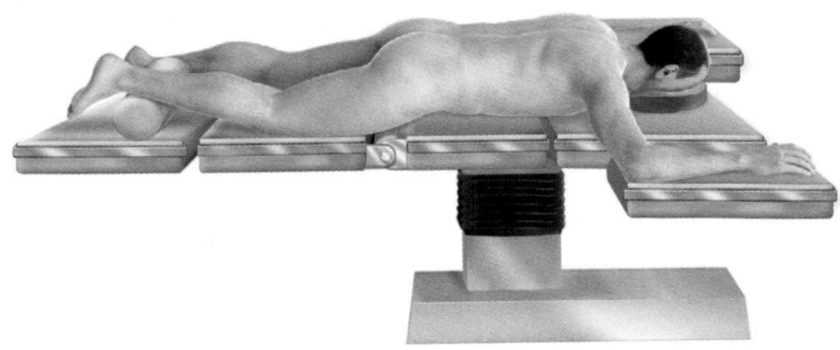

FIGURE 3 ● Patient position for popliteal dissection. Note that the operative leg (right) is slightly flexed.

SURGICAL MANAGEMENT

Preoperative Planning

- In the preoperative area, a focused history and physical examination should be repeated, and the patient's prior pathology and imaging studies should be reviewed.
- The patient should be marked to confirm laterality.
- Although there are no data that specifically address the wound infection rate in popliteal dissection, we favor the administration of a dose of preoperative antibiotics, particularly if concomitant inguinal dissection is planned.

Positioning

- The patient is placed prone, with pressure points padded and the operative knee slightly flexed (**FIGURE 3**). The operative leg should be prepped circumferentially from above the midthigh to below the midcalf.
- If a concomitant inguinal dissection is planned, the popliteal dissection is usually performed first.

TECHNIQUES

PLACEMENT OF INCISION

- There are two options for the incision for popliteal dissection (**FIGURE 4**). The incision should be planned such that a prior incision for sentinel lymph node biopsy can be excised.
  - The S-shaped incision was described by Karakousis[7] in his initial report of the technique of popliteal dissection. This incision typically extends from approximately 10 cm proximal to the joint crease along the lateral thigh overlying the biceps femoris muscle, crosses the joint transversely, and extends approximately 10 cm distal to the joint crease along the medial calf overlying the medial aspect of the gastrocnemius muscle (**FIGURE 4A**). A mirror image of this incision, extending from the medial thigh to the lateral

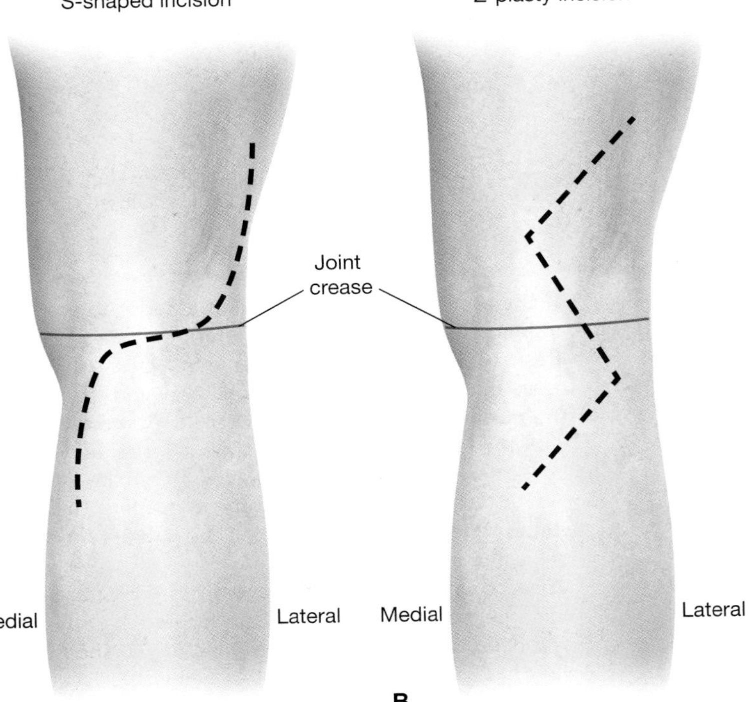

FIGURE 4 ● Incisions for popliteal dissection (right leg). **A,** S-shaped incision. **B,** Z-plasty incision.

calf, is also acceptable and may be preferable depending on the orientation of any previous incisions.

- We prefer a Z-plasty incision that allows for optimal exposure and heals without joint contracture.[8] Again, the orientation is typically superolateral to inferomedial. The width and length of the Z is relative to the size of the lower thigh, usually with an interior angle ranging from 100° to 120° (**FIGURE 4B**).

SKIN INCISION AND RAISING OF FLAPS

- The incision is sharply made, and dissection is carried down through the subcutaneous tissues. Medial and lateral flaps are raised while traction is maintained with skin hooks. The flaps should extend to all the boundaries of the popliteal fossa, remaining above the deep fascia.
- The lesser saphenous vein is exposed inferiorly; it should be ligated and divided (**FIGURE 5**).

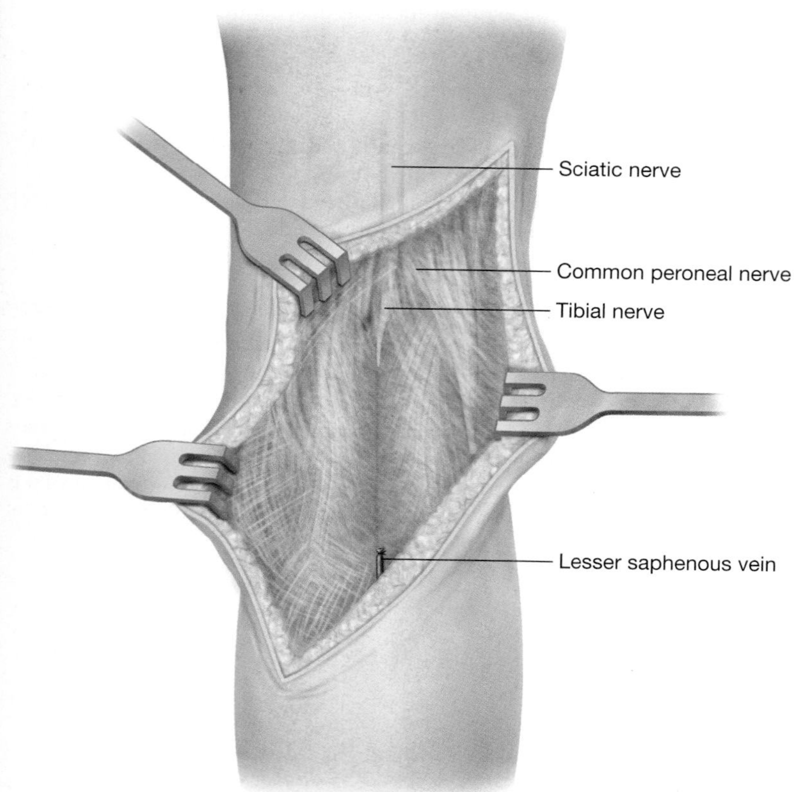

FIGURE 5 ● Medial and lateral skin flaps are raised, and the lesser saphenous vein is divided (right leg).

INCISION OF THE DEEP FASCIA AND IDENTIFICATION OF STRUCTURES TO BE PRESERVED

- The deep fascia is incised vertically with great care not to injure underlying structures; the nerves are very superficial (**FIGURE 6**).
- The common peroneal nerve runs laterally in the field, just medial to the biceps femoris muscle. The lateral sural nerve branches medially from it and eventually connects inferiorly with the medial sural nerve to form the sural nerve. The lateral sural nerve may be sacrificed if necessary; no significant deficit is appreciated as long as the medial sural nerve remains intact.
- The tibial nerve is the most superficial midline structure. It lies lateral to the popliteal vessels at the superior aspect of the popliteal fossa then courses anterior to the vessels and lies medial to them at the inferior aspect of the popliteal fossa. The medial sural nerve branches off the tibial nerve and descends in the groove between the heads of the gastrocnemius muscle to where it connects inferiorly with the lateral sural nerve. The medial sural nerve should be preserved if possible; however, it can be divided if greater access to deeper structures is needed. The patient will experience sensory loss along the lateral aspect of the ankle and foot.
- Upon opening the fibrinous sheath of the popliteal vessels, the popliteal artery will be located slightly medial and deep to the popliteal vein (**FIGURE 7**). The popliteal vein has several small tributaries below the level of the lesser saphenous vein branch, which can cause bothersome bleeding.

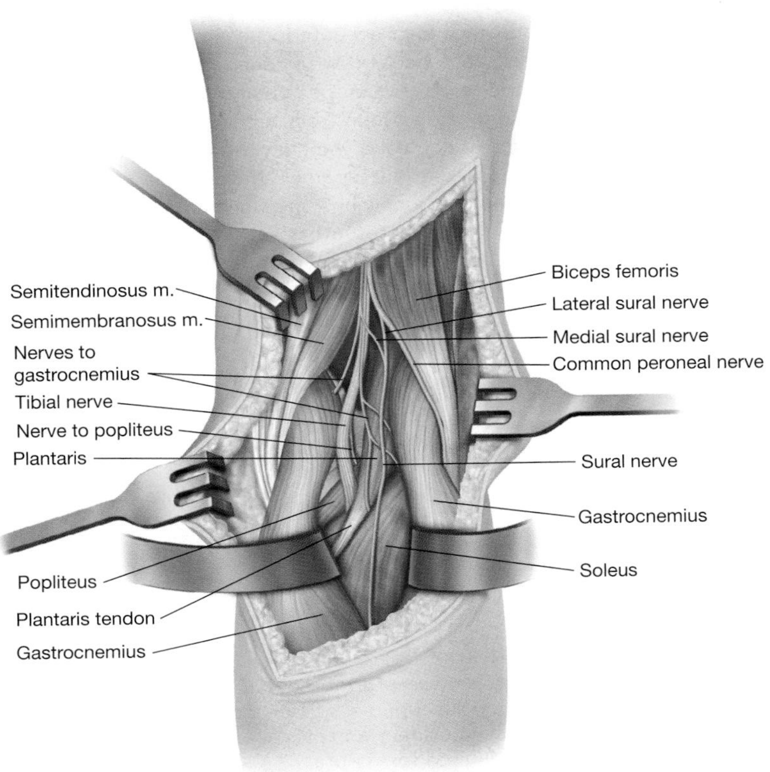

FIGURE 6 ● Upon opening the deep fascia and entering the popliteal fossa, the nerves are exposed (right leg).

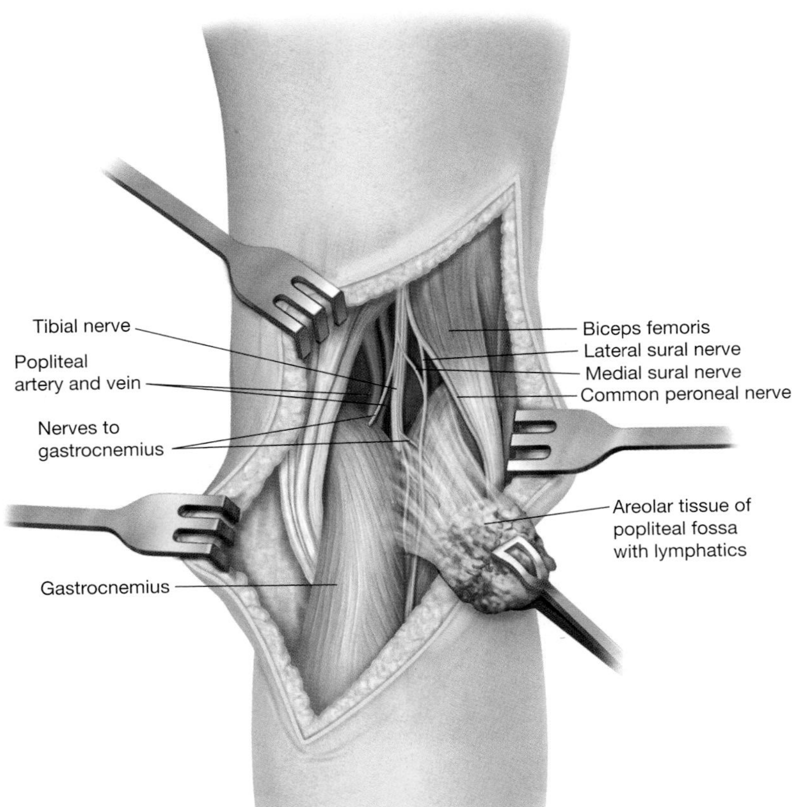

FIGURE 7 ● The nodal specimen is swept away from the nerves and vessels (right leg). Careful attention must be paid to the space between the popliteal vessels and the knee joint (anterior/deep to the vessels) as one to two lymph nodes are commonly located here and are easily overlooked.

DISSECTION OF FIBROFATTY NODE–BEARING TISSUE AWAY FROM NERVES AND VESSELS

- The fibrofatty node–bearing tissue is dissected sharply away from the nerves and vessels and is removed in continuity, with care to preserve all important structures (**FIGURES 7** and **8**).
- It is important to recognize that one or two lymph nodes are frequently located in the space between the popliteal artery and the knee joint (ie, anterior to the popliteal artery from the anatomic perspective or deep to the popliteal artery from the perspective of the operating surgeon). These lymph nodes are often overlooked; this space should be carefully dissected to not leave lymphatic tissue behind.
- After removal of the specimen, the popliteal fossa should be evaluated thoroughly by inspection and palpation to ensure that all lymphatic tissue has been resected, especially any grossly abnormal or enlarged lymph nodes.
- The specimen is sent to pathology for permanent section.

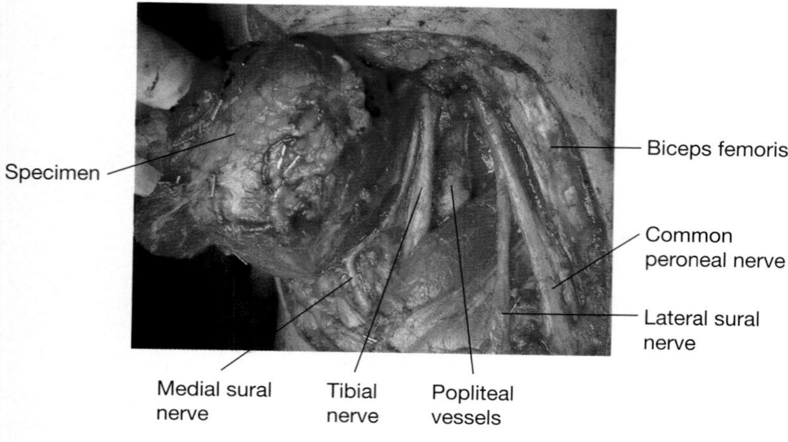

FIGURE 8 ● Photograph depicting resection of bulky disease in the popliteal fossa (right leg). Skin and subcutaneous tissue were resected en bloc with the specimen, and plastic surgical reconstruction was required for closure.

CLOSURE

- Hemostasis is achieved. The wound is irrigated copiously with saline.
- A 15-Fr round fluted, closed suction drain is placed into the wound and brought out through a separate stab incision (usually inferiorly; **FIGURE 9**).
- The incision is closed using absorbable suture for the deep dermis and a subcuticular stitch for the skin. A sterile dressing is applied.

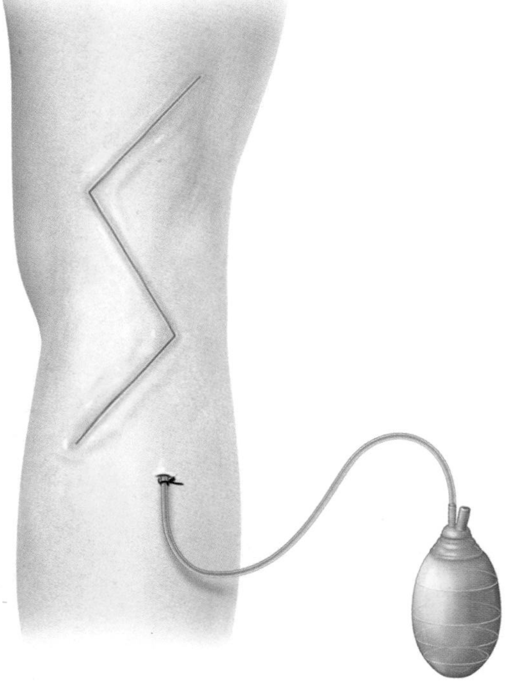

FIGURE 9 ● The drain is brought out through a separate stab wound inferiorly (right leg).

PEARLS AND PITFALLS

Indications	■ Clinically palpable lymph nodes may be difficult to appreciate in the popliteal fossa because of thick overlying fascia. ■ Most patients currently undergo popliteal lymph node dissection for failure to respond to systemic therapy.
Incision	■ Options are S-shaped and Z-plasty to preserve joint function. ■ Orient incision so that any prior biopsy scar is excised (usually superolateral to inferomedial).
Raising of medial and lateral flaps	■ Extend flaps to boundaries of popliteal fossa. ■ Ligate and divide lesser saphenous vein inferiorly.
Incision of the deep fascia and identification of structures to be preserved	■ Take care as fascia is incised; important structures lie directly beneath it. ■ Identify common peroneal nerve, tibial nerve, medial sural nerve, lateral sural nerve, popliteal artery, and popliteal vein. ■ Division of lateral sural nerve alone results in no significant deficit. ■ Division of medial sural nerve results in sensory loss.
Dissection of fibrofatty node–bearing tissue away from nerves and vessels	■ Remember to dissect the space between the popliteal artery and the knee joint (ie, anterior or deep to the artery), as one or two lymph nodes are frequently identified in this location and are easily overlooked.
Closure	■ Place a drain.

POSTOPERATIVE CARE

- The patient remains hospitalized at least overnight, but perhaps for several days, depending on the extent of other lymphadenectomies that may have been performed during the same operation. A posterior knee splint (knee immobilizer) is used for the first few postoperative days to allow for wound healing prior to returning to full mobility. Ambulation is often initially difficult; physical therapy is useful. The drain may be removed when output falls below 30 mL/d for two consecutive days. Typically, this is a relatively short interval compared with drain times for axillary or inguinal dissections.

OUTCOMES

- Lymphedema is rare after popliteal dissection, and the functional outcome of the knee is usually excellent.
- The popliteal fossa is historically reported to contain 6 to 7 lymph nodes.[7] However, contemporary experience suggests that finding far fewer nodes is more common.[8] In a recent study of 15 patients who underwent popliteal sentinel lymph node biopsy, the mean number of popliteal lymph nodes harvested was 1.4 (range was 1-3); however, in six patients who subsequently underwent completion popliteal dissection, the mean number of lymph nodes in the popliteal dissection specimen was 0.3, with four of the six patients' specimens yielding no additional (nonsentinel) lymph nodes.[2]
- With the advances in systemic immunotherapy and targeted therapy for melanoma, and the omission of routine completion lymphadenectomy for positive SLN melanoma, it is difficult to comment on the anticipated outcomes for popliteal dissection in the contemporary era. Overall, the 5-year survival for patients with stage III melanoma (lymph node–positive disease) ranges widely (14%-85%), with the 5-year survival of a patient with a single microscopically positive lymph node approximating 70%.[9,10] For patients with clinically apparent lymph node metastases, 5-year survival is much worse, on the order of 30% to 50% without adjuvant therapy, with high rates of systemic metastases.[9,11] Adjuvant therapy with immune checkpoint inhibitors in these patients improves survival.[12,13]
- Presumably, popliteal dissection should only be performed in rare clinical circumstances, for patients who have persistent disease isolated to the popliteal lymph node basin after adequate systemic immunotherapy or targeted therapy. It is our opinion that there is a role for operative lymphadenectomy in these patients, but the outcomes for these particular situations will need to be evaluated as experience with this indication grows. For patients presenting with clinically apparent lymph node metastases in the popliteal fossa, we would encourage consideration of enrollment in neoadjuvant therapy trials, since this approach is likely our most promising treatment for this high-risk patient population.[14,15]

COMPLICATIONS

- Common complications of popliteal dissection include wound infection (cellulitis or abscess), seroma, and hematoma.
- Injury to the common peroneal nerve results in postoperative foot drop and sensory loss or paresthesia over the dorsum of the foot (including the space between the great and second toes) and lateral shin.
- Injury to the tibial nerve results in postoperative loss of plantar flexion of the foot, loss of flexion of the toes, weakened inversion of the foot, and sensory loss or paresthesia over the posterior aspect of the leg and the sole of the foot.

REFERENCES

1. Thompson JF, Hunt JA, Culjak G, et al. Popliteal lymph node metastasis from primary cutaneous melanoma. *Eur J Surg Oncol.* 2000;26:172-176.
2. Steen ST, Kargozaran H, Moran CJ, et al. Management of popliteal sentinel nodes in melanoma. *J Am Coll Surg.* 2011;213:180-187.
3. Menes TS, Schachter J, Steinmetz AP, et al. Lymphatic drainage to the popliteal basin in distal lower extremity malignant melanoma. *Arch Surg.* 2004;139:1002-1006.

4. Uren RF, Howman-Giles R, Thompson JF. Patterns of lymphatic drainage from the skin in patients with melanoma. *J Nucl Med.* 2003;44:570-582.
5. Marone U, Caraco C, Chiofalo MG, et al. Resection in the popliteal fossa for metastatic melanoma. *World J Surg Oncol.* 2007;5:8.
6. Nijhuis AAG, de AO Santos Filho ID, Uren RF, et-al. Clinical importance and surgical management of sentinel lymph nodes in the popliteal fossa of melanoma patients. *Eur J Surg Oncol.* 2019;45:1706-1711.
7. Karakousis CP. The technique of popliteal node dissection. *Surg Gynecol Obstet.* 1980;151:420-423.
8. Sholar A, Martin RCGII, McMasters KM. Popliteal lymph node dissection. *Ann Surg Oncol.* 2005;12:189-193.
9. Balch CM, Gershenwald JE, Soong SJ, et al. Multivariate analysis of prognostic factors among 2,313 patients with stage III melanoma: comparison of nodal micrometastases versus macrometastases. *J Clin Oncol.* 2010;28:2452-2459.
10. Morton DL, Thompson JF, Cochran AJ, et al. Sentinel-node biopsy or nodal observation in melanoma. *N Engl J Med.* 2006;355:1307-1317.
11. Khosrotehrani K, van der Ploeg AP, Siskind V, et al. Nomograms to predict recurrence and survival in stage IIIB and IIIC melanoma after therapeutic lymphadenectomy. *Eur J Cancer.* 2014;50:1301-1309.
12. Eggermont AMM, Blank CU, Mandala M, et al. Adjuvant pembrolizumab versus placebo in resected stage III melanoma. *N Engl J Med.* 2018;378:1789-1801.
13. Weber J, Mandala M, Del Vecchio M, et al. Adjuvant nivolumab versus ipilimumab in resected stage III or IV melanoma. *N Engl J Med.* 2017;377:1824-1835.
14. Blank C, Rozeman E, Fanchi L, et al. Neoadjuvant versus adjuvant ipilimumab plus nivolumab in macroscopic stage III melanoma. *Nat Med.* 2018;24:1655-1661.
15. Amaria R, Reddy S, Tawbi H, et al. Neoadjuvant immune checkpoint blockade in high-risk resectable melanoma. *Nat Med.* 2018;24:1649-1654.

Chapter 39 Robotic Pelvic Node Dissection

Jeffrey S. Montgomery and Michael S. Sabel

DEFINITION

- The robotic-assisted transperitoneal approach to the pelvic lymph node dissection (PLND) is widely used for the staging and treatment of urologic and gynecologic malignancies. It can also be used in patients with melanoma in the pelvic lymph nodes.
- The robotic-assisted pelvic lymph node dissection allows for excellent exposure and visualization of the pelvis. Compared to the open approach, it minimizes postoperative pain and improves recovery time. It also allows for improved visualization of the iliac and obturator nodes.
- While pelvic lymph node dissection can be performed with a strictly laparoscopic approach, the robotic approach has the advantage of 3D visualization, ergonomic, intuitive control, and wristed instruments with more precise movements. This is advantageous given the close proximity to the iliac vessels and obturator nerve.

ANATOMY

- See **FIGURE 1**.
- The pelvic nodes include several groups that receive lymphatic drainage from the lower extremity and pelvic organs. These include the external iliac nodes, internal iliac nodes, common iliac nodes, obturator and presacral nodes.
- The pelvic lymph node dissection for melanoma primarily involves the external iliac and obturator nodes—the node-bearing tissue that is in direct communication with the inguinal nodes. The sacral nodes and common iliac nodes are not routinely included in the melanoma dissection as these are generally considered stage IV disease, although they may be excised in more extensive dissections.
- The *external iliac nodes* are located above the pelvic brim, along the external iliac vessels, and receive drainage from the inguinal lymph nodes. There are packets of nodes lateral to the artery, medial to the vessels, as well as above the external iliac artery and between the artery and vein.
- The *obturator node*s are situated in the obturator fossa in close proximity to the obturator internus muscle and obturator nerve.
- The *internal iliac nodes* form a cluster around the anterior and posterior divisions of the internal iliac artery. In addition to the inferior pelvic organs, they receive drainage from the external iliac nodes. The internal iliac nodes can also receive drainage from the perineum, buttock, and back of the thigh.

INDICATIONS

- For patients presenting with clinically evident inguinofemoral disease, the performance of concomitant PLND was controversial, as the prevalence of positive iliac/obturator nodes is around 30%. PLND was considered for patients at higher

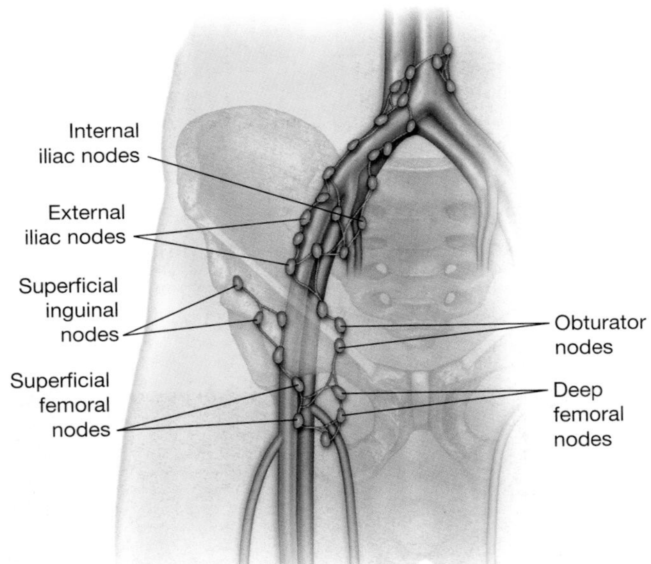

FIGURE 1 ● Anatomy of the pelvic lymph nodes.

risk of pelvic disease (>3 inguinal nodes, positive Cloquet node) or with radiographic suspicion of pelvic disease.

- Today, the majority of melanoma patients are clinically node negative, with nodal disease identified through intraoperative lymphatic mapping (IOLM) and sentinel lymph node (SLN) biopsy. Prior to the publication of the Multicenter Selective Lymphadenectomy Trial II (MSLT-II), patients with a positive inguinal SLN returned to the operating room (OR) for an inguinofemoral lymph node dissection. After the publication of MSLT-II, the majority of patients with positive SLN are observed with ultrasound surveillance of the groin. Lymph node dissection is reserved for patients who present with clinically evident disease, or have a regional recurrence after SLN biopsy, without evidence of distant metastases.
- While many patients recur with disease isolated to the inguinal region, others may recur only in the pelvis, or in both locations. Iliac/obturator nodal metastases should not be thought of as stage IV disease, with 5-year survival rates after complete resection ranging from 25% to 40%, prior to the immunotherapy era.
- Given the improved visualization of the pelvic nodes and the decreased postoperative pain, the retroperitoneal pelvic lymph node dissection (rPLND) is the preferred approach for patients with isolated pelvic recurrence. Patients with extensive prior abdominal or pelvic surgery may be better candidates for the open approach.

IMAGING AND OTHER DIAGNOSTIC STUDIES

- See **FIGURE 2**.
- Staging to rule out stage IV disease is imperative; however, the majority of melanoma patients with iliac/pelvic adenopathy will be detected on thorough imaging, either CT scan of the chest, abdomen, and pelvis, or positron emission tomography (PET) scan. This might include patients with metastases to the inguinal lymph nodes (either clinically detected inguinal lymph nodes or a positive SLN) undergoing initial staging studies, or on surveillance imaging.
- A thorough history and physical exam, and blood tests including a complete blood count, comprehensive metabolic profile and serum lactate dehydrogenase (LDH) level, should be performed to rule out signs or symptoms of stage IV disease that may require additional, more directed imaging. If not already done, an MRI of the brain to rule out brain metastases, even in asymptomatic patients, should also be performed.
- While some patients may have already undergone an inguinal lymph node dissection, many patients with positive inguinal SLN may have opted for nodal observation with ultrasound as an alternative to LND, as per the MSLT-II results. For patients who have not had an inguinal lymph node dissection, physical exam and adequate imaging (CT scan including the inguinal basin or PET scan) are critical to determine whether patients have simultaneous inguinal recurrence.
- For patient with both inguinal and external iliac disease, the iliac nodes can be excised along with the inguinofemoral nodes by dividing the inguinal ligament (which provides excellent exposure of the distal external iliac nodes), or through a retroperitoneal approach through a separate incision (which provides higher exposure and avoids the morbidity of a divided inguinal ligament) as described in Part 5, Chapter 35.
- For patients with inguinofemoral and more extensive pelvic disease, an inguinal lymph node dissection (ILND) may be performed (either open or minimally invasive) in conjunction with a robotic pelvic node dissection.
- Image-guided core biopsy to establish a diagnosis of iliac/pelvic node involvement is strongly recommended. Enlarged or "hot" iliac pelvic nodes can occasionally be false positive, reactive nodes following biopsy or surgery.
- For patients who have not had prior systemic therapy, neoadjuvant therapy should be strongly considered for patients presenting with iliac or pelvic node involvement. This may include neoadjuvant immunotherapy with PD-1 blocking antibodies, or for patients harboring activating mutations in the BRAF V600 gene, neoadjuvant therapy with BRAF/MEK inhibition. For patients who have a complete clinical response, omission of the node dissection is presently being investigated in clinical trials. Outside of clinical trials, patients undergoing neoadjuvant therapy should still undergo PLND following treatment, even if a complete clinical response on CT or PET is noted. For patients who have had prior systemic therapy and have iliac/pelvic recurrence, multidisciplinary discussion regarding options for neoadjuvant therapy vs proceeding directly to surgery.

SURGICAL MANAGEMENT

Operating Room Setup and Patient Positioning

- Positioning must be done with consideration of conversion to open and for inguinofemoral dissection if this is being performed as a combined procedure.

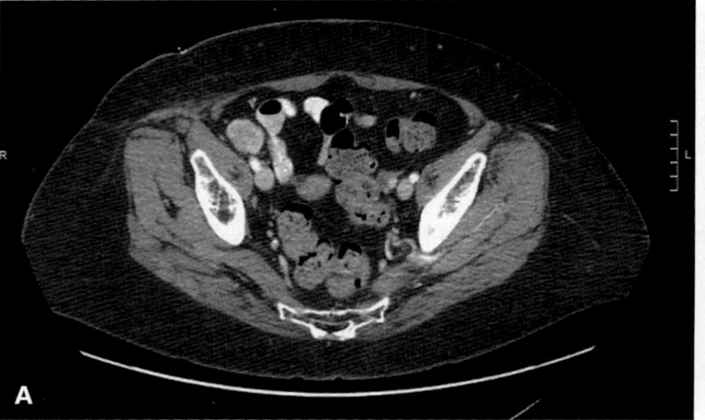

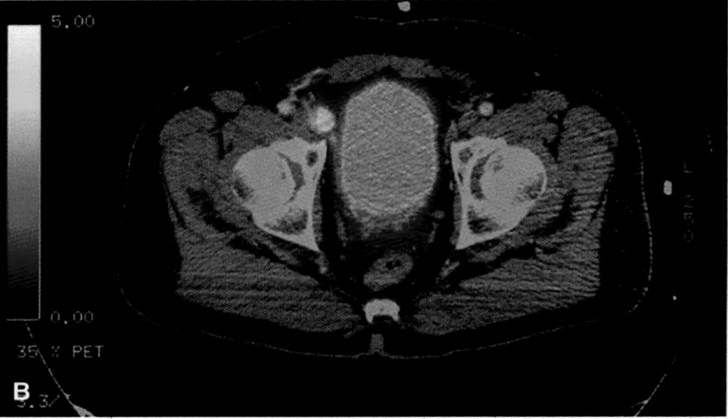

FIGURE 2 ● CT scan of the pelvis demonstrating an enlarged pelvic node.

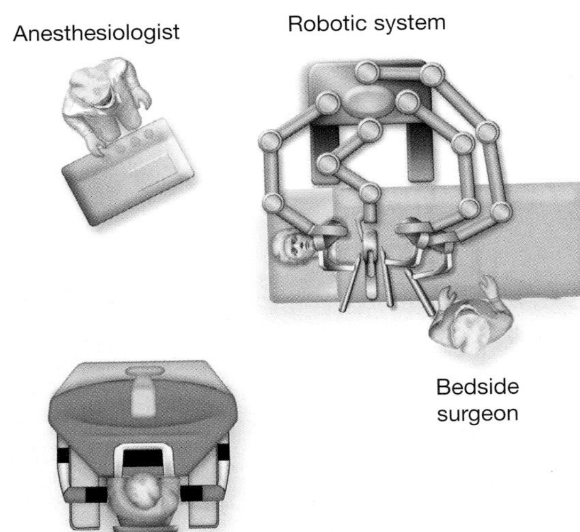

FIGURE 3 ● Docking of the robot to the side of the patient.

- If rPLND is being done in conjunction with ILND, the order in which the two procedures are completed is not important, understanding that some minor leg repositioning will be necessary. The rPLND extends distally under the inguinal ligament so that, with an inguinofemoral dissection, the inguinal and pelvic node spaces are connected, removing all possible nodes. In so doing, the inguinal ligament is left intact.
- For the rPLND, the patient is placed in the Trendelenburg position—approximately 30° from horizontal. Depending on the system, the robot is either docked between the legs of the patient or side-docked (**FIGURE 3**).

PORT PLACEMENT

- See **FIGURE 4**.
- An 8-mm port is placed 1 to 2 cm above the umbilicus in the midline.
- Two 8-mm robotic ports are placed on the left side, the most medial port approximately 10 cm directly lateral from the top of the umbilicus, the most lateral 8 cm lateral and inferior from this port.
- A 12-mm assistant port is placed 2 cm above and slightly medial of the measured midline between the camera port and the most medial left sided port.
- An 8-mm robotic port is placed 8 cm directly lateral from the top of the umbilicus on the right.

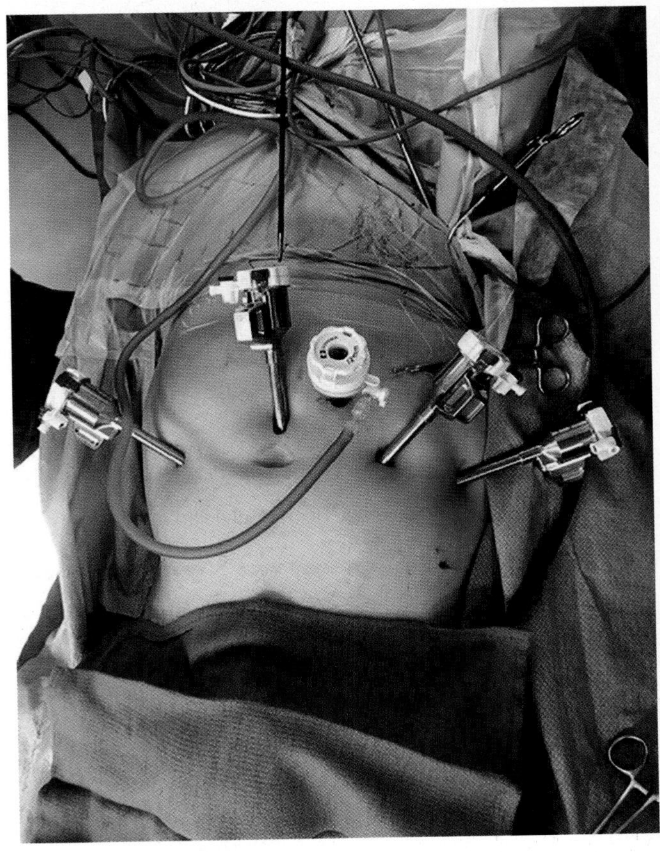

FIGURE 4 ● Port placement.

EXPOSURE

- The abdominal cavity is assessed for any evidence of distant metastases. Exposure of the pelvis is obtained to view the relevant anatomy. Adhesions are lysed as needed to gain full exposure of the pelvis on the side the dissection (**FIGURE 5**).
- The peritoneum is incised over the external iliac artery from the common iliac artery to the level of the vas deferens or round ligament at the internal ring (**FIGURE 6**). The ureter can often be seen coming over the common iliac artery. Depending on the patient's age and desire to preserve fertility, fulgurating and transecting the vas deferens or round ligament allows more freedom to open the lateral vesical space. Otherwise, these structures can be preserved. Using both blunt and sharp dissection, the lateral vesical space is developed fully exposing the iliac vessels (external iliac artery and vein, internal iliac artery and vein and the distal common iliac vessels) and pelvic nodal packets (**FIGURE 7**).
- The lymph node packets can then be isolated and dissected free from the surrounding structures. It is important to note that given the inflammatory nature of melanoma, involved lymph nodes are often densely adherent to vessels and nerves. Great care must be taken when dissecting on these structures to avoid injury and rupturing of any metastatic nodes. There are times when the surgeon must decide if possible injury to the pelvic vessels is oncologically worth a complete resection. Alternatively, the surgeon could elect to leave the inflamed outer nodal rind on the vessels vs aborting the procedure.
- Some surgeons elect to use clips during dissection to assure lymphostasis. Given the fact that the peritoneum is open to the abdominal cavity as a peritoneal window, the use of clips is not essential. Patients very rarely develop symptomatic lymphoceles that require management after pelvic lymph node dissection.

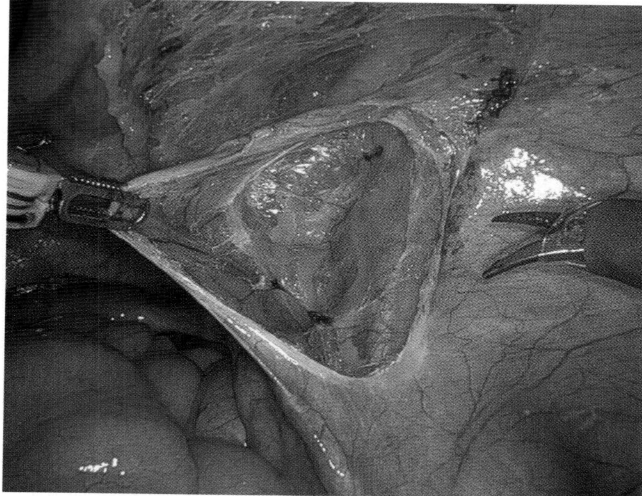

FIGURE 6 ● Incision of the peritoneum over the external iliac artery.

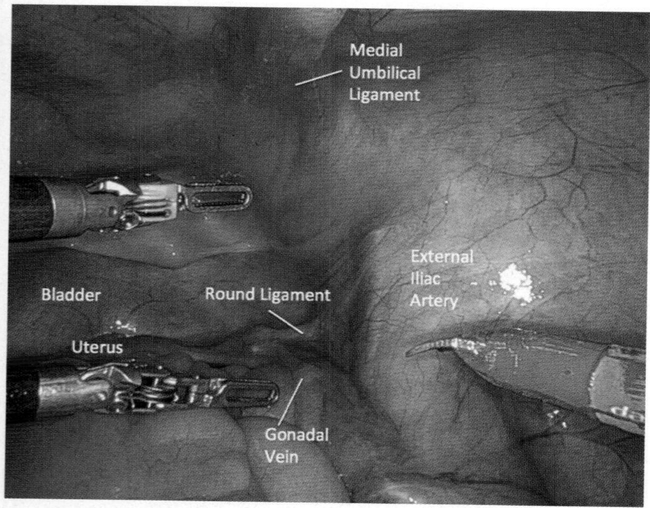

FIGURE 5 ● Exposure of the pelvic anatomy.

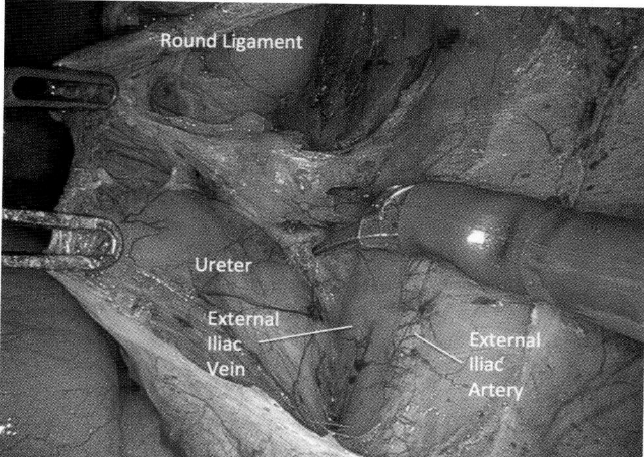

FIGURE 7 ● The iliac vessels are fully exposed revealing the pelvic lymph node packets.

EXTERNAL ILIAC DISSECTION

- The lymph node packet lateral to and overlying the external iliac artery and vein is dissected from underneath the inguinal ligament to the iliac bifurcation (**FIGURE 8**). This can be extended superiorly to include the common iliac lymph nodes if indicated.
- Depending on the adherence of any involved nodes to the vessels, the adventitia and areolar tissue overlying the vessels should be left on the vessels. Removing the entire nodes is important, but this does not require stripping the vessels of their adventitia.
- The lateral side of the lymph node packet is dissected off the psoas muscle.

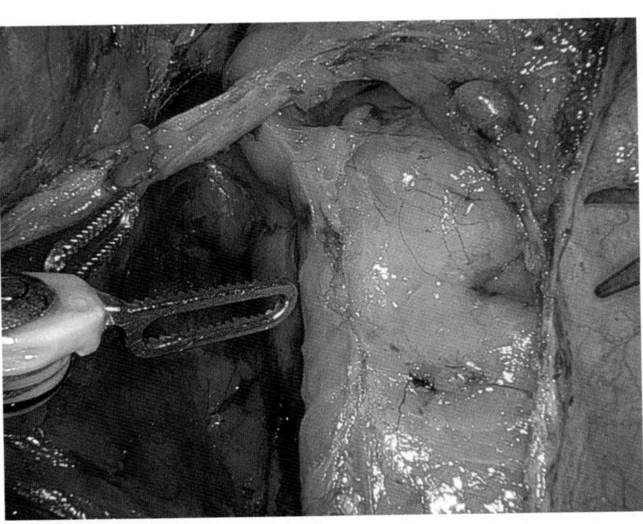

FIGURE 8 ● Developing the external iliac node packet.

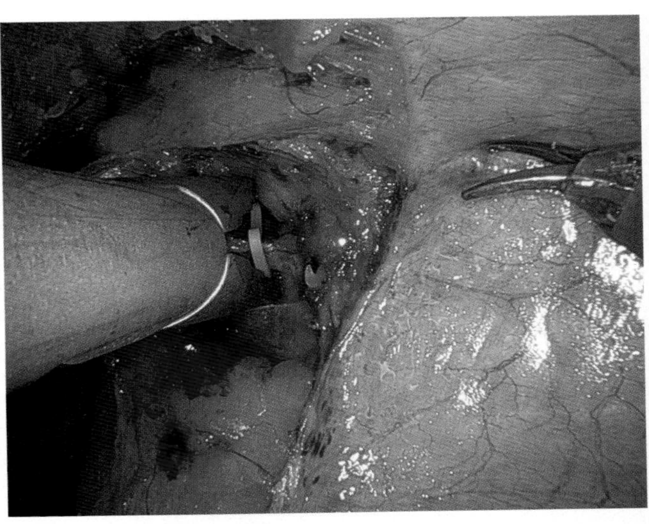

FIGURE 9 ● Clipping the distal lymphatics of the external iliac node packet.

- If possible, it is best to begin with the distal dissection under the inguinal ligament. This allows gravity to help retract the nodal tissue off of the vessels. If a prior inguinal dissection has been completed, a clip during this dissection may indicate that the nodal tissue communicating with the inguinal nodal station has been included in your dissection. Alternatively, if the inguinofemoral dissection will follow, leaving a clip at the distal extent of the pelvic dissection aids in identifying a complete nodal resection.
- During this distal dissection, the origin of the inferior epigastric artery and vein may be intimately adherent to the nodal packet. If possible, these vessels should be preserved, but occasionally they need to be sacrificed for a complete dissection of involved nodes. It is preferred to clip these vessels prior to fulguration and transection to secure hemostasis.
- There are several small branches of the genitofemoral nerve that travel through the external iliac nodal packet. It is impossible to preserve these branches. The patient should be counseled that they may have numbness of the medial thigh after surgery as a result of transecting these nerve branches. This numbness may diminish over several months or may be permanent. The main genitofemoral nerve running lateral to the external iliac artery should be preserved, though, if at all possible.
- Any vessels or lymphatics feeding the node packet can be clipped or cauterized and transected (**FIGURE 9**).
- Once free from the artery and muscle, the tissue is dissected off of the vein. The areolar tissue connecting the nodal packet to the vein can be safely excised with sharp dissection (**FIGURE 10**).
- Once freed, this node packet can be placed in the lateral vesical space or elsewhere in the pelvis to be bagged and extracted after the remaining dissection is completed (**FIGURE 11**).

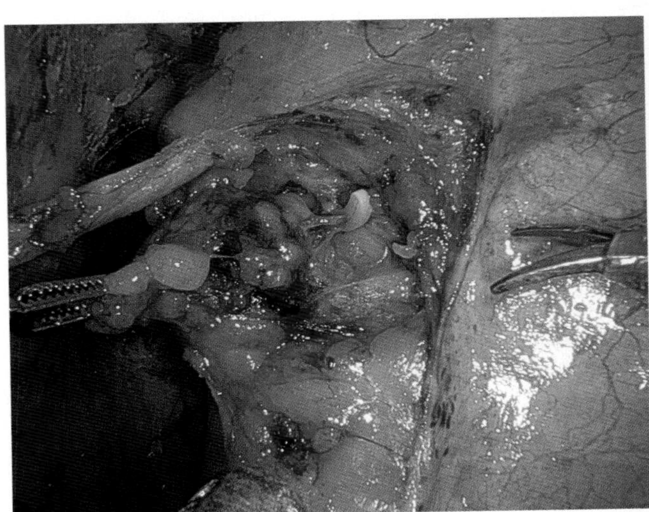

FIGURE 10 ● Dark lymph nodes containing melanoma are visualized within the external iliac node packet.

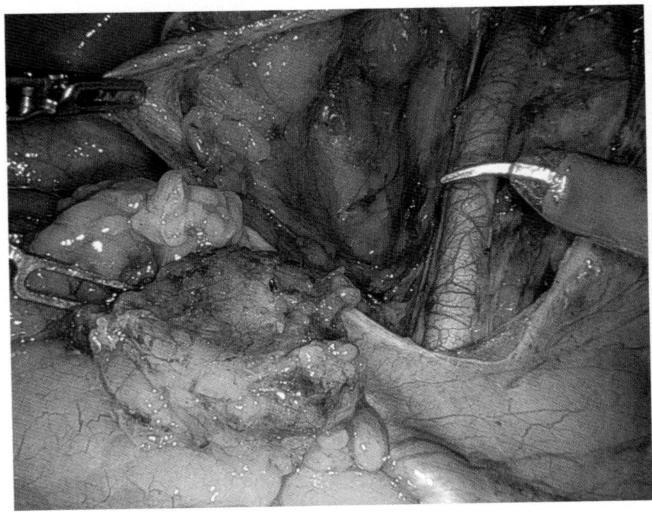

FIGURE 11 ● External iliac node packet resected free.

OBTURATOR DISSECTION

- The iliac vein is retracted superiorly. Again, the distal-most dissection should be completed under the inguinal ligament. The nodal packet either needs to be split and rolled off of the obturator vein, or alternatively, this vein can be fulgurated and/or clipped and transected without consequence (**FIGURES 12** and **13**).
- The obturator nerve and vessels should be identified early in the dissection at the posterior aspect of the obturator node packet. Care should be taken to avoid injury of these structures (**FIGURE 14**).
- The lymph node packet is dissected off of the obturator muscle. There is fatty tissue and small vessels between these structures that can be controlled and transected with cautery.
- At the superior base of the dissection, the nodal packet dives lateral to the obturator nerves and inferior to the external iliac vein. There are often significant vessels feeding the nodal packet at this proximal portion. This tissue should be isolated as pedicles that can be controlled and transected with cautery, freeing the packet.
- The nodes can then be collected in a laparoscopic sack (**FIGURE 15**). This can often be removed via the 12-mm assistant port. If there is significant nodal bulk, the sack should be removed via the midline camera port after extending the skin and fascial incisions.

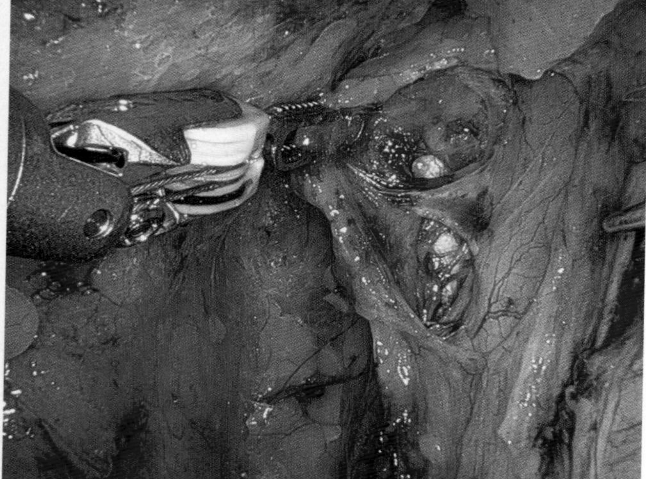

FIGURE 12 ● The obturator nodes and obturator vein. The nodal packet can be split and brought under the obturator vein, or the vein can be ligated.

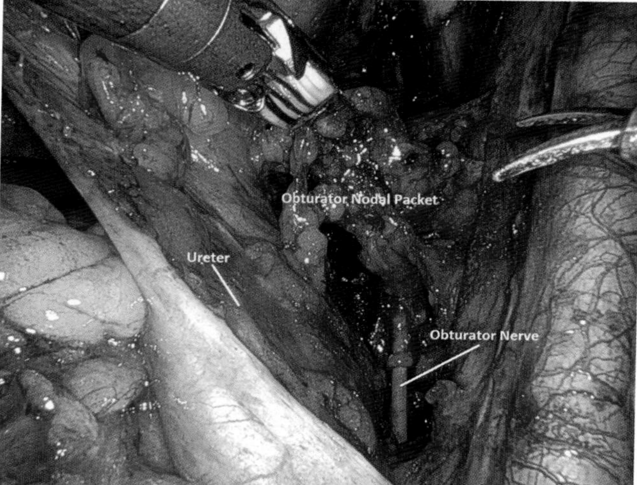

FIGURE 14 ● Taking great care, the obturator nodal packet is dissected free from the obturator nerve and vessels.

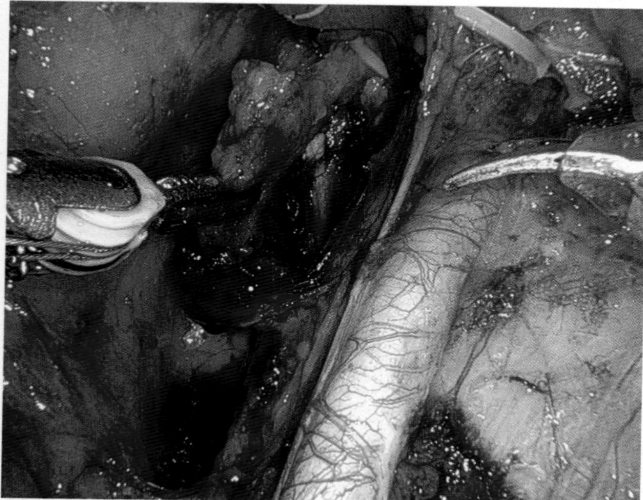

FIGURE 13 ● The lymphatics leading to the distal obturator nodes are clipped.

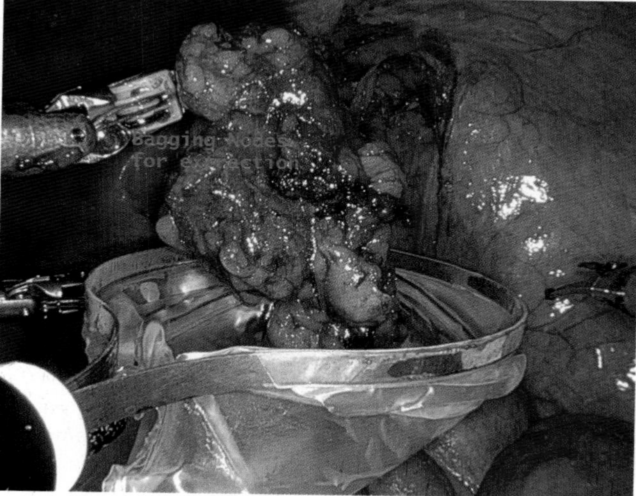

FIGURE 15 ● The external iliac and obturator nodes are placed into a laparoscopic sack.

CLOSURE

- The robot is undocked and the case is converted to laparoscopy, using the robotic camera as a laparoscope.
- The 12-mm assistant port can be closed with a 0-Vicryl suture in a figure-of-eight fashion under direct vision using the Carter-Thomason device.
- If it was necessary to extract the nodal tissue via an extended midline abdominal incision, the fascia is closed with interrupted 1-Vicryl sutures in a figure-of-eight fashion.
- After irrigation of the subcutaneous fat, the skin is closed with a running Monocryl and surgical glue. Injection of the peri-incisional skin with local anesthetic prior to closure is helpful for managing postoperative pain.

PEARLS AND PITFALLS

Indications and preoperative evaluation	■ Complete history and physical examination, blood work, CT scan or PET scan and brain MRI to rule out stage IV disease. ■ Strongly consider neoadjuvant immunotherapy or targeted therapy prior to PLND. ■ Patients with both inguinal and iliac/pelvic disease can undergo open inguinal-iliac dissection or ILND (open or minimally invasive) with robotic pelvic node dissection.
Patient selection	■ Patients with extensive prior abdominal or pelvic surgery may be better suited to the open approach.
Abdominal exploration	■ Assess the abdominal cavity for evidence of stage IV disease not seen on staging CT or PET.
Visualization of neurovascular structures	■ In addition to the vessels, great care is needed to identify and preserve the ureter, genitofemoral nerve, obturator nerve. ■ The inferior epigastric artery and vein can be preserved, but may need to be sacrificed for complete dissection. ■ Depending on the patient's age and preferences, transecting the vas deferens or round ligament may improve visualization and access to the lateral vesical space.
Dissection	■ Sharp dissection is favored over blunt when the inflamed metastatic nodes are densely adherent to the vessels. ■ To avoid serious injury to the iliac vessels and/or obturator nerve, the inflamed rind of the metastatic node can be left on the structure. ■ Assure that you dissect the external iliac and obturator node packets anterior to the pubic arch and as far distally under the inguinal ligament as possible. Leave clips at the most distal extent of these node packets for easy identification if a ILND is to follow.

POSTOPERATIVE CARE

- If the rPLND was performed without complication, the patients can be discharged same day from the recovery room.
- For patients undergoing rPLND in conjunction with an inguinofemoral dissection, the patient is typically admitted for 23-hour observation.
- Pain is typically well controlled with over-the-counter acetaminophen and/or a nonsteroidal anti-inflammatory drug.
- Once the pathology report returns, patients will require postoperative consultation with medical oncology for adjuvant therapy (or continuation of systemic therapy begun in the neoadjuvant setting). In select cases, adjuvant radiation therapy may be considered, particularly if systemic therapy options are limited. Presentation at a multidisciplinary tumor board is strongly recommended.

COMPLICATIONS

- Surgical site infection
- Abscess
- Postoperative bleeding
- Small bowel obstruction
- Urinary dysfunction
- Urinary infection
- Obturator nerve injury/paralysis

Chapter 40 Epitrochlear Dissection

Adil Ayub and Douglas Tyler

DEFINITION

Epitrochlear Lymph Node Dissection

- Epitrochlear lymph node involvement occurs in a minority of patients with hand, wrist, and forearm melanoma. The epitrochlear nodes typically consist of one to four lymph nodes located in the distal medial upper arm and the medial antecubital fossa and form an integral part of the superficial lymphatic system.[1] The epitrochlear lymph node basin, which is also referred to as the "epitrochlear triangle," is roughly defined by the medial head of triceps muscle, the short head of biceps muscle, and the medial epicondyle[2] (**FIGURE 1**).
- Possible indications for epitrochlear lymph node dissection include either a clinically detected, biopsy-proven node or a positive epitrochlear sentinel lymph node biopsy (SLNB).[3]
- Since the advent of lymphatic mapping and sentinel lymph node biopsy, there appeared to be an increase in performance of epitrochlear dissections.[4] Today, with the publication of two prospective randomized trials showing equivalent melanoma-specific survival for patients with a positive sentinel lymph node randomized to either completion lymphadenectomy or observation with serial clinical examinations and nodal ultrasonography, patients with a positive epitrochlear SLN may be followed with serial ultrasounds of the epitrochlear and axillary basins, with complete dissection reserved for patients who experience a regional recurrence.[5,6]
- Understanding the anatomy of the epitrochlear triangle is crucial especially for surgeons who deal with melanomas.

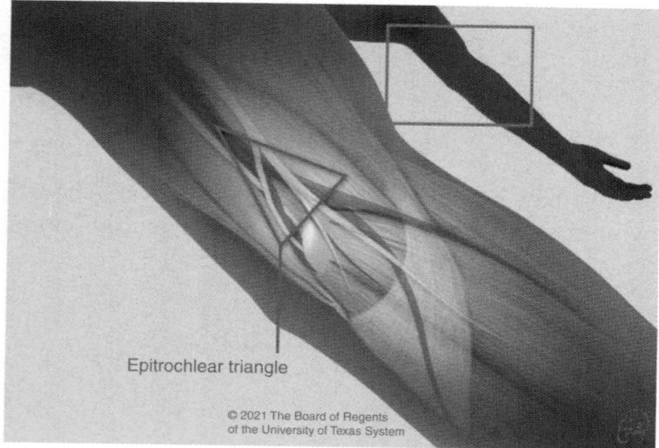

FIGURE 1 ● Epitrochlear triangle: Roughly defined by the medial head of triceps muscle, the short head of biceps muscle, and the medial epicondyle. (Copyright used with the permission of The Board of Regents of the University of Texas System through The University of Texas Medical Branch.)

PATIENT HISTORY AND PHYSICAL FINDINGS

- A thorough history and physical examination should be performed. Examination should include comprehensive skin exam including bilateral lymph node basins (supraclavicular, cervical, axillary, epitrochlear, and inguinal nodes) to rule out any other abnormal skin lesions or nodes that may require further workup.

IMAGING AND OTHER DIAGNOSTIC STUDIES

- The majority of patients with upper extremity melanomas do not present with clinically obvious epitrochlear nodes. Therefore, lymphoscintigraphy forms an integral part in workup to identify involvement of epitrochlear and/or axillary lymph node. Patient with epitrochlear nodes identified on lymphoscintigraphy should undergo SLNB of the epitrochlear basin.
- For clinically palpable epitrochlear nodes, image-guided biopsy should be performed for diagnosis. Melanoma patients with clinically evident disease or disease recurrence are often recommended to undergo complete staging. This should include magnetic resonance imaging (MRI) of the brain and body imaging, either with a computed tomography scan (CT) or positron emission tomography (PET/CT).
- Other imaging techniques such as an ultrasound, CT scan, or MRI may be used in selected cases to delineate the anatomy and study characteristics of the nodes including the number, size, concerning features, and proximity to adjacent neurovascular structures.

SURGICAL MANAGEMENT

Preoperative Planning

- Prior to surgery, all imaging especially lymphoscintigraphy should be reviewed, and any involvement of axillary lymph node basin should be noted as this may affect decision making to do concomitant axillary lymph node dissection.

Positioning

- The patient is positioned supine with the target arm abducted and extended on an arm board. Foam padding is placed on the arm board to elevate the arm and to prevent hyperextension injury. We generally recommend a circumferential arm prep with a stockinette on the hand. The prep should also include the chest wall and axilla on the ipsilateral side (**FIGURE 2**). If a simultaneous axillary lymph node dissection or sentinel lymph node biopsy is planned, the scapula should be elevated using a bump and prepped as well.

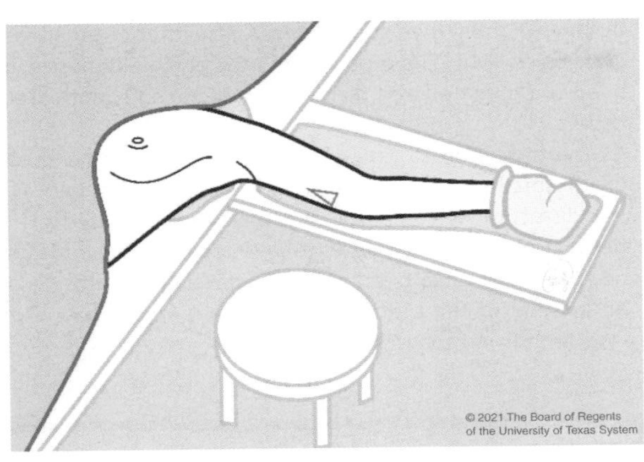

FIGURE 2 ● Patient positioning and prep (including the chest, the axilla, and the whole arm and forearm up to the wrist). (Copyright used with the permission of The Board of Regents of the University of Texas System through The University of Texas Medical Branch.)

INCISION

- A longitudinal incision is made starting from a point approximately 5 cm proximal to the medial epicondyle (**FIGURE 3**). The incision is extended distally and curved medially and transversely across the antecubital region to the medial edge of the brachioradialis muscle. If a prior scar/incision is present, it should be included in the incision.

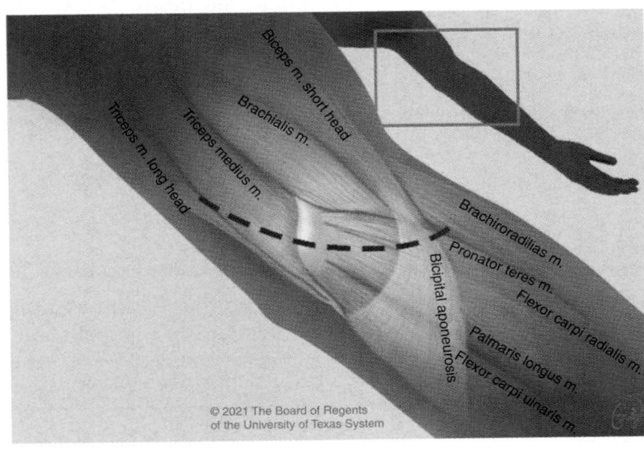

FIGURE 3 ● Incision is made starting from a point approximately 5 cm proximal to the medial epicondyle and extended distally and curved medially and transversely across the antecubital region to the medial edge of the brachioradialis. (Copyright used with the permission of The Board of Regents of the University of Texas System through The University of Texas Medical Branch.)

DISSECTION

- Small skin flaps are raised to optimally expose the fascia. The fascia is divided longitudinally to identify the underlying muscles (biceps, short head of triceps, brachioradialis, and flexor carpi radialis) (**FIGURE 4**). Self-retaining retractors are used for exposure. The epitrochlear lymph nodes lie just beneath the muscular fascia and bicipital aponeurosis (**FIGURE 5**). The subcutaneous and lymphatic tissue deep to the bicep aponeurosis is carefully dissected. Dissection then proceeds proximally, with en bloc resection of the lymphoareolar tissue found within the confines of the epitrochlear triangle (bordered by the biceps muscle, the triceps muscle, and the medial epicondyle). The proximal extent of the lymphadenectomy is where the brachial artery crosses the medial intermuscular septum. The inferior aspect is defined by the

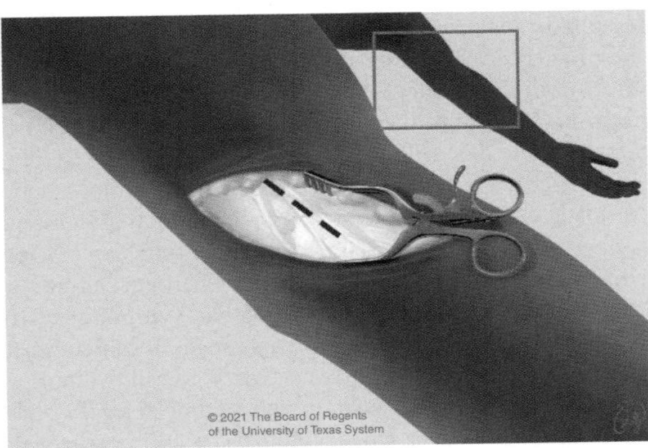

FIGURE 4 ● Fascial incision. (Copyright used with the permission of The Board of Regents of the University of Texas System through The University of Texas Medical Branch.)

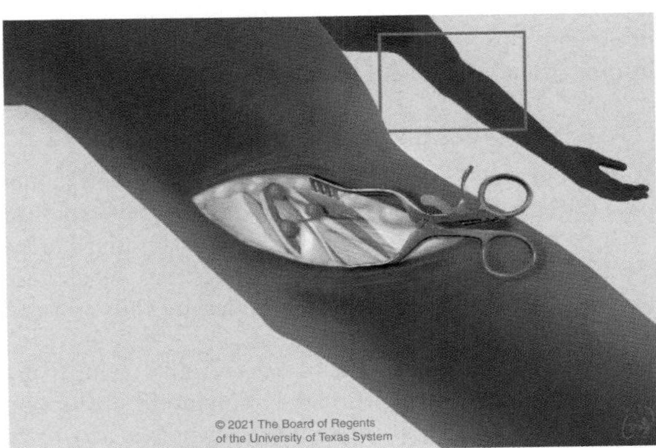

FIGURE 5 ● Use of self-retaining retractors for exposure. (Copyright used with the permission of The Board of Regents of the University of Texas System through The University of Texas Medical Branch.)

proximal lateral edge of the pronator teres and flexor carpi radialis and the medial edge of the brachioradialis. The base of the epitrochlear space is the brachialis muscle.

- During the dissection, the superficial branches of the basilic vein are ligated. An attempt is made to preserve the basilic vein and the branches of the median antebrachial cutaneous nerve by retracting these structures. The median nerve and the brachial artery lie deep to the bicep muscle and their location should be identified by palpation. Typically, the exposure of median nerve and brachial artery is not required unless there is concern for involvement of these structures by clinical nodal metastatic disease. The inferior ulnar collateral vessels, which lie superficial to the brachialis muscle, may need to be ligated and divided to remove all lymphoareolar tissue.
- As the dissection is undertaken, small clips can be used to divide small lymphatic vessels and small blood vessels. Once the dissection is complete, the specimen is passed off the field. Occasionally, superior cubital fossa lymph nodes may be found at or just deep to the bicipital aponeurosis at the bifurcation of the brachial artery. These nodes may also be resected during the dissection.

CLOSURE

- Once the dissection is completed, hemostasis is achieved. The wound is irrigated with saline and closed in layers. A small, closed suction drain can be left in the basin. The wound is dressed with Kerlix and an ACE wrap.

PEARLS AND PITFALLS

Preoperative care	■ Perform a complete skin and bilateral nodal basin examination. Review imaging and if axillary nodes are involved, prep the axilla and ipsilateral chest as well.
Placement of incision	■ If a prior scar is present, consider including it within the incision.
Dissection	■ Care should be taken to dissect carefully around neurovascular structures especially preserving branches of median antecubital brachial nerve, brachial artery and median nerve.
Closure	■ If the dissection is extensive, consider leaving a small, closed suction drain to prevent seroma formation. Consider doing ipsilateral axillary lymph node dissection in selected situations.

POSTOPERATIVE CARE

- After the procedure, patients are generally discharged same day. Compressive dressing is left for 24 to 48 hours to help with hemostasis and relieve tension on the skin closure. Drain is usually removed when output is less than 20 mL/d.

DATA AND OUTCOMES

- Most melanomas of the distal upper extremity tend to metastasize to the axillary basin lymph nodes. However, occasionally they may drain to the epitrochlear basin and failure to detect affected epitrochlear lymph nodes may be a cause of tumor relapse.[7,8] The epitrochlear nodes are thus considered an "in-transit" target.[1]
- The overall incidence of in-transit sentinel lymph nodes in patients undergoing sentinel lymph node evaluation is around 2% to 10%. Of these in-transit nodes, 5% to 25% are found to be in the epitrochlear nodes.[4,9-11] The reported incidence of metastases in these epitrochlear lymph node ranges from 2.4% to 18%.[3,8,12,13]
- When performing lymphatic mapping of the upper extremity and an epitrochlear lymph node lights up, we generally recommend also mapping the axilla to identify a sentinel lymph node there as well. Some lymphatic channels can bypass the epitrochlear system and go directly to the axilla. At the time of surgery, we prefer to dissect out the axillary sentinel lymph node first before removing the epitrochlear sentinel lymph node to minimize any disruption of the lymph flow (carrying blue dye and radiolabeled colloid) to the axilla.
- Historically, when a positive epitrochlear lymph node is identified, a completion epitrochlear lymph node dissection was performed. Current data from the Multicenter Selective Lymphadenectomy Trial II (MSLT-II) and German Dermatologic Cooperative Oncology Group-Selective Lymphadenectomy Trial (DeCOG-SLT) randomized trials suggest that completion lymph node dissection is not necessary for individuals with small volume tumor burden in the sentinel lymph node.[5,14] However, what defines small volume is a little controversial, but we generally consider this to be less than 1 cm diameter of tumor deposit. For disease greater than 1 cm, or that is clinically

palpable, consideration of neoadjuvant treatment with either a target therapy or systemic immunotherapy should be considered. Several recent trials have suggested that this approach prior to surgical resection, is associated with improved disease-free survival in stage III patients.[15-18]

- Another question that arises in patients who undergo epitrochlear lymph node dissection due to the presence of metastatic disease is whether axillary lymph node dissection should also be performed. To this direction, research data remain controversial. If the epitrochlear lymph node is clinically positive or has a tumor deposit greater than 1 cm, some groups advocate that these patients undergo a concurrent axillary dissection, at the time of their complete epitrochlear dissection.[8] However, other studies conclude that in the absence of clinical or radiographically positive axillary lymph nodes, an axillary dissection is not required.[1,10] Therefore, the clinical decision making should be catered to every case; however, special consideration should be given to patients with palpable epitrochlear nodal metastases, because up to 50% of these patients have subclinical involvement of their axillary nodes[3]

COMPLICATIONS

- Seroma
- Hematoma
- Wound infection/cellulitis
- Damage to neurovascular structures in the proximity (median nerve, median antebrachial cutaneous nerve, brachial artery, basilic vein)

REFERENCES

1. Karantonis F-F, Vakis G, Papadopoulos O. *Epitrochlear lymph node dissection*. In: *Non-Melanoma Skin Cancer and Cutaneous Melanoma*: Springer; 2020:747-749.
2. Tanabe KK. Lymphatic mapping and epitrochlear lymph node dissection for melanoma. *Surgery*. 1997;121(1):102-104.
3. Wong SL, Tyler DS, Balch CM, Thompson JF, McMasters KM. Axillary and epitrochlear lymph node dissection for melanoma. *Cutaneous Melanoma*. 2020:657-667.
4. Hochwald SN, Kissane N, Grobmyer SR, Lopes J. Epitrochlear lymph node dissection. *Ann Surg Oncol*. 2011;18(2):505.
5. Faries MB, Thompson JF, Cochran AJ, et al. Completion dissection or observation for sentinel-node metastasis in melanoma. *N Engl J Med*. 2017;376(23):2211-2222.
6. Leiter U, Stadler R, Mauch C, et al. Final analysis of DeCOG-SLT trial: no survival benefit for complete lymph node dissection in patients with positive sentinel node. *J Clin Oncol*. 2019;27:3000-3008.
7. Catalano O, Nunziata A, Saturnino PP, Siani A. Epitrochlear lymph nodes: anatomy, clinical aspects, and sonography features. Pictorial essay(). *J Ultrasound*. 2010;13(4):168-174.
8. Kidner TB, Yoon JL, Faries MB, Morton DL. Epitrochlear sentinel lymph nodes in melanoma: interval or independent?. *Am Surg*. 2012;78(6):702-705.
9. Uren RF, Howman-Giles RB, Thompson JF. Failure to detect drainage to the popliteal and epitrochlear lymph nodes on cutaneous lymphoscintigraphy in melanoma patients. *J Nucl Med*. 1998;39(12):2195.
10. McMasters KM, Chao C, Wong SL, et al. Interval sentinel lymph nodes in melanoma. *Arch Surg*. 2002;137(5):543-547; discussion 547-549.
11. Carling T, Pan D, Ariyan S, Narayan D, Truini C. Diagnosis and treatment of interval sentinel lymph nodes in patients with cutaneous melanoma. *Plast Reconstr Surg*. 2007;119(3):907-913.
12. Smith TJ, Sloan GM, Baker AR. Epitrochlear node involvement in melanoma of the upper extremity. *Cancer*. 1983;51(4):756-760.
13. Hunt JA, Thompson JF, Uren RF, Howman-Giles R, Harman CR. Epitrochlear lymph nodes as a site of melanoma metastasis. *Ann Surg Oncol*. 1998;5(3):248-252.
14. Leiter U, Stadler R, Mauch C, et al. Complete lymph node dissection versus no dissection in patients with sentinel lymph node biopsy positive melanoma (DeCOG-SLT): a multicentre, randomised, phase 3 trial. *Lancet Oncol*. 2016;17(6):757-767.
15. Moschos SJ, Edington HD, Land SR, et al. Neoadjuvant treatment of regional stage IIIB melanoma with high-dose interferon alfa-2b induces objective tumor regression in association with modulation of tumor infiltrating host cellular immune responses. *J Clin Oncol*. 2006;24(19):3164-3171.
16. Eggermont AM, Chiarion-Sileni V, Grob JJ, et al. Prolonged survival in stage III melanoma with ipilimumab adjuvant therapy. *N Engl J Med*. 2016;375(19):1845-1855.
17. Amaria RN, Reddy SM, Tawbi HA, et al. Neoadjuvant immune checkpoint blockade in high-risk resectable melanoma. *Nat Med*. 2018;24(11):1649-1654.
18. Huang AC, Orlowski RJ, Xu X, et al. A single dose of neoadjuvant PD-1 blockade predicts clinical outcomes in resectable melanoma. *Nat Med*. 2019;25(3):454-461.

Chapter 41

Intralesional Injection of Melanoma In-Transit Metastases

Danielle K. DePalo, Kelly M. Elleson, Michael J. Carr, and Jonathan S. Zager

DEFINITION

- Melanoma in-transit metastases (ITM) are metastases located within the subdermal and dermal lymphatics, between the primary melanoma site and draining lymph node basin. ITM are considered non-nodal locoregional metastases, along with microsatellite and satellite metastases, which only differ by distance from the primary tumor according to the American Joint Committee on Cancer (AJCC). ITM are located >2 cm from the primary melanoma.[1]
- It is estimated that ITM may develop in up to 13% of melanoma patients. Tumor characteristics associated with higher risk of development of ITM include location of the primary tumor, Breslow depth, presence of ulceration, and age older than 50 years.[2,3]

DIFFERENTIAL DIAGNOSIS

- The diagnosis of ITM is usually clinical. They can have a varied presentation including flat lesions, nodules, or blisters, most of which are typically but not always pigmented (**FIGURE 1**). The number of lesions may range from a single lesion to hundreds of nodules and size varies from 1 to 2 mm to very large masses.
- Melanoma ITM present at a median time of 18 months after primary excision.[3] Differential diagnosis could include an additional primary melanoma, local recurrence, nonmelanoma skin cancer, benign skin lesions, and trauma to the skin, subcutaneous fat, and underlying soft tissues.

PATIENT HISTORY AND PHYSICAL FINDINGS

- When a patient presents with a dermal, subcutaneous, or deeper soft tissue nodule, it is imperative to review their history of sun exposure and skin cancers, especially a history of melanoma in the vicinity of the new possible in-transit nodules. For patients with a history of melanoma, it is important to determine the time from diagnosis and review prior pathology reports and treatment regimens.
- A total-body skin exam and lymph node evaluation should be performed on all patients presenting with a new in-transit nodule. Focused attention should be given to any abnormalities in close proximity to a prior melanoma resection site.
- Number of lesions, size, and site should be assessed to guide treatment options, including resection, and properly photo documented to monitor response. While surgical resection is the first-line treatment for isolated in-transit metastases, it may not be appropriate for patients with unresectable or numerous nodules, those with significant comorbidities, or those who are rapidly recurring with new lesions despite resections to negative margins.[4]

IMAGING AND OTHER DIAGNOSTIC STUDIES

- Any suspicious findings on physical exam, especially in close proximity to a previous melanoma, or between the location of the previous primary wide excision and the drainage

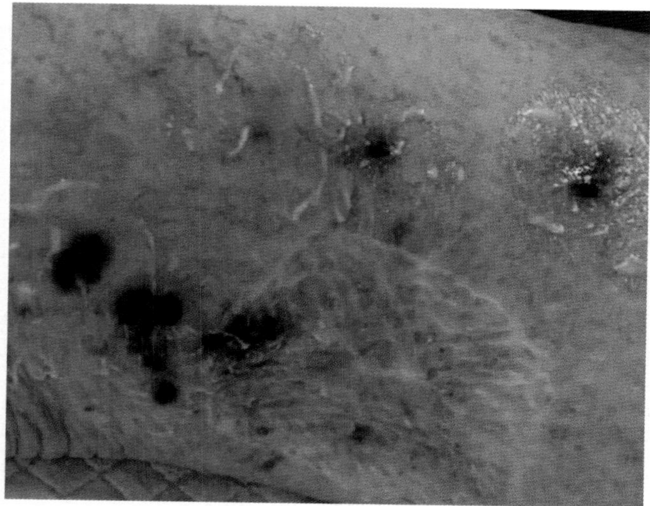

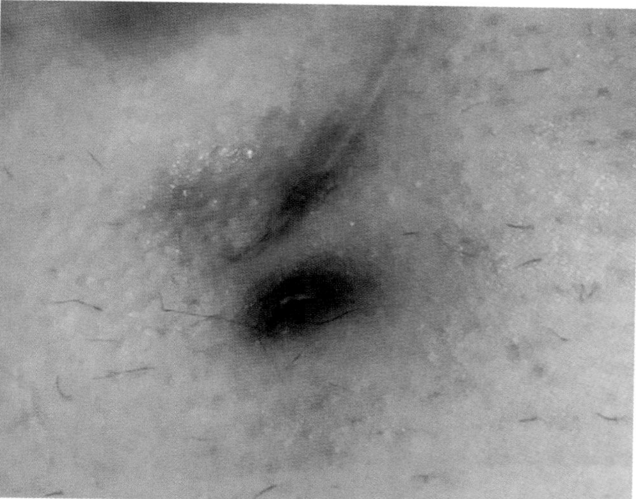

FIGURE 1 ● In-transit metastases. (Courtesy of Jonathan S. Zager, MD, Moffitt Cancer Center.)

regional nodal basin, should be evaluated pathologically by shave or core biopsy or fine needle aspiration. Excisional biopsy may be indicated in certain circumstances.[3,4]

- Regional nodal or distant disease may be synchronous or develop in up to 75% of patients with ITM.[5] Therefore, it is recommended that patients presenting with biopsy-proven ITM undergo total-body computed tomography (CT) imaging (neck, chest, abdomen, and pelvis), full body positron emission tomography (PET), and brain magnetic resonance imaging (MRI). CT of the brain may be performed if MRI is contraindicated.[3,4]

SURGICAL MANAGEMENT

Preprocedure Planning

Intralesional Injection Planning

- Available imaging and pathology should be reviewed prior to injection to ensure the patient is an appropriate candidate for intralesional injection and to determine if ultrasound guidance is needed for deeper lesions. Imaging can also help identify what lesions to inject in cases where in-transit metastases are too numerous for all to be injected. When there are many lesions present, focusing on the largest lesions is usually the best approach as discussed further in the "Technique and Steps" section. Additionally, allergies, medical history, and current medications should be reviewed.
- Patients should be counseled on the process of intralesional injection, the schedule of injections (which differs for various intralesional agents), recovery, side effects, risks, and benefits.
- The appropriate intralesional therapy should be selected after review of risks, benefits, and alternatives with the patient, as well as review of all available clinicopathologic data and imaging. Intralesional therapy may also be combined with systemic therapy (at this current time off protocol or on a clinical trial).
- Historically, Bacillus Calmette-Guerin (BCG) and cytokines including interleukin-2 (IL-2), interferon-a2b (IFN-a2b), and interferon-b (IFN-b), and granulocyte-macrophage colony-stimulating factor (GM-CSF) have been used as intralesional injections, but have fallen out of favor due to side effect profiles, treatment cost, injection frequency, and efficacy.[6-12]
- Talimogene laherparepvec (TVEC) is an oncolytic viral therapy created from live-attenuated herpes simplex virus type 1 that has been modified to express human GM-CSF.[13] It is, at this time, the preferred local therapy for unresectable ITM and is FDA approved for this indication.[4] **FIGURE 2** demonstrates baseline appearance and complete response of ITM to 6 months of TVEC therapy.
  - In the randomized open-label phase III OPTiM trial, which compared TVEC to GM-CSF in patients with unresectable stage IIIB-IVM1c melanoma, the primary end point of durable response rate (DRR, objective response lasting >6 months) was 16.3% and 2.1%, respectively. When examining all disease stages, overall survival (OS) was not significantly improved on TVEC compared to GM-CSF. However, when analyzed by stage of disease, a significant improvement in OS was found in stage IIB, IIC, and IVM1a disease in patients treated with TVEC compared to GM-CSF.[14]
  - The efficacy of TVEC at a single institution after it was made commercially available was retrospectively evaluated by Perez et al, finding an overall response rate (ORR) of 56.5% in 23 patients with a follow-up of at least 8 weeks and median 8.6 months. Complete response (CR) was seen in 43.5%, partial response (PR) in 13.1%, and stable disease (SD) in 21.7%.[15]

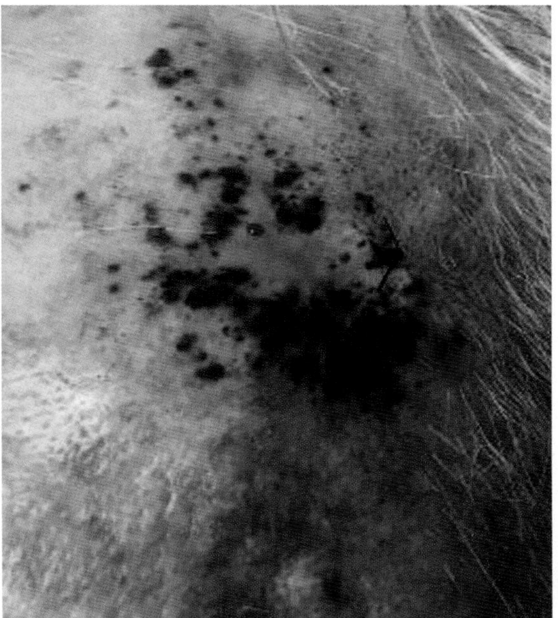
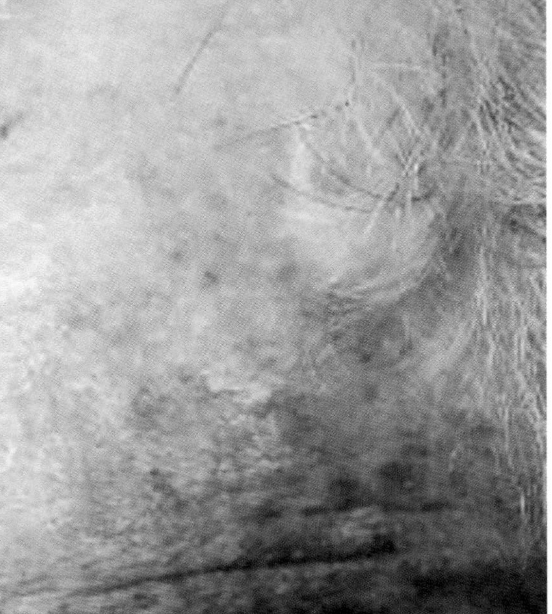

FIGURE 2 ● In-transit metastases at baseline and complete response after 6 months TVEC. (Courtesy of Jonathan S. Zager, MD, Moffitt Cancer Center.)

    - This real-world experience was expanded upon by Louie et al in a multi-institutional review of 121 patients who received commercially available TVEC. Of the 80 patients with treatment response data, CR was seen in 39%, with no evidence of disease (NED) at last follow-up in 37% of the complete responders, and PR was seen in 18% at a median follow-up of 9 months.[16]
    - COSMUS-1 was a multi-institutional observational study that sought to evaluate the role of TVEC in the modern real-world setting since the use of immunotherapies and targeted therapies became standard practice after the OPTiM trial closed to accrual in 2011. Of the 76 patients reviewed, 19.7% completed TVEC treatment with pathologic CR or no remaining injectable lesions. One-year OS was 76.7% in stage IIIB-IVM1a and 64.6% in stage IVM1b-c disease. In this study, checkpoint inhibitors were used prior to or concurrent with TVEC in 43.4% of patients while 22.4% were treated with TVEC alone. Median TVEC therapy duration was shorter in the COSMUS-1 review than compared to OPTiM, 3.0 vs 5.8 months, respectively.[17]
    - COSMUS-2 further evaluated the real-world use of TVEC with the use of checkpoint inhibitors, specifically anti-PD-1. Of the 83 patients, 26.5% received TVEC after anti-PD-1, 38.6% received TVEC concurrent with anti-PD-1, and 34.9% did not receive anti-PD-1. Of all patients, 25.3% completed treatment with no remaining injectable lesions in a median time of 4 months. However, efficacy was not evaluated by COSUMS-2.[18]
    - The efficacy of TVEC specifically after failure of immunotherapy was examined in 112 patients by Carr et al. In this multi-institutional retrospective review, the authors found an ORR of 51% with a 37% CR and 14% PR. The addition of TVEC to immunotherapy (concurrent), or sequential use of TVEC after immunotherapy did not appear to alter the ORR.[19]
  - PV-10, a 10% solution of rose bengal disodium, is a xanthene dye that was found to preferentially enter melanoma cell lysosomes and is theorized to cause release of proteases and subsequent melanoma cell death while sparing normal tissue.[20]
    - A phase II trial by Thompson et al injected PV-10 4 times over 16 weeks, ORR was 51% and complete response rate (CRR) was 26% in target lesions over 52 weeks of follow up.[21]
    - A phase III randomized controlled trial comparing PV-10 alone vs systemic dacarbazine, systemic temozolomide, or intralesional TVEC in patients who are not candidates for checkpoint blockade (CB) is ongoing (NCT02288897).
    - PV-10 in combination with pembrolizumab immunotherapy is being evaluated in a phase 1b/2 study in both CB naïve and refractory patients (NCT02557321). Preliminary data on 21 CB naïve patients revealed an ORR of 67% with 10% CR and 57% PR, PFS estimated at 11.7 months.[22] Preliminary results on 14 CB refractory patients revealed a 29% ORR with 7% CR and 21% PR.[23]
- There are numerous additional experimental intralesional agents currently being studied in clinical trials.[24,25] These include toll-like receptor (TLR) agonists, immunocytokines, and oncolytic viruses; some of the more established experimental therapies currently in clinical trials at this time are outlined below.
  - TLR agonists
    - Tilsotolimod, a TLR9 agonist, acts like endogenous TLR9 to activate Th1-type immune response, increase local antigen-presenting cell (APC) maturation, and increase expression of PD-1 and CTLA4 among other immune checkpoints.[26] The effect of systemic ipilimumab CTLA4 inhibition in combination with intratumoral tilsotolimod is under investigation in phase I/II trial ILLUMINATE-204.[27] In the 49 patients who received the recommended phase 2 dose, ORR was 22.4% with CR in 4% and PR in 18.4%.
    - SD-101 is a synthetic cytidine-phospho-guanosine (CpG) oligonucleotide that acts as a TLR9 agonist.[28] It has been evaluated in combination with pembrolizumab in a phase 1b trial, in 9 patients who were naïve to prior anti-PD-1/L1, ORR was 78% with 22% CR and 56% PR.[29] In the 13 patients who had received prior anti-PD-1/L1 therapy, 15% had ORR, all of those were PR.
    - CMP-001 is similar to SD-101 in that it is a TLR9 agonist that is an oligodeoxynucleotide CpG-A DNA coated in a virus-like particle.[30] A phase 1b trial in combination with pembrolizumab (NCT02680184) and phase 2 trial in combination with nivolumab (NCT03618641) are ongoing.
    - Other investigational TLR agonists include TLR9 agonists AST-008 (NCT03684785) and MGN1703 (NCT02668770), TLR7/8 agonists NKTR-262 (NCT03435640) and CV8102 (NCT03291002), and TLR7 agonist LHC165 (NCT03301896).[24,30-32]
  - Immunocytokines
    - Tavokinogene telseplasmid (Tavo), a plasmid encoding IL-12, intratumoral injection followed by electroporation increased the expression of IL-12 and IFN-γ and subsequent activation of the innate and adaptive immune system.[33,34] Electroporation is a tool for plasmid DNA delivery that acts to increase the cell membrane permeability and facilitate plasmid uptake.[35] In a phase II trial of Tavo with electroporation (Tavo-EP), ORR was 35.7% with CR in 17.9% of the 28 patients.[34] Tavo-EP in combination with pembrolizumab in anti-PD-1 refractory patients is actively being evaluated in KEYNOTE 695, a phase II clinical trial (NCT03132675). On interim analysis of 54 patients, ORR was 30% with CR in 6% and PR in 24%.[36]
    - Daromun is a combination immunocytokine of monoclonal L19 antibody fused with IL-2 and TNF-α. L19 has been shown to selectively bind to tumor cells through extradomain B of fibronectin, an extracellular matrix component present in newly formed blood vessels and neoplastic tissue.[37] The combination of L19TNF and L19IL-2 was found to act synergistically through both direct tumor cell necrosis and induction of a systemic antitumor response.[38] This was evaluated in a phase II trial, of 20 patients 5% experienced CR and 50% PR in treated ITM lesions at 12 weeks.[39] The neo-DREAM trial is an ongoing

phase III trial evaluating neoadjuvant Daromun vs surgery alone in surgically resectable IIIb/c melanoma (NCT03567889).[40]

- Oncolytic viral therapies
  - Canerpaturev (C-REV, previously HF10) is a HSV1 strain, HF10, with a naturally occurring genomic structure of deletions, insertions, and frame-shift mutations that allows it to preferentially infect and replicate in tumor cells, causing cytolysis and infiltration of intratumoral CD4, CD8, and natural killer cells.[41] A phase II trial of C-REV in combination with ipilimumab as a second line or later treatment had an ORR of 11%, all PR, in 27 patients at 48 weeks.[42] Neoadjuvant C-REV in combination with nivolumab is being evaluated in an ongoing phase II trial (NCT03259425).
  - Coxsackievirus A21 (CVA21, CAVATAK commercially) is an enterovirus that naturally preferentially infects neoplastic cells though its ability to bind intracellular adhesion molecule-1 (ICAM-1) as well as decay-accelerating factors (DAF), both receptor types are overexpressed on melanoma cells.[43] A phase II trial of CAVATAK in Late Stage Melanoma (CALM) found that in 57 patients, ORR was 28.1% with 75.4% 1-year survival.[44] Additional phase 1b trials of CAVATAK in combination with ipilimumab (NCT02307149) and pembrolizumab (NCT02565992) are awaiting publication.

Positioning

- Patients do not require general anesthesia for intralesional injection and are typically able to participate in positioning. Positioning will vary dependent upon the location of the ITM and the patient may need to be repositioned throughout the injection process to access multiple ITM.

- Once the patient is appropriately positioned, the area should be prepared with antiseptic solution and topical or local anesthetic may be applied.
- Most intralesional injectables follow a similar technique as per below with the exception of how many lesions can or should be injected and how often the ITMs are injected. We have chosen the FDA-approved TVEC to highlight the intralesional technique.

TVEC SPECIFIC TECHNIQUE

See **Video 1**.

- TVEC is initially dosed with a concentration of 10^6 pfu/mL to seroconvert HSV-seronegative patients (**FIGURE 3A**). Patients then return 3 weeks later for a second dose of 10^8 pfu/mL. Subsequent doses are at 10^8 pfu/mL every 2 weeks.[13,14]
- The injection volume should be limited to 4.0 mL per session. At the initial visit, largest lesions should be injected first, and the remaining dose should be injected into progressively smaller lesions until 4.0 mL is administered or until all lesions are injected. At subsequent visits, injection of new lesions should be prioritized, followed by the largest lesions.
- The recommended lesion injection volume is proportional to lesion size: >5 cm lesions should receive up to 4 mL, >2.5 to 5 cm lesions should receive up to 2 mL, >1.5 to 2.5 cm lesions should receive up to 1 mL, >0.5 to 1.5 cm lesions should receive up to 0.5 mL, and ≤0.5 cm should receive up to 0.1 mL (**FIGURE 3B**).
- Each lesion should be injected by using a fanning out technique through a single injection site to evenly disperse the medication and prevent the TVEC from leaking out of additional injection sites in the lesion. A new needle should be used for every new insertion.
- Treatment should be continued for at least 4 to 6 months unless there are no longer injectable ITM or alternative treatment is required.

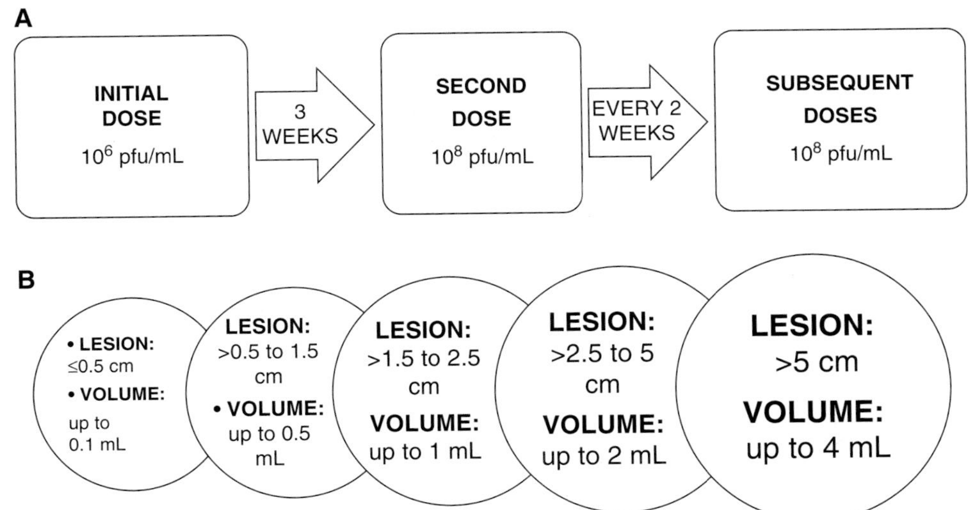

FIGURE 3 • TVEC dosing regimen **(A)** and volume **(B)**.

PEARLS AND PITFALLS

Injection technique	▪ Application of topical EMLA cream, instead of local infiltration of lidocaine, will minimize the number of puncture sites in each lesion. This reduces the possibility of the compound leaking out of the ITM through additional needle tracks. ▪ Inject each lesion using a fanning out technique from a single puncture to minimize injection sites. ▪ Prioritize largest lesions at first injection. At subsequent injections, new lesions should be prioritized, then additional lesions should be injected in order of descending size, unless specifically stated in the Instructions for Use (IFU).
Safety	▪ PPE, including a face shield, should be worn while performing injections. ▪ When it is time to remove the dressing at least 7 d after injection, the patient should do so using gloves and ensure it is disposed of in a sealed bag.

POSTOPERATIVE CARE

- After intralesional injection, apply pressure and gentle massage to the injection site for 30 seconds. The sites should be cleansed with alcohol and a dry sterile absorbent and occlusive dressing can be placed for a specific duration of time per IFU (TVEC dressings stay on for 7 days). The site should remain covered per IFU until there is no evidence of drainage from the injection site.

COMPLICATIONS

- Complications may vary based upon the intralesional therapy used but are usually local reactions, including injection site pain and mild to moderate short-term flu-like illnesses. For TVEC, common complications include:
  - Systemic: chills, pyrexia, fatigue, flu-like illness, and nausea that are usually mild and occur within 72 hours of injections. These symptoms seem to abate over time and become less common and less severe.
  - Local: injection site pain.[13,14]

REFERENCES

1. Gershenwald JE, Scolyer RA, Hess KR, et al. Melanoma staging: evidence-based changes in the American Joint Committee on Cancer eighth edition cancer staging manual. *CA Cancer J Clin*. 2017;67(6):472-492.
2. Patel A, Carr MJ, Sun J, Zager JS. In-transit metastatic cutaneous melanoma: current management and future directions. *Clin Exp Metastasis*. 2022;39(1):201-211.
3. Perone JA, Farrow N, Tyler DS, Beasley GM. Contemporary approaches to in-transit melanoma. *J Oncol Pract*. 2018;14(5):292-300.
4. National comprehensive cancer network clinical practice guidelines in oncology, melanoma: cutaneous version 2.2021. 2021.
5. Pawlik TM, Ross MI, Johnson MM, et al. Predictors and natural history of in-transit melanoma after sentinel lymphadenectomy. *Ann Surg Oncol*. 2005;12(8):587-596.
6. Robinson JC. Risks of BCG intralesional therapy: an experience with melanoma. *J Surg Oncol*. 1977;9(6):587-593.
7. Cohen MH, Elin RJ, Cohen BJ. Hypotension and disseminated intravascular coagulation following intralesional bacillus Calmette-Guerin therapy for locally metastatic melanoma. *Cancer Immunol Immunother*. 1991;32(5):315-324.
8. Byers BA, Temple-Oberle CF, Hurdle V, McKinnon JG. Treatment of in-transit melanoma with intra-lesional interleukin-2: a systematic review. *J Surg Oncol*. 2014;110(6):770-775.
9. Miura JT, Zager JS. Intralesional therapy as a treatment for locoregionally metastatic melanoma. *Expert Rev Anticancer Ther*. 2018;18(4):399-408.
10. Testori A, Faries MB, Thompson JF, et al. Local and intralesional therapy of in-transit melanoma metastases. *J Surg Oncol*. 2011;104(4):391-396.
11. Nasi ML, Lieberman P, Busam KJ, et al. Intradermal injection of granulocyte-macrophage colony-stimulating factor (GM-CSF) in patients with metastatic melanoma recruits dendritic cells. *Cytokines Cell Mol Ther*. 1999;5(3):139-144.
12. Hoeller C, Michielin O, Ascierto PA, Szabo Z, Blank CU. Systematic review of the use of granulocyte-macrophage colony-stimulating factor in patients with advanced melanoma. *Cancer Immunol Immunother*. 2016;65(9):1015-1034.
13. *IMLYGIC (talimogene laherparepvec) [package insert]*. Amgen Inc.; 2019.
14. Andtbacka RH, Kaufman HL, Collichio F, et al. Talimogene laherparepvec improves durable response rate in patients with advanced melanoma. *J Clin Oncol*. 2015;33(25):2780-2788.
15. Perez MC, Miura JT, Naqvi SMH, et al. Talimogene laherparepvec (TVEC) for the treatment of advanced melanoma: a single-institution experience. *Ann Surg Oncol*. 2018;25(13):3960-3965.
16. Louie RJ, Perez MC, Jajja MR, et al. Real-world outcomes of talimogene laherparepvec therapy: a multi-institutional experience. *J Am Coll Surg*. 2019;228(4):644-649.
17. Perez MC, Zager JS, Amatruda T, et al. Observational study of talimogene laherparepvec use for melanoma in clinical practice in the United States (COSMUS-1). *Melanoma Manag*. 2019;6(2):MMT19.
18. Sun J, Gastman BR, McCahon L, et al. Observational study of talimogene laherparepvec use in the anti-PD-1 era for melanoma in the US (COSMUS-2). *Melanoma Manag*. 2020;7(2):MMT41.
19. Carr MJ, Sun J, DePalo D, et al. Talimogene Laherparepvec (TVEC) for the treatment of advanced locoregional melanoma after failure of immunotherapy: a multi-institutional experience. *Ann Surg Oncol*. 2021. (in press).
20. Mousavi H, Zhang X, Gillespie S, Wachter E, Hersey P. Rose Bengal induces dual modes of cell death in melanoma cells and has clinical activity against melanoma. *Melanoma Res*. 2006;16:S8.
21. Thompson JF, Agarwala SS, Smithers BM, et al. Phase 2 study of intralesional PV-10 in refractory metastatic melanoma. *Ann Surg Oncol*. 2015;22(7):2135-2142.
22. Agrawala SS, Ross MI, Zager JS, et al. *A Phase 1b Study of Rose Bengal Disodium and Anti-PD-1 in Metastatic Cutaneous Melanoma: Results in Patients Naive to Immune Checkpoint Blockade*. Poster presented at: ESMO Virtual Congress; September 17-20, 2020; (Virtual).
23. Zager JS, Sarnaik AA, Pilon-Thomas S, et al. *Response for Combination of PV-10 Autolytic Immunotherapy and Immune Checkpoint Blockade in Checkpoint-Refractory Patients*. Oral presentation at: Melanoma Bridge; December 3-5, 2020; (Virtual).
24. Zawit M, Swami U, Awada H, Arnouk J, Milhem M, Zakharia Y. Current status of intralesional agents in treatment of malignant melanoma. *Ann Transl Med*. 2021;9(12):1038.

25. Hamid O, Ismail R, Puzanov I. Intratumoral immunotherapy-update 2019. *Oncol.* 2020;25(3):e423-e438.
26. Wang D, Jiang W, Zhu F, Mao X, Agrawal S. Modulation of the tumor microenvironment by intratumoral administration of IMO-2125, a novel TLR9 agonist, for cancer immunotherapy. *Int J Oncol.* 2018;53(3):1193-1203.
27. Haymaker C, Johnson DH, Murthy R, et al. Tilsotolimod with ipilimumab drives tumor responses in anti-PD-1 refractory melanoma. *Cancer Discov.* 2021;11(8):1996-2013.
28. Wang S, Campos J, Gallotta M, et al. Intratumoral injection of a CpG oligonucleotide reverts resistance to PD-1 blockade by expanding multifunctional CD8+ T cells. *Proc Natl Acad Sci U S A.* 2016;113(46):E7240-E7249.
29. Ribas A, Medina T, Kummar S, et al. SD-101 in combination with pembrolizumab in advanced melanoma: results of a phase ib, multicenter study. *Cancer Discov.* 2018;8(10):1250-1257.
30. Adamus T, Kortylewski M. The revival of CpG oligonucleotide-based cancer immunotherapies. *Contemp Oncol.* 2018;22(1A):56-60.
31. Weihrauch MR, Richly H, von Bergwelt-Baildon MS, et al. Phase I clinical study of the toll-like receptor 9 agonist MGN1703 in patients with metastatic solid tumours. *Eur J Cancer.* 2015;51(2):146-156.
32. Ziegler A, Soldner C, Lienenklaus S, et al. A new RNA-based adjuvant enhances virus-specific vaccine responses by locally triggering TLR- and RLH-dependent effects. *J Immunol.* 2017;198(4):1595-1605.
33. Curtsinger JM, Mescher MF. Inflammatory cytokines as a third signal for T cell activation. *Curr Opin Immunol.* 2010;22(3):333-340.
34. Algazi A, Bhatia S, Agarwala S, et al. Intratumoral delivery of tavokinogene telseplasmid yields systemic immune responses in metastatic melanoma patients. *Ann Oncol.* 2020;31(4):532-540.
35. Heller LC, Jaroszeski MJ, Coppola D, Heller R. Comparison of electrically mediated and liposome-complexed plasmid DNA delivery to the skin. *Genet Vaccines Ther.* 2008;6:16.
36. Fernandez-Penas P, Carlino MS, Tsai KK, et al. *Durable Responses and Immune Activation with Intratumoral Electroporation of pIL-12 Plus Pembrolizumab in Actively Progressing Anti-PD-1 Refractory Advanced Melanoma: KEYNOTE 695 Interim Data.* Poster presented at: Society for Immunotherapy of Cancer Annual Meeting; November 9-14, 2020; (Virtual).
37. Carnemolla B, Borsi L, Balza E, et al. Enhancement of the antitumor properties of interleukin-2 by its targeted delivery to the tumor blood vessel extracellular matrix. *Blood.* 2002;99(5):1659-1665.
38. Pretto F, Elia G, Castioni N, Neri D. Preclinical evaluation of IL2-based immunocytokines supports their use in combination with dacarbazine, paclitaxel and TNF-based immunotherapy. *Cancer Immunol Immunother.* 2014;63(9):901-910.
39. Danielli R, Patuzzo R, Di Giacomo AM, et al. Intralesional administration of L19-IL2/L19-TNF in stage III or stage IVM1a melanoma patients: results of a phase II study. *Cancer Immunol Immunother.* 2015;64(8):999-1009.
40. Miura JT, Zager JS. Neo-DREAM study investigating Daromun for the treatment of clinical stage IIIB/C melanoma. *Future Oncol.* 2019;15(32):3665-3674.
41. Eissa IR, Naoe Y, Bustos-Villalobos I, et al. Genomic signature of the natural oncolytic herpes simplex virus HF10 and its therapeutic role in preclinical and clinical trials. *Front Oncol.* 2017;7:149.
42. Yokota K, Isei T, Uhara H, et al. *Final Results from Phase II Combination with Canerpaturev (Formerly HF10), an Oncolytic Viral Immunotherapy, and Ipilimumab in Unresectable or Metastatic Melanoma in 2nd or Later Line Treatment.* Poster presented at: European Society for Medical Oncology Congress; September 27-October 1, 2019.
43. Bradley S, Jakes AD, Harrington K, Pandha H, Melcher A, Errington-Mais F. Applications of coxsackievirus A21 in oncology. *Oncolytic Virother.* 2014;3:47-55.
44. Andtbacka RHI, Curti BD, Kaufman H, et al. Final data from CALM: a phase II study of Coxsackievirus A21 (CVA21) oncolytic virus immunotherapy in patients with advanced melanoma. *J Clin Oncol.* 2015;33(15_suppl):9030-9030. doi:10.1200/jco.2015.33.15_suppl.9030.

Chapter 42

Isolated Limb Infusion

Betzaira Getzemani Childers, Jeffrey J. Sussman, and Joseph S. Giglia

DEFINITION

Isolated limb infusion is the term that is commonly used to indicate a minimally invasive, low-flow-rate, nonoxygenated perfusion of a limb with chemotherapy to effect control of a cancer within that extremity[1] (**FIGURE 1**). It is a more recent modification of a more traditional technique commonly referred to as *isolated limb perfusion* whereby larger arterial and venous catheters are used to achieve higher flow rates, extracorporeal oxygenation is used, and vascular access is obtained via an open approach (see Part 5, Chapter 43). Isolated limb perfusion is considered a minimally invasive approach with percutaneous access and lower systemic leakage rates and is more amendable to repeat dosing. Given numerous differences in patient selection, superior response rates attributed to limb perfusion in nonrandomized comparisons should be made with caution,[2,3] and even if modestly improved, isolated limb perfusion entails a higher severe adverse complication risk without a survival benefit. The evolution of systemic therapies for metastatic melanoma and intralesional treatments of in-transit disease have decreased the use of limb infusion/perfusion surgery over the last several years. However, there may be a role for combined therapeutic strategies to include isolated limb infusion techniques in advanced or refractory cases.[4]

PATIENT HISTORY AND PHYSICAL FINDINGS

- The most common indication for this procedure is a patient with in-transit melanoma restricted to an extremity whose lesions are too numerous or recurrent to be amenable to simple excision. It should be thought of as a limb salvage technique to treat regionally advanced disease and has no proven systemic benefit. Therefore, it is not commonly used in the face of distant metastasis unless regional control/palliation is the central goal.
- The minimally invasive nature of this technique is well tolerated by older and more frail patient populations.[5]
- Common malignancies treated in this manner include melanoma and Merkel cell carcinoma. Other histologies treated less commonly include squamous cell carcinoma and sarcoma.

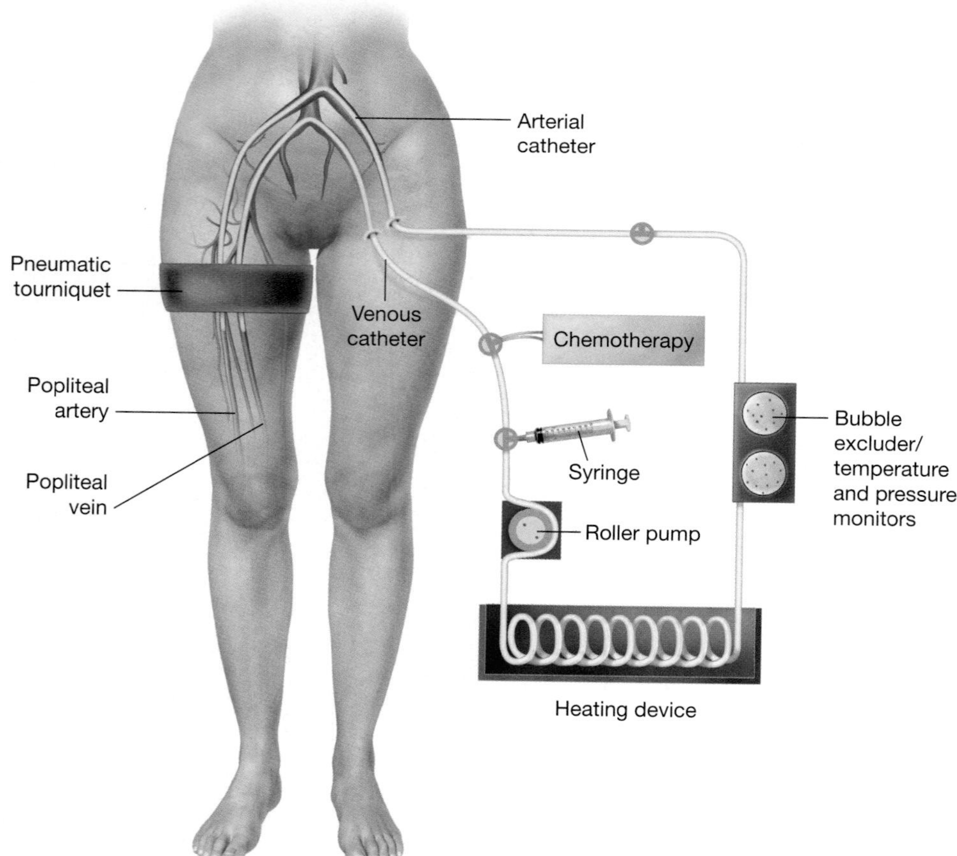

FIGURE 1 ● Schematic of circuit used for isolated limb infusion. Roller pump is optional.

- A through history and physical should be performed with attention to documenting location and extent of extremity disease, limb function, edema, vascular examination, and evaluation of draining nodal basins.
- Limb volume is estimated by water displacement.
  - Sequential circumferential measurements or computed tomography (CT) volumetric measurements have been described as alternatives.
  - The contralateral limb should be measured if the involved limb is edematous.
  - The limb is submerged in a water tank up to level anticipated to be at bottom of tourniquet. The water level is marked, and then after removal of the limb, the tank is filled with a measured amount of water to reach the marked level.
- Patients should have nonoccluded arterial and venous systems to allow catheter placement and chemotherapy infusion.
- The extent of disease needs to be distal enough in the extremity to be able to place a tourniquet proximally.
  - In selected cases, this may require resection of limited more proximal disease combined with infusion of greater distal disease burden distally.
  - Isolated limb infusion can be combined with a lymph node dissection with direct placement of the catheters in the exposed vessels.

IMAGING AND OTHER DIAGNOSTIC STUDIES

- Arterial and venous duplex ultrasound to establish arterial and venous patency. With adequate collaterals, limb infusion has been described even when superficial vessels are occluded.
- Imaging to evaluate limb disease burden if lesions are deep seated and difficult to appreciate and measure on examination.
- Imaging to evaluate for distant disease including brain magnetic resonance imaging (MRI); whole body positron emission tomography (PET)/CT; and/or chest, abdomen, pelvis contrast-enhanced CT scans.

SURGICAL MANAGEMENT

- Patients should be discussed in multidisciplinary fashion to consider alternatives to isolated infusion including isolated limb perfusion; intralesional therapy; simple excision; radical excision, including circumferential excision and grafting or amputation; radiation; or systemic cytotoxic, immunotherapeutic, and other biologic therapies as well as clinical trial eligibility.

Preoperative Planning

- Who and where vascular access is to be obtained should be determined preoperatively and may be institution specific. Possible methods include the following:
  - Interventional radiology. Vascular access can be performed in the interventional radiology suite, with the patient then transported to the operating room (OR) with the arterial and venous catheters in place.
  - Vascular surgery. Some vascular surgeons have the training, experience, and interest to perform the vascular access as an alternative to the interventional radiologist. Access can be obtained in the OR directly if appropriately equipped with fluoroscopic capabilities. Although additional OR time is required if done in the OR, the catheters can more easily be manipulated later, as needed. Moreover, access can be obtained under general anesthesia and risk of dislodgement during transport/bed transfer is eliminated.
  - Chemotherapy. Melphalan and dactinomycin are prepared just prior to the procedure. The calculated drug dosage is often reduced if the patient's actual body weight exceeds ideal body weight by multiplying the calculated drug dose by the ratio of ideal to actual body weight.
  - Melphalan dose is 7.5 mg/L volume for lower extremity infusions (maximum dose of 100 mg) or 10 mg/L volume for the upper extremity (maximum dose 50 mg).
  - Dactinomycin dose is 1% of the melphalan dose (maximum 0.5 mg).
  - The drugs are mixed together in 400 mL normal saline lower extremity (200 mL upper extremity) and delivered to OR for administration.

Positioning

- The patient is positioned supine on a fluoroscopy-capable OR bed for vascular access or in case catheter manipulation is needed.
- The room should be prewarmed.
- A heated circulating water blanket is placed around the affected extremity, or an external radiant heater is utilized (**FIGURES 2** and **3**).
- Heated air blankets are placed on the patient's trunk and head, or an external radiant heater is used.

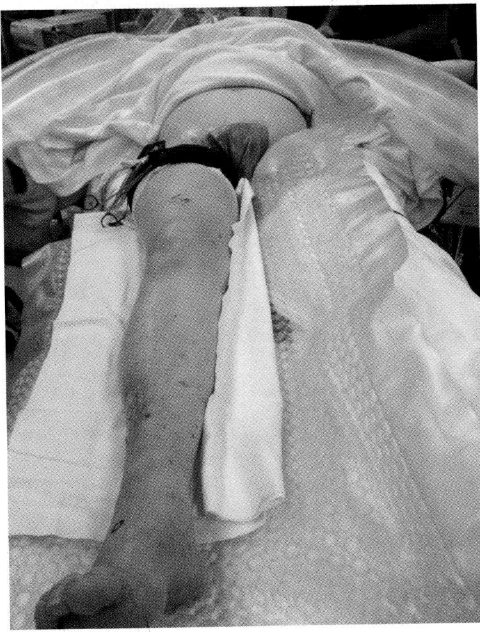

FIGURE 2 • Exposed affected limb with tourniquet proximally.

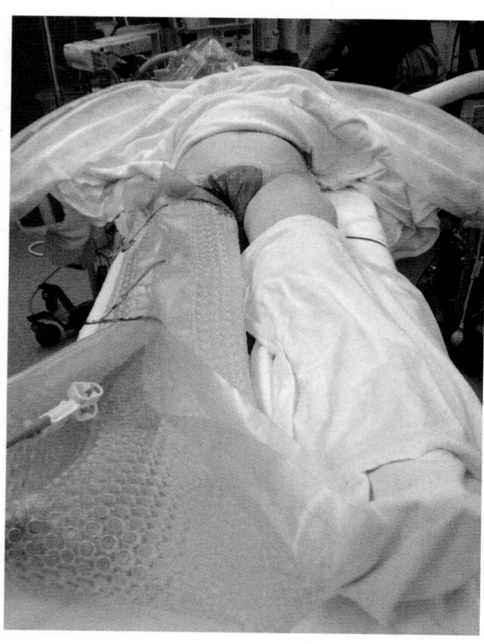

- A pneumatic tourniquet is placed on the proximal aspect of the extremity with the lower edge marked with a radiopaque hemostat. For distal-only infusions, the tourniquet can be placed lower.
- Needle temperature probes are inserted into deep and superficial locations within the proximal and distal limb locations.
- Baseline activated clotting time (ACT) is obtained.

FIGURE 3 ● Affected limb wrapped in water blanket.

VASCULAR ACCESS

- Venous and arterial access is obtained in the contralateral lower limb using the Seldinger technique with ultrasound and fluoroscopic guidance.
- After placing a vascular access sheath, a 5- or 6-Fr 100-cm catheter is introduced into the external iliac artery retrograde and manipulated across the iliac bifurcation and down the index limb arterial system to a point beyond the lower edge of the tourniquet. Similarly, a 7- to 8-Fr catheter is placed through the venous system and positioned below the tourniquet (**FIGURE 4**).
- In upper extremity cases, the catheter tip is placed in the brachial artery and basilic vein above the elbow.
- The patient is heparinized at 200 to 300 U/kg to obtain an ACT of 400.

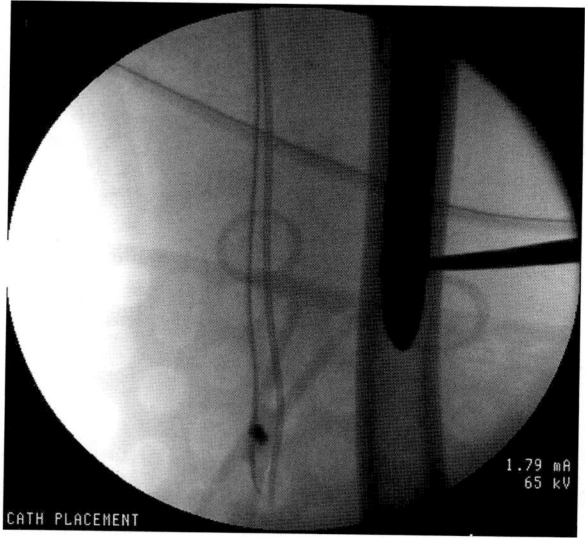

FIGURE 4 ● Radiograph of extremity with catheters in place below lower edge of pneumatic tourniquet. Note, wire in arterial catheter will be removed prior to infusion.

INFUSION CIRCUIT

- The catheters are connected to sterile 1/4″ pump tubing with high-flow stopcock connectors and a 20-mL syringe as a hand pump or through a single roller pump (**FIGURES 5** and **6**).
- The circuit then passes through a heat exchange unit or heated water bath set to heat the fluid to 41 °C followed by a bubble excluder before connecting to the arterial catheter. The circuit is primed with saline.
- Inflate the tourniquet to 250 to 300 mm Hg.
- Adequate flow is obtained by hand pumping the syringe and using the three-way stopcock to pull from the venous catheter and infuse toward the arterial catheter. Alternatively, a roller pump can be used at rate approximately 100 mL/min.

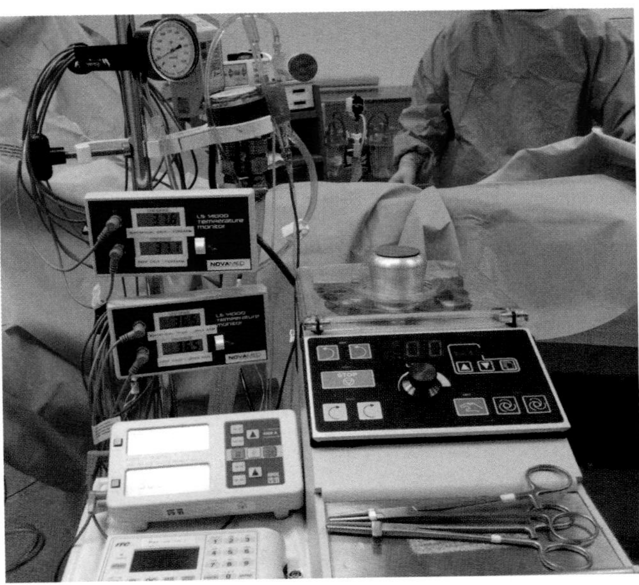

FIGURE 5 ● Photograph of roller pump workstation with temperature monitors, heat exchanger (water bath not depicted), ACT monitor, pressure gauge, and patient in background.

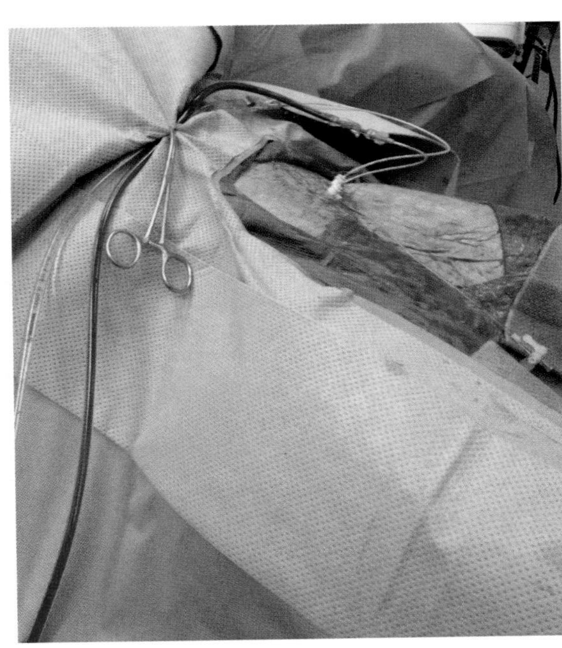

FIGURE 6 ● Contralateral groin with catheters in place connected to infusion circuit.

CHEMOTHERAPY INFUSION

- If the hand or foot is not to be perfused, an Esmarch bandage is tightly wrapped around the hand or foot to exclude the chemotherapy.
- Papaverine (60 mg for the lower extremity, 30 mg for the upper extremity) is infused into the circuit for vasodilatory effects to optimize cutaneous flow.
- The chemotherapy drug and dosage is double checked and then infused into the circuit.
- Chemotherapy and blood are circulated for 30 minutes by hand pump syringe or roller pump method.
- Temperature, flow rate, pressure, and extremity are monitored. Blood gas and ACT are checked at 10- to 15-minute intervals.

CHEMOTHERAPY WASHOUT

- The venous tubing is disconnected from circuit and allowed to gravity drain blood into a waste container.
- One liter of lactated Ringer solution (500 mL upper extremity) is infused into the arterial circuit.
- Repeat interval isolated limb infusion can be performed given that there is less systemic leakage and fewer systemic side effects from infusion compared with perfusion.

CONCLUSION

- The tourniquet is released after notification to anesthesiologist of possible electrolyte and volume changes.
- The catheters are removed while leaving sheaths in place. Esmarch bandage, if used, is removed.
- Vascular examination of infused extremity is assessed and, if baseline, protamine is given to reverse the heparin.
- Once ACT is corrected, the sheaths are removed with pressure applied for hemostasis at the vascular puncture sites.

PEARLS AND PITFALLS

Drug dosing	■ If no ideal body weight correction, overall response rate may be increased; however, toxicity is also increased without clear improvement in complete response rate.
Poor venous return	■ Catheter may be up against valve, vein sidewall, or pulled back under the tourniquet. ■ With heating, limb may vasodilate leading to relative intravascular volume loss. Infusing extra 500 mL saline into limb through arterial circuit may help.
Proximal disease	■ An Esmarch bandage can be used as a tourniquet high on the limb to allow for greater volume of leg infused.
Limb temperature	■ Pumping heated blood through circuit prior to chemotherapy administration can heat up limb internally to greater than 37 °C in 5-15 min.
Antiemetics	■ Steroids should not be used as antiemetics during or after anesthesia as they have an unknown effect on response rate.
Residual melanin pigmentation	■ Response may continue over several months. In-transit lesions may flatten but retain pigment. Biopsy may indicate melanin-laden macrophages without viable tumor.

POSTOPERATIVE CARE

- The patient is routinely extubated and admitted to an appropriate care unit capable of frequent neurovascular extremity monitoring for the first 24 hours. Baseline serum creatinine phosphokinase (CPK), complete blood count, and chemistry panel are obtained.
- The extremity should be elevated when in bed, but the patient is allowed to get out of bed after 24 hours if extremity toxicity is not evident and vessel access sites are okay.
- Twice-daily physician examination should be performed, checking for vascular access complications, vascular and neurologic examination, and compartment syndrome. Daily CPK is obtained, as muscle injury will routinely occur to some extent.
- CPK levels are expected to rise, peaking on postoperative days 4 and 5. Once levels begin to decrease and the extremity is stable, then the patient may be discharged. If the patient is reliable and has immediate health care access, it may be possible to discharge patient sooner with careful outpatient follow-up and instructions as most often inpatient care after the first day is for toxicity monitoring.
- If the CPK levels rapidly rise sooner than day 4 and/or exceed 1000 IU/L, then the patient is in danger of developing a compartment syndrome and potential limb loss. Steroids can ameliorate associated inflammation and decrease risk of requiring operative intervention. Dexamethasone can be given at 4 mg every 6 hours with rapid taper when the CPK drops below 1000 IU/L.

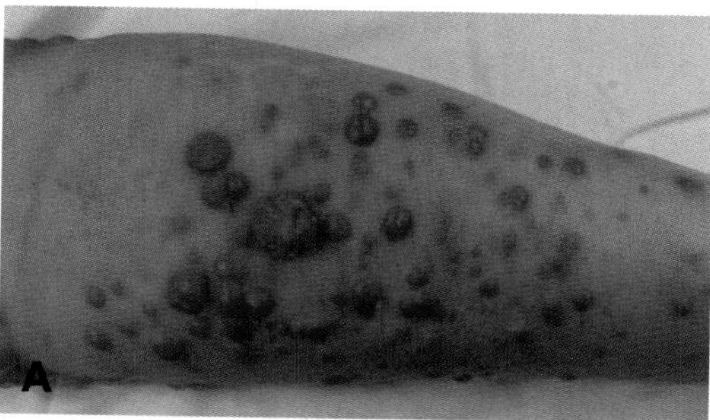

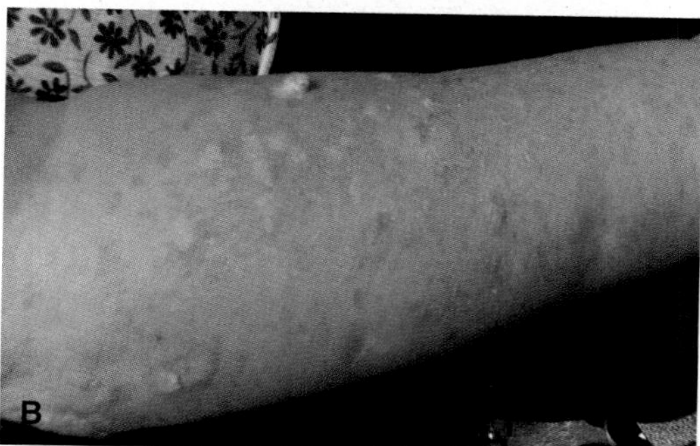

FIGURE 7 ● **A,** Photograph of limb with in-transit disease. **B,** Photograph of same limb 4 weeks following isolated limb infusion.

OUTCOMES

- A complete clinical response is seen in 30% to 40% of patients after a single isolated limb infusion with another 30% to 50% of patients experiencing a partial response. Complete and partial responses are 60% to 70% with overall survival of 38 months.[6-10] Complete responses are often durable, whereas partial responses are usually not (**FIGURE 7A** and **B**). Response may take 2 to 6 weeks to be seen clinically. Limb salvage is obtained in the vast majority of patients, whereas 5-year overall survival is approximately 30% due to distant disease progression. Nearly all patients will develop some mild side effects from the procedure, including skin erythema and lymphedema. Approximately half of patients will report return to baseline limb function by 3 months and the remainder by a year.
- Response rates in octogenarians and older patients appear similar to that of younger patients.[11]
- Isolated limb infusion is better tolerated with less toxicity as compared with isolated limb perfusion, is technically easier to perform, and appears to have similar response rates.

Table 1: Wieberdink Extremity Toxicity Scale

Grade I	No reaction
Grade II	Slight erythema and/or edema
Grade III	Considerate erythema and/or edema with some blistering; slightly disturbed motility permissible
Grade IV	Extensive epidermolysis and/or obvious damage to the deep tissues, causing definite functional disturbances; threatening or manifest compartmental syndromes
Grade V	Reaction that may necessitate amputation

Reprinted from Wieberdink J, Benckhuysen C, Braat RP, et al. Dosimetry in isolated perfusion of the limbs by assessment of perfused tissue volume and grading of toxic tissue reactions. Eur J Cancer Clin Oncol. 1982;18(10):905-910. Copyright © 1982 Elsevier. With permission.

COMPLICATIONS

- Potential complications related to vascular access include hematoma, pseudoaneurysm, dissection, and embolization. Stroke can be a complication of upper extremity arterial access transversing the arch.
- Toxicity from the isolated limb infusion of chemotherapy into the extremity skin and soft tissue are classified by the Wieberdink grading scale (**TABLE 1**).[12] Grade V or limb loss occurs in less than 1% of cases.
- Systemic toxicity from the chemotherapy should be rare but might include nausea and bone marrow suppression.

REFERENCES

1. Thompson JF, Kam PCA, Waugh RC, Harman CR. Isolated limb infusion with cytotoxic agents: a simple alternative to isolated limb perfusion. *Semin Surg Oncol.* 1998;14(3):238-247. 10.1002/(SICI)1098-2388(199804/05)14:3<238::AID-SSU8>3.0.CO;2-9
2. Kroon HM, Thompson JF. Isolated limb infusion and isolated limb perfusion for melanoma: can the outcomes of these procedures be compared? *Ann Surg Oncol.* 2019;26(1):8-9. 10.1245/s10434-018-7067-4
3. Testori A, Verhoef C, Kroon HM, et al. Treatment of melanoma metastases in a limb by isolated limb perfusion and isolated limb infusion. *J Surg Oncol.* 2011;104(4):397-404. 10.1002/jso.22028
4. Ariyan CE, Brady MS, Siegelbaum RH, et al. Robust antitumor responses result from local chemotherapy and CTLA-4 blockade. *Cancer Immunol Res.* 2018;6(2):189-200. 10.1158/2326-6066.CIR-17-0356
5. Noorda EM, Vrouenraets BC, Nieweg OE, van Geel AN, Eggermont AMM, Kroon BBR. Safety and efficacy of isolated limb perfusion in elderly melanoma patients. *Ann Surg Oncol.* 2002;9(10):968-974. 10.1007/BF02574514
6. Kroon HM, Moncrieff M, Kam PCA, Thompson JF. Outcomes following isolated limb infusion for melanoma. A 14-year experience. *Ann Surg Oncol.* 2008;15(11):3003-3013. 10.1245/s10434-008-9954-6
7. McClaine RJ, Giglia JS, Ahmad SA, McCoy SJ, Sussman JJ. Quality of life outcomes after isolated limb infusion. *Ann Surg Oncol.* 2012;19(5):1373-1378. 10.1245/s10434-012-2239-0
8. Miura JT, Kroon HM, Beasley GM, et al. Long-term oncologic outcomes after isolated limb infusion for locoregionally metastatic melanoma: an international multicenter analysis. *Ann Surg Oncol.* 2019;26(8):2486-2494. 10.1245/s10434-019-07288-w
9. Beasley GM, Sharma K, Wong J, et al. A multi-institution experience comparing the clinical and physiologic differences between upper extremity and lower extremity melphalan-based isolated limb infusion. *Cancer.* 2012;118(24):6136-6143. 10.1002/cncr.27676
10. Beasley GM, Caudle A, Petersen RP, et al. A multi-institutional experience of isolated limb infusion: defining response and toxicity in the US. *J Am Coll Surg.* 2009;208(5):706-715. 10.1016/j.jamcollsurg.2008.12.019
11. Teras J, Kroon HM, Miura JT, et al. International multicenter experience of isolated limb infusion for in-transit melanoma metastases in octogenarian and nonagenarian patients. *Ann Surg Oncol.* 2020;27(5):1420-1429. 10.1245/s10434-020-08312-0
12. Wieberdink J, Benckhuysen C, Braat RP, Van Slooten EA, Olthuis GAA. Dosimetry in isolation perfusion of the limbs by assessment of perfused tissue volume and grading of toxic tissue reactions. *Eur J Cancer Clin Oncol.* 1982;18(10):905-910. 10.1016/0277-5379(82)90235-8

Chapter 43

Isolated Limb Perfusion

Omgo E. Nieweg, Oscar V. Imhof, Hidde M. Kroon, and Bin B. R. Kroon

DEFINITION

- Compared with other cancer types, melanoma has a peculiar biology in various respects. In-transit dissemination is typical of this disease and occurs in 4% to 6% of patients.[1] In-transit metastases grow from tumor cells that are stuck in a lymph vessel in the skin or in the subcutaneous tissue. Such metastases are preferably excised, but they tend to recur in larger numbers (**FIGURE 1**).
- With the advent of effective systemic therapies and intralesional treatments of in-transit disease (Part 5, Chapter 41), the use of limb infusion or perfusion has decreased over the last several years. However, there may be a role for combined therapeutic strategies to include isolated limb infusion techniques in advanced or refractory cases. Isolated perfusion can be considered when in-transit lesions are situated on a limb and are refractory to other therapies, or those therapies are contraindicated. Soft tissue sarcoma, Merkel cell carcinoma, and squamous cell carcinoma are other malignancies that are occasionally treated in this manner.
- Isolated limb perfusion (ILP) enables administration of a high dose of cytostatic drugs to the upper or lower limb without exposing the remainder of the body to this treatment. This is accomplished by isolating the limb from the body's circulation and creating a separate oxygenated blood circuit. This is in contrast to isolated limb infusion (ILI), a low-flow, nonoxygenated perfusion that is described in Part 5, Chapter 42. See also **TABLE 1**. ILP and ILI are therapeutic options for patients with locally or regionally advanced melanoma who would otherwise require a more debilitating operation, for example, amputation.

PATIENT HISTORY AND PHYSICAL FINDINGS

- After treatment of their primary melanoma, patients are instructed to regularly examine the scar of the excision for local recurrence and to check the skin and subcutaneous tissue around this area up to the regional lymph node basin for visible or palpable satellite and in-transit metastases.

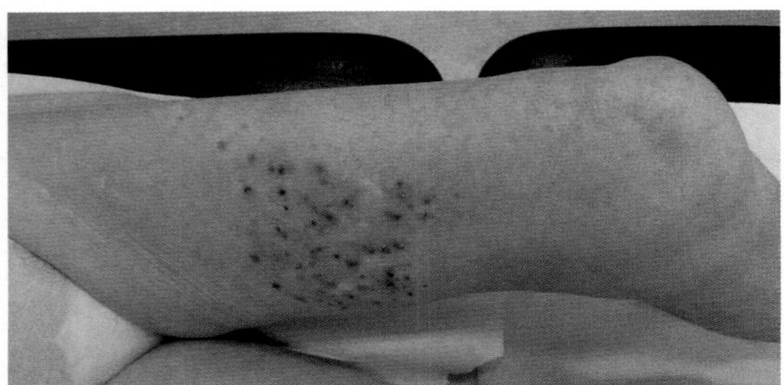

FIGURE 1 ● Extensive in-transit metastases on the left thigh.

- The physician who follows the patient inquires about new regional lesions.
- Physical examination of patients with melanoma is aimed at detecting local recurrence, satellite metastases, in-transit metastases, regional lymph node involvement, and a subsequent primary melanoma. A detailed examination of the skin, the regional subcutaneous tissue, and the regional node field is warranted.
- At an early stage, in-transit metastases can look quite innocuous. The detection of the more subtle ones requires the expertise and suspicious mind of an experienced surgeon. Patients themselves detect about half of the recurrences.
- If ILP is contemplated, a detailed history should be obtained to assess the general condition of the patient and to be informed about other relevant ailments, allergies, and medication.
- The vascular situation of the limb is assessed. The presence of peripheral arterial pulsations needs to be sufficient to allow for ILP.

IMAGING AND OTHER DIAGNOSTIC STUDIES

- The presence of advanced melanoma in the extremity should be confirmed by biopsy.
- In addition to the routine preoperative tests, screening for metastases elsewhere is appropriate as their presence may change the treatment plan. Whole-body positron emission tomography with computed tomography (PET/CT) or computed tomography (CT) and magnetic resonance imaging (MRI) of the brain are frequently used for this purpose.
- Arteriography is indicated if the arterial blood supply is questionable. A complete obstruction in the target artery or a major impediment downstream renders perfusion impossible. Extensive arterial calcification per se is not a contraindication.
- An elevated tumor marker such as the TA90 glycoprotein antigen or the S100 protein provides an opportunity to monitor the course of the disease.

SURGICAL MANAGEMENT

Rationale and Contraindications

- Extensive involvement limited to a certain region is typical for melanoma.
- Patients with complex regional cancer in a limb are discussed in a multidisciplinary meeting. Local and regional treatment options that can be considered *in lieu* to ILP are excision, cryotherapy, electrocoagulation, topical agents, electrochemotherapy, CO_2 laser, intralesional drug injection, ILI, and radiotherapy.
- In the presence of distant metastases, systemic therapy is the preferred first option.
- New immunotherapy and targeted drugs are effective in patients with advanced stage III and IV disease.[2,3] As a result, there is now a greater role for systemic therapy in patients in whom ILP would normally have been considered in the past.

Table 1: Differences Between Isolated Limb Perfusion and Isolated Limb Infusion

Isolated limb perfusion	Isolated limb infusion
Technically complex	Technically simple
Open catheter insertion	Percutaneous catheter insertion by radiologist
4 to 6 hours duration	1 h in radiology department + 1 h in theater
Perfusionist required	No additional staff required
Complex and expensive equipment needed	Equipment requirements modest
Not possible when artery occluded	Can be performed when artery occluded
Challenging to perform repeat procedure	Easy to repeat
Higher perfusion pressures predispose to systemic leakage	Low-pressure system, effective vascular isolation with tourniquet
High-flow blood circulation	Low-flow circulation system
Limb tissues oxygenated with normal blood gases maintained	Progressive hypoxia and acidosis
Hyperthermia (>41 °C can be achieved)	Usually not possible to raise limb temperature above 40 °C
General anesthesia required	Possible with regional anesthesia
Can treat proximal limb disease	Not applicable for proximal limb
Easy to combine with regional node dissection	Regional node dissection is separate procedure
Higher reported complete and overall response rates	Lower reported complete and overall response rates
Established as procedure since 1958	Established as procedure since 1994

- The rationale for ILP is that melanoma is sensitive to cytotoxic drugs but effective treatment requires a higher dosage compared with various other cancer types. In contrast to the vital organs, the normal tissues in the extremities tolerate such a high dose. ILP with cytotoxic medication may improve regional tumor control while limiting the systemic side effects.
- The procedure makes it possible to vary physiologic conditions such as blood flow, temperature, and oxygenation.
- ILP can be carried out safely at an advanced age.[4]
- The presence of regional node involvement is not a contraindication, as this procedure can be combined with a regional node dissection.
- Perfusion can provide good regional palliation in the presence of blood-borne metastases refractory to other treatment modalities.
- ILP is not indicated as an adjuvant in patients with excised high-risk primary melanoma without evidence of regional metastases.[5]
- The contraindications are listed in **TABLE 2**. A major vascular obstruction may prevent access to the artery and precludes the operation.
- Diabetes mellitus with severe peripheral vascular disease is a contraindication.
- ILP should not be performed in children as it may damage the epiphyseal plates.
- Previous radiotherapy is a relative contraindication as perfusion may cause necrosis of prior irradiated skin.
- A large superficial tumor with major tendon involvement is a relative contraindication as a firm response may leave tendons exposed.
- Brain metastases tend to bleed, and their presence is a relative contraindication in view of the anticoagulant that is administered during ILP.
- An infected wound or ulcer is another relative contraindication.

Anatomy

- For advanced disease of the leg, ILP can be performed at the femoral or iliac level. The arm can be treated at the brachial level or through the axilla.

Preoperative Planning

- ILP requires a perfusionist and a nuclear medicine worker in addition to the customary operating room team.
- Melphalan and tumor necrosis factor α (TNF-α) are the standard drugs used in current practice. The dosage of melphalan is adjusted to the need of the individual patient. The volume of the extremity is an often-used parameter to calculate the required dose. The volume can be determined using a water reservoir (**FIGURE 2**). Adjustments to the dosage can be made based on risk factors for regional toxicity like female gender and obesity.

Table 2: Absolute and Relative Contraindications to Isolated Limb Perfusion

Absolute contraindications
Obstruction of major artery
Diabetes with serious peripheral vascular disease
Child with open epiphyseal plates
Relative contraindications
Previous radiotherapy
Large superficial tumor with major tendon involvement
Brain metastases
Infected wound or ulcer

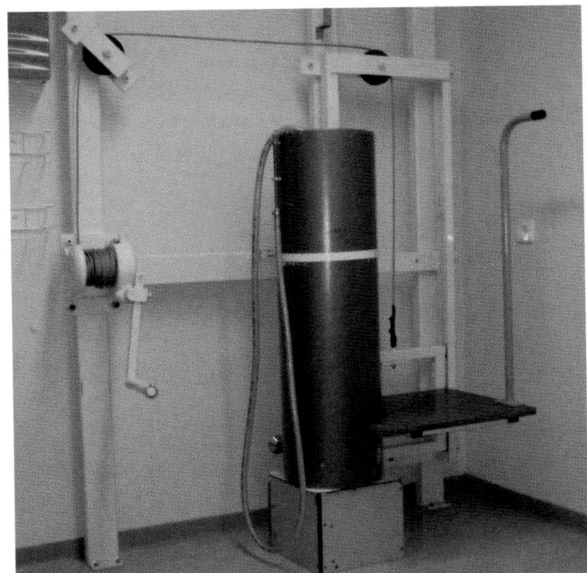

FIGURE 2 ● Water reservoir for measuring the volume of a limb. On the right is the elevator to bring the patient up to the required height. The elevator handle is on the left.

- TNF induces apoptosis of tumor endothelial cells and is particularly beneficial in patients with bulky tumor nodules.[6] It causes thrombosis and increased melphalan penetration.
- ILP requires sophisticated technology. The surgeon should verify the availability of the required drugs and ensure that the necessary equipment and materials are present and in good working order.
- General anesthesia is required. Epidural anesthesia is to be avoided as it induces vasodilation and predisposes to leakage of blood from the systemic circulation to the perfusion circuit.
- Preoperative antibiotics are not necessary.

ISOLATED FEMORAL PERFUSION

Positioning

- The patient is placed on the operating table in a supine position. The leg may be slightly exorotated.
- The leg is prepped in its entirety, and the operative field is draped in a sterile fashion.
- A pneumatic tourniquet is positioned around the upper thigh, but it is not inflated yet.
- A heating blanket is wrapped around the knee and the lower leg.
- A cotton doughnut is positioned underneath the heel to prevent decubitus.
- The operating table is tilted toward the surgeon.

Incision

- A longitudinal incision of approximately 10 cm is made starting just below the pneumatic tourniquet (**FIGURE 3**). The incision runs over the sartorius muscle. The skin and the subcutaneous tissue are divided and, subsequently, the fascia. Adson retractors are placed (**FIGURE 4**).

Access to the Superficial Femoral Vessels and Cannulation

- The external femoral vessels run behind the sartorius muscle. The vessels are reached either medially or laterally from the muscle. The thin fascia covering the vessels (**FIGURE 5**) is incised, exposing the superficial femoral artery. The artery is mobilized over the exposed length (**FIGURE 6**). Small arteries branching from this vessel are ligated and divided. A vessel loop facilitates the dissection. The accompanying vein is identified when the artery is pulled aside (**FIGURE 7**). The vein is mobilized over the exposed length. Attributing branches are ligated at the confluence and divided.
- Heparin is administered in a quantity of 150 U/kg body weight.
- Open access to the saphenous vein at the level of the ankle is gained to measure the venous pressure. The venous pressure is monitored throughout the procedure and should not

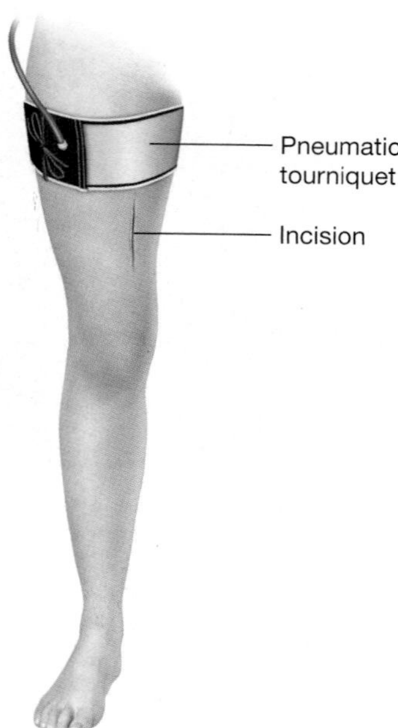

FIGURE 3 ● The incision is made over the inner thigh just below the pneumatic tourniquet.

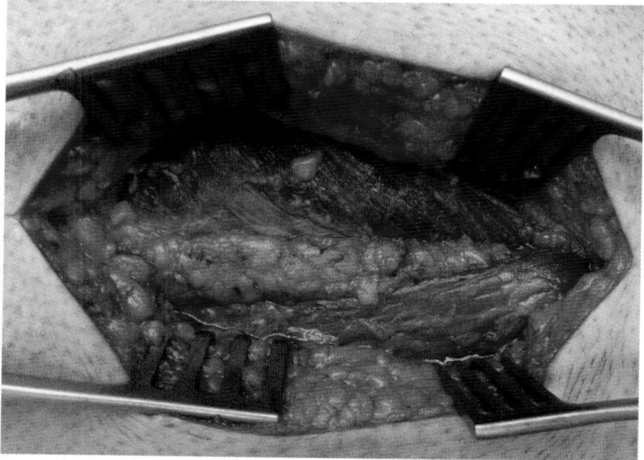

FIGURE 4 ● The long adductor muscle (above) and the sartorius muscle (below) are exposed. The superficial femoral vessels lie behind the sartorius muscle.

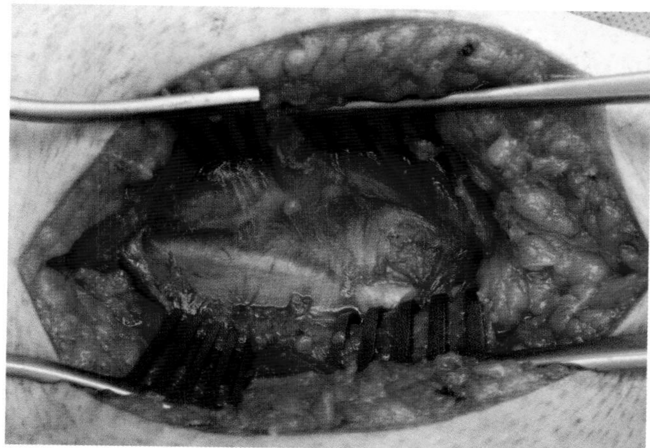

FIGURE 5 ● The superficial femoral artery can be seen through the thin fascia that covers the vessels.

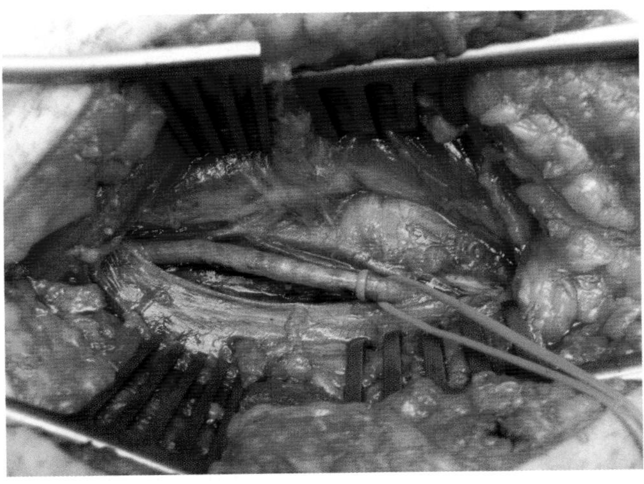

FIGURE 6 ● The superficial femoral artery is mobilized.

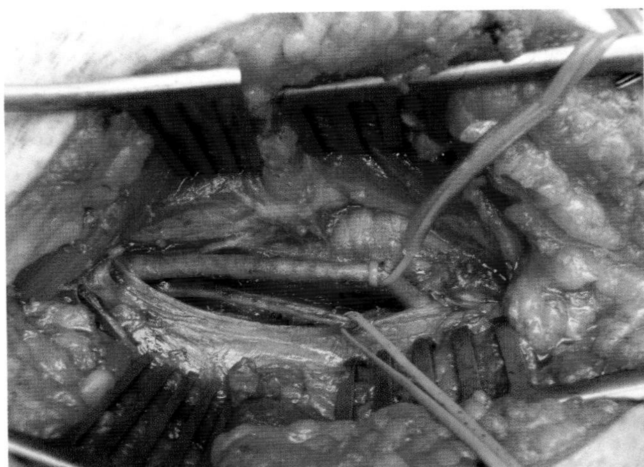

FIGURE 7 ● The superficial femoral artery is pulled aside (red vessel loop), and the accompanying vein is identified and dissected (blue vessel loop).

deviate more than 10 mm H_2O from the initial assessment. An increase is associated with postoperative morbidity.

- The appropriate diameter of arterial and venous cannulae for the perfusion is determined. The cannulae are tunneled subcutaneously underneath the tourniquet to the open wound to prevent kinking.
- The vein is clamped cranially and caudally. A transverse venotomy of a few millimeters is performed. The cannula is inserted caudally and secured with a vessel loop (**FIGURE 8A** and **B**). The cannula is hooked up to the extracorporeal circuit, and 300 mL of blood is tapped for the perfusion circuit. Subsequently, the arteriotomy is performed in a similar fashion and the arterial cannula is introduced and secured. The circuit is now complete (**FIGURE 9**).

Establishing the Perfusion

- The perfusion device consists of a reservoir to collect the venous blood, an oxygenator, a heat exchanger, and a roller pump (**FIGURE 10**). In addition to the patient's own blood, the perfusion fluid consists of 100 mL of a crystalloid solution (lactated Ringer solution), 200 mL 6% hydroxyethyl starch solution, and 2500 units of heparin. The hematocrit is approximately 30%. The flow should be generous, but it should not increase the venous pressure in the limb. The flow is typically 30 to 60 mL/L lower extremity volume/min. The venous blood is recollected by gravity.
- Thermistor probes are inserted in the subcutaneous tissue and a muscle compartment of the lower leg and the thigh. At this point, the temperature of the leg is found to be around 34 °C.

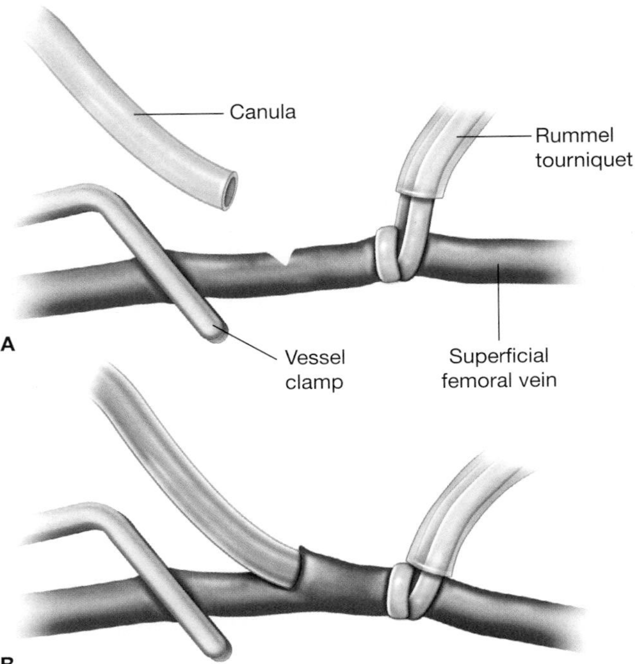

FIGURE 8 ● **A** and **B,** Insertion of cannula in superficial femoral vein.

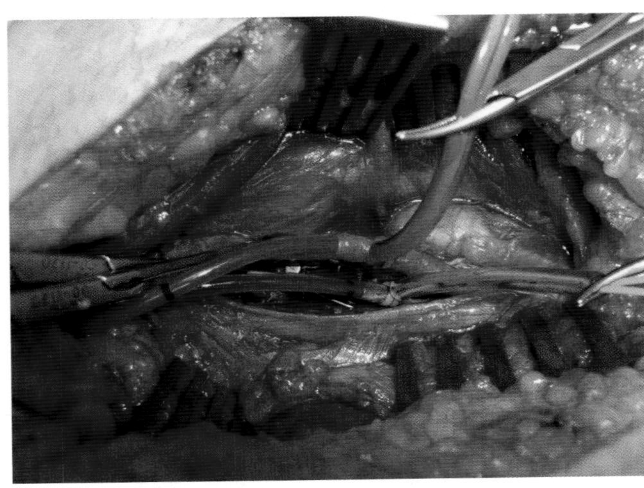

FIGURE 9 ● The cannulae in the superficial femoral artery and vein are secured with vessel loops tightened through Rummel tourniquets.

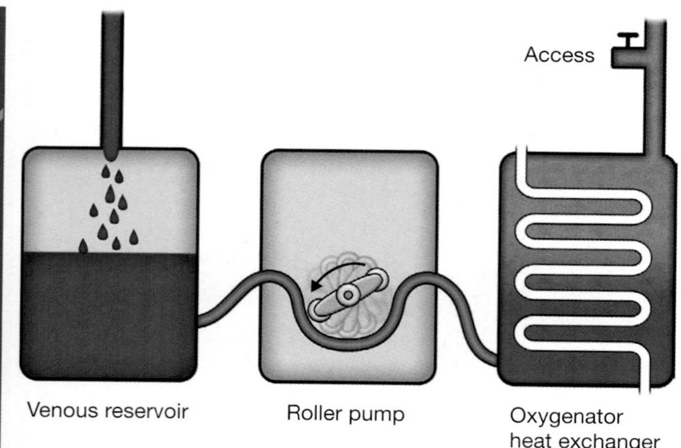

FIGURE 10 ● The perfusion device contains a venous inflow reservoir, a roller pump, an oxygenator annex heat exchanger, and access to the circuit for tapping blood and administration of drugs.

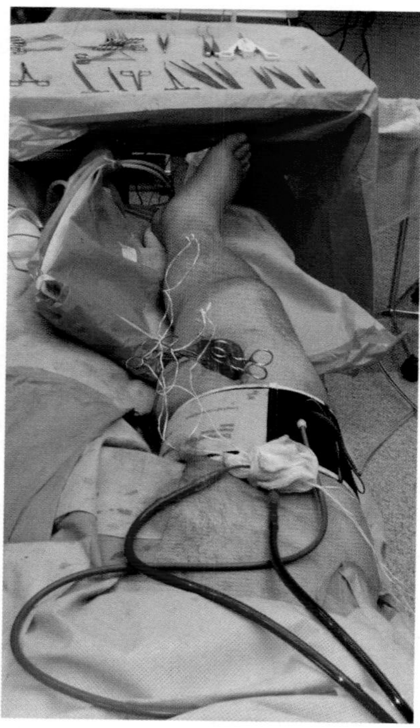

FIGURE 11 ● From top to bottom, note the cotton doughnut under the heel to prevent decubitus, the thermistors with the white cords to monitor the tissue temperatures, the blue warming blanket that is folded open for the picture, the open wound that would normally be covered with a wet gauze to prevent the vessels from drying out, the pneumatic tourniquet around the root of the thigh, and the arterial **(left)** and venous cannulae tunneled subcutaneously underneath the tourniquet.

- The heating blanket is another tool to attain the desired temperature of >37 °C.
- The tourniquet is inflated to a pressure of 350 mm Hg, if necessary higher. This occludes the collateral vessels to and from the systemic circulation in the skin, the subcutaneous tissue, and muscles. **FIGURE 11** shows the setup at this point.

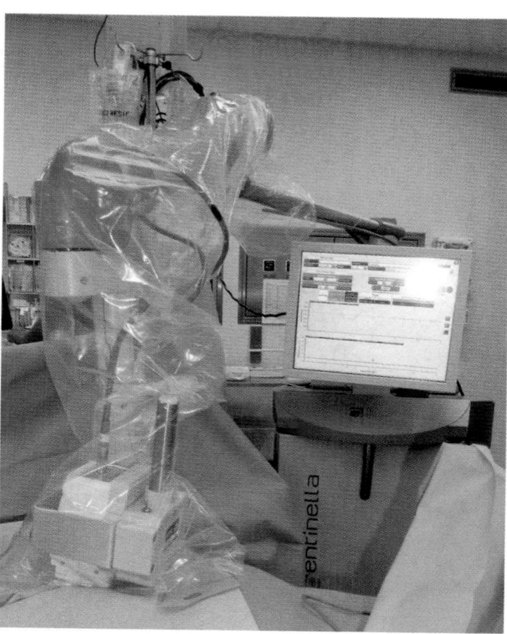

FIGURE 12 ● Mobile gamma-ray detector with screen to assess leakage.

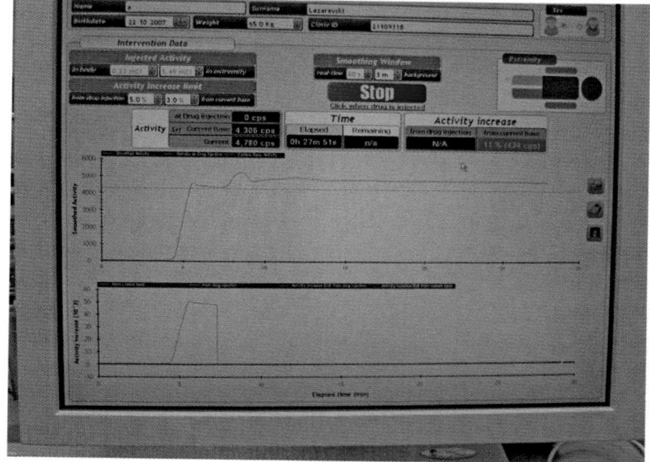

FIGURE 13 ● The green curve reflects the leakage. Note steep increase when background radiopharmaceutical is administered to the systemic circulation and subsequent two bumps up when the main dose initially passes through the perfusion circuit. The curve is flat thereafter, indicating adequate isolation during the perfusion.

- Escape of the drugs from the limb to the main circulation is to be avoided. Leakage can be monitored continuously by administering a small dose of a radiopharmaceutical such as technetium-99m-labeled serum human albumin to the perfusion circuit.[7] An even smaller background dose is administered intravenously into the systemic circulation. A gamma-ray detector is placed over the heart (**FIGURE 12**). The percentage of leakage can be calculated when the number of counts increases after correction for the physical half-life of the radionuclide (**FIGURE 13**).

- Substantial leakage either way can also be detected by assessing the fluid level in the venous return reservoir.
- A dose of 2 mg of TNF is administered when the flow and venous pressure are stable, when the tissue temperatures are around 37 °C, and when there is no leakage. Melphalan is added 10 minutes later. The dosage of melphalan is 10 mg/L of perfused volume with adjustments based on risk factors for morbidity. The dose should not exceed 150 mg.
- The limb is exposed to the combination of the two drugs for another 50 minutes.
- The temperature of the leg is increased to a maximum of 39.5 °C in the last half hour. At this time, most of the melphalan has been accumulated in the tissues, which limits potential heat-induced toxicity.
- Parameters to monitor are flow, venous and arterial blood gas values, activated clotting time, venous and arterial pressure in the perfusion circuit, leakage to or from the systemic circulation, and venous pressure and tissue temperature in the limb.
- There is considerable variation in the perfusion technique between institutions. Some surgeons use body weight (0.5-1.5 mg/kg) or another parameter to calculate the melphalan dose instead of the volume of the leg. Some surgeons use other drugs than the ones described here, such as dactinomycin or cisplatin. TNF is not registered throughout the world. If available, the dosage used ranges between 0.5 and 4 mg. Despite its obvious advantages, few surgeons use autologous blood for the perfusion circuit. Temperatures up to 43 °C have been used for the leg, but these higher temperatures tend to severely increase the postoperative morbidity. The venous pressure is not always measured to guide the flow. The duration of the perfusion in different institutions ranges from 45 to 90 minutes. Judging by the published response rates, one technique is not necessarily better than another.

Terminating the Perfusion

- After the leg has been exposed to the drugs for the intended duration, the perfusate is washed from the leg using a colloid or a similar fluid followed by a lactated Ringer solution. Massaging the leg helps to clear the less well-perfused tissues. The leg will be seen to turn pale.
- Meanwhile, the temperature probes and the venous pressure cannula are removed. The saphenous vein is ligated.
- The flushing is terminated when the fluid returning from the leg is clear. The tourniquet is deflated and taken off. The cannulae are removed from the superficial femoral artery and vein and the distal vessel clamps are reapplied.
- The vein is closed with a running Prolene 6-0 suture (**FIGURE 14**) and the clamps are removed. The artery is closed with horizontal mattress sutures using double-armed Prolene 6-0 (**FIGURE 15**).
- The clamps from the artery are removed and the leg assumes a pinkish hue. The nuclear medicine worker will now see an upward turn in the curve, and the leakage, which typically is 0% during the perfusion, ends up being 2% or 3%.
- A vacuum drain is inserted and the wound is closed in layers.
- Protamine administration to counter the heparin is optional.

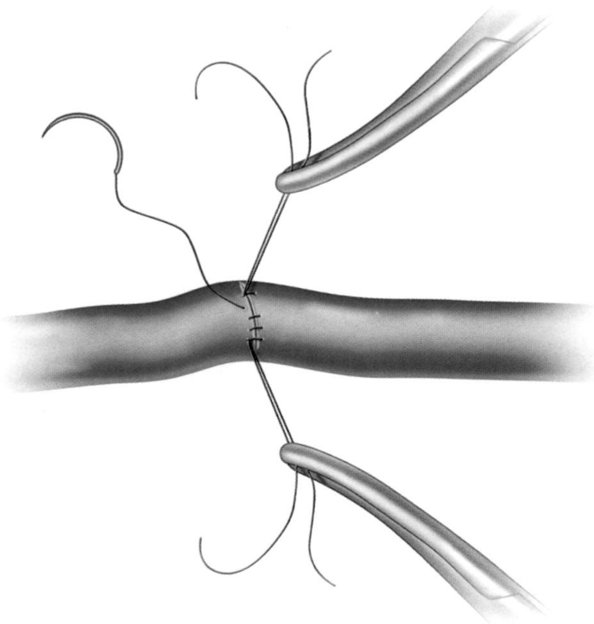

FIGURE 14 ● The vein is closed with a running Prolene 6-0 suture.

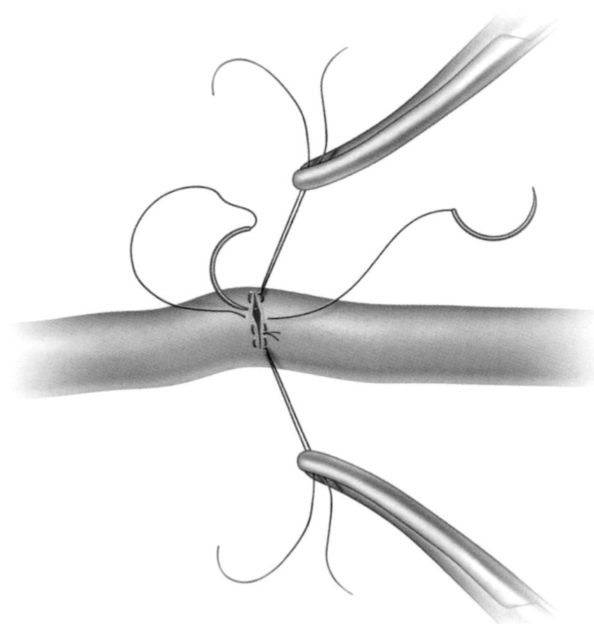

FIGURE 15 ● The artery is closed with double-armed Prolene 6-0. Horizontal mattress sutures evert the edges of the arterial wound in order to appose the endothelium layers.

ISOLATED ILIAC PERFUSION

Aspects Specific to Isolated Iliac Perfusion

- Isolated perfusion at the external iliac level is performed if the disease involves the upper thigh. Specific points inherent to this procedure that are different from femoral perfusion are described here.
- The approach to the external iliac vessels is extraperitoneal. The Bookwalter retractor provides an excellent exposure. An external iliac and obturator lymph node dissection is carried out first (see Part 5, Chapter 35). These nodes may contain metastasis, but even if this is not the case, their dissection is worthwhile because they can become involved later on and a retroperitoneal approach after perfusion is challenging. Also, an iliac and obturator node dissection results in little morbidity.
- Arterial branches and venous tributaries of the external iliac vessels are ligated and divided. The obturator artery and vein are ligated and also other vessels that connect to the thigh, as they may be the source of leakage. The internal iliac vessels may be clamped temporarily.
- The cannulae are inserted in the external iliac vessels, and the tips are positioned in the common femoral vessels.
- The generous diameter of the iliac vein permits a longitudinal venotomy without fear of stenosis after suturing.
- Occlusion of collateral vessels is obtained by wrapping an Esmarch rubber bandage around the thigh through the groin, anchored by a Steinmann pin in the iliac crest. The Steinmann pin is inserted before the heparin is administered.
- Prolene 5-0 is used for closing the vessels.

ISOLATED BRACHIAL PERFUSION

Aspects Specific to Isolated Brachial Perfusion

- Isolated perfusion at the brachial level is performed if the disease is limited to the forearm. Some specific points inherent to this procedure are described here.
- The patient is placed on the operating table in a supine position. The arm is placed in 90% abduction.
- A pneumatic tourniquet is wrapped around the proximal upper arm.
- Microvascular instruments are used.
- An 8-cm longitudinal incision is made over the medial aspect of the upper arm, caudally from the tourniquet. The cannulae are led through a subcutaneous tunnel underneath the tourniquet to avoid kinking.
- There may be two brachial veins. Both can be cannulated if the venous return from a single one is insufficient.
- The quantity of autologous blood needed to prime the extracorporeal circuit is 200 mL.
- Venous pressure measurement is performed using the cephalic vein at the wrist (**FIGURE 16**).
- The tourniquet is inflated to a pressure of 250 mm Hg.
- The dosage of melphalan is 13 mg/L of perfused volume if the volume of the arm exceeds 3.5 L, with adjustments based on risk factors for morbidity. Otherwise, 10 mg/L of perfused volume is given. The dosage of TNF is 1 mg.
- For the upper limb, the temperature in the tissue is kept between 37 and 38 °C throughout the procedure.

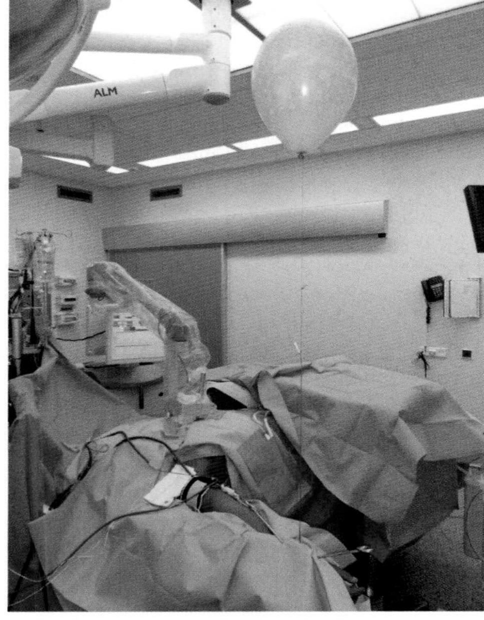

FIGURE 16 ● Helium-filled balloon keeping up the venous pressure line in a brachial perfusion.

- Prolene 6-0 sutures are used for closing the vessels. Alternatively, the vein(s) may be ligated because there is sufficient collateral circulation.

ISOLATED AXILLARY PERFUSION

Aspects Specific to Isolated Axillary Perfusion

- Isolated perfusion at the level of the axilla is performed if the disease involves the upper arm. Some specific points inherent to this procedure and differing from the brachial perfusion are described here.
- The axilla is approached via an incision along the lateral margin of the major pectoral muscle. Axillary lymph node dissection is optional (see Part 5, Chapter 34).
- The axillary vein is exposed and dissected. The axillary artery lies amid the brachial plexus and is mobilized. Branches are ligated and divided.
- Occlusion of collateral vessels is obtained by wrapping an Esmarch rubber bandage around the upper arm through the axilla anchored by a Steinmann pin in the humeral head. A cotton pad underneath the bandage protects the brachial plexus from undue pressure.[8]
- The dosage of the drugs is as for the brachial perfusion.

PEARLS AND PITFALLS

Volume measurement	▪ If the limb is edematous, the volume of the contralateral limb, if normal, should be measured to guide the melphalan dosage.
Drug dosage	▪ A sufficient dose for the desired effect is warranted, but an excessive dose can be associated with limb-threatening morbidity. The surgeon threads a thin line, and this implies a careful calculation of the drug dose and attention to the details of the procedure.
Prevention of systemic side effects	▪ Extremely high doses of cytotoxic drugs are used, and the toxicity in case of leakage of the drugs to the systemic circulation can be life threatening. Therefore, painstaking occlusion of collateral vessels and meticulous measuring of leakage are of the essence.
Insertion of the cannula in the femoral vein	▪ Valves in the femoral vein may prevent accurate positioning of the venous cannula. A high arterial inflow and temporary clamping of the vein create a generous outflow, which opens the valves and facilitates advancing the cannula. Alternatives are abduction of the leg or cannula insertion over a Fogarty catheter.
Perfusion	▪ The hand and foot are particularly sensitive to the side effects of melphalan. Their exposure to the drug can be limited by temporarily excluding them from the perfusion circuit. This can be accomplished by wrapping the hand or foot in a tight Esmarch rubber bandage for the first 30 minutes of the melphalan perfusion.
Major tendon involvement is a contraindication	▪ A large superficial tumor mass with substantial tendon involvement intuitively appears as an appropriate indication for perfusion. However, a complete response will expose necrotic tendons, which may necessitate amputation.
Autologous blood	▪ Most surgeons use allogeneic blood, but autologous blood obtained at the beginning of the procedure is cheaper and safer.
Elderly patients	▪ In contrast to what is often suggested in the literature, advanced age is not a contraindication, as ILP is effective and quite safe in elderly patients.[4]
Palliation	▪ In the presence of refractory blood-borne metastases, ILP can provide valuable palliation for patients with otherwise unmanageable limb disease that is bothersome because of pain, recurrent bleeding, or fungating infection.

POSTOPERATIVE CARE

- Overnight monitoring of the distal arterial pulsations is obligatory as arterial occlusion at the level of the sutured arteriotomy is a complication that is threatening in the first few hours and requires immediate intervention.
- Postoperatively, the leg is kept elevated on a Braun frame to limit development of edema. The vacuum drain is removed the next day. Muscle-setting exercises are initiated, but bed rest is maintained until the inflammatory signs subside. Patients experience surprisingly little pain.
- Creatine phosphokinase is checked daily. An increase in the first few days is normal, but an excessive level may indicate muscle necrosis due to a compartment syndrome.
- Responding dermal in-transit metastases may be seen to wrinkle, shrink, and develop a crust. Subcutaneous metastases typically soften, and fluctuation is noticed on physical examination.
- The patient is mobilized when the inflammatory signs subside and discharged when fully mobilized, usually within a week.
- An anticoagulant is given for the duration of 3 months.

OUTCOMES

- There appears to be no relationship between limb toxicity and tumor response to the treatment.[9,10]
- A response may become evident as early as on the operating table but may also take up to 9 months. ILP with melphalan alone results in a complete response in 54% of the patients.[11] The complete response is durable in half of them. In an additional 30% of patients, a partial response is obtained. Their remaining lesions can be excised later. The complete response rate when melphalan plus TNF is used is around 70%,[12] but the end result is not better than with melphalan alone. Ten-year survival in patients with a complete response is 49%.[13]
- Long-term survivors have a better quality of life than comparable control individuals.[14]
- The Wieberdink classification is used to quantify the limb morbidity (**TABLE 3**).[15]

Table 3: Wieberdink Classification of Postoperative Limb Morbidity

1	No skin reaction
2	Redness, edema
3	Blisters
4	Superficial necrosis, damage to deep tissues causing functional impairment, threatening or manifest compartmental syndrome
5	Necrosis requiring amputation

Reprinted from Wieberdink J, Benckhuysen C, Braat RP, et al. Dosimetry in isolated perfusion of the limbs by assessment of perfused tissue volume and grading of toxic tissue reactions. Eur J Cancer Clin Oncol. 1982;18:905-910. Copyright © 1982 Elsevier. With permission.

- Acute regional toxicity determines long-term morbidity. One year after treatment, 44% of the patients show some degree of morbidity: recurrent infections, 3%; neuropathy, 4%; pain, 8%; muscle atrophy or fibrosis, 11%; limb malfunction, 15%; or lymphedema, 28%.[16] The lymphedema can be attributed to concomitant lymph node dissection.
- Postoperative toxicity necessitates amputation in 0.9% of the patients.[17] Amputation for intractable recurrence is required in 2.4% of the patients.[18]
- Given the success in patients with stage III melanoma, it seems reasonable to explore the targeting drugs and immunotherapy as adjuvant in case of a complete response to ILP.[19,20]

COMPLICATIONS

- Perioperative mortality is less than 1%.[17,21]
- If tumor necrosis factor is used, some of the drug inevitably remains in the body and may cause a slight fever immediately after the operation.
- Serious postoperative complications associated with ILP are rare, but they demand urgent intervention. Arterial thrombosis looms in the first few hours and requires thrombectomy. A venous patch is often necessary to ensure a sufficient flow.
- Excessive swelling of the muscles in the limb compresses the vessels, which may decrease the blood supply and lead to a compartmental syndrome. Excruciating pain suggests this diagnosis, and it can be confirmed by measuring the intracompartmental pressure. Timely fasciotomy of the involved muscle compartments prevents permanent damage.
- In the first few days, an inflammatory response typically develops and the leg becomes red, warm, and slightly edematous.
- Over a period of 2 to 3 weeks, the edema and redness subside and give way to a tan discoloration that gradually disappears over the course of several months.

REFERENCES

1. Mitchell TC, Karakousis G, Schuchter L. Melanoma. In: Niederhuber JE, Armitage JO, Doroshow JH, Kastan MB, Tepper JE, eds. *Abeloff's Clinical Oncology*. 6th ed. Elsevier, 2020.
2. Long GV, Stroyakovskiy D, Gogas H, et al. Dabrafenib and trametinib versus dabrafenib and placebo for Val600 BRAF-mutant melanoma: a multicentre, double-blind, phase 3 randomised controlled trial. *Lancet*. 2015;386:444-451.
3. Hodi FS, Chiarion-Sileni V, Gonzalez R, et al. Nivolumab plus ipilimumab or nivolumab alone versus ipilimumab alone in advanced melanoma (CheckMate 067): 4-year outcomes of a multicentre, randomised, phase 3 trial. *Lancet Oncol* 2018;19:1480-1492.
4. Noorda EM, Vrouenraets BC, Nieweg OE. Safety and efficacy of isolated limb perfusion in elderly melanoma patients. *Ann Surg Oncol*. 2002;9:968-974.
5. Schraffordt Koops H, Vaglini M, Suciu S, et al. Prophylactic isolated limb perfusion for localized, high-risk limb melanoma: results of a multicenter randomized phase III trial. European Organization for Research and Treatment of Cancer Malignant Melanoma Cooperative Group Protocol 18832, the World Health Organization Melanoma Program Trial 15, and the North American Perfusion Group Southwest Oncology Group-8593. *J Clin Oncol*. 1998;169:2906-2912.
6. Deroose JP, Eggermont AM, van Geel AN, et al. Isolated limb perfusion for melanoma in-transit metastases: developments in recent years and the role of tumor necrosis factor alpha. *Curr Opin Oncol*. 2011;23:183-188.
7. Klaase JM, Kroon BBR, van Geel AN, et al. Systemic leakage during isolated limb perfusion for melanoma. *Br J Surg*. 1993;80:1124-1126.
8. Vrouenraets BC, Eggermont AM, Klaase JM, et al. Long-term neuropathy after regional isolated perfusion with melphalan for melanoma of the limbs. *Eur J Surg Oncol*. 1994;20:681-685.
9. Beasley GM, Tyler DS. Optimizing regional therapy for melanoma. *Ann Surg Oncol*. 2009;16:1095-1097.
10. Vrouenraets BC, Hart GA, Eggermont AM, et al. Relation between limb toxicity and treatment outcomes after isolated limb perfusion for recurrent melanoma. *J Am Coll Surg*. 1999;188:522-530.
11. Vrouenraets BC, Nieweg OE, Kroon BBR. Thirty-five years of isolated limb perfusion for melanoma: indications and results. *Br J Surg*. 1996;83:1319-1328.
12. Alexander HR, Fraker DL, Bartlett DL, et al. Analysis of factors influencing outcome in patients with in-transit malignant melanoma undergoing isolated limb perfusion using modern treatment parameters. *J Clin Oncol*. 2010;28:114-118.
13. Sanki A, Kam PC, Thompson JF. Long-term results of hyperthermic, isolated limb perfusion for melanoma: a reflection of tumor biology. *Ann Surg*. 2007;245:591-596.
14. Noorda EM, Van Kreij RHJ, Vrouenraets BC, et al. The health-related quality of life of long-term survivors of melanoma treated with isolated limb perfusion. *Eur J Surg Oncol*. 2007;33:776-782.
15. Wieberdink J, Benckhuysen C, Braat RP, et al. Dosimetry in isolation perfusion of the limbs by assessment of perfused tissue volume and grading of toxic tissue reactions. *Eur J Cancer Clin Oncol*. 1982;18:905-910.
16. Vrouenraets BC, Klaase JM, Kroon BBR, et al. Long-term morbidity after regional isolated perfusion with melphalan for melanoma of the limbs. The influence of acute regional toxic reactions. *Arch Surg*. 1995;130:43-47.
17. Cavaliere R, Di Filippo F, Giannarelli D, et al. Hyperthermic antiblastic perfusion in the treatment of local recurrence or "in-transit" metastases of limb melanoma. *Semin Surg Oncol*. 1992;8:374-380.
18. Kapma MR, Vrouenraets BC, Nieweg OE, et al. Major amputation for intractable extremity melanoma after failure of isolated limb perfusion. *Eur J Surg Oncol*. 2005;31:95-99.
19. Long GV, Hauschild A, Santinami M, et al. Adjuvant Dabrafenib plus Trametinib in stage III BRAF-mutated melanoma. *N Engl J Med*. 2017;377:1813-1823.
20. Eggermont AMM, Blank CU, Mandala M, et al. Adjuvant Pembrolizumab versus placebo in resected stage III melanoma. *N Engl J Med*. 2018;378:1789-1801.
21. Sonneveld EJ, Vrouenraets BC, Van Geel AN, et al. Systemic toxicity after isolated limb perfusion with melphalan for melanoma. *Eur J Surg Oncol*. 1996;22:521-527.

Chapter 44 Principles of Extremity/Trunk Sarcoma Resection

Paul J. Gagnet, Janet Sybil Biermann, and Geoffrey W. Siegel

DEFINITION

- Soft tissue sarcomas are rare malignancies that originate from mesenchymal cells with an incidence of roughly 13,000 cases per year in the United States.[1] Soft tissue sarcomas are classified as low or high grade with higher-grade sarcomas having a higher predilection for metastasis and recurrence. Owing to their rarity sarcomas are best treated at a sarcoma center through a multidisciplinary approach with a team consisting of medical oncologists, radiation oncologists, musculoskeletal radiologists, musculoskeletal pathologists, and a surgeon specializing in oncologic resections. Current recommendations suggest a referral to a sarcoma center if the mass is enlarging and greater than 5 cm in size.[2,3]
- Proper workup of soft tissue sarcomas is essential. Sarcomas that are believed to be benign masses on presentation and resected without adequate preoperative workup or an intent to achieve wide margins are termed ***unplanned resections***. Unplanned resections can lead to morbid reresections necessitating soft tissue coverage procedures or potential limb loss.[4] Unfortunately, soft tissue sarcomas are diagnosed 25% to 40% of the time after having undergone an unplanned resection.[5-7] Proper workup for soft tissue sarcomas includes preoperative magnetic resonance imaging (MRI) with and without intravenous (IV) contrast, initial staging studies, and biopsy. Chest imaging should follow any biopsy diagnosis of sarcoma if not obtained preoperatively. Preoperative biopsy provides a definitive diagnosis and can guide perioperative treatment including radiation and chemotherapy when warranted (**FIGURE 1**).

DIFFERENTIAL DIAGNOSIS

- The differential for soft tissue masses can range from benign to malignant. Benign lesions include lipomas, atypical lipomatous tumors, ganglion cysts, vascular malformations, desmoid tumors, giant cell tumor of tendon sheath, myxomas, and benign neural tumors. Malignant lesions include sarcomas and malignant peripheral nerve sheath tumors. Benign and malignant lesions can be distinguished from each other based on imaging and biopsy findings.

PATIENT HISTORY AND PHYSICAL FINDINGS

- Physical examination findings can aid in the workup of soft tissue masses. Visual inspection should be performed as overlying skin changes can be observed in some vascular tumors and cutaneous sarcomas. Palpation of the mass should be performed. Firm masses that are adherent to the surrounding tissue have a higher likelihood of malignancy. Soft and mobile masses are more frequently associated with benign diagnoses. Masses that are deep to the subcutaneous layer and greater than 5 cm in size have a high likelihood of being malignant and should always prompt further workup.
- Regional lymphatic examination should also be performed as there are several sarcomas that can spread via lymphatics. Lymphoma can also present as a soft tissue mass, and enlarged lymph nodes can help direct further laboratory testing. Neurovascular examination of the extremity should also be performed to assess for potential nerve or vascular involvement of the tumor.

IMAGING AND OTHER DIAGNOSTIC STUDIES

- Preoperative workup of soft tissue masses is essential. For small masses less than 5 cm that are subcutaneous, ultrasound can be very useful in determining probable benign and malignant features. In a small superficial mass with ultrasound findings consistent with a benign lesion, excision can be performed without referral to a sarcoma center. The specimen should always be sent for pathologic confirmation.
- For masses that are greater than 5 cm or deep to the subcutaneous tissue, MRI with IV contrast is the gold standard for workup. Malignant lesions will show postcontrast enhancement with gadolinium (**FIGURE 1**).
- Masses that cannot be definitively diagnosed as a benign lesion on imaging or have malignant features will require a preoperative biopsy. Biopsy should be preferentially performed via core needle biopsy with or without the aid of image guidance (**FIGURE 2**). Core needle biopsy has been shown to be able to diagnose soft tissue sarcoma histiotypes with a sensitivity of 88% and specificity of 93% while having lower complication rates compared with open biopsy.[8] Open surgical biopsies should be reserved for rare instances when image-guided biopsies are nondiagnostic or the mass is inaccessible by core needle approach. Biopsy should be performed at a sarcoma center by a musculoskeletal radiologist familiar with sarcoma biopsy or by the treating oncologic surgeon. The oncologic surgeon will choose to excise the biopsy tract during resection of the tumor to remove any remnant tumor cells seeded within the tract. It becomes especially difficult to excise the tract if it is not placed in the area of the planned surgical incision. Improperly placed biopsy tracts can risk contaminating surrounding structures such as adjacent muscle or neurovascular structures if not properly planned, resulting in increased morbidity of subsequent resection.
- Staging scans to include chest imaging should be obtained prior to any definitive surgery. Presumptive evidence of metastasis may require histologic confirmation and local surgical management may be deferred in favor of systemic approaches or palliative radiotherapy in selected cases.

SURGICAL MANAGEMENT

Preoperative Planning

- Preoperative planning is essential for obtaining negative margins. Wide resection should always be performed in

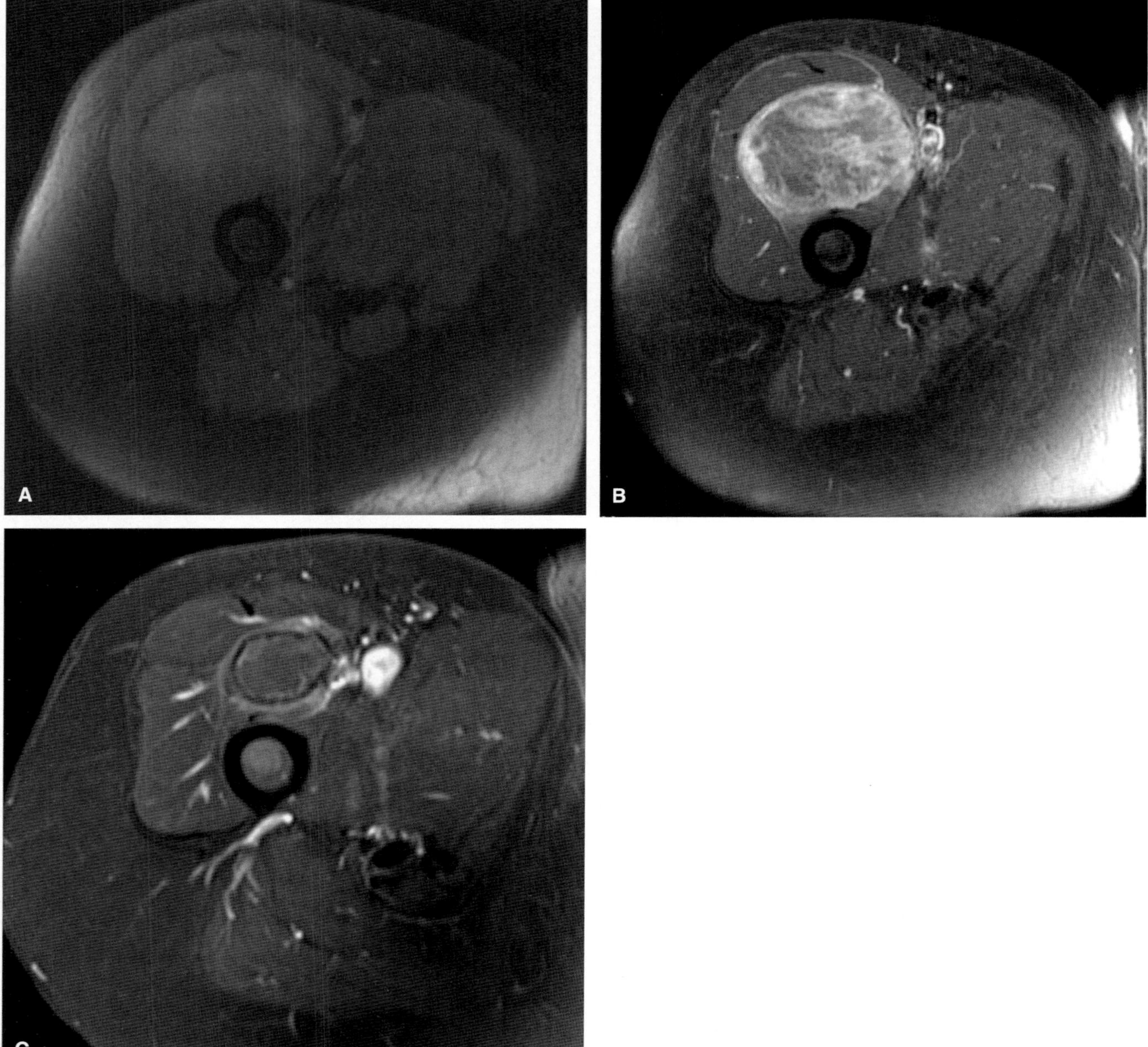

FIGURE 1 ● **A,** MRI T1 fat suppression image showing precontrast sequence with large mass within the vastus medialis. **B,** T1 fat suppression sequence after administration of gadolinium showing heterogenous uptake within the mass. **C,** Postcontrast T1 fat suppression imaging in same patient status post chemotherapy with dramatic treatment response and shrinking of the tumor.

sarcoma resections. Intralesional excision should never be performed as it contaminates the soft tissues with tumor cells leading to an almost assured recurrence especially in high-grade sarcomas. The surgeon should plan to leave an intact cuff of tissue surrounding the lesion whether that be adipose tissue, fascia, or muscle to obtain negative margins. Preoperative cross-sectional imaging is essential to facilitate accurate surgical planning.

- Incisions should always be made longitudinal and not transverse. This is important in cases of recurrence requiring reresection in the future as it allows the surgeon to ellipse the previous incision during resection and assists in closure of the wound. Longitudinal incisions also allow a more extensile approach if the original incision is not large enough and facilitate reresection in the case of local recurrence.

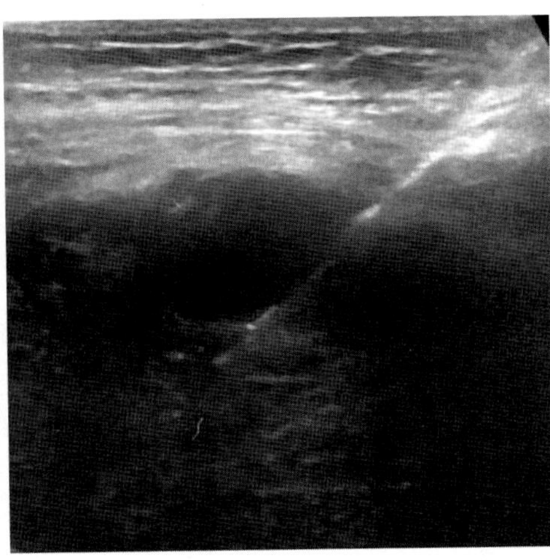

FIGURE 2 ● Ultrasound-guided biopsy showing insertion of the core needle into a soft tissue mass of the anterior thigh.

- Adjacent neurovascular structures should be identified on preoperative imaging. If the involvement of critical structures cannot be made on imaging the surgeon should be prepared to send frozen sections to pathology to determine if a structure can be spared or has to be sacrificed to obtain adequate margins.
- Standard preincision antibiotic prophylaxis should be employed.

Positioning

- Positioning of the patient is dependent upon location of the lesion and can vary from case to case. If operating on a limb the entire limb should be completely draped with access to the large vessels proximally if needed. The mass should be palpated and the incision marked. In cases where sarcoma resection is sufficiently distal that a tourniquet may be applied without compressing the tumor, gravity exsanguination should be used rather than an Esmarch bandage.

- Longitudinal approaches should be made directly over the mass (**FIGURE 3**). Electrocautery is used to dissect through the subcutaneous tissues, and vessels are coagulated along the way. A dissecting hemostat is used to create a dissection plane and pull a thin cuff of tissue superficially, with electrocautery used to divide the tissue between the tines of the hemostat (**FIGURE 4**). This helps ensure that the surgeon does not cut into the tumor or any other important neurovascular structures. In cases of prior radiation therapy, electrocautery is used in cut mode to prevent thermal injury to radiated tissue that could potentially hamper wound healing. The electrocautery is switched to coagulate mode when a small vessel is encountered. Any large vessels that are identified are clamped and tied off with a silk suture on a passer (**FIGURE 5**). Sharp retraction should be avoided on the tumor side of the resection.
- If the mass is sitting on the superficial aspect of the fascia, then the fascia should be incised circumferentially around the mass to be included as the deep margin.
- If the mass is deep in the muscle tissue, then the fascia should be incised and a cuff of normal muscle should be included as the surrounding tumor margin. Frequent palpation of the mass should be performed to ensure that the tumor is not penetrated (**FIGURE 6**).
- If the mass is involving a nerve, the nerve should be identified proximal and distal to the tumor and transected sharply utilizing a scalpel.
- Intraoperative margins should be assessed with frozen sections. It is customary to take several deep sections from the tumor bed and utilize a "clock face" to label the remaining frozen sections from the periphery of the wound bed such as a 12-, 3-, 6-, and 9-o'clock section as well as a deep margin. It is appropriate to take more if needed or if there is a particular area with abnormal appearing tissue. If margins come back positive then further wide resection should be performed in that area until the frozen section comes back negative for tumor cells.

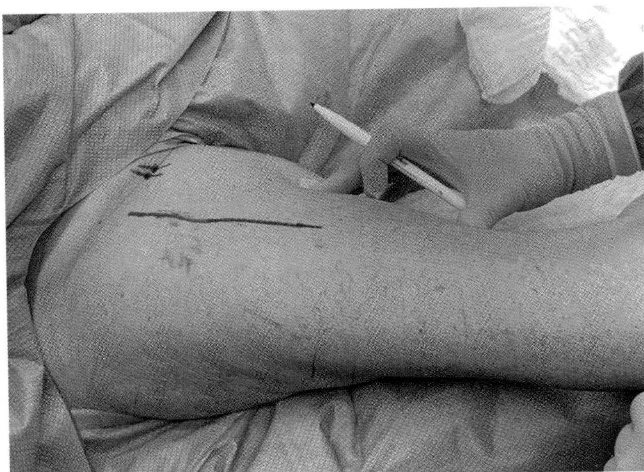

FIGURE 3 ● Longitudinal incision centered over the mass.

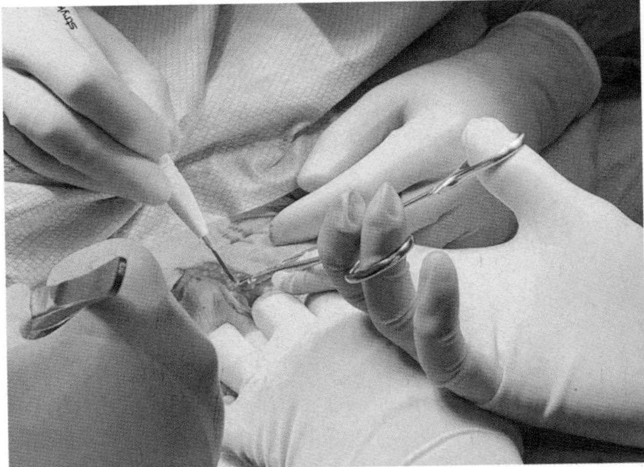

FIGURE 4 ● Electrocautery dissection between the dissecting hemostat tines.

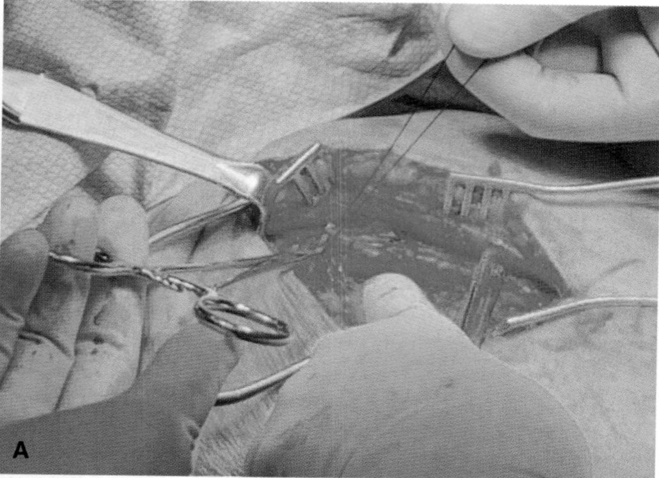

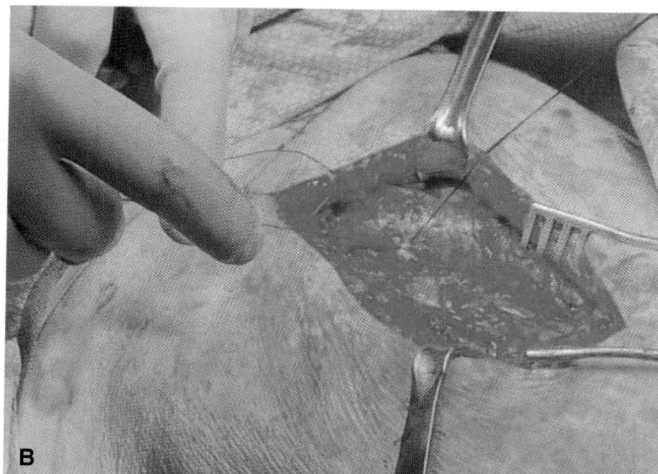

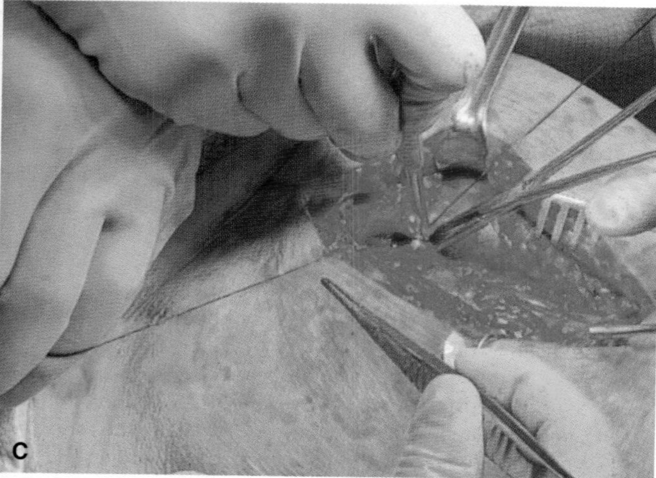

FIGURE 5 ● **A,** Tying of a clamped vessel. **B,** Tying of two sutures that have been passed under a crossing vessel followed by incision of the vessel between the two sutures in **(C)**.

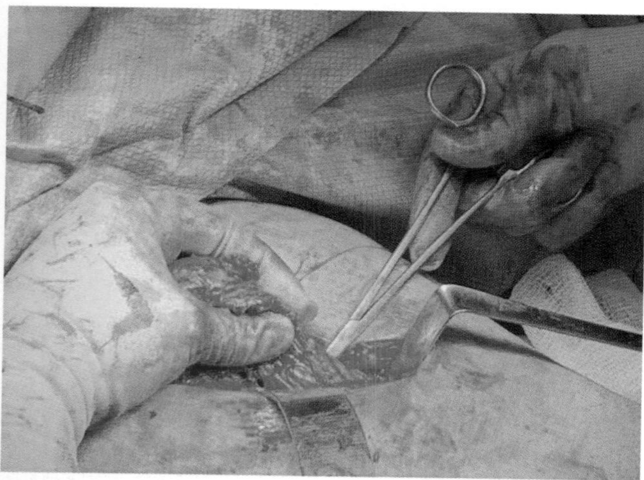

FIGURE 6 ● Demonstrating the mass contained in the left hand encompassed by a healthy layer of muscle tissue. The remaining muscular attachments free from tumor are elevated with the dissecting hemostat for incision with electrocautery.

- The tumor is taken to the back table, and the 12-, 3-, 6-, and 9-o'clock margins of the tumor are tagged with color-coded suture (**FIGURE 7**). The specimen is then taken to pathology and the deep margin is inked (**FIGURE 8**).
- Surgical clips are placed at the 12-, 3-, 6-, and 9-o'clock positions and deep portions of the tumor bed to aid in radiation therapy simulation should it be indicated postoperatively.
- The wound should be copiously irrigated with saline.
- Meticulous hemostasis is very important in sarcoma resections. If any tumor cells are left behind and a large hematoma forms, the entire area of hematoma is then seeded or contaminated with tumor cells. Following irrigation the entire wound bed is sprayed with thrombin to aid in hemostasis. A glove is placed into the wound and then pressure is held over the wound either manually or with a sterile ACE wrap for 10 minutes (**FIGURE 9**). The purpose of the glove instead of a lap sponge is that it does not rip any clot off with it upon removal. One to two channel drains are placed depending on the size of the wound. Drains should be placed in line with the incision in near proximity (**FIGURE 9**). This is done in case there are positive margins seen on final pathology requiring

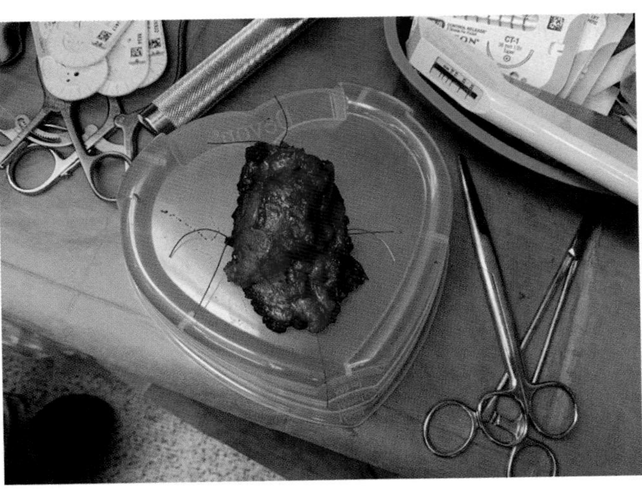

FIGURE 7 ● Tumor encased in healthy surrounding muscle tissue and marked with color-coded suture.

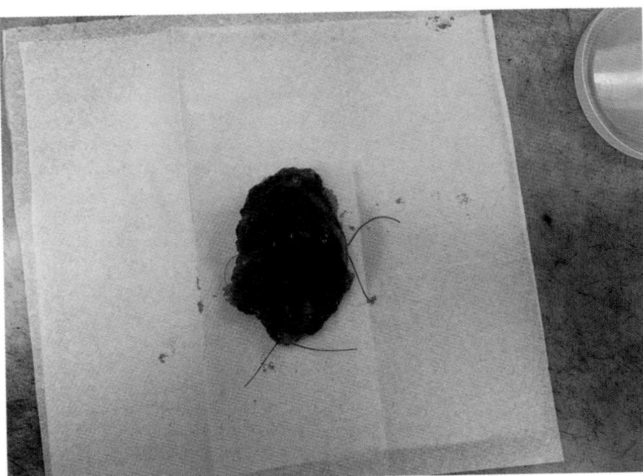

FIGURE 8 ● Inking of the deep margin for final pathology.

a re-excision. The drain tract would be considered contaminated and need to be excised on re-excision.

- Depending on how much resection is performed it is possible that complex closure with tissue rearrangement may be required. Ideally, this is arranged preoperatively. If plastic surgery coverage is planned, this can be performed in a staged fashion, which allows for definitive pathologic interpretation of the margins. If margins are positive a reresection can be performed prior to the closure procedures at the second date,

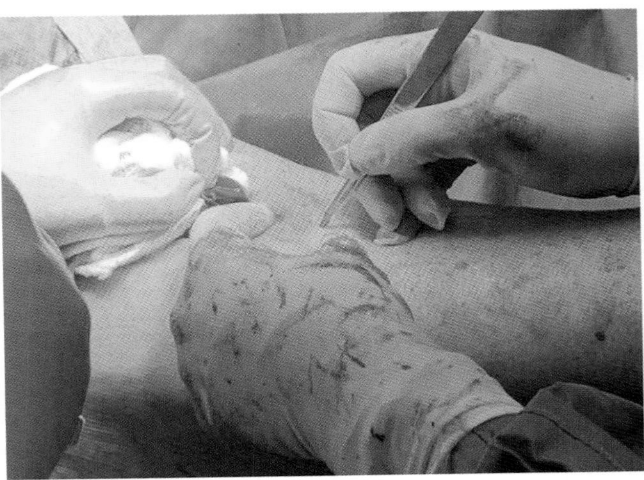

FIGURE 9 ● Gloves in the wound with pressure being held. Incision for drain placement is being made in line with the surgical incision.

avoiding the difficulty of assessing positive margin location in a bed with complex rearrangement.[9] Temporary wound coverage is accomplished with either irradiated homograft or artificial skin substrate. The patient is taken back to the operating room for final coverage following confirmed margins on pathology.

- If plastic surgery is not required for wound closure the surgeon should perform a layered wound closure. Any adjacent muscle bellies should be reapproximated with nonabsorbable suture to decrease dead space for possible hematoma formation. The fascia is closed with thick absorbable suture. The subcutaneous tissue is closed with absorbable suture. The skin is then closed with staples, and the drains are sutured into place. Wound closure is very important in patients with cancer due to possible nutritional deficiencies or preoperative radiation putting them at risk for delayed wound healing.
- Xeroform is placed over the incision followed by gauze. Three gauze bandage rolls are unrolled and "fluffed" and placed over the incision. This is followed by an ABD and an elastic bandage wrap. The purpose of the gauze roll fluffs is to place a slight and even amount of pressure on the wound to help prevent hematoma formation. A vacuum assisted incisional wound dressing may be considered for patients at high risk for wound complications, including preoperative radiation, morbid obesity, or those with extensive resection and removal of fascia.

PEARLS AND PITFALLS

Preop evaluation	■ Masses greater than 5 cm have a higher likelihood of being malignant.
Imaging	■ Preoperative cross-sectional imaging ideally with IV contrast should always be obtained for large deep masses. ■ In highly suspicious cases, obtaining an MRI prior to biopsy is often recommended as a hematoma from a core biopsy can distort the imaging findings.

Biopsy	▪ Should be performed at a sarcoma center by a musculoskeletal radiologist or the oncologic surgeon planning to perform the resection to ensure proper placement. ▪ Core needle biopsy is favored as a first-line diagnostic approach over open surgical biopsy.
Incision	▪ Longitudinal and directly over the tumor.
Excision	▪ Ensure adequate margins and send frozen sections if needed.
Closure	▪ Ensure meticulous hemostasis and place a drain.

POSTOPERATIVE CARE

- For lower extremity sarcomas in the thigh and knee area the patient is placed in a knee immobilizer postoperatively until staple removal for wound rest and to prevent increased tension on the wound due to knee flexion. For upper extremity sarcomas in the shoulder or upper arm the patient will be placed in a sling to rest the wound until staple removal. The drains remain in until there is less than 30 mL of output over 24 hours. Staples are generally left in for 3 weeks if the patient has had preoperative radiation to ensure adequate wound healing.
- A first-generation cephalosporin is given until the drains are removed.

COMPLICATIONS

- Recurrence
- Hematoma
- Infection
- Nerve palsy
- Vascular injury

REFERENCES

1. Siegel RL, Miller KD, Jemal A. Cancer statistics, 2018. *CA Cancer J Clin*. 2018;68(1):7-30.
2. Siegel GW, Biermann JS, Chugh R, et al. The multidisciplinary management of bone and soft tissue sarcoma: an essential organizational framework. *J Multidiscip Healthc*. 2015;8:109-115.
3. Dangoor A, Seddon B, Gerrand C, et al. UK guidelines for the management of soft tissue sarcomas. *Clin Sarcoma Res*. 2016;6:20.
4. Gagnet P, Nelson J, Wallace N, et al. Analysis of the effect of the size and grade of soft tissue sarcoma on rates of unplanned resection, metastatic disease, mortality, and morbid Re-resection over 20 years. *Orthopedics*. 2021;44(3):166-171.
5. Potter BK, Adams SC, Pitcher JD, Temple HT. Local recurrence of disease after unplanned excisions of high-grade soft tissue sarcomas. *Clin Orthop Relat Res*. 2008;466(12):3093-3100.
6. Goodlad JR, Fletcher CD, Smith MA. Surgical resection of primary soft-tissue sarcoma. Incidence of residual tumour in 95 patients needing re-excision after local resection. *J Bone Joint Surg Br*. 1996;78(4):658-661.
7. Noria S, Davis A, Kandel R, et al. Residual disease following unplanned excision of soft-tissue sarcoma of an extremity. *J Bone Joint Surg Am*. 1996;78(5):650-655.
8. Birgin E, Yang C, Hetjens S, et al. Core needle biopsy versus incisional biopsy for differentiation of soft-tissue sarcomas: a systematic review and meta-analysis. *Cancer*. 2020;126(9):1917-1928.
9. Siegel GW, Kuzon WM, Hasen JM, Biermann JS. Staged soft tissue reconstruction following sarcoma excision with anticipated large cutaneous defects: an oncologically safe alternative. *Iowa Orthop J*. 2016;36:104-108.

Chapter 45

Principles of Retroperitoneal Sarcoma Resection

Kerry M. Madison and Christina V. Angeles

DEFINITION

- Soft tissue sarcomas are rare malignant tumors of mesenchymal cell origin that can arise from any location. Retroperitoneal (RP) sarcomas comprise 15% to 20% of all soft tissue sarcomas and are a distinct entity compared to extremity sarcomas with differences in workup, management, and treatment.
- The anatomic retroperitoneum (**FIGURE 1**) is a three-dimensional space containing several key structures including the adrenal glands, aorta, inferior vena cava (IVC), second and third portions of the duodenum, pancreas, kidneys and ureters, the ascending and descending colon, and the rectum. RP sarcomas can involve any intra-abdominal or retroperitoneal structures. They frequently distort normal anatomy and obscure key structures, landmarks, and planes, requiring careful assessment of both preoperative imaging and intraoperative assessment.
- One of the challenges of studying and treating sarcomas is that there are over 70 different histologic subtypes, the most

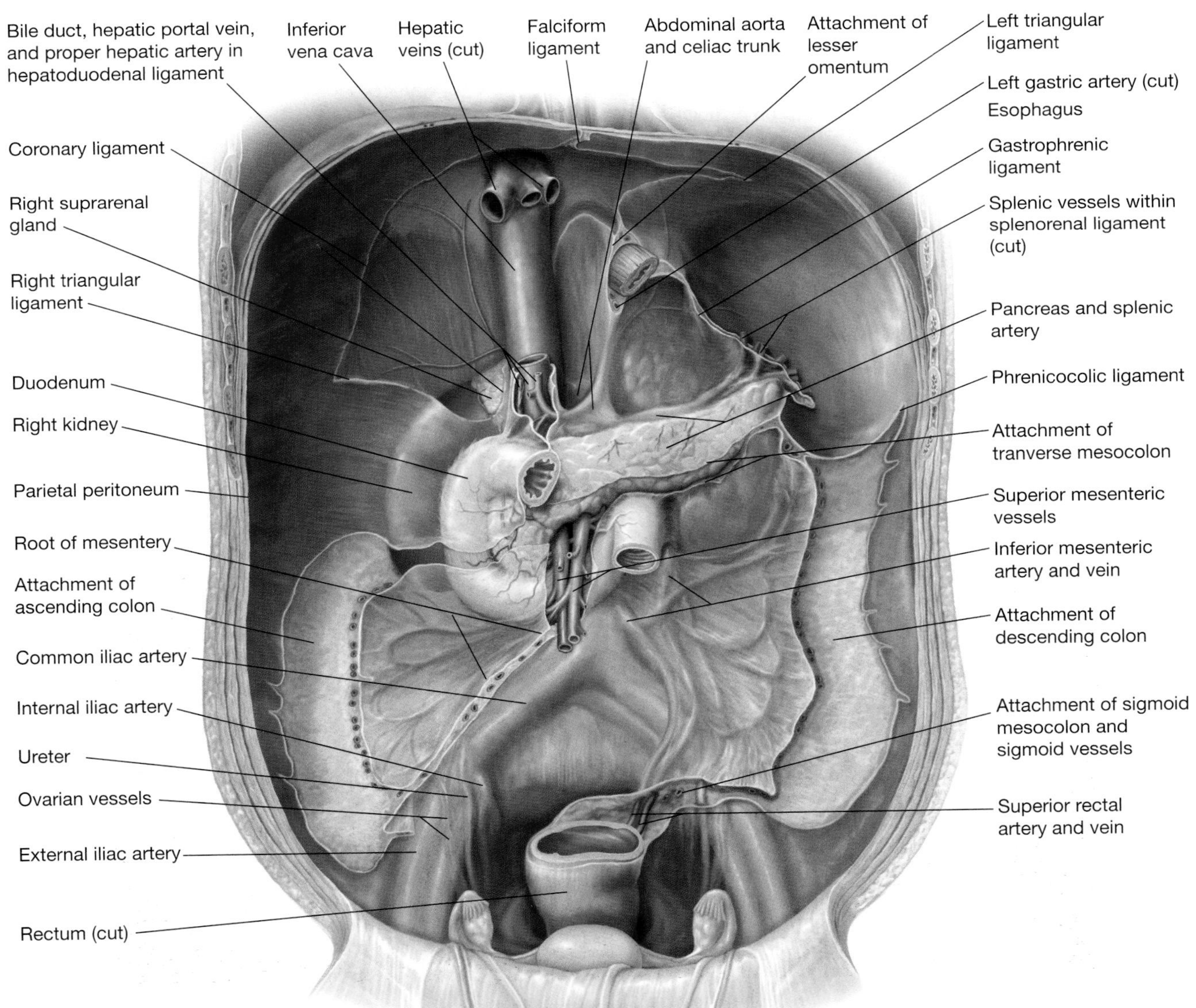

FIGURE 1 ● Retroperitoneal anatomy.

common being liposarcoma (60%) and leiomyosarcoma (20%), each with different biological behaviors and recurrence patterns.

- Prognosis is largely dictated by the ability to achieve complete surgical resection. Other factors that affect prognosis are histologic grade, tumor size, and patient age.

DIFFERENTIAL DIAGNOSIS

- The majority of RP masses are malignant; however, only about one-third of these are sarcomas. The differential diagnosis includes germ cell tumors, lymphomas, primary RP solid organ neoplasms, benign nerve sheath tumors, and metastatic lesions. Before approaching a RP mass like a sarcoma, it is important to confirm the diagnosis since several of the entities on the differential are not surgical diseases.

PATIENT HISTORY AND PHYSICAL FINDINGS

- Patients with RP sarcoma commonly present with vague symptoms. Often, the masses are identified incidentally on cross-sectional imaging performed for other reasons. Unfortunately, given the nonspecific symptoms, diagnosis is often delayed, and tumors are often larger than 10 cm at the time of initial diagnosis.
- Presenting symptoms can include abdominal or back pain, weight loss, or symptoms secondary to mass effect on surrounding structures. Patients may have early satiety if there is mass effect on the stomach, lower extremity edema secondary to venous obstruction from compression of the IVC or iliac vessels, or neurologic symptoms including foot drop if the tumor involves the psoas muscle or femoral and/or obturator nerves.
- It is important to perform a thorough physical exam, which may provide clues as to which structures are involved and help narrow the different diagnoses. Physical exam should include the abdomen as patients may have a palpable abdominal mass, lymph nodes, scrotum, and extremities in order to pick up signs of nerve or vessel involvement.

IMAGING AND OTHER DIAGNOSTIC STUDIES

- All patients require cross-sectional imaging of the abdomen and pelvis. Some histologic subtypes of RP sarcomas have characteristic radiological features. For example, a homogeneous fat dense mass is suggestive of a well-differentiated liposarcoma (WDLPS) (**FIGURE 2A**), while a heterogenous mass with both fat dense and solid components is more concerning for a dedifferentiated liposarcoma (**FIGURE 2B**). A noncalcified heterogenous enhancing mass with necrosis or cystic degeneration is highly suggestive of a leiomyosarcoma. Guided core-needle biopsy is necessary to confirm the diagnosis and direct management plan. Fine needle aspiration is inadequate for sarcoma diagnosis.
- When imaging is pathognomonic for benign lipomatous mass or WDLPS, preoperative biopsy is unlikely to change management and may be deferred. If the patient is being considered for neoadjuvant chemotherapy or radiation, pretreatment biopsy is required.
- Sarcomas most commonly metastasize to the lungs, therefore, once diagnosis is confirmed, patients need to be evaluated for pulmonary metastasis. This is done with chest radiograph or cross-sectional imaging with CT scan if the subtype of sarcoma is considered high risk for metastasis.
- Laboratory studies are not routinely used in the diagnosis of RP sarcomas. They should be obtained selectively to evaluate for alternative diagnoses. Consider obtaining serum and/or urine metanephrines if concern for pheochromocytoma or paraganglioma, lactate dehydrogenase (LDH) for lymphoma, or germ cell tumor markers (eg, alpha-fetoprotein [AFP], beta-human chorionic gonadotrophin [β-hCG]) for germ cell tumors.

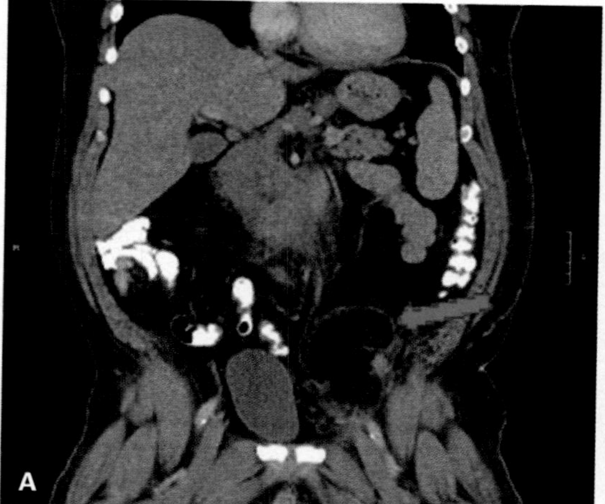

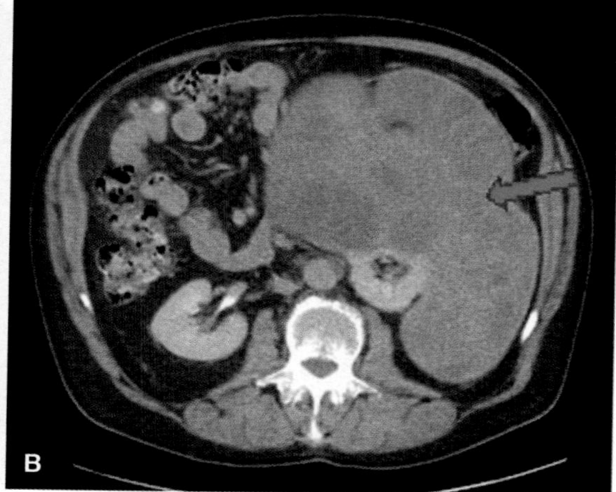

FIGURE 2 ● Contrasted computed tomography (CT) scan of well-differentiated liposarcoma (WDLPS), coronal view **(A)** and dedifferentiated liposarcoma (DDLPS), axial view **(B)**. *Red arrow* denotes liposarcoma.

SURGICAL MANAGEMENT

Preoperative Planning

- RP sarcoma is a complex disease and all cases require evaluation and presentation at a multidisciplinary sarcoma tumor board prior to initiating any treatment. Neoadjuvant chemotherapy and/or radiation therapy should be considered for high-risk tumors given the unsatisfactory outcomes with resection alone. Overall survival is increased by 20% when patients are treated at specialized sarcoma centers.[1]
- Preoperative imaging should be carefully reviewed to determine resectability. A tumor is deemed unresectable if it involves critical vascular structures (eg, superior mesenteric artery, portal vein, or the root of the mesentery), invades the spinal cord, if there are peritoneal implants, or if complete removal would result in unacceptable morbidity. This last point often requires joint decision-making between the patient and their provider. For example, if complete resection would require a nephrectomy in a patient at risk of becoming dialysis-dependent, the team must determine if this aligns with the patient's goals of care.
- Overall survival after an R2 resection (gross residual disease) or unresectable disease is equal[2]; therefore, surgical debulking is not recommended. Unresectable disease is managed as stage IV disease. For patients with intractable symptoms, operative bowel diversion or other palliative procedures may be pursued.
- Imaging should be reviewed to plan on what, if any, additional organs are likely going to need to be resected en bloc along with the tumor. For example, if a nephrectomy is considered, a renal perfusion scan should be obtained to ensure adequate contralateral kidney function. If a splenectomy is anticipated, patients should receive appropriate preoperative vaccinations.
- For patients with RP sarcoma, the first surgery is the most important; if a complete resection is achieved, outcomes are improved.[3] With this in mind, it is important to discuss with necessary specialists preoperatively to plan approach and confirm availability on the day of surgery. For example, involving urology for ureteral reimplantation or vascular surgery for vascular reconstruction.

Intraoperative Planning and Positioning

- Appropriate preoperative antibiotic coverage for skin and bowel flora should be administered prior to the induction of anesthesia to decrease the risk of surgical site infection.
- After induction, a Foley catheter and nasogastric/orogastric tubes are placed. Depending on the size, location, and extent of the tumor, placement of uni- or bilateral ureteral stents should be considered.
- Extent of resection and anticipated blood loss should be discussed with the anesthesia team prior to starting. If the tumor is large and with vascular involvement, blood products should be readily available in the operating room. Appropriate vascular access is needed with multiple large bore peripheral IVs or a central line especially if there is major vascular involvement (example, IVC).
- Patient positioning is dictated by placement of skin incision and approach. The goal is to optimize exposure to allow for complete en bloc resection and vascular control. The optimal approach should be determined preoperatively and depends on the size and location of the mass.
- Commonly, patients are positioned supine with their arms out and a midline laparotomy (**FIGURE 3A**) incision is used. This allows for adequate exposure for mobilization and can easily be re-entered should the patient develop a recurrence.
- For tumors that extend high into the upper left or right quadrants or if there is diaphragm involvement, a thoracoabdominal incision (**FIGURE 3B**) can be used. In these instances, the patient is be positioned laterally (full or sloppy) with the bed flexed. When positioning patients laterally, it is important to pad pressure points appropriately and leave access to the abdominal wall in case an ostomy is needed.
- When tumors are concentrated in the lower RP or pelvis, a transverse flank incision (patient positioned laterally) (**FIGURE 3A**) or a Gibson incision (patient placed supine) (**FIGURE 3A**) can be used.
- If the tumor extends into the femoral or inguinal canal, this may require an additional inguinal incision (**FIGURE 3A**).

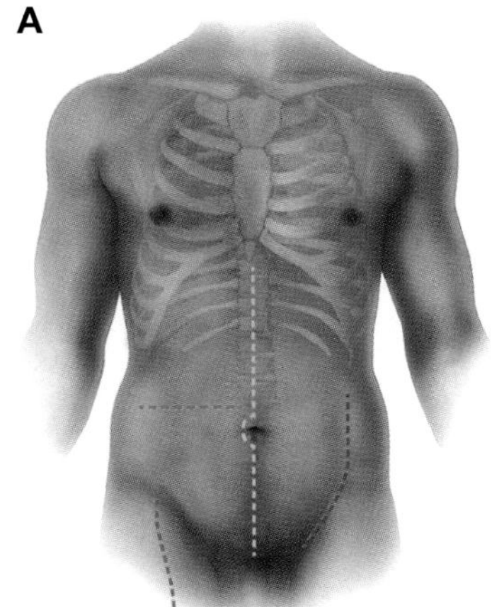

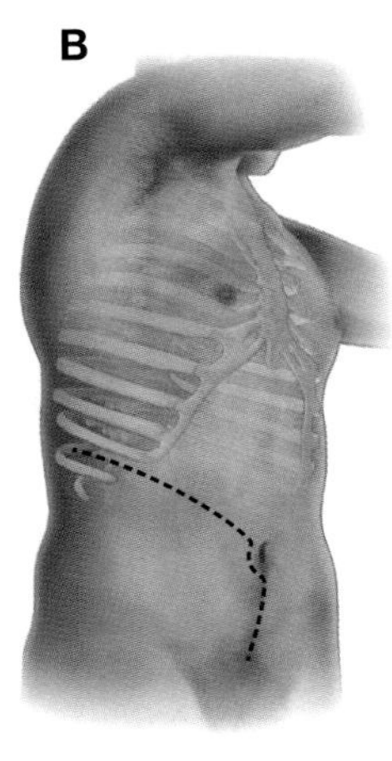

FIGURE 3 • Surgical incisions. **A,** Midline Laparotomy (denoted by green line). Inguinal counter incision (denoted by red line). Gibson incision (denoted by purple line). Transverse incision (denoted by blue line). **B,** Thoracoabdominal incision.

- Surgical resection with negative margins continues to be the mainstay of treatment for RP sarcoma as it is the only potential curative option. However, given the significant heterogeneity of the disease, every case will be different; however, adhering to basic principles can help achieve the goal of complete en bloc resection.
  - Upon entering the retroperitoneum, thorough inspection is performed to confirm and ensure resectability. Structures such as mesentery, ureters, and major vessels should not be divided until resection is known to be possible.
  - Next, further dissection should be carried out to visualize and expose the entire mass and ensure ability to obtain vascular control. Large tumors often distort anatomy, so it is very important to identify all structures using surrounding landmarks for verification before dividing structures.
  - Once the mass is fully exposed (**FIGURE 4**) and anatomy is fully ascertained, proceed with resection noting that this may require removal of multiple organs.
  - Metal clips are placed in the resection bed in areas of closest margin for identification if postoperative radiation is recommended. Reconstruction is completed and the abdomen is closed.
  - Lymphadenectomy is not routinely performed due to the low incidence of nodal metastasis.
  - Consider directly orienting tumor with the pathologist to ensure accurate margin assessment, especially areas of closest margin.
  - Use of routine intraoperative frozen section is not recommended.
  - Throughout the operation, is important to handle the tumor with care to minimize risk of rupture or capsule tearing.
- The location and extent of RP sarcomas vary greatly. Surgical resection is not one size fits all, and the approach must be tailored to each patient. Below, we have outlined some anatomic considerations that may be encountered during resection:
  - RP sarcoma resection commonly requires mobilization of the colon with resection of portions with bowel wall or vascular supply involvement.
  - The kidneys are retroperitoneal organs and are often surrounded or involved by tumor. Depending on involvement of parenchyma or renal vessels, nephrectomy may be required (refer to Part 7, Chapter 30 for necessary steps). If the renal parenchyma has not been invaded, you can consider a capsulectomy in low-grade sarcomas. Additionally, if the ureter is involved and the kidney and its vascular supply are completely free of tumor, kidney sparing resection with reimplantation of the ureter can be considered.
  - For left sided tumors, splenectomy and/or distal pancreatectomy may be required (Part 3, Chapters 37 and 47). The spleen should be removed if the tumor involves the splenic vessels or its parenchyma. Ideally, proximal control of the splenic artery should be performed prior to ligating venous outflow. If distal pancreatectomy is performed, there is a high risk of postoperative pancreatic leak in a normal residual soft pancreas. Drain placement should be considered.
  - A subset of RP sarcomas arises from and/or involves the IVC (**FIGURE 5**). The IVC can be divided into anatomic thirds: the lower section (the confluence of iliac veins to the renal veins), the middle section (the renal veins to the hepatic veins), and the upper section (the hepatic veins to the right atrium). Exposure of the inferior IVC can be accomplished using the Kocher (**FIGURE 6A**) or Cattell-Braasch maneuvers (**FIGURE 6B**). For tumors involving the retrohepatic middle IVC, concurrent hepatic resection and/or venous-venous bypass may be required. Similarly, tumors involving the upper segment of the IVC, if deemed resectable, may require cardiopulmonary bypass and/or hypothermic circulatory arrest. While the use of intraoperative frozen sections is not routinely recommended

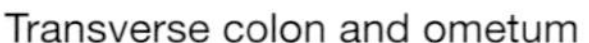

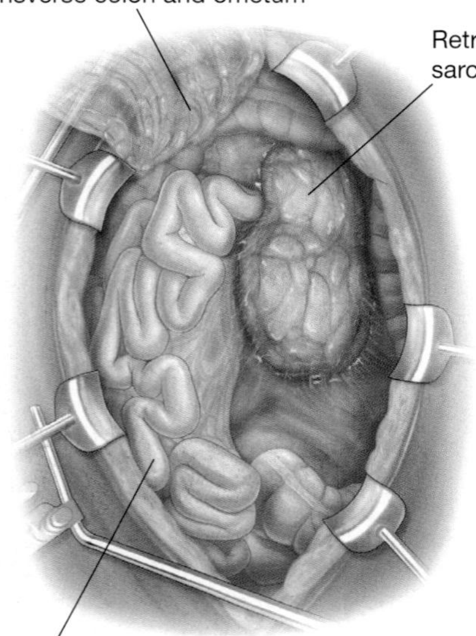

FIGURE 4 ● Exposure of retroperitoneal sarcoma via midline laparotomy using Thompson retractor.

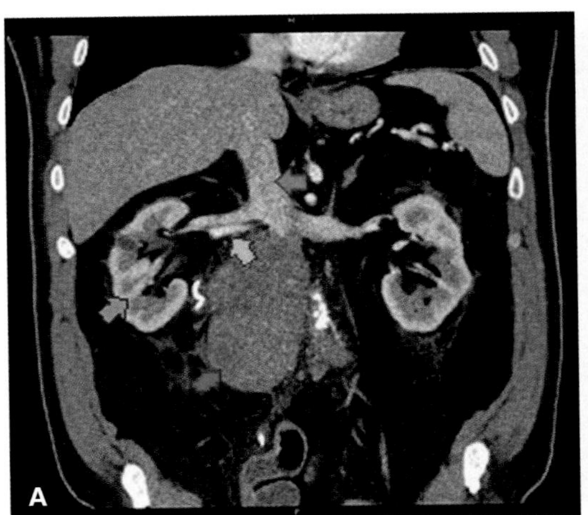

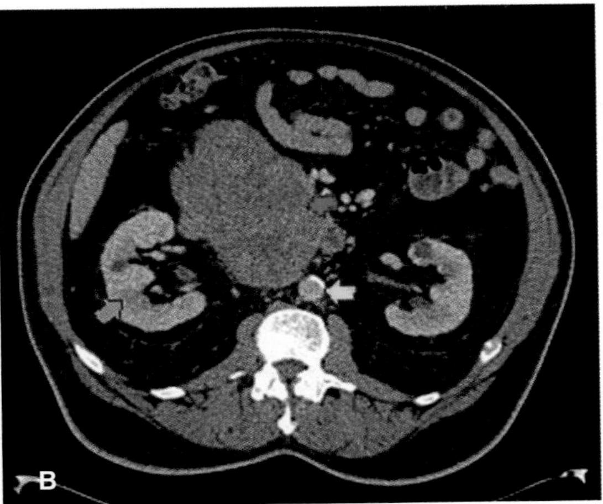

FIGURE 5 ● Computed tomography (CT) scan of retroperitoneal leiomyosarcoma involving inferior vena cava, coronal **(A)** and axial **(B)** views. *Red arrow* denotes sarcoma. *Blue arrow* denotes inferior vena cava. *Yellow arrow* denotes abdominal aorta. *Orange arrow* denotes right renal artery. *Green arrow* denotes right kidney.

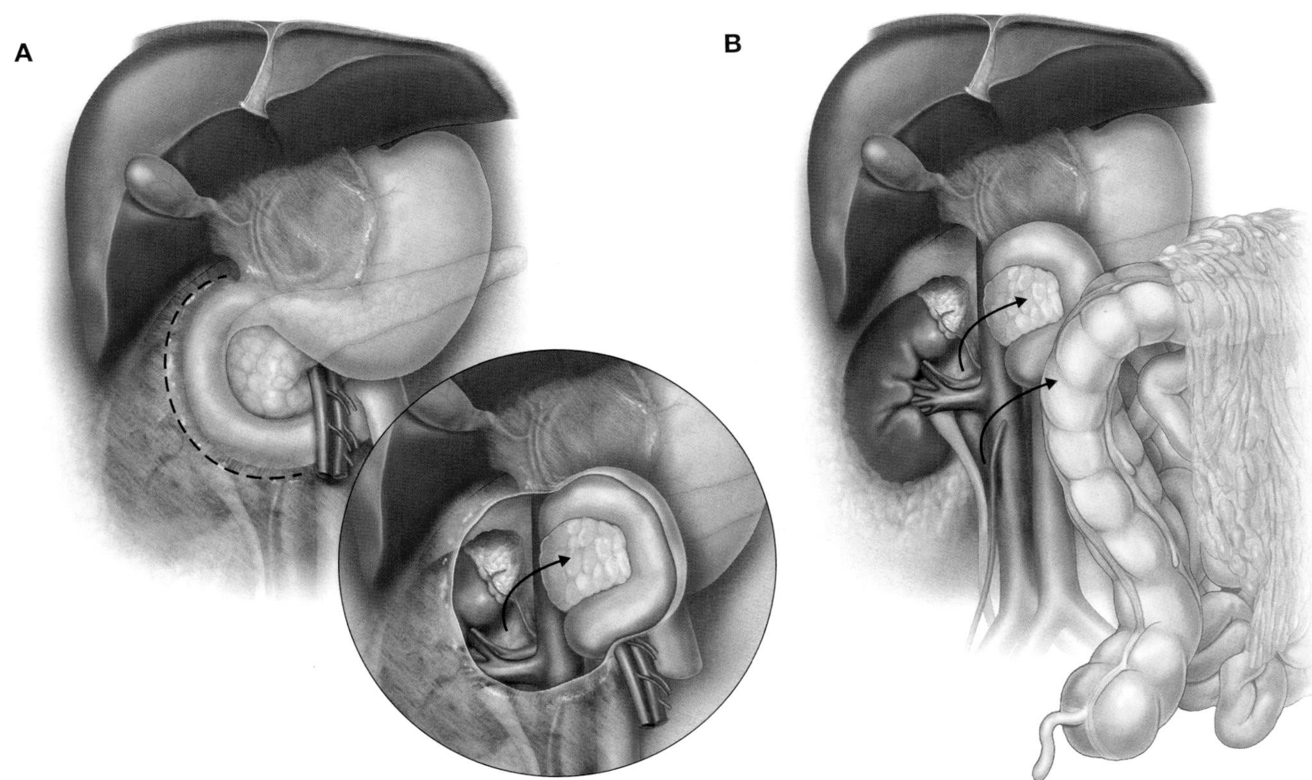

FIGURE 6 ● Inferior vena cava exposure. **A,** The Kocher maneuver involves mobilizing the duodenum and head to the pancreas medially to expose the inferior vena cava. **B,** The Cattell-Braasch maneuver requires extension of the dissection to rotate the ascending colon medially.

for the majority of RP sarcoma resections, they should be performed for the IVC tumor margin. IVC reconstruction is steered by specific clinical situation and intraoperative findings; options include synthetic tube grafts, autologous patch repair, and, if chronically occluded/compressed with sufficient intact collaterals (eg, gonadal and adrenal veins), you can consider ligation.

- Bowel resection is commonly required as part of the en bloc resection. Operative reports should document whether the ileocecal valve remains intact and how much small intestine was resected and how much is remaining. This is important to note due to risk of short gut if additional resections are required.

EXTENT OF RESECTION

- Standard removal of only contiguously involved organs vs compartmental resection (removal of all adjacent and uninvolved organs) continues to be debated. Studies show decrease in local recurrence with compartmental resection but no improvement in overall survival.[4,5]
- Aggressive histology is the most important predictor of local recurrence so a wider margin may be beneficial in these patients.
- Consideration of the most limiting margin will help determine the overall extent of resection.

PEARLS AND PITFALLS

Preoperative planning	■ Inadequate review of preoperative imaging to determine involvement of major structures can result in inadequate resection and poor outcomes.
Incision	■ Placement of incision is crucial for optimal exposure in a field with limited exposure due to size of tumor.
Resectability	■ Critical structures should not be divided until resection is known to be possible.
Tumor capsule	■ Great care must be taken to ensure resection without capsular intrusion during the index operation.
Debulking	■ The cornerstone of treatment is complete surgical resection. Debulking does not improve survival and should not be performed. Palliative procedure can be considered for symptomatic control.
Lack of follow-up	■ Recurrence rates are high. Patients should be followed closely with cross-sectional imaging and clinical evaluation.

POSTOPERATIVE CARE

- Some of the specifics and nuances of postoperative care are dictated by the extent of resection. However, all patients should receive adequate analgesia, aggressive pulmonary toilet, early ambulation, and deep vein thrombosis (DVT) prophylaxis, which are continued for 30 days postoperatively regardless of length of hospital stay.
- For larger tumors, patients tend to have sizable fluid shifts and should be appropriately monitored and resuscitated.
- Even if no bowel resection was required, patients tend to have prolonged postoperative ileus so consideration of nasogastric tube placement and removal and diet advancement should be done cautiously.

Neoadjuvant and Adjuvant Therapies

- Because of the high rates of local recurrence, ranging from 22% to 84%, radiation therapy may be considered in patients with high-grade subtypes and those with planned or known close margins. However, while some data demonstrate a favorable effect on recurrence-free interval, more recent data from a randomized controlled trial examining neoadjuvant radiation vs surgery alone do not show benefit.[6] Postoperative radiation is typically not recommended given the toxicity to the organs in the tumor bed and re-resection is favored over radiation if feasible.
- Chemotherapy is typically not used for patients with resectable disease due to the high rates of chemoresistance among common sarcoma subtypes. Adjuvant (or neoadjuvant) chemotherapy can be considered for chemosensitive histologies such as extraskeletal Ewing sarcoma, myxoid liposarcoma, rhabdomyosarcoma, and synovial sarcoma.

Surveillance

- The National Comprehensive Cancer Network (NCCN) Guidelines recommend surveillance with physical exam and cross-sectional imaging of the chest, abdomen, and pelvis every 3 to 6 months for 2 to 3 years, and then every 6 months until year 5, then annually.[7]

Outcomes

- RP sarcomas are a distinct entity from those of the trunk and extremity and have an overall worse prognosis. The reasons behind this difference are multifactorial and include differences in histology, large size, and multiorgan involvement including critical structures.
- Despite a complete macroscopic resection, local recurrence rates for RP sarcoma remain as high as 84%. Local recurrence is the leading cause of death in patients with RP sarcoma.[8] Given poor response to systemic therapy, surgical resection remains the best treatment option. However, reoperation and more extensive resection is associated

with higher morbidity and mortality and must be carefully weighed against potential benefit.

COMPLICATIONS

- Bleeding/hematoma
- Bowel anastomotic leak or fistula
- Abscess
- Wound infection
- Acute kidney injury and need for long-term hemodialysis
- Ileus
- Pancreatic leak
- Deep vein thrombosis or pulmonary embolism

REFERENCES

1. Gronchi A, Strauss DC, Miceli R, et al. Variability in patterns of recurrence after resection of primary retroperitoneal sarcoma (RPS): a report on 1007 patients from the multi-institutional collaborative RPS working group. *Ann Surg*. 2016;263(5):1002-1009.
2. Kirane A, Crago AM. The importance of surgical margins in retroperitoneal sarcoma. *J Surg Oncol*. 2016;113:270-276.
3. Schwartz PB, Vande Walle K, Winslow ER, et al. Predictors of disease-free and overall survival in retroperitoneal sarcomas: a modern 16-year multi-institutional study from the United States Sarcoma Collaboration (USSC). *Sarcoma*. 2019;2019:5395131.
4. Gronchi A, Lo Vullo S, Fiore M, et al. Aggressive surgical policies in a retrospectively reviewed single-institution case series of retroperitoneal soft tissue sarcoma patients. *J Clin Oncol*. 2009;27:24-30.
5. Bonvalot S, Rivoire M, Castaing M, et al. Primary retroperitoneal sarcomas: a multivariate analysis of surgical factors associated with local control. *J Clin Oncol*. 2009;27:31-37.
6. Bonvalot S, Gronchi A, Le Péchoux C, et al. Preoperative radiotherapy plus surgery versus surgery alone for patients with primary retroperitoneal sarcoma (EORTC-62092: STRASS) – a multicentre, open-label, randomised, phase 3 trial. *Lancet Oncol*. 2020;21:1366-1377.
7. National Comprehensive Cancer N. *Sarcoma (Version 2.2021)*. Accessed September 2021. 2021. https://www.nccn.org/professionals/physician_gls/pdf/sarcoma.pdf
8. Trans-Atlantic RPSWG. Management of recurrent retroperitoneal sarcoma (RPS) in the adult: a consensus approach from the trans-Atlantic RPS working group. *Ann Surg Oncol*. 2016;23:3531-3540.

Chapter 46 Thyroidectomy

Hunter J. Underwood and David T. Hughes

DEFINITION

- Total thyroid lobectomy is defined as the surgical removal of an entire thyroid lobe and isthmus. It can be used as a diagnostic or a therapeutic procedure.
- Total thyroidectomy is a therapeutic procedure that involves removal of all thyroid tissue, including both lobes and the isthmus.
- Thyroid disease requiring a lobectomy is most often due to the presence of a thyroid nodule. The prevalence of thyroid nodules among adults is high and varies depending on the mode of discovery. Approximately 2% to 6% of nodules are discovered by palpation, whereas 19% to 35% are found incidentally on unrelated imaging studies (eg, CT neck for trauma, screening carotid duplex).[1]
- The most common indications for a thyroid lobectomy are:
  - A thyroid nodule with diagnostic uncertainty
  - A symptomatic thyroid nodule (eg, compressive unilateral goiter or autonomous toxic nodule)
  - Low-risk papillary thyroid cancer (eg, <4 cm, no evidence of extrathyroidal extension, no evidence of lymph node metastasis)
- The most common indications for a total thyroidectomy include:
  - Graves disease
  - In general, total thyroidectomy is indicated for most thyroid cancers, other than low-risk papillary thyroid cancer. Patients may also need a concomitant central lymph node dissection (Part 5, Chapter 51)
  - Multinodular goiter

ANATOMY

- The thyroid gland has a right and left lobe bridged by a narrow isthmus and is located in the central compartment of the anterior neck, below the thyroid cartilage. The thyroid cartilage forms the laryngeal prominence known as the "Adam's Apple."
- The thyroid lobes lie medial to the carotid sheaths and sternocleidomastoid muscles (**FIGURE 1**).
- The anterolateral surface of the gland is covered by the sternothyroid and sternohyoid muscles.
- The "thyroid sheath" is a connective tissue expansion of the pretracheal fascia and envelops the thyroid, condensing posteromedial into the ligament of Berry.
- The thyroid gland receives its blood supply from the superior and inferior thyroid arteries. The superior thyroid artery arises from the ipsilateral external carotid artery and the superior thyroid vein runs with the artery. The inferior thyroid artery originates from the thyrocervical trunk. The middle thyroid vein drains into the ipsilateral internal jugular vein.
- The left recurrent laryngeal nerve (RLN) arises from the vagus at the level of the aortic arch and loops around the ligamentum arteriosum; the right RLN loops around the right subclavian artery (**FIGURE 2**). The right RLN may be nonrecurrent in 0.5% to 1% of individuals.
- The RLN innervates all the intrinsic muscles of the larynx except the cricothyroid muscles.
- The internal branch of the superior laryngeal nerve is the sensory nerve for the supraglottic larynx. The external branch of the superior laryngeal nerve lies on the inferior pharyngeal constrictor muscle and descends alongside the superior thyroid vessels before innervating the cricothyroid muscle.
- The superior parathyroid glands are generally located posterior to the superior thyroid lobe and the RLN. The inferior parathyroid locations are more variable but oftentimes are located anterior to the inferior thyroid lobes and RLN or on the inferolateral aspect of the lobes.

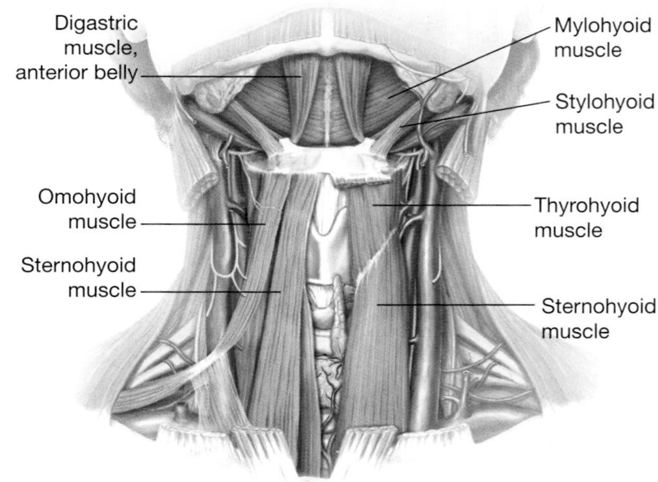

FIGURE 1 • Strap muscles of the neck.

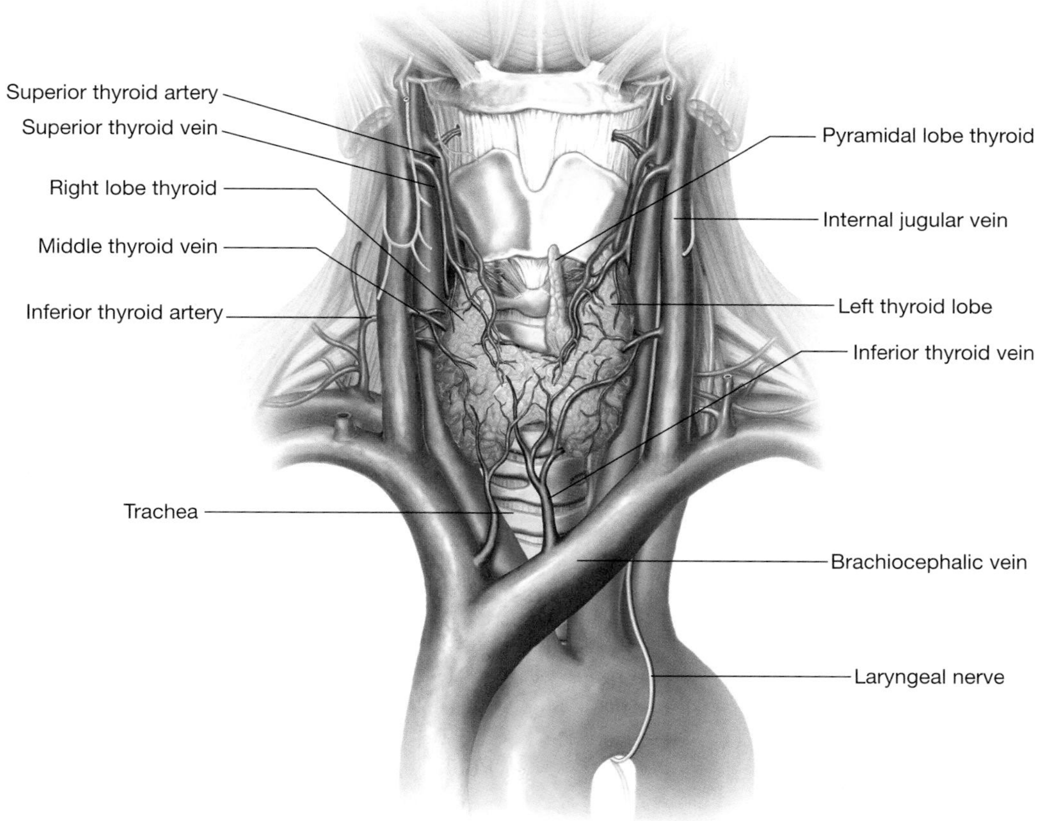

FIGURE 2 ● Anatomic location of thyroid gland and vascular anatomy.

PATIENT HISTORY AND PHYSICAL FINDINGS

- Although thyroid nodules are common, most of them are benign. A thorough patient history can assist the clinician in determining which thyroid nodules may require surgical management. Previous radiation to the neck, a rapidly growing mass, hoarseness, associated lymphadenopathy, or a family history of cancer may raise the suspicion of malignancy. Dysphagia, choking, tightness, or intolerance to things around the neck may suggest local compressive symptoms from a large thyroid nodule.
- The physical exam should focus on characteristics of the thyroid such as size, firmness, and the presence of multiple nodules. The neck should be palpated for associated lymphadenopathy.

IMAGING AND OTHER DIAGNOSTIC STUDIES

- **Thyroid function studies.** A thyroid-stimulating hormone (TSH) can assess the biochemical status of the patient's thyroid.
- **Ultrasonography.** Neck ultrasound is a highly sensitive, but user-dependent adjunct to the physical exam in the evaluation of the thyroid. Ultrasonographic evidence of extrathyroidal extension of the thyroid nodule or suspicious cervical lymphadenopathy or morphologically abnormal appearing lymph nodes should raise suspicion of more advanced thyroid cancer, which would necessitate total thyroidectomy and lymph node dissection of the involved lymph node basins followed by radioactive iodine treatment.
- **Biopsy.** Fine-needle aspiration (FNA) is indicated for thyroid nodules based on ultrasonographic appearance and patient-related risk factors (eg, family history or radiation exposure). FNA cytology results are categorized according to the Bethesda system,[2] which can then be used to recommend thyroidectomy or surveillance with ultrasound. FNA can also be used to confirm the presence of metastatic cervical lymph nodes.
- **Molecular testing.** Bethesda III and IV nodules are often referred to as "indeterminate thyroid nodules" and convey a risk of malignancy of 6% to 18% and 10% to 40%, respectively. Traditionally, diagnostic lobectomy was

recommended for indeterminate thyroid nodules; however, most patients ultimately did not have cancer on final pathology. Molecular testing can be a useful adjunct to stratify cancer risk in patients with indeterminate biopsy results.

- **Computed tomography** (CT). A preoperative neck or chest CT is usually not necessary except in specific situations:
  - Malignancy—A neck CT may suggest local invasion of the thyroid into surrounding structures such as the carotid artery, internal jugular vein, or trachea, which could potentially modify the operative approach. A CT scan of the neck can also provide a detailed map of cervical lymphadenopathy. A chest CT can evaluate for pulmonary metastatic disease.
  - Large goiters—A neck and chest CT scan can help determine the degree of tracheal obstruction or substernal extension of large goiters, which is difficult to determine on ultrasound. If the inferior extent of the thyroid gland or nodule is not visible on ultrasound or palpable on exam, cross-sectional imaging of the chest can determine the degree of substernal extension and help predict the need for sternotomy for removal.
- **Laryngoscopy.** Flexible laryngoscopy should be performed on all patients with hoarseness or a previous history of neck surgery to evaluate the function of the recurrent laryngeal nerves. This provides a current assessment and baseline evaluation of bilateral vocal cords prior to surgery.

SURGICAL MANAGEMENT

- Thyroid lobectomy is therapeutic for patients with symptomatic unilateral goiter or a solitary toxic nodule.
- Thyroid lobectomy is diagnostic and can potentially be therapeutic for patients with indeterminate thyroid nodules (Bethesda III and IV) or molecular testing, which is suspicious for malignancy depending on the final surgical pathology.
- Thyroid lobectomy is therapeutic for patients with low-risk papillary thyroid cancer, which is defined by a tumor size less than 4 cm and absence of extrathyroidal extension and lymph node or distant metastasis.[3,4]
- Total thyroidectomy should be considered in other cases of thyroid cancer, cases of suspicious or definite malignant nodules where there is a history of head and neck irradiation, Graves disease, large or substernal goiter (see Part 5, Chapter 47), or symptomatic goiter (dysphagia, pressure, dyspnea).
- When going to the OR for a thyroid lobectomy, the patient and surgeon should be prepared for conversion to a total thyroidectomy if intraoperative findings display unexpected evidence of high-risk features such as gross extrathyroidal extension, unexpected central neck lymph node metastases, or inability to obtain a grossly negative margin.

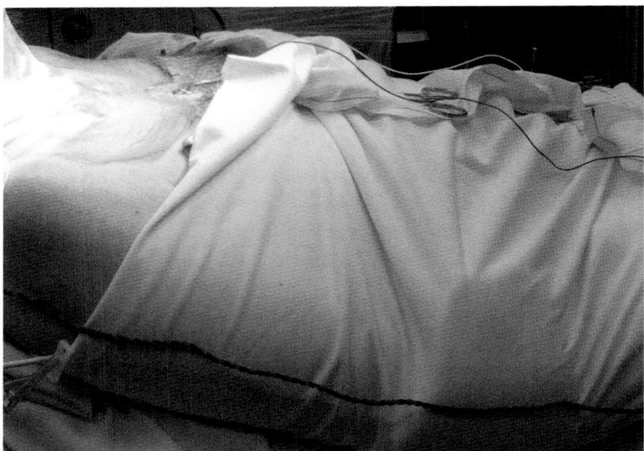

FIGURE 3 ● Patient positioning. The arms should be padded and can be tucked to the side with a sheet using a towel clip.

Preoperative Planning

- Thyroidectomy is performed under a general anesthesia, but locoregional anesthetic with sedation may be adequate for lobectomy in select patients. Short-acting paralytic, for example, succinylcholine, should be used for induction if using a recurrent laryngeal nerve monitoring system.
- Routine use of preoperative antibiotics is not common as wound infections after thyroidectomy are rare.

Positioning

- The patient is placed in the supine position with the arms padded and tucked at the side (**FIGURE 3**). A shoulder roll can be placed to help extend the neck; however, care should be taken to cause excessive extension as this can cause postoperative discomfort. The operative table may also be placed in the semi-fowler or beach-chair position to further extend the neck.

SKIN INCISION AND FLAP CREATION

- A low collar incision is placed at the midline symmetrically across the neck regardless of sidedness. The incision can be placed anywhere above the sternal notch and below the cricoid cartilage and in a natural skin crease to aid in cosmesis (**FIGURE 4**). If no skin crease is appropriate, Langer's lines provide an adequate guide. This location provides good exposure to the entire gland and particularly the superior pole.

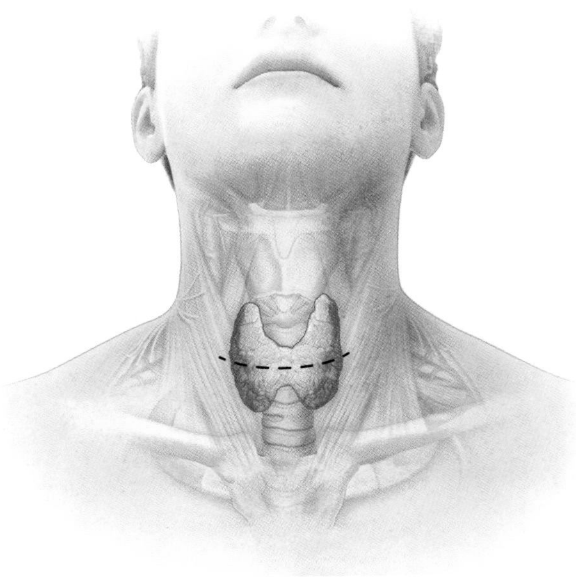

FIGURE 4 ● Incision anatomy. The sternal notch and cricoid cartilage are palpated to help determine the incision site.

GLAND EXPOSURE

- The incision is carried through the subcutaneous tissue and platysma. Subplatysmal flaps are created to enhance exposure (**FIGURE 5**). These flaps should extend to the thyroid cartilage superiorly and the suprasternal notch inferiorly. Care should be taken to avoid injury to the anterior jugular veins during flap creation as bleeding from these veins can be profuse. If injury is noted, definitive control should be obtained prior to proceeding.
- The midline raphe between the strap muscles is opened and dissection extends down to the level of the thyroid isthmus (**FIGURE 6**).
- The sternohyoid and, subsequently, the sternothyroid muscles are dissected off the thyroid and retracted laterally. The strap muscles can be divided in case of very large thyroid nodules to aid in exposure and are then reapproximated at the conclusion of the lobectomy.
- The thyroid lobe is then retracted medially with a finger or hemostatic clamp. The space between the thyroid and the carotid sheath is opened bluntly until the prevertebral fascia is encountered (**FIGURE 7**). During this portion of the dissection, the middle thyroid veins are controlled and ligated.

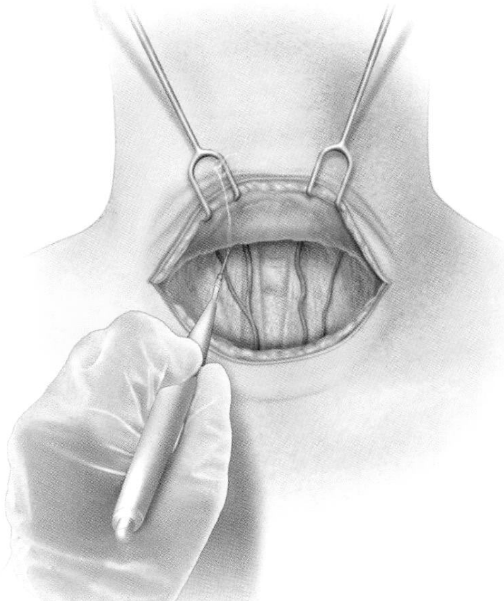

FIGURE 5 ● Creation of subplatysmal flaps. Adequate retraction helps creation of the subplatysmal flaps and prevents buttonholing the skin.

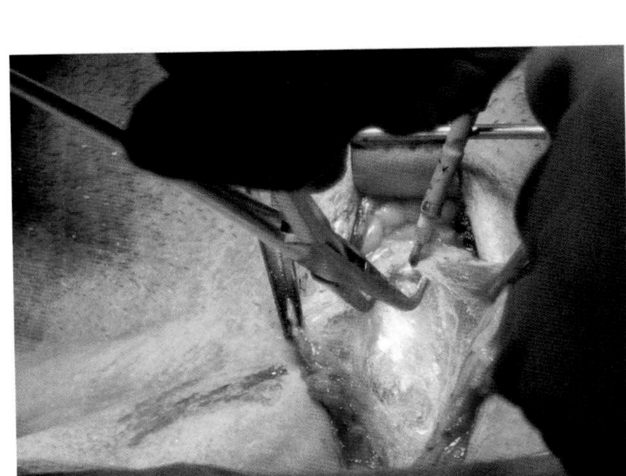

FIGURE 6 ● Exposure of the thyroid. The midline raphe between the strap muscles is avascular and provides access to the thyroid when opened.

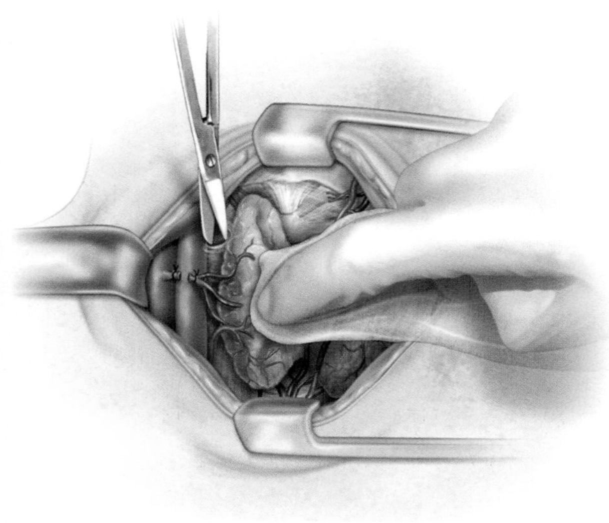

- Dissection of the isthmus can help mobilize the thyroid gland. The superior suspensory ligament and associated vessels at the superior border of the isthmus should be divided. A pyramidal lobe can be dissected and divided if present. The inferior vessels and attachment to the trachea along the inferior border of the isthmus should also be divided.
- Dissection on the contralateral side should be avoided to prevent scar formation in the event the patient requires completion thyroidectomy in the future.

FIGURE 7 ● Exposure of the posterior thyroid. The thyroid is retracted toward the midline and the middle thyroid vein is divided. The areolar tissue behind the thyroid can be bluntly dissected with scissors.

SUPERIOR POLE DISSECTION

- The cricothyroid space is an avascular space between the cricothyroid muscle and superior pole of the thyroid gland. This space can be bluntly opened posteriorly to the prevertebral fascia. Retraction of the superior pole of the thyroid in the inferior and lateral directions can facilitate this dissection (**FIGURE 8**).
- The external branch of the superior laryngeal nerve may be identified during this dissection and should be preserved. The nerve is vulnerable to injury as it crosses the vessels close to the superior pole of the thyroid prior to its insertion into the muscle. The anatomic variations of the nerve in relation to the superior thyroid vessels are best described by Cernea et al[5] (**FIGURE 9**).
- The superior pole vessels are divided at the level of the thyroid capsule to prevent injury of the nerve.
- A superior parathyroid gland may be identified in this area and should be dissected off the gland attempting to preserve its blood supply, which can originate from the inferior thyroid artery or the superior thyroid arteries.

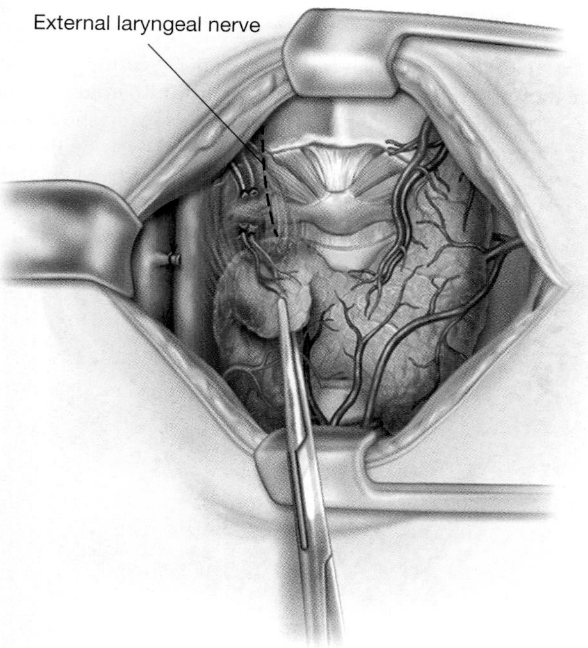

FIGURE 8 ● Exposure of the superior pole. The cricothyroid space is opened up bluntly. Retraction of the superior pole in a lateral and inferior direction helps to minimize the risk of injury to the external branch of the superior laryngeal nerve (dotted line).

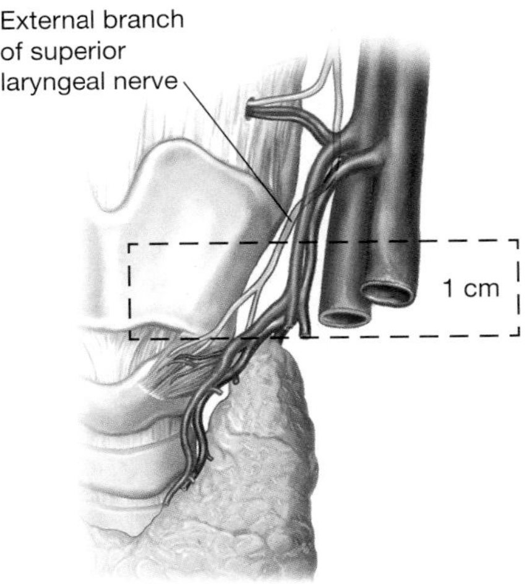

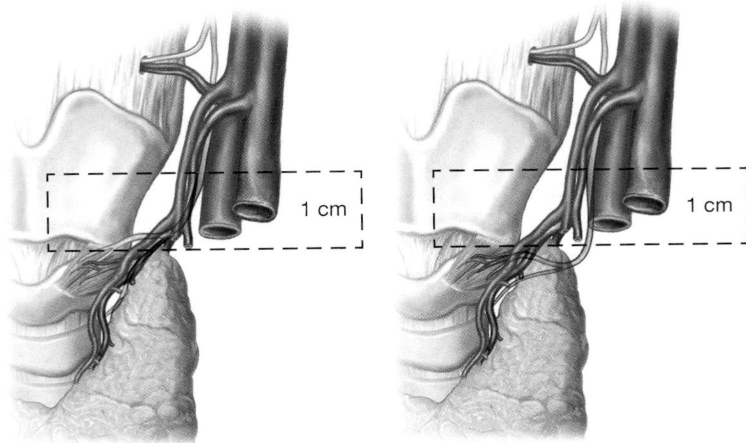

FIGURE 9 ● Anatomic variations of the external branch of the superior laryngeal nerve. The nerve crosses the vessels greater than a centimeter from the superior pole in type 1 anatomy. Type 2 anatomy places the nerve at higher risk of injury during dissection because it crossed less than a centimeter from the superior pole (type 2a) or even below it (type 2b). (From Cernea CR, Ferraz AR, Nishio S, et al. Surgical anatomy of the external branch of the superior laryngeal nerve. *Head Neck*. 1992;14(5):380-383. Copyright © 1992 Wiley Periodicals, Inc. Reprinted by permission of John Wiley & Sons, Inc.)

LATERAL LOBE DISSECTION

- Once the superior pole is mobilized, the lateral and inferior aspect of the thyroid can be dissected. The thyroid lobe should be retracted medially and elevated anteriorly off the paraesophageal space. An assistant should retract the strap muscles and carotid sheath laterally to open the parathyroidal space.
- The identification and preservation of the recurrent laryngeal nerve is critical to the dissection. The nerve should be identified early and can often be found in the tracheoesophageal groove below the inferior thyroid pole and then dissected cranially where it passes either superior or inferior to the inferior thyroid artery up to its cricothyroid insertion. The nerve is most vulnerable in this area due to traction of the thyroid and the attachments of the ligament of Berry.
- The tertiary vessels of the inferior thyroid artery are divided at the level of the thyroid capsule (**FIGURE 10**). This capsular dissection helps decrease the risk of nerve injury and devascularization of the parathyroid glands.
- The attachments of the thyroid to the trachea are freed by dividing the ligament of Berry.

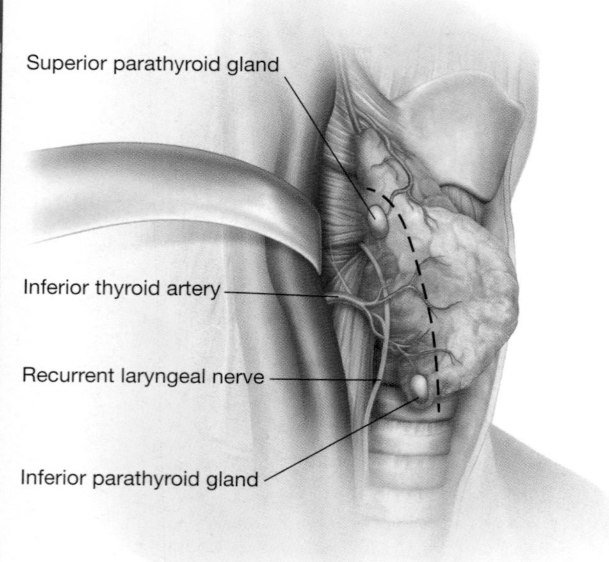

FIGURE 10 ● Division of the inferior thyroid artery. The tertiary branches of the inferior thyroid artery are ligated at the thyroid capsule to prevent injury to the recurrent laryngeal nerve and the blood supply to the parathyroid glands. The *dotted line* denotes the area of dissection.

PARATHYROID PRESERVATION

- The inferior and superior parathyroid glands should be identified and preserved. This is accomplished by careful dissection and reflection of them in a posterolateral direction away from the thyroid. The main trunk of the inferior thyroid artery should not be ligated far away from the thyroid capsule as it typically provides the blood supply to both parathyroid glands.

TRANSECTION OF THE THYROID FOR TOTAL THYROID LOBECTOMY

- If a total thyroidectomy is being performed, the contralateral lobe is resected in an identical fashion and the isthmus is separated from the underlying trachea (**FIGURE 11**).
- A thyroid lobectomy requires transection of the thyroid at the junction of the isthmus and contralateral lobe. If this junction is small, an energy device or cautery can transect this area while providing good hemostasis. If the area is bulky, a clamp can be placed across the area of transection. A knife is then used to transect the thyroid and the specimen is removed (**FIGURE 12**). A running absorbable suture can be placed as a hemostatic stitch underneath the clamp.

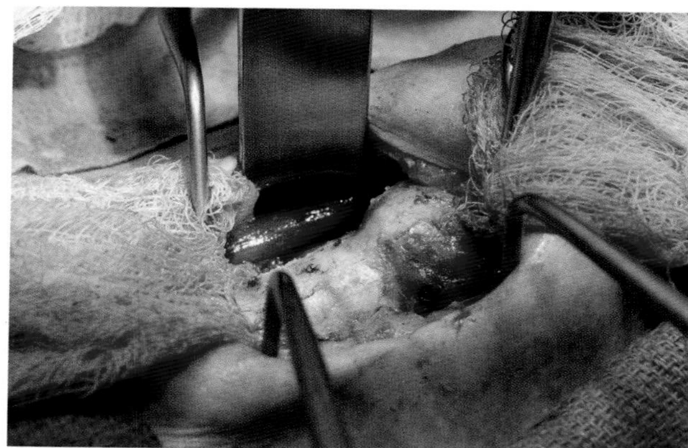

FIGURE 11 ● After a total thyroidectomy, the trachea is left exposed.

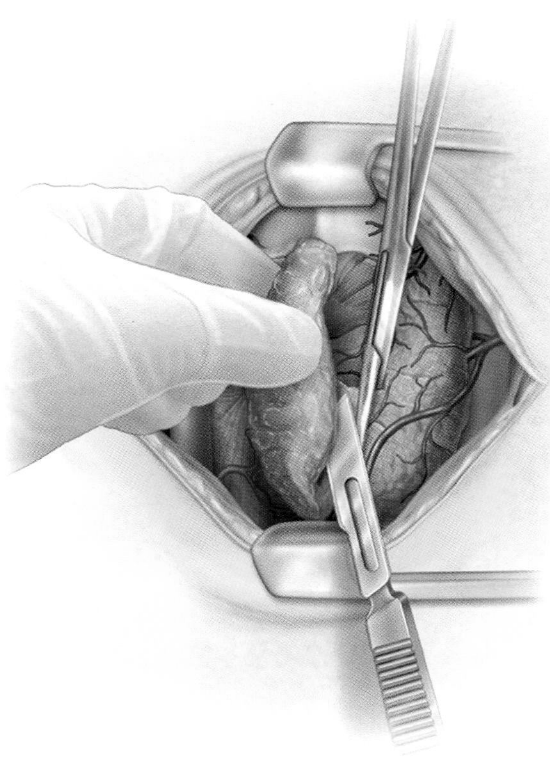

FIGURE 12 ● Transection of the thyroid. The junction between the isthmus and contralateral lobe is transected to remove the specimen.

CLOSURE

- Prior to closure, the surgical field is meticulously evaluated for hemostasis. Small occult bleeding can lead to clinically significant neck hematomas if not controlled.
- The parathyroid glands are evaluated once more for viability. Additionally, the lobectomy specimen should be examined for the inadvertent removal of a normal parathyroid gland. If either situation arises, the parathyroid gland should be minced up and implanted into the ipsilateral sternocleidomastoid. Frozen section can be helpful in confirming the presence of parathyroid tissue prior to reimplantation.
- The recurrent laryngeal nerve is examined with visual inspection or nerve monitoring to ensure an intact motor function. Previous literature has suggested that the benefit of intraoperative nerve monitoring in preventing nerve damage is similar to visual inspection; however, more contemporary studies have shown the use of nerve monitoring to be independently associated with reduced risk of injury.[5]
- After adequate hemostasis and inspection, the strap muscles are reapproximated with absorbable interrupted sutures (**FIGURE 13**). Placement of these sutures requires care to avoid injury to the anterior jugular veins.
- The platysma is reapproximated with buried interrupted absorbable sutures (**FIGURE 14**).
- The skin can be closed in a variety of ways including subcuticular suture, skin glue, and/or steri strips (**FIGURE 15**). If the wound appears to be under tension during closure, removal of the shoulder roll can help.

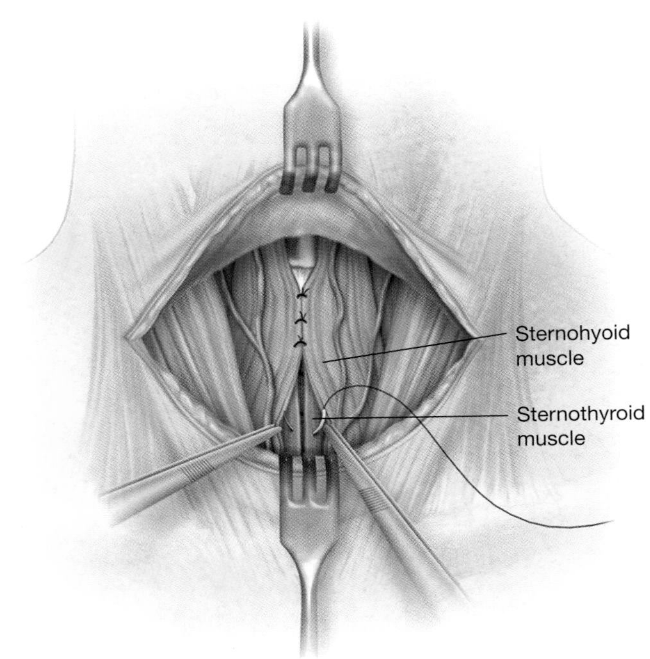

FIGURE 13 ● Closing the strap muscles. The strap muscles are reapproximated with interrupted sutures.

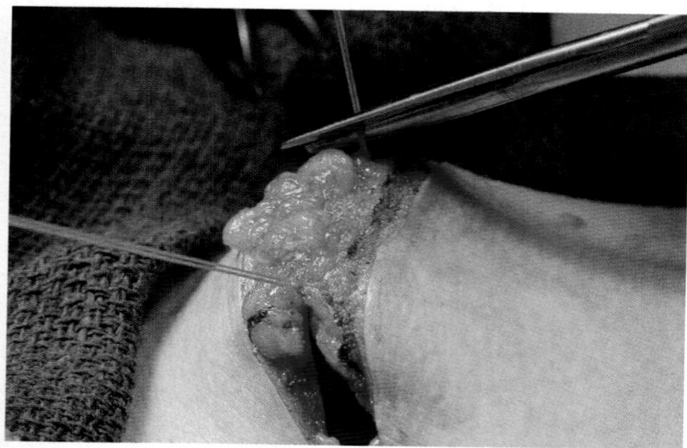

FIGURE 14 ● Platysmal muscle layer reapproximated with interrupted absorbable sutures.

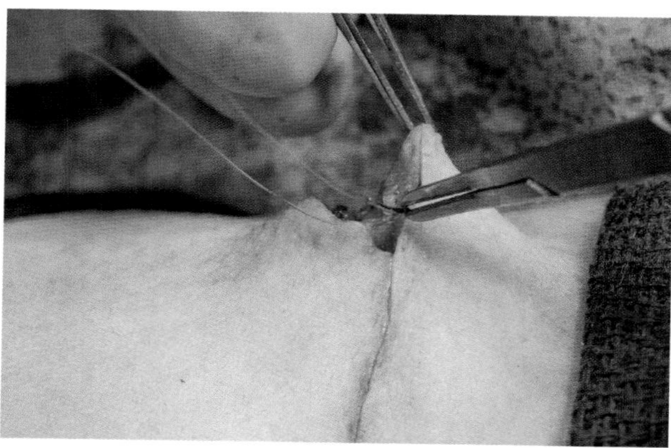

FIGURE 15 ● Subcuticular running suture technique.

PEARLS AND PITFALLS

Incision aesthetics	■ A natural skin crease should be used if present. ■ An incision too cephalad is more noticeable with normal clothing as opposed to a lower neck incision. ■ An incision too caudal on the upper chest can increase the risk of keloid formation.
Parathyroid preservation and autotransplantation	■ If a parathyroid gland cannot be preserved, it should be placed into cold saline for preservation. ■ A small portion of the parathyroid gland can be sent for frozen section to confirm the presence of normal parathyroid tissue. ■ The gland should then be minced into small pieces and implanted into the ipsilateral sternocleidomastoid. ■ A clip or permanent suture can mark the autograft sites.
Hemostasis	■ Hemostasis can be evaluated under Valsalva maneuver after irrigation to look for occult bleeding. ■ Drains are rarely needed and are never a substitute for adequate hemostasis. ■ Electrocautery should be avoided in the area of the recurrent laryngeal nerve.
Large substernal goiter	■ Most substernal goiters located above the brachiocephalic vein can be removed through a cervical collar incision. ■ Dissection of the superior pole and early transection of the isthmus can provide added mobility needed to pull up a goiter from behind the sternum. ■ The patient should be counseled, and the chest prepped in case a sternotomy is needed.
Intraoperative recurrent laryngeal nerve injury	■ If loss of signal on nerve monitor is identified, the nerve should be completely exposed to determine if it is anatomically intact and to release any areas of traction. ■ If the nerve is intact, the loss of signal may be attributable to excessive traction on the nerve at the insertion point during medial retraction of the thyroid gland and will often recover over time postoperatively. ■ If the nerve is noted to be disrupted upon further inspection a primary anastomosis or ansa cervicalis graft can be performed.

POSTOPERATIVE CARE

- The patient should be monitored in the postoperative area for a few hours to ensure no hematoma develops. Most clinically significant hematomas occur within the first several hours postoperatively. If a clinically significant hematoma occurs, the patient should return to the operating room to drain the hematoma and control bleeding.
- An ice pack may be placed over the neck to assist with pain and swelling. Once the patient is sufficiently awake, the diet may be advanced as tolerated.
- After a period of monitoring, most patients may be safely discharged home after a thyroid lobectomy. Large goiters, those with substernal extension, or patients at higher risk of bleeding may be observed overnight.
- Except in those with previous removal of the contralateral lobe, a unilateral lobectomy will not cause hypoparathyroidism and therefore no calcium monitoring or calcium supplementation is required.
- Patients should expect to resume their normal activities within a few days of surgery.

- Approximately 15% to 30% of patients will require thyroid hormone after lobectomy; thus thyroid hormone levels should be checked 6 weeks after surgery to ensure adequate function of the remaining lobe.[6]

COMPLICATIONS

- Hematoma
- Hypocalcemia (only in setting of completion thyroid lobectomy)
- Hoarseness
- Vocal cord paralysis
- Wound infection

ACKNOWLEDGMENTS

The authors would like to thank Dr. Amy C. Fox, Dr. Paul Gauger, Dr. Said C. Azoury, and Dr. Martha A. Zeigler for their prior contributions to this textbook.

REFERENCES

1. Tamhane S, and Gharib H. "Thyroid nodule update on diagnosis and management." *Clin Diabetes Endocrinol*. 2016;2(1):1-10.
2. Cibas ES, and Ali SZ. "The 2017 Bethesda system for reporting thyroid cytopathology." *Thyroid*. 2017;27(11):1341-1346.
3. Haugen BR, Alexander EK, Bible KC, et al. "2015 American Thyroid Association management guidelines for adult patients with thyroid nodules and differentiated thyroid cancer: the American Thyroid Association guidelines task force on thyroid nodules and differentiated thyroid cancer." *Thyroid*. 2016;26(1):1-133.
4. Patel KN, Yip L, Lubitz CC, et al. "The American Association of Endocrine Surgeons guidelines for the definitive surgical management of thyroid disease in adults." *Ann Surg*. 2020;271(3):e21-e93.
5. Kim J, Graves CE, Jin C, et al. "Intraoperative nerve monitoring is associated with a lower risk of recurrent laryngeal nerve injury: a national analysis of 17,610 patients." *Am J Surg*. 2021;221(2):472-477.
6. Wilson M, Patel A, Goldner W, et al. "Postoperative thyroid hormone supplementation rates following thyroid lobectomy." *Am J Surg*. 2020;220(5):1169-1173.

Chapter 47 Thyroidectomy for Substernal Goiters

Andrew G. Shuman and Ashok R. Shaha

DEFINITION

- A goiter refers to any abnormal thyroid enlargement secondary to nutritional deficiency, endocrine disease, or neoplasm. In general terms, substernal goiter applies to conditions in which most of the thyroid volume lies below the thoracic inlet.

PATIENT HISTORY AND PHYSICAL FINDINGS

- A comprehensive medical history is obligatory, including assessment of the indications for surgery, consideration of medical comorbidities, and ensuring that patients are medically optimized and risk-stratified for surgery. Any prior operative records and pathology reports should be reviewed in advance.
- A detailed physical examination is mandatory, including consideration of upper airway patency and visualization of the larynx to assess vocal fold mobility.
- Flexible fiberoptic laryngoscopy is helpful in evaluating glottic function and assessing the airway.

IMAGING AND OTHER DIAGNOSTIC STUDIES

- Cross-sectional imaging (usually computed tomography) is invaluable in defining the intrathoracic anatomic extent of the mass and its relationship to critical cervical and intrathoracic structures.[1]
- Intravenous contrast may delay the ability to use radioactive iodine but should be used whenever anatomic considerations may affect the surgical planning or technique.
- Ultrasound may also be employed but is of limited use in assessing the intrathoracic extent of disease.
- A thoughtful approach to the airway is necessary. In addition to history, physical examination, and imaging studies, exclusion of cardiopulmonary factors affecting respiration is important.
- Evaluation by speech pathology with a video swallow study can elucidate if extrinsic esophageal compression is contributing to patient-reported dysphagia.
- Spirometry and flow-volume loops are useful adjuncts in order to understand the underlying respiratory physiology. However, surgical decisions are made based on functional and anatomic considerations rather than strictly physiologic tests.
- Preoperative laboratory studies should include thyroid function testing and thyroglobulin.
- In the case of a thyroid mass or nodule, fine needle aspiration (preferably image-guided) with cytologic evaluation should be attempted prior to surgery.

SURGICAL MANAGEMENT

- Consideration for removal of substernal goiters is multifactorial.[2]
- Indications for an operation may relate to the need to make a diagnosis, extirpate malignancy, ameliorate compression of the upper aerodigestive tract, or relieve venous outflow obstruction (superior vena cava syndrome).
- In most patients meeting criteria for surgery, medical options other than watchful waiting are limited.
- Given that most goiter operations are elective, prudent and deliberate preoperative planning and counseling are essential. The indications, risks, benefits, and alternatives of surgery vs expectant management should be discussed.[3]

Preoperative Planning

- Preoperative communication with anesthesia is critical. Although most patients can be readily intubated, airway compression or deviation must be considered. Atraumatic intubation is necessary.[4]
- The endotracheal tube cuff should be well below the vocal folds to avoid both glottic trauma and inadvertent extubation, as the endotracheal tube has a tendency to be displaced with movement during surgery.
- Thoracic surgeons should provide preoperative input and be available to assist in cases in which their presence may be needed.
- Options such as small endotracheal tubes, endotracheal tubes facilitating nerve monitoring, and/or fiberoptic bronchoscopy/intubation should be discussed prior to induction with anesthesia.
- Recurrent laryngeal nerve (RLN) monitoring may be of added technical assistance to locate the nerve and maintain its continuity in complex surgical procedures. Continuous vagal monitoring may help avoid traction injury to the RLN. Superior laryngeal nerve monitoring may be of assistance as well as the nerve can be intimately associated with an enlarged superior thyroid pole.
- Fiberoptic intubation is rarely necessary, although adjunctive technologies, such as the GlideScope, may be useful.

Positioning

- The patient is positioned supine with gentle neck extension. Effort should be made to prepare and drape in a manner that facilitates some movement of the head and neck while preserving the sterile field.
- Overextension of the neck may put the RLNs under tension and make them more difficult to identify. The right RLN is more vulnerable during substernal thyroidectomies.[5]
- Even if sternotomy is not planned, the chest should be prepped for access in case of either an emergency or the inability to free the gland transcervically.

Anatomy

- The tuberculum of Zuckerkandl is a posterolateral prominence of thyroid tissue that frequently approximates the location of the RLN.[6]
- Berry ligament is a condensation of the pretracheal fascia that attaches the thyroid to the airway. Small vessels run along the ligament, and it may be in close proximity to the RLN, requiring careful attention in order to ensure preservation of the nerve when the thyroid is being mobilized.
- In general, the substernal component of the thyroid gland originates from one lobe. Left substernal goiters are anteriorly displaced by the aortic arch. Right substernal goiters are frequently nestled between the superior vena cava and the prevertebral muscles (**FIGURE 1**).
- Posterior mediastinal goiters are rare, but when present, the RLN may be anteriorly displaced.
- In rare cases, substernal goiters may not be contiguous with the cervical thyroid gland.

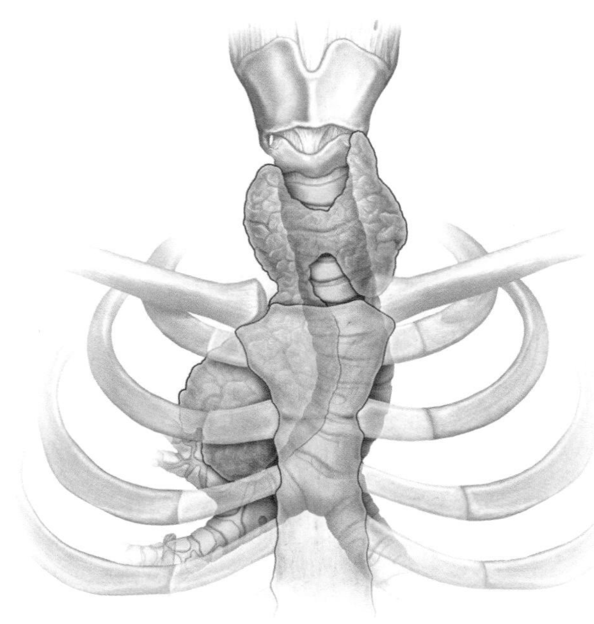

FIGURE 1 • Anatomy of substernal goiter. The substernal component of the thyroid gland usually originates from one lobe. Left substernal goiters are anteriorly displaced by the aortic arch. Right substernal goiters (pictured) are frequently nestled between the superior vena cava and the prevertebral muscles.

Approach

- The cervical vascular supply, anterior position, and rarity of bilateral intrathoracic extension typically facilitate complete removal of substernal goiters transcervically.[7]
- Less than 10% of substernal goiters require sternotomy or thoracotomy.
- Relative indications for sternotomy include the following:
  - Prior mediastinal surgery
  - Retroesophageal/posterior mediastinal location
  - Goiter abutting the carina
  - Intrathoracic malignancy with extrathyroidal extension
  - Intimate association with the great vessels
  - Massive substernal goiters that physically cannot be removed through the neck
- When sternotomy is indicated, a "T" incision is frequently preferred.
- Transcervical dissection and ligation of vessels occur prior to opening the chest. However, in cases with venous obstruction, sternotomy precedes vessel ligation in order to limit intrathoracic venous distension.
- The sternotomy may be partial or complete. Division of the interclavicular ligament may improve access without the need for a sternal split.
- Care is necessary in order to identify and manage aberrant mediastinal vascular tributaries supplying the thyroid gland.
- The intrathoracic trajectory of the RLNs can be identified and preserved under direct vision.
- Lateral thoracotomy typically provides suboptimal visualization of critical structures but may be preferred in specific cases.
- Video-assisted thoracic surgery may also be considered and may help avoid sternotomy in selected cases.

INCISION AND EXPOSURE

- Exposure is critical, as satisfactory access facilitates appropriate visualization. Thus, a generous transverse neck incision is planned within an existing neck crease, approximating the level of the cricoid cartilage.
- The strap muscles are identified and divided along the midline raphe. In order to obtain sufficient access, the strap muscles are transected at least on the side of intrathoracic extension (**FIGURE 2**).

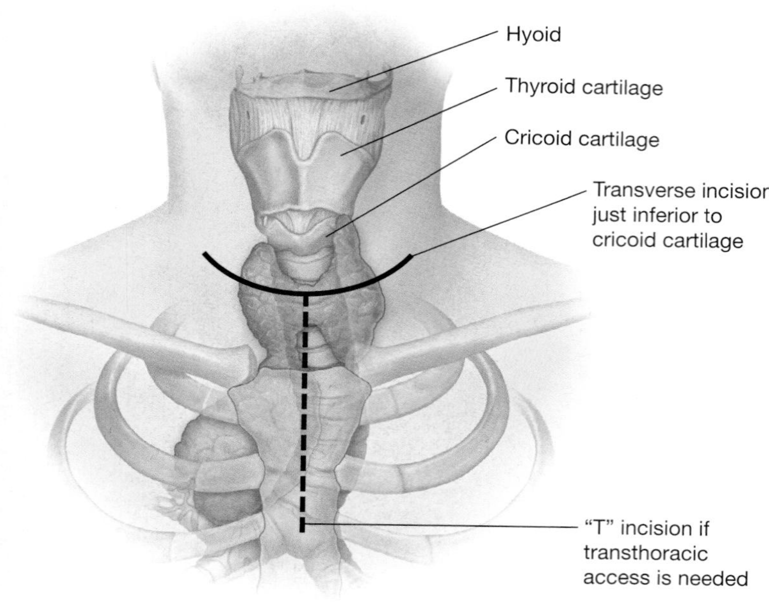

FIGURE 2 ● Incision and exposure. The patient is positioned supine with gentle neck extension. A generous transverse neck incision is planned within an existing neck crease, approximating the level of the cricoid cartilage. The chest should be prepped within the field. When sternotomy is indicated, a "T" incision is preferred.

MOBILIZATION OF THYROID GLAND

- As the thyroid is gently and bluntly freed from surrounding areolar tissue, meticulous attention is necessary to ensure extracapsular dissection in order to maintain a bloodless field.
- The middle thyroid vein is isolated and divided.
- The superior parathyroid gland is identified and preserved, given that the inferior glands are at higher risk for injury during dissection of the substernal extent of the thyroid gland.
- When necessary, devascularized or excised parathyroid glands may be autotransplanted into the sternocleidomastoid muscle. Perform frozen section confirmation of histology prior to reimplantation.
- The superior thyroid pedicle is isolated and divided close to the superior pole, taking care not to injure the superior laryngeal nerve or superior parathyroid gland.

IDENTIFICATION OF RECURRENT LARYNGEAL NERVE

- The RLN is identified. The size and bulk of the thyroid gland may make this dissection difficult, and the nerve may be displaced from its standard anatomic position. In general, its entry into the larynx at the cricothyroid joint is the most consistent and reliable location for identification.
- The RLN is traced and exposed inferiorly. In cases in which the substernal goiter is posteriorly positioned, the nerve is likely to be displaced anteriorly, putting it at higher risk for injury.
- In some cases, the thyroid gland will need to be displaced in order to facilitate nerve dissection, which involves retrograde dissection of the RLN from the cricothyroid joint inferiorly while displacing the thyroid gland anteromedially ("toboggan approach") (**FIGURE 3**).
- The RLN may branch prior to its entry into the larynx, and such anatomic variations should be expected. Anterior divisions of the nerve are more likely to be motor branches.

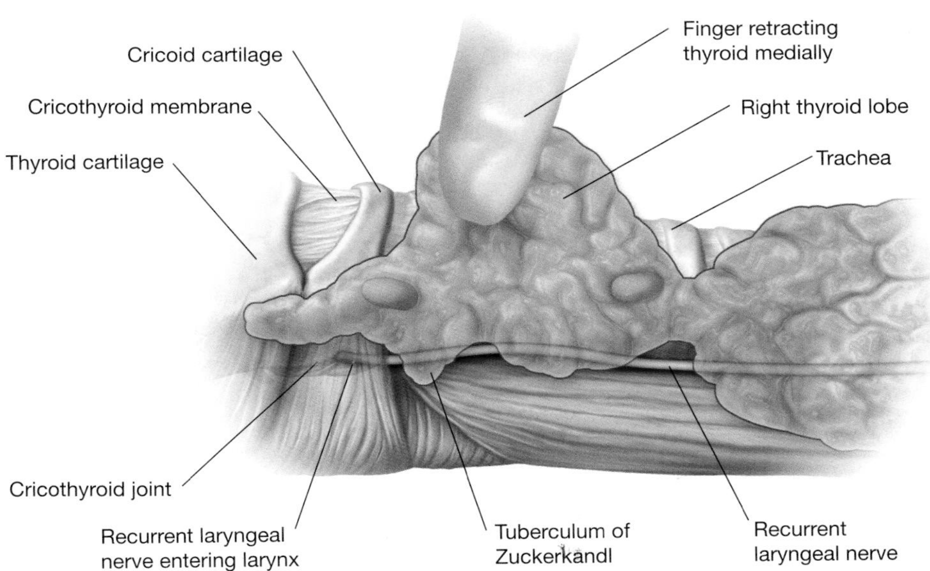

FIGURE 3 ● Identification of recurrent laryngeal nerve (RLN). The RLN's entry into the larynx at the cricothyroid joint is the most consistent and reliable location for identification. The RLN is traced and exposed inferiorly. In some cases, the thyroid gland will need to be displaced in order to facilitate nerve dissection, which involves retrograde dissection of the RLN from the cricothyroid joint inferiorly while displacing the thyroid gland anteromedially ("toboggan approach").

LIGATION OF THE INFERIOR PEDICLE AND MOBILIZATION

- The inferior thyroid vessels are isolated and divided meticulously. Damage to these vessels during mobilization can cause intrathoracic hemorrhage not amenable to transcervical hemostasis.
- Gentle, blunt substernal dissection should commence laterally, under the sternocleidomastoid muscle, and progress medially. It may be useful to divide the sternal head of this muscle to improve access. Small venous tributaries are frequently encountered and divided.
- Hemoclips, LigaSure, Harmonic, or other hemostatic adjunctive devices may be employed at the surgeon's discretion and may be particularly helpful for superior mediastinal small veins which may be otherwise difficult to ligate (**FIGURES 4** and **5**).

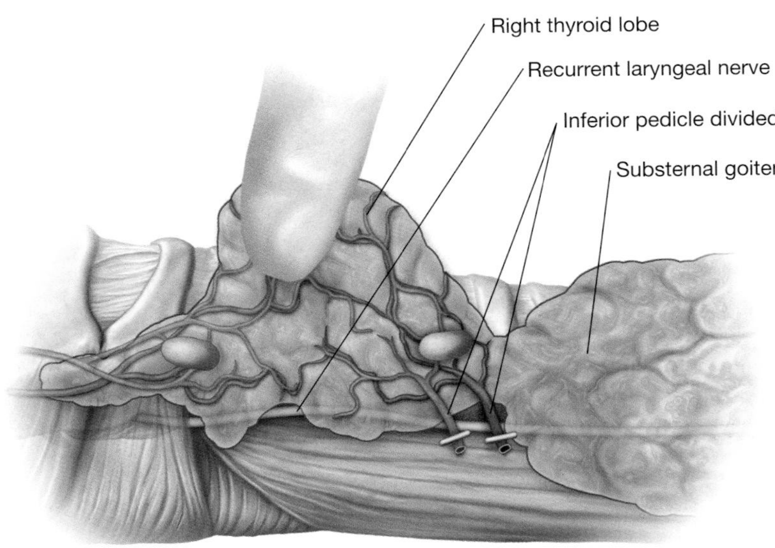

FIGURE 4 ● Ligation of the inferior pedicle. The inferior thyroid vessels are isolated and divided meticulously. Damage to these vessels during mobilization can cause intrathoracic hemorrhage not amenable to transcervical hemostasis. It may be difficult to visualize and preserve the ipsilateral inferior parathyroid gland.

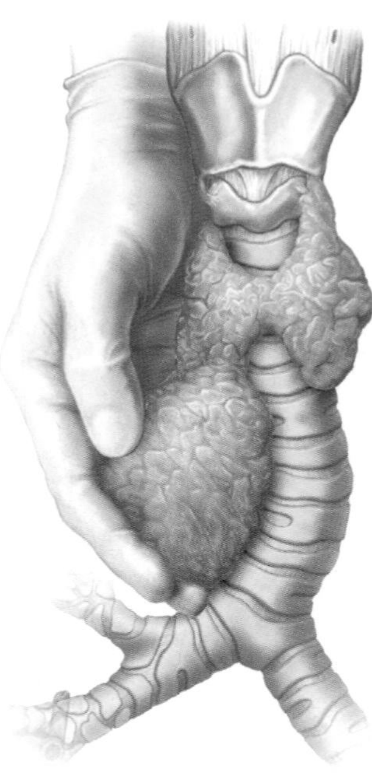

FIGURE 5 ● Mobilization of substernal goiter. Gentle, blunt substernal finger dissection should commence laterally, under the sternocleidomastoid muscle, and progress medially.

CONTRALATERAL DISSECTION

- The procedure is repeated on the other thyroid lobe.
- Typically, the lobe with substernal extension is removed first in order to ensure that the RLN is preserved prior to contralateral dissection. If the nerve monitor is being used, it is appropriate to test the dissected nerve's integrity prior to contralateral surgery.
- Care should be taken when freeing the gland off of the cricothyroid joint and Berry ligament, as small vessels can cause bleeding that obscures visualization of the RLN.

CLOSURE

- Closed suction drain placement is frequently indicated due to the large potential space created by expansive substernal goiters.
- Wound closure is performed in the standard manner, taking care to reapproximate divided muscles (sternocleidomastoid and straps). The midline raphe between the strap muscles should be loosely approximated to facilitate egress of blood and transudate and to mitigate airway compression in the case of an expansile hematoma.
- The method of skin closure is at the discretion of the surgeon (**FIGURE 6**).
- Smooth extubation and anesthetic emergence is important in order to limit sudden increases in intrathoracic pressure. If airway concerns are present, delayed extubation can be considered.

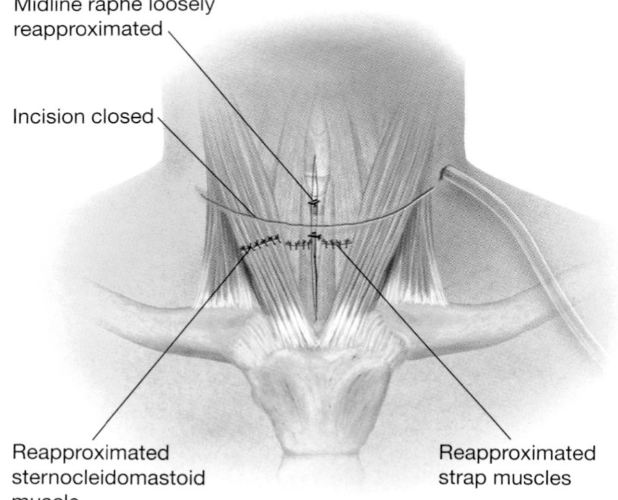

FIGURE 6 ● Closure. Take care to reapproximate divided muscles (sternocleidomastoid and straps). The midline raphe between the strap muscles should be loosely approximated to facilitate egress of blood and transudate. Closed suction drain placement is frequently indicated.

PEARLS AND PITFALLS

Indications	■ Given that most goiter operations are elective, prudent and deliberate preoperative planning and counseling are essential.
Approach	■ Sternotomy is rarely necessary for removal of a substernal thyroid gland.
Positioning	■ The patient should be placed supine with gentle neck extension and draped in a manner that facilitates movement of the head and neck.
Airway	■ Although most patients can be readily intubated, airway compression or deviation must be considered. Because the endotracheal tube has a tendency to become displaced during surgical manipulation, confirm that the cuff is well below the vocal folds.
Exposure	■ Satisfactory access is critical for safety and visualization. Use a generous transverse neck incision and consider dividing strap muscles at least on the side of intrathoracic extension.
Plane of dissection	■ As the thyroid is mobilized, meticulous attention is necessary to ensure extracapsular dissection in order to maintain a bloodless field.
Management of parathyroid glands	■ The inferior glands are at higher risk for injury or devascularization during dissection of the substernal extent of the thyroid gland. Thus, make sure to identify and preserve the superior parathyroid glands.

POSTOPERATIVE CARE

- Check postoperative serum calcium levels. The use of intraoperative and/or postoperative parathyroid hormone levels is optional. Decisions regarding calcium supplementation and further laboratory studies should be based on individual circumstances, laboratory findings, and clinician preferences.
- Patients should be informed to call 911 if they develop any sudden difficulty breathing or neck swelling.
- Patients should be encouraged to ambulate early and perform pulmonary toilet, although they should restrict from strenuous physical activity and heavy lifting for a few weeks.

COMPLICATIONS

- Rates of complications are higher for substernal goiters compared to standard thyroidectomies, but in experienced hands, substernal thyroidectomy is a safe operation.[8]
- Surgical site infection—In general, strict adherence to aseptic technique and maintenance of the sterile field assures that surgical site infections are uncommon in patients without underlying risk factors. Perioperative antibiotics should be administered in accordance with established guidelines.[9]
- Seroma—Some degree of seroma formation within the operative bed is inevitable. Intervention rarely becomes necessary.
- Intraoperative hemorrhage—Meticulous techniques including limiting shearing/tearing vessels and maintaining an intact thyroid capsule are critical. Rarely, uncontrolled intrathoracic hemorrhage will require emergent sternotomy and/or aggressive resuscitation.
- Hematoma—Approximately 1% to 3% of cases will develop a postoperative hematoma that requires intervention. All cases of expansile hematomas require consideration of airway compression and prompt attention.
- Nerve injury—The RLNs are susceptible to injury both within the neck and chest. Rates of injury are slightly higher in cases of substernal goiter than in standard thyroidectomies.
- Hypoparathyroidism—Inferior parathyroid glands are more difficult to identify and preserve with substernal goiters, making identification and meticulous preservation of superior glands critical.
- Hemothorax/pneumothorax—Intrathoracic complications are quite rare. Routine postoperative chest X-ray should be considered.
- Tracheomalacia—Despite frequent tracheal deviation and/or compression, clinically significant tracheomalacia is rare. The adult airway is quite resilient, and even long-standing compression will not often be problematic.

REFERENCES

1. Netterville JL, Coleman SC, Smith JC, et al. Management of substernal goiter. *Laryngoscope*. 1998;108:1611-1117.
2. Katlic MR, Wang C, Grillo HC. Substernal goiter. *Ann Thorac Surg*. 1985;39:391-399.
3. Hanson MA, Shaha AR, Wu JX. Surgical approach to the substernal goiter. *Best Pract Res Clin Endocrinol Metab*. 2019;33(4):101312.
4. Newman E, Shaha AR. Substernal goiter. *J Surg Oncol*. 1995;60(3):207-212.
5. Alvim Fiorelli RK, Vasconcelos Duarte AJ, Teixeira AQ, Montenegro TS, Portari Filho PE, Santos Morard MR, da Silva Ascenção AM,Basílio Oliveira CA, Novellino P. Anatomical and developmental aspects of iatrogenic injury to the right recurrent laryngeal nerve in surgical resections of substernal goiter. *Anat Rec*. 2021;304(6):1242-1254. doi:10.1002/ar.24629
6. Mohebati A, Shaha AR. Anatomy of thyroid and parathyroid glands and neurovascular relations. *Clin Anat*. 2012;25(1):19-31.
7. Mack E. Management of patients with substernal goiters. *Surg Clin North Am*. 1995;75(3):377-394.
8. Simó R, Nixon IJ, Vander Poorten V, et al. Surgical management of intrathoracic goiters. *Eur Arch Oto-Rhino-Laryngol*. 2019;276(2):305-314.
9. Ríos A, Rodríguez JM, Balsalobre MD, et al. The value of various definitions of intrathoracic goiter for predicting intra-operative and postoperative complications. *Surgery*. 2010;147(2):233-238.

Chapter 48 Subtotal Thyroidectomy for Graves Disease

Edwin L. Kaplan and Raymon H. Grogan

DEFINITION

- Subtotal thyroidectomy means the removal of most of both lobes of the thyroid, but some thyroid tissue is intentionally left on one or both sides of the neck.
  - Thyroid lobectomy or total thyroidectomy alone or with appropriate neck dissections is the procedure of choice for most thyroid cancers and is discussed in Part 5, Chapters 46 and 51.
  - Thyroid lobectomy is used for some unilateral benign colloid nodules or goiters and for many indeterminate thyroid lesions; that is, when the fine needle aspirate demonstrates a possible follicular neoplasm or a follicular lesion of undetermined significance (FLUS) that requires operation (see Part 5, Chapter 46).
  - Subtotal thyroidectomy is frequently used in the treatment of *benign* thyroid diseases such as nontoxic or toxic multinodular goiters, especially when the disease is bilateral and commonly in the treatment of Graves disease, although near-total or total thyroidectomy may be more appropriate in some patients.
  - The purpose of subtotal thyroidectomy is to reduce the incidence of postoperative complications of total thyroidectomy—permanent hypoparathyroidism and recurrent laryngeal nerve injury—and to leave functional thyroid tissue in the neck of some patients. Although the rate of complications of total thyroidectomy is low in the hands of expert thyroid surgeons, most surgeons would agree and most studies have demonstrated a lower incidence of complications when subtotal thyroidectomy is performed.
  - This section will briefly discuss the diagnosis and preoperative assessment of patients with benign thyroid conditions and will illustrate the preoperative management and surgical technique when performing *a subtotal thyroidectomy for Graves disease.*

DIFFERENTIAL DIAGNOSIS

- A short list of common benign thyroid conditions:
  - Thyroid abnormalities associated with normal thyroid function or hypothyroidism
    - Single colloid nodule or cyst
    - Single microfollicular or macrofollicular adenoma
    - Multinodular goiter
    - Hashimoto thyroiditis
  - Thyroid abnormalities associated with thyrotoxicosis
    - Toxic adenoma
    - Toxic multinodular goiter
    - Graves disease
      - Graves disease is an autoimmune disease characterized by a goiter, thyrotoxicosis, and exophthalmic eye disease. Less commonly, pretibial myxedema is also present. It is closely related to Hashimoto thyroiditis, which usually presents with hypothyroidism.
      - It was described first in the English language by Caleb Perry (1755-1822) but commonly bears the name of the Irish physician, Robert Graves. On the European continent, it is called Basedow disease.
      - As an autoimmune thyroid disease, it exhibits both antibodies and cell-mediated immunity directed to thyroid peroxidase (TPO) and thyroglobulin (TG) as well as stimulating antibodies against the TSH receptor (called TSab or TSI, but formerly called long-acting thyroid stimulator [LATS]). Antibodies against eye muscle and fibroblasts are also found in the serum of same patients with severe Graves ophthalmopathy.
      - Incidence of Graves disease
        - Found in women 5 to 8 times more commonly than in men
        - Thirty cases per 108,000 population annually in Olmsted County, Minnesota
        - Increases in incidence during each decade from adolescence to 60 years of age
        - Six percent of all Americans have autoimmune thyroid disease.

PATIENT HISTORY AND PHYSICAL FINDINGS

- In order to differentiate these benign thyroid conditions, a careful history and physical examination are first necessary.
- History: Of greatest importance is a previous history of low-dose (or high-dose) radiation to the neck, which is associated with an increased risk of thyroid cancer. Also important are the metabolic status of the patient and whether or not there are symptoms of respiratory impairment, pressure on the trachea, or difficulty swallowing from an enlarged thyroid or from thyroid nodules.
  - Major symptoms of hypothyroidism
    - Severe fatigue, weight gain, dry skin, irregular menstrual periods, constipation, depression, hair loss, brittle nails, feeling cold, slowness of speech, and puffiness. In its most severe form, hypothyroid coma may rarely occur.
  - Major symptoms of hyperthyroidism (thyrotoxicosis)
    - Weight loss despite a normal or an increased appetite, rapid or irregular heartbeat, nervousness, anxiety, irritability, tremor, sweating, changes in menstrual pattern, increased sensitivity to heat, more frequent bowel movements, fatigue, muscle weakness, difficulty sleeping, and fine brittle hair. In its most severe form, thyroid storm might occur.
  - Respiratory and compressive changes and difficulty swallowing
    - Nodules of the thyroid or an enlarged thyroid (goiter) may cause pain and tenderness in the neck as well as trouble breathing. As the thyroid enlarges, the trachea can be compressed and narrowed and eventually

respiratory impairment may occur resulting in coughing, shortness of breath, and stridorous breathing. Rarely, an enlarged goiter can result in recurrent laryngeal nerve impairment with hoarseness. Pressure from a goiter or from thyroid nodules can also result in trouble swallowing.

- Physical findings
  - The physician should assess the size of the thyroid gland and the size, consistency, number, and position of any thyroid nodules; whether or not the trachea is deviated; and if any enlarged and abnormal lymph nodes are present in the central or lateral neck. Finally, the physician should assess whether there are any signs of thyrotoxicosis in general or evidence of manifestations of Graves disease such as exophthalmos, pretibial myxedema, and a diffuse goiter with a bruit.

IMAGING AND OTHER DIAGNOSTIC STUDIES

- Thyroid function tests
  - Almost all patients with hypothyroidism have an elevated thyrotropin (TSH) level with low free thyroxine (FT4) and triiodothyronine (T3) values.
  - Almost all thyrotoxic patients have a suppressed TSH with elevated FT4 and T3 values.
- Tests for autoimmunity
  - In Hashimoto disease and Graves disease, antibodies to thyroid peroxidase (anti-TPO antibodies) are found in up to 90% of patients, whereas antithyroglobulin (anti-TG) antibodies are found in approximately 50%. Elevated anti-TSH receptor antibodies (TSab) are also commonly detected in patients with Graves disease and these thyroid-stimulating immunoglobulins (TSI) are the cause of the thyrotoxicosis of Graves disease.
- Imaging and nuclear uptake scanning
  - The thyroid uptake of radioiodine or technetium isotopes is usually increased in toxic multinodular goiter, toxic adenoma, and Graves disease.
  - Nuclear scans may help to differentiate each of these diseases.
    - With toxic multinodular goiter, an enlarged thyroid gland is noted with one or more "hot" areas usually among other "cold" areas.
    - Toxic adenoma. A single "hot" area, which corresponds to the thyroid nodule, is clearly seen. The remaining thyroid tissue is suppressed and barely visualized on the scan.
    - Graves disease. Both lobes of the thyroid demonstrate increased uptake of isotope on the scan.
  - Other imaging studies
    - Ultrasound examinations are commonly used to evaluate the thyroid for nodules and to identify abnormal lymph nodes and have replaced a nuclear scan unless a hot nodule is suspected.
    - Computed tomography (CT) scan and magnetic resonance imaging (MRI) exams are helpful to evaluate the presence or absence of tracheal compression; abnormal lymph nodes; or the presence, size, and anatomic location of a substernal goiter. These are often reserved for goiters that extend below the clavicle or if significant.
    - Tracheal narrowing is of concern.
- Fine needle aspiration (FNA)
  - The most important test to evaluate a thyroid nodule is an FNA with cytologic examination. This exam should be used liberally. Usually, it is performed under ultrasound guidance in order to be certain that the nodule in question has correctly been sampled.

SURGICAL MANAGEMENT

- A thyroidectomy is usually indicated for the following reasons:
  - To treat thyroid malignancies and some benign thyroid nodules
  - To establish a definitive diagnosis when diagnosis by FNA is equivocal, nondiagnostic, or indeterminate
  - To alleviate pressure symptoms or respiratory difficulties associated with a malignant or a benign process
  - To remove a substernal goiter
  - To remove an unsightly goiter
  - As definitive therapy for individuals with thyrotoxicosis—selected patients with hot nodules, toxic multinodular goiter, and Graves disease
- Preparation for surgery
  - Most patients undergoing a thyroid operation are euthyroid and require no specific preoperative preparation related to their thyroid gland. Determination of serum calcium and parathyroid hormone (PTH) levels may be helpful. Endoscopic or indirect laryngoscopy might be helpful for all patients preoperatively but definitely should be done in those who are hoarse or who have had a change in voice and in others who have had a prior thyroid, parathyroid, carotid, lateral neck, anterior cervical disc, or upper chest operation in order to detect the possibility of a recurrent laryngeal nerve injury.
- Hypothyroidism
  - Modest hypothyroidism is of little concern when treating a surgical patient; however, severe hypothyroidism can be a significant risk factor. Severe hypothyroidism can be diagnosed clinically by myxedema as well as by slowness of affect, speech, and reflexes. Circulating thyroxine and triiodothyronine values are low. The serum TSH level is high in all cases of hypothyroidism that are not caused by pituitary insufficiency. In the presence of *severe* hypothyroidism, both the morbidity and the mortality of surgery are increased as a result of the effects of both the anesthesia and the operation. Such patients have a higher incidence of perioperative hypotension, cardiovascular problems, gastrointestinal hypomotility, prolonged anesthetic recovery, and neuropsychiatric disturbances. They metabolize drugs slowly and are very sensitive to all medications. Therefore, when severe myxedema is present, it is preferable to defer elective surgery until a euthyroid state is achieved.
- Hyperthyroidism
  - Toxic multinodular goiter and a toxic adenoma are usually treated to a euthyroid state with an antithyroid medication such as methimazole (Tapazole) or propylthiouracil (PTU), and the possible use of a beta-adrenergic blocker such as propranolol. Radioiodine therapy may sometimes be used as definitive therapy.

- Operative therapy for a toxic multinodular goiter is usually a subtotal or total thyroidectomy. For a toxic adenoma, enucleation of the nodule or a thyroid lobectomy is curative because a hot nodule is almost always benign. This can be confirmed preoperatively by FNA evaluation. Furthermore, because most of the thyroid tissue remains after enucleation, the majority of patients become euthyroid postoperatively without the need for thyroid hormone replacement.
- Treatment of patients with Graves disease
  - In the United States, most patients with thyrotoxicosis have Graves disease. Furthermore, in the United States, over 90% of all patients with Graves disease are treated with radioiodine therapy.
  - Operative indications for Graves disease may include very young patients, others with very large goiters, some pregnant women, and those with suspicious thyroid nodules or severe ophthalmopathy.
  - In patients with severe thyroid eye disease, thyroidectomy rather than radioiodine therapy has often been chosen because radioiodine treatment has been shown to worsen the eye problems in some patients.
  - Recently, a new drug infusion teprotumumab-trbw (Tepezza), an insulin-like growth factor-1 receptor inhibitor, is being used to medically treat patients with severe thyroid eye disease. This therapy has been shown to decrease proptosis and double vision in many patients and may reduce the need for thyroidectomy in some patients with severe thyroid eye disease associated with Graves disease.
  - For greatest safety, patients with Graves disease should be treated preoperatively with PTU or methimazole and iodine drops to restore a euthyroid state and to prevent *thyroid storm*. Beta blockers should also be used liberally. Thyroid storm is the name for the most severe manifestations of thyrotoxicosis including a very rapid heart rate or cardiac arrhythmias, fever, disorientation, hypotension, coma, and even death. In the past, mortality of thyroid storm was very high, but now, with the use of beta-blockers, antithyroid medications, iodine, oxygen, glucose, possibly adrenocortical steroids, and intensive care measures, the death rate has been greatly reduced. Both anesthesia and operation on a poorly prepared thyrotoxic patient are the leading precipitating factors for this event. Furthermore, operation on an unprepared Graves gland can be more difficult because severe bleeding may occur because the thyroid is often soft and very vascular. With proper preoperative preparation, however, operation on the thyroid gland in Graves disease can be performed safely.
- Preparation of Graves patient for operation
  - In *mild* cases of thyrotoxicosis with Graves disease, iodine therapy alone has been used for preoperative preparation, although we do not recommend this approach routinely. Lugol's solution or a saturated solution of potassium iodide (SSKI), two or three drops twice daily, is given for 8 to 10 days preoperatively. This medication is taken in milk or orange juice to make it more palatable. Iodine therapy suppresses thyroid hormone release only in Graves disease and should not be given to patients with toxic nodular goiter or toxic adenoma.
  - Most patients with Graves disease are treated initially with antithyroid drugs, PTU or more commonly, methimazole (Tapazole) until they approach a euthyroid state. Then iodine is added to the regimen for 8 to 10 days before surgery. The iodine decreases the vascularity and increases the firmness of the thyroid gland. Sometimes, thyroxine is added to this regimen to prevent hypothyroidism and to decrease the size of the gland. Beta-adrenergic blockers such as propranolol (Inderal) are used commonly with the antithyroid drugs to decrease the pulse rate and eliminate the tremor. Other preoperative protocols using propranolol alone or with Lugol's solution are sometimes necessary, especially when allergic reactions to antithyroid medications have occurred. However, we do not use these routinely because they appear to be less safe. It should be emphasized again that iodine drops are only used in preparation for operation for Graves disease and not in patients with a toxic nodular goiter or a toxic adenoma.

TECHNIQUES

OPERATION

- Following general anesthesia, the patient is placed in a supine position with the neck extended. A low collar incision is made, usually in a skin crease, and carried down through the subcutaneous tissue and platysma muscle. Currently, small incisions are the rule unless a large goiter is present.
- Superior and inferior subplatysmal flaps are developed, and the strap muscles are divided vertically in the midline and retracted laterally. Often, a large pyramidal lobe is present in patients with Graves disease (**FIGURE 1, left**).
- The thyroid isthmus is clamped and divided early in the course of operation for most patients with Graves disease (**FIGURE 1, right**). Alternatively, an energy device can be used to transect the isthmus.
- The isthmus on each side is then sharply dissected from the front of the trachea in order to improve mobilization of the gland. The isthmus on each side is oversewn for hemostasis (**FIGURE 2**). The medial side of the thyroid lobe to be operated on first is then carefully dissected in a superficial plane toward the upper pole, developing a plane between the thyroid lobe and the cricothyroid muscle. Care is taken to preserve and not damage the external branch of the superior laryngeal nerve and the cricothyroid muscle.
- The thyroid lobe to be operated on first is mobilized by dividing the areolar tissue and any small vessels along its lateral surface.
- The upper pole vessels are then individually ligated along the front surface of the upper pole and not more cephalad in the neck. The right angle is kept "pointing out laterally" to prevent damage to the external branch of the superior laryngeal nerve (**FIGURE 2**). This nerve can often be visualized if the area is carefully evaluated.

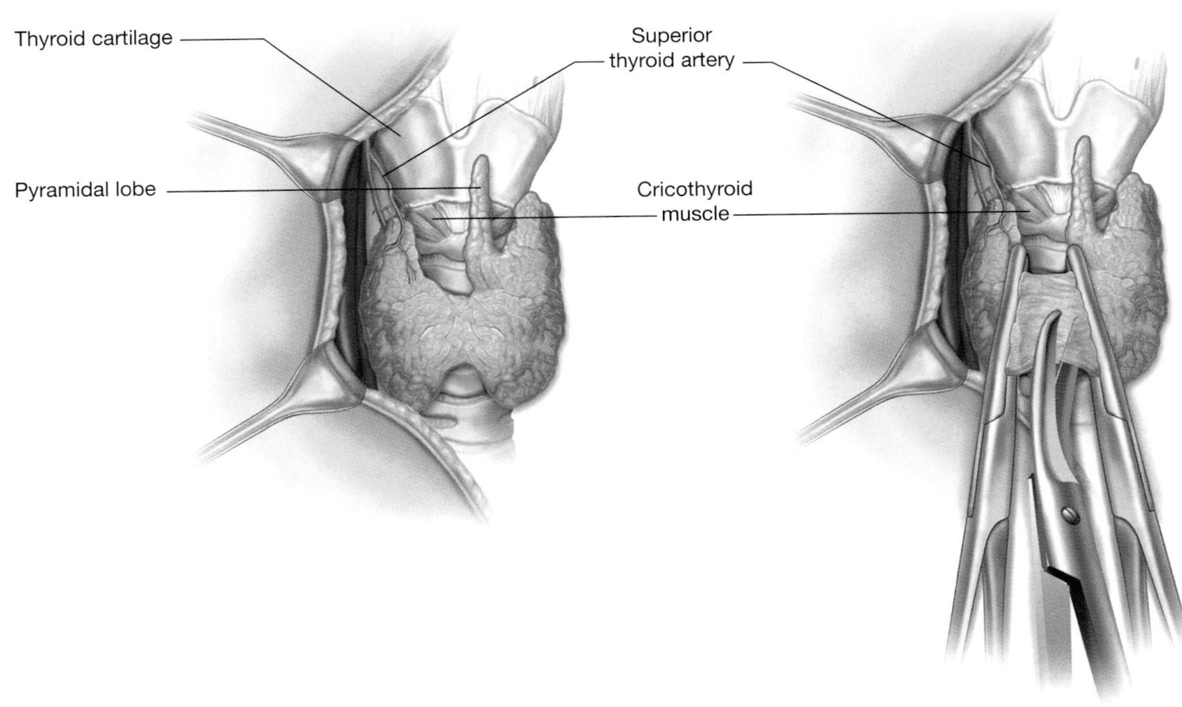

FIGURE 1 ● **Left:** An enlarged thyroid gland of Graves disease is usually quite vascular and often exhibits a large pyramidal lobe. **Right:** The isthmus is mobilized from the anterior trachea using a right angle clamp and the plane between the thyroid and the cricothyroid muscle is carefully developed. Then, the isthmus is divided between clamps or by use of an energy device.

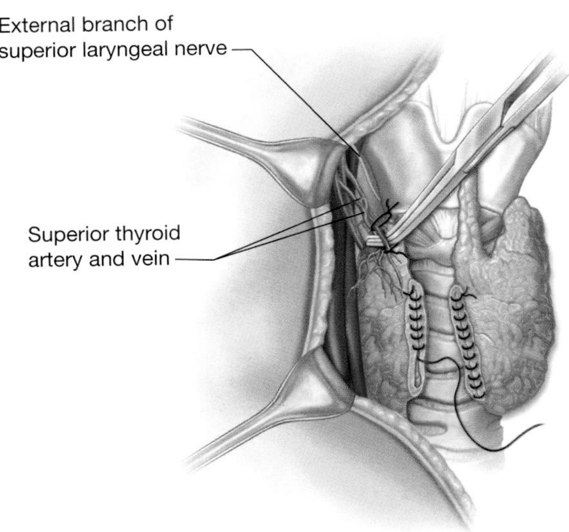

FIGURE 2 ● If the isthmus was clamped, it is oversewn by a running horizontal mattress suture behind the hemostat followed by a "baseball stitch" for hemostasis. The upper pole vessels are individually ligated on the anterior surface of the upper thyroid pole and divided. The points of the right angle should face away from the trachea and care is taken to identify the external branch of the superior laryngeal nerve when possible and not to injure it.

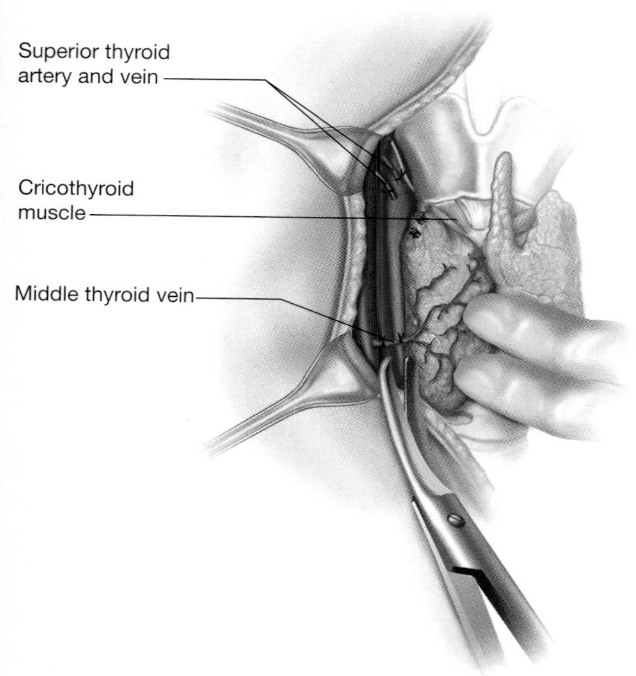

FIGURE 3 ● The thyroid lobe is retracted medially and care is taken to clearly identify the middle thyroid vein and to ligate and divide it. Be certain that the vein is separate from other structures before dividing it in order to avoid injury to the recurrent laryngeal nerve.

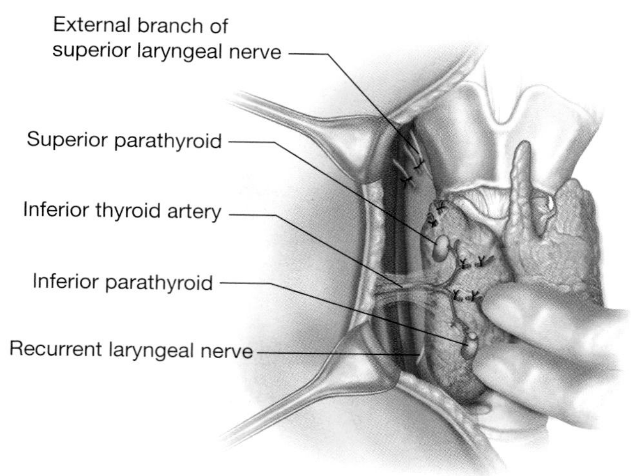

FIGURE 4 ● With further blunt dissection, the inferior thyroid artery, which runs transversely toward the thyroid lobe, is identified and the recurrent nerve is visualized. The inferior thyroid artery is not ligated as a single trunk but rather individual branches of it are ligated and divided on the surface of the lobe, and the lower parathyroid gland is moved off the thyroid lobe with its blood supply intact.

- The thyroid lobe is then retracted medially again and the middle thyroid vein is identified, ligated, and divided (**FIGURE 3**). This vein is usually in a plane superficial to the inferior thyroid artery and to the recurrent laryngeal nerve, but all structures should be carefully evaluated before ligation.
- The inferior thyroid artery, a branch of the thyrocervical trunk that runs medially and enters the field deep to the carotid artery, as well as the recurrent laryngeal nerve are now carefully identified (**FIGURE 4**). Whenever possible, the inferior thyroid artery is not ligated as a single trunk because this might devascularize the parathyroid glands. Rather, the small branches of the artery are individually ligated and divided along the surface of the thyroid lobe. The inferior parathyroid gland, which often is present high along the lower thyroid lobe, is mobilized with its intact blood supply and moved more posteriorly and laterally off the thyroid lobe.
- The carotid artery is now retracted laterally and the recurrent laryngeal nerve is more carefully identified, usually in the lower neck, and followed in an inferior to superior direction by "unroofing" the tissues from the front of the nerve (**FIGURE 5**). Remember that on the right side, the recurrent laryngeal nerve takes an oblique course from lateral to medial and from deep to superficial. On the left side, the nerve usually runs straight upward and is usually found in the lower neck much more medially than on the right side within or near the tracheoesophageal groove.
- If a subtotal lobectomy is to be done, before any clamps are placed on the thyroid lobe, the surgeon must be certain that the recurrent nerve has been identified and followed in a cephalad direction to near the ligament of Berry and that the nerve and parathyroid glands are clearly posterior and away from the sites to be clamped. Then, hemostats are applied to the tissue and most of the lobe is resected (**FIGURE 5**). The remaining small thyroid remnant is oversewn for hemostasis. This resection can also be accomplished by using an energy device if one is far enough from the nerve so the heat does not damage it. Do not perform a subtotal thyroid lobectomy without visualizing the recurrent laryngeal nerve, for this is unsafe.
- At the end of the procedure for Graves disease (**FIGURE 6**), a small, well-vascularized remnant of thyroid tissue can be left on each side, a procedure called bilateral subtotal lobectomies. In other instances, to achieve the same result, a lobectomy can be performed on one side with a subtotal lobectomy on the other side, often called a Dunhill operation from the Australian surgeon who popularized this technique. Whichever operation is performed, it is important to leave small thyroid remnants especially in young patients in order to prevent a recurrence of disease. When severe ophthalmopathy is present, a total thyroidectomy may be most appropriate and many surgeons recommend total thyroidectomy instead of subtotal thyroidectomy more commonly for patients with Graves disease. However, always remember that Graves disease is a benign disorder and our aim is to do an operation that does not cause a nerve injury or hypoparathyroidism.
- Many surgeons find a recurrent laryngeal nerve monitor to be helpful to identify the recurrent nerve; although in current practice, its use is not mandatory.
- Finally, as stated, instead of suturing the thyroid, an energy device may be used. However, be careful when using these instruments, especially near the recurrent laryngeal nerve for the heat generated may damage it.

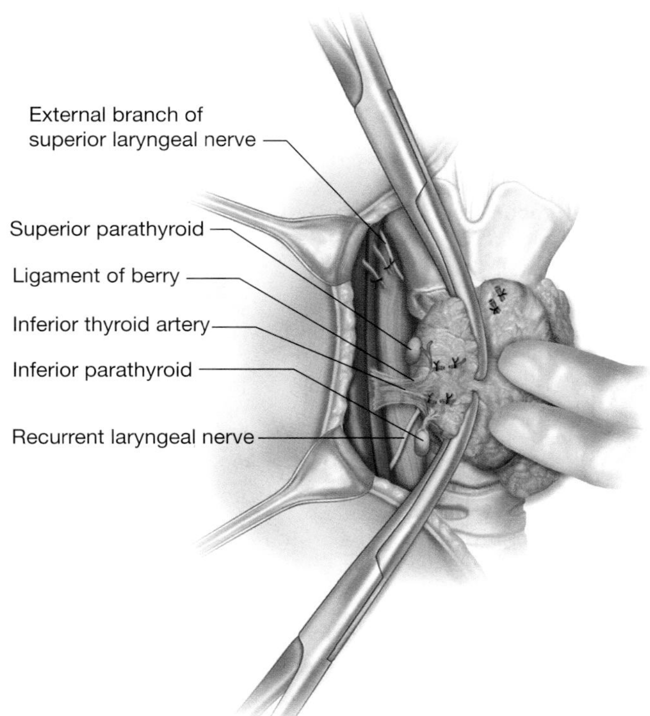

FIGURE 5 ● The recurrent laryngeal nerve should be visualized and followed up toward the ligament of Berry. The nerve should be treated gently and tissues "unroofed" from its anterior surface. Clamps are then applied (or an energy device used) only after the recurrent laryngeal nerve and parathyroids are seen to be safely preserved.

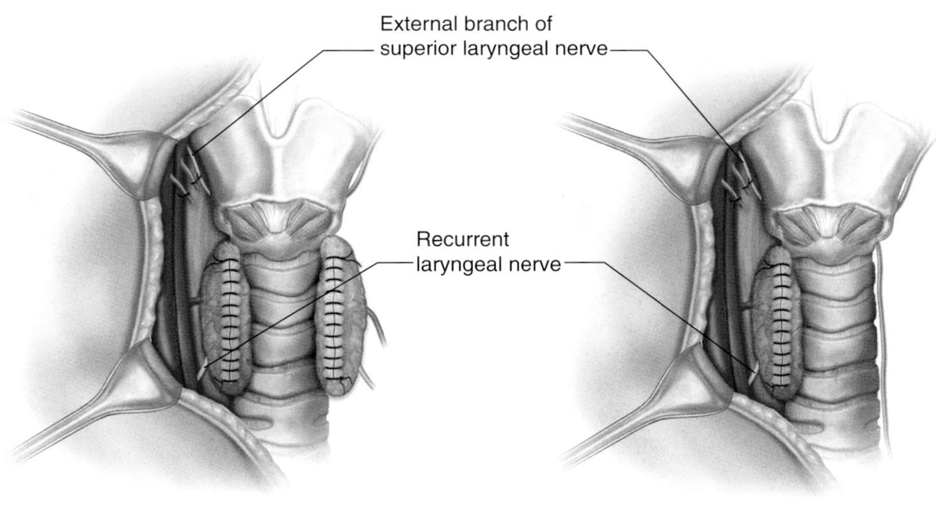

FIGURE 6 ● At the end of an operation for Graves disease, each recurrent laryngeal nerve has been identified and preserved, and the parathyroid glands have been spared. Either small thyroid remnants are left bilaterally **(left)** or a total lobectomy and contralateral subtotal lobectomy **(right)** are performed, often called a "Dunhill operation."

PEARLS AND PITFALLS

Preoperative considerations	■ When operating on the thyroid, some surgeons raise the head of the bed. Although this may seem attractive because it decreases venous bleeding, it is more dangerous because it increases the chance of an air embolism if a major vein is opened during the dissection. ■ The operation for Graves disease is often more difficult than for colloid nodular disease because of an increase in vascularity and "stickiness" in some cases. Treatment with iodine preoperatively has been shown to decrease the blood flow to the thyroid. ■ Although it may be best to check the vocal cords preoperatively in all patients, the surgeon must be sure that both vocal cords are moving well in any patient who has had a previous neck or chest operation or in others who are hoarse.
Recurrent laryngeal nerve	■ Always visually identify the recurrent laryngeal nerve, carefully "unroof" it, and gently follow its course. Although temporary nerve injuries may occur when this practice is followed, rarely will the injury be permanent. ■ Remember that nonrecurrent recurrent laryngeal nerves may occur especially on the right side of the neck. Each is associated with a vascular anomaly. ■ Use of a recurrent laryngeal nerve monitor may be helpful especially in a reoperative thyroidectomy. However, this technique has not been shown to reduce nerve injuries and sometimes can be misleading to the casual user. ■ If the nerve monitor demonstrates the loss of recurrent laryngeal nerve function on the first side of the neck, one should strongly consider halting the operation or limiting the contralateral resection in order to prevent the possibility of a bilateral nerve injury if one proceeds.
Parathyroid	■ Carefully search for and try to save each parathyroid gland with a good blood supply. ■ Do not ligate the inferior thyroid artery as a single trunk. Rather, ligate small branches on the surface of the thyroid lobe in order to preserve the delicate blood supply to the parathyroid glands. ■ Autotransplant each parathyroid gland that looks devascularized if it does not bleed well on biopsy or if it is accidently removed.
Postoperative care	■ Do not hesitate to use a drain if the wound is not completely dry before closure. ■ Observe patients carefully postoperatively. Delayed bleeding with a hematoma can occur. ■ A postoperative neck hematoma is an emergency that requires rapid return to the operating room or opening of the wound at the bedside if respiratory symptoms are present. ■ In the postoperative care of a patient with Graves disease, one cannot reliably use the TSH value alone to assess thyroid function, for the TSH value may stay suppressed even for weeks postoperatively if the patient was still thyrotoxic at the time of operation. The FT4 is usually a better indicator of function in the early postoperative course.

POSTOPERATIVE CARE

- In the recovery room, the patient should be observed for difficulty breathing and for swelling of the neck, which might indicate postoperative bleeding or hematoma. Return the patient to the operating room as an emergency if an expanding hematoma is recognized. Some surgeons advise endoscopic evaluation of the vocal cords in each patient; however, this should definitely be done if respiratory impairment is present.
- A serum calcium and PTH value is helpful. Some obtain a PTH in the recovery room; however, the authors generally wait until the morning of the first operative day to routinely obtain these results. Patients with Graves disease may be more prone to manifesting hypocalcemia than others, partly due to bone hunger.
- Severe symptomatic hypocalcemia may require intravenous calcium therapy postoperatively followed by oral calcium and vitamin D therapy. However, most patients are treated with oral calcium alone, which is given liberally and do very well. Thyroid replacement is given to many patients soon after surgery unless they are still thyrotoxic with a tachycardia. Although TSH is usually the best indicator of thyroid function, the FT4 is often a better indication in Graves patients postoperatively because their TSH value may be suppressed for a considerable period of time.

OUTCOMES

- Although radioiodine therapy is the usual treatment, thyroidectomy is a very successful treatment for the thyrotoxicosis of Graves disease in selected patients (**TABLE 1**). A major benefit is the rapid return to a euthyroid state, which is much quicker than following radioiodine therapy. It can be used in very young patients and during pregnancy if necessary. In each of these instances, radioiodine therapy is contraindicated. Thyroidectomy removes the goiter and any thyroid nodules which are present. Finally, in patients with severe ophthalmopathy, many studies have shown improvement of eye changes or stabilization in others following total thyroidectomy, whereas following radioiodine, the eye changes in some patients become worse.

Table 1: Ablative Treatment of Graves Disease With Thyrotoxicosis

Method	Dose or extent of surgery	Onset of response	Complications	Remarks
Surgery	Subtotal excision of gland	Immediate	Mortality <1% Permanent hypothyroidism 20%-30% or greater[a] Recurrent hyperthyroidism <15%[a] Vocal cord paralysis approximately 1% Hypoparathyroidism approximately 1%	Applicable in young patients, pregnant women, large goiter, or nodular gland
Radioiodine 5–10 mCi		Several weeks to months	Permanent hypothyroidism, at least 50%=70%, often with delayed onset; multiple treatments sometimes necessary in large goiters	Avoid in children or pregnant women

[a]Depends on size of thyroid remnant which is left in neck. As more tissue is removed, the incidence of hypothyroidism is increased but recurrence rate is diminished.

- In summary, in the United States more than 90% of patients with Graves disease are treated with radioiodine therapy. In young individuals, pregnant women, and those with very bad thyroid eye disease, large goiters, and nodules which are suspicious for cancer, thyroidectomy may be appropriate. These operations are often difficult because of increased vascularity, fibrosis, and "stickiness" of the gland.
- Over the years, subtotal thyroidectomy has been the operation of choice for Graves disease, for it offers safety and very good, but not perfect, cure rates. Near-total or total thyroidectomy has been reserved for young patients and for those with very aggressive thyroid eye disease. However, long-term follow up studies have demonstrated that recurrence of Graves disease occurs in some patients over time after subtotal thyroidectomy.
- To prevent such problems, there is a trend by expert thyroid surgeons to perform near-total or total thyroidectomy in all patients with Graves disease who are operated upon, for they are able to do these operations with a low incidence of recurrent laryngeal nerve injury or hypoparathyroidism. For less experienced surgeons, subtotal thyroidectomy remains the best choice for patients with Graves disease, for it has been shown that complications are greater when more extensive thyroid operations are performed by these surgeons.

COMPLICATIONS

- Thyroid storm
- Postoperative hemorrhage (with respiratory distress)
- Injury to the external branch of the superior laryngeal nerve
- Unilateral or bilateral recurrent laryngeal nerve injury
- Temporary or permanent hypoparathyroidism

SUGGESTED READINGS

1. Behar R, Arganini M, Wu TC, et al. Graves' disease and thyroid cancer. *Surgery*. 1986;105:1121-1126.
2. Campbell MJ, McCoy KL, Shen WT, et al. A multi-institutional international study of risk factors for hematoma after thyroidectomy. *Surgery*. 2013;154(6):1283-1289.
3. Cheetham T, Bliss R. Treatment options in the young patient with Graves' disease. *Clin Endocrinol*. 2016;85(2):161-164.
4. DeGroot LJ. Diagnosis and treatment of Graves' disease. Thyroid Disease Manager Website. http://www.thyroidmanager.org
5. DeGroot LJ. Graves' disease and the manifestations of thyrotoxicosis. Thyroid Disease Manager Website. http://www.thyroidmanager.org
6. Douglas RS, Kahaly GJ, Patel A, et al. Teprotumumab for the treatment of active thyroid eye disease. *N Engl J Med*. 2020;382:341-352.
7. Jitpratoom P, Ketwong K, Sasanakietkul T, Anuwong A. Transoral endoscopic thyroidectomy vestibular approach (TOETVA) for Graves' disease: a comparison of surgical results with open thyroidectomy. *Gland Surg*. 2016(6):546-552.
8. Kaplan EL, Angelos P, Grogan RH. *Surgery of the thyroid gland. Thyroid Disease Manager Website*. http://www.thyroidmanager.org/thyroidbook.htm
9. Kaplan EL, Angelos P. Surgery of the thyroid. In: DeGroot LJ, Jameson JL, eds. *Endocrinology*. 6th ed. Elsevier; 2009.
10. Kaplan EL, McCaffrey K. Subtotal thyroidectomy in the treatment of Graves' disease. In: Thompson NW, ed. *Endocrine Surgery Update*. Grune & Stratton; 1983:43-57.
11. Kaplan EL. The place of subtotal thyroidectomy in the treatment of Graves' disease. *Surg Rounds*. 1984;7(1):22-31.
12. Klementschitsch P, Shen KL, Kaplan EL. Reemergence of thyroidectomy as treatment for Graves' disease. *Surg Clin North Am*. 1979;59:35-42.
13. Smithson M, Asban A, Miller J, Chen H. Considerations for thyroidectomy as treatment for Graves' disease. *Clin Med Insights Endocrinol Diabetes*. 2019;12:1179551419844523.
14. Sridama V, Reilly M, Kaplan EL, et al. Long-term follow-up study of compensated low dose 131–I therapy for Graves' disease. *N Engl J Med*. 1984;311:426-432.

Chapter 49 Minimally Invasive Video-Assisted Thyroidectomy

Paolo Miccoli and Gabriele Materazzi

DEFINITION

- Minimally invasive video-assisted thyroidectomy (MIVAT) is an endoscopic procedure characterized by the use of external retraction, avoiding any gas inflation, in order to create an operative space in the neck.
- This approach to the thyroid has been used at our Department of Surgery for the last 20 years on more than 5000 patients with results that can successfully rival those of standard open surgery.[1]
- This is not an appropriate operation for any patient with thyroid disease; patients must be strictly selected. Only 10% to 30% of the cases[2] are appropriate for a MIVAT procedure.
- In appropriately selected patients, MIVAT produces results comparable with that of open surgery with improved cosmetic outcomes.[3-5]

PATIENT HISTORY AND PHYSICAL FINDINGS

- The inclusion criteria and the main contraindications are summarized in the following text. The most significant limit is represented by the size of both the nodule(s) and/or the gland as measured by means of an accurate ultrasonographic study obtained preoperatively. In countries where goiter is endemic, the gland volume can be relevantly independent from the nodule volume, and this aspect might be responsible for the necessity of converting the procedure.
- Ultrasonography can also be useful to exclude the presence of thyroiditis, which might make the dissection troublesome. In case ultrasonography only gives the suspicion of thyroiditis, autoantibodies should be measured in the serum. If thyroiditis is diagnosed preoperatively, this is a consideration to MIVAT.
- One of the most controversial aspects regarding the appropriateness of MIVAT is in the treatment of malignant thyroid disease. "Low-risk" papillary carcinoma constitutes an ideal indication for MIVAT,[6-8] but it is important to take into account the possibility of lymph node involvement in the neck. Great caution should be taken when there is the possibility of either metastatic lymph nodes or extracapsular invasion of the gland, both of which represent a contraindication to the minimally invasive endoscopic procedure.
- Indications
  - Multinodular goiter (thyroid volume less than 25 mL and nodules smaller than 3 cm)
  - Low-risk papillary carcinoma
  - Graves disease
  - Microfollicular/Hürthle cell adenoma
  - *RET* gene mutation carriers (familial medullary thyroid carcinoma)
- Contraindications
  - Absolute
    - Previous neck surgery
    - Acute thyroiditis
    - Metastatic carcinoma (levels II to VI)
    - Locally advanced carcinoma
    - Sporadic medullary carcinoma
  - Relative
    - Previous neck irradiation
    - Short neck in an obese patient
    - Chronic thyroiditis

IMAGING AND OTHER DIAGNOSTIC STUDIES

- All patients should undergo (1) neck ultrasound in order to evaluate thyroid gland total volume (this should be less than 25 mL) and diameter of nodule/s (these should be less than 3 cm); (2) fine needle aspiration cytology of suspicious nodules; (3) blood tests in order to exclude thyrotoxicosis and acute thyroiditis before surgery; (4) basal serum calcitonin dosage is strongly suggested in order to exclude medullary carcinoma, which is a contraindication to MIVAT; (5) routine preoperative laryngoscopy is strongly recommended in all patients in order to identify asymptomatic vocal cord palsy.

TECHNIQUES

POSITIONING OF THE PATIENT AND DRAPING

- The patient is positioned in supine position without neck extension (**FIGURE 1**). Hyperextension must be avoided because it would reduce the operative space. Conventional neck preparation and draping is obtained. The skin is protected by means of a sterile film (Tegaderm).

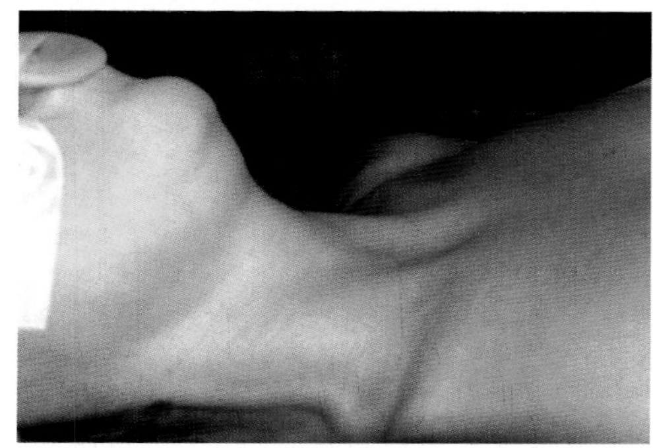

FIGURE 1 ● Position of the patient on the operative table: Neck is not extended and skin is covered by sterile drapes.

POSITIONING OF THE SURGICAL TEAM

- Operation is performed by four surgeons: The first surgeon is on the right side of the table; the first assistant is on the left side of the table. The second assistant, who is holding the retractors, is at the head of the table. The third assistant, who is holding the endoscope, is on the left side of the table. The scrub nurse is behind the surgeon on the right side of the table (**FIGURE 2**).

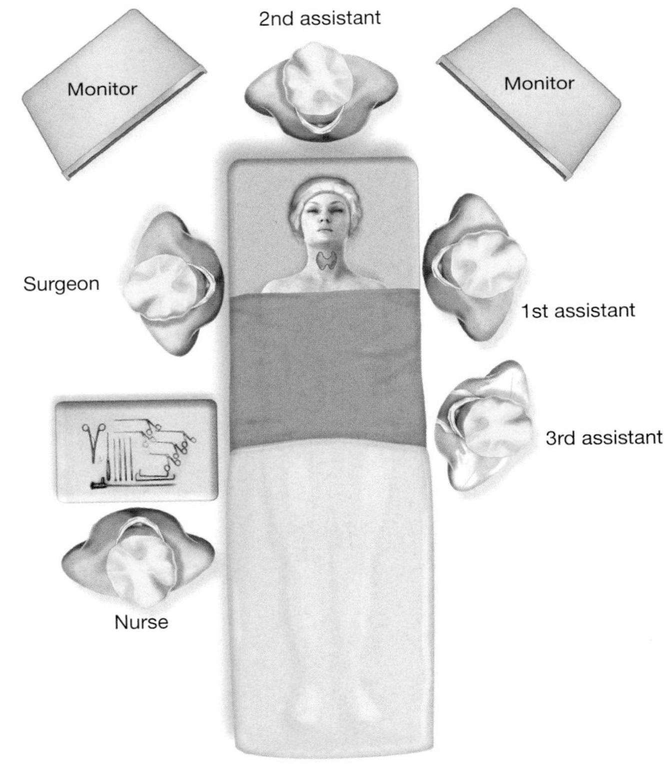

FIGURE 2 ● Operating room setup: Team.

- The surgeon is on the right side of the table.
- The first assistant is on the left side of the table (opposite the surgeon).
- The second assistant is at the head of the table.
- The third assistant is on the left side of the table.
- The scrub nurse is behind the surgeon on the right side of the table.

INSTRUMENTATION

- Forward-oblique telescope 30°, diameter 5 mm, length 30 cm; suction dissector with cutoff hole, with stylet, blunt, length 21 cm; ear forceps, very thin, serrated, working length 12.5 cm; conventional tissue retractor army navy type; small tissue retractor, double ended, length 12 cm; clip applier for vascular clips; straight scissors, length 12.5 cm, energy device (ultrasound or radiofrequency); electrocautery (monopolar) (**FIGURE 3**).

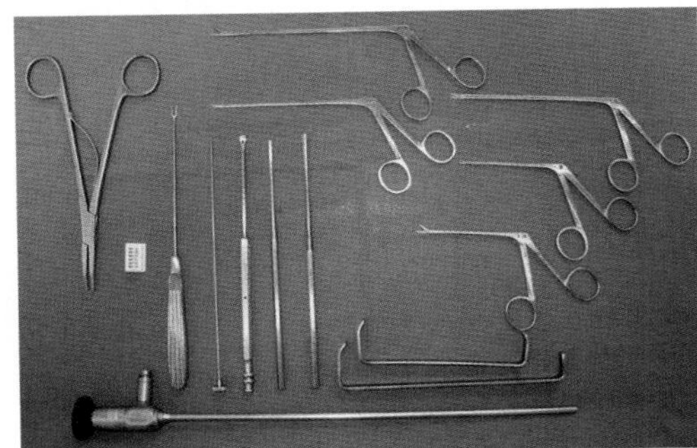

FIGURE 3 ● Instrumentation for MIVAT.

INCISION AND PREPARATION OF THE OPERATIVE SPACE

- A 1.5-cm horizontal skin incision is performed 2 cm above the sternal notch in the central cervical area (**FIGURE 4**). Subcutaneous fat and platysma are carefully dissected so as to avoid any minimum bleeding.
- Two small retractors are used to expose the midline, which has to be incised for 2 to 3 cm in an absolutely bloodless plane (**FIGURE 5**).
- The blunt dissection of the thyroid lobe from the strap muscles is performed through the skin incision by gentle retraction and using tiny spatulas. When the thyroid lobe is almost completely dissected from the strap muscles, larger and deeper retractors (army navy type) can be inserted and they will maintain the operative space during all the endoscopic part of the procedure (**FIGURE 6**).
- Then, a 30°, 5-mm or 7-mm endoscope is introduced through the skin incision: From this moment on, the procedure is entirely endoscopic until the extraction of the lobe of the gland. Preparation of the thyrotracheal groove is completed under endoscopic vision by using small (2 mm in diameter) instruments such as spatulas, forceps, spatula-sucker, and scissors.

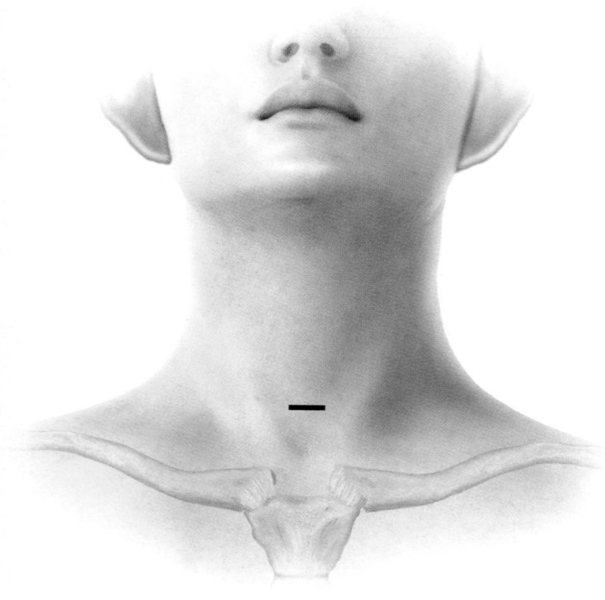

FIGURE 4 ● A 1.5-cm horizontal skin incision is performed 2 cm above the sternal notch in the central cervical area.

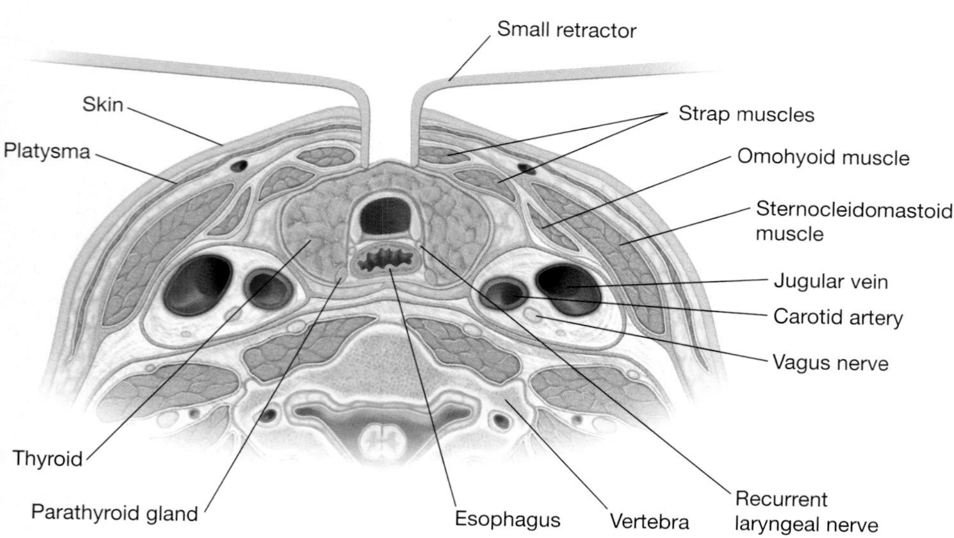

FIGURE 5 ● Two small retractors are used to expose the midline, which has to be incised for 2 to 3 cm on an absolutely bloodless plane.

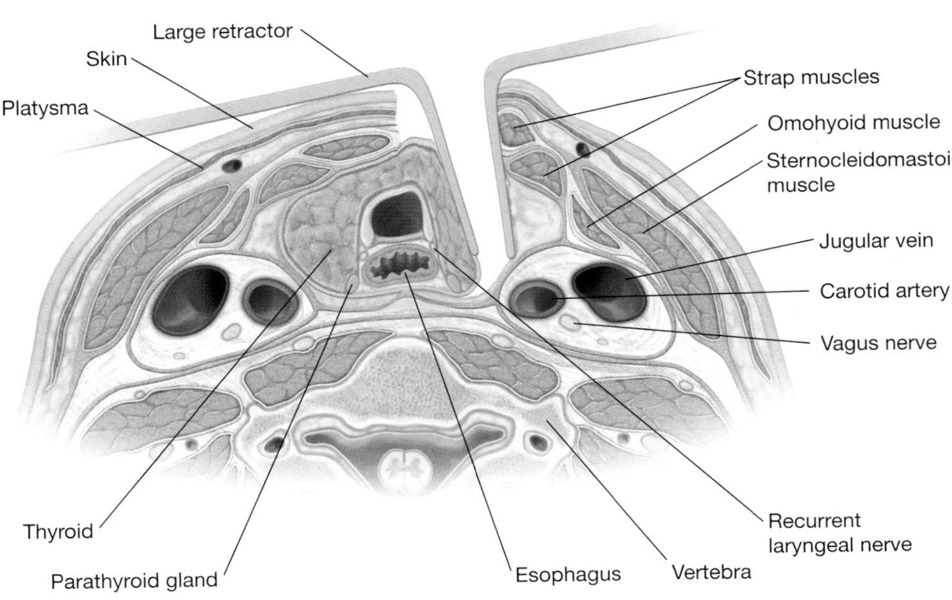

FIGURE 6 ● Access to the operative space during MIVAT: when the thyroid lobe is almost completely dissected from the strap muscles, larger and deeper retractors (army navy type) can be inserted and they will maintain the operative space during all the endoscopic part of the procedure.

SECTION OF THE MAIN THYROID VESSELS

- The first vessel to be ligated is the middle vein, when present, or the small veins between jugular vein and thyroid capsule. This step allows a better preparation of the thyrotracheal groove where the recurrent nerve will be later searched.
- During this step, the endoscope has to be held inside the camera with the 30° tip looking downward and in an orthogonal axis with the thyroid lobe and trachea.
- A further step is represented by the exposure of the upper pedicle, which must be carefully prepared, until an optimal visualization of the different branches is achieved. During this step, the endoscope should be rotated to 180° with the 30° tip looking upward (**FIGURE 7**) and held in a parallel direction with the thyroid lobe and trachea in order to better visualize the upper portion of the operative space where the superior thyroid vein and artery are running.
- The upper pedicle is then prepared by retracting downward and medially the thyroid lobe by means of the retractor and the spatula. A further spatula can be used to pull the vessels laterally. This will allow the external branch of the superior laryngeal nerve to be easily identified during most procedures (**FIGURE 8**). Its injury can be avoided by keeping the energy device at least 5 mm far from the nerve so as to not transmit the heat to this delicate structure. At this point in time, section of the upper pedicle can be obtained by the energy device en bloc or selectively, depending on the diameter of the single vessels and/or the anatomic situation (**FIGURE 9**).

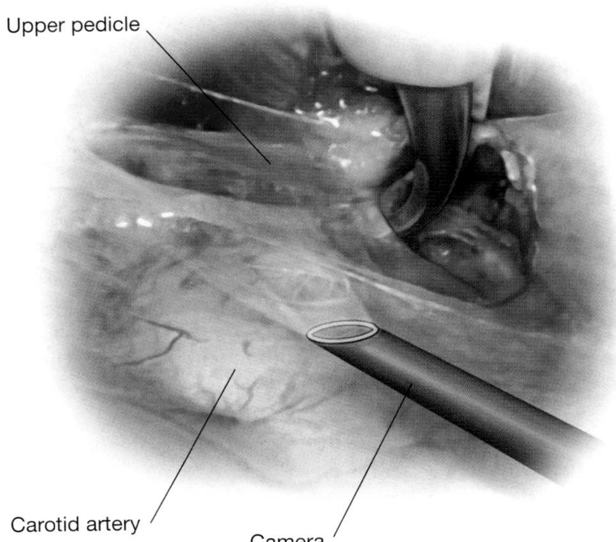

FIGURE 7 ● Upper pole section: During this step, the endoscope should be rotated to 180° with the 30° tip looking upward and held in a parallel direction with the thyroid lobe and trachea in order to better visualize the upper portion of the operative space where the superior thyroid vein and artery are running.

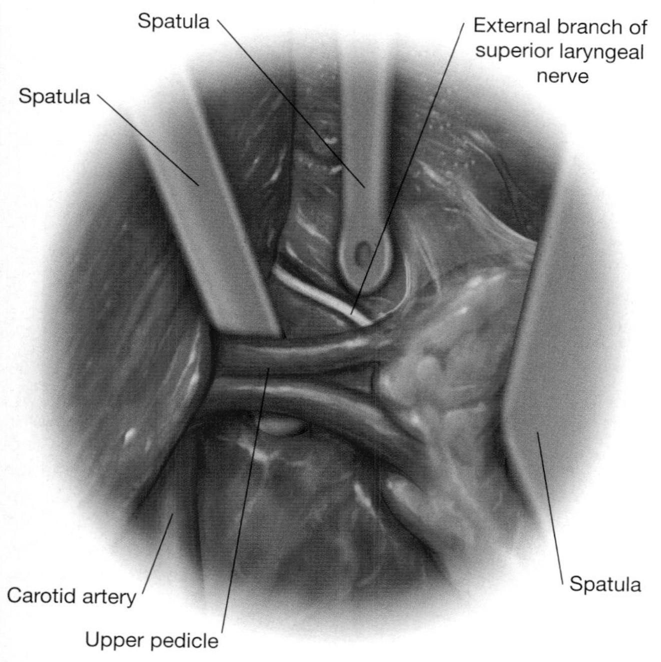

FIGURE 8 ● Identification of the external branch of the superior laryngeal nerve: The vessels (right side) are prepared by retracting downward and medially the thyroid lobe by means of the retractor and the spatula. A further spatula can be used to pull the vessels laterally. This will allow the external branch of the superior laryngeal nerve (SLN) to be easily identified during most procedures.

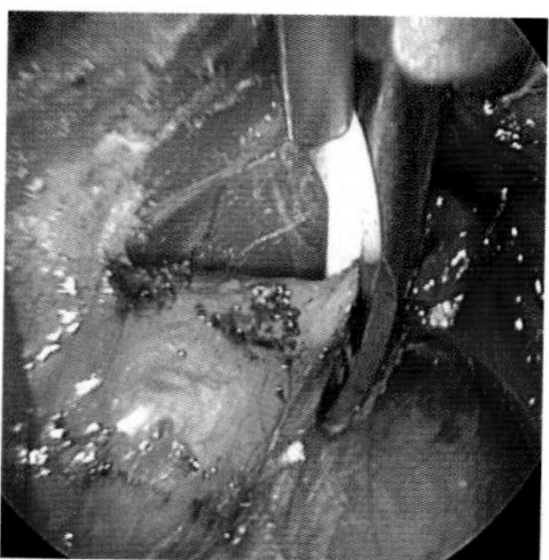

FIGURE 9 ● Section of the upper pedicle (left side) by energy device. The blade must be 5 mm from laryngeal muscles and the superior laryngeal nerve in order to avoid any injury to these structures.

INFERIOR LARYNGEAL NERVE AND PARATHYROID GLANDS IDENTIFICATION AND DISSECTION

- After retracting medially and lifting up the thyroid lobe, the fascia can be opened by a gentle spatula retraction. During this step, the endoscope should be repositioned in an orthogonal axis with the thyroid lobe and trachea, looking downward with its 30° (**FIGURE 10**). The recurrent laryngeal nerve appears generally at this point in time, lying in the thyrotracheal groove, posterior to the Zuckerkandl tuberculum (posterior lobe), which is an important landmark in this step. This way, the recurrent nerve and the parathyroid glands are dissected and freed from the thyroid (**FIGURE 11A** and **B**).
- Dissection of the entire nerve from the mediastinum to its entrance into the larynx is not mandatory and might result in a time waste during the endoscopic phase. It is correct and very safe to identify the laryngeal nerve, to free it from the thyroid capsule as much as possible, but it is important to stress that the complete dissection of the nerve can be more easily obtained during the subsequent step, under direct vision, when the thyroid lobe has already been extracted.
- Both parathyroid glands are generally easily visualized during the endoscopic step; thanks to the camera magnification.

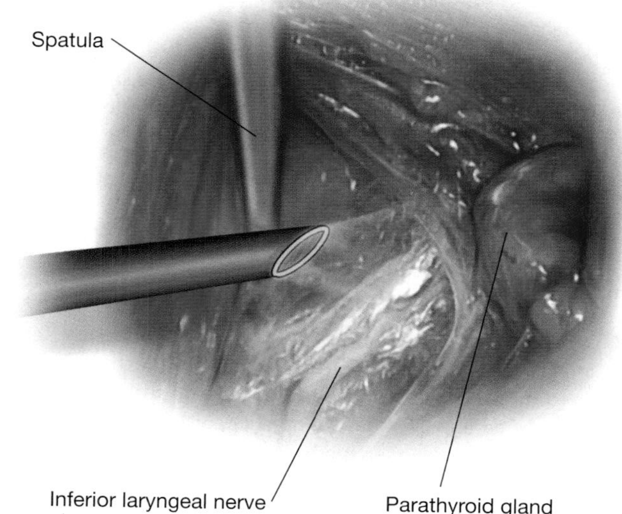

FIGURE 10 ● Inferior laryngeal nerve and parathyroids dissection: During this step, the endoscope should be repositioned in an orthogonal axis with the thyroid lobe and trachea, looking downward with its 30° angle.

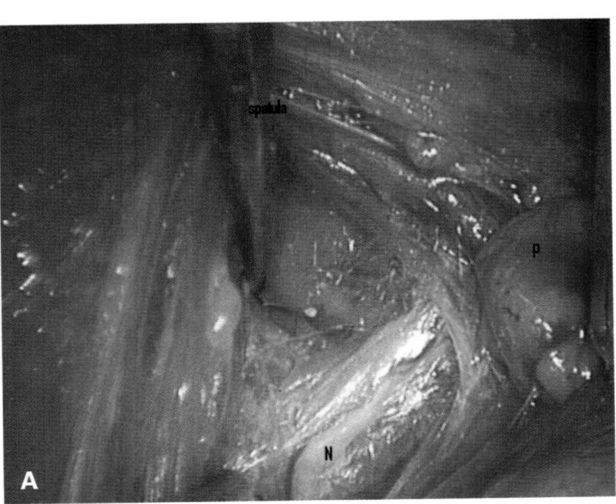

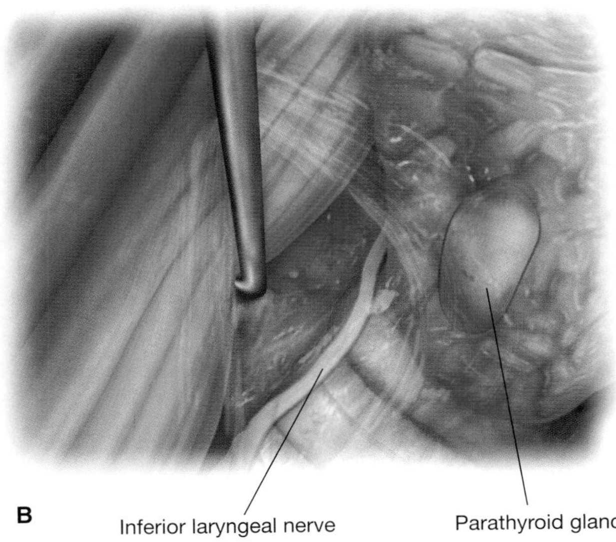

FIGURE 11 ● **A,** Endoscopic vision: dissection of the inferior laryngeal nerve. The recurrent laryngeal nerve *(n)* appears lying in the thyrotracheal groove. Parathyroid gland is also well visible *(p)*. **B,** Illustration of this step.

Their vascular supply is preserved by selective division of the branches of the inferior thyroid artery. During dissection, when dealing with large vessels or small vessels close to the nerve, hemostasis can be achieved by 3-mm titanium vascular clips.

EXTRACTION OF THE LOBE AND RESECTION

- At this point in time, the lobe is completely freed. The endoscope and the retractors can be removed and the upper portion of the gland rotated and pulled out using conventional forceps. A gentle traction over the lobe allows the complete exteriorization of the gland (**FIGURE 12**). The operation is now conducted as an open surgery under direct vision. The lobe is freed from the trachea by ligating the small vessels and dissecting the Berry ligament. It is very important to check once again the laryngeal nerve at this point in time, so as to avoid its injury before the final step. The isthmus is then dissected from the trachea and divided. After completely exposing the trachea, the lobe is finally removed.

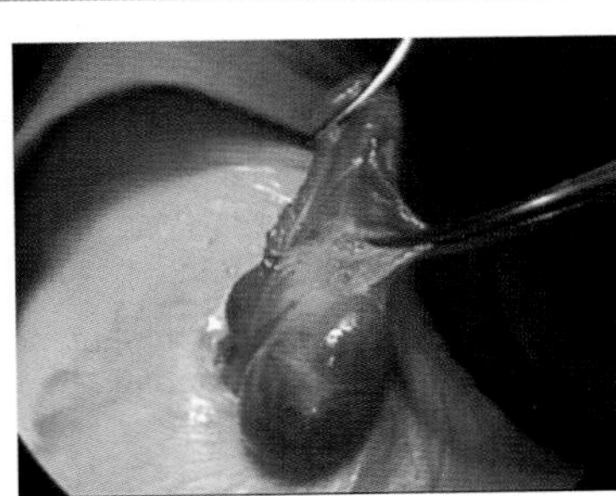

FIGURE 12 ● Thyroid lobe extraction. A gentle traction over the lobe allows the complete exteriorization of the gland.

CLOSURE

- Drainage is not necessary. The midline is then approached by a single stitch; platysma is closed by a subcuticular suture, and a cyanoacrylate sealant is used for the skin (**FIGURES 13** and **14**).

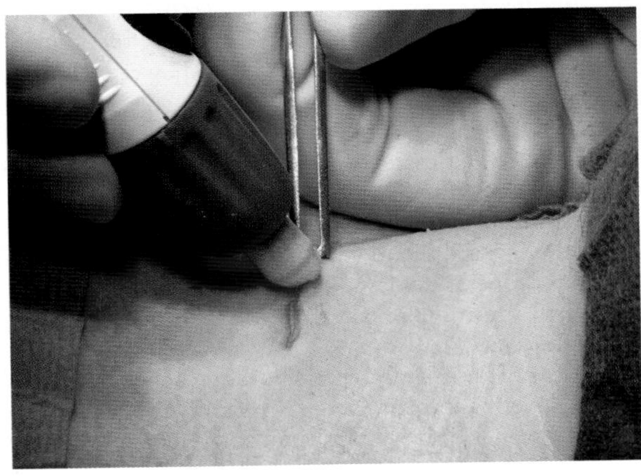

FIGURE 13 ● Skin is reapproximated and closed by means of glue.

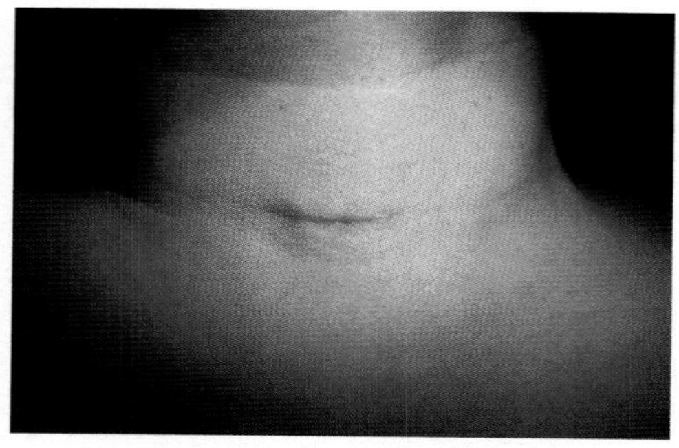

FIGURE 14 ● MIVAT: final result.

PEARLS AND PITFALLS

Indications	■ Perform preoperative ultrasound in order to evaluate thyroid volume (less than 25 mL) and nodule diameter (< 3 cm). ■ Exclude thyrotoxicosis and acute thyroiditis. ■ Exclude locally advanced or metastatic carcinoma.
Incision	■ Create a central cervical incision two fingers above the sternal notch in order to easily allow for eventual conversion to cervicotomy. ■ Use a thin film of sterile drape on the electrocautery blade, leaving just the tip able to coagulate, in order to avoid damage to the skin or the superficial planes. ■ Avoid any bleeding from the anterior jugular veins.
Section of upper pedicle	■ The correct position of the retractors (both the first one on the strap muscles and the second one on the upper part of the thyroid lobe) is very important during this step, in order to obtain the best visualization of the vessels. ■ The endoscope should be rotated 180° with the 30° tip looking upward.
Recurrent laryngeal nerve dissection	■ Avoid electrocautery (bipolar or monopolar) until both laryngeal nerves have been exposed. The energy device is used for almost all the vascular structures, but if the vessel is running particularly close to the inferior laryngeal nerve, then hemostasis is achieved by means of small vascular clips.
Closure	■ Close the midline with one single stitch, leaving some space in between the strap muscles, allowing quick blood evacuation in case of compressive hematoma.

POSTOPERATIVE CARE

- After surgery, patients undergoing MIVAT require strict observation during the first 5 to 10 hours on the ward. Dysphonia, airway obstruction, and neck swelling must be carefully checked. No drain is left, so careful surveillance for postoperative hematomas is required during the immediate postoperative period. Postoperative bleeding risk is very low and dramatically decreases after 5 hours.
- In case of postoperative hematoma, if compressive symptoms and airway obstruction are present, reintervention and immediate hematoma evacuation is required.
- Patients can start oral intake on the evening of the operative day and will be discharged the day after. On the first and second postoperative days, serum calcium must be checked in order to control hypoparathyroidism by substitutive therapy, as described in **TABLE 1**.
- Wound care is not really necessary after MIVAT because of the glue covering the skin, and postoperative pain will be controlled by means of both intravenous (IV) or oral analgesics.

Table 1: Management of Postoperative Hypocalcemia

Management of hypocalcemia following thyroidectomy on the first Postoperative day	
Acute symptomatic	Calcium gluconate IV
Asymptomatic calcium ≤7.5 mg/dL[a]	Calcium (3 g) + vitamin D (0.5 μg) per os daily
Asymptomatic calcium 7.5–7.9 mg/dL	Calcium (1.5 g) per os daily

[a]*Normal range: 8 to 10 mg/dL.*

- Voice impairments and subjective or objective dysphonia requires an immediate postoperative vocal cord check by an otolaryngologist. In the case of a normal postoperative course, a vocal cord check can be delayed until after 3 months.

COMPLICATIONS

- Transient hypoparathyroidism and definitive hypoparathyroidism

- Transient monolateral inferior laryngeal nerve palsy and definitive monolateral inferior laryngeal nerve palsy
- Transient bilateral inferior laryngeal nerve palsy and definitive bilateral inferior laryngeal nerve palsy
- Hematoma (subcutaneous-conservative treatment; below strap muscles-reoperation):
  - Seroma
  - Wound infection

REFERENCES

1. Miccoli P, Biricotti M, Matteucci V, Ambrosini CE, Wu J, Materazzi G. Minimally invasive video-assisted thyroidectomy: reflections after more than 2400 cases performed. *Surg Endosc*. 2016;30(6):2489-2495. doi:10.1007/s00464-015-4503-4
2. Miccoli P, Fregoli L, Rossi L, et al. Minimally invasive video-assisted thyroidectomy (MIVAT). *Gland Surg*. 2020;9(suppl 1):S1-S5. doi:10.21037/gs.2019.12.05
3. de Vries LH, Aykan D, Lodewijk L, Damen JAA, Borel Rinkes IHM, Vriens MR. Outcomes of minimally invasive thyroid surgery—a systematic review and meta-analysis. *Front Endocrinol*. 2021;12:719397. doi:10.3389/fendo.2021.719397
4. Alesina PF, Wahabie W, Meier B, et al. Long-term cosmetic results of video-assisted thyroidectomy: a comparison with conventional surgery. *Langenbeck's Arch Surg*. 2021;406(5):1625-1633. doi:10.1007/s00423-021-02196-8
5. Sahm M, Otto R, Pross M, Mantke R. Minimally invasive video-assisted thyroidectomy: a critical analysis of long-term cosmetic results using a validated tool. *Ann R Coll Surg Engl*. 2019;101(3):180-185. doi:10.1308/rcsann.2018.0178
6. Miccoli P, Elisei R, Materazzi G, et al. Minimally invasive video assisted thyroidectomy for papillary carcinoma: a prospective study about its completeness. *Surgery*. 2002;132:1070-1074.
7. Miccoli P, Pinchera A, Materazzi G, et al. Surgical treatment of low- and intermediate-risk papillary thyroid cancer with minimally invasive video-assisted thyroidectomy. *J Clin Endocrinol Metab*. 2009;94(5):1618-1622.
8. Miccoli P, Matteucci V. Video-assisted surgery for thyroid cancer patients. *Gland Surg*. 2015;4(5):365-367. doi:10.3978/j.issn.2227-684X.2015.04.17

Chapter 50

Transoral Endoscopic Thyroidectomy and Parathyroidectomy

Robin M. Cisco and Dana T. Lin

DEFINITION

- Transoral Endoscopic Thyroidectomy, Vestibular Approach (TOETVA) is a remote-access thyroidectomy with access to the central neck via endoscopic ports placed within the oral vestibule.
- Standard endoscopic instruments including a 10 mm, 30° endoscope, dissecting graspers, and a 5-mm energy device of choice (LigaSure or Harmonic Scalpel) are used.
- The procedure was first described in 2014 by Anuwong and colleagues.[1]
- In a standard TOETVA procedure, the only incisions are on the oral mucosa of the lower lip. The procedure is therefore a form of Natural Orifice Transluminal Endoscopic Surgery (NOTES). This same remote-access approach may be applied to parathyroidectomy.
- The primary advantage of TOETVA is the absence of a visible skin scar. Hypertrophic or keloid scar is reported in up to 12.5% of thyroidectomy patients, and low scar satisfaction is associated with decreased quality of life for these patients.[2]
- Compared with other remote-access approaches to thyroidectomy, advantages of TOETVA include the short distance between the mouth and the central neck, allowing a short length of soft tissue dissection. In addition, the procedure may be performed using standard endoscopic instruments available at most facilities for routine laparoscopy.

PATIENT HISTORY AND PHYSICAL FINDINGS

There are various eligibility criteria described for this procedure.[3] Ours include:

- Benign single nodule **<6 cm**
- Malignant tumor **<2 cm with or without need for central neck dissection**
- Total thyroid lobe **<10 cm**
- Multinodular goiter
- Graves' disease
- Localized primary hyperparathyroidism

Criteria will likely expand as experience with this technique grows.

Exclusion Criteria Include

- Medically unfit for surgery/anesthesia
- Substernal goiter
- Large PTC with local invasion
- Prior neck surgery or radiation
- Active dental infection (relative)

IMAGING AND OTHER DIAGNOSTIC STUDIES

- Preoperative Ultrasound—All patients should have a preoperative thyroid ultrasound to characterize the thyroid pathology and evaluate for any adenopathy.
- Computed tomography (CT)- Patients with suspicion of substernal extension of the thyroid should have cross-sectional imaging such as CT, as substernal extension is a contraindication to this approach.
- Intraoperative ultrasound is useful in allowing the surgeon to confirm the pathology and mark an appropriate location for incision to be prepared for conversion to an open procedure.

SURGICAL MANAGEMENT

Preoperative Planning

- All preoperative imaging is reviewed. Any oral or dental concerns should be addressed.
- Benefits and risks of the transoral procedure versus the traditional open approach, as well as criteria for conversion to an open procedure are discussed with the patient.
- We discuss risks of laryngeal nerve injury, neck hematoma, and hypoparathyroidism as common to any thyroidectomy approach. We also discuss the risk of lip numbness related to mental nerve injury, skin numbness, and the rare risk of tracheal injury as unique to the transoral endoscopic approach.
- Peridex mouthwash is given in the preoperative holding area.
- Preoperative antibiotics are administered to cover oral flora. We typically use Ampicillin/Sulbactam (Unasyn).
- We do not give subcutaneous heparin preoperatively. Sequential compression devices (SCDs) are utilized.
- Route of intubation should be discussed with the anesthesiologist preoperatively. Although the procedure was initially developed with nasotracheal intubation, many surgeons, including those at our institution, now use orotracheal intubation. This does require securing the head to the table and careful immobilization of the endotracheal tube so that it is not inadvertently displaced during the procedure.

Patient Positioning, Preparation, and Draping

- The patient is positioned supine, with both arms tucked, and a small gel roll is placed under the shoulders for moderate neck extension.
- Oral or nasal intubation is performed with a nerve monitoring endotracheal tube (Nerveäna, *Neurovision Medi*cal) placed under direct visualization to ensure placement of the nerve monitoring electrodes at the vocal cords.

- A Foley catheter is placed, if appropriated based on the anticipated length of the operation.
- Pressure points are padded and eye protection goggles are placed on the patient.
- The operating table is turned 180°, so that the anesthesia machine is at the at foot of the table.
- A transparent adhesive drape is placed at the upper lip.
- Chlorhexidine-based skin prep solution is applied from the lower lip past the clavicles bilaterally.
- The mouth, lips, tongue, and teeth are prepped with an oral chlorhexidine solution using swabs.
- Two split sheets are used to drape with exposure of the lower face, neck, and upper chest.
- The endotracheal tube is well secured and padded to immobilize and reduce the risk of displacement during the procedure.

Positioning of the Surgical Team

- The operating surgeon stands at the head of the table and faces the main monitor, which is located directly ahead at the foot of the bed (**FIGURE 1**).
- The first assistant navigates the endoscope and stands next to the operating surgeon. The second assistant is on the same side of the table as the thyroid lobe that is being removed, holding traction sutures anteriorly and laterally.
- The scrub nurse stands on the opposite side of the second assistant.

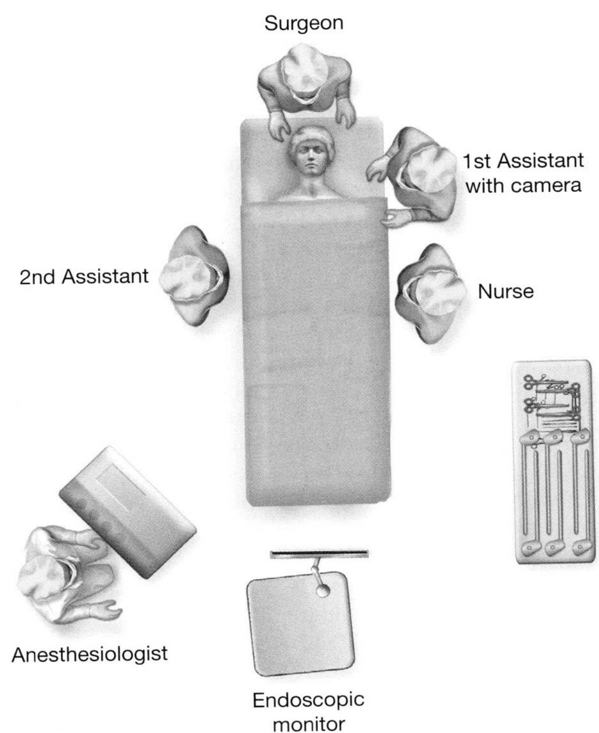

FIGURE 1 ● Positioning of the surgical team.

PORT PLACEMENT AND CREATION OF THE WORKING SPACE

- A 10-mm transverse incision is made within the oral vestibule anterior to the frenulum (**FIGURE 2**).
- A small clamp is used to dissect to the chin.
- The Veress needle is advanced through this incision and over the chin while injecting a hydrodissection solution of 1 mg epinephrine in 500 mL NS. The Veress needle is advanced in the subplatysmal plane at the midline and then to the right and left of midline, injecting both while inserting and withdrawing the needle. The skin of the anterior neck is lifted and tented upwards as the hydrodissection needle is advanced.
- After hydrodissection, a blunt-curved Kelly clamp is inserted through the opening and over the chin into the subplatysmal space. The clamp is gently spread to enlarge the tract.
- A dilator or vascular tunneler (we a use Kelly-Wick tunneler with an 8-mm tip) is introduced through the 10-mm incision into the subplatysmal space. It is advanced toward the sternal notch and then directed to the right and left of midline. Approximately 10 to 15 excursions of the dilator are made to begin to create the subplatysmal space.

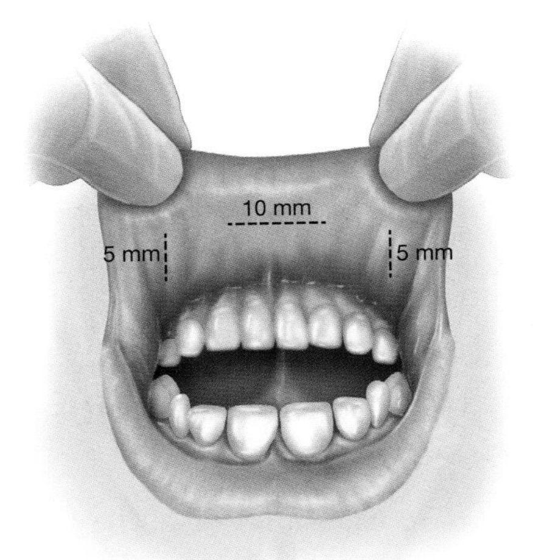

FIGURE 2 ● Placement of incisions within the oral vestibule. Three incisions are made within the oral vestibule.

- A 10-mm bladeless trocar is then placed through the midline transoral incision into the subplatysmal space. Use of a bariatric length 10-mm trocar may be helpful in preventing the hub of the trocar from bumping against the 5-mm trocars during the dissection.

- Insufflation is initiated to 6 mm Hg. This low pressure insufflation reduces the risk of subcutaneous emphysema.
- Smoke evacuation at low setting is helpful in maintaining clear visualization during the procedure.
- An external traction suture is placed in the skin just inferior to the tip of the 10-mm trocar to lift the skin and platysma anteriorly.
- Two 5-mm lower lip incisions are made anterior and lateral to the canine on either side of the mouth. These are vertically oriented. The Veress needle with hydrodissection solution is then advanced through these 5-mm incisions over the jaw and into the subplatysmal space. A 5-mm bladeless trocar is inserted into each incision following the tract created by the Veress needle. Countertraction is provided against the jaw to facilitate trocar entry. Once inserted, the trocars can be quite superficial just under the skin (**FIGURE 3**).
- A standard 10 to 30 laparoscope is introduced via the 10-mm midline trocar. Dissecting graspers are advanced into the subplatysmal space via the two 5-mm trocars. Bridging muscle fibers and connective tissue are divided with L-hook monopolar cautery in a dome shape around the trachea to create a working space (**FIGURE 4**).
- Dissection extends inferiorly until the sternal notch is reached. The dissection should extend laterally to the anterior borders of the sternocleidomastoid. Care is taken throughout to avoid thermal injury to the overlying skin.
- The strap muscles are opened along the median raphe with cautery or an energy device of choice. We prefer the L-hook cautery or a 5-mm LigaSure. Cautery and blunt dissection are used to separate the strap muscles from the thyroid capsule, exposing the desired thyroid lobe. When the strap muscles are adequately mobilized, a hanging silk suture is placed through the skin, around the strap muscles and back out through the skin for retraction. An assistant retracts this suture anteriorly and laterally to improve the working space and exposure of the thyroid.

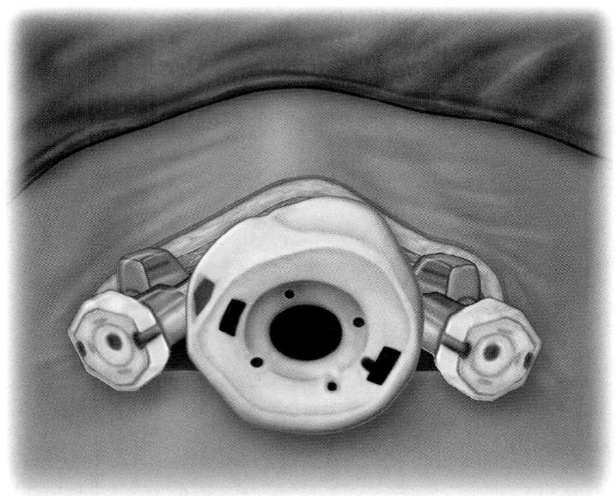

FIGURE 3 • Port placement in TOETVA. One 10-mm and two 5-mm bladeless trocars are used. The patient is intubated via orotracheal approach.

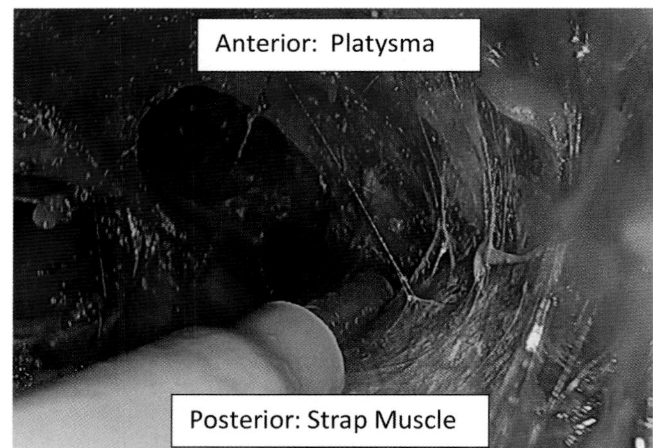

FIGURE 4 • Initial view when creating the working space. The subplatysmal working space is created by dividing bridges of muscle and connective tissue between the platysma and the strap muscles. L-hook monopolar cautery is used. The view is toward the sternal notch.

DIVIDING THE ISTHMUS AND MOBILIZING THE UPPER POLE

- The isthmus is isolated and divided with LigaSure, taking care to mobilize any pyramidal lobe.
- The superior pole is exposed, grasped, and retracted anteriorly and inferiorly. The superior thyroid vessels are ligated with LigaSure (**FIGURE 5**). We fire the LigaSure twice on any larger superior thyroid vessels.
- Perithyroidal tissue, often containing the upper parathyroid gland, is gently swept posteriorly with a closed grasper as upper pole mobilization progresses.

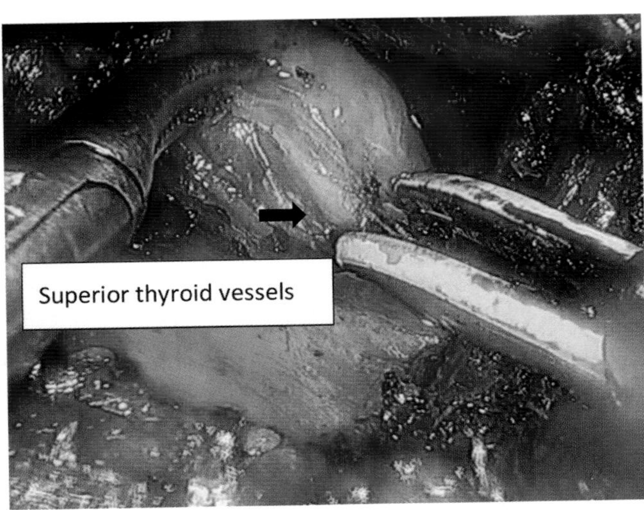

FIGURE 5 ● Mobilization of the superior pole of the thyroid. The right upper pole is retracted anteriorly and inferiorly with a grasper. The LigaSure device is used to ligate the superior thyroid vessels.

IDENTIFICATION OF THE RECURRENT LARYNGEAL NERVE AND CONTROL OF THE INFERIOR THYROID VESSELS

- When the upper pole is fully mobilized, it is retracted anteriorly.
- The tissue posterior to the junction of the upper pole and the remainder of the thyroid lobe is gently interrogated with a Maryland grasper to identify the recurrent laryngeal nerve (**FIGURE 6**).
- Nerve monitoring is used routinely to confirm identification of the recurrent laryngeal nerve and monitor its course and function throughout the procedure. Once the nerve is seen, one jaw of the open Maryland dissecting grasper may be carefully run between the nerve and the adjacent thyroid tissue to gently free the recurrent laryngeal nerve.
- After the nerve is identified, the inferior thyroid vessels are ligated with LigaSure. The lower parathyroid gland is freed from the thyroid tissue and preserved.

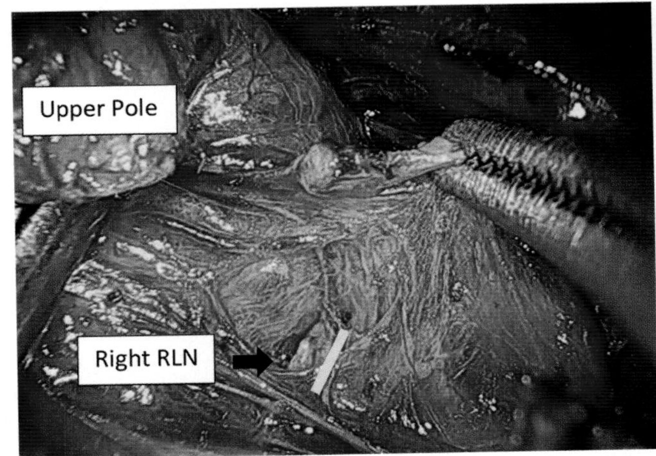

FIGURE 6 ● Identification of the recurrent laryngeal nerve. An atraumatic grasper is used to grasp the right thyroid lobe, retracting it anteriorly and medially. A dissecting grasper is used to spread posterior to the right lobe, and then to retract the perithyroidal tissue, exposing the right recurrent laryngeal nerve. The yellow line indicates the trajectory of the right recurrent laryngeal nerve.

DIVIDING THE LIGAMENT OF BERRY

- The contralateral atraumatic grasper is used to gently grasp the entire thyroid lobe transversely, so that it may be retracted anteriorly. This optimizes exposure of the recurrent laryngeal nerve and puts the Ligament of Berry on tension, so that it may be divided with bipolar cautery or careful use of LigaSure.
- Use of energy devices near the recurrent laryngeal nerve should be brief and intermittent.
- Once free, the specimen is placed in an extraction bag and removed through the 10 mm port site. We use a standard extraction bag, which is removed from the delivery device. Gentle spreading through the 10-mm incision, extending over the chin, may be needed to facilitate removal of the specimen.

TECHNIQUES

TRANSORAL ENDOSCOPIC PARATHYROIDECTOMY

- We use the same approach for port placement and creation of the working space that is used during TOETVA when performing Transoral Endoscopic Parathyroidectomy.
- At our institution, this remote-access approach is primarily reserved for cases of focused parathyroidectomy, in which a single abnormal gland has been identified on preoperative localizing imaging.
- The localized parathyroid gland is identified intraoperatively and excised with gentle spreading and use of LigaSure (**FIGURE 7**). We send intraoperative parathyroid hormone levels at 10 and 20 minutes post excision of the abnormal gland.
- Whether or not to proceed to a four-gland exploration via a transoral approach or an open approach is an important preoperative discussion with the patient.
- Some surgeons do perform routine four-gland parathyroid explorations via a transoral vestibular approach.

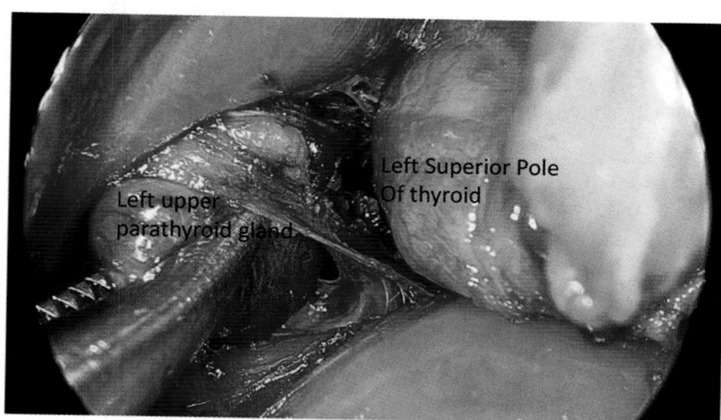

FIGURE 7 ● Excision of the left upper parathyroid gland during transoral endoscopic parathyroidectomy.

CLOSURE

- The thyroid bed is irrigated with normal saline and hemostasis is assured. Tisseel is placed into the thyroid bed. Closure of the strap muscles is optional. The 10-mm port site is closed in two layers with Vicryl and chromic suture. The 5-mm sites are closed with interrupted chromic suture.

PEARLS AND PITFALLS

Positioning	■ Secure the patient's head to the table with foam tape in order to avoid unwanted movement during surgery.
Trocar placement	■ During hydrodissection, dilation, and port insertion, use your nondominant hand to tent the overlying skin anteriorly to avoid inadvertent penetration through the skin. ■ Provide countertraction against the jaw as you insert the 5-mm trocars.
Dissection	■ After insertion of the 5-mm lateral trocars, create a clear and open tract to the working space by cauterizing the soft tissue around the trocars using hook cautery. This will facilitate the entry and removal of multiple endoscopic instruments, nerve probe, suction, and irrigation.
Nerve monitoring	■ Use Neurovision's long DryTouch probe via the 5-mm trocar to stimulate the recurrent laryngeal nerve. This probe is compatible with the Nerveäna nerve monitoring system.

POSTOPERATIVE CARE

- Postoperatively, patients are given a soft diet for 3 days.
- They rinse with Peridex mouthwash three times daily.
- For the first 2 days after surgery, we ask them to brush the upper teeth only; after that, they may brush teeth normally.
- We treat with antibiotics (amoxicillin/clavulanate, *Augmentin*) for 3 days postoperatively, although some institutions have discontinued this practice.

COMPLICATIONS

- Complications include those for any thyroidectomy approach: bleeding, infection, recurrent laryngeal nerve injury, superior laryngeal nerve injury, and parathyroid gland injury.
- Adverse outcomes specific to transoral thyroidectomy include mental nerve injury, inadvertent skin penetration during port insertion, and rare tracheal injury. Bruising along the chin and jawline is common and usually resolves within 1 to 2 weeks.

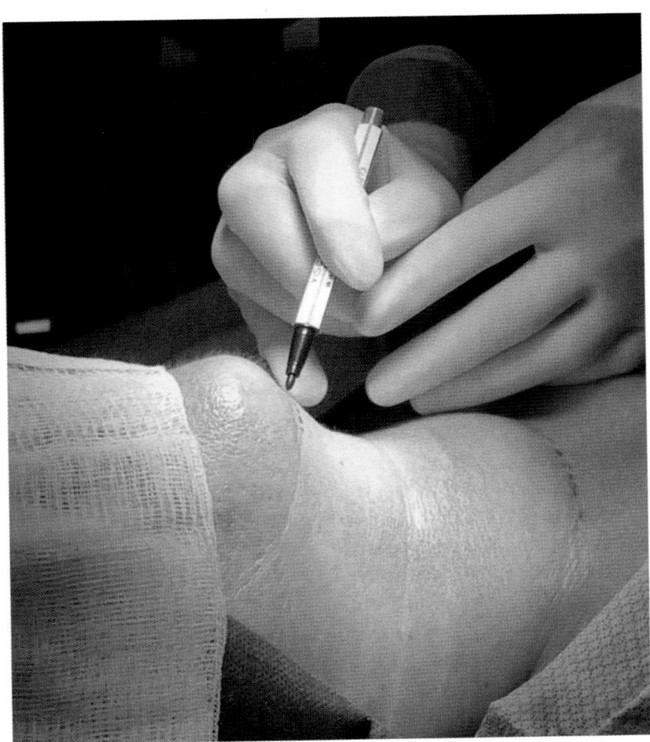

FIGURE 8 ● Submental incision for TOAST. The surgeon marks a 10-mm incision 1 mm posterior to the submental crease in a patient undergoing TOAST.

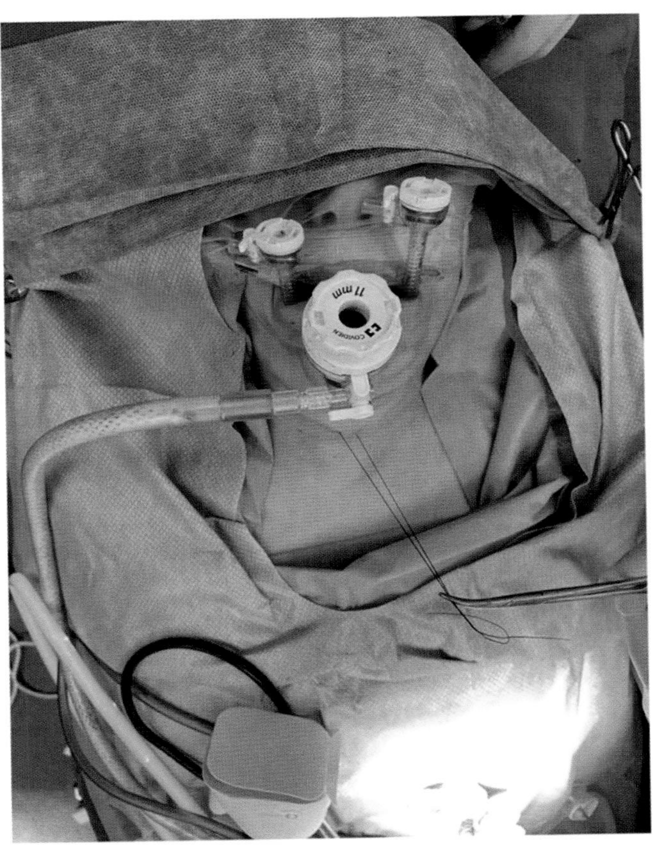

FIGURE 9 ● Trocar placement in a patient undergoing TOAST. The 10-mm trocar is placed via a submental incision rather than an incision within the oral vestibule.

VARIATIONS

Transoral and Submental Thyroidectomy (TOAST)[4]

The TOAST approach differs from the original TOETVA approach in that the midline 10-mm port is placed through a 10-mm submental incision. This avoids the morbidity associated with a 10-mm vestibular incision and the need to pull larger specimens over the chin and through a small lip incision for extraction. It therefore improves the ability to remove a larger thyroid specimen intact.

Placement of 10-mm Incision for TOAST

- A 10-mm midline incision is made 1 mm posterior to the natural submental crease (**FIGURE 8**).
- The platysma is divided with cautery.
- A Kelley clamp is used to dissect into the subplatysmal plane. The Veress needle with hydrodissection fluid is advanced into the subplatysmal space.
- From this point, the procedure proceeds as with the TOETVA approach. **FIGURE 9** shows trocar placement in the TOAST approach.

REFERENCES

1. Anuwong A. Transoral endoscopic thyroidectomy vestibular approach: a series of the first 60 human cases. *World J Surg*. 2016;40(3):491-497. doi:10.1007/s00268-015-3320-1
2. Arora A, Swords C, Garas G, et al. The perception of scar cosmesis following thyroid and parathyroid surgery: a prospective cohort study. *Int J Surg*. 2016;25:38-43. doi:10.1016/j.ijsu.2015.11.021
3. Grogan RH, Suh I, Chomsky-Higgins K, et al. Patient eligibility for transoral endocrine surgery procedures in the United States. *JAMA Netw Open*. 2019;2(5):e194829. doi:10.1001/jamanetworkopen.2019.4829
4. Suh I, Viscardi C, Chen Y, et al. Technical innovation in transoral endoscopic endocrine surgery: a modified the United States. *J Surg Res*. 2019;243:123-129. doi:10.1016/j.jss.2019.05.019

Chapter 51 Lymph Node Dissection in Thyroid Cancer

Gerard M. Doherty

DEFINITION

- Most thyroid cancer develops from the follicular cells of the thyroid gland (differentiated thyroid cancer includes papillary and follicular subtypes).
- Rare thyroid cancers develop from the C cells of the thyroid gland (medullary thyroid cancer).
- Thyroid cancer of any subtype can be associated with lymph node metastases in the neck.
- Clinical circumstances can indicate the need for cervical lymphadenectomy, either as a therapeutic intervention for known metastases or as a prophylactic procedure for the diagnosis or therapy of occult metastases.
- The lymph node compartments of the neck are divided into "levels" to allow communication of the affected and dissected areas (**FIGURE 1**).
  - Level 6 is also known as the central neck and includes the lymph nodes medial to the carotid sheath on each side, bounded by the hyoid bone superiorly and the sternum inferiorly.
  - Levels 1 through 5 are also known as the lateral neck and include all of the node compartments lateral to the carotid sheath on each side.

PATIENT HISTORY AND PHYSICAL FINDINGS

- Thyroid cancer lymph node metastases can be palpable or more often nonpalpable but identifiable by imaging. Very small foci of thyroid cancer in lymph nodes may only be evident at microscopic pathology examination.

IMAGING AND OTHER DIAGNOSTIC STUDIES

- Patients with thyroid cancer should each have a staging ultrasound examination prior to operation.[1] This allows for the mapping of the lymph node status of each compartment in the neck (**FIGURE 2**).
- The Level 6 lymph nodes are the most difficult to evaluate by ultrasound when the thyroid gland is still present, as these structures are in the same compartment.
- Patients with large tumors or gross adenopathy may be best studied by computed tomography scan with contrast or magnetic resonance scanning, as these modalities allow better examination of the areas low in the neck that may be obscured by gross disease on ultrasound (**FIGURE 3**).

SURGICAL MANAGEMENT

- Dissection of the Level 6 lymph nodes is generally performed in conjunction with total thyroidectomy.
- The Level 6 lymph nodes are removed by clearing the soft tissue that surrounds the thyroid gland. No additional incision or mobilization is necessary.
- Clearing these Level 6 nodes involves additional manipulation of the soft tissue and vascular supply that surrounds the parathyroid glands. With these glands at additional risk of being damaged during operation, the performance of parathyroid autograft is particularly important to avoid permanent hypoparathyroidism[2,3] (**FIGURE 4**).

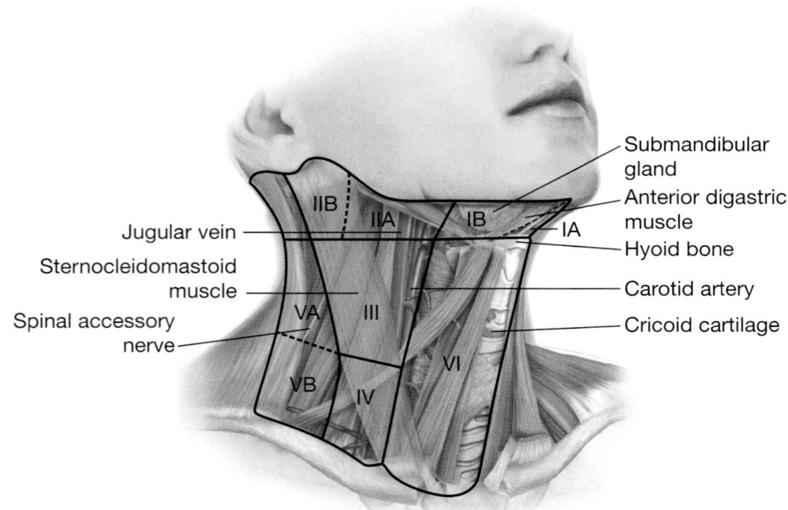

FIGURE 1 • Lymph node levels in the neck.

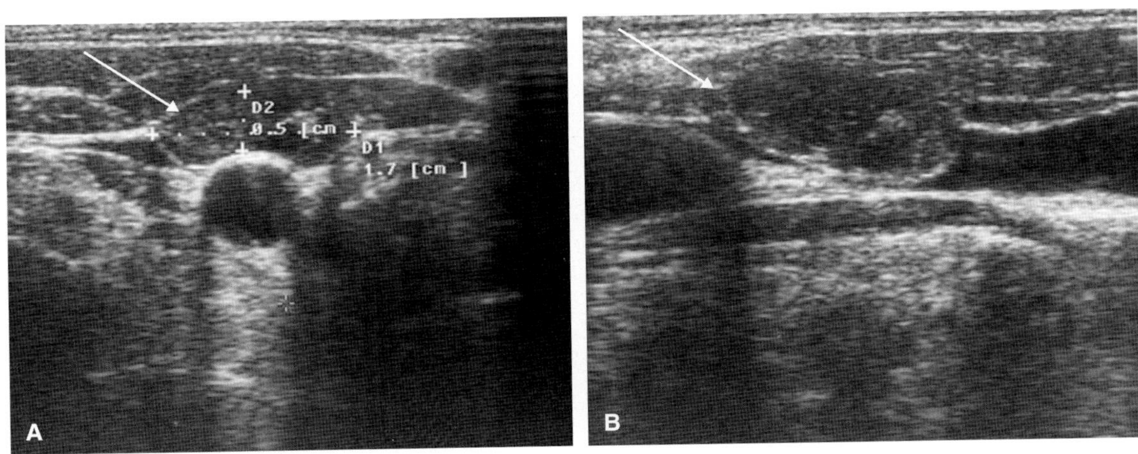

FIGURE 2 ● Ultrasound demonstration of metastatic lymph nodes in thyroid cancer. Panel **(A)** shows a transverse view, and panel **(B)** shows the longitudinal view.

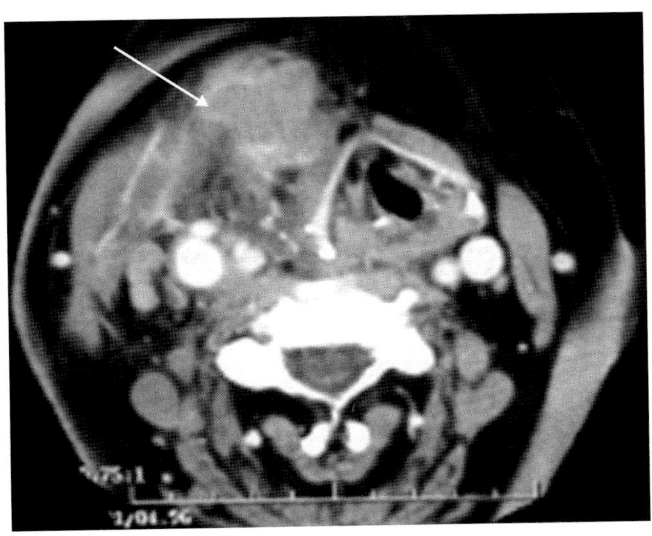

FIGURE 3 ● Computed tomography (CT) scan of recurrent nodal disease in the lateral neck impinging upon the central compartment. CT is useful in this instance as ultrasound cannot completely define the anatomy.

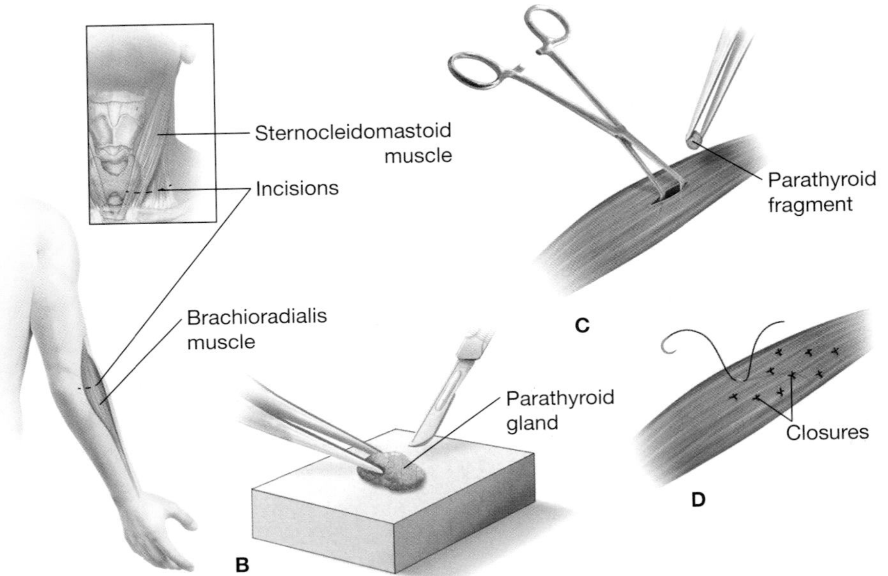

FIGURE 4 ● Schematic of parathyroid autograft. If a parathyroid gland has been devascularized during dissection, then the best management is parathyroid autograft. **A,** Parathyroid glands can be grafted into any muscle; common choices include the neck muscles for normal glands, and the brachioradialis muscle for abnormal glands. **B,** The gland should be minced into small pieces (1-2 mm in each dimension). **C** and **D,** The fragments are placed into individual muscle pockets. The pockets are secured with a stitch. The grafts typical require 10 to 12 before measurable function.

Preoperative Planning

- Review of the preoperative ultrasound findings is critical to the proper inclusion of all suspicious lymph nodes.
- Especially in re-operations, ultrasound in the operating room after the induction of anesthesia and positioning can be helpful to localize small lymph nodes.
- A nerve stimulating and monitoring system can be helpful and is commonly used to identify and to test function of motor nerves during dissection. Testing of the vagus nerve is probably best accomplished by using a specialized nerve stimulator that includes EMG monitoring pads on the endotracheal tube to detect vocalis muscle contraction. Testing of motor nerves for which the enervated muscle is visible can be done with a simple nerve stimulator.

Positioning

- The patient should be supine, and the head may be raised above the heart to decrease venous congestion in the neck (**FIGURE 5**).
- Airway management is of particular concern. Preoperative anesthesiology consultation should alleviate positioning concerns while ensuring proper airway safety during the procedure.
- A towel roll or thyroid air pillow can be placed beneath the shoulder blades to facilitate neck extension.
- Arms should be tucked.

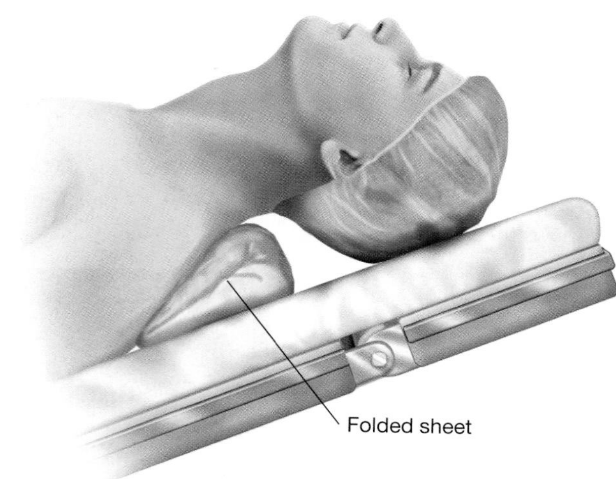

FIGURE 5 ● Position of the neck should emphasize extension, but support. Overextension of the neck or lack of support for the head and neck can cause avoidable posterior neck stiffness postoperatively.

TECHNIQUES

INCISION

- If a thyroidectomy is performed during the same anesthetic, the incision is extended laterally toward the posterior aspect of the neck; if not, then the dissection can generally be completed through a transverse incision at the level of the lower edge of the cricoid cartilage from the edge of the trachea to the anterior border of the trapezius muscle. The goal is to provide exposure of the anterolateral neck and posterior triangles.

RAISING SKIN AND PLATYSMA MUSCLE FLAPS

- Flaps are made superiorly, inferiorly, and posteriorly (**FIGURE 6**). The flaps should be in a plane superficial to the external jugular vein and should extend broadly over the compartments to be dissected. The facial vein can be divided and retracted superiorly. This has some benefit to retract and protect the marginal mandibular branch of the facial nerve. Erb's point can be identified as the area where the greater auricular nerve comes around the posterior edge of the sternocleidomastoid muscle. This site is important to identify in order to protect the superficial sensory nerves that converge at that site.

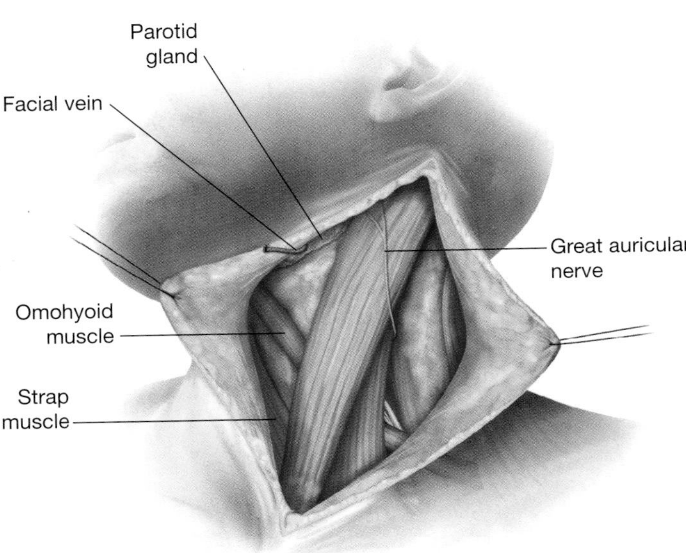

FIGURE 6 ● The subplatysmal flaps should be generous to avoid struggling at the margins of dissection later in the case.

MOBILIZING THE STERNOCLEIDOMASTOID MUSCLE

- The fascia over the middle of the sternocleidomastoid muscle is incised longitudinally with careful preservation of the greater auricular nerve (**FIGURE 7**).
- The fascia is then stripped from the muscle over a broad area, unwrapping the muscle and following the fascial plane around the front edge of the muscle to its deep surface. The plane is continued deep to the muscle back to its posterior edge.
- The sensory nerves at Erb's point (greater auricular, lesser occipital, transverse cervical and supraclavicular) are all preserved.
- The sternocleidomastoid muscle is encircled with a Penrose drain for traction to provide exposure.
- The omohyoid muscle is divided to improve exposure of the underlying nodal packet.

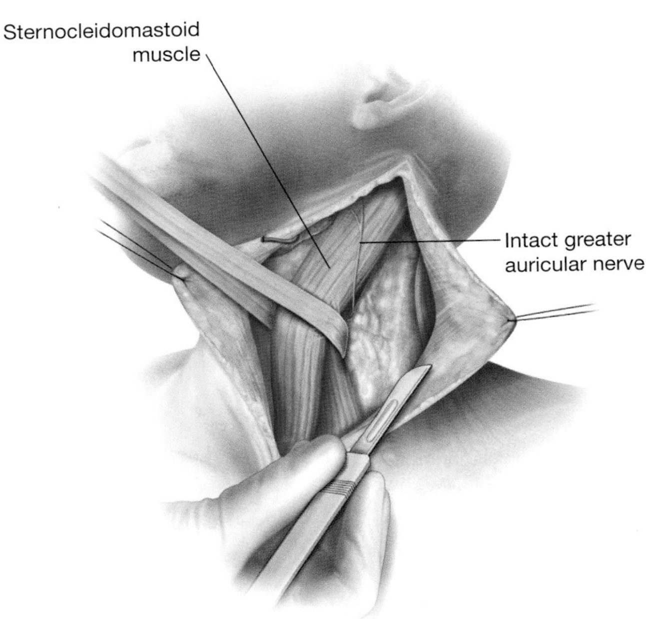

FIGURE 7 ● Once the sternocleidomastoid muscle has been mobilized, the fascia over the node packet can be incised laterally. This will allow separation of the fatty soft tissue from the anterior edge of the trapezius muscle. Great care is needed to identify the spinal accessory nerve without injury.

DISSECTION OF SOFT TISSUE SPECIMEN

- Dissection of the nodal packet can be initiated in a number of places (**FIGURE 8**). The posterior triangle is a common choice. The superficial fascia along the anterior edge of the trapezius muscle is carefully incised along the muscle edge to avoid inadvertent division of the spinal accessory motor nerve.
- The nodal packet attachments to the trapezius are taken down initially with blunt dissection, especially prior to identification of the spinal accessory nerve. Unless there is direct involvement of the nerve by tumor, the nerve should be preserved.
- The specimen is dissected from lateral to medial with attention to the underlying structures.

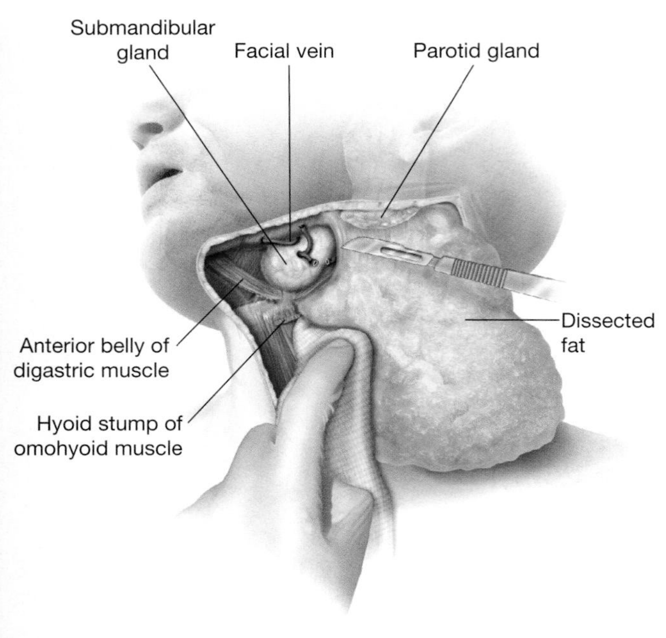

FIGURE 8 ● The dissection progresses with mobilization of the soft tissues away from the jugular vein.

- The supraclavicular sensory nerves fan out from Erb's point and divide the Level 5 specimen into superficial and deep components. Removal of all nodes with preservation of the major branches of these nerves requires recognition of this and careful dissection.
- Once the dissection reaches the area deep to the sternocleidomastoid muscle, the jugular nodes (Levels 2-3-4) are dissected either starting from the top (Level 2) or the bottom (Level 4) of the jugular chain, removing these nodes en bloc with the posterior triangle specimen.
- The jugular vein is generally preserved unless there is involvement of the vein by direct invasion or tumor thrombus. If the vein cannot be preserved, it is included in the specimen. There is no morbidity of including this in a unilateral dissection.
- The specimen is removed en bloc, marked, and prepared for pathologic examination.

INSPECTION AND CLOSURE

- Once the specimen has been removed, the field is **carefully inspected for residual soft tissue** that can be removed (**FIGURE 9**). Nerves are tested for confirmation of function, and hemostasis is ensured. Special inspection at the base of the jugular vein should ensure that there is no evidence of chyle leak.
- A small drain is often placed to remove serum or chyle that could accumulate. If the operation has been straightforward and the disease burden low, then this may be omitted.
- The wound is closed in two layers, the platysma muscle layer with interrupted absorbable suture and the skin by whatever cosmetically advantageous method the surgeon chooses.

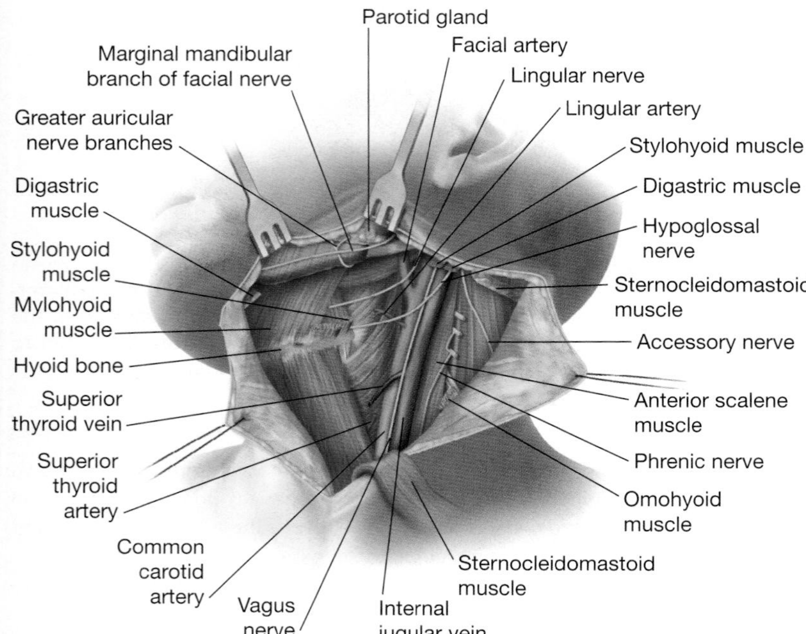

FIGURE 9 ● Anatomy of the neck after the node-bearing soft tissues have been removed.

PEARLS AND PITFALLS

Indications	Prophylactic lateral neck dissection is not generally indicated for thyroid cancer.
Raising of flaps	The flaps plane must be accurately placed deep to platysma and superficial to external jugular vessels.
Mobilizing sternocleido-mastoid muscle	Avoid injury to the sensory nerves at Erb's point.
Dissecting specimen	Identify the spinal accessory nerve early to avoid injury.
Ensuring hemostasis	Small venous branches in the soft tissue deep to the clavicle, at the inferior margin of the dissection, can cause bothersome bleeding.
Avoiding chyle leak	Pay careful attention to clear fluid welling up near the inferior-most visible portion of the jugular vein, on either side, but especially the left.

POSTOPERATIVE CARE

- Drains should be inspected for lymphatic leak, and patients instructed on drain care.
- Drains should be removed once output decreases to 30 mL or less per day.

OUTCOMES

- Functional outcomes are excellent if nerves are preserved.
- A minority of patients requires physical therapy to regain full range of shoulder motion.

COMPLICATIONS

- Nerve injury: spinal accessory nerve; vagus or recurrent laryngeal nerve injury (if central neck dissection is included in the procedure); brachial plexus.
- Vascular injury: internal jugular vein; carotid artery causing neck hematoma, which can progress to airway compromise.
- Thoracic duct injury leading to lymphatic leak, possibly requiring operative intervention for thoracic duct ligation.
- Regional disease recurrence.

REFERENCES

1. Haugen BR, Alexander EK, Bible KC, et al. American thyroid association management guidelines for adult patients with thyroid nodules and differentiated thyroid cancer: the American thyroid association guidelines task force on thyroid nodules and differentiated thyroid cancer. *Thyroid*. 2016;26:1-133.
2. Doherty GM. Complications of thyroid and parathyroid surgery. In: Mulholland MW, Doherty GM, eds. *Complications in Surgery*, 2nd ed. Lippincott Williams & Wilkins; 2011:550-566.
3. Patel KN, Yip L, Lubitz CC, et al. The American association of endocrine surgeons guidelines for the definitive surgical management of thyroid disease in adults. *Ann Surg*. 2020 March;271(3):e21-e93.

Chapter 52 Open Neck Exploration for Primary Hyperparathyroidism

Christopher R. McHenry

DEFINITION

- Primary hyperparathyroidism (HPT) is caused by autonomous overproduction of parathyroid hormone (PTH) by a single or multiple parathyroid glands and is most often characterized by an elevated serum calcium with an elevated or an inappropriately normal, nonsuppressed serum PTH level (normohormonal HPT). There is also a normocalcemic variant of primary HPT, but this is less common.
- An open neck exploration for primary HPT is defined as exposure of an abnormal parathyroid gland or glands using standard operative techniques through a single incision without videoscopic assistance. This includes bilateral neck exploration for patients with multiglandular disease and unilateral focused parathyroidectomy with intraoperative PTH monitoring for a single adenoma localized preoperatively.

DIFFERENTIAL DIAGNOSIS

- Primary HPT and malignancy account for 80% of all causes of hypercalcemia.
- Primary HPT accounts for 50% to 60% of all cases of hypercalcemia diagnosed in an ambulatory setting and approximately 30% of cases diagnosed in a hospital setting.
- There are many less common causes for hypercalcemia (**TABLE 1**).
- In patients with primary HPT, 85% to 90% will have a single adenoma, 5% to 10% hyperplasia, 3% to 4% double adenoma, and less than 1% carcinoma.

Table 1: Causes of Hypercalcemia

Hyperparathyroidism
Primary and tertiary
Malignancy
Osteolytic bone metastases
Tumor production of PTH-related polypeptide:
Squamous cell carcinoma of the lung
Renal cell carcinoma
Bladder cancer
Hematologic malignancies:
Leukemia
Lymphoma
Multiple myeloma
Granulomatous disease
Tuberculosis
Sarcoidosis
Fungal infection
Medications
Calcium
Vitamin A or D intoxication
Lithium
Thiazides
Milk-alkali syndrome
Miscellaneous
Hyperthyroidism
Paget disease
Immobilization
Familial hypocalciuric hypercalcemia

PTH, parathyroid hormone.

PATIENT HISTORY AND PHYSICAL FINDINGS

- Primary HPT occurs in 1 out of every 500 women and 1 out of every 2000 men. It most commonly occurs in women between the ages of 50 and 60 years.
- The incidence of primary HPT increases with age and the prevalence is approximately 1% in postmenopausal women and 0.86% of the general population.[1]
- Most patients with primary HPT are diagnosed as a result of the incidental hypercalcemia detected on blood work that is obtained for an unrelated medical problem. Patients often have nonspecific symptoms such as fatigue, weakness, constipation, and depression.
- Patients with primary HPT may present with plethora of clinical manifestations (**TABLE 2**). Nephrolithiasis is the most common metabolic complication of primary HPT occurring in 15% to 20% of patients; however, only 2% to 5% of patients with kidney stones have primary HPT.

Table 2: Clinical Manifestation of Primary Hyperparathyroidism

Renal
Nephrolithiasis
Nephrocalcinosis
Polyuria
Renal insufficiency
Skeletal
Generalized bone or joint pain
Osteopenia
Osteoporosis
Gout
Pseudogout
Pathologic bone fracture
Osteitis fibrosa cystica
Gastrointestinal
Constipation
Peptic ulcer disease
Pancreatitis
Nausea
Vomiting
Abdominal pain
Psychiatric
Depression
Lethargy
Memory loss
Confusion
Hallucinations
Coma
Neuromuscular
Fatigue
Weakness
Malaise
Cardiovascular
Exacerbation of hypertension
Cardiac calcification
Left ventricular hypertrophy
Shortened QT interval
Conduction abnormalities
Heart block

Table 3: Familial Hyperparathyroidism

A. Familial isolated hyperparathyroidism
B. MEN I
- Primary hyperparathyroidism
- Gastroenteropancreatic neuroendocrine tumors
- Pituitary adenoma
- Adrenocortical and thyroid tumors
- Lipomas
- Meningiomas
- Facial angiofibromas
- Bronchial and thymic neuroendocrine tumors

C. MEN IIA
- Medullary thyroid cancer
- Pheochromocytoma
- Primary hyperparathyroidism
- Lichen planus amyloidosis
- Hirschsprung disease

D. Hyperparathyroidism–jaw tumor syndrome
- Ossifying fibromas of the mandible or maxilla
- Renal cysts, hamartomas, and Wilms tumor
- Uterine adenosarcoma, adenofibroma, leiomyoma, adenomyosis, and endometrial hyperplasia

- Approximately 3% of patients may present with hyperparathyroid crisis manifested by severe hypercalcemia (serum calcium > 14 mg/dL), nausea, vomiting, dehydration, and central nervous system dysfunction including coma.[2]
- Primary HPT is associated with a higher risk of cardiovascular disease and mortality that decreases after parathyroidectomy.[3]
- A prior history of head or neck radiation in childhood, radioiodine treatment, and long-term lithium therapy are associated with a greater prevalence of primary HPT.
- In 5% of patients, primary HPT is an inherited syndrome, underscoring the importance of obtaining a thorough family history. Familial HPT is inherited as an autosomal dominant syndrome with primary HPT occurring as an isolated entity or as part of multiple endocrine neoplasia (MEN) I, MEN IIA, or the HPT–jaw tumor syndrome (**TABLE 3**). Patients with HPT–jaw tumor syndrome have more severe hypercalcemia and a 10% to 15% incidence of parathyroid cancer.
- In most patients with primary HPT, the physical examination is normal. Less than 5% of patients with primary HPT will have a palpable parathyroid tumor. Patients with hyperparathyroid crisis are more likely to have a palpable neck mass.
- A palpable neck mass in patients with primary HPT should raise suspicion for parathyroid cancer or an associated thyroid nodule.
- Rare patients may have band keratopathy, a condition characterized by calcium phosphate deposition in the cornea, which can be identified by slit lamp examination.

IMAGING AND OTHER DIAGNOSTIC STUDIES

- A diagnosis of primary HPT is made by an elevated serum calcium level and an elevated or inappropriately normal, nonsuppressed serum intact PTH level.
- Up to 20% of patients have normocalcemic primary HPT with a serum calcium level in the normal range. Most patients with normocalcemic primary HPT are diagnosed as a result of evaluation for kidney stones, osteoporosis, or osteopenia. Vitamin D deficiency, excess phosphate intake, low calcium set point, and hypo- or hypermagnesemia may be contributory factors to normocalcemic HPT.
- Patients with primary HPT may have low or low normal serum phosphate and high serum chloride, alkaline phosphatase, and uric acid levels. Alkaline phosphatase is elevated in patients with bone disease.
- Patients may also have a mild metabolic acidosis, which occurs because of the inhibitory effect of PTH on phosphorus and bicarbonate reabsorption in the kidney.
- Prior to the introduction of sensitive immunoradiometric and chemiluminescence assays for measurement of intact PTH levels, a chloride to phosphorus ratio greater than 33:1 was used to make the diagnosis of primary HPT.
- Blood urea nitrogen, serum creatinine, and glomerular filtration rate should be measured and followed, because renal insufficiency is a known complication of primary HPT.
- Bone mineral density should be measured at the lumbar spine, hip, and distal radius using dual energy x-ray absorptiometry.
- A calcium:creatinine clearance ratio should be determined if familial hypocalciuric hypercalcemia (FHH) is suspected. FHH is a rare autosomal dominant disorder characterized by asymptomatic hypercalcemia, hypocalciuria, and variable PTH elevation that results from a higher renal set point for calcium secretion. Patients with FHH have one or more first-degree relatives with hypercalcemia, a calcium:creatinine clearance less than 0.01, and a 24-hour urine calcium less than 100 mg. Parathyroidectomy is not indicated.
- Once a diagnosis of primary HPT has been established, imaging should be performed to localize an abnormal parathyroid gland or glands. When an abnormal parathyroid gland can be localized preoperatively, a focused parathyroidectomy can be performed with intraoperative PTH measurement to confirm cure of the primary HPT. This minimizes dissection, shortens the operation, and reduces cost.
- Localization studies should only be performed once a diagnosis of HPT has been established and a decision to proceed with surgical therapy has been made. The role of localization studies is to help determine the site of the incision and where in the neck to begin the exploration.
- Office-based, high-resolution ultrasonography is the initial imaging study performed. A parathyroid adenoma appears as a homogeneous, hypoechoic, oval- or bean-shaped mass posterior to the thyroid gland (**FIGURE 1**). Occasionally, a parathyroid adenoma may be multilobulated. Ultrasound is also of value in identifying concomitant nodular thyroid disease.
- Technetium-99m sestamibi with single-photon emission computed tomography (SPECT) is a combined functional and anatomic imaging study, which is obtained prior to operation. It is particularly beneficial for identifying ectopic parathyroid glands (**FIGURE 2**).
- Four-dimensional computed tomography is another imaging study used to help localize abnormal parathyroid glands. In some institutions, it has become the preferred imaging modality for parathyroid localization. It requires intravenous contrast and its associated with a high radiation dose.
- Recently, positron emission computed tomography using radiolabeled fluorocholine has been shown to have a high

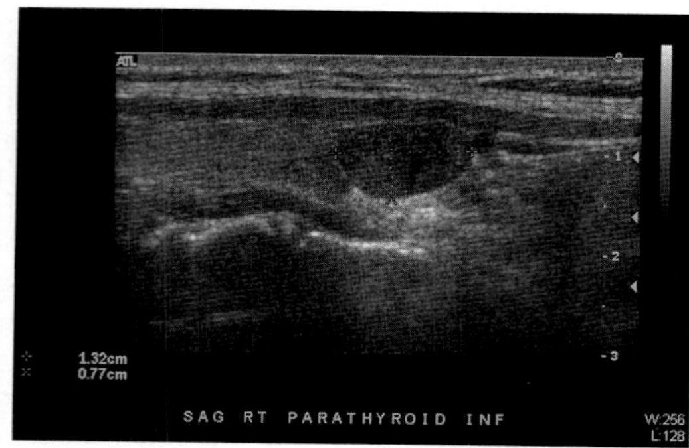

FIGURE 1 ● High-resolution ultrasound image of 1.32 × 0.77 cm homogenous, hypoechoic mass inferior to the right lobe of the thyroid gland in a sagittal view. At operation, this was confirmed to be a right inferior parathyroid adenoma.

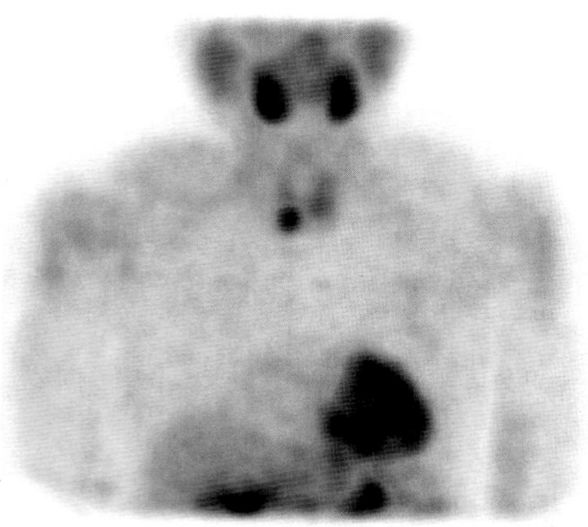

FIGURE 2 ● Technetium-99m sestamibi image demonstrating abnormal radiotracer accumulation inferior to the inferior pole of the right lobe of the thyroid gland.

accuracy for parathyroid localization and is a promising new imaging modality that is currently under investigation by the Food and Drug Administration for use in the United States.

- Intraoperative PTH monitoring is used in combination with image-focused parathyroidectomy in order to try and reduce operative failure rates.

SURGICAL MANAGEMENT

- All patients with primary HPT should be presented with the option of surgical therapy, because parathyroidectomy is the only curative treatment. The classical symptoms of primary HPT (nephrolithiasis, nephrocalcinosis, osteoporosis, osteitis fibrosa cystica, fragility fracture, and neuromuscular dysfunction) are well-established indications for surgery.
- In patients with asymptomatic primary HPT, indications for surgical therapy have been defined by the 2014 revised consensus guidelines sponsored by the National Institutes of Health[4] (**TABLE 4**). Parathyroidectomy is recommended in all patients younger than 50 years of age because at least 25% will develop one or more complications of HPT during their lifetime, which can be irreversible. Significant hypercalcemia (>1 mg/dL above the upper limit of the normal range for serum calcium), impaired renal function (glomerular filtration rate <60 mL/min), reduction in bone mineral density (T score of −2.5 or less at lumbar spine, femoral neck, hip, or distal radius), vertebral compression fracture, hypercalciuria with increased stone risk (24 hour urine calcium >400 mg/dL), and inability or unwillingness to participate in subsequent medical surveillance and follow-up are other indications for parathyroidectomy in patients with asymptomatic primary HPT.

Table 4: Indications for Surgical Therapy in Patients With Asymptomatic Primary Hyperparathyroidism as Established by the 2014 Revised National Institutes of Health Consensus Guidelines

Serum calcium >1 mg/dL above the upper limit of the normal range
Glomerular filtration rate <60 mL/min
Decreased bone density: T score of −2.5 or less at lumbar spine, femoral neck, hip, or distal radius
Age < 50 y
Vertebral compression fracture on spine imaging
24 hour urine calcium > 400 mg/dL
When routine follow-up and medical surveillance is problematic or not possible

- Open neck exploration for primary HPT is performed as an outpatient procedure under general anesthesia or local anesthesia with sedation. Various intraoperative adjuncts may be used including ultrasound, PTH monitoring, radioguidance, and near-infrared fluorescence (NIR).
- Intraoperative ultrasound may be used to help determine the best site for the incision.
- Intraoperative PTH monitoring may be used to help determine that all hyperfunctioning parathyroid tissue has been excised and to confirm cure of primary HPT.
- Administration of technetium-99m sestamibi prior to operation and use of a gamma probe intraoperatively is used by some surgeons to help localize abnormal parathyroid tissue and confirm ex vivo that a sestamibi-avid parathyroid gland has been removed and that no sestamibi-avid glands remain in the neck. Some of the limitations of this technique include that hyperplastic parathyroid glands are most often not sestamibi-avid, and thyroid nodules may also retain sestamibi, producing false-positive results.
- NIR detection is being used intraoperatively to help identify parathyroid adenomas. A variety of imaging devices are available for NIR autofluorescence detection. One NIR autofluorescence system consists of a fiber optic probe connected to a console containing a NIR light source and an interactive display (PTeye, AiBiomed, Santa Barbara, CA). The probe provides visual and auditory feedback when the probe makes contact with a parathyroid gland. A second system consists of a handheld camera that contains a NIR light source to illuminate the tissues and then autofluorescence signals are converted to grayscale images on a display monitor (Fluobeam 800 and Fluobeam LX, Fluoptics, France). Contrast-enhanced NIR fluorescence using indocyanine green (ICG) is also being used as an adjunct for real-time identification of parathyroid glands during parathyroidectomy (**FIGURE 3**). Parathyroid glands are highly vascularized and are surrounded by adipose tissue or thymus, which are not well vascularized. ICG is able to enhance the contrast

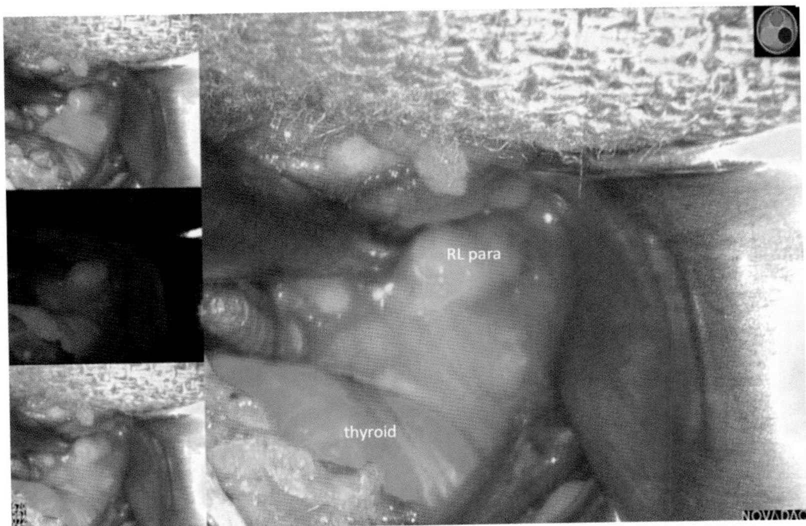

FIGURE 3 ● (*Upper left*) Bright light image of the operating field. (*Middle left*) The operative field in the grayscale fluorescent mode. (*Lower left*) Fluorescent mode with computer-generated overlay where green color saturation is proportional to the intensity of the fluorescent signal. (*Right*) Fluorescent mode with thyroid gland and the right inferior parathyroid gland in the superior cervical thymus. (Figure provided by Eren Berber, MD.)

between the well-vascularized parathyroid gland and the poorly vascularized adipose tissue or thymus.[5,6]

- For a single adenoma localized preoperatively, a unilateral focused parathyroidectomy with intraoperative PTH monitoring to confirm cure of primary HPT is performed.
- Bilateral neck exploration is indicated for patients with negative or discordant preoperative imaging or when bilateral disease is detected preoperatively and for patients with a higher likelihood of multiglandular disease such as patients with MEN I, MEN IIA, or lithium-associated HPT. It may also be necessary for patients with associated thyroid disease. Bilateral neck exploration may also be preferentially used in all patients with primary HPT.
- Patients with a double adenoma are treated with resection of the two enlarged glands.
- Patients with parathyroid hyperplasia are preferentially treated with subtotal parathyroidectomy, leaving a well-vascularized parathyroid remnant that approximates the weight and size of one normal parathyroid gland. A bilateral transcervical thymectomy is also performed because of a 5% to 15% incidence of supernumerary parathyroid glands, which are most commonly found in the thymus. Alternatively, a total parathyroidectomy and parathyroid autotransplantation into the brachioradialis muscle of the nondominant forearm may be performed (see Part 5, Chapter 53).
- Patients with parathyroid cancer are treated with an en bloc resection of the tumor and the surrounding structures that are invaded. This usually involves resection of the lobe of the thyroid gland and the strap muscles.
- Patients with parathyroid cancer usually present with marked elevation in serum calcium and PTH levels and they may have a palpable neck mass. Parathyroid cancer typically has a gray-white appearance and diagnosis is confirmed by the presence of local invasion of surrounding structures, lymph node metastases, or systemic metastases (**FIGURE 4**).

Preoperative Planning

- Serum levels of 25-hydroxy-vitamin D and alkaline phosphatase are measured preoperatively. Patients with low 25-hydroxy-vitamin D and elevated alkaline phosphatase levels are at increased risk for symptomatic postoperative hypocalcemia.
- A sequential compression device is preferably used for prophylaxis against deep vein thrombosis to minimize the risk of postoperative neck hematoma, which may occur with the use of subcutaneous heparin or Lovenox. Routine surgical antimicrobial prophylaxis is unnecessary.
- No special preoperative preparation is required except for patients who present with hyperparathyroid crisis. Hydration with a saline infusion, furosemide to induce calciuresis, bisphosphonate therapy, and/or a calcimimetic agent are used to correct severe life-threatening hypercalcemia before proceeding with parathyroidectomy.[2]

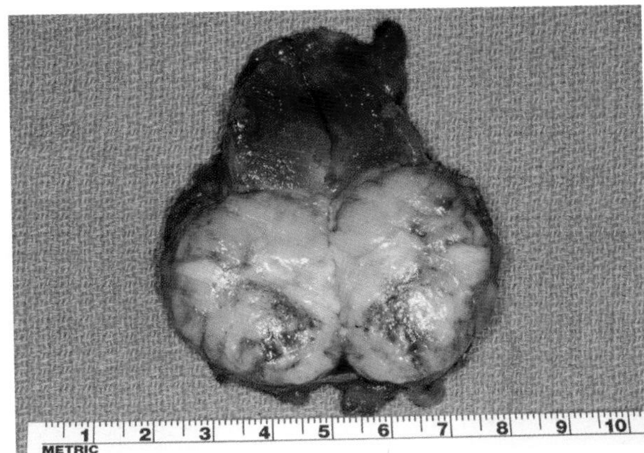

FIGURE 4 ● A parathyroid cancer with its typical gray-white appearance and the lobe of the thyroid gland, which was invaded by the cancer.

POSITIONING

- The patient is positioned on the operating table with a roll placed lengthwise beneath the shoulders, the neck extended, and the head on a soft foam headrest. The patient's arms are tucked at the side (**FIGURE 5**).
- The bed is placed in slight reverse Trendelenburg position to reduce venous pressure. The ventilatory tubing is directed off the back of the operating table to optimize the working space for the surgeon and assistants (**FIGURE 5**).
- The surgical field is widely prepped with ChloraPrep and allowed to dry for 3 minutes before sterile drapes are applied.

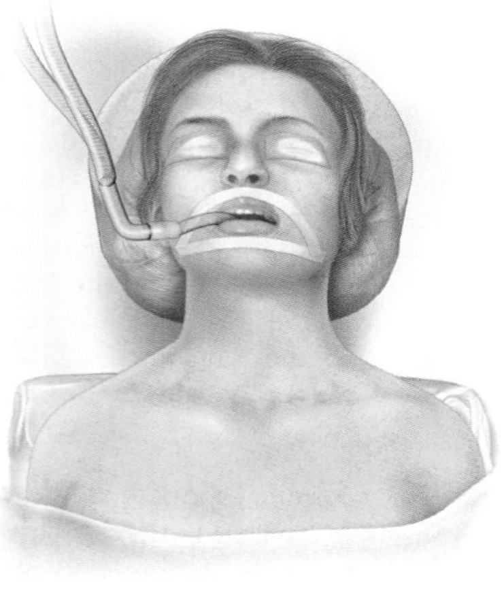

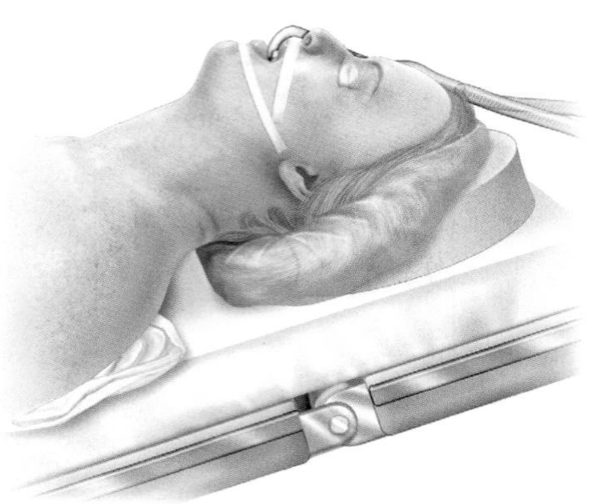

FIGURE 5 ● **(A)** Anteroposterior and **(B)** lateral views of patient who is positioned for parathyroid surgery. The patient's neck is extended with a soft roll placed beneath the shoulder blades and their head positioned on a soft foam pillow. The bed is placed in approximately 30° of reverse Trendelenburg. The ventilator tubing is passed of the head of the bed.

INCISION

- The surface anatomy of the neck is identified before determining the site of the skin incision (**FIGURE 6**). For the best cosmetic result, the site of the skin incision is preferably placed in a normal skin crease. A curvilinear incision is made in the midline of the neck between the cricoid cartilage and the sternal notch.
- The site of the incision is based on preoperative localizing scans, the patient's natural skin creases, and other cosmetic considerations. Intraoperative ultrasound may sometimes be of help to decide the placement of the incision.
- A midline incision is cosmetically preferable and it allows easy access to both sides of the neck for exploration.
- Applying gentle pressure to the neck using a 0 silk suture marks the site of the incision. This is important to maintain symmetry and ensure a curvilinear incision (**FIGURE 6**).
- The midpoint of the incision is marked on the skin using the midpoint of the sternal notch as a landmark.
- A 3- to 5-cm incision in the midline of the neck is used for parathyroidectomy (**FIGURE 6**). Patients with a short, thick neck and/or morbid obesity may require a longer incision to improve exposure.
- 0.5% Bupivacaine is used to anesthetize the site of the incision prior to making the incision to establish preemptive analgesia (**FIGURE 6**). This helps enhance patient comfort postoperatively.
- A no. 15 blade scalpel is used to incise the skin. The electrocautery is used to divide the subcutaneous tissue and the platysma muscle.

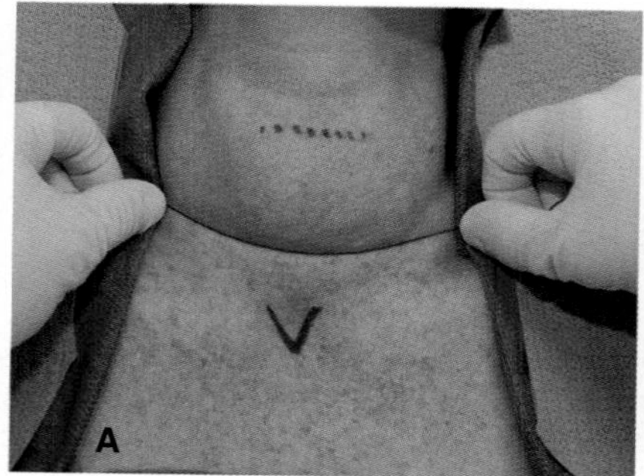

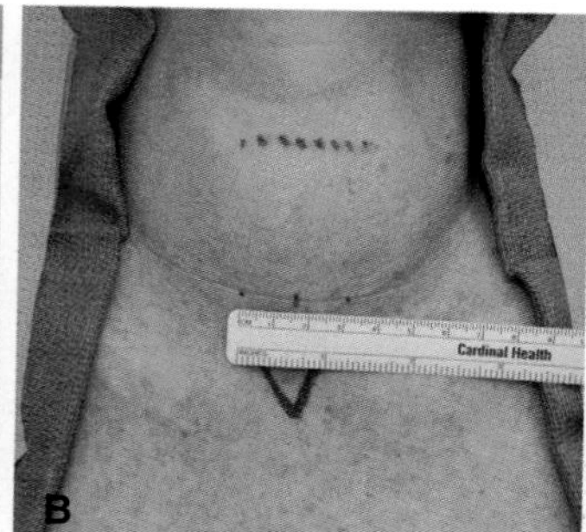

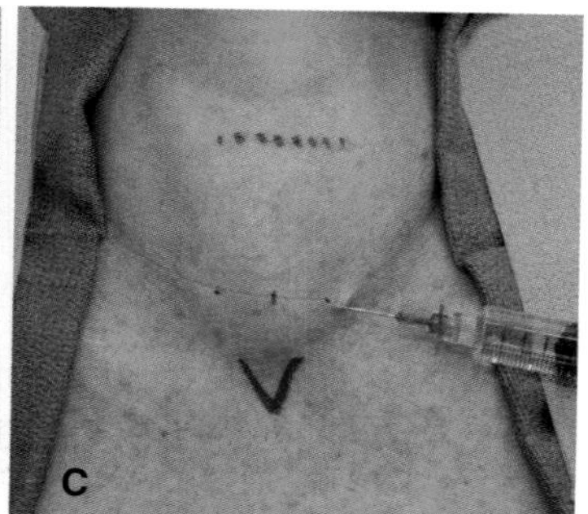

FIGURE 6 ● **A,** The sternal notch and cricoid cartilage are marked to help decide the most appropriate site for the incision. A 0 silk suture is used to mark the site of the incision. **B,** A 3-cm incision is marked in the midline. **C,** 0.5% Marcaine is used to anesthetize the site of the incision prior to making the incision to establish preoperative analgesia.

CREATION OF A WORKING SPACE

- Skin flaps are raised in a subplatysmal plane using skin hooks and small Richardson retractors to elevate the skin (**FIGURE 7**).
- The anterior jugular veins are identified and the plane of dissection is established immediately anterior to the veins (**FIGURE 7**).
- The superior skin flap is raised to the prominence of the thyroid cartilage and the inferior skin flap is raised to the sternal notch.
- The sternal heads of the sternocleidomastoid muscle are exposed laterally.

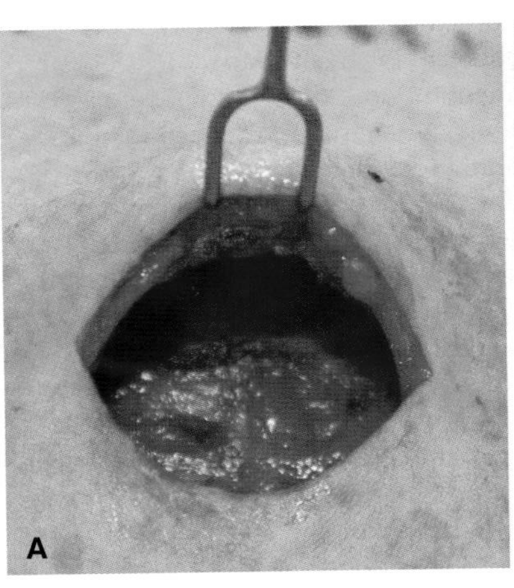

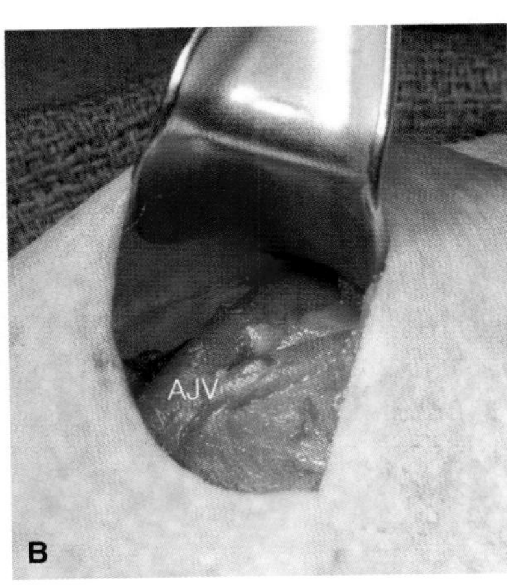

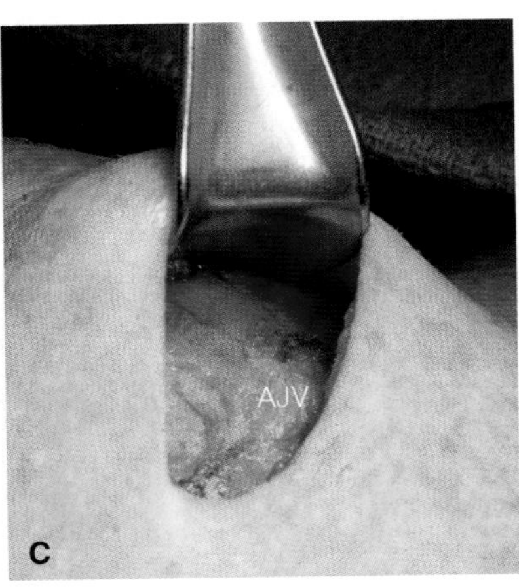

FIGURE 7 ● **A,** Superior skin flaps raised in a subplatysmal plane using the anterior jugular veins (**B** and **C**) to create the plane of dissection.

EXPOSURE OF THE THYROID GLAND

- The sternohyoid muscles are separated in the midline along the median raphe with the electrocautery from the thyroid cartilage superiorly to the sternal notch inferiorly (**FIGURE 8**). The median raphe is an avascular plane consisting of the investing fascia of the thyroid gland.
- Separation of the sternohyoid muscles exposes the thyroid gland.
- The sternothyroid muscle is then dissected and elevated from the surface of the thyroid lobe (**FIGURE 9**). This is accomplished by blunt and sharp dissection of the intervening loose areolar tissue.

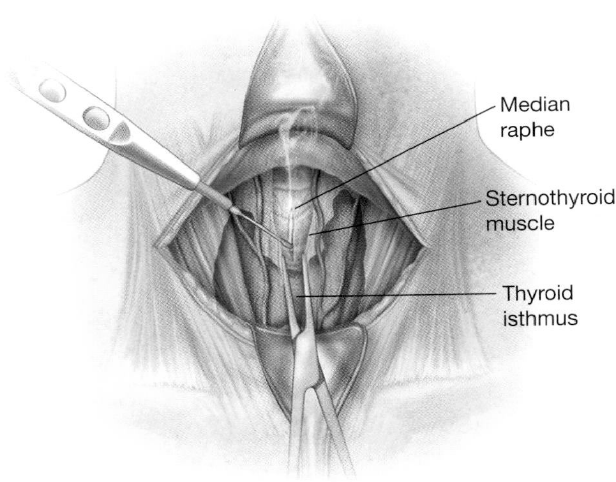

FIGURE 8 ● The sternothyroid muscles are separated along the median raphe to expose the underlying thyroid gland.

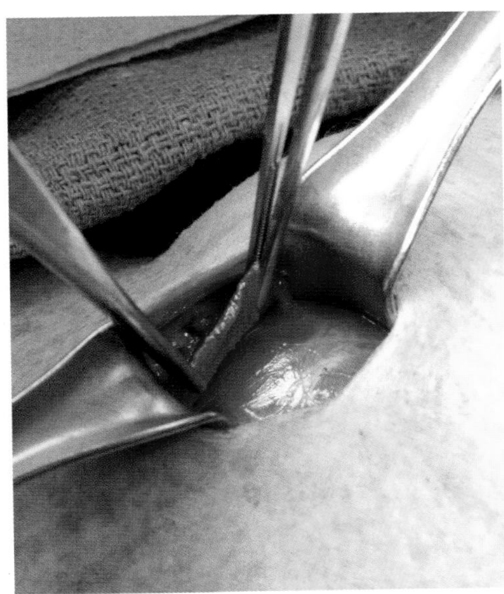

FIGURE 9 ● The sternothyroid muscle is gently retracted with forceps and is freed from the underlying thyroid lobe.

MOBILIZATION OF THE THYROID LOBE AND EXPOSURE OF AN ABNORMAL PARATHYROID GLAND

- The sternothyroid and the sternohyoid muscles are retracted laterally.
- The lobe of the thyroid gland is elevated anteriorly and medially. An Allis clamp applied to the thyroid lobe facilitates retraction and optimizes exposure in a small working space.
- After mobilization of the thyroid lobe anteriorly and medially, some surgeons choose to use NIR fluorescence to help identify a parathyroid adenoma (**FIGURE 3**).
- The middle thyroid vein is identified. It may be divided if necessary for improved exposure.

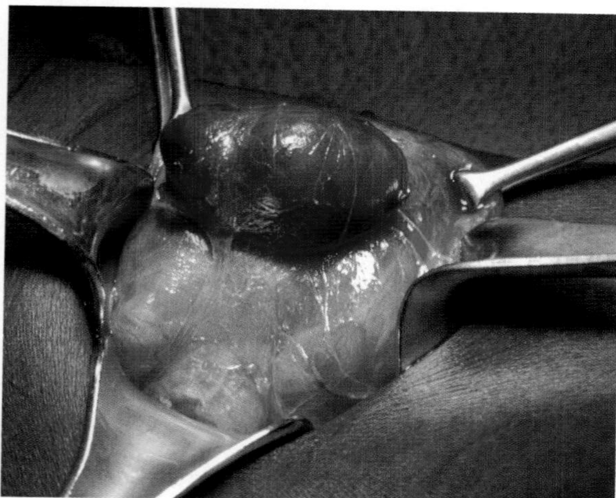

FIGURE 10 ● Anteromedial rotation of the lobe of the thyroid gland to expose a large abnormal parathyroid gland that is firm and dark in color.

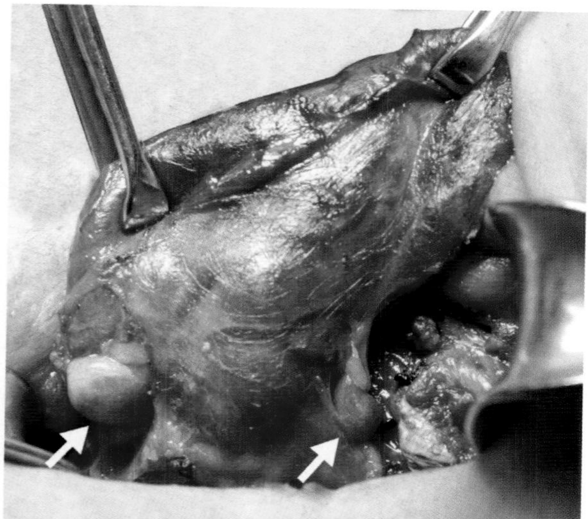

FIGURE 11 ● Two normal parathyroid glands are seen in their normal anatomic position (*arrows*). Both have a typical yellow-tan color and are oval in shape. The superior parathyroid gland is surrounded by the adipose tissue.

- It is important to maintain a bloodless field. Blood staining of the tissues can make it more difficult to identify normal and abnormal parathyroid tissue.
- The initial search for an abnormal parathyroid gland is based on preoperative localization studies. Exploration of the normal anatomic location for a superior or inferior parathyroid gland is completed first.
- Abnormal parathyroid glands are larger, more firm, and darker in color than normal parathyroid glands (**FIGURE 10**).
- In adults, a normal parathyroid gland is yellow-tan in color and oval-, spherical-, or bean-shaped. It is usually 5 mm in maximum dimension and, on average, weighs 35 to 50 mg (**FIGURE 11**). In general, there is no need to biopsy a normal-appearing parathyroid gland.
- The normal location for a superior parathyroid gland is posterior and superior to the recurrent laryngeal nerve. It is approximately 1 cm cephalad to the junction of the inferior thyroid artery and the recurrent laryngeal nerve where the recurrent laryngeal nerve enters the larynx posterior to the inferior pharyngeal constrictor muscle (**FIGURE 12**).
- The normal location for an inferior parathyroid gland is approximately 1 cm caudal to the junction of the inferior thyroid artery and the recurrent laryngeal nerve on the posterior lateral aspect of the inferior pole of the thyroid

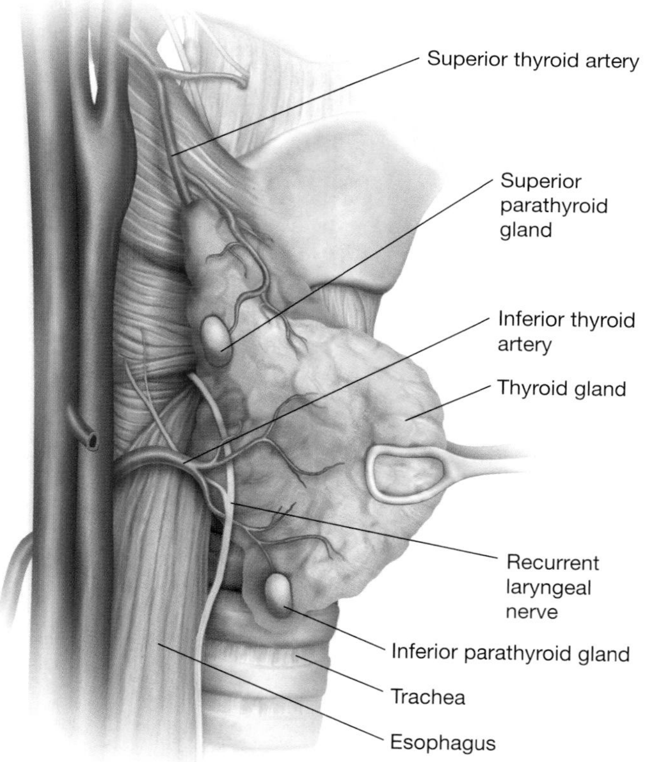

FIGURE 12 ● Anteromedial rotation of the lobe of the thyroid gland to expose the normal superior and inferior parathyroid glands seen with the right lobe of the thyroid gland retracted anteriorly and medially.

lobe. It is usually anterior to the recurrent laryngeal nerve (**FIGURE 12**).

- Approximately 16% of patients with primary HPT will have ectopic parathyroid glands.[7] The inferior parathyroid gland is more likely to be in an ectopic location related to its more extensive embryologic migration.
- When a parathyroid gland is not found in its normal anatomic location, a search for an ectopic gland should be completed.
- The most common location for an ectopic inferior parathyroid gland is in the thymus. Other ectopic locations are the thyrothymic ligament, the anterior superior mediastinum, intrathyroidal, the carotid sheath, and undescended in a submandibular location (see Part 5, Chapters 53 and 56).
- The most common location for an ectopic superior parathyroid gland is the tracheoesophageal groove. Other ectopic locations are retroesophageal, retropharyngeal, posterior mediastinal, and intrathyroidal.
- A transcervical thymectomy is performed to resect an intrathymic parathyroid adenoma. This is accomplished by exposing the cervical tongue of the thymus beneath the sternothyroid muscle. The thymus is anterior to the inferior thyroid veins and is often immediately adjacent to the inferior pole of the thyroid lobe. The recurrent laryngeal nerve is routinely exposed and dissected into the chest to avoid injury. The connective tissue anterior to the thymus is divided. The thymic veins, which drain into the innominate veins, are divided with an electrothermal bipolar vessel-sealing system. Gentle traction is applied to the cervical tongue of the thymus with a right-angle clamp, progressively elevating more and more of the retrosternal thymic tissue into the operative field.

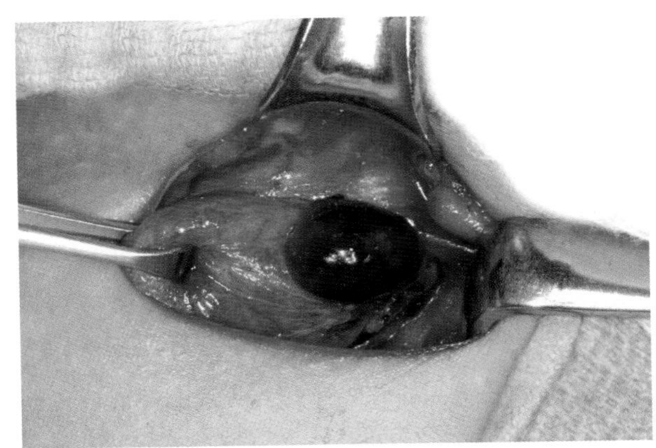

FIGURE 13 ● Enucleation of an intrathyroidal parathyroid adenoma.

- An intrathyroidal parathyroid adenoma (**FIGURE 13**), found in approximately 1% of patients with primary HPT, can usually be enucleated and does not require resection of the lobe of the thyroid gland.
- Division of the superior pole vessels may be helpful when a superior parathyroid gland is not found in its normal anatomic location and it is necessary to search ectopic sites.
- For patients who undergo bilateral neck exploration for multiglandular disease, parathyroid gland location is most often symmetrical.

RESECTION OF AN ABNORMAL PARATHYROID GLAND

- Initially, the enlarged parathyroid gland is dissected anteriorly, laterally, and posteriorly. The medial dissection is left until the end (**FIGURE 14**).
- An enlarged parathyroid gland is gently mobilized by separating it from the surrounding areolar tissue using blunt dissection with a fine curved hemostat until all that remains is the vascular pedicle.

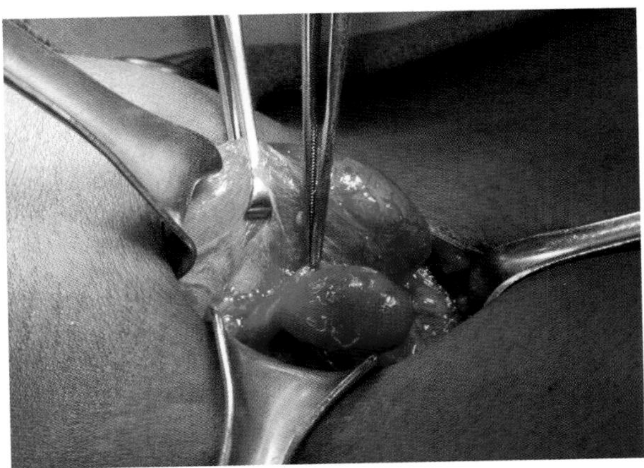

FIGURE 14 ● A large, superior parathyroid adenoma that has been completely mobilized and all that remains is the medial vascular pedicle.

- Care should be taken to avoid violation of the capsule of the abnormal parathyroid gland, which can lead to parathyroid cell deposition into the soft tissue or parathyromatosis, which is a cause for recurrent HPT.
- The surgeon should always be aware of the recurrent laryngeal nerve, but it is not necessary to routinely expose it nor is nerve monitoring necessary during parathyroidectomy. This is left up to surgeon discretion.
- Care should be taken to stay close to the enlarged parathyroid gland when it is being dissected to avoid injury to the recurrent laryngeal nerve.
- Exposure of the recurrent laryngeal nerve is more often necessary when searching for and removing an enlarged superior parathyroid gland. The superior parathyroid gland is usually posterior to the recurrent laryngeal nerve and the nerve may need to be dissected to resect the gland.
- After mobilization of a parathyroid adenoma has been completed and prior to ligating the vascular pedicle, 3 mL of blood is obtained from the internal jugular vein, a peripheral vein, or an arterial line for intraoperative PTH monitoring (**FIGURE 15**). The vascular pedicle is then ligated and divided and the enlarged parathyroid gland is weighed and submitted to pathology for paraffin evaluation. An additional 3 mL of blood is obtained 5 and 10 minutes after resection of an abnormal parathyroid gland for intraoperative PTH measurement.

- A greater than 50% decline in PTH compared to the preexcision or preoperative PTH value is predictive of cure, although a greater than 50% decline compared to the preoperative value and a level that is in the normal range is preferred before deciding that no additional exploration is necessary. Because of some variability in the half-life of intact PTH, which is normally between 3 and 5 minutes, it may be necessary to obtain an additional intact PTH level before making a decision to proceed with additional exploration. Intact PTH levels that fail to decline by more than 50% suggest that there is persistent hyperfunctioning parathyroid tissue.
- Frozen section examination of an excised parathyroid adenoma is unnecessary if intraoperative PTH monitoring is used. Frozen section examination may be of value to distinguish normal or hyperplastic parathyroid tissue from nodal or thyroid tissue. It may also be useful in patients who undergo thyroidectomy for a nodule with an inconclusive fine needle aspiration biopsy or an incidentally discovered thyroid nodule that has not been previously biopsied.

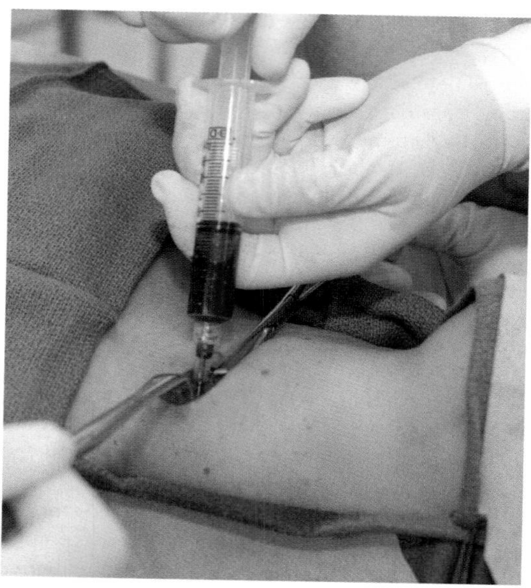

FIGURE 15 ● Blood is obtained from the internal jugular vein for intraoperative parathyroid hormone monitoring. The thyroid lobe is retracted with an Allis clamp. The strap muscles are retracted laterally and the common carotid artery is identified. The internal jugular vein is anterior and lateral to the common carotid artery.

SURGICAL SITE CLOSURE

- The surgical site is closed while awaiting the results of the intraoperative PTH measurements, which have a minimum 20-minute turnaround time. The wound is examined for hemostasis. Venipuncture sites in the internal jugular vein close with some brief packing with a sponge gauze.
- The sternohyoid muscles are reapproximated in the midline with a running absorbable suture, leaving a 3-cm opening at the inferior aspect of the incision (**FIGURE 16**). This is done to prevent blood from collecting in an enclosed space if bleeding should occur postoperatively. It allows the blood to drain into the subcutaneous space, delaying the onset of respiratory compromise, which occurs from impairment of the venous return from the larynx and laryngeal edema.
- The subcutaneous tissue is reapproximated with absorbable suture. The skin is closed with absorbable suture placed in a subcuticular fashion and Mastisol and Steri-Strips or alternatively Dermabond is applied (**FIGURE 17**).

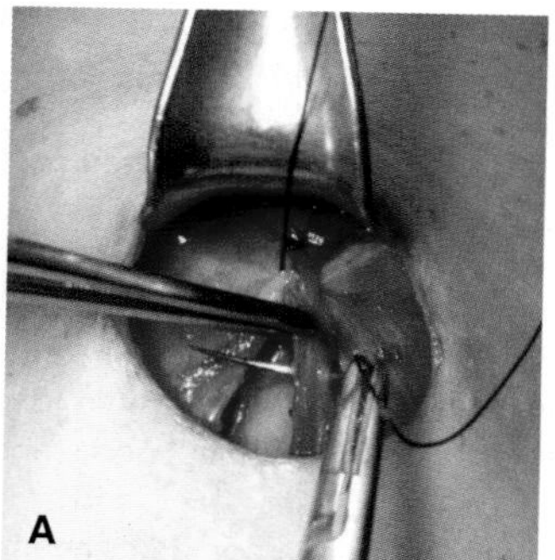

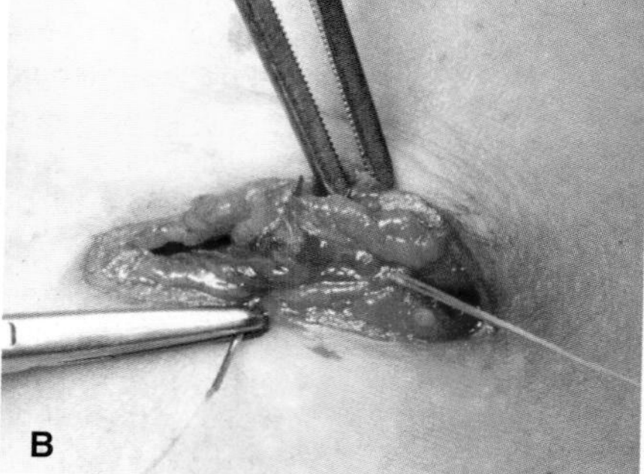

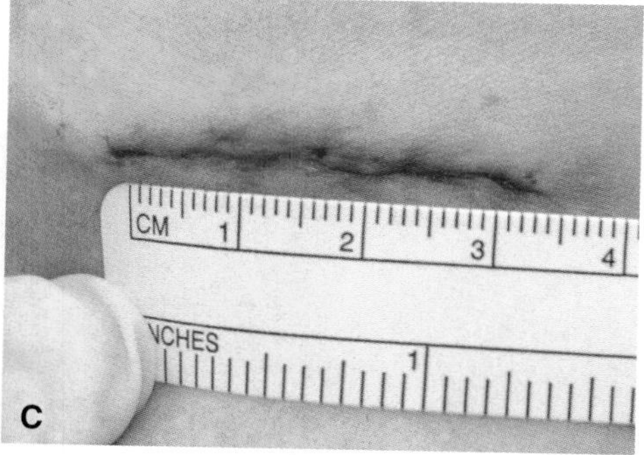

FIGURE 16 ● **A,** The sternohyoid muscles are reapproximated in the midline with a running absorbable suture. **B,** The subcutaneous tissue is reapproximated in the midline with interrupted absorbable suture. **C,** The skin is closed with an absorbable suture placed in a subcuticular fashion.

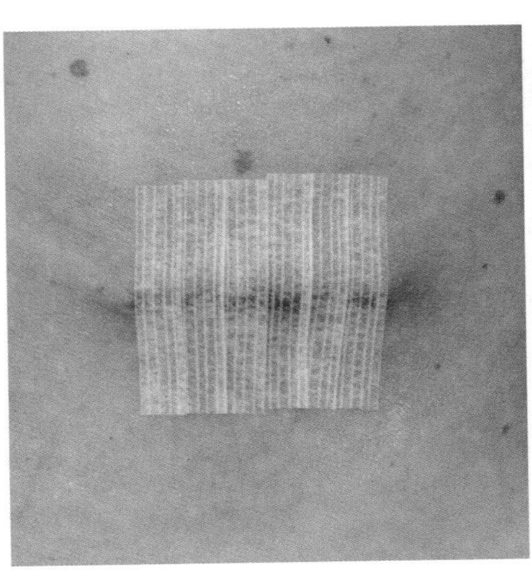

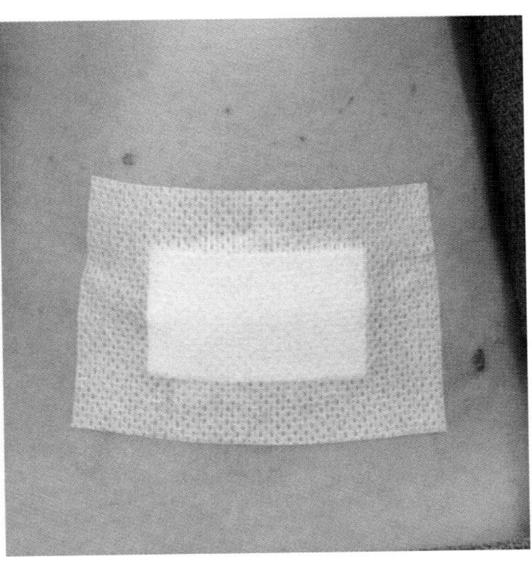

FIGURE 17 ● Mastisol, Steri-Strips, and a dressing are applied. Alternatively, Dermabond may be used.

PEARLS AND PITFALLS

Incision	■ For the best cosmetic result, the skin incision is made within a normal skin crease. Mark the site of the incision with a 0 silk suture to ensure that the incision is curvilinear and symmetric.
Raising skin flaps	■ Use the anterior jugular veins to help develop the skin flaps. For the most part, the plane just anterior to the veins is avascular.
Mobilization of the thyroid lobe	■ Use an Allis clamp to apply traction and elevate the thyroid lobe anteromedially. This will allow you to optimize exposure and use a smaller incision.
Parathyroid dissection	■ An enlarged parathyroid gland is surrounded by areolar tissue anteriorly, laterally, and posteriorly. The vascular pedicle is medial in location. The gland is mobilized primarily by blunt dissection, staying close to the gland to avoid the recurrent laryngeal nerve. The vascular pedicle is ligated last. The capsule of the parathyroid gland should not be violated. This can lead to parathyroid cell implantation in the soft tissues (parathyromatosis) and recurrent HPT.
Ectopic parathyroid glands	■ A gland that is described as inferior on a localizing scan may actually be a superior gland that has descended posteriorly from its normal anatomic location. The most common location for a supernumerary or an ectopic inferior parathyroid gland is in the thymus and is resected by performing a transcervical thymectomy. The most common location for an ectopic superior parathyroid gland is in the tracheoesophageal groove. An intrathyroidal parathyroid adenoma can usually be enucleated and normally does not require thyroid lobectomy.
Multiglandular disease	■ Parathyroid glands are most often symmetrical in location.

POSTOPERATIVE CARE

- Patients are discharged home after routine recovery in the post anesthesia care unit. They are instructed to keep their dressing on for 48 hours and keep the Steri-Strips on until they return for their first follow-up visit in 2 weeks.
- Patients are instructed about the potential for neck hematoma and symptoms of hypocalcemia. They are told to come directly to the emergency department if they experience neck swelling that is out of the ordinary or they have difficulty breathing. They are asked to call if they develop symptoms of hypocalcemia and are told to begin oral calcium 500 to 1000 mg three times daily.
- A serum calcium level is obtained at their first follow-up visit and in 6 months to confirm curative parathyroidectomy. Patients are followed yearly thereafter with a serum calcium level to assess for recurrent disease.

OUTCOMES

- The cure rate for primary HPT with parathyroidectomy performed by an experienced surgeon is 95% to 99%.
- Parathyroidectomy for primary HPT results in improvement in health quality-of-life measures including energy level, muscle strength, fine motor skills, and neurocognitive deficits.[8-10]

- Parathyroidectomy for primary HPT results in improvement of bone density.[11]
- After parathyroidectomy, there is complete resolution of the skeletal abnormalities associated with osteitis fibrosa cystica and the reduced concentrating ability of the renal tubules. In 90% of patients, kidney stone formation resolves.
- Although renal insufficiency and nephrocalcinosis do not resolve, parathyroidectomy may halt progressive decline in renal dysfunction. It may also help prevent progression of hypertension, although hypertension is unlikely to remit.
- The increased cardiovascular mortality associated with primary HPT is reversed with parathyroidectomy.[3]
- Recurrent HPT, defined as hypercalcemia with an elevated or inappropriately normal, nonsuppressed serum PTH level that develops after greater than 6 months of normocalcemia, following curative parathyroidectomy, occurs in 1% to 3% of patients.
- Approximately 25% of patients have postparathyroidectomy secondary HPT manifested by a normal serum calcium level with an elevated serum PTH level following curative parathyroidectomy. The pathogenesis is not completely understood. Low vitamin D levels, impaired kidney function, and bone remineralization have been suggested as contributory factors. This entity is important to recognize because it can be confused with recurrent disease, but it is rarely of clinical significance.

COMPLICATIONS

- The potential complications from parathyroidectomy include bleeding with neck hematoma that can lead to acute respiratory compromise, hypocalcemia, permanent hypoparathyroidism, recurrent laryngeal nerve injury, transient thyrotoxicosis, and persistent HPT.
- Recurrent laryngeal nerve injury and significant bleeding and neck hematoma are rare following parathyroidectomy, occurring in less than 1% of patients. They occur less often than in patients who undergo thyroidectomy because there is less tissue dissection—most of which is blunt—and no major vessels are ligated and divided.
- Symptomatic hypocalcemia is uncommon after resection of a single adenoma. Patients with elevated preoperative alkaline phosphatase levels are at higher risk for symptomatic hypocalcemia from "bone hunger" following parathyroidectomy. Patients who undergo subtotal or total parathyroidectomy are at higher risk for developing symptomatic postparathyroidectomy hypocalcemia and permanent hypoparathyroidism.
- Permanent hypoparathyroidism may occur in patients following subtotal parathyroidectomy when the remnant fails and total parathyroidectomy when the autotransplant fails.
- Persistent HPT may occur as a result of an ectopic adenoma, a supernumerary parathyroid gland, unrecognized multiglandular disease in patients with false-positive intraoperative PTH results (>50% decline), and an adenoma in a normal anatomic position unrecognized as a result of surgeon inexperience.
- Transient thyrotoxicosis may occur in one-third of patients following parathyroidectomy. It is thought to be the result of thyroid gland manipulation and it is self-limited. Beta-blocker therapy may be used for patients who are symptomatic.
- Recurrent HPT occurs in 1% to 3% of patients and should raise concern for MEN I or MEN IIA.

REFERENCES

1. Wilhelm SM, Wang TS, Ruan DT, et al. The American Association of Endocrine Surgeons guidelines for definitive management of primary hyperparathyroidism. *JAMA Surg*. 2016;151:959-968.
2. Phitayakorn R, McHenry CR. Hyperparathyroid crisis: the use of bisphosphonates as a bridge to parathyroidectomy – a case series and review of the literature. *J Amer Coll Surg*. 2008;206:1106-1115.
3. Nilsson IL, Yin L, Lundgren E, et al. Clinical presentation of primary hyperparathyroidism in Europe: nationwide cohort analysis on mortality from nonmalignant causes. *J Bone Miner Res*. 2002;17(suppl 2):N68-N74.
4. Bilezikian JP, Brandi ML, Eastell R, et al. Guidelines for the management of asymptomatic primary hyperparathyroidism: summary statement from the fourth international workshop. *J Clin Endocrinol Metab*. 2014;99:3561-3569.
5. Solorzano CC, Giju T, Berber E, et al. Current state of intraoperative use of near infrared fluorescence for parathyroid identification and preservation. *Surgery*. 2021;169:868-878.
6. DeLong JC, Ward EP, Lwin TM, et al. Indocyanine green fluorescence-guided parathyroidectomy for primary hyperparathyroidism. *Surgery*. 2018;163:388-392.
7. Phitayakorn R, McHenry CR. Incidence and location of ectopic abnormal parathyroid tissue. *Am J Surg*. 2006;191:418-423.
8. Pasieka JL, Parsons LL. Prospective surgical outcome study of relief of symptoms following surgery in patients with primary hyperparathyroidism. *World J Surg*. 1998;22:513-519.
9. Roman SA, Sosa JA, Mayes L, et al. Parathyroidectomy improves neurocognitive deficits in patients with primary hyperparathyroidism. *Surgery*. 2005;138:1121-1128; discussion 1128-1129.
10. Edwards ME, Rotramel A, Beyer T, et al. Improvement in the health-related quality-of-life symptoms of hyperparathyroidism is durable on long-term follow up. *Surgery*. 2006;140:655-663.
11. Rubin MR, Bilezikian JP, McMahon DJ, et al. The natural history of primary hyperparathyroidism with or without parathyroid surgery after 15 years. *J Clin Endocrinol Metab*. 2008;93(9):3462-3470.

Chapter 53

Subtotal Parathyroidectomy or Total With Autologous Graft

Rolfy A. Perez Holguin and Brian D. Saunders

DEFINITION

- Parathyroidectomy is a functional surgical procedure performed to remove all or nearly all of a patient's hyperactive parathyroid tissue.
- Primary hyperparathyroidism is the most common pathologic entity requiring parathyroidectomy. Although roughly 80% of primary hyperparathyroidism involves a single overactive parathyroid gland, there are somatic, as well as inherited, conditions that result in multiglandular parathyroid pathology.[1] Furthermore, secondary and occasionally tertiary hyperparathyroidism may require surgical resection of more than one parathyroid gland.
- Subtotal parathyroidectomy is the removal of all but a small portion of one parathyroid gland from the neck. This usually equates to removing three and a half parathyroid glands. The remnant portion of parathyroid tissue is left on its native blood supply and in its normal anatomic position. An alternative to a subtotal resection of parathyroid tissue is a total or complete removal of parathyroid tissue (eg, all four glands) and the immediate transplantation of autologous parathyroid tissue into a heterotopic position.

DIFFERENTIAL DIAGNOSIS

- The necessity for a multiglandular resection of parathyroid tissue may be recognized preoperatively or intraoperatively. There are a number of etiologies for hyperparathyroidism that are always multiglandular in nature and, as such, would warrant preoperative planning for either a subtotal parathyroidectomy or a total parathyroidectomy with parathyroid autotransplantation. These include multiple endocrine neoplasia (MEN) type I– and type IIa–related primary hyperparathyroidism and secondary hyperparathyroidism related to renal failure. Other pathophysiologic conditions leading to hyperparathyroidism may involve the overactivity of more than one gland. Intraoperative recognition of multiple enlarged glands, or recognition through intraoperative parathormone monitoring data, may lead the surgeon to subtotally resect the parathyroids or perform a total parathyroidectomy with immediate transplant. These include sporadic primary hyperparathyroidism due to multiglandular hyperplasia, lithium-related primary hyperparathyroidism, tertiary hyperparathyroidism, and CDC73-related causes of hyperparathyroidism.[2] This latter category is a familial hyperparathyroidism caused by germline mutations in the CDC73 gene (also known as HRPT2 or parafibromin) and includes familial, isolated hyperparathyroidism and hyperparathyroidism–jaw tumor syndrome.[3]

PATIENT HISTORY AND PHYSICAL FINDINGS

- Hyperparathyroidism is a biochemical diagnosis. The evaluation of a patient for hyperparathyroidism may begin with an incidental note of an elevated calcium level on a laboratory report or with interrogating a patient's calcium level based on the patient's presenting signs or symptoms. Patients with recurrent nephrolithiasis (especially calcium-based kidney stones) or osteoporotic (eg, fragility or nontraumatic) bone fractures should be evaluated for hypercalcemia and hyperparathyroidism. Other, less specific, symptoms that may warrant a biochemical investigation for hyperparathyroidism include fatigue; sleep disturbances; musculoskeletal aches and pains; neurocognitive decline; mood lability; abdominal pain; and recurrent, otherwise unexplained, pancreatitis.
- A detailed family history should be sought to evaluate the possibility of an inherited cause of hyperparathyroidism. The patient should be queried about family members with pituitary tumors, other cases of parathyroid disease, medullary thyroid cancer, pheochromocytomas, enteropancreatic neuroendocrine tumors (especially gastrin-producing tumors), and ossifying fibromas of the mandible.
- Patients with suspected inherited causes of hyperparathyroidism should be counseled to seek genetic counseling and testing as this may impact operative planning, future disease surveillance, and the health of relatives.
- Renal-related secondary hyperparathyroidism is a constant and expected biochemical finding in all patients with chronic kidney dysfunction. The degree of hyperparathormonemia is routinely followed by treating nephrologists, especially in patients who have progressed to some form of renal replacement therapy (peritoneal or hemodialysis). National management guidelines exist for the target parathyroid hormone (PTH) level for each stage of chronic kidney disease.[4]
- Physical examination findings for patients with hyperparathyroidism are uncommon. Certainly, the neck of each patient proposed for a parathyroidectomy should be thoroughly examined. The identification of a palpable mass would warrant further imaging investigation. It is distinctly unusual to palpate a parathyroid adenoma. A palpable mass with severe hyperparathyroidism should raise the specter of the unusual entity of parathyroid carcinoma. Often, though, a palpable central neck mass in a patient with hyperparathyroidism is an incidentally discovered thyroid nodule.
- For patients who planned to undergo a total parathyroidectomy with immediate autologous parathyroid transplantation, a detailed inspection of the forearms should be undertaken. It is important to note the handedness of the patient, as the parathyroid autograft is usually placed in the nondominant forearm. In patients with preexisting or impending renal failure, note should be made of arteriovenous fistula position. Great care should be taken to avoid injuring a functional fistula or disturbing the bed of a soon-to-be constructed fistula.

IMAGING AND OTHER DIAGNOSTIC STUDIES

- Hyperparathyroidism (whether primary, secondary, or tertiary) is a biochemical diagnosis. This must be made to the satisfaction of the surgeon prior to contemplating any

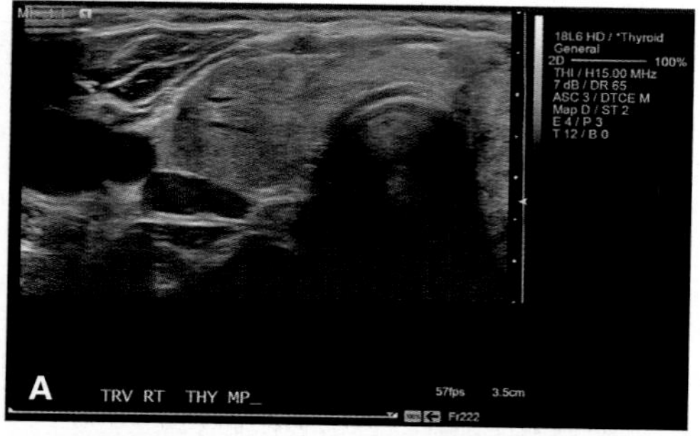

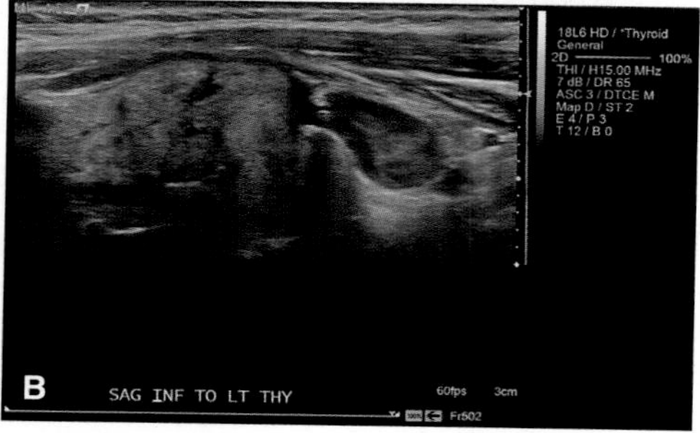

FIGURE 1 ● High-resolution cervical ultrasound demonstrating clear parathyroid adenomata. **A,** Right thyroid lobe with a hypoechoic right upper parathyroid adenoma in the tracheoesophageal groove. **B,** Sagittal ultrasound view of the left thyroid lobe with a hypoechoic left inferior parathyroid adenoma.

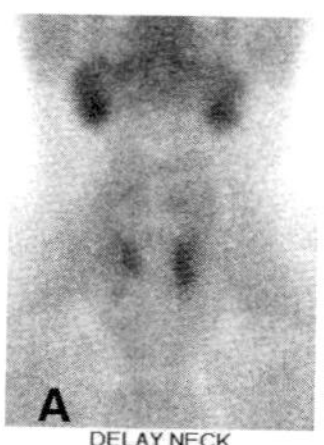

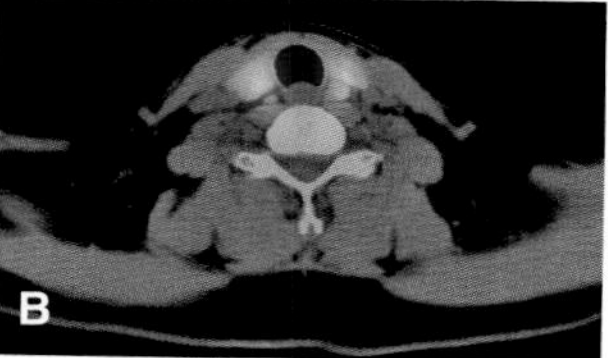

FIGURE 2 ● Nuclear medicine parathyroid scan. **A,** A 2-hour delayed planar view showing bilateral parathyroid adenomata. **B,** Fused sestamibi-SPECT/CT scan showing bilateral sestamibi-avid parathyroid lesions posterior to each lobe of the thyroid gland.

procedure. The surgeon should consider imaging studies only after a diagnosis has been secured and the need for an operation has been established.

- Known multiglandular parathyroid disease processes that will require preoperative planning for a subtotal parathyroidectomy or a total parathyroidectomy with autologous graft do not require parathyroid imaging as both sides of the neck will need to be explored and all four of the parathyroid glands identified.
- High-resolution ultrasonography of the neck (whether performed by the surgeon or a radiologist) is an excellent modality to attempt to localize enlarged parathyroid glands. Parathyroid adenomas appear as hypoechoic, ovoid masses that are separable from the thyroid gland. Upper parathyroid adenomas that lie in the tracheoesophageal groove will often be mobile with graded compression of the ultrasound probe (**FIGURE 1A** and **B**). Parathyroid adenomas adjacent to the thyroid can usually be well seen, although ectopic parathyroid adenomas (eg, posterior to the clavicular heads) may be difficult to visualize due to limitations of the ultrasound waves in traveling through bone. Ultrasonography will also aid in the identification of concurrent thyroid pathology, which may then be dealt with at the time of the parathyroid operation.
- Nuclear medicine parathyroid scans using technetium sestamibi as a tracer can accurately identify overactive parathyroid glands about 85% of the time, in patients with single-gland disease.[5] When performed with a concurrent single-photon emission computed tomography (SPECT)/computed tomography (CT) scan, this overlay of functional and structural imaging provides an excellent anatomic map of disease localization invaluable to the operating surgeon (**FIGURE 2A** and **B**). One caveat is that small parathyroid adenomas in close association with the thyroid gland may be difficult to visualize with this imaging technique.
- Neck CT scan or magnetic resonance imaging (MRI) is occasionally used to image parathyroid glands. CT scan imaging protocols are becoming more widespread, such as 4D CT scans; the phases commonly used are noncontrast, contrast enhanced, arterial, and venous delayed. This takes advantage of the timing of the intravenous (IV) contrast bolus, the vascularity of the parathyroid tumors, and the delayed washout of hyperactive parathyroid lesions. 4D CT scans can identify single-gland disease in over 90% of cases.[6]
- More invasive modalities of parathyroid localization include selective venous sampling for PTH measurement. This technique requires experienced interventional radiologists and is best reserved for the reoperative setting.
- Imaging prior to reoperative parathyroid surgery is essential to minimize exploration in a scarred operative field and to minimize iatrogenic morbidity. It is ideal to have two concordant imaging studies prior to all reoperative parathyroid surgery (see Part 5, Chapter 56).

SURGICAL MANAGEMENT

Preoperative Planning

- Prior to any parathyroid operation, all diagnostic biochemical data should be reviewed to conform to the surgeon's satisfaction that a diagnosis of surgically correctable hyperparathyroidism is present in the patient.
- If an autologous parathyroid transplant is planned, confirmation with the patient as to which upper extremity will be the recipient site should be sought.
- The wound classification for parathyroid surgery is clean. It is rare for parenteral antibiotics to be indicated prior to parathyroid surgery. Individual patient characteristics (eg, cardiac valvular lesions, implanted prosthetic hardware), however, should always be considered.
- Local or general anesthesia may be used.

Positioning

- The patient is positioned supine on the operating room (OR) table with the arms tucked either at the sides or lying on the abdomen. A sheet, fastened with towel clips, is used to secure the arms next to the patient and to allow for removal of the arm boards from the OR table (**FIGURE 3**).
- If a parathyroid transplant is planned to the patient's forearm, this arm can be extended from the patient and reprepped and draped at the time of that portion of the procedure (after the parathyroid tissue has been removed from the neck).
- A towel roll or other small bump is placed behind the patient's shoulder to aid in extension of the neck.
- The bed is positioned with the head up, the feet down, and in some slight Trendelenburg. This is known as the semi-Fowler position or the beach chair position.
- Some surgeons will rotate the OR table 90° to have the head of the patient away from the anesthesia providers and thus more accessible to the surgical team.

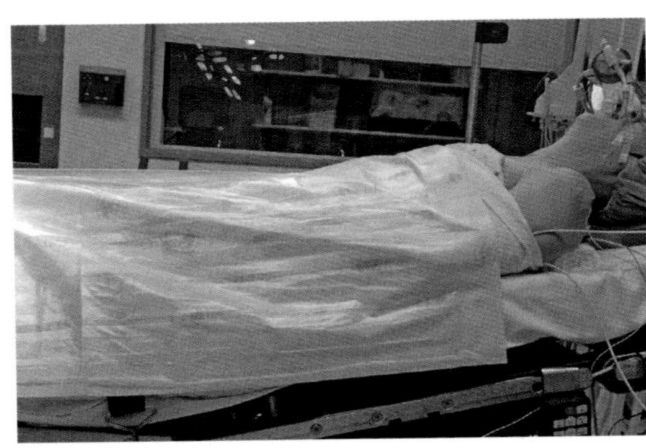

FIGURE 3 ● The patient is positioned on the OR table with the arms tucked, a roll behind the shoulders, and the head elevated.

TECHNIQUES

PLACEMENT OF INCISION

- A transverse incision is made in the line of a skin crease roughly 1 cm caudal to the cricoid cartilage or two finger-breadths cephalad to the suprasternal notch. The incision may be between 3 and 5 cm in length and is centered on the midline of the neck (**FIGURE 4**). Some surgeons will infiltrate the region of the incision with a local anesthetic combined with epinephrine. Placement of the incision within a natural skin line or crease of the neck is more important for postoperative cosmesis than the length of the incision (**FIGURE 5**).

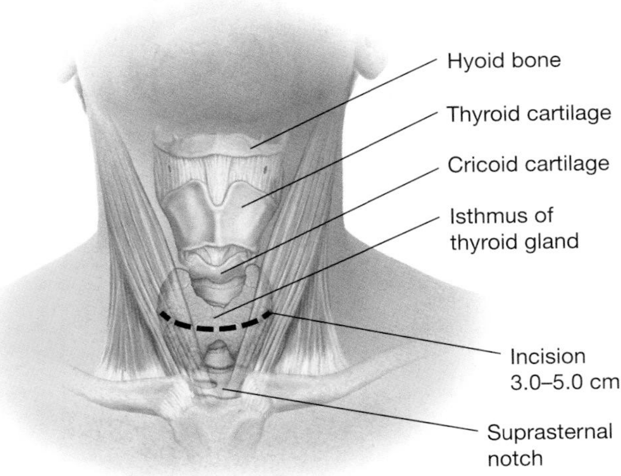

FIGURE 4 ● Surface anatomy and relationships for parathyroid incision placement.

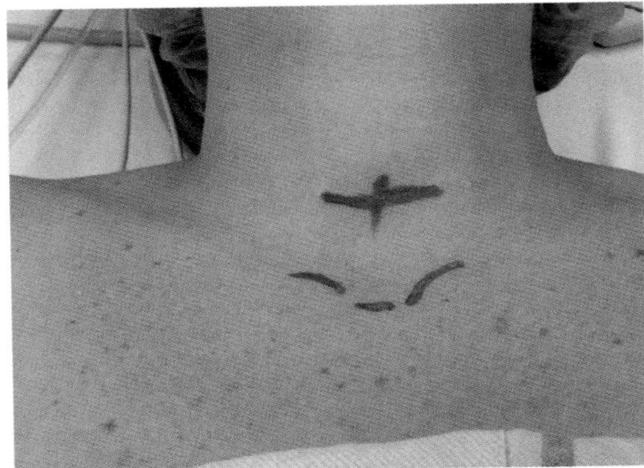

FIGURE 5 ● Diagram of planned parathyroidectomy incision, with clavicular heads and sternal notch marked for reference.

CREATION OF FLAPS

- Dissection is deepened through the subcutaneous tissues and through the platysma muscle with electrocautery. Subplatysmal flaps are created superiorly, inferiorly, and laterally with a combination of electrocautery and blunt dissection (**FIGURE 6**).
- Care must be taken to avoid injury to the paired anterior jugular veins. Should a rent be made in one of these veins, it is best to ligate the vein rather than attempt to cauterize the vein.
- The superior flap should extend to the level of the thyroid cartilage and the inferior flap down to the sternal notch.

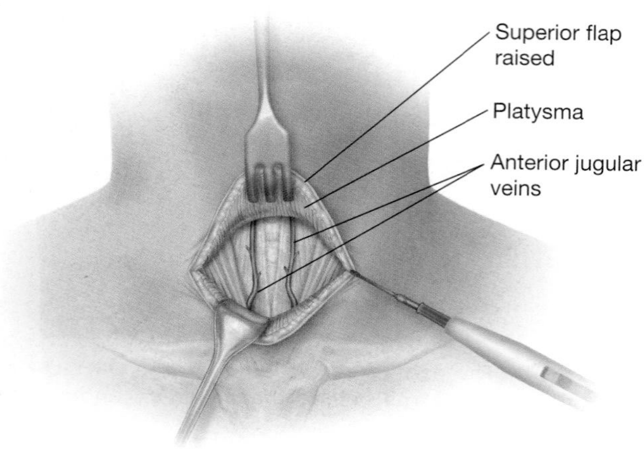

FIGURE 6 ● Myocutaneous flaps are raised superiorly, inferiorly, and laterally to facilitate skin retraction and to expose the various sites to be explored.

ENTRY INTO THE DEEP CENTRAL NECK SPACE

- The avascular, midline raphe between the sternohyoid and sternothyroid muscles on each side is entered with electrocautery. This midline is best identified by digital palpation of the midline of the underlying trachea. These strap muscles should be separated to expose the underlying thyroid isthmus (**FIGURE 7**).
- The layers of the strap muscles are separated into two by dividing the connective tissue in the layer between the sternohyoid and the sternothyroid muscles. The lateral extent of this dissection is the lateral borders of these muscles and the carotid sheath. This exposes the internal jugular vein, a site from which to draw a baseline blood sample for intraoperative PTH monitoring[7] (**FIGURE 8**).
- An alternate site for PTH sampling is a peripheral venipuncture (often in the lower extremity) performed by the anesthesiologist. If an arterial catheter is present for anesthetic monitoring, it is acceptable to use an arterial blood sample for PTH monitoring.
- The space between the sternothyroid muscle and the thyroid lobe is developed with a combination of blunt dissection and electrocautery. The operation must necessarily begin on one side of the neck, but an identical procedure will be done on the contralateral side of the neck to identify all four parathyroid glands. This space lateral to the thyroid lobe and medial to the carotid artery is developed back to the level of the prevertebral fascia. The crossing middle thyroid vein may need to be divided. This may be accomplished with metallic clips or suture or through any of the available powered surgical devices (**FIGURE 9**). Caution must be taken to avoid searching for parathyroid tissue too soon, as it is possible for the tumor to be more posterior than one has opened, or remaining with either the thyroid or the carotid sheath.
- The recurrent laryngeal nerve may be identified at this point, coursing cephalad in the tracheoesophageal groove (**FIGURE 10**).

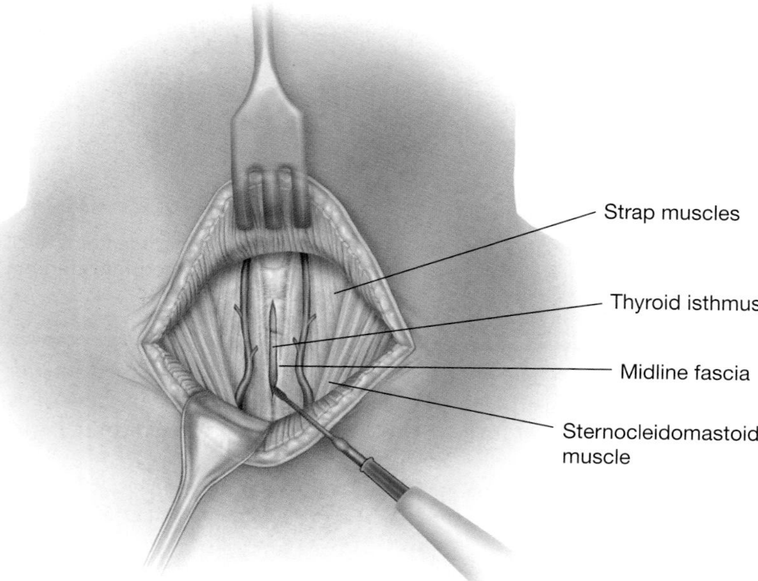

FIGURE 7 ● The strap muscles (sternohyoid and sternothyroid) are separated in the midline with electrocautery to expose the underlying thyroid isthmus.

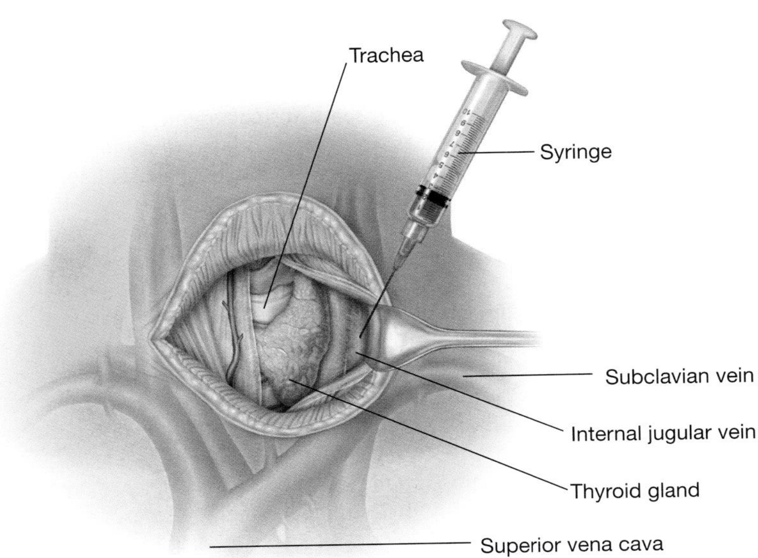

FIGURE 8 ● Blood is drawn from the internal jugular vein to test for PTH levels.

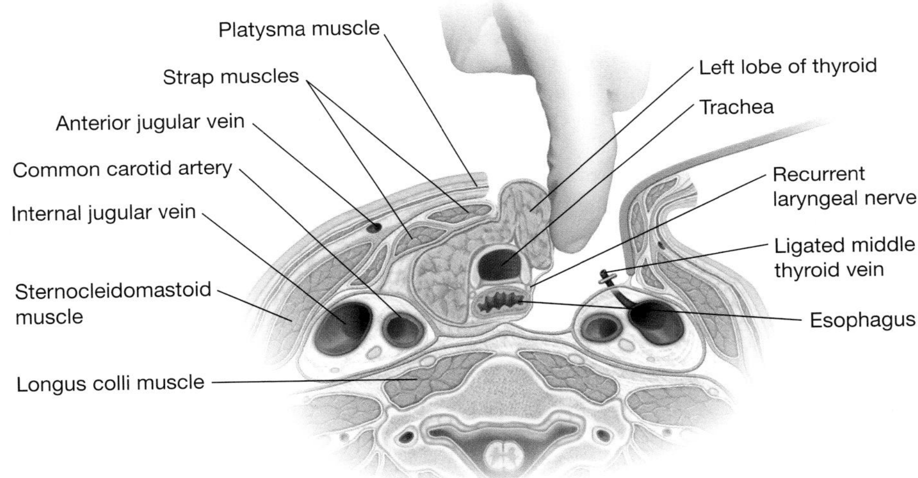

FIGURE 9 ● Initial dissection for a parathyroidectomy includes separating the strap muscles off the underlying thyroid lobe. The plane just medial to the carotid sheath is followed posteriorly to the level of the spine. The only transversely crossing structure is the middle thyroid vein, which can be ligated. All soft tissue, along with the thyroid lobe, is kept under the surgeon's finger.

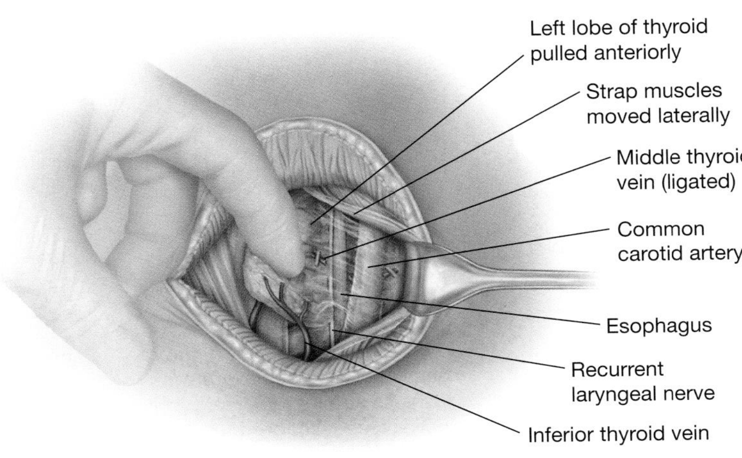

FIGURE 10 ● The recurrent laryngeal nerve courses superiorly in the tracheoesophageal groove and can often be identified most easily at the level of the inferior pole of the thyroid gland.

IDENTIFICATION OF SUPERIOR PARATHYROID GLANDS

- The superior parathyroid glands lie posterior to the upper pole of the thyroid lobe. To explore this space, the thyroid lobe is rolled anteromedially using one's finger or a Kittner dissector. The superior parathyroid glands are posterior to the recurrent laryngeal nerve as it passes underneath the tubercle of Zuckerkandl and just posterolateral to the ligament of Berry (**FIGURE 11**). Their position is more constant than that of the inferior parathyroid glands. There is often symmetry between sides of the neck, and if one cannot locate a superior parathyroid gland on one side, it is often advisable to locate it on the contralateral side.
- Owing to limited space for enlargement, superior parathyroid adenomas often grow caudad and ultimately lie in a pseudoectopic position in the tracheoesophageal groove, low in the neck. The blood supply, however, remains in the eutopic position near the upper pole of the thyroid lobe. Caution must be taken elevating these low-lying superior parathyroid adenomas out of the tracheoesophageal groove as they often lie with the recurrent laryngeal nerve draped over them.
- Ectopic positions for the superior parathyroid glands include low in the tracheoesophageal groove, retroesophageal, retrotracheal, within the carotid sheath, and within the thyroid gland.
- Exploration of the carotid sheath begins with retraction of the sternothyroid muscle laterally to expose the carotid artery. Gentle blunt dissection anterior to the carotid artery allows separation of the carotid artery from the internal jugular vein just lateral to it. Posterior in the carotid sheath is the vagus nerve. Exposure of the carotid sheath for about 5 to 6 cm in a cephalocaudal direction allows one to search for a soft, brown nodule consistent with a parathyroid adenoma (**FIGURE 12**). Care must be taken not to mistake nodules posterior to the carotid sheath for parathyroid adenomas as these may in fact be ganglia of the sympathetic chain.
- Once identified, the parathyroid tumor should be dissected back to its single vascular pedicle. Great care should be taken to avoid entry into the parathyroid capsule and the potential for spilling and seeding parathyroid tumor cells in the central neck space (known as parathyromatosis).
- Any uncertainty in the visual identification of parathyroid tissue should prompt a biopsy sent for frozen section analysis. A small fragment of tumor can be taken with a pair of scissors. Gentle pressure can control any slight ooze from the biopsied gland.
- Once the superior gland has been identified, it should remain in place until the inferior gland has been identified.
- This same procedure will be used to identify the superior parathyroid glands on each side of the neck.

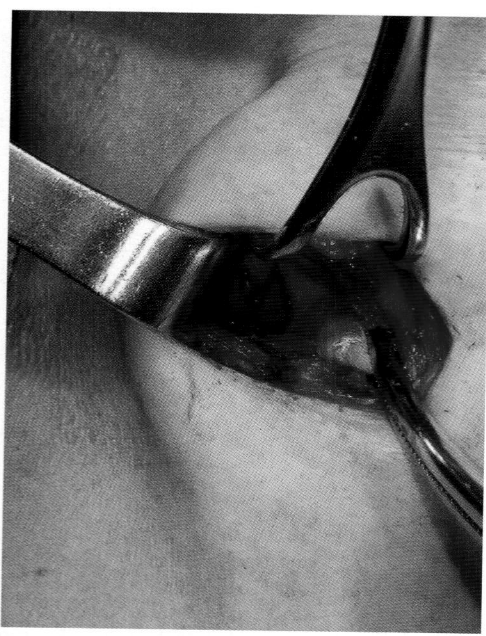

FIGURE 11 ● Right superior parathyroid adenoma lying posterior to the right thyroid lobe (rolled anteriorly with Kittner dissector). The right strap musculature is seen retracted laterally.

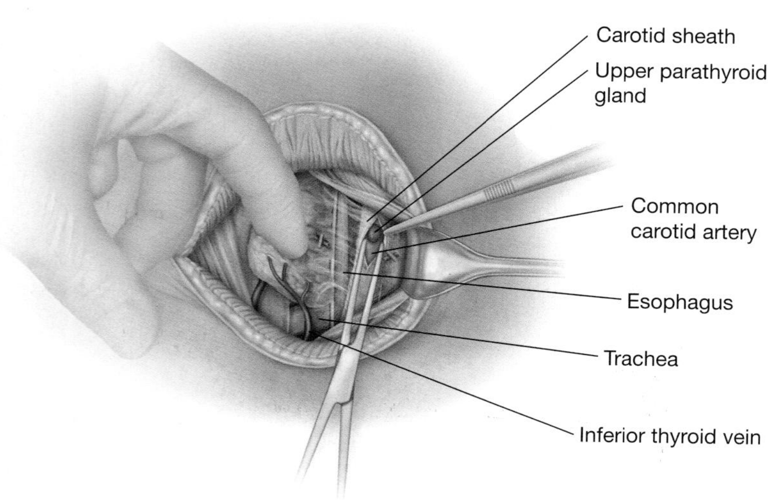

FIGURE 12 ● Exploration of the carotid sheath for a missing or ectopic superior parathyroid gland. The soft tissue covering the carotid artery is opened, and this space can be explored from the retropharyngeal region into the posterior superior mediastinum.

IDENTIFICATION OF INFERIOR PARATHYROID GLANDS

- The inferior parathyroid glands have a slightly more variable location than the superior parathyroid glands related to the greater distance of migration during embryologic development. The typical location for these glands is just caudal and slightly posterior to the inferior tip of the lower pole of the thyroid lobe. The inferior parathyroid glands often lie in a plane equal to the trachea. They are uniformly anterior to the recurrent laryngeal nerve (**FIGURE 13**).

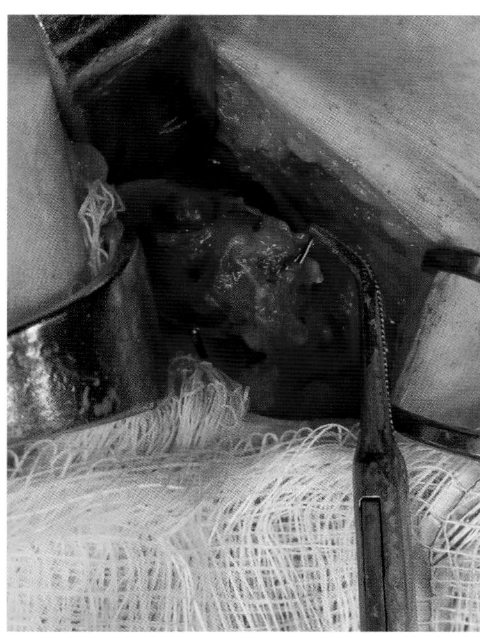

FIGURE 13 ● Left inferior parathyroid adenoma retracted away from the inferior pole of the thyroid gland.

- As the inferior parathyroid gland enlarges, it may descend with gravity into the fatty tissue caudal to the thyroid lobe and into the anterior superior mediastinum. Gentle dissection in this region can allow for identification of a parathyroid adenoma without causing bleeding.
- The inferior parathyroid glands may lie in the connective tissue ligament that attaches the lower pole of the thyroid to the cervical horn of the thymus (the so-called thyrothymic ligament).
- Ectopic positions for the inferior parathyroid glands include the thyrothymic ligament, the cervical portions of the thymus, the intrathoracic thymus, undescended within the neck, and with the thyroid gland itself. Each of these spaces needs to be examined for a missing parathyroid gland. There is often symmetry of location of the inferior parathyroid glands, and inability to find one inferior parathyroid gland should prompt attempts at identification of the contralateral inferior parathyroid gland as a guide.
- A transcervical thymectomy may be done to identify missing or ectopically located inferior parathyroid glands. This procedure is begun by dissecting the fatty tissue in the anterior superior mediastinum just posterior to the clavicular head and just lateral to the trachea. A search is undertaken for the canary yellow color of the remnant thymus. Gentle traction in a cephalad direction will allow one to extract the thymus from the mediastinum. An encasing membrane will often need to be opened to fully allow the thymus to be removed. The cervical thymic remnant will thin out to a small attachment often containing a blood vessel that should be clipped or suture ligated (**FIGURE 14**).
- Once the inferior parathyroid adenoma is identified, it should be dissected back to its vascular pedicle. Any question as to its identity should prompt a small sample to be taken with scissors for frozen section biopsy.
- An identical procedure will be followed to identify the inferior parathyroid tumor on the contralateral side.

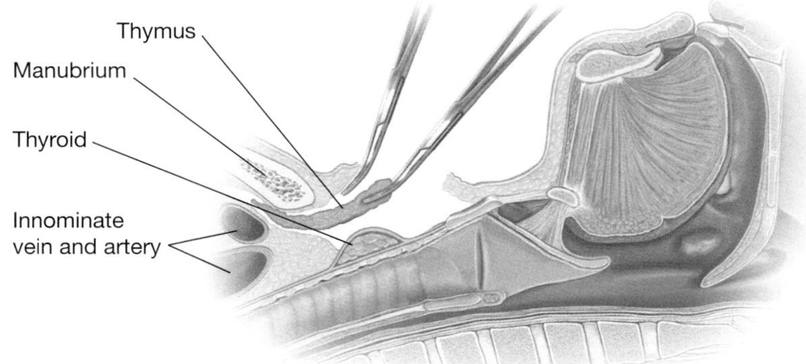

FIGURE 14 ● A transcervical thymectomy can be accomplished to identify ectopic inferior parathyroid glands that lie caudal to the sternal notch. The thymic tissue is grasped and gently pulled up from the mediastinum and into the cervical incision.

FROZEN SECTION PATHOLOGIC ANALYSIS

- It is often advisable to confirm the identity of the four parathyroid glands identified with frozen section.
- Frozen section is used to confirm identification as parathyroid tissue more so than to quantify cellularity of the parathyroid gland. It is nearly impossible to reliably determine parathyroid hyperplasia from a parathyroid adenoma on frozen section (**FIGURE 15A** and **B**).

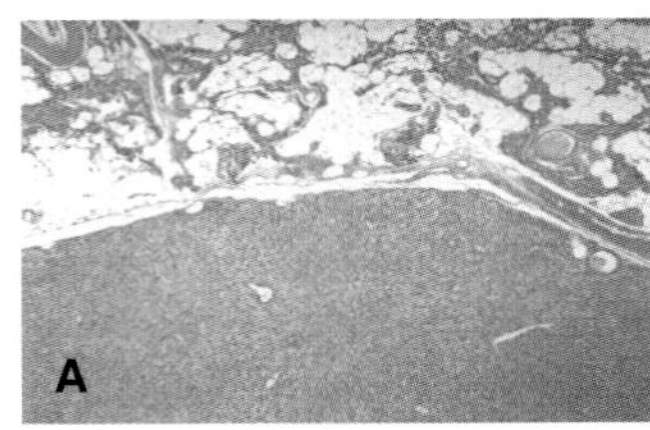

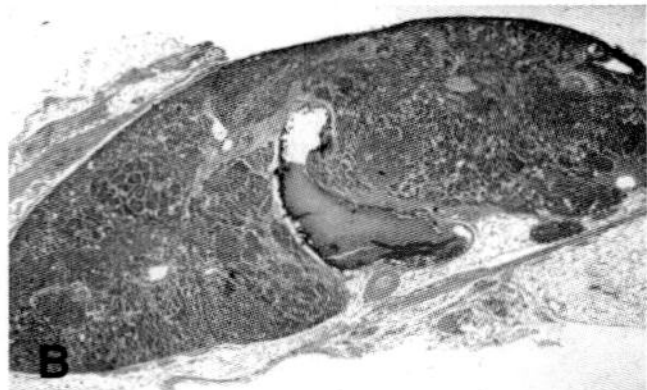

FIGURE 15 ● Low-power photomicrographs of **(A)** a parathyroid adenoma and **(B)** a hyperplastic parathyroid gland. The adenoma has a characteristic compressed rim of normal parathyroid tissue, with admixed adipocytes and parathyroid chief cells.

SUBTOTAL RESECTION OF PARATHYROIDS

- If a subtotal resection of the parathyroid glands is to be done, one plans to resect three and a half of the four glands. This is best done by dividing one of the glands first and continually checking on its viability as the resection of the second through fourth glands ensues to avoid an inadvertent total parathyroidectomy.
- In general, the remnant of parathyroid gland to remain on its native blood supply in the neck should be a portion of the most normal-appearing gland of the four identified.
- If possible, a remnant inferior gland should be left, as this remnant will sit more anterior, and anterior to the recurrent laryngeal nerve, making it easier to reoperate upon if necessary.
- A sufficient parathyroid remnant is about 30 to 50 mg of tissue or the size of a normal parathyroid gland.
- The parathyroid remnant is created by placing a metallic clip or clips across the gland and sharply dividing the distal segment of the gland away from the remnant (**FIGURE 16**).
- The remnant may also be tagged with a Prolene suture to aid in future identification if a reoperation becomes necessary. Great care should be taken when placing this marking stitch to avoid injury to the end arteriole feeding the parathyroid gland.
- The second through fourth glands are removed by dividing the vascular pedicle of the gland. The vascular pedicle can be clipped or tied as per surgeon preference.

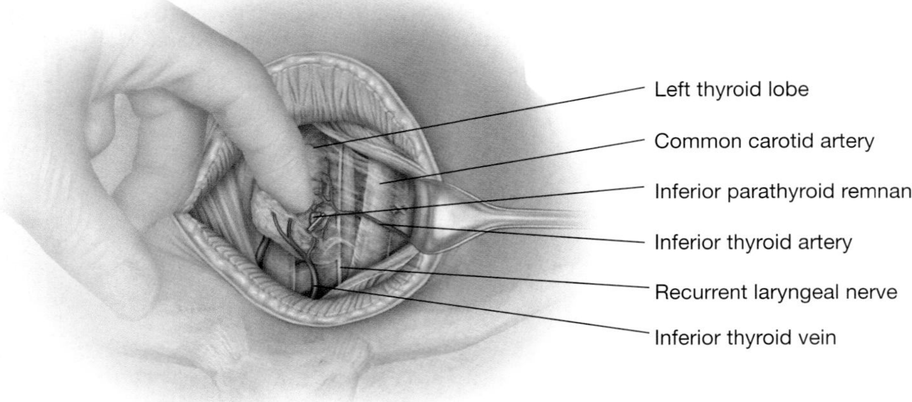

FIGURE 16 ● A remnant of a left lower parathyroid gland is left on its native blood supply. A metallic surgical clip is placed to divide the gland and to mark in the case that a future reoperative parathyroid surgery becomes necessary. Great care must be taken to ensure that the clip is not placed across the blood supply to the parathyroid remnant.

TOTAL PARATHYROIDECTOMY

- A total parathyroidectomy involves the removal of all parathyroid tissue (usually four glands) from the neck.
- Each gland is fully dissected back to its vascular pedicle, which is clipped or ligated and then divided.
- The parathyroid tissue to be transplanted is identified and kept moist. Great care should be taken to avoid this tissue from mistakenly being handed off the sterile field (**FIGURE 17**).

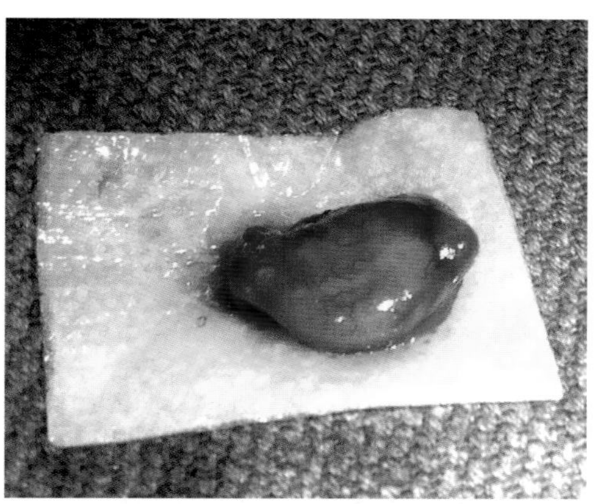

FIGURE 17 ● Ex vivo right superior parathyroid adenoma.

INTRAOPERATIVE PARATHYROID HORMONE MONITORING

- If intraoperative PTH monitoring is being used, a postresection PTH value should be drawn and sent at 5, 10, or 15 minutes post resection of all parathyroid tissue. Timing is per the surgeon's protocol. Longer time points (15 minutes) are usually used if the PTH specimen is being drawn from a central vein (internal jugular). Shorter time points may be used if the specimen is from a peripheral venipuncture or a radial arterial line.[6]
- Resolution of hyperparathyroidism and long-term eucalcemia is well predicted by postresection PTH values that are at least 50% of the baseline value and into the normal range (<40 pg/mL).[8]

HEMOSTASIS

- Careful attention to hemostasis is of paramount importance throughout the entire parathyroidectomy to ease in parathyroid identification.
- Postoperative neck hematomas are a rare but potentially disastrous complication following parathyroidectomy.
- Prior to wound closure, a Valsalva maneuver is requested to decrease venous return and to identify any slight bleeding in the operative bed.
- Topical hemostatic agents may be placed in the tracheoesophageal groove and inferior to the thyroid lobes.
- Routine placement of closed suction drains is not required.

WOUND CLOSURE

- The two layers of strap musculature are closed in the midline in either one layer or two separate layers. Three to four interrupted, absorbable stitches are sufficient to reapproximate these muscles.
- The platysma muscle layer is reapproximated with interrupted, buried, absorbable sutures.
- The skin edges are brought together with a 3-0 Prolene suture in a subcuticular stitch.
- Skin glue is applied to the wound, and once dry, the Prolene suture may be removed immediately. No further dressings are required.

IMMEDIATE PARATHYROID AUTOTRANSPLANTATION

- If a total parathyroidectomy has been performed, one must reimplant autologous parathyroid tissue to avoid permanent hypoparathyroidism.
- Roughly 30 to 50 mg of parathyroid tissue should be transplanted.
- The upper extremity in which the parathyroid graft is to be placed is extended out from the patient and supported on an arm board (**FIGURE 18**).
- The transplant site is into the brachioradialis muscle on the dorsal aspect of the forearm (usually the nondominant forearm). Again, thought must be given to the location of a current or future hemodialysis access in those patients on chronic renal replacement therapy.
- The dorsal forearm is prepped and draped in the usual fashion.
- A 3- to 4-cm longitudinal incision is made, and dissection is deepened through the subcutaneous tissue to the fascia overlying the brachioradialis muscle (**FIGURE 19A** and **B**).
- The fragment of parathyroid tissue to be transplanted is then cut into 1-mm^3 fragments, totaling about 15 fragments (**FIGURE 20**).
- A small muscle pocket is made in the brachioradialis muscle with the tip of a dissecting instrument, and a single fragment

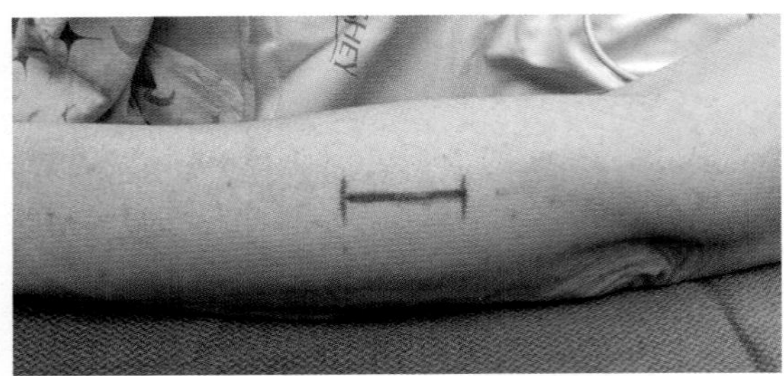

FIGURE 18 ● The heterotopic transplant site is marked prior to surgical prepping and draping. The transplant site is the brachioradialis muscle of the nondominant forearm.

of parathyroid tissue is placed into this pocket. The edges of the pocket are loosely approximated with an absorbable suture or a metallic clip.

- This procedure is repeated until each fragment of parathyroid tissue has been placed into a separate muscle pocket (**FIGURE 21**).
- Great care needs to be taken to avoid any bleeding in these muscle pockets as the initial nutrient supply of the parathyroid graft requires contact with the vascularized muscle.
- The wound is then closed in layers, using interrupted, absorbable sutures to close the deep dermal layers and tissue adhesive to reapproximate the skin edges (**FIGURE 22**).

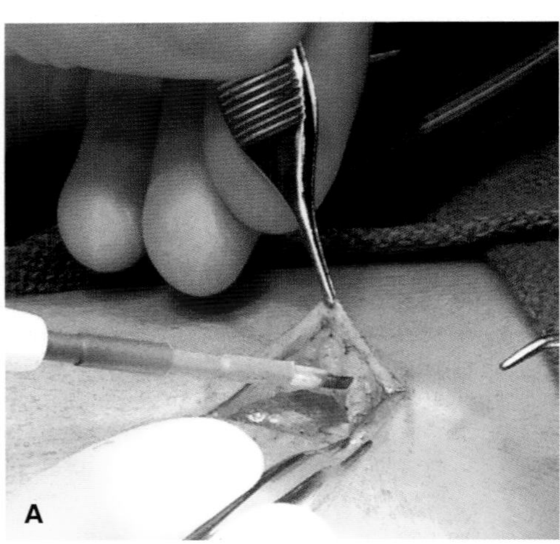

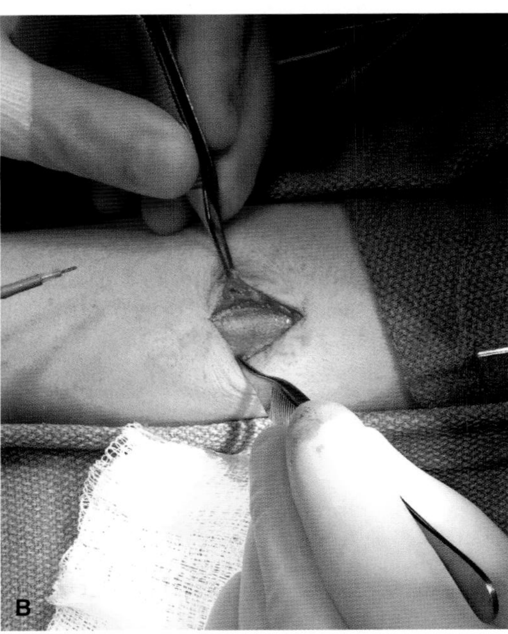

FIGURE 19 ● Preparing the recipient site for parathyroid tissue. **A,** Dissection through subcutaneous tissue to the level of the brachioradialis muscle. **B,** Exposed brachioradialis muscle.

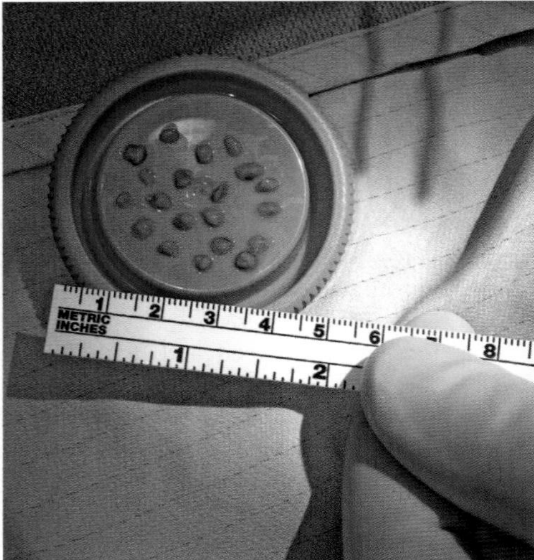

FIGURE 20 ● Minced parathyroid to be transplanted. Numerous 1-mm^3 fragments of parathyroid tissue await placement into individual muscle pockets.

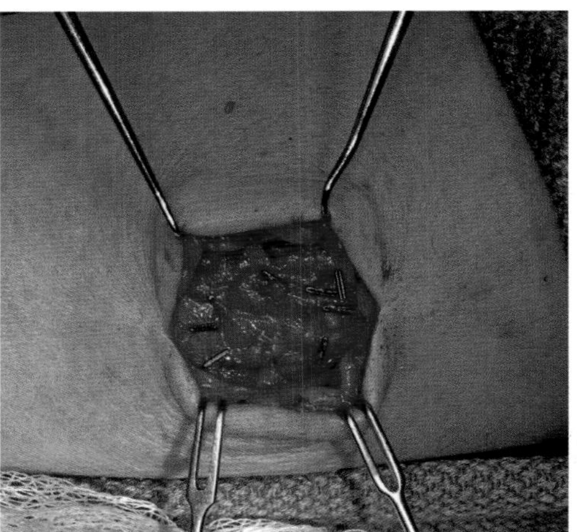

FIGURE 21 ● Parathyroid autotransplantation completed, with muscle pockets loosely approximated with metallic clips.

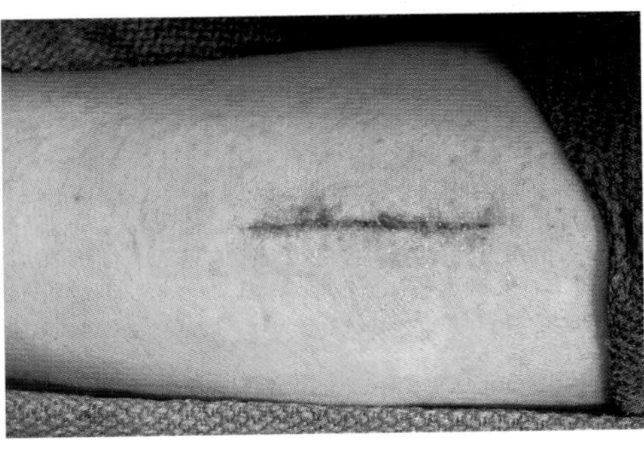

FIGURE 22 ● The transplant incision is closed with skin glue.

PEARLS AND PITFALLS

Indications	■ Hyperparathyroidism is a biochemical diagnosis, and this needs to be secured prior to cervical imaging or planning an operation.
Identification of parathyroids	■ Dissection in the central neck space should free the carotid sheath medially and include all the tissue down to the prevertebral fascia.
Excision of parathyroid adenomas	■ Parathyroid glands have a singular blood supply and should be dissected back to this vessel prior to ligation and division to avoid injury to critical adjacent structures such as the recurrent laryngeal nerve.
Hemostasis	■ A bloodless field greatly aids in the identification of parathyroid glands from their surrounding tissue. ■ A hematoma at the site of a parathyroid transplant greatly jeopardizes the viability of the autologous graft.
Placement of autologous graft	■ The parathyroid autotransplant may be placed in either the dorsal forearm or the presternal area.
Postoperative hypocalcemia	■ Anticipate and aggressively treat the hypocalcemia that accompanies either a subtotal parathyroidectomy or certainly a total parathyroidectomy with autologous graft.

POSTOPERATIVE CARE

- Patients undergoing subtotal parathyroidectomy or total parathyroidectomy with autologous graft should be admitted for at least 1 day to monitor postoperative calcium and PTH levels.
- Patients having undergone a forearm parathyroid transplant should have a limb alert placed, and blood pressures, IV sites, and venipunctures should be avoided in the transplant arm.
- Acetaminophen or ibuprofen is often sufficient for the pain related to the procedure. Occasionally, opioid agents are needed for a short time postoperatively.
- Endocrinology consultation can be sought as needed by the surgical team.
- Oral calcium and possibly vitamin D (in the form of calcitriol) should be started immediately and titrated if hypocalcemia occurs.
- Patients having undergone a total parathyroidectomy will have an obligate period of hypoparathyroidism until their autograft begins to function.
- Parenteral calcium should be restricted to severely low serum calcium levels and/or patients with symptomatic hypocalcemia.
- Symptoms of hypocalcemia include perioral and digital numbness or tingling, muscle aches/spasms, carpopedal spasms, facial nerve hyperactivity (Chvostek sign), respiratory muscle insufficiency, and tetany.

OUTCOMES

- The long-term outcome as measured by eucalcemia from a subtotal parathyroidectomy and a total parathyroidectomy with immediate parathyroid autotransplantation are very similar. Both have a small rate of recurrent hyperparathyroidism (as a result of the natural history of the parathyroid disease). This recurrence may occur 10 to 20 years after the index operation.[9]
- Immediate transplantation of autologous parathyroid tissue has successful engraftment approximately 95% of the time. Most parathyroid grafts will gain function in about 8 weeks.[10]

COMPLICATIONS

- Compressive cervical hematoma
- Laryngeal nerve injuries (external branch of the superior laryngeal nerve or recurrent laryngeal nerve)
- Sympathetic chain/stellate ganglion injury
- Prolonged or permanent hypoparathyroidism
- Inability to extirpate all hyperactive tissue with resultant persistent hyperparathyroidism

- Tracheal injury
- Esophageal injury
- Lymph or chylous leak
- Wound infection
- Unsightly neck or arm scarring

REFERENCES

1. Bilezikian JP, Bandeira L, Khan A, Cusano NE. Hyperparathyroidism. *Lancet*. 2018;391(10116):168-178.
2. Saunders BD, Saunders EFH, Gauger PG. Lithium therapy and hyperparathyroidism: an evidence-based assessment. *World J Surg*. 2009;33(11):2314-2323.
3. Pichardo-Lowden AR, Manni A, Saunders BD, et al. Familial hyperparathyroidism due to a germline mutation of the CDC73 gene: implications for management and age-appropriate testing of relatives at risk. *Endocr Pract*. 2011;17(4):602-609.
4. Kidney Disease: Improving Global Outcomes (KDIGO) CKD-MBD Update Work Group. KDIGO 2017 clinical practice guideline update for the diagnosis, evaluation, prevention, and treatment of chronic kidney disease-mineral and bone disorder (CKD-MBD). *Kidney Int Suppl (2011)*. 2017;7(1):1-59.
5. Wong KK, Fig LM, Gross MD, Dwamena BA. Parathyroid adenoma localization with 99mTc-sestamibi SPECT/CT: a meta-analysis. *Nucl Med Commun*. 2015;36(4):363-375.
6. Yeh R, Tay YD, Tabacco G, et al. Diagnostic performance of 4D CT and sestamibi SPECT/CT in localizing parathyroid adenomas in primary hyperparathyroidism. *Radiology*. 2019;291(2):469-476.
7. Woodrum DT, Saunders BD, England BG, et al. The influence of sample site on intraoperative PTH monitoring during parathyroidectomy. *Surgery*. 2004;136(6):1169-1175.
8. Heller KS, Blumberg SN. Relation of final intraoperative parathyroid hormone level and outcome following parathyroidectomy. *Arch Otolaryngol Head Neck Surg*. 2009;135(11):1103-1107.
9. Richards ML, Wormuth J, Bingener J, et al. Parathyroidectomy in secondary hyperparathyroidism: is there an optimal operative management? *Surgery*. 2006;139(2):174-180.
10. Feldman AL, Sharaf RN, Skarulis MC, et al. Results of heterotopic parathyroid autotransplantation: a 13-year experience. *Surgery*. 1996;126(6):1042-1048.

Chapter 54

Minimally Invasive Parathyroidectomy

Peter Angelos and Raymon H. Grogan

DEFINITION

- Although there is no uniformly agreed upon definition of a "minimally invasive parathyroidectomy" (MIP), most surgeons accept that this term refers to an operation to remove the parathyroid gland that is a focused or unilateral exploration done through a small incision.[1] Some surgeons stress that MIP should also refer to an operation done without general anesthesia in an outpatient setting. However, we believe that because the choice of anesthesia and determination of whether a patient is discharged on the day of surgery is dependent on the patient (and not always the operation), we do not limit MIP to outpatient procedures without general anesthetic.[2] We believe that MIP is the treatment of choice for primary hyperparathyroidism (HPT) when the location of the abnormal parathyroid gland has been well localized preoperatively.[3,4]
- MIP is effective and recommended for the treatment of sporadic primary HPT but not in cases of familial HPT (eg, multiple endocrine neoplasia type 1 or 2), secondary HPT, or tertiary HPT. In all of the latter categories, the high likelihood of multigland disease necessitates the exploration of all four glands.
- Although MIP is effective in both primary operations as well as in reoperative cases, we will focus on primary operations in the following description. The decision making for reoperative parathyroidectomy is complicated by the scarring that will be present in the neck and the potential difficulty with performing a four-gland exploration. For this reason, preoperative localization becomes much more important in reoperative cases and is beyond the scope of this chapter.

DIAGNOSIS AND INDICATIONS FOR SURGERY

- The diagnosis of HPT is made by the finding of an elevated calcium level with an elevated intact parathyroid hormone (iPTH) level. It is possible to have normocalcemic HPT if the calcium level is at the upper range of normal but the iPTH is elevated. Alternatively, patients sometimes have elevated calcium levels with the iPTH level being inappropriately in the high normal range.[5] It is important when making the diagnosis of HPT to assess both calcium and iPTH levels so that the relative values of these tests can be compared. In a patient with normally functioning parathyroid glands, a high calcium should be associated with a low iPTH level.
- In order to confirm the diagnosis of HPT and rule out familial benign hypocalciuric hypercalcemia (FBHH), a 24-hour urine calcium should be obtained. In FBHH, the urinary calcium is expected to be very low. A normal or elevated 24-hour urine calcium level effectively rules out FBHH. An elevated 24-hour urine calcium increases the risk of kidney stones.
- The indications for surgery in HPT are well described in several National Institutes of Health (NIH) consensus conferences over the last few decades.[6] In addition, the American Association of Endocrine Surgeons recently published guidelines that have been widely adopted.[7] Most surgeons and endocrinologists currently agree that patients with HPT who are symptomatic or have marked elevations in serum calcium should have surgery. A history of kidney stones and the presence of osteoporosis are widely accepted as indications for surgery. It is common for patients with HPT to have additional symptoms that may be associated with the disease, including low energy, bone pain, decreased proximal extremity muscle strength, decreased ability to concentrate, and reductions in short-term memory. Although all of these symptoms may be caused by conditions other than HPT, they are very common in patients with HPT and may influence the decision to recommend surgery.
- The diagnosis of HPT in a young patient (<50 years old) also is a relative indication for parathyroidectomy because such patients will have more years to develop osteoporosis and other problems associated with HPT. In addition, for women of childbearing age, HPT also appears to increase the risks of spontaneous abortion.
- There is currently no approved medical treatment for primary HPT. For this reason, the choice for patients and physicians is between parathyroidectomy and continued observation.

IMAGING AND OTHER DIAGNOSTIC STUDIES

- Once the decision is made to proceed to surgical treatment, localization studies to attempt to identify the location of the abnormal parathyroid gland are indicated. We recommend the routine use of technetium-99m (Tc-99m) sestamibi scan and ultrasound evaluation of the thyroid gland.[8]
- Sestamibi scanning has high rates of sensitivity and specificity and is effective in localizing parathyroid adenomas not only in the neck but also in ectopic locations such as undescended glands in the neck or intrathoracic glands. Unfortunately, in cases of multigland disease, sestamibi scanning is least likely to identify the location of abnormal glands. Sestamibi is taken up by both thyroid and parathyroid cells. It is more rapidly cleared from thyroid cells than from abnormal parathyroid cells. For this reason, a comparison of early and delayed scans often reveals the presence of a persistent focus of increased activity in the abnormal parathyroid gland. With the use of fused sestamibi–computed tomography (CT) scanning or three-dimensional single photon emission computed tomography (SPECT) reconstructions, it is often possible to determine whether the focus of uptake is anterior in the neck (at or near the level of the thyroid lobe) or more posterior. Because the superior parathyroid gland is located posterior to the recurrent laryngeal, posterior parathyroid glands on scans are most likely superior glands, whereas anterior glands are more likely to be inferior glands.

- Ultrasonography is an effective noninvasive means of identifying abnormal parathyroid glands. The study can be performed in the radiology department or by surgeons in the clinic or operating room. Ultrasonography is effective in identifying enlarged parathyroid glands that are close to the thyroid gland. Abnormal parathyroid glands usually appear as hypoechoic lesions either posterior or inferior to the thyroid gland. Parathyroid glands that are located posterior to the esophagus and those in the mediastinum are less likely to be visualized on ultrasound.
- Ultrasound is very effective at identifying thyroid nodules, which may be a source of increased uptake on sestamibi scans. We believe that thyroid nodules meeting size and/or imaging characteristics to be concerning for thyroid cancer should be evaluated with fine needle aspiration cytology prior to planned parathyroidectomy. This strategy limits the chances of missing a nonpalpable thyroid malignancy and thus reduces the likelihood for reoperative neck surgery.
- In cases of primary HPT when patients have negative preoperative localization studies, we recommend proceeding with surgery and planning on a four-gland exploration (see Part 5, Chapter 52). Some surgeons would obtain a four-dimensional CT scan of the neck and chest prior to exploring the patient. The decision on whether to proceed with a four-gland exploration or pursue additional imaging with four-dimensional CT scanning prior to surgery should be made based on the surgeon's comfort level with four-gland exploration.

SURGICAL MANAGEMENT

- MIP can be performed either with local anesthesia and sedation or with general anesthesia, depending on surgeon and patient preference. We have found that because inferior parathyroid adenomas are located more anteriorly in the neck, these glands are more amenable to resection without using general anesthesia. Large posteriorly located superior parathyroid adenomas often are more challenging to remove without general anesthetic because of the need to rotate the thyroid lobe medially to gain access to the space posterior to the esophagus. Although it is possible to access these glands even when the patient is not asleep, surgeons should be cognizant of the challenge and choose the appropriate patient for such an approach.
- Identification of the optimal skin crease for a cosmetic incision is best done with the patient sitting up while awake. Although extending the neck in the operating room may change the location of skin creases, marking them prior to entering the operating room increases the likelihood of a good cosmetic result.
- After the patient has been either intubated or appropriately sedated, a superficial cervical plexus block may be used to facilitate local anesthesia if the patient has not received a general anesthetic or to improve postoperative pain control if a general anesthetic is used.
- The superficial cervical plexus block is a safe, effective technique to provide cutaneous anesthesia to the C2, C3, and C4 dermatomes. We perform a two-point (transverse and inferior), bilateral superficial blockade to allow complete local anesthesia of the midline Kocher incision, which, if done correctly, will last for several hours after the procedure. Anecdotally, this should also allow for reduced general anesthesia intraoperatively, particularly for superficial lower parathyroidectomies. We use 10 mL of 0.25% bupivacaine without epinephrine for each side of the neck.
- After induction of general anesthesia, the patient's neck is extended with a beanbag or shoulder roll. The midpoint of the posterior border of the sternocleidomastoid muscle is identified, and a 22-gauge needle is inserted subcutaneously (no more than 1 cm) at this anatomic landmark (**FIGURE 1**). Check to be sure the needle is not inserted into a vein by pulling back on the plunger of the syringe. First, 5 mL of anesthetic is injected straight toward the midline of the neck (transverse injection) just posterior to the muscle. The needle is then repositioned without removing it from the skin so that it is now pointing at the sternal notch. The remaining 5 mL of anesthetic is then injected inferiorly along the posterior border of the muscle (inferior injection). The other side of the neck is then injected in a similar manner.
- If done correctly, there is minimal risk associated with this technique. The main risk of this procedure occurs if the injection is done too deep. If injected too deep into the neck, branches of the brachial plexus can be anesthetized, and the patient may have a temporary paralysis of the ipsilateral upper extremity. A deep injection can also anesthetize the phrenic nerve and lead to temporary diaphragmatic paralysis. For this reason, if the injection is being done without general anesthetic while the patient is awake, it is important that bilateral blockade is not performed simultaneously on both sides of the neck. Finally, if the injection infiltrates superiorly, the greater auricular branch of the plexus will be blocked and the patient will have numbness of the skin overlying the parotid and the earlobe. This is a common side effect that the patient should be told to be aware of in the immediate postoperative period.

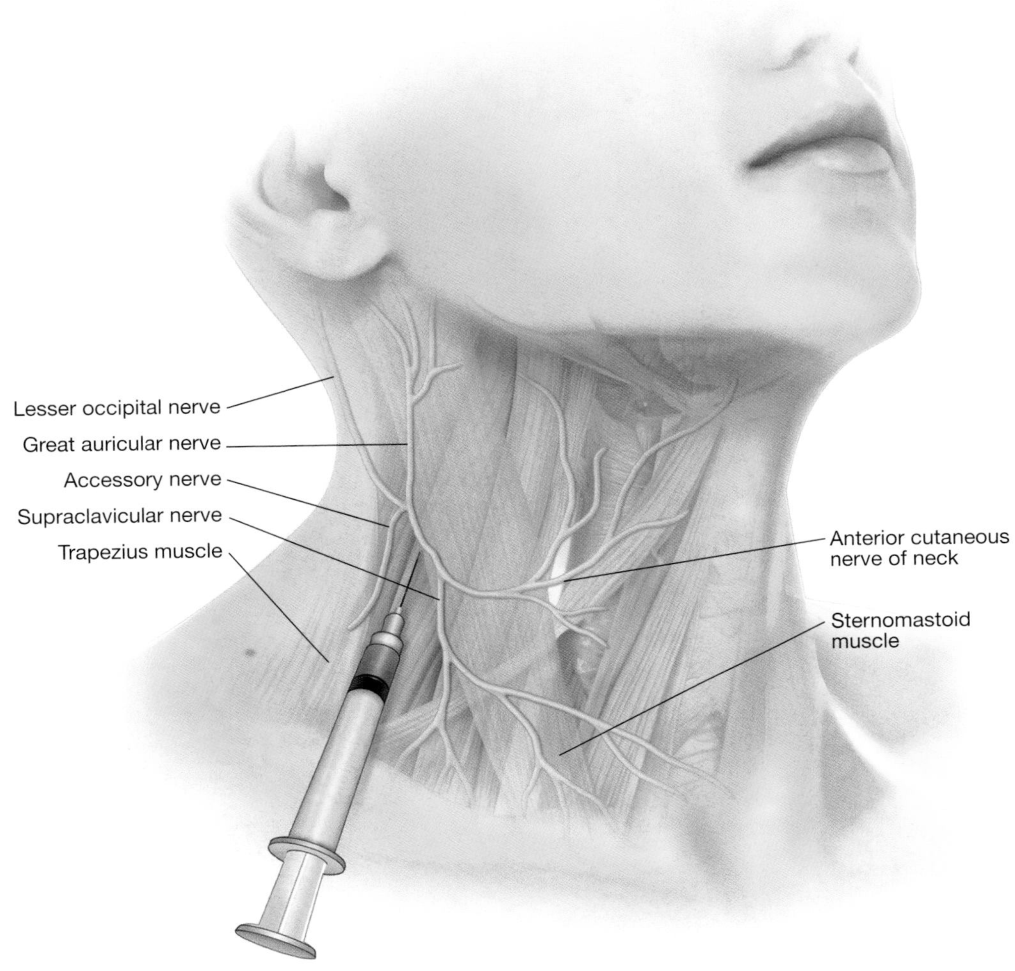

FIGURE 1 ● A 22-gauge needle is inserted no more than 1 cm subcutaneously at the midpoint of the posterior border of the sternocleidomastoid muscle. After assuring the needle is not in a vein, 5 mL of anesthetic is injected toward the midline of the neck (transverse injection). The needle is repositioned without removing it toward the sternal notch. The remaining 5 mL of anesthetic is then injected inferiorly along the posterior border of the muscle (inferior injection).

- Optimal positioning for parathyroidectomy is with the patient's neck gently extended but well supported. Prior to prepping the skin, we routinely perform an intraoperative ultrasound of the neck to ensure the choice of the optimal location for the skin incision (**FIGURE 2**). In addition, intraoperative ultrasound often allows the surgeon to confirm the location of the adenoma and focuses the subsequent surgical exploration.
- After prepping the skin, it is critical that, if the patient has not received a general anesthetic, care must be taken when placing drapes to ensure that the operative field is fully separated from the space below the drapes. Patients who are receiving sedation and local anesthesia usually are also given supplemental oxygen by the anesthesiologist during the operation. This is commonly done with a nasal cannula and results in relatively high oxygen concentrations below the drapes. If that oxygen comes in contact with a spark from electrocautery used during the performance of the parathyroidectomy, the risk of fire is increased. For this reason, when draping the patient, an occlusive dressing or adherent drapes are important to separate the operative field from the space below the drapes (**FIGURE 3**).
- A small (2-3 cm) incision in the midline is made in a skin crease. Although some surgeons prefer an incision shifted toward the side of the parathyroid adenoma, we prefer using a midline incision so that, if it becomes necessary to explore both sides, the same incision can often be used. If it is necessary to lengthen the incision, this is usually only a minimal increase in incision size.
- Small subplatysmal flaps are created with electrocautery to allow the skin incision to be moved up or down depending on where the abnormal gland is located. The midline strap

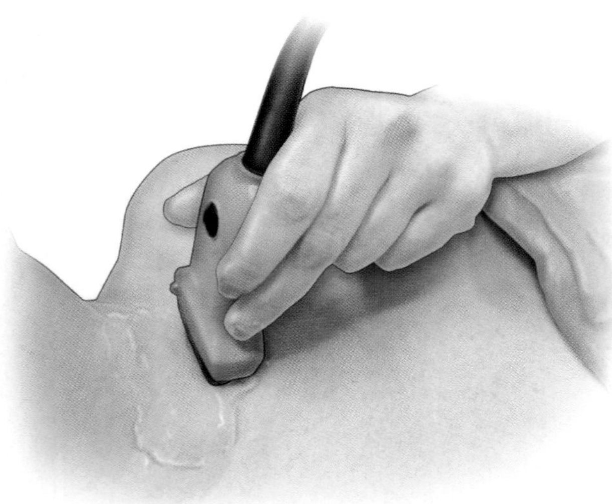

FIGURE 2 ● Ultrasound of the neck is performed prior to prepping the patient's neck. The ultrasound is particularly useful in determining the optimal location for the small neck incision.

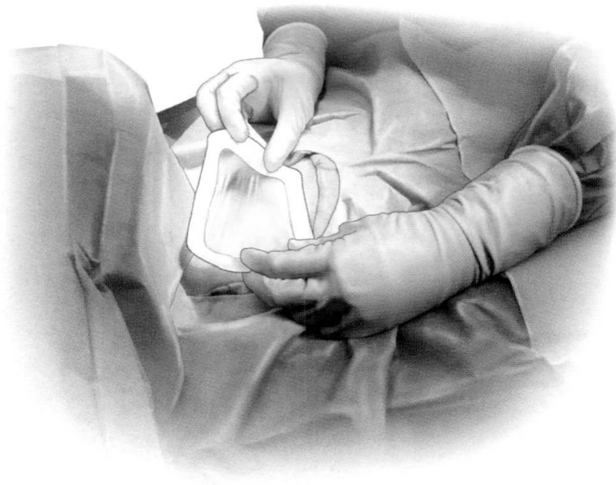

FIGURE 3 ● Occlusive barrier dressing being placed. This is very important if the patient is not intubated and supplemental oxygen is used. The barrier dressing separates the space under the drapes from the operative field and reduces the risk of fire.

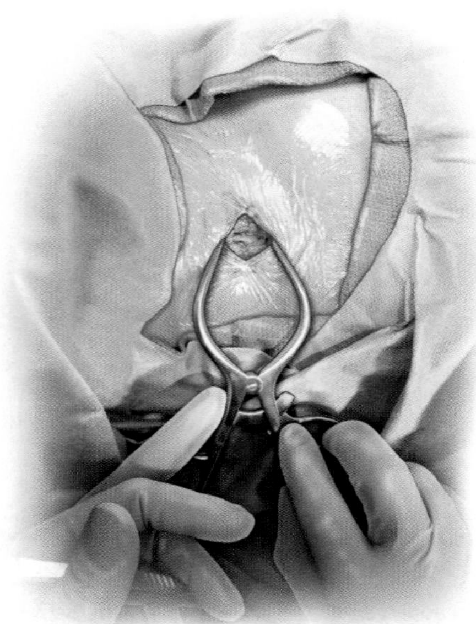

FIGURE 4 ● Small skin incision after the subplatysmal flaps have been created and the midline strap muscles have been separated to expose the thyroid gland below.

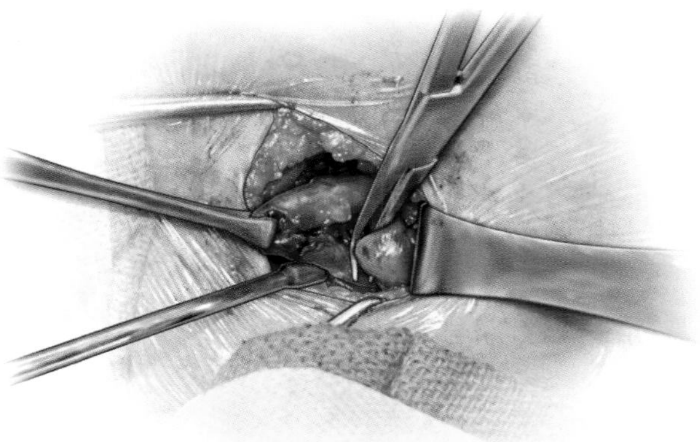

FIGURE 5 ● Parathyroid adenoma is identified in proximity to the thyroid gland. The parathyroid adenoma is separated from the surrounding tissue, taking care not to enter the capsule of the gland. The vascular pedicle is identified, ligated, and divided.

muscles are then separated in the midline so that the thyroid lobe on the involved side can be rotated medially (**FIGURE 4**). If, based on preoperative imaging, the abnormal parathyroid appears to be the inferior parathyroid, then the dissection is focused on the area near the inferior pole of the thyroid or in the thyrothymic tract where inferior parathyroid glands are most commonly located. If the abnormal parathyroid gland appears to be a superior gland, then dissection is focused on the more posterior tissue. The entire thyroid lobe is mobilized medially such that the space posterior to the esophagus can be adequately explored.

- Once an abnormal parathyroid gland is identified, the vascular pedicle should be carefully identified, ligated, and divided (**FIGURE 5**). Once adequate hemostasis is achieved, the incision is closed.

INTRAOPERATIVE DECISION MAKING WITH INTRAOPERATIVE PARATHYROID HORMONE

- We believe that intraoperative PTH assay is an important component of any MIP. iPTH has such a short half-life that, if the abnormal parathyroid gland is removed and the other glands are normal, the PTH levels will drop by more than 50% in 5 to 10 minutes for the vast majority of patients. In most circumstances, a second peripheral intravenous catheter is placed prior to positioning the patient. Blood samples are then drawn through this intravenous catheter, taking care to ensure adequate blood is drawn to avoid a dilute sample from the intravenous fluid. We routinely draw four samples. The first is drawn after the skin preparation prior to making an incision ("preincision"). The second is drawn after finding the parathyroid adenoma prior to dividing its blood supply ("preexcision"). Postexcision levels are then drawn at 5 and 10 minutes after removing the parathyroid adenoma.
- Although many papers have been written on identifying the optimal criteria for intraoperative drop in PTH, we believe that a drop of 50% from the first baseline level at 5 or 10 minutes post excision, as long as the value is within normal range, is strongly predictive of a successful operation.[9] If the preincision PTH level is very high and the preexcision level is even higher, it is sometimes necessary to draw levels beyond 10 minutes post excision in order to see an adequate drop in PTH levels. We believe that, with positive preoperative localization studies and a dramatic drop in PTH after excising the adenoma, the likelihood of a second abnormal parathyroid gland is exceedingly low and a four-gland exploration is not indicated.

CLOSURE

- As long as the skin incision is located in a skin crease or at least in line with skin creases, the likelihood of a cosmetically appealing scar is very high. We routinely close the skin with an absorbable suture in the platysma and subdermal level to take tension off the skin edges. The skin is closed with a 5-0 monofilament subcuticular suture with no knots. If an absorbable suture is used, Steri-Strips are applied and the suture is then cut flush with the skin. If a nonabsorbable suture is used, skin glue is placed over the incision prior to pulling the subcuticular stitch out in the operating room. Most patients have excellent cosmetic results.

POSTOPERATIVE CARE

- Assuming no other medical issues, many patients can be discharged after a successful MIP. Because a focused exploration has been undertaken, only one side of the neck has been dissected. Patients are generally given extra oral calcium for several days to prevent transient symptomatic hypocalcemia while the remaining parathyroid glands recover from having been suppressed. The extra calcium can be rapidly weaned. Patients are allowed to shower the day after surgery, and the only restriction in activity is to avoid driving a car until there is no neck pain in turning and the patient is off pain medication.

OUTCOMES

- The outcomes after MIP have been shown to be excellent in several large series.[10,11] Patients recover rapidly, and many have improvements in energy level with decreased bone pain in the weeks to months after surgery. The long-term risks of recurrent HPT are not different in many large series when comparing MIP with four-gland exploration.

COMPLICATIONS

- The primary risk of MIP is the small possibility of recurrent laryngeal nerve injury resulting in hoarseness. The risk of permanent hoarseness is in the 1% to 2% range in most large series of parathyroidectomies. Use of MIP in comparison with four-gland exploration does not seem to affect risk of recurrent laryngeal nerve injury. By contrast, the risk of permanent hypoparathyroidism, which is approximately 1% with a four-gland exploration, is eliminated with an MIP approach.
- Other potential complications of MIP include bleeding and infection. Both of these risks are extremely low with a parathyroidectomy and are not increased by use of MIP.

REFERENCES

1. Grant CS, Thompson G, Farley D, et al. Primary hyperparathyroidism surgical management since the introduction of minimally invasive parathyroidectomy: Mayo Clinic experience. *Arch Surg*. 2005;140(5):472-478; discussion 478-479.
2. James BC, Kaplan EL, Grogan RH, Angelos P. What's in a name? Providing clarity in the definition of minimally invasive parathyroidectomy. *World J Surg*. 2015;39(4):975-980.
3. Udelsman R, Lin Z, Donovan P. The superiority of minimally invasive parathyroidectomy based on 1650 consecutive patients with primary hyperparathyroidism. *Ann Surg*. 2011;253(3):585-591.
4. Kuntsman JW, Udelsman R. Superiority of minimally invasive parathyroidectomy. *Adv Surg*. 2012;46:171-180.
5. Applewhite MK, White MG, Tseng J, et al. Normohormonal primary hyperparathyroidism is a distinct form of primary hyperparathyroidism. *Surgery*. 2017;161(1):62-69.
6. Bilezikian JP, Khan AA, Potts JT Jr. Guidelines for the management of asymptomatic primary hyperparathyroidism: summary statement from the third international workshop. *J Clin Endocrinol Metab*. 2009;94(2):335.
7. Wilhelm SM, Wang TS, Ruan DT, et al. The American Association of Endocrine Surgeons guidelines for definitive management of primary hyperparathyroidism. *JAMA Surg*. 2016;151(10):959-968.
8. Siperstein A, Berber E, Mackey R, et al. Prospective evaluation of sestamibi scan, ultrasonography, and rapid PTH to predict the success of limited exploration for sporadic primary hyperparathyroidism. *Surgery*. 2004;136(4):872-880.
9. Chiu B, Sturgeon C, Angelos P. Which intraoperative parathyroid hormone assay criterion best predicts operative success? A study of 352 consecutive patients. *Arch Surg*. 2006;141:483-487.
10. McGill JF, Sturgeon C, Kaplan S, et al. How does the operative strategy for primary hyperparathyroidism impact the findings and cure rate? A comparison of 800 parathyroidectomies. *J Am Coll Surg*. 2008;207:246-249.
11. Zanocco K, Angelos P, Sturgeon C. Cost-effectiveness analysis of parathyroidectomy for asymptomatic primary hyperparathyroidism. *Surgery*. 2006;140:874-881; discussion 881-882.

Chapter **55**

Endoscopic Parathyroidectomy by Lateral Approach

Nunzia Cinzia Paladino, Frédéric Sebag, and Henry Jean François

DEFINITION

- A minimally invasive parathyroidectomy (MIP) may be defined as an operation requiring a small and discrete incision for a very direct access to the parathyroid glands, resulting in a focused dissection. MIP may be divided in two groups: open MIP performed under direct vision via a small cervical incision[1] and various endoscopic MIP performed partially or totally with the help of an endoscope.
- Today, three different types of endoscopic parathyroidectomies can be considered to be an option for surgeons:
  - (1) Video-assisted parathyroidectomy (MIVAP),[2] which is a mini-open procedure performed partially with the help of the endoscope.
  - (2) Endoscopic techniques using an extracervical approach. These techniques have the advantage of leaving no scar in the neck area but cannot reasonably be described as minimally invasive as they require more dissection than conventional open surgery. Among these extracervical approaches, the access to the parathyroid gland is obtained through the mouth, anterior chest wall, breast, or axilla with or without robotic assistance.[3] These techniques, such as transoral endoscopic parathyroidectomy vestibular approach (TOEPVA), have developed particularly in Asia for cultural reasons; TOEPVA is a parathyroidectomy performed through a 10-mm central incision in the lower lip's vestibule using laparoscopic instruments[4] (see Part 5, Chapter 50).
  - (3) Pure endoscopic techniques using a cervical access. These operations are performed totally with the help of the endoscope and include constant gas insufflation. Two pure endoscopic techniques have been described: the endoscopic parathyroidectomy by midline approach[5] and the endoscopic parathyroidectomy by lateral approach (EPLA).[6] EPLA develops the plane between the carotid sheath laterally and the strap muscles medially. This "back-door route" does not require complete dissection of the thyroid lobe from the strap muscles. It allows direct access to the posterior aspect of the thyroid lobe and does not require anterior and medial retraction of the thyroid lobe during the entire procedure.

DIFFERENTIAL DIAGNOSIS

- Today, the diagnosis of primary hyperparathyroidism can be made with near certainty by documenting an increased serum intact parathormone (iPTH) level in a patient with increased ionized or total calcium. It is therefore necessary to eliminate all other causes of hypercalcemia and iPTH elevation. As for iPTH elevation, renal dysfunction and vitamin D deficiency are well known. Among causes of hypercalcemia, thought should be given to the syndrome of benign familial hypocalciuric hypercalcemia, where the hypercalcemia is associated with normal or slightly raised levels of iPTH coexisting with hypocalciuria.

PATIENT HISTORY AND PHYSICAL FINDINGS

- The patient must be carefully selected. Not all patients presenting with HPT are candidates for an EPLA, as EPLA does not allow for a bilateral exploration.[7] Patients who are suspected to have multiglandular disease (MGD), including patients with secondary hyperparathyroidism (HPT) or patients with familial primary HPT, are not eligible for this procedure. Suspicion of parathyroid carcinoma is also an absolute contraindication. A history of neck irradiation, the presence of a large goiter, and previous surgery in the thyroid vicinity are relative contraindications. EPLA can be performed in patients who have previously undergone a contralateral neck operation (**TABLE 1**).
- When considering EPLA, the adenoma must be solitary and clearly localized by preoperative imaging studies. Whether preoperative localizations techniques can rule out MGD with sufficient accuracy is questionable. Therefore, as with other minimally invasive techniques, the risk of missing MGD justifies the use of a quick intraoperative parathormone assay (QPTH).[8] The less definitive the localizations studies, the more imperative the need for QPTH.
- When patients are selected on the basis of the abovementioned criteria, no more than 50% of patients are eligible for this procedure (**FIGURE 1**).
- EPLA is technically more challenging than standard cervical exploration, and its performance should be confined to tertiary centers. The surgeon must be experienced in conventional parathyroid surgery. Mentoring by a surgeon who has experience with endoscopic neck procedures is also recommended.

Table 1: Absolute and Relative Contraindications for Endoscopic Parathyroidectomy by Lateral Approach

Absolute contraindications
Suspicion of parathyroid carcinoma
Large goiter
Secondary or tertiary HPT
Familial HPT
Suspicion of MGD
No localization
Relative contraindications
Previous surgery
History of neck irradiation
Large tumor (>3 cm)
Inferior adenoma located anteriorly

HPT, hyperparathyroidism; MGD, multiglandular disease.

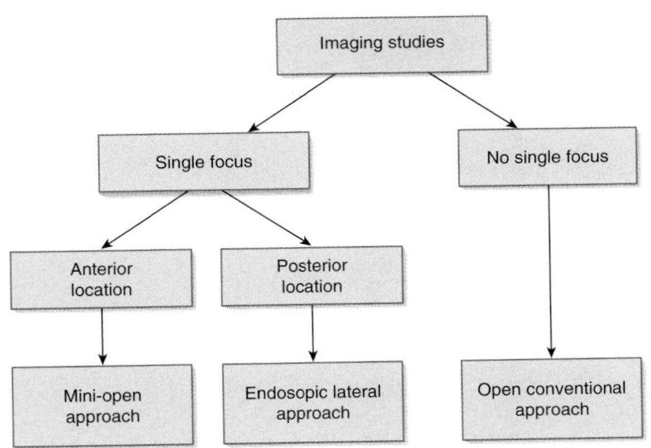

FIGURE 1 ● Algorithm for the surgical management of patients eligible for an endoscopic parathyroidectomy by lateral approach.

IMAGING AND OTHER DIAGNOSTIC STUDIES

- Only noninvasive tests should be considered. When these tests are negative, EPLA is not indicated and the traditional open cervicotomy is preferable. The topographic diagnosis should ideally be established by convergence of the results of two different investigations, one providing good anatomic information and the other providing functional information.
- High-resolution ultrasonography (US) and technetium-99m (Tc-99m) sestamibi scan are used most commonly in combination.[9] US can only assess the cervical region but gives good anatomic information, including useful information about the thyroid gland. The patient should be examined in the supine position with the neck in hyperextension. A pillow can be placed under the shoulders if the patient has a short neck. A high-frequency linear transducer (7.5-10 MHz) is used to obtain optimal depth penetration of 3 to 4 cm. A bilateral and comparative scan should be performed in transverse section, then in longitudinal section. In transverse section, the examination concentrates on an area defined by the longus colli muscles posteriorly, the thyroid gland anteriorly, the trachea medially, and the carotid artery laterally. The scan is then performed in cranial and caudal directions. An additional scan can be performed with the head of the patient turned away to the side and during deglutition to optimize the lateroesophageal images. The anterosuperior mediastinum is examined by inclining the transducer deeply in a retrosternal direction. The examiner should note the precise location with respect to surrounding structures, particularly to the thyroid gland, and the depth from the skin. Finally, a color flow Doppler or a power flow Doppler will be performed to test the vascularization of the area and define the artery branches involved.
- Mediastinal or posterior glands could be missed by US. Parathyroid scintigraphy has several advantages over US: it can detect major parathyroid ectopias, is more specific, and enables fusion of scintigraphic images with computed tomography for better resolution and localization.[10] Two protocols for sestamibi scanning can be used: the single isotope dual phase protocol and the subtraction protocol. The dual protocol requires early (15 minutes postinjection) and delayed images (at 1 and 2-3 hours, depending on thyroid washout). In cases of multinodular thyroid disease, additional further delayed images are sometimes needed. When a subtraction protocol is used, Tc-99m sestamibi is used in conjunction with another radionuclide specific to the thyroid. Tc-99m pertechnetate and ^{123}I are the most widely used radioisotopes for thyroid scintigraphy. The main advantage of using ^{123}I is that thyroid and parathyroid images can be acquired simultaneously in a dual energy window setup. The disadvantage is the cost of the protocol related to ^{123}I. Parathyroid scintigraphy should include views of the neck and the mediastinum. Single-photon emission computed tomography (SPECT) can be helpful for more precise localization of adenomas, as it provides simultaneous three-dimensional (3-D) information on both neck and superior mediastinum. The combination of ^{123}I/99mTc-sestamibi pinhole acquisition with subtraction and SPECT/CT offers the optimal information on parathyroid location and guides surgical strategy.[10]
- Instead of US and Tc-99m sestamibi scan, four-dimensional computed tomography (4D-CT)[11] or the use of computed axial tomography-methoxyisobutyl isonitrile (MIBI) image fusion,[12] when available, may be preferable.
- Recently 18F-fluorocholine PET/CT has gained an increased role in preoperative imaging workup of primary hyperparathyroidism, but its role is limited to situations with doubtful or discordant imaging findings.[13]
- Consideration for EPLA depends on the results of preoperative imaging. EPLA should be strongly considered when the parathyroid adenoma is in close proximity to the recurrent laryngeal nerve, as the nerve is at risk during MIP. Therefore, EPLA is the procedure of choice in all cases where the parathyroid adenomas are deeply located in the neck.
- Three locations of parathyroid adenomas with regard to the recurrent laryngeal nerve can be described (**FIGURE 2**).[6] Location 1 is posterior to the two superior thirds of the thyroid lobe (**FIGURES 3** and **4**). These adenomas are superior glands. Location 2 is at the level of or below the inferior pole of the thyroid lobe but in a plane posterior to it (**FIGURES 5** and **6**). These adenomas may be either a superior gland that has migrated posteriorly and in a downward direction or an inferior gland that has fallen posteriorly. These glands can also migrate into the superior and posterior mediastinum. Location 3 is at the level of or below the inferior pole of the thyroid lobe but in a superficial plane (**FIGURES 7** and **8**). These adenomas are always inferior glands and can be found in close contact with the tip of the inferior pole of the thyroid lobe and also along the thyrothymic ligament or into the superior pole of the thymus.
- Adenomas in locations 1 and 2 are deeply located and are in the vicinity of the recurrent laryngeal nerve. The nerve is at risk, and its clear identification during the procedure is recommended. The lateral view, provided by EPLA, permits its easy identification and allows a secure dissection. On the other hand, adenomas in location 3 are at distance from the nerve, which runs more deeply. Its identification is not essential. An anterior mini-open approach without the help of the endoscope is indicated.
- In conclusion, the need to know preoperatively when the nerve is at risk reinforces the role of preoperative imaging studies. Depending on whether the patient has a deep-seated

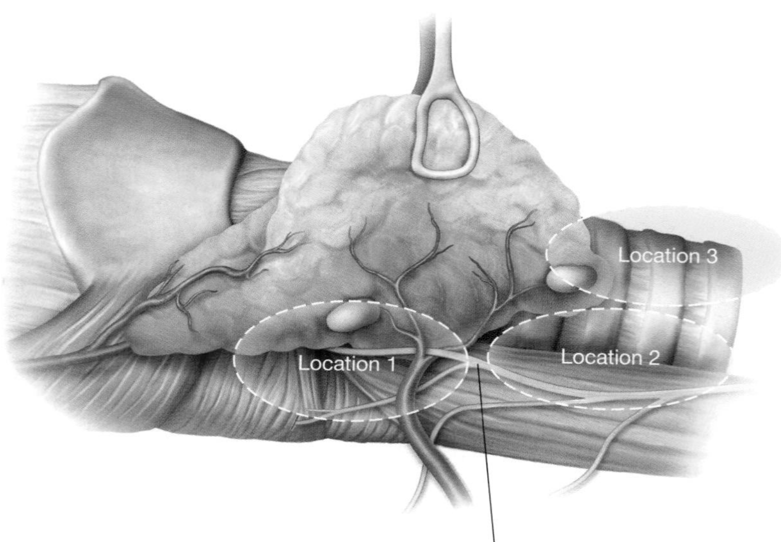

FIGURE 2 ● The three different locations of parathyroid adenomas with regard to the recurrent laryngeal nerve. Location 1, posterior to the two superior thirds of the thyroid lobe; location 2, at the level of or below the inferior pole of the thyroid lobe but in a plane posterior to it; location 3, at the level of or below the inferior pole of the thyroid lobe but in a superficial plane.

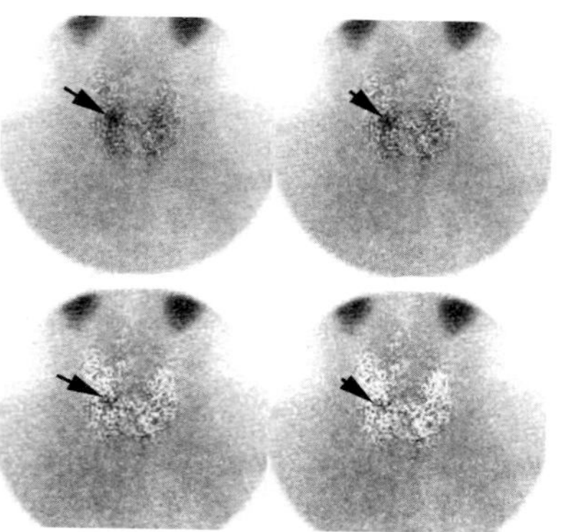

FIGURE 3 ● Parathyroid Tc-99m sestamibi scintigraphy; subtraction protocol. The subtraction image demonstrates a right parathyroid adenoma at the level of the middle third of the right thyroid lobe *(arrow)*.

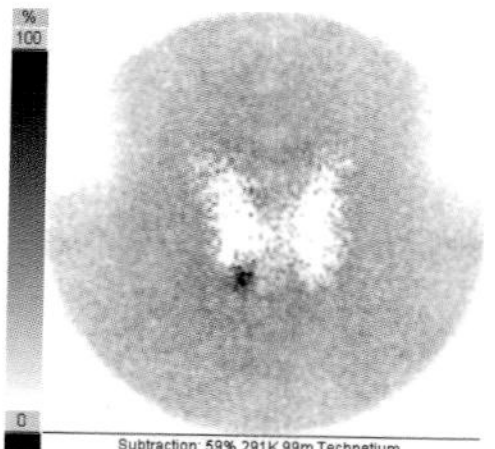

FIGURE 5 ● Parathyroid Tc-99m sestamibi scintigraphy; subtraction protocol. The subtraction image demonstrates a right parathyroid adenoma at the level of the inferior third of the right thyroid lobe.

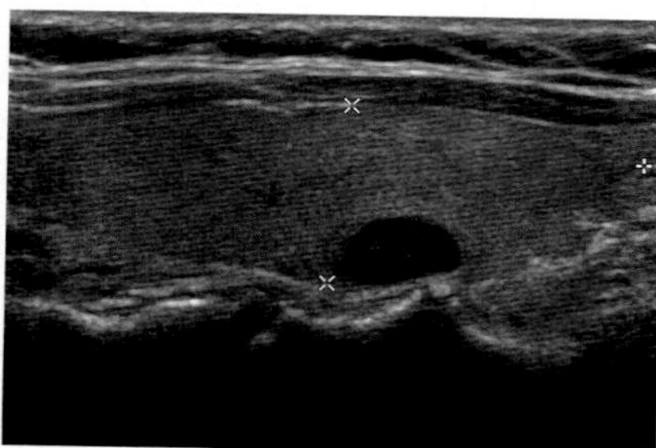

FIGURE 4 ● Ultrasound (same patient as in **FIGURE 3**). Right parathyroid adenoma posterior to the middle third of the thyroid lobe: right superior parathyroid adenoma in location 1. EPLA is indicated.

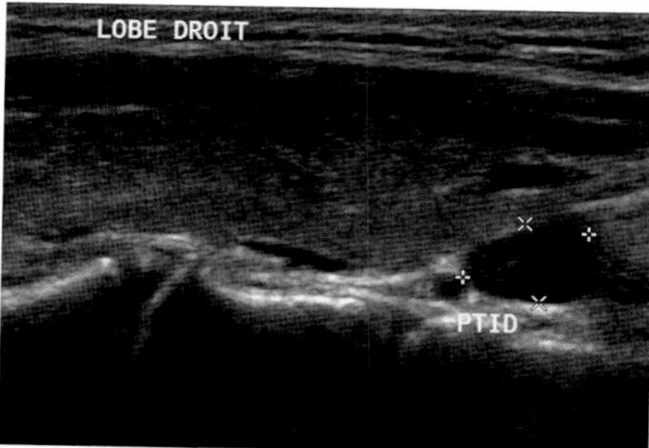

FIGURE 6 ● Ultrasound (same patient as in **FIGURE 5**). Right parathyroid adenoma posterior to the inferior third of the thyroid lobe: right, more probably inferior, parathyroid adenoma in location 2. EPLA is indicated.

adenoma or a superficial-seated adenoma, the surgeon can choose between EPLA and an anterior mini-open approach.

- The main interest of using an endoscope is not that one can perform a parathyroidectomy through a small incision but that one can perform a safe parathyroidectomy through a small incision.
- The interest of this approach is also the posterior mediastinum parathyroid ectopia that, although rare, would require a larger scar and more extensive dissection when performed by traditional techniques.[14]

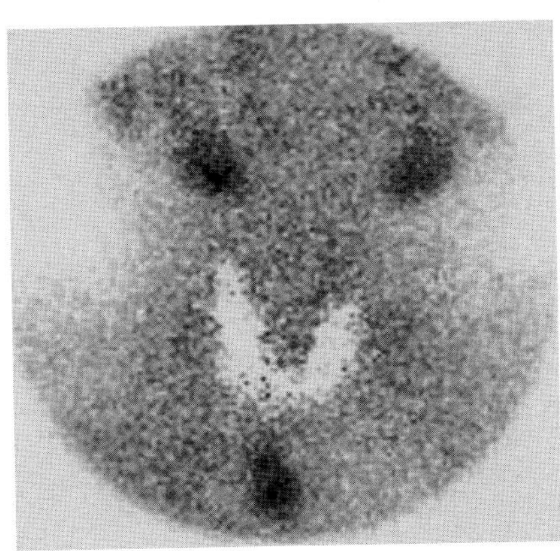

FIGURE 7 ● Parathyroid Tc-99m sestamibi scintigraphy; subtraction protocol. The subtraction image demonstrates a right parathyroid adenoma below the inferior pole of the thyroid lobe.

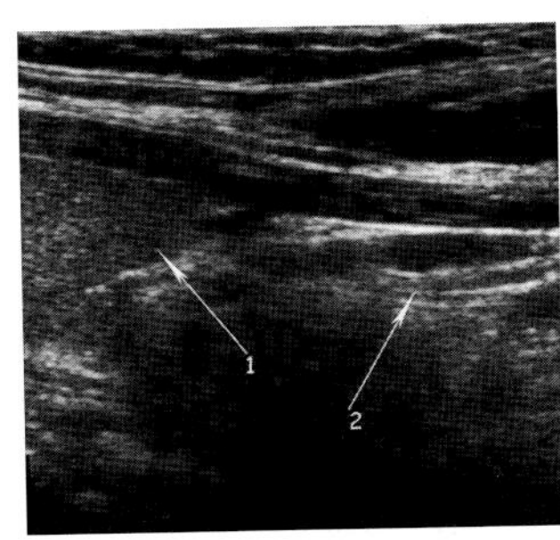

FIGURE 8 ● Ultrasound (same patient as in **FIGURE 7**). The adenoma *(2)* is in the superficial plane, below the inferior pole of the thyroid lobe *(1)*, along the thyrothymic tract: right inferior parathyroid adenoma in location 3. There is no need for the endoscope. A mini-open procedure is indicated.

SURGICAL MANAGEMENT

Preoperative Planning

- Prior to surgery, the patient undergoes a vocal cord check.
- The procedure is performed under general anesthesia with endotracheal intubation. Trocars are poorly tolerated by patients under local or regional anesthesia. In addition, swallowing and spontaneous breathing present impediments when dissecting in a small operative space.
- The surgical instruments required include a 10-mm trocar, which will accommodate a 0° fiberoptic endoscope, and two 3-mm trocars, which will receive a series of purpose-made instruments (Medtronic Xomed, MicroFrance) including blunt-tipped dissectors, graspers, scissors, a diathermy hook, and an aspiration canula. These instruments measure 25 cm in length (**FIGURE 9**).
- In patients presenting with small parathyroid adenomas less than 2 cm in diameter, a 5-mm trocar and a 5-mm 0° endoscope can be used.
- QPTH assays are performed before and at the time of incision, directly before parathyroid excision and, subsequently, 5 and 15 minutes after parathyroid excision. Parathyroidectomy is considered successful when QPTH value falls by greater than 50% with respect to the highest pre-excision level and into normal range (10-65 pg/mL).[7]
- The surgical team consists of the operator, first assistant, and a scrub nurse. The surgeon and first assistant stand on the side of the diseased gland, with the scrub nurse facing them.

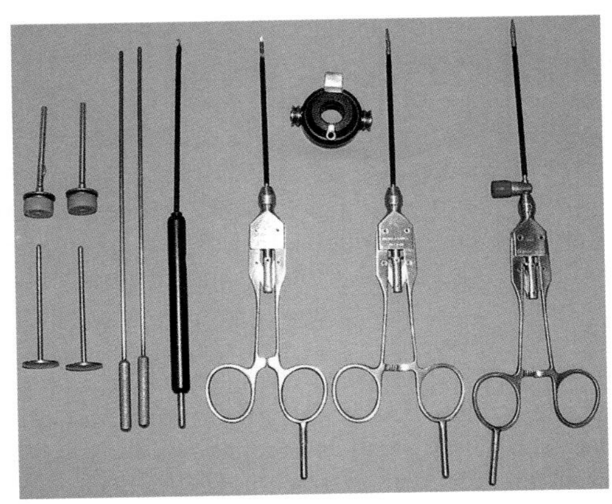

FIGURE 9 ● Instruments of 3-mm trocars (Medtronic Xomed, MicroFrance, Saint Aubin Le Monial, France).

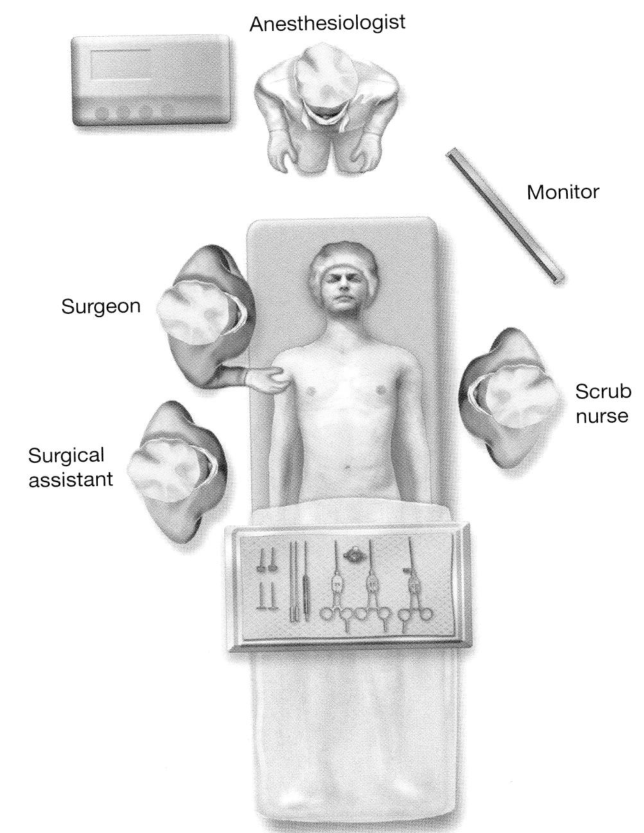

FIGURE 10 ● Operating room organization.

The monitor is placed next to the scrub nurse and directly in front of the surgeon (**FIGURE 10**).

Positioning

- The patient is positioned in the supine position. The head is placed in a neutral position without hyperextension to avoid tensing the sternocleidomastoid muscle (SCM) and the strap muscles. Complete relaxation and suppleness of these muscles are essential to prevent narrowing down the operative space given that this is maintained with low-pressure gas insufflation. The patient is prepped and draped as for standard parathyroid surgery.

THE BACK-DOOR APPROACH

- An initial 12- to 15-mm transverse skin incision (optic trocar incision) is made on the anterior border of the SCM, at the level of the thyroid isthmus (**FIGURE 11**). It will permit the creation of a space through which the 10-mm trocar will be introduced. This incision is placed such that, in the event of conversion, it can be extended medially to result in a symmetric collar incision.
- After division of the platysma, the anterior border of the SCM is identified and the investing layer of cervical fascia is incised. This allows access to the plane of dissection between the SCM laterally and the strap muscles medially, just inferior to the omohyoid muscle (**FIGURE 12**).
- The fascia connecting the posterior aspect of the thyroid lobe medially to the carotid sheath laterally is gently divided with scissors (**FIGURE 13**). A middle thyroid vein may be encountered. It is ligated without any difficulty through the incision.
- A small moist gauze is then inserted through the incision and packed deeply in an upward and downward direction into the initially created space (**FIGURE 14**). This blind maneuver enlarges the cavity and permits a surprisingly quick, efficient, and bloodless exposure of the operative field.

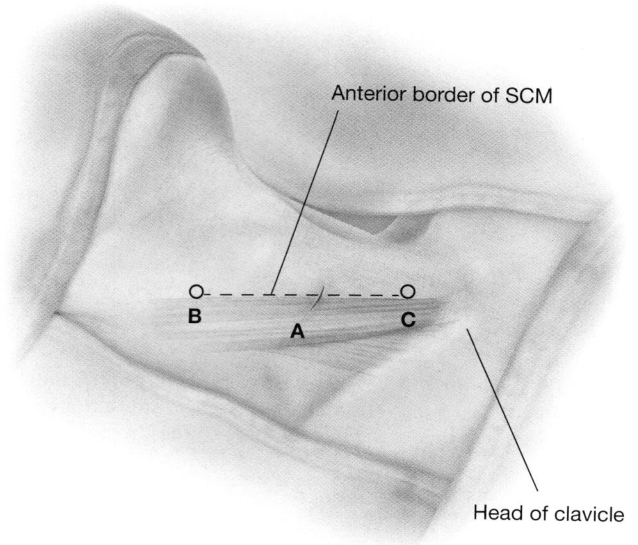

FIGURE 11 ● Trocar sites. All three trocars are positioned on the line of the anterior border of the SCM. The main trocar *(A)* is placed at the level of the thyroid isthmus. Trocars *B* and *C* should be 3 to 4 cm apart and will be used for the 2-mm instruments. SCM, sternocleidomastoid muscle.

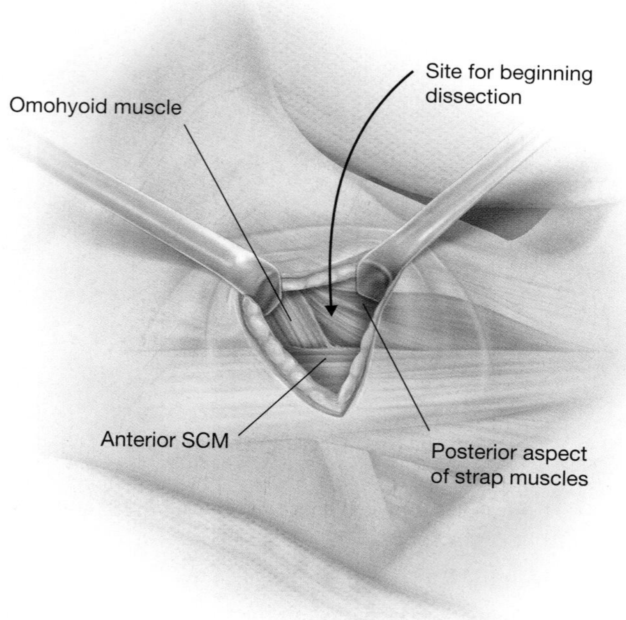

FIGURE 12 ● The access to the plane of dissection between the SCM laterally and the strap muscles medially is just inferior to the omohyoid muscle. SCM, sternocleidomastoid muscle.

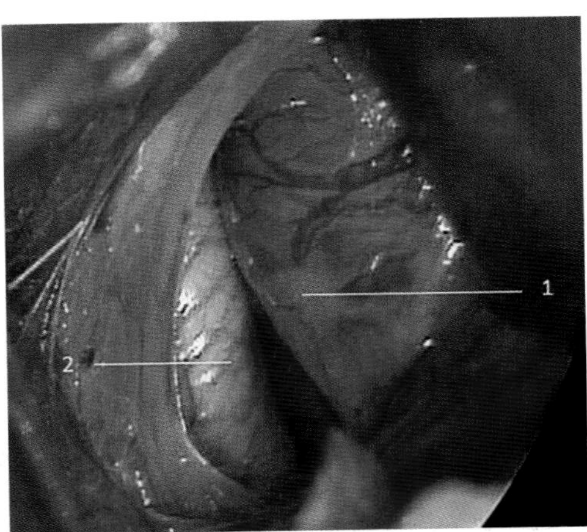

FIGURE 13 ● The back-door approach uses the plane between the posterior aspect of the thyroid lobe medially *(1)* to the carotid sheath laterally *(2)*.

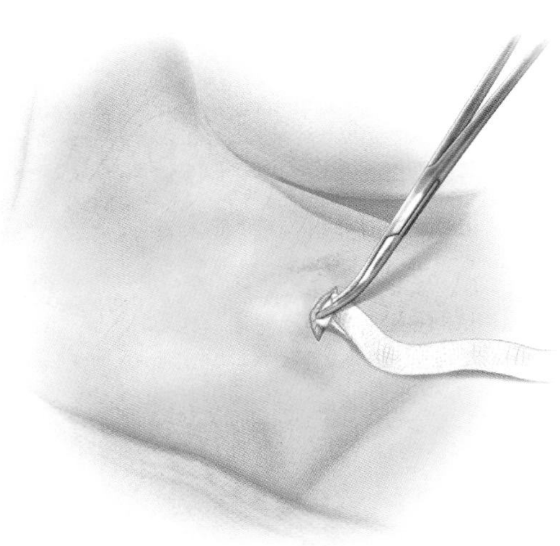

FIGURE 14 ● Creating space for endoscopic exploration. A small moist gauze roll is inserted through the incision and packed deeply into the initially created space.

INSTALLATION OF THE TWO 3-MM WORKING TROCARS (▶ VIDEO 1)

- The two 3-mm trocars are placed on the line situated along the anterior border of the SCM, in their respective positions, above (5-6 cm) and below (3-4 cm) the main optic trocar incision. Safe trocar placement is achieved by tunneling a 2.5-mm drain introducer needle inserted from within the main incision through to the skin. The direction this guide takes must follow the anterior border of the SCM. During this maneuver, one must constantly be aware of the internal jugular vein situated posteriorly, the external jugular vein situated cranially, and the anterior jugular vein situated caudally. The 3-mm trocar is placed over the tip of the introducer needle, which has pierced the skin from inside out and railroaded into the operative space (**FIGURE 15**). Each appropriately positioned 3-mm trocar is then loosely fixed to the skin with a nonabsorbable monofilament stitch to prevent involuntary removal.

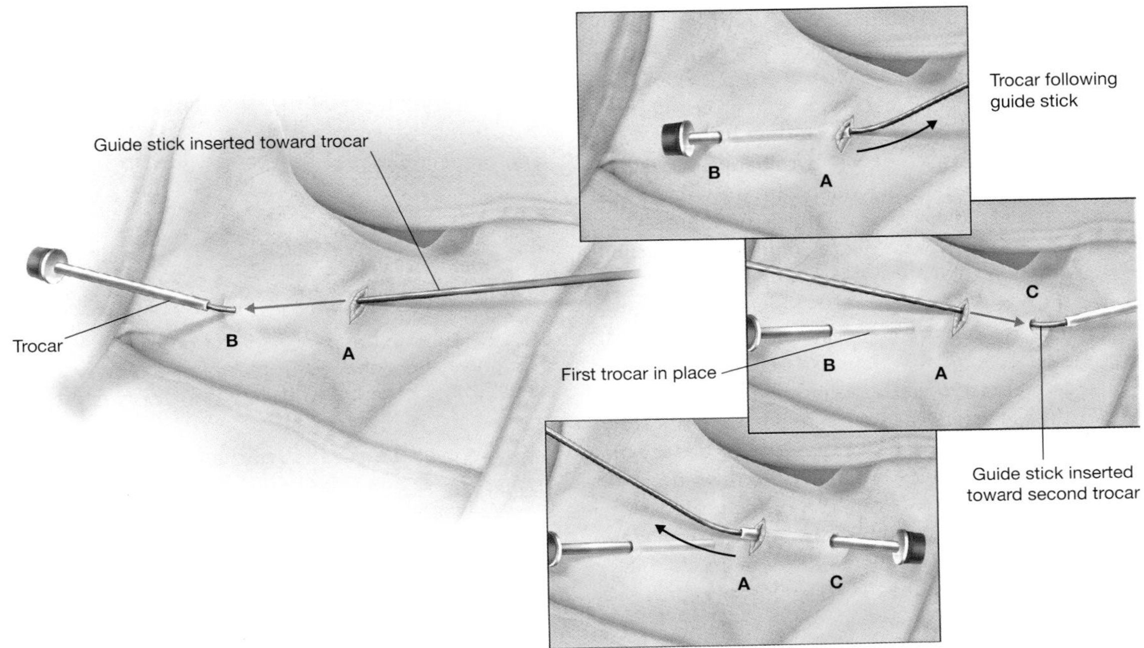

FIGURE 15 ● Installation of the 3-mm trocars. The transparietal path of both trocars is made through the incision *(A)*, from the inside to the outside, using a guide stick. The pathway of the guide stick must follow the anterior border of the SCM. Then, the 3-mm trocar is placed over the tip of the guide stick and railroaded into the operative space.

INSTALLATION OF THE 10-MM OPTIC TROCAR

- A purse-string stitch is placed around the main wound. It incorporates not only the skin but also the anterior border of the SCM laterally and the posterior border of the sternothyroid muscle medially. At this stage, the gauze roll is removed and the 10-mm trocar inserted and held in position with the purse-string suture.
- The purse string is subsequently threaded through an eyelet mounted on a specifically designed device encircling the trocar and secured to this (**FIGURE 16**). This arrangement guarantees air tightness, allows the amplification of the operative space, and prevents the trocar from slipping out of the wound.
- The three trocars are now positioned. The assistant takes care of the endoscope, and the surgeon works through the other two trocars (**FIGURE 17**).

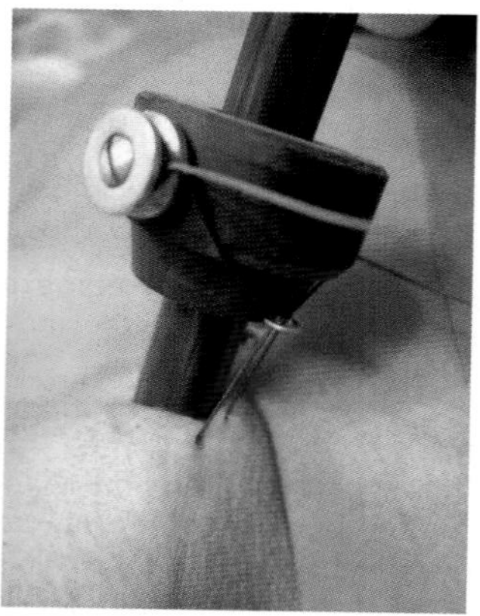

FIGURE 16 ● Installation of the main trocar. A purse-string stitch is placed around the main wound and is tied on a specifically designed device encircling the main trocar.

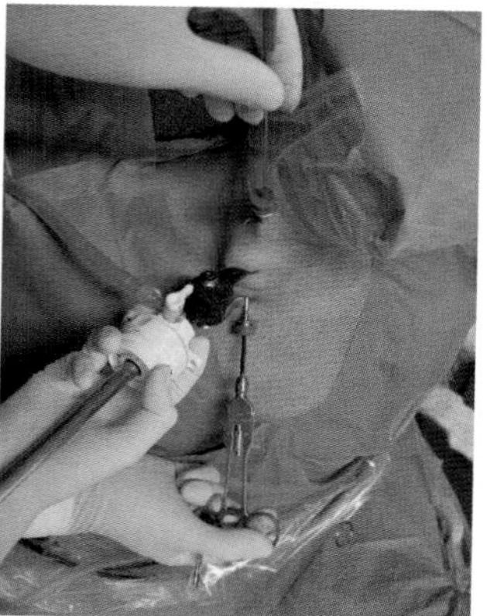

FIGURE 17 ● The three trocars are positioned. Insufflation (8 mm Hg) is installed. The assistant holds the camera, and the operator works through the other two 3-mm trocars. Endoscopic exploration can start.

ENDOSCOPIC PARATHYROID EXPLORATION

- A pneumocervicotomy is established using insufflation with carbon dioxide (CO_2) at low pressure (8 mm Hg). The gas not only maintains the working operative space but also may tamponade off minor bleeders. First, the carotid must be identified. Then, the space between the carotid laterally and the posterolateral aspect of the thyroid lobe medially is developed. The dissection is performed with the help of two blunt-tipped metallic dissectors. Ligatures or clip applications are not necessary. The combination of blunt dissection and gas insufflation allows easy separation of structures, minimizing the need for sharp dissection. This facilitates identification of the key structures and landmarks that will permit a safe dissection. The inferior thyroid artery and, of course, the recurrent laryngeal nerve must be identified first. The inferior thyroid artery is a useful landmark for locating the recurrent laryngeal nerve. The easiest site to identify the nerve is at the level of the lower pole of the thyroid gland, just caudally to the trunk of the artery. On the left side, the nerve ascends at the depth of the tracheoesophageal groove. On the right side, the nerve courses more obliquely. The magnification allowed by the endoscope provides improved visualization of the vasa nervorum running along the nerve and helps its identification.
- Very often one can observe that the nerve branches far below its laryngeal entry point (**FIGURE 18**). Also, small extralaryngeal branches extending to the adjacent trachea and esophagus are easily seen.

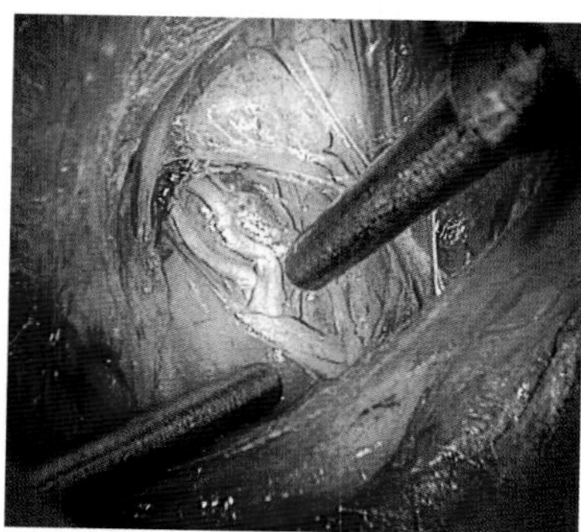

FIGURE 18 ● Endoscopic exploration on the right side: identification of the right recurrent laryngeal nerve. In this case, the nerve branches far below its laryngeal entry point.

IDENTIFICATION OF THE PARATHYROID ADENOMA

- Based on the results of the preoperative imaging studies, the surgeon may suspect an adenoma in location 1 or 2.
- All glands in location 1 are superior parathyroid adenomas. The search for them requires the dissection of the upper two-thirds of posterior aspect of the thyroid lobe (**FIGURE 19**). Small superior adenomas usually remain located in their orthotopic site, floating in a loose, fatty setting immediately adjacent to the inferior thyroid artery. Large superior adenomas tend to migrate posteriorly and downward. Therefore, if they are not found in immediate contact with the thyroid capsule, they should be sought beside or behind the esophagus.
- Glands in location 2 may be also superior parathyroid adenomas. Their migration may drag them down very low, well below the inferior thyroid artery, behind whose trunk they cross during their descent. Endoscopic exploration behind the inferior thyroid artery, along the esophagus, and down into the posterior mediastinum can be easily accomplished by this back-door approach. These adenomas are revealed by their vascular pedicle, which is easily dissected at the level of the inferior thyroid artery. They emerge with simple traction on it, and their elongated shape is amenable to expeditious extraction.
- The search of inferior parathyroid adenomas in location 2 requires the exploration of the lower third of the posterior aspect of the thyroid lobe. Sometimes, they are identified immediately after introducing the endoscope. They tend to descend posteriorly and in a downward direction to acquire a paratracheal or a paraesophageal position. It is in these cases that they become intimate with the recurrent laryngeal nerve. Their posterior surface may adhere to the nerve. In these cases, the lateral view allows a secure dissection of the nerve.
- Although searching for the ipsilateral gland is not mandatory, it can often be identified when it is in location 1 or 2 (**FIGURE 20**).

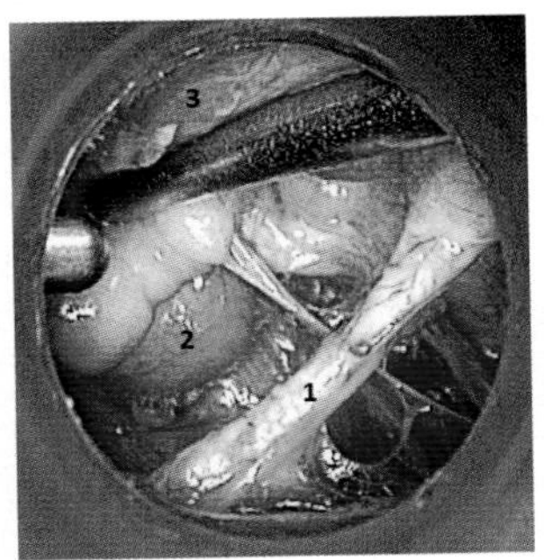

FIGURE 19 ● Endoscopic exploration on the right side: inferior thyroid artery *(1)*, superior parathyroid adenoma *(2)* posterior to the middle third of the thyroid lobe *(3)*. The adenoma is located in location 1.

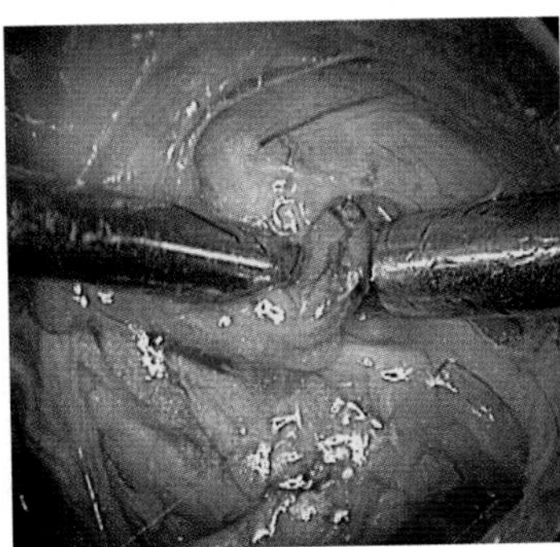

FIGURE 20 ● Identification of the ipsilateral inferior parathyroid gland. The gland is normal.

DISSECTION OF THE PARATHYROID ADENOMA

- The adenoma must never be grasped to avoid parathyroid fracture and potential risk of parathyromatosis. The adenoma is progressively freed from adjacent structures by blunt dissection with the help of two blunt-tipped metallic dissectors (**FIGURE 21**). One dissector retracts the adenoma, providing tension, while the other instrument is used to dissect the gland away from surrounding structures and loose areolar tissue until complete mobilization is achieved. When the pedicle is isolated (**FIGURE 22**), the terminal vascular branches are grasped, skeletonized, and electrocoagulated with the 3-mm diathermy hook (**FIGURE 23**).

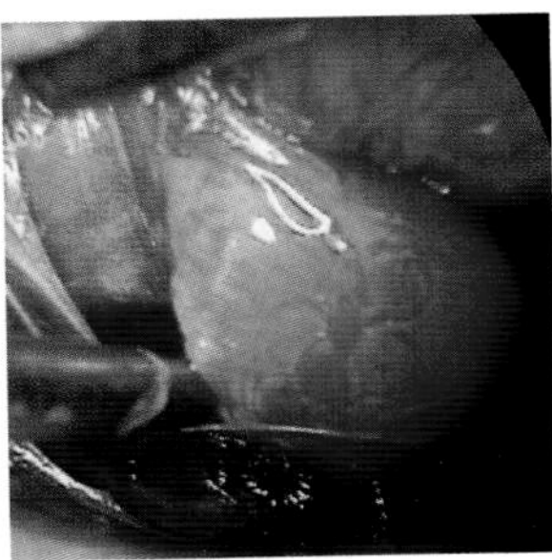

FIGURE 21 ● Endoscopic dissection of the superior parathyroid adenoma with the help of two blunt-tipped dissectors. The gland should not be grasped to avoid capsular disruption.

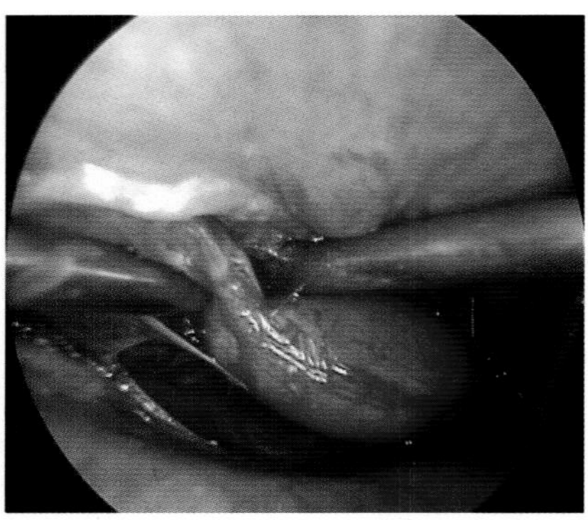

FIGURE 22 ● Dissection of the vascular pedicle of the superior parathyroid adenoma.

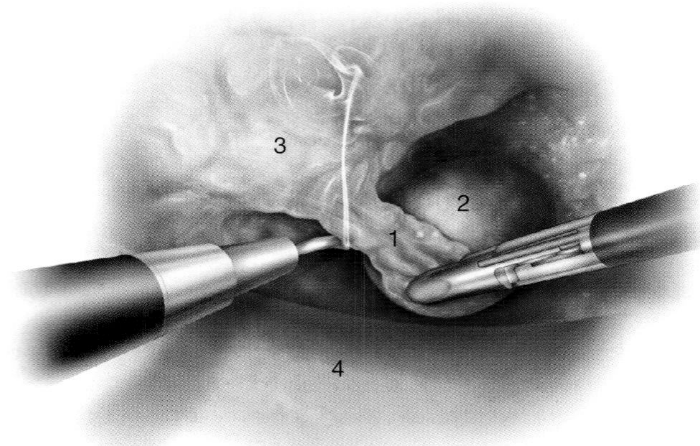

FIGURE 23 ● Electrocoagulation of the terminal vascular branches *(1)* of the superior parathyroid adenoma *(2)* with the 3-mm diathermy hook. *3*, Thyroid lobe; *4*, carotid artery.

EXTRACTION OF THE PARATHYROID ADENOMA

- Most parathyroid adenomas can be extracted through the 10-mm trocar. In performing this step, after removing the 10-mm endoscope, a grasper and a 5-mm lens are simultaneously introduced into the 10-mm trocar. The pedicle of the adenoma is grasped and the adenoma is drawn into the trocar (**FIGURE 24**); the trocar containing the specimen is then removed.
- Larger adenomas that cannot be drawn into the 10-mm trocar are extracted directly through the trocar site under direct vision. There is no need to place them in a sterile plastic bag during this maneuver. After checking hemostasis, the two 3-mm trocars are removed.

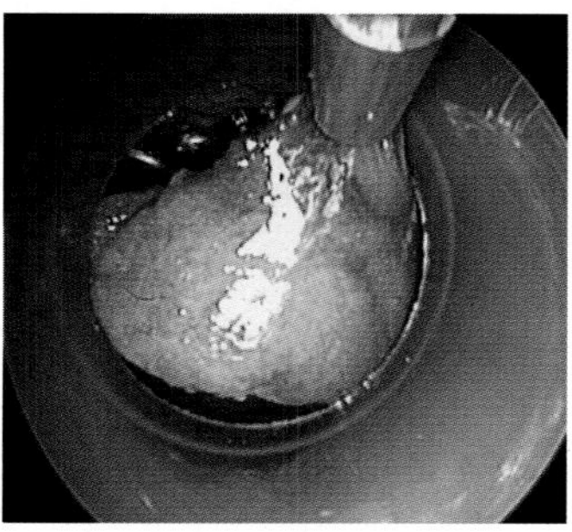

FIGURE 24 ● Extraction of the parathyroid adenoma. The pedicle of the adenoma is grasped and the adenoma is drawn into the trocar.

CLOSURE

- A surgical drain is not necessary. The platysma is sutured. The skin incision and the two 3-mm trocars sites are closed with fibrin glue (**FIGURE 25**). No dressing is required.

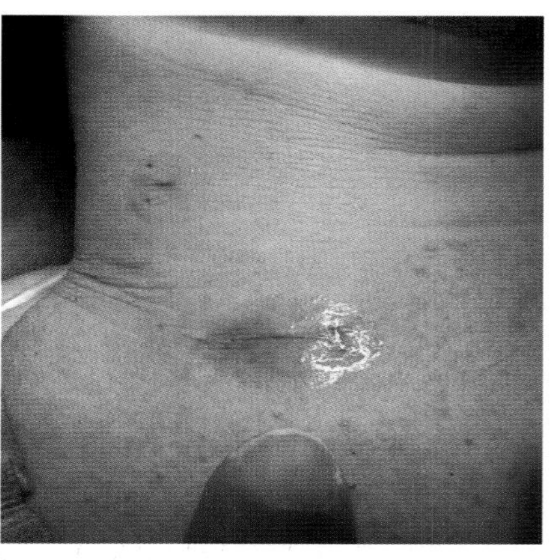

FIGURE 25 ● Fibrin glue is used to close the skin.

PEARLS AND PITFALLS

Indications	■ Only patients with sporadic primary HPT, in whom a single adenoma has been clearly localized by preoperative imaging studies, are potential candidates for EPLA. ■ Based on the results of preoperative imaging studies, EPLA should be reserved for patients presenting with parathyroid adenomas deeply located in the neck.
QPTH assay	■ The availability of the QPTH assay is of utmost importance. This test is especially useful when localization studies are less certain.
Installation of trocars	■ Place all three trocars on the line of the anterior border of the SCM and fix them to the skin to prevent involuntary removal. ■ Optic trocar incision should be created such that, in the event of conversion, it can be extended medially to result in a traditional cervicotomy. ■ The transparietal path of the working trocars should be made through the optic trocar incision, from the inside to the outside.
Working space	■ Place the head in a neutral position to avoid tensing the SCM and the strap muscles. ■ In order to enlarge the working area, before introducing the optic trocar, stuff a small moist gauze, upward and downward, deeply into the initially created space, and then remove it.
Endoscopic exploration	■ Bear in mind that, because the working space is very small, the endoscope is very close to the anatomic structures, which will therefore appear highly magnified. There is a definite risk of removing a normal gland that appears enlarged under endoscopic vision.
Endoscopic dissection	■ Never grasp the adenoma to avoid parathyroid fracture. The dissection can be performed entirely with the two blunt-tipped palpators.

POSTOPERATIVE CARE

- The patient may remain in the operating room or, in case of long processing for the QPTH assay, may be transferred to the postanesthesia care unit after extubation. In this latter case, if the results of QPTH are not consistent with successful removal of parathyroid adenoma, the patient must be returned to the operating room. In both cases, conversion to bilateral neck exploration is performed if the QPTH value does not fall by greater than 50% and into normal range (10-65 pg/mL).
- Patients have determination of serum parathyroid hormone (PTH) 4 hours after excision of the adenoma, then on day 1 and day 8 after surgery. Calcemia and phosphoremia are also systematically evaluated on day 1 and day 8.
- The serum PTH level reaches its nadir 4 hours after excision of the adenoma and, in most patients, the serum calcium reaches its lowest level within 48 to 72 hours after surgery. Because the parathyroid exploration is unilateral, postoperative hypoparathyroidism is not observed. However, postoperative hypocalcemia can be observed in patients with severe skeletal depletion of calcium, resulting in "bone hunger." If symptoms appear, calcium and vitamin D derivatives should be administrated.
- Usually, patients are discharged the day after surgery.
- Postoperative vocal cord evaluation must be performed systematically.

OUTCOMES

- After EPLA, more than 95% of patients are normocalcemic. However, it should be kept in mind that these excellent results are obtained in a group of carefully selected patients.[6]
- EPLA does not appear to be clearly superior to other MIP techniques in terms of recurrent disease or postoperative complications.[15]
- As with other techniques of single-gland excision through a limited neck exploration, EPLA does not lead to an increased incidence of persistent/recurrent HPT[15]; it is associated with a better postoperative course in terms of pain and produces better cosmetic results compared with bilateral neck exploration[16] (**FIGURE 26**). Prevalence and severity of postoperative hypocalcemia are lowered.[17]
- EPLA is feasible and reproducible by surgeons with specific skills in parathyroid surgery, allows one to obtain results comparable with those of the classical open surgery[18]

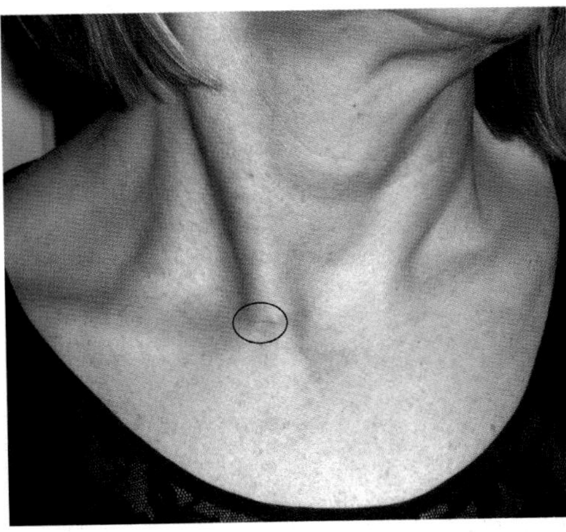

FIGURE 26 ● Cervical scar 1 month after surgery.

with minimal tissue dissection, and is associated with less postoperative pain and a higher level of patient satisfaction. The scar is smaller than in open techniques; it is also widely appreciated[19] and does not compromise a possible reintervention. Today, this technique is beginning to be less widely used in favor of open minimally invasive focused approaches, although these require a more extensive dissection. However, EPLA remains a safe approach whose best results are achieved when the procedure is performed by experienced surgeons.

COMPLICATIONS

- Hematoma
- Inferior laryngeal nerve injury
- Parathyroid adenoma not found: conversion
- Capsular rupture of adenoma
- False-positive result of preoperative imaging studies
- False-negative result of QPTH assay

REFERENCES

1. Udelsman R, Donovan PI, Sokoll LJ. One hundred consecutive minimally invasive parathyroid explorations. *Ann Surg.* 2000;232:331-339.
2. Miccoli P, Bendinelli C, Vignali E, et al. Endoscopic parathyroidectomy: report of an initial experience. *Surgery.* 1998;124:1077-1080.
3. Ohgami M, Ishii S, Arisawa Y, et al. Scarless endosocpic thyroidectomy: breast approach for better cosmesis. *Surg Laparosc Endosc Percutan Tech.* 2000;10(1):1-4.
4. Bhandarwar A, Gala J, Arora E, et al. Endoscopic parathyroidectomy: a retrospective review of 27 cases. *Surg Endosc.* 2021;35(3):1288-1295.
5. Gagner M, Rubino F. Endoscopic parathyroidectomy. In: Schwartz AE, Pertsemlidis D, Gagner M, eds. *Endocrine Surgery.* Marcel Dekker; 2004:289-296.
6. Henry JF, Sebag F, Cherenko M, et al. Endoscopic parathyroidectomy: why and when? *World J Surg.* 2008;32:2509-2515.
7. Mihai R, Barczynski M, Iacobone M, et al. Surgical strategy for sporadic primary hyperparathyroidism: an evidence-based approach to surgical strategy, patient selection, surgical access, and reoperations. *Langenbeck's Arch Surg.* 2009;394:785-798.
8. Harrison BJ, Triponez F. Intraoperative adjuncts in surgery for primary hyperparathyroidism. *Langenbeck's Arch Surg.* 2009;394:799-809.
9. Mihai R, Simon D, Hellman P. Imaging for primary hyperparathyroidism: an evidence-based analysis. *Langenbeck's Arch Surg.* 2009;394:765-784.
10. Asseeva P, Paladino NC, Guerin C, et al. Value of 123 I/99m Tc-sestamibi parathyroid scintigraphy with subtraction SPECT/CT in primary hyperparathyroidism for directing minimally invasive parathyroidectomy. *Am J Surg.* 2019;217(1):108-113.
11. Rodgers SE, Hunter GJ, Hamberg LM. Improved preoperative planning for directed parathyroidectomy with 4-dimensional computed tomography. *Surgery.* 2006;140:932-941.
12. Profanter C, Prommegger R, Gabriel M, et al. Computer axial tomography-MIBI image fusion for preoperative localization in primary hyperparathyroidism. *Am J Surg.* 2004;187:383-387.
13. Quak E, Blanchard D, Houdu B, et al. F18-choline PET/CT guided surgery in primary hyperparathyroidism when ultrasound and MIBI SPECT/CT are negative or inconclusive: the APACH1 study. *Eur J Nucl Med Mol Imaging.* 2018;45(4):658-666.
14. Martos-Martínez JM, Sacristán-Pérez C, Pérez-Andrés M, María Durán-Muñoz-Cruzado V, Pino-Díaz V, Padillo-Ruiz FJ. Prevertebral cervical approach: a pure endoscopic surgical technique for posterior mediastinum parathyroid adenomas. *Surg Endosc.* 2017;31(4):1930-1935.
15. Bergenfelz OA, Hellman P, Harrison B, et al. Positional statement of the European Society of Endocrine Surgery on modern techniques in pHPT surgery. *Langenbeck's Arch Surg.* 2009;394:761-764.
16. Henry JF, Raffaeli M, Iacobone M, et al. Video-assisted parathyroidectomy via the lateral approach vs conventional surgery in the treatment of sporadic primary hyperparathyroidism. *Surg Endosc.* 2001;15:1116-1119.
17. Westerdalh J, Bergenfelz A. Unilateral versus bilateral neck exploration for primary hyperparathyroidism: five-year follow-up of a randomized controlled trial. *Ann Surg.* 2007;246:976-980.
18. Vidal-Pérez O, Valentini M, Baanante-Cerdeña JC, Ginestà-Martí C, Fernández-Cruz L, García-Valdecasas JC. Endoscopic lateral parathyroidectomy as surgical treatment for patients with primary hyperparathyroidism. *Cir Cir.* 2016;84(1):15-20.
19. Baudouin R, Simon F, Denoyelle F, Couloigner V, Irtan S. Lateral endoscopic parathyroidectomy in children. *Eur Ann Otorhinolaryngol Head Neck Dis.* 2021;138(2):103-106.

Chapter 56 Reoperative Parathyroidectomy

Barnard J. A. Palmer and William B. Inabnet III

DEFINITIONS

- Reoperative parathyroid surgery occurs in multiple clinical settings but is most frequently performed as the result of failed exploration, recurrent or persistent hyperparathyroidism.
- Persistent hyperparathyroidism is defined as hypercalcemia that remains or recurs within 6 months of an initial parathyroid operation.
- Recurrent hyperparathyroidism is the reappearance of hypercalcemia after a period of 6 months of postoperative normocalcemia following successful surgery.
- Patients undergoing reoperative surgery carry additional complexities and require significant preoperative planning prior to exploration.

PATIENT HISTORY AND PHYSICAL FINDINGS

- A detailed history of the patient's disease should be performed, focusing on the management to date. Patients with familial disease are more likely to have multigland disease.
- Biochemical confirmation of persistent or recurrent hyperparathyroidism is the initial step in management. A 24-hour collection for calcium is recommended.[1,2]
- The benefits of reoperation must be weighed against the risks of continued hyperparathyroidism and the surgical complications for each individual patient. Nonsurgical management can be considered if the sequela of continued parathyroid disease is relatively low risk or the risk of operation is high.
- Surgical history is an essential component of reoperative parathyroid surgery. The surgeon must understand reasons for initial operative failure, which include unidentified, ectopic, or supernumerary glands and multigland disease.[3]
- Operative and pathology reports should be carefully reviewed, focusing on the extent of exploration, glands identified and removed, whether confirmed by biopsy, if marked, and if reimplanted.

IMAGING AND OTHER DIAGNOSTIC STUDIES

- Extensive preoperative planning is key to successful reoperative surgery.
- Previous operative reports, imaging, and pathology results should be obtained and reviewed to understand the cause of failure.[2]
- Localization studies are an essential portion of preoperative planning and should be performed in all reoperative parathyroid patients. Ultrasound, sestamibi, computed tomography (CT) (parathyroid protocol, 4-D) (**FIGURE 1**), single-photon emission computed tomography, and fluorodeoxyglucose-positron emission tomography can be used for localization and to rule out multigland disease. Preoperative location of abnormal glands can significantly alter the operative approach particularly if aberrant glands lie in the mediastinum.
- Fine needle aspiration with measurement of parathyroid hormone (PTH) can confirm parathyroid tissue in questionable lesions or parathyroid adenomatosis identified by ultrasound.
- Invasive localization studies such as selective venous sampling (**FIGURE 2**) or arteriography can be useful when noninvasive localizing studies are indeterminate.[4]

SURGICAL MANAGEMENT

Preoperative Planning

- The imaging must be thoroughly reviewed to plan the operative approach.
- Prior operative notes are reviewed, and a map of the neck is created. The operative plan and steps must be determined prior to reexploration.
- Positively localized lesions lend themselves to focused reexplorations, whereas more extensive exploration is required for multigland or nonlocalized diseases. Reexplorations for

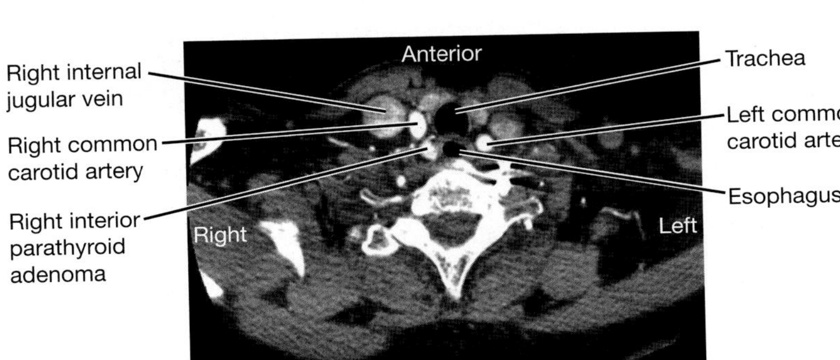

FIGURE 1 ● 4-D Parathyroid CT demonstrates a contrast-enhancing lesion posterior to the right common carotid artery, posterolateral to the trachea, and lateral to the esophagus, representing a right inferior parathyroid adenoma.

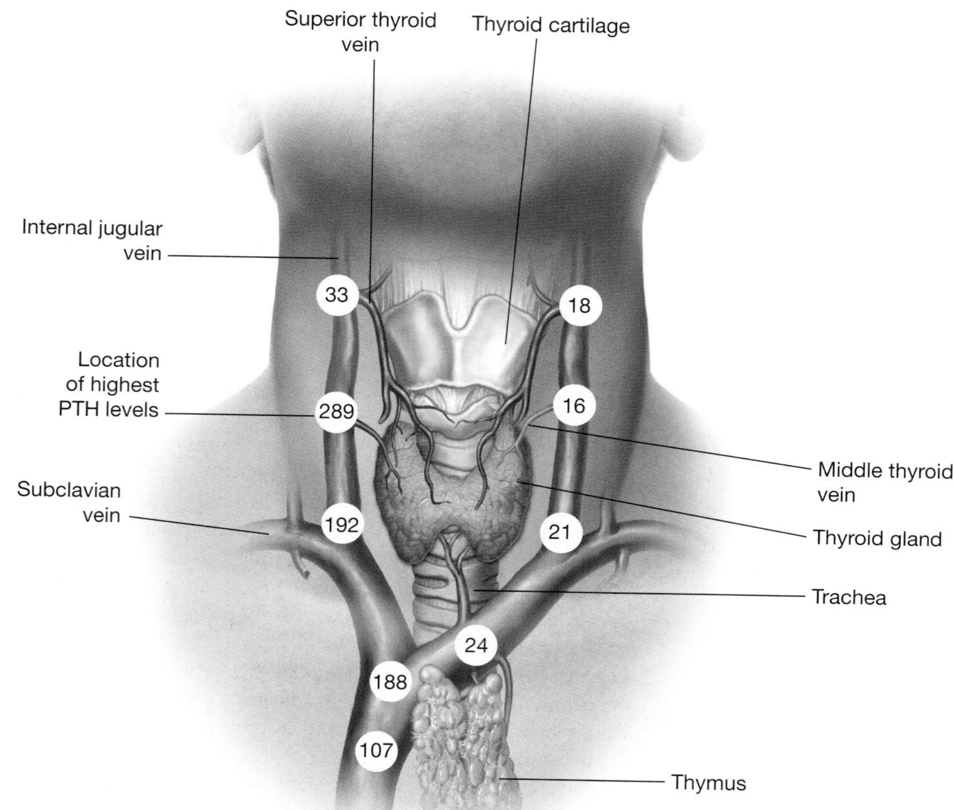

FIGURE 2 ● Selective venous sampling schematic lists PTH levels at different anatomic locations and is consistent with a right midlobe parathyroid adenoma.

nonlocalized lesions should only be performed when the need for cure is compelling.

- Preoperative flexible laryngoscopy is recommended prior to reoperative surgery to document vocal cord function and guide the extent of surgery.
- Frozen section and intraoperative PTH assays are useful adjuncts to confirm parathyroid identification and biochemical cure.

Positioning

- The patient is positioned supine or in the semi-Fowler position. Both arms are tucked and neck extension is achieved with a shoulder roll (**FIGURE 3**).
- General endotracheal anesthesia permits the use of intraoperative nerve monitoring.
- Draping that allows the surgeon to stand at the head facilitates dissection in the craniocaudal direction when accessing the inferior neck and superior mediastinum.
- Surgical prep must be wide enough to allow access superiorly to angle of mandible and inferiorly to xiphoid in the instance that sternotomy is necessary.

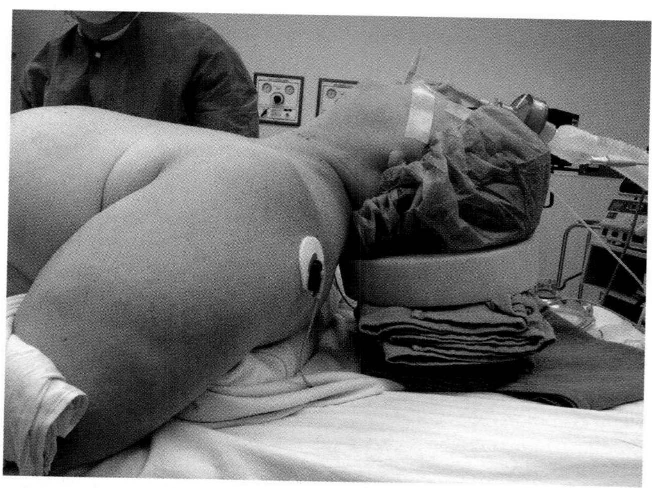

FIGURE 3 ● The patient is placed supine with both arms tucked. A shoulder roll provides additional neck extension, which elevates the trachea anteriorly and superior mediastinal structures cephalad.

CERVICAL REEXPLORATION

Incision and Flap Elevation

- Skin incisions are placed as indicated by the preoperative localizing studies, preferably in a natural cervical skin crease or the old incision unless the scar is too superior or inferior. Width of incision is dependent on depth of neck and extent of dissection but is large enough to allow access superiorly to the level of the hyoid bone and inferiorly to the anterior mediastinum (**FIGURE 4**).
- Skin and platysma are divided, and subplatysmal flaps superficial to the anterior jugular veins are elevated superiorly to the thyroid notch, inferiorly to the sternal notch, and laterally to anterior borders of the sternocleidomastoid muscles (SCMs).
- Limited incisions may be placed over the site of pathology for a directed approach if preoperatively localized.

Cervical Approach[3]

- Surgical approach to the reoperative neck is done via focused exploration or by classic midline, posterolateral, or thyrothymic ligament approaches.
- Focused explorations for preoperatively localized ectopic glands not accessible via prior cervicotomy should be adjusted to location and surgeon experience with incisions placed according to imaging.
- Revision cervicotomy is indicated when multigland disease is suspected or when abnormal glands are not localized preoperatively. The previous incision is used and the cervical scar revised prior to opening the midline raphe by vertical separation of strap muscles.

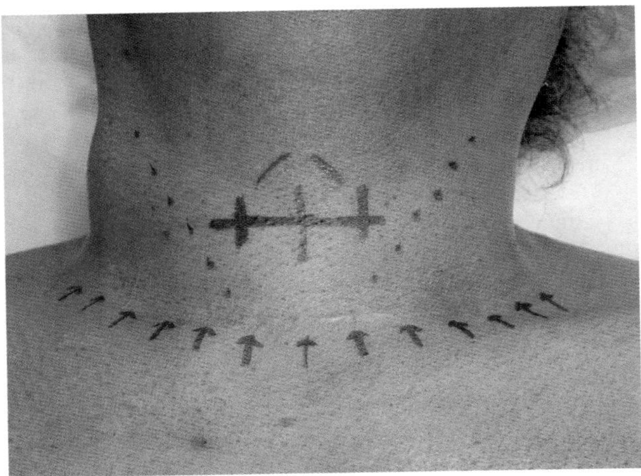

FIGURE 4 ● Skin incisions are placed in a natural skin crease and are adjusted according to preoperative localization and planned approach. Classic, large, inferior incisions have been substituted by more superior smaller incisions or incisions directly over parathyroid lesions. Lateral incisions can be made for a posterolateral approach with entry between the anterior border of the sternocleidomastoid and lateral border of the strap muscles. *Upward arrows* on the pictures show a classic incision vs a small superior incision as indicated by the *solid transverse line markings*.

- The ***posterolateral*** approach should be considered when there is extensive scar tissue or when seeking a posteriorly localized gland. The lateral portion of a prior wound is used and entry to the neck is achieved between the lateral aspect of the straps and medial border of the SCM (**FIGURE 5**).
- The ***thyrothymic*** ligament approach should be considered when adenomas are localized anteriorly along the inferior thyroid pole or thyrothymic ligament. Infrahyoid muscles may be divided as inferiorly as possible to allow direct access to the thyrothymic ligaments, avoiding dissection between the strap muscles and thyroid capsule.
- Once deep to the strap muscles, retraction of the thyroid involves elevation of the strap muscles off the gland and medial thyroid rotation. A Kittner, thyroid clamp, or figure-of-eight suture assists thyroid retraction.
- The recurrent laryngeal nerve (RLN) is then identified and preserved.

Exploration

- Based on preoperative imaging, steps are systematically planned including initiation and extent of exploration.
- If an abnormal gland is localized preoperatively, commence with focused exploration.
- Start by exploring the normal locations of the missing glands. The superior glands are generally at the mid to upper one-third of the thyroid in the expected position 85% of the time, at the inferior border of the thyroid cartilage posterior to the RLN and the superior portion of the inferior thyroid artery.
- The inferior glands are classically located near the posterior aspect of the thyroid pole, anterior to the RLN from the inferior thyroid artery to the inferior thyroid pole or along the thyrothymic ligament.
- If unable to locate in normal positions, search expected aberrant positions.
- Ectopic superior glands are generally displaced posteriorly or inferiorly, becoming more posterior as they travel inferiorly.
- Search circumferentially around the superior thyroid pedicle and visceral sheath of the thyroid capsule with thyroid palpation.
- Follow the tracheoesophageal groove inferiorly down to the posterior mediastinum (**FIGURE 6**).
- Inferior glands have a greater range of position but nearly 25% are along the thyrothymic ligament or upper pole of the thymus. They are rarely posterior and become more anterior the lower they are.
- Search and digitally explore the posterior and inferior thyroid gland.
- Inspect the thyrothymic ligament, incise the thymic sheath, and pull the thymic lobe cephalad to inspect the thymus (see **FIGURE 8**).
- Explore the carotid sheath up to the angle of the mandible (**FIGURE 7**).

Gland Identification and Excision

- Normal parathyroids are approximately 3 × 2 × 4 mm and tan in appearance.
- Parathyroid confirmation can be achieved through histologic examination. Biopsy of the antihilar tip of the gland using

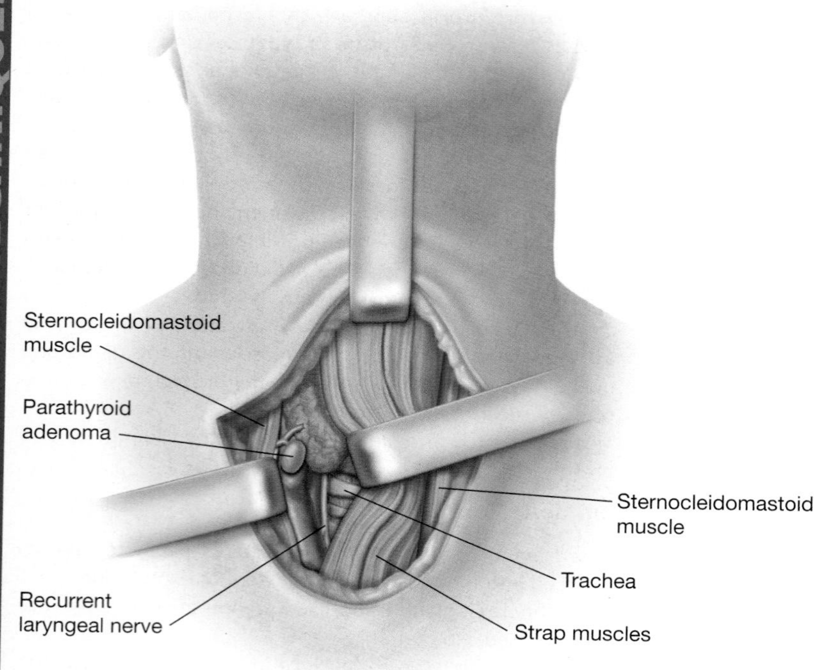

FIGURE 5 ● The posterolateral approach to the neck is similar to the classic approach except that subsequent access is achieved along the medial border of the SCM and lateral to the strap muscles, minimizing dissection through midline scar. The omohyoid muscle is divided as necessary.

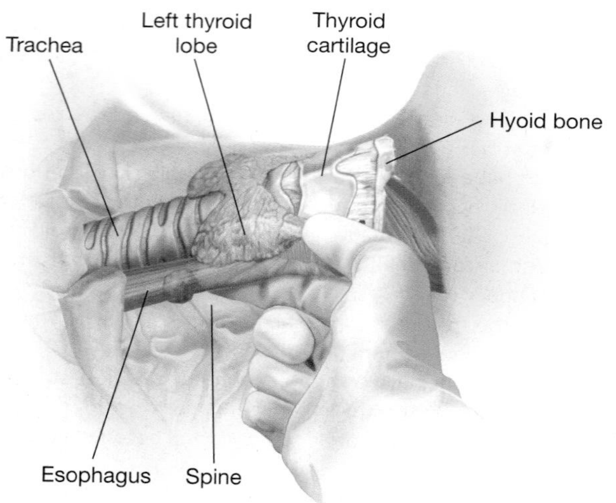

FIGURE 6 ● The lateral wall of the esophagus and the tracheo-esophageal groove are exposed from the hypopharynx superiorly down to the mediastinum. Missing glands may be found in the prevertebral space, and the search for parathyroids in this region is augmented by digital palpation.

sharp dissection is performed with care to not disturb the fragile blood supply.

- Abnormal glands have a characteristic rubbery feel and reddish brown appearance.
- They are freed from the surrounding tissue and the vascular pedicle is clamped and divided.
- Intraoperative PTH monitoring improves the cure rate and guides the extent of exploration.
- A drop in PTH by 50% of baseline and within normal limits at 10 minutes is indicative of cure. If operating for multigland disease (as opposed to a missed adenoma), the PTH level at 10 minutes should also be within normal limits.
- Exploration continues if levels do not fall precipitously and the process is repeated until an appropriate drop is achieved.

Intraoperative Imaging

- Technetium-99m sestamibi, 20 mCi, can be injected 1 hour prior to the procedure in patients who have positive preop sestamibi imaging to help guide the dissection with use of an intraop gamma probe.
- Intraoperative ultrasound helps identify abnormal parathyroids and aids in localization of intrathyroidal lesions.
- Indocyanine green (ICG) fluorescence facilitates identification of parathyroids. Intravenous ICG, 1 mL, is injected and can be visualized using near infrared imaging. A second injection of 1 mL can be repeated if the parathyroid is not highlighted after 5 to 7 minutes (**FIGURE 8**).

Additional Maneuvers

- Bilateral jugular venous sampling intraoperatively as the case commences has benefit in lateralizing parathyroid lesions.
- Inferior adenomas are usually displaced into the anterior aspect of superior mediastinum and may be intimately associated with the thymus gland. Cervical thymectomy may be performed in the case of absent glands (**FIGURE 9**). Gentle traction cephalad with sequential grasps and blunt mobilization are used to deliver the thymus into the cervical wound

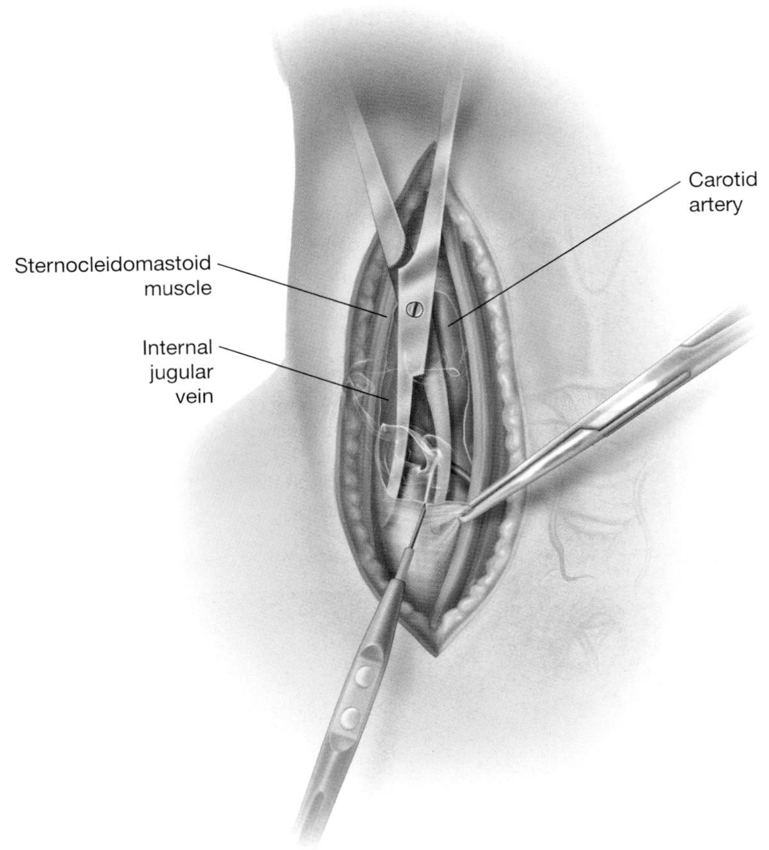

FIGURE 7 ● If the search fails to disclose an adenoma, the carotid sheath is opened.

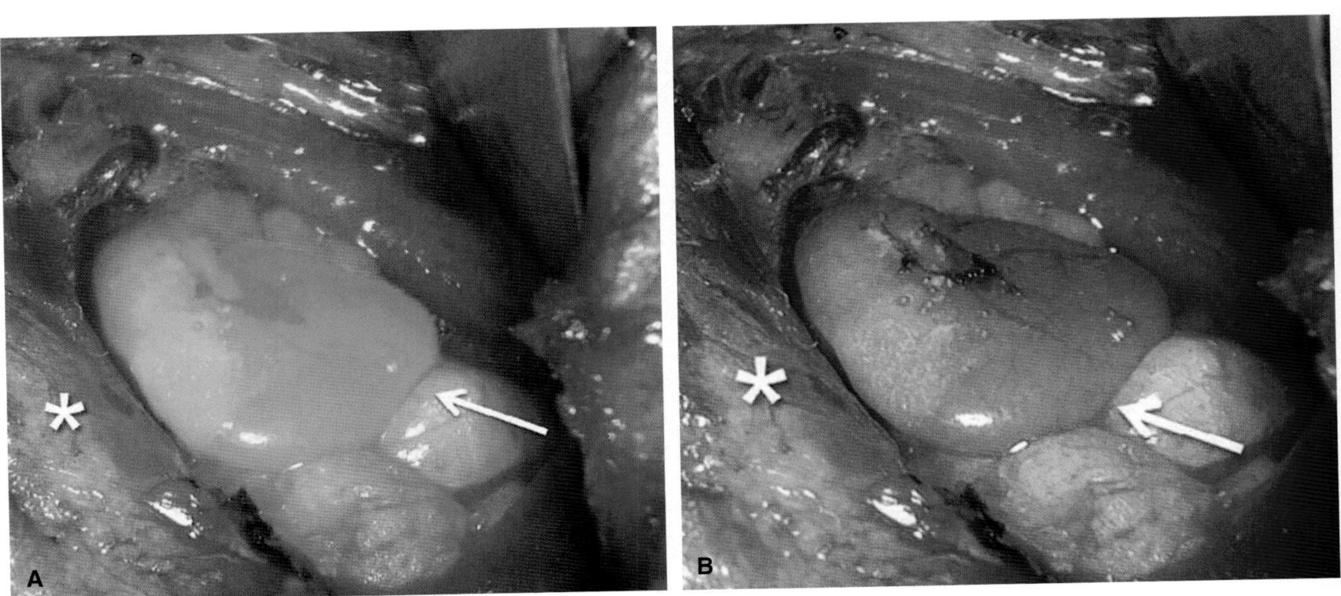

FIGURE 8 ● Intraoperative image of ICG fluorescence for a parathyroid adenoma **(A)** compared with the operative field **(B)**. Arrow designates a parathyroid gland, * designates thyroid gland. (Reprinted from DeLong JC, Ward EP, Lwin TM, et al. Indocyanine green fluorescence-guided parathyroidectomy for primary hyperparathyroidism. *Surgery*. 2017;163(2):388-392. Copyright © 2017 Elsevier. With permission.)

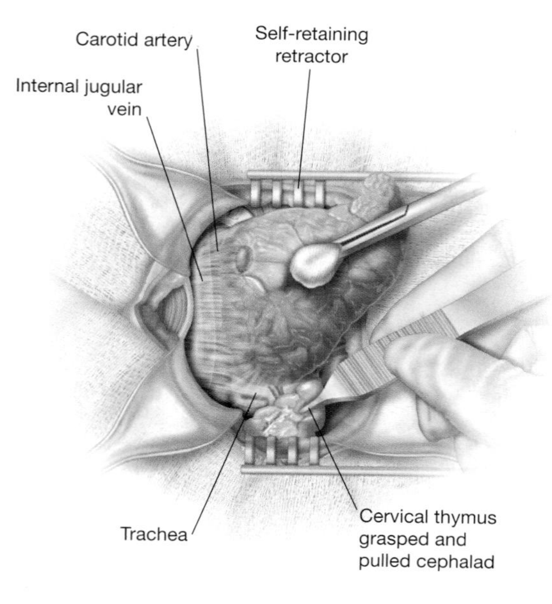

with the aim of removal of thymus tissue to the level of the innominate vein.

- Thyroid lobectomy on the side of a missing parathyroid may be performed.
- Staged procedures are common with nonlocalized reoperative parathyroid surgery. Closure and relocalization should be performed if the offending gland cannot be found.

Closure

- Meticulous hemostasis is achieved. Strap muscles are reapproximated in midline (or to SCM if lateral approach done), followed by platysma reapproximation and skin closure.
- Drains are not regularly used unless there is extensive dissection or exploration.

FIGURE 9 ● Cervical thymectomy may be performed in the case of a missing gland. The superior aspect of the thymus is grasped and pulled by continuous traction from the chest. It can be grabbed sequentially and lifted cephalad until the often single posterior vessel is seen and divided.

MEDIASTINAL EXPLORATION[1,3]

Approach

- Mediastinal exploration should not be performed without localization evidence of an ectopic parathyroid in the mediastinum. Preferably, two different correlating studies should identify gland location prior to surgery (**FIGURE 10**).
- Most adenomas in the posterior mediastinum or anterior mediastinum above the aortic arch can be initially approached and excised through neck.
- Those deep in the anterior mediastinum or in the middle mediastinum require a thoracic approach (**FIGURE 11**).
- Precise localization is paramount and may allow less invasive approaches of anterior mediastinotomy or thoracoscopy rather than partial or median sternotomy (**FIGURE 12**).
- Choice of approach depends on gland location and surgeon expertise.

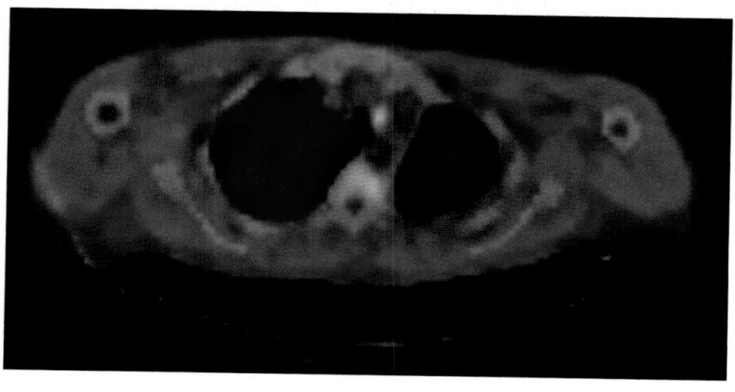

FIGURE 10 ● Single-photon emission computed tomography image of a parathyroid adenoma localized to the mediastinum.

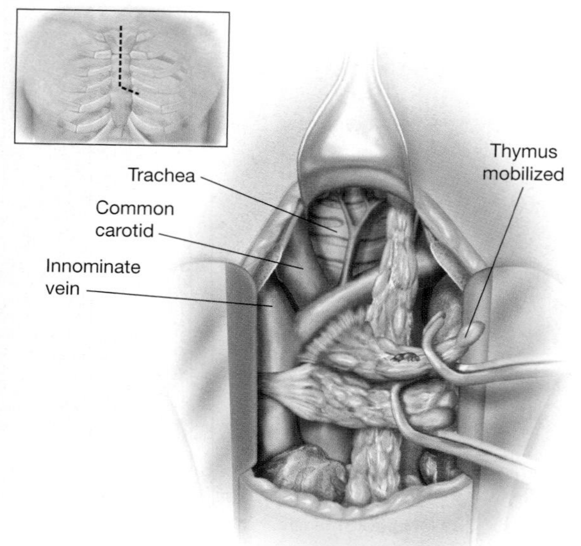

FIGURE 11 ● Median sternotomy or partial sternotomy to 3 cm below the predicted level of the adenoma provides access to the mediastinum (inset shows where the incision would be on the chest). The area of exploration is bound by the innominate vein superiorly and the pericardium inferiorly. Adenomas commonly lie in the thymic remnant in the anterior mediastinum.

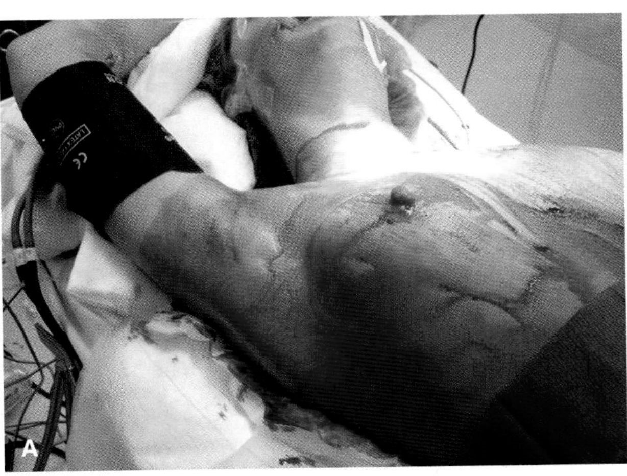

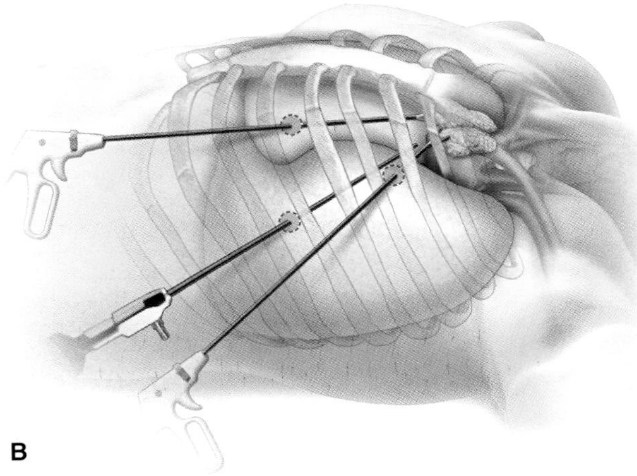

FIGURE 12 ● Thoracic approaches should not be performed without positive localization studies. **A,** Positioning for a thoracoscopic approach. The patient is supine, with the ipsilateral arm elevated above the head to allow transthoracic access between ribs. **B,** Placement of thoracoscopic trocars.

PARATHYROID REIMPLANTATION

Procedure

- For multigland disease or when the vasculature of normal parathyroids is compromised, parathyroid reimplantation may be performed to preserve function. Grafts have a high success rate but may take several weeks to function.
- Approximately 50 mg of the most normal-appearing parathyroid tissue is minced into 1-mm pieces and placed into muscular pockets in the forearm. Alternatively, it may be placed in the subcutaneous tissue overlying the forearm or anterior chest wall (**FIGURE 13**).

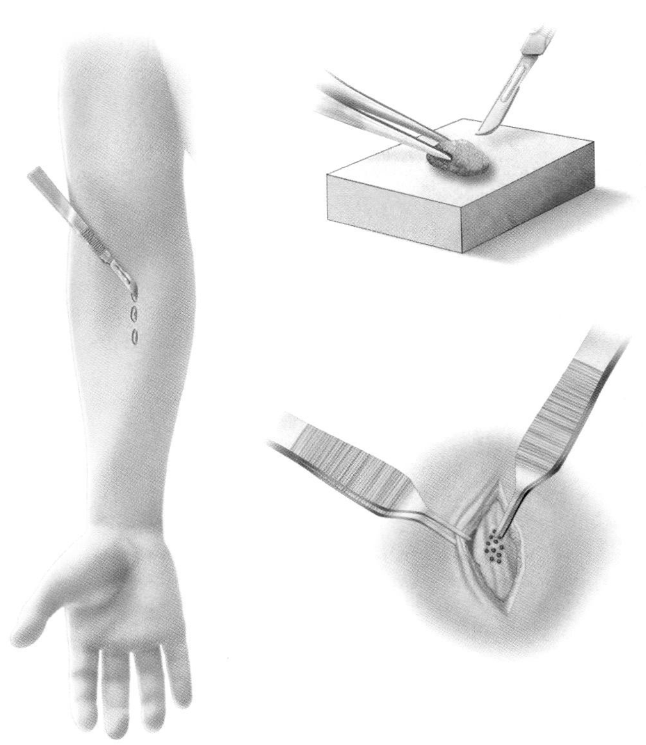

FIGURE 13 ● Parathyroid tissue to reimplant is minced into 1-mm pieces and placed into intramuscular pockets in the forearm as seen in the figure. Alternatively, they can be placed subcutaneously in the forearm or on the anterior chest wall.

PEARLS AND PITFALLS

Indications	■ Complete history and physical with symptoms and severity of hypercalcemia should be obtained. Biochemical diagnosis of recurrent or persistent hyperparathyroidism must be confirmed.
Preoperative planning	■ Review of initial operative notes and pathology is required to create a map for reoperative surgery. ■ Preoperative localization is critical as nonlocalized patients should only be explored when indications are compelling.

Placement of incision	■ Incisions are created, keeping in mind the localization of pathology and the operative plan. ■ Cosmesis is improved when placed in a natural skin crease.
Cervical approach	■ Entry into the neck may be via focused, posterolateral, thyrothymic ligament, or revision midline cervicotomy approach.
Exploration	■ Normotopic locations for superior and inferior glands should first be searched. ■ Exploration in expected ectopic sites along the tracheoesophageal groove, carotid sheath, thyrothymic ligament, cervical thymus, and intrathyroid should follow.
Mediastinal lesions	■ Accurate preoperative localization allows the least invasive procedure for lesions in the mediastinum, which may be approached via cervicotomy, sternotomy, or thoracoscopy.
Intraoperative imaging Additional maneuvers	■ Intraoperative ultrasound. ■ Preoperatively injected technetium-99m sestamibi permits localization with a gamma probe. ■ Injection of ICG highlights parathyroids using near infrared fluorescence imaging. ■ Intraoperative jugular venous sampling can help lateralize pathology to the right or left neck. ■ Cervical thymectomy or ipsilateral thyroid lobectomy can be performed when an offending gland cannot be located. ■ Parathyroid reimplantation provides a useful adjunct to patients with multigland disease.
Closure	■ Layered closure without drain.

POSTOPERATIVE CARE

- Patients should be monitored for respiratory compromise in the immediate postoperative period.
- Patients with reimplantation, extensive dissection, gland or vascular manipulation, or multiple gland removal are at increased risk of postoperative hypoparathyroidism.
- Postoperative hypocalcemia can be mitigated with calcium and vitamin D prophylaxis vs expectant monitoring of serum calcium and PTH. Calcium supplements are generally continued for 3 to 6 months to avoid reactive secondary hyperparathyroidism from a chronic hypocalcemic state.

OUTCOMES

- Success rates between 82% and 98% are expected of reoperative parathyroid surgery, with rates as low as 37% to 73% in multigland disease.
- RLN injury ranges from 0% to 2.7%, whereas permanent hypocalcemia rates vary from 1% to 18%.

COMPLICATIONS

- Neck seroma
- Hematoma
- Infection
- Voice change
- RLN injury
- Hypocalcemia, hypoparathyroidism
- Failure of cure, recurrence

REFERENCES

1. Hubbard JGH, Inabnet WB, Lo C-Y. *Endocrine Surgery: Principles and Practice*. Springer-Verlag; 2009.
2. Inabnet WB, Lee JA. Parathyroid disease, syndromes and pathophysiology. In: Lennard TWJ, ed. *Endocrine Surgery: A Companion to Specialist Surgical Practice*. 4th ed. Saunders Elsevier; 2009:1-20.
3. Henry JF, Sebag F. Operative strategy for the management of parathyroid disease. In: Lennard TWJ, ed. *Endocrine Surgery: A Companion to Specialist Surgical Practice*. 4th ed. Saunders Elsevier; 2009:20-38.
4. Zolin S, Crawford K, Rudin AV, et al. Selective parathyroid venous sampling in reoperative parathyroid surgery: a key localization tool when noninvasive tests are unrevealing. *Surgery*. 2021;169(1):126-132.

Chapter 57 Adrenalectomy: Open Anterior

D. Brock Hewitt and Barbra S. Miller

DEFINITION

- Adrenal masses may be functional or nonfunctional and benign or malignant. Most are incidentally discovered when imaging is obtained for other reasons. Laparoscopic adrenalectomy is the gold standard for appropriately sized benign adrenal masses and for some metastatic tumors to the adrenal gland (see Part 5, Chapters 60 and 61). If adrenocortical carcinoma is a concern, adrenalectomy by an open approach should be performed.[1] Several genetic syndromes are associated with adrenal abnormalities and appropriate testing should be obtained if indicated.

DIFFERENTIAL DIAGNOSIS

- Adenoma
- Metastatic cancer
- Pheochromocytoma
- Ganglioneuroma
- Primary adrenocortical carcinoma
- Cyst
- Adjacent paraganglioma
- Soft tissue tumor

PATIENT HISTORY AND PHYSICAL FINDINGS

- All adrenal abnormalities should be evaluated in a systematic fashion, including a thorough history and physical examination investigating the possibility of a hormone-secreting mass. This includes the possibility of a pheochromocytoma, Cushing syndrome, primary hyperaldosteronism, and hypertestosteronemia. Specifically, the patient should be questioned regarding poorly controlled hypertension, diabetes, edema, diaphoresis, tachycardia, palpitations, sudden severe headaches, flushing, and easy bruising. The physical examination should look for evidence of central obesity, edema, peripheral wasting, core muscle weakness, a buffalo hump, striae, thin skin, and facial plethora as well as hirsutism or virilization in women and recent onset gynecomastia in men. Because the adrenal gland is situated in the retroperitoneum, unless it is extremely large, palpation of the mass is usually unable to be achieved.

IMAGING AND OTHER DIAGNOSTIC STUDIES

- All adrenal masses should undergo appropriate biochemical testing (**TABLE 1**). Selective testing according to signs or symptoms of hormone excess is to be avoided as up to 25% found to have autonomous adrenal hormone secretion are "asymptomatic." Urine steroids may help differentiate benign from malignant adrenocortical tumors. In those with a malignant adrenal tumor, hormone levels (intermediaries in the steroid pathway as well as end products) can serve as tumor markers.
- Imaging studies should include an adrenal protocol computed tomography (CT) scan (to assess imaging characteristics and calculate washout percentage of contrast from the tumor) or magnetic resonance imaging (MRI) (to assess for loss of signal intensity between in-phase and out-of-phase images) and a positron emission tomography (PET) scan if malignancy is questioned (**FIGURE 1**).

Table 1: Adrenal Biochemical Evaluation

Glucocorticoid excess	• 1 mg dexamethasone suppression test • Alternatively, late-night salivary cortisol or serum bedtime cortisol • 24-h urine cortisol if overt clinical signs of cortisol excess to quantify degree of excess • Basal plasma ACTH • DHEA-S
Sex steroids	• Androstenedione • Testosterone (only in women) • 17-Beta-estradiol (only in men and postmenopausal women)
Mineralocorticoid excess	• Potassium • Aldosterone • Renin
Catecholamine excess	• Fractionated plasma metanephrines and normetanephrines or 24-h urine
Other steroid pathway intermediaries	• 11-Deoxycortisol • 17-Hydroxyprogesterone

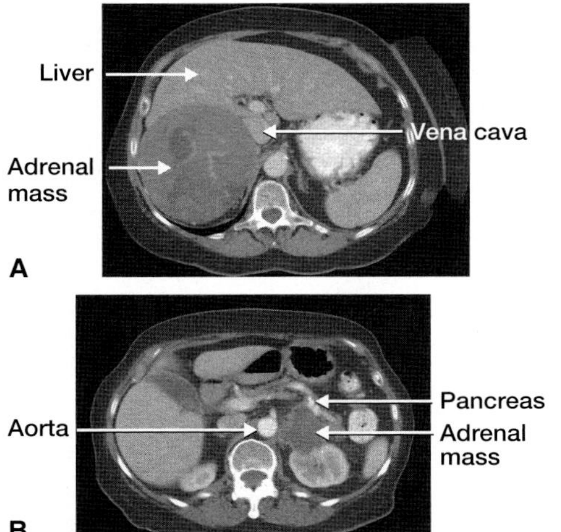

FIGURE 1 ● **A,** Computed tomography (CT) scan showing large heterogeneous right adrenal mass concerning for adrenocortical carcinoma. **B,** CT scan showing a large left adrenal mass.

- Additional imaging studies may be required depending on the functionality of the tumor (metaiodobenzylguanidine [MIBG] or 68Ga-DOTATATE-PET/CT for pheochromocytoma in select cases, adrenal vein sampling for hyperaldosteronism, etc.). A chest CT should be obtained preoperatively to assess for evidence of metastatic disease if the adrenal mass is indeterminate by imaging criteria or known to be malignant.
- Fine needle aspiration or core biopsy is not recommended if adrenocortical carcinoma is suspected, but may be useful if metastasis to the adrenal gland is in the differential and the adrenal tumor is the most accessible site of metastasis for biopsy in the setting of multiple sites of metastatic disease. If biopsy is performed, it is imperative to first biochemically rule out a pheochromocytoma.

SURGICAL MANAGEMENT

- Adrenal tumors, if benign appearing by imaging criteria, nonfunctional, and therefore not requiring resection, should be reevaluated with at least one additional CT scan or MRI 6 to 12 months after the initial imaging study to ensure stability in size and internal imaging characteristics. Some advocate for a longer period of follow-up imaging for 2 years with reevaluation of biochemistry for 4 more years.[2]
- Functional tumors leading to hormone excess are often removed, although may be medically treated depending on the situation and the number of adrenal glands involved. Those with indeterminate or growing adrenal masses and those with suspected of being adrenocortical carcinoma or isolated metastatic disease from another primary tumor without evidence of widespread metastatic disease are most often offered surgery.

Preoperative Planning

- The surgeon must evaluate available imaging studies for tumor involvement of adjacent organs, vessels, and lymphadenopathy. Invasion of major vessels (vena cava) or adjacent organs may require additional teams or different approaches to the tumor as en bloc resection is encouraged when feasible. As CT tends to overestimate invasion of adjacent vessels, MRI with magnetic resonance venogram can be especially helpful to assess for vena cava invasion or venous tumor thrombus.
- The risks, benefits, and alternatives to surgery are discussed with the patient, including potential need for steroid supplementation in the postoperative setting. Patients with pheochromocytomas should be adequately alpha blocked and volume replete. Beta blockade may also be necessary. In patients with hyperaldosteronism, a potassium level should be checked the morning of surgery and treated if necessary.
- Routine prophylactic antibiotics and deep vein thrombosis prophylaxis is administered prior to surgery, and sequential compression devices are applied.
- General endotracheal anesthetic is administered, and an epidural is often placed for postoperative pain management.
- Common to all approaches, skin preparation with clipping rather than shaving is preferred, and the surgical area is prepped and draped in a sterile fashion.

Positioning

- The patient is placed supine with the arms out. Multiple incisions may be utilized. The subcostal incision is the most commonly utilized incision and provides excellent access to the adrenal gland and surrounding organs and is optimal when multivisceral resection or vascular resection is needed (**FIGURE 2**).

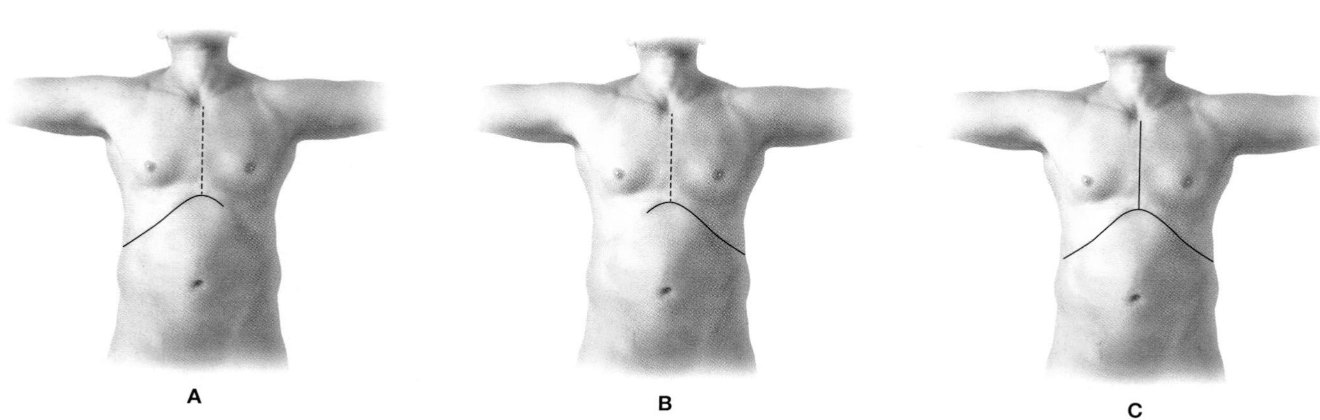

FIGURE 2 ● Multiple incisions can be made to access the adrenal gland depending on the laterality, situation, and planned operation. (**A** and **B**) Subcostal; (**C**) bilateral subcostal; (**D**) Midline; (**E**) Makuuchi—two options—the more superior horizontal line allowing for extension between the ribs if desired; (**F** and **G**) Thoracoabdominal; (**H** and **I**) Flank extending between ribs. Dashed line indicates possible extension of incision.

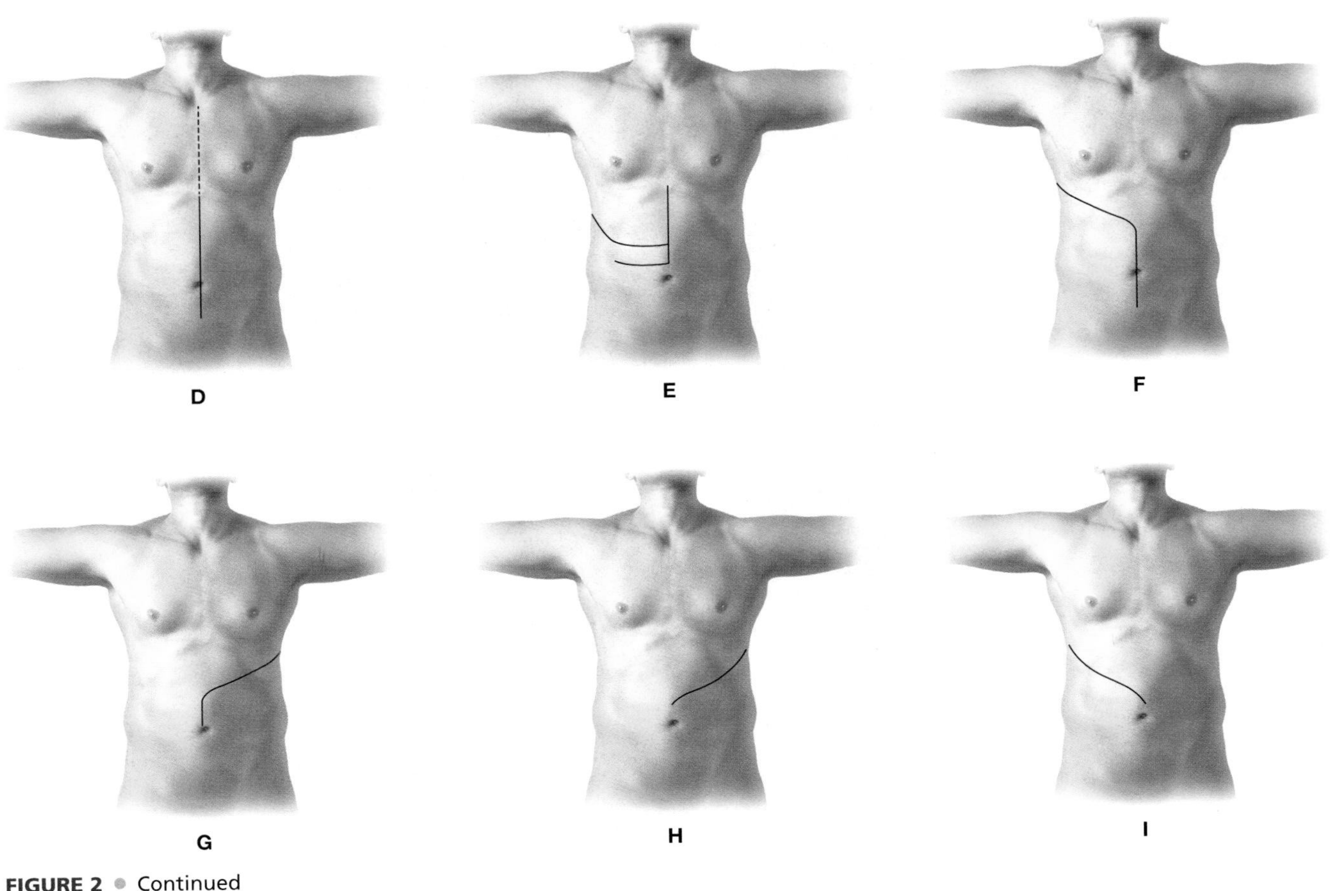

FIGURE 2 ● Continued

RIGHT ADRENALECTOMY

Exposure

- A wide right subcostal incision is made and carried across the midline to the mid-left abdomen. The subcutaneous fat, fascia, abdominal wall musculature, and posterior fascia are incised with cautery. The peritoneum is entered sharply with scissors and the incision opened to its full length. The ligamentum teres is divided between sutures and the peritoneal cavity is inspected in a systematic manner, assessing for evidence of metastatic disease or other abnormalities. The falciform ligament, triangular, and coronary ligaments of the left and right lobes of the liver are divided to allow for full mobility of the liver during retraction (**FIGURES 3** and **4**).
- Ultrasound of the liver is also performed to assess for metastatic disease not identified on preoperative imaging, and the vena cava may also be evaluated sonographically for evidence of intracaval tumor thrombus or direct tumor invasion.
- The hepatic flexure of the colon may need to be mobilized, and if a Kocher maneuver is needed, it should be done at this time. The right lobe of the liver is retracted medially to expose the retroperitoneum and allow access to the area of the tumor and vena cava. A retractor system is placed. The Omni retractor provides excellent retraction as well as the critically important ability to retract the costal margin and ribs as superiorly and anteriorly as possible. A large saline-soaked towel is placed against the bowel with retractors to not only provide exposure but also to exclude the rest of the peritoneal cavity and minimize potential seeding of the peritoneal cavity by a malignant tumor (**FIGURE 5**).

Dissection

- A number of critical elements of dissection have been described for dissection of tumors concerning for malignancy (indeterminate by imaging characteristics or obviously invasive)[3]
  1. To achieve a microscopically complete (R0) resection of the primary tumor without tumor capsule violation, the surrounding retroperitoneal fat, Gerota fascia, and peritoneum should be resected en bloc.
  2. For an adrenal tumor with direct invasion of the inferior vena cava, renal vein, or renal artery, the vascular structure(s) should be resected en bloc with the primary adrenal tumor when technically feasible.
  3. Routine prophylactic locoregional lymphadenectomy is not recommended in patients with adrenal cancer. However, in patients with clinically suspicious lymphadenopathy, nodal dissection of the affected lymph node basin(s) should be performed.

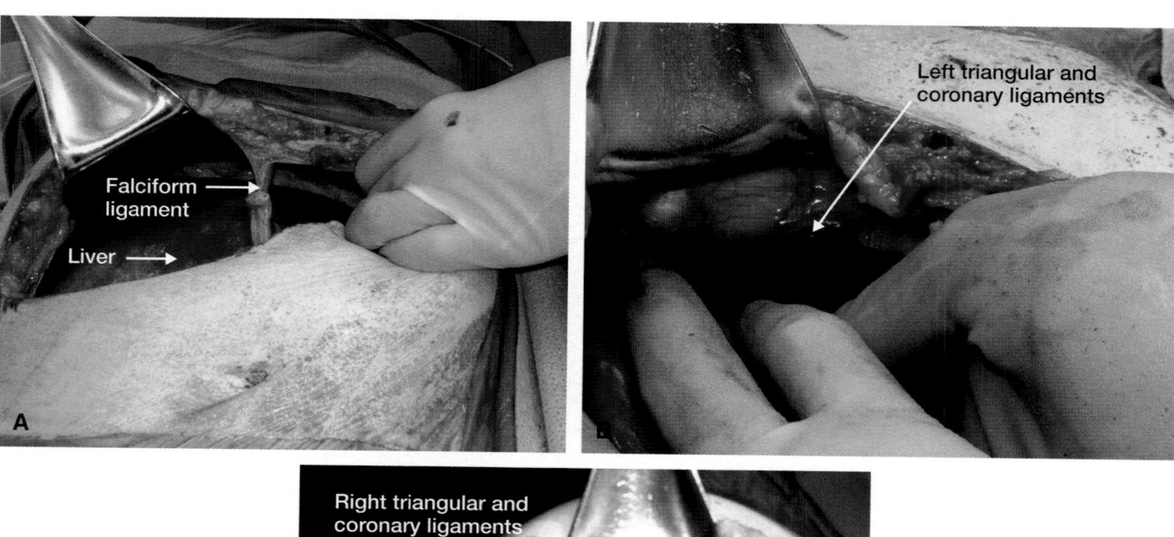

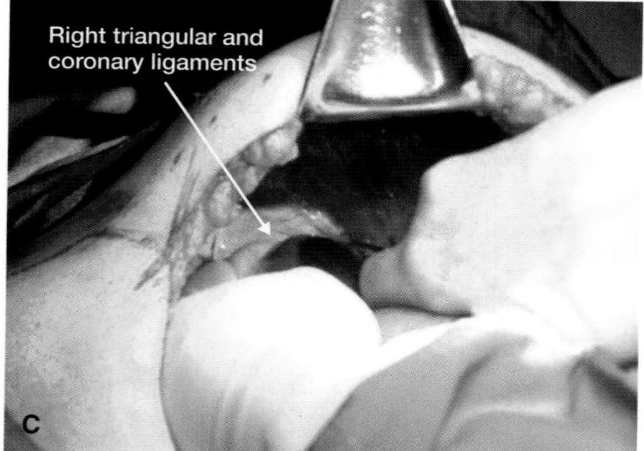

FIGURE 3 ● **A-C,** The falciform ligament and left and right triangular and coronary ligaments are divided.

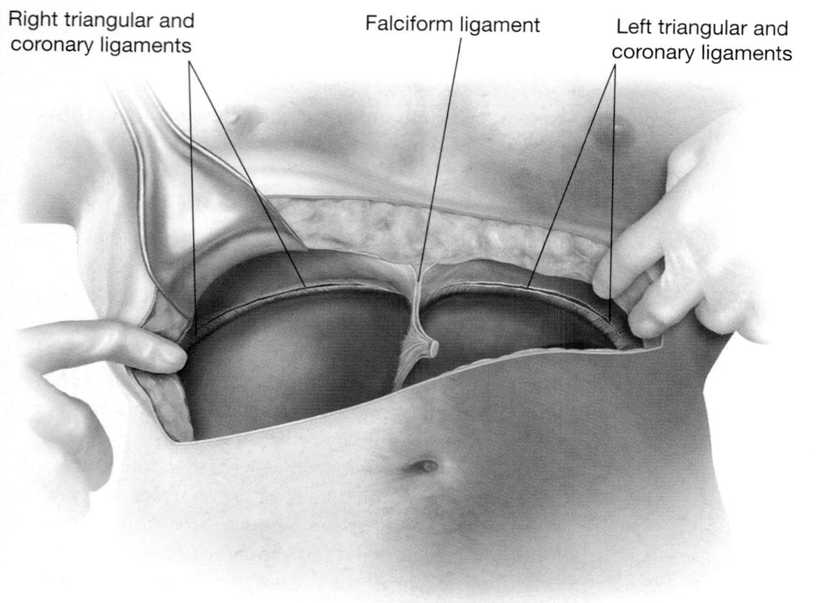

FIGURE 4 ● With the ligamentum teres, falciform ligament, and triangular and coronary ligaments divided, this allows adequate retraction of the liver and access to the tumor and vena cava.

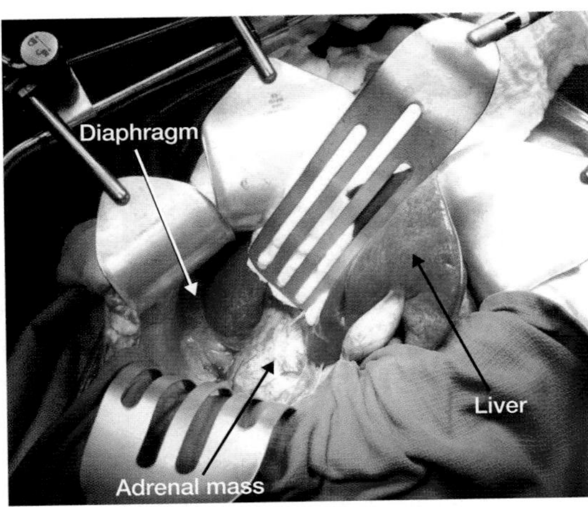

FIGURE 5 ● A retractor system is placed to retract the ribs superiorly and anteriorly and to retract the liver medially. A moist towel is placed inferiorly to retract the bowel and exclude the rest of the peritoneal cavity.

- The posterior peritoneal lining over the retroperitoneum is incised over the superior half of the right kidney and carried from medial to lateral out to the side of the abdominal wall. Medial dissection should proceed carefully to the vena cava, making sure not to divide branches of the renal artery supplying the upper portion of the kidney or venous branches draining to the renal vein. Small branches supplying and draining the adrenal gland should be carefully ligated and divided. Any abnormal appearing lymph nodes posterior to the renal hilum should be included in the dissection (**FIGURES 6** and **7**).
- The fat overlying and just superior to the kidney is mobilized from inferior to superior, making this tissue the inferior margin, using cautery, silk sutures, and other hemostatic devices as needed, making sure not to create a nonexistent plane between the inferior aspect of the tumor and the superior aspect of the kidney. The peritoneal lining should remain intact over the anterior aspect of the tumor to serve as the anterior margin if not already invaded by the tumor (**FIGURE 8A** and **B**).

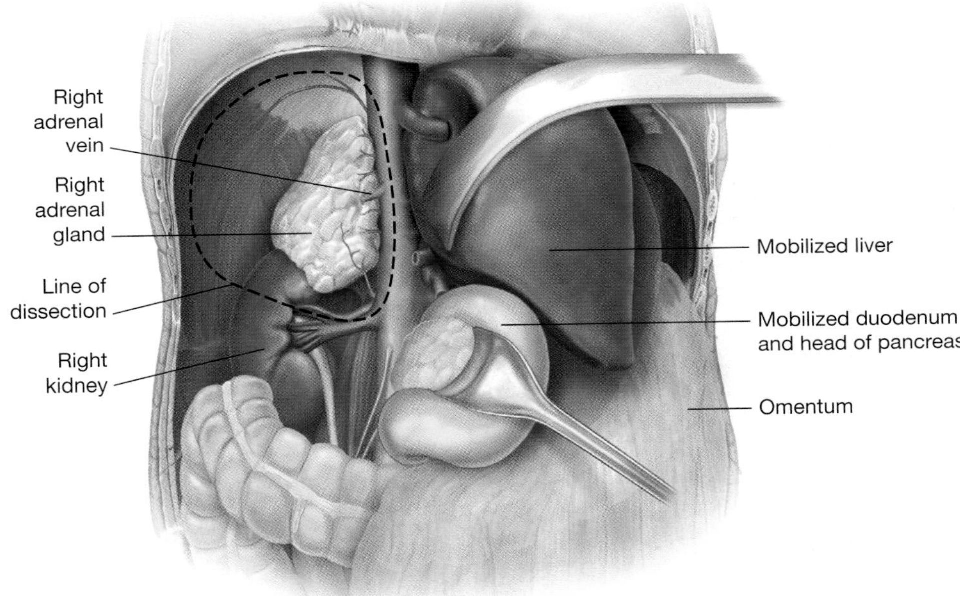

FIGURE 6 ● With the liver retracted medially, the adrenal vein and inferior vena cava are exposed. The *dotted line* demonstrates the intended line of dissection.

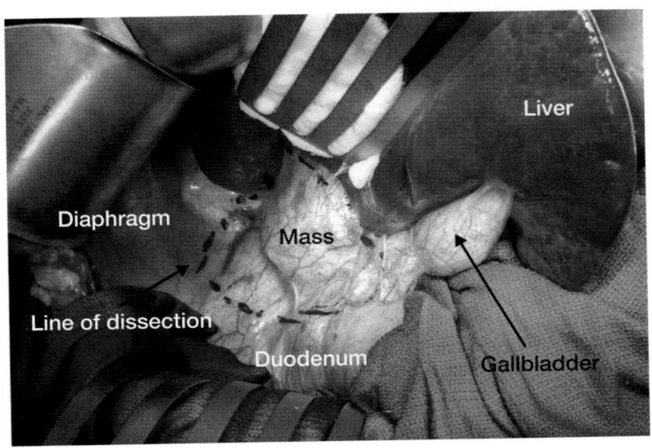

FIGURE 7 ● The intended line of dissection to include the tumor and all retroperitoneal soft tissue is marked.

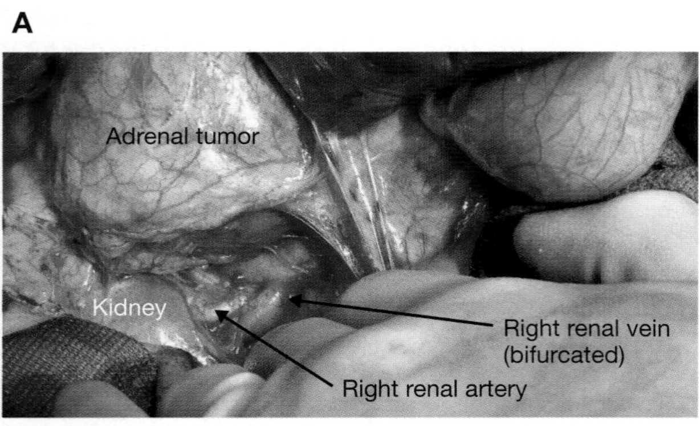

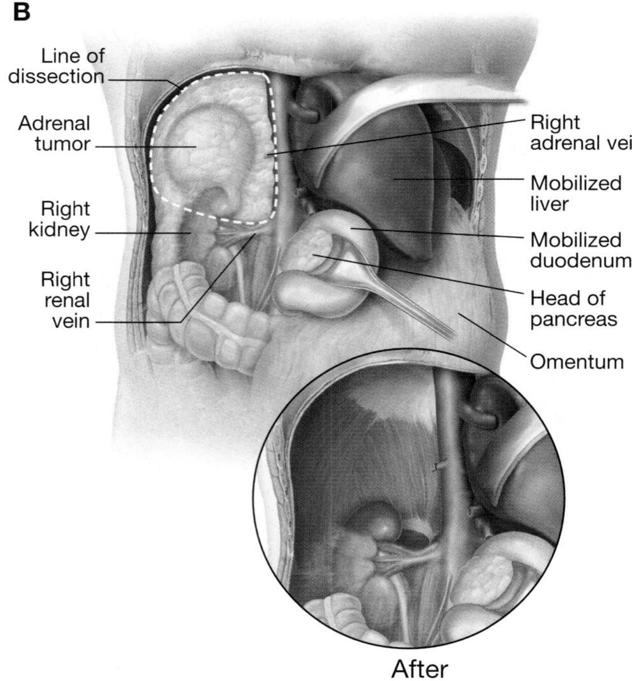

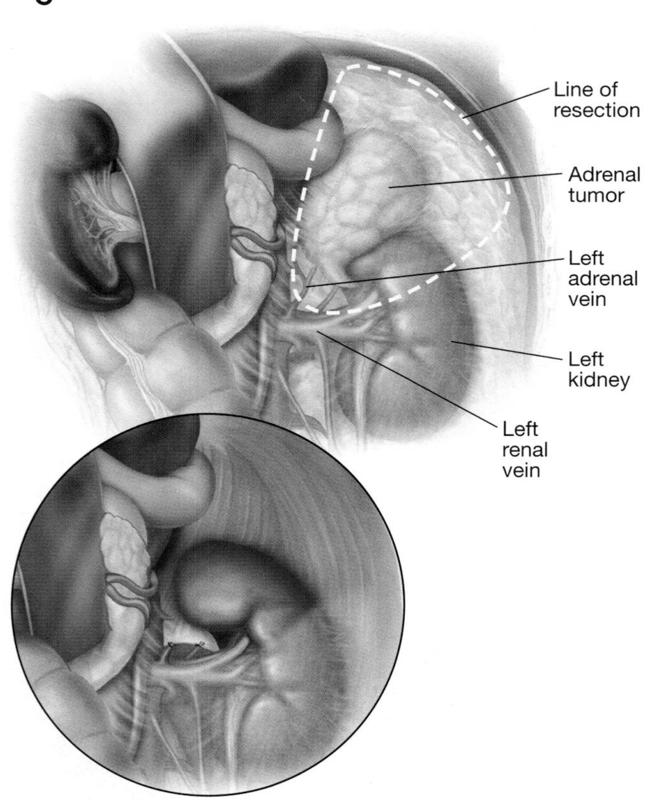

FIGURE 8 ● **A,** The inferior portion of the dissection is shown. A branch of the right renal artery is seen between two branches of the right renal vein. **B,** Exposure and line of dissection before and after for right adrenalectomy for adrenal cancer, including the periadrenal fat. **C,** Exposure and line of dissection before and after for left adrenalectomy for adrenal cancer.

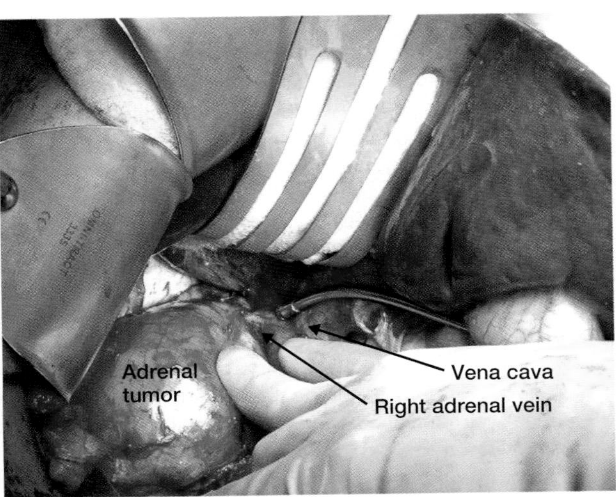

FIGURE 9 ● The right adrenal vein has been dissected free of its attachments. More superiorly along the vena cava, a second vein from the adrenal to the inferior vena cava has been clipped and divided.

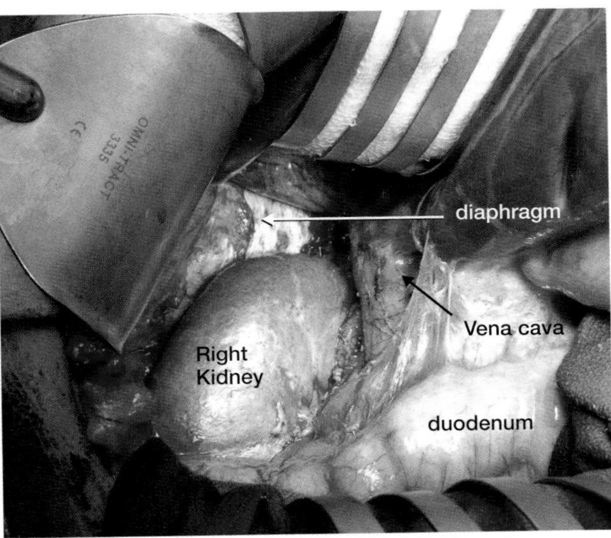

FIGURE 10 ● The adrenal tumor and all retroperitoneal soft tissue has been removed en bloc. The right kidney has migrated superiorly against the diaphragm to fill the space.

- The dissection continues superiorly along the diaphragm, making sure to ligate and divide any feeding vessels, most commonly branches from the inferior phrenic vessels.
- Posterior dissection should proceed from lateral to medial, making sure to remove all fat posterior to the tumor in an en bloc fashion. If the tumor invades the muscle, a portion of the muscle should be included with the tumor to ensure negative margins.
- The anterior surface of the vena cava should be identified and the peritoneal lining overlying this should be incised along its length. Using a vein retractor to retract the vena cava medially, soft tissue attachments medial to the gland and posterior to the vena cava, including lymphatics, are ligated and divided. As the midpoint of the adrenal gland is reached, the right adrenal vein should be identified, ligated, and divided (**FIGURE 9**). The vein should be inspected and carefully palpated to assess for any tumor thrombus so that the tumor thrombus can be included with the specimen in an en bloc fashion. Advanced techniques for managing large tumor thrombi within the vena cava are beyond the scope of this chapter. If removing a pheochromocytoma, the anesthesiologist should be warned well in advance prior to ligating the adrenal vein in anticipation of ensuing hypotension. The dissection is continued superiorly until all medial attachments have been released (**FIGURE 10**).

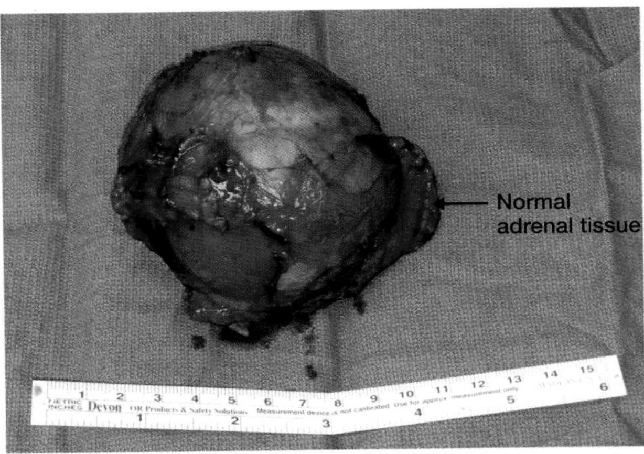

FIGURE 11 ● A small portion of normal adrenal tissue remains and is seen at the right side of the gland in this image. Surrounding soft tissue and the overlying anterior peritoneal lining remain on the anterior surface of the gland.

- The adrenal gland and the periadrenal soft tissue are removed, marked with orienting sutures for the pathologist, and sent to the pathology lab (**FIGURE 11**).

Closure

- A small amount of water should be used for irrigation and final hemostasis is achieved. The area encompassed by the dissection should be marked with large clips to assist with postoperative external beam radiation therapy if needed.
- A drain may be placed if desired but is not required in most cases.
- The retractor system is removed, the organs are replaced in their normal anatomic positions, and the abdominal wall musculature is closed in two separate layers. The subcutaneous tissue may be reapproximated with interrupted absorbable sutures if needed and the skin is closed with staples or suture. A sterile dressing is applied.

LEFT ADRENALECTOMY

Exposure

- A wide left subcostal incision is made and carried across the midline to the midright abdomen (**FIGURE 12**). The subcutaneous fat, fascia, abdominal wall musculature, and posterior fascia are incised with cautery. The peritoneum is entered sharply with scissors and the incision is opened to its full length. The ligamentum teres is divided between sutures and the peritoneal cavity is inspected in a systematic manner, assessing for evidence of metastatic disease or other abnormalities.

- Ultrasound of the liver is also performed to assess for metastatic disease and the vena cava may also be evaluated for evidence of intracaval tumor thrombus from the left adrenal and renal veins.
- The falciform ligament and left triangular and coronary ligaments of the left lobe of the liver are divided to allow for mobility of the liver during retraction (**FIGURE 13**).
- The descending colon is mobilized along the line of Toldt and the colon is reflected medially. The mobilization is continued superiorly to divide the splenic attachments to the abdominal sidewall and the diaphragm. The spleen, stomach, pancreas, splenic flexure, and colon should be reflected medially, allowing exposure of the left retroperitoneum (**FIGURE 14**). A retractor system is placed. A large saline-soaked towel with retractors is placed against the bowel, pancreas, and spleen to not only provide exposure but also to exclude the rest of the peritoneal cavity to minimize potential seeding of the peritoneal cavity by a malignant tumor. The left side of the aorta should be clearly appreciable if the exposure is adequate.

Dissection

- Because the peritoneal covering on the left has been reflected with the spleen and pancreas, the surgeon should make every effort to manipulate the tumor surface as little as possible (no-touch technique). The soft tissue overlying the superior half of the left kidney is incised and carried from medial to lateral out to the side of the abdominal wall. Inferior dissection should proceed carefully to the aorta medially along the left renal vein, making sure not to divide branches of the posteriorly situated renal artery supplying the upper portion of the kidney or venous branches draining to the renal vein. Small branches supplying and draining the adrenal gland should be carefully ligated and divided. Any lymph nodes posterior to the renal hilum should be included in the dissection.
- The left adrenal vein will be identified at the medial aspect of the left renal vein as it courses anterior to the aorta (**FIGURE 15**). It generally enters the adrenal gland in the 7-o'clock position. It should be ligated and divided. The adrenal vein and renal vein should be inspected and carefully palpated to assess for any tumor thrombus so that the tumor thrombus can be included with the specimen in an en bloc fashion. Advanced techniques for managing large

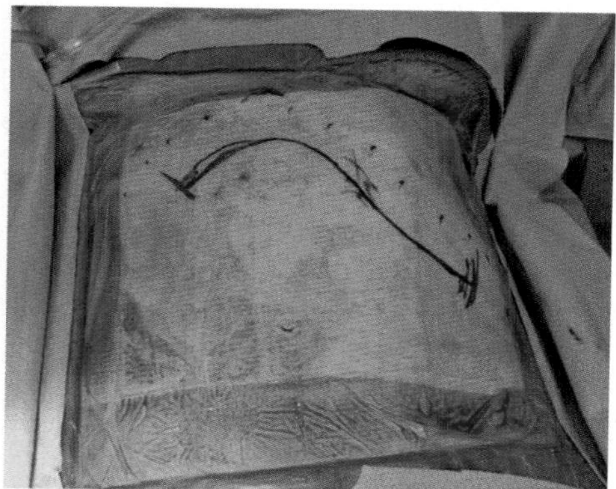

FIGURE 12 ● The patient is placed supine on the table with arms out. Pressure points are padded. A wide left subcostal incision is marked 2 cm inferior to the costal margin and carried across the midline to the right abdomen to facilitate exposure.

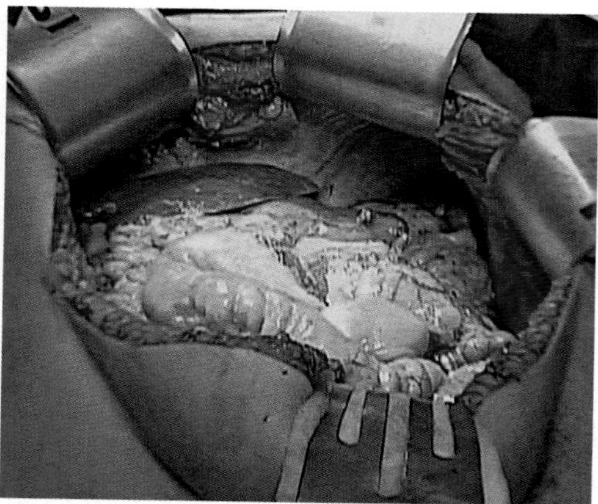

FIGURE 13 ● The falciform ligament and left triangular and coronary ligaments are divided, allowing exposure of the left upper abdomen and mobility of the liver.

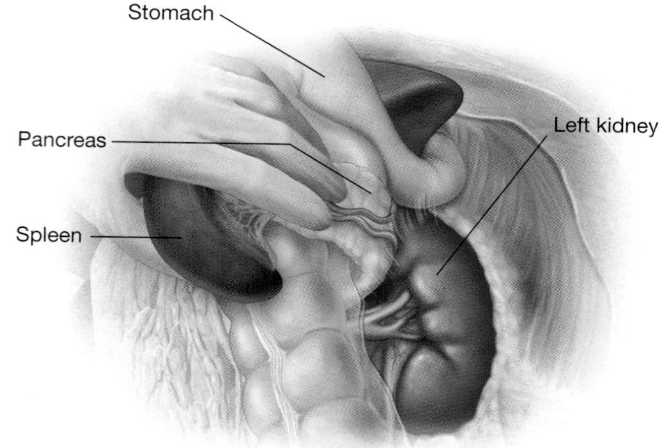

FIGURE 14 ● The spleen, stomach, and pancreas are mobilized medially.

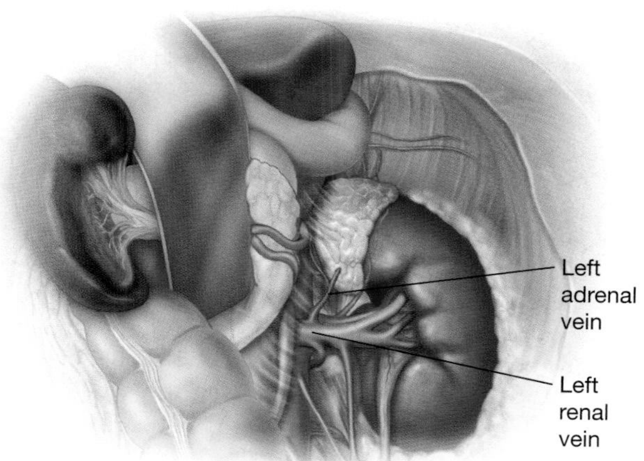

FIGURE 15 ● With retractors in place, the left retroperitoneum is exposed and excluded from the rest of the peritoneal cavity. The left side of the aorta, renal vein, and adrenal vein are visualized, with the left adrenal vein identified at the medial aspect of the left renal vein. The adrenal vein can be ligated and divided at its junction with the renal vein.

tumor thrombi within the renal vein and vena cava are not discussed in this chapter.

- The fat overlying and just superior to the kidney is mobilized from inferior to superior, making this tissue the inferior margin, using cautery, silk sutures, and other hemostatic devices as needed, making sure not to create a nonexistent plane between the inferior aspect of the tumor and the superior aspect of the kidney (**FIGURE 8C**).
- Lateral dissection should continue along the abdominal sidewall. The dissection continues superiorly along the diaphragm, making sure to ligate and divide any feeding vessels, most commonly branches from the inferior phrenic vessels.
- Posterior dissection should proceed from lateral to medial, making sure to remove all fat and any involved muscle posterior to the tumor in an en bloc fashion.
- The left lateral surface of the aorta should be identified, and the soft tissue attachments including small vessels and lymphatics are ligated and divided. If removing a pheochromocytoma, the anesthesiologist should be warned well in advance prior to ligating the adrenal vein in anticipation of ensuing hypotension. The dissection is continued superiorly until all medial attachments have been released. Any lymph nodes along the aorta or identified near the superior mesenteric artery or celiac axis should be included with the specimen.
- The adrenal gland and the periadrenal soft tissue are removed, marked with orienting suture for the pathologist, and sent to the pathology lab.

Closure

- A small amount of water should be used for irrigation and final hemostasis is achieved. The area encompassed by the dissection should be marked with large clips to assist with postoperative external beam radiation therapy if needed. A drain may be placed.
- The retractor system is removed, the organs are replaced in their normal anatomic position, and the abdominal wall musculature is closed in two separate layers. The subcutaneous tissue may be reapproximated with interrupted absorbable sutures if needed and the skin is closed with staples or suture. A sterile dressing is applied.

TECHNIQUES

PEARLS AND PITFALLS

Bleeding—arterial and venous	■ May result from disruption of the vena cava, renal vein or artery, and aorta. Kitner dissectors, sponge sticks, and vascular clamps are helpful. Obtain proximal and distal control prior to potentially dangerous maneuvers.
Liver mobilization	■ Mobilize right and left lobes to obtain best exposure for right adrenalectomy. Mobilize left lobe to obtain best exposure for left adrenalectomy.
Tumor capsule penetration	■ Tumor capsule violation leads to peritoneal spread, which will result in recurrence and often shortened survival compared to alternate sites of recurrence. En bloc resection is critical to the prevention of creating a plane through microscopically positive tumor margins.

POSTOPERATIVE CARE

- Most patients will not need intensive care unit (ICU) care, although pheochromocytoma patients often need closer monitoring for the first 24 hours, depending on intraoperative stability and volume status.
- Hydrocortisone should be given administered to patients with overt Cushing syndrome. A cosyntropin stimulation test can be performed the morning after surgery in subclinical or mild Cushing cases if there is a question about the requirement for steroid supplementation.
- Electrolytes should be checked the morning after surgery. Patients undergoing surgery for primary hyperaldosteronism may experience rebound hyperkalemia.
- After bilateral adrenalectomy, intravenous hydrocortisone should be weaned to a daily replacement dose of oral hydrocortisone. Fludrocortisone (usually 0.1 mg daily) is often required to balance sodium and potassium.
- Antihypertensive medications are withheld in the immediate postoperative setting and reinstituted as needed.
- Routine postoperative care is pursued, and patients are discharged 3-7 days after surgery.
- Follow-up is typically 1-2 weeks after surgery with endocrine testing as needed.

OUTCOMES

- Although laparoscopic surgery has become the gold standard for benign adrenal disease due to decreased bleeding, infection, pain, and hospital stay, open adrenalectomy is still performed if conversion from laparoscopic adrenalectomy is required for various reasons, for very large adrenal tumors, and when adrenocortical carcinoma is in the differential diagnosis, as some studies have found a significantly higher incidence of incomplete positive margin resections, a higher incidence of and shorter time to tumor bed and peritoneal cavity recurrence, and decreased survival compared to laparoscopic surgery.[4-6] A greater number of oncologic principles of resection can be respected with open surgery for adrenal cancer compared to a laparoscopic approach.

COMPLICATIONS

- Bleeding
- Infection
- Adrenal insufficiency in those with Cushing syndrome
- Postoperative hypotension in those with pheochromocytoma
- Rebound hyperkalemia in those with Conn syndrome

- Lymphatic leak
- Pneumothorax
- Neurogenic pain
- Abdominal wall laxity

REFERENCES

1. Miller BS, Gauger PG, Hammer GD, et al. Resection of adrenocortical carcinoma is less complete and local recurrence occurs sooner and more often after laparoscopic adrenalectomy than after open adrenalectomy. *Surgery*. 2012;152(6):1150-1157.
2. Young WF. The incidentally discovered adrenal mass. *N Engl J Med*. 2007;356:601-610.
3. Adrenalectomy including multivisceral resection. In: Katz MHG, Hunt KK, Veeramachaneni N, et al, eds. *Operative Standards for Cancer Surgery, Volume 3: Sarcoma, Adrenal, Neuroendocrine, Peritoneal Malignancies, Urothelial, Hepatobiliary*. Wolters Kluwer; 2022:83-102; chap 3.
4. Gonzalez RJ, Shapiro S, Sarlis N, et al. Laparoscopic resection of adrenal cortical carcinoma: a cautionary note. *Surgery*. 2005;138:1078-1085.
5. Leboulleux S, Deanderis D, Al Ghuzian A, et al. Adrenocortical carcinoma: is the surgical approach a risk factor of peritoneal carcinomatosis? *Eur J Endocrinol*. 2010;162:1147-1153.
6. Porpiglia F, Miller BS, Manfredi M, et al. A debate on laparoscopic versus open adrenalectomy for adrenocortical carcinoma. *Horm Cancer*. 2011;2(6):372-377.

Chapter 58 Adrenalectomy: Open Thoracoabdominal

Barbra S. Miller

DEFINITION

- Adrenal masses may be benign or malignant. If adrenocortical carcinoma is a concern, adrenalectomy by an open approach should be performed. Adrenal masses may be functional or nonfunctional with regard to excess hormone secretion. Several genetic syndromes are associated with adrenal abnormalities and should be evaluated if indicated.

DIFFERENTIAL DIAGNOSIS

- Primary adrenal adenoma
- Primary adrenocortical carcinoma
- Cyst
- Metastatic cancer
- Pheochromocytoma
- Ganglioneuroma
- Adjacent paraganglioma
- Soft tissue tumor

PATIENT HISTORY AND PHYSICAL FINDINGS

- All adrenal abnormalities should be evaluated in a systematic fashion, including a thorough history and physical examination investigating the possibility of a hormone-secreting mass. This includes the possibility of a pheochromocytoma, Cushing syndrome, primary hyperaldosteronism, and hypertestosteronemia. Specifically, the patient should be questioned regarding poorly controlled hypertension, diabetes, edema, diaphoresis, tachycardia, palpitations, sudden severe headaches, flushing, and easy bruising. The physical examination should look for evidence of central obesity, edema, peripheral wasting, core muscle weakness, a buffalo hump, striae, thin skin, and facial plethora as well as hirsutism or virilization in women and recent onset gynecomastia in men. Because the adrenal gland is situated in the retroperitoneum, unless it is extremely large, palpation of the mass is usually unable to be achieved.

IMAGING AND OTHER DIAGNOSTIC STUDIES

- All adrenal masses should undergo appropriate biochemical testing. Selective testing according to signs or symptoms even in the absence of signs or symptoms of hormone excess is to be avoided as up to 25% found to have autonomous adrenal hormone secretion are "asymptomatic." Urine steroids may help differentiate benign from malignant adrenocortical tumors. In those with a malignant adrenal tumor, hormone levels (intermediaries in the steroid pathway as well as end products) can serve as tumor markers.
- Imaging studies (**FIGURES 1** and **2**) should include an adrenal protocol computed tomography (CT) scan (noncontrast, contrast, 15-minute delayed scan to calculate washout percentage of contrast from the tumor) or magnetic resonance imaging (MRI) (to assess for loss of signal intensity between in-phase and out-of-phase images) and a positron emission tomography (PET) scan if malignancy is questioned.
- Additional imaging studies may be required depending on the functionality of the tumor (metaiodobenzylguanidine [MIBG] or 68Ga-DOTATATE-PET/CT for pheochromocytoma in select cases, adrenal vein sampling for hyperaldosteronism, etc.). A chest CT should be obtained preoperatively to assess for evidence of metastatic disease if the adrenal mass is indeterminate by imaging criteria or known to be malignant. Fine needle aspiration or core biopsy is not recommended if adrenocortical carcinoma is possible but may be useful if metastasis to the adrenal gland is in the differential and the adrenal tumor is the most accessible site of

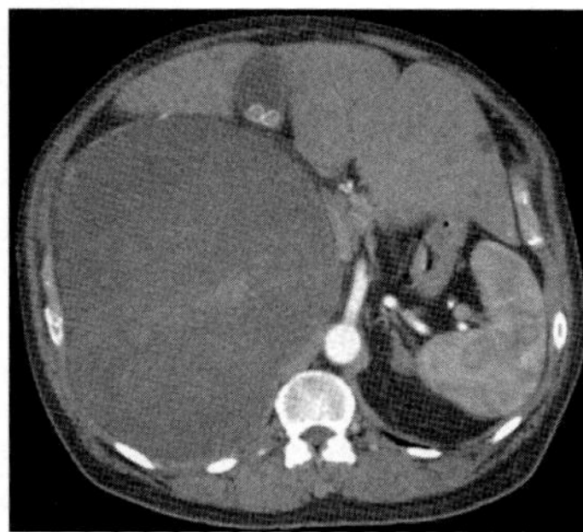

FIGURE 1 • Computed tomography image (axial cut) showing large heterogeneous right adrenal mass concerning for adrenocortical carcinoma.

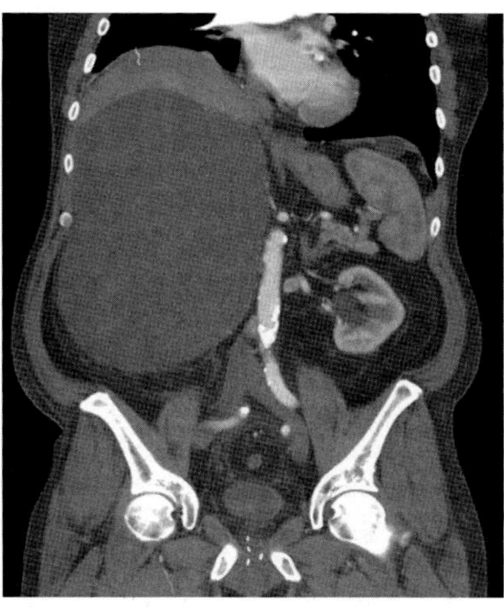

FIGURE 2 • Computed tomography image (coronal cut) showing large heterogeneous right adrenal mass concerning for adrenocortical carcinoma.

metastasis in the setting of multiple sites of metastatic disease. If biopsy is performed, it is imperative to first biochemically rule out pheochromocytoma as a diagnosis.

SURGICAL MANAGEMENT

- Adrenal tumors, if benign appearing by imaging criteria and hormonally nonfunctional, should be reevaluated with at least one additional CT scan or MRI 6 to 12 months after the initial imaging study to ensure stability in size and internal imaging characteristics. Some advocate for a longer period of follow-up imaging for 2 years with reevaluation of biochemistry for 4 more years.[1]
- Functional tumors leading to hormone excess are often removed, although may be medically treated depending on the situation and the number of adrenal glands involved. Those with indeterminate or growing adrenal masses and those with suspected of being adrenocortical carcinoma or isolated metastatic disease from another primary tumor without evidence of widespread metastatic disease are most often offered surgery. Adrenalectomy may be performed by anterior, posterior, or thoracoabdominal approach. The thoracoabdominal approach is particularly useful for providing excellent exposure and access to large adrenal tumors.[2-5] Although excellent exposure can be achieved by an anterior approach in most cases, the thoracoabdominal approach is most beneficial in patients who have undergone prior abdominal or adrenal surgery, have had the liver previously mobilized, have disease involving the diaphragm or thoracic cavity, or when there is need for control of the vena cava superior to the liver.

Preoperative Planning

- The surgeon must evaluate available imaging studies for possible involvement of adjacent organs and vessels and lymphadenopathy. Invasion of major vessels (vena cava) or adjacent organs may require additional teams or different approaches to the tumor as en bloc resection is encouraged when feasible. As CT tends to overestimate invasion of adjacent vessels, MRI with magnetic resonance venogram can be especially helpful to assess for vena cava invasion or venous tumor thrombus.
- The risks, benefits, and alternatives to surgery are discussed with the patient including potential need for steroid supplementation in the postoperative setting. Patients with pheochromocytomas should be adequately alpha blocked and volume replete. Beta blockade may also be necessary. A potassium level should be checked the morning of surgery and treated as necessary in patients with hyperaldosteronism.
- Routine prophylactic antibiotics and deep vein thrombosis prophylaxis are administered prior to surgery, and sequential compression devices are applied.
- A general endotracheal anesthetic is administered. A dual lumen endotracheal tube may be placed for improved exposure but in general is not required.
- An epidural is often placed for postoperative pain management.
- Common to all approaches, skin preparation with clipping rather than shaving is prepared, and the surgical area is prepped and draped in a sterile fashion.

Positioning

- For a right adrenalectomy, the patient is placed in semi-left lateral decubitus position on a beanbag with an axillary roll beneath the left axilla. The right arm is held in a place parallel over the left arm with a thoracic arm holder (**FIGURE 3**). For a left adrenalectomy, the opposite setup is performed. The pelvis remains flat. This allows access to the chest and abdomen. The bed is flexed to increase the space between the ribs and the pelvis.
- All pressure points are padded appropriately.
- The patient is prepped and draped.

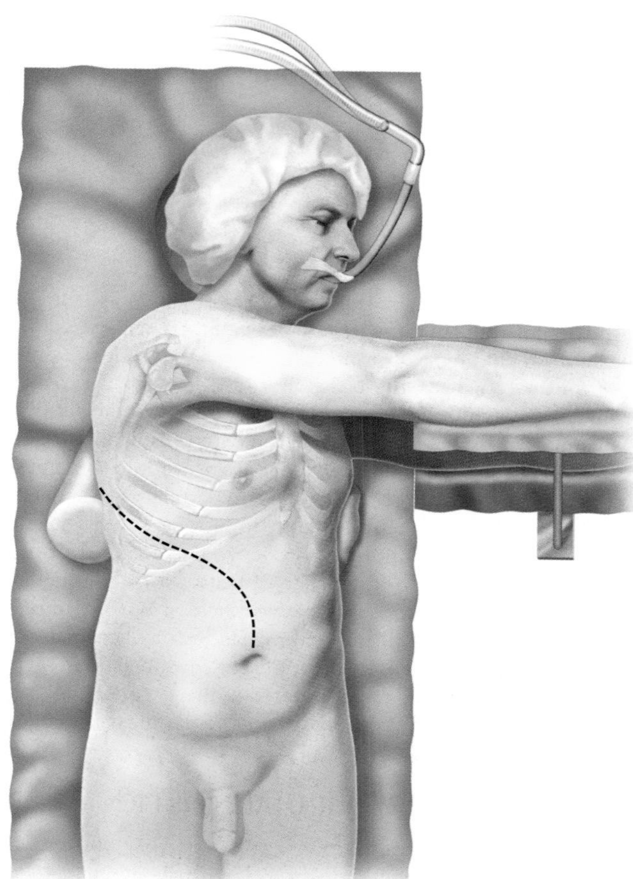

FIGURE 3 • The patient is placed in semi-left lateral decubitus position on a beanbag with an axillary roll beneath the left axilla. The chest is nearly fully lateral, and the pelvis remains flat (corkscrew twist). The right arm is held in place parallel over the left arm with a thoracic arm holder.

RIGHT ADRENALECTOMY

Exposure

- An incision is made 2 cm inferior to the tip of the right scapula and extended to a point midway between the xiphoid process and the umbilicus (**FIGURE 4**). If necessary, the incision can then be carried inferiorly along the midline of the abdomen. The subcutaneous tissue and muscle are divided, sparing the latissimus dorsi and incising the serratus anterior. The chest is entered at the eighth intercostal space, the pulmonary ligament divided, and the lung retracted superiorly. The diaphragm is incised 2 to 4 cm from its attachments, sparing the phrenic nerve. Several marking stitches should be placed intermittently on either side of the divided diaphragm to aid with reapproximation at the end of the case (**FIGURE 5**). The costochondral cartilage is divided. A portion may be excised. The abdominal incision is extended and the peritoneal cavity is entered. A self-retaining retractor system can be placed.
- The diaphragmatic attachments to the right lobe of the liver are released with electrocautery as is the falciform ligament. The ligamentum teres is ligated and divided with silk ligatures. If the adrenal tumor is adherent to the diaphragm, that portion of the diaphragm should be removed en bloc with the tumor and can be reconstructed with mesh or other material. Inspection of the peritoneal cavity is performed as much as possible in a systematic fashion and an ultrasound of the liver is performed. The right lobe of the liver is retracted toward the left side, allowing access to the retrohepatic inferior vena cava (**FIGURE 6**).

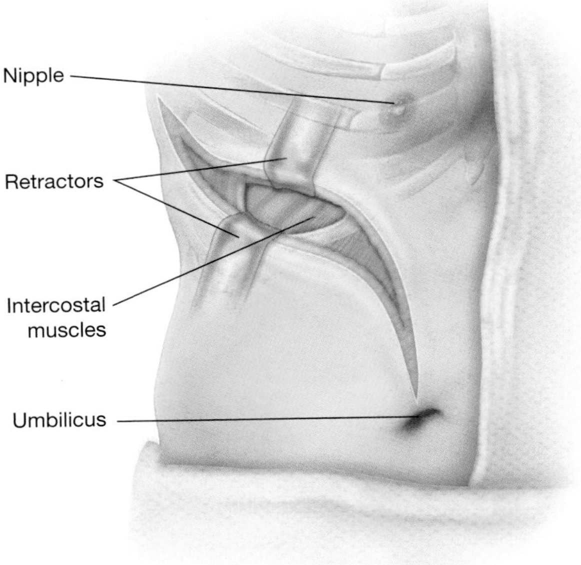

FIGURE 4 ● An incision is made 2 cm inferior to the tip of the right scapula and extended to a point midway between the xiphoid process and the umbilicus. The incision can then be carried inferiorly along the midline of the abdomen. The subcutaneous tissue and muscle are divided, sparing the latissimus dorsi and incising the serratus anterior. The chest is entered at the eighth intercostal space.

Dissection

- A number of critical elements of dissection have been described for dissection of tumors concerning for malignancy (indeterminate by imaging characteristics or obviously invasive)[6]
  1. To achieve a microscopically complete (R0) resection of the primary tumor without tumor capsule violation, the surrounding retroperitoneal fat, Gerota fascia, and peritoneum should be resected en bloc.
  2. For an adrenal tumor with direct invasion of the inferior vena cava, renal vein, or renal artery, the vascular structure(s) should be resected en bloc with the primary adrenal tumor when technically feasible.
  3. Routine prophylactic locoregional lymphadenectomy is not recommended in patients with adrenal cancer. However, in patients with indeterminate adrenal masses or known adrenal cancer and clinically suspicious lymphadenopathy, nodal dissection of the affected lymph node basin(s) should be performed.
- The posterior peritoneal lining over the retroperitoneum in incised over the superior half of the right kidney and carried from medial to lateral out to the side of the abdominal wall (**FIGURE 7**). Medial dissection should proceed carefully to the vena cava, making sure not to divide branches of the renal artery supplying the upper portion of the kidney or venous branches draining to the renal vein. Small branches supplying and draining the adrenal gland should be carefully ligated and divided. Any lymph nodes posterior to the renal hilum should be included in the dissection.
- The fat overlying and just superior to the kidney is mobilized from inferior to superior, making this tissue the inferior margin, using cautery, silk sutures, and other hemostatic devices as needed, making sure not to create a nonexistent plane between the inferior aspect of the tumor and the superior aspect of the kidney. The peritoneal lining should remain intact over the anterior aspect of the tumor to serve as the anterior margin if not already invaded by the tumor. The dissection continues superiorly along the diaphragm, making sure to ligate and divide any feeding vessels, most commonly branches from the inferior phrenic vessels. Posterior dissection should proceed from lateral to medial, making sure to remove all fat posterior to the tumor in an en bloc fashion. If the tumor invades the muscle, a portion of the muscle should be included with the tumor to ensure negative margins.

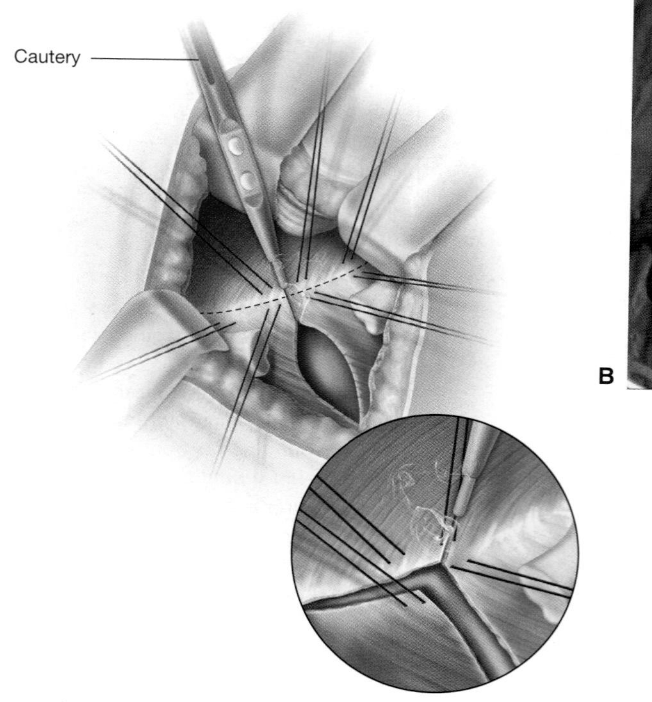

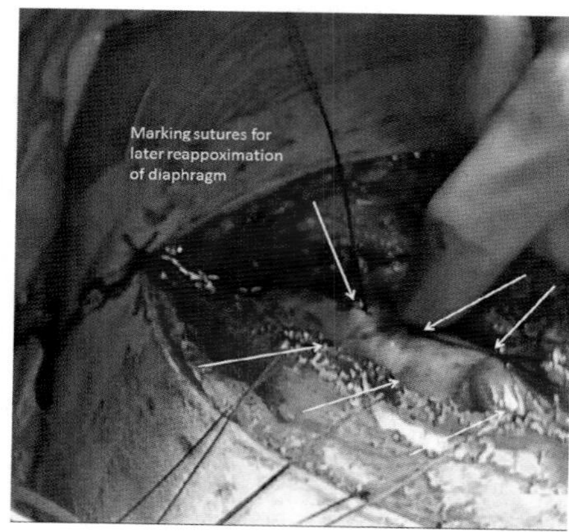

FIGURE 5 ● **A,** The diaphragm is incised 2 to 4 cm from its attachments, sparing the phrenic nerve. **B,** Several marking stitches (*arrows*) can be placed intermittently on either side of the divided diaphragm to aid with reapproximation at the end of the case.

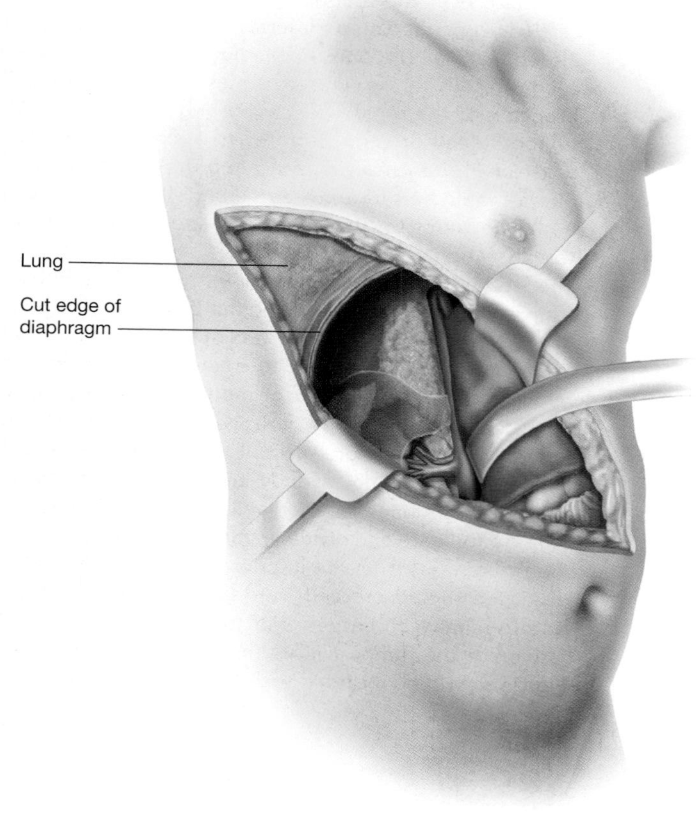

FIGURE 6 ● The diaphragmatic attachments to the right lobe of the liver are released with electrocautery as is the falciform ligament. Both lobes of the liver are mobilized. A portion of the diaphragm should be removed en bloc with any adherent tumor.

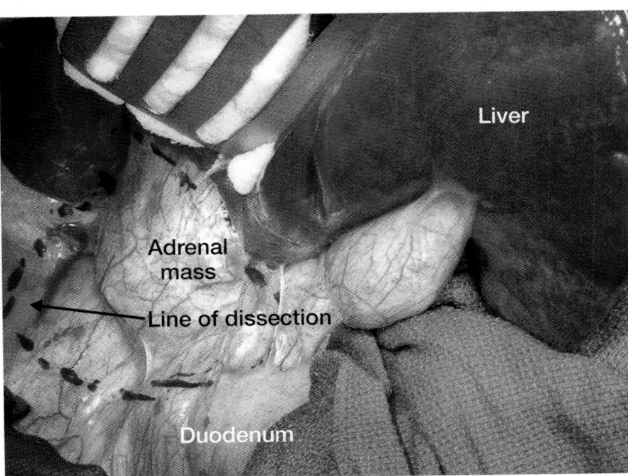

FIGURE 7 ● The posterior lining over the retroperitoneal fat and kidney is incised over the superior half of the right kidney and carried from medial to lateral out to the side of the abdominal wall.

- The anterior surface of the vena cava should be identified and the peritoneal lining overlying this should be incised along its length. Using a vein retractor to retract the vena cava medially, soft tissue attachments, including small vessels and lymphatics, are ligated and divided. As the midpoint of the adrenal gland is reached, the right adrenal vein should be identified, ligated, and divided. The vein should be inspected and carefully palpated to assess for any tumor thrombus so that the tumor thrombus can be included with the specimen in an en bloc fashion. Advanced techniques for managing large tumor thrombi within the vena cava are not discussed in this chapter. If removing a pheochromocytoma, the anesthesiologist should be warned well in advance prior to ligating the adrenal vein in anticipation of ensuing hypotension. The dissection is continued superiorly until all medial attachments have been released. Retraction of the vena cava allows access to posterior tissue, which should be removed as well. The adrenal gland and the periadrenal soft tissue are removed, marked with orienting suture for the pathologist, and sent to the pathology lab.

Closure

- A small amount of water should be used for irrigation and final hemostasis is achieved. The area encompassed by the dissection should be marked with large clips to assist with postoperative external beam radiation therapy if needed. A drain may be placed in the adrenal bed, and a chest tube is placed.
- Closure is begun, and the bed is taken out of the flexed position. A chest tube is placed. The diaphragm is repaired with no. 1 polydioxanone (PDS) suture in a running locking or interrupted fashion.
- At the junction of the diaphragm and abdominal fascia, a no. 2 Vicryl figure-of-eight suture is used to reapproximate the tissue en masse. If a portion of the costochondral cartilage has not been excised, it may be reapproximated using a microdrill and a no. 2 Vicryl suture. The ribs are also reapproximated with no. 2 Vicryl sutures, with or without the microdrill (**FIGURES 8** and **9**). A rib approximator device helps decrease the tension required to tie the sutures. The abdominal midline is reapproximated with running no. 1 PDS suture. The chest wall musculature is closed in two separate layers using no. 1 Vicryl suture. The skin is closed with staples and a sterile dressing is applied (**FIGURE 10**).

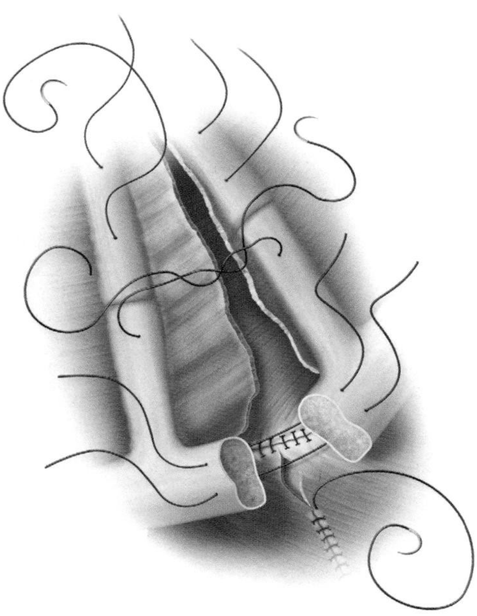

FIGURE 8 ● A portion of the costal margin can be excised to minimize postoperative rubbing of the ends and costochondritis. If a portion of the costochondral cartilage has not been excised, it may be reapproximated using a microdrill and a no. 2 Vicryl suture. The ribs are reapproximated with no. 2 Vicryl sutures, with or without the microdrill.

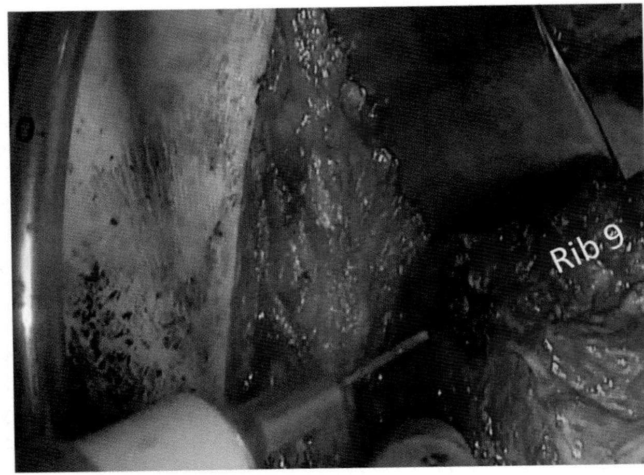

FIGURE 9 ● The microdrill is used to help reapproximate the ribs.

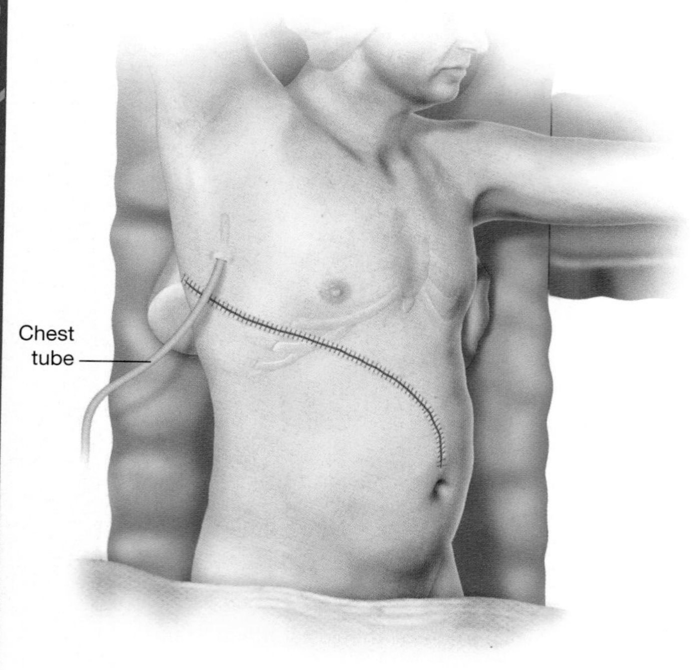

FIGURE 10 ● During closure, a chest tube is inserted. The abdominal midline is reapproximated in a single layer. The chest wall musculature is closed in several layers. The skin is closed with staples and a sterile dressing is applied.

LEFT ADRENALECTOMY

Exposure

- An incision is made 2 cm inferior to the tip of the right scapula and extended to a point midway between the xiphoid process and the umbilicus (**FIGURES 11** and **12**). If necessary, the incision can then be carried inferiorly along the midline of the abdomen. The subcutaneous tissue and muscle are divided, sparing the latissimus dorsi and incising the serratus anterior. The chest is entered at the eighth intercostal space, the pulmonary ligament divided, and the lung retracted superiorly. The diaphragm is incised 2 to 4 cm from its attachments, sparing the phrenic nerve. Several marking stitches should be placed intermittently on either side of the divided diaphragm to aid with reapproximation at the end of the case. The costochondral cartilage is divided. A portion may be excised if needed. The abdominal incision is extended and the peritoneal cavity is entered. A self-retaining retractor system is placed.
- The diaphragmatic attachments to the spleen are released with electrocautery and reflected toward the right side along with the stomach and pancreas. If the adrenal tumor is adherent to the diaphragm, that portion of the diaphragm should be removed en bloc with the tumor and can be reconstructed with mesh or other material. The splenocolic attachments will require release and the omentum is released from the colon. The ligamentum teres is ligated and divided with silk ligatures.
- Inspection of the peritoneal cavity is performed as much as possible in a systematic fashion, and an ultrasound of the liver is performed.
- The left lobe of the liver is retracted toward the right side, allowing for better mobilization of the stomach, spleen, and pancreas.

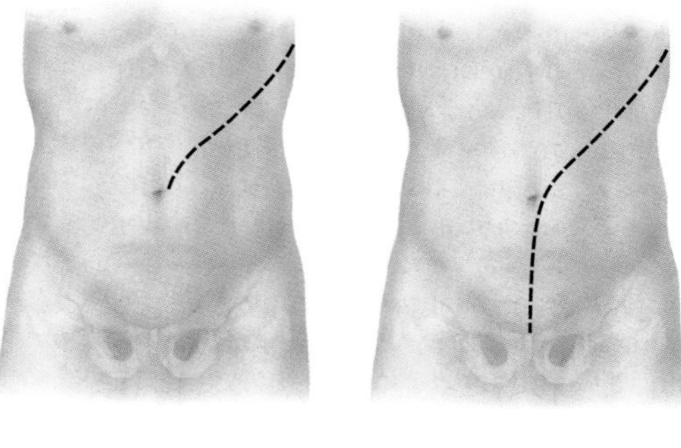

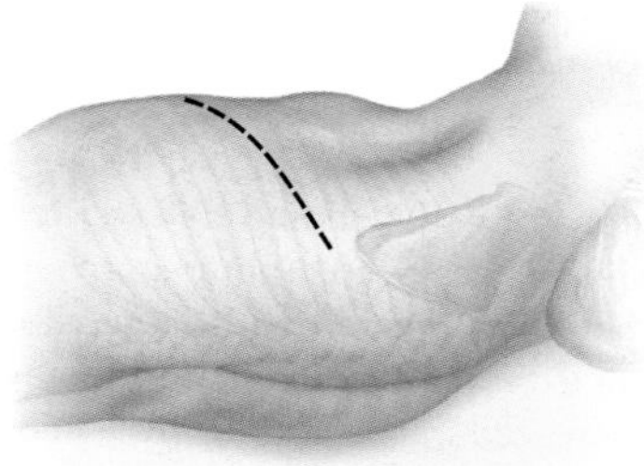

FIGURE 11 ● Options for left thoracoabdominal incision for adrenalectomy.

- A large saline-soaked towel with retractors is placed against the bowel, pancreas, and spleen to not only provide exposure but also to exclude the rest of the peritoneal cavity to minimize potential seeding of the peritoneal cavity. The left side of the aorta should be appreciable if the exposure is adequate (**FIGURE 13**).

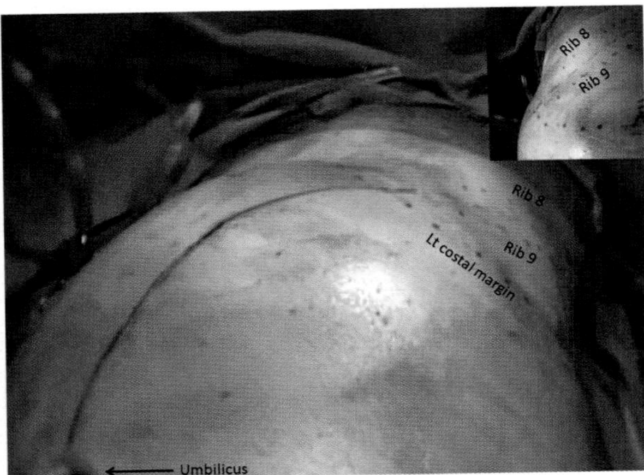

FIGURE 12 ● An incision is made 2 cm inferior to the tip of the right scapula and extended to a point midway between the xiphoid process and the umbilicus.

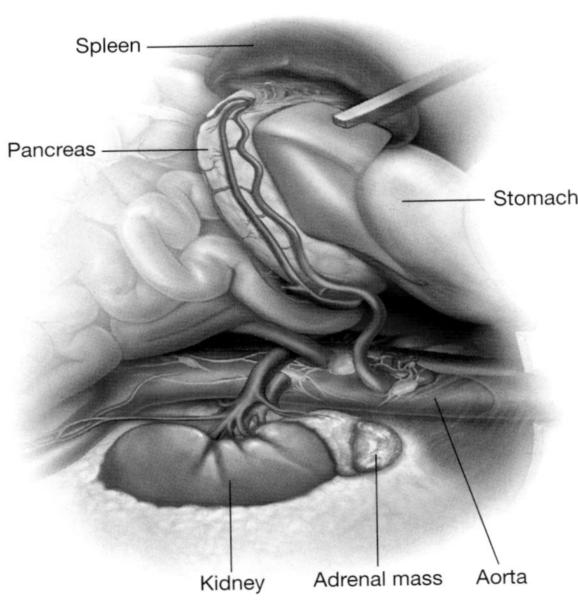

FIGURE 13 ● With the stomach, pancreas, and spleen retracted medially, the aorta, adrenal mass, and kidney are exposed and excluded from the rest of the peritoneal cavity.

Dissection

- Because the peritoneal covering on the left has been reflected with the spleen and pancreas, the surgeon should make every effort to manipulate the tumor surface as little as possible (no-touch technique). The soft tissue overlying the superior half of the left kidney is incised and carried from medial to lateral out to the side of the abdominal wall. Inferior dissection should proceed carefully to the aorta medially along the left renal vein, making sure not to divide branches of the posteriorly situated renal artery supplying the upper portion of the kidney or venous branches draining to the renal vein. Small branches supplying and draining the adrenal gland should be carefully ligated and divided. Any lymph nodes posterior to the renal hilum should be included with the dissection. The left adrenal vein will be identified at the medial aspect of the left renal vein as it courses anterior to the aorta. It generally enters the adrenal gland in the 7-o'clock position. It should be ligated and divided. The adrenal vein and renal vein should be inspected and carefully palpated to assess for any tumor thrombus so that the tumor thrombus can be included with the specimen in an en bloc fashion. Advanced techniques for managing large tumor thrombi within the renal vein and vena cava are not discussed in this chapter. The fat overlying and just superior to the kidney is mobilized from inferior to superior, making this tissue the inferior margin, using cautery, silk sutures, and other hemostatic devices as needed, making sure not to create a nonexistent plane between the inferior aspect of the tumor and the superior aspect of the kidney. Lateral dissection should continue along the abdominal sidewall. The dissection continues superiorly along the diaphragm, making sure to ligate and divide any feeding vessels, most commonly branches from the inferior phrenic vessels. Posterior dissection should proceed from lateral to medial, making sure to remove all fat posterior to the tumor in an en bloc fashion. If the tumor invades the muscle, a portion of the muscle should be included with the tumor to ensure negative margins. The left lateral surface of the aorta should be identified, and the soft tissue attachments including small vessels and lymphatics are ligated and divided. If removing a pheochromocytoma, the anesthesiologist should be warned well in advance prior to ligating the adrenal vein in anticipation of ensuing hypotension. The dissection is continued superiorly until all medial attachments have been released. Any lymph nodes along the aorta or identified near the superior mesenteric artery or celiac axis should be included with the specimen. The adrenal gland and the periadrenal soft tissue is removed, marked with orienting suture for the pathologist, and sent to the pathology lab.

Closure

- A small amount of water should be used for irrigation and final hemostasis achieved. The area encompassed by the dissection should be marked with large clips to assist with postoperative external beam radiation therapy if needed. A drain may be placed in the adrenal bed, and a chest tube is placed. Closure is begun, and the bed is taken out of the flexed position. The diaphragm is repaired with no. 1 PDS suture in a running locking or interrupted fashion. At the junction of the diaphragm and abdominal fascia, a no. 2 Vicryl figure-of-eight suture is used to reapproximate the tissue en masse. If a portion of the costochondral cartilage has not been excised, it may be reapproximated using a microdrill and a no. 2 Vicryl suture. The ribs are also reapproximated with no. 2 Vicryl sutures, with or without the microdrill. A rib approximator device helps decrease the tension required to tie the sutures. The abdominal midline is reapproximated with running no. 1 PDS suture. The chest wall musculature is closed in two separate layers using no. 1 Vicryl suture. The skin is closed with staples and a sterile dressing is applied.

PEARLS AND PITFALLS

Atelectasis	▪ Ensure excellent respiratory care and pulmonary toilet due to increased pain limiting respiratory effort.
Bleeding	▪ Access to the suprahepatic inferior vena cava is improved during left adrenalectomy with this approach, allowing for easier vascular control.
Pain	▪ Thoracoabdominal incisions are associated with greater pain than other incisions. Local anesthetic blocks may be helpful.
Neurovascular bundle of the rib	▪ Avoid transection of the bundle and damage to the nerve by incising along the superior border of the rib.
Phrenic nerve palsy	▪ Take care to stay away from the phrenic nerve when incising the diaphragm.

POSTOPERATIVE CARE

- Most patients will need intensive care unit (ICU) care for 24 to 48 hours, either for pulmonary care or for resuscitation. The chest tube may be managed in standard fashion and removed when appropriate.
- Hydrocortisone should be administered to patients with overt Cushing syndrome. A cosyntropin stimulation test can be performed the morning after surgery in subclinical or mild Cushing cases if there is a question about the requirement for steroid supplementation. After bilateral adrenalectomy, high-dose intravenous hydrocortisone should be weaned to replacement dose oral hydrocortisone and fludrocortisone 0.1 mg daily. Electrolytes should be checked the morning after surgery. Patients undergoing surgery for primary hyperaldosteronism may experience rebound hyperkalemia. Antihypertensive medications are withheld in the immediate postoperative setting and reinstituted as needed. Routine postoperative care is pursued and patients are discharged approximately 5 to 7 days after surgery. Follow-up is typically 1 to 2 weeks after surgery with endocrine testing as needed.

OUTCOMES

- Excellent outcomes can be expected with low morbidity if aggressive respiratory care and pain control is initiated early in the postoperative period.

COMPLICATIONS

- Prolonged atelectasis: 21%
- Prolonged ileus: 9%
- Phrenic nerve injury and diaphragmatic paralysis
- Chronic pain

REFERENCES

1. Young WF. The incidentally discovered adrenal mass. *N Engl J Med*. 2007;356:601-610.
2. Gusani NJ, Avella D, Staveley-O'Carroll KF, et al. Thoracoabdominal incision: a forgotten tool. *Oper Tech Gen Surg*. 2008;10(2):107-110.
3. Karakousis CP, Pourshahmir M. Thoracoabdominal incisions and resection of upper retroperitoneal sarcomas. *J Surg Oncol*. 1999;72:150-155.
4. Lumsden AB, Colborn GL, Sreeram S, et al. The surgical anatomy and technique of the thoracoabdominal incision. *Surg Clin North Am*. 1993;73(4):633-644.
5. Yang M, Zhao X. Retrospective study of the efficacy and complication of thoracoabdominal incision for nephrectomy: a comparison with flank approach. *Front Med China*. 2009;3(2):191-196.
6. Oltmann S. Chapter 3: Adrenalectomy including multivisceral resection. In: Katz MHG, Hunt KK, Veeramachaneni N, et al., eds. *Operative Standards for Cancer Surgery, Volume 3: Sarcoma, Adrenal, Neuroendocrine, Peritoneal Malignancies, Urothelial, Hepatobiliary.* Wolters Kluwer; 2022: 83-102.

Chapter 59 Adrenalectomy: Open Posterior

Barbra S. Miller

DEFINITION

- Adrenal masses may be benign or malignant and functional or nonfunctional with regard to excess hormone secretion. An open posterior approach should be considered if:
  - An anterior, lateral, or posterior retroperitoneoscopic approach is not feasible in a patient with a benign or metastatic adrenal tumor.
  - An open anterior approach is not feasible in patients who have undergone previous extensive upper abdominal surgery and are presumed to have dense adhesions limiting access.
  - Conversion from a retroperitoneoscopic posterior approach to an open approach is required.
  - Both adrenals need to be removed and repositioning of the patient during the case is to be avoided.

DIFFERENTIAL DIAGNOSIS

- Primary adrenal adenoma
- Primary adrenocortical carcinoma
- Cyst
- Metastatic cancer
- Pheochromocytoma
- Ganglioneuroma
- Adjacent paraganglioma
- Soft tissue tumor

PATIENT HISTORY AND PHYSICAL FINDINGS

- All adrenal abnormalities should be evaluated in a systematic fashion, including a thorough history and physical examination investigating the possibility of a hormone-secreting mass. This includes the possibility of a pheochromocytoma, autonomous cortisol secretion, primary hyperaldosteronism, and hypertestosteronemia. Specifically, the patient should be questioned regarding poorly controlled hypertension, diabetes, edema, diaphoresis, tachycardia, palpitations, sudden severe headaches, flushing, and easy bruising. The physical examination should look for evidence of central obesity, edema, peripheral wasting, core muscle weakness, a buffalo hump, striae, thin skin, facial plethora, hirsutism, or virilization in women or recent onset gynecomastia in men. Because the adrenal gland is situated in the retroperitoneum, unless it is extremely large, palpation of the mass is usually unable to be achieved.

IMAGING AND OTHER DIAGNOSTIC STUDIES

- All adrenal masses should undergo appropriate biochemical testing (see Part 5, Chapter 57). Even in the absence of signs or symptoms, patients should have at a minimum: potassium, aldosterone, renin, plasma fractionated metanephrines (followed by 24-hour urine metanephrines and normetanephrines, catecholamines, and vanillylmandelic acid [VMA] if plasma values are abnormal), adrenocorticotropic hormone (ACTH), dehydroepiandrosterone sulfate (DHEA-S), and 1 mg dexamethasone suppression test. Other biochemical tests are also often obtained.
- Imaging studies should include an adrenal protocol computed tomography (CT) scan (to assess imaging characteristics and calculate washout percentage of contrast from the tumor) or magnetic resonance imaging (MRI) (to assess decrease in signal between in-phase and out-of-phase images) and 18F-fluorodeoxyglucose (18FDG) positron emission tomography (PET) CT if malignancy is questioned (**FIGURE 1**).
- Additional imaging studies may be required depending on the functionality of the tumor (metaiodobenzylguanidine [MIBG] or 68Ga-DOTATATE-PET/CT for pheochromocytoma patients, adrenal vein sampling for hyperaldosteronism, etc.).
- Fine needle aspiration (FNA) or core biopsy is not recommended if adrenocortical carcinoma is questioned. FNA may be useful if metastasis to the adrenal gland is in the differential and the adrenal tumor is the most accessible site of metastasis in the setting of multiple sites of metastatic disease. If biopsy is performed, it is imperative to first biochemically rule out pheochromocytoma.

SURGICAL MANAGEMENT

- Adrenal tumors, if benign appearing by imaging criteria, nonfunctional, and therefore not requiring resection, should be reevaluated with at least one additional CT scan or MRI 6 to 12 months after the initial imaging study to ensure stability

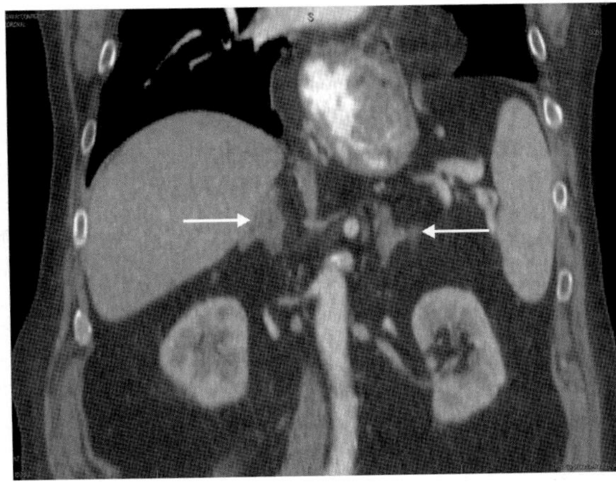

FIGURE 1 ● Bilateral hyperplastic adrenal glands (*arrows*) with benign imaging characteristics are shown in an obese patient with Cushing disease requiring bilateral adrenalectomy.

in size and internal imaging characteristics. Some advocate for a longer period of follow-up imaging for 2 years with reevaluation of biochemistry for 4 years.[1]

- Functional tumors leading to hormone excess are often removed, although may be medically treated depending on the situation and the number of adrenal glands involved. Those with growing benign adrenal masses are most often offered surgery. Indeterminate masses or masses known to be adrenocortical carcinoma are removed by an open anterior approach. Open posterior approaches are most often selected for benign tumors when other approaches to the adrenal gland are not feasible.[2]

Preoperative Planning

- The surgeon must evaluate available imaging studies for possible adrenocortical carcinoma or tumor involvement of adjacent organs, vessels, and lymphadenopathy. An open posterior approach is not optimal for removing adrenocortical carcinomas or large tumors, as the working space is limited by the rib cage and does not allow for multivisceral resections. These types of tumors should be approached by an open anterior or thoracoabdominal approach.
- The surgeon should evaluate the position of the adrenal gland with respect to the overlying rib that will need to be resected as well as any visible vasculature supplying or draining the adrenal gland.
- The risks, benefits, and alternatives to surgery are discussed with the patient including potential need for steroid supplementation in the postoperative setting. Patients with pheochromocytomas should be adequately alpha blocked and volume replete. Beta blockade may also be necessary. A potassium level should be checked the morning of surgery and treated as necessary in patients with Conn syndrome (hyperaldosteronism).

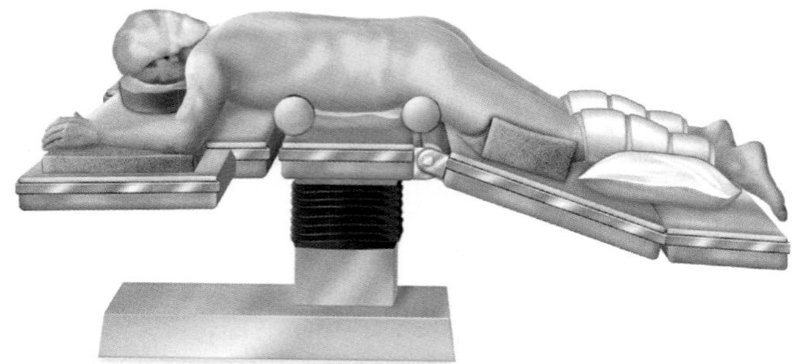

FIGURE 2 • The patient is placed in a modified prone position. Pressure points are padded.

- Routine prophylactic antibiotics and deep vein thrombosis prophylaxis are administered prior to surgery, and sequential compression devices are applied.
- A general endotracheal anesthetic is administered.
- Common to all approaches, skin preparation with clipping rather than shaving is prepared, and the surgical area is prepped and draped in a sterile fashion.

Positioning

- Patients are intubated and a Foley catheter is placed prior to placing the patient in a modified prone position. Several methods for positioning may be used, including use of the Wilson frame, the Cloward surgical saddle, gel rolls, and flexion of the table (**FIGURE 2**). All of these have the common goal of creating a gentle flexion of the spine. Space is also created for the abdominal contents to shift away from the retroperitoneum.
- All pressure points are padded appropriately.

TECHNIQUES

LEFT ADRENALECTOMY

Exposure

- A curvilinear incision is made from a paramedian position (4-5 cm from the spine) over the left 10th rib and carried inferolaterally toward the iliac crest. Alternatively, a straighter incision over the 11th or 12th rib, depending on the position of the gland on CT scan, with a more vertical upward incision medially may be made (**FIGURES 3** and **4**).
- The subcutaneous tissue and musculature (latissimus dorsi and lumbodorsal fascia) are divided. The sacrospinalis is retracted medially with a handheld retractor. The 12th rib (and occasionally the 11th rib) is cleared of its attachments in a subperiosteal fashion using cautery and a doyen or periosteal elevator, making sure to preserve the neurovascular bundle (**FIGURES 5** and **6**). The rib is transected as far medially as possible with bone cutters and removed in its entirety. Bone wax may be used to assist with hemostasis.
- Entrance into the diaphragm and pleura should be avoided and the diaphragm is reflected superiorly. The retroperitoneal fat will be evident (**FIGURE 7**).

Dissection

- Using retractors to separate the tissue and rib(s), Gerota fascia is incised after identifying the upper pole of the kidney. The surgeon's hand places downward (inferior and toward the peritoneal cavity) pressure on the kidney to facilitate exposure of the adrenal gland (**FIGURE 8**).
- The inferior, lateral, superior, and medial attachments may be divided in a similar fashion to the standard open anterior approach, but the peritoneum overlying the anterior surface of the gland as described in the anterior open approach is not included with the specimen. The inferior attachments should be left until last, as they assist in retraction and exposure of the gland.
- The left adrenal vein should be ligated and divided when encountered during the course of dissection of the

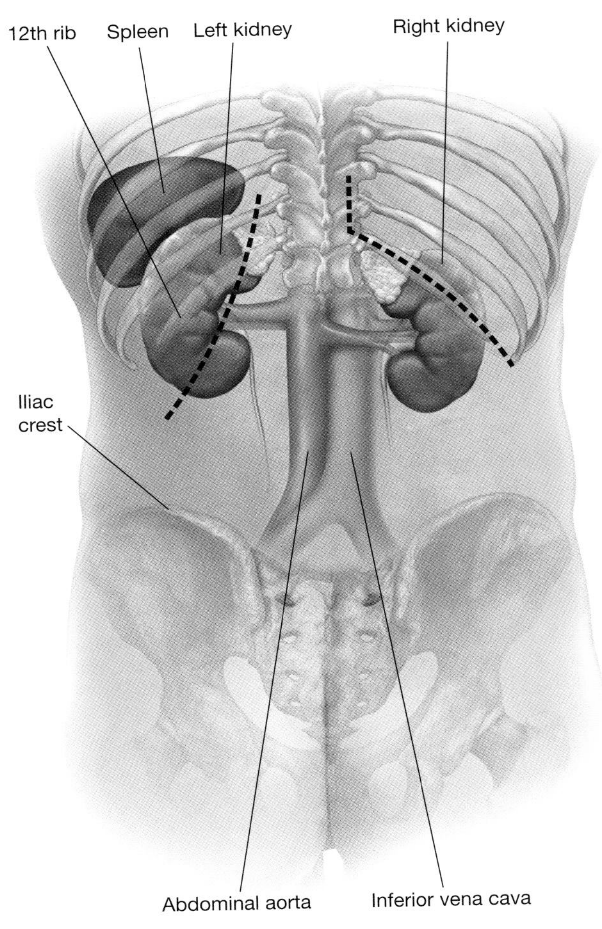

FIGURE 3 ● The incision can be made in a linear or curvilinear fashion to facilitate access to the 11th and 12th ribs.

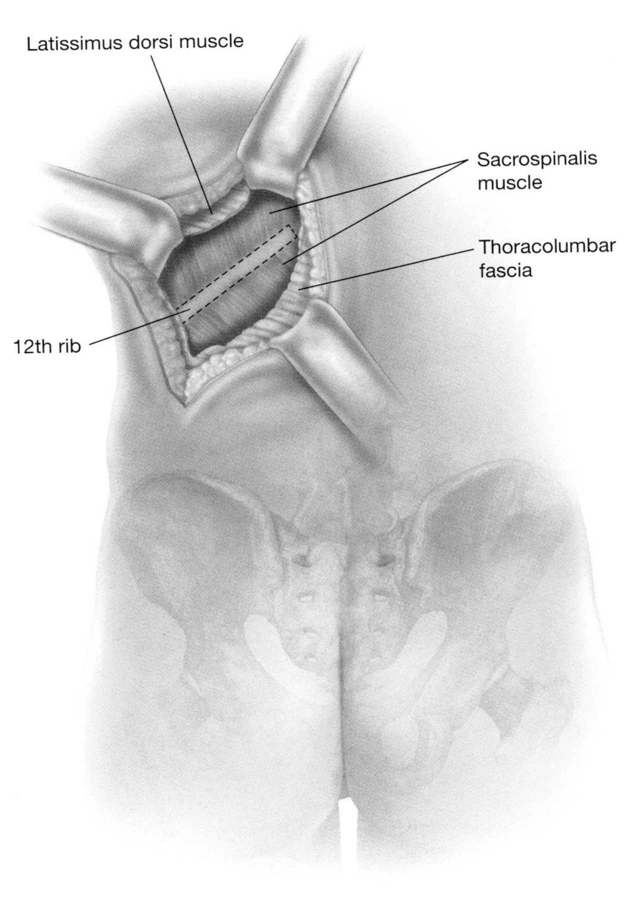

FIGURE 5 ● Schematic of exposure of the 12th rib that is cleared of its attachments in a subperiosteal fashion using cautery and a doyen or periosteal elevator, making sure to preserve the neurovascular bundle.

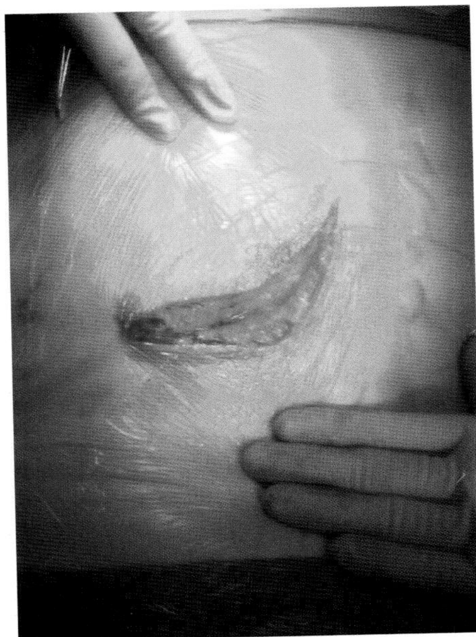

FIGURE 4 ● Intraoperative image of curvilinear incision carried from 10th rib medially across the 11th rib and inferior to the 12th rib laterally.

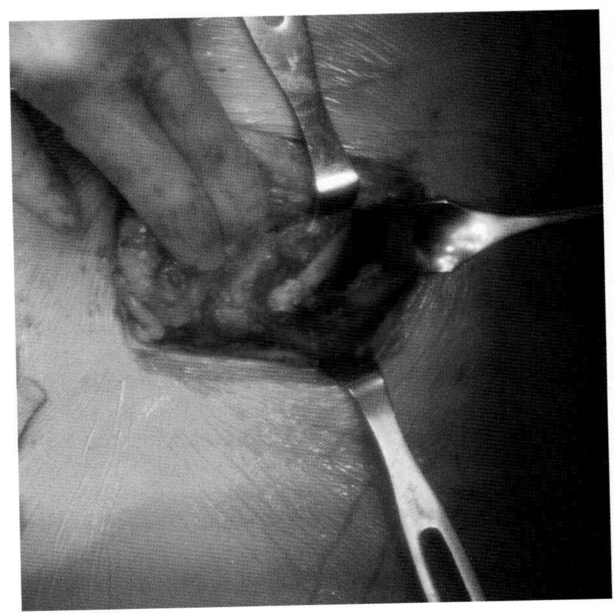

FIGURE 6 ● Intraoperative photo showing exposure of the 12th rib.

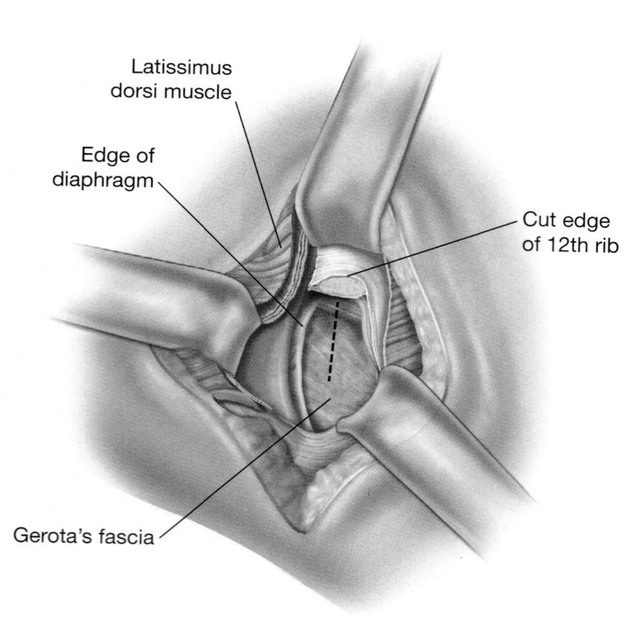

FIGURE 7 ● After removal of the 12th rib, Gerota fascia and the retroperitoneal fat is evident.

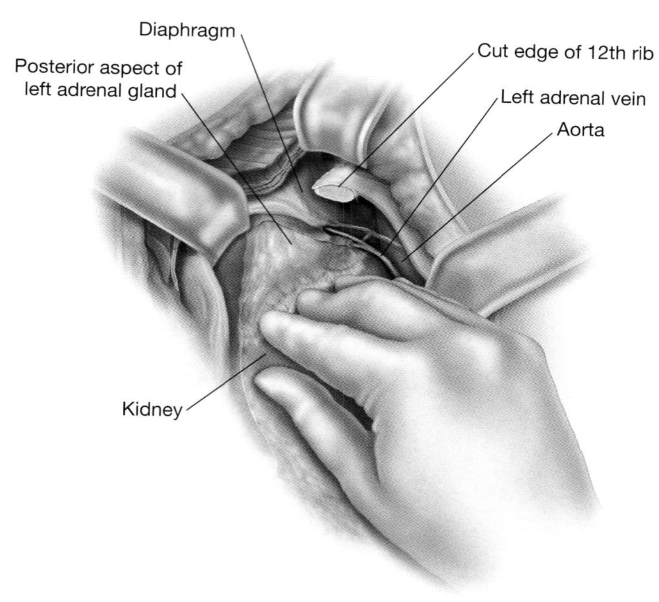

FIGURE 8 ● The left adrenal gland is best exposed using retractors and downward retraction using the hand on the upper pole of the kidney. The left adrenal vein is located in a 5-o'clock position.

inferior attachments and will be found medially near the junction of the superior aspect of the left renal vein with the lateral aspect of the aorta in a 5-o'clock position due to the prone position. The left adrenal vein will be slightly posterior while in the prone position beneath some of the fatty attachments between the adrenal gland and left renal vein.

- The adrenal gland with the periadrenal soft tissue is removed en bloc, marked with orienting sutures for the pathologist, and sent to the pathology lab.

Closure

- A small amount of water should be used for irrigation and final hemostasis is achieved. A drain may be placed if desired but is not required in most cases.
- The musculature and subcutaneous tissues are closed in layers and the skin is closed with staples or suture. A sterile dressing is applied.

RIGHT ADRENALECTOMY

Exposure

- A curvilinear incision is made from a paramedian position (4-5 cm from the spine) over the right 10th rib and carried inferolaterally toward the iliac crest. Alternatively, a straighter incision over the 11th or 12th rib, depending on the position of the gland on CT scan, with a more vertical upward incision medially may be made.
- The subcutaneous tissue and musculature (latissimus dorsi and lumbodorsal fascia) are divided. The sacrospinalis is retracted medially with a handheld retractor. The 12th rib (and occasionally the 11th rib) is cleared of its attachments in a subperiosteal fashion using cautery and a doyen or periosteal elevator, making sure to preserve the neurovascular bundle. The rib is transected as far medially as possible with bone cutters and removed in its entirety. Bone wax may be used to assist with hemostasis.
- Entrance into the diaphragm and pleura should be avoided and is reflected superiorly. The retroperitoneal fat will be evident.

Dissection

- Using retractors to separate the tissue and rib(s), Gerota fascia is incised after identifying the area of the upper pole of the kidney. The surgeon's hand places downward (inferior and toward the peritoneal cavity) pressure on the kidney to facilitate exposure of the adrenal gland (**FIGURE 9**).
- The right adrenal vein will be found along the medial aspect of the gland in a more anterior position off of the inferior vena cava due to the prone position of the patient and should be ligated and divided.

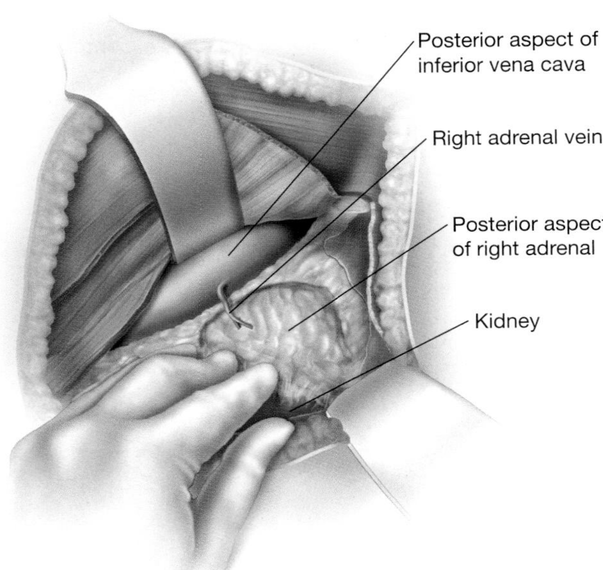

FIGURE 9 ● The right adrenal gland is best exposed using retractors and downward retraction using the hand on the upper pole of the kidney. The right adrenal vein is located in a 9-o'clock position.

- The inferior, lateral, superior, and medial attachments may be divided in a similar fashion to the standard approach, but the peritoneum overlying the anterior surface of the gland as described in the anterior open approach is not included with the specimen. The inferior attachments should be left until last, as they assist in retraction and exposure of the gland.
- The adrenal gland with the periadrenal soft tissue is removed en bloc, marked with orienting sutures for the pathologist, and sent to the pathology lab.

Closure

- A small amount of water should be used for irrigation and final hemostasis is achieved.
- A drain may be placed if desired but is not required in many cases.
- The musculature and subcutaneous tissues are closed in layers and the skin is closed with staples or suture. A sterile dressing is applied.

PEARLS AND PITFALLS

Bleeding—arterial and venous	■ May result from the disruption of the vena cava, renal vein or artery, and aorta. A laparoscopic knot pusher, Allis clamp, and/or Kitner may be helpful given limited access due to the overlying ribs.
Diaphragmatic penetration	■ May occur upon entry to the retroperitoneum. May be closed in standard fashion.
Neurovascular bundle injury	■ Chronic pain may result if care is not taken to spare the bundle when removing the rib or upon closure of the wound.

POSTOPERATIVE CARE

- Most patients will not need intensive care unit (ICU) care, although pheochromocytoma patients often need closer monitoring for the first 24 hours, depending on intraoperative stability and volume status.
- Hydrocortisone should be given to patients with overt Cushing syndrome. A cosyntropin stimulation test can be performed the morning after surgery in subclinical or mild Cushing cases if there is a question about the requirement for steroid supplementation.
- Electrolytes should be checked the morning after surgery. Patients undergoing surgery for primary hyperaldosteronism may experience rebound hyperkalemia.
- After bilateral adrenalectomy, high-dose intravenous hydrocortisone should be weaned to replacement dose oral hydrocortisone and fludrocortisone 0.1 mg daily.

- Routine postoperative care is pursued. Diets may be begun early, as ileus is not usually an issue due to the entirely retroperitoneal dissection. Patients are discharged 2 to 3 days after surgery.
- Follow-up is typically 1 to 2 weeks after surgery with endocrine testing as indicated.

OUTCOMES

- Outcomes in general are quite good. Hospital stay is generally 2 to 3 days. Outcomes and cost are somewhere between laparoscopic and open anterior approaches.[2,3]
- Neurologic changes due to injury of the neurovascular bundle coursing along the inferior aspect of the rib can be problematic.

COMPLICATIONS

- Bleeding
- Infection
- Adrenal insufficiency in those with Cushing syndrome
- Postoperative hypotension in those with pheochromocytoma
- Rebound hyperkalemia in those with Conn syndrome
- Lymphatic leak
- Pneumothorax
- Neurogenic pain
- Laxity of flank musculature

REFERENCES

1. Young WF. The incidentally discovered adrenal mass. *N Engl J Med*. 2007;356:601-610.
2. Miller BS. "Old fashioned" open adrenalectomy. *World J Surg*. 2019; 44(2):618-621.
3. Thompson GB, Grant CS, van Heerden JA, et al. Laparoscopic versus open posterior adrenalectomy: a case-control study of 100 patients. *Surgery*. 1997;122(6):1132-1136.

Chapter 60

Laparoscopic Retroperitoneal Adrenalectomy

Eric James Kuo, Michael Gwynne Johnston, and James A. Lee

DEFINITION

Indications

- Adrenalectomy is indicated for a variety of different clinical scenarios, including patients with (1) a functional tumor; (2) a solid adrenal mass larger than 3 to 4 cm, due to increasing risk of adrenocortical carcinoma; (3) growth of 0.5 cm or greater in 6 months based on serial cross-sectional imaging, again due to a risk of adrenocortical carcinoma; and (4) isolated metastasis from a remote primary malignancy.
- Laparoscopic adrenalectomy is now considered standard practice due to its shorter duration of postoperative pain, shorter hospitalization, and faster return to work compared to an open procedure.
- Contraindications to the transabdominal laparoscopic approach include severe cardiopulmonary disease and coagulopathy. Relative contraindications include prior intra-abdominal surgery and very large tumor size.
- The laparoscopic retroperitoneal approach is based on the historical open posterior approach. This approach is gaining popularity as it offers advantages over a laparoscopic transabdominal approach. These advantages include faster operating times, potentially less postoperative pain, a lower risk of complications (especially of incisional hernia), and improved intraoperative hemostasis as the surgeon has the ability to increase the insufflation pressure to 30 mm Hg (a maneuver not feasible in a laparoscopic transabdominal approach given the negative impact on central venous return and renal perfusion).
- The laparoscopic retroperitoneal approach does have some potential drawbacks. There is a slightly longer learning curve associated with the nontraditional "back-door" anatomic view. This approach may also be more difficult in patients with large tumors or who are morbidly obese.
- The posterior approach is the ideal approach for bilateral procedures because it eliminates the need for patient repositioning. It is also preferable for patients who have had previous transabdominal operations.
- Absolute contraindications to the laparoscopic retroperitoneal approach include the need to explore the rest of the abdomen and coagulopathy.
- Relative contraindications include an adrenal mass greater than 8 cm due to the smaller working space and morbid obesity due to the patient's pannus and visceral fat compressing the retroperitoneal working space. Patient body mass index greater than 45 and indicators of adiposity on axial imaging such as the distance from the skin to renal parenchyma at the level of the 12th rib are associated with increased operative times. Severe cardiopulmonary disease is also a relative contraindication but may be less of an issue than for the transabdominal laparoscopic approach, as the diaphragm is not compressed to the same extent. Theoretically, increased ocular pressures are also a relative contraindication, as an extended time in a prone position would put the optic nerve at risk. This is usually only a problem for very long operations, however, and the vast majority of laparoscopic retroperitoneal adrenalectomies should not threaten the optic nerve.

SURGICAL MANAGEMENT

Preoperative Planning

- As with any endocrine disease, the workup of adrenal disease typically follows a logical progression, from making a biochemical diagnosis to localizing the lesion to determining the indications for an operation. In deciding if an operation is indicated, the two principal questions to be answered are (1) "Is the mass functional?" and (2) "What is the risk for cancer (either primary or metastatic disease)?" Most functional tumors and most malignant lesions should be considered for resection, taking into account the patient's overall health, prognosis, and preferences.
  - Aldosteronoma: Ideally, the potassium level should be normalized preoperatively. Potassium supplements and/or aldosterone antagonists may be employed to achieve this goal. Maintain or optimize the antihypertensive regimen preoperatively.
  - Pheochromocytoma: Give the patient an α-blocker such as phenoxybenzamine. Start at 10 mg twice daily and increase the frequency and dose as tolerated until the patient becomes slightly symptomatic (including mild orthostasis and stuffy nose). A selective α-blocker is a good alternative in an older male patient due to less reflex tachycardia and potential prostatism benefits. In addition, some patients may be candidates for calcium channel therapy instead. As α-blockade proceeds, it is critical to replete the intravascular space with liberal fluid and some additional salt intake preoperatively. β-Blockade may be started a few days prior to the operation if the patient becomes tachycardic. Do *not* start β-blockade prior to adequate α-blockade or the resulting unopposed α-mediated vasoconstriction may cause stroke, myocardial infarction, and even death. Close communication with the anesthesia team is critical throughout the operation as manipulation of the tumor may cause wide swings in hemodynamics. Ensure that the anesthesia team is equipped with short-acting vasoactive agents to control or support intraoperative blood pressure as needed.
  - Cortisol-producing tumor: Give stress-dose steroids prior to induction. The patient will require a careful steroid taper postoperatively and endocrinology consultation is recommended. Although no level I data are available, perioperative antibiotics should be considered due to the relative immunosuppressed state in a patient with cortisol excess.

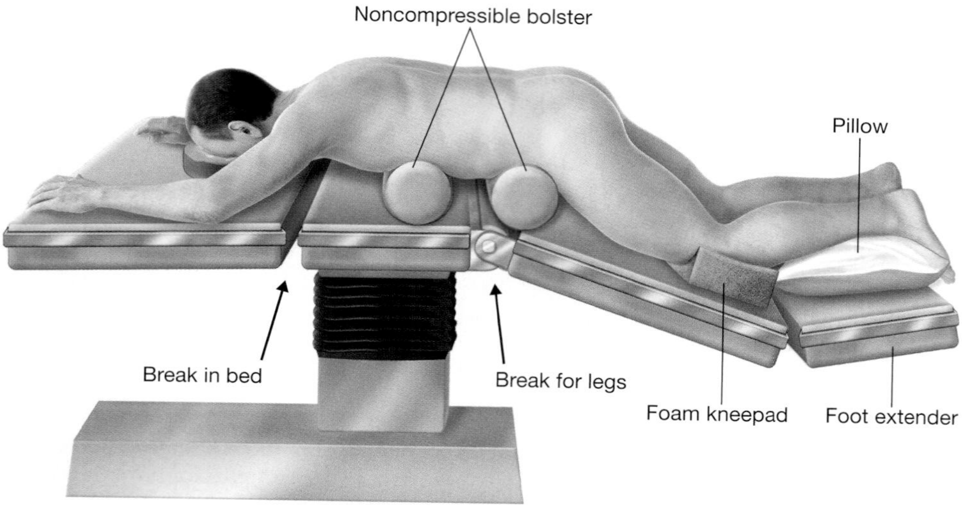

FIGURE 1 ● Patient positioning for a laparoscopic retroperitoneal adrenalectomy.

- Adrenocortical carcinoma: Primary adrenal cancers may manifest any or all of the biochemical irregularities found in the aforementioned tumors and should be addressed as appropriate. It is important to assess the vasculature for evidence of venous invasion and tumor thrombus, ideally with a magnetic resonance venogram or formal venogram. The laparoscopic retroperitoneal approach should not be used in cases of very large or locally invasive adrenal tumors.

Anatomy

- The retroperitoneal space is bounded by the peritoneum laterally, the paraspinous muscle medially, the rib cage posteriorly (ie, away from the table), the kidney/adrenal gland/peritoneum anteriorly (ie, toward the table), and the diaphragm superiorly.
- The superior pole of the kidney and the paraspinous muscle serve as the major landmarks.

Patient Positioning

- A modification of the "Walz position."
- Intubate, obtain intravenous/arterial access as indicated, and place a urinary catheter while patient is still on stretcher. Administer stress-dose steroids and perioperative antibiotics if indicated.
- Place patient prone on two noncompressible bolsters with the lower bolster positioned at the break in the operating room (OR) table. The hips rest on the lower bolster. The lower rib cage rests on the upper bolster. The pannus should hang freely in between the bolsters to allow for the greatest amount of retroperitoneal working space. Place the operative side of the patient flush with that side of the table so that the table will not hinder the full range of motion of instruments, especially in the lateral-most port. If performing a bilateral adrenalectomy, the only patient repositioning necessary will be to shift the patient to the other edge of the bed (**FIGURE 1**).
- The lower back should be in a completely horizontal plane. This can be accomplished by lowering the leg portion of the OR table as much as possible to stretch the back and counter the natural convexity of the lower back.
- Raising the leg extension with the knees flexed and lower legs horizontal/parallel to the floor will help to prevent the patient from slipping further down on the bed.
  - Flex arms at elbows, pad pressure points, and secure patient in place. Prep from midchest to just above buttocks.

PORT PLACEMENT

- Three ports (lateral, middle, and medial) (**FIGURE 2**):
  - Medial: 5-mm "pediatric" or short port. Place this just lateral to paraspinous muscle and a few centimeters inferior to the costal margin.
  - Middle: 10-mm port with a "donut" balloon. Place this halfway in between the medial and lateral ports.
  - Lateral: 5-mm pediatric or short port. Place this as laterally as possible.
- The middle port is placed first via a direct cutdown by making a transverse incision just large enough to admit a finger immediately inferior to the tip of 12th rib or the costal margin. The position of this port is determined as discussed earlier.
- Dissection proceeds through the subcutaneous tissue to the muscle just inferior to the costal margin by spreading with a Metzenbaum scissors. The retroperitoneal space is entered by blunt dissection with the Metzenbaum scissors through the fascia and muscle using a technique similar to placing a chest tube (except that the hole is made directly *inferior* to the costal margin). Feeling the smooth undersurface of the ribs provides confirmation that the correct space has been entered. Use blunt dissection with the finger both laterally and medially to develop space for the placement of the subsequent 5-mm ports under direct palpation. Dissection should not be carried superiorly as this can make entering Gerota fascia more challenging.
- Place the medial port 3 to 4 cm inferior to the costal margin just lateral to the paraspinous muscle entering the

retroperitoneal space on a bias/angle cephalad of approximately 45° such that the port enters the retroperitoneal space just inferior to the inferior margin of 12th rib. This angling of the port will improve visualization, obviating the need to torque the port.

- Place the lateral port just inferior to the costal margin as far laterally as possible.
- Place a balloon port in the middle port site to form a seal for the retroperitoneal insufflation.
- Single incision technique
  - A single 20-mm incision inferior to the tip of the 12th rib is made in the same location as the middle port as described earlier and blunt dissection is used to develop a space in a subfascial plane.
  - A GelPort device is introduced to accommodate a 5-mm 30° camera, blunt grasper, and vessel sealing device through three short 5-mm ports.
  - Dissection proceeds in a similar fashion to the three-port technique as described below.
  - An additional 5-mm lateral port in the traditional location as described earlier can be placed in a hybrid two-port modification to aid in dissection.

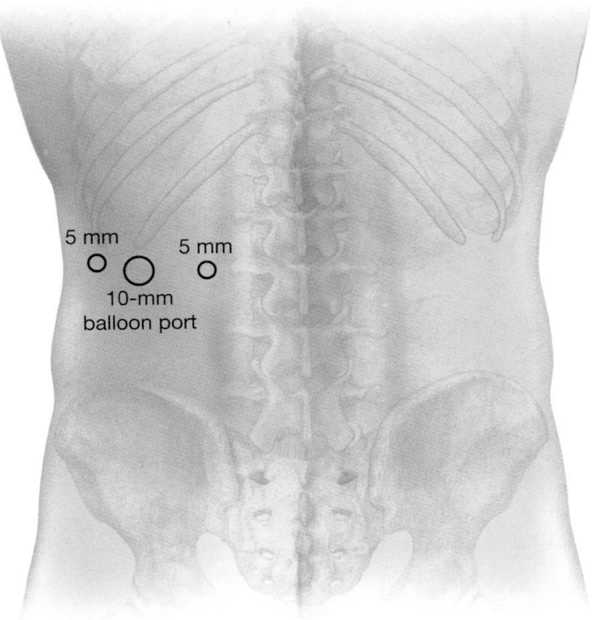

FIGURE 2 ● Right-sided port placement.

DISSECTION OF THE RETROPERITONEAL SPACE

- Insufflate to 20 mm Hg, liberally increasing as needed to a maximum of 30 mm Hg.
- Place camera into the middle port and a sealing device into the lateral port.
- Enter Gerota fascia bluntly and open it widely from left to right.
- Sweep the filmy posterior attachments of the periadrenal and perirenal fat anteriorly (ie, toward the table). Continue this dissection to expose the peritoneum laterally, paraspinous muscle medially, and peritoneum superiorly.
- Switch camera to medial port and place a grasper into the middle port (**FIGURE 3**).
- Identify the superior border of the kidney. Starting laterally, divide the adrenal-renal connections using a combination of blunt and sharp dissection. Carry this dissection toward the paraspinous muscle following the superior contour of the kidney, which will allow the kidney to be retracted inferomedially.

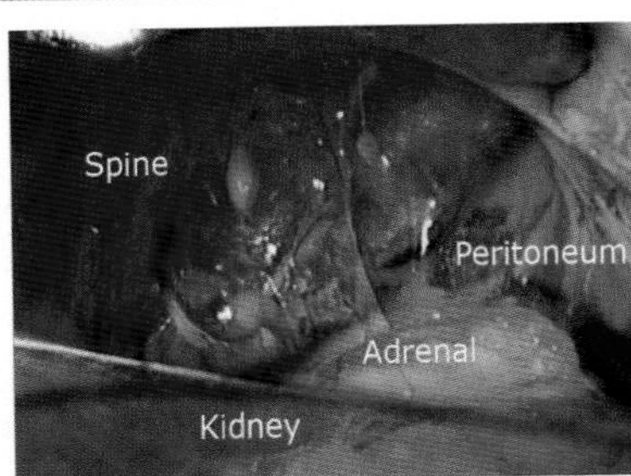

FIGURE 3 ● Retroperitoneoscopic view of the spatial relationships during initial dissection of a right adrenal gland.

- Carefully dissect the filmy plane between the adrenal gland and the paraspinous muscle medially to allow identification of the inferior vena cava during a right adrenalectomy or the inferior phrenic vein during a left adrenalectomy. The adrenal arteries will be in a plane that is posterior (ie, away from the table) to the level of the adrenal vein. These arteries may be ligated with a sealing device.

IDENTIFICATION OF THE ADRENAL VEIN

- Right adrenal vein (**FIGURE 4**): Once the inferior vena cava is identified, follow the cava superiorly. The adrenal vein can typically be found entering the adrenal gland at the junction of the middle and superior third of the adrenal gland. The adrenal vein enters the adrenal gland anteriorly (ie, toward the table). Divide the vein with clips or a sealing device.
- Left adrenal vein (**FIGURE 5**): Identify the adrenal vein either by tracing the inferior phrenic vein from superiorly to inferiorly or by dissecting the inferior border of the adrenal gland from lateral to medial until the confluence of the adrenal vein and inferior phrenic vein is encountered. Ensure that the inferior-medial border of the adrenal gland is fully dissected from the surrounding tissue, as there is often a tongue of adrenal tissue extending toward

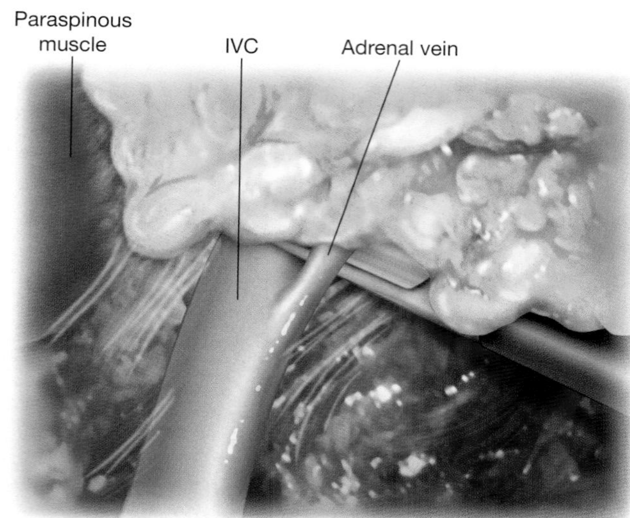

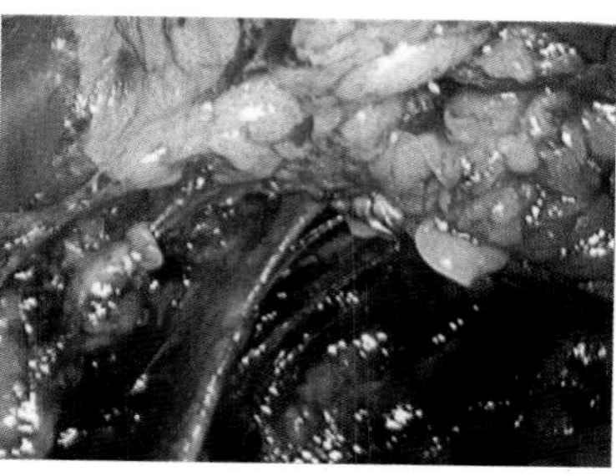

FIGURE 4 ● The short right adrenal vein is seen here at the end of the instrument in the middle of the picture. Note the relatively flat inferior vena cava due to the insufflation pressure.

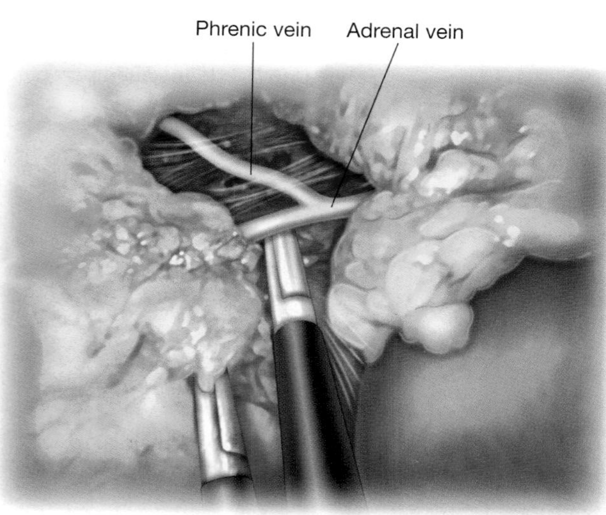

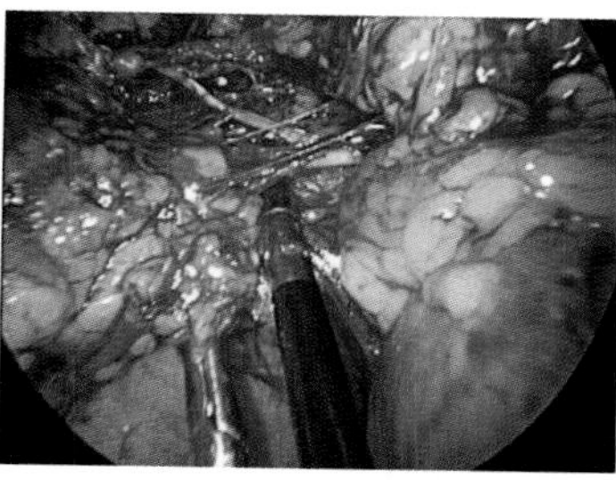

FIGURE 5 ● The left adrenal gland (notable for its distinct color that differentiates it from surrounding retroperitoneal fat) seen here at the end of the left adrenal vein (directly above the instrument in the middle of the picture). The left phrenic vein joins at an angle from above and can often be spared. The red-toned structure in the right foreground is the paraspinous muscle.

the renal hilum. Divide the left adrenal vein with clips or a sealing device. The inferior phrenic vein may be either ligated or spared.

- Once the vein is divided, the remainder of the adrenal gland can be dissected with mostly blunt dissection and a minimum of sharp dissection.

SPECIMEN EXTRACTION

- The adrenal gland can be placed in a specimen bag and removed through the middle port site, usually without the need to enlarge this site.
- Replace the middle port and inspect for hemostasis. Decrease insufflation to 5 to 7 mm Hg to assist in identification of bleeding.
- A closed suction drain is not normally necessary.
- Remove the ports and close the middle port site fascia with a single absorbable figure-of-eight stitch, taking care to avoid the subcostal nerve.
- Close the skin with subcuticular stitches.

PEARLS AND PITFALLS

Patient positioning	▪ Proper patient positioning is critical. ▪ Make sure the rib cage and hips rest on the bolsters with the pannus hanging freely. ▪ Place the operative side flush with the side of the table. ▪ Lower the leg portion of the OR table to stretch the back so it is completely horizontal. Then raise the leg extension with the knees flexed to prevent the patient slipping down the bed.
Port placement and insufflation	▪ The middle port is placed just inferior to the tip of 12th rib. Use blunt dissection with Metzenbaum scissors and fingers to enter the correct plane and allow the other two ports under direct palpation. ▪ Make liberal use of increased insufflation pressures (20-30 mm Hg) to improve visualization and hemostasis.
Dissection	▪ Due to the nontraditional view of the anatomy, there may be a longer learning curve associated with this approach. ▪ Dissecting the superior pole of the kidney from lateral to medial, ensuring the superior attachments of the adrenal are not divided too early, provides countertraction for inferomedial retraction of the kidney which in turn allows for the best exposure of the adrenal gland and adrenal vein.

POSTOPERATIVE MANAGEMENT

- Remove the urinary catheter 4 to 6 hours postoperatively.
- Patients may ambulate and eat a regular diet on the day of surgery.
- Aldosteronoma: Draw potassium, aldosterone, and renin levels the morning after surgery. Stop potassium supplements and aldosterone antagonists. Implementation of the antihypertensive regimen differs from patient to patient. Some clinicians will choose to stop all antihypertensives and add them back as needed, whereas others will cut the patient's typical doses in half and add them back as needed. Typically, β-blockers are continued postoperatively.
- Pheochromocytoma: Monitor hemodynamics closely and treat as indicated until stabilized. Stop all α-blockade. After removal of a pheochromocytoma, the major hemodynamic change to watch for is hypotension.
- Cortisol-producing tumor: Begin steroid taper. Consider keeping patients in-house for a day or two to begin the steroid taper under observed conditions.

COMPLICATIONS

- Bleeding: Significant bleeding occurs in less than 1% of cases. Increasing insufflation pressures as high as 30 mm Hg often tamponades small bleeding sites. Even with a significant caval injury, increasing the insufflation pressure can cause tamponade that allows time either to repair the injury laparoscopically or to convert to an open procedure.
- Significant intraoperative hypertension occurs in 1% to 2% of cases.
- Conversion to an open operation occurs in approximately 1% of cases. Emergent conversion (such as for significant bleeding) should be done through a posterior approach, obviating the need for patient repositioning and minimizing the dissection needed to get to the affected area. Resection of the 12th rib improves exposure to the retroperitoneal space significantly. If conversion is not emergent, conversion to a laparoscopic transabdominal adrenalectomy or an open lateral approach should be considered.
- Incisional hernia, pneumothorax, and wound infection occur in less than 1% of cases.
- Hyperesthesia and abdominal wall laxity occur in approximately 5% to 8% of cases but are usually temporary.

RESULTS

- Walz et al. reported in 2006 a prospective study of 560 laparoscopic retroperitoneal adrenalectomies on 520 patients, demonstrating a 2% conversion rate, a median operating time of 55 minutes that decreased throughout the study, and a median intraoperative blood loss of 10 mL.
- More recently, Dickson et al. reported a prospective series of 118 laparoscopic retroperitoneal adrenalectomies on 109 patients. A conversion rate of 6.6% was reported, mainly due to a failure to maintain an adequate working space with CO_2 insufflation, not due to uncontrolled bleeding.

SUGGESTED READINGS

1. Dickson PV, Jimenez C, Chisholm GB, et al. Posterior retroperitoneoscopic adrenalectomy: a contemporary American experience. *J Am Coll Surg*. 2011;212:659-667.
2. Giebler RM, Walz MK, Peitgen K, et al. Hemodynamic changes after retroperitoneal CO_2 insufflation for posterior retroperitoneoscopic adrenalectomy. *Anesth Analg*. 1996;82(4):827-831.
3. Lindeman B, Gawande AA, Moore FD Jr, Cho NL, Doherty GM, Nehs MA. The posterior adiposity index: a quantitative selection tool for adrenalectomy approach. *J Surg Res*. 2019;233:26-31. doi:10.1016/j.jss.2018.07.003

4. Perrier ND, Kennamer DL, Bao R, et al. Posterior retroperitoneoscopic adrenalectomy: preferred technique for removal of benign tumors and isolated metastasis. *Ann Surg*. 2008;248:666-674.
5. Sho S, Yeh MW, Li N, Livhits MJ. Single-incision retroperitoneoscopic adrenalectomy: a North American experience. *Surg Endosc*. 2017;31(7):3014-3019.
6. Silberfein E, Perrier ND. Management of pheochromocytomas. In: Cameron JL, ed. *Current Surgical Therapy*. 10th ed. Elsevier; 2011:579-584.
7. Walz MK, Alesina PF, Wenger FA, et al. Laparoscopic and retroperitoneoscopic treatment of pheochromocytomas and retroperitoneal paragangliomas: results of 161 tumors in 126 patients. *World J Surg*. 2006;30(5):847-853.
8. Walz MK, Alesina PF, Wenger FA, et al. Posterior retroperitoneoscopic adrenalectomy—results of 560 procedures in 520 patients. *Surgery*. 2006;140:943-950.
9. Walz MK, Gwosdz R, Levin SL, et al. Retroperitoneoscopic adrenalectomy in Conn's syndrome caused by adrenal adenomas or nodular hyperplasia. *World J Surg*. 2008;32(5):847-853.

Chapter **61**

Laparoscopic Adrenalectomy—Lateral Approach

Anna Kundel and Geoffrey B. Thompson

DEFINITION

- Lateral laparoscopic adrenalectomy is defined as a minimally invasive procedure to remove all or part of an adrenal gland via a lateral transperitoneal approach with the patient in a nearly full decubitus position.

ANATOMY

- The adrenal glands lie partially anterior, medial, and superior to the upper pole of the kidneys. The caudal limb of the left adrenal gland often lies in close proximity to the left renal hilum.
- The left adrenal vein frequently joins with the medially located inferior phrenic vein to form a common channel entering the left renal vein. This anatomic configuration, resulting in hormonal dilution within the common channel, is very important in understanding and interpreting the results of adrenal venous sampling (**FIGURE 1**).
- The right adrenal vein is short, often wide, and empties directly into the posterolateral aspect of the inferior vena cava. On occasion, additional right adrenal veins may drain directly into the inferior vena cava or the right hepatic vein. Arterial inflow to the adrenals is less predictable but generally arises as small arteries originating from the renal artery (inferior adrenal artery), the aorta (middle adrenal artery), and the inferior phrenic artery (superior adrenal artery).
- Paired small veins may accompany these arteries. It is these anatomic findings that allow for cortical-sparing adrenalectomy in familial pheochromocytoma syndromes, such as von Hippel-Lindau (vHL), neurofibromatosis type 1 (NF1), and multiple endocrine neoplasia type 2 (MEN-2) (**FIGURE 2**).
- Rarely, small rests of adrenocortical tissue may be found at sites near the adrenal bed or within the gonads. This has particular importance when treating corticotropin-dependent hyperadrenocorticism.

PATHOGENESIS

- Pheochromocytomas, aldosteronomas, and cortisol-secreting tumors produce catecholamines and hormones in an uncontrolled fashion, resulting in potentially life-threatening hormonal sequelae. Some of these tumors are seen in familial cases (MEN, vHL, NF1); most occur sporadically.

NATURAL HISTORY

- Untreated functional tumors can lead to death and disability. Undiagnosed adrenocortical carcinomas are most often fatal.

PATIENT HISTORY AND PHYSICAL FINDINGS

- Laparoscopic adrenalectomy is used for small functional and nonfunctional adrenal tumors, the latter being removed because of suspicion of underlying malignancy (either primary or metastatic).
- Adrenal incidentalomas are incidentally discovered (asymptomatic) adrenal masses, typically picked up on cross-sectional imaging studies performed for some other reason. For example, a patient comes to the emergency room with renal colic and a computed tomography (CT) with stone protocol is performed, revealing a ureteral calculus and an incidentally discovered 4-cm right adrenal mass.
- Indications for removal of an adrenal incidentaloma include (1) a functional lesion because of the risk associated with excess hormonal sequelae; (2) a growing lesion or a lesion greater than 4 cm in diameter because of the risk of

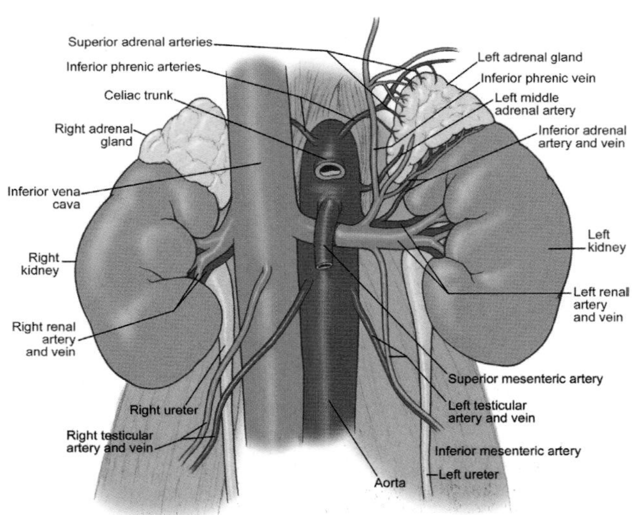

FIGURE 1 • Vascular anatomy of the adrenal glands.

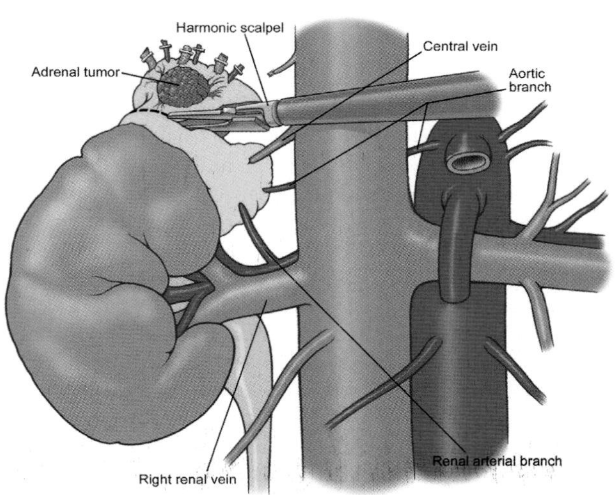

FIGURE 2 • Cortical-sparing adrenalectomy.

Table 1: Absolute Contraindications to the Laparoscopic Approach

Obvious, large adrenocortical carcinomas
Pheochromocytomas > 8 cm or clearly malignant pheochromocytomas associated with direct invasion, nodal metastases, or distant metastases
Extensive upper abdominal surgery in which the surgeon should consider a posterior endoscopic approach (see Part 5, Chapter 49)

adrenocortical malignancy; or (3) an abnormal radiographic phenotype, which can be an indicator of an underlying malignancy.

- Absolute contraindications to the lateral laparoscopic approach are described in **TABLE 1**.

IMAGING AND OTHER DIAGNOSTIC STUDIES

Diagnostic Studies

- Evaluation of an adrenal incidentaloma should include a 24-hour urine collection for fractionated catecholamines and total metanephrines or plasma metanephrines and normetanephrines.
- In patients who are hypertensive, regardless of their serum potassium level, plasma aldosterone concentration (PAC) divided by plasma renin activity (PRA) should be calculated to screen for primary aldosteronism. In the case of a high PAC:PRA ratio, confirmation of primary aldosteronism is obtained by salt loading and demonstration of a failure to suppress urinary aldosterone in a 24-hour sample. Autonomous cortisol secretion should be ruled out with an overnight 1 mg or 8 mg dexamethasone suppression test. The demonstration of autonomous cortisol secretion is confirmed by a 2-day low-dose dexamethasone suppression test.
- Other studies available include a 24-hour urinary free cortisol level or demonstration of loss of diurnal variation between a.m. and p.m. plasma cortisol levels.
- Midnight salivary cortisol levels are also being used with increasing frequency for case detection of cortisol hypersecretion.
- Studies for estrogen and androgen excess are obtained when clinically indicated but are not routinely done.

Imaging

- Imaging of pheochromocytomas (**FIGURE 3**), aldosteronomas, cortisol-secreting tumors, and adrenocortical carcinomas is best performed with CT or magnetic resonance imaging (MRI). Tumors that are round, homogeneous, and low in Hounsfield units on CT scan with rapid washout of intravenous contrast are thought to represent lipid-rich cortical adenomas (**FIGURE 4**).
- Malignancies tend to be large and heterogeneous, with areas of hemorrhage or necrosis associated with high Hounsfield units on CT and delayed washout of intravenous contrast (**FIGURE 5**). These lesions appear bright on T2-weighted MRI images.
- Approximately 25% of lesions 6 cm and greater are likely to be malignant, whereas 6% of lesions between 4 and 6 cm turn out to be primary malignancies. It is for this reason that the 4-cm cutoff is used. This avoids taking out an excessive amount of nonfunctional cortical adenomas while missing very few adrenocortical carcinomas.

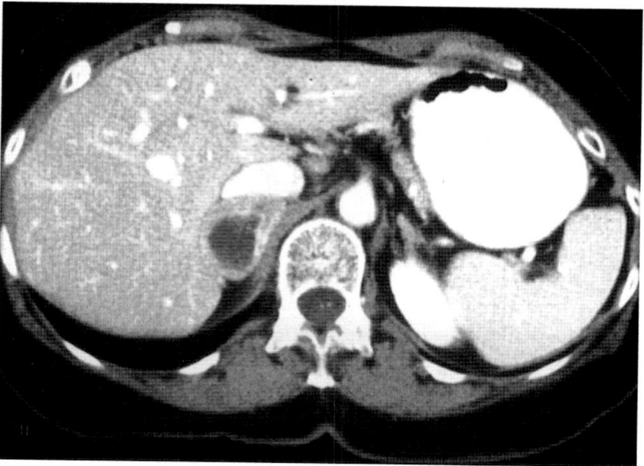

FIGURE 3 ● CT scan of pheochromocytoma.

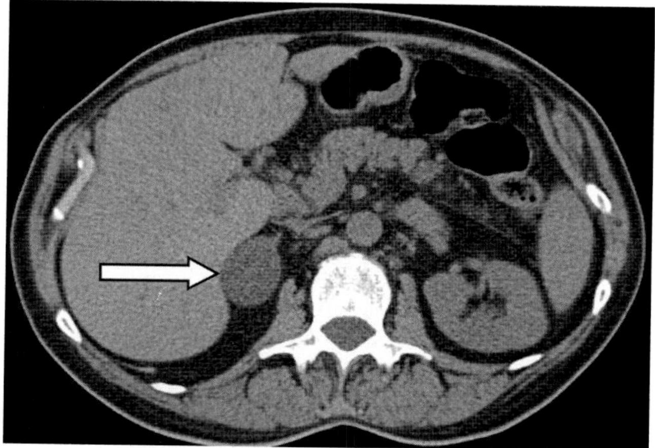

FIGURE 4 ● CT scan of benign cortical adenoma (arrow).

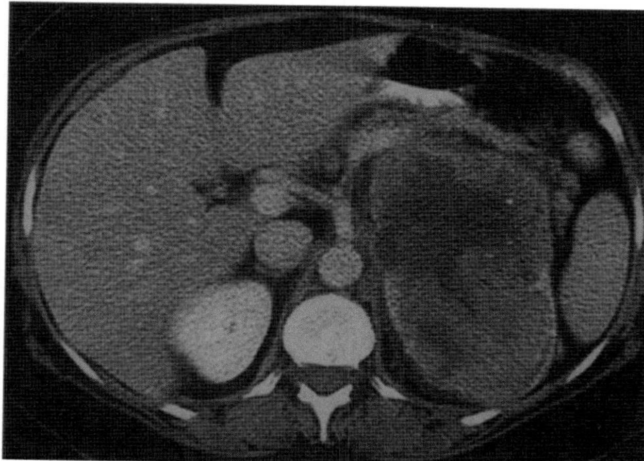

FIGURE 5 ● CT scan of left adrenocortical carcinoma.

- CT imaging is also valuable in picking up small aldosteronomas, but because of the high incidence of nonfunctional incidentalomas in patients older than 50 years, adrenal venous sampling has become the localizing procedure of choice for determining lateralization of an aldosterone-producing adenoma or hyperplasia.

- Metaiodobenzylguanidine scanning is useful for detecting occult pheochromocytomas, paragangliomas, metastatic disease, and multiple tumors in familial cases.

NONOPERATIVE MANAGEMENT

- Pheochromocytomas can be managed, albeit less effectively, with medical blockade (α-blockers). Aldosteronomas can be treated with mineralocorticoid receptor blockers, but this is not an ideal choice for younger patients.

SURGICAL MANAGEMENT

Preoperative Considerations

- Laparoscopic adrenalectomy via a lateral approach is indicated in the following circumstances:
  - All benign, functional adrenal masses less than 6 cm in maximal diameter (aldosteronomas, cortisol-secreting tumors) and pheochromocytomas less than 8 cm in diameter
  - All nonfunctional adrenocortical tumors greater than 4 cm but less than 6 cm in diameter
  - All nonfunctional tumors less than 4 cm in diameter demonstrating interval growth by cross-sectional imaging (CT or MRI)
  - All tumors regardless of size with a worrisome radiographic phenotype (high Hounsfield units on noncontrast CT, poor washout of intravenous contrast on CT, bright image on T2-weighted MRI)

Preoperative Preparation

- For pheochromocytomas, pharmacologic blockade (α-blockade for 7 to 10 days, then β-blockade for 24 to 48 hours preoperatively for atrial tachyarrhythmias and calcium channel blockers) is instituted. Effective circulating volume is restored using salt loading and increased fluid intake over a period of 10 to 14 days. α-Methyl-para-tyrosine, Demser (Valeant Pharmaceuticals International, Inc, Montreal, Quebec, Canada), can be added in refractory cases.
- When treating aldosteronomas, optimal blood pressure control must be achieved and hypokalemia should be corrected. Mineralocorticoid receptor blockade is often instituted.
- The patient with Cushing syndrome undergoes perioperative steroid preparation as well as prophylaxis for deep venous thrombosis, stress ulcer, and opportunistic infection.

Table 2: Equipment Typically Recommended to Perform a Lateral Laparoscopic Adrenalectomy

Three 5-mm trocars
One 10-, 11-, or 12-mm trocar
An OptiView port
Five-millimeter scopes, both straight and 30° (occasionally 45° scopes are necessary)
Insufflator, light source, and camera
Two monitors: Stryker 1688 AIM MIS Tower (Stryker Endoscopy, San Jose, CA)
Five-millimeter Harmonic scalpel
L cautery tip
Five-millimeter clip applier
Suction/irrigation apparatus

Surgical Equipment

- The equipment typically used to perform a lateral laparoscopic adrenalectomy in my practice is shown in **TABLE 2**.

Preoperative Steps

- In addition to one or two large-bore peripheral intravenous lines, a radial artery line should also be placed preoperatively. A central line should be used in the elderly, the infirmed, and select patients with pheochromocytoma.
- General endotracheal anesthesia is used. Antibiotics and deep venous prophylaxis are administered.
- Nitroprusside, labetalol, nicardipine, and intravenous pressors should be readily available for patients with pheochromocytoma.
- An orogastric tube is placed.

Positioning and Port Placement

- The patient is placed in (near-complete) lateral decubitus position with the side of the tumor facing.
- Three to four ports are placed on the left; the fourth port is used for a fan retractor in obese patients, and the most medial port is used for a liver retractor for right-sided tumors. The ports should be spread out between the midaxillary line and the midabdomen, approximately two to three fingerbreadths below the costal margin.
- The OptiView (Ethicon Endo-Surgery, Cincinnati, OH) system and a straight scope are used for introduction of the first trocar, typically along the anterior axillary line.
- Patient pressure is maintained between 14 and 18 mm Hg.

LEFT ADRENALECTOMY

- The splenic flexure is mobilized using the L cautery or Harmonic scalpel with caudal displacement of the large bowel (**FIGURE 6**).
- The lateral splenic attachments are divided with medial rotation of the spleen and body and tail of the pancreas, exposing Gerota fascia and the adrenal gland.
- The surgeon opens the avascular plane between the posterior aspect of the pancreas and the adrenal gland, much like opening a book. The adrenal vein often can be found directly across the "valley" from the splenic vein.
- The adrenal vein, inferior phrenic vein, and common channel are exposed.
- No attempts should be made to dissect out the renal artery and vein.
- The surgeon doubly clips the veins and divides them (**FIGURE 7**).
- The caudal tip of the adrenal gland is elevated away from the area of the renal hilum; very often, renal artery pulsation is visible.

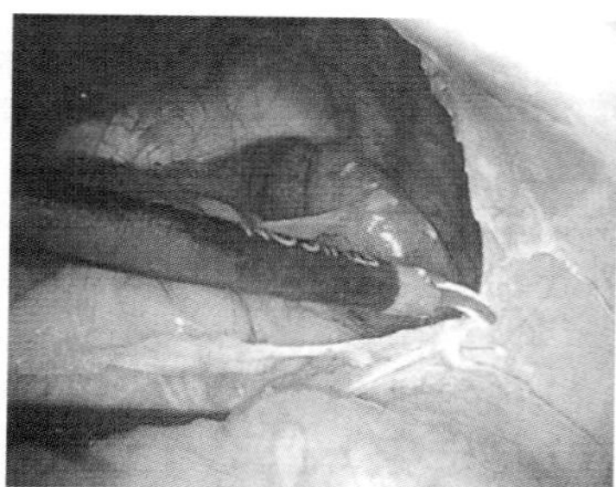

FIGURE 6 ● Mobilization of splenic flexure.

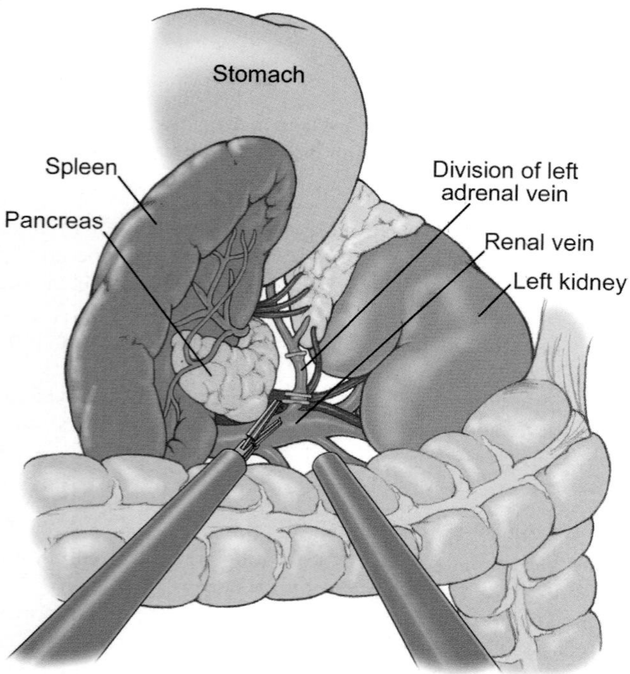

FIGURE 7 ● Division of left adrenal vein.

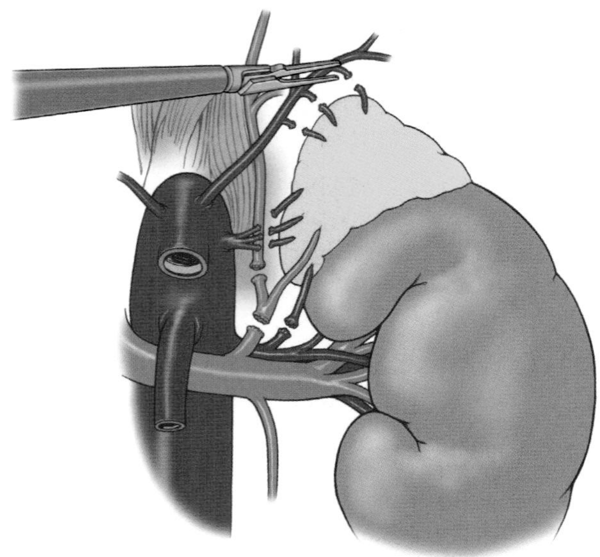

FIGURE 8 ● Division of arterial tributaries.

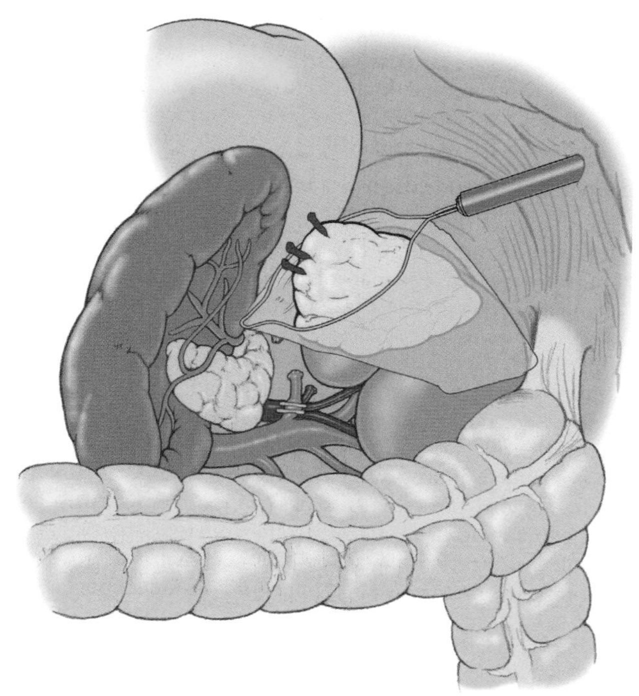

FIGURE 9 ● Retrieval of resected adrenal gland.

- The surgeon dissects up along the medial aspect of the gland using the Harmonic scalpel. If the inferior phrenic vein does not fall away from the dissection, it may require further division between clips at this level.
- Arterial tributaries from the aorta can be divided using the Harmonic scalpel as can the inferior phrenic artery tributaries, as dissection is carried around the superior aspect of the gland (**FIGURE 8**).
- The plane between the adrenal gland and the kidney is dissected using the Harmonic scalpel. This can be performed just outside the edge of the adrenal gland or, when thin, just inside Gerota fascia.
- The gland is then elevated anteriorly, and a small arterial branch from the renal artery, often present, is divided with the Harmonic scalpel.
- Any remaining areolar attachments are divided, and the gland is removed using a commercially available retrieval device (**FIGURE 9**).
- The adrenal bed is irrigated and aspirated completely, and hemostasis is ensured. A sheet of a topical hemostatic agent can be left within the adrenal bed for added hemostasis.
- If bladeless ports are used and dilation was not necessary for specimen retrieval, no deep fascial sutures are placed.
- Dilated port sites undergo fascial closure with interrupted suture, using a fascial closure device.
- Skin incisions are closed in a subcuticular fashion with an absorbable suture and are covered with Steri-Strips.
- Sterile dressings are applied.

RIGHT ADRENALECTOMY

- Attachments to the right lobe of the liver are divided using the Harmonic scalpel so as to allow the liver to be fully retraced medially. This brings the adrenal gland and inferior vena cava into view (**FIGURE 10**).
- The peritoneum overlying the lateral border of the inferior vena cava is incised using the L cautery on a low setting.
- If possible, the right renal vein is exposed to define the lower limit of the dissection.
- A blunt-ended instrument is used to gently retract the adrenal gland away from the inferior vena cava (**FIGURE 11**).
- Using the L cautery or Harmonic scalpel, the areolar tissue posterior and lateral to the inferior vena cava is divided. This may contain arterial tributaries directly from the aorta.
- The dissection is carefully carried out along the lateral border of the inferior vena cava up to the level of the adrenal vein (**FIGURE 12**).
- If the adrenal vein is easily exposed at this stage, it can be doubly clipped and divided; otherwise, it can be done later when visualization is optimal (**FIGURES 13** and **14**).

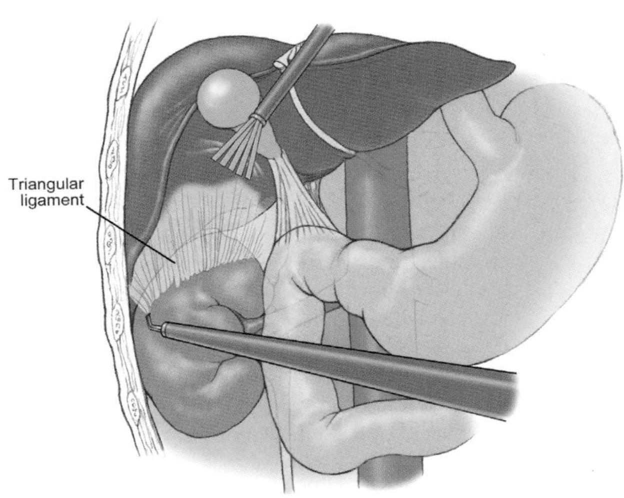

FIGURE 10 ● Liver retractor placement and division of triangular ligament.

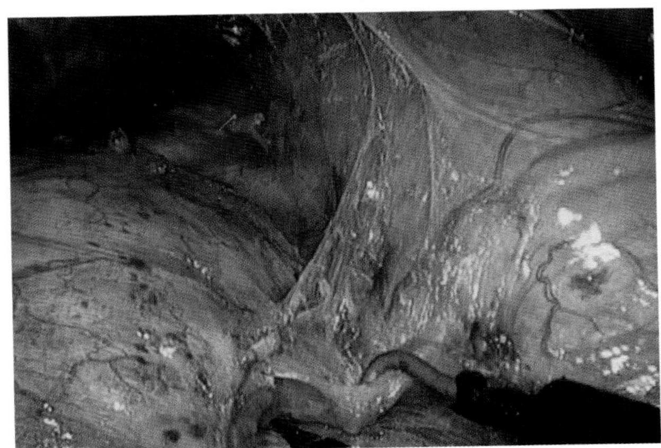

FIGURE 11 ● A right-sided pheochromocytoma is separated from the inferior vena cava.

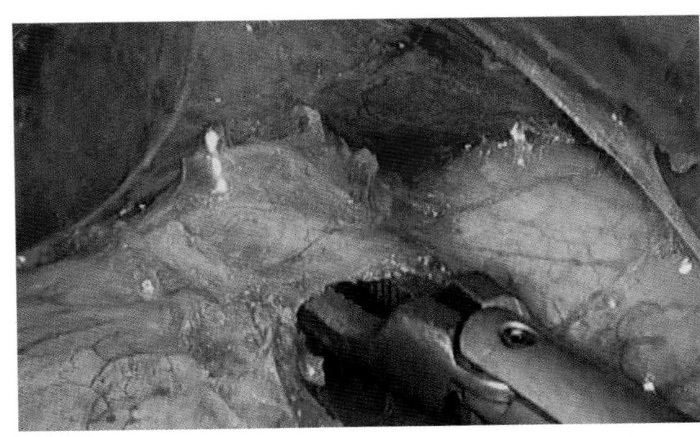

FIGURE 12 ● The right adrenal vein is encircled.

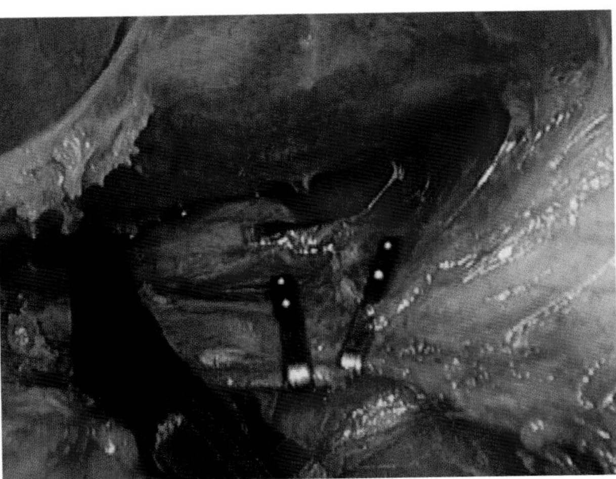

FIGURE 13 ● The right adrenal vein is doubly clipped and divided.

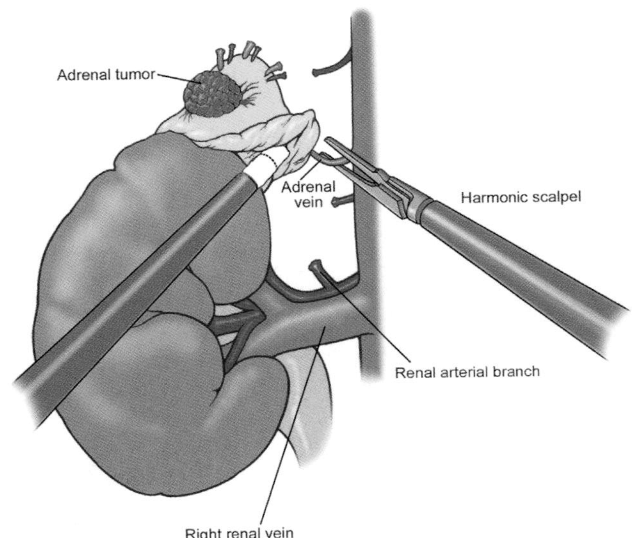

FIGURE 14 ● Division of right adrenal vein.

- In a larger pheochromocytoma, the adrenal vein really should be divided after the gland has been mobilized to avoid venous congestion and bleeding.
- The superior pole, including its inferior phrenic artery branches, is mobilized using the Harmonic scalpel to free the gland from the diaphragm posteriorly. Care must be taken to control additional veins at the junction of the medial and superior portions of the gland.
- Using the distal right renal vein as a landmark, the caudal aspect of the gland is exposed, dissected, and elevated, often revealing a renal artery branch to the adrenal, which is divided using the Harmonic scalpel.
- Final step in the dissection is freeing the lateral aspect of the gland from the kidney using cautery or Harmonic scalpel.

See also **Video 1**.

PEARLS AND PITFALLS

Adrenal vein	■ The adrenal vein does not have to be ligated as a first step in adrenalectomy; do it when it is safe and easy, even in patients with pheochromocytoma.
Accessory renal arteries	■ When dissecting on the posterior aspect of the adrenal gland, watch out for accessory renal arteries. If a large vessel is present, follow its course before considering ligation.
Low-pressure bleeding	■ If bleeding occurs, remember that most of the time, it is low-pressure bleeding. Pack the area with a sheetlike hemostatic agent. Work above and below the area, in which case, oftentimes, the bleeding site will become clear and manageable.
Renal hilum	■ Once the adrenal vein has been divided on the left side, never dissect caudally or posterior to the plane of the adrenal vein stump. This will avoid injury to the renal hilum.

POSTOPERATIVE CARE

Pheochromocytoma

- Patients with pheochromocytoma (**FIGURE 15**) will often be mildly hypotensive, with systolic blood pressures in the 90s for 8 to 12 hours postoperatively. Greater or more prolonged falls in blood pressure accompanied by oliguria or tachycardia should prompt investigation for bleeding.
- All blood pressure medications should be stopped after the morning preoperative doses have been administered, the exception being β-blockers used long-term for ischemic heart disease. Rarely, pressors may be required, although volume replacement may be all that is necessary for a short period of time.
- Plasma metanephrines and normetanephrines are drawn prior to dismissal.

Primary Aldosteronism

- Patients with primary aldosteronism (**FIGURE 16**) may require decreasing antihypertensive agents for weeks and will need careful monitoring.
- Potassium supplements should be withheld and only given on an as-needed basis because severe hyperkalemia may otherwise ensue with ongoing supplementation.
- PAC is collected prior to dismissal, and serum potassium levels are checked weekly for the first month.

Cushing Syndrome

- Patients with Cushing syndrome (**FIGURE 17**) are released on a tapering steroid dose to be monitored and adjusted by their endocrinologist.
- Resumption of oral intake is rapid.
- Dismissal usually occurs within 24 to 48 hours after surgery.

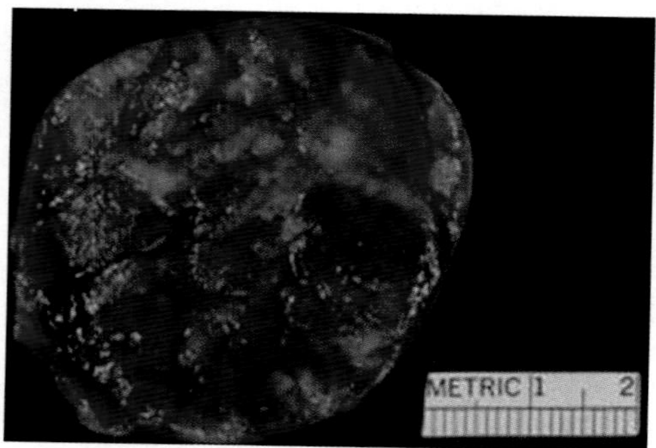

FIGURE 15 ● Pheochromocytoma.

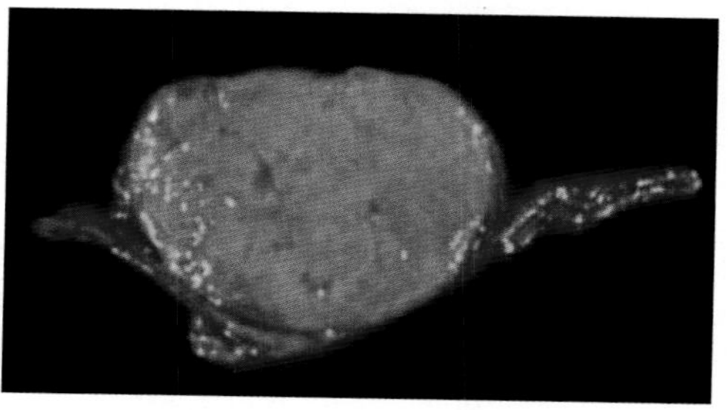

FIGURE 16 ● Aldosteronoma.

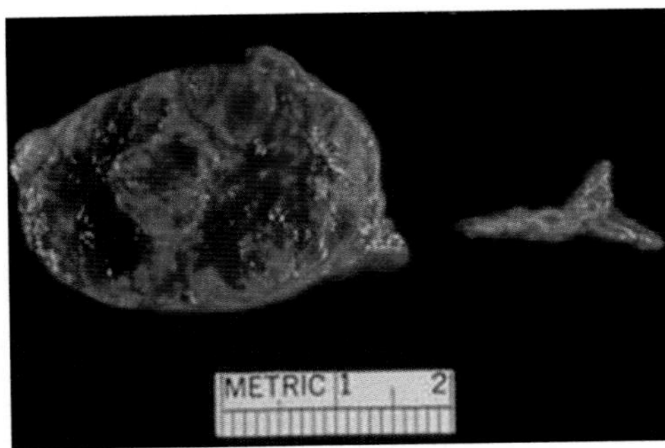

FIGURE 17 ● Cortical-secreting tumor.

- Hemoglobin, electrolytes, and creatinine are checked the day after surgery, along with a serum amylase in left adrenal gland patients to rule out pancreatic injury.
- Patients undergoing bilateral adrenalectomy for adrenocorticotropic hormone (ACTH)-dependent Cushing syndrome require lifelong replacement of glucocorticoids and mineralocorticoids, with increased doses during times of stress (illness, trauma, surgery).

OUTCOMES

- Outcomes for laparoscopic adrenalectomy are no different from those for open procedures with regard to cure rates. Morbidity is certainly less (pain, return to work, paresthesias, hypesthesias, and bulging flank muscles).

COMPLICATIONS

- Bleeding
- Spleen, pancreatic, renal, colon, and gastric injury (rare)
- Diaphragmatic injury (pneumothorax)

SUGGESTED READINGS

1. Brunt ML. Laparoscopic adrenalectomy. In: Eubanks WS, Swanstrom LL, Soper NJ, eds. *Mastery of Endoscopic and Laparoscopic Surgery*. Lippincott Williams & Wilkins; 2000:320-329.
2. Dy BM, Wise KB, Richards ML, et al. Operative intervention for recurrent adrenocortical cancer. *Surgery*. 2013;154(6):1292-1299.
3. Kiernan CM, Solórzano CC. Surgical approach to patients with hypercortisolism. *Gland Surg*. 2020;9(1):59-68.
4. McManus C, Kuo JH. Surgical approach to patients with primary aldosteronism. *Gland Surg*. 2020;9(1):25-31.
5. Patel D. Surgical approach to patients with pheochromocytoma. *Gland Surg*. 2020;9(1):32-42.
6. Porpiglia F Miller BS, Manfredi M, et al. A debate on laparoscopic versus open adrenalectomy for adrenocortical carcinoma. *Horm Cancer*. 2011;2:372-377.
7. Strajina V, Dy BM, Farley DR, et al. Surgical treatment of malignant pheochromocytoma and paraganglioma: retrospective case series. *Ann Surg Oncol*. 2017;24(6):1546-1550. doi:10.1245/s10434-016-5739-5

Chapter 62 Insulinomas

Douglas L. Fraker

DEFINITION

- Insulinomas are neoplasms arising from the beta cells of the pancreas. The vast majority are benign, sporadic, and unifocal.[1,2] These neoplasms release insulin in a dysregulated manner and therefore cause decreased blood sugar, resulting in neuroglycopenic symptoms. Surgical excision uniformly provides long-term cure for the majority of benign insulinomas and corrects all of the associated symptoms.

ANATOMY

- The beta cells of the pancreas are distributed among the pancreatic islets uniformly throughout the pancreas. For this reason, insulinomas can occur in all areas of the pancreas. Virtually all large series of insulinomas demonstrate that there is a uniform distribution related to the volume of pancreatic tissue.[3-5] Half of insulinomas occur in the pancreatic head, neck, and uncinate process, and the other half are distributed across the body and tail of the pancreas. Most series report insulinomas only occurring within the parenchyma of the pancreas. They can be exophytic and extend off the surface, and these exophytic lesions may not be appreciated by standard cross-sectional imaging. There are reports of less than 2% of insulinomas being located outside of the pancreas parenchyma.[1] Virtually all of these lesions are found in the wall of the duodenum, and presumably, they occur within embryologic pancreatic rest tissue that is physically separate from the pancreatic parenchyma, such that the insulinoma occurs within the duodenal wall with a similar appearance to duodenal gastrinomas.
- In most surgical series, insulinomas are small, measuring under 2 cm in cross-sectional diameter. Because symptomatology is caused by release of hormone and not by direct effects of tumor mass, lesions as small as 5 to 6 mm may present with significant clinical symptoms. In most series, 90% to 97% of insulinomas are benign. The average size of malignant insulinomas is over 6 cm, and the majority of those present with concurrent regional lymph node or hepatic metastases.[1,2]

NATURAL HISTORY

- Insulinomas cause virtually all of their symptoms due to excess circulation of insulin and the subsequent hypoglycemic effects. The first clinical case of insulinoma was described in 1927 when a patient who had severe hypoglycemic episodes had an abdominal operation with a large tumor of the pancreas and lymph node and liver metastases.[2] Extracts of this tumor actually were injected into animals and caused hypoglycemia. Allen Whipple described the triad carrying his name that is known to define the symptoms of insulinoma in 1938. *Whipple's triad* consists of hypoglycemia, documentation of hypoglycemia during periods of fasting, and relief of symptoms with administration of glucose. On analysis, this constellation of signs and symptoms is not truly a distinct triad but rather makes a single point of symptoms related to low blood sugar.[6]
- The majority of symptoms experienced by patients relate to lack of blood glucose to the central nervous system. These are called *neuroglycopenic symptoms* and can range from mild confusion to coma. Patients may experience visual disturbances and there are numerous reports in the literature of insulinoma being misdiagnosed as an epileptic seizure. A second set of symptoms relate to the sympathetic nervous system release of adrenaline due to the effects of the hypoglycemia. This catecholamine release leads to palpitations, diaphoresis, and tremors. In most series, the onset of symptoms initially noted by the patient may be years before the specific time of diagnosis of the insulinoma. The average interval from onset of symptoms to diagnosis is between 2 and 3 years, but sometimes symptoms may exist for over 10 years. Patients adapt and know that when they experience their symptoms, intake of food, particularly carbohydrates, provide rapid relief; however, this practice of glucose intake may not be elicited when taking a clinical history. Although the majority of patients exhibit weight gain in the anabolic state of hyperinsulinemia, some patients maintain a normal weight.
- The vast majority of patients with insulinoma have sporadic tumors with no family history. A small proportion is associated with multiple endocrine neoplasia type 1 (MEN-1).[5] The most common functional neuroendocrine tumor in MEN-1 is gastrinoma, outnumbering insulinoma by three- or fourfold. Insulinoma is the second most common pancreatic tumor in this syndrome. Because patients with MEN-1 may have multifocal nonfunctional neuroendocrine tumors throughout the pancreas, it may be difficult to distinguish the lesion making insulin vs other tumors. Typically, the dominant neuroendocrine tumor is the insulinoma, but occasionally, patients will have multiple large lesions. Intraoperative measurement of insulin from direct tumor aspiration has been reported as an adjunct to insulinoma identification in this unusual situation.

LABORATORY DIAGNOSIS

- The key to diagnosis of insulinoma is not with imaging but rather with biochemical testing. The cornerstone of diagnosing hypoglycemia is detecting glucose levels typically below 40 mg/dL. Additional blood tests that should be obtained are insulin levels, proinsulin levels, and C-peptide levels.[7] Virtually all patients will have a plasma insulin concentration greater than 5 μU/mL at the time of low blood glucose. The vast majority of patients have insulin levels greater than 10 μU/mL. The insulin to glucose ratio can define hypoglycemia due to insulinoma as opposed to other causes with high specificity and sensitivity.[8] The measurements of proinsulin levels and C-peptide are helpful in eliminating the diagnosis of surreptitious insulin abuse. The majority of patients have a proinsulin to insulin ratio greater than 25% and a C-peptide concentration greater than 1.7 ng/mL.

- The gold standard for confirming the diagnosis of an insulinoma is a monitored 48-hour or 72-hour fast.[9,10] Patients are typically in the inpatient setting given intravenous normal saline without glucose or allowed to drink noncaloric compounds while monitored for clinical symptoms and sequential blood analysis. The vast majority of patients who truly have an insulinoma causing hypoglycemia become symptomatic within the first 24 hours of the fast and virtually 100% of patients will become symptomatic by 72 hours. As time progresses, patients' symptoms include decreased mental acuity, confusion, or other neuroglycopenic symptoms, which are documented by the nursing staff and physicians during the monitored fast. When symptoms reach a significant level, blood is drawn for glucose, insulin, and proinsulin before administering glucose to relieve the neurologic symptoms.

DIFFERENTIAL DIAGNOSIS

- The differential diagnosis of hypoglycemia includes surreptitious use of either insulin or oral hypoglycemic agents and noninsulinoma pancreatogenous hypoglycemia syndrome (NIPHS).[7,11] In general, blood tests for proinsulin, C-peptide, as well as specific tests for sulfonylureas can eliminate the use of surreptitious agents. NIPHS is distinguished from insulinoma by the timing of hypoglycemia. These patients often do not become symptomatic during a 72-hour monitored fast but will become profoundly hypoglycemic after ingesting glucose orally.[7] Pathology often shows significant beta cell hypertrophy but does not show a mass on imaging.

IMAGING

- The vast majority of insulinomas are small and are located within the substance of the pancreatic parenchyma. The three choices of imaging that have been highly specific for identifying the insulinoma are contrast-enhanced computed tomography (CT) scan, magnetic resonance imaging (MRI) scan, and endoscopic ultrasound.[12,13] Insulinomas are hypervascular with very well-defined margins and have a classic appearance on enhanced CT and MRI scans (**FIGURES 1** and **2**). They are oval and well marginated and show a characteristic vascular blush.[12] The limitations of imaging relate to the size of the lesions. Again, insulinomas may cause symptoms that mandate surgical resection for correction with sizes smaller than 5 to 6 mm. Small insulinomas are ones that would be potentially missed on cross-sectional imaging studies. Also, exophytic lesions that may not be surrounded by pancreatic parenchyma may be a challenge to identify on CT or MRI, particularly if they are small. Insulinomas located near the tip of the pancreatic tail are the most common location for false-negative imaging; insulinomas may be incorrectly identified as lymph nodes, accessory spleens, and splenic vessels.
- Since the early 1990s, a variety of institutions with large experience in insulinoma have used endoscopic ultrasound as the primary imaging technique.[12,13] Endoscopic ultrasound allows for direct imaging in three dimensions with very close field ultrasonography of the head, neck, and uncinate process. The pancreatic body is less well imaged as it can only be seen from the placement of the ultrasound probe within the stomach, and depending on the patient's body habitus, the tail may be a blind zone for endoscopic ultrasound. The ultrasound appearance of insulinoma is an oval hypoechoic mass with well-defined margins (**FIGURE 3**). Endoscopic ultrasound also allows a relatively straightforward fine needle aspiration biopsy, which would produce neuroendocrine cells on cytology to confirm the diagnosis. Positive imaging may occur with identification of peripancreatic lymph nodes that are often embedded on the surface of the pancreas or accessory spleen, which can be found on the surface or actually within the parenchyma of the pancreas primarily in the tail region. Standard fluorodeoxyglucose-positron emission tomography (FDG-PET) scans have been shown to be of limited value in insulinomas as these may not be particularly hypermetabolic lesions.[14] A recent report showed a specific targeting agent of indium-labeled glucagonlike peptide-1 receptor that was sensitive for insulinomas and also

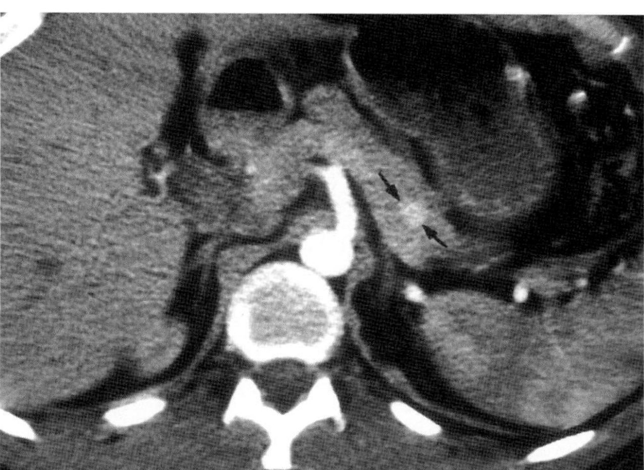

FIGURE 1 • Axial cut of MRI scan demonstrating an insulinoma in the body tail junction of the pancreas (marked by *arrows*). The insulinoma is small, oval, and hypervascular compared with the surrounding pancreas.

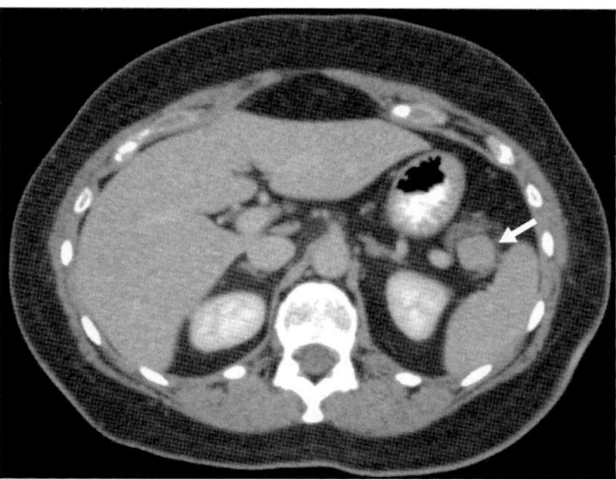

FIGURE 2 • Axial cut of a CT scan demonstrating a 2-cm insulinoma in the tail of the pancreas (marked by *arrow*). This scan, an MRI scan, and an endoscopic ultrasound all reported this lesion to be an accessory spleen as it was exophytic off the pancreas tail and had identical imaging characteristics as the spleen on all three imaging modalities.

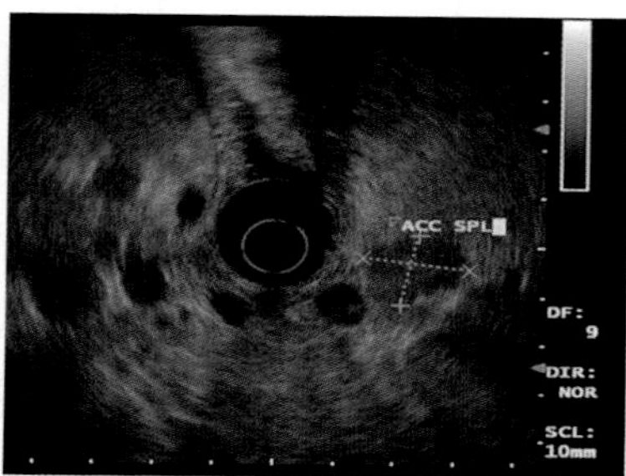

FIGURE 3 ● Endoscopic ultrasound image of the same patient in **FIGURE 2**. The insulinoma is oval and hypoechoic. The gastroenterologist has incorrectly labeled the insulinoma as accessory spleen.

could allow the use of a handheld intraoperative probe to detect these lesions.[15] This technique is being developed in Switzerland and has not been widely adapted elsewhere.

- Despite the high sensitivity of cross-sectional imaging and endoscopic ultrasound, a portion of patients with well-documented biochemical insulinoma may have no lesions imaged.[16,17] Historically, an interventional radiology invasive procedure called portal venous sampling was used in which a transhepatic portal vein cannulation was performed and blood was drawn from various regions and tributaries from the portal vein and assayed for insulin.[18,19] Portal venous sampling has now been replaced by intra-arterial calcium stimulation with hepatic vein sampling. In this technique, two catheters are placed: one in the right hepatic vein and a second standard arterial angiogram catheter advanced into arterial branches feeding the pancreas. Calcium is injected into branches of the splenic artery supplying the body or tail or branches of the superior pancreaticoduodenal artery off the gastroduodenal artery or the inferior pancreaticoduodenal artery off the superior mesenteric artery. Blood is drawn from the right hepatic vein at 0 second, 30 seconds, and 60 seconds after calcium infusion, and an increased gradient of greater than twofold in the hepatic vein insulin levels is significant.[18] This procedure does not image insulinoma but rather identifies the region of production of insulin. It is a highly specific test and may be helpful in focusing efforts in the operating room to one area or the other. It may justify performance of a blind distal pancreatectomy for patients without imaged lesions that have gradient in the body and tail, but a blind pancreaticoduodenectomy is virtually never indicated.

NONOPERATIVE MANAGEMENT

- The choices for nonoperative management include diet modification or hypoglycemic agents. One approach for management of hypoglycemic symptoms is small frequent meals, particularly of slowly absorbed carbohydrates to provide more of a steady level particularly while patients are sleeping.[2,5] Diazoxide is a benzothiazide analog with antihypertensive effects but also with potent hyperglycemic effects. It inhibits insulin release from the beta cells and enhances glycogenolysis to also contribute to elevation of blood sugar. Side effects include sodium retention causing edema and some patients have nausea. A second agent that has been used for control of hypoglycemic symptoms in insulinoma is somatostatin analogs. However, due to relatively low expression of somatostatin receptors on most well-differentiated insulinomas, these have not been markedly effective.

TECHNIQUES

PREOPERATIVE PLANNING

- The cornerstone to performing an insulinoma resection is being absolutely certain the patient has the disease proven by definitive biochemical workup. In patients who have imaged lesions, particularly if they are biopsied as neuroendocrine tumors or have classic appearance on CT or MRI, this provides very good evidence that the patient has the disease. In patients who have no definitive imaging of the site of the lesion, the surgeon has to review in detail the preoperative blood chemistries. This analysis includes reviewing the data related to a 72-hour fast, looking at concurrent glucose, insulin, and proinsulin levels as described earlier.
- It is very important for patients to either be the first case of the day or to be admitted to the hospital and have dextrose solution running so that they do not suffer from severe hypoglycemia while they are nil per os (NPO) prior to general anesthesia. In general, for abdominal procedures, anesthesiologists do not administer glucose-containing fluids as they are infused at a relatively rapid rate and patients are catabolic. When operating on patients with insulinoma, it is very important to communicate to the anesthesia team that dextrose needs to be administered often and frequent analysis of glucose levels need to be performed.

SURGICAL APPROACH AND PATIENT POSITIONING

- Over the past few decades, the majority of patients in most surgical series have been treated with an open surgical technique. There have been many recent reports of laparoscopic excision of insulinomas, particularly in the body and tail, with high success rate. We will describe primarily identification and resection of insulinomas using an open technique and also provide information on laparoscopic approaches.
- The approach for the open resection of an insulinoma is performed with the patient lying supine with either an upper midline incision or a bilateral subcostal incision. The vast majority of the substance of the pancreas can be assessed with an upper midline incision with the exception of the far distal tail, which may be somewhat difficult particularly in obese patients. For patients with a well-localized insulinoma in the head and neck, uncinate process, or proximal body, a midline incision is preferred if the patient's body habitus is appropriate. Any patient can be approached with a bilateral subcostal incision.

EXPOSURE OF THE PANCREAS

- The initial step of an insulinoma resection is to briefly assess the liver, although insulinoma is a benign disease in the vast majority of patients, and if liver metastases existed, they should have been identified on preoperative imaging. The next step is exposure of the pancreas parenchyma. Exposure of the head and neck of the pancreas as well as uncinate process can be achieved with a Kocher maneuver (**FIGURE 4**). The duodenum and head of the pancreas are brought up from the retroperitoneal location to allow bimanual palpation for mass lesions as well as visual inspection of both the anterior and posterior surfaces of the pancreatic head. The greater omentum is taken off the transverse colon along its entire length using energy devices with the omentum reflected superiorly, pulling the stomach off the pancreas. There are avascular attachments of the posterior stomach to the anterior pancreas that can be divided sharply. There is always a bridge of vascular tissue from the right gastroepiploic to the middle colic vessels, which crosses anterior to the neck and proximal pancreatic body that needs to be controlled with either energy devices or suture ligation. By dissection along the inferior border of the pancreatic body and tail, the posterior surface can be exposed and the majority of the substance of the pancreatic body and tail can be palpated between two digits (**FIGURE 5**). By doing these maneuvers, 95% of the pancreatic parenchyma is accessible for palpation and virtually all of the anterior surface and most of the posterior surface of the body and proximal tail are accessible for visual inspection as well. The only inaccessible area is the very tip of the tail of the pancreas, which may be located completely behind the spleen and require dividing the lateral margins of the splenic ligaments to reflect the spleen medially and expose that area of the very tip of the pancreatic tail.
- Insulinomas are identified by a combination of visual inspection, palpation, and intraoperative ultrasound. Insulinomas are uniformly red-brown in color against the yellow-gray background of the pancreas, and lesions near the surface or exophytic lesions can be easily identified by visual inspection (**FIGURE 6**). Neuroendocrine tumors have a classic ultrasound appearance, and intraoperative ultrasound is a key to management (**FIGURE 7**). Even in patients with lesions of the head and uncinate process of the pancreas that are well seen by preoperative endoscopic ultrasound, it is mandatory to have intraoperative ultrasound available. The reason for having intraoperative ultrasound available is because if the small lesion is deep within

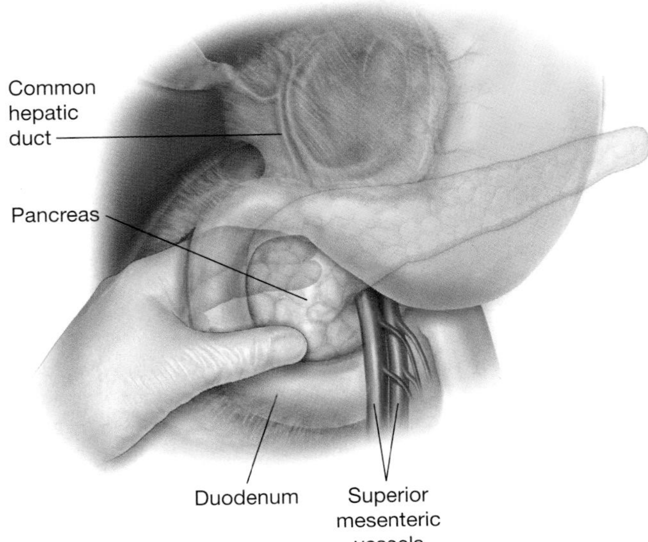

FIGURE 4 ● The lateral retroperitoneal attachments of the duodenum are divided along the entire length of the duodenum from the pylorus to the superior mesenteric vessel. By doing the Kocher maneuver, the entire head and uncinate process can be palpated between two fingers. By clearing the surface, all of the anterior head and uncinate process and most of the posterior surface can be visually inspected.

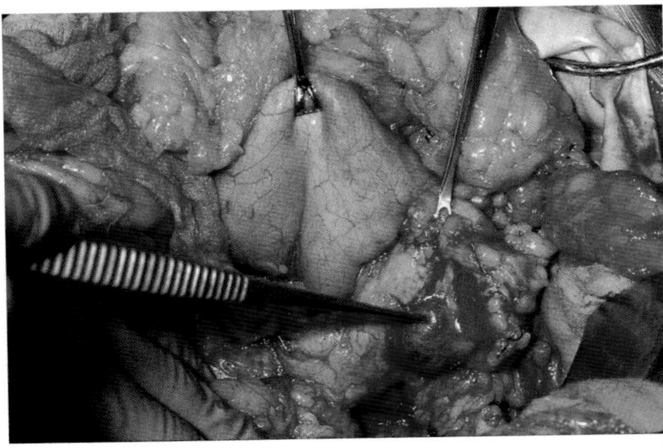

FIGURE 5 ● The lesser sac is exposed by reflecting the stomach and omentum superiorly and the transverse colon inferiorly. By dividing the retroperitoneum at the inferior edge of the pancreatic body and tail, the posterior surface of the pancreas is visualized as well. A large posterior body insulinoma is seen pointed at by the forceps.

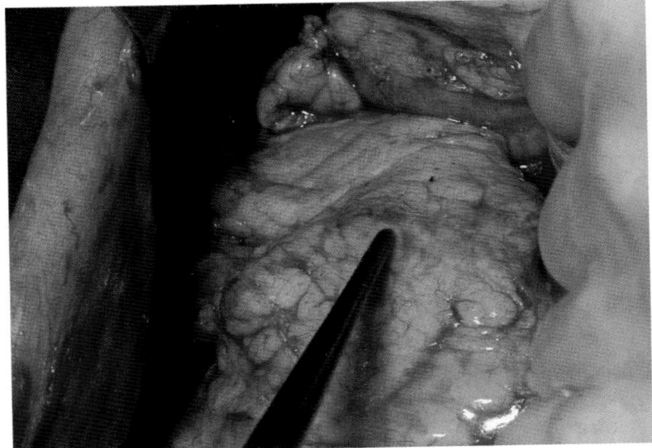

FIGURE 6 ● The anterior surface of the body and tail of the pancreas is skeletonized and exposed by retracting the stomach superiorly (posterior stomach on the left side of the picture) and the transverse colon inferiorly (retracted by the hand on the right side of the picture). The forceps is pointing at a red-brown insulinoma near the surface of the body of the pancreas.

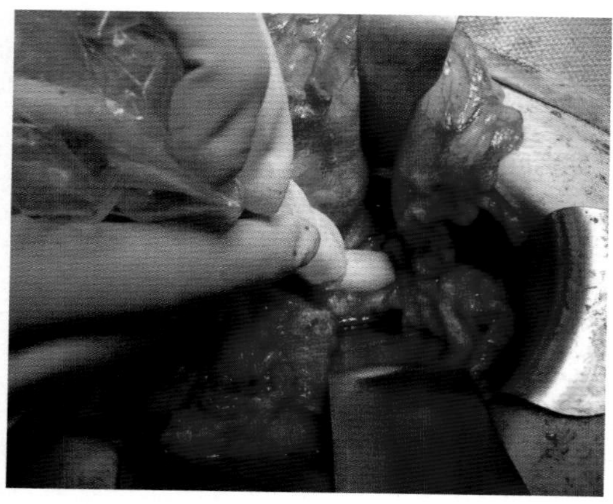

the parenchyma of the pancreas, it is essential to know exactly where the insulinoma is located so an appropriate enucleation can be performed. It is impossible to use preoperative imaging alone to know where to cut into the pancreas in the same way breast surgeons need intraoperative localizing techniques to remove nonpalpable breast tumors.

FIGURE 7 ● The head, neck, body, tail, and uncinate process of the pancreas are exposed and the intraoperative ultrasound probe is placed directly on the pancreatic surface. Ultrasound not only identifies the insulinoma but can also demonstrate precise relationships to the pancreatic duct and main vessels.

EXCISION OF THE INSULINOMA

- After exposure and identification of the insulinoma, the choices for excision of the lesion are enucleation vs a segmental pancreatic resection. In most surgical series, the majority of insulinomas are removed by enucleation, with one-third or more removed by distal pancreatectomy with or without splenic preservation, and a very small fraction removed with pancreaticoduodenectomy or a Whipple procedure. The ability to enucleate an insulinoma relates to how close the insulinoma is located to the pancreatic duct. For patients who have their lesion identified by preoperative imaging, the proximity of the insulinoma to the main pancreatic duct is known prior to surgery. The pancreatic duct generally runs along the length of the midline of the pancreas slightly superior and slightly toward the dorsal or deep side of the pancreas. The duct can virtually always be identified on intraoperative ultrasound as a tubular structure with no vascular flow within on color Doppler. Even in the case of insulinomas that are well localized on the pancreatic surface, routine use of intraoperative ultrasound is helpful, partly to look for additional lesions and mostly to identify the proximity of the insulinoma to the duct.
- For lesions that are on the surface or visible from the surface, enucleation is relatively straightforward (**FIGURE 8**). The reddish brown color of the insulinoma is easily differentiated from the glandular tissue of the pancreas. The plane on the capsule of the insulinoma is quite distinct and easily separated from the parenchyma with gentle traction. The attachment of the insulinoma to the pancreatic tissue can be controlled with ties, clips, or use of energy device such as a Harmonic scalpel. The large bleeding vessels could be treated with a suture ligature. Even lesions as large as 4 to 5 cm when they are exophytic off the surface can be enucleated as long as they are not near the main pancreatic duct such that all exocrine pancreas duct branches are controlled to prevent postoperative fistula.
- Enucleation of an insulinoma that is deep in the parenchyma and not seen by inspection requires continuous use of intraoperative ultrasound. Generally, insulinomas are softer in terms of their substance compared with the tissue density of the normal pancreas, and therefore, unless lesions are quite large, they cannot be felt by manual palpation with a finger behind and a finger in front of the pancreas. Ultrasound is used to mark the precise location of the lesion, and the distance from the pancreatic surface to the closest margin of the insulinoma can be accurately measured to know exactly how deep to go for an enucleation (**FIGURE 9**). In general, a cruciate incision centered right over the mass is made using an energy device such as a Harmonic scalpel. Any sizable vessels are controlled with small hemoclips or ties as needed. Ultrasound is continuously used to monitor the progress of the enucleation to make certain the defect in the pancreas is aimed toward the tumor until the capsule of the insulinoma is seen. Once a small surface area of the tumor is definitely visualized, ultrasound becomes unnecessary as the tumor enucleation is completed, staying right on the capsule of the lesion just as for lesions located on the surface (**FIGURE 10**). Again, specific knowledge of the main pancreatic duct anatomy is crucial as an injury to the main duct by either making a defect in it or transecting it may lead to a significant pancreatic or cutaneous fistula that may require reoperation.

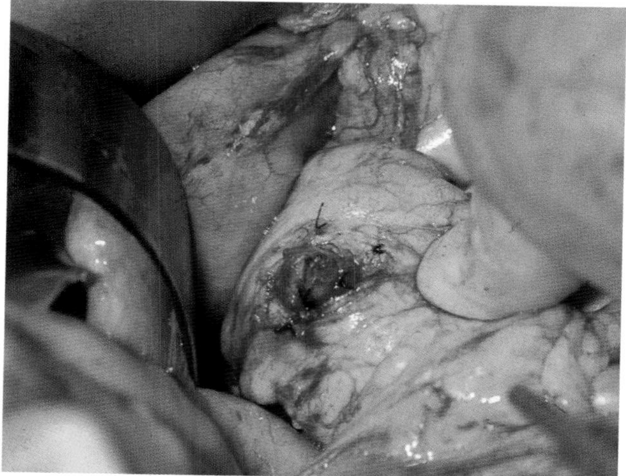

FIGURE 8 ● Enucleation of the insulinoma seen in **FIGURE 6**. Ultrasound confirms the lesion does not abut the pancreatic duct and the insulinoma is enucleated on the capsule of the tumor.

- For larger lesions or lesions that abut or distort the main pancreatic duct located in the body and tail of the pancreas, there

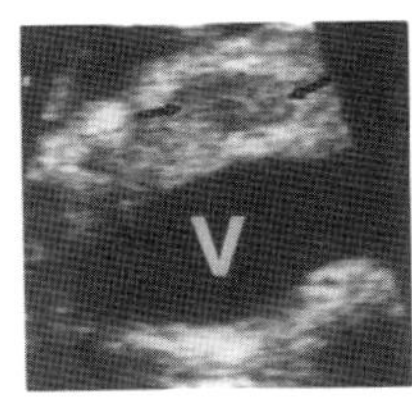

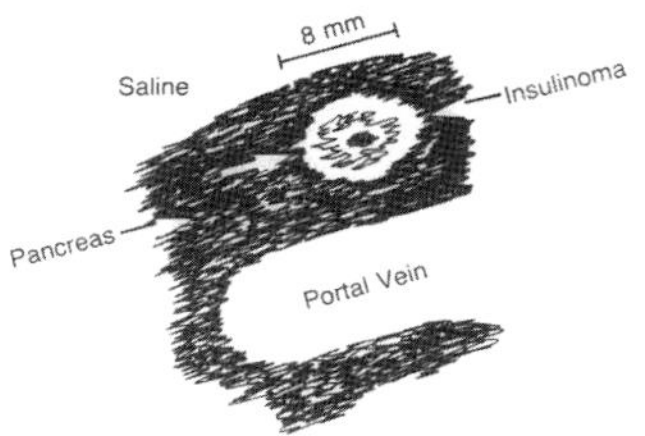

FIGURE 9 ● The *top panel* shows an image from an intraoperative ultrasound demonstrating the hypoechoic insulinoma indicated by the *black arrows*. The drawing on the *lower panel* shows the 8-mm insulinoma and the precise distance between the tumor and the underlying portal vein.

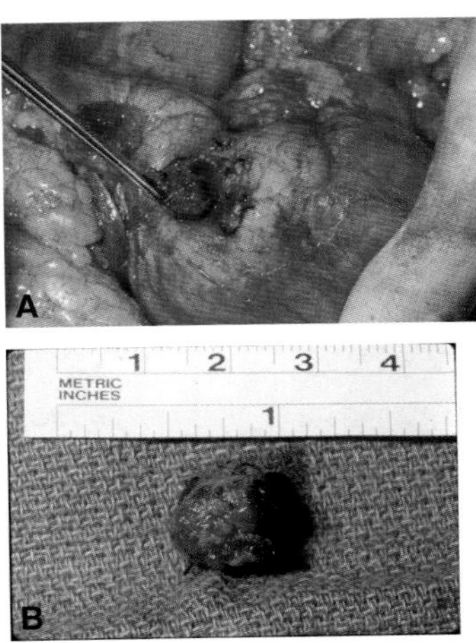

FIGURE 10 ● **A,** Enucleation of an insulinoma from the deep tissue of the head of the pancreas. Once the capsule of the insulinoma is seen, intraoperative ultrasound is no longer needed to guide the dissection. **B,** Intact pancreatic head insulinoma after enucleation. Small amounts of pancreatic parenchyma are attached to the lesion.

is no question that the appropriate operation is a distal pancreatectomy (**FIGURE 11**). Again, intraoperative ultrasound is used to map the transection of the pancreas to the right of the lesion to get a margin. This resection can be either spleen preserving or a distal pancreatectomy plus splenectomy, depending on the preference of the operating surgeon. There are some minor advantages of preserving the spleen in adult patients, but the incidence of postsplenectomy sepsis is exceedingly rare. Again, the location of the lesion is mapped out or, if it is not visible on the surface, mapped using ultrasound. Distal pancreatectomy is generally done by dissecting the short gastric vessels along the greater curvature of the stomach using an energy device. At this point, when doing a distal pancreatectomy plus splenectomy, a large silk tie is placed around the splenic artery at the site of pancreatic transection to control blood inflow to the spleen. The lateral

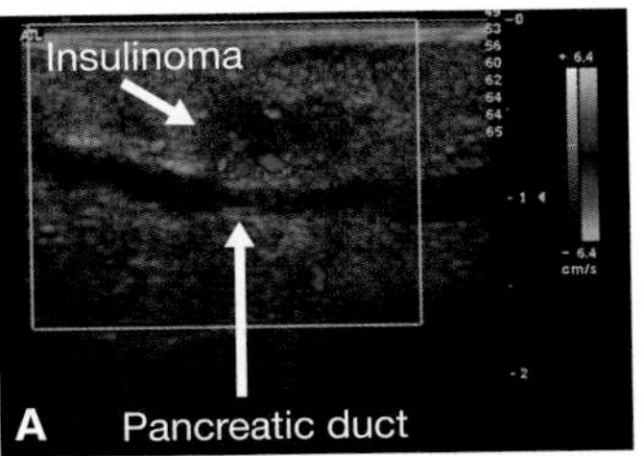

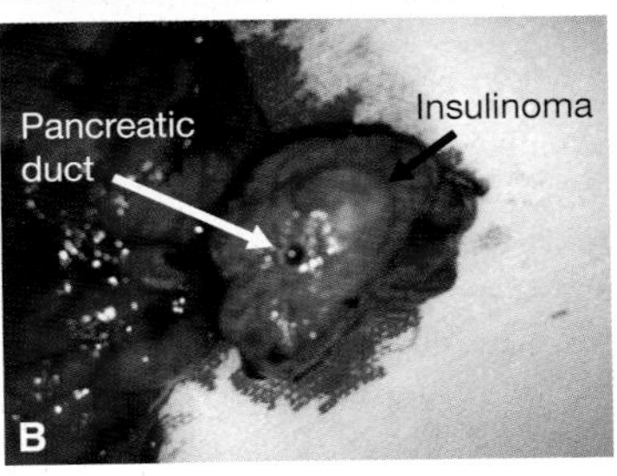

FIGURE 11 ● The patient had a small midbody insulinoma seen by CT scan. Intraoperative ultrasound **(A)** shows the insulinoma clearly but it indents the main pancreatic duct. Color Doppler ultrasound identifies the duct as there is no blood flow and the insulinoma is hypervascular. Owing to the proximity of the main pancreatic duct to the insulinoma, a distal pancreatectomy was performed. **(B)** shows the insulinoma bordering a mildly dilated pancreatic duct. If the insulinoma was enucleated, there would be a high likelihood of a significant pancreatic leak.

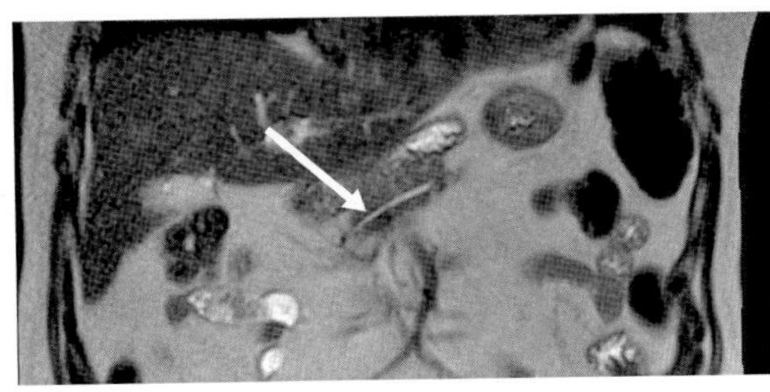

FIGURE 12 ● A coronal MRI scan shows a 2-cm insulinoma in close proximity to the main pancreatic duct in the head of the pancreas *(white arrow)*. After confirmation of the duct by intraoperative ultrasound, a pylorus-preserving pancreaticoduodenectomy was performed.

margins of the spleen are divided, and the spleen and tail of the pancreas are reflected medially. The spleen and tail and body of the pancreas are reflected up and to the right off the left adrenal gland to the point of the targeted pancreatic transection line. The artery is then double ligated and divided, and the splenic vein is either stapled separately with vascular staples or stapled with the stapling device used to transect the pancreas. A gas-powered stapler in which pressure can slowly be applied over 30 to 60 seconds to close the jaws of the stapling device minimizes fracturing the pancreatic parenchyma before firing the stapler load. Always inspect the margin and ensure complete excision of the insulinoma either by cutting into the pancreas on the back table or by having the pathologist do a gross evaluation of the specimen.

- Only for very large lesions in the head of the pancreas that abut the main pancreatic duct would a pancreaticoduodenectomy be performed for a benign insulinoma (**FIGURES 11** and **12**). A Whipple procedure for insulinoma is a generally relatively straightforward procedure in terms of the resection portion as major vascular structures are virtually never invaded and can be done with pylorus-preserving technique. It may be somewhat more challenging to do the reconstruction as these patients typically have normal-sized pancreatic duct and bile duct, as even large insulinomas do not cause ductal obstruction, as well as a soft normal pancreas increasing the incidence of pancreatic leak.

- The most challenging situation for a surgeon is to be in the operating room and to be unable to identify the insulinoma.[17] Understanding the correct interpretation of the biochemical diagnosis of insulinoma should avoid the pitfall of operating on a patient who does not have the disease, which is a procedure obviously destined for failure. Historically, performance of a stepwise blind distal pancreatectomy with interval checks of blood glucose was advocated by some. In the era of high-resolution ultrasound, this blind resection of tissue should never be done. The key to success in this situation is the use of intraoperative ultrasound and evaluation of areas where small insulinomas may be difficult to identify. Specifically, the very tip of the pancreatic tail lateral to the spleen, the uncinate process adjacent to the superior mesenteric vein, and the neck of the pancreas under the vascular bridge between the right gastroepiploic middle colic vessels should be closely examined.
- In the unusual or rare case of a malignant insulinoma, tumor debulking may be very beneficial in terms of controlling hypoglycemic symptoms. In general, this would require either a pancreaticoduodenectomy or distal pancreatectomy to remove the primary lesion and lymph node metastases. If there is limited number of liver metastasis, simultaneous liver resection or ablation may be performed. Chemoembolization also has benefit in controlling the hormone output from these hypervascular lesions and benefits the patients in terms of hypoglycemic control.

LAPAROSCOPIC RESECTION OF INSULINOMAS

- Although the majority of insulinomas are excised using standard open techniques described earlier, several surgeons have reported successful excision of insulinomas using laparoscopic techniques over the past 2 decades.[19-21] The precise location of the insulinoma and the success of preoperative localization studies are the keys to patient selection for laparoscopic excision.
- Insulinomas located in the body and proximal tail are the ones that are best approached by laparoscopy. Patients are positioned supine, and a 30° scope is used in a central periumbilical port. The gastrocolic ligament is divided and the omentum and stomach are retracted superiorly to expose the pancreas at the base of the lesser sac. Laparoscopic ultrasound is used in an identical manner to intraoperative ultrasound in open procedures to identify both the insulinoma and the main pancreatic duct. Either enucleation or distal pancreatectomy is chosen based on tumor location again with the same decision-making process as in open procedures.
- Several studies, including a meta-analysis, have confirmed that laparoscopic removal of insulinomas is safe and has advantages over open excision. In institutional comparative studies, there was no difference in operative time, overall cure rate (which is uniformly 100%), and the incidence of pancreatic fistula. Length of hospital stay and blood loss generally favor laparoscopic excision. For surgeons who have experience in managing insulinomas and who have advanced laparoscopic skills, selected patients should have their insulinomas resected laparoscopically. However, as opposed to adrenalectomy in which video-assisted techniques are absolutely the standard of care, insulinoma procedures are much less common and the majority of procedures are still done with an open technique.

PEARLS AND PITFALLS

Indications	▪ Confirm definitive biochemical diagnosis by review of primary laboratory reports including glucose levels with simultaneous insulin, proinsulin, and C-peptide levels. ▪ Insist on a 72-hour monitored fast with appropriate documentation of symptoms and biochemical disease in patients with equivocal diagnosis and negative imaging.
Imaging	▪ Obtain cross-sectional imaging with either contrast-enhanced CT scan or MRI scan to look for hypervascular lesion. ▪ For image-negative patients, have endoscopic ultrasound performed by skilled invasive gastroenterologist. ▪ If definitive diagnosis and negative imaging by CT and endoscopic ultrasound (EUS), consider calcium-stimulated angiogram with hepatic vein sampling.
Exposure of pancreas	▪ Expose head and uncinate process by doing a complete Kocher maneuver all the way to the fourth portion of the duodenum. ▪ Expose body and tail by dividing gastrocolic ligament and reflecting omentum and stomach superiorly and colon inferiorly. ▪ Expose tip of pancreatic tail by dividing lateral attachments of the spleen.

Resection	■ Be certain to have intraoperative ultrasound available to evaluate the insulinoma and the proximity of the main pancreatic duct. ■ Decide between enucleation vs segmental pancreatectomy based on tumor size and relationship to the pancreatic duct.
Enucleation techniques	■ For surface lesions, stay right on the capsule of the insulinoma using energy device or clips to divide and seal tissue. ■ For deep lesions, continuously monitor progress with intraoperative ultrasound as pancreatic parenchyma is divided.

POSTOPERATIVE MANAGEMENT AFTER INSULINOMA RESECTION

- After excision of the entire insulinoma, patients recover almost instantaneously in terms of their glucose metabolism. Typically, blood sugars may rise to between 150 and 200 mg/dL or higher in the recovery room and for the first 24 to 48 hours, patients should be placed on appropriate sliding scale of insulin. It is certainly possible and has been reported that resection of an insulinoma may unmask a patient who has developed diabetes, but the majority of these patients correct and normalize their glucose metabolism within 2 to 3 days.[22,23]
- The major postoperative complication from either a distal pancreatectomy or enucleation, either laparoscopic or open, is a pancreatic fistula.[24] The standard practice is to leave a closed suction drain adjacent to the enucleation site or the staple line and to leave that in until the patient is eating at least a low-fat diet. The color and character of the drain fluid can be monitored. If it is a serosanguineous color, it is likely to have a low pancreatic amylase content. Pancreatic fistulas normally present with a dishwater-gray discoloration and can be confirmed by measuring drain content amylase levels. Standard maneuvers to decrease pancreas secretion including nonfat diets or even using total parenteral nutrition should decrease pancreatic fistula outputs.

OUTCOMES AND ALTERNATIVE TREATMENT TO SURGERY FOR TREATMENT OF INSULINOMA

- In virtually all of the surgical series resecting insulinoma, there is uniformly a 100% long-term cure rate after excision of these small benign lesions.[3,4,25] The only exception would be inability to identify an occult insulinoma resulting in immediate operative failure. Because the vast majority of patients are cured by surgery, there has been no impetus to use nonsurgical treatments. Two percutaneous or endoscopic techniques have been reported.
- Ethanol injection to ablate insulinomas[26] and radiofrequency ablation[27] of lesions may provide nonsurgical resolution of hypoglycemic symptoms. Only for very selected patients who are poor surgical candidates should these ablative techniques be offered.

REFERENCES

1. Okabayashi T, Shima Y, Sumiyoshi T, et al. Diagnosis and management of insulinoma. *World J Gastroenterol*. 2013;19(6):829-837.
2. Mathur A, Gorden P, Libutti SK. Insulinoma. *Surg Clin North Am*. 2009;89:1105-1121.
3. Zhao YP, Zhan HX, Zhang TP, et al. Surgical management of patients with insulinomas: result of 292 cases in a single institution. *J Surg Oncol*. 2011;103:169-174.
4. Nikfarjam M, Warshaw AL, Axelrod L, et al. Improved contemporary surgical management of insulinomas. A 25-year experience of the Massachusetts General Hospital. *Ann Surg*. 1008;247:165-172.
5. Krampitz GW, Norton JA. Pancreatic neuroendocrine tumors. *Curr Prob Surg*. 2013;50:509-545.
6. Van Heerden JA, Edis AJ, Service FJ. The surgical aspects of insulinomas. *Ann Surg*. 1979;189(6):677-682.
7. Service FJ. Diagnostic approach to adults with hypoglycemic disorders. *Endocrinol Metab Clin N Am*. 1999;28(3):519-532.
8. Nauck MA, Meler JJ. Diagnostic accuracy of an "amended" insulin-glucose ratio for the biochemical diagnosis of insulinoma. *Ann Int Med*. 2012;157:767-775.
9. Van Bon A, Benhadi N, Endert E, et al. Evaluation of endocrine tests. D: the prolonged fasting test for insulinoma. *Neth J Med*. 2009;67(7):274-278.
10. Hirshberg B, Livi A, Bartlett DL, et al. Forty-eight hour fast: the diagnostic test for insulinoma. *J Clin Endocrinol Metab*. 2000;85(9):3222-3226.
11. Thompson GB, Service FJ, Andrews JC, et al. Noninsulinoma pancreatogenous hypoglycemia syndrome: an update in 10 surgically treated patients. *Surgery*. 2000;128:937-945.
12. McAuley G, Delaney H, Colville J, et al. Multimodality preoperative imaging of pancreatic insulinomas. *Clin Radiol*. 2005;60:1039-1050.
13. Atiq M, Bhutani MS, Bektas M, et al. EUS-FNA for pancreatic neuroendocrine tumors: a tertiary cancer center experience. *Dig Dis Sci*. 2012;57:791-800.
14. Tessonnier L, Sebag F, Ghander C, et al. Limited value of 18F-F-DOPA PET to localize pancreatic insulin-secreting tumors in adults with hyperinsulinemic hypoglycemia. *Endocrinol Metab*. 2010;95:303-307.
15. Christ E, Wild D, Forrer F, et al. Glucagon-like peptide-1 receptor imaging for localization of insulinomas. *J Clin Endocrinol Metab*. 2009;94:3298-4405.
16. Abboud B, Boujaoude J. Occult sporadic insulinoma: localization and surgical strategy. *World J Gastroenterol*. 2008;15(5):657-665.
17. Rostambeigi N, Thompson GB. What should be done in an operating room when an insulinoma cannot be found? *Clin Endocrinol*. 2009;70:512-515.
18. Guettier JM, Kam A, Chang R, et al. Localization of insulinomas to regions of the pancreas by intraarterial calcium stimulation: the NIH experience. *J Clin Endocrinol Metab*. 2009;94:1074-1080.
19. Hu M, Zhao G, Luo Y, et al. Laparoscopic versus open treatment for benign pancreatic insulinomas: an analysis of 89 cases. *Surg Endosc*. 2011;25:3831-3837.
20. Richards ML, Thompson GB, Farley DR, et al. Setting the bar for laparoscopic resection of sporadic insulinoma. *World J Surg*. 2011;35:785-789.
21. Su AP, Ke NW, Zhang Y, et al. Is laparoscopic approach for pancreatic insulinomas safe? Results of a systematic review and meta-analysis. *J Surg Res*. 2014;186:126-134.
22. Crippa S, Zerbi A, Boninsegna L, et al. Surgical management of insulinomas. Short- and long-term outcomes after enucleations and pancreatic resections. *Arch Surg*. 2012;147(1):261-266.

23. Roland CL, Lo CY, Miller BS, et al. Surgical approach and perioperative complications determine short-term outcomes in patients with insulinoma: results of a bi-institutional study. *Ann Surg Oncol.* 2008;15(12):3532-3537.
24. Zhao YP, Zhan HX, Cong L, et al. Risk factors for postoperative pancreatic fistula in patients with insulinomas: analysis of 292 consecutive cases. *Hepatobiliary Pancreat Dis Int.* 2012;11:102-106.
25. Placzkowski KA, Vella A, Thompson GB, et al. Secular trends in the presentation and management of functioning insulinoma at the Mayo Clinic, 1987-2007. *J Clin Endocrinol Metab.* 2009;94(4):1069-1073.
26. Levy MJ, Thompson GB, Topazian MD, et al. US-guided ethanol ablation of insulinomas: a new treatment option. *Gastrointest Endosc.* 2012;75(1):200-206.
27. Procházka V, Hlavsa J, Andrašina T, et al. Laparoscopic radiofrequency ablation of functioning pancreatic insulinoma: video case report. *Surg Laparosc Endosc Percutaneous Tech.* 2012;22(5):e312-315.

Chapter **63** **Surgery for Glucagonoma**

Richard A. Prinz, Mark S. Talamonti, Melissa E. Hogg, Charles C. Vining, and Erin C. MacKinney

DEFINITION

- Glucagonomas are pancreatic neuroendocrine tumors (PNETs) that arise from the glucagon-secreting alpha islet cells of the pancreas. They are very rare with an estimated incidence of 0.01 to 0.1/1,000,000/year and represent only 5% to 7% of functional PNETs.[1-3] Most are sporadic, but 10% are associated with multiple endocrine neoplasia type 1 (MEN-1) syndrome.[4] Most glucagonomas are large (>5 cm) at diagnosis, with 50% to 90% of patients presenting with metastatic disease.[5,6] Operative treatment of a glucagonoma involves resection of the primary tumor as well as metastatic disease for cure when possible or to palliate hormonal or local symptoms.

PATIENT HISTORY AND PHYSICAL FINDINGS

- The most common presenting age range is 40 to 60 years.[7]
- Glucagonoma is classically associated with the four "Ds": dermatitis, diabetes, depression, and deep vein thrombosis.
- The skin lesions associated with a glucagonoma are termed necrolytic migratory erythema and are pathognomonic for glucagonoma. It is a pruritic rash that occurs in the lower abdomen, lower extremities, perineum, perioral area, and feet (**FIGURES 1** and **2**). It is seen in 50% to 70% of patients and may be the initial presentation of the tumor.[3,8]
- Glucose intolerance is often mild, and insulin administration usually is not required.
- Weight loss is often out of proportion to the amount of tumor burden and is due to the catabolic effect of excess glucagon and through glucagon-like peptides such as GLP-1.
- Stomatitis, glossitis, anemia, and diarrhea are other frequent findings.
- Psychiatric manifestations may include depression, anxiety, and psychoses.
- Glucagonoma creates a hypercoagulable state, 4% to 30% of patients may experience a thromboembolic event.[3,9]
- A thorough personal and family history should be taken, with particular interest in other endocrinopathies because glucagonomas may be associated with MEN-1. Glucagonomas may also secrete secondary hormones, which may lead to Zollinger-Ellison syndrome in up to 10% of patients. Less commonly, they may secrete vasoactive intestinal polypeptide, pancreatic polypeptide, somatostatin, or adrenocorticotropic hormone.[10]

DIAGNOSIS

- Diagnosis is confirmed by high levels of fasting serum glucagon (>1000 pg/mL; normal, <150 pg/mL). Other conditions that cause hyperglucagonemia include hepatic insufficiency, stress, sepsis, and starvation, but levels rarely reach beyond 500 pg/mL.

IMAGING AND OTHER DIAGNOSTIC STUDIES

- Glucagonomas are typically greater than 5 cm at time of diagnosis and are easier to localize preoperatively than most PNETs. Most glucagonomas are located in the body or tail

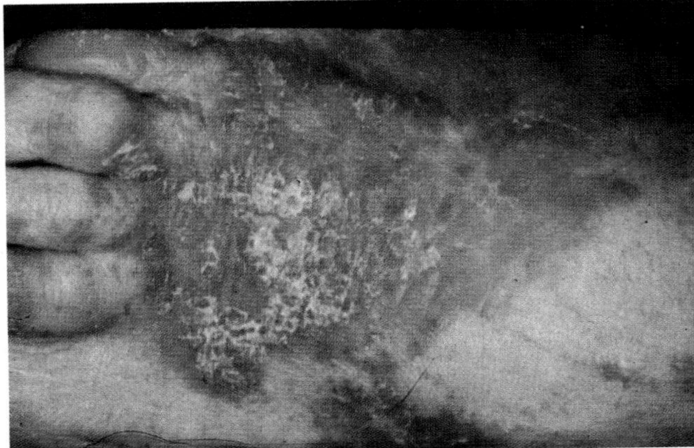

FIGURE 1 ● Necrolytic migratory erythema of the lower extremity.

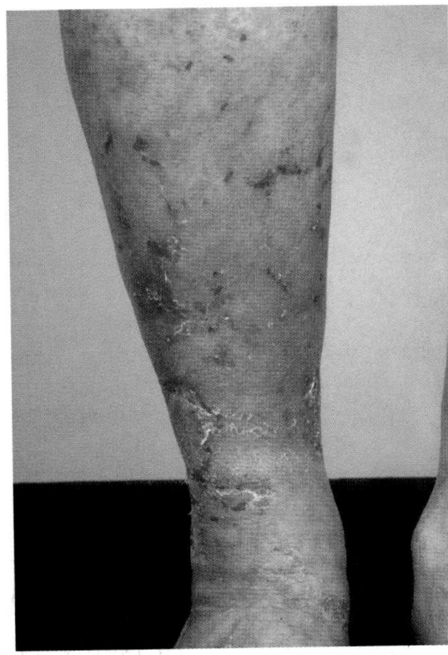

FIGURE 2 ● Necrolytic migratory erythema of the lower extremity.

of the pancreas. Rarely, they may be located outside the pancreas in the duodenal wall, accessory pancreatic tissue, or the kidney.
- Triple-phase computed tomography (CT) scan is often the first study. Somatostatin receptor scintigraphy, ^{68}Ga-DOTATATE, and ^{18}F-FDG PET/CT can also be used and can identify extra-abdominal spread to lymph nodes and liver.
- Endoscopic ultrasound, visceral angiography, and portal venous sampling may be required for glucagonomas that are difficult to identify, but this is very unusual.

SURGICAL MANAGEMENT

- The goal of operative management of glucagonoma is an R0 resection including the primary tumor and all metastases. Patients who cannot undergo R0 resection benefit from tumor debulking because it can palliate symptoms due to excess glucagon by decreasing the levels of circulating hormone.
- If the tumor is limited to the pancreas, surgical resection can completely reverse all clinical manifestations of a glucagonoma. This demands a formal pancreatic resection due to the large size of the tumors, usually a distal pancreatectomy with or without splenectomy. Pancreaticoduodenectomy is required for tumors in the head of the gland. Resection should include peripancreatic lymph node dissection. Although smaller tumors may be technically amenable to enucleation, the high malignant potential of these tumors suggests caution with this approach (**FIGURE 3**).
- All nodal and hepatic metastases that can be safely removed should be excised. Hepatic metastases may be managed by either wedge resection or formal hepatic resection.
- Tumor debulking leads to a dramatic improvement in symptoms, and the hormonal manifestations of glucagonoma may be diminished for years. Repeat debulking of recurrent disease may also prolong survival.
- In patients with MEN-1, consideration must be given to the presence of other functional and nonfunctional PNETs. If hyperparathyroidism is present as a component of the MEN-1 syndrome, it should be treated before addressing the pancreatic tumor to avoid problems with postoperative hypercalcemia.

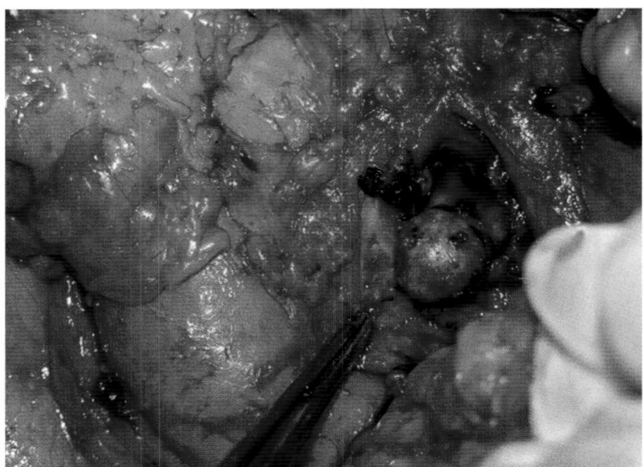

FIGURE 3 ● Small glucagonomas (<2 cm) with no malignant features can be enucleated from the pancreas using cautery or an energy device to control bleeding. Intraoperative ultrasound should be used to avoid injury to the pancreatic duct.

Preoperative Planning

- Preoperative management is focused on treating the metabolic effects of excess glucagon and preventing or treating venous thromboembolism.
- Somatostatin analogue therapy with octreotide is titrated to symptomatic improvement. Total parenteral nutrition may be needed if marked cachexia is present and may also help ameliorate necrolytic migratory erythema.
- Hyperglycemia and diabetes, when present, should be controlled.
- Patients should receive anticoagulation with Coumadin or low-molecular-weight heparin at the time of diagnosis. Preoperative placement of an inferior vena cava (IVC) filter may be necessary in patients with a history of thrombosis.

TECHNIQUES

POSITIONING

- As most patients present with metastatic disease and may require both pancreatic and hepatic resection, an open approach is preferred. For tumors confined to the pancreas, a minimally invasive approach may be possible. The open approach will be described first.
- The patient is placed supine with arms either extended laterally or tucked according to surgeon preference.

INCISION

- Midline laparotomy, extended left subcostal, chevron, or a combination of these are all acceptable approaches to the abdomen and should be chosen based on surgeon preference and experience, the body habitus of the patient, and the possible need for hepatic or other organ resection.

DISTAL PANCREATECTOMY WITHOUT SPLENECTOMY

- After the abdomen has been explored, the lesser sac is entered by separating the greater omentum from the transverse colon. The short gastric vessels must be preserved to provide blood flow to the spleen.
- Mobilize the posterior wall of the stomach off the anterior surface of the pancreas and retract the stomach cephalad. The stomach may be held in place with retractors or stay sutures. The anterior body and tail of the pancreas should now be fully exposed (**FIGURE 4**).
- Incise the peritoneum along the inferior border of the pancreas along the length of the body and tail. Gently elevate the pancreas off the retroperitoneum using blunt dissection along the avascular plane.
- The splenic artery and vein, which run along the superior border of the pancreas (the vein runs posterior to the artery), will be elevated along with the rest of the pancreas.
- Determine the point of transection for the pancreas. This should be just to the left of the superior mesenteric vein in the pancreatic neck.
- Bluntly develop a plane between the splenic vessels and the pancreas at the point of transection. Place vessel loops around the splenic vessels to facilitate retraction and provide vascular control (**FIGURE 5**).
- Ligate the splenic artery and vein individually—ligatures, suture ligatures, or a vascular stapler (as shown) can be used according to surgeon preference (**FIGURE 6**).
- Divide the pancreas using a stapler with a vascular load. Multiple firings may be required (**FIGURE 7**). If there is bleeding from the staple line, place 2-0 sutures in a figure-of-eight pattern at the superior and inferior borders of the pancreas to secure the gastropancreatic arteries.
- Ligate, clip, or use an energy device to control the numerous small, short vessels connecting the splenic vessels to the pancreas along the entire body and tail. Control any bleeding that occurs on the splenic artery or vein with fine Prolene sutures.
- As the splenic vessels approach the hilum, they will branch into multiple tributaries. Care must be taken to avoid injury to these branches along the tail of the pancreas. The hilum of the spleen may be directly abutting or within 1 cm of the tail of the pancreas. Once fully dissected off the vessels, the specimen may be removed.
- Check the surgical bed for hemostasis. Omentum may be placed over the pancreatic stump. Placement of a closed suction drain is our preference.

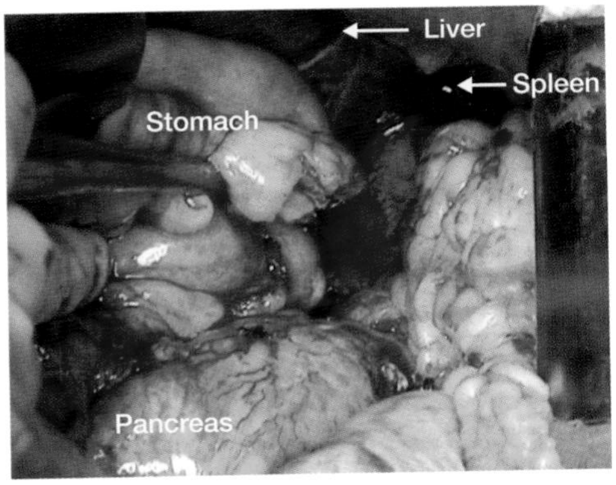

FIGURE 4 ● The anterior surface of the body and tail of the pancreas is exposed by entering the lesser sac through the gastrocolic omentum and retracting the stomach cephalad.

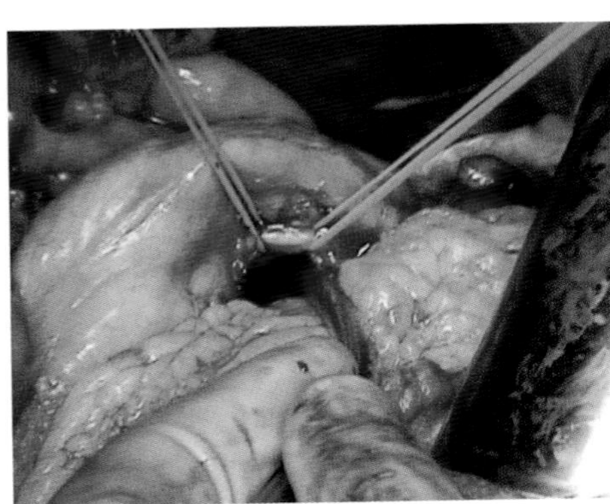

FIGURE 5 ● A plane is developed between the superior border of the pancreas and the splenic flexure at the point of transaction. Vessel loops are placed around the splenic vessels for retraction and vascular control.

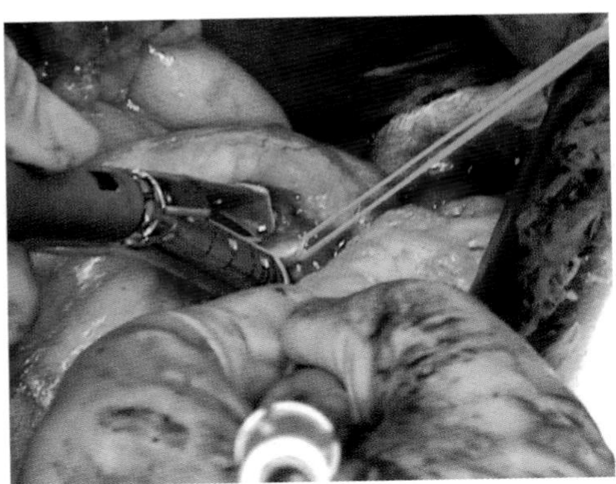

FIGURE 6 ● The splenic artery and vein are ligated with a vascular stapler as shown. Ligatures or suture ligatures may also be used according to surgeon preference.

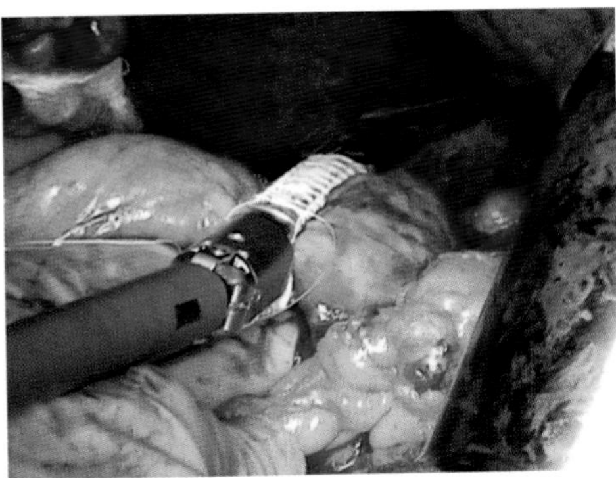

FIGURE 7 ● The pancreas is divided using a stapler with a vascular load.

DISTAL PANCREATECTOMY WITH SPLENECTOMY

- The exposure and mobilization of the pancreas proceed as described earlier.
- Divide the short gastric vessels.
- Mobilize the splenic flexure of the colon and retract it inferiorly.
- Divide the splenophrenic and splenocolic ligaments, and reflect the spleen and pancreatic body and tail up from the retroperitoneum.
- Once the point of transection of the pancreas has been determined, carefully isolate the splenic artery and vein and ligate them individually.
- Mobilize the splenic vessels along with the superior border of the pancreas.
- Divide the pancreas using a stapler with a vascular load. Multiple firings may be required. If there is bleeding from the staple line, place 2-0 sutures in a figure-of-8 pattern at the superior and inferior borders of the pancreas to secure the gastropancreatic arteries.

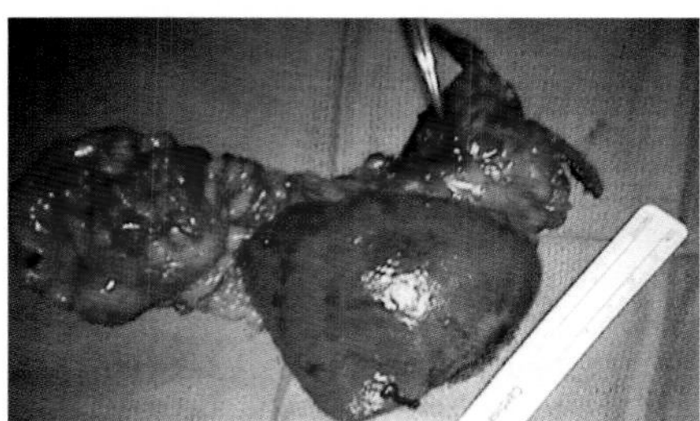

FIGURE 8 ● The body and tail of the pancreas have been removed en bloc. The instrument points to the tumor.

- The pancreas and spleen are then removed as specimen (**FIGURE 8**).
- Check the surgical bed for hemostasis. Omentum may be placed over the pancreatic stump. Placement of a closed suction drain is our preference.

MINIMALLY INVASIVE DISTAL PANCREATECTOMY

Overview

- A laparoscopic or robotic distal pancreatectomy is a suitable approach for patients with localized disease confined to the pancreas.
- Based on consensus guidelines, if a surgeon is technically proficient, minimally invasive distal pancreatectomy is considered standard of care if anatomically possible.[11]
- The estimated learning curve for robotic distal pancreatectomy ranges from 5 to 40 cases.[12-15]
- Educational training programs for minimally invasive distal pancreatectomy have been described such as the LAELAPS-1 and the University of Pittsburg Medical Center educational curriculum.[16]
- The LEOPARD-1 and DIPLOMA trials demonstrated reduced blood loss, length of stay, and time to functional recovery with minimally invasive distal pancreatectomy compared with open with no difference in median overall survival, 90-day mortality, and overall rate of complications[17,18]

Robotic Positioning and Port Placement

- The patient is placed supine on the operating table, in the split-leg position with the arms out. Foot boards are placed to prevent sliding while in steep reverse Trendelenburg position. Sufficient foam padding is used on the legs and arms to prevent pressure injuries (**FIGURE 9**).
- Using an optical trocar, a 5-mm port is placed in the left upper quadrant robotic port location.
- A diagnostic laparoscopy and laparoscopic ultrasound of both the pancreas and liver is performed to evaluate for evidence of local invasion and metastatic disease.
- Suspicious lesions are biopsied and sent for frozen section analysis. If metastatic disease or invasion into surrounding organs is identified, conversion to an open procedure should be considered.
- The remaining ports are placed. Four 8-mm robotic ports are placed, one 5-mm port is placed for liver retraction, and two assistant ports (one 5 mm and one 12 mm) are placed as shown in the figure (**FIGURE 10**).

Robotic Distal Pancreatectomy and Splenectomy Technique

- Once the robot is docked, the stomach is retracted anteriorly, and the lesser sac is entered through the gastrocolic ligament using an energy device.
- The short gastric vessels are divided with an energy device to free the greater curvature of the stomach from the spleen.
- The splenic flexure of the colon is mobilized inferiorly and the transverse mesocolon is separated from the inferior border of the pancreas, allowing visualization of the anterior surface of the pancreas and splenic hilum.
- The robotic drop-in ultrasound probe is used to delineate the extent of the tumor and identify the proximal pancreatic transection location.
- The hepatic artery lymph node is dissected free from the hepatic artery, and the portal vein is identified inferior and dorsal to the hepatic artery.
- The peritoneum on the inferior edge of the pancreas is incised and dorsal dissection is performed over the neck of the pancreas to identify the superior mesenteric vein and splenic vein confluence (**FIGURE 11**).
- A window posterior to the pancreas and anterior to the splenic vein is created.
- The robotic or laparoscopic stapler is placed in the window dorsal to the pancreas, ventral to the splenic vein and the pancreas is divided (**FIGURE 12**).
- The splenic artery to the left of the hepatic artery is isolated and circumferentially dissected at the proposed transection site.

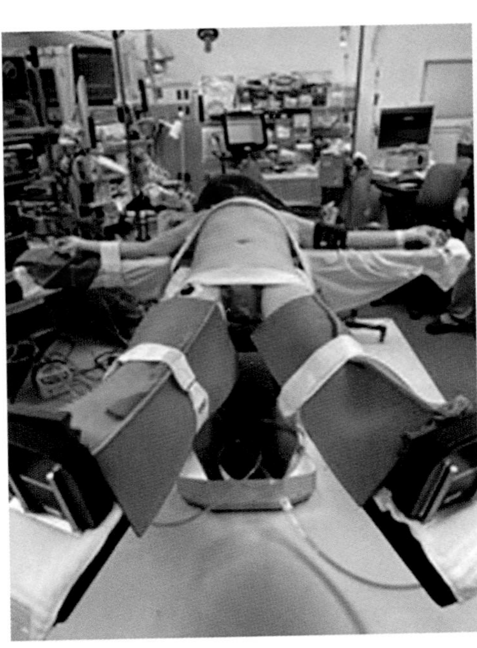

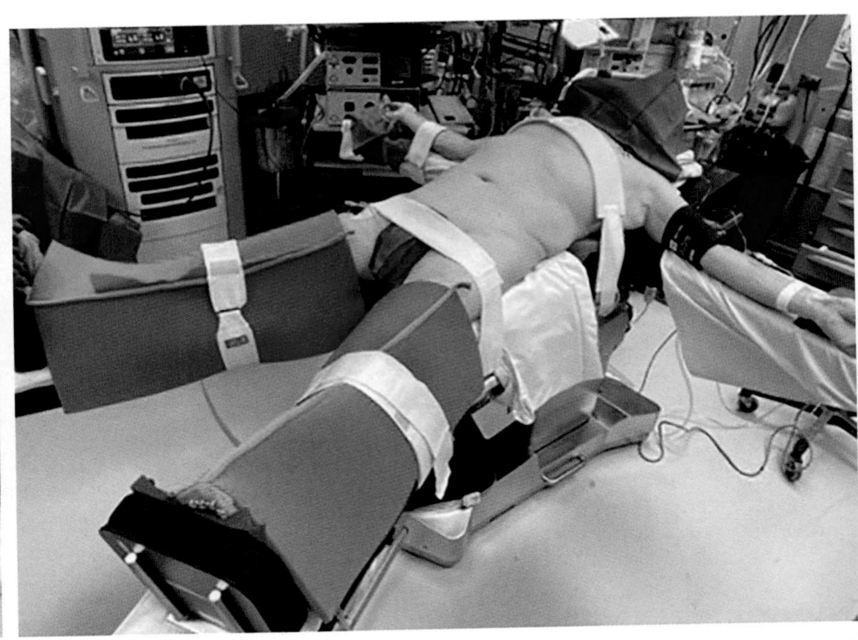

FIGURE 9 ● Positioning for robotic distal pancreatectomy and splenectomy. Supine, split-let, arms out position with foot boards, both chest and pelvis straps, and ample padding.

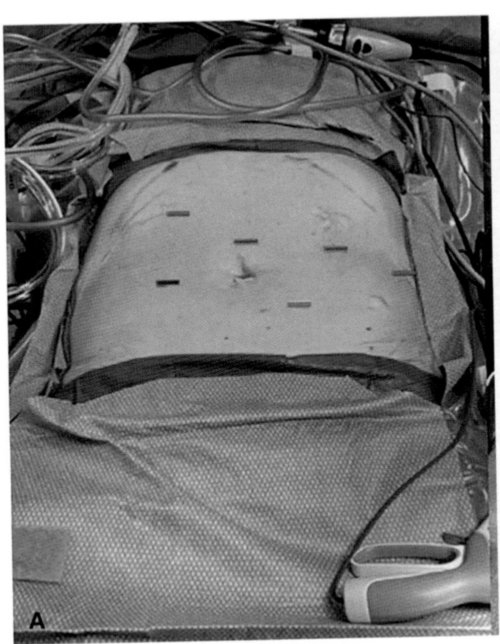

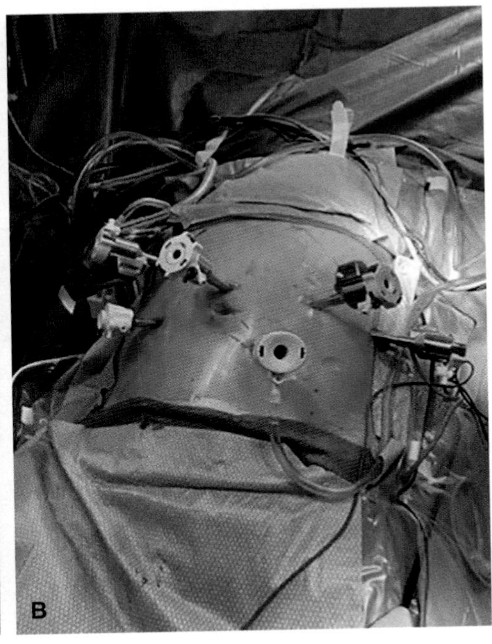

FIGURE 10 ● Location and size of port placement for robotic distal pancreatectomy and splenectomy (blue line represents 8-mm robotic port; green line represents 5-mm assistant port; red line represents 12-mm assistant port). Panel A demonstrates the location and size of the ports. Panel B demonstrates the ports placed.

- The splenic artery is divided using either a robotic or laparoscopic vascular stapler (**FIGURE 13**).
- Following division of the splenic artery, a window dorsal to the splenic vein is created and the splenic vein is divided with a vascular load laparoscopic or robotic stapler (**FIGURE 14**).
- The pancreas, splenic artery, and splenic vein are mobilized ventral and to the left.
- The specimen is placed in a plastic retrieval bag, and a port incision is extended to allow removal of the specimen (**FIGURE 15**).
- A closed suction drain is placed through the most left lateral port to the pancreatic transection line and is secured to the skin with sutures.
- All robotic ports are removed under direct vision, and the skin is closed with absorbable sutures.

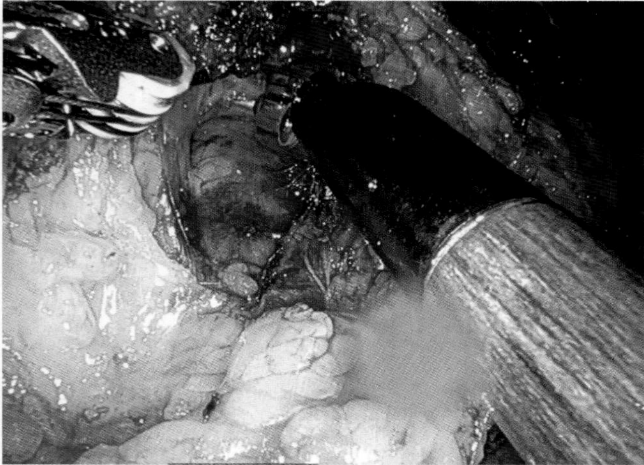

FIGURE 11 ● Peritoneum on the inferior boarder of the pancreas is incised at the neck to identify the superior mesenteric vein.

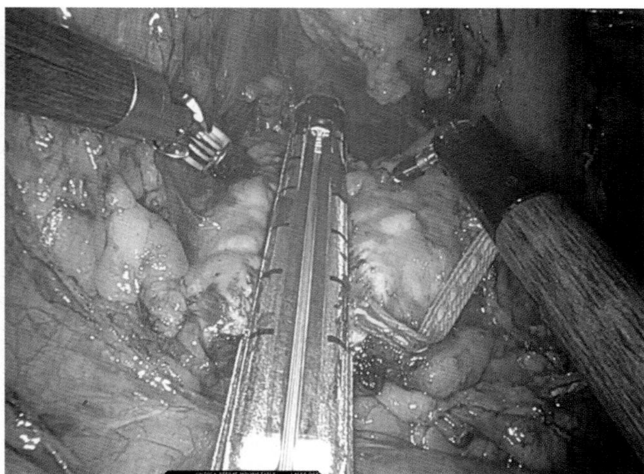

FIGURE 12 ● The neck of the pancreas is divided using a robotic or laparoscopic stapler.

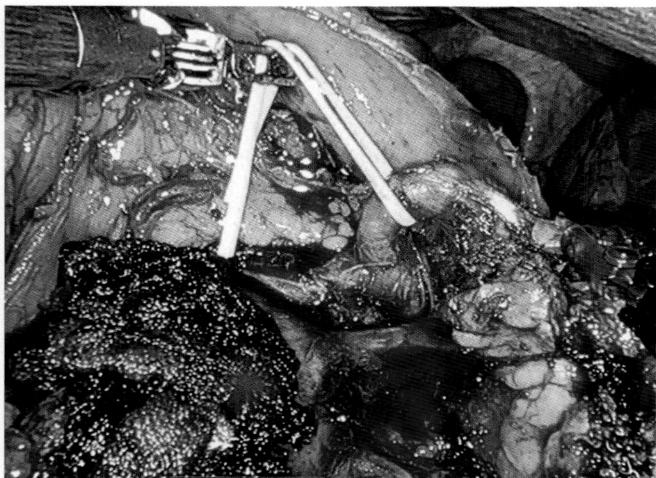

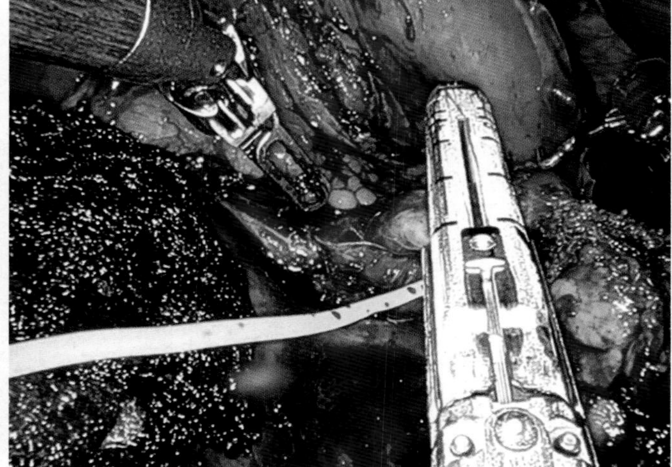

FIGURE 13 ● The splenic artery is encircled and divided using a robotic or laparoscopic stapler.

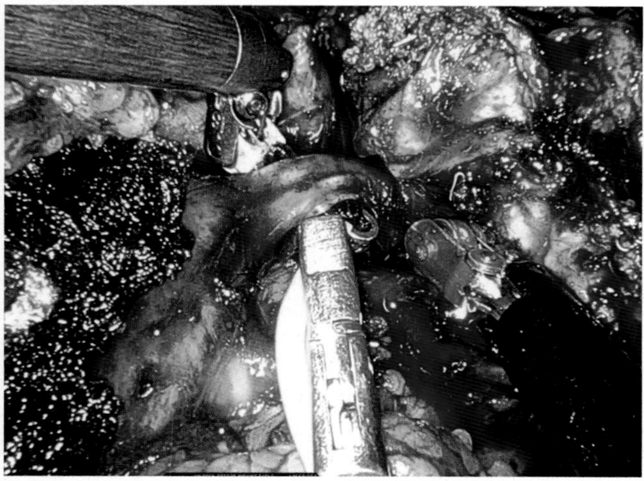

FIGURE 14 ● The splenic vein divided with a laparoscopic or robotic stapler.

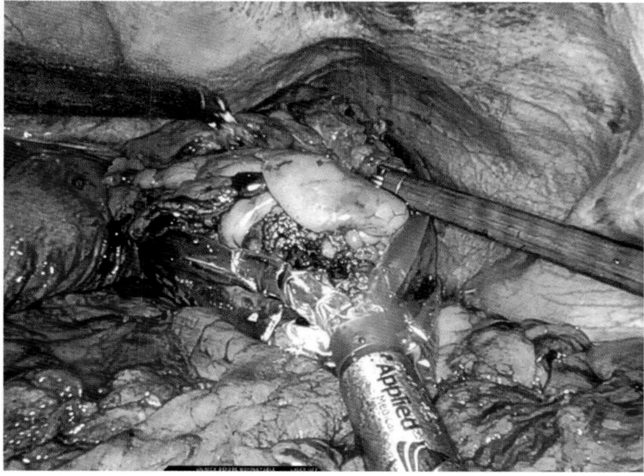

FIGURE 15 ● The specimen is placed in a plastic retrieval bag.

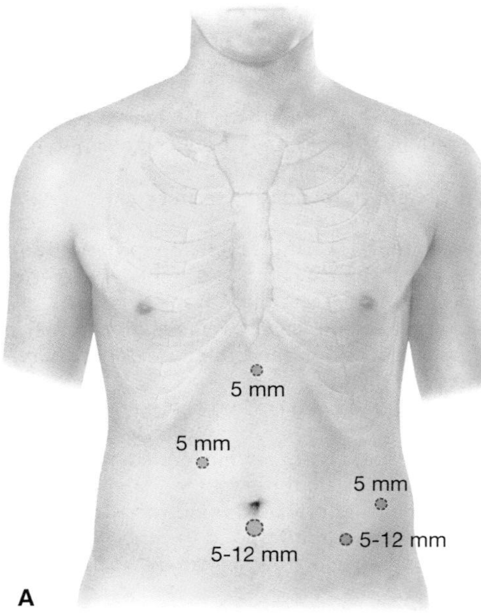

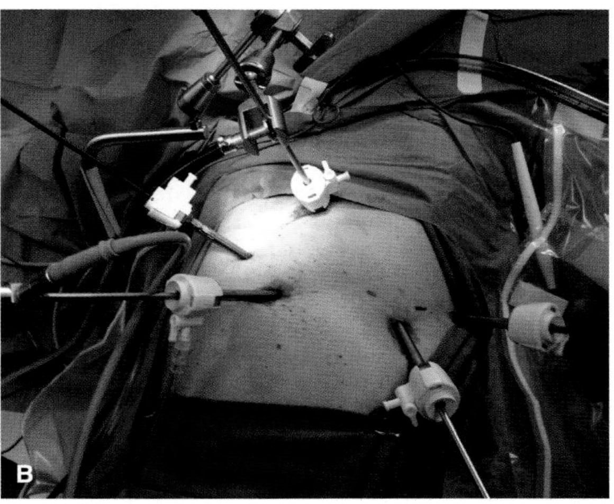

FIGURE 16 ● **A** and **B,** The position of the trocars for laparoscopic distal pancreatectomy is shown. A 5- to 12-mm trocar is placed at the umbilicus. A 5-mm trocar is placed subxiphoid for retraction. An optional assistant working port (5 mm) is placed in the right upper quadrant. Two working trocars, one 5 to 12 mm and another 5 mm, are placed in the left abdomen as shown. Trocar placement may be individualized for the patient.

Laparoscopic Distal Pancreatectomy and Splenectomy Technique

- Similar to the robotic approach, the patient is placed supine.
- A 5- to 12-mm port is placed infraumbilically, and a diagnostic laparoscopy is performed.
- Additional trocars are as shown in the figure (**FIGURE 16**).
- The technique of laparoscopic distal pancreatectomy is similar to that of robotic distal pancreatectomy.

Management of Hepatic Metastases

- Both curative intent resection and palliative intent resection are recommended for malignant glucagonoma (**FIGURE 17**). Other treatment options include hepatic artery occlusion or embolization, radiofrequency ablation, and cryoablation.
- Regional lymphadenectomy should be considered because lymph node metastases are common.

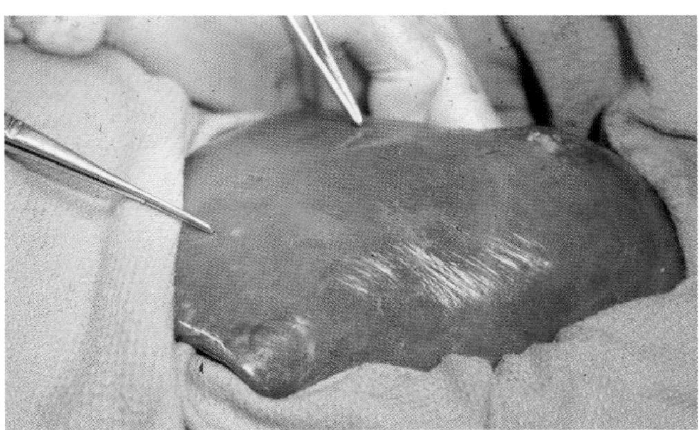

FIGURE 17 ● Glucagonoma metastases to the liver.

PEARLS AND PITFALLS

Minimally invasive distal pancreatectomy	■ For optimal outcomes, a surgeon performing minimally invasive distal pancreatectomy should be skilled in both open and minimally invasive techniques and beyond the learning curve required for proficiency.[19] ■ An experienced team in the operating room (including the circulating nurse, scrub technicians, and operative assistants) is essential for a timely and safe procedure. ■ Barriers to proficiency in robotic pancreatectomy include lack of platform familiarity, absence of tactile feedback, and complex navigation within the abdomen.

Glucagonomas	■ Patients with MEN-1 with glucagonomas should have hyperparathyroidism addressed before surgical treatment for glucagonoma. Failure to do so may lead to uncontrolled hypercalcemia postoperatively. ■ Although some tumors may be amenable to enucleation, formal pancreatic resection is preferred due to the high malignant potential of glucagonomas. ■ Glucagonomas are associated with hypercoagulability, and 30% of patients will have a deep vein thrombosis (DVT). Anticoagulation is recommended, and serious consideration should be given to IVC filter placement preoperatively. ■ Even if an R0 resection is not possible, patients may benefit tremendously from extensive debulking for palliation of symptoms. ■ When performing a spleen-preserving distal pancreatectomy, care must be taken to avoid trauma to branches off the splenic vessels as you approach the tail of the pancreas. Remember, if extensive bleeding is encountered, the procedure can be changed to a distal pancreatectomy with splenectomy. ■ Large tumors in the body of the pancreas may involve the splenic vein. In this situation, it may be helpful to divide the pancreatic neck early to better visualize the splenoportal confluence. If necessary, the splenic vein may be ligated flush with the superior mesenteric vein (SMV). ■ The left adrenal may be located more superiorly than expected and may be injured by excessive medial retraction of the pancreas and spleen. ■ Laparoscopic pancreatectomy without laparoscopic ultrasound is not recommended. Failure to use a laparoscopic ultrasound may result in a specimen that lacks part or all of the tumor. ■ Pancreatic stump leak/fistula is one of the most common postoperative complications and may occur in up to 30% of patients. Consider octreotide for patients who do not respond to closed suction drainage or have high-output fistula. However, routine use of perioperative octreotide will not reduce the rate of fistula.

POSTOPERATIVE CARE

- Admission to the intensive care unit is not mandatory and should be decided on a patient-by-patient basis. Management of pain, nasogastric intubation, and diet is similar to most major abdominal resections.
- Closed suction drain output should be tested for amylase before removal to evaluate for evidence of a postoperative pancreatic fistula.
- For locally advanced unresectable or metastatic disease, several treatment options exist including targeted therapy with Everolimus and Sunitinib, cytotoxic chemotherapy with capecitabine and temozolomide, and peptide receptor radionucleotide therapy.[20-23]
- Continued symptoms of excess glucagon after the operation should be treated with a somatostatin analog. However, routine perioperative use of octreotide therapy is not necessary and will not reduce the rate of pancreatic fistula.

OUTCOMES

- There is a paucity of outcomes data for glucagonoma. According to one study of patients with MEN-1, 10-year survival is approximately 50%.[24] In another, 5-year survival is approximately 50% following operative resection and adjuvant chemotherapy.[25]

COMPLICATIONS

- Patients may experience any postoperative complication associated with general anesthesia and major abdominal surgery such as superficial or deep wound infection, urinary tract infection, pneumonia, and cardiac dysrhythmia or ischemia.
- The risk of venous thromboembolism is elevated in patients with glucagonoma, and the physician should remain vigilant about detection and treatment of thromboembolic events.
- Postoperative pancreatic fistula occurs in up to 30% of patients undergoing distal pancreatectomy. This is managed by continued closed suction drainage in the stable patient. In a patient showing signs of infection, a CT scan should be obtained to look for abscess or an inadequately controlled fistula. This can usually be treated with an additional percutaneous drain placed with image guidance. Consider octreotide therapy for persistent high-output fistulas. Operative drainage, endoscopic sphincterotomy, or stent placement may be necessary in patients not responding to percutaneous drainage.

REFERENCES

1. Jensen RT, Cadiot G, Brandi ML, et al. ENETS Consensus Guidelines for the management of patients with digestive neuroendocrine neoplasms: functional pancreatic endocrine tumor syndromes. *Neuroendocrinology*. 2012;95(2):98-119. doi:10.1159/000335591
2. Zaidi MY, Lopez-Aguiar AG, Poultsides GA, et al. The impact of failure to achieve symptom control after resection of functional neuroendocrine tumors: an 8-institution study from the US Neuroendocrine Tumor Study Group. *J Surg Oncol*. 2019;119(1):5-11. doi:10.1002/jso.25306
3. Kindmark H, Sundin A, Granberg D, et al. Endocrine pancreatic tumors with glucagon hypersecretion: a retrospective study of 23 cases during 20 years. *Med Oncol*. 2007;24(3):330-337. doi:10.1007/s12032-007-0011-2
4. Stacpoole PW, Jaspan J, Kasselberg AG, et al. A familial glucagonoma syndrome. Genetic, clinical, and biochemical features. *Am J Med*. 1981;70:1017-1026.
5. Economopoulos P, Christopoulos C. Glaucagonoma. *Ann Gastroenterol*. 2001;14(2):99-108.
6. Wei J, Song X, Liu X, et al. Glucagonoma and glucagonoma syndrome: one center's experience of six cases. *J Pancreat Cancer*. 2018;4(1):11-16. doi:10.1089/pancan.2018.0003
7. Qu Y, Li H, Wang X, et al. Clinical characteristics and management of functional Pancreatic neuroendocrine neoplasms: a single institution 20-year experience with 286 Patients. *Int J Endocrinol*. 2020;2020:1030518. doi: 10.1155/2020/1030518. PMID: 33204258; PMCID: PMC7665912.

8. Wermers RA, Fatourechi V, Wynne AG, et al. The glucagonoma syndrome. Clinical and pathologic features in 21 patients. *Medicine (Baltim)*. 1996;75:53.
9. Stacpole PW. The glucagonoma syndrome: clinical features, diagnosis, and treatment. *Endocr Rev*. 1981;2:347.
10. Wynick D, Williams SJ, Blooms SR. Symptomatic secondary hormone syndromes in patients with established malignant pancreatic endocrine tumors. *N Engl J Med*. 1998;319:605-607.
11. Asbun HJ, Moekotte AL, Vissers FL, et al. The miami international evidence-based guidelines on minimally invasive pancreas resection. *Ann Surg*. 2020;271(1):1-14. doi:10.1097/SLA.0000000000003590
12. Takahashi C, Shridhar R, Huston J, Meredith K. Outcomes associated with robotic approach to pancreatic resections. *J Gastrointest Oncol*. 2018;9:936-941. doi:10.21037/jgo.2018.08.04
13. Napoli N, Kauffmann EF, Perrone VG, Miccoli M, Brozzetti S, Boggi U. The learning curve in robotic distal pancreatectomy. *Updat Surg*. 2015;67:257-264. doi:10.1007/s13304-015-0299-y
14. Shyr BU, Chen SC, Shyr YM, Wang SE. Learning curves for robotic pancreatic surgery-from distal pancreatectomy to pancreaticoduodenectomy. *Medicine (Baltim)*. 2018;97:e13000. doi:10.1097/MD.0000000000013000
15. Shakir M, Boone BA, Polanco PM, et al. The learning curve for robotic distal pancreatectomy: an analysis of outcomes of the first 100 consecutive cases at a high-volume pancreatic centre. *HPB*. 2015;17:580-586. doi:10.1111/hpb.12412
16. de Rooij T, van Hilst J, Boerma D, et al. Impact of a nationwide training Program in minimally invasive distal Pancreatectomy (LAELAPS). *Ann Surg*. 2016;264(5):754-762. doi:10.1097/SLA.0000000000001888
17. de Rooij T, van Hilst J, van Santvoort H, et al. Minimally invasive versus open distal Pancreatectomy (LEOPARD): a multicenter Patient-blinded randomized controlled trial. *Ann Surg*. 2019;269(1):2-9. doi:10.1097/SLA.0000000000002979
18. van Hilst J, de Rooij T, Klompmaker S, et al. Minimally invasive versus open distal pancreatectomy for ductal adenocarcinoma (DIPLOMA): a pan-european propensity score matched study. *Ann Surg*. 2019;269(1):10-17. doi:10.1097/SLA.0000000000002561
19. Vining CC, Hogg ME. How to train and evaluate minimally invasive pancreas surgery. *J Surg Oncol*. 2020;122(1):41-48. doi:10.1002/jso.25912
20. Yao JC, Shah MH, Ito T, et al. Everolimus for advanced pancreatic neuroendocrine tumors. *N Engl J Med*. 2011;364(6):514-523. doi:10.1056/NEJMoa1009290
21. Raymond E, Dahan L, Raoul JL, et al. Sunitinib malate for the treatment of pancreatic neuroendocrine tumors. *N Engl J Med*. 2011;364(6):501-513. doi:10.1056/NEJMoa1003825
22. Strosberg JR, Fine RL, Choi J, et al. First-line chemotherapy with capecitabine and temozolomide in patients with metastatic pancreatic endocrine carcinomas. *Cancer*. 2011;117(2):268-275. doi:10.1002/cncr.25425
23. Strosberg J, El-Haddad G, Wolin E, et al. Phase 3 trial of ^{177}Lu-dotatate for midgut neuroendocrine tumors. *N Engl J Med*. 2017;376(2):125-135. doi:10.1056/NEJMoa1607427
24. Levy-Bohbot N, Merle C, Goudet P, et al. Prevalence, characteristics, and prognosis of MEN 1-associated glucagonomas, VIPomas, and somatostatinomas: study from the GTE (Group de Tumeurs Endocrines) registry. *Gastroenterol Clin Biol*. 2004;28(11):1075-1081.
25. Lepage C, Ciccolallo L, DeAngelis R, et al. European disparities in malignant digestive endocrine tunmours survival. *Int J Cancer*. 2010;126(12):2928-2934.

Part 6 Operative Techniques in Vascular Surgery

SECTION I: CEREBROVASCULAR ARTERIAL SURGERY/INTERVENTION

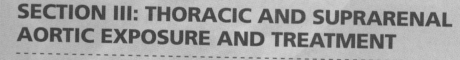

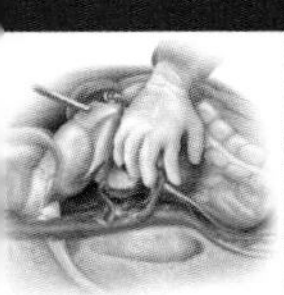

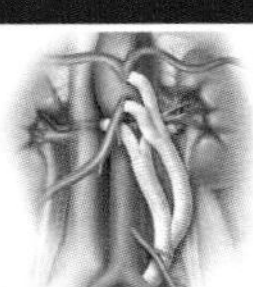

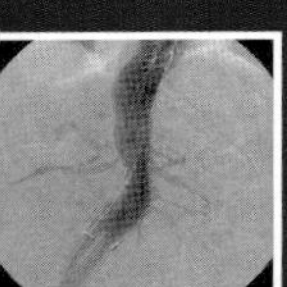

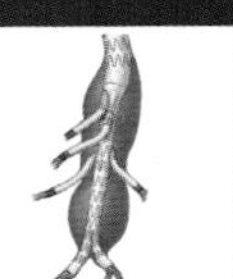

SECTION IV: VISCERAL AND RENAL ARTERY DISEASE MANAGEMENT

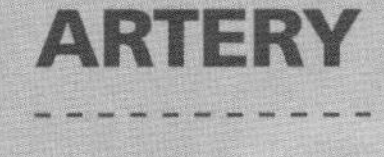

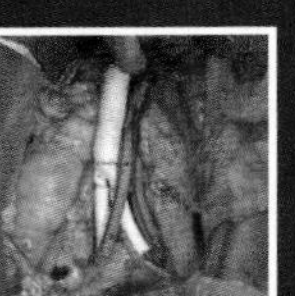

SECTION V: INFRAINGUINAL ARTERIAL DISEASE MANAGEMENT

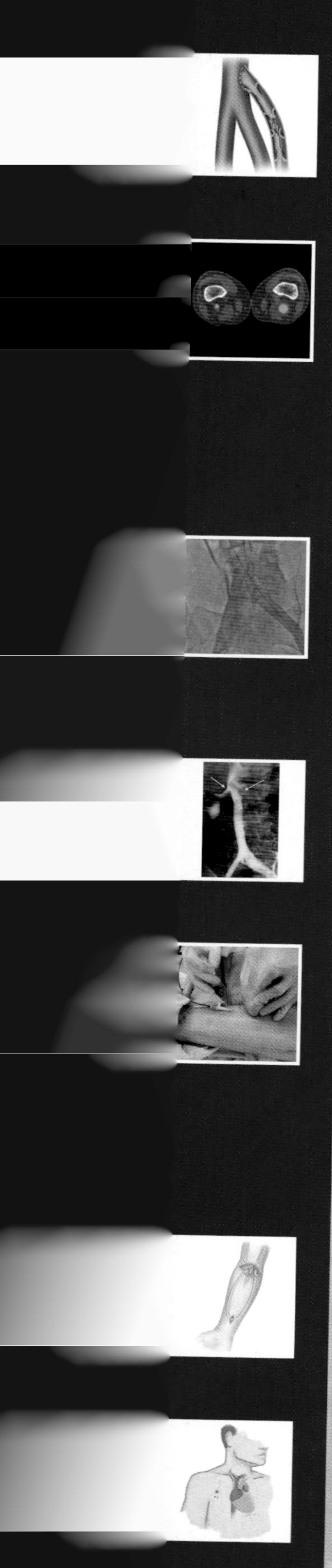

SECTION I: Cerebrovascular Arterial Surgery/ Intervention

Chapter 1 Arch and Great Vessel Revascularization and Reconstruction

Matthew P. Sweet and Christopher Burke

DEFINITION

- The aortic arch is defined as the segment from the proximal end of the innominate artery ostium through the distal end of the left subclavian ostium (Ishimura Zones 1-3). This segment is a dynamic and complex anatomic structure: with compliance that augments coronary blood flow during diastole; a high degree of curvature as the aorta takes a 180° turn from an ascending to descending direction; and critical branch vessels. Rarely occurring in isolation, aneurysms of the arch are often extensions of aneurysms present in the ascending or descending thoracic aorta. The proximal and mid-arch is best approached surgically via a median sternotomy while the more distal arch is often best approached via a high posterolateral left thoracotomy. Given these anatomic and physiologic factors, surgical intervention on the arch necessitates a specific set of techniques.
- This chapter will focus on the management of aortic arch aneurysm and will attempt to combine the approaches utilized by both cardiac and vascular surgeons, each of whom bring discrete tools to approach these lesions. Leading aortic centers of excellence are moving toward multidisciplinary team-based approach with both cardiac and vascular surgeons and in varying circumstances interventional cardiologists, anesthesiologists, geneticists, and other team members to engage in care of these patients. This multidisciplinary approach facilitates individualization of the surgical approach without regard to which specialty drives the operation, integrates open and endovascular tools, improves comprehensive assessment and risk factor modification, and importantly helps anticipate future needs of the patient so that the operative approach may facilitate future care. Institutional infrastructure required to safely care for these patients includes fixed angiographic imaging, cardiac anesthesia, cardiac intensive care, and endovascular inventory.

PATHOPHYSIOLOGY

- Aortic arch aneurysms can occur from a variety of causes, most commonly atherosclerotic degeneration and degeneration of residual aortic dissection after prior ascending aortic repair for a type A dissection (DeBakey 1).
- Patients with genetic aortopathy (eg, Marfan syndrome) are an important group as they require disease-specific treatment. Genetic aortopathies run a wide spectrum of severity, and familial aortopathies without specifically identified genetic abnormality have worse outcomes than patients without family history.[1] Awareness of a potential genetic cause for aortic pathology can significantly affect treatment decisions and should be a routine component of patient evaluation.
- Less frequent etiologies include inflammatory (eg, giant cell arteritis), traumatic pseudoaneurysm (iatrogenic or traumatic), mycotic infectious aneurysm, and saccular aneurysms associated with penetrating atherosclerotic ulcers.

PATIENT HISTORY AND PHYSICAL FINDINGS

- As with any surgical practice, patient assessment begins with a thorough history and physical examination. History should include any prior chest or neck surgery or radiation, concomitant coronary or peripheral vascular disease, aortic insufficiency, smoking history, chronic obstructive pulmonary disease (COPD), and a thorough family history of aneurysm, dissection, or unexplained sudden death.
- Beyond the routine history and physical examination, we place particular importance on two factors: physiologic fitness and anatomic fitness.

Physiologic Fitness

- Physiologic assessment is a composite assessment of patient age, activity level, medical comorbid illness, and frailty. A young, active patient with few comorbidities who is not frail is more likely to tolerate an open operation and benefit from its long-term effectiveness and durability. Conversely, an older patient with more comorbidities and/or frailty may benefit from a less invasive approach and accept a less well-defined long-term effectiveness. Although age, in and of itself, is a poor metric of wellness, it is often used as a surrogate for anticipated remaining life expectancy, which is a critical concept when determining whether to proceed with prophylactic aneurysm repair. That said, octogenarians are clearly considered higher risk for open repair in general and except in very selected cases would typically be offered endovascular or hybrid repair.
- In terms of medical illness, specific attention needs to be paid to coronary artery disease, heart failure, heart valvular function, renal disease, liver disease, and pulmonary function. Concomitant coronary or valvular heart disease may require treatment at the time of open arch intervention or prior to endovascular therapy. Advanced nonischemic cardiomyopathy and severe COPD are conditions that would portend poor outcome from an open operation, particularly if cardiopulmonary bypass (CPB) is utilized.

- Frailty is different from medical comorbid illness. It is a multifactorial clinical syndrome associated with loss of metabolic reserve, physical capability, cognitive ability, and the ability to withstand physiologic stress. We use the Clinical Frailty Scale (CFS).[2] Open repair is generally considered problematic when the CFS is >4. This constellation of age, comorbid illness, and frailty can be used to classify patients as being at standard, increased, or prohibitive risk for both endovascular and open repair.

Anatomic Fitness

- To assess operative risk, one must understand the anatomic suitability of endovascular treatment and the technical feasibility of open repair.
- Each endovascular device has specific anatomic constraints as outlined in their instructions for use (IFU). Deviation from IFU is associated with a high risk of treatment failure. Similar to physiologic assessment, anatomic fitness can be assessed as standard, increased, or prohibitive risk. Features putting a patient at increased risk include calcific atherosclerosis of the arch vessels, small/diseased iliac access vessels, or significant aortic tortuosity. Prohibitive risk features include severe mural atheroma at the arch vessel ostia (aka "shaggy aorta"), absence of a suitable landing zone, or a dominant intercostal artery (artery of Adamkiewicz) where endovascular coverage might confer a very high risk of spinal cord injury. Furthermore, a patient with multiple moderate risk factors might, collectively, be considered prohibitive risk.
- Analogous anatomic risk factors influence the patient's suitability for open repair. Prior sternotomy with high-risk reentry anatomy, coronary bypass grafts, calcified aorta, and other factors may alter the patient's overall suitability for an open operation.
- To assess anatomic suitability, a computed tomography (CT) angiogram with 3D reconstruction on a workstation (eg, TeraRecon, 3mensio, or other) is essential.

IMAGING AND OTHER DIAGNOSTIC STUDIES

Imaging

- Contrast-enhanced fine-cut CT with arterial phase imaging (CTA) is the most important diagnostic test and is essential for any patient being considered for arch operation. ECG gated CTA is an useful tool when assessing the arch as it improves clarity by capturing images in the same phase of the cardiac cycle. Contrast is essential to assess for vessel patency, the presence of mural atheroma, dissection, wall thickening, and device sizing.
- The standard of care is to utilize a 3D workstation to evaluate the CT images. Two-dimensional imaging can be misleading as device sizing is based on the orthogonal plane (the plane that is perpendicular to the centerline of the aorta.)
- Moving from cranial to caudal, specific anatomic assessments for an endovascular approach include the following:
  - Arch branch vessels: patency, atherosclerotic disease, dissection, and aberrant anatomy (hemi-bovine trunk, left vertebral origin from the arch, etc.). For arch branch devices, one must also know the diameter, length, and quality of the innominate, left common carotid, and/or left subclavian arteries to determine if they will serve as suitable landing zones.
  - Aortic landing zones: defined as a segment of healthy, parallel aortic tissue with a <10% change in diameter or surgical graft without a sharp kink. One needs to assess diameter, presence of atherosclerosis, dissection, and atheroma. One also needs to assess the distance from the leading edge of the stent graft to the aortic valve. If the deployment needs to occur low in Zone 0, then the wire might need to cross the aortic valve to accommodate the nosecone.
  - Gantry angles: views with the fluoroscopy machine to optimize visualization of the arch and target vessels.
  - Aortic arch shape: a steep "gothic" arch may complicate stent graft delivery.
  - Distal aortic disease: occlusive disease, dissection, atheroma burden, or tortuosity that might complicate stent graft delivery to the arch.
  - Iliofemoral arterial access: Suitability of access for appropriately sized sheath (based on device sizing).
- Specific to an open operation:
  - Evaluation of the aortic root and valve for concomitant pathology.
  - Space between the posterior table of the sternum and the aorta, to determine the safety of redo sternotomy.
  - Anterior-posterior orientation of the arch, to assess the accessibility of the left subclavian artery (LSA) and distal sewing cuff.
  - Presence of aberrant arch vessel anatomy.
  - Presence of prior coronary bypass grafts, valvular operation, or other prior cardiac intervention.
  - Location of healthy, nondissected arterial cannulation site.

Other Diagnostic Studies

- Magnetic resonance imaging is useful as a screening tool, but the detail is insufficient for operative planning.
- Carotid duplex ultrasound can be helpful in the setting of concomitant cerebrovascular occlusive disease or prior stroke.
- Transthoracic echocardiogram is routinely ordered. It is required in patients with any clinical history of congestive heart failure, genetic aortopathies, or disease of the aortic root.
- Pulmonary function testing is not routinely obtained, but it is indicated in patients with a heavy smoking history or known COPD in whom an open approach is being considered.
- For patients being considered for open repair, a preoperative left heart catheterization is needed to assess for concomitant coronary artery disease requiring revascularization.

SURGICAL MANAGEMENT

- There are two general approaches to treatment of aortic arch aneurysmal disease, open and endovascular. Combinations of these techniques are termed "hybrid repairs."
- Open repair replaces the diseased aortic segment with a fabric surgical graft (typically Dacron). Open repair requires suitable exposure, use of CPB and often deep hypothermic circulatory arrest (DHCA), control of blood flow to the heart, brain, and viscera, and tissue adequate to sew to.
- Endovascular repair serves to reline the diseased aortic segment. The stent graft seals at either end in healthy aortic tissue or prior surgical graft, serving as a bridge across the diseased aorta. Just as with a bridge across a river with

foundations laid in a sand bar, a stent graft landed into diseased tissue may look good at completion of the procedure but will have poor durability. The depressurization of the aneurysm takes away the risk of rupture and often leads to aortic "remodeling" around the stent graft. This basic conceptual framework is essential as endovascular repair cannot be successful without adequate healthy tissue or graft to land the device within, where the device can both seal and fixate. In evaluating a patient with arch pathology, understanding their treatment options is entirely dependent on a comprehensive and quantitative assessment of their aortic anatomy.

This chapter will describe three options for aortic arch aneurysm repair, progressing from the most to the least invasive.

TECHNIQUES

OPEN ARCH REPLACEMENT (WITH OR WITHOUT FROZEN ELEPHANT TRUNK AKA "FET")

- Meticulous preoperative planning and patient selection is critical to successful open aortic arch replacement. In general, these procedures are performed via a median sternotomy with the use of CPB and various DHCA techniques. Fundamentally, operative strategy is divided into the following aspects:
    - Assessment of reentry into the mediastinum, in the case of a reoperative median sternotomy (need for peripheral cannulation, cooling prior to reentry, need for left ventricular (LV) venting if significant aortic insufficiency is present, etc.).
    - CPB cannulation strategy.
    - Proximal and distal aortic extent of operation.
    - Cerebral protection strategy and temperature management (antegrade vs retrograde cerebral perfusion, or hypothermia only).
- The importance of thorough preoperative CTA evaluation of the aorta cannot be overemphasized. This is especially true in the reoperative setting. Cross-sectional imaging shows the position of critical structures to the posterior table of the sternum (innominate vein, right ventricle, aorta, bypass grafts, etc.). In the case of an aortic aneurysm that is in close proximity to the sternum, this can lead to a lethal situation if the aneurysm is injured on reentry. This is especially true if significant aortic insufficiency is present, as efforts to place on CPB and cool will result in LV distension if/when ventricular fibrillation occurs. In this circumstance, peripheral CPB cannulation is often performed. Lidocaine is given and the patient slowly cooled prior to sternotomy. Depending on risk, a LV vent can be placed directly by utilizing a small left anterior thoracotomy.
- The next critical aspect of preoperative planning is CPB strategy. Effective CPB facilitates a bloodless surgical field and allows cooling for DHCA and aortic arch reconstruction. Certain CPB strategies also allow convenient antegrade cerebral protection (ACP) during DHCA. The most commonly used strategy in this regard is right axillary artery cannulation. By placing clamps on the innominate and left common carotid artery (LCCA) during DHCA, ACP can be given via the right axillary artery to perfuse the brain during arch replacement (**FIGURE 1**). Other arterial cannulation options for CPB include central aortic, femoral, and various much less commonly used sites (eg, left axillary artery, innominate artery, etc.).
- The surgeon must have a clear, defined plan for the proximal and distal aortic extent of the operation. Proximal extent varies from aortic root replacement to supracoronary graft anastomosis. This decision rests on whether root pathology is present. Regarding aneurysmal disease, in general any aortic root with a maximum diameter in the sinus segment of greater than 4.5 cm warrants root replacement. This can be accomplished with associated aortic valve replacement (AVR) (Bentall procedure) or with a valve sparing root replacement (David or Yacoub procedure). In rare cases of asymmetric root aneurysms or sinus of Valsalva aneurysms, selective sinus replacement is possible, most commonly performed in the noncoronary sinus.

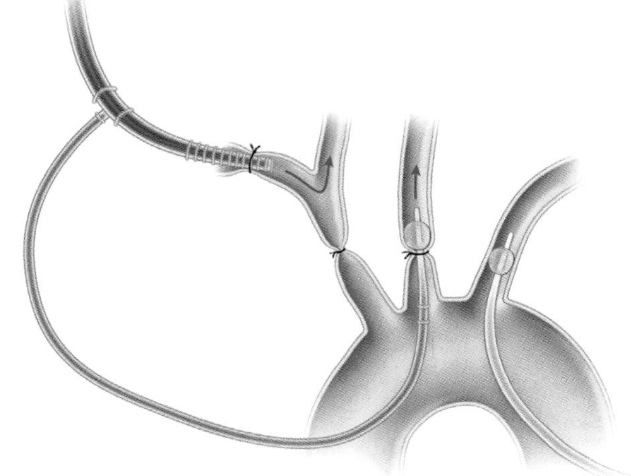

FIGURE 1 ● Antegrade cerebral perfusion via axillary cannulation and left common carotid artery (LCA) and left subclavian artery (LSA) cannulation.

- The distal extent of the aortic operation is driven by the pathology being treated. Options include a hemiarch (**FIGURE 2**), which involves resection of the lesser curvature of the aorta and a single aortic anastomosis performed under circulatory arrest, or a variety of more extensive transverse arch operations including several hybrid strategies (**FIGURE 2**). A repair extended to Zone 2 can be performed with a thoracic endovascular aortic repair (TEVAR) stent graft deployed distally across the distal arch and into the descending aorta. The stent graft is then incorporated into the distal surgical anastomosis. This operation is a called a "frozen elephant trunk" as it fixates the TEVAR device and creates a strong platform from which to extend the repair distally in the aorta at a subsequent operation. Recently, due to the emergence of single-side branch aortic arch TEVAR, enthusiasm has increased for a Zone 2 arch replacement concept with creation of a TEVAR landing zone followed by interval endovascular therapy of Zone 3 or the

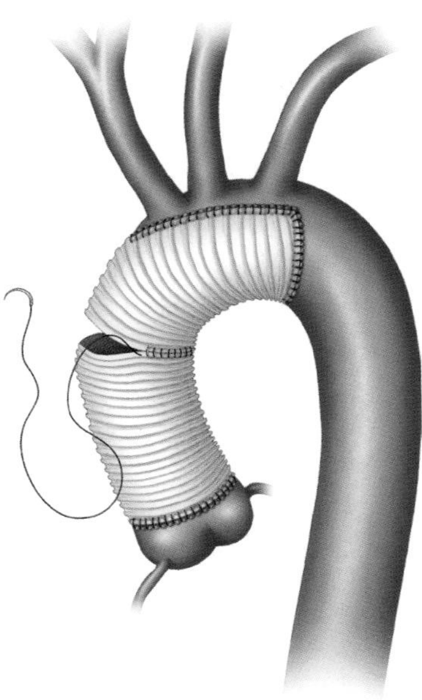

FIGURE 2 ● Ascending aorta and hemiarch reconstruction.

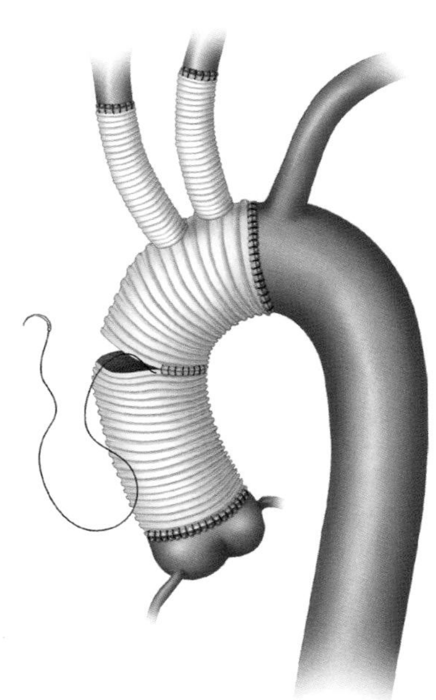

FIGURE 3 ● Ascending aorta and Zone 2 arch reconstruction.

arch as well as DTA (**FIGURE 3**).[3] This allows the surgeon a relatively straightforward arch operation with limited DHCA times.

- Cerebral protection strategies and temperature management are intimately associated. In general, the single most important cerebral protection strategy performed during open arch surgery is hypothermia. Temperature management most commonly varies from moderate hypothermia (MHCA, 22-28 °C) to DHCA (18-22 °C). However, most surgeons in contemporary practice will include cerebral perfusion techniques to supplement hypothermia. These include the antegrade (ACP, via the arterial system) and retrograde (RCP, infused through the venous system, most often the SVC) strategies. Advantages of ACP are the ability to provide nutritive blood flow to the cerebral circulation during periods of circulatory arrest. This also facilitates performance of arch operations at MHCA especially if straightforward repair is being pursued. As mentioned previously, right axillary artery cannulation provides a convenient strategy and is an excellent choice during arch reconstruction. Another option is to use balloon tipped cannulas down the carotid arteries. ACP strategies can be given unilaterally or bilaterally, although no difference in neurologic outcome has been shown between the two techniques. An exception would be when a precipitous fall in left-sided cerebral head saturations during right-sided unilateral ACP, which should mandate addition of LCCA ACP. Retrograde cerebral perfusion involves infusing cold blood into the SVC during periods of DHCA. RCP techniques are commonly used, though not necessarily limited, to straightforward arch reconstructions (hemiarch) and performed at deep hypothermic conditions. Advantages to this technique include the ability to "uniformly" keep the brain cool during circulatory arrest and may provide an "antiembolic" flushing function as well. No significant difference has been shown in outcomes between ACP and RCP techniques, though there may be some evidence of lower rates of cerebral embolic events during hemiarch with RCP as compared to ACP.[4]
- Left carotid-subclavian (CS) revascularization: The left SCA can be approached in several ways. For complete arch replacement, routine revascularization is indicated to mitigate the risk of perioperative stroke. We generally perform transposition of the LSA to the LCCA in a staged fashion from a supraclavicular approach.[5] Staging the operation simplifies the open arch operation and is of particular importance when the LSA ostium is located more posteriorly, there is a separate origin of the left vertebral from the arch (seen in 5% of cases), or there has been prior open surgical intervention of the distal arch. The transposition also serves as a "stress test" for those patients of uncertain fitness for open repair. If a patient does not tolerate a transposition well, they are unlikely to withstand the stress of an open arch with DHCA and CPB. If the LSA ostium is located anteriorly in the chest making it more easily accessible during sternotomy, the patient has had prior left neck surgery/radiation, the case is urgent, or the logistics of a staged approach are otherwise problematic we tend to do the operation concomitantly with the arch (**FIGURE 4**).

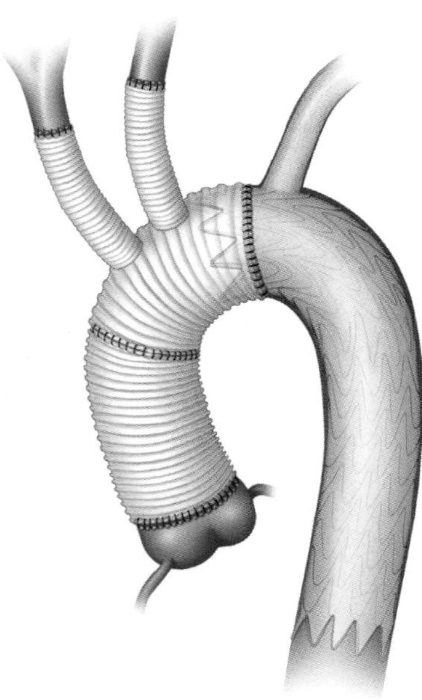

FIGURE 4 ● Ascending aorta and Zone 2 arch reconstruction with Zone 2 gore thoracic branched endograft.

HYBRID ARCH DEBRANCHING

- Hybrid arch debranching was an approach that was developed for patients with a healthy ascending aorta and distal arch disease in whom total arch repair was considered to be too stressful. Via median sternotomy, a side-biting clamp is used to control the ascending aorta, from which a 10-mm Dacron graft is sewn on a steep upgoing bevel. This graft is then taken to the innominate artery. An 8-mm Dacron graft is sewn at a 90° angle from the more distal aspect of the 10-mm graft and taken to the LCCA. Following this debranching, a TEVAR procedure is done landing the proximal end of the stent graft in the distal ascending aorta (**FIGURES 5-7**). Several factors have led to a reduction in the use of this approach. First, the majority of patients with arch aneurysms have concomitant abnormalities of the ascending aorta, thereby necessitating a more extensive open operation. Among patients with a healthy ascending aorta or prior graft who are deemed high risk for open arch replacement, the advent of totally branched arch stent grafts has created a far less stressful, safe, and effective treatment option that obviates the need for sternotomy. The third reason is that as multidisciplinary teams have evolved, this operation has fallen out of favor. The appeal of the hybrid operation was that it could be done without CPB, but experience has shown that most patients are well treated with either a definitive arch operation or a branched stent graft, with the exception being the rare patients with severe arch vessel occlusive disease and otherwise healthy ascending aortic tissue.

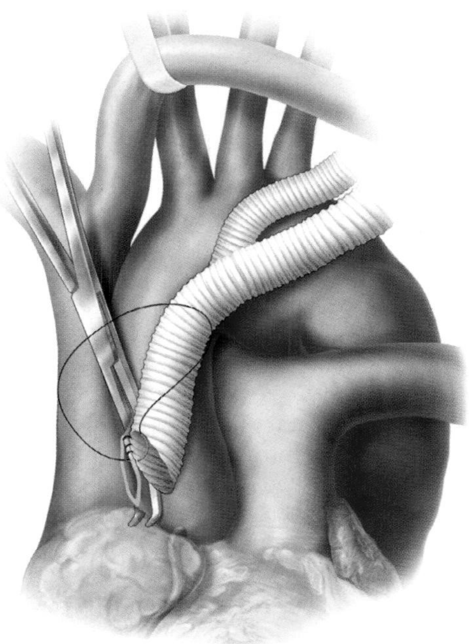

FIGURE 5 ● An aortic side-biting clamp is placed on the right anterolateral side (convexity) of the ascending aorta, as low as possible. The proximal end of the larger (10 or 12 mm) graft is beveled and sewn end-to-side to the ascending aorta with a running 3-0 or 4-0 polypropylene suture.

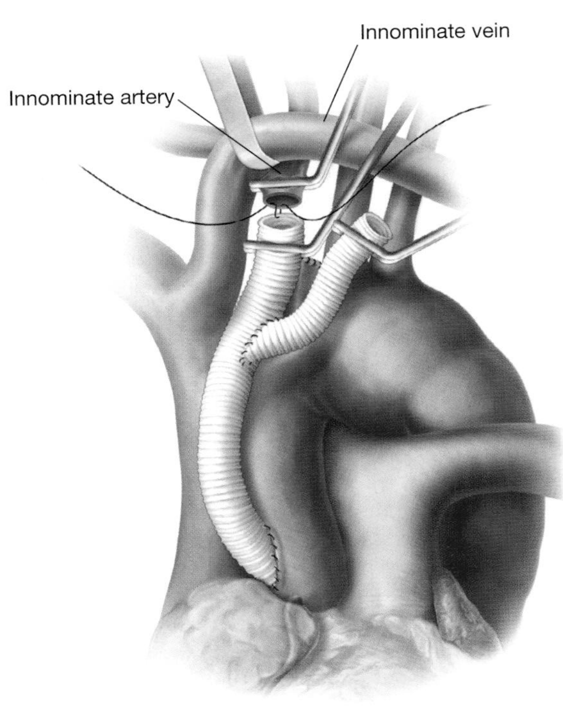

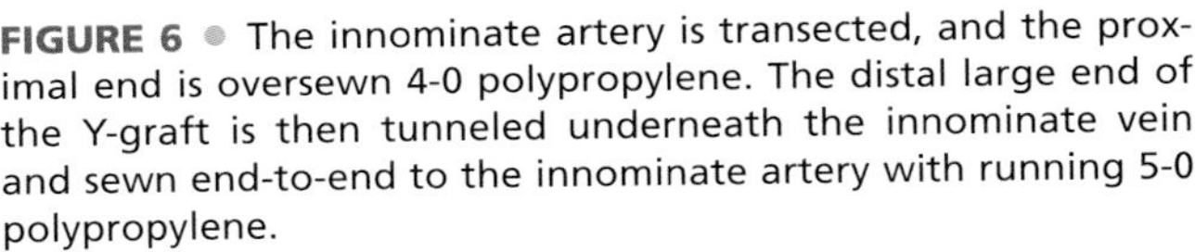
FIGURE 6 ● The innominate artery is transected, and the proximal end is oversewn 4-0 polypropylene. The distal large end of the Y-graft is then tunneled underneath the innominate vein and sewn end-to-end to the innominate artery with running 5-0 polypropylene.

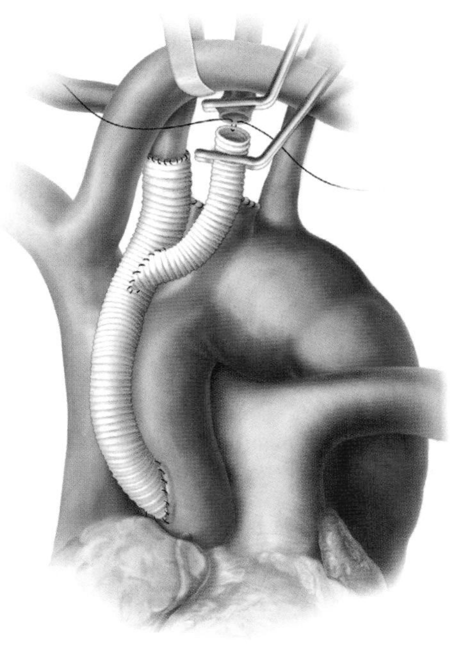

FIGURE 7 ● The left common carotid artery is transected, and the proximal end of the carotid artery is oversewn with 4-0 polypropylene. The distal smaller end of the Y-graft is tunneled underneath the innominate vein and sewn end-to-end to the carotid artery with running 5-0 polypropylene.

TOTAL ENDOVASCULAR ARCH REPAIR

- Currently, there are no FDA-approved commercially available arch stent grafts in the United States. Several devices are in use outside the United States and trials for multiple devices are ongoing in the United States. Device design is primarily a function of device curvature to accommodate the arch and Zone 0 landing zone, delivery control, as well as branch and branching stent design. Given the consistency of arch anatomy, standard branch position(s) can accommodate most patients, obviating the need for customization.[6]
- Endovascular treatment of the arch requires several anatomic features:
  - suitable iliofemoral access or the ability to use a surgical iliac conduit
  - a healthy proximal landing zone in Zone 0, with either nondilated tissue or a prior surgical graft
  - distal landing zone in Zones 3 to 5 (or a surgical plan for a staged endovascular repair of the arch and thoracoabdominal aneurysm, which is beyond the scope of this chapter)
  - a thoracic stent graft with one or more side branches
  - patent and nondiseased great vessels to serve as a suitable distal landing zone
  - a strategy for cervical debranching

Access and Landing Zones

- First-generation arch graft technology requires large delivery systems as the branch adds significant material to the device. Current investigational devices run in the 22 to 26F range. It is possible that those sizes will come down as lower profile systems come forward.
- The proximal landing zone is one of the biggest limitations for endovascular arch repair. As described earlier, most patients with arch aneurysms have diseased ascending aorta. Ascending aorta diameters >38 mm is associated with significant increase in adverse events as the landing zone is ecstatic and intrinsically unhealthy. Prior surgical repair of the ascending aorta, as is typical for patients with postdissection arch aneurysms, can provide an excellent landing zone. The primary difficulty with ascending grafts is if they are kinked, leaving a short segment of parallel graft or when they are so short and/or distant from the the innominate origin that the stent graft cannot reach the surgical graft when appropriately positioned adjacent to the arch vessels.
- The distal landing zone can be more flexible than the proximal. A grossly aneurysmal descending thoracic aorta will not provide seal, but separate surgical management of the distal aorta can be carried distal to the arch device.

Branched Arch Device

- There are two configurations for arch TEVAR devices: branches and fenestrations.
- A branched device utilizes a manufactured gate or cuff built into the main body of the device. The branching stent then has a 15 to 20 mm length of graft-to-graft interface with the main aortic stent graft, providing a stable and secure connection.
- Fenestrations are simply holes in the graft which can be manufactured with sewn reinforcement, or created using a technique of in situ fenestration with laser perforation and balloon dilation of a hole in the graft.
- There are two problems with the use of fenestrations in the aortic arch.
  - First, fenestrations must be located exactly to align with the target vessel, as malalignment will result in "shuttering" and failure of branch stent placement or excessive torquing on the interface between the branching stent and the aortic stent. Fenestrations for renal targets work well as there is usually a high degree of device rotational control in the abdominal aorta. That rotational control is gone when the device reaches the arch, so trying to align targets in the arch can require multiple attempts to withdraw and advance the device to rotate it in the more distal aorta. These manipulations are a risk factor for stroke and often are ineffective.
  - Secondly, fenestrations provide a very short length of interface between the branching stent and the main body, and as such, they provide a less stable interface. In the setting of in situ fenestration in particular, the repeated movement of the aorta during the cardiac cycle puts a significant stress on the device-to-device interface which likely cause tears in the TEVAR device with uncertain medium- to long-term durability.
- Given these limitations, all commercial arch devices under development in the United States use variations of a branched construct. Branched devices accommodate imperfect rotational alignment and create robust and durable interface between the aortic stent and the bridging stent.

Cervical Revascularization

- Cervical revascularization has been done using a myriad of surgical strategies.
- Our approach is to do a right common carotid to left common carotid bypass with 8-mm Dacron graft in a retropharyngeal tunnel with a concomitant left common carotid to left subclavian end-to-end transposition (**FIGURE 8**).
  - The patient is placed supine with a shoulder roll and their head at the very top of the OR table. The endotracheal tube and associated monitors are taken over the patient's nose/forehead and padded carefully.
  - On the left, a curved supraclavicular incision is taken from the midline for about 10 to 12 cm. Subplatysmal flaps are elevated. The heads of the sternocleidomastoid muscle are separated. The omohyoid is divided. The carotid sheath is then incised longitudinally. Care must be taken to watch for the vagus nerve which sits anterior in the carotid sheath in about 10% of cases. The vein and nerve are retracted laterally and the carotid artery medially. Lymphatic tissues are ligated with silk ligatures, carrying the dissection down to the medial border of the anterior scalene muscle, best identified by palpation as a firm/full structure in the midlateral base of the wound. The entire operation should be done lateral to the strap muscles. It can be difficult to palpate the subclavian artery, as the arch pulsation is transmitted throughout the wound, so I find that following the medial border of the anterior scalene is the best landmark to follow. The left vertebral vein will usually be the last structure to sit on the LSA, again this is ligated with silk ties. Generous use of silk ties is recommended to avoid lymph leak from what may be smaller lymphatic tributaries. The dissection is then taken down on the LSA to ensure exposure proximal to the vertebral ostium.
  - On the right, a 6-cm symmetrical incision is made centered over the anterior border of the sternocleidomastoid muscle, leaving a 1 to 2 cm of intact skin just right of midline of the neck. A similar dissection is performed, but it is necessary to control just a few centimeters of the right common carotid artery (CCA) so a far more limited dissection is required.
  - Once both dissections are complete, the retropharyngeal tunnel is created. To do so, create a small incision on the investing fascia overlying the anterior aspect of the cervical vertebrae. Use finger dissection from both sides, pushing hard against the anterior spinal ligament, to move across the retropharyngeal space. This tunnel is only 2 to 3 cm in length. During this dissection, it is imperative to stay as posterior as possible. One cannot damage the anterior spinal ligament with finger dissection, but you can injury the esophagus/pharynx if the dissection deviates anteriorly.
  - An 8-mm rifampin-soaked nonreinforced Dacron graft is then passed through the tunnel. Heparin is administered. The right CCA is then clamped and the proximal anastomosis created in an end-to-side fashion to the posteromedial aspect of the vessel. Once this is flushed/back-bled, flow is restored to the right CCA and the graft is clamped in the right neck.
  - The distal anastomosis is then created to the mid-left CCA in a symmetrical fashion.
  - Once this is complete, the LSA is ligated proximal to the origin of the left vertebral artery.
  - The LCCA is similarly ligated at the base of the wound.
  - The LCCA and LSA vessels are then anastomosed in an end-to-end fashion.
- This approach definitively deals with the proximal LCCA and LSA and avoids any risk of a stump syndrome. This reconstruction keeps the length of the bypass short and provides a clean and definitive reconstruction.
- This reconstruction is not suitable for a patient with a prior CABG and a left internal mammary artery (LIMA) bypass. In that case, the graft is taken end to side from the right CCA to end to side to the LSA and the LCCA is reimplanted end to side to the graft with ligation of the proximal LCCA. The proximal LSA is then coil embolized after the cervical revascularization is complete (**FIGURE 8**).
- A spectrum of approaches have been used for cervical revascularization, each with advantages and disadvantages.
  - Some surgeons use a ministernotomy and do the bypass in the anterior mediastinum. This minimizes the risk of

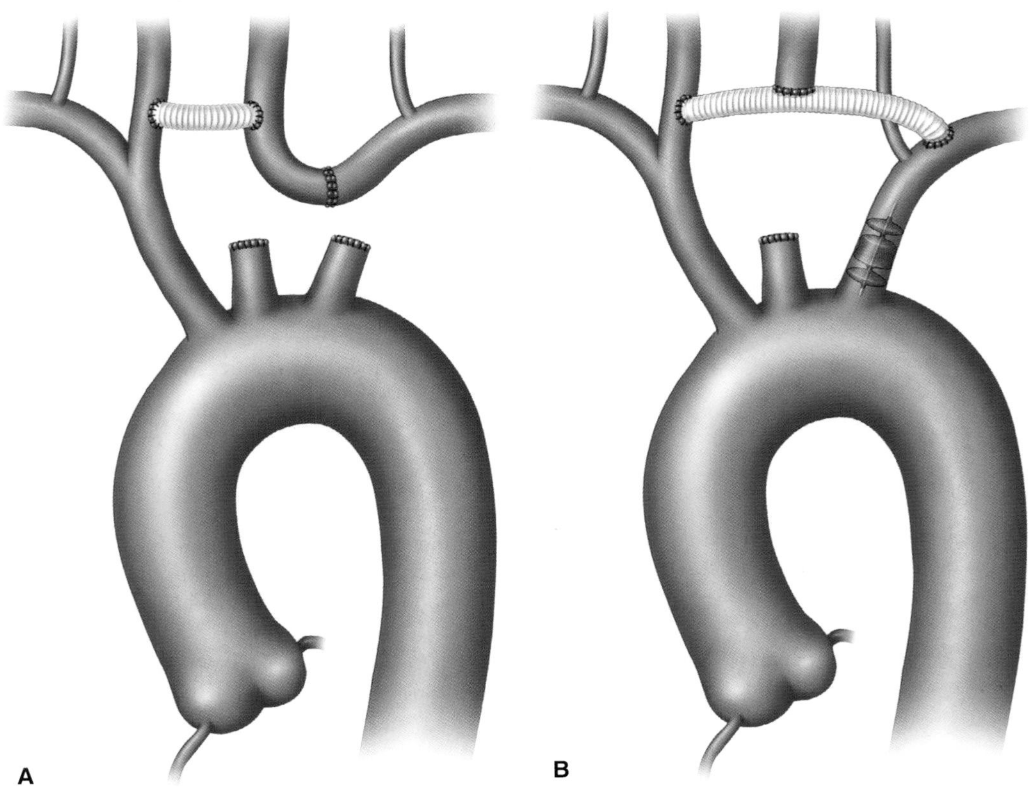

FIGURE 8 ● **A,** Right to left carotid-carotid bypass with left carotid-subclavian transposition. The carotid-carotid bypass with a retropharyngeal tunnel minimizes the length of prosthetic graft and definitively deals with the left carotid and subclavian stumps. This does require a deeper neck dissection on the left to control the proximal subclavian and is not appropriate for patients with prior LIMA bypass. **B,** Right carotid to left subclavian bypass with reimplantation of the left carotid. This approach allows for *continued* flow in the LIMA, so is appropriate for patients with a prior CABG and patent LIMA graft. This operation also avoids deep exposure of the left neck but requires endovascular occlusion of the left subclavian ostium during the endovascular portion of the operation.

cranial nerve injury and creates a "near-anatomical" reconstruction, but one primary advantage of endovascular repair is to avoid sternotomy altogether, and this approach is unnecessarily invasive.

- Axillary to axillary collar bypass is a preferred approach by some centers in Japan. This is advocated as it has no risk of cranial nerve injury. Long subcutaneous extra-anatomic bypasses, however, have increased risk of thrombosis and infection in other anatomic locations. There are no data to inform that risk in this setting, but these are potentially catastrophic disadvantages to this approach.
- The retropharyngeal bypass has the advantages of a very short prosthetic bypass that is well protected from the surface within healthy vascularized tissue. Although some authors have expressed concern about dysphagia from a retropharyngeal bypass, this does not happen with nonreinforced Dacron, which will simply ovalize to fit the space. There are anecdotal reports of ringed PTFE used in the retropharyngeal space causing postoperative dysphagia which can be seriously problematic, although other surgeons have advocated for use of this bypass material.

CHALLENGES TO ENDOVASCULAR REPAIR

Stroke

- Stroke remains the greatest concern for total endovascular repair of the arch. Clinical trials have strict inclusion/exclusion criteria and may not reflect the "real-world" risk of this devastating complication. Factors of greatest concern include arch atheroma, diseased arch vessels, aorta-iliac tortuosity, and patients with prior stroke. There is no effective way to mitigate the stroke risk from atheroma at this time. Good case planning should minimize the device manipulation in the arch, but severe tortuosity can be troublesome. In that situation, using a 65-cm DrySeal Sheath (WL Gore) to try to straighten out the iliac and distal aortic tortuosity can help. Generous device flushing, including CO_2 flushing, will also reduce the number of MRI detected cerebral ischemic events.[7]

Aortic Valve

- An AVR is a major difficulty. A bioprosthetic valve can be more difficult to obtain wire access across. A mechanical AVR is essentially a strong contraindication as wire/catheter manipulation in the ascending/root can damage the valve with immediate unfixable aortic insufficiency.

Coronary Arteries

- Current first-generation arch branched endografts are designed to land in the distal 30% to 60% of the ascending aorta. In some cases, such as a patient with prior CABG or a prior short ascending interposition graft, the arch graft may extend in close proximity to a coronary ostium. In this case, it is helpful to consult with interventional cardiology and consider prewiring the coronaries.

Spinal Cord Injury

- Spinal cord injury due to coverage of thoracic intercostal arteries occurs in 2% to 3% of patients requiring treatment of the arch. The incidence rises with increased coverage of the descending thoracic aorta. Prevention is directed at maintaining higher systemic perfusion pressure and treatment uses the same plus lumbar drains to relieve pressure on the injured cord.

PEARLS AND PITFALLS

Endovascular repair

- A written step-by-step operative plan should be shared with team members ahead of the operation. This case plan facilitates each step by outlining the needed devices/wires/catheters/balloons and gantry views. This keeps the surgeon on track without distraction/skipping any steps, serves to remind the team of concerning aspects of the case, and helps the OR team prepare for each step in advance.
- Review the case plan with each operator knowing their role ahead of time. As deployment often requires several operators, it's essential that all team members are coordinated and understand the deployment sequence and their responsibilities during the case.
- Minimize wire/catheter/device manipulation in the arch. Accept "good enough" alignment of the device with the arch vessel rather than worry about "perfect" alignment.
- Cross the aortic valve with an atraumatic floppy wire and exchange for a dedicated intraventricular wire used for transcatheter AVR (eg, Safari wire).
- The device nosecone will often cross the aortic valve, which can cause temporary aortic insufficiency; therefore, the deployment process needs to occur smoothly and expeditiously. Communication with the anesthesia team is essential.
- Generous flushing of all devices/catheters to remove air is critical. Consider CO_2 flushing.
- Post-deployment trans-esophageal echocardiogram (TEE) can help ensure that the ascending aorta and aortic valve are functioning properly.
- Keep track of the length of time the large sheaths are in the femoral arteries. If the case proceeds slowly, these sheaths can be occlusive and cause pelvic and/or limb ischemia with devastating complications.

POSTOPERATIVE CARE

The care of open patients is beyond the scope of this chapter. A contemporary aortic center of excellence will have a dedicated cardiovascular intensive care unit experienced in the care of patients with both open and endovascular repair. Established protocols for neurologic monitoring for stroke and postoperative spinal cord injury in the setting of more extensive aortic coverage should be used to avoid variation in practice.

SUMMARY

- Five steps to proper arch aneurysm repair:
  1. Proper patient selection
  2. Proper case planning, device sizing, and team preparation
  3. Proper technical conduct of the operation
  4. Proper postoperative care, with the ability to recognize complications and "rescue" patients when complications occur
  5. Proper long-term follow-up surveillance and reintervention
- Attention is often focused on step 3, but successful patient treatment requires each of these steps.

REFERENCES

1. Shalhub S, Rah JY, Campbell R, Sweet MP, Quiroga E, Starnes BW. Characterization of syndromic, nonsyndromic familial, and sporadic type B aortic dissection. *J Vasc Surg*. 2021;73:1906-1914.
2. Rockwood K, Song X, MacKnight C, et al. A global clinical measure of fitness and frailty in elderly people. *CMAJ*. 2005;173:489-495.
3. Desai ND, Hoedt A, Wang G, et al. Simplifying aortic arch surgery: open zone 2 arch with single branched thoracic endovascular aortic repair completion. *Ann Cardiothorac Surg*. 2018;7:351-356.
4. Leshnower BG, Rangaraju S, Allen JW, Stringer AY, Gleason TG, Chen EP. Deep hypothermia with retrograde cerebral perfusion versus moderate hypothermia with antegrade cerebral perfusion for arch surgery. *Ann Thorac Surg*. 2019;107(4):1104-1110.
5. Morasch MD. Technique for subclavian to carotid transposition, tips, and tricks. *J Vasc Surg*. 2009;49:251-254.
6. Bosse C, Kolbel T, Mougin J, Kratzberg J, Fabre D, Haulon S. Off-the-shelf multibranched endograft for total endovascular repair of the aortic arch. *J Vasc Surg*. 2020;72:80-811.
7. Charbonneau P, Kolbel T, Rohlffs F, et al. On behalf of STEP collaborators. Silent brain infarction after endovascular arch procedures: preliminary results from the STEP registry. *Eur J Vasc Endovasc Surg*. 2021;61:239-245.

Chapter 2

Extrathoracic Revascularization (Carotid–Carotid, Carotid–Subclavian Bypass and Transposition)

Kyle B. Reynolds, Edward Y. Woo, and Steven D. Abramowitz

DEFINITION

- Extrathoracic revascularization of the proximal great vessels, including carotid–subclavian and carotid–carotid bypass, is characterized by arterial bypass outside of the chest cavity. Initially described for treatment of cerebrovascular and upper extremity occlusive disease, these procedures are also now employed to create a proximal seal zone for the endovascular treatment of thoracic aortic disease by "debranching" the aortic arch.
- Carotid–subclavian bypass is accomplished by creating a conduit between the mid-common carotid artery and the ipsilateral subclavian artery.
- Subclavian artery transposition divides the subclavian artery proximal to the vertebral artery origin and transposes the vessel onto the ipsilateral common carotid artery. It is an alternative means to revascularize the subclavian artery without the use of prosthetic conduit.[1]
- Carotid–carotid bypass provides flow from one common carotid artery to the contralateral common carotid artery.
- Carotid–carotid bypass performed in a right-to-left manner and in conjunction with carotid–subclavian bypass preserves the blood flow to the left brain while allowing for proximal extension of a thoracic endovascular aortic repair (TEVAR) to the distal margin of the innominate artery.

PATIENT HISTORY AND PHYSICAL FINDINGS

- The patient history should be focused on the identification of underlying cerebrovascular disease. A focused review of systems seeks to identify the presence of symptomatic cerebrovascular lesions. The medical history should be reviewed for prior head, neck or carotid surgery, as well as an external beam radiation to the head, neck, or upper chest region. A history of coronary revascularization, specifically with the use of the left internal mammary artery as the inflow, should also be identified due to the impact surgical revascularization may have on coronary flow.
- The physical examination should be focused on the detection of inflow segment atherosclerotic disease. Bilateral upper extremity blood pressures should be obtained; a difference of greater than 15 mm Hg indicates the potential presence of preexisting occlusive disease. Likewise, the presence of carotid bruits, delayed carotid upstrokes, or abnormal upper extremity pulses suggests arterial occlusive disease that should be delineated prior to extrathoracic reconstruction.
- Special attention should be directed toward a baseline examination of the cranial nerves and vocal cord function, particularly in patients with prior cervical surgical procedures. Indirect laryngoscopy should be performed preoperatively in patients with hoarseness or in whom a preexisting vocal cord or cranial nerve deficit had been noted.
- Neck mobility and the presence of cervical spinal disease should be assessed, as neck extension and rotation are required for adequate operative exposure. Patients with significant neck immobility may be poorly suited for these procedures.

IMAGING AND OTHER DIAGNOSTIC STUDIES

- Carotid duplex scanning should be used to identify carotid artery stenosis prior to bypass procedures. Failure to identify and address stenoses at the carotid bifurcation may lead to postoperative steal phenomenon resulting in neurologic sequelae. Manipulation of a diseased carotid artery may also increase the risk of intraoperative stroke. In these circumstances, concomitant or staged carotid intervention may be warranted.
- Computed tomographic (CT) angiography of the aortic arch and extracranial carotid arteries provides the anatomic detail necessary to plan for safe carotid–subclavian bypass, subclavian artery transposition, or carotid–carotid bypass. This study is complementary to duplex scanning, as it provides an anatomic, rather than hemodynamic, assessment of the vessels. For example, CT is helpful in visualizing the distortion caused by a large arch aneurysm to the course of the subclavian artery in relationship to the clavicle. This also allows for the preoperative identification of any aberrant anatomy.

SURGICAL MANAGEMENT

Preoperative Planning

- Neuromonitoring is a useful adjunct to ensure adequacy of cerebral perfusion via contralateral cerebral circulation via collaterals while the ipsilateral common carotid artery is clamped. Numerous modalities exist for neuromonitoring, such as electroencephalography, transcranial Doppler, cerebral oximetry, and somatosensory evoked potentials. Stump pressure measurement has also been shown to be effective in predicting adequate cerebral blood flow. A temporary shunt may be routinely placed prophylactically to maintain ipsilateral blood flow or selectively placed when monitoring indicates cerebral perfusion is inadequate after clamping. Inadequate collateral flow is infrequently encountered, as during these procedures only the common carotid is occluded allowing for retrograde flow from the external carotid artery.
- Invasive continuous arterial pressure monitoring should be routinely employed, with care to place the line relative to

the laterality of the procedure. Typically, the arterial line is placed in the contralateral limb or in a femoral artery.

Positioning

- The patient is positioned supine with the head rotated away from the operative side. A roll or pneumatic pillow is placed below the shoulders to allow for neck extension. Careful attention must be paid to achieve maximum neck extension while still supporting the occiput. The bed may be placed in a semi-Fowler position (supine with back of bed up at 30°) to reduce venous pressure and minimize bleeding.
- For carotid–carotid bypass, the head is positioned midline to facilitate bilateral dissection.

TECHNIQUES

CAROTID–SUBCLAVIAN BYPASS

Exposure of the Subclavian Artery

- An incision is made from the lateral aspect of the clavicular head of the sternocleidomastoid (SCM) muscle laterally across the supraclavicular fossa. This is further developed through the subcutaneous tissue and platysma with electrocautery. If the external jugular vein is encountered, it should be ligated and divided.
- The clavicular head of the SCM may be divided to allow for adequate medial exposure. Up to one-half of the sternal head of the SCM may be divided if needed, but this is rarely necessary. The scalene fat pad is visualized and divided. It is preferable to divide and dissect the fat pad near its inferior and medial border so that most of the fat pad can be preserved and reclosed to cover the reconstruction. Care must be taken to identify and preserve the phrenic nerve as it courses over the anterior scalene muscle deep to the fat pad. The thoracic duct is easily identified. It should be ligated in the field of dissection to prevent significant morbidity from a postoperative lymphatic leak that can occur if unintentional injury occurs during dissection or retraction.
- Once the fat pad has been mobilized and the phrenic nerve identified and protected, the anterior scalene muscle is divided to reveal the subclavian artery (**FIGURE 1**). It is best to divide the muscle slowly and in layers to prevent injury to the underlying vessel. The subclavian artery is dissected circumferentially and controlled with vessel loops. Care must be taken when manipulating this vessel, as the subclavian artery is significantly more fragile and prone to injury than lower extremity arteries of comparable diameter (eg, femoral or popliteal). Depending on the method of reconstruction and location of the planned anastomosis, the thyrocervical trunk, inferior mammary, and vertebral arteries may need to be individually controlled (**FIGURE 2**).

Exposure of Carotid Artery

- In the medial aspect of the wound, the lateral border of the internal jugular vein is identified and dissected. The vein is then retracted posteriorly, and the carotid sheath is entered from the posterolateral margin. Care must be taken to identify the vagus nerve, as its usual posterior position places it immediately in the field of dissection as the sheath is opened from this approach.

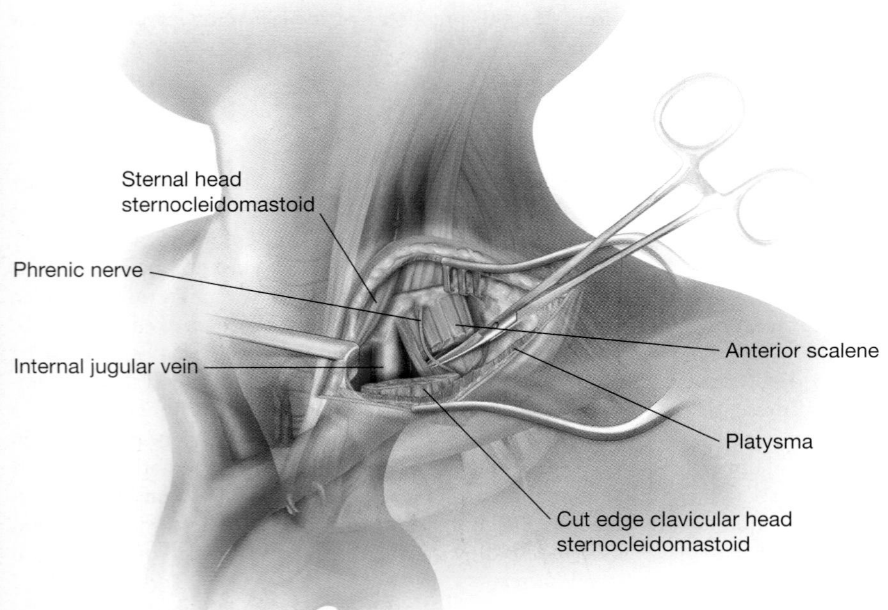

FIGURE 1 • The skin incision is placed in the supraclavicular fossa over the clavicular head of the sternocleidomastoid muscle. The subclavian artery lies directly beneath the anterior scalene muscle. Care must be taken to identify and preserve the phrenic nerve when dividing the anterior scalene muscle.

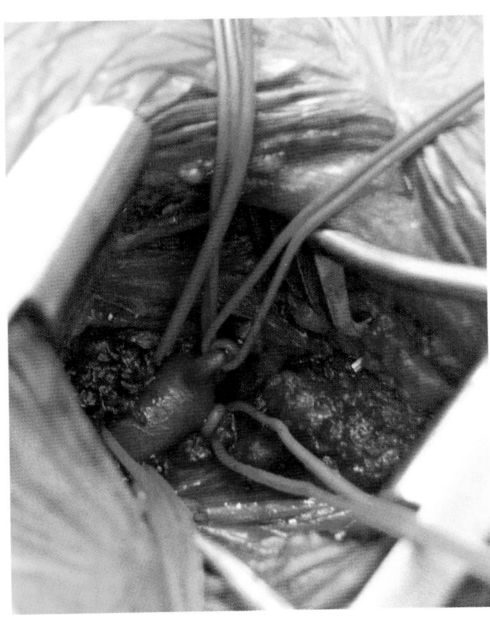

FIGURE 2 ● The subclavian artery and its branches are circumferentially dissected and controlled with vessel loops.

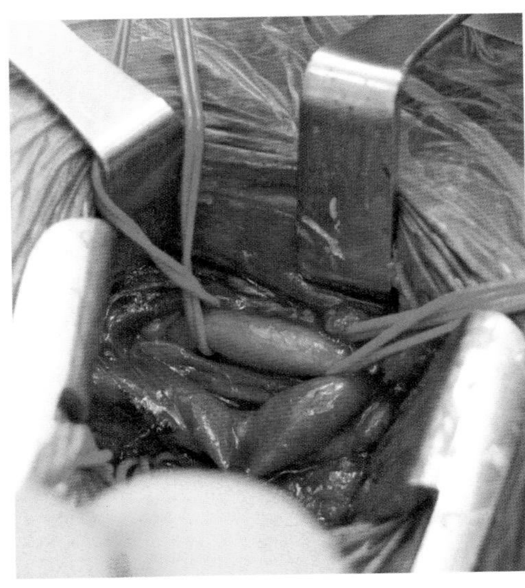

FIGURE 3 ● The carotid artery is dissected circumferentially after entering the carotid sheath from its posterior lateral margin. The internal jugular vein can be seen retracted out of the way. The vagus nerve is running parallel to the artery between it and the nerve.

- The common carotid artery is dissected circumferentially (**FIGURE 3**). Only 5 cm of artery needs to be isolated to allow for surgical control and to perform the anastomosis. The dissection should remain proximal to the carotid bulb, thus minimizing the risk of cerebral embolization and injury to more distal nerves.

Bypass

- Dacron or polytetrafluoroethylene (PTFE) grafts can be used as conduits for extrathoracic bypass with no difference in outcomes such as patency or infection.[2] Autogenous vein grafts should be avoided, however, as their long-term patency is inferior to prosthetic in this location.[3]
- Prior to arterial clamping, systemic anticoagulation is achieved with intravenous heparin administration. The activated clotting time should be monitored and additional heparin administered throughout the procedure to maintain adequate anticoagulation.
- The subclavian anastomosis is performed first. Arterial control (vessel loops or clamps) is obtained and the vessel is opened with a longitudinal arteriotomy. The anastomosis should be fashioned in the position most favorable to the anatomic course of the planned graft. The graft is beveled and trimmed so that the graft lies at an approximately 60° angle to the artery. A running Prolene suture is used to perform the anastomosis with completion of the back wall first. Once the anastomosis is complete, the graft is clamped, and flow restored to the arm after flushing the inflow and outflow segments through the graft to remove any potential embolic debris. The graft should also be flushed with heparinized saline and clamped near the anastomosis to avoid thrombosis within the stagnant blood column contained within the graft. If repairs are needed for hemostasis, control is restored and pledgeted sutures are used to avoid injury to the fragile artery.
- The graft is tunneled in a retrojugular fashion. It is then tailored to the appropriate length to prevent redundancy and kinking. If beveling, the heel of the anastomosis should lie proximally on the carotid artery. As the common carotid artery is clamped, special attention should be paid to the patients' mean arterial pressure or systolic blood pressure as well as to any neuromonitoring being used. Shunt placement would be performed during this stage of the procedure. A longitudinal arteriotomy is performed and the proximal anastomosis completed with running Prolene suture, again starting with the back wall (**FIGURES 4** and **5**).
- The final sequence of clamp removal is important to prevent embolism to the brain. Proximal subclavian artery control is again obtained, and the clamp is removed from the graft. The proximal carotid clamp is then removed to allow "flushing" down the arm rather than to the brain. After a few cardiac cycles, the distal carotid clamp is also removed. The proximal subclavian artery clamp is then released.
- When performed in anticipation of thoracic aortic stent grafting, the subclavian artery must be ligated proximal to the origin of the vertebral artery. This can involve dissection deep into the mediastinum, which may be associated with significant morbidity and potentially catastrophic bleeding. Alternatively, the proximal subclavian artery can be occluded via placement of an intra-arterial occlusion device (eg, Amplatzer plug), by endovascular access to the carotid–subclavian bypass or after subsequent stent graft placement via a left radial or brachial artery percutaneous approach.[4]

Closure

- If a pneumatic pillow was used to provide exposure, it is deflated prior to wound closure in order to reduce neck extension and assist in closing the incision without tension from extension.

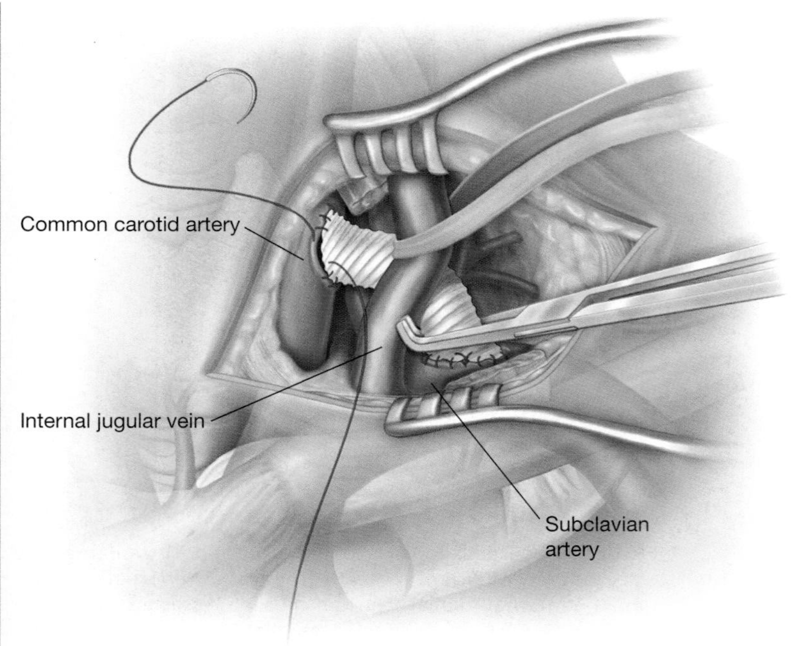

FIGURE 4 ● After completing the distal anastomosis, the graft and the subclavian artery are all controlled and the proximal anastomosis is performed in a running fashion. The graft can be tunneled superficial or deep to the internal jugular vein depending on patient anatomy and surgeon preference.

- A closed suction drain may be left in the deep wound and brought out through a separate stab incision, depending on surgeon preference.
- In order to provide coverage for the graft, the scalene fat pad is returned to its anatomic location and sutured in place. The SCM is reapproximated with running absorbable sutures.
- The platysma and subcutaneous tissues are closed in separate layers in a running fashion and the skin is reapproximated with a running dermal suture.

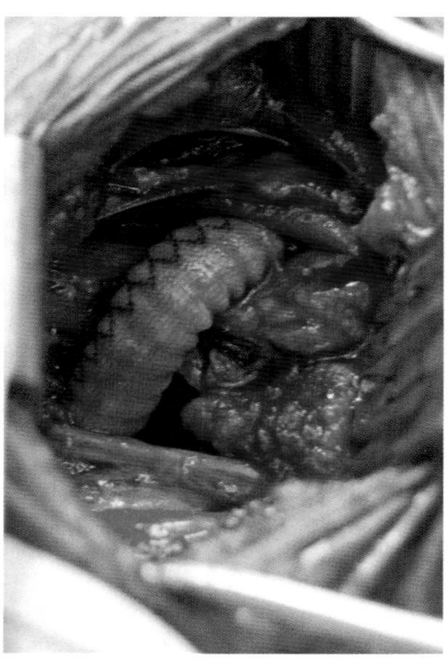

FIGURE 5 ● The completed bypass graft can course anterior or posterior to the internal jugular vein. The phrenic nerve is seen in the lower field.

SUBCLAVIAN ARTERY TRANSPOSITION

Exposure

- The subclavian artery is exposed as previously described. The dissection must be carried proximal to the vertebral artery and enough artery must be exposed proximally to allow sufficient length for the anastomosis as well as control of the proximal stump. This can be difficult as an aortic aneurysm can occupy a significant portion of the mediastinum limiting vessel manipulation.
- The carotid artery is exposed in the same manner as described in the previous section.

Division of the Subclavian Artery

- Systemic heparin is administered, and maximum arterial length is obtained by advancing a Cooley clamp as deeply as possible into the mediastinum along the subclavian artery. A distal atraumatic clamp is then applied, typically in the mid-subclavian artery, with the more proximal branches individually controlled with vessel loops. There must be adequate distance between the proximal clamp and the vertebral artery to allow for proximal control, transposition, and anastomosis. Prior to transection, stay sutures, such as pledgeted 5-0 Prolene sutures, are placed on each side of the proximal artery to ensure that if clamp control is lost for any reason, the open, bleeding artery does not retract into the mediastinum (**FIGURE 6**).

- The proximal subclavian artery is then oversewn. Hemostasis is confirmed by slowly releasing clamp control while maintaining traction on the stay sutures. Once hemostasis is ensured, the stay sutures are divided, and the proximal subclavian artery is allowed to retract into the mediastinum.

Carotid–Subclavian Anastomosis

- The subclavian artery, having been freed circumferentially, is then mobilized toward the carotid artery. It may be tunneled either anterior or posterior to the internal jugular vein depending on the length of the mobilized artery. The carotid artery is then clamped proximally and distally and the anastomosis performed in the standard running fashion. Prior control of the subclavian artery is maintained (**FIGURE 7**). As the anastomosis is completed, the unclamping sequence should be repeated as described in the preceding section to prevent inadvertent air or particulate embolization to the brain.

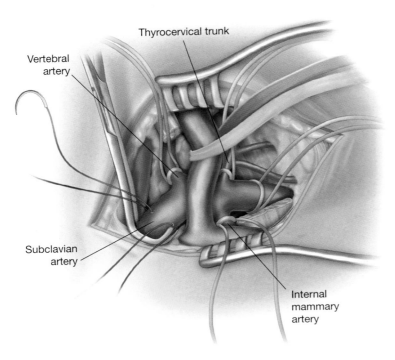

FIGURE 6 ● The subclavian artery and its branches are controlled individually with vessel loops and clamps. A Cooley clamp is used proximally on the subclavian artery. Stay sutures of 5-0 Prolene are placed in both ends of the subclavian artery proximal to the transection line.

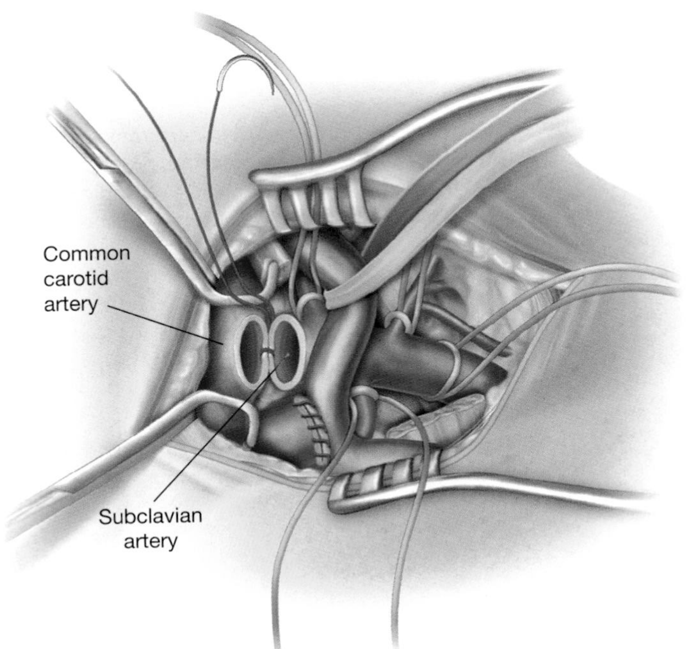

FIGURE 7 ● The subclavian artery is mobilized so that it may reach to the carotid artery and the end-to-side anastomosis is performed in the standard running fashion, starting along the back wall. The thyrocervical trunk may be divided if necessary to facilitate mobilization.

Closure

- As described in the section on carotid–subclavian bypass, the wound is closed in multiple layers. A closed suction drain may also be used.

CAROTID–CAROTID BYPASS

Exposure of the Bilateral Carotid Arteries

- Incisions are made over the anterior border of the SCM at the base of the neck bilaterally. The subcutaneous tissues and platysma are then divided and the anterior border of the SCM identified.
- The SCM is mobilized laterally by carrying the dissection down toward the internal jugular vein; this exposes the carotid sheath. Any bridging veins encountered can be divided. Dissection should not extend above the level of the facial vein, as this marks the carotid bifurcation. This limits the risk of injury to adjacent structures and stroke when exposing or manipulating the carotid bifurcation. To obtain sufficient proximal exposure, the omohyoid muscle may need to be divided bilaterally.
- The carotid sheath is entered sharply on its anterior surface. The vagus nerve must be identified within the carotid sheath and protected as the common carotid artery is exposed and controlled.

Graft Tunneling and Anastomosis

- Once the bilateral common carotid arteries are sufficiently exposed and controlled, the appropriate graft tunnel can be created. Tunneling is achieved via blunt finger dissection from both sides of the neck to avoid injuries to these critical structures. The graft may be tunneled either between the trachea and esophagus or behind the esophagus, depending on surgeon preference (**FIGURE 8**). We preferentially create a retroesophageal tunnel, dissecting just anterior to the prevertebral fascia. Placement of an orogastric or nasogastric tube prior to creation of the dissection plane can be helpful for identifying the esophagus.
- Once the tunnel has been developed, the graft is passed and patient systemically anticoagulated with intravenous heparin administration.
- The anastomoses are performed in the standard running fashion; either one may be performed first. Careful attention must be paid to neuromonitoring as the carotid artery is clamped.
- Once the first anastomosis is complete, the graft is clamped and carotid artery flow restored on that side. Prior to removing the distal carotid artery clamp, the distal artery can be back-bled and the proximal artery flushed out the open graft. As with the subclavian artery, the graft should be flushed with heparinized saline and clamped close to the anastomosis to avoid a long stagnant column of blood within the prosthetic graft.

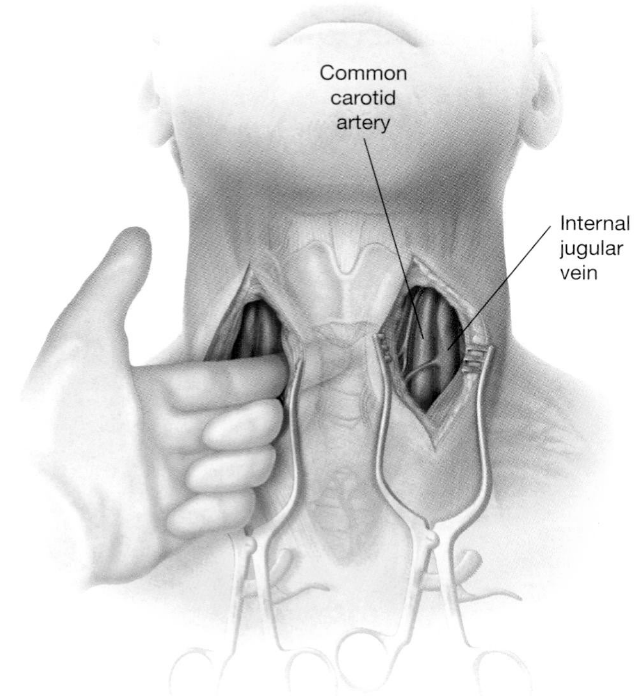

FIGURE 8 ● After isolating both common carotid arteries, a retropharyngeal tunnel is fashioned using blunt finger dissection. The placement of a nasogastric or orogastric tube allows for easy identification and protection of the esophagus.

- The contralateral anastomosis is then performed in the same fashion (**FIGURE 9**). The graft should be flushed with heparinized saline and the graft, proximal carotid artery, and distal carotid artery should be vigorously flushed prior to completion.

Closure

- Hemostasis is obtained. The neck wounds are closed in layers, first taking care to reapproximate the SCM in its anatomic position with interrupted absorbable sutures.
- A closed suction drain may be left in each surgical bed.
- The platysma and subcutaneous tissues are closed with running absorbable sutures and the skin reapproximated with a running deep dermal suture.

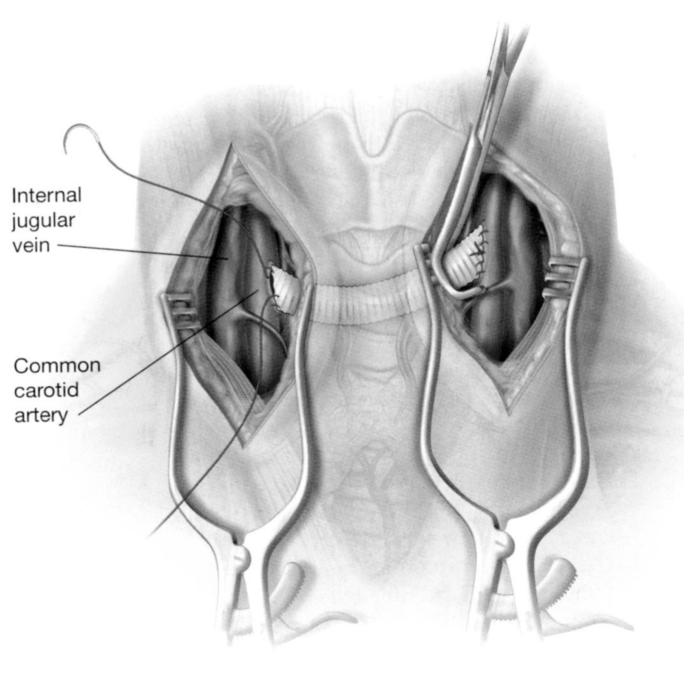

FIGURE 9 • The distal anastomosis is performed in the standard running fashion starting with the back wall. Prior to completing the anastomosis, the carotid arteries and graft should be back-bled and flushed with heparinized saline.

PEARLS AND PITFALLS

Positioning	■ When inflating the pneumatic pillow or placing a shoulder roll, care must be taken to ensure that the occiput is adequately supported. Failure to adequately support the head may result in cervical spine and neurologic injuries.
Thoracic duct	■ Great care must be taken to avoid injuring the thoracic duct when exposing the subclavian artery. All lymphatic tissue encountered should be ligated before being divided as the ensuing lymphatic leak can be quite troublesome for the patient and the surgeon.
Subclavian artery control	■ The subclavian artery can be controlled either with vessel loops or with atraumatic vascular clamps, depending on which helps to better deliver the artery into the wound without undue tension.
Subclavian artery anastomosis	■ In comparison to other peripheral arteries, the subclavian artery is fragile and exceedingly friable, requiring careful handling. Bleeding may best be controlled with pledgeted sutures.
Tunneling	■ The prosthetic graft in a carotid-to-carotid bypass is typically retrojugular. Tunneling in a carotid-to-subclavian bypass is typically posterior to the internal jugular.
Proximal subclavian control during transposition	■ The use of stay sutures on the proximal subclavian artery in subclavian artery transposition is crucial. Once the stay suture on the proximal end of the artery is released, the artery may retract deep into the mediastinum. Uncontrolled bleeding may lead to fatal complications. As such, the proximal oversewn subclavian artery must be hemostatic prior to release of the stay sutures.
Common carotid artery exposure	■ It is neither necessary nor advisable to expose or manipulate the carotid bifurcation in performing these bypasses unless a concomitant CEA is necessary, or the bifurcation is situated unusually low in the neck. These procedures are performed on the common carotid artery, and exposing the bifurcation only increases the risk of cranial nerve injury and stroke.
Closure	■ The pneumatic pillow should be deflated prior to closure to assist in bringing the tissue together without tension.

POSTOPERATIVE CARE

- Careful attention should be paid to both systolic and mean arterial blood pressure in the postoperative period. Invasive arterial monitoring is usually maintained for the first 24 hours. When carotid–subclavian bypass or subclavian artery transposition is performed, blood pressure should be monitored in the contralateral arm.
- Neurologic status and distal pulses should be followed closely in the postoperative period. Any pulse changes need to be rigorously investigated as they may indicate the presence of either graft occlusion or distal embolization.
- When carotid–subclavian bypass is performed as a debranching procedure prior to thoracic aortic stent grafting and the proximal subclavian artery is not ligated, the timing of the endovascular procedure is important. In these patients who tend not to have concomitant occlusive disease, there is competitive flow via the native circulation, putting the newly placed graft at risk of thrombosis. In the absence of complications or other mitigating circumstances, the endovascular aortic procedure should be performed within 3 to 5 days of the debranching bypass.
- Patients should be placed on aspirin therapy and followed at regular intervals with duplex ultrasonography.

OUTCOMES

- A review of the American College of Surgeons National Surgical Quality Improvement Program (ACS-NSQIP) database from 2005 to 2010 demonstrates that extrathoracic revascularization carries a 3.5% risk of stroke and 3.3% risk of death in the immediate perioperative period.[5] Over this time period, 918 procedures were performed, with 10% of them as part of a staged approach to thoracic aortic stent grafting.
- A recent review focusing on outcomes of carotid–subclavian bypass performed in the setting of TEVAR from 2005 to 2016 showed a primary patency of 97% at 5 years.[6]
- Carotid–subclavian bypass has excellent durability. In a series of 284 consecutive patients, Takach and colleagues[2] reported 5-, 10-, and 15-year primary patency rates of 94%, 88%, and 86%, respectively. These results have subsequently been replicated by other large, multiple-decade series.[7] Subclavian artery transposition has similarly outstanding long-term patency, with rates as high as 99% reported at 5 years.[7,8]
- Symptom-free survival following revascularization is likewise excellent, with long-term results approaching 88% to 99% at 5 years.[7,8]

COMPLICATIONS

- The thoracic duct lies at the medial aspect of the field of dissection when dissecting in the supraclavicular fossa. This can be easily injured and remain undetected during the course of the operation. Continued or milky drainage is a clear sign of duct injury. The oral administration of cream can be used to promote chyle flow, and if a leak is present, it will promptly increase drain output. When this occurs, a closed suction drain should be left in place, the patient kept fasting, and parenteral nutrition instituted. With conservative management, some of these injuries may close without further intervention. The complete management of this complication is beyond the scope of this text; however, it should be mentioned that re-exploration of the wound in the early period is relatively straightforward and may represent the best way to resolve the problem. Late re-exploration can be fraught with difficulty finding the leak as the tissue becomes fixed. A muscle flap may then be needed to close the space. The main concern with a persistent leak is the potential for graft infection. Unfortunately, early wound re-exploration significantly increases the risk of prosthetic graft infection.
- The vagus, phrenic, and recurrent laryngeal nerves, as well as the brachial plexus, can all be injured as a result of carotid and subclavian artery exposure. Most injuries are due to traction rather than transection, and conservative therapy will generally resolve symptoms over the course of months to a year. In the case of a staged bilateral subclavian revascularization, it is important to ensure that any vagus or phrenic nerve injury has resolved prior to contralateral intervention, as bilateral injuries can lead to tracheal obstruction and acute respiratory failure.
- Although uncommon, significant bleeding from the wound should mandate immediate re-exploration. More commonly, minor wound hematomas may develop that can be observed. Judgment regarding the need for re-exploration of a neck hematoma is similar to that required during any other neck procedure.
- Infection of the wound can be devastating if prosthetic is involved. Local cellulitis should be treated aggressively with early institution of antibiotics in order to prevent deeper infection. Upon removal of the drain, it is important that the drain site does not continue to leak, as continued leakage may act as an entry point for bacterial contamination. Simple suture closure should resolve this. Prosthetic graft infection necessitates graft removal, which is extremely difficult and beyond the scope of this chapter.
- Although uncommon, stroke is a complication of any carotid procedure. Taking the precautions outlined previously in this chapter should minimize these risks.

REFERENCES

1. Morasch MD. Technique for subclavian to carotid transposition, tips, and tricks. *J Vasc Surg*. 2009;49(1):251-254.
2. Takach TJ, Duncan JM, Livesay JJ, et al. Contemporary relevancy of carotid-subclavian bypass defined by an experience spanning five decades. *Ann Vasc Surg*. 2011;25(7):895-901.
3. Ziomek S, Quiñones-Baldrich WJ, Busuttil RW, et al. The superiority of synthetic arterial grafts over autologous veins in carotid-subclavian bypass. *J Vasc Surg*. 1986;3(1):140-145.
4. Woo EY, Bavaria JE, Pochettino A, et al. Techniques for preserving vertebral artery perfusion during thoracic aortic stent grafting requiring aortic arch landing. *Vasc Endovasc Surg*. 2006;40(5):367-373.
5. Madenci AL, Ozaki CK, Belkin M, et al. Carotid-subclavian bypass and subclavian-carotid transposition in the thoracic endovascular aortic repair era. *J Vasc Surg*. 2013;57(5):1275-1282.
6. Voigt SL, Bishawi M, Ranney D, et al. Outcomes of carotid-subclavian bypass performed in the setting of thoracic endovascular aortic repair. *J Vasc Surg*. 2019;69(3):701-709.
7. Cinà CS, Safar HA, Laganà A, et al. Subclavian carotid transposition and bypass grafting: consecutive cohort study and systematic review. *J Vasc Surg*. 2002;35(3):422-429.
8. Berguer R, Morasch MD, Kline RA, et al. Cervical reconstruction of the supra-aortic trunks: a 16-year experience. *J Vasc Surg*. 1999;29(2):239-246; discussion 246-248.

Chapter 3

Carotid Surgery: Interposition/ Endarterectomy (Including Eversion)/Ligation

Peter DeVito Jr. and Wei Zhou

DEFINITION

- Annually, approximatively 795,000 people experience a new or a recurrent stroke.[1]
- In 2019, stroke was the 5th leading cause of death, accounting for 37 out of 100,000 deaths.[2]
- Pivotal studies have shown the efficacy of carotid endarterectomy (CEA) for stroke prevention in both symptomatic and asymptomatic patients with internal carotid artery (ICA) stenosis vs medical therapy alone.[3,4]
- More recently, there are questions regarding the benefit of intervention on asymptomatic patients primarily due to changes in more modern medical management. However, studies still demonstrate a benefit of intervention in low-risk patients with the high grade stenosis.[5,6]
- CEA is defined as the surgical excision of atherosclerotic lesions of the intima and tunica media of the carotid artery.
- On rare occasions, ICA ligation and/or interposition bypass may be indicated for stroke prevention.

PATIENT HISTORY AND PHYSICAL FINDINGS

- In the United States, most CEA procedures are performed on asymptomatic patients. Symptoms of cerebroembolic disease originating from the carotid bifurcation, when present, may include dysarthria, dysphasia, aphasia, hemiparesis, hemisensory deficit, or amaurosis fugax. Symptoms that resolve within 24 hours are defined as transient ischemic attacks regardless of severity; symptoms that persist past the first day constitute a stroke.
- For patients at risk for cerebroembolic disease, a thorough vascular history is obtained including modifiable risk factors such as smoking, hyperlipidemia, hypertension, and diabetes management. Prior to surgery, antiplatelet therapy is initiated and continued indefinitely following intervention. Blood pressure control at or below 140 mm Hg systolic and 90 mm Hg diastolic is the single most important medical intervention to reduce stroke risk.[7] Sufficient β-blockade to stabilize resting heart rate at 60 to 80 bpm is also instituted prior to surgery to limit perioperative myocardial oxygen demand unless contraindicated.[8]
- Cervical auscultation is performed in both the supraclavicular and mandibular regions. Bruits appreciated at the mandibular angle usually indicate ICA or bifurcation disease. More proximal bruits may indicate common carotid artery (CCA) disease or radiating heart sounds.
- A full neurologic assessment including mental status, speech, facial symmetry, and extremity strength must be obtained and documented prior to surgery.

IMAGING AND OTHER DIAGNOSTIC STUDIES

- All patients exhibiting symptoms of carotid territory ischemia need appropriate vascular imaging studies. Screening is not recommended to detect asymptomatic disease in the general population; patients with atherosclerotic risk factors (age > 65, coronary artery disease, peripheral occlusive disease, tobacco use, hypercholesterolemia)[9] or those with a bruit on physical examination should be evaluated when clinical circumstances warrant.
- Carotid duplex ultrasound provides a reliable and accurate noninvasive tool to identify predicted stenosis and is the initial diagnostic study of choice. Peak systolic velocity (PSV) higher than 125 cm per second predicts angiographic stenosis more than 50% and higher than 230 cm per second predicts more than 70% stenosis. However, a combination of PSV, end diastolic velocity, and the PSV ratio of ICA to CCA is more accurate in estimating significant carotid stenosis. In general, end diastolic velocity higher than 100 cm per second correlates to more than 80% carotid stenosis.
- When duplex imaging is not definitive, as is the case in the setting of extensive carotid bifurcation calcification, additional cross-sectional imaging (computed tomography angiography or magnetic resonance angiography) may be necessary to quantify the degree of stenosis. When accurate velocity information is obtainable, duplex imaging provides the most accurate and physiologically relevant estimates of percent diameter reduction.

SURGICAL MANAGEMENT

Indications

Endarterectomy

- The Society for Vascular Surgery recommends that neurologically symptomatic patients with greater than 50% stenosis or asymptomatic patients with greater than 70% stenosis should be offered CEA to reduce risk of recurrent or initial stroke, respectively.[9]
- Surgical endarterectomy is the procedure of choice for good-risk surgical patients with normal cervical anatomy.[9] For selected high-risk patients, such as those with a tracheal stoma, previously radiated neck, prior cranial nerve injury, or for lesions proximal to the clavicle or distal to the C2 vertebral body endovascular interventions can be considered.[9] These include transcatheter angioplasty and stenting, generally from a transfemoral approach, and TCAR (transcarotid artery revascularization), placement of a stent via open exposure of the proximal CCA.
- Indications and technical guidelines for carotid angioplasty/stenting and TCAR procedures are covered in Part 6, Chapter 4.

Carotid Artery Interposition Bypass

- Reconstruction for extensive bifurcation disease, injury to the bifurcation during endarterectomy, or aggressive restenosis following previous intervention (endarterectomy or stent placement) is best accomplished by carotid resection and interposition grafting. Other indications include the following:
  - Significant diffuse CCA and ICA disease
  - Radiation-induced stenosis or other forms of arteritis involving long arterial segments
  - Aneurysms (degenerative or traumatic) and invasive carotid body tumors.

Ligation

- Ligation and resection of the proximal ICA may be indicated in the setting of carotid stump syndrome, when persistent distal embolization from the "cul-de-sac" of the occluded ICA into the external carotid artery (ECA) circulation and ultimately into the cerebral circulation via reversed flow in the ophthalmic artery.

Preoperative Planning

- Similar overall outcomes are achieved with general anesthesia or regional anesthesia.
- The use of a shunt during CEA is dependent on operator preference. Most surgeons either shunt selectively or use a shunt for all cases. Surgeons should develop the methods they feel most comfortable with to optimize outcome. Objective measures used in selective shunting include stump pressure measurement, electroencephalographic monitoring, and transcranial Doppler assessment. Data supporting use of these adjuvants are inconsistent, and strategy used should be based on surgeon comfort and local expertise.
- Optimal neck extension is obtained by placing a towel or gel roll behind the scapula. The head is rotated contralateral to the operative side. In patients with limited neck movement or prior cervical fusions, it is critical to carefully pad and support the neck to prevent hyperextension injury. The chin, angle of the mandible, lower earlobe, and sternal angle are prepped and preliminarily draped within the operative field. The bed itself can be flexed with the head in relative extension to aid in positioning (**FIGURE 1**).
- Arterial blood pressure monitoring is necessary for optimal anesthetic management. If endarterectomy is performed with regional anesthesia, an audible squeeze device is placed in the patient's contralateral hand for indirect neurologic monitoring. Preoperative antibiotics are administered routinely.
- Aspirin therapy is initiated well in advance of surgery and continued throughout the perioperative period. Evidence suggests that statin therapy initiated preoperatively reduces postoperative neurologic events and mortality.[10]

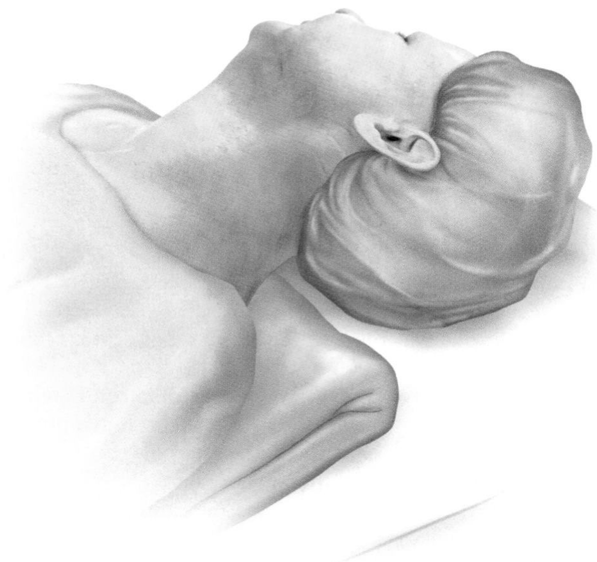

FIGURE 1 ● Recommended patient position for a carotid endarterectomy procedure.

CAROTID ENDARTERECTOMY—PATCH ANGIOPLASTY

Incision

- The skin incision is optimally placed along the anterior border of the sternocleidomastoid muscle. This should be curved posterolaterally near the angle of the mandible to avoid dissection into the parotid gland.
- Alternatively, a more transverse incision can be made at the level of the carotid bifurcation. Although providing an improved cosmetic result, exposure of the distal ICA may be compromised with this approach (**FIGURE 2**).

Carotid Exposure and Control

- As the incision is extended through the platysma muscle, the anterior border of the sternocleidomastoid muscle is visualized and retracted posterolaterally. The greater auricular nerve should be identified and protected at the superior extent of the incision.
- Following fascial incision, the facial vein is identified and securely ligated. This vein usually transverses the CCA near the bifurcation. Failure to adequately secure this vein may lead to bleeding and airway compromise during postoperative cough spells or Valsalva maneuvers.
- Within the carotid sheath, the vagus nerve usually extends posterior to, and parallel with, the artery and vein. However, this position relative to the other contents of the carotid sheath may vary, and the vagus should always be identified and protected in the course of the dissection. An anterior vagus nerve can be found in as many as 5% of patients.[11] The ansa cervicalis nerve is commonly much smaller than the vagus and runs anterior to the carotid bifurcation. When completely isolated, the proximal ansa arises from the ipsilateral hypoglossal (XII) cranial nerve. The ansa cervicalis can be divided to improve exposure if

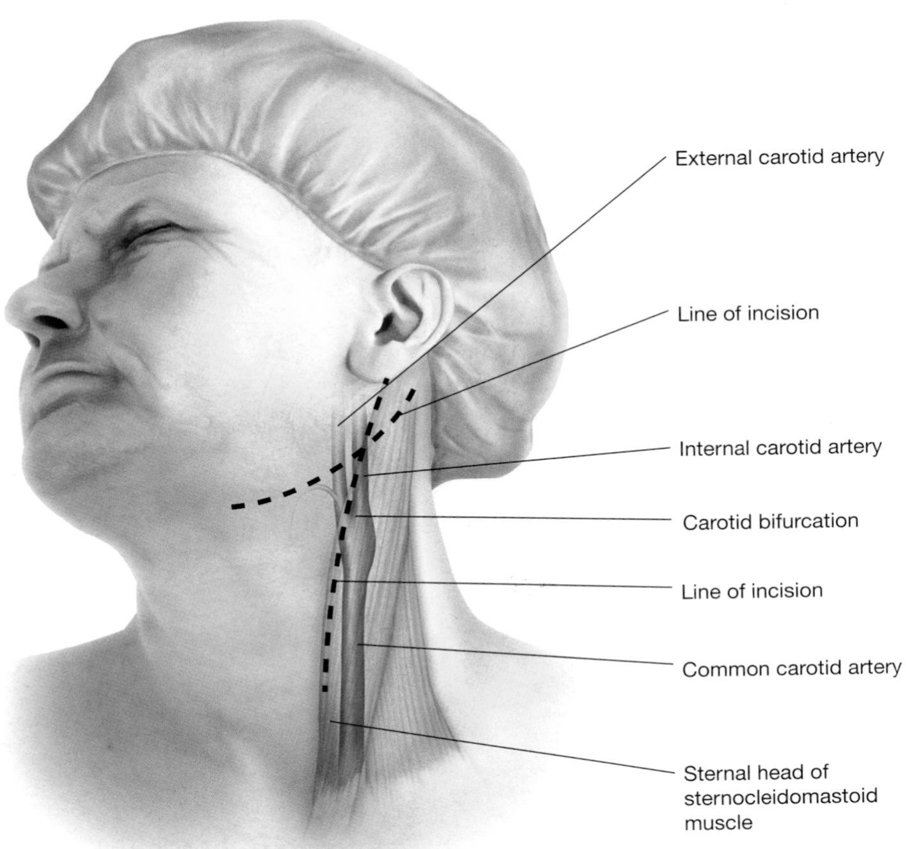

FIGURE 2 ● The incision along the anterior border of sternocleidomastoid muscle is the most commonly used incision for a carotid endarterectomy procedure. A transverse incision along a skin crease in the vicinity of the carotid bifurcation is an alternative incision for a better cosmetic result.

necessary or mobilized sufficiently to be gently retracted out of the operative field.

- The CCA is circumferentially dissected from surrounding structures in sufficient length to provide adequate exposure for proximal clamping and control. Passing silastic loops around the CCA can provide temporary control if needed.
- Following common carotid exposure, the dissection is extended cranially and posteriorly along the posterolateral border of the ICA. Development of the dissection plane posterolaterally along the proximal ICA minimizes the risk of hypoglossal nerve injury. This dissection is also performed with minimal displacement and instrumentation of the ICA to reduce intraoperative embolization risk (**FIGURE 3**).
- To complete the necessary exposure, the ECA is dissected and mobilized to at least the level of the superior thyroidal artery. The superior laryngeal nerve may also be encountered posterior to the carotid bifurcation in this area.
- Following dissection, and prior to clamp placement, sufficient unfractionated heparin is administered intravenously to obtain an activated clotting time of more than 200 seconds. With normal circulation times, this is usually accomplished within 2 or 3 minutes of injection.
- Clamping of ICA is performed first, followed by clamping of the external and common carotid arteries. This sequence is followed to minimize embolization risk associated with clamping. When necessary, measurement of ICA stump pressure is obtained at this juncture by cannulation of the carotid bifurcation and selective removal of the internal carotid clamp. The CCA is optimally ultimately controlled by placement of an appropriately sized, atraumatic vascular clamp such as a Gregory profunda clamp, engaged to the minimal force necessary for control.

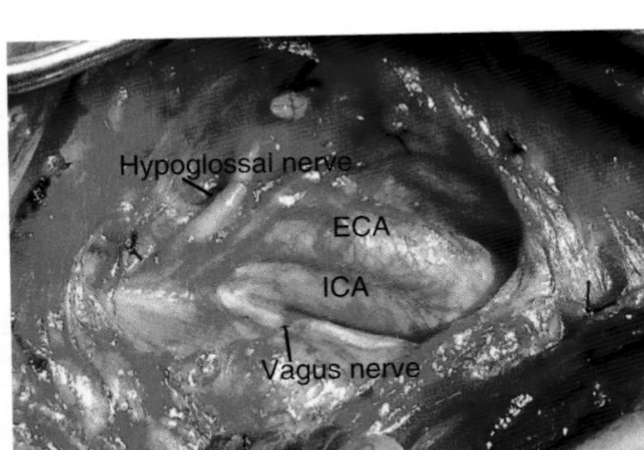

FIGURE 3 ● Exposure of carotid bifurcation. Vagus nerve and hypoglossal nerve are the most commonly encountered nerves during carotid dissection. ECA, external carotid artery; ICA, internal carotid artery.

Conventional Endarterectomy

- The arteriotomy is initiated in a soft, uninvolved proximal segment of the CCA and extended cephalad with Potts scissors. It should be positioned on the anterior-lateral surface of the ICA to avoid the flow divider (**FIGURE 4A**).

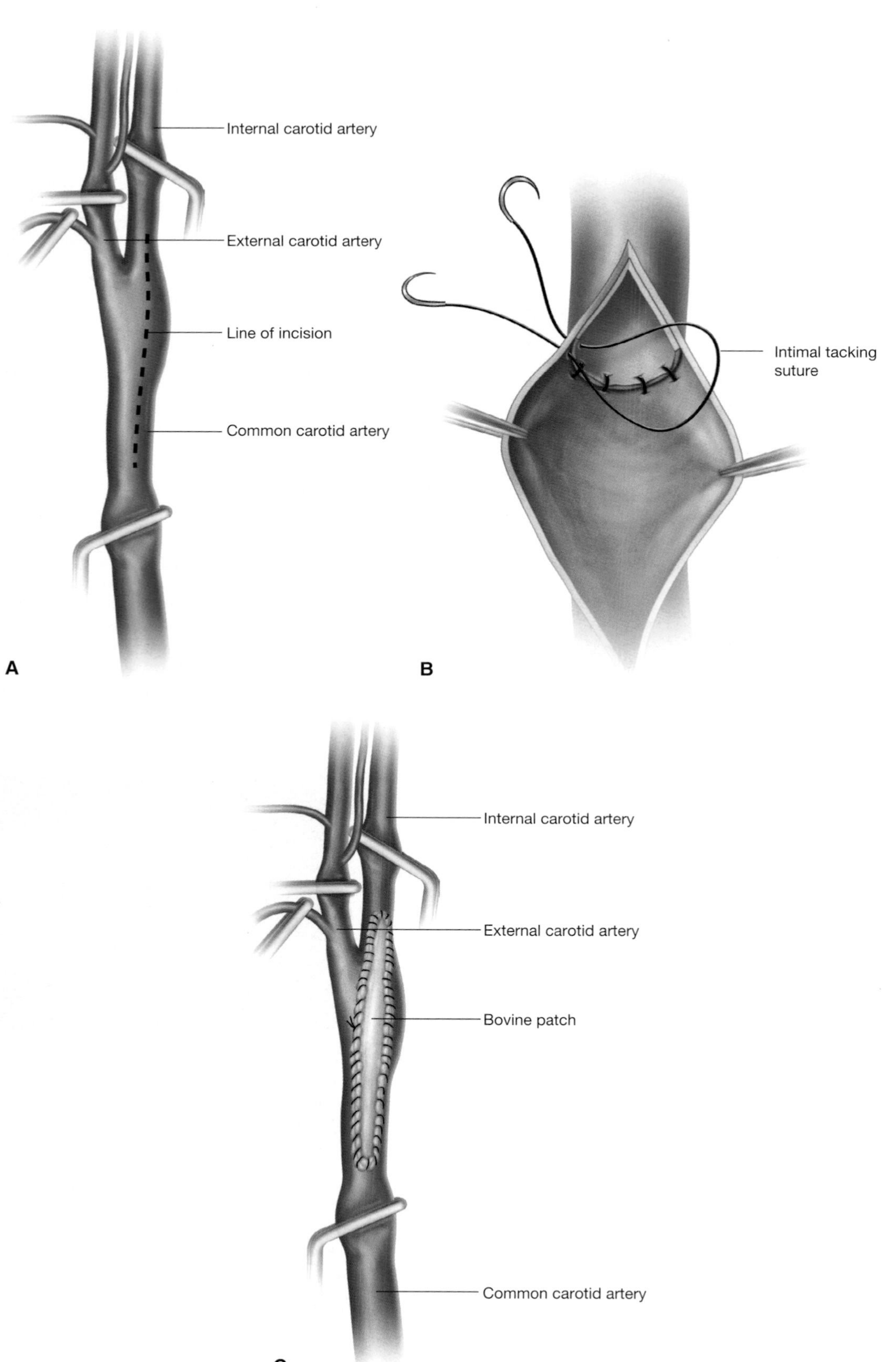

FIGURE 4 • Arteriotomy is extended from the anterior surface of common carotid artery to the anterior surface of internal carotid artery distal to the lesion **(A)**. Intimal flap is tacked down to ensure smooth distal endpoint **(B)**. Arteriotomy is closed with a patch **(C)**.

- When an indwelling shunt is used, the distal tapered end is carefully inserted into the ICA under direct vision. There are multiple shunts available for the purpose including Sundt, Javid, Argyle, Pruitt-Inahara, Brener, and Furui. Each is utilized primarily based on operator preference and familiarity.
- We prefer the Pruitt-Inahara shunt, which has pilot balloons at both ends to maintain shunt position and hemostasis. Once the distal end is inserted, the distal balloon is inflated with less than 1 mL of air until the "pop-off" balloon inflates on the pilot tube. Familiarity with this shunt prior to insertion is essential; if the inflation override cuff covers the "pop-off" balloon on the pilot tube, overinflation may injure or rupture the distal ICA. Following distal ICA cannulation and balloon inflation, the shunt is back-bled to confirm luminal placement and decant air. With the shunt actively back-bleeding, the proximal end is inserted into the CCA followed by proximal clamp removal into the unobstructed lumen. The proximal pilot tube is inflated with the provided syringe until the cuff is palpable in the CCA, after which a prepositioned Rumel tourniquet is gently cinched around the artery. When performed quickly, with concurrent digital control of the CCA following clamp removal and prior to shunt insertion, minimal bleeding ensues. When saline is applied to the shunt tubing, pulsatile flow is appreciable with handheld Doppler insonation.
- At the site of maximal atherosclerotic disease in the CCA, a Penfield dissector or Freer elevator is employed to identify and develop the appropriate endarterectomy plane within the medial layer. When the correct plane is identified, the plaque is easily and rapidly elevated from the underlying adventitia. In areas containing intraplaque hemorrhage, inflammation may increase adherence of the plaque to the adventitia, and care should be taken not to extend the dissection plane into the adventitia itself.
- At the distal extent of the plaque, sufficient exposure should be present to create a defined endpoint, allowing placement of tacking sutures if necessary, ensuring that no further potentially mobile plaque remains. It is essential to "feather" the plaque at the distal endpoint to minimize risk for distal dissection or thrombus accumulation. If the plaque extends past the point where feathering is feasible, a distal endpoint should be determined and created sharply with scissors or a no. 15 blade (**FIGURE 4B**). Tacking sutures, placed circumferentially, can control distal plaque at the transection site. Care should be taken to place the minimal number of sutures necessary to prevent dissection or consider extending the arteriotomy and endarterectomy to identify a more suitable termination site. Successful suture placement requires circumferential dissection and optimal visualization.
- Once the distal endpoint is determined, residual plaque is removed from the ECA by eversion into the CCA and circumferential dissection and traction. Sufficient back-bleeding is performed to remove any luminal debris within the ECA.
- Direct visualization of the endarterectomy bed following plaque removal commonly identifies loosely attached residual medial elements. These are best removed with fine forceps under magnification. Complete removal is facilitated by continuous irrigation to identify mobile medial elements. Integrity of the distal and proximal endpoints is also verified using this technique.

Patch Placement

- An appropriately sized bovine pericardial or prosthetic patch is selected and trimmed as necessary for closure-assisted angioplasty. Both bovine pericardial and prosthetic patches have chirality considerations; one surface is preferred for luminal apposition. Please consult the accompanying instructions for use prior to implantation.
- An autogenous vein patch can be utilized in select cases concerning for infection or in repeat operation with concerns regarding thrombogenicity of the patch.
- Closure is secured with running 6-0 polypropylene suture initiated at the cephalad extent of the arteriotomy and continued proximally along the long axis of the patch.
- After 90% or more of the circumference of the patch is secured, flushing is accomplished by sequential clamp removal and luminal irrigation with heparinized saline. Closure is then completed prior to restoration of flow.
- The declamping sequence is of critical importance. The CCA is released first, followed by the ECA clamp. After several cardiac cycles have ensued, the distal ICA is released (**FIGURE 4C**).
- It is essential to perform a completion assessment prior to closure. We perform intraoperative completion duplex imaging of the endarterectomy site as well as the proximal and distal carotid arteries, with purpose-designed, miniaturized 7 MHz probes. Completion duplex scanning is quick, efficient, highly reproducible, and effective at identifying significant residual luminal defects.[12] Detailed description of the characteristics of significant luminal defects identified by completion ultrasonography is beyond the scope of this chapter. Alternatively, intraoperative insonation can be performed; however, it is not possible through extruded polytetrafluoroethylene (ePTFE) patches. Furthermore, a completion angiogram can also be considered.

Closure

- Following adequate duplex imaging and endpoint determination, anticoagulation may be reversed with protamine sulfate. Some practitioners are reluctant to reverse anticoagulation due to uncertainty regarding thrombogenicity at the endarterectomy site; however, this is unfounded in literature.[13] In our experience, technical issues at the endarterectomy site are most predictive of postoperative neurologic events, and these are efficiently identified and corrected with completion ultrasonography.
- Following reversal, the entire wound is inspected for venous or arterial bleeding. The entirety of the patch angioplasty suture line is reinspected for periodicity of suture placement and potential leaks. Reinforcing sutures are applied liberally as needed to ensure hemostasis, but with experience and even suture spacing, the need for additional sutures should be rare. Bleeding lymph nodes should be sutured and removed from the operative field. Once hemostasis is achieved, the platysma is reapproximated with running absorbable suture followed by skin closure. We usually also perform a Valsalva maneuver to identify occult venous injuries that may not be apparent with positive pressure ventilation prior to closure.

CAROTID ENDARTERECTOMY—EVERSION ENDARTERECTOMY

- The incision, dissection, and control of the carotid artery for eversion endarterectomy are identical to that for CEA with patch angioplasty.
- Once distal and proximal clamps are placed on the carotid artery, an oblique or circumferential incision is made at the junction of the bulbous portion of the ICA and CCA (**FIGURE 5A**).
- The ICA adventitia is grasped with fine forceps and everted away, as gentle traction is placed on the plaque within the artery. This maneuver is extended distally until the feathered endpoint identifies itself. Tacking sutures are not possible using this approach, which can be a deterrent to adoption by surgeons trained with conventional endarterectomy.
- Common and external carotid plaque is subsequently removed by the Penfield dissector or Freer elevator as indicated. The proximal CCA arteriotomy may be extended as possible to ensure complete removal (**FIGURE 5B**).

Anastomosis

- The ICA is reverted and anastomosed end-to-end to the proximal CCA (**FIGURE 5C**).
- If redundant residual ICA is present following plaque removal, the ICA spatulation is extended, as is the CCA arteriotomy, and the two ends are further advanced over each other prior to closure. Alternatively, a portion of the redundant ICA may also be excised. This can prove ideal in circumstances with a kinked ICA.

Closure

- Completion imaging and closure of the incision is identical to that for standard endarterectomy.

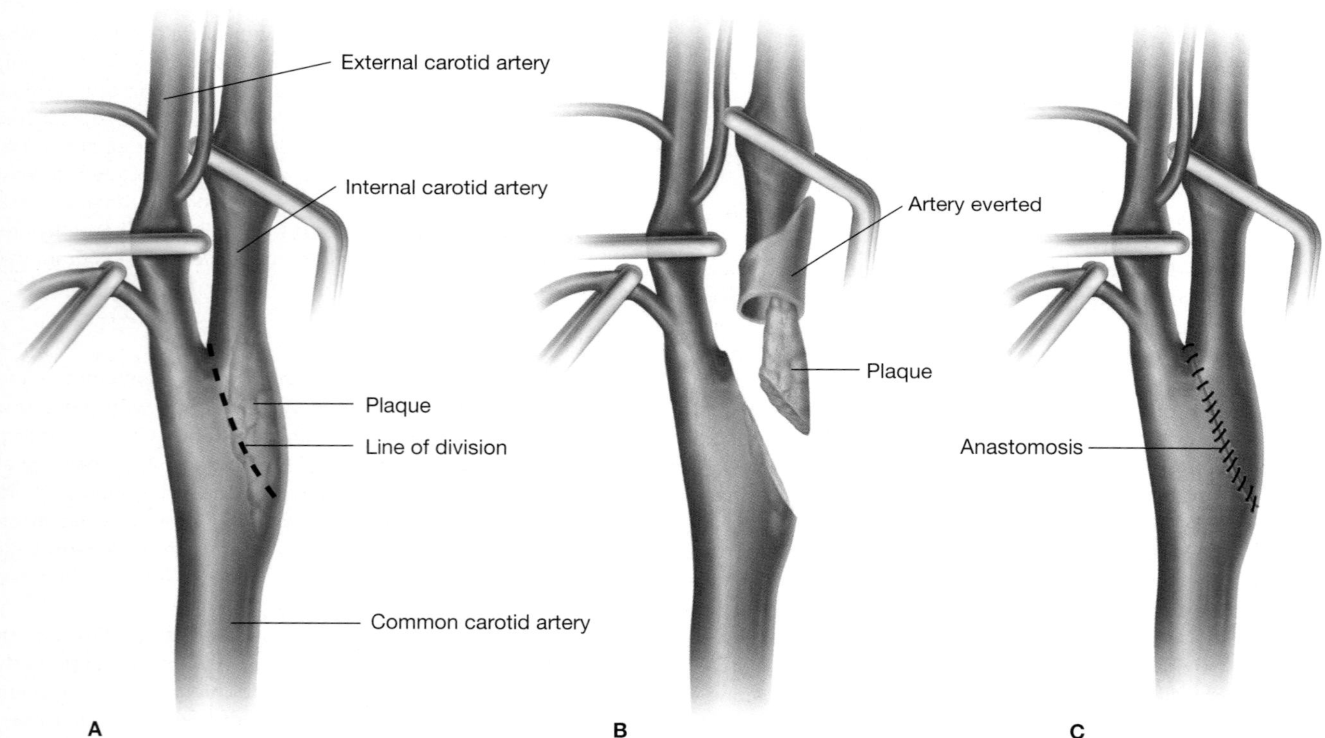

FIGURE 5 ● Carotid eversion endarterectomy. The internal carotid artery (ICA) is divided from the common carotid artery (CCA) in an oblique line **(A)**. The divided ICA is everted on itself until the plaque endpoint is encountered and the plaque is removed from the ICA **(B)**. Following endarterectomy, the ICA is reverted and reattached to the CCA **(C)**.

CAROTID ARTERY INTERPOSITION BYPASS

Incision, Dissection, and Control of the Carotid Artery

- The incision, dissection, and control of the carotid artery are identical for a carotid artery interposition bypass as it is for a CEA.
- Although reversed autogenous vein is the preferred conduit when available, ePTFE provides a suitable alternative when necessary.[14]

Anastomosis

- The diseased segment of the carotid artery is resected. Commonly, the ECA is oversewn as well.
- End-to-end anastomoses are performed in standard fashion. Typically, the proximal anastomosis is completed first. Upon completion, a clamp is placed on the bypass and the CCA clamp is removed to test the integrity of the anastomosis.
- Prior to completion of the distal anastomosis, flushing maneuvers are done to evacuate particular matter or residual air (**FIGURE 6**).
- Completion duplex imaging is suggested for this approach as well.

Closure

- Completion imaging and closure of the incision is identical to that for standard CEA.

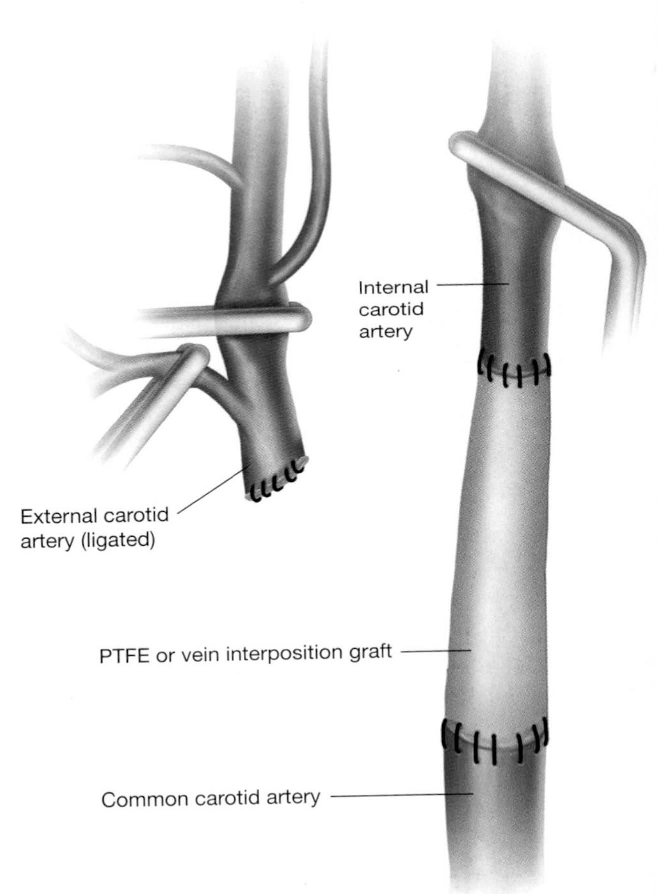

FIGURE 6 ● Carotid interposition graft. Following resection of the diseased segment, a prosthetic graft or a segment of reversed greater saphenous vein is used to bridge the common carotid artery and internal carotid artery in an end-to-end fashion.

CAROTID ARTERY LIGATION (CAROTID STUMP SYNDROME)

Incision, Dissection, and Control of the Carotid Artery

- The incision, dissection, and control of the carotid artery are identical in this procedure as it is for CEA.

Endarterectomy

- The technique is similar to that for standard ICA endarterectomy, the difference being the arteriotomy being carried out on the distal CCA into the ECA (**FIGURE 7A**).
- The thrombosed ICA is resected, ideally in line with the common and external carotid arteriotomies. Closure is accomplished via patch angioplasty (**FIGURE 7B** and **C**).

Closure

- The completion imaging and closure is identical to that for standard endarterectomy.

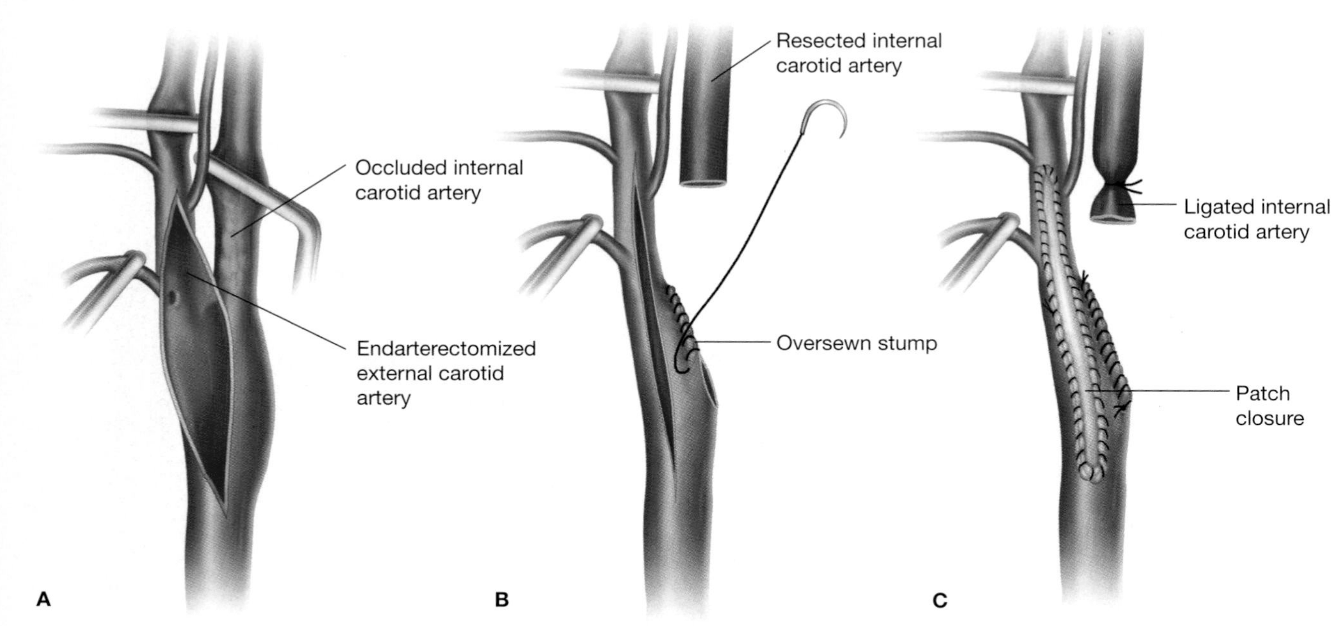

FIGURE 7 ● Carotid ligation. The occluded internal carotid artery (ICA) is amputated and removed **(A)**, and the ICA stump is oversewn **(B)**. The plaque in the common carotid artery and external carotid artery is removed, and the arteriotomy is closed with a patch **(C)**.

PEARLS AND PITFALLS

Incision	■ On-table duplex scanning optimizes incision placement, particularly for transverse exposure to localize the bifurcation.
Identifying the vagus nerve and hypoglossal nerve	■ Vagus nerve is located posterolateral to the carotid artery, within the carotid sheath and between carotid artery and internal jugular vein. Hypoglossal nerve typically crosses ICA anteroinferiorly to posterosuperiorly. Following the ansa cervicalis will lead to the hypoglossal nerve.
Clamping	■ A "robin blue" hue is often seen in the distal ICA, which signifies a soft area for safe clamp placement.
Shunting	■ Be prepared in all cases for potential shunt placement. This should be flushed and prepared on the back table prior to performing the arteriotomy.
Conventional endarterectomy	■ Lavage the arterial lumen with heparinized saline to identify and remove luminal debris.
Eversion endarterectomy	■ Use caution in patients with high bifurcation (difficulty visualizing and securing distal endpoint), those who require a shunt, or those with a small ICA. These procedures are best suited for patients with redundant ICAs.
Interposition bypass	■ Use the anastomotic suture line to tack down distal residual plaque as necessary to prevent antegrade dissection.
Ensuring technical perfection	■ A completion imaging study, an on-table angiogram, a carotid duplex, or doppler insonation, must be performed prior to skin closure.
Closure	■ If a closed suction drain is placed, it should be removed on postoperative day 1.

POSTOPERATIVE CARE

- Patients should be placed on continuous monitoring to assess for blood pressure lability. Patients generally are discharged on postoperative day 1.
- A postoperative duplex should be obtained at initial postoperative visit to assess the reconstruction, provide a new baseline for long-term surveillance, and monitor wound healing and plaque incorporation. Serial ultrasounds should be obtained to identify and manage restenosis, which most commonly occurs in the first 2 years following endarterectomy.

OUTCOMES

- The North American Symptomatic Carotid Endarterectomy Trial (NASCET) demonstrated the 30-day CEA stroke and death rate of 5.5% for symptomatic patients. For symptomatic patients with moderate (50%-69%) stenosis, reduced 5-year stroke rate from 22.2% with BMT (best medical therapy) to 15.7% with BMT and CEA.[3]
- The Asymptomatic Carotid Atherosclerosis Study (ACAS) demonstrated a combined 30-day CEA stroke and death rate of 2.3%. For asymptomatic patients with >60% stenosis, reduced 5-year stroke rate from 11% with BMT to 5.1% with BMT and CEA.[4]
- In 2010, the Carotid Revascularization Endarterectomy vs Stenting Trial (CREST) demonstrated the 30-day stroke, death, or rate of myocardial infarction (MI) to be 5.4% in symptomatic patients and 3.6% in asymptomatic patients, and the 30-day death and stroke rates were found to be 3.2% in symptomatic patients and 1.4% in asymptomatic patients undergoing CEA. In the periprocedural period, there is a lower rate of stroke with CEA vs stenting (2.3% vs 4.1%) but a higher rate of MI (2.3% vs 1.1%). Mortality rates are similar.[15]

COMPLICATIONS

- Cervical hematoma
- Hemodynamic instability
- Cerebral hyperperfusion syndrome manifested by severe headache
- Cranial nerve palsy
- Stroke/MI
- Thrombosis (early)
- Recurrent stenosis (late)

REFERENCES

1. Virani SS, Alonso A, Benjamin EJ, et al. Heart disease and stroke statistics—2020 update: a report from the American Heart Association. *Circulation*. 2020;141(9):e139-e596.
2. Kochanek KD, Xu JQ, Arias E. *Mortality in the United States, 2019. NCHS Data Brief, No 395*. National Center for Health Statistics; 2020.
3. North American Symptomatic Carotid Endarterectomy Trial Collaborators. Beneficial effect of carotid endarterectomy in symptomatic patients with high-grade carotid stenosis. *N Engl J Med*. 1991;325:445-453.
4. Walker MD, Marler JR, Goldstein M. Endarterectomy for asymptomatic carotid artery stenosis. Executive committee for the asymptomatic carotid Atherosclerosis study. *JAMA*. 1995;273:1421-1428.
5. Goessens BMB, Visseren FLJ, Kappelle LJ, Algra A, Van Der Graaf Y. Asymptomatic carotid artery stenosis and the risk of new vascular events in patients with manifest arterial disease: the SMART study. *Stroke*. 2007;38(5):1470-1475. doi:10.1161/STROKEAHA.106.477091
6. Howard DPJ, Gaziano L, Rothwell PM. Risk of stroke in relation to degree of asymptomatic carotid stenosis: a population-based cohort study, systematic review, and meta-analysis. *Lancet Neurol*. 2021;20(3):193-202. doi:10.1016/S1474-4422(20)30484-1
7. Brott TG, Halperin JL, Abbara S, et al. 2011 ASA/ACCF/AHA/AANN/AANS/ACR/ASNR/CNS/SAIP/SCAI/SIR/SNIS/SVM/SVS guideline on the management of patients with extracranial carotid and vertebral artery disease: executive summary. A report of the American college of cardiology foundation/American heart association task force on practice guidelines, and the American stroke association, American association of neuroscience nurses, American association of neurological surgeons, American college of radiology, American society of neuroradiology, congress of neurological surgeons, society of Atherosclerosis imaging and prevention, society for cardiovascular angiography and interventions, society of interventional radiology, society of NeuroInterventional surgery, society for vascular medicine, and society for vascular surgery. *Circulation*. 2011;124(4):489-532.
8. American College of Cardiology Foundation/American Heart Association Task Force on Practice Guidelines, American Society of Echocardiography, American Society of Nuclear Cardiology, et al. 2009 ACCF/AHA focused update on perioperative beta blockade incorporated into the ACC/AHA 2007 guidelines on perioperative cardiovascular evaluation and care for noncardiac surgery. *J Am Coll Cardiol*. 2009;54:e13-e118.
9. AbuRahma AF, Avgerinos ED, Chang RW, et al. Society for vascular surgery clinical practice guidelines for management of extracranial cerebrovascular disease. *J Vasc Surg*. 2021;75(1S):4S-22S.
10. Mcgirt MJ, Perler BA, Brooke BS, et al. 3-Hydroxy-3-methylglutaryl coenzyme A reductase inhibitors reduce the risk of perioperative stroke and mortality after carotid endarterectomy. *J Vasc Surg*. 2005;42:829-835.
11. Kawahara I, Shiozaki E, Soejima K, et al. Unusual course of the vagus nerve passing anterior to the internal carotid artery during carotid endarterectomy. *Surg Neurol Int*. 2021;12:278.
12. Ascher E, Markevich N, Kallakuri S, Schutzer RW, Hingorani AP. Intraoperative carotid artery duplex scanning in a modern series of 650 consecutive primary endarterectomy procedures. *J Vasc Surg*. 2004;39(2):416-420. doi:10.1016/j.jvs.2003.09.019
13. Newhall KA, Saunders EC, Larson RJ. Use of protamine for anticoagulation during Carotid Endarterectomy: a meta-analysis. *J Vasc Surg*. 2016;63(6):1662-1663. doi:10.1016/j.jvs.2016.04.017
14. Dorafshar AH, Reil TD, Ahn SS, et al. Interposition grafts for difficult carotid artery reconstruction: a 17-year experience. *Ann Vasc Surg*. 2008;22(1):63-69.
15. Mantese VA, Timaran CH, Chiu D, et al. The Carotid Revascularization Endarterectomy versus Stenting Trial (CREST): stenting versus carotid endarterectomy for carotid disease. *Stroke*. 2010;41(suppl 10):S31-S34.

Chapter 4

Transcarotid Artery Revascularization (TCAR)

Jeffrey Jim

DEFINITION

- Endovascular treatment of carotid artery stenosis was first described in 1997. Carotid angioplasty and stenting (CAS) is typically done through percutaneous access at the common femoral artery. Transfemoral CAS is considered an alternative to traditional carotid endarterectomy (CEA) due to the less invasive nature of this procedure. However, the available clinical evidence has demonstrated this technique to be associated with an increased rate of perioperative neurologic events.[1] As such, CAS is typically reserved for patients considered to be at high risk for complications during a CEA.
- Transcarotid artery revascularization (TCAR) combines open surgical principles with less invasive endovascular techniques. Direct surgical exposure of the common carotid artery (CCA) allows stent delivery to the carotid bifurcation lesion while neuroprotection is provided by creating a reversal of flow through the internal carotid artery (ICA). This technique was first described in small cases series. In 2015, the publication of the results of the ROADSTER clinical trial using the ENROUTE Transcarotid Neuroprotection System (NPS) demonstrated the clinical efficacy of this technique in successfully treating carotid artery stenosis.[2]

PATIENT HISTORY AND PHYSICAL FINDINGS

- A thorough history should be obtained from the patient prior to any intervention. The presence and duration of lateralizing neurologic symptoms (eg, amaurosis fugax, facial droop, slurred speech, paresthesia/paralysis of any extremity) should be elicited. Any underlying cardiovascular risk factors (eg, hypertension, diabetes, smoking history) should be documented and an evaluation of the patient's current medications (including antiplatelet agents, anticoagulation, and statin therapy) should be recorded. A thorough physical examination should be performed with careful attention to any residual neurologic deficits. The presence of a carotid bruit or heart murmur is noted. The presence of prior surgical scars (especially head and neck) as well as effects of radiation therapy should also be documented.

IMAGING AND OTHER DIAGNOSTIC STUDIES

- The presence of carotid artery stenosis is first evaluated using duplex ultrasonography. This diagnostic study has been shown to be reliable in determining the presence of underlying carotid plaque as well as associated level of stenosis. However, the presence of significant calcification as well as vessel tortuosity may limit reliability.
- Catheter-based diagnostic angiography is considered the "gold standard" in determining carotid artery stenosis. However, this is an invasive procedure with associated risks of periprocedural complications. With continued advance in noninvasive axial imaging, patient evaluation with computed tomographic angiography (CTA) or magnetic resonance angiography (MRA) has largely supplanted the need for catheter angiography. In our practice, a CTA of the head and neck is performed with images starting at the aortic arch at the chest and proceed cranially to include the intracranial circulation. This will allow evaluation of the aortic arch, disease at the carotid bifurcation, as well as the presence of intracranial disease (**FIGURE 1**).

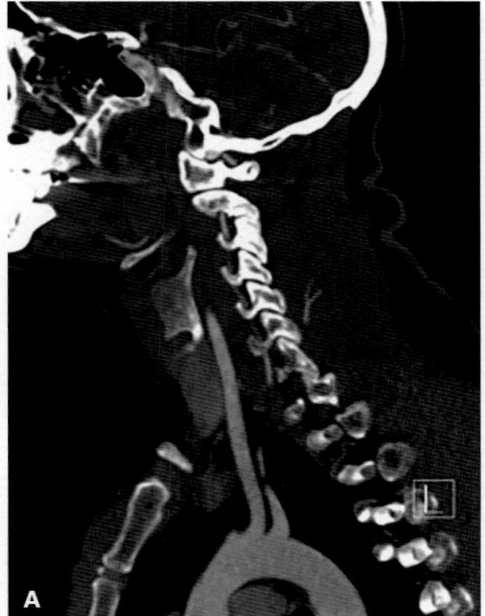

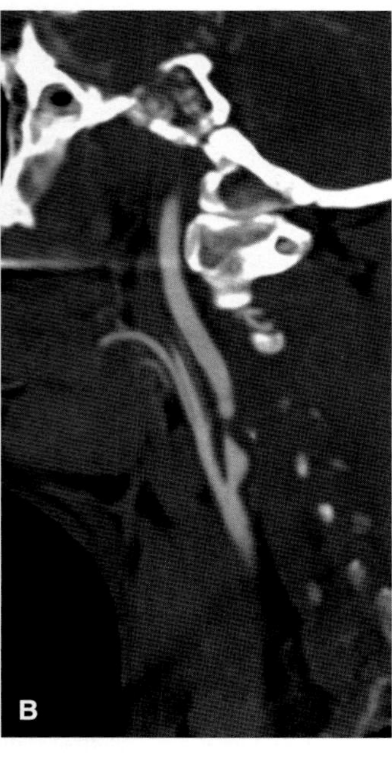

FIGURE 1 • Computed tomographic angiography showing the arterial anatomy. **A,** Sagittal reconstruction demonstrates the aortic arch. **B,** Sagittal reconstruction showing a severe left internal carotid artery stenosis.

SURGICAL MANAGEMENT

- The indication for carotid revascularization depends primarily on the presence of underlying neurologic symptoms as well as the degree of stenosis in the corresponding carotid artery.[3] It is generally accepted that for patients with symptomatic carotid disease, intervention is warranted if the stenosis is between 70% and 99% in severity. Treatment is offered to appropriate patients without prohibitive periprocedural risks. The anticipated periprocedural stroke/death risk must be <6%. The choice to intervene on a patient with severe carotid stenosis without associated neurologic symptoms is less clear. Data from the clinical trials in the 1990s suggest benefit of surgical revascularization in asymptomatic patients with >60% stenosis. However, with advances in medical care (eg, statin medications) and overall decreasing stroke rates in the general population, most physicians typically reserve intervention now for people with much more severe disease. In our practice, we reserve intervention to asymptomatic patients only if they are otherwise healthy with a minimum life expectancy of 3 to 5 years and the presence of a severe >80% stenosis. The anticipated periprocedural stroke/death risk should be well below the recommended 3% standard.

Preoperative Planning

- The instructions for use for TCAR NPS include several anatomic requirements. The patient's anatomy must adhere to three requirements:

1. ≥5 cm distance between arterial access site to the proximal aspect of lesion
2. ≥6 mm CCA diameter
3. CCA free of significant disease (eg, calcification/thrombus) at access site and occlusive site

- While measurements can be obtained through analysis of the CTA, more appropriate measurements may be obtained by performing an ultrasound while the patient is in the surgical position (neck extended and turned). Furthermore, the carotid lesion should be free of acute mobile thrombus or significant calcification that precludes stent placement.[4]
- All patients undergoing TCAR must be on dual antiplatelet therapy (DAPT) prior to the procedure. The most common DAPT regimen includes daily doses of aspirin (81-325 mg) and clopidogrel (75 mg). In cases of urgent intervention, a loading dose may be administered at minimum 4 hours prior to the procedure. Alternative P2Y12 inhibitors (eg, ticagrelor or prasugrel) may also be utilized in place of clopidogrel. Due to the prevalence of clopidogrel resistance in the general population, platelet function testing should be performed if available. It should be noted that systemic anticoagulation (eg, warfarin or direct oral anticoagulants) are not substitutes for DAPT for TCAR. The patient should also be on statin therapy prior to the procedure.
- While fixed fluoroscopic imaging in a hybrid operating room is preferred, the procedure can also be performed in a standard operating room with a mobile fluoroscopy C-arm unit.

ANESTHESIA CONSIDERATIONS

- A TCAR procedure can be done under either general or local anesthesia with moderate sedation. The choice of anesthesia should be determined jointly by the proceduralist, patient, and the anesthesia team. Intraoperative neuromonitoring can be utilized at the physician's discretion but is not considered as mandatory.
- The patient should have a radial arterial line to allow for continuous hemodynamic monitoring during the entire procedure. During the procedure, the patient will be administered a bolus dose (100 U/kg) of heparin to achieve systemic anticoagulation. This is typically given immediately after the surgical incision is made. The target activated clotting time (ACT) is >250 and additional heparin is administered as necessary. The patient should also be given glycopyrrolate (0.2-0.4 mg) to try to mitigate bradycardia/hypotension during balloon angioplasty. During the period of CCA occlusion to establish reversal of flow, the systolic blood pressure should be maintained between 140 to 160 mm Hg and heart rate above 70 beats per minute. The anesthesia team should be ready with necessary vasoactive agents (eg, phenylephrine drip) to maintain the desired hemodynamic parameters during the procedure.

PERCUTANEOUS FEMORAL VENOUS SHEATH PLACEMENT

- It is preferred to obtain venous access in the common femoral vein contralateral to the carotid lesion. This is done using standard ultrasound guidance with a micropuncture system.
- Once the micropuncture sheath is placed into the vein, the NPS 8 French venous sheath should be inserted over an access wire. The sheath is secured to the patient's skin using a 2-0 silk suture.

COMMON CAROTID EXPOSURE

- The patient is positioned similar to a standard carotid endarterectomy. The head should be tilted away from the side of the lesion and a shoulder roll can be placed underneath the patient to elevate the neck and chest. We typically perform a repeat ultrasound to identify the anatomic landmarks (**FIGURE 2**).
- We clearly delineate the two heads of the sternocleidomastoid (SCM) as well as the clavicle. The location of the CCA is identified with ultrasound, with careful attention to the depth of the vessel at the base of the neck and its relation to the internal jugular vein (IJV) (**FIGURE 3**).
- A short transverse skin incision (typically between 2 and 4 cm) is made about a fingerbreadth above the clavicle and

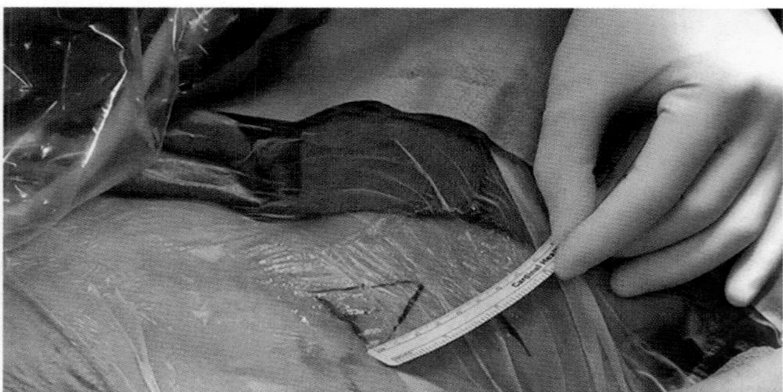

FIGURE 2 ● Intraoperative photograph demonstrating preoperative skin marking. The marked triangle is bordered by the clavicle and sternal and clavicular heads of the sternocleidomastoid muscle. A ruler is utilized to confirm adequate distance between the common carotid artery access site and the carotid lesion to be treated.

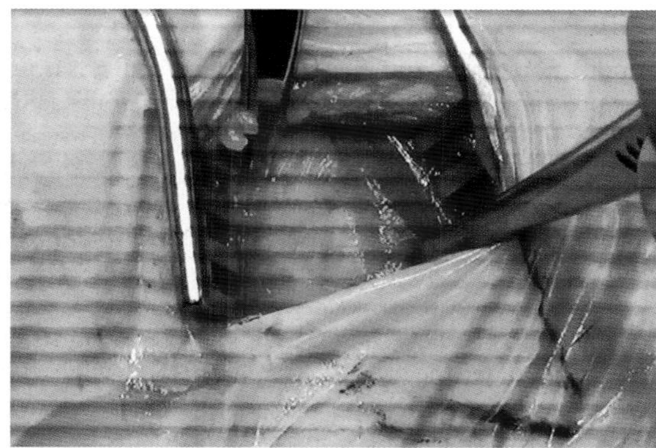

FIGURE 4 ● Intraoperative photograph demonstrating the avascular plane between the two heads of the sternocleidomastoid muscle.

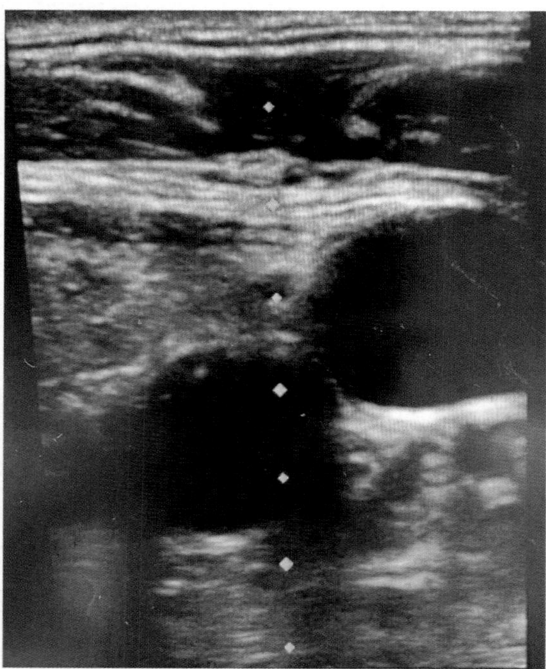

FIGURE 3 ● Ultrasound of the base of the neck demonstrating the location of the common carotid artery (bottom left) in relation to the internal jugular vein (upper right). The two heads of the sternocleidomastoid muscle are also identified and the avascular plane is centered at the top of the image.

centered between the two heads of the SCM. Subcutaneous dissection allows identification of the platysma, which is divided utilizing electrocautery. Subplatysmal planes are then developed superiorly and inferiorly. Gentle blunt dissection is utilized to identify the avascular plane between the two heads of the SCM and a self-retaining retractor is placed (**FIGURE 4**).

- There often is a large venous branch coming off medially from the IJV, which may be divided between ties. The proximal CCA is identified and dissected using sharp dissection. The vagus nerve, which usually courses posterior to the CCA, is identified and preserved. The proximal CCA is encircled using a silastic loop close to the clavicle to ensure adequate distance away from the lesion. It is our practice to utilize a 16-gauge vessel loop for retraction and occlusion during the procedure. Alternatively, an umbilical tape can be used for retraction and a surgical clamp for vessel occlusion. The anterior surface of the CCA is dissected clean. A "U-stitch" is then placed and left in place at the intended arterial access puncture site utilizing a 5-0 Prolene suture.

COMMON CAROTID ARTERIAL SHEATH PLACEMENT

- Prior to arterial access, we perform fluoroscopy to ensure that the surgical field is clear of radiopaque materials that may obstruct visualization. Using an ENHANCE Transcarotid Access kit, we puncture the CCA at the site of the U-stitch stitch placement. A key to success is maintaining stability of the CCA during arterial access. This can be done by apply slight caudal retraction of the vessel with retraction of the vessel loop while avoiding CCA occlusion. Once there is adequate blood return from the access needle, the microwire is inserted into the CCA for between 3 and 5 cm using the markings on the wire. The microsheath is then inserted over the wire into the CCA lumen between 2 and 3 cm. With the microsheath in place, an angiogram is performed to delineate the location of the carotid bifurcation.

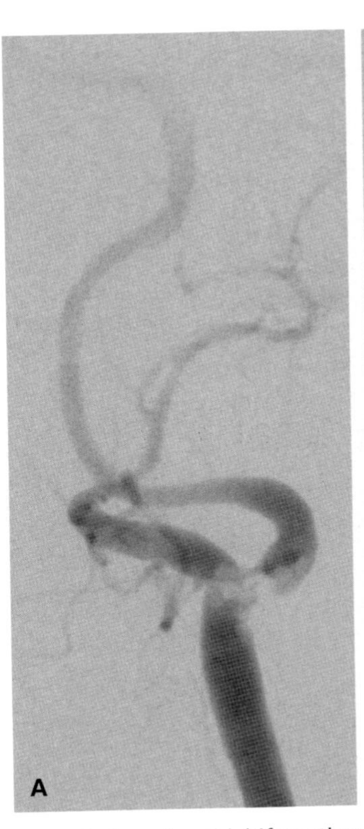

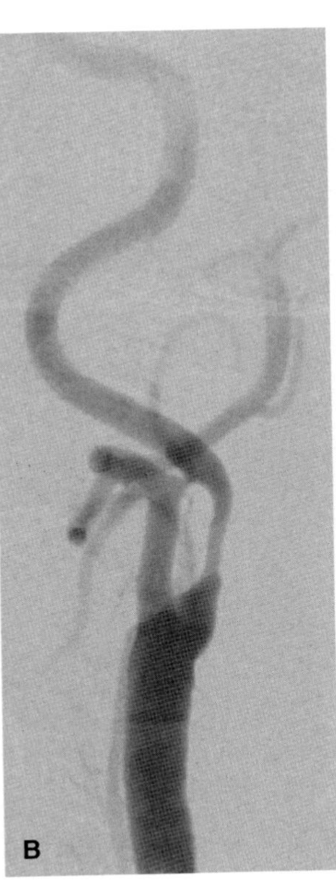

FIGURE 5 ● Carotid bifurcation anatomy and arterial sheath insertion technique. **A,** "Stop short" technique is utilized in the presence of disease involving the distal common carotid artery. **B,** "Engage EC" is utilized when the external carotid artery is free of disease and can accommodate wire insertion.

"Stop short" Technique

- In patients with distal CCA involvement or a diseased external carotid artery (ECA), we employ the "stop short" technique to place the arterial sheath (**FIGURE 5A**).
- After the initial angiogram, the provided 0.035″ stiff wire is inserted into the CCA under fluoroscopic guidance. Care should be taken to ensure that the wire does not engage the carotid lesion during sheath insertion. With clear verbal communication between the operators, the microsheath is removed and the arterial sheath is then placed into the CCA by the operator while the assistant maintains caudal retraction of the CCA. The arterial sheath is placed into the CCA until the footplate is placed directly onto the outer wall of the CCA.

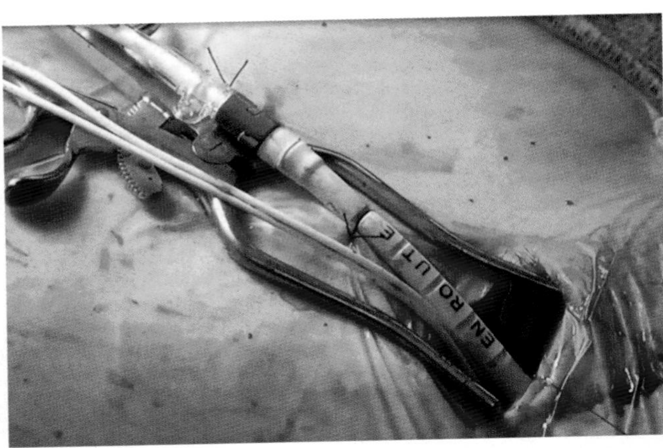

FIGURE 6 ● Intraoperative photograph demonstrating the arterial sheath in place after insertion in the common carotid artery. The silastic vessel loop is in place for later vessel occlusion to establish flow reversal. The sheath is secured to the patient at two locations (shaft of sheath and islet of sheath) with sutures.

- The retraction on the CCA is relaxed and the arterial sheath is then secured in place utilizing 2 separate 2-0 silk sutures (**FIGURE 6**). One is placed around the body of the sheath at the base of the neck and the other is placed at the islet of the arterial sheath. The dilator and wire are then removed, leaving the distal 2.5 cm tip of the arterial sheath in the CCA lumen. The NPS flow controller is first connected to the arterial sheath. After appropriate flushing maneuvers to deair the flow controller, the sheath is then connected to the venous sheath and flow between the sheaths is initiated. A "saline bolus test" is performed by infusing heparinized saline into the venous sheath and visualizing the clearance of saline by the patient's blood in the tubing.

"Engage external carotid" Technique

- In patients with a healthy ECA, we employ the "engage EC (external carotid)" technique to place the arterial sheath (**FIGURE 5B**). After the initial angiogram, the microwire is inserted back into the microsheath and the ECA is carefully selected with the wire under fluoroscopy. The microsheath along with the dilator is then inserted into the ECA. The provided 0.035″ stiff wire is then inserted into the ECA. The arterial sheath is then placed into the CCA as above in the "stop short" technique.

ANGIOGRAM AND "TCAR TIMEOUT"

- It is important to point out that there remains antegrade flow through the CCA to the brain during this portion of the procedure. As such, there is no cerebral protection until the CCA is occluded during the angioplasty and stent portion of the procedure. Angiography is performed to further assess the arterial anatomy. This requires a minimum of two angiograms in orthogonal views to identify any possible access site complications (eg, dissection) and to confirm proper positioning of the arterial sheath tip. The images should also clearly delineate the flow channel through the lesion as well as the petrous portion of the ICA (typically represented by a 90° turn of the distal carotid as it enters the skull) (**FIGURE 7A**).
- Once the desired images are obtained, the positions of the patient and image intensifier are locked. The tip of the intervention 0.014″ wire is then shaped as necessary to help facilitate crossing the carotid stenosis. The tip of the wire is inserted into the sheath with care to not engage the lesion with the wire. The predilation angioplasty balloon is then inserted over the wire into the arterial sheath. The balloon should be sized to the nominal ICA diameter. In our practice,

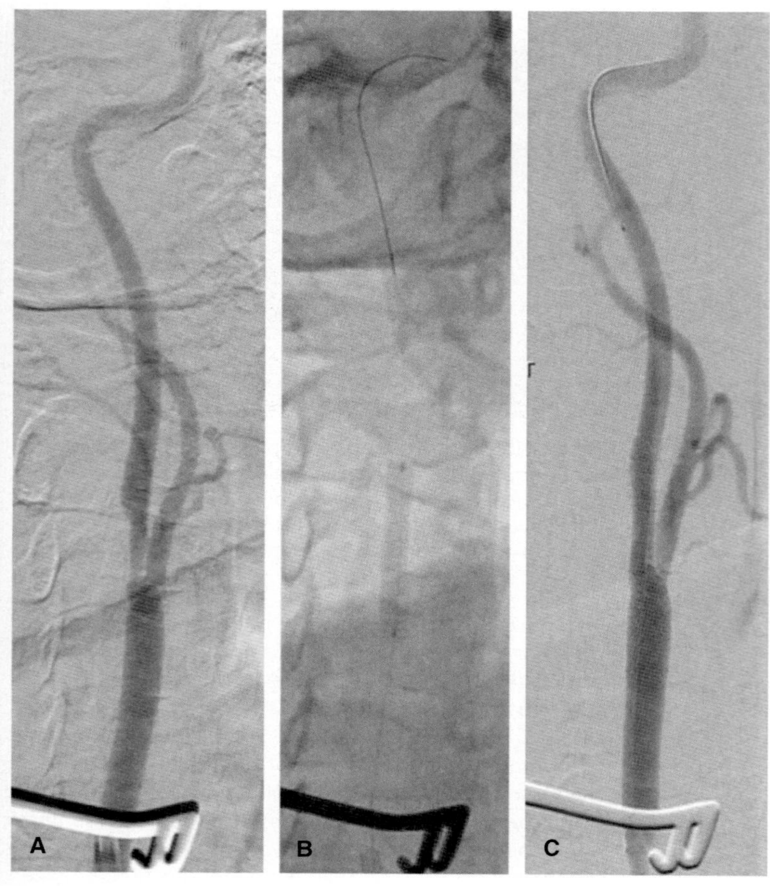

FIGURE 7 ● Intraoperative angiograms. **A,** Preintervention angiogram demonstrating carotid stenosis at proximal internal carotid artery. **B,** Balloon angioplasty while under neuroprotection with reversal of flow. **C,** Completion angiogram after stent placement.

we routinely use a 5.5 × 30 mm angioplasty balloon. Once the wire and balloon are in place, a "TCAR timeout" is then performed. This is a second surgical pause (in addition to the standard preincision surgical timeout) to confirm all members of the surgical and anesthesia teams are ready for CCA occlusion. The anesthesia team should confirm adequate blood pressure, appropriate ACT level, and premedication to prevent bradycardia/hypotension during carotid angioplasty. The surgical team should confirm the proper positioning of the wire and balloon in the arterial sheath. The carotid stent should be open, prepped, and ready for use. The stent is typically sized to be 1 to 2 mm greater than the size of the carotid bulb. In our practice, we routinely use 40-mm long stents.

CAROTID ANGIOPLASTY AND STENT PLACEMENT

- After the "TCAR timeout," the common carotid artery is occluded. This can be done by tightening the double looped vessel loop or by placing a surgical clamp. A repeat "saline bolus test" is performed to monitor the rate of saline clearance. Once adequate flow is ensured, the 0.014″ wire is passed through the carotid lesion and the distal tip of the wire is placed at the petrous portion of the ICA. The angioplasty balloon is then placed at the desired location and a predilatation is then performed (**FIGURE 7B**).
- Even though appropriate premedication has been administered, anesthesia personnel should be alert and ready to treat (with atropine administration) any potential bradycardia and hypotension that arise. The balloon is removed, and the stent is then placed at the desired location and subsequently deployed. The degree of residual stenosis can be ascertained with plain fluoroscopic analysis of the stent architecture in orthogonal views (**FIGURE 8**). Postdilatation of the lesion may be performed as necessary, but we typically tolerate a residual stenosis of <30%. After waiting for 2 to 3 minutes of additional flow reversal after the last manipulation, completion angiograms are performed in at least two orthogonal views (**FIGURE 7C**). This is done to ensure adequate flow through the ICA. The wire is then removed and antegrade flow through the CCA is restored by releasing the occlusion (loosening vessel loop or removing clamp).

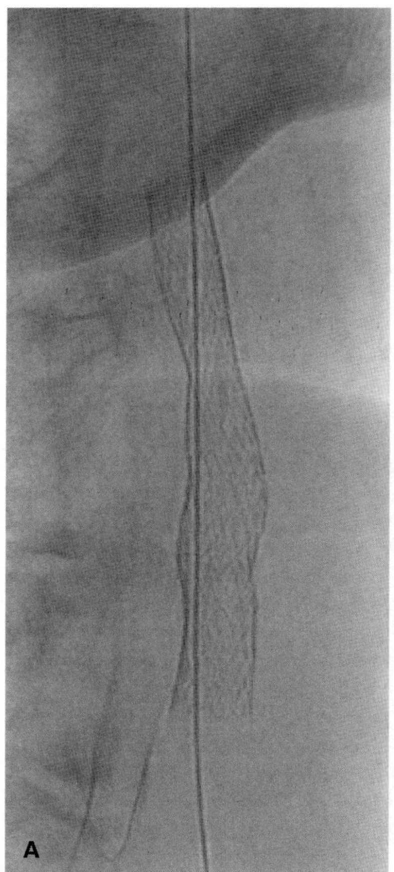

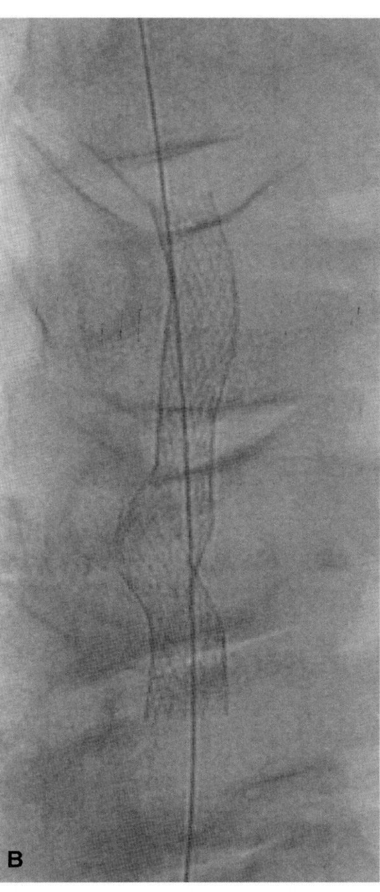

FIGURE 8 ● **A** and **B,** Intraoperative plain fluoroscopic images in orthogonal views to demonstrate no significant stenosis based on stent architecture.

NPS REMOVAL AND COMPLETION OF PROCEDURE

- To conclude the procedure, the flow controller is disconnected from the arterial sheath and blood returned to the patient's circulation through the venous sheath. The flow controller is then disconnected from the venous sheath. The filter within the flow controller can be removed and examined to evaluate for the presence of debris (**FIGURE 9**).
- The venous sheath is flushed with heparinized saline and attention is directed back to the neck. The silk sutures securing the arterial sheath are cut. The arterial sheath is removed and the arteriotomy repaired by tying off the previously placed 5-0 Prolene suture. Protamine (typically 40 mg) is routinely administered at this time. After ensuring adequate hemostasis, the platysma is reapproximated utilizing a 3-0 Vicryl suture. The skin is then reapproximated utilizing a subcuticular suture followed by Dermabond. The femoral sheath is removed and manual pressure is utilized for hemostasis.

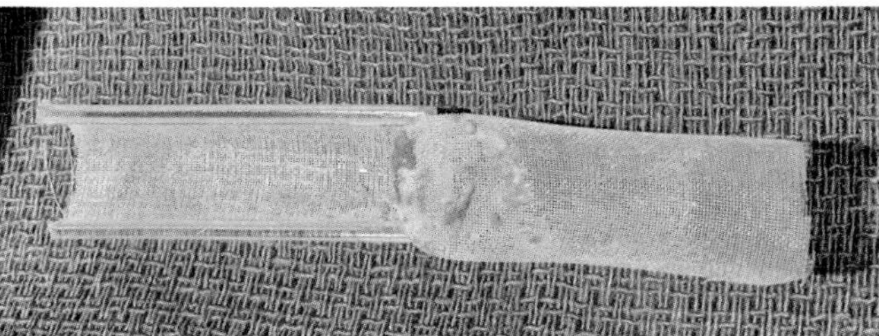

FIGURE 9 ● Filter after a TCAR procedure showing the presence of atherosclerotic debris.

PEARL AND PITFALLS

Access site dissection	■ Maintain constant verbal communication between proceduralist and assistant during procedure. ■ Provide slight caudal retraction of CCA to provide stability during needle access. ■ Wire insertion should be gentle and avoid the use of force. ■ Utilize "engage EC" maneuver (if anatomy permits) to provide more wire access/stability during arterial sheath insertion. ■ Careful interrogation of access site with angiography.
Neck hematoma	■ Utilize preoperative ultrasound to identify location of two heads of SCM and depth of CCA. ■ Identify avascular plane during dissection and utilize gentle blunt dissection to identify CCA. ■ Routinely administer protamine after removal of arterial sheath and closure of CCA arteriotomy.
Calcification/ thrombus	■ Obtain high-quality thin cuts (<1 mm) CTA of the head and neck. ■ Carefully perform duplex ultrasound to examine proximal CCA for arterial access/occlusion. ■ Do not perform TCAR in patients with intraluminal thrombus. ■ Avoid stent placement in patients with circumferential (>50%) or thick (>3 mm) calcific burden.
Hypotension	■ Encourage adequate hydration on the night prior to procedure. ■ Hold selected antihypertensive medications day of surgery (continue beta blockers). ■ Appropriate premedication with glycopyrrolate prior to TCAR timeout. ■ Have vasoactive agents prepared and ready for infusion during the procedure. ■ Encourage early ambulation in the postprocedure period.

POSTOPERATIVE CARE

- A neurologic evaluation is performed at the completion of the procedure. The patient should have close neurologic as well as hemodynamic monitoring during the postprocedure period.
- The arterial line is typically left in for a minimum of 4 to 6 hours to determine the need of vasoactive agents. The systolic blood pressure is kept between 100 to 140 mm Hg (20% above baseline). Due to the stent exerting pressure on the carotid bulb, the presence of hypotension after stent placement is more frequent than with CEA. This can be treated with intravenous vasoactive agents (eg, phenylephrine infusion) or with oral medications (eg, pseudoephedrine).
- The patient should remain on bedrest for 1-2 hours due to the presence of the femoral venous puncture. The groin puncture site as well as the surgical wound at the neck will need to be monitored for bleeding/hematoma. Upon discharge, the patient should be maintained on DAPT and statin therapy for a minimum of 1 month. A carotid duplex is obtained at the 1 month follow-up visit to establish a new baseline for long-term monitoring.

OUTCOMES/COMPLICATIONS

- The ROADSTER trial is the first multicenter prospective clinical trial evaluating TCAR using the NPS system.[2] The study enrolled 141 pivotal phase patients between 2012 and 2014 with either symptomatic >50% or asymptomatic >70% stenosis considered to be at "high risk" for complications from CEA. In the pivotal cohort, the all-stroke rate was 1.4% (2 of 141), stroke/death was 2.8% (4 of 141), and stroke/death/MI was 3.5% (5 of 141). These data subsequently led to Food and Drug Administration approval in the United States in 2015.
- The ROADSTER 2 trial is a prospective multicenter postapproval registry for patients undergoing TCAR between 2015 and 2019.[5] The study enrolled 692 "high risk" patients with symptomatic stenosis >50% or asymptomatic stenosis >80% at 43 sites. As 60 cases had major study protocol violations, this left 632 patients (per protocol [PP] population) adhering to the FDA-approved protocol. The technical success occurred in 99.7% of all cases. The primary end point of procedural success (technical success plus the absence of stroke, MI, or death within the 30-day postoperative period) was 97.9% in the PP population. In the PP population, there were strokes in four patients (0.6%), death in one patient (0.2%), and MI in six patients (0.9%) leading to a composite 30-day stroke/death rate of 0.8% and stroke/death/MI rate of 1.7%. In the 60 patients with protocol violations, 11 were for not adhering to the inclusion/exclusion criteria of the study. The remaining 49 patients either did not start or discontinued their DAPT and statin. In this group of 60 patients, there were 11 additional stroke and two additional deaths, emphasizing the detrimental effect of medication noncompliance with the TCAR procedure.
- Data from >95% of TCAR procedures are entered into the TCAR Surveillance Project (TSP), a database created to allow for an evaluation of "real-world" TCAR outcomes compared to CEA.[6] Using data from the TSP and comparing outcomes between 1182 TCAR and 10,797 CEA patients, TCAR patients were older, more likely to be symptomatic, and had more medical comorbidities. On unadjusted analysis, TCAR had similar rates of in-hospital stroke/death (1.6% vs 1.4%) and stroke/death/MI (2.5% vs 1.9%) compared with CEA. There was no difference in the rates of stroke (1.4% vs 1.2%), in-hospital death (0.3% vs 0.3%), 30-day death (0.9% vs 0.4%), or MI (1.1% vs 0.6%). However, TCAR procedures were 33 minutes shorter than CEA and TCAR patients were less likely to incur cranial nerve injuries (CNI) (0.6% vs 1.8%) and less likely to have a postoperative length of stay >1 day (27% vs 30%). On adjusted analysis, there was no difference in terms of stroke/death, stroke/death/MI, or the individual outcomes.
- In an analysis of 86,027 patients that underwent carotid revascularization from over 400 centers in North America between 2015 and 2019, it was shown that the number of centers performing both TCAR and CEA increased from 15

to 247, a more than 16-fold increase.[7] The proportion of all carotid procedures that were TCAR increased from 0.7% to 17.0%, a 24-fold increase. In addition to increased adoption, the study also demonstrated that availability of TCAR at a hospital was associated with a decrease in the likelihood of perioperative major adverse cardiovascular events (MACE). Centers that adopted TCAR had a 10% decrease in the likelihood of MACE at 12 months after TCAR adoption vs if those centers had continued to perform CEA alone.

REFERENCES

1. Brott TG, Hobson RWII, Howard G, et al. Stenting versus endarterectomy for treatment of carotid artery stenosis. *N Engl J Med*. 2010;363:11-23.
2. Kwolek CJ, Jaff MR, Leal JI, et al. Results of the ROADSTER multicenter trial of transcarotid stenting with dynamic flow reversal. *J Vasc Surg*. 2015;62:1227-1235.
3. AbuRahma AF, Avgerinos ED, Chang RW, et al. Society for Vascular Surgery clinical practice guidelines for management of extracranial cerebrovascular disease. *J Vasc Surg*. 2022;75:4S-22S.
4. Kokkosis AA, MacDonald S, Jim J, et al. Assessing the suitability of the carotid bifurcation for stenting: anatomic and morphologic considerations. *J Vasc Surg*. 2021;74:2087-2095.
5. Kashyap VS, Schneider PA, Foteh M, et al. Early outcomes in the ROADSTER 2 study of transcarotid artery revascularization in patients with significant carotid artery disease. *Stroke*. 2020;51:2620-2629.
6. Schermerhorn ML, Liang P, Dakour-Aridi H, et al. In-hospital outcomes of transcarotid artery revascularization and carotid endarterectomy in the Society for Vascular Surgery Vascular Quality Initiative. *J Vasc Surg*. 2020;71:87-95.
7. Columbo JA, Martinez-Camblor P, O'Malley J, et al. Association of adoption of transcarotid artery revascularization with center-level perioperative outcomes. *JAMA Netw Open*. 2021;4:e2037885.

Chapter 5

Carotid Surgery: Distal Exposure and Control Techniques and Complication Management

Cheong Jun Lee

DEFINITION

- The carotid artery typically bifurcates at the level of the C3-C4 cervical spine. Distal internal carotid artery (ICA) exposure for control is required in high carotid bifurcations and lesions that extend to the C1-C2 level. Access to the distal ICA is impeded by the mastoid process and the angle of the mandible and furthermore by its intimate relationship to the hypoglossal and glossopharyngeal nerves. As such, exposure of the vessel cephalad to C3 poses technical challenges that may increase the perioperative risk of stroke and cranial nerve injury.
- To better ascertain the risk of distal ICA exposure, Vang et al subdivided the artery into three anatomic zones based on lesion extent and its relationship to the vertebral body[1]: the proximal segment of the ICA to the level of C3 body is designated Zone 1; Zone 2 extends from the C2 vertebral body but remains below C1; and Zone 3 is the segment of ICA above the C2 vertebral body (**FIGURE 1**).
- Ideally, the need for distal access in carotid surgery should be anticipated preoperatively with appropriate imaging. Familiarity of the anatomy and various exposure techniques are necessary for safe distal carotid control. The optimal level of distal control and which control techniques are employed depends strongly on the underlying pathology as aneurysmal conditions often require higher exposure compared to atherosclerotic disease.[2]

PATIENT HISTORY AND PHYSICAL FINDINGS

- As with any medical therapy, the clinician must first clearly define the goals of treatment and the indication for intervention, as well as thoroughly review the operative risk with the patient.
- An evidence-based approach to the treatment of atherosclerotic carotid disease has been reviewed previously; however, optimal medical therapy must be instituted prior to intervention (eg, antiplatelet agent, statin, appropriate antihypertensive agents).[3-5]
- Patients with hostile neck anatomy, such as those with history of high-dose neck radiation or severe systemic comorbidities contraindicating general or cervical block anesthesia, should be offered carotid angioplasty and carotid stenting (CAS) as an alternative procedure.
- Patients with prior contralateral carotid revascularization procedures should have laryngeal, hypoglossal, and glossopharyngeal nerve function documented prior to ipsilateral dissection and exposure. When evidence of prior injury to CN IX, X, or XII is evident, CAS should be considered as an alternative. If CAS is not feasible under these circumstances, the potential need for tracheostomy to manage postoperative airway obstruction should be reviewed with the patient.

IMAGING AND OTHER DIAGNOSTIC STUDIES

- Although duplex scanning provides accurate and reproducible assessment of the presence and severity of carotid stenosis, precise anatomic detail required for surgical planning is better obtained from computed tomographic angiography (CTA) or magnetic resonance arteriography (MRA). Localization of the carotid bifurcation in regard to cervical landmarks, as well as the distal extent of ICA disease, is best assessed by high-resolution CTA or MRA.
- CTA and MRA have enabled highly accurate characterization of plaque morphology, which may provide useful guidance regarding risk of distal embolization or intimal fractures leading to dissection during operative manipulation.

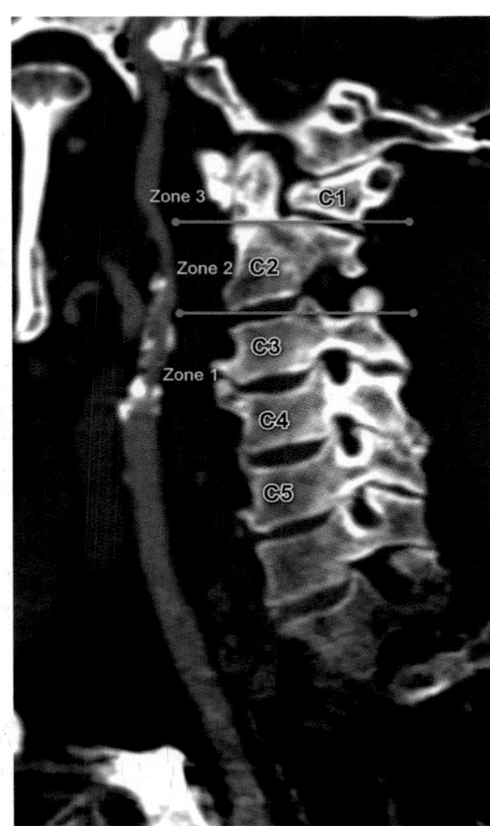

FIGURE 1 • The carotid artery can be divided into three zones respective to the cervical spine. A critical atherosclerotic plaque extending to Zone 1 is pictured in this reformatted computed tomography scan. Lesions that extend Zone 2 and above are deemed high and will require additional surgical maneuvers for exposure and control.

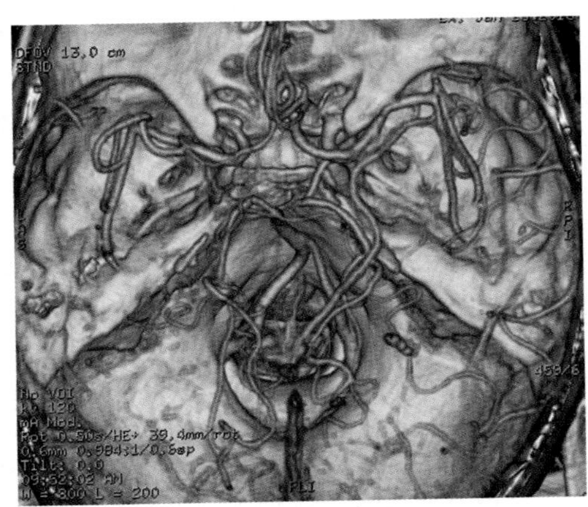

FIGURE 2 ● Rendered computed tomographic angiography demonstrating incompetency of the circle of Willis.

- CTA and MRA also provide essential information regarding potential collateral arterial flow through the circle of Willis and the need for adjuvant maneuvers such as shunt placement during carotid revascularization (**FIGURE 2**).

SURGICAL MANAGEMENT

Preoperative Planning for Distal Cervical Carotid Exposure

- "Forewarned is forearmed."
- The degree of difficulty in distal carotid exposure is exacerbated in patients who have a short neck or high carotid bifurcation. As mentioned, for atherosclerotic disease specifically, CAS should be considered when lesion extent is high. However, in select patients with severe ICA tortuosity or heavy calcification, CAS will not be a good option. In these circumstances, CEA remains a safe and viable treatment modality. Nevertheless, being prepared for a challenging endpoint during CEA by having endovascular rescue options readily available is prudent.
- Knowledge of patient-specific cervical spine anatomy and potential patient tolerance for variable neck positioning is important. If neck flexion or extension is not feasible, more invasive maneuvers such as nasotracheal intubation or mandibular subluxation may be required as simple cephalad extension of the cervical incision may not offer significant distal exposure or maneuverability of key anatomic structures.
- Nasotracheal intubation and a chin-up position is an effective method to allow exposure of the distal ICA. Weiss et al. as well as others have described this method allowing operators to obtain as much as 2.5 cm of more distal exposure.[6,7] When recognized as necessary, specifying nasotracheal, rather than orotracheal, intubation for general endotracheal anesthesia is a simple and practical maneuver to improve exposure. Nasotracheal intubation allows the mouth to stay closed during surgery, providing more room between the ramus of the mandible and mastoid process for distal dissection.
- Temporomandibular subluxation may further advantage carotid exposure cephalad to the C2 cervical spine.[8] This technique is more invasive in that it requires subluxation of the ipsilateral mandibular condyle, performed via intraoral wiring. Mandibular subluxation with the addition of mandibular osteotomy and resection of the mastoid process are alternate strategies to obtain additional exposure from the infratemporal ICA to the skull base. Subluxation is distinguished from dislocation, which is more injurious and can potentiate long-term temporomandibular joint pain syndromes. The technique requires craniomaxillofacial surgery or otolaryngology colleagues for assistance. Though rarely utilized in atherosclerotic carotid disease management, anticipation of its application is realized in high extension of carotid body tumors and ICA aneurysms.
- Once the procedure is underway, however, neither nasotracheal intubation nor mandibular subluxation strategies can be used and other exposure methods will need to be considered.

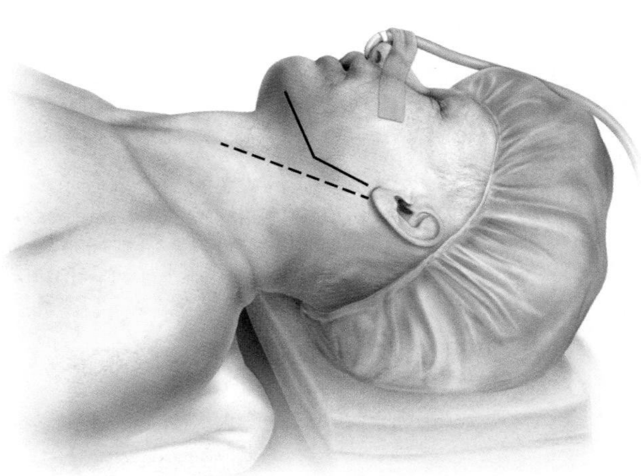

FIGURE 3 ● Nasotracheal intubation facilitates exposures of the distal internal carotid artery by opening the angle between the mastoid process and the mandible (*black lines*).

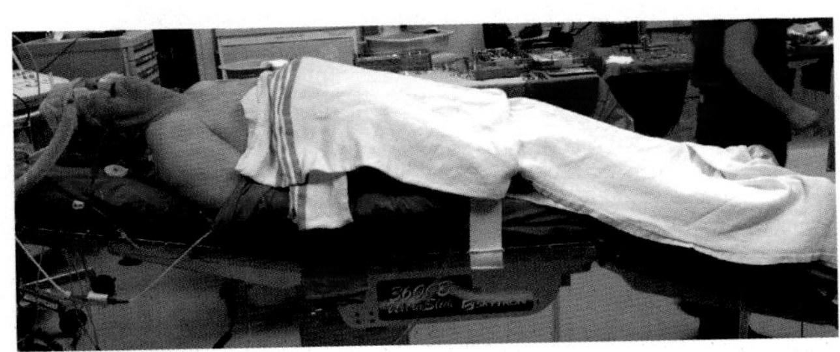

FIGURE 4 ● Patient in the "beach chair" position.

Positioning

- The patient is positioned supine, with the head extended and rotated away from the operative site. Shoulder rolls and appropriate padding are placed to stabilize the neck and optimize extension. The nasotracheal tube is secured over the head (**FIGURE 3**).
- Arms are tucked to the patient's side to allow the operator and the assistant to maneuver and stand comfortably. This position also facilitates C-arm positioning when needed.
- The patient is placed in the "beach chair" position to limit venous hypertension (**FIGURE 4**).

ANTERIOR APPROACH TO THE DISTAL INTERNAL CAROTID ARTERY

Incision

- A longitudinal incision along the anterior margin of the sternocleidomastoid muscle (SCM), rather than a transverse cervical incision is recommended for optimal distal ICA access (**FIGURE 5**).

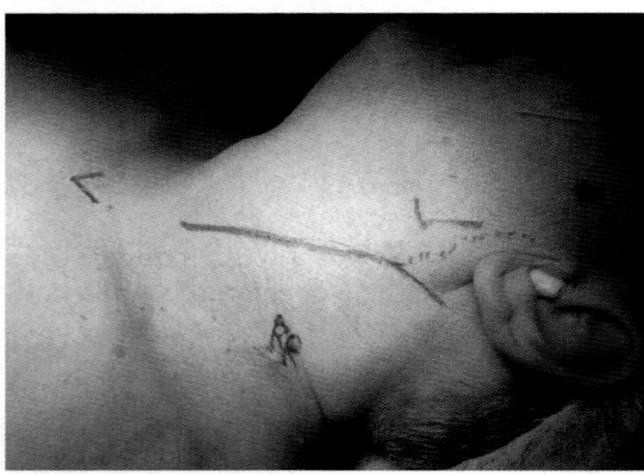

FIGURE 5 ● Anatomic landmarks for carotid exposures include the mastoid process, the angle of the mandible, and the sternal notch. Skin incision for carotid exposures is placed anterior to the sternocleidomastoid muscle (*solid line*). If distal exposure is anticipated, the incision can be carried in front of the ear (*dotted line*).

- The incision can be extended anterior to the ear for distal exposure if needed but may require mobilization of the parotid gland in later stages of the dissection when lesion extent is significant.
- At the upper edge of the platysma and SCM, attention must be paid to the great auricular nerve. This nerve exits at the lateral border of the SCM, crosses over the surface of the SCM, and courses to the parotid gland and inferior part of the auricle.

Exposure of the Internal Carotid Artery Distal to the Bifurcation

- Key structures that lie superior to the carotid bifurcation are the posterior belly of the digastric muscle, the hypoglossal nerve, crossing veins from the SCM to the internal jugular vein, and muscular arterioles of the posterior branches of the external carotid artery (ECA) (**FIGURE 6**).
- The hypoglossal nerve is identified safely using a posterolateral to anteromedial dissection of the ICA. Moving cephalad, the hypoglossal nerve is dissected free from the medial surface of the digastric muscle. Crossing artery and veins of the SCM often tether this nerve closer to the bifurcation. Meticulous identification and controlled division of these tethering vessels will enable mobilization of the nerve. Tracing the course of the descending branch of the ansa cervicalis back to the hypoglossal itself provides positive confirmation of the location and course of the nerve (**FIGURE 7**).

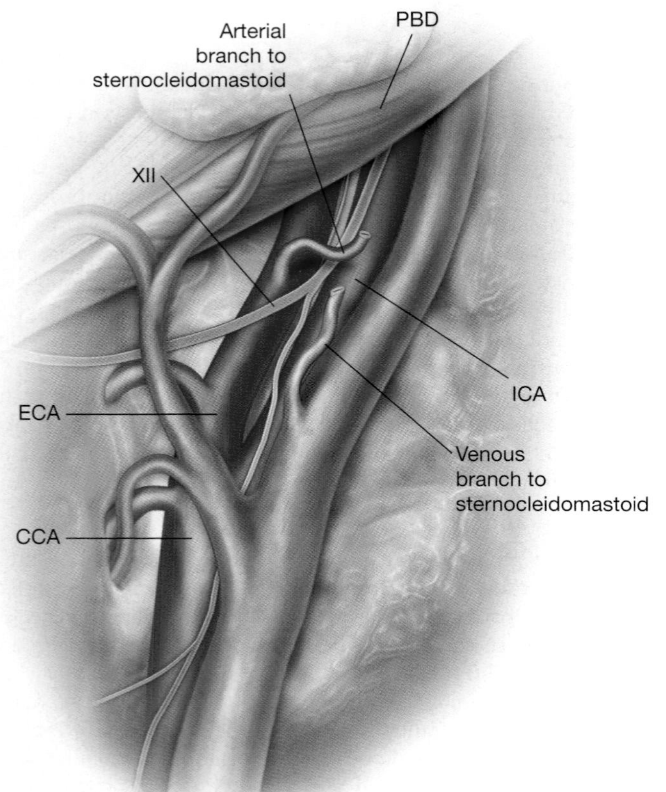

FIGURE 6 ● Once the carotid sheath is entered, exposure of the distal internal carotid artery (ICA) from an anterior approach begins with identification and dissection of the hypoglossal nerve (XII), the posterior belly of the digastric muscle (PBD), and the crossing veins and arteries to the sternocleidomastoid muscle. CCA, common carotid artery; ECA, external carotid artery.

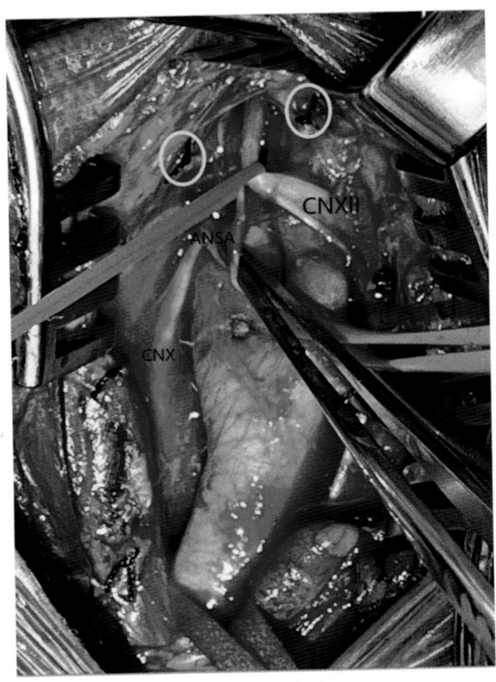

FIGURE 7 ● To further facilitate hypoglossal mobilization, the occipital artery coming off the external carotid artery has been ligated and divided. The ansa cervicalis (ANSA) can be ligated to further mobilize the hypoglossal nerve for distal carotid exposure.

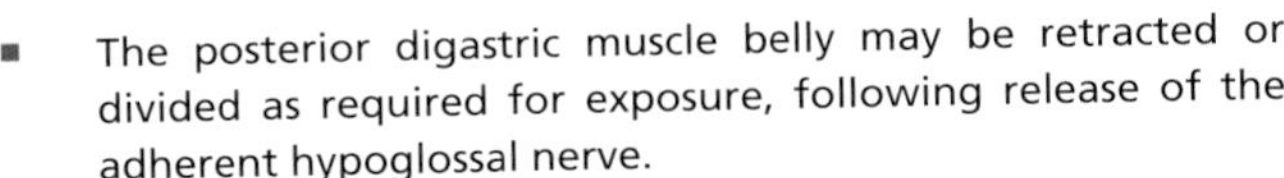

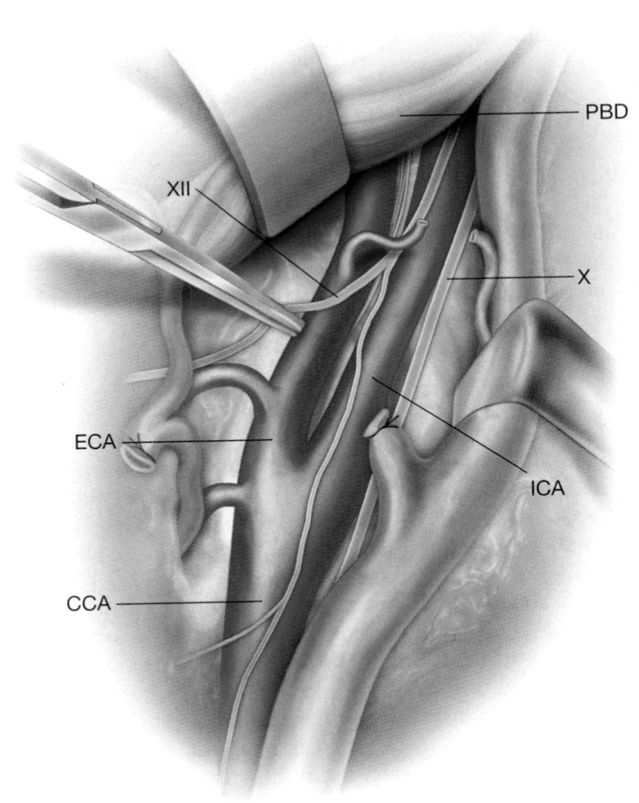

FIGURE 8 ● Mobilization of the hypoglossal nerve (XII) allows exposure of the distal internal carotid artery (ICA). CCA, common carotid artery; ECA, external carotid artery; PBD, posterior belly of the digastric muscle.

- The posterior digastric muscle belly may be retracted or divided as required for exposure, following release of the adherent hypoglossal nerve.
- Additional cephalad exposure at this juncture requires division of the occipital branch of the ECA. This further releases the hypoglossal nerve. This maneuver also requires division of the styloid musculature (styloglossus, stylopharyngeus).
- Continued cephalad dissection exposes the glossopharyngeal nerve, seen as a single or double trunk crossing the ICA anteriorly and coursing posterior to the external carotid. Care must be taken in separating the hypoglossal and glossopharyngeal nerves, as small motor fibers exiting the vagus nerve also course in this plane. Damage to these nerves or the glossopharyngeal can cause swallowing dysfunction. Classically, injury to the glossopharyngeal nerve in this region may impair the ability of the soft palate to rise sufficiently with swallowing to prevent nasopharyngeal liquid reflux.
- When these steps are safely completed, the ICA may be adequately exposed for reconstruction up to the level of C2 (**FIGURE 8**). Further exposure to the level of C1 following this course requires styloidectomy and/or preoperative mandibular subluxation.
- Distal dissection may also be facilitated by mobilization of the parotid gland and facial nerve. This is most safely accomplished with assistance from otolaryngologists or craniomaxillofacial surgeon. To provide this method of exposure, the skin incision is carried cephalad, anterior to the ear (**FIGURE 9**). This enables mobilization of the parotid gland superiorly and medially.

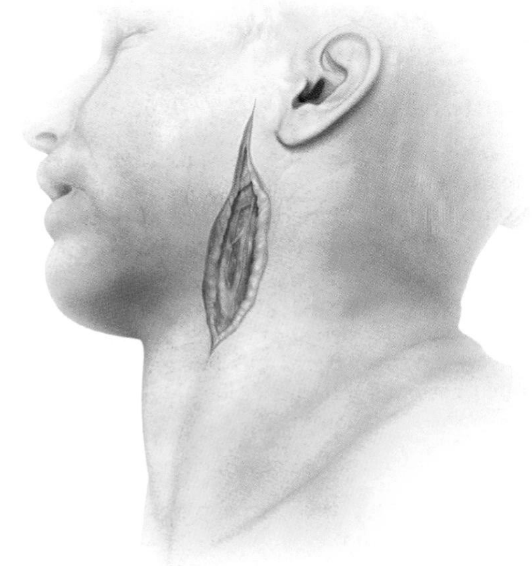

FIGURE 9 ● If further exposure of the internal carotid artery (ICA) is required and mandibular subluxation is not feasible, incision can be carried in front of the ear for mobilization of the parotid gland.

- The parotid fascia is entered and the branches of the facial nerve are dissected, identified, and protected before dividing the posterior belly of the digastric muscle.
- Care is again taken to identify the glossopharyngeal nerve and the motor fibers of the vagus nerve (**FIGURE 10**).
- Distal control of the ICA at high C1-C2 level may require specialized instrumentation. Small detachable occluding clamps (such as the Heifetz or Yasargil clips) may provide improved exposure compared to traditional "handled" vascular clamps in this region. When used, however, care must be taken to avoid clamp dislodgement in this crowded and moving field, which when it does happen, it usually does so at the maximally inconvenient time.
- As an alternative to distal clamp control, short occluding intraluminal catheters can be used, such as a #2 Fogarty embolectomy catheter with stopcock. Extreme care must be taken in positioning and deploying embolectomy balloons in this area, however, as inflation within the petrous portion or overinflation in any region may precipitate dissection, arterial rupture, or thrombosis. Only the lowest amount of inflation required to prevent back-bleeding should be used. The carotid artery is thin-walled at this level and easily traumatized by balloon inflation. Late complications also include pseudoaneurysm or arteriovenous fistula formation. The inflated catheter should be secured to prevent its migration. Stay sutures may be placed in the distal carotid to maintain access should control be lost due to reflux of the balloon from the distal artery or balloon puncture during suture closure of the anastomosis.

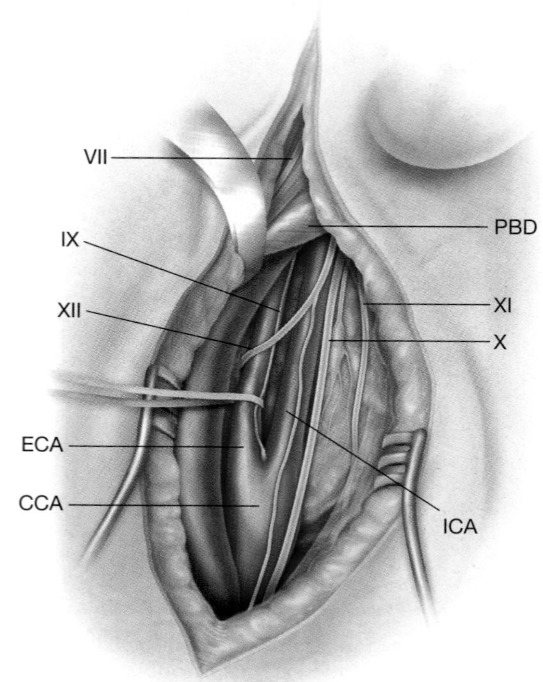

FIGURE 10 • Once the parotid fascia is entered, the branches of the facial nerve (VII) are identified followed by the division of the posterior belly of the digastric muscle (PBD). CCA, common carotid artery; ECA, external carotid artery. Dissection is then carried anterior to the internal carotid artery (ICA) from the hypoglossal nerve (XII) distally to identify the glossopharyngeal nerve (IX). Motor fibers from the vagus nerve (X) are carefully identified and preserved.

RETROJUGULAR APPROACH TO THE DISTAL INTERNAL CAROTID ARTERY

Retrojugular Dissection

- A third approach to the distal ICA is provided by retrojugular access. The internal jugular (IJ) vein angles anteriorly as it ascends from the base of the neck to the base of the skull and overlies the distal ICA as the artery approaches the transverse process of C1.
- Using the posterior approach, dissecting behind the IJ vein, obviates the need for hypoglossal exposure and relocation, as that nerve passes anteriorly over the ICA. This approach is ideal when performing bypass rather than endarterectomy for an extensive ICA lesion.

Identification of the Spinal Accessory Nerve

- The retrojugular dissection uses the same incision as other approaches to the distal internal carotid, with the incision made longitudinally, anterior to the SCM muscle.
- Using this approach, it is essential to identify the spinal accessory nerve where it exits 2 to 3 cm below the edge of the mastoid process, anterior to the SCM. The SCM is fully mobilized to facilitate this exposure.
- Once the spinal accessory nerve is identified and isolated, the IJ vein is dissected along its posterior border. The vagus nerve is identified and reflected anteriorly. With the vein and vagus nerve mobilized anteriorly, the hypoglossal nerve remains anterior to the distal ICA (**FIGURE 11**).

Identification of the Superior Laryngeal Nerve

- In the retrojugular space, the ICA can be dissected along its posterior lateral wall superiorly whereupon the superior laryngeal nerve will be encountered exiting the vagus nerve and looping around the distal ICA. Often, the superior cervical ganglion can be identified just lateral to this looping point (**FIGURE 12**).
- For added exposure, the nerve is carefully lifted from the ICA adventitia.

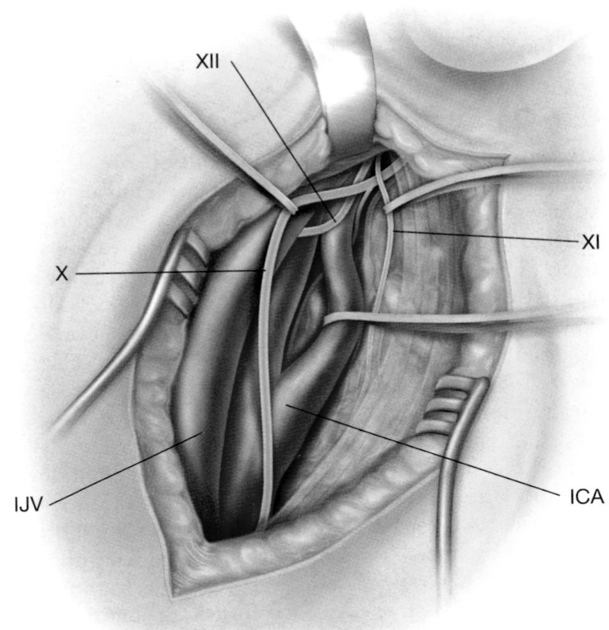

FIGURE 11 ● Retrojugular exposure of the internal carotid artery (ICA): Dissection is carried behind the internal jugular vein (IJV) and the vagus nerve (X) mobilized anterior to the ICA. Care is taken in identifying the spinal accessory nerve (XI) at the superior aspect of the dissection. This approach avoids mobilization of the hypoglossal nerve (XII) as the plane of dissection remains posterior to the nerve.

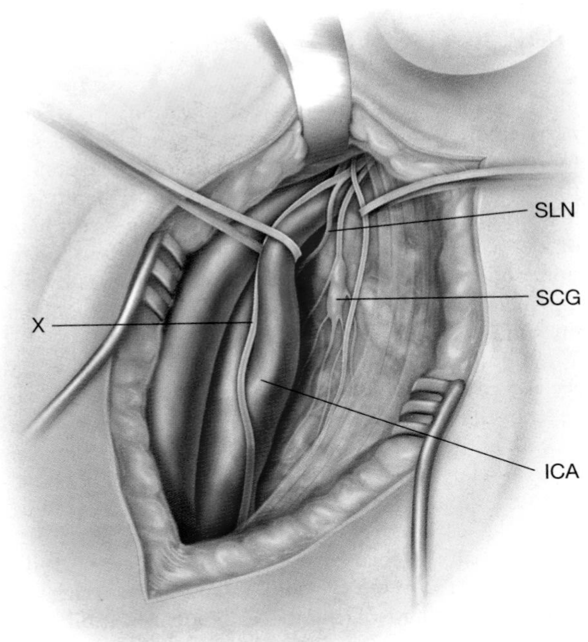

FIGURE 12 ● At the distal aspect of this retrojugular space, the internal carotid artery (ICA) will be looped by the superior laryngeal nerve (SLN) as it comes off the vagus nerve (X). Often, the superior cervical ganglion (SCG) serves as a landmark for where the SLN emanates.

PEARLS AND PITFALLS

Indications	■ Make note of significant radiation or surgery to the neck, which may inform the choice of procedure (surgery vs CAS). ■ Make certain the patient's cranial nerve status is documented, especially in the setting of prior neck operations.
Imaging	■ High-resolution cross-sectional imaging (CTA/MRA) is essential for anticipating complex exposures and strategizing reconstructive techniques. ■ The status of the circle of Willis should be defined in the course of preoperative planning.
Technique	■ For lesions extending to the C1-C2 cervical spine, consider at a minimum nasotracheal intubation. ■ In extreme situations, mandibular subluxation may provide critical additional degrees of freedom. ■ Mandibular dislocation is not recommended and should not be performed to assist carotid surgery. ■ *Knowledge of cranial nerve anatomy is the most important determinant of success as these are the structures most vulnerable to injury.* ■ Any neural tissue crossing anterior to the carotid bifurcation and the ICA should *not* be divided. ■ Mobilization of diseased arterial segments, including the carotid bifurcation, should be avoided and handling minimized prior to heparinization. ■ Anterior distal ICA exposure is dependent on the extent to which the hypoglossal nerve can be safely mobilized. ■ Posterior, retrojugular exposure requires early identification of the spinal accessory nerve and anterior reflection of the vagus nerves to visualize the superior laryngeal nerve encircling the distal internal carotid. ■ Balloon occlusion may facilitate far distal carotid control, but overadvancement and overinflation are real risks that must be considered. ■ Placement of stay sutures on the distal ICA will facilitate control maneuvers.

POSTOPERATIVE CARE AND COMPLICATION MANAGEMENT

- Cranial nerve injury during distal carotid exposure is the most frequently encountered complication. Most of these nerve injuries are transient; however, permanent deficits are more likely to occur with distal exposures.[1] The majority of these injuries are due to excessive retraction; therefore sharp dissection of the nerve and vessels, avoiding direct handling of any nerve tissue by grasping perineural tissue for retraction, and removal of excessive tension on nerves by detaching them from the surrounding tissues are recommended preventative strategies.
- If the endpoint of the CEA remains questionable despite the use of adjunct maneuvers, endovascular rescue should be considered.[9] Intraoperative CAS can be performed by extending the skin incision inferiorly to allow for placement of a vascular sheath in the supraclavicular common carotid artery.
- Following carotid revascularization, the immediate postoperative care is focused on close neurologic surveillance. Patients are recovered typically in an intensive care unit or monitored setting to facilitate ready identification of evolving neurologic deficits.
- Careful blood pressure monitoring and management is also essential. Following carotid revascularization, patients need to avoid the extremes of blood pressure, which may lead to development of hemodynamic stroke and cerebral reperfusion syndromes that can result in devastating intracerebral hemorrhage.
- Immediate postoperative (<24 hours) neurologic deficits should be assumed to be thromboembolic in nature, most commonly associated with a technical (surgical) error. Further imaging studies are unlikely to alter decision-making and should not delay immediate re-exploration. Neurologic deficits arising later in the postoperative period (>24 hours) may be due to intracranial hemorrhage; in these cases, computed tomography (CT) or magnetic resonance (MR) imaging may assist the decision-making process and should be considered when etiologic circumstances are less certain.
- Bleeding complications following carotid surgery are rare but potentially serious or fatal. These typically occur during the first several hours after surgery or even later, particularly in patients resuming anticoagulation therapy for existing conditions early in the postoperative period. Recognition and expeditious control of the airway is of utmost importance as a wound hematoma develops, as cord and airway edema rapidly worsen in response to reduced venous and lymphatic drainage. Reopening a carotid incision prior to anesthetic induction may facilitate emergency endotracheal intubation; however, this dramatic maneuver is best performed in a controlled environment with resuscitation equipment available should complications ensue. Ideally, preparations are made for wound decompression as endotracheal intubation is being attempted, with the wound being opened as a last step maneuver prior to emergency cricothyroidotomy. Cord edema in these circumstances may be profound, however, and visualization may not improve sufficiently after hematoma evacuation to enable orotracheal or nasotracheal intubation. Therefore, cricothyroidotomy may become necessary in extreme circumstances, and all carotid surgeons should be facile in this maneuver as a matter of course.

OUTCOMES

- Surgical outcomes of distal carotid exposure are dependent on the nature of disease vs lesion extent. Equivalent surgical mortality and neurologic outcomes are seen in patients undergoing CEA regardless of the extent of disease involvement.[1,10] Permanent cranial nerve injuries, however, are more realized with higher lesions. When distal carotid/skull base exposure appears to be necessary to safely manage an occlusive lesion, consideration should again be given to CAS as a lower risk alternative technique to open endarterectomy or interposition grafting.[10]
- Data describing the outcome of distal (base of skull) carotid reconstruction and bypass for aneurysmal disease or tumors are based on more limited, institution-specific case series. In these circumstances, outcomes are more difficult to benchmark. One recent series reported that one of five patients requiring a distal ICA bypass for aneurysm repair suffered a stroke; 60% suffered varying degrees of cranial nerve deficit.[11] The largest experience reported to date is that of Sessa et al,[12] who reported a 3% and 6% rate of perioperative stroke and restenosis at 1 year, respectively.

COMPLICATIONS

- Cranial nerve injury
- Stroke
- Horner syndrome
- Seroma
- Infection

REFERENCES

1. Vang S, Hans SS. Carotid endarterectomy in patients with high plaque. *Surgery*. 2019;166(4):601-606. doi:10.1016/j.surg.2019.06.017. Epub 2019 Aug 9. PMID: 31405580.
2. Attigah N, Hyhlik-Dürr A, Hakimi M, Allenberg JR, Böckler D. Der hohe Zugang zur Arteria carotis interna [High exposure of the distal internal carotid artery]. Article in German. *Chirurg*. 2010;81(2):155-159. doi: 10.1007/s00104-009-1784-y. PMID: 19711019.
3. North American symptomatic carotid endarterectomy trial. Methods, patient characteristics, and progress. *Stroke*. 1991;22:711-720.
4. Endarterectomy for asymptomatic carotid artery stenosis. Executive Committee for the asymptomatic carotid atherosclerosis study. *JAMA*. 1995;273:1421-1428.
5. Randomised trial of endarterectomy for recently symptomatic carotid stenosis: final results of the MRC European Carotid Surgery Trial (ECST). *Lancet*. 1998;351:1379-1387.
6. Weiss MR, Smith HP, Patterson AK, Weiss M. Patient positioning and nasal intubation for carotid endarterectomy. *Neurosurgery*. 1986;19(2):256-257.
7. Takigawa T, Yanaka K, Yasuda M, Asakawa H, Matsumaru Y, Nose T. Head and neck extension-fixation with a head frame for exposure of the distal internal carotid artery in carotid endarterectomy–technical note. *Neurol Med Chir (Tokyo)*. 2003;43:271-273. discussion 273, 2003.
8. Capoccia L, Montelione N, Menna D, et al. Mandibular subluxation as an adjunct in very distal carotid arterial reconstruction: incidence of peripheral and cerebral neurologic sequelae in a single-center experience. *Ann Vasc Surg*. 2014;28:358-365.

9. Tameo MN, Dougherty MJ, Calligaro KD. Carotid endarterectomy with adjunctive cephalad carotid stenting: complementary, not competitive, techniques. *J Vasc Surg*. 2008;48(2):351-354. doi:10.1016/j.jvs.2008.03.054. PMID: 18644483.
10. Kondo T, Ota N, Göhre F, et al. High cervical carotid endarterectomy-outcome analysis. *World Neurosurg*. 2020;136:e108-e118. doi: 10.1016/j.wneu.2019.12.002. Epub 2019 Dec 9. PMID: 31830599.
11. Eliason JL, Netterville JL, Guzman RJ, et al. Skull base resection with cervical-to-petrous carotid artery bypass to facilitate repair of distal internal carotid artery lesions. *Cardiovasc Surg*. 2002;10:31-37.
12. Sessa CN, Morasch MD, Berguer R, et al. Carotid resection and replacement with autogenous arterial graft during operation for neck malignancy. *Ann Vasc Surg*. 1998;12:229-235.

Chapter 6 Vertebral Transposition Techniques and Stenting

Mark D. Morasch

DEFINITION

- Treatment for occlusive lesions involving the origin of the vertebral artery (V1 segment) is undertaken to relieve posterior brain circulation ischemia, otherwise known as vertebrobasilar insufficiency. Revascularization options include open surgical and endovascular techniques. The most common operation is a proximal vertebral to common carotid transposition. Endoluminal treatment includes balloon angioplasty and (typically) stenting.

DIFFERENTIAL DIAGNOSIS

- Other medical conditions mimicking posterior circulation ischemia include postural hypotension, cardiac arrhythmias, anemia, brain tumors, and benign vertiginous states. A thorough investigation consists of ruling out (1) inner ear pathology, (2) cardiac arrhythmias, (3) internal carotid artery stenosis/occlusion, and (4) complications of excessive blood pressure control (**TABLE 1**).
- Evaluation of patients with posterior circulation ischemia requires defining the precise circumstances that elicit symptoms. Vertigo, instability, and occasional loss of consciousness often accompany positional changes and standing in older individuals due to reduced sympathetic venous tone. This is particularly common in patients with diabetes. The presence of orthostatic hypotension should be evaluated as a common alternative cause for vertebrobasilar symptoms. Any decreases in basilar artery perfusion pressure may precipitate hemodynamic symptomatology, with or without concomitant vertebral occlusive disease.
- The next most common cause of brainstem ischemia is reduced cardiac output. When suspected, evaluation includes 24-hour Holter monitoring and echocardiography. In patients with vertebrobasilar insufficiency, palpitations may be noted with the onset of symptoms. Transesophageal echocardiography may be necessary to rule out structural heart issues.
- Inner ear pathology, including rare cerebellopontine angle tumors, produces symptoms suggestive of vertebrobasilar insufficiency. Benign vertiginous states should also be considered. Physical examination can alert the physician to the possibility of subclavian steal syndrome in patients with differences in brachial blood pressure greater than 25 mm Hg or with diminished left upper extremity pulses. Reversed flow in the ipsilateral vertebral artery demonstrated on duplex scanning is pathognomonic for subclavian steal physiology and subclavian steal syndrome in patients with appropriate symptoms at rest or following exercise in the ipsilateral upper extremity.
- Patients may relate symptoms of vertebrobasilar insufficiency to positional changes, including turning or extending their head. These dynamic symptoms usually appear when turning the head to one side. In this circumstance, symptoms may be elicited by extrinsic compression of the dominant or sole vertebral artery (in the case of unilateral occlusion) by adjacent arthritic bone spurs.[1]

Table 1: Nonvascular and Cardiac Conditions That Mimic Vertebrobasilar Ischemia

Cardiac arrhythmia
Pacemaker malfunction
Cardioemboli
Antihypertensive medications
Labyrinthine dysfunction
Cerebellopontine angle tumors
Cerebellar degeneration
Myxedema
Electrolyte imbalance
Hypoglycemia

PATIENT HISTORY AND PHYSICAL FINDINGS

- In general, ischemic mechanisms in vertebrobasilar insufficiency can be categorized as hemodynamic or embolic. Symptoms of vertebrobasilar insufficiency include dizziness, vertigo, drop attacks, diplopia, perioral numbness, alternating paresthesia, tinnitus, dysphasia, dysarthria, and ataxia. When two or more of these symptoms are present, vertebrobasilar ischemia is more likely to be the inciting cause. Unlike other regions of the brain, strokes in the posterior circulation territory occur due to large artery occlusive diseases.
- Patients with "hemodynamic" ischemia experience transient vertebrobasilar symptoms due to inadequate vertebral artery inflow or collateral circulation. Symptoms are typically short lived, repetitive, somewhat predictable, and rarely result in stroke. Postural hypotension may precipitate serious traumatic injury, however, when patients lose their balance with standing.
- Embolic events may also precipitate vertebrobasilar ischemia as well as cerebellar and brainstem infarction. Microemboli from the heart, aortic arch, or any arteries leading directly to the basilar artery may arise from atherosclerotic lesions, intimal defects, repetitive trauma, fibromuscular dysplasia lesions, aneurysms, or dissections. Although much less

common than hemodynamic vertebrobasilar insufficiency, when present, microemboli are much more likely to cause fatal events or debilitating infarcts.[2-4]

- Timing of the onset of symptoms following positional changes may help differentiate vertebrobasilar insufficiency from labyrinthine disorders. In the latter circumstance, rapid head movement invokes immediate symptoms. In the case of vertebrobasilar insufficiency, however, a short delay usually precedes the onset of symptoms, including nystagmus.

IMAGING AND OTHER DIAGNOSTIC STUDIES

Duplex ultrasound, an otherwise excellent tool for the assessment of extracranial cerebrovascular disease, has limitations in the diagnosis of vertebral artery pathology. Direct visualization of the second portion is obscured by the transverse processes of C2-C6. As previously mentioned, however, duplex imaging reliably identifies subclavian steal physiology, as well as detects proximal velocity increases consistent with orificial vertebral or proximal subclavian stenosis.[5]

- Magnetic resonance imaging (MRI) provides safe, noninvasive, and detailed evaluation of the aortic arch and great vessels, the extracranial and intracranial arterial vasculature, as well as the presence of mass lesions, fluid collections, or parenchymal defects in the posterior fossa. Contrast-enhanced magnetic resonance angiography (MRA), with three-dimensional reconstruction and maximum image intensity techniques, provides excellent image quality in high resolution (**FIGURE 1**). As in other applications, however, in low-flow circumstances, excessive signal dropout may result in overestimation of lesion severity based on signal intensity alone.
- In contrast to computed tomographic (CT) imaging, transaxial MRI readily diagnoses both acute and chronic brain infarctions in the posterior fossa. Brainstem infarctions are typically small and as such may be overlooked with noncontrast CT imaging. Brain MRI is performed in symptomatic patients prior to vertebral artery intervention to identify infarctions when they are present and provide baseline images for future comparison.
- Evaluation of vertebral anatomy via catheter-based, contrast arteriography requires acquisition of images in multiple projections to fully evaluate the entire extent of both vertebral arteries. Evaluation begins with the aortic arch to determine the origin of the bilateral vertebral arteries. Anomalous origin of the left vertebral artery, arising directly from the aorta proximal to the left subclavian, is present in 6% of patients. Much less frequently, the right vertebral artery originates from the innominate or right common carotid artery. This anomaly often accompanies an aberrant right subclavian artery, which itself may precipitate symptoms of dysphagia lusoria.
- Usually, right and left posterior oblique projections are sufficient to comprehensively evaluate the V1 (first) vertebral artery segment from the origin to the transverse process of C6. In most patients, the left artery is usually dominant, but a number of normal variants may be encountered, including congenital atresia of either vertebral artery.
- The vertebral artery origin may not be visualized adequately with either duplex ultrasonography or MRA. Oblique projections are required during arteriography due to superimposition of the subclavian artery over the vertebral origin. Additional projections, including craniocaudal tube angulation, may also be required to optimize visualization. The presence of a poststenotic dilatation in the first centimeter of the vertebral artery is a clue that should prompt further projections to isolate the origin from the overlying subclavian artery.
- Dynamic arteriography, incorporating provocative positioning, may be required to assess the possibility of extrinsic vertebral artery compression. Finally, delayed imaging may demonstrate reconstitution of patent distal extracranial vertebral arteries through cervical collaterals when the origin initially appears occluded.

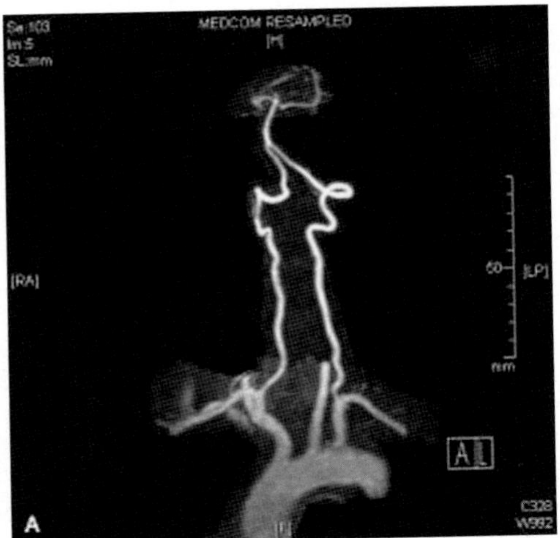

FIGURE 1 • Vertebral MRA (with the carotid image subtracted).

SURGICAL MANAGEMENT

- Some degree of vertebral artery orificial stenosis is present in 20% to 40% of patients with other manifestations of cerebrovascular disease.[2] A number of operative approaches will satisfactorily address V1 segment disease and orificial stenosis.[6,7] Vertebral transposition or repositioning of the origin of the vertebral artery onto the adjacent common carotid artery is the most common. Endoluminal dilatation, with or without stenting, is also appropriate in selected circumstances.

Vertebral to Common Carotid Transposition

- General endotracheal anesthesia is preferred. Positioning supine, with the back of the table slightly elevated toward a chair position with the head rotated away from the planned incision site facilitates additional deep mediastinal exposure when required.
- Proximal vertebral artery exposure is similar to that required for subclavian-to-carotid transposition. One fingerbreadth above the clavicle, a transverse incision is created directly over the two heads of the sternocleidomastoid muscle (SCM). Between the SCM heads, the omohyoid muscle is identified and divided. Lateral retraction of the internal jugular vein and vagus nerve exposes the carotid sheath medially. Maximal proximal carotid artery exposure, facilitated by positioning of the primary operator at head of the patient, is necessary to ensure an optimal result (**FIGURE 2**).
- The sympathetic ganglia are identified running behind and parallel to the carotid artery. On the left side, the thoracic duct is divided between ligatures to minimize lymphatic leaks. The proximal end should be doubly ligated, avoiding

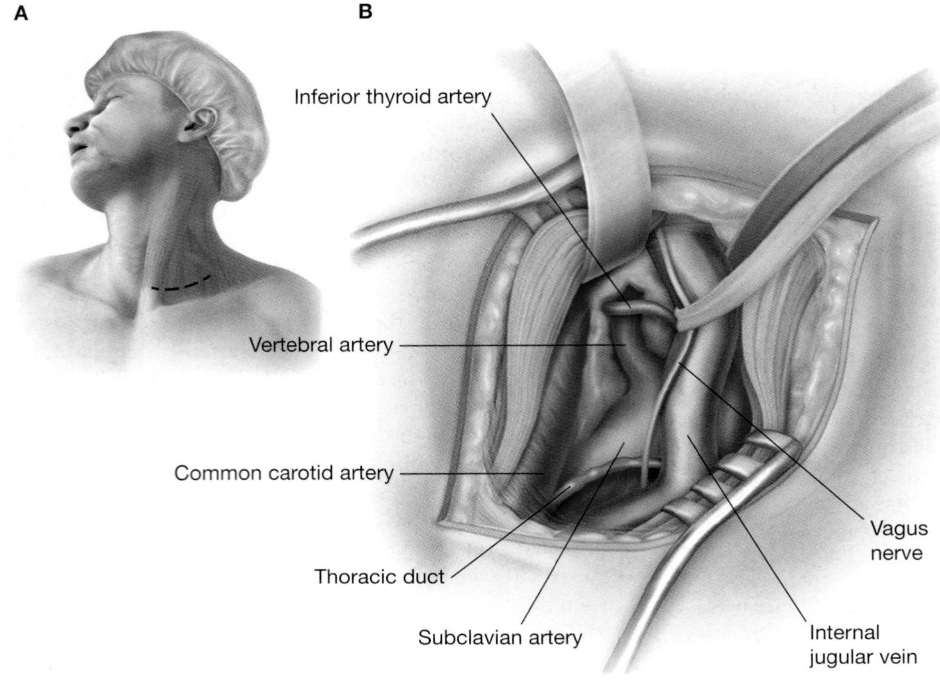

FIGURE 2 ● **A,** Access to the proximal vertebral artery between the sternocleidomastoid muscle bellies. **B,** Transposition of the proximal vertebral artery to the posterior wall of the common carotid artery.

transfixion sutures. Accessory lymph ducts—often seen on the right side—should also be ligated and divided when identified. The entire dissection is confined medial to the prescalene fat pad covering the scalenus anticus muscle and phrenic nerve. These latter structures are left unexposed lateral to the field. The inferior thyroid artery, running transversely across the field, is also ligated and divided.

- The vertebral vein is next identified emerging from the angle formed by the longus colli and scalenus anticus and overlying the vertebral artery and, at the bottom of the field, the subclavian artery. Unlike its sister artery, the vertebral vein has branches. It is ligated in continuity and divided. Below the vertebral vein lies the vertebral artery. It is important to identify and avoid injury to the adjacent sympathetic chain. The vertebral artery is dissected superiorly to the tendon of the longus colli and inferiorly to its origin in the subclavian artery. The vertebral artery is freed from the sympathetic trunk resting on its anterior surface without damaging the trunk or the ganglionic rami. Preserving the sympathetic trunks and the stellate or intermediate ganglia resting on the artery usually requires freeing the vertebral artery from these structures, and after dividing its origin, the latter is transposed anterior to the sympathetics.
- Once the artery is fully exposed, an appropriate site for reimplantation in the common carotid artery is selected. The patient is systemically anticoagulated with intravenous heparin. The distal portion of the V1 segment of the vertebral artery is clamped below the edge of the longus colli with a microclip placed vertically to indicate the orientation of the artery and to avoid axial twisting during its transposition. The proximal vertebral artery is closed by transfixion with 5-0 polypropylene suture immediately above the stenosis at its origin. The artery is divided at this level, and its proximal stump is further secured with a hemoclip. The artery is then brought to the common carotid artery and its free end is spatulated for anastomosis.
- The carotid artery is then crossclamped. An elliptical 5- to 7-mm arteriotomy is created in the posterolateral wall of the common carotid artery with an aortic punch. The anastomosis is performed in open fashion with a continuous 6-0 or 7-0 polypropylene suture while avoiding any tension on the vertebral artery, which tears easily. Before completion of the anastomosis, any slack in the suture is tightened appropriately with a nerve hook, standard flushing maneuvers are performed, and the suture is tied to reestablish flow (**FIGURE 3**).

Vertebral Artery Angioplasty and Stent Placement

- In the past decade, endovascular treatment of vertebral artery disease has gained increasing acceptance. For endovascular intervention, patients are pretreated with dual antiplatelet therapy (aspirin and clopidogrel). The procedure is usually performed with local anesthesia and conscious sedation, enabling continuous neurologic monitoring of the patient. The patients are positioned supine and prepped to allow percutaneous entry into the chosen access vessel. Most cases are performed from a femoral approach (93%), although transbrachial (3%) and transradial (5%) access has also been used as noted in one recent review.[8] The stenotic lesions are crossed and then dilated with 0.014- or 0.018-in guidewires and small coronary-diameter balloons. If a stent is chosen, these are usually bare metal type, but drug elution has also been used. The same 0.014- or 0.018-in guidewires are used as platforms over which the stents are delivered and then deployed. Postdeployment angioplasty may be necessary in selected cases. Procedures can be performed with or without the assistance of embolic protection, although most vertebral arteries are too small to accommodate most distal protection devices.

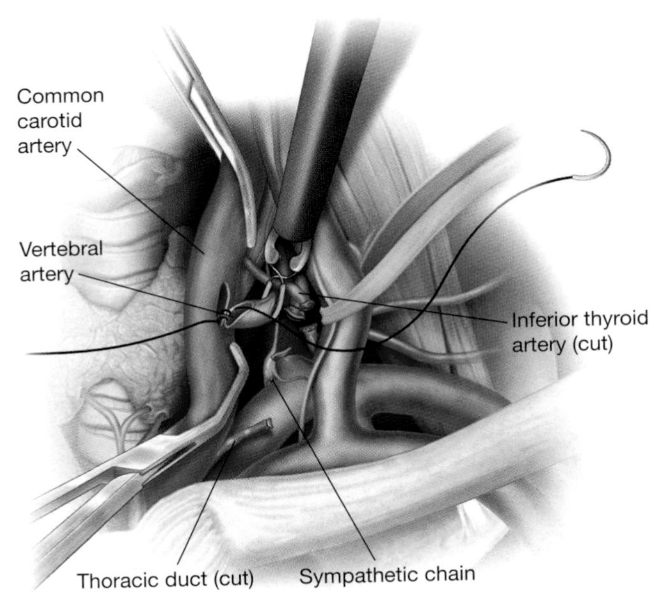

FIGURE 3 ● Proximal vertebral-to-common carotid transposition.

PEARLS AND PITFALLS

Placement of incision	■ It is important to place the incision medially enough to dissect between the heads of the sternocleidomastoid. An approach lateral to this structure will make the transposition challenging, if not impossible, to complete.
Orientation	■ Enough of the V1 segment of the vertebral artery, up to near where it disappears into the transverse process of C6, needs to be mobilized. Also, plan ahead and see where on the carotid is best to reimplant the vertebral before creating the carotid arteriotomy.
Closure	■ A drain is usually helpful, especially on the left side where the thoracic duct crosses the exposure, just in case a tie comes off of a large lymphatic. The drain allows for early diagnosis of this complication.

POSTOPERATIVE CARE

- Following surgical transposition, absent significant lymphatic drainage from the wound, the patient may be safely discharged on the first or second postoperative day. Similarly, after endoluminal therapy, patients are kept overnight to ensure neurologic stability.

OUTCOMES

- After proximal vertebral-to-common carotid transposition, patency rates at 5 and 10 years equal or exceed 95% and 91%, respectively. When selected appropriately, more than 80% of patients will experience symptomatic relief following proximal surgical reconstruction.[9]
- Appropriate reconstruction and subsequent reperfusion of the brainstem in patients experiencing hemodynamic vertebrobasilar symptoms may also improve hypertension management.
- Overall, retrospective reviews suggest that endoluminal vertebral artery intervention is reasonably safe, although a selection bias exists. A 2005 Cochrane review identified 313 interventions for vertebral artery stenosis, with just over half using stent placement as part of the treatment. The technical success rate was 95%, and the 30-day stroke and death rate was 6.4%.[10]
- Despite high technical success rates, vertebral artery angioplasty alone, especially when used for the treatment of disease at the origin of the vessel, appears to have an unacceptably high rate of restenosis. Adjuvant stent placement adds to the clinical durability but adds potential morbidity such as malposition or potential fracture. In their series of 105 patients who underwent endovascular stenting for symptomatic vertebral artery disease, Jenkins et al[11] achieved 100% radiographic improvement (residual stenosis ≤30%). The authors reported immediate (30-day) periprocedural risk of death of 1% and periprocedural complication rate of 4.8%. Complications included transient ischemic attack, flow-limiting dissection, hematoma, and catheter-access-site problems. At 1 year of follow-up, six patients had died and five had experienced a vertebrobasilar stroke, and at approximately 2.5 years of follow-up, 70% of patients remained symptom-free, but 13% of patients had restenosis requiring retreatment.[11]
- A recent systematic review of the available literature noted a weighted mean technical success rate of 97%. The authors estimated mean periprocedural stroke and death rate from combined angioplasty and stenting to be around 1.1%.

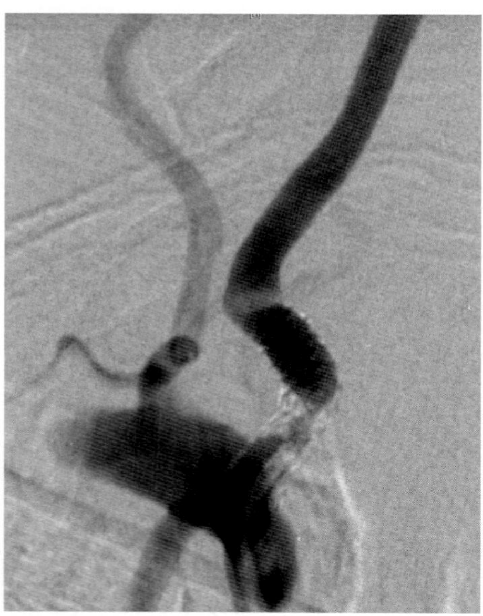

FIGURE 4 ● Vertebral artery stent with fracture and in-stent restenosis. (Reprinted from Cronenwett JL, Johnston KW, eds. *Rutherford's Vascular Surgery*. 7th ed. Saunders; 2010. Copyright © 2010 Elsevier. With permission.)

Transient ischemic events occurred in 1.5% of patients. Recurrent symptoms occurred in 8% of patients within a reported range of follow-up of 6 to 54 months and greater than 50% restenosis developed in 23% of the subset of patients who underwent follow-up imaging.[8]

COMPLICATIONS

- Proximal vertebral to common carotid transposition has been reported to have a combined stroke and death rate of 0.9%.[9] Among patients undergoing this operation, in one report, there were no deaths or strokes in those who underwent only a vertebral reconstruction. Berguer and coauthors reported four instances of immediate postoperative thrombosis (1.4%). Three of the four patients had vein grafts interposed between the vertebral artery and the common carotid because of a short V1 segment. The grafts kinked and thrombosed. Other complications that are particular to proximal reconstruction include vagus and recurrent laryngeal nerve palsy (2%), Horner syndrome (8.4%-28%), lymphocele (4%), and chylothorax (0.5%).
- Periprocedural risks for angioplasty and stenting include access complications, distal embolization and stroke, arterial rupture, stent malposition, and vessel thrombosis or dissection. Later, restenosis and stent fracture are not uncommon (**FIGURE 4**).

REFERENCES

1. Bauer R. Mechanical compression of the vertebral arteries. In: Berguer R, Bauer R, eds. *Vertebrobasilar Arterial Occlusive Disease: Medical and Surgical Management*. Raven; 1984:45-71.
2. Caplan LR, Wityk RJ, Glass TA, et al. New England medical center posterior circulation registry. *Ann Neurol*. 2004;56:389-398.
3. Caplan L, Tettenborn B. Embolism in the posterior circulation. In: Berguer R, Caplan L, eds. *Vertebrobasilar Arterial Disease*. Quality Medical; 1992:52-65.
4. Pessin M. Posterior cerebral artery disease and occipital ischemia. In: Berguer R, Caplan L, eds. *Vertebrobasilar Arterial Disease*. Quality Medical; 1992:66-75.
5. Berguer R, Higgins R, Nelson R. Noninvasive diagnosis of reversal of vertebral-artery blood flow. *N Engl J Med*. 1980;302:1349-1351.
6. Edwards WH, Mulherin JL Jr. The surgical approach to significant stenosis of vertebral and subclavian arteries. *Surgery*. 1980;87:20-28.
7. Roon AJ, Ehrenfeld WK, Cooke PB, et al. Vertebral artery reconstruction. *Am J Surg*. 1979;138:29-36.
8. Antoniou GA, Murray D, Georgiadis GS, et al. Percutaneous transluminal angioplasty and stenting in patients with proximal vertebral artery stenosis. *J Vasc Surg*. 2012;55:1167-1177.
9. Berguer R, Flynn LM, Kline RA, et al. Surgical reconstruction of the extracranial vertebral artery: management and outcome. *J Vasc Surg*. 2000;31:9-18.
10. Coward LJ, Featherstone RL, Brown MM. Percutaneous transluminal angioplasty and stenting for vertebral artery stenosis. *Cochrane Database Syst Rev*. 2005;2005(2):CD000516.
11. Jenkins JS, Patel SN, White CJ, et al. Endovascular stenting for vertebral artery stenosis. *J Am Coll Cardiol*. 2010;55(6):538-542.

Chapter 7

Neurogenic Thoracic Outlet Syndrome Exposure and Decompression: Supraclavicular

Robert W. Thompson and Esmaeel Reza Dadashzadeh

DEFINITION

- Thoracic outlet syndrome (TOS) is a group of conditions caused by compression of one of the neurovascular structures that serve the upper extremity.[1-3] Neurogenic TOS (NTOS) is the most frequent of these, occurring in 85% to 90% of patients. It is caused by compression and irritation of the brachial plexus nerves within the supraclavicular scalene triangle and/or underneath the pectoralis minor muscle tendon in the subcoracoid space (**FIGURE 1**). NTOS tends to occur between the ages of 15 and 40 years and typically results in neck and upper extremity pain, paresthesia, and functional limitations. Although relatively uncommon, clinical recognition and appropriate treatment of NTOS are crucial to prevent disability in young active individuals.
- The causes of NTOS include anatomical variations (anomalous scalene musculature, aberrant fibrofascial bands, and/or cervical ribs) and previous neck or upper extremity injury, which has resulted in scalene/pectoralis muscle spasm, fibrosis, and other pathological changes. These muscular alterations, in turn, lead to compression and irritation of the adjacent brachial plexus nerves. The presence of a cervical rib is often cited as a predisposing factor in the development of NTOS; however, few patients with NTOS (approximately 10%) exhibit a definable cervical rib and the development of NTOS symptoms is rare, even in patients with a cervical rib, in the absence of additional injury.[4]
- NTOS often occurs in individuals engaged in occupational or recreational activities that involve repetitive overhead use of the arms and/or heavy lifting and may develop following various types of injury (eg, motor vehicle collisions or falls upon the outstretched arm). It may also arise as a consequence of low-grade repetitive strain injury (eg, prolonged keyboard use), poor posture, and dysfunctional shoulder girdle mechanics.
- Surgical treatment for NTOS may be effectively accomplished by several different approaches, including transaxillary first rib resection and anterior (supraclavicular) decompression. The supraclavicular approach has long been a mainstay in the surgical treatment of NTOS, providing excellent exposure for

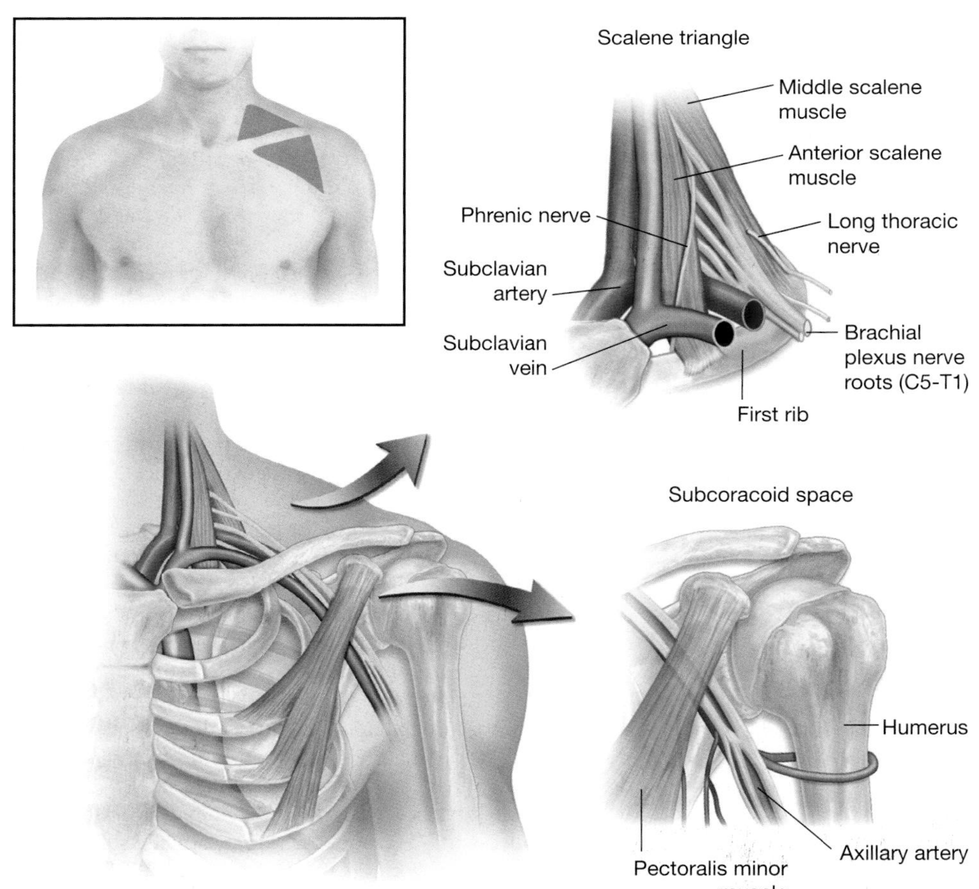

FIGURE 1 ● Anatomy of the thoracic outlet, with emphasis on the supraclavicular scalene triangle and the infraclavicular subcoracoid space.

safe and definitive decompression of the relevant neurovascular structures and the flexibility to manage the entire spectrum of circumstances that may be encountered.[5-7]

DIFFERENTIAL DIAGNOSIS

- NTOS produces symptoms that can mimic or overlap those observed in other upper extremity neurological and musculoskeletal disorders, producing a particularly broad differential diagnosis (**TABLE 1**).[2,8-10] Clinical evaluation requires differentiation of NTOS from other cervical-brachial syndromes and optimal selection of patients for different forms of treatment.
- NTOS should be readily differentiated from venous TOS, which produces marked arm swelling, cyanotic discoloration, and distention of subcutaneous veins around the shoulder and chest wall, and often presents with axillary-subclavian vein "effort thrombosis" (Paget-Schroetter syndrome).[2] NTOS should also be distinguished from arterial TOS, which causes either fixed subclavian artery obstruction, resulting in cramping muscular fatigue with arm use similar to intermittent claudication, or poststenotic subclavian artery aneurysm formation, which can cause thromboembolism, hand ischemia, rest pain, and/or digital ulceration and necrosis.[2]
- Some patients with NTOS exhibit severe upper extremity pain and hypersensitivity, with digital swelling and discoloration, suggesting the presence of sympathetic nerve overactivity. In such cases, the possibility of reflex sympathetic dystrophy (complex regional pain syndrome) should be considered and evaluated using a temporary cervical sympathetic (stellate ganglion) anesthetic block.

PATIENT HISTORY AND PHYSICAL FINDINGS

- Symptoms attributable to brachial plexus nerve compression include pain, numbness, and tingling (paresthesia) in the neck, shoulder, arm, and hand. The distribution of symptoms in the hand often extends beyond that expected for either the median or ulnar nerves, involving all fingers. Patients with NTOS attributable to compression at the pectoralis minor tendon often describe upper anterior chest and axillary pain. The intensity of symptoms of NTOS can vary with the extent of upper extremity activity and is usually reliably exacerbated with arm elevation and abduction.[2,8-10]
- Many patients with NTOS have relatively mild symptoms, with a slow gradual progression interspersed by occasional exacerbations. Others exhibit a steady progression in the severity of symptoms leading to increasing and significant disability. Hand muscle weakness and atrophy (Gilliatt-Sumner hand) are rare and occur when there is particularly advanced and longstanding brachial plexus compression, associated with a cervical rib or other bony anomaly.
- Physical examination of patients with NTOS usually reveals well-localized tenderness to palpation over the supraclavicular scalene triangle and/or the infraclavicular subcoracoid space, associated with reproduction of upper extremity symptoms[2,8-10] (**FIGURE 2**).
- Most patients with NTOS exhibit rapid reproduction of upper extremity symptoms with provocative positional maneuvers, such as the upper limb tension test or the 3-minute elevated arm stress test (**FIGURE 2**). Positional dampening of the radial artery pulse at the wrist during arm abduction and external rotation (Adson test) is nonspecific and inaccurate and is not useful in establishing or excluding a diagnosis of NTOS.[2,11]
- Physical examination should include assessment for potential cervical spine degenerative disease and peripheral nerve compression (carpal tunnel and cubital canal syndromes), as well as any evidence of arterial or venous compromise to the upper extremity. Signs of upper extremity sympathetic overactivity should also be sought (mild digital swelling and discoloration, and skin hypersensitivity or allodynia).
- Documentation of patient-reported symptoms and quantification of the level of disability prior to treatment are facilitated by the use of various survey forms and other outcome measurement tools, such as the Disabilities of the Arm, Shoulder and Hand and quality-of-life instruments.[2,9,10,12] Repeated use of these instruments at various intervals before and following treatment has become increasingly important to assess the outcomes of different management strategies.[13]

Table 1: Differential Diagnosis of Neurogenic Thoracic Outlet Syndrome

Acromioclavicular arthropathy	Fibromyalgia and fibromyositis
Arterial atheroembolism	Nerve sheath neoplasm
Brachial plexus (stretch) injury	Pancoast tumor (lung apex)
Carpal tunnel syndrome (median nerve)	Parsonage-Turner syndrome
Cervical dystonia	Psychogenic syndrome
Cervical spine degenerative arthritis	Radial nerve compression (extensor forearm)
Complex regional pain syndrome	Raynaud syndrome
Cervical spine degenerative disc disease	Rotator cuff tendinitis
Cervical spine (muscular) strain	Scleroderma
Cubital canal syndrome (ulnar nerve)	Vasculitis

IMAGING AND OTHER DIAGNOSTIC STUDIES

- Although imaging and other diagnostic studies may provide helpful ancillary information, there are none with sufficient sensitivity or specificity to confirm or exclude the diagnosis of NTOS. Identification of NTOS thereby remains a clinical diagnosis dependent on experienced pattern recognition.[14]
- Plain anteroposterior chest radiographs may be useful to determine the presence or absence of a cervical rib. Other types of imaging studies of the brachial plexus are not specifically helpful in diagnosis or planning treatment (**FIGURE 3**).
- Conventional electrophysiological tests (electromyography and nerve conduction studies) are often performed to exclude peripheral nerve compression disorders or cervical radiculopathy. These tests are usually negative or nonspecific in NTOS and cannot be used to establish or exclude the diagnosis.[2]
- Vascular laboratory studies (Duplex ultrasound) are often performed to detect alterations in upper extremity blood flow that can be attributed to subclavian artery compression during arm elevation. However, positional subclavian artery compression may only be an incidental and unrelated vascular finding and does not establish a diagnosis of NTOS, nor does it represent arterial TOS. Vascular laboratory studies do not assess brachial plexus compression and are therefore of little specific value in the evaluation of patients with suspected NTOS.[11]
- Imaging-guided anterior scalene muscle and/or pectoralis minor muscle blocks with a local anesthetic can provide support for the clinical diagnosis of NTOS.[15-18] A positive block, characterized by a temporary relief or improvement in the presenting symptoms, is almost always attributable to NTOS. A positive

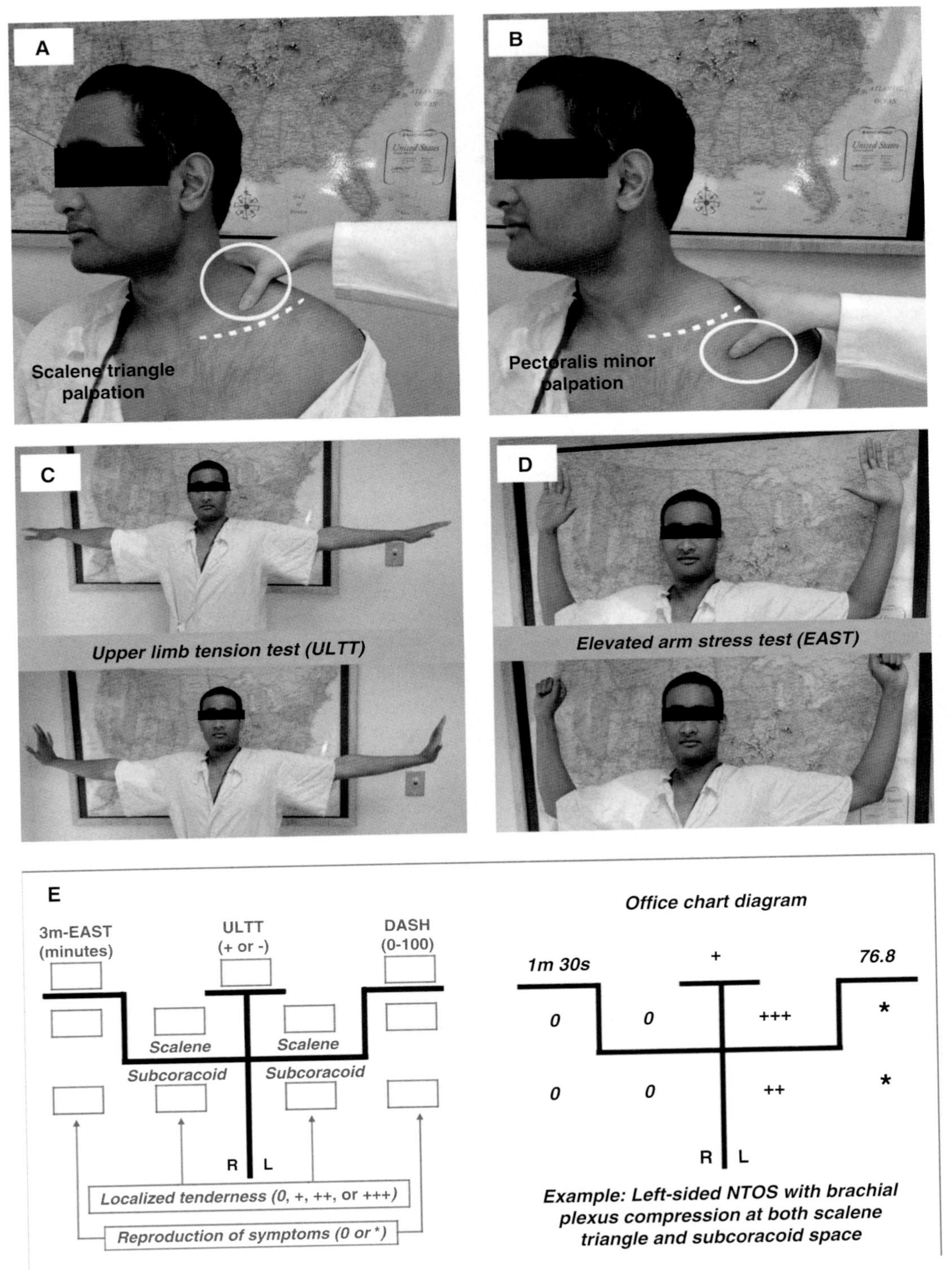

FIGURE 2 ● Physical examination reveals localized tenderness to palpation over the supraclavicular scalene triangle **(A)** and/or the infraclavicular subcoracoid space **(B)**. The upper limb tension test (ULTT) **(C)** and the 3-minute elevated arm stress test (EAST) **(D)** utilize provocative positional maneuvers that rapidly elicit reproduction of upper extremity symptoms in patients with neurogenic thoracic outlet syndrome (NTOS). An office chart diagram is used to easily summarize physical examination findings for patients being evaluated for NTOS **(E)**.

muscle block can also help predict the reversibility of symptoms with treatment and is therefore useful in prognosis. In contrast, a negative anterior scalene/pectoralis minor muscle block is not sufficiently interpretable to exclude a diagnosis of NTOS or to preclude consideration of patients for surgical treatment.

- Initial treatment for NTOS is based on physical therapy to relieve scalene/pectoralis minor muscle spasm, improve postural disturbances, enhance functional limb mobility, strengthen associated shoulder girdle musculature, and diminish repetitive strain exposure in the workplace.

Incorrect approaches to physical therapy can result in worsening of symptoms and premature failure of conservative management. In most patients with mild NTOS or with symptoms of short duration, significant improvement is usually observed within the initial 4 to 6 weeks of physical therapy. Because NTOS is often a chronic condition subject to occasional "flare-ups" of acute symptoms (often related to overuse activities or new injury), such patients should continue regular physical therapy exercises during long-term follow-up. Patients that have not improved with an appropriate trial of physical therapy and other conservative measures are considered candidates for surgical treatment.[2,13]

SURGICAL MANAGEMENT

- Supraclavicular decompression (scalenectomy, first rib resection, and brachial plexus neurolysis) is a recommended treatment option when there is (1) a sound clinical diagnosis of NTOS, (2) substantial disability (symptoms interfering with daily activities and/or work), and (3) an insufficient response to targeted physical therapy.[5-7,13,19] Supraclavicular decompression is also ideal for patients with persistent or recurrent symptoms of NTOS following a previous operation, when there has been no response to appropriate conservative measures.

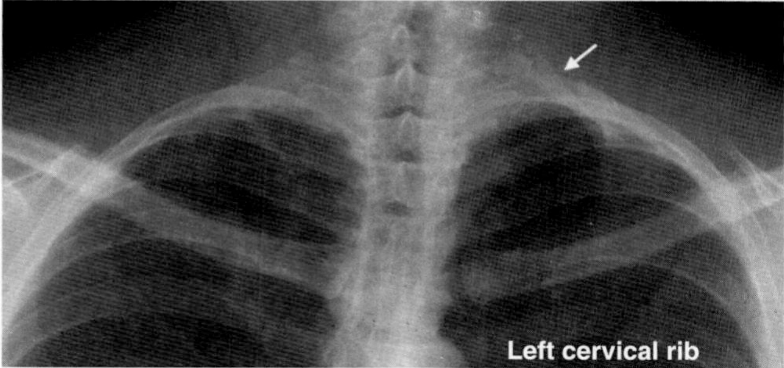

FIGURE 3 • A left-sided cervical rib identified by plain chest radiography (*arrow*).

- For patients with symptoms of NTOS referable to the subcoracoid space, pectoralis minor tenotomy is an important addition to supraclavicular thoracic outlet decompression. Pectoralis minor tenotomy may also be performed as an isolated procedure when the subcoracoid space is the dominant location of nerve compression symptoms.[20,21]
- Surgical treatment should be staged for patients with bilateral NTOS. The initial supraclavicular decompression, with or without pectoralis minor tenotomy, is performed on the side with the most severe symptoms or for the dominant upper extremity. If contralateral symptoms persist or progress, supraclavicular decompression on the second side may be recommended at least 6 to 12 weeks later. Normal phrenic nerve function should be verified on the side of the previous procedure, by chest fluoroscopic examination, before proceeding with a contralateral operation.

Preoperative Planning

- The supraclavicular surgical site is marked in the preoperative holding area, being sure to include the subcoracoid space if concomitant pectoralis minor tenotomy is planned. Prophylactic antibiotics are administered within an hour of the planned procedure.
- An erector spinae plane local anesthetic block is placed in the preoperative holding area as a useful adjunct to help manage postoperative pain.[22]

Positioning

- After the induction of general endotracheal anesthesia, the patient is positioned supine with the head of the operating table elevated 30°. The neck is extended and turned to the opposite side, a small inflatable pillow is placed behind the shoulders, and the neck, chest, and affected upper extremity are prepped into the field. The arm is wrapped in stockinette to permit free range of movement during the operation and then held comfortably across the abdomen (**FIGURE 4**). Lower extremity sequential compression devices are used for thromboprophylaxis. Neuromuscular blocking agents are not used following the initial induction of anesthesia.

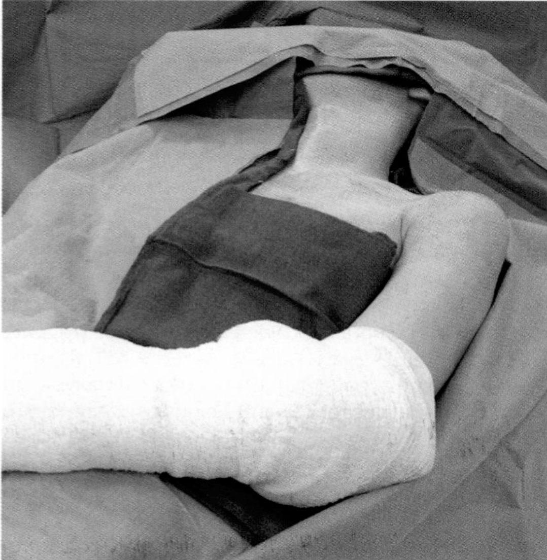

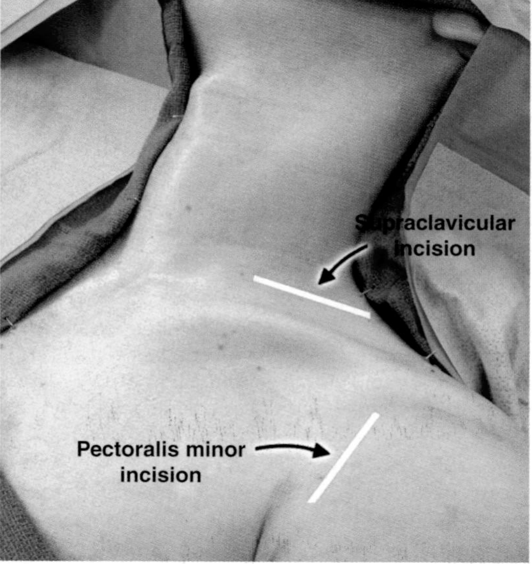

FIGURE 4 • Patient position and planned incisions for left-sided supraclavicular thoracic outlet decompression with pectoralis minor tenotomy.

SUPRACLAVICULAR DECOMPRESSION

Incision and Mobilization of the Scalene Fat Pad

- A transverse neck incision is made parallel to and just above the clavicle, beginning at the lateral edge of the sternocleidomastoid muscle and extending to the anterior edge of the trapezius muscle. The incision is carried through the subcutaneous layer, the platysma muscle is divided, and subplatysmal flaps are developed to expose the scalene fat pad. The sternocleidomastoid muscle is retracted medially, but is not divided (**FIGURE 5**).
- One of the keys to simplifying the supraclavicular exposure is proper mobilization and lateral reflection of the scalene fat pad. This begins with the detachment of the fat pad along the lateral edge of the internal jugular vein and the superior edge of the clavicle, with ligation of small blood vessels and lymphatic tissues. The thoracic duct, usually observed near the junction of the internal jugular and subclavian veins on the left side (a prominent accessory thoracic duct may also exist on the right side), may be ligated and divided. The omohyoid muscle is routinely divided (**FIGURE 5**).
- The scalene fat pad is progressively elevated in a medial to lateral direction, by gentle fingertip dissection over the surface of the anterior scalene muscle. The phrenic nerve is observed passing in a lateral to medial direction as it descends along the muscle surface. Gentle manipulation of the phrenic nerve produces a "dartle" (diaphragmatic startle) response.

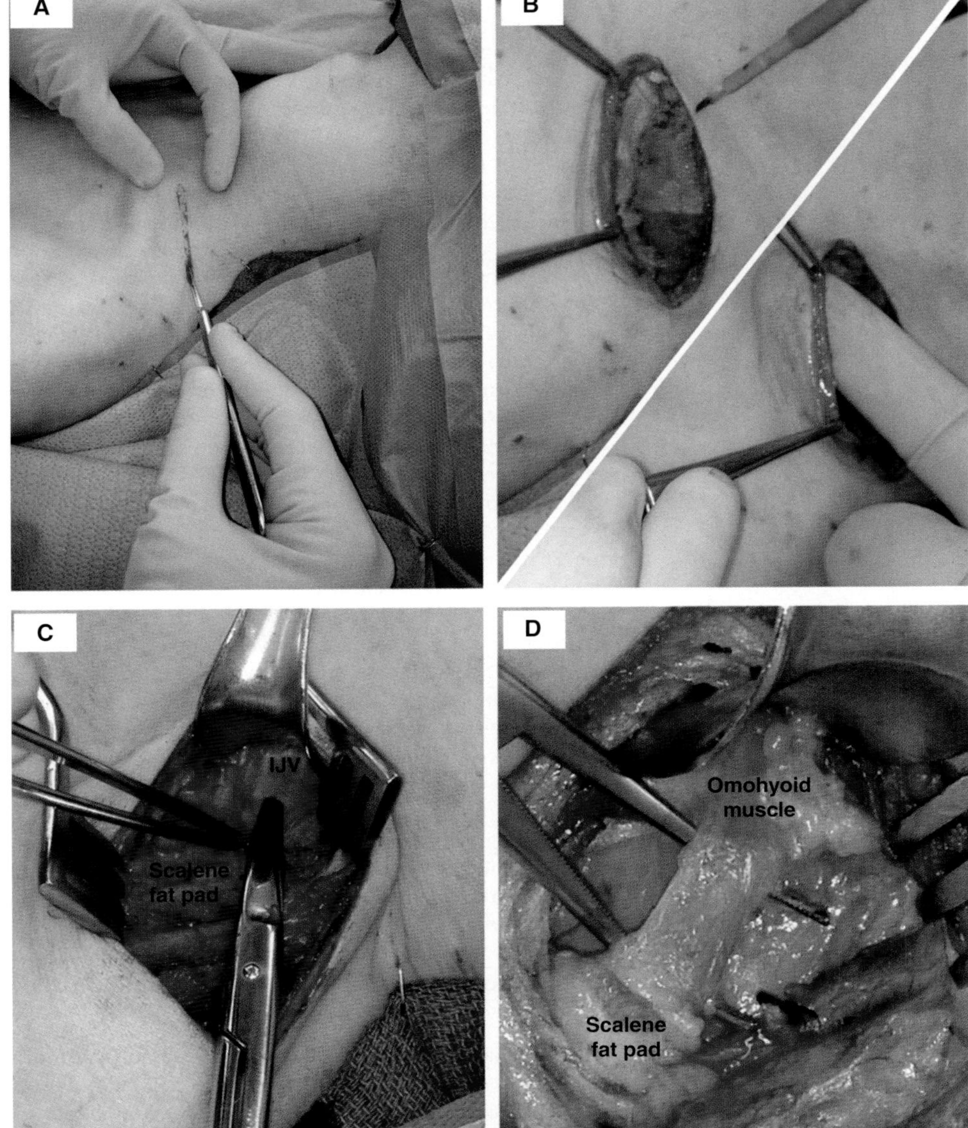

FIGURE 5 ● The skin incision is made just above and parallel to the clavicle, extending from the lateral border of the sternocleidomastoid muscle to the anterior border of the trapezius muscle **(A)**. Subplatysmal flaps are created to expose the underlying scalene fat pad **(B)**. The scalene fat pad is mobilized, beginning with its medial attachments to the internal jugular vein (IJV) **(C)**, and the omohyoid muscle is divided **(D)**.

Table 2: Critical Views Obtained During Supraclavicular Thoracic Outlet Decompression

1. View of the operative field after lateral reflection of the scalene fat pad with visualization of the internal jugular vein, anterior scalene muscle, phrenic nerve, brachial plexus, subclavian artery, middle scalene muscle, and long thoracic nerve.
2. View of the lower part of the anterior scalene muscle where it attaches to the first rib with space sufficient to allow a finger to pass behind the anterior scalene muscle and in front of the brachial plexus and subclavian artery prior to division of the anterior scalene muscle insertion from the top of the first rib.
3. View of the upper part of the anterior scalene muscle at the level of the C6 transverse process in relation to the C5 and C6 nerve roots prior to division of the anterior scalene muscle origin.
4. View of the insertion of the middle scalene muscle on the first rib with each of the five nerve roots of the brachial plexus and the subclavian artery retracted medially and the long thoracic nerve retracted laterally prior to division of the middle scalene muscle insertion from the top of the lateral first rib.
5. View of the posterior neck of the first rib with the T1 nerve root passing from underneath the rib to join the C8 nerve root to form the inferior trunk of the brachial plexus prior to division of the posterior first rib.
6. View of the anterior portion of the first rib with placement of the rib shears medial to the scalene tubercle prior to division of the anterior first rib.

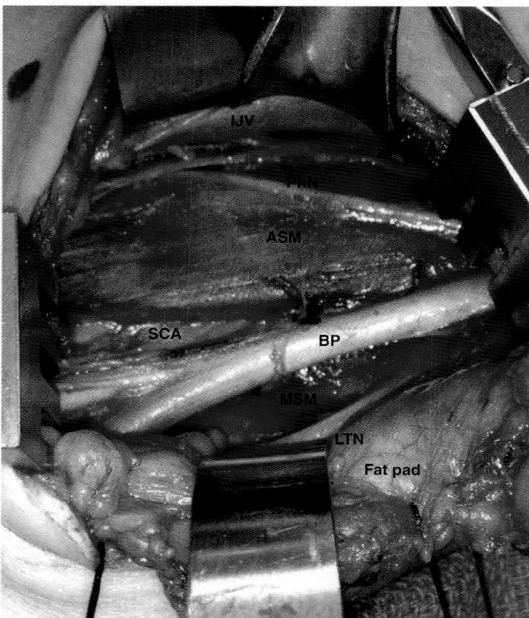

FIGURE 6 ● Following lateral reflection of the scalene fat pad, direct visualization is obtained of the internal jugular vein (IJV), anterior scalene muscle (ASM), phrenic nerve (PhN), brachial plexus (BP), subclavian artery (SCA), middle scalene muscle (MSM), and long thoracic nerve (LTN).

- Upon further lateral rotation of the scalene fat pad, the brachial plexus nerve roots (posterior and lateral to the anterior scalene muscle) and the middle scalene muscle (behind the brachial plexus) are brought into view. The lateral aspect of the first rib is palpated and visualized, and the long thoracic nerve is identified as it emerges from the body of the middle scalene muscle to course past the lateral part of the first rib. The scalene fat pad is then held in position with several silk retraction sutures and the exposure is maintained with a Henley self-retaining retractor (using the third arm to hold the edge of the sternocleidomastoid muscle). The resulting exposure represents the first and most important of six "critical views" to be obtained during supraclavicular decompression (**TABLE 2**) (**FIGURE 6**).

Anterior Scalenectomy

- Attention is turned to the insertion of the anterior scalene muscle on the first rib. At the lower lateral edge of the anterior scalene muscle, the subclavian artery and brachial plexus are carefully mobilized until a fingertip can easily pass behind the muscle just above the first rib, thereby displacing the neurovascular structures posterolaterally. Blunt fingertip dissection is continued behind the muscle to its medial edge, taking care to avoid the phrenic nerve. Once the insertion of the anterior scalene muscle onto the first rib has been isolated under direct vision to protect the phrenic nerve, the subclavian artery, and the brachial plexus, it is sharply divided from the anterior surface of the bone with scissors (**FIGURE 7**).
- The end of the divided anterior scalene muscle is elevated and its attachments to the underlying extrapleural fascia are sharply divided (electrocautery is not used to avoid inadvertent nerve injury). Muscle fibers extending from the posterior surface of the muscle often pass around the subclavian artery to form a tethering "sling" and should also be resected to fully release the artery. Any scalene minimus muscle fibers found to be present (passing between the roots of the brachial plexus) are divided as the anterior scalene muscle is mobilized. As the anterior scalene muscle is lifted further, it is passed underneath and medial to the phrenic nerve, and its posterior attachments are divided with direct visualization and protection of the upper brachial plexus nerve roots. Dissection of the muscle is carried superiorly to its origin on the C6 transverse process, which is easily palpated in the upper aspect of the operative field (the apex of the "scalene triangle"). The anterior scalene muscle is then divided with scissors from its origin on the transverse process under direct vision and the entire muscle is removed, with a typical specimen weighing 5 to 10 g. Any minor bleeding from the edge of the divided muscle origin is controlled with small polypropylene sutures rather than electrocautery, given the proximity of the nerve roots (**FIGURE 7**).
- Anomalous fibrofascial bands may be observed after anterior scalene muscle resection, typically passing in front of the lower brachial plexus nerve roots. These structures are also resected as they are encountered to ensure thorough decompression and full nerve root mobility.

Mobilization of the Brachial Plexus and Middle Scalenectomy

- The brachial plexus nerve roots are next separated from the front edge of the middle scalene muscle. Blunt fingertip dissection along the lateral aspect of the nerves is used to extend the exposure deeper, to the inner curve of the first rib and the extrapleural space, and a small malleable retractor is placed between the brachial plexus nerves and the middle

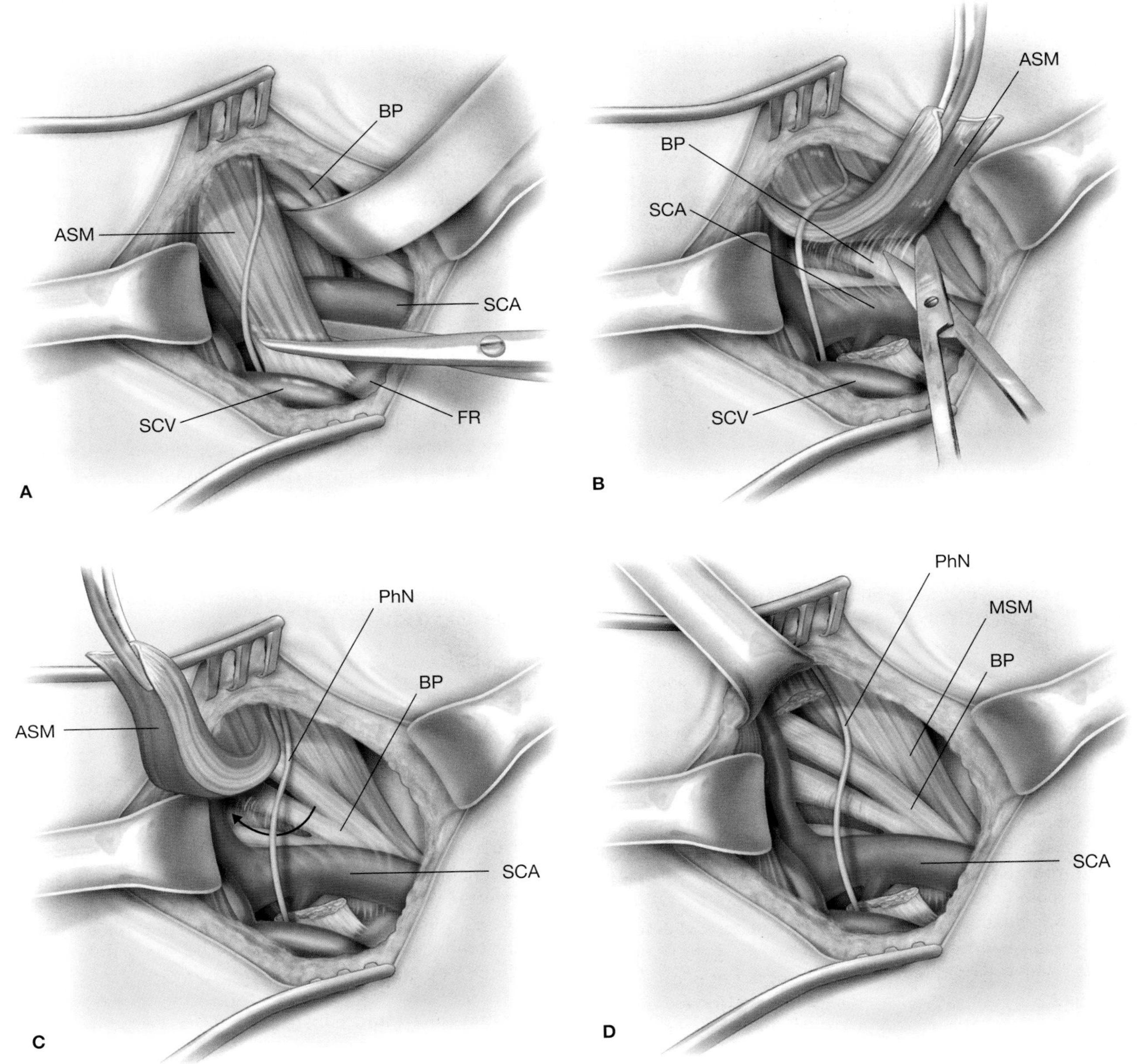

FIGURE 7 ● The anterior scalene muscle (ASM) insertion is isolated by displacing the underlying subclavian artery (SCA) and brachial plexus (BP), using blunt fingertip dissection behind the muscle, and the muscle is sharply divided from the top of the first rib (FR) **(A)**. The end of the divided anterior scalene muscle is lifted and sharply dissected free of structures lying behind the muscle, including the subclavian artery **(B)**. As it is mobilized, the anterior scalene muscle is passed underneath and to the medial side of the phrenic nerve (PhN) **(C)**. The dissection is carried up to the level of the C6 transverse process, where the anterior scalene muscle can be safely divided from its origin and removed **(D)**. MSM, middle scalene muscle; SCV, subclavian vein.

scalene muscle. With gentle medial retraction of the brachial plexus, each nerve root from C5 to T1 is sequentially identified (**FIGURE 8**).

- The transverse cervical artery and vein should be ligated and divided where they pass through the brachial plexus and middle scalene muscle as they are at risk for avulsion during retraction.
- A second malleable retractor is placed lateral to the middle scalene muscle and first rib, to displace the long thoracic nerve posteriorly. The oblique attachment of the middle scalene muscle along the top of the posterolateral first rib is exposed. This muscle insertion is carefully divided from the surface of the bone with the electrocautery, using a periosteal elevator as the dissection proceeds posteriorly, extending to a point on the first rib that is parallel with the underlying T1 nerve root. The bulk of the middle scalene muscle anterior to the long thoracic nerve is then sharply excised, with a typical specimen weighing 3 to 8 grams (**FIGURE 9**). Minor bleeding

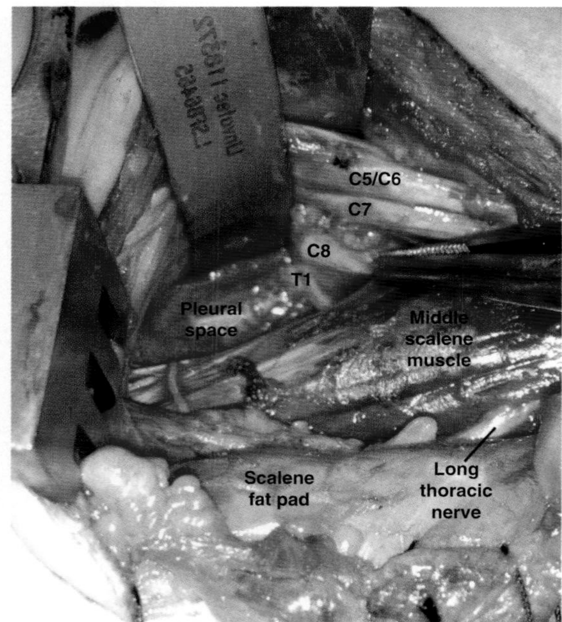

FIGURE 8 ● The brachial plexus is separated from the anteromedial border of the middle scalene muscle down to the level of the first rib and extrapleural fascia and gently retracted medially to visualize all five nerve roots (C5 to T1).

from the cut edge of the middle scalene muscle should be controlled with figure-of-eight silk sutures rather than the electrocautery, to avoid thermal injury to the C8 nerve root or long thoracic nerve.

First Rib Resection

- Once the scalenectomy has been completed, the intercostal muscle attached to the lateral edge of the first rib is separated from the bone with the electrocautery. The first rib is fully exposed posteriorly, where the T1 nerve root emerges from underneath the bone to join the C8 nerve root in forming the lower trunk of the brachial plexus. A large right-angle clamp is passed underneath the posterior neck of the first rib and gently spread to detach additional intercostal tissues. A modified Stille-Giertz rib cutter is inserted around the neck of the first rib. After verifying protection of the C8 and T1 nerve roots, the bone is sharply divided. A Kerrison bone rongeur is used to smooth the posterior end of the bone, to a level medial to the underlying T1 nerve root, and the end of the bone is sealed with bone wax (**FIGURE 9**).
- The free end of the divided posterior first rib is elevated, and blunt fingertip dissection is used to separate the remaining extrapleural fascia and intercostal muscle attaching to the undersurface of the rib, progressing anteriorly to the level of the scalene tubercle (the previous site of attachment of the anterior scalene muscle). No effort is made to avoid opening the pleura during first rib resection, as the opened pleural space will allow better drainage of postoperative fluids away from the brachial plexus (which might otherwise promote perineural adhesions).
- The soft tissues underneath the clavicle, including the subclavian vein, are elevated with a small Richardson retractor. The posterior first rib is displaced inferiorly with fingertip pressure to open the anterior costoclavicular space, and the subclavian artery and brachial plexus are displaced laterally with a small malleable retractor. The Stille-Giertz rib cutter is placed around the anterior first rib, immediately medial to the scalene tubercle (**FIGURE 10**). The first rib is then divided under direct vision, and the intact specimen is extracted from the operative field (**FIGURE 11**). The remaining anterior end of the first rib is remodeled to a smooth surface with a bone rongeur, to a level well underneath the clavicle. Oxidized cellulose fabric (Surgicel, Ethicon, Inc.) is placed within the bed of the resected first rib as a topical hemostatic agent.
- Cervical ribs arise within the plane of the middle scalene muscle, posterior to the brachial plexus and subclavian artery, and anterior to the long thoracic nerve. Incomplete cervical ribs typically have a ligamentous extension to the first rib, whereas complete cervical ribs attach to the lateral first rib in the form of a true joint. The posterior portion of a cervical rib is thereby readily encountered during dissection of the middle scalene muscle and is divided in a manner similar to the posterior first rib. The anterior attachment of the cervical rib is then divided and the bone is removed, prior to first rib resection. When there is a true joint between a complete cervical rib and the first rib, the anterior portion of the cervical rib is left attached while the first rib resection is completed, and the two are removed together as a single specimen (**FIGURE 11**).

Brachial Plexus Neurolysis

- The last step of supraclavicular decompression is to fully mobilize each of the individual nerve roots contributing to the brachial plexus. Each nerve root from C5 to T1 is meticulously dissected free of any adherent perineural fibrous scar tissue that might impair mobility (external neurolysis). Inspection of the most proximal aspect of the C8 and T1 nerve roots will often reveal a small fibrofascial band overlying these nerves, which should be specifically sought out and resected. This step of the operation is not considered complete until each of the five nerve roots and three trunks of the brachial plexus has been completely cleared throughout its course in the operative field (**FIGURE 12**).

Drain Placement and Closure

- Upon the completion of supraclavicular decompression, the apex of the pleural membrane is opened to promote postoperative drainage of fluid into the chest cavity, away from the brachial plexus. A #19 closed suction drain is placed through a separate stab wound into the operative field, placed posterior to the brachial plexus with its tip extending into the posterior pleural space. To minimize postoperative perineural fibrosis, the brachial plexus is loosely wrapped with either a bioresorbable polylactide film (SurgiWrap; Mast Biosurgery) or a gluteraldehyde-free preparation of decellularized bovine pericardium membrane (Photofix; CryoLife, Inc.), held in place with several 5-0 polypropylene sutures. The scalene fat pad is restored to its anatomic position overlying the brachial plexus and held in place with several tacking sutures to the edge of the sternocleidomastoid muscle and to the periclavicular subcutaneous fascia. The platysma muscle layer is reapproximated with interrupted sutures and the skin is closed with an absorbable subcuticular stitch.

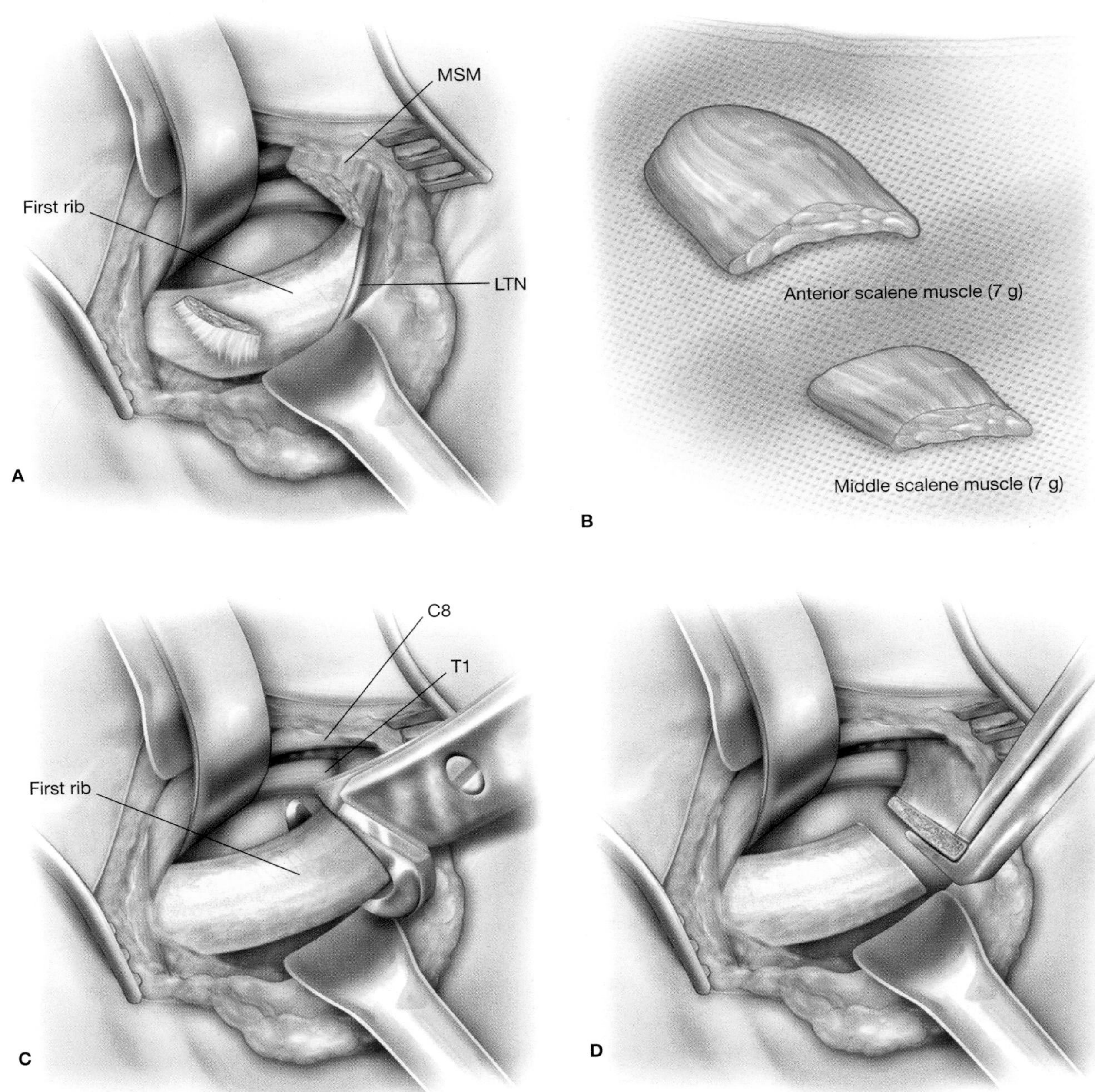

FIGURE 9 ● After detaching the middle scalene muscle (MSM) from the top of the posterolateral first rib using the electrocautery, the muscle tissue lying anterior to the long thoracic nerve (LTN) is excised **(A)**. Typical operative specimens of the anterior and middle scalene muscles **(B)**. The posterior first rib is exposed with visualization of the C8 and T1 nerve roots, and the rib is divided with a modified Giertz-Stille rib cutter **(C)**. The posterior edge of the first rib is further remodeled with a Kerrison rongeur to obtain a smooth edge, immediately medial to the T1 nerve root **(D)**.

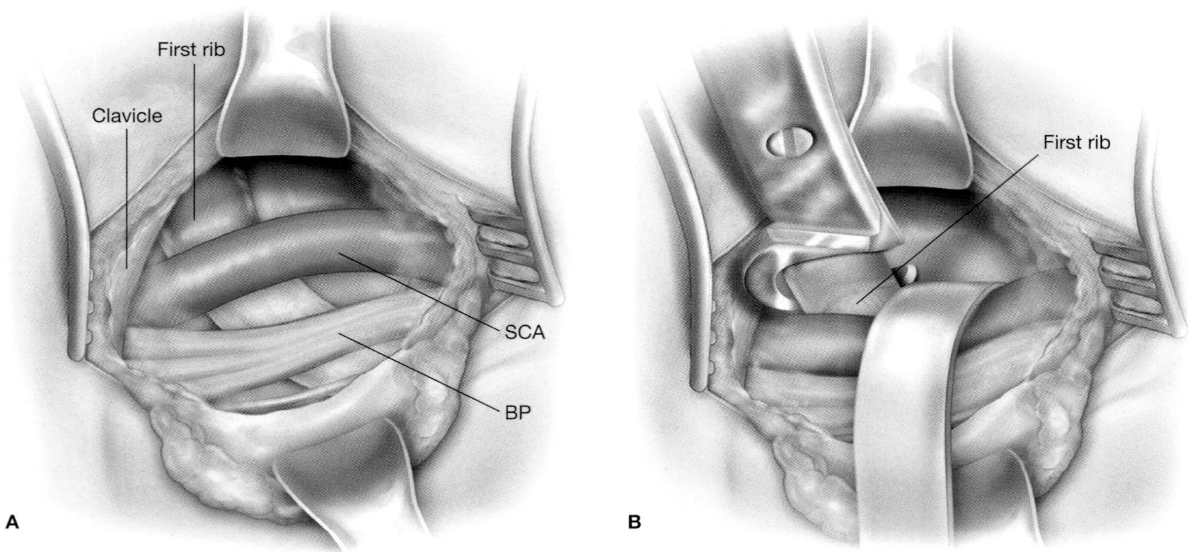

FIGURE 10 ● With the posterior end of the first rib pushed downward to open the anterior costoclavicular space, the anterior portion of the first rib is exposed underneath the clavicle and the subclavian vein **(A)**. The subclavian artery (SCA) and brachial plexus (BP) are protected, and the anterior first rib is divided with a rib cutter immediately medial to the scalene tubercle **(B)**.

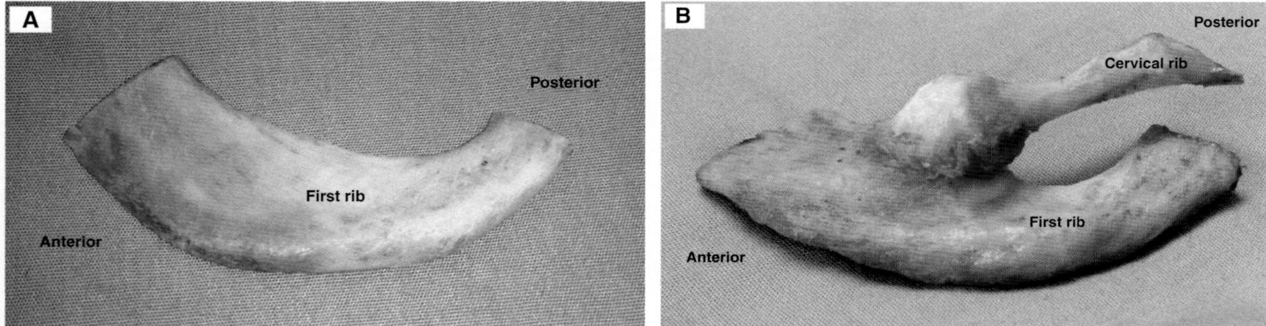

FIGURE 11 ● Operative specimens following first rib resection **(A)** and following combined resection of a cervical rib and first rib **(B)**.

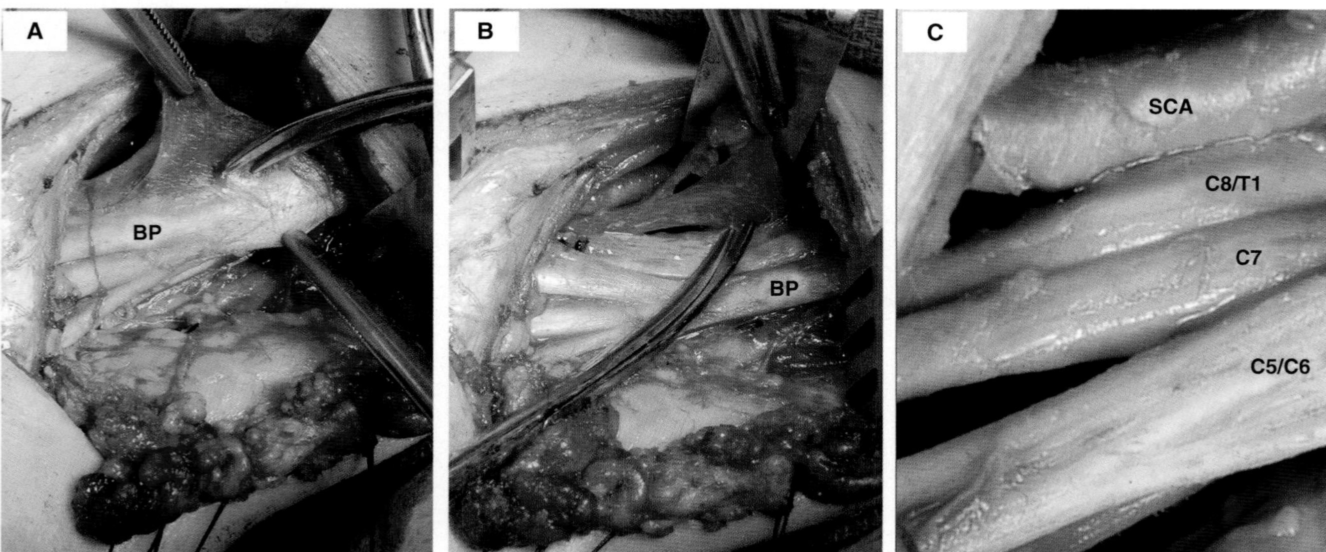

FIGURE 12 ● Fibrous scar tissue is removed from each of the brachial plexus (BP) nerve roots and trunks by external neurolysis **(A-C)**. SCA, subclavian artery.

PECTORALIS MINOR TENOTOMY

Incision and Exposure

- A short vertical incision is made in the deltopectoral groove, beginning at the level of the coracoid process. The deltoid and pectoralis major muscles are gently separated and the plane of deeper dissection is carried medial to the cephalic vein. The lateral edge of the pectoralis major muscle is gently lifted with a small Deaver retractor, and the plane underneath the muscle is separated from the underlying fascia by blunt fingertip dissection. The fascia over the pectoralis minor muscle is exposed, where the muscle can be easily identified by palpation (**FIGURE 13**).

Division of the Pectoralis Minor Muscle Tendon

- The pectoralis minor muscle tendon is identified where it extends from the anterior chest wall to the coracoid process. The fascia along its medial border is opened and the muscle is encircled using blunt fingertip dissection. The fascia along the lateral border of the pectoralis minor muscle is opened to ensure its separation from the short head of the biceps muscle, which also inserts on the coracoid process. Taking care to protect the underlying neurovascular bundle, the pectoralis minor tendon is then elevated with umbilical tape or rubber tubing and its insertion on the coracoid process is exposed with a small Richardson retractor. A finger is placed behind the muscle to prevent thermal injury to the neurovascular structures and the insertion of the pectoralis minor tendon is divided with electrocautery. After the pectoralis minor muscle has been divided, the lower edge will retract inferiorly to release any compression of the neurovascular bundle (**FIGURE 14**).
- The remaining clavipectoral fascia is also incised to the level of the clavicle, along with any other anomalous fascial bands that might be present over the brachial plexus, such as Langer axillary arch, but no further dissection of the brachial plexus nerves or the axillary vessels is performed. The wound is irrigated and closed in layers without a drain.

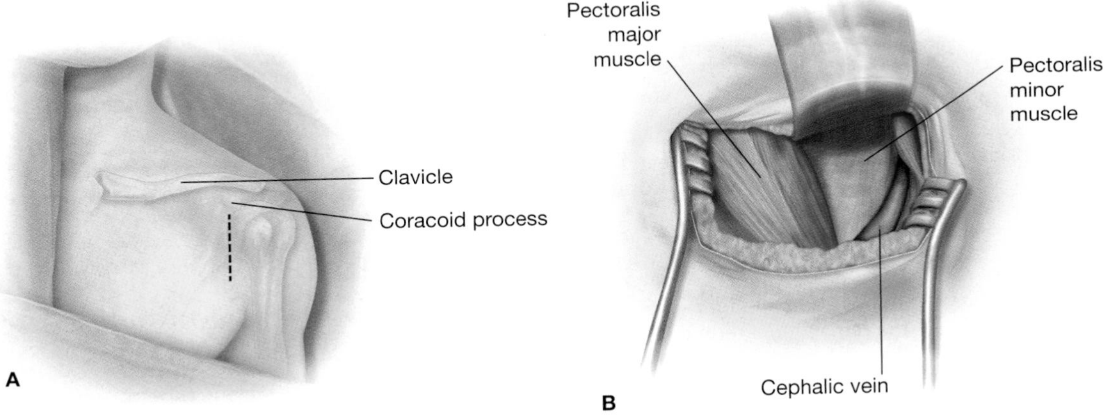

FIGURE 13 ● Pectoralis minor tenotomy is performed through a short vertical incision in the deltopectoral groove, just below the coracoid process **(A)**. The plane of dissection is carried medial to the cephalic vein, and the pectoralis major muscle is lifted to expose the fascia over the pectoralis minor muscle **(B)**.

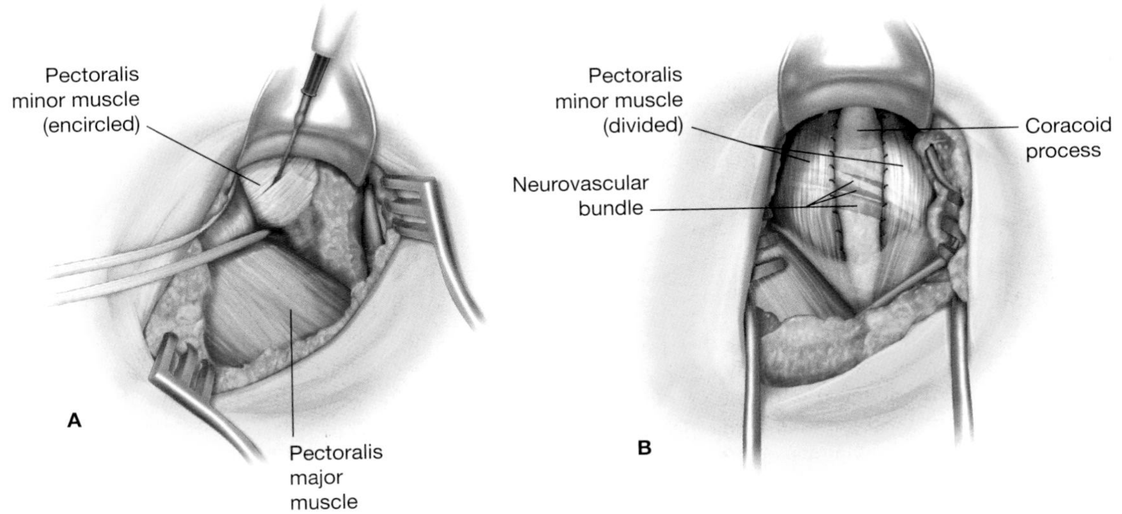

FIGURE 14 ● The pectoralis minor muscle is encircled near its insertion on the coracoid process and then divided with the electrocautery **(A)**. The retracted edge of the divided pectoralis minor muscle is oversewn with a continuous suture **(B)**.

PEARLS AND PITFALLS

Indications	▪ Operative treatment of NTOS should be based on a sound clinical diagnosis, a substantial level of disability, and failure of symptoms to improve with an adequate trial of conservative management. ▪ Imaging studies, electrophysiological tests, and vascular laboratory examinations add little in the evaluation of NTOS, but may be useful in excluding other conditions. ▪ A positive anterior scalene muscle block is a useful adjunct to support the clinical diagnosis of NTOS and indicates a strong likelihood of responsiveness to surgical treatment. ▪ Assess the potential contribution of brachial plexus compression at the level of the subcoracoid space and include pectoralis minor tenotomy if present.
Mobilization of the scalene fat pad	▪ Avoid division of the sternocleidomastoid muscle. ▪ Proper mobilization and lateral reflection of the scalene fat pad is a key step in simplifying supraclavicular exposure for thoracic outlet decompression. This permits the critical view to be obtained in which all of the relevant structures can be visualized in the same operative field (internal jugular vein, phrenic nerve, anterior scalene muscle, brachial plexus, middle scalene muscle, first rib, and long thoracic nerve). ▪ Ligate and divide the thoracic duct if necessary to prevent postoperative lymph leak. ▪ Visualize and protect the phrenic nerve.
Anterior scalenectomy	▪ Divide all fibers passing from the posterior aspect of the anterior scalene muscle to the subclavian artery and extrapleural fascia. ▪ Divide any scalene minimus muscle encountered. ▪ Pass the anterior scalene muscle underneath the phrenic nerve to facilitate dissection of the muscle up to its superior origin on the C6 transverse process.
Mobilization of the brachial plexus	▪ Visualize all five nerve roots and three trunks of the brachial plexus. ▪ Ligate and divide the transverse cervical vessels where they pass through the brachial plexus and middle scalene muscle.
Middle scalenectomy	▪ Visualize and protect the long thoracic nerve. ▪ Control minor bleeding from the cut edge of the muscle with silk sutures rather than the electrocautery.
First rib resection	▪ Visualize the T1 and C8 nerve roots at the level of the posterior first rib, prior to division of the bone, to avoid nerve injury. ▪ Remove a small segment of the divided posterior first rib to facilitate fingertip dissection underneath the remaining lateral and anterior portions of the bone. ▪ Do not try to avoid opening the pleura. ▪ Divide the anterior first rib at a level immediately medial to the scalene tubercle, underneath the clavicle and subclavian vein, while protecting the subclavian artery and brachial plexus. ▪ Resect any cervical rib present along with the first rib.
Brachial plexus neurolysis	▪ Thoroughly remove fibrous scar tissues from around each nerve root (C5 to T1) and trunk of the brachial plexus, to avoid one of the causes of persistent symptoms. ▪ Resect any small fibrofascial bands overlying the proximal aspect of the C8 and T1 nerve roots.
Drain placement and closure	▪ Wrap the brachial plexus to minimize perineural fibrosis. ▪ Place a closed suction drain behind the brachial plexus with its tip extending into the pleural space.
Pectoralis minor tenotomy	▪ Include pectoralis minor tenotomy as part of the supraclavicular decompression if there are concomitant symptoms of NTOS referable to the subcoracoid space. ▪ Divide the pectoralis minor tendon close to its insertion on the coracoid process. ▪ It is not necessary to place a separate drain in the subcoracoid space.

POSTOPERATIVE CARE

- An upright chest radiograph is performed in the recovery room and each morning for 3 days, and any small air or pleural fluid collections are observed with the expectation of spontaneous resolution. Postoperative analgesia is provided by patient-controlled intravenous opiates, until adequate pain control is achieved by oral medications alone. Oral narcotics, a muscle relaxant, and a nonsteroidal anti-inflammatory agent are routinely prescribed at hospital discharge and for at least several weeks following surgery. Postoperative hospital stay is typically 4 to 5 days. The closed suction drain is removed when its output is less than 50 to 100 mL/d, usually 3 to 4 days after surgery.
- Physical therapy is resumed the day after surgery to maintain range of motion and limit muscle spasm. The patient is allowed to use the extremity as tolerated, with no use of a sling or other restraint. Physical therapy is continued after hospital discharge, with advice to avoid excessive reaching

overhead or heavy lifting with the affected upper extremity, and other activities that might result in muscle strain, spasm and significant pain in the sternocleidomastoid, trapezius, and other neck muscles. Further rehabilitation is overseen by a physical therapist with expertise in the management of NTOS, usually in conjunction with a physical therapist located near the patient, emphasizing a gradual steady return to normal use of the upper extremity.

- The majority of patients are permitted cautious light-duty work activities by 4 to 6 weeks. Restrictions on upper extremity activity are progressively lifted between 6 and 12 weeks, when recovery from surgery is typically considered complete. Patients are seen in follow-up every 3 months in the first year to assess long-term results. Physical therapy and other aspects of care are continued as long as necessary to achieve an optimal level of function.

OUTCOMES

- In properly selected patients with disabling NTOS, approximately 85% to 90% can expect a substantial improvement in symptoms and increased functional use of the upper extremity within several months of supraclavicular decompressio n.[5-7,13,19] This estimate is higher in those who exhibited a positive anterior scalene/pectoralis minor muscle block prior to treatment. Factors that tend to diminish responsiveness to treatment include extremely longstanding (>5 years) and debilitating symptoms, widespread pain syndromes, multiple previous operations (cervical spine, shoulder, or peripheral nerves), depression, older age (>50 years), and preexisting use of opiate pain medications.[13,19]
- Patients with longstanding NTOS often display residual symptoms that may not be completely eliminated by thoracic outlet decompression. While these symptoms may be tolerable and are expected to gradually improve, the surgeon must provide continuing support and reassurance during the prolonged period of recovery and rehabilitation.
- Patients in the adolescent age group (<21 years) tend to have even better outcomes than adults, based on assessment of patient-reported survey instruments and postoperative use of opiate pain medications.[19] Patients that have been selected for isolated pectoralis minor tenotomy can exhibit early outcomes similar to those of patients that have undergone combined supraclavicular decompression and pectoralis minor tenotomy, but require ongoing follow-up for recurrent symptoms to determine if supraclavicular decompression may be warranted at a later time.[20,21]
- Recurrent symptoms of NTOS that warrant reoperation occur in 5% to 6% of patients, usually within the first 2 years of treatment. Reoperations for NTOS are generally performed using the supraclavicular approach, because this provides the most complete exposure of the anatomy with the greatest margin of safety.[23,24] Following lateral reflection of the scalene fat pad, the brachial plexus nerve roots are carefully exposed and mobilized. Great care must be taken during this dissection to avoid nerve and blood vessel injury, given the dense fibrous scar tissue that is usually present within the operative field. Any structures that were retained at the initial operation are then resected, including the scalene muscles, anomalous fibrofascial bands, and/or the first rib. A complete brachial plexus neurolysis is performed and the nerves are protected with a biological wrap and soft tissue coverage with the scalene fat pad.

COMPLICATIONS

- Persistent pain, numbness, and/or paresthesias
- Postoperative bleeding, localized hematoma, or hemothorax
- Wound infection (cellulitis or abscess)
- Pleural effusion (serosanguinous)
- Persistent lymph leak, chylothorax
- Brachial plexus nerve dysfunction (temporary or sustained)
- Phrenic nerve dysfunction (temporary or sustained)
- Long thoracic nerve dysfunction (temporary or sustained)
- Recurrent NTOS

REFERENCES

1. Thompson RW. Thoracic outlet syndrome: neurogenic. In: Sidawy AN, Perler BA, eds. *Rutherford's Vascular Surgery and Endovascular Therapy*. 9th ed. Elsevier; 2018:1619-1638.
2. Illig KA, Donahue D, Duncan A, et al. Reporting standards of the Society for Vascular Surgery for thoracic outlet syndrome. *J Vasc Surg*. 2016;64(3):e23-e35.
3. Illig KA, Thompson RW, Freischlag JA, et al, eds. *Thoracic Outlet Syndrome (TOS)*. 2nd ed. Springer Nature; 2021.
4. Sanders RJ, Hammond SL. Management of cervical ribs and anomalous first ribs causing neurogenic thoracic outlet syndrome. *J Vasc Surg*. 2002;36(1):51-56.
5. Reilly LM, Stoney RJ. Supraclavicular approach for thoracic outlet decompression. *J Vasc Surg*. 1988;8:329-334.
6. Sanders RJ, Hammond SL. Supraclavicular first rib resection and total scalenectomy: technique and results. *Hand Clin*. 2004;20:61-70.
7. Thompson RW, Ohman JW. Surgical techniques: operative decompression using the supraclavicular approach for neurogenic thoracic outlet syndrome. In: Illig KA, Thompson RW, Freischlag JA, et al, eds. *Thoracic Outlet Syndrome (TOS)*. 2nd ed. Springer Nature; 2021:265-285.
8. Sanders RJ, Hammond SL, Rao NM. Diagnosis of thoracic outlet syndrome. *J Vasc Surg*. 2007;46(3):601-604.
9. Jordan SE, Ahn SS, Gelabert HA. Differentiation of thoracic outlet syndrome from treatment-resistant cervical brachial pain syndromes: development and utilization of a questionnaire, clinical examination and ultrasound evaluation. *Pain Physician*. 2007;10(3):441-452.
10. Thompson RW. Diagnosis of neurogenic thoracic outlet syndrome: 2016 consensus guidelines and other strategies. In: Illig KA, Thompson RW, Freischlag JA, et al, eds. *Thoracic Outlet Syndrome (TOS)*. 2nd ed. Springer Nature; 2021:67-97.
11. Goeteyn J, Pesser N, van Sambeek MRHM, Thompson RW, van Neunen BFL, Teijink JAW. Duplex ultrasound studies are neither necessary or sufficient for the diagnosis of neurogenic thoracic outlet syndrome. *Ann Vasc Surg*. Published online November 11, 2021. doi:10.1016/j.asvg.2021.09.048
12. Balderman J, Holzem K, Field BJ, et al. Associations between clinical diagnostic criteria and pretreatment patient-reported outcomes measures in a prospective observational cohort of patients with neurogenic thoracic outlet syndrome. *J Vasc Surg*. 2017;66(2):533-544.
13. Balderman J, Abuirqeba AA, Pate C, et al. Physical therapy management, surgical treatment, and patient-reported outcomes measures in a prospective observational cohort of patients with neurogenic thoracic outlet syndrome. *J Vasc Surg*. 2019;70:832-841.
14. Raptis CA, Sridhar S, Thompson RW, Fowler K, Bhalla S. Imaging of the patient with thoracic outlet syndrome. *Radiographics*. 2016;36(4):984-1000.
15. Jordan SE, Machleder HI. Diagnosis of thoracic outlet syndrome using electrophysiologically guided anterior scalene blocks. *Ann Vasc Surg*. 1998;12(3):260-264.
16. Torriani M, Gupta R, Donahue DM. Sonographically guided anesthetic injection of anterior scalene muscle for investigation of neurogenic thoracic outlet syndrome. *Skeletal Radiol*. 2009;38(11):1083-1087.

17. Braun RM, Shah KN, Rechnic M, Doehr S, Woods N. Quantitative assessment of scalene muscle block for the diagnosis of suspected thoracic outlet syndrome. *J Hand Surg Am*. 2015;40(11): 2255-2261.
18. Weaver ML, Hicks CW, Fritz J, Black JHIII, Lum YW. Local anesthetic block of the anterior scalene muscle increases muscle height in patients with neurogenic thoracic outlet syndrome. *Ann Vasc Surg*. 2019;59:28-35.
19. Caputo FJ, Wittenberg AM, Vemuri C, et al. Supraclavicular decompression for neurogenic thoracic outlet syndrome in adolescent and adult populations. *J Vasc Surg*. 2013;57(1):149-157.
20. Sanders RJ, Rao NM. The forgotten pectoralis minor syndrome: 100 operations for pectoralis minor syndrome alone or accompanied by neurogenic thoracic outlet syndrome. *Ann Vasc Surg*. 2010;24:701-708.
21. Vemuri C, Wittenberg AM, Caputo FJ, et al. Early effectiveness of isolated pectoralis minor tenotomy in selected patients with neurogenic thoracic outlet syndrome. *J Vasc Surg*. 2013;57(5):1345-1352.
22. Guffey R, Abuirqeba AA, Wolfson M, et al. Erector spinae plane block versus perineural local anesthetic infusion for postoperative pain control after supraclavicular decompression for neurogenic thoracic outlet syndrome: a matched case-control comparison. *Ann Vasc Surg*. Published online August 26, 2021. doi:10.1016/j.avsg.2021.05.067
23. Ambrad-Chalela E, Thomas GI, Johansen KH. Recurrent neurogenic thoracic outlet syndrome. *Am J Surg*. 2004;187(4):505-510.
24. Jammeh ML, Ohman JW, Vemuri C, Abuirqeba AA, Thompson RW. Anatomically complete supraclavicular reoperation for recurrent neurogenic thoracic outlet syndrome: clinical characteristics, operative findings, and long-term outcomes. *Hand (NY)*. Published online January 27, 2021. doi:10.1177/1558944720988079

Chapter **8**

Neurogenic Thoracic Outlet Syndrome Exposure and Decompression: Transaxillary

Gabriela Velazquez-Ramirez, Lauren N. West-Livingston, Misty D. Humphries, and Julie Ann Freischlag

DEFINITION

- In 1821, Sir Astley Cooper recognized the constellation of neurovascular symptoms involving the thoracic outlet. Ochsner called this the *scalenus anticus syndrome* in 1936 and described the presence of muscle abnormalities secondary to repetitive trauma. The first report of symptoms consistent with this condition was conveyed by Rogers in 1949. Rob and Standeven narrowed down the characterization in 1958. Peet assigned this condition its contemporaneous moniker *thoracic outlet syndrome* (*TOS*) in 1966.[1-4]
- TOS is a condition defined as a group of disorders that involve compression of one or more of the neurovascular structures contained within the thoracic outlet.[5]
- There are three important anatomic spaces that are part of the thoracic outlet: the scalene triangle, the costoclavicular space, and the pectoralis minor space.
  - Scalene triangle—this space is bordered by the anterior scalene muscle, the middle scalene muscle, and the first rib. Important anatomical structures that traverse this space include the brachial plexus and subclavian artery. Cervical ribs may impede on this space, causing compression leading to TOS.[6]
  - Costoclavicular space—this is the space between the clavicle and first rib. Important anatomical structures found in this space include the subclavian artery, the subclavian vein, and the brachial plexus. This is the most common site of compression of the subclavian vein.
  - Pectoralis minor space—this is the space between the anterior pectoralis minor and the posterior chest wall. This is a common site of compression causing neurovascular TOS.[7]
- From the surgeon's point of view the thoracic outlet can be visualized as an anatomic triangle: the two sides being the anterior and middle scalene muscles with the first rib serving as the base of the triangle. The scalene muscles, which originate from the lower cervical spine, may hypertrophy with repetitive neck motion or minor trauma. This hypertrophy is believed to contribute to compression of thoracic outlet structures.
- TOS is subdivided into three discrete etiologies[5,8]: neurogenic, venous, and arterial. In this chapter, we will focus on transaxillary exposure decompression for neurogenic TOS.
  - Neurogenic (over 90% of cases)
  - Venous (3%-5% of cases)
  - Arterial (1%-2% of cases)
- Appropriate classification of the type of TOS is important in guiding perioperative management, as well as surgical approach. This chapter focuses on transaxillary decompression and first rib resection for neurogenic TOS.

PATIENT HISTORY AND PHYSICAL FINDINGS

- A careful history and physical examination enables proper classification of TOS.
- **Neurogenic TOS**, which is more prevalent in women, include paresthesia, pain, and impaired strength in the affected shoulder, arm, or hand along with occipital headaches and neck discomfort.[9] There is commonly an antecedent history of hyperextension neck injury or repetitive neck trauma. Patients frequently manifest tenderness on palpation in the supraclavicular fossa over the anterior scalene muscle. A careful vascular physical examination should confirm the presence of normal circulation.[5,10]
  - Three physical examination maneuvers support the diagnosis of neurogenic TOS:
    - Rotation of the neck and tilting of the head to the opposite side elicit pain in the affected arm.
    - The upper limb tension test, in which the patient first abducts both arms to 90° with the elbows in a locked position, then dorsiflexes the wrists, and finally tilts the head to the side. Each subsequent step imparts greater traction on the brachial plexus, with the first two positions causing discomfort on the ipsilateral side and the head-tilt position causing pain on the contralateral side.
    - During the elevated arm stress test (EAST), the patient raises both arms directly above the head and repeatedly opens and closes the fists. Characteristic upper extremity symptoms arise within 60 seconds in patients with neurogenic TOS.
- **Venous TOS** is also called Paget-von Schroetter syndrome or effort vein thrombosis when the entrapped subclavian vein has progressed to thrombosing. Patients typically present with acute onset of dull aching pain of the upper extremity associated with arm edema and cyanosis. Paresthesias may be present but are due to hand swelling instead of thoracic outlet nerve involvement. A history of strenuous and repetitive work or athletics involving the affected extremity is common, and most patients are young. Some patients will present less acutely with nonthrombotic subclavian vein occlusion or stenosis manifested by intermittent swelling with activity. Regardless, the etiology of venous TOS is mechanical, and treatment is ultimately aimed at eliminating not only the venous obstruction but also the muscular bands and ligaments that have entrapped and damaged the vein.[5]
- **Arterial TOS** typically presents in one of the three ways: (1) asymptomatic, (2) arm claudication, and (3) critical ischemia of the hand. The majority of these patients have a cervical rib, which may or may not be fused to the first rib and is most commonly posterior to the subclavian artery.[6] The etiology is chronic repetitive injury to the subclavian artery as it exits the thoracic outlet. This injury may cause subclavian artery stenosis but more commonly leads to ectasia or a true aneurysm.[11]
  - In asymptomatic patients, a pulsatile mass or supraclavicular bruit can be detected on physical examination.

- Arm claudication is caused by areas of stenosis which may be static due to long-standing repetitive injury or dynamic, occurring only with arm abduction or extension.
- Critical ischemia is due to emboli of fibrin platelet aggregates that originate from an ulcerated mural thrombus in the aneurysmal segment.

DIFFERENTIAL DIAGNOSIS

- Carpal tunnel syndrome
- Ulnar nerve compression
- Rotator cuff tendinitis
- Pectoralis minor syndrome
- Cervical spine strain
- Cervical disc disease
- Cervical arthritis
- Brachial plexus injury
- Fibromyositis

PREOPERATIVE EVALUATION AND OTHER DIAGNOSTIC STUDIES

- Preoperative presentation of neurogenic TOS may be classic; however, it is always important to obtain a good history specifically looking for history of neck trauma or known cervical disease. In these cases, magnetic resonance imaging (MRI) is a valuable study.[12]
- A chest X-ray will show presence of cervical ribs as well as other bony abnormalities that could be contributing to the neurogenic presentation. This is imperative to determine if the cervical rib is complete or incomplete.
- Duplex ultrasound of the subclavian artery or vein may be needed in instances of combined types of TOS. This would specifically evaluate for subclavian artery aneurysm as well as patency of subclavian vein. Preoperative physical therapy should be attempted for at least 8 weeks in all patients with a diagnosis of neurogenic TOS. The aims of therapy are to improve posture and achieve greater range of motion. Patients with persistent symptoms of neurogenic TOS despite physical therapy merit surgical intervention. At least 60% of patients will improve with physical therapy and lifestyle alterations.
- A radiographically guided anterior scalene block with local anesthetic (lidocaine) injection may provide a few hours of symptomatic relief. Patients with suspected neurogenic TOS often present with a wide constellation of physical complaints, not all of which are directly attributable to the disorder. A scalene block not only helps confirm the diagnosis but also simulates the expected postoperative result, especially in older patients.[13] This provides the patient and the surgeon reassurance that surgical intervention will be of benefit and demonstrates which symptoms can be reliably expected to improve.
- Other options include Botox (Allergan, Irvine, CA) injection which takes approximately 2 weeks to effect symptom improvement and can be done several times. This may provide symptomatic relief for 2 to 3 months, allowing participation in physical therapy. Importantly, not all TOS patients respond to Botox. This practice is most helpful in patients who have had cervical spine fusions or shoulder operations as it allows them to strengthen the muscles of their neck and back, which may alleviate the TOS symptoms.
- Nerve conduction studies are typically normal in neurogenic TOS but may be useful in ruling out nerve compression such as carpal tunnel or cubital compression syndrome.

SURGICAL MANAGEMENT

Surgical Approach

- The transaxillary decompression is our preferred approach due to its low-risk profile and documented improvement in patients' quality of life.[4,5] This approach effectively decompresses the thoracic outlet and is generally reserved for patients with neurogenic or venous TOS.
- If vessel reconstruction is anticipated, a different approach should be considered as the transaxillary approach limits vessel exposure.

Surgical Anatomy

- The subclavian artery and the five nerve roots (C5–T1) to the brachial plexus are located within the thoracic outlet. The artery courses anterior to the brachial plexus nerve roots and exits the mediastinum in its course over the first rib behind the posterior border of the anterior scalene muscle. The cervical spine nerve roots join to form the initial trunks of the brachial plexus within the thoracic outlet and are located posterior to the subclavian artery. Subsequent merging and branching of these trunks into divisions, cords, and terminal nerves occurs outside the thoracic outlet.
- Other significant nerves within the thoracic outlet are the phrenic and long thoracic nerves.
  - The phrenic nerve receives fibers from C3–C5 and courses in a descending oblique direction from the lateral to the medial edge of the middle portion of the anterior scalene muscle. The phrenic nerve approaches the mediastinum posterior to the subclavian vein.
  - The long thoracic nerve, composed of nerve fibers from C5 to C7, passes through the center of the middle scalene muscle and heads toward the chest wall to innervate the serratus anterior muscle.
- The subclavian vein technically does not course through the thoracic outlet. It passes over the first rib anterior to the anterior scalene muscle. However, the middle segment of the vein remains susceptible to compression between the anteromedial first rib, clavicle, and the subclavius muscle (**FIGURE 1**). Hypertrophy of the subclavius muscle and tendon may occur in athletes and is often implicated in venous TOS.
- Several anatomic anomalies are relevant to the surgeon, as they predispose patients to the development of TOS.

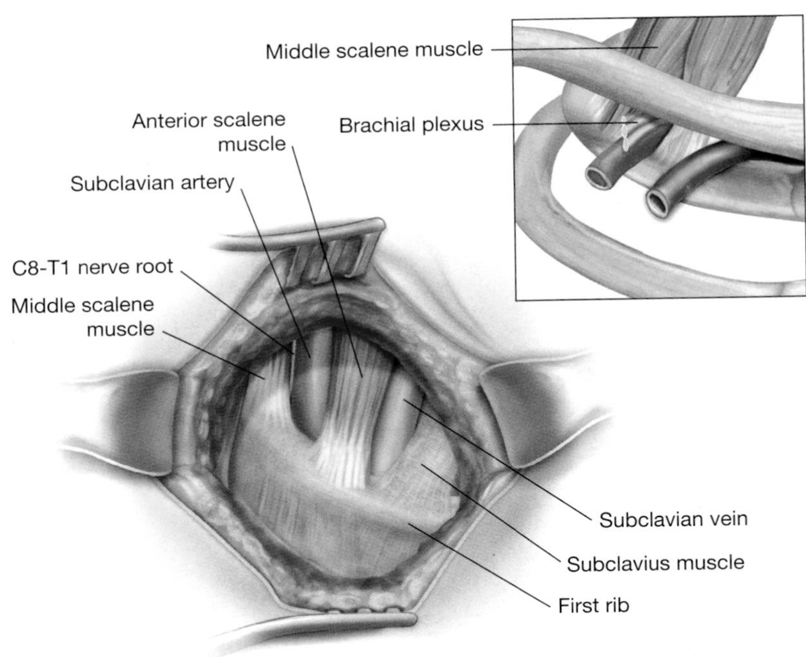

FIGURE 1 ● Right-sided thoracic outlet anatomy from the surgeon's perspective as viewed through the operative field in a transaxillary approach. *Inset*, normal anatomic relationships of important thoracic outlet structures.

- The most common is a cervical rib, and a preoperative chest radiograph is adequate for its detection. When present, cervical ribs appear as extensions of the transverse process of C7. Cervical ribs may be complete or partial, with the anterior end attaching to the first rib or floating freely. Additionally, the anterior end may be fibrous and not calcified and thus not completely visualized on chest radiograph. By rigidly confining the thoracic outlet, cervical ribs render the neurovascular structures more prone to compression. Although present in the general population with an incidence of 0.5% to 1%, they are found in 5% to 10% of all TOS patients. A recent meta-analysis demonstrated that while the prevalence of a cervical rib in healthy patient populations was roughly 1%, the prevalence in individuals with TOS was 29.5%. Furthermore, 51.3% of symptomatic patients with a cervical rib had vascular TOS, while 48.7% had neurogenic TOS.[6]
- A prominent C7 transverse process or bifid first rib is also associated with TOS.

Anesthesia

- TOS surgeries are performed under general anesthesia, though since the case is relatively short, a Foley catheter is often not needed.
- Neuromuscular blocking agents should be limited at the time of induction due to proximity of the surgical procedure to the brachial plexus.
- Of note, a pectoralis block can be done after surgery is completed for postoperative pain control purposes.

Positioning

- General endotracheal anesthesia is induced and sequential compression devices are applied.
- The patient is then moved to the lateral decubitus position with affected arm up.
- A bean bag is used to hold the patient and axillary roll should be placed under the down arm. Patient is padded properly to protect bony prominences.
- The entire arm is prepped into the field, we use the Machleder retractor which is extremely helpful.
  - Care should be taken to pad the dependent axilla and support the head. The sterile field incorporates the arm, axilla, and shoulder.
- An adjustable Machleder arm support is affixed to the operating table with the vertical support bar attached to the operating table at the level of the patient's chin.
  - Generous padding around the patient's arm prior to placement in the arm holder protects the median and ulnar nerves from compression as they cross the elbow joint (**FIGURE 2**).

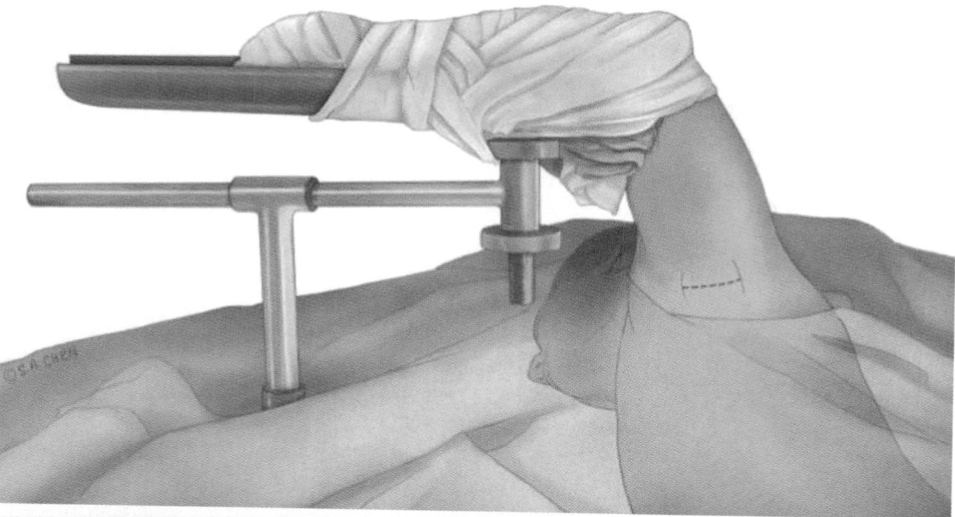

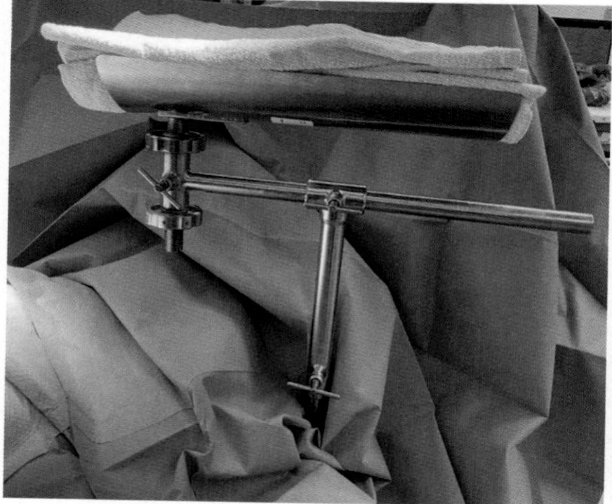

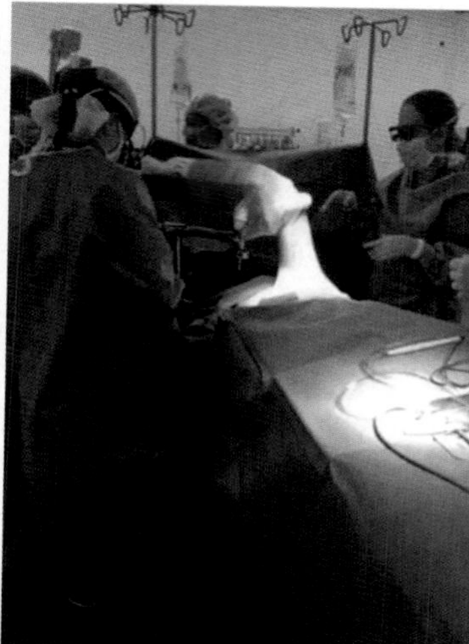

FIGURE 2 ● An illustration and photograph depicting proper patient positioning for right transaxillary first rib resection and use of the Machleder arm support with generous padding to prevent compression nerve injury. A padded axillary roll is placed under the dependent axilla, and the patient is stabilized in the left lateral decubitus with the aid of a bean bag. The *dashed line* indicates the preferred location of the skin incision.

INCISION AND EXPOSURE

- After securing the arm in the retractor, the surgeon identifies the anterior border of the latissimus dorsi muscle and the posterior surface of the pectoralis major muscle.
- A transverse skin line incision should be made in the inferior axillary hairline extending between these two muscle borders.
- Electrocautery is used to divide the subcutaneous tissue until thin areolar tissue superficial to the chest wall is encountered. A self-retaining Cerebellar or Weitlaner retractor is then inserted into the wound. Upon encountering the chest wall—and if in the correct anatomic plane—gentle blunt dissection with the surgeon's fingers or a pair of Kittner or peanut dissectors easily separates the soft tissues from the chest wall. Once the chest wall is encountered, the arm is lifted in the retractor system and the connective tissue over the thoracic outlet is bluntly dissected. Raising the Machleder arm support allows for optimal access to the first rib and the thoracic outlet. The arm is lifted with the retractor at 15-minute intervals, releasing the arm down intermittently prevents any nerve stretching injury. The intercostobrachial nerve is located in the second intercostal space. Although frequently difficult to avoid, care should be taken not to impart excess traction as injury results in numbness or dysesthesia of the medial aspect of the proximal arm.
- The aid of fiber optic–lighted Deaver retractors facilitates visualization during this portion of the dissection. Alternatively, the surgeon should wear a headlight (**FIGURE 3**).
- The first rib is identified near its insertion at the sternoclavicular joint and generally encountered higher than anticipated. A Kittner or peanut dissector is then used to gently sweep away the loose fibrous tissue overlying the first rib partially exposing the brachial plexus, subclavian artery and vein, and scalene muscles. There is occasionally a small branch of the subclavian artery that must be ligated and divided in order to fully expose the operative field.
- The next step is to fully expose the rib. Depending on the patient's anatomy, it generally is the easiest to first clear off the intercostal muscles laterally. A periosteal elevator works

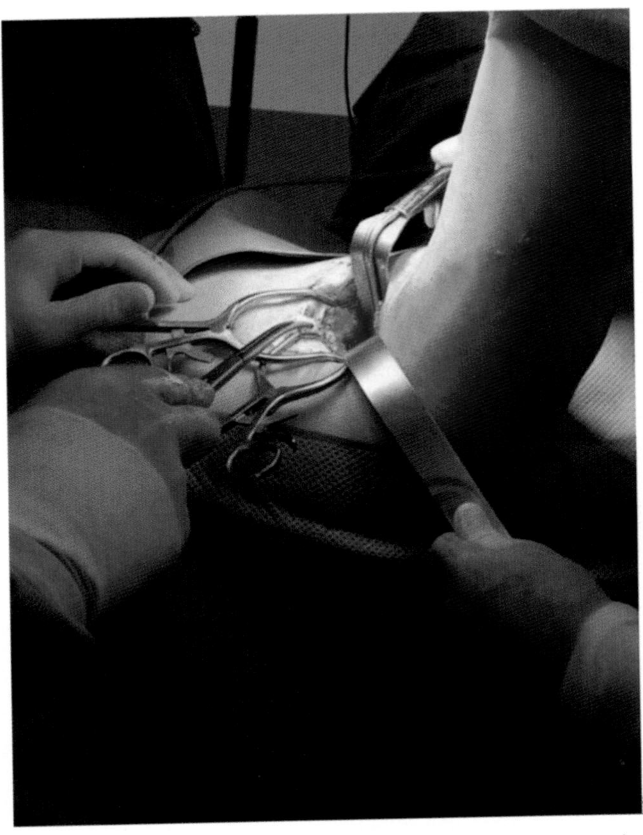

FIGURE 3 ● A lighted retractor and Deaver retractor are used to give good visualization of the surgical field.

best, but any type of long elevator may be used (**FIGURE 4**). The dissection proceeds in the anterior and posterior directions until all the intercostal muscle attachments are divided from the rib. The elevator can then be used to elevate the first rib, thus separating the rib from the underlying parietal pleura. This mobilization should continue from behind the brachial plexus in the posterior direction to beyond the subclavian vein in the anterior direction.

- Attention is then directed to the superior border of the first rib, where the periosteal elevator is used to bluntly detach the scalene medius fibers from the rib. The long thoracic nerve courses along the lateral edge of the scalene medius muscle but is generally not visualized. Avoiding sharp dissection and closely adhering to the surface of the rib during blunt dissection prevents injury to the long thoracic nerve.
- The anterior scalene muscle should now be clearly identified as it arises from the medial superior aspect of the first rib (**FIGURE 5**). A right-angled clamp is passed behind the anterior scalene muscle Neurogenic Thoracic Outlet Syndrome Exposure and Decompression: Transaxillarynear its insertion on the scalene tubercle. Gently lifting the anterior scalene with the right-angled clamp protects the subclavian artery as it courses posterior to the muscle (**FIGURE 6**). It is important to free several centimeters of the muscle prior to dividing it with Metzenbaum scissors (**FIGURE 7**). This maneuver facilitates resection of a portion of the anterior scalene muscle, which has been shown to reduce recurrence rates when compared with division at its insertion point on the rib.
- Lastly, the subclavius muscle will appear as a crescent-shaped ligamentous attachment to the first rib adjacent to the subclavian vein. With care not to injure the subclavian vein, the subclavius muscle is sharply divided with scissors.

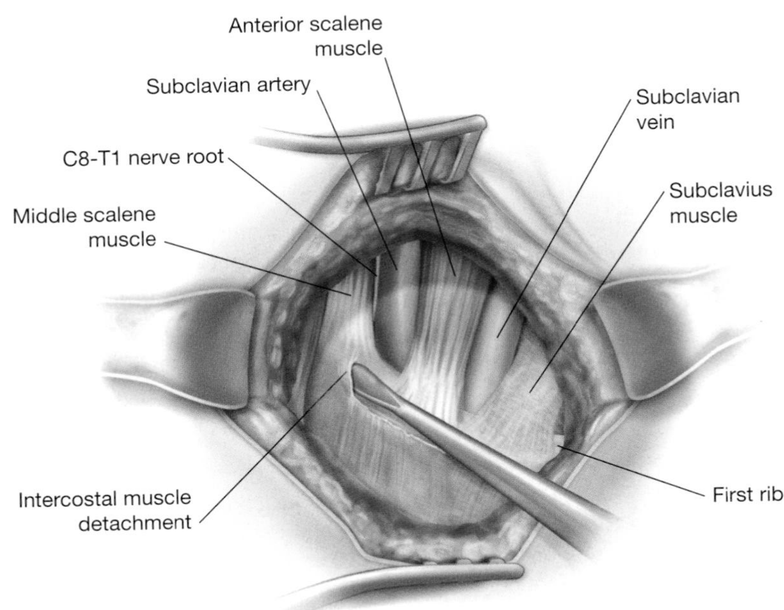

FIGURE 4 ● A periosteal elevator is used to dissect along the superior surface of the first rib in order to divide intercostal muscle attachments.

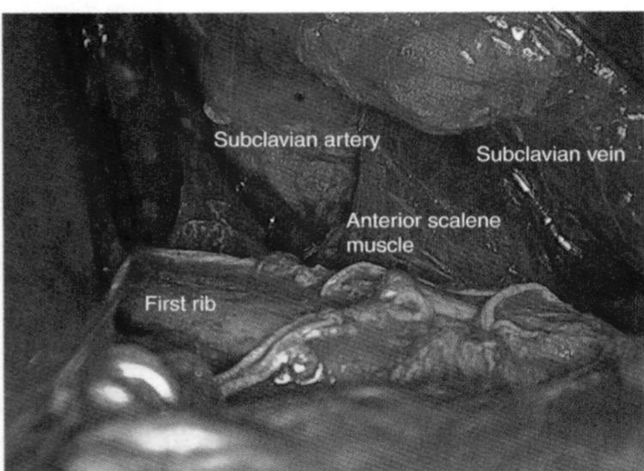

FIGURE 5 ● An image of the gross anatomy from a close-up perspective of the right-sided thoracic outlet. The important relationships between the first rib, anterior scalene muscle, and subclavian vessels can be seen. (Reprinted from Arnaoutakis G, Freischlag JA, Reifsnyder T. Transaxillary rib resection for thoracic outlet syndrome. In: Cambria R, Chaikof E, eds. *Atlas of Vascular and Endovascular Surgery: Anatomy and Technique*. Elsevier; 2014:193-203. Copyright © 2014 Elsevier. With permission.)

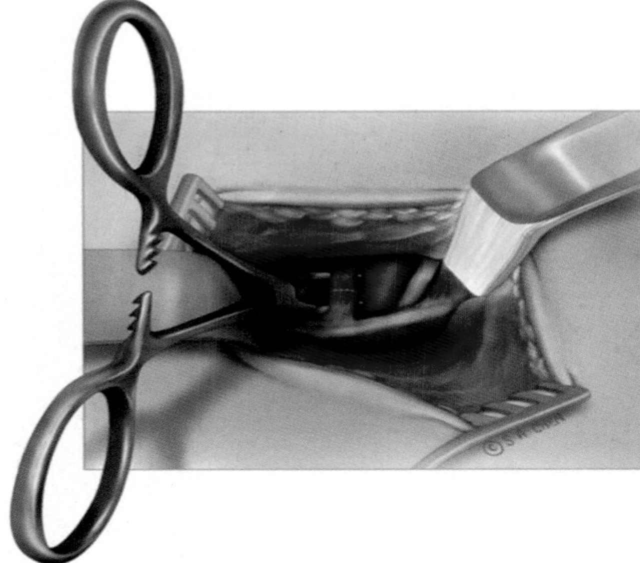

FIGURE 6 ● A right-angled clamp is insinuated behind the anterior scalene muscle. Gentle elevation pulls the muscle away from the underlying subclavian artery, thereby protecting the artery prior to dividing the muscle with scissors. The subclavius muscle is a crescent-shaped ligamentous attachment to the first rib adjacent to the subclavian vein. The subclavius muscle is sharply divided with scissors with care not to injure the subclavian vein. (Images illustrated by S.A. Chen, made for Dr. Julie Freischlag, http://www.sarahachen.com/.)

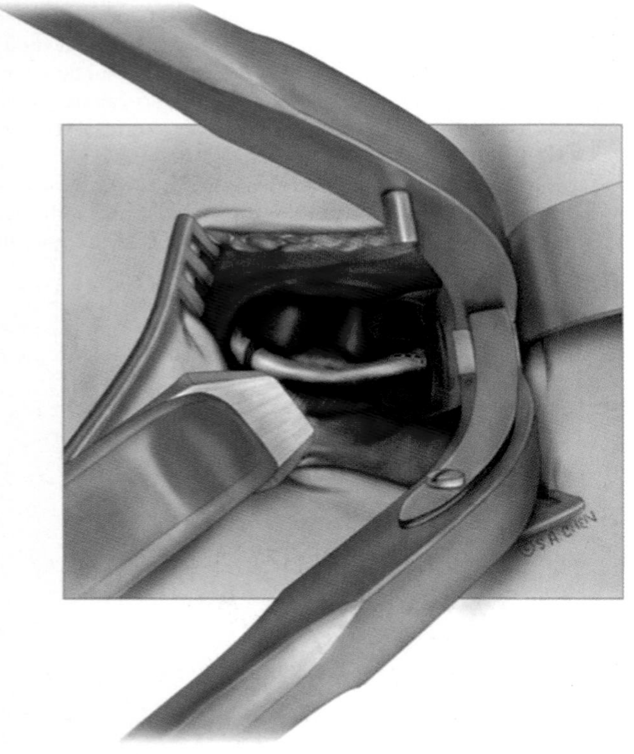

FIGURE 7 ● The first rib is seen in the illustration of a left first rib resection. Metzenbaum scissors are used to sharply divide the anterior scalene muscle, with the right-angled clamp elevating the muscle to protect the subclavian artery as it courses behind the muscle. The divided ends of the tendinous anterior scalene fibers can be seen. (Images illustrated by S.A. Chen, made for Dr. Julie Freischlag, http://www.sarahachen.com/.)

RIB RESECTION

- Once the subclavius and anterior scalene muscles are divided and the rib completely mobilized, a periosteal elevator can be used again to free up the reminder intercostal muscle fibers along the lateral aspect of the first rib, and a bone cutter is then used to divide the rib. Generally, it is divided anteriorly and then posteriorly; however, the patient's body habitus may make the reverse order easier (**FIGURE 8**).
- In its anterior extent, the rib is divided adjacent to the subclavian vein, and in the posterior direction, it is divided just anterior to the brachial plexus; this ensures that the nerve roots are not inadvertently injured. The rib is then removed. It is important to always identify the tips of the bone cutter so that they are free of other structures to prevent injuries.
- A bone rongeur is used to remove residual rib and to smooth the cut ends until there is no residual nerve impingement. A Ross retractor or similar instrument may be used to protect the nerves during use of the rongeur (**FIGURE 9**).

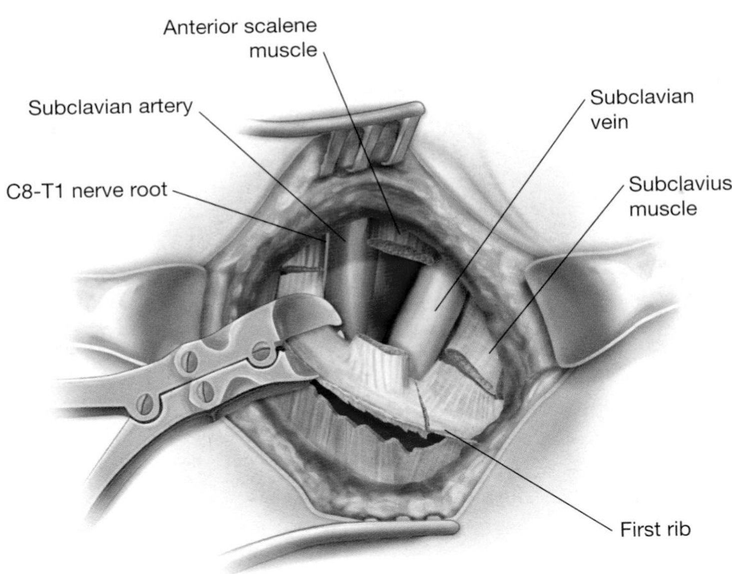

FIGURE 8 ● A bone cutter is used to divide the first rib in its anterior and posterior direction. Once removed, the rongeur is used to achieve smooth rib edges.

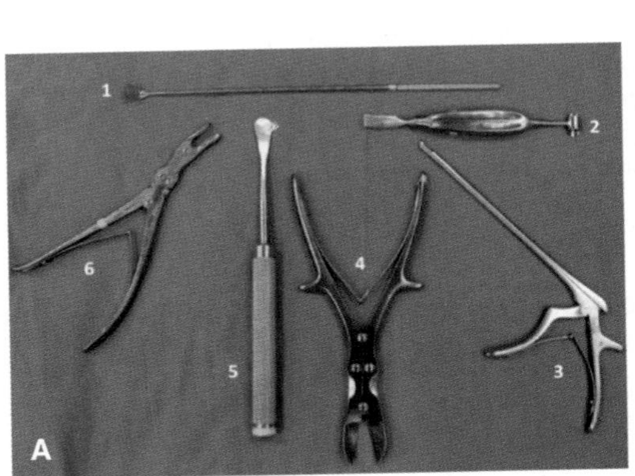

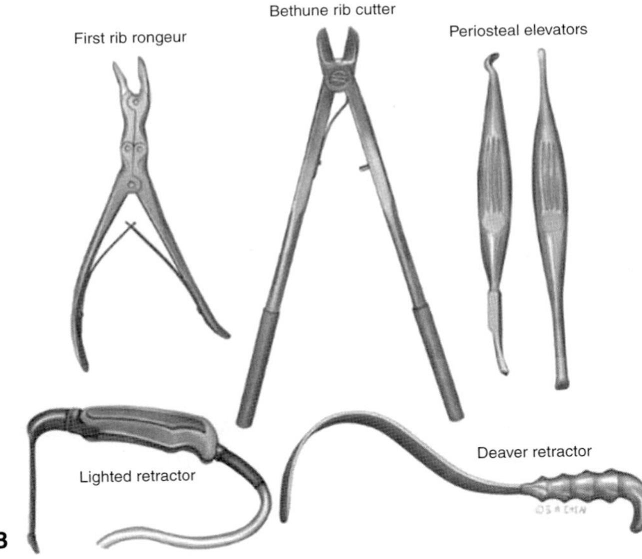

FIGURE 9 ● **A,** From the top of the image in the clockwise direction, the instruments depicted are *(1)* Roos retractor, *(2)* Alexander periosteotome, *(3)* Kerrison punch upbiting instrument, *(4)* double-action bone cutter, *(5)* Cobb periosteal elevator, and *(6)* Rongeur. **B,** From the top of the image in the clockwise direction, the instruments depicted are (1) first rib rongeur, (2) Bethune rib cutter, (3) periosteal elevators, (4) Deaver retractor, (5) lighted retractor. **A,** (Reprinted from Arnaoutakis G, Freischlag JA, Reifsnyder T. Transaxillary rib resection for thoracic outlet syndrome. In: Cambria R, Chaikof E, eds. *Atlas of Vascular and Endovascular Surgery: Anatomy and Technique*. Elsevier; 2014:193-203. Copyright © 2014 Elsevier. With permission.)

- It is important to ensure that the rib be removed all the way to the spine, and that there are no residual fibers from the anterior scalene muscle crossing beneath the subclavian artery and inserting onto the thickened surface at the apex of the pleura, known as Sibson fascia. Any such fibers should be identified and divided (**FIGURE 10**).
- New approaches to TOS surgery have been described in the literature, such as rib-sparing scalenectomy.[14] Recent advances in technology include robotic first rib resections. Recent studies demonstrate symptom relief as well as less frequent complications with the robotic approach relative to the supraclavicular approach, though further investigation is necessary into this emerging approach.[15,16] We continue to advocate for complete decompression of the thoracic outlet with first rib resection and scalenectomy.

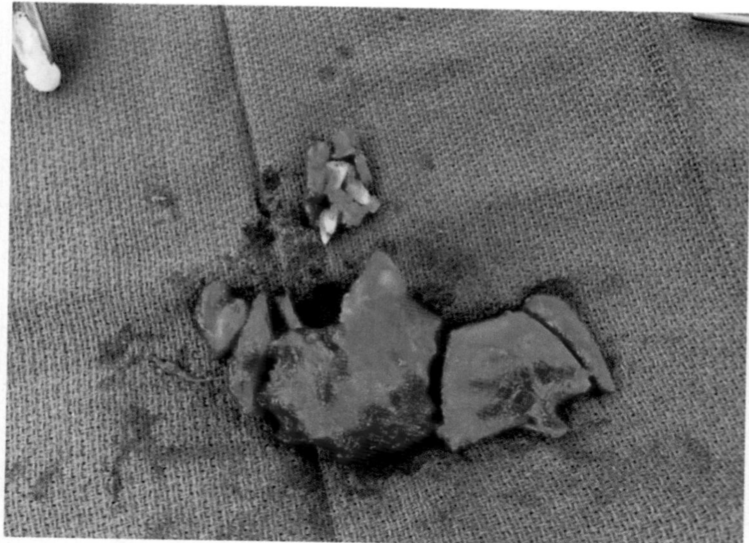

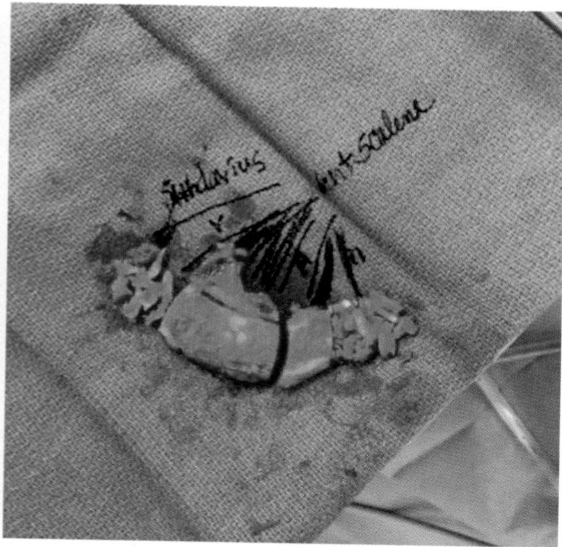

FIGURE 10 ● Resected rib labeled with previous anatomical attachments and relationships.

CLOSURE

- The surgical field is next inspected for bleeding. Temporarily packing the wound reliably controls minor bleeding. The wound is then reinspected, and hemostasis is completed with judicious use of electrocautery.
- The wound is then filled with saline. Several positive pressure ventilations are administered with saline left in the wound to assess for an air leak indicative of a postoperative pneumothorax. If an air leak is present, a small caliber (12 French [Fr]) chest tube is warranted prior to closure.
- If the irrigation drains into the pleural space but there is no air leak, the pleura has been breached, but a chest tube may not be necessary. In this situation, a 12-Fr or 14-Fr red rubber catheter is placed into the bed of the first rib and attached to gentle suction. The Machleder arm holder is lowered to facilitate a tension-free closure. The subcutaneous fascia is then closed around the tube. While suction is applied to the red rubber catheter, the anesthesia team provides a sustained Valsalva and the fascial suture is tied as the suction tube is rapidly removed. This maneuver generally avoids a clinically significant postoperative pneumothorax.
- Closure is performed with absorbable 2-0 suture in the fascia and a 4-0 subcuticular skin closure.

PEARLS AND PITFALLS

Operative mantra	▪ Look twice and cut once. Always double-check placement of the bone cutters before dividing the first rib.
Incorrect diagnosis	▪ A successful operation hinges on an accurate preoperative diagnosis. A thorough history and physical and the anterior scalene block help to identify patients likely to benefit from first rib resection.
Brachial plexus injury	▪ Proper positioning and careful retraction help prevent excessive traction and injury to the brachial plexus.
Misidentification of the first rib	▪ During initial exposure, the second rib is often mistaken for the first rib. The cephalad surface of the first rib is flat unlike the second, which is more concave.
Incomplete first rib resection	▪ Incomplete first rib resection has been associated with recurrent TOS. After cutting and removing the rib, take your time to trim back the ends with the rongeur.
Hemostasis	▪ To keep a clean operative field, pack a 4 × 4 gauze into the wound, lower the arm retractor, and wait a couple of minutes. This often aids in hemostasis.

POSTOPERATIVE CARE

- A chest X-ray is obtained in the recovery room only in instances when a chest tube was placed or there was a pleural tear identified.
  - Small, clinically asymptomatic pneumothoraces may be observed with a follow-up chest X-ray the next morning.
- Postoperative pain control is one of the most important aspects of postoperative care.
- Patients are typically discharged from the hospital when adequate oral analgesia has been achieved.
- Activity is restricted by the amount of postoperative pain. Occasionally, a sling is required for patient comfort, but it is preferable to have the arm as mobile as tolerated.
- Physical therapy should be prescribed after 2 weeks in all patients undergoing transaxillary first rib resection, regardless of the cause, to restore range of motion and strength.

OUTCOMES

- Improvement after surgery for neurogenic TOS is somewhat subjective and based on the patient's perception of disability before and after decompression. Improvement in symptoms exceeds 90%.[17,18]
- Over time, the durability of these results may decrease, reinforcing the need for close follow-up of these patients beyond 2 years.[19,20]
- Factors that predict surgical failure include major depression, chronic symptoms, work-related injury, lack of response to anterior scalene muscle blocks, and a short segment of divided anterior scalene muscle.[21]
- The Quick Disabilities of the Arm, Shoulder, and Hand (QuickDASH) survey and the Cervical-Brachial Symptom Questionnaire (CBSQ) have increasingly been used to evaluate symptoms and functions preoperatively and postoperatively.[22,23]

CONTRAINDICATIONS AND COMPLICATIONS

Contraindications

- The primary contraindication to the transaxillary approach is vascular reconstruction. Scher class 2 and 3 subclavian artery aneurysm reconstructions are specifically contraindicated in the transaxillary approach, due to the inability to repair the subclavian vein with patch angioplasty.
- While dialysis access maintenance is not an absolute contraindication to the transaxillary approach, this surgical procedure should be approached with caution in this setting.

Vascular Injury

- A national query identified injury to the subclavian vessels as the most common complication following transaxillary rib resection for neurogenic TOS, occurring in 1% to 2% of cases.[24,25]
- Patients experiencing a vascular injury have greater lengths of stay as well as increased hospital charges.
- It is difficult to obtain proximal control of these vessels from the transaxillary approach, and therefore, the surgeon should exercise extreme caution when dissecting near these vessels.
- The prevalence of vascular injury is equal in the transaxillary and supraclavicular surgical approaches.[26]

Nerve Injury

- Major nerve injury has been traditionally regarded as the most common complication following surgery for TOS. However, large contemporary series disprove this belief, with rates of brachial plexus injury for patients undergoing transaxillary first rib resection approaching 0%.[20,24]
- Temporary or permanent numbness of the upper medial arm due to excessive traction or division of the intercostobrachial nerve occurs in up to 10%. Frequently, these symptoms will improve over time.
- Transient brachial plexus injury is more common in the transaxillary approach than in the supraclavicular approach, but not in a statistically significant fashion.[26]

Pneumothorax

- This complication occurs in 2% to 10% of patients.[20] Accordingly, an upright chest X-ray is routinely performed in the recovery room.
- Radiographically detected pneumothoraces only require a chest tube if symptomatic or enlarging.
- Adhering closely to the inferior surface of the first rib during blunt dissection will help protect against postoperative pneumothorax.
- The prevalence of pneumothorax is equal between the transaxillary and supraclavicular surgical approaches.[26]

Persistent Pain

- Persistent pain and symptoms are more common in the transaxiallary approach compared to the supraclavicular approach in a statistically significant fashion.[26]

Recurrence

- Symptoms of TOS recur in 10% to 20% of patients.[27-29]
- There may be functional impairment despite clinical improvement of symptoms.[30]
- Two intraoperative factors are known to reduce recurrence rates.
  - Resecting a significant portion (2-3 cm) of the anterior scalene muscle as opposed to simply dividing it at its insertion point
  - Ensuring that the posterior edge of the first rib is resected sufficiently so as to leave as short a rib stump as technically feasible
- Patients with spontaneous recurrence compared to those that are reinjured have worse outcomes when reoperation is performed.

REFERENCES

1. Roos DB. Transaxillary approach for first rib resection to relieve thoracic outlet syndrome. *Ann Surg*. 1966;163:354-358.
2. Kaplan J, Kanwal A. "*Thoracic Outlet Syndrome*." *StatPearls*. StatPearls Publishing; 2020. https://www.ncbi.nlm.nih.gov/books/NBK557450/.
3. Li N, Dierks G, Vervaeke HE, et al. Thoracic outlet syndrome: a narrative review. *J Clin Med*. 2021;10(5):962.
4. Chang MC, Kim DH. Essentials of thoracic outlet syndrome: a narrative review. *World J Clin Cases*. 2021;9(21):5804.
5. Jones MR, Prabhakar A, Viswanath O, et al. Thoracic outlet syndrome: a comprehensive review of pathophysiology, diagnosis, and treatment. *Pain Ther*. 2019;8(1):5-18.
6. Henry BM, Vikse J, Sanna B, et al. Cervical rib prevalence and its association with thoracic outlet syndrome: a meta-analysis

of 141 studies with surgical considerations. *World Neurosurg*. 2018;110:e965-e978.
7. Hussain MA, Aljabri B, Al-Omran M. *Vascular thoracic outlet syndrome*. In *Seminars in Thoracic and Cardiovascular Surgery*. Vol 28, No. 1. WB Saunders; 2016:151-157.
8. Illig KA, Rodriguez-Zoppi E, Bland T, Muftah M, Jospitre E. The incidence of thoracic outlet syndrome. *Ann Vasc Surg*. 2021;70:263-272.
9. Ferrante MA, Ferrante ND. The thoracic outlet syndromes: Part 1. Overview of the thoracic outlet syndromes and review of true neurogenic thoracic outlet syndrome. *Muscle Nerve*. 2017;55(6):782-793.
10. Povlsen S, Povlsen B. Diagnosing thoracic outlet syndrome: current approaches and future directions. *Diagnostics*. 2018;8(1):21.
11. Vemuri C, McLaughlin LN, Abuirqeba AA, Thompson RW. Clinical presentation and management of arterial thoracic outlet syndrome. *J Vasc Surg*. 2017;65(5):1429-1439.
12. Raptis CA, Sridhar S, Thompson RW, Fowler KJ, Bhalla S. Imaging of the patient with thoracic outlet syndrome. *Radiographics*. 2016;36(4):984-1000.
13. Lum YW, Brooke BS, Likes K, et al. Impact of anterior scalene lidocaine blocks on predicting surgical success in older patients with neurogenic thoracic outlet syndrome. *J Vasc Surg*. 2012;55:1370-1375.
14. Johansen K. Rib-sparing scalenectomy for neurogenic thoracic outlet syndrome: early results. *J Vasc Surg*. 2021;73(6):2059-2063.
15. Kocher GJ, Zehnder A, Lutz JA, Schmidli J, Schmid RA. First rib resection for thoracic outlet syndrome: the robotic approach. *World J Surg*. 2018;42(10):3250-3255.
16. Burt BM, Palivela N, Cekmecelioglu D, et al. Safety of robotic first rib resection for thoracic outlet syndrome. *J Thorac Cardiovasc Surg*. 2021;162(4):1297-1305.
17. Roos DB. The place for scalenectomy and first-rib resection in thoracic outlet syndrome. *Surgery*. 1982;92:1077-1085.
18. Peek J, Vos CG, Ünlü Ç, van de Pavoordt HD, van den Akker PJ, de Vries JP. Outcome of surgical treatment for thoracic outlet syndrome: systematic review and meta-analysis. *Ann Vasc Surg*. 2017;40:303-326.
19. Rochlin DH, Gilson MM, Likes KC, et al. Quality-of-life scores in neurogenic thoracic outlet syndrome patients undergoing first rib resection and scalenectomy. *J Vasc Surg*. 2013;57:436-443.
20. Altobelli GG, Kudo T, Haas BT, et al. Thoracic outlet syndrome: pattern of clinical success after operative decompression. *J Vasc Surg*. 2005;42:122-128.
21. Axelrod DA, Proctor MC, Geisser ME, et al. Outcomes after surgery for thoracic outlet syndrome. *J Vasc Surg*. 2001;33:1220-1225.
22. Beaton DE, Wright JG, Katz JN; Upper Extremity Collaborative Group. Development of the QuickDASH: comparison of three item-reduction approaches. *JBJS*. 2005;87(5):1038-1046.
23. Ruopsa N, Ristolainen L, Vastamäki M, Vastamäki H. Neurogenic thoracic outlet syndrome with supraclavicular release: long-term outcome without rib resection. *Diagnostics*. 2021;11(3):450.
24. Thompson RW. *Complications of surgery for thoracic outlet syndrome*. In *Vascular and Endovascular Complications*. CRC Press; 2021:233-245.
25. Chang DC, Rotellini-Coltvet LA, Mukherjee D, et al. Surgical intervention for thoracic outlet syndrome improves patient's quality of life. *J Vasc Surg*. 2009;49:630-635; discussion 635-637.
26. Hosseinian MA, Loron AG, Soleimanifard Y. Evaluation of complications after surgical treatment of thoracic outlet syndrome. *Korean J Thorac Cardiovasc Surg*. 2017;50(1):36.
27. Mingoli A, Feldhaus RJ, Farina C, et al. Long-term outcome after transaxillary approach for thoracic outlet syndrome. *Surgery*. 1995;118:840-844.
28. Mingoli A, Sapienza P, di Marzo L, et al. Role of first rib stump length in recurrent neurogenic thoracic outlet syndrome. *Am J Surg*. 2005;190:156.
29. Sanders RJ, Haug CE, Pearce WH. Recurrent thoracic outlet syndrome. *J Vasc Surg*. 1990;12:390-398; discussion 398-400.
30. Peek J, Vos CG, Ünlü Ç, Schreve MA, Van de Mortel RH, De Vries JP. Long-term functional outcome of surgical treatment for thoracic outlet syndrome. *Diagnostics*. 2018;8(1):7.

Chapter 9

Venous and Arterial Thoracic Outlet Syndrome

Kathryn Lambeth DiLosa and Misty D. Humphries

DEFINITION

- Venous thoracic outlet syndrome (vTOS), also known as effort thrombosis or Paget-Schroetter syndrome, involves repetitive subclavian vein compression resulting in endothelial injury and intermittent stasis. This damage ultimately contributes to acute thrombosis of the axillosubclavian veins. The external compression of the vein occurs between the clavicle/subclavius muscle from above, the first rib inferiorly, and the anterior scalene muscle insertion (**FIGURE 1**).
- Arterial thoracic outlet syndrome (aTOS) is the least common form of TOS, accounting for less than 1% of overall cases. Extrinsic subclavian artery compression results in poststenotic dilatation, aneurysmal degeneration, and subsequent distal embolization.[1] In aTOS, the arterial compression is caused by bony or muscular abnormalities including a cervical rib, anomalous first rib, anterior or middle scalene muscle bands, or hypertrophic callus from a healed clavicular injury or fracture.[2] The higher preponderance of cervical ribs in women translates to an increased incidence of aTOS among women.[3]

DIFFERENTIAL DIAGNOSIS

- Patients with vTOS present with upper extremity swelling and a differential diagnosis is elicited by a thorough history. Secondary axillosubclavian thrombosis due to iatrogenic catheterization or prior instrumentation of the upper extremity veins is far more common and should be considered first. In patients who do not perform repetitive overhead movements or play high-performance sports, malignancy or underlying hypercoagulable state should be ruled out.[4,5]
- In patients with hand or digit ischemia, a thorough workup for a cardiogenic source should be sought before assigning the etiology to aTOS. Cardiac etiology is far more common than embolization of thrombus from a subclavian aneurysm due to underlying aTOS. Paradoxical emboli, a patent foramen ovale, axillary artery branch aneurysms, congenital vascular abnormalities, or traumatic injuries/arterial dissection of the axillosubclavian arterial system should be ruled out.

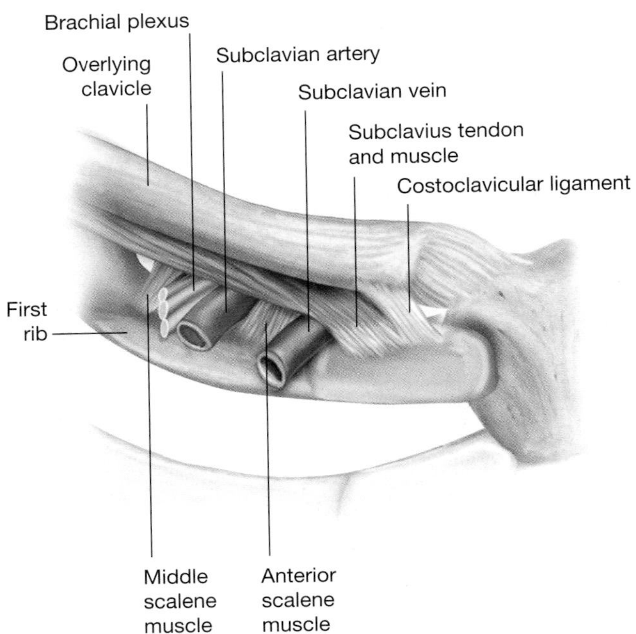

FIGURE 1 ● Normal structures in the thoracic outlet that can contribute to venous compression.

PATIENT HISTORY AND PHYSICAL FINDINGS

- Patients with vTOS are often young men, healthy, and athletically inclined who present with the abrupt onset of unilateral arm swelling in their dominant arm after repetitive, strenuous use for sport, work, or recreation.[6] Athletes who require their arms to hyperabduct and extend repeatedly, such as swimmers and baseball pitchers, are most commonly affected. The characteristic swelling present in the shoulder, arm, and hand and can be accompanied by aching, throbbing, or tightness that worsens with activity. The severity of venous thrombosis also correlates with symptomatology. Because most patients are otherwise young and healthy, orthopedic causes such as strain, muscle pull, or joint injury are often considered initially. Range of motion in the affected extremity can be impeded due to discomfort, further suggesting, albeit incorrectly, a musculoskeletal cause. Cyanosis of the affected extremity, chest wall venous collaterals, or progressively worsening symptoms indicate a vascular etiology and should prompt referral to a TOS comprehensive care center. On exam, the arm will appear edematous, tender to palpation, warm, and often has visible superficial collaterals that track onto the anterior chest wall (**FIGURE 2**).
- aTOS patients present with mild to severe hand ischemia arising from embolization. Frequently, there is long-standing embolization leading to small vessel thrombosis and this can manifest as digital ischemia or present with splinter hemorrhages. The diagnosis is often delayed as these patients have no typical atherosclerotic risk factors and are frequently young and athletic. A bruit or pulsatile mass may be palpable in the supraclavicular fossa and a bony prominence in that region may imply the presence of a cervical rib or muscular abnormality. Symptoms often are gradual and unnoticed by patients until the vessels thrombose or there is embolization to the brachial bifurcation and the patient presents with critical upper extremity ischemia.

IMAGING AND OTHER DIAGNOSTIC STUDIES

- Patients with suspected vTOS should undergo duplex ultrasound of the affected extremity. Depending on the chronicity of the lesion, well-developed collaterals can be mistaken for the subclavian vein. Color flow duplex, phasicity of flow with respiration, and augmentation with provocative maneuvers can all aid in confirming the diagnosis of deep venous thrombosis (DVT). An experienced vascular sonographer and interpreter can make the diagnosis with a high degree of accuracy based on the duplex alone. Cross-sectional imaging with magnetic resonance imaging (MRI) or computed tomography (CT) venography is rarely needed or indicated in the workup of vTOS. Catheter-based venography can confirm diagnosis and document the extent of vTOS while allowing for thrombolysis and reduction of clot burden; however, long-term studies have not supported that thrombolysis improves outcomes after first rib resection.[7]

- Patients presenting with digital ischemia suspicious for aTOS should undergo plain radiographic imaging to assess for a cervical rib (**FIGURE 3**). Digital photoplethysmography (PPG) of the bilateral upper extremities can be performed to visualize blood flow to each finger and can rule out Raynaud type etiologies but offers no anatomic evaluation of the artery for aneurysmal degeneration. When combined with provocative arm elevation, PPG will demonstrate dampening of waveforms, though this is nonspecific for the diagnosis of aTOS.[5] Similar results can be observed with duplex ultrasound when combined with provocative maneuvers. It is imperative to also understand that subclavian artery compression can be seen in up to a quarter of the population, and simple arterial compression is not diagnostic of aTOS.[6] CT angiography (CTA) of the neck or chest and upper extremity provides the most definitive visualization of the subclavian artery and thoracic outlet, confirming the presence of the cervical rib, delineating the amount of thrombus in the subclavian aneurysm, and documenting the proximal and distal vasculature for preoperative planning (**FIGURE 4A** and **B**). Arm elevation with CTA can obscure the course of the artery, thus should be done only in combination with neutral position imaging. While magnetic resonance angiography (MRA) can also be used to identify aTOS, the longer imaging acquisition times and bony artifact can fail to delineate the specific arterial anatomy for surgical planning.

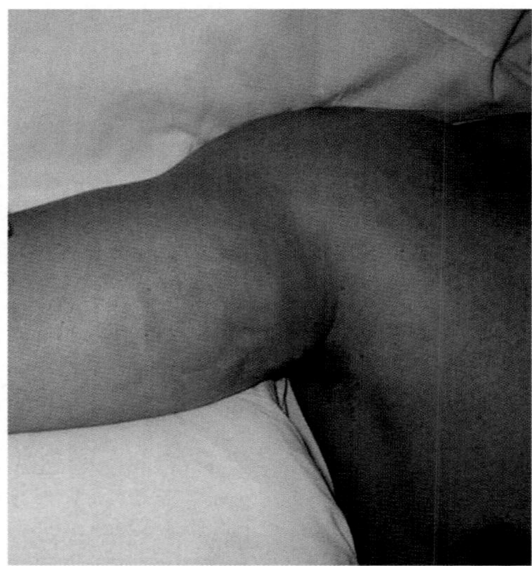

FIGURE 2 • Physical exam appearance of a patient with venous TOS and venous collaterals from long standing subclavian vein compression.

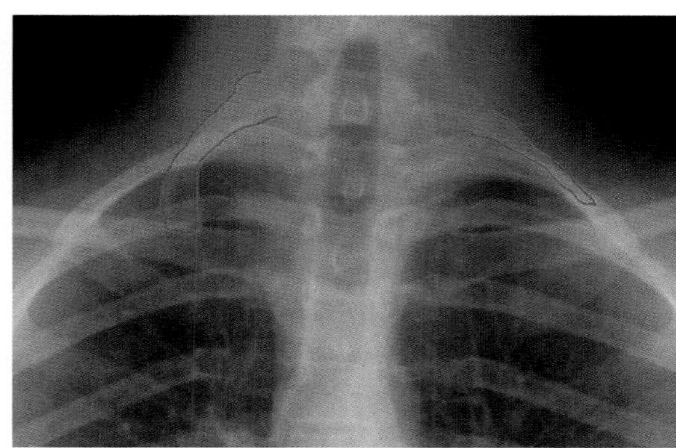

FIGURE 3 • Young patient with bilateral asymmetric cervical ribs (outlined in red).

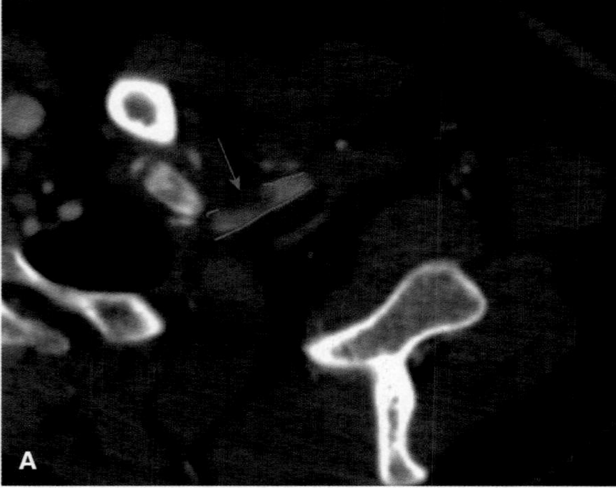

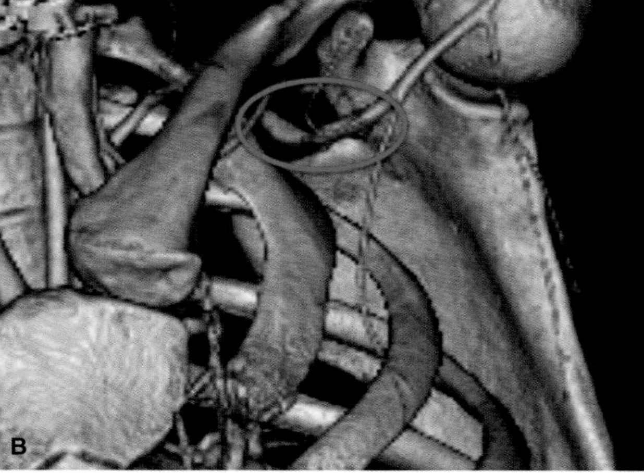

FIGURE 4 • **A,** Axial CT image of a left subclavian artery aneurysm (outlined in red) with evidence of thrombus (*blue arrow*). **B,** Three dimensional rendering of the left subclavian artery aneurysm (*red circle*) in relation to the left cervical rib and first rib.

COMPREHENSIVE CARE MODELS

- Chronic pain symptoms are common with neurogenic TOS, but outcomes for patients undergoing treatment for TOS have been shown to be better and more consistent when patients receive care from a coordinated care center.[8] Comprehensive TOS centers are more likely to use tools that adhere to the Society for Vascular Surgery Reporting Standards and collect long-term outcomes for patients with TOS, which are necessary for further advances in treatment methods.[9] These centers are also able to provide tailored pre and postoperative care for optimal recovery and prevention/management of recurrent symptoms.

SURGICAL MANAGEMENT

Preoperative Planning

- Patients with mild to moderate vTOS symptoms can be managed with anticoagulation.[10] Young patients and high-performance athletes have better long-term outcomes with surgical decompression of the thoracic outlet.[11] When patients present with severe symptoms of swelling, pain, and numbness, thrombolysis should be performed. Successful thrombolysis can involve a combination of chemical and mechanical thrombectomy and is effective in decreasing clot burden and reducing long-term sequelae of upper extremity chronic DVT (**FIGURE 5A** and **B**).[12] Technical details of thrombolysis are well described and can be performed with minimal morbidity.
- Definitive therapy after thrombolysis involves thoracic outlet decompression, consisting of anterior scalenectomy, resection of the subclavius tendon, first rib resection, and venolysis. Venous reconstruction is an option, but with increased endovascular techniques; this is frequently not necessary.
- The timing of surgery after thrombolysis remains somewhat controversial and is limited by anecdotal reports and various surgeon biases. Successful outcomes can be achieved with definitive thoracic outlet decompression performed during the same hospitalization as the thrombolysis and up to 3 months after.[10] Management of anticoagulation during this time also impacts decisions about planning surgery, as intolerance to blood thinners or difficulty with maintaining adequate anticoagulation can affect the urgency of the required definitive decompression. The use of direct oral anticoagulants (DOACs) has limited most intolerance issues previously seen with anticoagulation.[13]
- aTOS in the presence of an ipsilateral cervical rib and a subclavian aneurysm is an indication for definitive surgical decompression and arterial reconstruction. Preoperative planning consists mainly of ensuring adequate and healthy vasculature proximal and distal to the aneurysmal segment, determining an appropriate bypass route, and choosing a conduit. Extra-anatomic bypass via a carotid-subclavian or carotid-axillary with interval ligation may be necessary, depending on the size and length of the subclavian aneurysm and extent of vascular thrombosis. Direct repair of the subclavian aneurysm with interposition grafting can be accomplished when there is a short segment aneurysm that limits itself to the visualized region in the supraclavicular

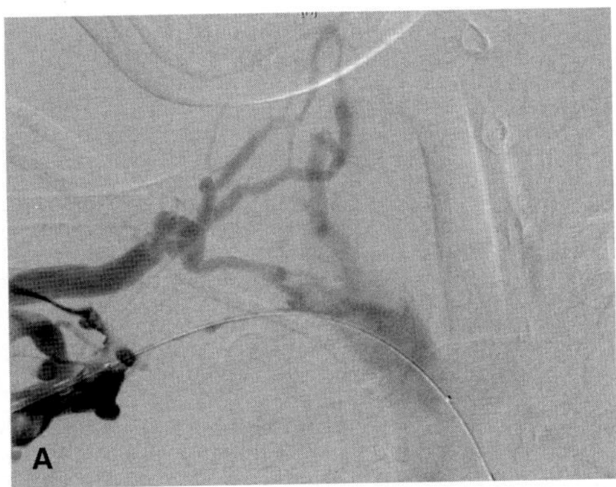

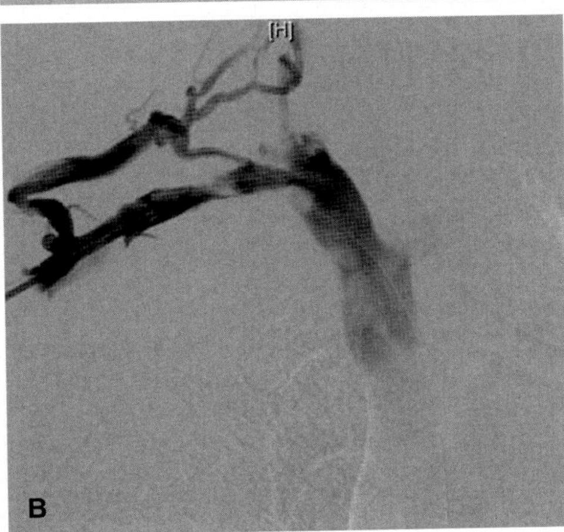

FIGURE 5 • **A,** Initial venogram demonstrating right axillosubclavian occlusion with large collateral development. Wire was passed through this region and pharmacomechanical thrombolysis initiated. **B,** Follow-up venogram 24 hours later with resolution of majority of thrombus load. Vein still shows signs of disease and scarring particularly in the region of compression.

fossa. Endovascular techniques such as stent grafting in the setting of aTOS are generally not recommended, given the young age of the typical patient, the compression that can occur from scarring even after surgical decompression, and the likely desire to resume prior activities in the postoperative period.

Positioning

- vTOS decompression can be achieved through an infraclavicular, paraclavicular, or transaxillary approach. The approach determines patient positioning. For the infraclavicular and paraclavicular approach, the patient is positioned supine with a small roll between the shoulder blades. The head of the bed is elevated to 30° to decrease venous return and the face turned away from the operative side. For the transaxillary approach, the patient is positioned laterally on a bean bag with the affected arm up. An axillary roll is placed underneath the arm that is down. In all approaches, the affected arm is prepped into the field so that it can be moved around to evaluate for residual compression. This affords anterior visualization of the first rib and particularly the subclavius muscle. The entire ipsilateral neck, shoulder, arm (and axilla for transaxillary), and anterior chest wall are prepped into the field as well as a region on the lateral chest wall should there be a small postprocedural pneumothorax necessitating a chest tube. For the transaxillary approach, the arm is placed in a sterile Machleder retractor after it is wrapped with Kerlix for padding (**FIGURE 6**).

- The approach for the treatment of aTOS is dependent on the potential need for subclavian artery reconstruction. A supraclavicular or combined supra and infraclavicular approach is used when arterial bypass is required, and the patient is positioned as above. When the subclavian artery is not damaged, but a cervical rib is identified, a transaxillary approach can be considered. When arterial reconstruction with a venous conduit is planned, preparations should be made for saphenous or femoral vein harvesting.

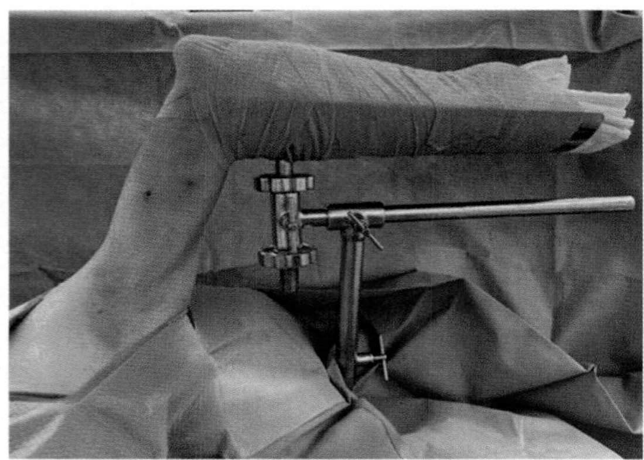

FIGURE 6 ● Positioning of the arm in the Machleder retractor for transaxillary first rib resection.

VENOUS TOS

Infraclavicular Approach

- A 5-cm transverse incision is made one fingerbreadth below the clavicle, starting along the edge of the sternum extending laterally. The dissection is carried through the subcutaneous tissue and pectoralis fascia to expose the upper fibers of the pectoralis major muscle (**FIGURE 7**). Gentle spreading between muscle fibers in this region exposes the anteromedial quadrant of the axillary fat pad and allows easy palpation of the first rib. Handheld or self-retaining retractors can be placed to fully expose the most anterior portion of the first rib beneath a layer of axillary fat (**FIGURE 8**).

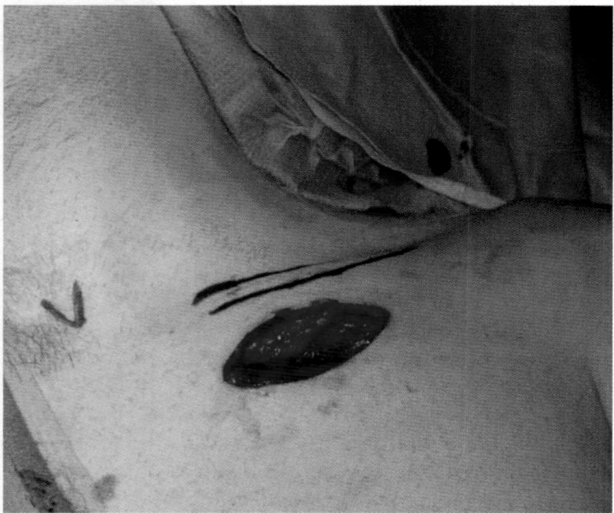

FIGURE 7 ● Infraclavicular incision is made one fingerbreadth below clavicle.

- Once the first rib is visualized, cautery is used to separate the inferior intercostal musculature from the rib. This dissection is carried superolateral along the C-curve of the rib (**FIGURE 9**). The lung pleura will be visualized immediately beneath the rib and care should be taken to not injure lung parenchyma. Along the inferior portion of the clavicle, the subclavius tendon is taken down with cautery to free up the anterior portion of the first rib from the overhanging clavicle. The costoclavicular ligament may also need to be taken down, as it can be a cause of venous compression.[14] Following along the superior aspect of the first rib, the anterior scalene fibers are also sharply taken down and further superior dissection takes place along the lateral edge of the first rib until palpation of the subclavian artery is noted. Often, moving the arm in a superior position facilitates more superior exposure of the first rib near the artery.

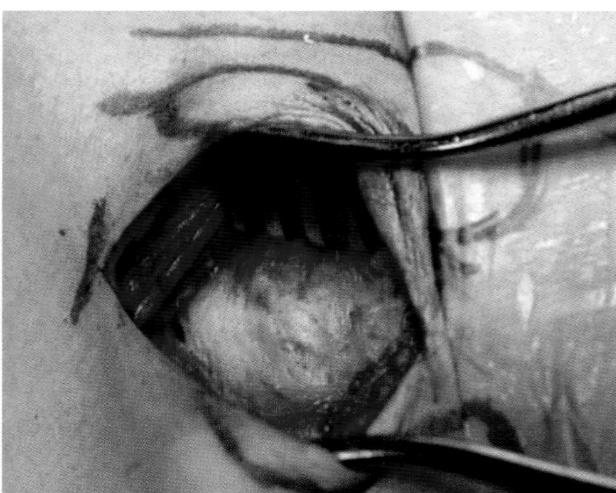

FIGURE 8 ● Incision is carried down through pectoralis fascia, then the muscle fibers are split until axillary fat that covers the first rib is reached.

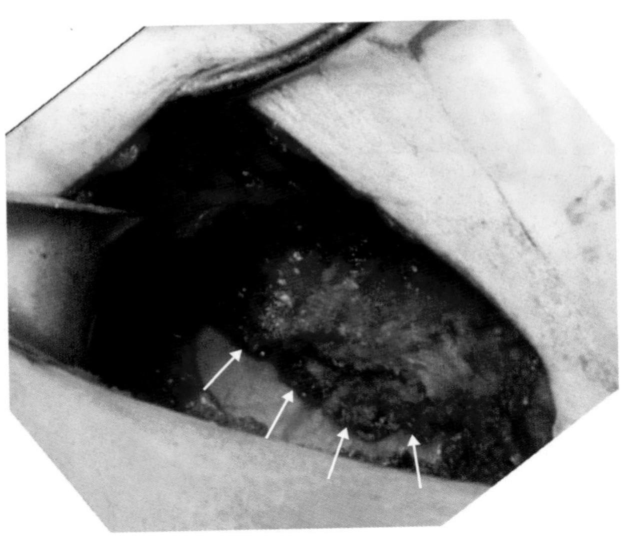

FIGURE 9 ● Further dissection around the 1st rib involves sharp dissection of intercostal musculature along inferior aspect of first rib (*arrows*).

- When the rib is clear on its superior, lateral, and inferior edge, a rib cutter can be inserted superiorly, taking care to visualize the jaws, and then the superior cut is made in the rib. The inferior cut is done near the manubrial junction, commonly with a power saw. As the rib is pulled away from the body, sharp cautery can be used to facilitate hemostasis of individual muscle fibers (intercostals, anterior and middle scalene) holding the first rib in place.
- Care should be taken to ensure that no anterior rib remnants remain, as this increases the risk for recurrent venous symptoms. Posterior rib remnants can result in the development of neurogenic symptoms as a result of brachial plexus compression.[11] Following surgical decompression, as many as 20% of patients may experience persistent recurrent symptoms, most commonly the result of residual first rib remnant left behind during the index operation.[12]

Transaxillary Approach (FIGURE 10)

- The external landmarks are marked out on the skin, including the pectoralis major muscle and the latissimus dorsi muscle. A skin incision is created 2 fingerbreadths from the apex of the axilla just above the base of the hairline between the two muscles. The subcutaneous tissues are dissected down to the chest wall using a combination of blunt dissection and electrocautery. The arm is then elevated in the retractor (**FIGURE 10A** and **B**).
- Using a peanut on a long Pean clamp, the tissues are dissected following the subclavian vein down to the thoracic outlet. The subclavius muscle/tendon attachments that come down to the first rib, anterior scalene, and subclavian artery are dissected as well. With the vein protected, once the subclavius tendon is dissected it can be cut with scissors. Next, the anterior scalene muscle is incised by passing a right angle clamp posterior and cutting the muscle piece by piece until the entire muscle is cut (**FIGURE 10C**).
- A periosteal elevator is used to free the intercostal muscles along the lateral aspect of the first rib. A smaller elevator is then passed under the rib to dissect the pleura away from the rib, allowing the rib to be cut anteriorly. The middle scalene muscle fibers are then dissected off the rib with the elevator. Once the posterior rib is free of muscle, a Bethune rib cutter can be used to cut the posterior rib, with care taken to ensure the inferior trunk of the brachial plexus is protected (**FIGURE 10D**).
- The residual rib is removed with a first rib rongeur both anteriorly and posteriorly. Once the rib is removed completely, the pleura is tested for a tear by instilling saline in the wound and having a Valsalva maneuver performed by the anesthesia team. If a tear is present, a 19 French Blake drain can be placed under direct visualization.

Endovascular Venous Treatment/Venous Reconstruction

- With the rib removed from the infraclavicular approach, the vein is often palpable in a bed of tissue and muscle fibers immediately below the clavicle. Venolysis consists of freeing up these muscle fibers to expose the vein (**FIGURE 11**). More proximal exposure of the vein can be accomplished via a transmanubrial extension of the infraclavicular incision to the center of the sternum and vertically up to the sternal notch (**FIGURE 12**). This can be necessary to obtain adequate vascular control for patching of chronically diseased venous segments. When a strictured segment of vein is localized, saphenous vein or bovine pericardial patching provides an excellent strategy for the restoration of luminal diameter and can be performed with adequate proximal and distal control of the vein under direct visualization (**FIGURE 13**).
- If an intraoperative venogram is to be performed, the arm is placed on an arm board out to the side and ultrasound guidance is used to access the basilic vein following decompression. In the event the basilic vein is thrombosed, a brachial vein should be accessed. This provides direct access for treatment of the axillary and subclavian vein. Once a sheath is placed, venography is performed to identify the area of stenosis within the vein. The stenosis is crossed with a Glidewire using a Bern or KMP style catheter for support. A working wire is then positioned in the superior vena cava to allow for balloon angioplasty.

Closure

- Careful attention should be paid to the bone edge for hemostasis, as well as the region of the vein after venolysis and/or reconstruction.
- If the pleura or lung parenchyma has been injured, a round drain (19F Blake) can be placed in the pleural space under direct visualization.

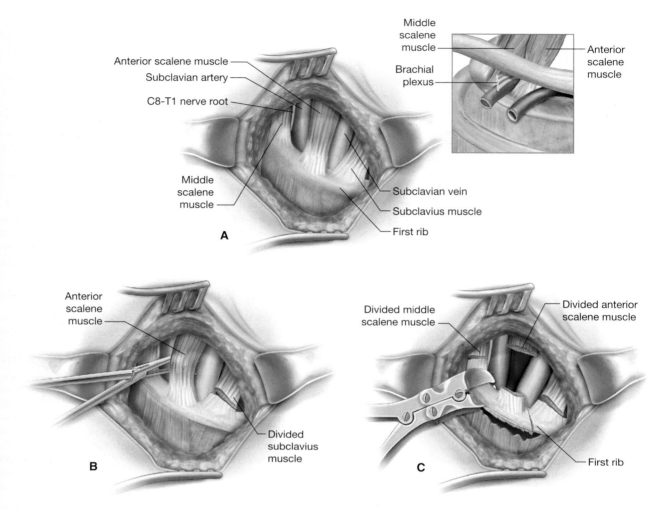

FIGURE 10 ● **A,** Transaxillary view of the relationship of the subclavian artery and vein with the scalene muscles. **B,** The anterior scalene is transected using a right angle and Bovie cautery to free up the first rib. The subclavian artery and vein are identified and preserved. The brachial plexus nerve roots are seen laterally in this view directly behind the middle scalene muscle. **C,** A periosteal elevator is used to free the intercostal muscles along the lateral aspect of the first rib. A smaller elevator is then passed under the rib to dissect the pleura away from the rib, allowing the rib to be cut anteriorly. The middle scalene muscle fibers are then dissected off the rib with the elevator. Once the posterior rib is free of muscle, a Bethune rib cutter can be used to cut the posterior rib, with care taken to ensure the inferior trunk of the brachial plexus is protected.

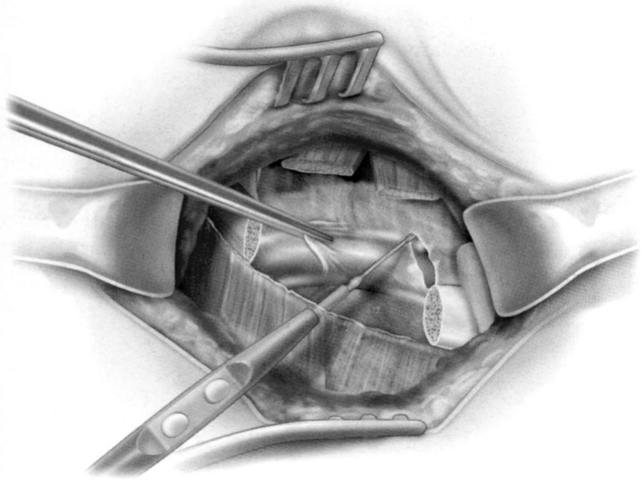

FIGURE 11 ● After first rib is resected, careful dissection around vein with venolysis and takedown of fibers surrounding vein allows adequate visualization to check for stenotic regions.

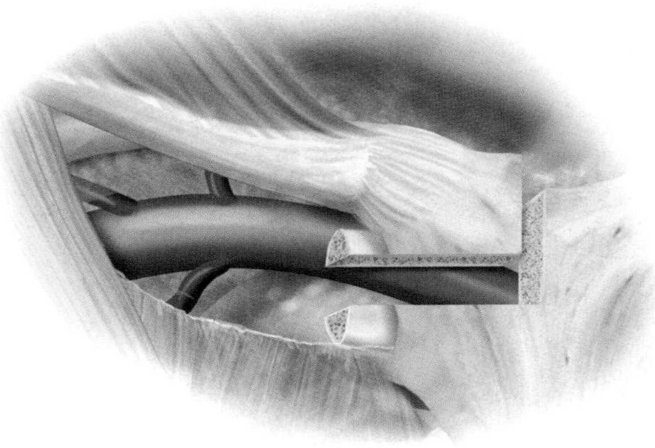

FIGURE 12 ● If more proximal exposure is needed to clamp for control, extension of the incision into the manubrium and toward sternal notch allows wider visualization of the origin of subclavian vein and junction with jugular into the innominate.

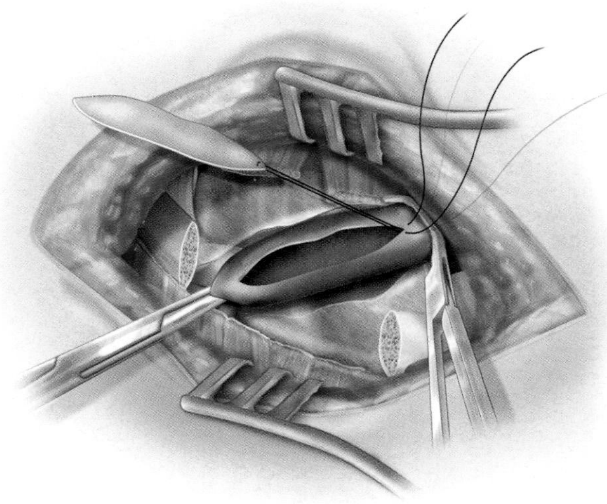

FIGURE 13 ● Stenotic region of the subclavian vein repaired with patch venoplasty using greater saphenous vein.

ARTERIAL THORACIC OUTLET SYNDROME

Supraclavicular Approach

- A 7-cm incision is made one fingerbreadth above the clavicle, starting lateral to the palpable edge of the sternal head of the sternocleidomastoid muscle and carried through the platysma. This exposes the clavicular head of the sternocleidomastoid, which is transected with a cuff to sew back together later, exposing the anterior scalene fat pad (**FIGURE 14**). The fat pad is dissected along three borders, inferiorly, laterally, and medially, to allow it to swing northward to expose the anterior scalene muscle and the phrenic nerve (**FIGURE 15**). When operating on the left side, extra care is taken to visualize the thoracic duct when present, which is suture ligated to prevent a postoperative chyle leak if it becomes injured.
- With the phrenic nerve slung and protected, transection of the anterior scalene muscle off the superior edge of the first rib is accomplished with the use of electrocautery. Care is taken to stay on the bone during this portion so as not to injure the underlying subclavian artery. After the inferior

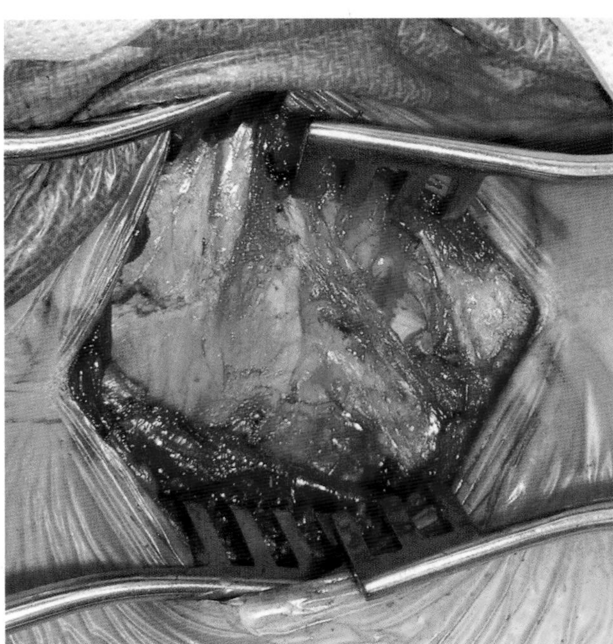

FIGURE 14 ● Supraclavicular incision one fingerbreadth above the clavicle continues after transecting clavicular head of the sternocleidomastoid and exposure of the anterior scalene fat pad.

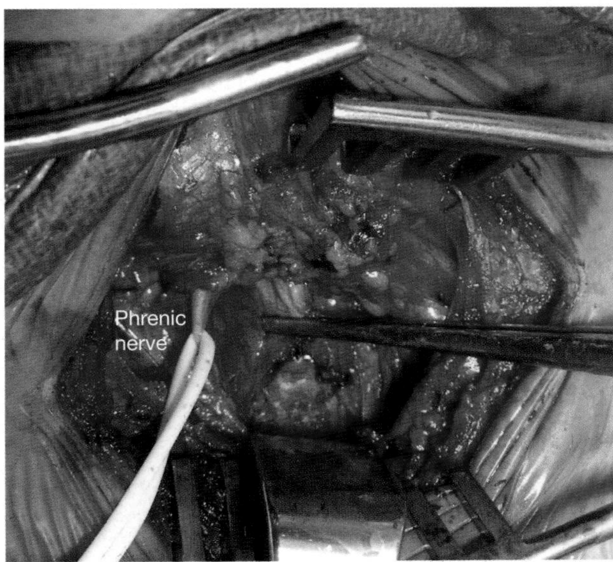

FIGURE 15 ● With the scalene fat pad retracted superiorly, the anterior scalene muscle and phrenic nerve are clearly seen. The nerve is slung with a silastic loop.

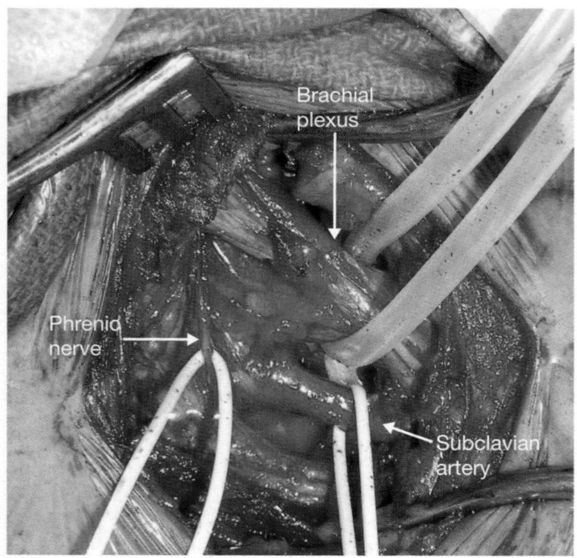

FIGURE 16 ● The first rib is cleared on both sides of the subclavian artery and the brachial plexus fibers, which are all slung to allow easy mobilization.

edge of the anterior scalene is removed, a portion of muscle can be transected to allow room for further visualization and subsequent dissection around the brachial plexus (**FIGURE 16**). The long thoracic nerve is identified laterally, and the brachial plexus structures are slung with a thick silastic loop.

- A cervical rib, when present, is often visualized at this time, with abnormal vasculature or musculature surrounding it, and can be fused to the first rib (**FIGURE 17**). Care is taken to dissect nerves and vessels away from the abnormal rib or its osseous portions that may not have been visualized on radiography.
- The first rib is visualized by maneuvering the subclavian artery and the nerve bundle back and forth while dissecting middle scalene fibers and intercostal musculature off the rib (**FIGURE 16**). This can be done sharply, with bipolar cautery, or by using a periosteal elevator. One should avoid the use of monopolar cautery in this area as it is likely to transmit to the brachial plexus or phrenic nerve.
- When the rib is clear from the region inferior to the subclavian artery and superior to the upper aspect of the brachial plexus, a power saw can be used to transect the rib. If there is a fused portion of the cervical rib, it should be removed as a single piece (**FIGURE 18**) to assure that all bony abnormalities have been freed up to allow for adequate decompression.
- The pleura is inspected to ensure there is no injury. If an injury is present, any air should be evacuated with a red rubber catheter underwater while the fat pad is replaced over

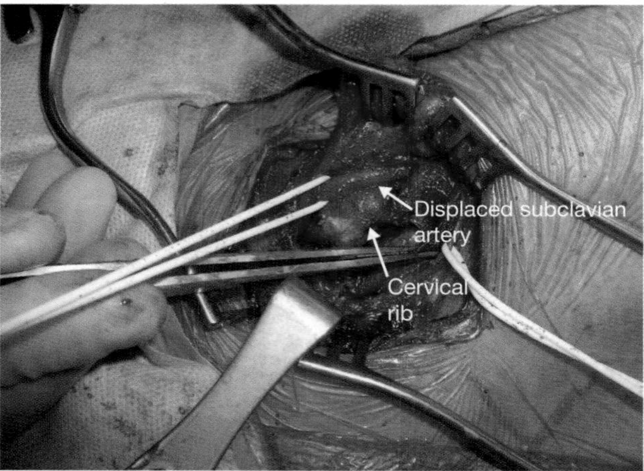

FIGURE 17 ● In this case, a fused cervical rib to the first rib is prominently tenting up the subclavian artery and brachial plexus fibers.

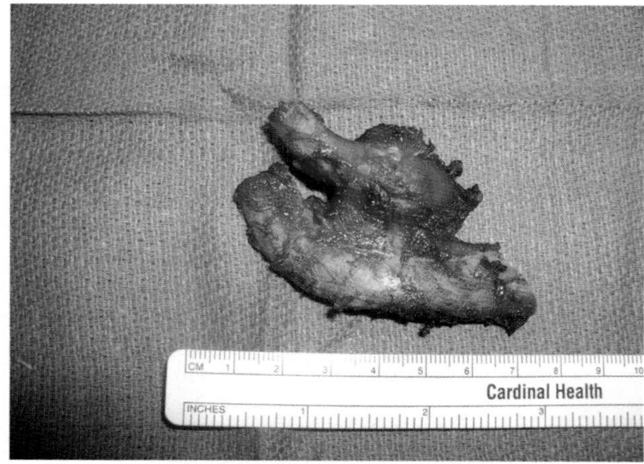

FIGURE 18 ● Removal of the congenitally fused cervical rib to the first rib as an en bloc piece, allowing the neurovascular bundle to return to its normal position without being kinked or displaced.

the outlet. A small 7 flat Jackson Pratt drain can then be placed.

Arterial Reconstruction

- Subclavian aneurysm resection, when needed, consists of appropriate bypass principles and replacement with an autogenous or prosthetic interposition graft or extra-anatomic bypass of carotid to distal subclavian or carotid to axillary graft. Typical sizes and types required for prosthetic grafts include 6- or 8-mm ringed polytetrafluoroethylene (PTFE) or Dacron.

PEARLS AND PITFALLS

Indications	▪ vTOS definitive therapy consists of prompt diagnosis, venography with thrombolysis, and appropriate selection of patients to undergo thoracic outlet decompression. ▪ aTOS patients often present with ischemic hand symptoms that will have some delay in management due to a wide differential. Efforts should be directed toward decreasing long-term sequelae by limiting ischemic time. Abnormal bony or muscular anatomy along with the presence of subclavian aneurysmal disease requires definitive repair including thoracic outlet decompression and arterial reconstruction.
Preoperative workup	▪ Venography and pharmacomechanical thrombolysis provide the optimal reduction of clot burden to restore functional venous patency in patients with vTOS. Timing of rib resection and definitive thoracic outlet decompression are somewhat variable, and the approach should be individualized. ▪ aTOS patients should undergo plain radiography to search for a cervical rib and CTA to determine the portions of the diseased subclavian artery that might require reconstruction.
Patient setup	▪ Prepping the affected arm in the vTOS patients affords the ability to move the arm and, from the infraclavicular approach, gain access to the rib that is responsible for venous compression. ▪ For cervical rib resection and arterial revascularization, the supraclavicular approach gives numerous options for reconstructive purposes as well as the possibility of the carotid artery as an inflow source for bypass.
Infraclavicular approach	▪ Visualization of the subclavius tendon and its fibers, as well as the costoclavicular ligament, is paramount in decompressing the region that compresses the subclavian vein in vTOS. ▪ Liberal patching of the subclavian vein and extensive venolysis provide the best long-term patency results after vTOS decompression.
Supraclavicular approach	▪ Carefully mobilizing the anterior scalene fat pad allows good visualization of the anterior scalene muscle and phrenic nerve. ▪ When performing left-sided supraclavicular TOS decompression, one must be careful to identify and ligate the thoracic duct to prevent a postoperative chyle leak. ▪ Slinging the subclavian artery and brachial plexus fibers allows gentle traction back and forth to expeditiously dissect free the entire first rib.
Transaxillary Approach	▪ When using a transaxillary approach, the phrenic nerve course is typically separate from the anterior scalene muscle above the level of the operative field. However, if it isn't separate, it may be injured when transecting the muscle. ▪ If the inferior trunk of the brachial plexus is adherent to the first rib, this can result in injury to the nerve during resection.

POSTOPERATIVE CARE

- At the conclusion of the procedure, patients are extubated. If there was no evidence of pleural tear by Valsalva at the time of surgery, a chest x-ray is not needed. For patients with a chest drain due to pleural injury, a chest x-ray is obtained. If a chest drain was placed for a pleural injury, it can be connected to a Pleur-evac. At 12 hours, we typically convert this to water seal unless an air leak is identified. The drain is removed on postoperative day 1.
- Patients do not need a sling for their arms. They are given range-of-motion exercises immediately to encourage strengthening and lessen compressive scar tissue formation. Patients with a transaxillary or infraclavicular incision can safely be discharged on postoperative day 1. Most patients will require a taper of muscle relaxant and opioid narcotics for pain control. Patients with a supraclavicular or paraclavicular incision should have their drains removed once it is clear that there is no evidence of a thoracic duct leak and can typically be discharged on postoperative day 2.
- Anticoagulation for vTOS patients is usually resumed 2 to 3 days postoperatively at home. If patients are to return for postoperative venography and venoplasty, there is no need to hold anticoagulation for this procedure.[15]
- Anticoagulation is not always needed for aTOS patients, especially if arterial reconstruction is performed. If the patient initially presented with arterial ischemia, it may be reasonable to continue the patient on anticoagulation. If the patient did not present with ischemia, but a reconstruction was performed, appropriate antiplatelet therapy should be initiated postoperatively.

OUTCOMES

- Patients treated for vTOS with lysis and subsequent thoracic outlet decompression have a very low recurrence rate of thromboembolic disease. Morbidity and mortality are minimal, as these are often young and healthy patients, but typically include wound issues and bleeding given the need for anticoagulation. Satisfactory quality of life scores and return to full function are reported in the 80% to 90% range, and most patients can be counseled to expect a near full return to sports.[16]
- aTOS and the cervical rib patients often have the most dramatic recovery, as they are often the most symptomatic at presentation. Results are uniformly positive with the resolution of ischemic hand symptoms and lack of significant disease recurrence.

COMPLICATIONS

- The most common perioperative complications related to both forms of thoracic outlet decompression revolve around lung injury and wound issues. Pneumothoraces are often self-limited and treated effectively with chest tubes. Wound complications can include chyle leaks, seromas, and skin breakdown. Most of these are managed expectantly.
- Brachial plexus injuries may also occur. These injuries are most commonly a function of not recognizing important anatomic structures or not providing sufficient exposure to eliminate collateral damage during rib transection and removal. Finally, scar tissue or first rib remnants can contribute to the development of persistent vTOS symptoms or the onset of new neurogenic TOS symptoms in up to a fifth of patients.
- Timing of restarting anticoagulation in vTOS patients can lead to postoperative bleeding, which can manifest as delayed hemothorax. The cause of this bleeding is often related to recent thrombolysis and raw surfaces of muscle and cut bone, and this has led to the general recommendation of holding anticoagulation until 2 to 3 days following surgery.

CONCLUSION

Though accounting for approximately 1% and 5% of all TOS cases, respectively, arterial and venous TOS can be effectively managed with minimal long-term morbidity and mortality.[15] In conjunction with a thorough history and physical exam, noninvasive imaging typically provides sufficient evidence to confirm the diagnosis in symptomatic patients, successfully ruling out more common diagnoses on the differential. More severe forms of vTOS and symptomatic aTOS should be evaluated for surgical decompression with lysis or vessel reconstruction to prevent long-term morbidity. Multiple approaches can be used to facilitate decompression of the thoracic outlet and revascularization of the extremity, with the optimal approach for each patient ultimately determined by preoperative imaging. Vascular surgeons remain the optimal caretaker of this unique population, with the knowledge and skill set to manage these patients most effectively. Comprehensive care centers are best situated to provide all-encompassing care both before and after surgery, along with safe and complete decompression of the thoracic outlet when surgery is indicated.

REFERENCES

1. Illig KA, Rodriguez-Zoppi E, Bland T, Muftah M, Jospitre E. The incidence of thoracic outlet syndrome. *Ann Vasc Surg*. 2021;70:263-272. doi:10.1016/j.avsg.2020.07.029
2. Sanders RJ, Pearce WH. The treatment of thoracic outlet syndrome: a comparison of different operations. *J Vasc Surg*. 1989;10(6):626-634. doi:10.1016/0741-5214(89)90005-0
3. Davidoviovi:626-634. doi:10.1016/0741-5214(89)9IB. Arterial complications of thoracic outlet syndrome. *Am Surg*. 2009;75(3):235-239.
4. Cassada DC, Lipscomb AL, Stevens SL, Freeman MB, Grandas OH, Goldman MH. The importance of thrombophilia in the treatment of Paget-Schroetter syndrome. *Ann Vasc Surg*. 2006;20(5):596-601. doi:10.1007/s10016-006-9106-z
5. Likes K, Rochlin D, Nazarian SM, Streiff MB, Freischlag JA. Females with subclavian vein thrombosis may have an increased risk of hypercoagulability. *JAMA Surg*. 2013;148(1):44-49. doi:10.1001/jamasurgery.2013.406
6. Illig KA, Doyle AJ. A comprehensive review of Paget-Schroetter syndrome. *J Vasc Surg*. 2010;51(6):1538-1547. doi:10.1016/j.jvs.2009.12.022
7. Guzzo JL, Chang K, Demos J, Black JH, Freischlag JA. Preoperative thrombolysis and venoplasty affords no benefit in patency following first rib resection and scalenectomy for subacute and chronic subclavian vein thrombosis. *J Vasc Surg*. 2010;52(3):658-662; discussion 662-663. doi:10.1016/j.jvs.2010.04.050
8. Lee JT, Dua MM, Chandra V, Hernandez-Boussard TM, Illig KA. RR18. Surgery for thoracic outlet syndrome: a nationwide perspective. *J Vasc Surg*. 2011;53(6):100S-101S. doi:10.1016/j.jvs.2011.03.195
9. Illig KA, Donahue D, Duncan A, et al. Reporting standards of the Society for Vascular Surgery for thoracic outlet syndrome. *J Vasc Surg*. 2016;64(3):e23-e35. doi:10.1016/j.jvs.2016.04.039
10. Goss SG, Alcantara SD, Todd GJ, Lantis JC. Non-operative management of paget-Schroetter syndrome: a single-center experience. *J Invasive Cardiol*. 2015;27(9):423-428.
11. Lee JT, Karwowski JK, Harris EJ, Haukoos JS, Olcott C. Long-term thrombotic recurrence after nonoperative management of Paget-Schroetter syndrome. *J Vasc Surg*. 2006;43(6):1236-1243. doi:10.1016/j.jvs.2006.02.005
12. Molina JE, Hunter DW, Dietz CA. Paget-Schroetter syndrome treated with thrombolytics and immediate surgery. *J Vasc Surg*. 2007;45(2):328-334. doi:10.1016/j.jvs.2006.09.052
13. Vedovati MC, Tratar G, Mavri A, Pierpaoli L, Agnelli G, Becattini C. Upper extremities deep vein thrombosis and DOAC treatment: a prospective cohort study. *Eur Heart J*. 2020;41(suppl 2). doi:10.1093/ehjci/ehaa946.2407
14. Gu G, Liu J, Lv Y, et al. Costoclavicular ligament as a novel cause of venous thoracic outlet syndrome: from anatomic study to clinical application. *Surg Radiol Anat*. 2020;42(8):865-870. doi:10.1007/s00276-020-02479-7
15. Ann Freischlag JA. Decade OF excellent outcomes after surgical intervention: 538 patients with thoracic outlet syndrome. *Trans Am Clin Climatol Assoc*. 2018;129:88-94.
16. Chandra V, Little C, Lee JT. Thoracic outlet syndrome in high-performance athletes. *J Vasc Surg*. 2014;60(4):1012-1017; discussion 1017-1018. doi:10.1016/j.jvs.2014.04.013

SECTION III: Thoracic and Suprarenal Aortic Exposure and Treatment

Chapter 10 Exposure and Open Surgical Reconstruction in the Chest: The Thoracoabdominal Aorta

Enrico Rinaldi, Diletta Loschi, and Germano Melissano

DEFINITION

- A thoracoabdominal aortic aneurysm (TAAA) involves the aorta at the diaphragmatic crura and extends variable distances proximally and/or distally from this point (**FIGURE 1**).[1] TAAAs can be classified in terms of their causes, the two most common being medial degeneration and dissection.
- Open treatment of TAAAs consists of graft replacement with reattachment of the main aortic branches: The inclusion technique was introduced by S. E. Crawford in the 1970s and refined by subsequent surgeons in the following decades. TAAA repair, especially in extensive aortic disease, is associated with greater operative risk than repair of other aortic segments. The main sources of morbidity are spinal cord (SC) ischemia and renal as well as respiratory and cardiac complications.
- Experienced surgical centers now report lower mortality and morbidity rates for TAAA repair,[2] largely due to multimodal approaches to reduce surgical trauma and maximize organ protection.[3]

IMAGING AND OTHER DIAGNOSTIC STUDIES

- To plan the best possible treatment strategy for each patient, the preferred modality is computed tomographic arteriography. The acquisition of computed tomography (CT) data has benefited from spectacular progress, including multirow detectors, higher rotation and translation speeds with reduced scan times (single breath-hold), cardiac cycle synchronization, and better postprocessing capabilities.
- Digital Imaging and Communications in Medicine (DICOM) slices of adequate thickness (≤1 mm) should be postprocessed on a digital workstation using a multiplanar reformatting tool to visualize a scan in which angulation matches that of the aorta or the vessel under investigation (**FIGURE 2**).
- Beyond analysis of aortic diameter and the extent of pathologic involvement, reformatted images are particularly useful for evaluating the presence, extension, and characteristics of dissection and thrombus, particularly at proposed

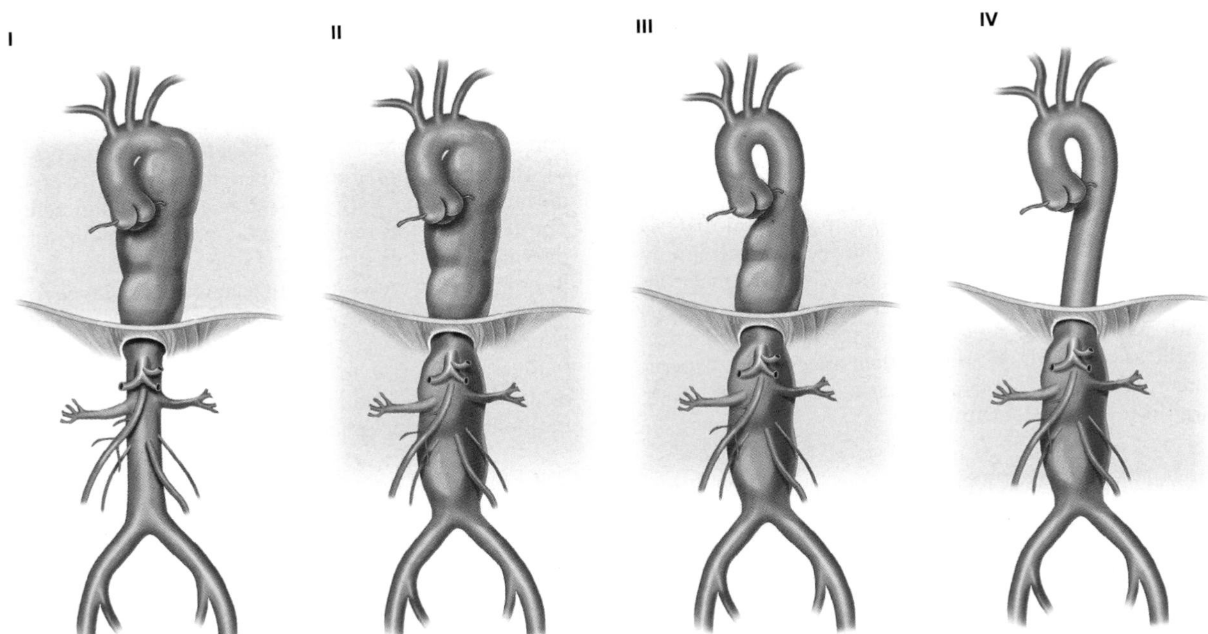

FIGURE 1 ● An aneurysm is defined as thoracoabdominal when the highlighted region is involved. Crawford classification was developed to improve stratification of perioperative paraplegia risk. Subclassifications include the following: Extent I includes the thoracic and abdominal aorta, from the left subclavian artery to the level of the renal arteries; Extent II includes the entire descending aorta from the level of the left subclavian artery to the aortic bifurcation; Extent III includes aorta beginning at the T6 level extending to the bifurcation or lower; Extent IV includes the entire abdominal aorta starting at the level of the diaphragm (T12) to the aortic bifurcation or lower.

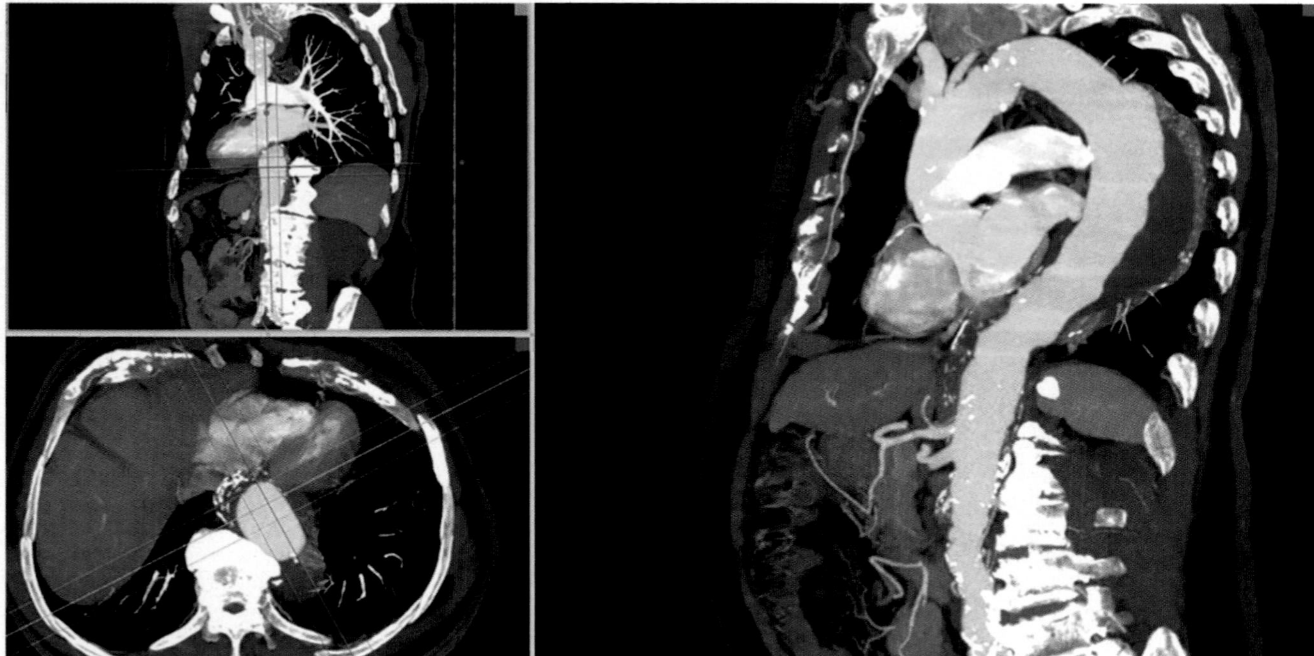

FIGURE 2 ● Multiplanar reformatting tools allow the sagittal reconstruction to properly follow the major axis of the thoracic aorta. In this reformatted image, the entire thoracoabdominal aorta is included despite significant tortuosity.

sites of clamp placement and the infradiaphragmatic aorta when direct aneurysm cannulation is considered for distal aortic perfusion. The exact location and geometry of aortic branches is obtained to reveal possible anatomic variations or anomalies, which are particularly common at the level of the renal arteries and arch vessels. Vessel patency is also routinely evaluated; in particular, obstruction of the superior and inferior mesenteric artery and the hypogastric arteries and dominance of one vertebral artery are assessed.

- Three-dimensional rendering tools produce realistic imaging of the anatomic structures that expand anatomic understanding including, for instance, the most appropriate intercostal space to perform thoracotomy (**FIGURE 3**).
- Perioperative SC ischemia may precipitate paraparesis or paraplegia. Prior knowledge of the SC arterial supply informs both procedural planning and risk stratification. During the last 2 decades a progressively increasing experience with noninvasive imaging techniques has allowed a better identification of preoperative patient-specific risk criteria for SC perfusion impairments, giving the possibility to tailor the surgical procedure[4] (**FIGURE 4**).

SURGICAL MANAGEMENT

Preoperative Workup and Patient Optimization

- Preoperative transthoracic echocardiography is a satisfactory noninvasive screening method to evaluate both valvular and biventricular function. Stress testing identifies patients who require coronary catheterization and possible intervention.[5] Electrocardiographically (EKG) gated CT has emerged as a less invasive method of visualizing coronary anatomy. For severe, symptomatic coronary disease requiring percutaneous transluminal angioplasty prior to aneurysm repair, use of drug-eluting stents requiring prolonged double antiplatelet therapy should be avoided to reduce subsequent perioperative bleeding.
- The use of estimated glomerular filtration rate (eGFR), rather than serum creatinine levels alone, is recommended to assess renal function.[6] Based on the eGFR metric, chronic kidney disease (CKD) has been shown to be a strong predictor of death following open or endovascular thoracic aneurysm repair, even in patients without other clinical evidence of preoperative renal disease.[7]
- Pulmonary function evaluation with arterial blood gases and spirometry is used to evaluate the respiratory reserve of all patients undergoing open surgery of the descending aorta. In patients with a forced expiratory volume in 1 second (FEV_1) of less than 1 L and a partial pressure of carbon dioxide (PCO_2) greater than 45 mm Hg, operative risk may be improved by cessation of cigarette smoking, treatment of chronic bronchitis (if present), weight loss, and participation in a supervised exercise program for a period of up to 6 months prior to surgery. However, in patients with aneurysm-related symptoms, this type of respiratory rehabilitation may not be practical or possible.

POSITIONING

- After inserting a cerebrospinal fluid drainage (CSFD)[8] catheter into the subarachnoid space between L2 and L3 or L3 and L4 (**FIGURE 5**), the patient is turned to a right lateral decubitus position, with the shoulders at 60° and the hips flexed back to 30°.
- Preparation should allow for access to the entire left thorax, abdomen, and both inguinal regions. Patient position is maintained with a moldable beanbag attached to a suction line for vacuum creation. A circulating water mattress is placed between the beanbag and the patient in order to modify body temperature as necessary.

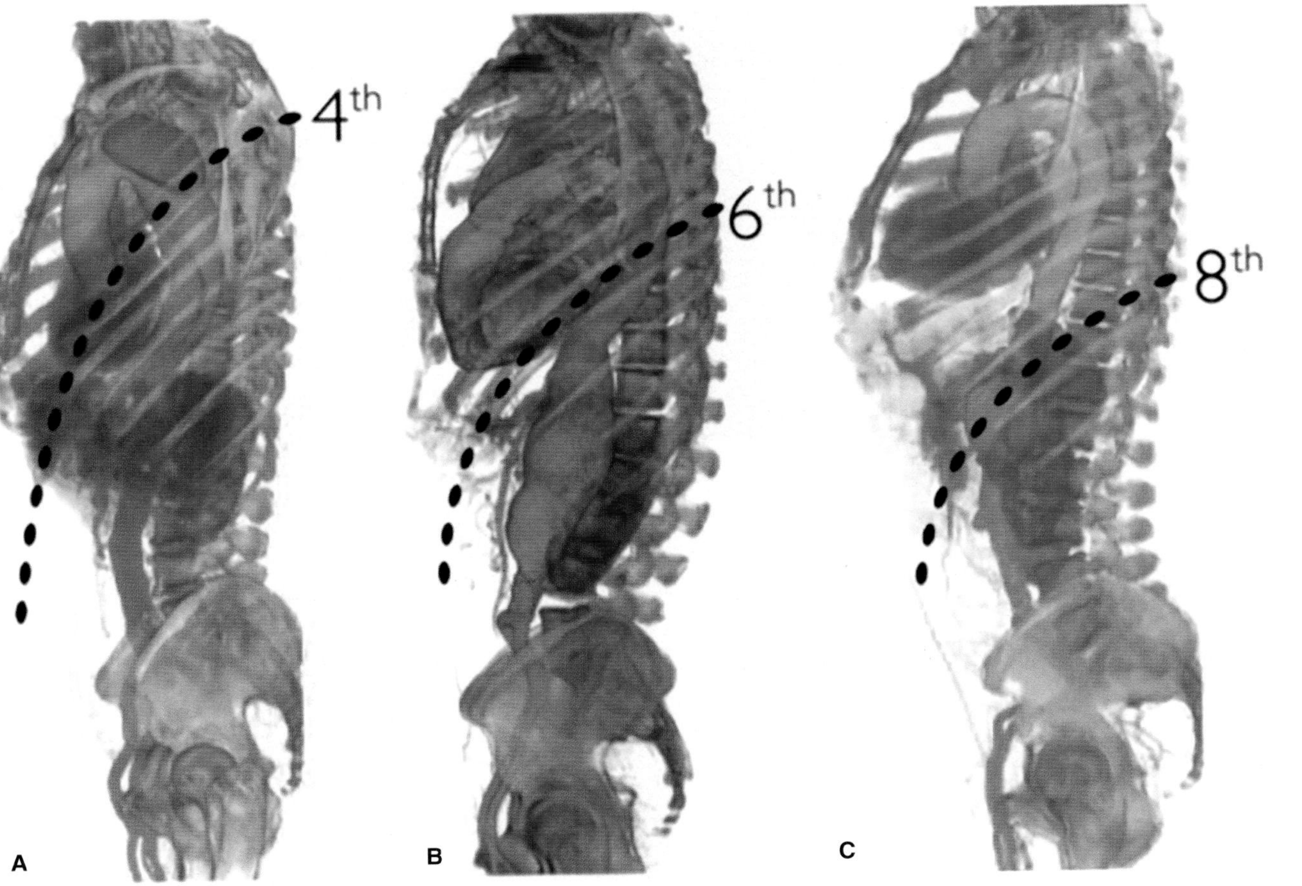

FIGURE 3 ● Beyond aortic imaging, computed tomography provides extensive anatomic information to guide exposure and surgical decision making. In case of Extent I thoracoabdominal aortic aneurysm (TAAA) **(A)**, a surgical access through the 4th intercostal space may be performed while an incision in the 6th intercostal space could be done in case of Extent III TAAA **(B)**. For an Extent IV TAAA **(C)**, a lower access through the 8th intercostal space is generally performed.

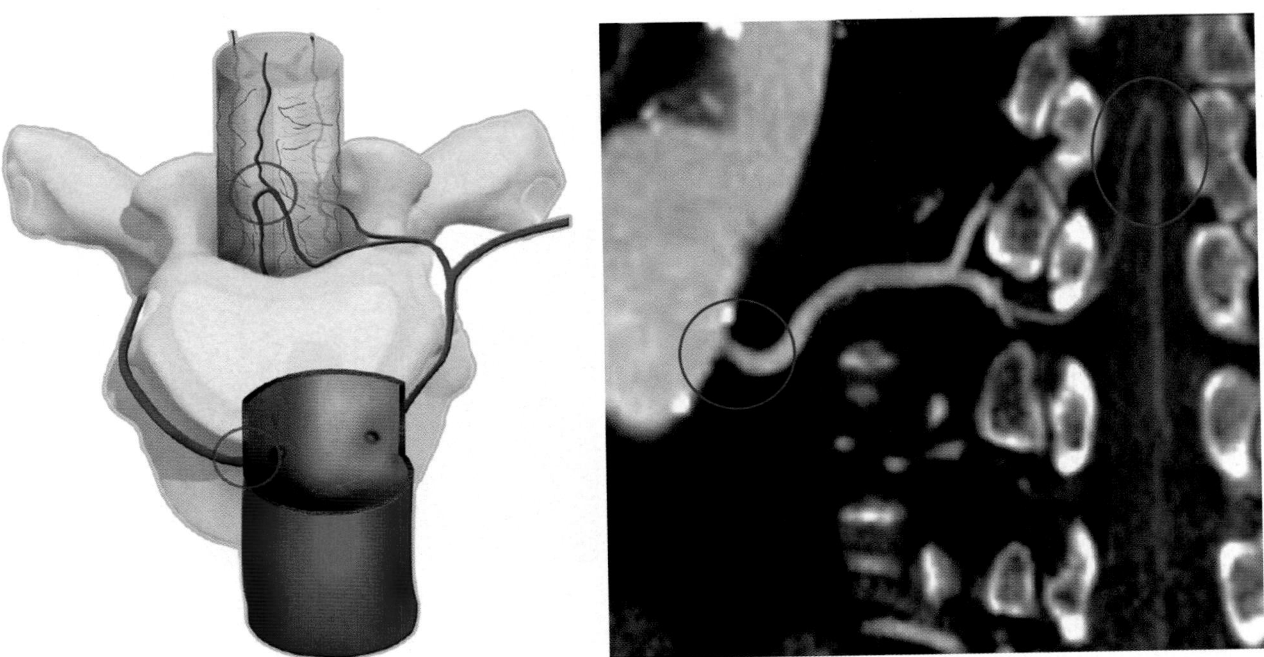

FIGURE 4 ● With preoperative computed tomography, using postprocessing tools, the whole path of the arterial feeder to the spinal cord (arteria radicularis magna) can be visualized, from the aorta to the anterior spinal artery.

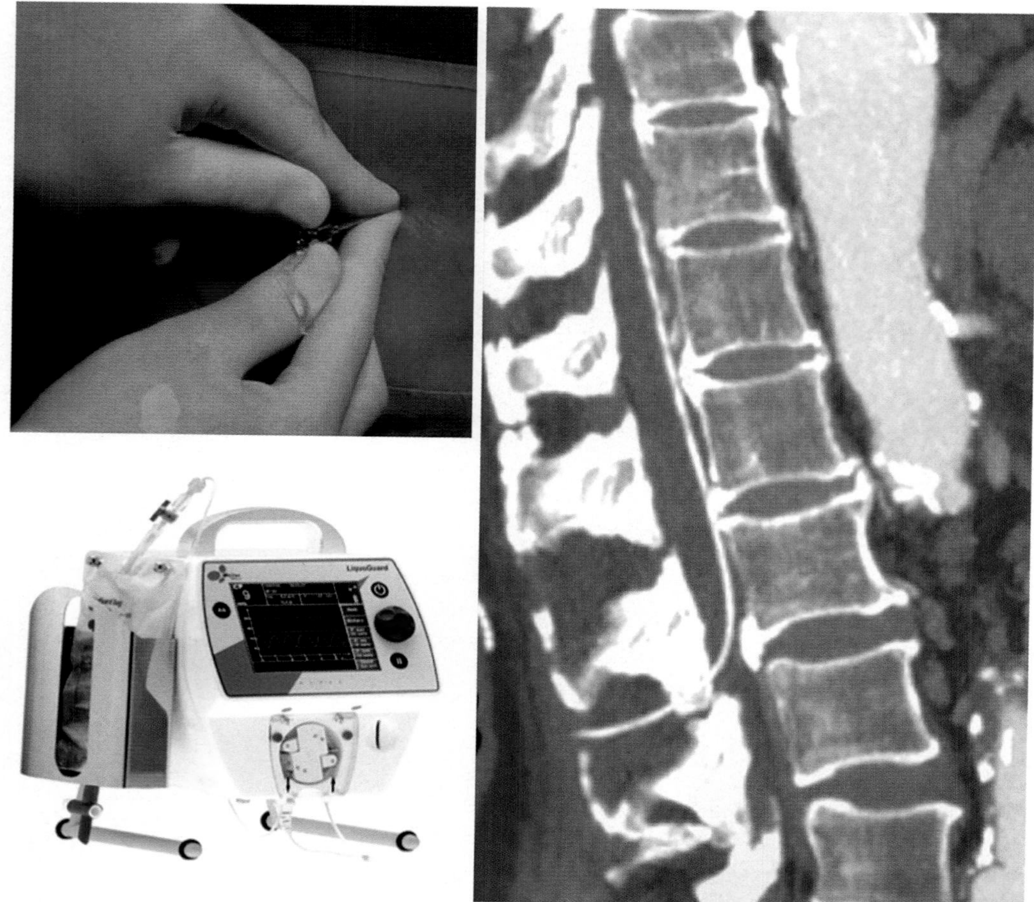

FIGURE 5 ● Once the dura has been punctured with the introducer needle, a drainage catheter is inserted 8 to 10 cm along the intradural space. The catheter is then connected to a pressure transducer, and the fluid is drained to keep the pressure below 10 cm H_2O. Automated systems are available for this purpose.

THORACOPHRENOLAPAROTOMY

- The thoracic incision varies in length and level, depending on exposure requirements. Usually, the 5th, 6th, or 7th intercostal space is employed according to the aneurysm anatomy. The posterior section of the ribs is gently spread to reduce thoracic wall trauma and fractures; anterolaterally, the incision curves gently as it crosses the costal margin to minimize subsequent tissue necrosis (**FIGURE 6**). The pleural space is entered after single right lung ventilation is initiated. Monopulmonary ventilation is maintained throughout thoracic aorta replacement.
- Thoracotomy incisions are painful and can lead to postoperative complications, such as pulmonary atelectasis and infections. Successful postoperative pain management allows early patient mobilization and may contribute to shorter hospital length of stay. Common analgesic methods include opioid pain medications and epidural catheters. Side effects of opioid use, including respiratory, central nervous system, and bowel function depression, are not uncommon.[9] In order to reduce the postoperative pain in patients undergoing TAAA open repair, electromyography-guided cryoablation of intercostal nerves has been introduced in some high volume centers. Cryoanalgesia induces a Wallerian degeneration of the axons within the intercostal nerve,[10,11] and its benefits in terms of postoperative pain relief after thoracotomies performed for general thoracic procedures are reported in the literature.[12-15] CryoICE (AtriCure, Inc, Mason, OH) is a nitrous oxide cryoablation probe originally indicated for cryoablation of the heart for arrhythmias and was approved for

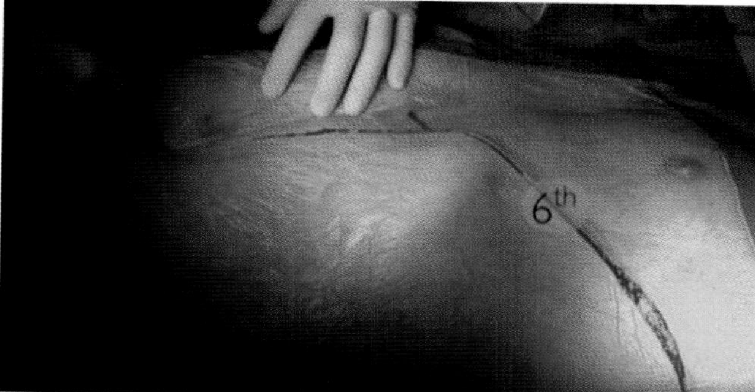

FIGURE 6 ● Prepping and draping for thoracoabdominal aortic aneurysm. Posterolateral aspects of the left thorax, abdomen, and left groin are included in the sterile operatory field. Thoracophrenolaparotomy in the 6th intercostal space, please note the gentle curvature of the line indicating the skin incision to avoid flap necrosis.

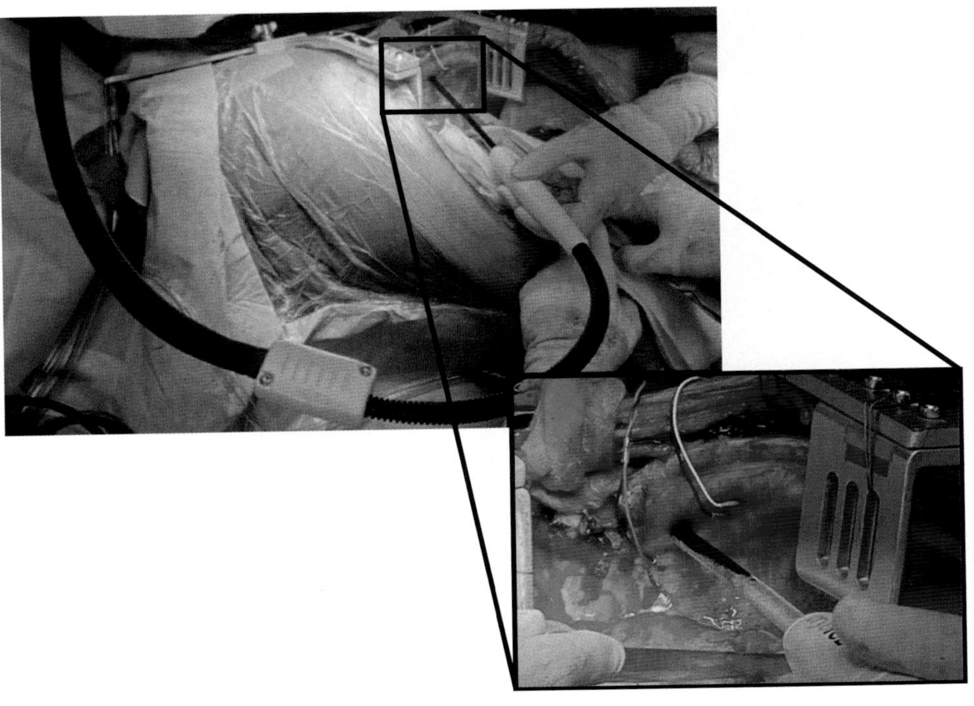

FIGURE 7 • CryoICE is a nitrous oxide cryoablation probe used to induce a Wallerian degeneration of the axons within the intercostal nerve in order to reduce thoracic postoperative pain. Cryoablation may be performed under electromyography-guidance in order to assess the effective ablation.

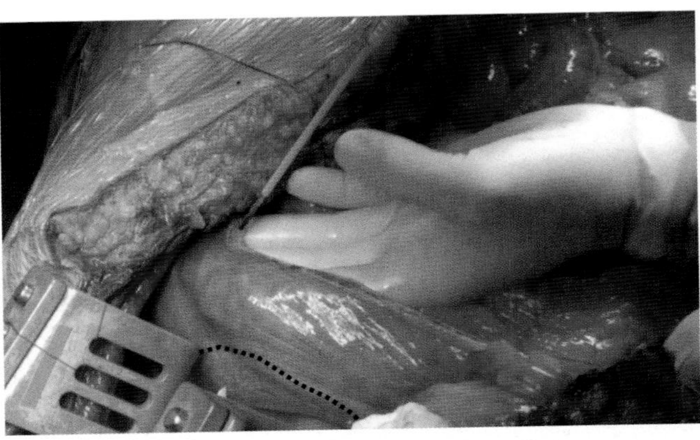

FIGURE 8 • The diaphragm is circumferentially divided, for several centimeters near its peripheral attachment to the anterior chest wall sparing the phrenic center (dotted line).

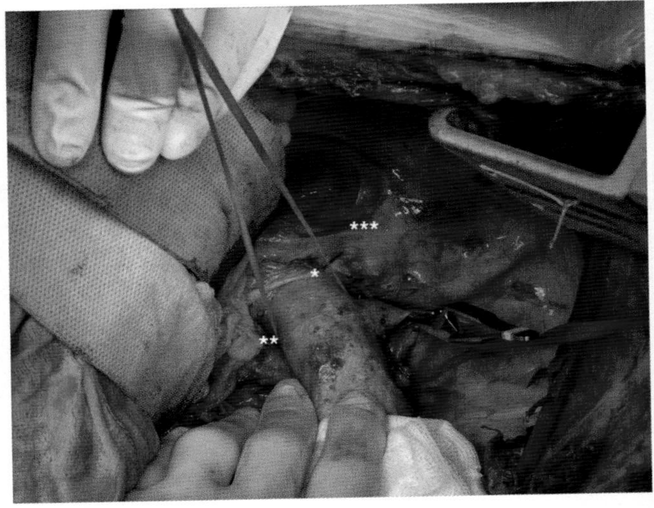

FIGURE 9 • The vagus nerve (*) and the origin of the recurrent laryngeal nerve (**) are mobilized and identified to prevent injury during aortic clamping maneuvers or suture placement. The phrenic nerve is also identified (***). In this case, an aortic cross-clamping between left carotid and subclavian artery is required, so prior selective clamping of the left subclavian artery is performed before arch manipulation to prevent possible embolization.

intercostal nerve cryoanalgesia by the US Food and Drug Administration in 2015. Two recent studies reviewed the operative technique and the intraoperative and postoperative outcomes in patients undergoing TAA and TAAA repairs with and without cryoanalgesia to evaluate its efficacy and feasibility.[16,17] In both studies, opioid use was significantly reduced in the cryoanalgesia group; incidence of other major postoperative complications was similar in both groups. This procedure required additional 20 to 25 minutes, but it did not increase postoperative complications.[16,17] Prospective investigations and long-term follow-up are needed in order to understand the efficacy of this technique (**FIGURE 7**).

- Paralysis of the left hemidiaphragm contributes to postoperative respiratory failure; therefore, a limited circumferential rather than radial section of the diaphragm is routinely performed, sparing the phrenic center. Under favorable anatomic conditions, this approach reduces respiratory weaning time[18] (**FIGURE 8**).
- Special care must be taken when isolating the proximal aneurysm neck. The insertion of a large caliber esophageal probe makes it easier to distinguish the esophagus at this level. The vagus nerve and the origin of the recurrent laryngeal nerve must also be identified because they can also be damaged during isolation and clamping maneuvers (**FIGURE 9**). Identification and clipping of some "high" intercostal arteries can sometimes facilitate the preparation for the proximal anastomosis, thus reducing aortic bleeding (**FIGURE 10**).

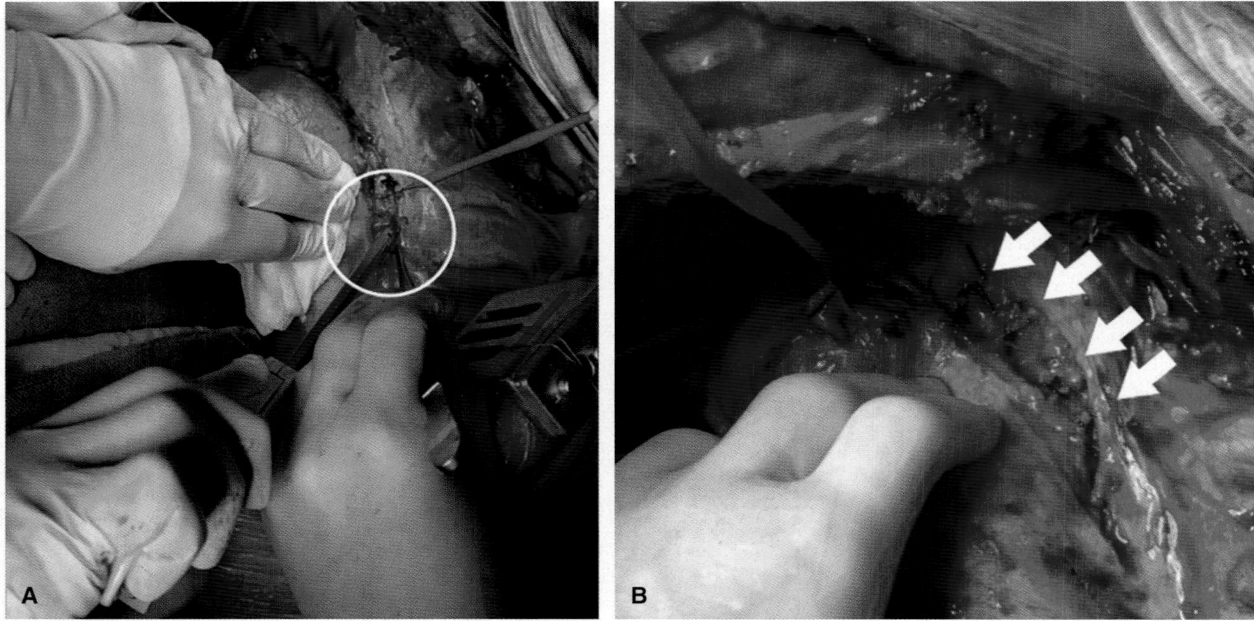

FIGURE 10 ● "High" noncritical intercostal arteries are identified during thoracic aortic exposure. These arteries are selectively clipped **(A)** in order to prevent back bleeding after the aortotomy. **B,** In this patient, four intercostal arteries were clipped at proximal thoracic aortic level.

- The upper abdominal aortic segment is exposed via a transperitoneal approach; after entering the peritoneum, medial visceral rotation is performed to retract the left colon, spleen, and left kidney anteriorly and to the right (**FIGURE 11**). Use of a transperitoneal approach allows direct assessment of the abdominal organs at the end of procedure. Extra care must be taken to avoid damage to the spleen, which is particularly prone to bleeding after capsular injuries regardless of size.

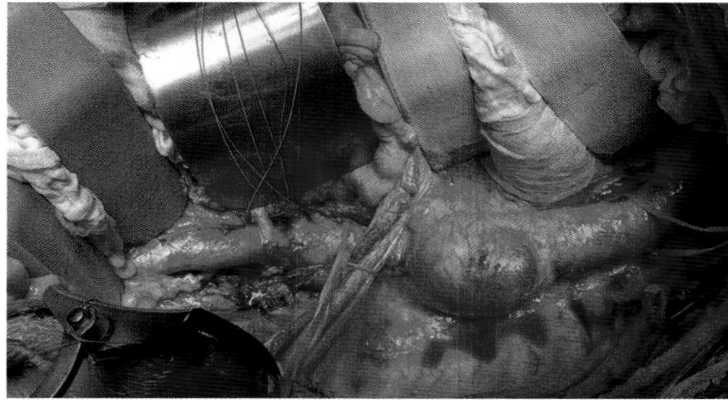

FIGURE 11 ● After thoracic aortic exposure, the abdominal aorta is also exposed throughout medial visceral rotation. With this approach, the origins of celiac trunk, superior mesenteric artery, and also left renal artery are identified and exposed.

DISTAL AORTIC PERFUSION

- Cross-clamping of the descending thoracic aorta produces immediate and significant increases in left ventricular afterload, myocardial oxygen consumption, and visceral and renal ischemia. Techniques incorporating distal aortic perfusion with left heart bypass (LHBP) have significantly improved outcomes in thoracic aortic surgery.[19] In preparation for LHBP and aortic cross-clamping, low-dose intravenous heparin is administered. If cessation of pump support is anticipated during the case, additional heparin should be administered at that time to provide full anticoagulation.
- The upper left pulmonary vein is usually cannulated for inflow of oxygenated blood, which is routed through a centrifugal pump (Bio-Medicus) into the left femoral artery. A "Y" connector included in the circuit provides two occlusion/perfusion catheters (9-Fr) for selective visceral perfusion when needed (**FIGURE 12**).

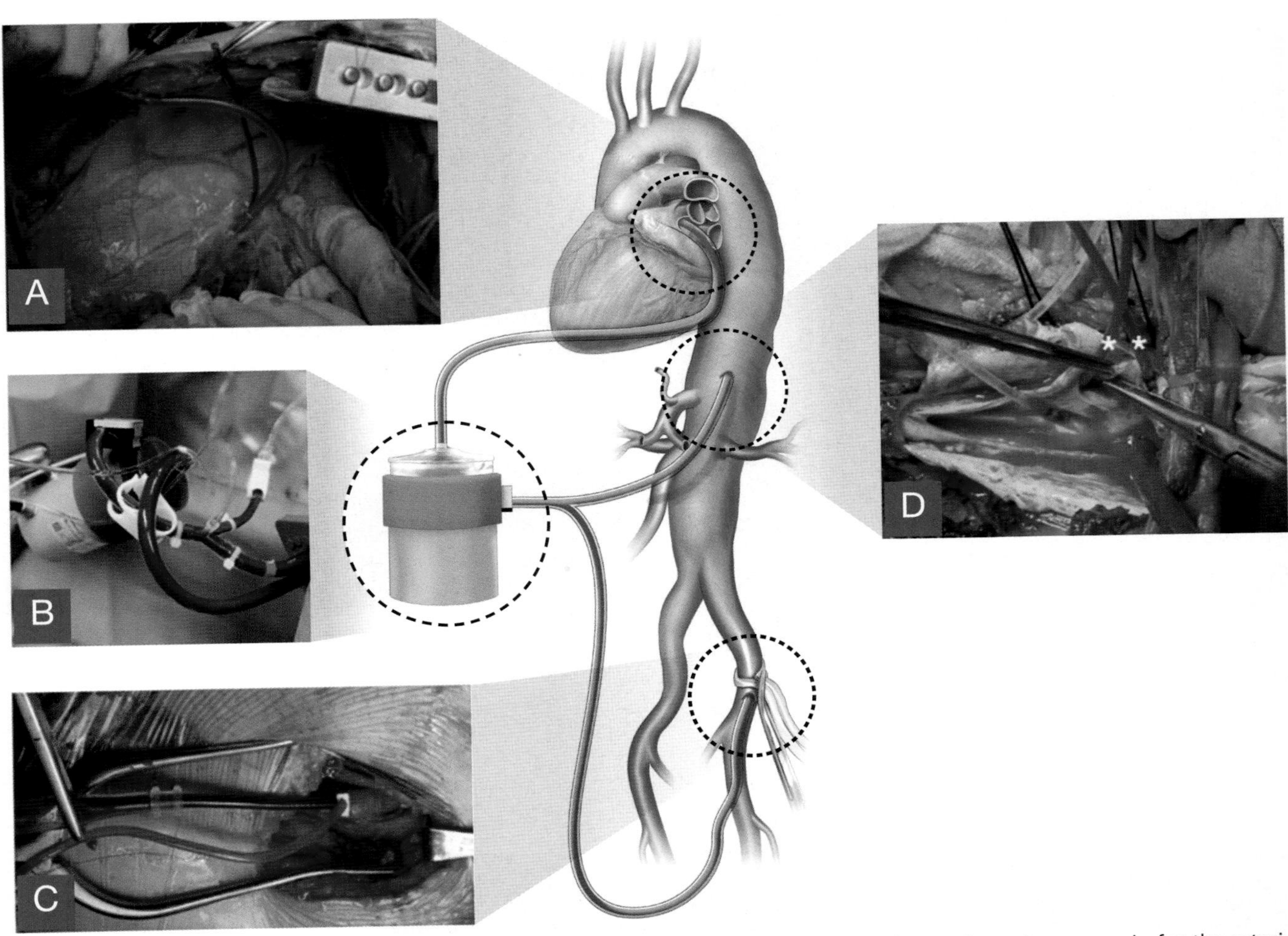

FIGURE 12 ● Schematic view of Left Heart Bypass (LHBP). A 20-Fr cannula is inserted in left superior pulmonary vein for the arterial blood drainage **(A)**. Through a centrifugal pump (Bio-Medicus) **(B)**, the oxygenated blood is routed into the left femoral artery for synchronous proximal and distal perfusion using a nonocclusive femoral cannula (14-18-Fr) **(C)**. **D**, A "Y" connector provides two occlusion/perfusion catheters (9-Fr) for selective visceral perfusion with blood (*).

AORTIC REPAIR

- Once the neck of the TAAA is isolated and controlled between clamps, the descending thoracic aorta is transected and separated from the esophagus (**FIGURE 13**). The graft is sutured proximally to the descending thoracic aorta using 2-0 polypropylene suture in a running fashion. The anastomosis is reinforced with Teflon felt (individual pledgets or single strip) (**FIGURE 14**). An additional aortic clamp is applied onto the abdominal aorta above the celiac axis before the proximal aortic clamp is removed (sequential cross-clamping).
- Intercostal artery reimplantation into the aortic graft plays a critical role in SC protection. Patent intercostal arteries from T7 to L2 are temporarily occluded to prevent back-bleeding/maximize cord perfusion pressure[20] and then selectively reattached to the graft by means of aortic patch or graft interposition (**FIGURE 15**). When ready, the distal clamp is moved below the renal arteries and the aneurysm is opened across the diaphragm. The centrifugal pump maintains visceral perfusion (400 mL per minute) following insertion of the 9-Fr irrigation-perfusion catheters (LeMaitre Vascular) into the celiac trunk and the superior mesenteric artery. Cold perfusion of Custodiol[21] (histidine-tryptophane-ketoglutarate) is directed into the renal arteries (**FIGURE 16**). For visceral artery reimplantation, a fenestration is created in the graft and the visceral vessels are reattached as a single patch. Usually, the left renal artery is reconnected with an 8-mm polyester interposition graft. If creation of the visceral patch requires retaining a large segment of native aorta, we prefer to place a multibranched graft instead. This prosthesis, although somewhat more time-consuming, significantly reduces the risk of recurrent aortic patch aneurysm (**FIGURES 17** and **18**). Finally, the distal end-to-end anastomosis with the distal aorta is performed, the graft flushed, and clamps removed.

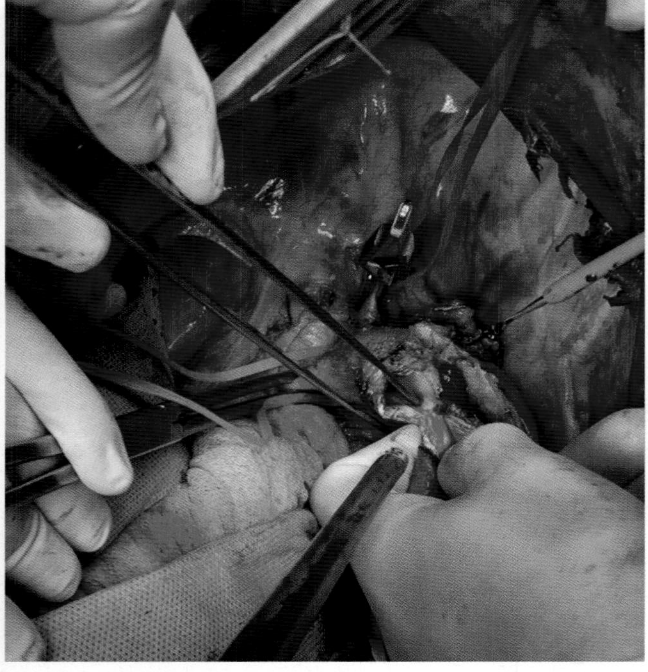

FIGURE 13 ● The proximal descending thoracic aorta is controlled and completely transected to avoid accidental injury to the adjacent esophagus.

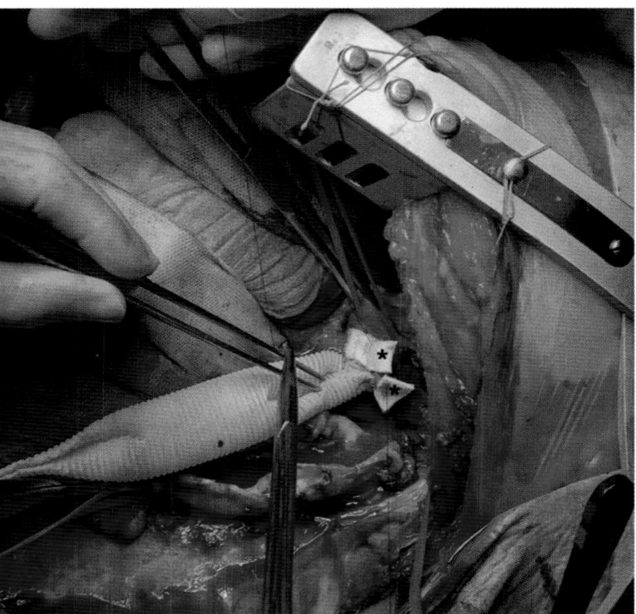

FIGURE 14 ● The proximal anastomosis is routinely reinforced with a Teflon strip (*).

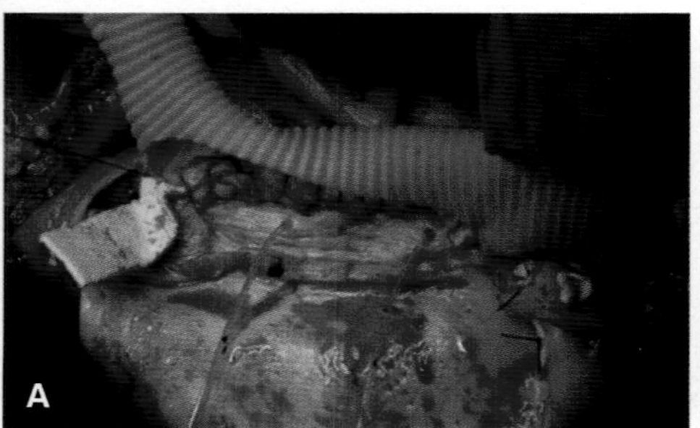

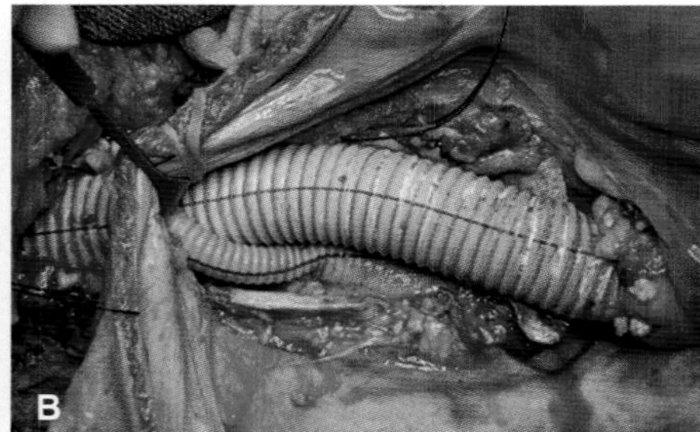

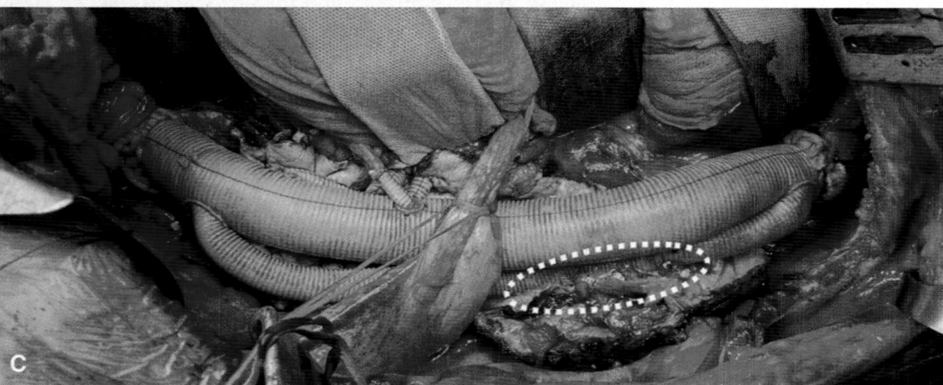

FIGURE 15 ● Critical intercostal arteries reattachment. Here visualized are three different techniques: **(A)** an aortic island including the origin of several intercostal arteries is reattached to a fenestration created on the aortic graft; **(B)** intercostal arteries are reattached selectively to the graft via 6/8-mm interposition grafts. **C,** Another possible way to reattach critical intercostal arteries is represented by the "loop graft." A 14/16-mm is anastomosed proximally and distally to the aortic graft. A fenestration is created in this loop graft to reattach the origin of multiple intercostal arteries (*dotted circle*).

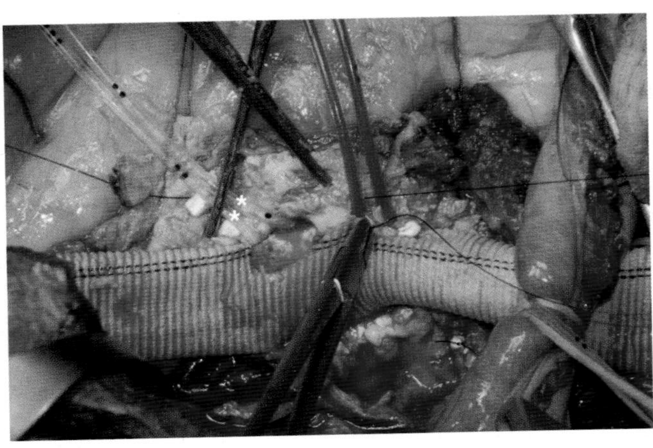

FIGURE 16 ● Visceral arteries perfusion with blood, renal perfusion with cold Custodiol solution (*) during branch artery reattachment.

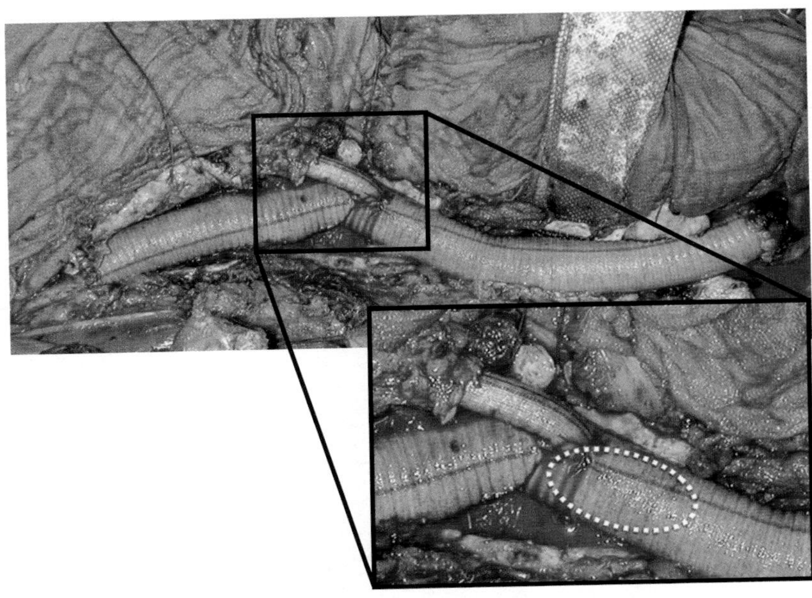

FIGURE 17 ● If creation of the visceral patch requires retaining a large segment of native aorta, a separate reattachment of the left renal artery may be performed. Celiac trunk ostia, superior mesenterica ostia, and right renal artery ostia are reattached using a standard Carrel patch (dotted circle) while a selective 6/8-mm bypass is used to reattach the left renal artery. This configuration significantly reduces the risk of recurrent aortic patch aneurysm.

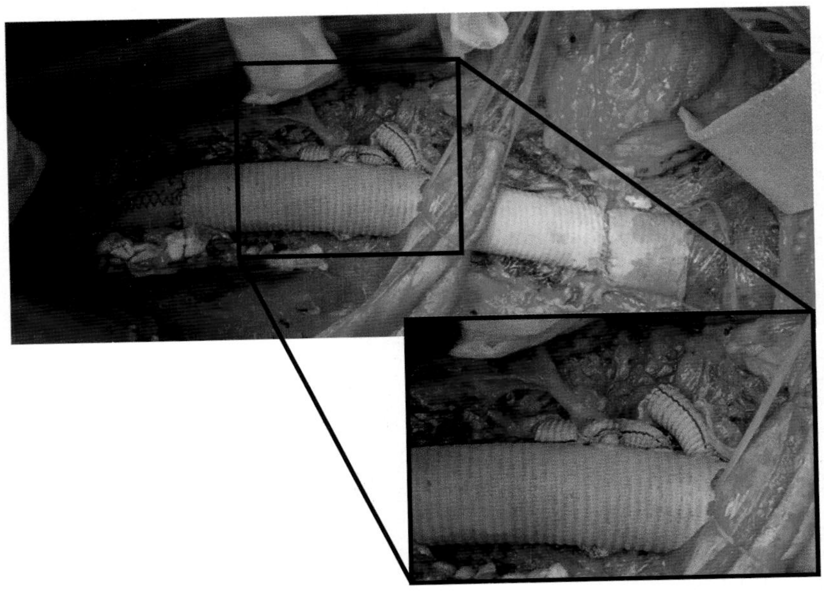

FIGURE 18 ● Visceral vessels and renal arteries could be reattached also separately by means of multibranched grafts. These prosthesis are used to reduce as much as possible the aortic native tissue and prevent recurrent aortic aneurysm formation, especially in patients with connective tissue disorders. In the white box, the selective reattachment of celiac trunk, superior mesenteric artery, and left renal artery are highlighted while the right renal artery bypass is located posteriorly and covered by the aortic graft. At the end of the aortic repair, radiopaque markers may be placed at the origin of the bypasses for an easier identification in case of possible late endovascular procedure.

RENAL PROTECTION

- Acute kidney injury (AKI) is a common complication in TAAA repair.[22-24] The incidence of postoperative AKI after TAAA repair varies depending on the patient's preoperative status and comorbidities, the surgical technique, and the disease extension. The duration of renal ischemia in determining the risk of postoperative AKI in aortic surgery is also important. Scores for postoperative AKI have been developed in order to objectively stratify the risk.[25-28] Postoperative AKI not only impairs renal function, but also confers a higher risk of morbidity and mortality in both the short- and long term, including an increased incidence of CKD at follow-up.[29-31] During TAAA open repair, temporary interruption of blood flow to the kidney is required, and the reduction of oxygenation after clamping in the proximal tubular cells induces an intracellular reduction of ATP and an increase in lactate. Prevention of renal hypoperfusion by maintaining both adequate cardiac output and mean arterial pressure (MAP) has been reported as effective in decreasing the incidence of postoperative AKI. Preventive pharmacological strategies have been also reported in the literature by the European Society of Intensive Care.[32] End-organ ischemia can be also prevented or reduced by means of perfusion strategies, such as active distal perfusion by partial cardiopulmonary bypass or LHBP during aortic cross-clamping. Selective renal perfusion during suture time may prevent ischemia/reperfusion injury.[33] Historically warm blood perfusion is the closest approach to physiologic perfusion that prevents cell membrane injury and intracellular edema; however, it requires a more complex setting in extracorporeal blood circuits and provides nonpulsatile blood flow. Until recently, clinical practice mainly involved crystalloid perfusion. Retrospective analysis of postoperative renal function in patients treated with renal cooling with crystalloid reported AKI in 7.6% of patients, temporary dialysis in 2%, and permanent dialysis in 0.66%.[34] Some studies reported renal damage with lactated Ringer solution.[35,36] Custodiol (Dr. Franz-Kohler Chemie GmbH, Bensheim, Germany) is another solution for organ protection, similar to intracellular fluid. Recently a single-center, randomized, double-blind, phase IV prospective study compared the efficacy of renal perfusion with Custodiol vs enriched Ringer solution during TAAA open repair.[37] A significantly lower AKI rate was found in patients who received Custodiol compared with patients who received Ringer solution for renal perfusion during open TAAA repair.

CLOSURE

- The entire aortic repair is inspected (**FIGURE 19**). All exposed aortic branch pulses are palpated after derotation and replacement of the abdominal viscera. Any bleeding or kinking of the aortic branches is addressed at this juncture. The atrial and femoral cannulae are removed; the purse-string sutures are tied and reinforced. Anticoagulation is reversed with protamine. The crus of the diaphragm is reapproximated to restore the aortic hiatus and the left hemidiaphragm loosely sutured with a running polypropylene suture. The left lung is temporarily inflated to check for air leakage.
- A closed suction abdominal drain is placed next to the aortic graft in the left retroperitoneal space, and two chest tubes are placed in the posteroapical and basal pleural space. Absorbable pericostal sutures are placed to approximate the ribs, and two steel wires are used to stabilize the costal margin. The lung is inflated, and the correct expansion of all the segments is carefully checked; the pericostal and diaphragmatic sutures are tightened and ligated. The steel wires are twisted and buried in the cartilaginous costal margin. The abdominal fascia is closed with a running suture. The abdominal and thoracic drains are connected to suction. The serratus and latissimus dorsi muscles are approximated with separate absorbable sutures. Subdermal layer is sutured, and the skin is closed with staples.

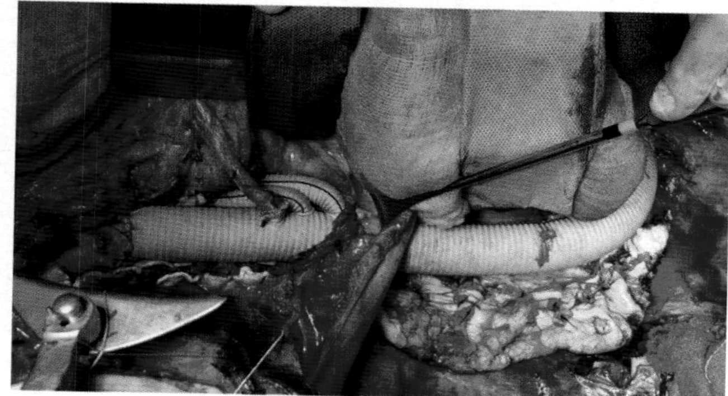

FIGURE 19 ● Final repair of a type II thoracoabdominal aortic aneurysm with selective reimplantation of visceral and renal vessels using a multibranched graft.

PEARLS AND PITFALLS

Indications	■ Aortic diameter and aneurysm morphology ■ Signs and symptoms of acute aortic syndrome
Preoperative planning	■ Level of intercostal incision ■ Graft selection ■ Identification of accessory renal arteries and other visceral anomalies (eg, horseshoe kidney) ■ Potential need for multibranch graft vs Carrel patch

Surgical access	■ Avoid skin flap necrosis ■ Rib section ■ Intercostal nerves cryoablation ■ Limited phrenotomy (circumferential diaphragmatic incision) ■ Transperitoneal approach ■ Careful and limited lung manipulation ■ Nonocclusive femoral cannulation
Technical adjuncts for organ protection	■ SC drainage ■ LHBP ■ Sequential aortic clamping ■ Critical intercostal artery reattachment ■ Visceral perfusion from LHBP cannulas ■ Renal perfusion with cold Custodiol

POSTOPERATIVE CARE

- The main focus of immediate postoperative management is the early detection of neurologic or cardiovascular complication as prompt intervention may prevent substantial long-term morbidity. As soon as baseline blood pressure and body temperature are restored, sedation is lightened regardless of ventilatory status. When SC or cerebral neurologic injury is suspected, CT imaging is performed immediately to address the possibility of intracranial or intradural SC hematoma. In case of paraparesis or paraplegia, MAP is chemically maintained above 80 mm Hg, CSFD is drained in order to lower the cerebrospinal fluid pressure below 10 mm Hg, and methylprednisolone (1 g bolus followed by 4 g per 24 hours continuous infusion) and 18% mannitol (5 mg/kg, four times a day) are administrated.
- If malperfusion develops in the lower limbs, renal or visceral circulation, efforts should be made to restore normal circulation immediately. For a precise visualization of visceral organ perfusion, emergency arteriography (catheter-based or CT) is required.
- Blood pressure fluctuations, including recalcitrant hypertension, is common in the early postoperative period, especially in the chronically hypertensive patient; prompt attention should be paid to regulating the MAP in a physiologic range. Immediate intervention may be required to reduce the risk of anastomotic bleeding, especially in the setting of dissection.
- In uncomplicated cases, drainage tubes are removed at 36 to 48 hours postoperatively, whereas the intrathecal CSFD catheter is removed usually after 72 hours. A prolonged requirement for ventilatory support is not unusual, especially after emergency operations, in patients with significant blood loss and after longer periods of circulatory arrest (if necessary for concurrent arch or ascending aortic reconstruction). In case of severe CKD, transient temporary renal replacement therapy may also be necessary in the early postoperative period.

COMPLICATIONS

- Bleeding
- Multiorgan failure
- Dialysis
- Paraplegia
- Stroke
- Death
- Aneurysm recurrence

REFERENCES

1. Johnston KW, Rutherford RB, Tilson MD, et al. Suggested standards for reporting on arterial aneurysms. Subcommittee on reporting standards for arterial aneurysms, Ad Hoc committee on reporting standards, society for vascular surgery and North American chapter, international society for cardiovascular surgery. *J Vasc Surg.* 1991;13:452-458.
2. Coselli JS, Bozinovski J, LeMaire SA. Open surgical repair of 2286 thoracoabdominal aortic aneurysms. *Ann Thorac Surg.* 2007;83:S862-S864.
3. MacArthur RG, Carter SA, Coselli JS, et al. Organ protection during thoracoabdominal aortic surgery: rationale for a multimodality approach. *Semin Cardiothorac Vasc Anesth.* 2005;9:143-149.
4. Melissano G, Civilini E, Bertoglio L, et al. Angio-CT imaging of the spinal cord vascularisation: a pictorial essay. *Eur J Vasc Endovasc Surg.* 2010;39:436-440.
5. Kieffer E, Chiche L, Baron JF, et al. Coronary and carotid artery disease in patients with degenerative aneurysm of the descending thoracic or thoracoabdominal aorta: prevalence and impact on operative mortality. *Ann Vasc Surg.* 2002;16:679-684.
6. Stevens LA, Coresh J, Greene T, et al. Assessing kidney function—measured and estimated glomerular filtration rate. *N Engl J Med.* 2006;354:2473-2483.
7. Mills JLSr, Duong ST, Leon LR Jr, et al. Comparison of the effects of open and endovascular aortic aneurysm repair on long-term renal function using chronic kidney disease staging based on glomerular filtration rate. *J Vasc Surg.* 2008;47:1141-1149.
8. Cina CS, Abouzahr L, Arena GO, et al. Cerebrospinal fluid drainage to prevent paraplegia during thoracic and thoracoabdominal aortic aneurysm surgery: a systematic review and meta-analysis. *J Vasc Surg.* 2004;40:36-44.
9. Senturk M. Acute and chronic pain after thoracotomies. *Curr Opin Anaesthesiol.* 2005;18:1-4.
10. Nelson KM, Vincent RG, Bourke RS, et al. Intraoperative intercostal nerve freezing to prevent postthoracotomy pain. *Ann Thorac Surg.* 1974;18:280-285.
11. Evans PJ, Lloyd JW, Green CJ. Cryoanalgesia: the response to alterations in freeze cycle and temperature. *Br J Anaesth.* 1981;53:1121-1127.
12. Law L, Rayi A, Derian A. *Cryoanalgesia.* In: *StatPearls* [Internet]. StatPearls Publishing; 2021.
13. Momenzadeh S, Elyasi H, Valaie N, et al. Effect of cryoanalgesia on post-thoracotomy pain. *Acta Med Iran.* 2011;49(4):241-245.
14. Maiwand O, Makey AR. Cryoanalgesia for relief of pain after thoracotomy. *Br Med J.* 1981;282:1749-1750.
15. Khanbhai M, Yap KH, Mohamed S, et al. Is cryoanalgesia effective for post-thoracotomy pain? *Interact Cardiovasc Thorac Surg.* 2014;18(2):202-209.
16. Clemence J Jr, Malik A, Farhat L, et al. Cryoablation of intercostal nerves decreased Narcotic usage after thoracic or thoracoabdominal aortic aneurysm repair. *Semin Thorac Cardiovasc Surg.* 2020;32(3):404-412.

17. Tanaka A, Al-Rstum Z, Leonard SD, et al. Intraoperative intercostal nerve cryoanalgesia improves pain control after descending and thoracoabdominal aortic aneurysm repairs. *Ann Thorac Surg*. 2020;109(1):249-254.
18. Engle J, Safi HJ, Miller CCIII, et al. The impact of diaphragm management on prolonged ventilator support after thoracoabdominal aortic repair. *J Vasc Surg*. 1999;29(1):150-156.
19. Schepens MA. Left heart bypass for thoracoabdominal aortic aneurysm repair: technical aspects. *Multimed Man Cardiothorac Surg*. 2016;2016:mmv039.
20. Etz CD, Homann TM, Plestis KA, et al. Spinal cord perfusion after extensive segmental artery sacrifice: can paraplegia be prevented? *Eur J Cardio Thorac Surg*. 2007;31(4):643-648.
21. Schmitto JD, Fatehpur S, Tezval H, et al. Hypothermic renal protection using cold histidine-tryptophan-ketoglutarate solution perfusion in suprarenal aortic surgery. *Ann Vasc Surg*. 2008;22(4):520-524.
22. Rocha RV, Lindsay TF, Friedrich JO, et al. Systematic review of contemporary outcomes of endovascular and open thoracoabdominal aortic aneurysm repair. *J Vasc Surg*. 2020;71(4):1396-1412.e12.
23. Coselli JS, Lemaire SA, Preventza O, et al. Outcomes of 3309 thoracoabdominal aortic aneurysm repairs. *J Thorac Cardiovasc Surg*. 2016;151(5):1323-1337.
24. Waked K, Schepens M. State-of the-art review on the renal and visceral protection during open thoracoabdominal aortic aneurysm repair. *J Vis Surg*. 2018;4:31.
25. Yuan SM. Acute kidney injury after cardiac surgery: risk factors and Novel biomarkers. *Braz J Cardiovasc Surg*. 2019;34(3):352-360.
26. Mehta RH, Grab JD, O'Brien SM, et al. Bedside tool for predicting the risk of postoperative dialysis in patients undergoing cardiac surgery. *Circulation*. 2006;114(21):2208-2216.
27. Ma MX, Chang Q, Yu CT, et al. Risk factors for acute renal failure after thoracoabdominal aortic aneurysm surgery. *Zhongguo Yi Xue Ke Xue Yuan Xue Bao*. 2020;42(2):147-153.
28. Pannu N, Graham M, Klarenbach S, et al. A new model to predict acute kidney injury requiring renal replacement therapy after cardiac surgery. *CMAJ (Can Med Assoc J)*. 2016;188(15):1076-1083.
29. Chertow GM, Burdick E, Honour M, et al. Acute kidney injury, mortality, length of stay, and costs in hospitalized patients. *J Am Soc Nephrol*. 2005;16(11):3365-3370.
30. Zeng X, McMahon GM, Brunelli SM, et al. Incidence, outcomes, and comparisons across definitions of AKI in hospitalized individuals. *Clin J Am Soc Nephrol*. 2014;9(1):12-20.
31. Doyle JF, Forni LG. Acute kidney injury: short-term and long-term effects. *Crit Care*. 2016;20(1):1-7.
32. Joannidis M, Druml W, Forni LG, et al. Prevention of acute kidney injury and protection of renal function in the intensive care unit: update 2017—expert opinion of the Working Group on Prevention, AKI section, European Society of Intensive Care Medicine. *Intensive Care Med*. 2017;43(6):730-749.
33. Wynn MM, Acher C, Marks E, et al. Postoperative renal failure in thoracoabdominal aortic aneurysm repair with simple cross-clamp technique and 4°C renal perfusion. *J Vasc Surg*. 2015;61(3):611-622.
34. Aftab M, Coselli JS. Renal and visceral protection in thoracoabdominal aortic surgery. *J Thorac Cardiovasc Surg*. 2014;148(6):2963-2966.
35. Lemaire SA, Jones MM, Conklin LD, et al. Randomized comparison of cold blood and cold crystalloid renal perfusion for renal protection during thoracoabdominal aortic aneurysm repair. *J Vasc Surg*. 2009;49(1):11-19.
36. Köksoy C, LeMaire SA, Curling PE, et al. Renal perfusion during thoracoabdominal aortic operations: cold crystalloid is superior to normothermic blood. *Ann Thorac Surg*. 2002;73(3):730-738.
37. Kahlberg A, Tshomba Y, Baccellieri D, et al. CURITIBA Investigators. Renal perfusion with histidine-tryptophan-ketoglutarate compared with Ringer's solution in patients undergoing thoracoabdominal aortic open repair. *J Thorac Cardiovasc Surg*. 2021:S0022-5223(21)00408-6.

Chapter 11

Thoracic Aortic Stent Graft Repair for Aneurysm, Dissection, and Traumatic Transection

Elizabeth Leigh George and Jason T. Lee

DEFINITION

- In 1994, Dake and colleagues[1] at Stanford University were the first to report the use of custom-designed thoracic aortic stent-grafts for the treatment of descending thoracic aortic aneurysms in patients deemed high risk for conventional open surgery. Each of these devices was delivered through peripheral arterial access, usually the femoral arteries, and, when successful, would exclude the aneurysm from systemic pressurization and possible rupture. This groundbreaking minimally invasive technique thereby avoided many of the physiologic insults associated with open surgery, including the need for thoracotomy, aortic cross-clamping, reperfusion injury, and acute hemodynamic changes.
- Results from the first multicenter US Food and Drug Administration–sponsored trial for thoracic aortic stent-grafts demonstrated significantly less perioperative mortality, respiratory failure, renal insufficiency, and spinal cord ischemia in patients after thoracic endovascular aortic repair (TEVAR) compared with a matched cohort of patients undergoing open descending thoracic aortic aneurysm repair.[2]
- After now nearly 3 decades of surgeon experience and endovascular technologic advancement, TEVAR has evolved to serve as a primary treatment strategy for an increasingly diverse group of acute and chronic aortic pathologies including thoracic aortic aneurysms, dissections, and traumatic transections.

DIFFERENTIAL DIAGNOSIS

- Depending on the type and extent of pathology, TEVAR may include the use of fenestrated or branched stent grafts, advanced snorkel/chimney/periscope or parallel graft techniques, or the need for hybrid debranching procedures. The decision to treat thoracic aortic pathology with stent grafts is based on individual patient comorbidity burden, detailed analysis of thoracic aortic anatomy, and physician experience.
- Acute thoracic aortic pathologies often present with chest pain and therefore must be considered in the workup for acute coronary syndrome. The ubiquitous use of computed tomography angiography (CTA) scanning for pain, shortness of breath, trauma, and to "rule out" many pathologies has led to an increase in the recognition of thoracic aortic pathology potentially benefitting from TEVAR technology.

PATIENT HISTORY AND PHYSICAL FINDINGS

- Thoracic aortic aneurysms (TAAs) are defined as localized (saccular) or diffuse (fusiform) dilation of 50% or more relative to the diameter of the adjacent normal-sized aorta. Common risk factors for aneurysmal degeneration include smoking, hypertension, chronic obstructive pulmonary disease, atherosclerosis, and connective tissue disorders. Indications for repair of descending TAAs are similar to those for conventional open repair: maximum aortic diameter greater than 6 cm, rapid aneurysmal growth (>5 mm of growth over 6 months), or symptoms such as persistent chest or back pain, rupture, or dissection. Most TAAs are diagnosed following routine imaging ordered for other reasons, and patients are typically asymptomatic when being considered for treatment.
- Aortic dissection occurs when an intimal tear in the aorta causes blood to flow between the layers of the wall of the aorta and most often presents as tearing chest pain that radiates to the back. Potential etiologic factors leading to aortic dissection include poorly controlled acute or chronic hypertension, connective tissue disorders, trauma, or vasculitis. Medical management of uncomplicated type B thoracic aortic dissection serves as the current standard of care, although there are high-risk anatomic and clinical factors that tend to favor more aggressive interventional therapy. These practice guidelines stem from the results of the INvestigation of STEnt grafts in patients with type B Aortic Dissection (INSTEAD) trial, the first prospective, multicenter randomized trial comparing optimal medical therapy (eg, blood pressure control) with TEVAR for uncomplicated type B dissection, and the follow-up INSTEAD-XL trial.[3,4] The first trial demonstrated no significant improvement in 2-year survival or adverse event rates with TEVAR despite favorable aortic remodeling, but the 5-year follow-up data with landmark analysis in INSTEAD XL trial suggest improved long-term survival in patients undergoing TEVAR. In contrast, for patients with complicated type B dissections involving rupture, malperfusion (eg, visceral or limb ischemia), or refractory back pain despite optimal medical management, TEVAR is indicated. The goal of TEVAR in this setting is to cover, or exclude, the primary entry tear and re-expand the true lumen while promoting thrombosis of the false lumen.
- Traumatic aortic transection results from a high-velocity or deceleration injury to the aorta. The tethering of the aorta by the ligamentum arteriosum makes this site most susceptible to shearing forces during sudden deceleration. A high index of suspicion is necessary to help make the diagnosis. Trauma workups most often involve whole-body CT scanning, which allows rapid triage for possible treatment. CTA commonly demonstrates an irregular outpouching beyond the takeoff of the left subclavian artery at the aortic isthmus, which corresponds to the presence of an aortic pseudoaneurysm caused by the traumatic event. Extent of blunt traumatic aortic injury and the corresponding physiologic insult may range from clinically occult intimal injury to life-threatening complete transection and rupture (**FIGURE 1**).[5]

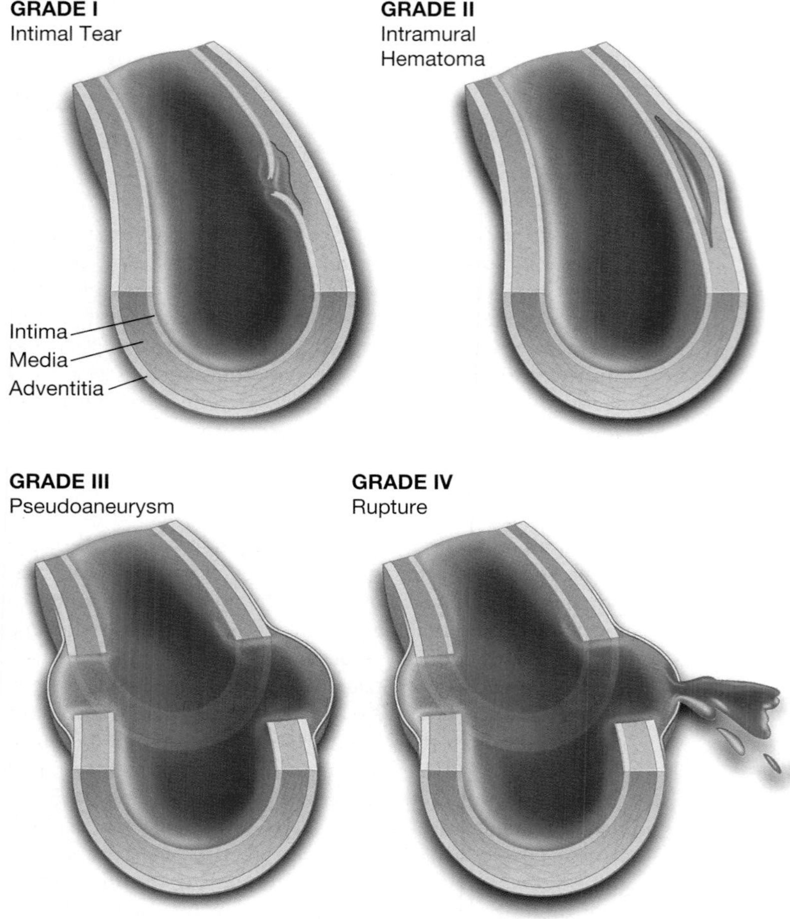

FIGURE 1 ● Society for Vascular Surgery classification of blunt traumatic aortic injury. (Adapted from Lee WA, Matsumura JS, Mitchell RS, et al. Endovascular repair of traumatic thoracic aortic injury: clinical practice guidelines of the Society for Vascular Surgery. *J Vasc Surg*. 2011;53:187-192.)

Early diagnosis and endovascular treatment is generally recommended for those presenting with a traumatic aortic transection, particularly when there is a contour abnormality visualized on cross-sectional imaging.

IMAGING AND OTHER DIAGNOSTIC STUDIES

- Transesophageal echocardiography (TEE) may serve as a useful imaging tool, particularly in the setting of acute thoracic aortic pathology. TEE can confirm the presence of aortic dissection, distinguish between types A and B dissections, identify involvement of supra-aortic vessels, and assess for contained rupture.
- High-resolution CTA with three-dimensional reconstructive software allows for the most complete anatomic analysis, including details regarding aneurysm morphology, diameter, dissection flap characterization, thrombus burden, calcification, angulation, and branch vessel orientation.
- Familiarity and routine usage of three-dimensional software on dedicated workstations and the ability to customize measurements provide an accurate road map to guide endovascular strategy, device selection, intraoperative maneuvers to best visualize pathology, and stent graft sizing.

SURGICAL MANAGEMENT

Preoperative Planning

- Patients scheduled for elective TEVAR undergo routine preoperative cardiac evaluation. Based on cardiovascular risk profile, symptomatology, and presence of electrocardiogram abnormalities, selected patients may need to undergo further evaluation in the form of an exercise stress test, dobutamine stress echocardiography, or Persantine thallium stress testing. Coronary angiography is pursued in cases involving extensive or symptomatic coronary artery disease.
- Aortic transections or symptomatic dissections and aneurysms should have early and aggressive blood pressure control using intravenous beta-blocker or calcium channel blocker medications. After obtaining a reliable clinical examination, refractory chest, back, or abdominal pain should be treated with narcotic analgesics.
- Renal protective strategies should be employed preoperatively to minimize the risk of contrast-induced nephropathy. Intravenous hydration is initiated preoperatively and, in the setting of baseline renal insufficiency, may warrant early hospital preadmission.
- Suspected blunt aortic injury should prompt a referral to a level I trauma center to facilitate early evaluation by an

endovascular specialist and other pertinent members of a multidisciplinary trauma team.

- Anesthetic choice is based on institution comfort, and can consist of general, regional, or local during TEVAR cases. Prophylactic lumbar cerebrospinal fluid (CSF) drainage is considered in every case based on the relative risk of spinal cord ischemia, hemodynamic status, and acuity of clinical presentation. Arterial monitoring is often performed via a right radial artery approach. Peripheral intravenous lines are typically adequate; however, more intensive central venous monitoring may be required in cases involving unstable traumatic transections, patients with significant baseline cardiovascular comorbidities, or any case involving hemodynamic instability.
- Preoperative imaging should be heavily scrutinized for the adequacy of iliofemoral access anatomy. An iliac conduit may be required in cases involving small-caliber, tortuous, or heavily calcified access vessels and can be done via a flank incision for an open bypass graft or via endovascular techniques with covered stenting of the iliac vessels.
- Numerous variables have been identified as risk factors for the development of spinal cord ischemia after TEVAR. Given that hypoperfusion represents the primary etiology of spinal cord injury following TEVAR, commonly cited risk factors involve those relating to the extent of impairment or exclusion of the collateral perfusion to the spinal cord. The European Collaborators on Stent/Graft Techniques for Aortic Aneurysm Repair (EUROSTAR) investigators reported results from the largest multicenter registry to date ($N = 606$).[6] In the EUROSTAR registry, the incidence of spinal cord ischemia was 2.5% and independent risk factors included left subclavian artery coverage without revascularization (odds ratio [OR], 3.9; $P = .037$), concomitant open abdominal aortic surgery (OR, 5.5; $P = .037$), and the use of three or more stent grafts (OR, 3.5; $P = .043$). Staging of TEVAR coverage for thoracoabdominal endovascular procedures should also be considered to allow for spinal conditioning.
- Based on the principle that spinal cord perfusion pressure is approximated by the difference between the mean arterial pressure (MAP) and CSF pressure, placement of a prophylactic lumbar drain has the potential to increase spinal cord perfusion pressure by decreasing CSF pressure and may be beneficial in select patients at high risk for spinal cord ischemia. Percutaneous drainage of CSF is performed by inserting a silastic catheter 10 to 15 cm into the subarachnoid space through a 14-gauge Tuohy needle at the L3-L4 vertebral interspace. The open end of the catheter is attached to a sterile closed-circuit reservoir, and the lumbar CSF pressure is measured with a pressure transducer zero-referenced to the midline of the brain. Lumbar CSF can be drained continuously or intermittently in the operating room to achieve target CSF pressures of 10 to 12 mm Hg. Postoperatively, intermittent or continuous CSF drainage can be continued in the intensive care unit for CSF pressures exceeding 10 mm Hg or at the first sign of lower extremity weakness. In the absence of neurologic deficits, the lumbar CSF drainage catheter can be clamped 24 hours post procedure followed by continued monitoring of CSF pressure together with serial neurologic assessments. The CSF drain can then be removed at 48 hours after operation. Although prophylactic or therapeutic lumbar CSF drainage has an established record of safety, complications have been reported to occur in approximately 1% of patients, which may include neuraxial hematoma, subdural hematoma, catheter fracture, meningitis, intracranial hypotension, chronic CSF leak, and spinal headache.

Selection and Sizing of Thoracic Stent Graft

Landing Zones

- Proximal and distal landing zones must be of sufficient length (usually at least 2 cm) to enable safe and accurate deployment bracketing the area of thoracic aortic pathology, which often includes the subclavian artery proximally or the celiac artery distally.
- Intentional coverage of the left subclavian artery is sometimes required due to a very proximal extent of aortic pathology, especially transections. Left subclavian artery revascularization may be required in select cases. The celiac artery rarely requires intentional coverage.
- Significant tortuosity, circumferential mural thrombus, and extensive calcification can compromise the proximal or distal landing zone, thereby predisposing to inadequate fixation and subsequent development of endoleak or migration. Site of proximal and distal landing zones should be selected to minimize the impact of these anatomic features, even if it requires extending the length of aortic coverage.
- A variety of anatomic measurements are taken from preoperative CTA imaging to assist in the sizing and selection of the thoracic stent-graft (**FIGURE 2**). Interventionalists should be proficient in accurate sizing and measuring of key thoracic aortic locations that influence device selection and ultimately determine patient outcomes.

Sizing of Stent Grafts

- The degree of stent graft oversizing can vary based on the indication for intervention. Stent-grafts are generally oversized by 10% to 20% based on the aortic diameter at the proximal and distal fixation sites for aneurysmal disease. Insufficient oversizing for the treatment of TAAs may predispose to inadequate exclusion and the potential for endoleak or migration. Aggressive oversizing, on the other hand, increases the risk for stent graft collapse, graft thrombosis, access arterial injury, and potential for peri- or postprocedural iatrogenic retrograde type A dissection.
- Chronic type B dissections are frequently characterized by a thick, nonmobile dissection flap, or septum, that separates true and false lumens into concave or convex discs of flow lumen. Such dissection flaps have limited compliance; therefore, minimal or no oversizing may be required to achieve a suitable proximal or distal seal.
- Aortic transections frequently occur in young trauma patients with normal or minimally diseased aortas. As such, minimal oversizing is needed to achieve an adequate seal and only recently did device manufacturers create devices meant for smaller-diameter aortas. Note also that underresuscitated patients on admission will have smaller aortic diameters on their CTA.
- Currently available stent-grafts range in diameter from 18 to 46 mm. Given the traditional 10% to 20% rule of device oversizing, these devices are designed to safely treat aortas with landing zones ranging from 16 to 43 mm in diameter.

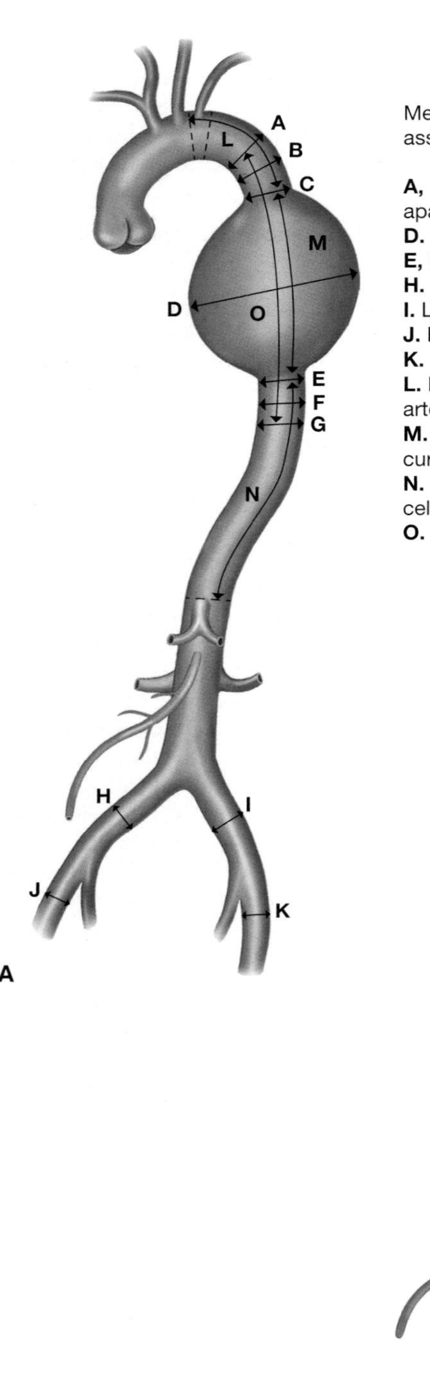

Measurements to be taken during the pretreatment assessment of isolated lesions are described below:

A, B, C. Proximal aortic neck diameter (minimum of 1 cm apart)
D. Maximum lesion diameter
E, F, G. Distal aortic neck diameter (minimum of 1 cm apart)
H. Right common iliac artery diameter
I. Left common iliac artery diameter
J. Right external iliac/femoral artery diameter
K. Left external iliac/femoral artery diameter
L. Distance between the left subclavian/left common carotid artery and the proximal end of the lesion (minimum of 2 cm)
M. Length of the lesion measured along the greater curvature of the flow lumen
N. Distance between the distal end of the lesion and the celiac axis (minimum of 2 cm)
O. Total treatment length

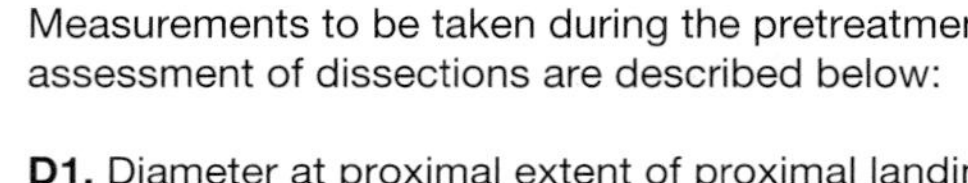

Measurements to be taken during the pretreatment assessment of dissections are described below:

D1. Diameter at proximal extent of proximal landing zone (must be in nondissected aorta)
D2. Maximum transverse aortic diameter (combined true and false lumen)
T1. Maximum true lumen diameter in DTA
T2. Minimum true lumen diameter in DTA
F. Maximum false lumen diameter in DTA
A1. Right access vessel diameter (common iliac, external iliac, femoral)
A2. Left access vessel diamter (common iliac, external iliac, femoral)
L1. Proximal landing zone length from proximal end of primary entry tear to left subclavian or left common carotid
L2. Distal neck length from distal end of primary entry tear to celiac
TTL. Total treatment length from left subclavian or left common carotid

B

FIGURE 2 ● Anatomic measurements to assist in thoracic stent graft device sizing and selection for the treatment of aneurysms **(A)** and dissections **(B)**. DTA, descending thoracic aorta.

Access Vessel Anatomy

- Current thoracic aortic stent-grafts require large-caliber delivery systems, ranging from 16 to 26 Fr in outer diameter. Depending on the manufacturer, some systems come with their own delivery systems. Small, tortuous, and heavily calcified iliofemoral arteries may prohibit sheath advancement and predispose to access site–related complications, including groin hematoma, dissection, or rupture.
- Careful evaluation of access vessel anatomy on preoperative imaging should be performed to assess the caliber, tortuosity, thrombus burden, and extent of calcification of the iliofemoral arteries. Such anatomic information will serve as the basis for deciding laterality of femoral access as well as to determine the need for an iliac conduit.
- Serial dilation may be attempted for patients with small iliofemoral vessels. Iliac atherosclerotic lesions may be pretreated with balloon angioplasty and/or stent-grafting (often with an iliac limb or peripheral stent-graft) to facilitate sheath advancement and introduction of the thoracic stent graft components.
- Iliac conduits serve as a safe and reliable technique to circumvent issues related to suboptimal access vessel anatomy. From either flank incision, a retroperitoneal exposure provides visualization of the common iliac artery or distal abdominal aorta. A 10- or 12-mm Dacron graft is commonly used as the conduit of choice. The conduit can be modified by creating a patch at the distal end to further facilitate the delivery of a large-caliber sheath and enable additional degrees of torqueability (**FIGURE 3**). This modification involves creating a patch by cutting the Dacron graft along its long access, thereby enlarging the transition zone from the graft to artery.

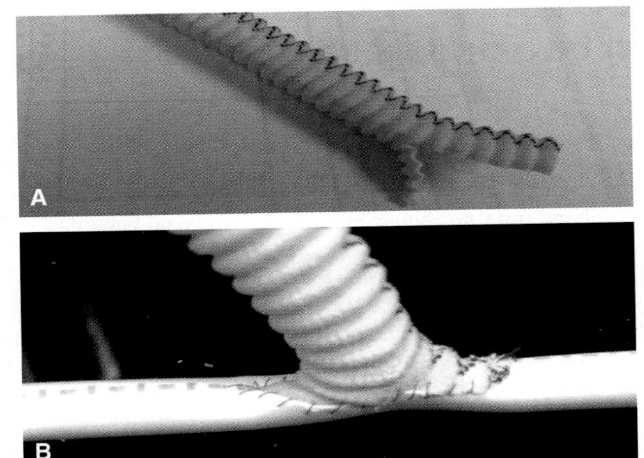

FIGURE 3 ● **A,** A 10-mm Dacron conduit bisected longitudinally to create a sewing patch. **B,** Dacron iliac conduit sewn to native iliac artery allows easy mobility of the conduit at multiple angles of entry for large-caliber device or sheath. (From Lee JT, Lee GK, Chandra V, et al. Comparison of fenestrated endografts and the snorkel/chimney technique. Published online April 27, 2014. *J Vasc Surg*. doi:10.1016/j.jvs.2014.03.255)

EARLY PROCEDURAL CONSIDERATIONS

Positioning

- The C-arm is typically configured in the "head" position. The left arm may be abducted to 75° to 90° and circumferentially prepped into the field if an embolization or snorkel/chimney procedure involving the left subclavian artery is anticipated. Axillary access can also be used and allows for the arms to be tucked. Some interventionalists prefer the right arm approach based on the design of their hybrid suite. The chest, abdomen, and bilateral groins should be prepped. As frequently only one groin access is required for the performance of a routine TEVAR, laterality of the operator position may vary based on surgeon preference or anticipated access site location.

Establishing Vascular Access

- The ipsilateral femoral artery is accessed either percutaneously or from an open exposure. Secondary access may be obtained from the contralateral femoral artery or brachial artery as needed for a 5-Fr sheath and flush catheter. Surgical exposure is obtained from a small oblique incision at the level of the inguinal ligament. The common femoral artery is exposed, with proximal control obtained at the level of the external iliac artery and distal control at the level of the femoral bifurcation or proximal superficial femoral and profunda femoral arteries. Heavy calcification may require preemptive endarterectomy and patch angioplasty to facilitate safe sheath placement.
- The femoral artery is punctured using a standard micropuncture set, and if arterial access is obtained percutaneously, a sheathogram is performed to confirm adequate puncture site location (mid–common femoral artery). A standard-length Bentson wire is inserted into the aorta through micropuncture sheath and exchange for a 7-Fr sheath is then performed using Seldinger technique. Wire exchange is then done for a 260-cm stiff Lunderquist wire. The Lunderquist wire should have a flexible, curved proximal end that should be advanced under fluoroscopy across the aortic arch to abut the aortic value. The location of the distal end of the Lunderquist wire should be marked on the operating table, and this wire position should be maintained throughout the procedure.
- Over the stiff Lunderquist wire platform, the 7-Fr sheath is removed and serial dilators are advanced to gradually enlarge the subcutaneous tract and arteriotomy site to accommodate either the stent-graft device itself or a larger 16- to 26-Fr introducer sheath required for device delivery.
- After placement of the larger sheath, systemic heparin is administered at a dose of 100 U/kg (goal activated clotting time of >250 seconds). Concomitant traumatic injuries, particularly intracranial hemorrhage, may alter the dose or decision to administer heparin.

INITIAL AORTOGRAM

- A 5-Fr 100-cm Omniflush or pigtail catheter is inserted into the aorta and advanced to the level of the aortic arch. This catheter may be advanced via a contralateral 5-Fr sheath or it may be inserted into an additional ipsilateral 5-Fr sheath placed distal to the arteriotomy for the main body delivery sheath.
- If satisfied with stent graft sizing based on available preoperative imaging, the thoracic aortic stent graft may be advanced over the Lunderquist wire and be positioned in the proximal to midportion of the thoracic aorta prior to initial aortogram.
- Optimal angiographic imaging of the aortic arch is obtained by placing the fluoroscopic C-arm in a left anterior oblique orientation, often 35° to 65°, and can be optimized by referencing the preoperative CTA. The location of the supra-aortic vessels, particularly the left subclavian artery, should be noted and marked on viewing monitors (**FIGURE 4A**). Many new advances with image overlay techniques have further allowed accurate stent-graft deployment and savings on branch catheterization time and radiation.
- Intravascular ultrasound (IVUS) is an important adjunct in cases involving dissection to assist in the identification of true and false lumens, as well as to gain additional information on aortic diameter, branch vessel location, and morphology of proximal and distal landing zones. IVUS also aids in limiting intravenous contrast exposure in those patients with baseline impaired renal function.
- If necessary to guide distal extent of stent graft placement, the celiac artery is best imaged from a full lateral projection. Additional structures to note are large, patent intercostal arteries at the level of the aortic hiatus. Efforts should be made to avoid covering these if at all possible during the course of the repair.

Device Deployment

- Precise proximal positioning of the stent graft is facilitated by either marking the location of the left subclavian artery on the viewing screen and/or using the road-mapping feature

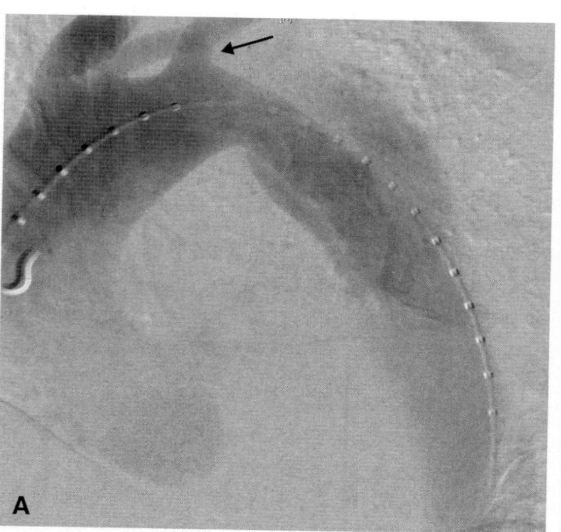

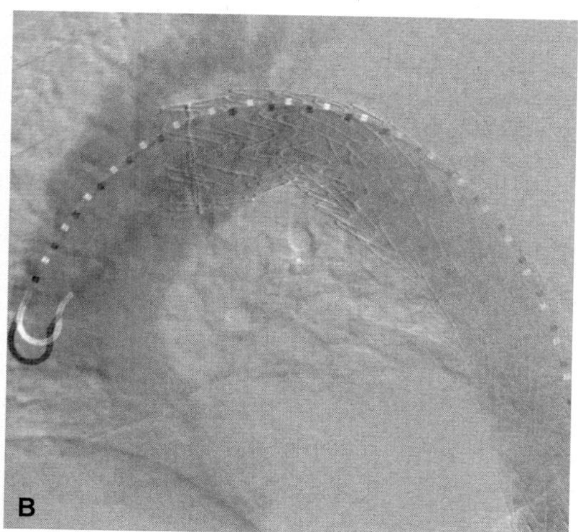

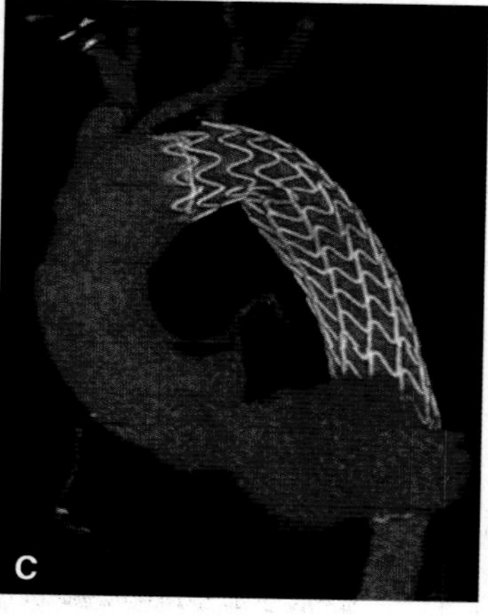

FIGURE 4 ● **A,** Initial thoracic aortogram performed with C-arm in a 45° left anterior oblique orientation in a case involving a type B aortic dissection. Note how clearly the origin of the subclavian (*arrow*) is seen to accurately decide if there is adequate proximal neck length. **B,** Aortogram following deployment of thoracic stent graft with coverage of the ostium of the left subclavian artery. **C,** Postoperative three-dimensional imaging demonstrating successful exclusion of the proximal entry dissection tear.

and/or using image overlay. The distal radiopaque line of the endotracheal tube seen on fluoroscopy at about 45° left anterior oblique can sometimes correlate to the position of the left common carotid artery, thereby serving as a convenient landmark in unstable cases requiring left subclavian artery coverage when bleeding must be expeditiously controlled.

- Immediately prior to stent graft deployment, systemic arterial blood pressure is reduced below 100 mm Hg to reduce risk of caudal migration.
- The stent-grafts are generally deployed in a proximal-to-distal sequence. However, a distal-to-proximal sequence may be preferred in cases involving precise deployment near the celiac artery or in aortas with significant diameter taper and a larger proximal landing zone compared with the distal landing zone (where devices of different diameter may need to be stacked up on each other).
- Deployed endografts will naturally extend toward the outer curvature of the aorta, and precision deployment is facilitated by gently providing forward traction on the wire toward the outer curve during deployment. This maneuver also facilitates straightening out of the transverse arch, which can be helpful in minimizing the "bird-beaking" effect at the proximal graft margin, where the device may not fully oppose to the "inner" aortic wall. Bird beaking, when present, can predispose to proximal type I endoleaks, endograft collapse, and potential aortic occlusion. Newer next-generation conformable devices and device modifications have significantly reduced this risk.
- Additional graft components are added, when necessary, by exchanging the first device over the Lunderquist wire. A minimum overlap of 5 cm between pieces is recommended to ensure adequate apposition and minimize risk of junctional (type III) endoleak.

Balloon Molding

- Balloon molding is often required in cases involving TAAs. Under fluoroscopic guidance, a noncompliant molding balloon (Coda [Cook Medical, Bloomington, IN, USA] or Tri-Lobe [W. L. Gore, Flagstaff, AZ, USA]) is advanced up to the proximal edge of the stent-graft and balloon molding is performed in a proximal-to-distal sequence. Balloon molding should be performed at the proximal and distal fixation sites, as well as at areas of stent-graft overlap in those cases requiring multiple stent-grafts.
- Aggressive ballooning can cause component fracture and aortic injury, and care must be taken during inflation with constant visualization and knowledge of the tension applied to the balloon.
- Balloon molding is not typically required in cases involving aortic dissection or transection, particularly in cases where no obvious endoleak is visualized. Balloon molding may increase risk for iatrogenic retrograde type A conversion if performed in a region of friable or fragile aorta and is generally not recommended during dissection cases.

COMPLETION AORTOGRAM

- After stent-graft deployment, the pigtail catheter is withdrawn along the outside of the deployed device(s) over a wire to below the level of the stent-graft. The catheter is then readvanced over a wire within the stent-graft lumen and positioned at the level of the aortic arch.
- Additional aortograms may be performed at this time as necessary in order to ensure adequate stent-graft position and patency of the supra-aortic and celiac arteries and to assess for the presence of endoleaks.

REMOVAL OF SHEATH AND ARTERIOTOMY CLOSURE

- In cases involving percutaneous access, the two previously placed Perclose ProGlide devices are used to close the arteriotomy site(s) (see Part 6, Chapter 23 for details). If open surgical exposure was obtained, proximal and distal vascular control is obtained in the respective groin. All wires and sheaths are removed. The arteriotomy is closed transversely using a polypropylene suture in either a running continuous or interrupted fashion. Antegrade and retrograde flushing maneuvers should be performed prior to completion of the arteriotomy closure.

LEFT SUBCLAVIAN ARTERY REVASCULARIZATION

- Endovascular procedures that require coverage of the left subclavian artery have the potential to increase the risk of spinal cord injury by compromising blood flow to the ipsilateral vertebral artery, an important collateral pathway for arterial flow to the anterior spinal artery. Subclavian artery revascularization therefore serves as an additional strategy to decrease the risk of spinal cord ischemia in select patients deemed high risk.
- Techniques to revascularize the left subclavian artery include transposition of the subclavian onto the left carotid artery or left carotid–subclavian bypass grafting with subsequent embolization of the left subclavian artery proximal to the bypass graft (**FIGURE 5**). These revascularization procedures may be performed as part of a staged repair or at the time of TEVAR. Laser in situ fenestrations and purpose-specific single side branch grafts are currently being studied as an alternative to extra-anatomic open revascularization.
- The existing clinical evidence to support the efficacy of routine left subclavian artery revascularization remains controversial; there are advocates for routine revascularization, selective revascularization, or no revascularization. A meta-analysis of published studies showed a trend toward increased risk of spinal cord ischemia when the left subclavian artery was covered, suggesting a potential benefit for left subclavian artery revascularization, but the finding was not statistically significant.[5-7]

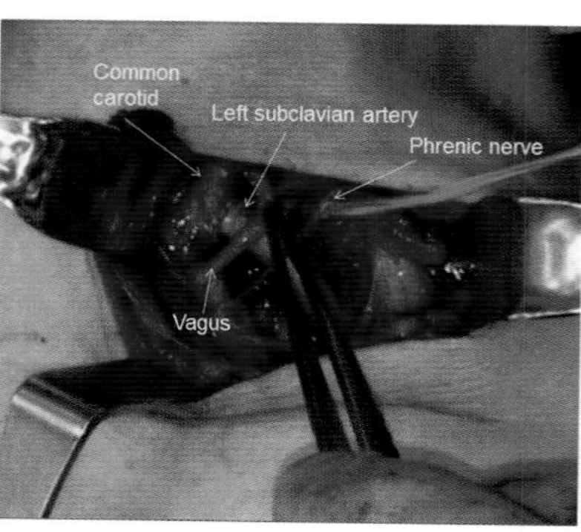

FIGURE 5 ● Left subclavian artery transposition is performed by ligating the left subclavian artery proximal to the vertebral artery and moving it cephalad in order to perform an end-to-side anastomosis between the left subclavian and left common carotid arteries. Alternatively, a Dacron graft can be used as a left carotid–subclavian bypass.

SPECIAL CONSIDERATIONS BASED ON AORTIC PATHOLOGY

Aortic Dissection

- The primary goal of TEVAR for the treatment of dissection is coverage of the proximal entry tear (**FIGURE 6A** and **B**). Stent-graft sizing is based on the diameter of the adjacent nondissected thoracic aorta. Minimal or no oversizing of the stent graft is recommended.
- In acute type B dissections, the septum is relatively mobile and compliant. Therefore, the diameter of the small true lumen in the dissected portion often returns to normal diameter following successful exclusion of the proximal entry tear.
- Chronic dissections have thicker, less compliant septa, which may limit expansion of the true lumen despite adequate entry tear coverage. Often, these patients have chronic false lumen aneurysmal dilation, and entry tear and fenestration covering serve simply to decrease false lumen pressurization and promote thrombosis.
- IVUS serves as a useful adjunct in dissection cases, both in terms of initial identification of true and false lumen, as well as assisting in precise positioning of the device.
- The placement of a distal noncovered stent in the manner of the STABLE trial in theory can lead to positive remodeling, and current outcomes are still in mid-term.[8]

Aortic Transection

- Traumatic aortic injuries are typically located along the inner curve of the proximal descending thoracic aorta (**FIGURE 7**). Given the proximal location, left subclavian artery coverage is sometimes needed.[5]
- In the absence of concomitant hemorrhage or brain injury, routine heparin is recommended.
- Trauma patients are frequently hypovolemic and, as a result, may have an underdistended aorta on preoperative cross-sectional imaging. Initial cross-sectional imaging can underestimate true aortic morphology at the region of the subclavian by as much as 10% to 20%. In such settings, IVUS may assist in more accurate stent graft sizing performed in vivo.[9]

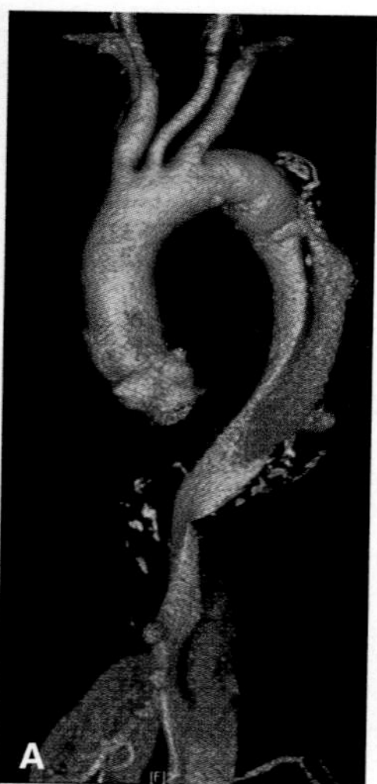

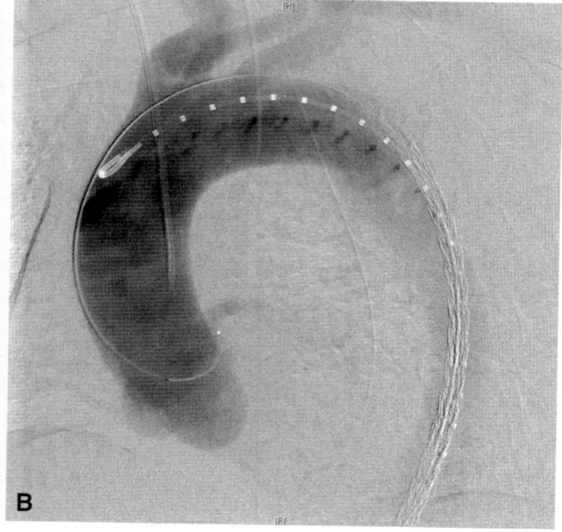

FIGURE 6 ● **A,** CTA reconstruction demonstrating complex thoracoabdominal aortic dissection with proximal entry tear located in the proximal descending thoracic aorta. **B,** Initial aortogram documenting position of the supra-aortic arteries. Note the stent graft has been advanced into approximate position but is not yet deployed.

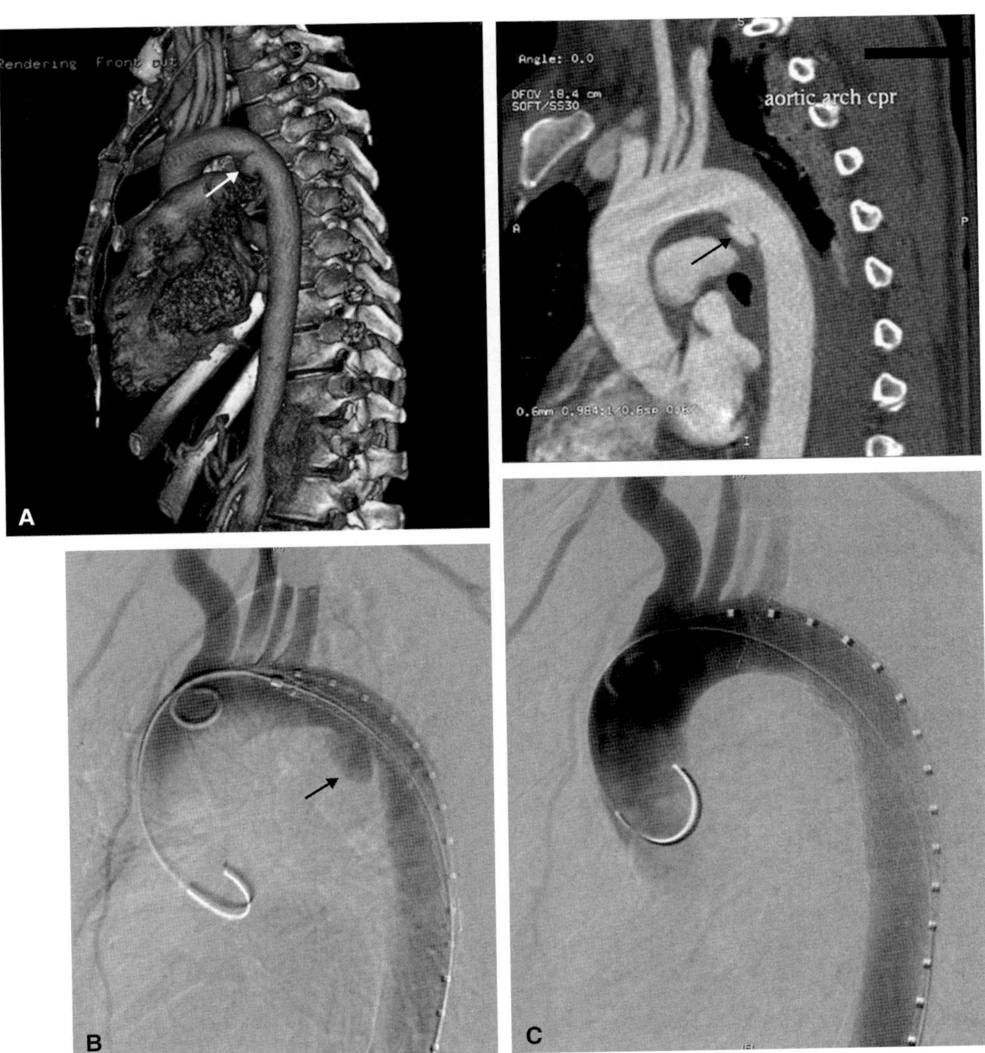

FIGURE 7 ● **A,** Three-dimensional reconstructed images showing the presence of traumatic aortic transection at the level of the ligamentum arteriosum (*arrow*). **B,** Aortogram showing focal outpouching (*arrow*) along the inner curve of the proximal descending thoracic aorta, correlating to the traumatic transection observed on preoperative imaging. Note that the stent graft has been advanced into the proximal descending thoracic aorta but is not yet deployed. **C,** Aortogram following thoracic stent graft deployment with successful exclusion of the transection site.

PEARLS AND PITFALLS

Indications	■ TEVAR follows general recommendations for elective repair of descending thoracic and thoracoabdominal aortic aneurysms and should be offered to good anatomic risk patients with aneurysms >6 cm. ■ Patient selection should take into account the need for regular interval clinical and radiologic follow-up in order to monitor for stent-graft–related complications and endoleaks.
Preoperative workup	■ High-quality imaging and ability to configure three-dimensional reconstructive software are essential for successful preoperative planning and device selection. ■ Pre- and perioperative hydration is a central part in the protection from contrast-induced nephropathy. ■ Patients should be stratified according to baseline risk of spinal cord ischemia. A prophylactic lumbar drain should be considered in those at high risk.
Patient setup	■ A hybrid endovascular suite provides optimal opportunity for accurate imaging and capability to perform necessary open surgical exposure or repair of access-related complications. ■ Anticipated adjunct procedures, including left subclavian artery embolization or revascularization, may require prepping the left neck and/or arm into the surgical field.

Thoracic aneurysms	■ Oversizing of stent-grafts by 10%-20% and balloon molding are generally recommended in order to maximize proximal and distal fixation. ■ Proximal and distal landing zones should be relatively free of stenosis, calcification, and thrombus to maximize durability of this minimally invasive technology.
Type B dissection	■ Accurate identification of true and false lumen is essential prior to deployment of the stent-graft. IVUS is a useful adjunct in this setting to confirm true or false lumen position. ■ Aggressive oversizing of stent-grafts is not recommended in patients with aortic dissection. Balloon molding is generally reserved only for those with type I or III endoleak on completion angiography and not against the region where there is a mobile septum.
Traumatic transection	■ Routine heparin is recommended unless contraindicated by concomitant intracranial or solid organ injury. ■ Similar to dissections, aggressive oversizing and balloon molding is not routinely performed during the treatment of transections.

POSTOPERATIVE CARE

- Patients are typically extubated if they had a general anesthetic immediately following the procedure unless prohibited by concomitant physiologic insults (eg, hemodynamic instability, trauma patient).
- Intensive care unit monitoring is required for patients who require a lumbar drain for 24 to 48 hours. Immediate and frequent neurologic assessments are critical in the early perioperative period to assess for spinal cord ischemia. Raising MAP goals are an additional way to minimize risk of cord ischemia.
- Durability of TEVAR is reliant on routine imaging to evaluate for stent-graft–specific complications postoperatively. Follow-up chest CTA and plain x-rays are typically obtained at 1, 6, and 12 months and at intervals thereafter. Consideration should be made between balancing risks for cumulative lifetime iodinated contrast and radiation exposure vs the necessity for serial graft monitoring. In stable patients, chest x-rays may suffice to confirm device position, with CT scanning reserved for those with migration suggested by CT or evidence of progressive aortic enlargement or onset of recurrent symptoms such as chest pain.

OUTCOMES

- The largest published series, which has reported 1-year follow-up, included 443 patients treated with TEVAR for a variety of indications, both emergent and elective, as follows: TAA (n = 249), thoracic aortic dissection (n = 131), traumatic aortic injury (n = 50), and false anastomotic aneurysm (n = 13).[10] Technical success was achieved in nearly 90% of patients, with an all-cause mortality among patients treated for aortic aneurysm and aortic dissection of 20% and 10%, respectively. In the most recent analysis of Medicare data, TEVAR for aneurysm has the best long-term survival after traumatic injury, with outcomes slightly worse in TAA and dissection, which has the highest reintervention rate.[11]
- No randomized trials comparing TEVAR with open surgery have been published to date. However, multiple nonrandomized comparisons suggest equivalent or better outcomes with TEVAR. In a single-center, retrospective study of over 700 patients who underwent either TEVAR or open surgery, mortality was not significantly different at 30-day (5.7% vs 8.3%, respectively) or 1-year (15.6% vs 15.9%, respectively) follow-up.[12] Two smaller studies demonstrated a reduction in 30-day perioperative mortality with TEVAR compared with open surgery (1.9% vs 5.7%).[13,14]

COMPLICATIONS

- Stroke continues to be a common complication following TEVAR and is associated with significant in-hospital mortality. Recent clinical series have reported an incidence of stroke after TEVAR to range from 2% to 8%.[15,16] The underlying mechanisms contributing to acute ischemic stroke after TEVAR and the temporal relationship of stroke to the procedure are not completely understood. However, the constellation of preoperative risk factors, neurologic examinations, and patterns of brain infarction observed in these patients has led most investigators to conclude that cerebral embolization and ischemic events are the primary mechanisms for perioperative stroke in TEVAR.[6,16,17] Embolic events are related to instrumentation of the aortic arch in patients with severe atheromatous disease, whereas ischemia is a result of the planned or inadvertent endovascular coverage of supra-aortic vessels. Flushing of devices is even thought to potentially contribute to embolic debris that can lead to cerebrovascular compromise.
- Spinal cord ischemia and subsequent acute or delayed paraplegia represents the most devastating complication of TEVAR. The pathogenesis of spinal cord injury after TEVAR is likely multifactorial but still poorly understood. The deployment of thoracic stent-grafts results in rapid complete exclusion of varying lengths of segmental collateral vessels without the ability to surgically reimplant or revascularize the intercostal arteries. Stent deployment and catheter manipulation can predispose patients to dislodgement of thrombotic or atheromatous debris from the aortic wall into segmental vessels, with subsequent distal embolization and occlusion of arteries supplying the spinal cord. Moreover, endovascular coverage of the left subclavian artery may compromise spinal cord perfusion in patients with a dominant left vertebral artery, solitary vertebral artery, carotid artery disease, or an incomplete circle of Willis. Access site injuries to the iliofemoral vessels may further increase the risk of spinal cord ischemia by compromising collateral flow to the anterior spinal artery through the hypogastric and pelvic vascular plexus. Lastly, pharmacologic measures aimed

at decreasing arterial blood pressure to enhance accuracy of device deployment in cases involving difficult aortic anatomy may lead to hypotension similar to that observed in open surgery.

- Due to the large sheath sizes required for the delivery of thoracic stent-grafts, small-diameter, tortuous, or heavily calcified access vessels can predispose to iliofemoral arterial injury. Postoperative CTA often documents arterial dissections and injury that can be followed with noninvasive duplex and managed expectantly until patients have claudication-like symptoms.
- Endoleaks are a relatively common finding after TEVAR, affecting nearly 15% of patients in the early or late postoperative periods. Type I or III endoleaks typically require additional stent placement or balloon molding in order to improve proximal, distal, or junctional fixation. Most type II endoleaks observed on completion angiogram or early follow-up cross-sectional imaging will resolve spontaneously. Persistent type II endoleaks, especially those with aneurysm sac expansion or failure to adequately seal a proximal entry tear or transection, warrant additional intervention. Retrograde flow from intercostal or left subclavian arteries can be treated using coil embolization or vascular plug placement.

REFERENCES

1. Dake MD, Miller DC, Semba CP, et al. Transluminal placement of endovascular stent-grafts for the treatment of descending thoracic aortic aneurysms. *N Engl J Med.* 1994;331:1729-1734.
2. Bavaria JE, Appoo JJ, Makaroun MS, et al. Endovascular stent grafting versus open surgical repair of descending thoracic aortic aneurysms in low-risk patients: a multicenter comparative trial. *J Thorac Cardiovasc Surg.* 2007;133:369-377.
3. Nienaber CA, Rousseau H, Eggebrecht H, et al. Randomized comparison of strategies for type B aortic dissection: the INvestigation of STEnt Grafts in Aortic Dissection (INSTEAD) trial. *Circulation.* 2009;120:2519-2528.
4. Nienaber CA, Kische S, Rousseau H, et al. Long-term results of the randomized investigation of stent grafts in aortic dissection trial. *Circ Cardiovasc Interv.* 2013;6:407-416.
5. Lee WA, Matsumura JS, Mitchell RS, et al. Endovascular repair of traumatic aortic injury: clinical practice guidelines of the Society for Vascular Surgery. *J Vasc Surg.* 2011;53:187-192.
6. Buth J, Harris PL, Hobo R, et al. Neurologic complications associated with endovascular repair of thoracic aortic pathology: incidence and risk factors. A study from the European Collaborators on Stent/Graft Techniques for Aortic Aneurysm Repair (EUROSTAR) registry. *J Vasc Surg.* 2007;46:1103-1110.
7. Rizvi AZ, Murad MH, Fairman RM, et al. The effect of left subclavian artery coverage on morbidity and mortality in patients undergoing endovascular thoracic aortic interventions: a systematic review and meta-analysis. *J Vasc Surg.* 2009;50:1159-1169.
8. Lombardi JV, Gleason TG, Panneton JM, et al. STABLE II clinical trial on endovascular treatment of acute, complicated type B aortic dissection with a composite device design. *J Vasc Surg.* 2020;71:1077-1087.
9. Pearce BJ, Jordan W. Using IVUS during EVAR and TEVAR: improving patient outcomes. *Semin Vasc Surg.* 2009;22:172-180.
10. Leurs LJ, Bell R, Degrieck Y, et al. Endovascular treatment of thoracic aortic diseases: combined experience from the EUROSTAR and United Kingdom Thoracic Endograft registries. *J Vasc Surg.* 2004;40:670-679.
11. Ho VT, Itoga NK, Tran K, et al. Mid-term survival after thoracic endovascular aortic repair by indication in the medicare population. *J Am Coll Surg.* 2021 01;232(1):46-53.e2.
12. Greenberg RK, Lu Q, Roselli EE, et al. Contemporary analysis of descending thoracic and thoracoabdominal aneurysm repair: a comparison of endovascular and open techniques. *Circulation.* 2008;118:808-817.
13. Matsumura JS, Cambria RP, Dake MD, et al. International controlled clinical trial of thoracic endovascular aneurysm repair with the Zenith TX2 endovascular graft: 1-year results. *J Vasc Surg.* 2008;47(2):247-257.
14. Bavaria JE, Appoo JJ, Makaroun MS, et al. Endovascular stent grafting versus open surgical repair of descending thoracic aortic aneurysms in low-risk patients: a multicenter comparative trial. *J Thorac Cardiovasc Surg.* 2007;133:369-377.
15. Feezor RJ, Martin TD, Hess PJ, et al. Risk factors for perioperative stroke during thoracic endovascular aortic repairs (TEVAR). *J Endovasc Ther.* 2007;14:568-573.
16. Gutsche JT, Cheung AT, McGarvey ML, et al. Risk factors for perioperative stroke after thoracic endovascular aortic repair. *Ann Thorac Surg.* 2007;84:1195-1200.
17. Fattori R, Nienaber CA, Rousseau H, et al. Results of endovascular repair of the thoracic aorta with the talent thoracic stent graft: the talent thoracic retrospective registry. *J Thorac Cardiovasc Surg.* 2006;132:332-339.

Chapter 12

Retroperitoneal Abdominal Aortic Exposure for Visceral Aortic Endarterectomy

Matthew W. Mell

DEFINITION

- Occasionally, patients may present with visceral aortic occlusive disease that is not conducive to endovascular repair or amenable to open repair through a transabdominal approach. Open thoracoabdominal surgical revascularization of the mesenteric or renal arteries remains a useful alternative for revascularization of symptomatic visceral artery occlusive disease.
- "Coral reef aorta" is one such example (**FIGURE 1**), whereby the atherosclerotic disease is calcified and encompasses the visceral aorta, extending into the celiac axis, superior mesenteric artery, and renal arteries. For this and related conditions, a thoracoretroperitoneal approach will provide adequate exposure to perform a transaortic endarterectomy to successfully restore flow to the visceral vessels and distal aorta. It has been shown that endarterectomy provides equivalent or superior durability to other open surgical approaches.[1]

Patient History and Physical Findings

- Patients to be considered for this procedure generally present with signs and symptoms of mesenteric ischemia, including postprandial abdominal pain, food fear, weight loss, and nausea, vomiting, or diarrhea. Persistent postprandial pain may lead to food fear in 30% to 50% of patients who ameliorate symptoms by avoiding meals.[2] Weight loss, thought to be due to both decreased caloric intake and reduced nutrient absorption, is present in nearly all patients and can be substantial. Diarrhea may be present in up to 30% of patients, and occurs because of intestinal malabsorption and subsequent increased osmotic load (REF).
- Renovascular hypertension accounts for only 1% of patients with hypertension. Suggestive clinical presentations may include refractory hypertension, hypertension with retinal artery hemorrhage, acute decompensation of otherwise stable hypertension, or flash pulmonary edema. Severe stenosis of the visceral aorta may manifest as bilateral claudication. Asymptomatic visceral artery stenosis is common; as such, the presence of symptoms is a requisite to recommending repair.
- It is imperative to perform and document a baseline vascular exam for postoperative comparison.

DIFFERENTIAL DIAGNOSIS

- The differential diagnosis of chronic mesenteric ischemia is broad, and includes peptic ulcer disease, acute cholecystitis and biliary colic, acute mesenteric ischemia, biliary obstruction, cholangitis, cholecystitis, gastritis, chronic pancreatitis, diverticulitis, irritable bowel syndrome, inflammatory bowel disease and others. It is not uncommon for there to be a delay in the diagnosis of chronic mesenteric ischemia in part due to its non-specific symptoms and its relative low incidence compared with other conditions.

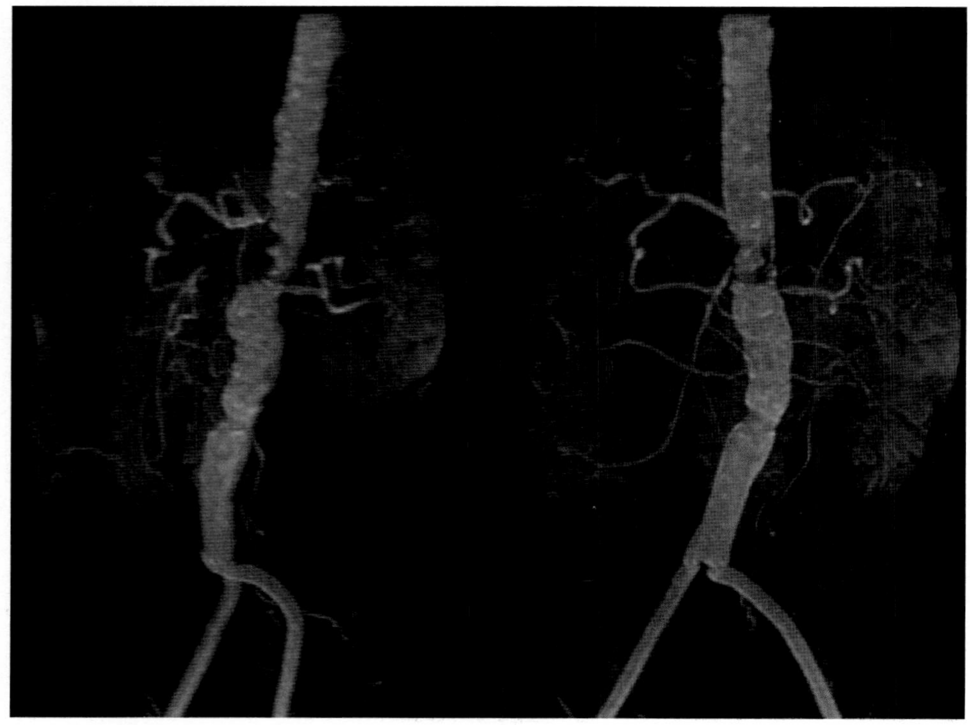

FIGURE 1 ● AP and oblique view of a coral reef aorta, with severe stenosis of the celiac origin and left renal artery origin, segmental occlusion of the superior mesenteric artery, and occluded right renal artery.

- Similarly, the differential diagnosis for hypertension is broad, and other more common causes of hypertension should be considered before attributing it to renal artery stenosis.

IMAGING AND OTHER DIAGNOSTIC STUDIES

- Duplex ultrasound and physiologic testing can identify significant stenosis of the visceral vessels as well as compromise of the lower extremity perfusion.
- Elevated plasma renin levels are consistent with symptomatic renal artery stenosis.
- High-definition computed tomographic angiography (CTA) has typically been performed as part of the workup of symptoms and to rule out other causes of abdominal pain, weight loss, nausea/vomiting, or diarrhea. CTA will confirm the anatomic disease and is essential in operative planning. Relevant information in addition to ruling out other causes includes the extent and degreed of atherosclerotic disease, the presence of occluded arteries, and the quality of the thoracic and abdominal aorta in regard to safe cross-clamping.
- Angiography is generally not required but can be helpful if the CTA cannot confirm the absence of completely occluded visceral arteries. For symptomatic patients with occluded visceral arteries, endarterectomy would not be the procedure of choice. For this anatomic pattern, an antegrade or retrograde bypass may be a more suitable option.

SURGICAL MANAGEMENT

Preoperative Planning

- When considering a thoracoabdominal approach, certain factors should be considered. Previous retroperitoneal surgery or left thoracic surgery or severe illness may preclude safe access.
- Cardiac and pulmonary function should be assessed prior to surgery. Severe pre-existing pulmonary disease may lead to pneumonia, ventilator dependence, or other pulmonary complications associated with thoracotomy. Cardiac function will need to be adequate to tolerate aortic cross-clamping at the supraceliac location.
- Many patients with severe visceral occlusive disease have had significant weight loss with an abnormally low body mass index (BMI), which provides for a technically more straightforward dissection; however, an increased BMI should not in itself be considered a contraindication to a thoracoretroperitoneal approach, as with positioning an abdominal pannus generally falls away from the incision and does not impede exposure.

Positioning

- Patients undergoing aortic endarterectomy should have adequate central intravenous access, a bladder catheter, and an arterial line (preferably place in the right arm). The need for transesophageal echocardiography and double-lumen endotracheal tube should discussed in collaboration with the anesthesia team. If it is not used a nasogastric or orogastric tube should be placed. A double lumen endotracheal tube may improve access to the thoracic aorta for cross-clamping. If exposure of only the distal thoracic aorta is required, a single lumen endotracheal tube with gentle retraction of the left lower lobe may provide sufficient exposure for cross-clamping.

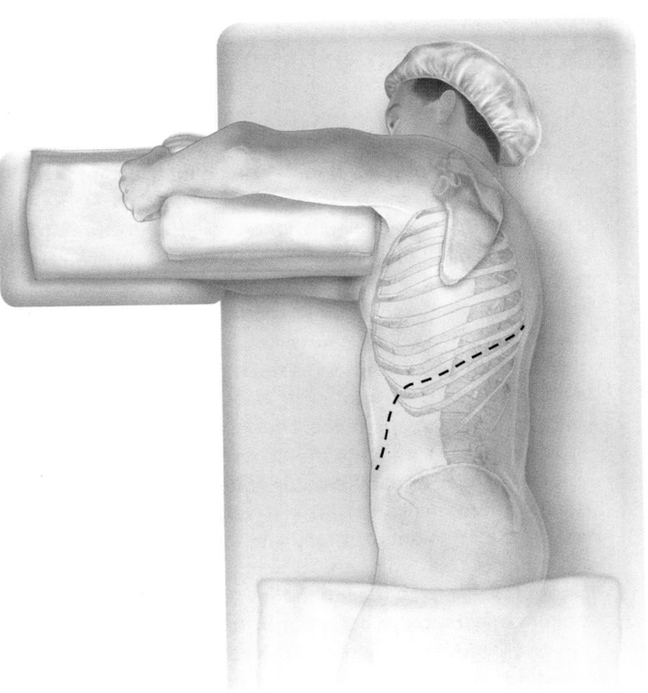

FIGURE 2 ● Patient position for thoracoabdominal exposure with incision in the 8th intercostal space (dotted line). Positioning is supported with a beanbag and right axillary roll.

- After monitoring lines have been placed and induction of general anesthesia, the patient should be positioned in a modified left lateral decubitus position, with the left arm supported over the right arm and the hips positioned as flat as possible (**FIGURE 2**). A beanbag or rolled towels placed on each side of the patient will stabilize the position. The hips should be placed over the break of the table which will improve exposure when the break is utilized. The goal of positioning is to have wide access to the entire left chest, scapula, abdomen, retroperitoneum, and both groins. Cell-saver suction should be used. Baseline vascular pulse exam should be confirmed.

OPERATIVE DETAILS

- The surgeon stands on the patient's left side. After positioning, the ribs can generally been counted from below to identify the 8th intercostal space. An oblique incision is made incorporating this space, from the lateral border of the rectus sheath at or just cephalad of the umbilicus to the mid- or posterior axillary line. The incision is carried down through Scarpa fascia with electrocautery.
- For the abdominal portion of exposure, the external oblique, internal oblique, and transversus abdominal muscles are divided with electrocautery, stopping at the preperitoneal layer. This layer can frequently be identified by a layer of yellow fat just deep to the abdominal muscles. With this approach, the peritoneum should not be entered and can be repaired with absorbable sutures if it is entered inadvertently.
- The retroperitoneal approach is developed with blunt dissection, first by working centrally and inferiorly to identify the psoas muscle. Laterally, the dissection is continued behind Gerota fascia, lifting the left kidney up (**FIGURE 3**). The peritoneum may be more adherent in the left upper quadrant, and care needs to be taken as it is taken off the diaphragm to avoid entry into the peritoneum or injury to the spleen. As exposure of the retroperitoneal space is developed the aorta will be exposed, as well as the left renal artery.
- For the thoracic exposure, the dissection is carried down to the latissimus dorsi. This muscle can be divided, or preserved by dissecting along its anterior border, developing a plane deep to the muscle, and retracting it posteriorly. Preserving the latissimus dorsi will add time to the dissection and save time from the closure, and may improve pain and pulmonary toilet postoperatively. The serratus anterior muscle is divided along its fibers, and the chest wall is exposed. At this time, the correct intercostal space can be confirmed. If more proximal thoracic aortic exposure is required, a more proximal intercostal space can be used.
- The chest is then entered by incising the intercostal space, which is opened posteriorly to the spinae erector muscles and anteriorly through the costal margin where the exposure is joined with retroperitoneal dissection.
- The inferior pulmonary ligament is identified and divided along its length to facilitate retraction of the left lower lobe. The thoracic aorta can then be dissected for proximal control. Circumferential control may not be necessary, and if obtained the esophagus and intercostal arteries must be avoided. The esophagus will be behind the aorta with this approach and can be avoided by palpating the TEE probe or NG tube during the dissection. The thoracic exposure is facilitated by cutting the eighth and or ninth ribs posteriorly and placing a Burford or Finochietto retractor.
- For complete exposure of the visceral aorta, the diaphragm should be divided circumferentially from the costal margin to the aortic hiatus (**FIGURE 4**). An effective approach is to start the division at the costal margin once the peritoneum has been dissected off the diaphragm and the costal margin divided. It is important to leave a rim of 2 to 4 cm attached to the chest wall and enough of the free edge dissected free to facilitate closure at the end of the case. Dividing the median arcuate ligament from the left chest will facilitate complete division of the diaphragm.

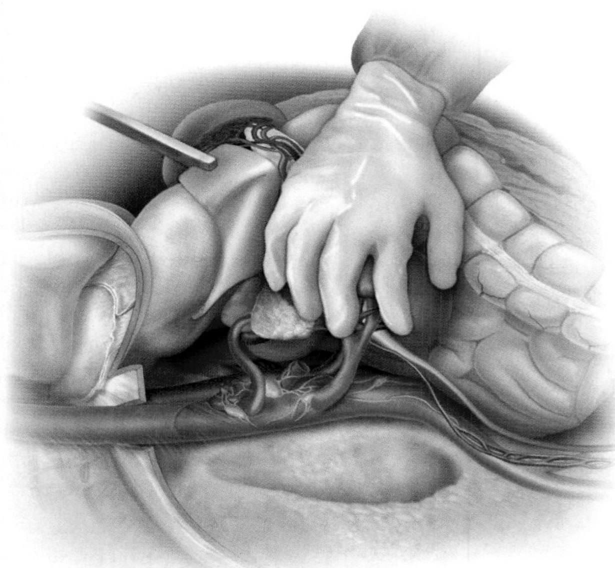

FIGURE 3 • Exposure of the visceral aorta with left kidney rotated anteriorly. This approach allows for additional exposure of the proximal superior mesenteric artery.

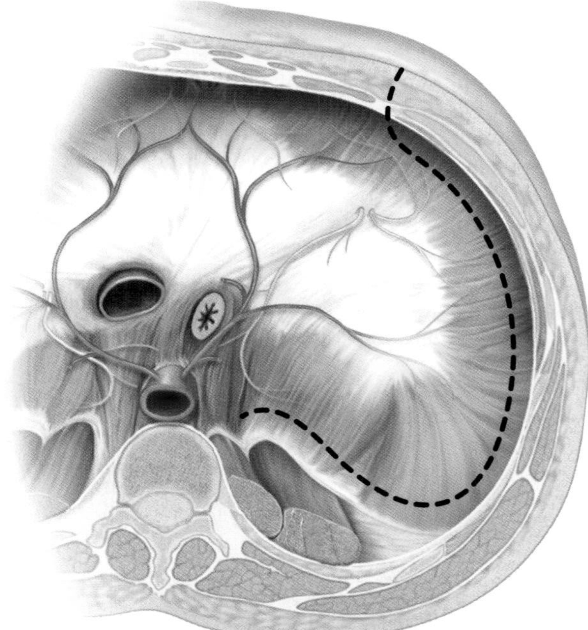

FIGURE 4 • The diaphragm is incised circumferentially (dotted line) to protect the phrenic nerve and thereby preserve diaphragmatic function. A 1 to 2 cm cuff of diaphragm is left attached to the chest was to aid in closure.

- With complete exposure of the visceral aorta the left renal artery, superior mesenteric artery (SMA), and celiac axis (CA) are addressed. If not already identified, the left renal artery is dissected and circumferentially controlled with a silastic loop. Depending on the extent of the atherosclerotic disease of the SMA and CA, a decision can be made to dissect these vessels and control them with silastic loops. If this is not performed, control can be obtained with occlusion balloons once the aorta is opened.
- At this point, the patient is given heparin (100 U/kg) to obtain an activating clotting time (ACT) of 250 to 300 seconds to be maintained throughout the cross-clamp, and 25 to 50 g of mannitol. After allowing for adequate circulation time, proximal and distal aortic clamps are placed.
- A longitudinal trap door incision is made in the aorta. This can be placed either anterior or posterior to the left renal artery orifice. Renal arteries should be cooled with 300-400 mL 4 °C saline for protection of renal function if not precluded by the plaque burden. The nondiseased left renal artery, SMA and CA are controlled with silastic loops or vascular clamps. A nondiseased right renal artery is controlled with an occlusion balloon. Control of diseased vessels requiring endarterectomy should not be initially obtained unless it can be done distal to the disease.
- The endarterectomy begins in the diseased aorta; it is performed circumferentially first at the proximal extent and then the distal extent. The plaque is transected sharply to obtain a satisfactory transition. The proximal transition generally does not require tacking sutures; distally the transition can be tacked with 5-0 prolene sutures if needed.
- The dissection plane is carried into the affected visceral vessels (**FIGURE 5**). At times, endarterectomy of these vessels may be simplified by first removing the aortic plaque, leaving postage stamp-sized aortic plaque at the orifices of the visceral vessels. This technique allows for endarterectomy of the branch vessels without the burden of the large aortic plaque and better control of the endarterectomy with feathering of the endpoints. As the atherosclerotic disease generally does not extend deep into the visceral vessels, the endpoint is generally easily obtained. If the feathering is inadequate, the plaque can be excised sharply and the transition tacked with 7-0 prolene sutures.
- When the endarterectomy is complete, there may be significant back-bleeding from the visceral arteries or lumbar arteries. Lumbar vessels, if they were occluded prior to the endarterectomy, can safely be suture-ligated for hemostasis without concern of spinal cord ischemia. Those that were patent should be preserved if possible. Significant back-bleeding from the left renal artery can be controlled with a vascular clamp or silastic loop. Back-bleeding from the right renal artery can be controlled with an occlusion balloon. Back-bleeding from the SMA and CA can be controlled with either technique. Control of these vessels also will protect from embolization when forward flow is re-established.
- The aortic incision is then closed directly with 3-0 or 4-0 running prolene, supported with pledgets if needed. Patch repair is generally not required. The shafts of the balloon occlusion catheters can be incorporated temporarily in the closure. Prior to completing closure, the visceral vessels and distal aorta are individually back flushed, and the proximal aorta is flushed. Flow is established serially to the visceral arteries and then distal aorta.
- Communication with the anesthesia team is key when preparing to re-establish antegrade flow, as blood pressure support will likely be required with volume and pressors. Flow should be established gradually to avoid uncontrolled hypotension.
- With closure complete the repair is inspected for hemostasis, and adequate flow in all vessels is confirmed with palpation and Doppler ultrasound. If concerns are present for the visceral vessels, intraoperative duplex can be performed to identify any anatomic obstruction to flow. Abnormalities if noted can be addressed with a variety of techniques, including embolectomy for thrombosis/embolization, excision with or without tacking for endothelial flaps, placement of visceral stents under direct vision, or bypass. If there is concern for

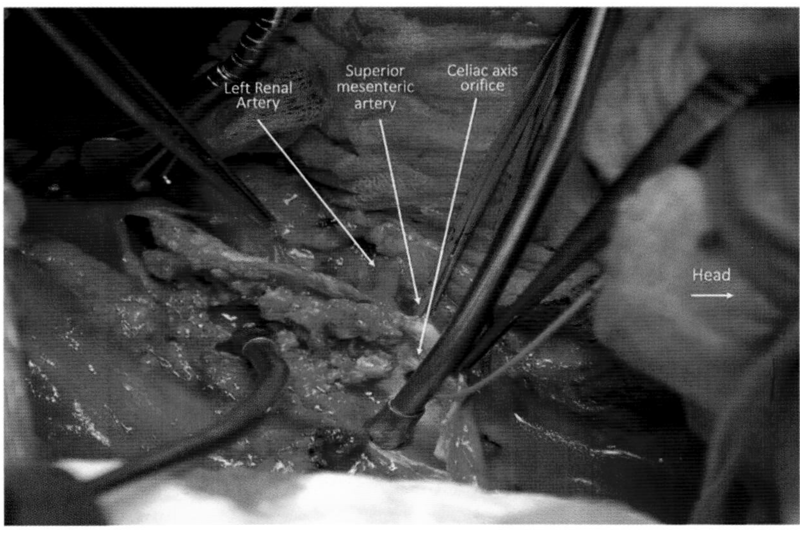

FIGURE 5 ● Intraoperative exposure and endarterectomy of a coral reef aortic plaque.

intestinal ischemia, the peritoneum can be opened and inspected directly.

- Once reconstruction is deemed adequate, heparin is reversed with an appropriate dose of protamine. Retractors are released and the operating table break is flattened. Two drains are placed through separate incisions in the thoracic cavity, one inferiorly and the other at the apex. The diaphragm is closed with PDS suture from the aortic hiatus to the costal margin. Usually, this can be done is a running fashion, at times facilitated with interrupted sutures reapproximating the costal margin. Absorbable interrupted sutures are placed to reapproximate the chest wall. The left lobe is inflated and the chest closed. This step may facilitate completing the diaphragmatic closure.
- The serratus anterior is reapproximated as is the latissimus dorsi if it was divided. The abdominal wall muscles are closed in layers. Scarpa fascia is reapproximated and the skin is closed.

PEARLS AND PITFALLS

Location of other visceral arteries	■ Identifying the left renal artery early can be helpful in orienting to the location of the other visceral arteries, and to identify and expose the infrarenal aorta for exposure and distal cross-clamping.
Exposure	■ If possible the retroperitoneal and thoracic exposure can be performed simultaneously by two teams. This strategy will allow for a more efficient dissection and provide for better exposure of the visceral aortic segment. ■ Self-retaining retractor systems will aid with exposure. Each (Buckwalter, Omni, Martin arm, etc.) has its benefits and limitations, and the decision of which to choose should be at the discretion, comfort, and human resources of the surgical team.
Positioning	■ With the patient in a lateral decubitus position, knowledge for the directionality of the visceral arteries will facilitate their safe exposure. The left renal artery origin will be directed toward the operating surgeon and toward the ceiling with the kidney retracted anteriorly, and will be found just caudal to where the median arcuate ligament was divided (ie, more cephalad than might be expected). The SMA and CA will be found on the anterior aortic surface, traveling up and away from the operating surgeon.
Equipment and tools	■ Compliant occlusion balloons with a stopcock are a convenient tool for direct endoluminal control of the visceral arteries. They can be left in place until the aortotomy closure is complete by placing throws on each size of the balloon shaft. Balloons can be slid out afterward, and any suture line bleeding from gaps caused by the balloon occlusion catheters can be repaired with interrupted prolene sutures.

POSTOPERATIVE CARE

- In addition to routine postoperative care, there are specific areas of focus when recovering these patients. This includes early and aggressive fluid resuscitation, as third-spacing may be significant in the first 48 hours. Generous urine output may not accurately reflect fluid status, as with the mannitol and the supraceliac clamping, urine output may reflect the osmotic load as well as mild nonoliguric acute kidney injury. It is common for the serum creatinine to rise over the first 2 days before trending to normal. When third-space fluid is mobilized, fluid requirements will decrease, and diuresis may be necessary.
- Routine vascular checks should be performed to confirm no decline from baseline. Patients with significant aortic lumen compromise can be expected to have an improved vascular exam postoperatively.
- Mesenteric revascularization after severe compromise can lead to hyperactive peristalsis, sometimes while the incision is still open. Under these circumstances, serial examination for bowel sounds in the first 24 hours can provide clues to the continued patency of the revascularization. Serial lactate levels can also be checked. Although immediate postoperative lactate levels are elevated, they should return to normal as the patient is warmed and resuscitated. Coagulation parameters may also be elevated initially in response to blood loss and transient hepatic ischemia. These parameters should be monitored and corrected for active bleeding; normal values are usually present by the first postoperative day.
- Chest tubes should be kept in place until any air leaks resolve and drainage decreases to less than 50 mL per shift, nasogastric tube removed with return of function, and bladder catheter until diuresis is complete and close monitoring of urine output is no longer necessary.

COMPLICATIONS

- In addition to the complications associated with a thoracoabdominal incision, complications specific to this procedure include embolization or thrombosis of the visceral arteries or embolization to the lower extremities.

- Thrombosis of a renal artery, unless it is quickly identified, generally leads to irreversible renal infarct.
- Thrombosis of the SMA or celiac artery may be asymptomatic; however, signs and symptoms of intestinal ischemia warrant urgent evaluation with CTA and intervention, either operative or endovascular depending on the anatomic defect, the interval between the index operation and the complication, and the likelihood of compromised bowel.
- Acute kidney injury is a potential but uncommon complication.[3-5] Contributing factors include hypoperfusion, hypovolemia, or renal artery thrombosis. Workup includes duplex ultrasound to identify reversible causes of acute kidney injury.
- While possible, spinal cord ischemia is unlikely with this procedure. As such, a spinal drain is typically not required unless there are other concerns such as subclavian artery occlusion or severe aortoiliac disease for compromised preoperative spinal cord circulation. Postoperative neurologic checks should be performed, focusing on both proximal and distal motor function of the lower extremities.

REFERENCES

1. Mell MW, Acher CW, Hoch JR, Tefera G, Turnipseed WD. Outcomes after endarterectomy for chronic mesenteric ischemia. *J Vasc Surg*. 2008;48(5):1132-1138.
2. ter Steege RW, Sloterdijk HS, Geelkerken RH, Huisman AB, van der Palen J, Kolkman JJ. Splanchnic artery stenosis and abdominal complaints: clinical history is of limited value in detection of gastrointestinal ischemia. *World J Surg*. 2012;36(4):793-799. doi:10.1007/s00268-012-1485-4. PMID: 22354487; PMCID: PMC3299959.
3. Kasirajan K, O'Hara PJ, Gray BH, et al. Chronic mesenteric ischemia: open surgery versus percutaneous angioplasty and stenting. *J Vasc Surg*. 2001;33(1):63-71.
4. Rapp JH, Reilly LM, Qvarfordt PG, Goldstone J, Ehrenfeld WK, Stoney RJ. Durability of endarterectomy and antegrade grafts in the treatment of chronic visceral ischemia. *J Vasc Surg*. 1986;3(5):799-806.
5. Weibull H, Bergqvist D, Bergentz SE, Jonsson K, Hulthen L, Manhem P. Percutaneous transluminal renal angioplasty versus surgical reconstruction of atherosclerotic renal artery stenosis: a prospective randomized study. *J Vasc Surg*. 1993;18(5):841-850; discussion 850-842.

Chapter 13 Hybrid Revascularization Strategies for Visceral/Renal Arteries

Benjamin W. Starnes

DEFINITION

- The term "hybrid" in vascular surgery traditionally refers to the use of *both* traditional open surgical and endovascular techniques for remedy of the vascular condition (**FIGURE 1**).
- Two hybrid approaches are described in this chapter:
  - Complete visceral debranching and endovascular tube graft repair
  - Partial visceral debranching and physician-modified fenestrated endovascular repair

DIFFERENTIAL DIAGNOSIS

- Paravisceral aortic aneurysms may develop due to the following conditions:
  - Degenerative aneurysm
  - Aortic dissection
  - Mycotic aneurysm
  - Paraanastomotic juxtarenal aneurysm
  - Connective tissue disorders (Marfan syndrome)
  - Behçet syndrome

PATIENT HISTORY AND PHYSICAL FINDINGS

- The majority of patients are asymptomatic and the diagnosis is made with imaging done for other reasons. Some patients will complain of mild to moderate abdominal and low back pain. Severe and unrelenting pain should raise the index of suspicion for a mycotic process which, if confirmed, would make hybrid approaches prohibitive.

IMAGING AND OTHER DIAGNOSTIC STUDIES

- Contrast-enhanced, axial thin-slice computed tomography arteriography (CTA) is the current standard for imaging paravisceral aneurysms. Detailed information can be gathered regarding the precise origin of the celiac, superior mesenteric artery (SMA), and renal arteries (**FIGURE 2**).
- Other important findings on CTA should be as follows:
  - Size and quality of access vessels for delivery of endovascular devices (>7 mm)
  - Location of left renal vein
  - Aberrant anatomy (eg, replaced right hepatic artery)
  - Quality of gastroduodenal artery for possible celiac artery ligation or sacrifice
  - Renal cortical thickness

SURGICAL MANAGEMENT

- Indications for repair include aortic aneurysms of more than 5.5 cm, symptoms, or evidence of rapid expansion (>0.5 cm per 6 months).

Preoperative Planning

- As formal open repair would often include a bicavitary incision (chest and abdomen, as in a formal thoracoabdominal repair), the standard preoperative assessment should focus on the patient's fitness to undergo major vascular surgery. This includes assessment of the heart, lung, and kidney function and reserve.

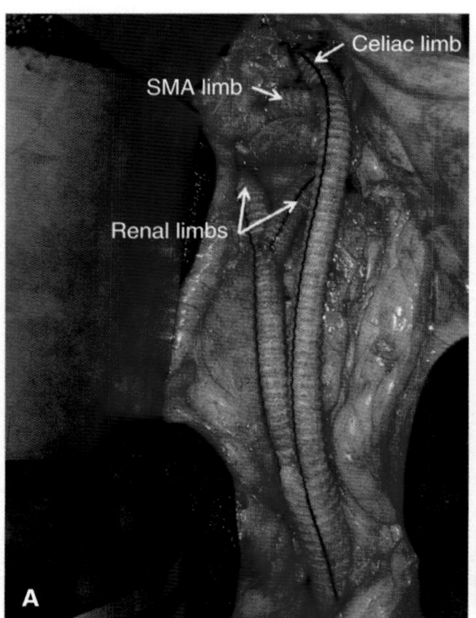

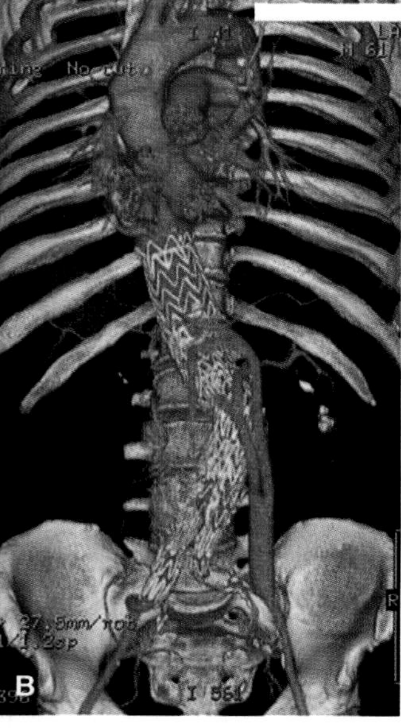

FIGURE 1 • "Hybrid repair" refers to the use of both traditional open surgical and endovascular techniques to manage the same problem. SMA, superior mesenteric artery. **A,** Intraoperative photo. **B,** Postoperative computed tomography arteriography after completed repair.

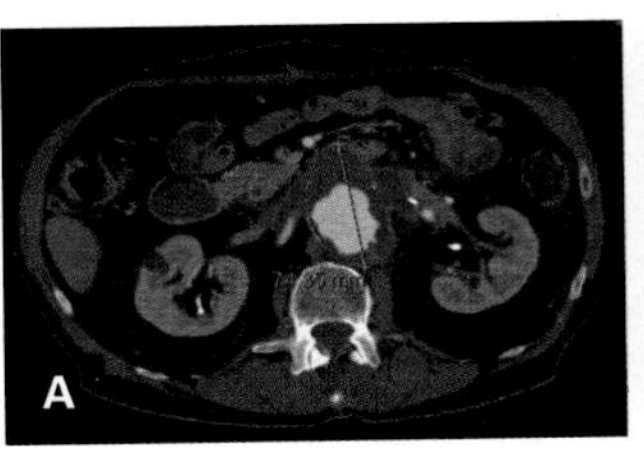

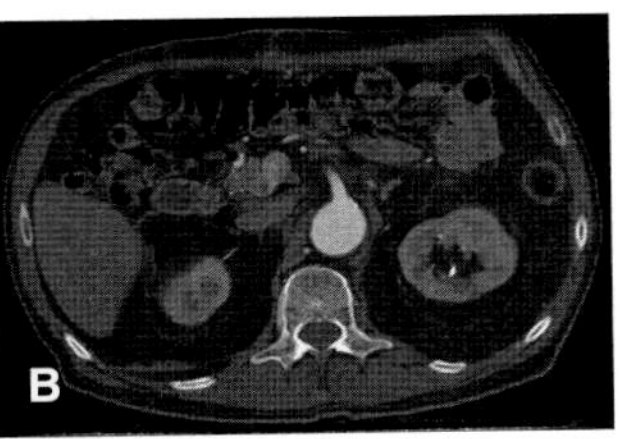

FIGURE 2 Computed tomography arteriography axial images depicting **(A)** a 7.4-cm paraanastomotic juxtarenal aortic aneurysm and **(B)** a healthy aortic segment in the region of the superior mesenteric artery.

Positioning

- Proper and precise positioning should be as follows (**FIGURE 3**):
  - Patient supine on standard operating room (OR) table or imaging table
  - Hair properly clipped over entire abdomen and both groins
  - Both arms tucked (option to have right arm at 90° if planning brachial access)
  - Foley under one leg and padded

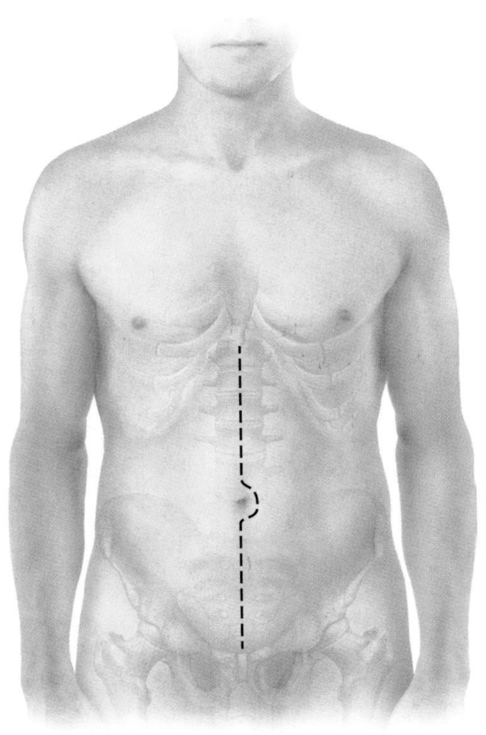

FIGURE 3 ● Depiction of positioning and intended incision in the midline.

COMPLETE VISCERAL DEBRANCHING AND ENDOVASCULAR TUBE GRAFT REPAIR—STAGE 1

First Step—Exposure

- Standard midline laparotomy and positioning of retractor system.
- Upon entry into the abdomen, the falciform ligament is divided between clamps and ligated. The triangular ligaments above the liver are divided to facilitate adequate exposure/retraction while minimizing risk of hepatic capsular injury, anticipating systemic anticoagulation later in the procedure.
- A nasogastric tube is positioned in the stomach to provide temporary decompression. The common hepatic artery is identified following division of the gastrohepatic ligament and traced back to origin of celiac artery. Once identified, the target artery is encircled with a silastic vessel loop. Space is created along the left side of the aorta with blunt/finger dissection, beginning at the level of the celiac artery, to create the retrograde bypass tunnel posterior to the pancreas (**FIGURE 4**).
- The colon and omentum are lifted in a cephalad direction, the small bowel swept to the patient's right and packed in moist towels. Self-retaining retractors (Omni or Bookwalter) should be positioned at this juncture to maintain exposure, with care taken to appropriately pad the retractor blades as necessary.
- The third and fourth portions of the duodenum are mobilized to the right following division of the ligament of Treitz, exposing the anterior surface of the aorta. The inferior mesenteric vein is ligated and divided as well and the dissection continued along the proximal aorta until the left renal vein is clearly identified (**FIGURE 5**).
- Widely mobilize the left renal vein sharply and encircle with a moist umbilical tape. The self-retaining renal vein retractor blade is used to retract the left renal vein cephalad as necessary to facilitate further exposure.
- The origin of the renal arteries is identified by careful posterolateral dissection around the aorta, just cephalad of the overlying renal vein. Exposure on the right is complicated somewhat by the overlying inferior vena cava/left renal vein confluence. At least 2 cm of renal artery should be exposed bilaterally. Encircle the renal arteries with silastic vessel loops. On the left, fingers dissect bluntly along the aorta in a cephalad fashion to complete the retropancreatic tunnel for the celiac limb of the bypass graft.
- The SMA is identified next by palpation within the base of the small bowel mesentery, directly anterior to the pancreas. Doppler ultrasonography may assist identification when the pulse is faint. Once identified, a 3-cm segment of SMA is isolated as proximal as possible to the root of the mesentery. Beginning with the middle colic artery, multiple mesenteric arteries quickly branch from the SMA as it emerges from the pancreas, underscoring the need for proximal identification and isolation. The SMA is controlled with vessel loops.
- The next step is to prepare the donor artery for hybrid bypass. The specific artery—most commonly the common or external iliac arteries—should be selected from the preoperative imaging study. The retroperitoneum is opened directly over

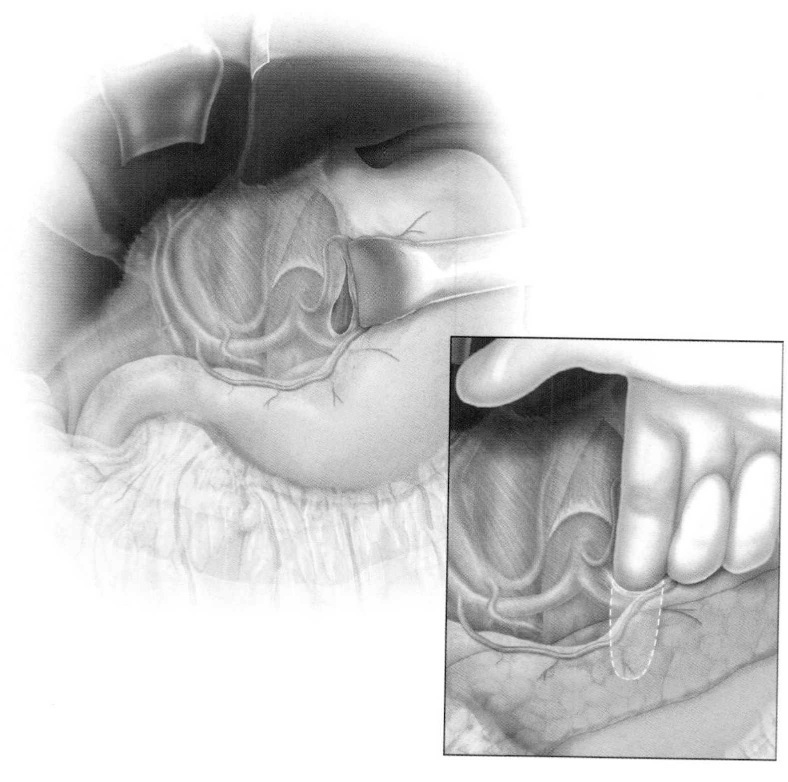

FIGURE 4 ● Drawing of exposure of the celiac artery through the lesser sac. Note the blunt finger dissection along the left side of the aorta and behind the pancreas.

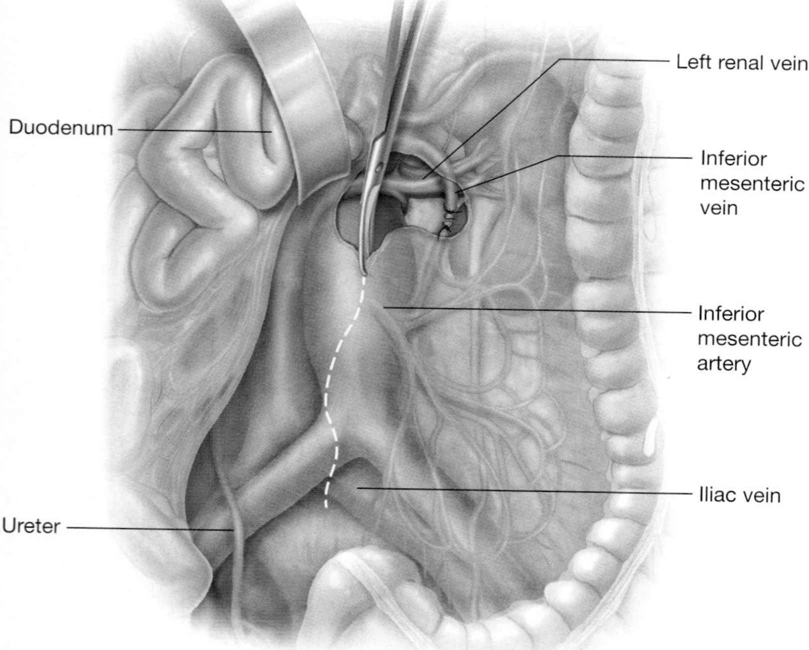

FIGURE 5 ● Drawing of exposure of the left renal vein and anterior surface of the aortic aneurysm. Dashed line depicts intended incision line to avoid nervi erigentes.

the selected donor artery, which is exposed while protecting the adjacent ureter. Alternatively, donor artery exposure may be achieved via medial-visceral rotation, developing the entire retroperitoneal plane on the left. The latter approach provides the added benefit of exclusion of the graft from the viscera and abdominal contents once the viscera are returned to their original position. This maneuver adds significantly more time to the case, however, and contributes to increased blood loss. Graft coverage can also be obtained without developing the entire retroperitoneal plane, either via direct tunneling along the preferred course of the graft or creation of an omental tongue affixed directly to the graft.

Second Step—Anticoagulation

- Systemic anticoagulation is achieved with a bolus injection of unfractionated heparin, 50 U/kg. Monitoring activated clotting time is a useful method of maintaining adequate anticoagulation during the procedure.

Third Step—Multivisceral Bypass

- Trifurcated grafts exist for the purpose of facilitating multivessel hybrid revascularization, but the use of these is limited by the tendency of the middle limb to occlude when "squeezed" between the outside limbs during graft routing and abdominal closure. In most circumstances, a standard 12 × 7 bifurcated, collagen-impregnated knitted polyester graft provides excellent conduits for bilateral renal revascularization, with a separate 8-mm limb connected to the celiac and SMA. Examples of bypass graft configurations are shown in **FIGURES 6** and **7**.
- The proximal (iliac/inflow) anastomosis is completed first with running 4-0 or 5-0 polypropylene suture.
- The next anastomosis to be completed should be one anticipated to be the technically most difficult, given exposure and graft routing issues. Most commonly, this is the right renal artery. This is divided following placement of a large clip at the origin. The appropriate graft limb is pulled to length and anastomosed end-to-end with 5-0 polypropylene suture. The limb and artery are flushed just prior to completion of the graft, after which the clamps are released to reperfuse the kidney. Following this sequence, warm renal ischemia time is generally less than 12 minutes. The stump of the right renal artery is then suture ligated; avoid clip dislodgement. Note: Excessive traction on the confluence of the left renal vein and vena cava may cause caval injury and massive hemorrhage during preparation and completion of the right renal artery anastomosis. Retractor positioning needs to account for potential venous injury during exposure and significantly relaxed following completion of the anastomosis.
- The left renal anastomosis is completed in nearly identical fashion, minus many of the exposure limitations present on the right.
- The SMA graft is carefully sized to length so that it follows a "C"-shaped configuration without kinking. Inflow can be obtained either from the many bodies of the graft or either of the completed renal limbs. The SMA graft anastomosis is completed end-to-side with interrupted or running 5-0 polypropylene suture. The end-to-side arteriotomy length is 1.5 to 2 times the width of the bypass graft (12-16 mm). Alternatively, end-to-end anastomotic configuration may reduce the likelihood of graft kinking depending on final configuration. Following completion of the anastomosis, the proximal SMA is ligated with a large clip or circumference suture. Again, ischemia time should be under 10 to 12 minutes.
- Typically, following SMA and renal graft completion, repositioning of the retraction system is necessary to reobtain and optimize celiac artery exposure. Prior to reexposing the celiac, a vascular clamp is repassed through the retropancreatic tunnel left of the aorta. This position is then maintained until the transverse colon and mesocolon are reduced to their usual location. This reexposes the "looped" celiac and common hepatic arteries previously isolated in the lesser sac. The

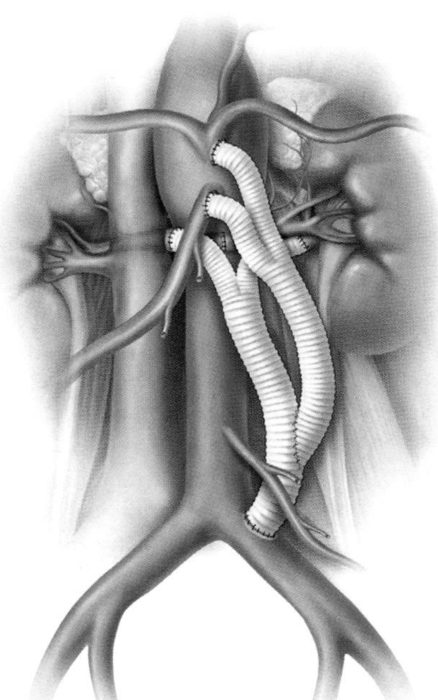

FIGURE 6 ● Drawing of a four-vessel debranching based on the left common iliac artery. Note that the left renal vein was divided in this case, and subsequently repaired, for better exposure of the renal arteries.

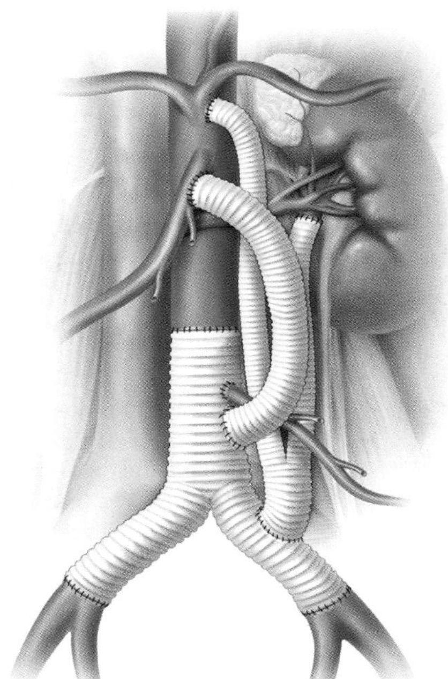

FIGURE 7 ● Aortobiiliac and subsequent debranching for a patient with a solitary left kidney and infrarenal aneurysm.

clamp tip exiting the retrohepatic tunnel is identified, and a moist umbilical tape is pulled through the tunnel. Following this, the celiac limb is tied to the umbilical tape, which is then pulled cephalad behind the pancreas and into position for either end-to-end or end-to-side anastomosis. Care again needs to be taken to optimize limb routing and length to minimize risk for kinking.

- After coverage of remaining exposed graft limbs with omentum or parietal peritoneum as appropriate, standard abdominal closure is performed.

COMPLETE VISCERAL DEBRANCHING AND ENDOVASCULAR TUBE GRAFT REPAIR—STAGE 2

First Step—Percutaneous Access

- Following the "debranching" procedure described in stage 1, endovascular aneurysm repair (EVAR) may be performed either at the same setting or within several weeks of the initial procedure. The risk of potential aneurysm rupture associated with a staged approach needs to be balanced with the additional operative risk inherent in the longer anesthetic time required to complete both stages in one sitting. For the EVAR procedure itself, standard percutaneous access to an appropriately sized access vessel is obtained using Seldinger technique and a wire advanced into the aorta under fluoroscopic guidance. In our practice, this is most commonly obtained percutaneously, using ultrasound guidance and preplacement of polypropylene suture prior to dilation of the access sites (also known as the "preclose" Perclose technique) (Abbott Vascular Inc., Redwood City, CA).[1] An 11-Fr standard sheath is placed into the common femoral artery and flushed with heparinized saline. Wire advancement from the femoral artery to the aortic arch must be visualized radiographically throughout its course, as the wire may preferentially enter the debranching graft and cause end-organ injury or hemorrhage without real-time position monitoring and guidance.

Second Step—Stiff Wire Exchange

- After wire advancement to the transverse aortic arch, standard wire exchange technique is used to position a 0.035-in stiff (eg, Lunderquist, Cook Medical, Bloomington, IN) wire through the abdominal and thoracic aorta. Optimal final wire positioning is at/just distal to the left subclavian artery orifice.

Third Step—Intravascular Ultrasound

- An 8.2-Fr Visions catheter (Volcano Therapeutics, Irvine, CA) is used to confirm appropriate proximal and distal landing zones for endovascular graft placement. The optimal graft size and configuration is determined by analysis of CTA images reformatted and visualized on a dedicated 3D image workstation (AquariusNet, TeraRecon, Inc., San Mateo, CA). Graft diameter should be oversized by 10% to 15% for this application.
- During advancement of the device, the origin of the debranching graft can also be visualized either through fluoroscopic confirmation of a metallic clip placed during the debranching procedure or under intravascular ultrasound (IVUS) real-time guidance. Using IVUS, the position of the IVUS catheter is marked on the fluoroscopic monitor when the catheter itself recognizes the orifice of the debranched graft. Alternatively, a contrast power injection can be performed through an appropriately positioned arteriographic catheter with 30 mL of contrast injected at 15 mL per second to confirm the proximal and distal landing zones.

Fourth Step—Endograft Deployment

- The endovascular graft is deployed following device-specific instructions for use (IFU), covering the native origins of the visceral vessels and excluding the aortic aneurysm. The femoral arteriotomy is then closed.

PARTIAL VISCERAL DEBRANCHING AND PHYSICIAN-MODIFIED ENDOVASCULAR REPAIR—STAGE 1

First Step—Exposure

- Standard midline laparotomy and positioning of retractor system.
- Upon entry into the abdomen, the falciform ligament is divided between clamps and ligated. The triangular ligaments above the liver are divided to facilitate adequate exposure/retraction while minimizing the risk of hepatic capsular injury, anticipating systemic anticoagulation later in the procedure.
- A nasogastric tube is positioned in the stomach to provide temporary decompression. The common hepatic artery is identified following division of the gastrohepatic ligament and traced back to origin of celiac artery. Once identified, the target artery is encircled with a silastic vessel loop. Space is created along the left side of the aorta with blunt/finger dissection, beginning at the level of the celiac artery, to create the retrograde bypass tunnel posterior to the pancreas.
- The colon and omentum are lifted in a cephalad direction, the small bowel swept to the patient's right and packed in moist towels. Self-retaining retractors (Omni or Bookwalter) should be positioned at this juncture to maintain exposure, with care taken to appropriately pad the retractor blades as necessary.
- The third and fourth portions of the duodenum are mobilized to the right following division of the ligament of Treitz, exposing the anterior surface of the aorta. The inferior mesenteric vein is ligated and divided as well and the dissection continued along the proximal aorta until the left renal vein is clearly identified.
- Widely mobilize the left renal vein sharply and encircle with a moist umbilical tape. The self-retaining renal vein retractor blade is used to retract the left renal vein cephalad as necessary to facilitate further exposure.
- The origin of the renal arteries is identified by careful posterolateral dissection around the aorta, just cephalad of the overlying renal vein. Exposure on the right is complicated somewhat

by the overlying inferior vena cava/left renal vein confluence. At least 2 cm of renal artery should be exposed bilaterally. Encircle the renal arteries with silastic vessel loops. On the left, finger dissect bluntly along the aorta in a cephalad fashion to complete the retropancreatic tunnel for the celiac limb of the bypass graft.

- The SMA is identified next by palpation within the base of the small bowel mesentery, directly anterior to the pancreas. Doppler ultrasonography may assist identification when the pulse is faint. Once identified, a 3-cm segment of SMA is isolated as proximal as possible to the root of the mesentery. Beginning with the middle colic artery, multiple mesenteric arteries quickly branch from the SMA as it emerges from the pancreas, underscoring the need for proximal identification and isolation. The SMA is controlled with vessel loops.
- The next step is to prepare the donor artery for hybrid bypass. The specific artery—most commonly the common or external iliac arteries—should be selected from the preoperative imaging study. The retroperitoneum is opened directly over the selected donor artery, which is exposed while protecting the adjacent ureter. Alternatively, donor artery exposure may be achieved via medial-visceral rotation, developing the entire retroperitoneal plane on the left. The latter approach provides the added benefit of exclusion of the graft from the viscera and abdominal contents once the viscera are returned to their original position. This maneuver adds significantly more time to the case, however, and contributes to increased blood loss. Graft coverage can also be obtained without developing the entire retroperitoneal plane, either via direct tunneling along the preferred course of the graft or creation of an omental tongue affixed directly to the graft.

Second Step—Anticoagulation

- Systemic anticoagulation is achieved with a bolus injection of unfractionated heparin, 50 units/kg. Monitoring activated clotting time is a useful method of maintaining adequate anticoagulation during the procedure.

Third Step—Multivisceral Bypass

- Trifurcated grafts exist for the purpose of facilitating multivessel hybrid revascularization, but the use of these is limited by the tendency of the middle limb to occlude when squeezed between the outside limbs during graft routing and abdominal closure. In most circumstances, a standard 12 × 7 bifurcated, collagen-impregnated knitted polyester graft provides excellent conduits for bilateral renal revascularization, with a separate 8-mm limb connected to the celiac and SMA. Examples of bypass graft configurations are shown in **FIGURES 6** and **7**.
- The proximal (iliac/inflow) anastomosis is completed first with running 4-0 or 5-0 polypropylene suture.
- The next anastomosis to be completed should be one anticipated to be the technically most difficult, given exposure and graft routing issues. Most commonly, this is the right renal artery. This is divided following the placement of a large clip at the origin. The appropriate graft limb is pulled to length and anastomosed end-to-end with 5-0 polypropylene suture. The limb and artery are flushed just prior to completion of the graft, after which the clamps are released to reperfuse the kidney. Following this sequence, warm renal ischemia time is generally less than 12 minutes. The stump of the right renal artery is then suture ligated; avoid clip dislodgement. Note: Excessive traction on the confluence of the left renal vein and vena cava may cause caval injury and massive hemorrhage during preparation and completion of the right renal artery anastomosis. Retractor positioning needs to account for potential venous injury during exposure and significantly relaxed following completion of the anastomosis.
- The renal anastomosis is completed in nearly identical fashion, minus many of the exposure limitations present on the right.

PARTIAL VISCERAL DEBRANCHING AND PHYSICIAN-MODIFIED ENDOVASCULAR REPAIR—STAGE 2[2]

First Step—Creation of a Fenestrated Graft for the Celiac and Superior Mesenteric Artery

- The appropriate endovascular device is chosen according to standard IFU sizing guidelines, typically incorporating 10% to 15% oversizing. The sterile graft is unsheathed on a dedicated sterile table in the OR and marked with the relative locations (length from proximal end and clockface measurements) of the celiac and SMA fenestrations as previously determined via TeraRecon workstation analysis. Minor adjustments are allowed to minimize strut overlap of planned fenestration locations. Fenestrations in the polyester endograft fabric are created with a disposable ophthalmic cautery to minimize fraying. The fenestrations are outlined and reinforced with 15-mm gold Amplatz Gooseneck snares (ev3 Endovascular, Inc., Plymouth, MN). These are hand sewn into place using 4-0 Prolene suture in a double row circumferentially (**FIGURE 8**). Diameter-reducing ties were then used to constrain the device along its posterior border (opposite the SMA and or celiac fenestration at 6-o'clock) by rerouting the existing proximal trigger wire through and through the graft material at the midportion of each of the top two Z stents. The constraining ties are then tied down into place over the trigger wire. The entire graft is then wetted with heparinized saline and then reloaded into the existing sheath.

Second Step—Percutaneous Access

- Standard percutaneous access to an appropriately sized access vessel is obtained using Seldinger technique. The initial guidewire is advanced into the aorta under fluoroscopic guidance. In our practice, this is most commonly obtained percutaneously, using ultrasound guidance and preplacement of polypropylene suture prior to dilation of the access sites (also known as the "preclose" Perclose technique) (Abbott Vascular Inc., Redwood City, CA).[1] An 11-Fr standard sheath is placed into the

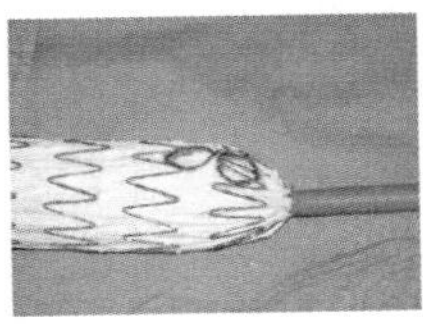

FIGURE 8 Photograph of a thoracic endograft with two fenestrations created for the celiac (struts present) and superior mesenteric artery (strut free), prior to resheathing and deployment.

common femoral artery and flushed with heparinized saline. Wire advancement from the femoral artery to the aortic arch must be visualized radiographically throughout its course, as the wire may preferentially enter the debranching graft and cause end-organ renal injury, rupture of Gerota fascia, and retroperitoneal hemorrhage without real-time position monitoring and guidance.

Third Step—Stiff Wire Exchange

- A standard 4-Fr or 5-Fr catheter is used to perform a wire exchange to a stiff 0.035-in Lunderquist wire (Cook Medical, Bloomington, IN). The wire is positioned so that its tip is just distal to the left subclavian artery.

Fourth Step—Marking of the Target Vessels and Graft Deployment

- A contrast power injection can be performed with 10 mL of contrast injected at 25 mL per second to mark the precise origins of the celiac and SMA (**FIGURE 9**). The modified graft is positioned over the target vessels, oriented, and deployed.

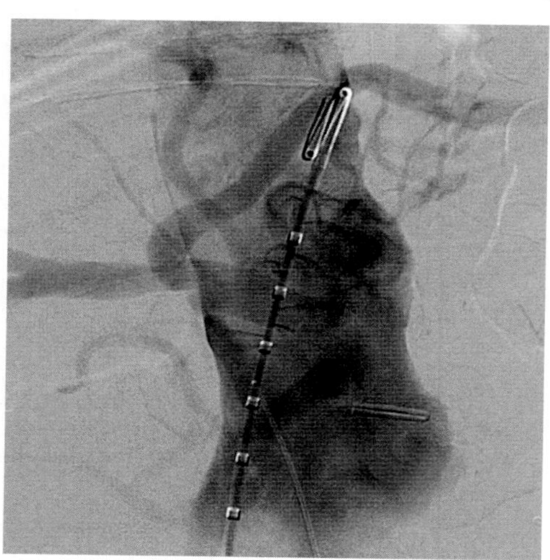

FIGURE 9 Note the double densities depicting the origins of the celiac and superior mesenteric artery on this flush aortogram.

Fifth Step—Cannulation of the Target Vessels

- An 18-Fr sheath is advanced from the contralateral groin and into the distal graft over a stiff wire. Two 7-Fr Raabe sheaths (Cook Medical, Bloomington, IN) are advanced together through the 18-Fr sheath. Working through these sheaths, the SMA and celiac vessels are selected through the fenestrations using standard catheter and guidewire techniques, with the sheaths ultimately advanced into the target vessels over stiff wires.
- After sheath advancement and confirmation of target vessel acquisition, the main body is distended flush with the surrounding aorta with a molding balloon (eg, Coda, Cook Medical, Bloomington, IN). This inflation represents the final opportunity to distend the endograft in the region of the visceral stents. Lateral positioning of the image intensifier guides stent placement into the SMA and celiac arteries (typically 8- to 9-mm stents; **FIGURE 10**). **FIGURE 11** shows follow-up computed tomography imaging of a patient 1 year after successful treatment with this technique.

Sixth Step—Access Site Closure

- The access sites are closed with the previously placed sutures.

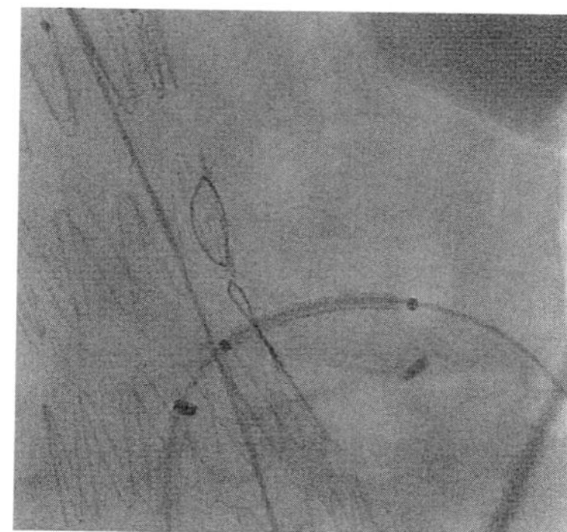

FIGURE 10 Lateral image depicting placement of a covered balloon-expandable stent into the superior mesenteric artery prior to deployment.

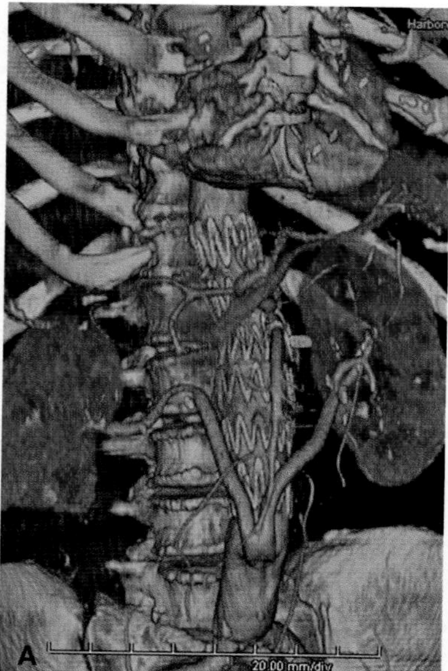

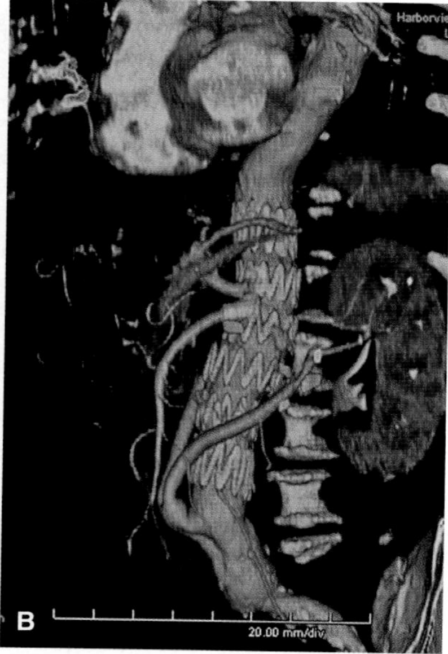

FIGURE 11 **A** and **B,** Follow-up computed tomography images of a patient successfully treated with partial visceral debranching and physician-modified endovascular fenestrated repair.

PEARLS AND PITFALLS

Choice of operating room (OR) table	■ Use standard OR tables for open surgical procedures and imaging tables for image-guided or hybrid procedures. Advanced planning is essential to optimize outcome. Never sacrifice exposure!
Exposure of common iliac artery	■ Identify and protect the ureter.
Placement of wires after debranching procedure	■ Pass guidewires under continuous fluoroscopic guidance following debranching. An advancing aortic wire may preferentially enter and traverse the debranching graft, causing end-organ injury, disorientation, and possible endograft maldeployment if not recognized.
Timing of stent graft balloon molding during fenestrated EVAR	■ Always seat the endograft with balloon inflation prior to placement of visceral bridging stents. Instrumentation or distention of the fenestrated endograft following branch vessel stenting may compromise stent positioning, integrity, and patency.

POSTOPERATIVE CARE

- Open aortic debranching procedures are not benign; almost all patients will require intensive care postprocedure. Spinal drainage is used selectively for aortic coverage extending more than 10 cm cephalad to the celiac artery. Postoperative anuria or persistent acidosis/rising lactate require immediate investigation to prove branch vessel patency.

OUTCOMES

- Contemporary hybrid debranching procedures for complex abdominal aortic aneurysmal disease are associated with a 13% operative mortality rate, 2% permanent paraplegia rate, and 1% stroke rate.[3]
- Hybrid approaches offer the advantage of versatility, avoidance of extensive operative exposures, and potentially offer a broader range of therapies to a patient population that would not otherwise be considered for aortic surgical repair.

COMPLICATIONS

- Access-related complications
- Hemorrhage requiring transfusion
- Paraplegia
- Stroke
- Renal failure
- Death

REFERENCES

1. Starnes BW, Andersen CA, Ronsivalle JA, et al. Totally percutaneous aortic aneurysm repair: experience and prudence. *J Vasc Surg*. 2006;43(2):270-276.
2. Starnes BW, Quiroga E. Hybrid-fenestrated aortic aneurysm repair: a novel technique for treating patients with para-anastomotic juxtarenal aneurysms. *Ann Vasc Surg*. 2010;24(8):1150-1153.
3. Starnes BW, Tran NT, McDonald JM. Hybrid approaches to repair of complex aortic aneurysmal disease. *Surg Clin North Am*. 2007;87(5):1087-1098, ix.

Chapter 14

Parallel Stenting for Visceral and Renal Protection During Complex Endovascular Aneurysm Repair

Matthew John Rossi and Javairiah Fatima

INTRODUCTION

- Endovascular aortic repair has been well established as a safe, and minimally invasive treatment for patients with anatomically suitable infrarenal aortic aneurysms.[1] Open repair and in select cases hybrid repair has traditionally been reserved for those with more complex anatomy including juxtarenal, pararenal, and thoracoabdominal aortic aneurysms. Over the past couple of decades, significant technological advances have occurred in the realm of endovascular aortic surgery to offer endovascular repair even in patients with such complex anatomy.
- Use of fenestrated and branched technology (F-/B-EVAR) has been a breakthrough to address complex aortic aneurysms while maintaining perfusion to the visceral and renal vessels. However, most of these devices require a lead time for customization to the individual patient anatomy or are currently still in trial phase with limited access, or to those with physician-sponsored investigational device exemptions, leaving a need for alternate techniques. One of these alternate approaches is the parallel graft technique (snorkels and chimneys) utilizing immediately available devices that can be readily used even in urgent or emergent settings. This technique encompasses placement of stents in the renal and visceral arteries that are extended parallel to the main aortic endograft to allow perfusion into the branches from above or below the excluded aneurysm.[2] Additionally, parallel stenting can be helpful as a bail out technique in inadvertent coverage of a renal artery during EVAR.[3]

DEFINITIONS

- Antegrade parallel stenting, or chimneys, extend cranially above the endograft (**FIGURE 1**) while retrograde parallel stenting, also known as periscopes, extend caudally below the endograft (**FIGURE 2**). Complex thoracoabdominal aneurysms may require thoracic coverage in conjunction with chimneys or snorkels; this type of repair is referred to as a snorkel sandwich (**FIGURE 3**).[4]

PATIENT HISTORY AND PHYSICAL FINDINGS

- Most aortic aneurysms are detected incidentally on imaging performed for other indications. Once diagnosed, repair is done prophylactically to prevent rupture, which can be fatal in over 90% of patients. In patients presenting in an elective setting, physiologic and anatomic considerations are the primary determinants of optimal repair for each patient. A thorough discussion should be held with the patient of the prophylactic nature of repair, risks, and benefits of continued surveillance vs open, hybrid, or various techniques of endovascular repair. It is important that patients understand what the undertaking entails perioperatively and in the long term, including need for continued imaging surveillance and potential future reinterventions. A discussion of the off-label use of the endografts as well as the anticipated radiation exposure should be had, and informed consent documented.

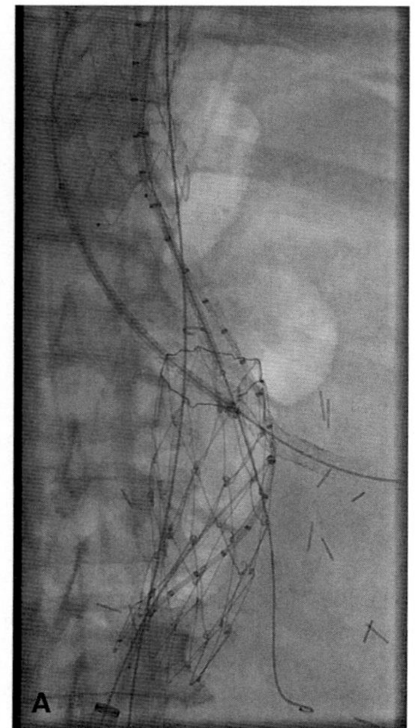

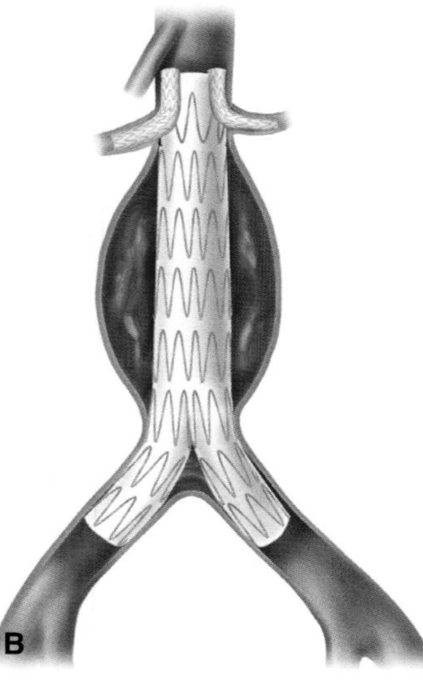

FIGURE 1 • Antegrade Parallel Stenting (Chimney) Repair with one renal stent, and superior mesenteric stent cannulation in preparation for stent placement. **A,** Placement of two renal chimneys for repair of a juxtarenal aortic aneurysm **(B)**.

- All patients should undergo history and physical exam, and evaluation of their comorbidities. A full cardiopulmonary evaluation should be undertaken to establish the patient's risk profile. Evaluation of potential renal or liver insufficiency is also necessary.

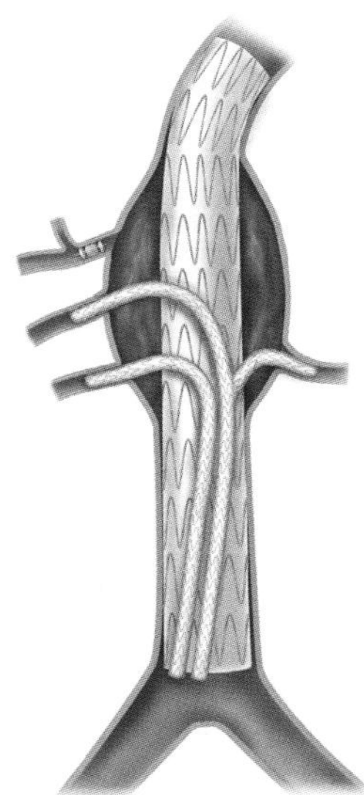

FIGURE 2 ● Retrograde Parallel Stenting (Periscope) Repair with a superior mesenteric and two renal stents and Amplatzer plug in the celiac axis.

IMAGING AND OTHER DIAGNOSTIC STUDIES

- Computed tomography angiography (CTA) of chest, abdomen, and pelvis with 1 to 2 mm slices is essential with virtual aortic reconstruction to allow for precise determination of lengths, diameters, angulation, and quality of the aortic landing zones and target vessels. It can help predict and plan for pitfalls and anatomic challenges preoperatively. The CTA is imported into three-dimensional reconstruction software for creation of centerline of flow to allow for precise anatomic evaluation and accurate operative planning and endograft selection.
- Given the use of axillary access for antegrade cannulation of target vessels, CTA should include upper extremity access vessels to look for kinks, dissection, aneurysm, or diseased artery that would preclude their use.

SURGICAL MANAGEMENT

Preoperative Planning

- Detailed review of preoperative imaging with 3D reconstruction and precise measurements must be completed ahead of time. A well-planned case is crucial for successful execution. A healthy, parallel aortic segment should be identified to provide an appropriate proximal seal zone. Thereafter, all necessary measurements of visceral and renal vessel diameters, lengths to branch points, and distances from planned proximal seal zone should be taken. An operative plan should be drawn out with any potential pitfalls discussed. Excessive tortuosity, calcifications, or thrombus burden

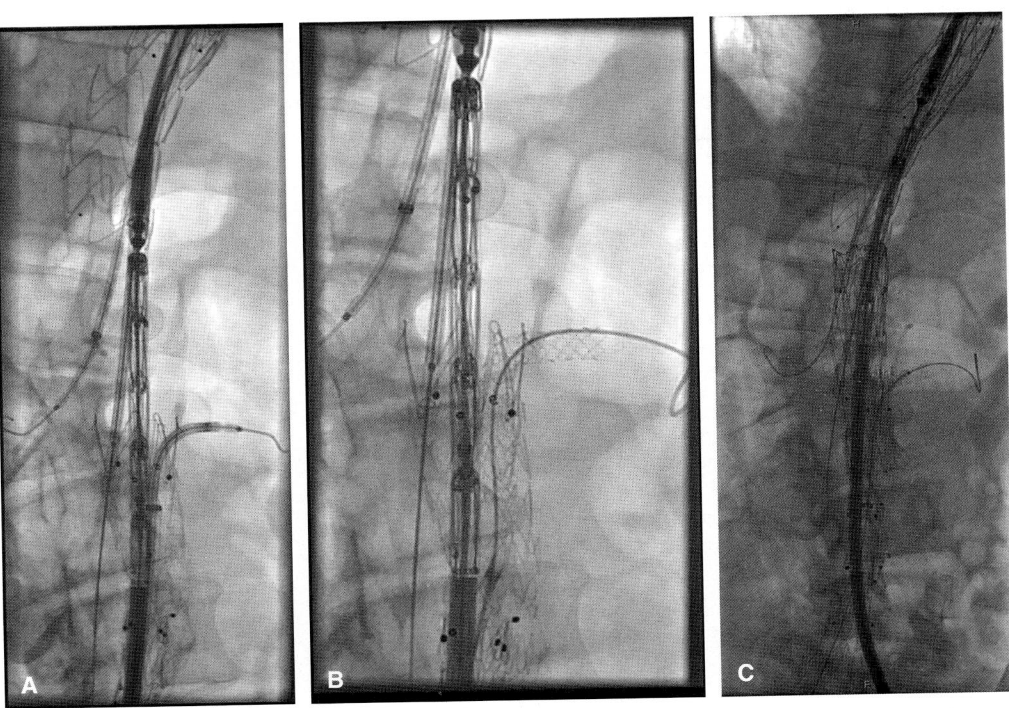

FIGURE 3 ● **A,** Pre-deployment placement of celiac antegrade and left renal retrograde stents **(B)** Post-deployment of left renal retrograde stent **(C)**. Complex thoracoabdominal aneurysms may require thoracic coverage in conjunction with chimneys and snorkels; this type of repair is referred to as a snorkel sandwich.

confer a formidable risk of stroke or distal embolization, rendering endovascular intervention prohibitive.

- The natural history of the aorta is to progressively degenerate, thus the plan should allow for room for proximal extension if needed in the future. Longer seal length will decrease the likelihood that the patient will require future intervention for a type Ia endoleaks. Given this likelihood, most parallel stenting procedures include the visceral vessels.
- Typically 25% to 30% oversizing to a healthy aortic segment is considered when selecting the aortic endograft to account for fabric infolding around the chimney/snorkel stent grafts. There are several carefully determined formulae that have been suggested to optimize seal and minimize gutter leaks.[5] It is also important for the renal arteries to be 4 to 8 mm in diameter to establish anatomic feasibility. An upward going renal artery is not amenable to chimney and is fraught with complications such as kinks and thrombosis with loss of renal artery. Such vessels would be best served by retrograde parallel stenting or prior debranching.

Operative Room Setup

- A hybrid room fixed imaging setup with CT fusion technology is ideal for complex aortic cases. This technology allows the preoperative imaging to overlay the images obtained intraoperatively, and can be used to delineate the anatomy and target vessels. Use of these tools minimizes the need for cine runs and significantly reduces contrast volume and radiation. Cone-beam CT should be considered at the end of procedures prior to removal of access sheaths to identify and address any kinks or suboptimal modular or stent architecture, thus preventing future reintervention.[6]
- Anesthesia/OR team: At our institution, a dedicated team of cardiovascular anesthesiologists are involved in all complex aortic cases. General anesthesia is preferred by our group given the length of the procedure, the ability to better control respiration during distal subtraction angiography, and often due to the need for access via axillary cutdown. Finally, the need for a spinal drain should be considered, especially if a long length of thoracic coverage is anticipated or any segment of aorta has been previously covered or replaced.[7,8]
- Intraoperative neurophysiologic monitoring of spinal cord somatosensory and motor-evoked potentials should be performed for elective cases and when available for nonelective cases when covering large segments of thoracic aorta, for early detection and intervention of spinal cord ischemia.
- A dedicated aortic scrub technician/nurse with knowledge and familiarity with the devices, procedure, and the surgeon's workflow allows the operation to proceed smoothly.

Positioning

- The patient is positioned supine with both arms tucked with the C-arm coming from the patient's left and the ability to position it at the patient's head as well. If two or more visceral/renal vessels will require access, then a right or left axillary cutdown is performed, depending on which offers the most trackability of sheaths to the descending thoracic aorta. There are conflicting data on whether right sided access to the arch confers a higher risk of stroke. In general, the optimal side for sheath trackability is chosen.[9,10]
- The patient is prepped from neck to knees, with a large piece of Ioban used to cover the prepped area, followed by draping in a sterile fashion. The primary operator is positioned on the patient's right with the second surgeon or first assistant at the head to facilitate axillary exposure and sheath/wire manipulations. Alternatively, when a left axillary approach is used, a sterile table may be directed laterally from the patients left arm to aid in maintaining sterility of the wires, catheters, and sheaths.

ANTEGRADE PARALLEL STENTING IN EVAR

Axillary Artery Access

- A 5-cm transverse incision is created 2 fingerbreaths below the mid clavicle. After dividing the subcutaneous tissue and pectoral fascia, the fibers of the pectoralis major are bluntly separated. Underneath, the clavipectoral fascia is divided. Approximately 5 to 6 cm of the axillary artery should be isolated, taking care to obtain control without damaging a branch.
- Starting proximally at 2-o'clock on the artery, micropuncture access is obtained and a purse-string suture using 4-0 polypropylene is placed. Approximately 15 mm distally and positioned in tandem to the first purse-string suture at 12-o'clock on the artery, the second access site is secured with a purse-string suture followed by the third at 10-o'clock (**FIGURE 4**). Alternatively, a 10-mm Dacron conduit can be sutured directly onto the axillary artery and access obtained through the conduit.
- A Cobra 2 catheter (Angiodynamics, Netherlands) is used to direct a Glidewire into the descending thoracic aorta, which can then be switched out under catheter protection to a stiffer wire such as an Amplatz (Cook, Bloomington, IN) to upsize to 6- or 7-French sheaths of appropriate length to

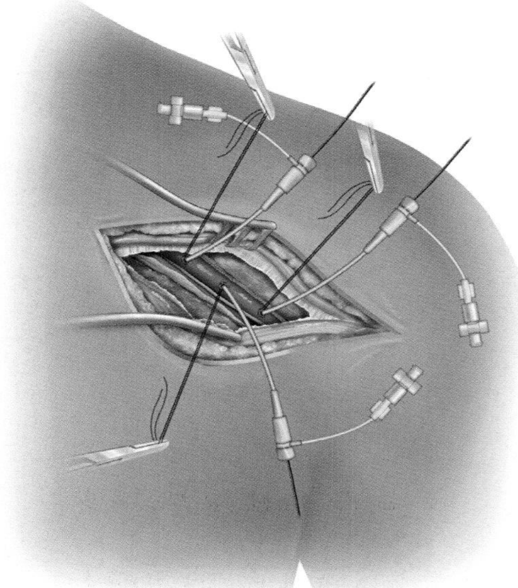

FIGURE 4 • Axillary cutdown with three strategically placed tandem access sites with Prolene purse-string sutures.

extend to the visceral/renal vessels. The patient is then systemically heparinized for a goal activated clotting time (ACT) of greater than 250 seconds. This is accomplished by ACT measurements every 30 minutes with appropriate redosing of IV unfractionated heparin.

Endograft Deployment

- Bilateral femoral artery access is obtained percutaneously under ultrasound guidance using a micropuncture kit. Perclose Proglide devices are placed for eventual closure. The access is then upsized to the appropriate sheath size for the main body of the selected device.
- While any endograft can be used for the main body, AFX (Endologix Irvine, CA) deserves a mention as the presence of the fabric outside of the stents in AFX, allows bellowing into the gutters than are inevitably formed with the use of the parallel stenting technique.
- Should you choose another endograft, the next step in the procedure is cannulation of the renal/visceral vessels.

Renal/Visceral Cannulation and Stent Positioning

- The appropriate length (typically 90 cm) 6- or 7-French sheath is advanced to the visceral segment. It is at this point that if the advanced software and C-arm is available, that a cone-beam CT scan is taken intraoperatively. Bony landmarks are then matched to the preoperative CTA imaging to allow for fusion of contrasted preoperative CT to overlay the bony landmarks to delineate the aortic, renal, and visceral anatomy, facilitating cannulation with less contrast and radiation. When CT fusion is not available, a digital subtraction angiography (DSA) is performed at the level of the visceral aorta, with the c-arm positioned at an angle perpendicular to the ostium of the desired vessel.
- Next, the target vessels are selectively catheterized using a selection catheter and a hydrophilic Glidewire (Terumo, Sunrise, FL). The Glidewire is exchanged for a Rosen wire (Cook, Bloomington, IN) with a floppy tip for renals and an Amplatz wire (Cook, Bloomington, IN) for mesenteric vessels (**FIGURE 5**). The sheaths are then advanced into the branch vessels and the catheters removed after angiographic confirmation of successful cannulation and vessel patency.
- If the parallel graft involves the celiac axis, it is not uncommon to establish the adequacy of gastroduodenal artery collaterals and then cover the celiac artery, precluding the need for a fourth parallel stent; one may consider placing an Amplatzer plug (Abbott) to prevent type II endoleaks in this setting. When this is performed, it is done prior to placement of parallel stents.
- A wide array of balloon expandable covered stents and self-expanding stent grafts are available to choose from for visceral and renal vessels. An ideal stent graft should offer a low-profile delivery system, incorporating flexibility

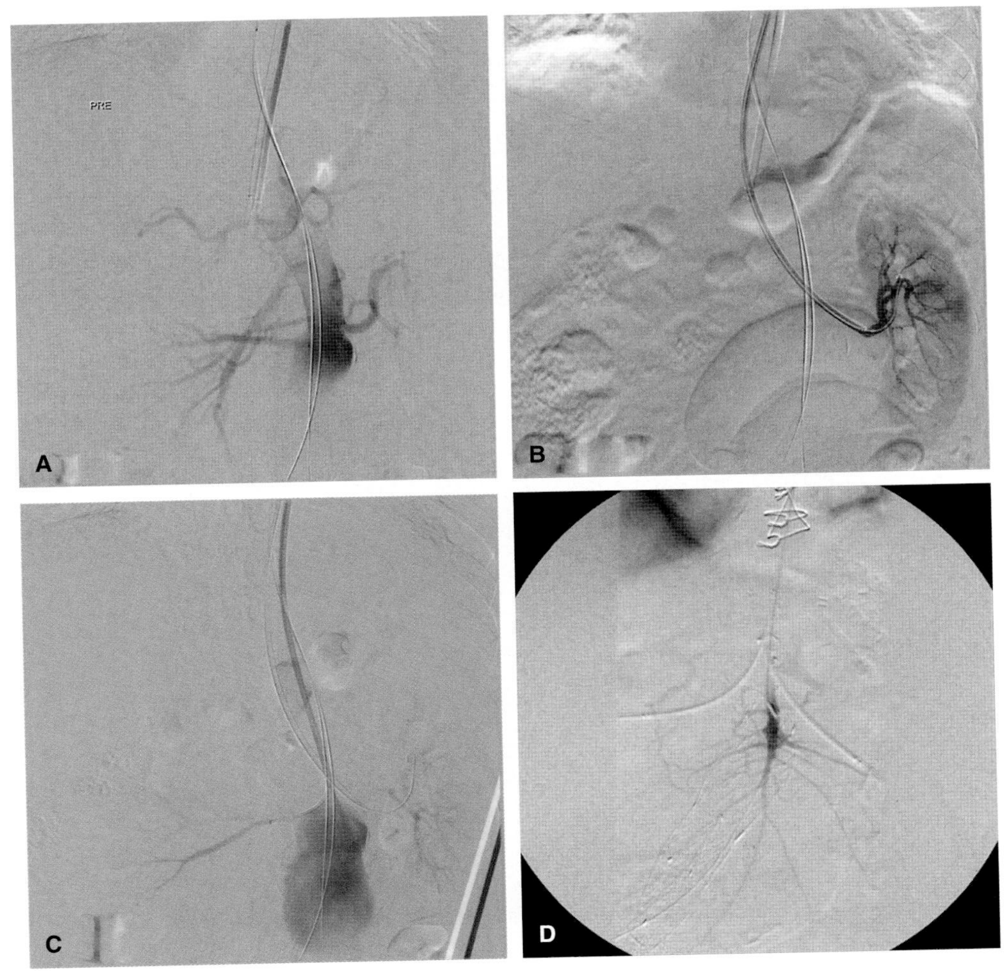

FIGURE 5 ● Angiography demonstrating pararenal aortogram. **A,** Selective catheterization of left renal artery with placement of a Rosen wire **(B)**, Selective catheterization of right renal artery with placement of a Rosen wire **(C)**, Selective catheterization of superior mesenteric artery **(D)**.

to conform to a wide range of target vessels and angulations. It is important to have a stent that can accommodate a wide range of diameters and lengths with minimal foreshortening, allowing predictable and precise stent deployment. Additionally, high radial strength with resistance to kinking is critical to achieve long-term patency, and resist migration, minimizing risk of endoleak.

- Viabahn (Gore, Flagstaff, AZ) offers high flexibility and kink-resistance; however, when high radial strength is needed as in tight orificial lesions, balloon expandable covered stents such as VBX (Gore, Flagstaff, AZ) or iCAST (Atrium Medical, USA) are advantageous given their increased radial strength as well as their ability to customize to a larger diameter with postdilatation. Additionally, the bidirectional deployment mechanism of Viabahn makes it suboptimal in short landing zones such as with early target vessel branching, where a balloon expandable stent graft may have a more predictable deployment. Ultimately, it is largely surgeon preference and experience that dictate the choice of stent graft.
- For renal/visceral stents, a minimum of 1.5 cm of length from the ostium should be covered to allow for appropriate fixation. Angiography is used to identify target vessel branches, which should be preserved whenever possible.

Endograft Positioning and Parallel Stent Deployment

- Once all the target vessel stent grafts are positioned within their respective sheaths, the main body aortic device is advanced and deployed at the desired level of seal. The sheaths of the branches are carefully walked back over the positioned stent grafts and the branch vessels stents are simultaneously deployed with caution to ensure the chimneys extend at least 1 cm proximal to the main body to maintain patency. With the balloons within parallel grafts still inflated, a CODA balloon is inflated in the aortic graft to achieve molding of the endograft fabric around the stent grafts (**FIGURE 6**). The CODA balloon is deflated prior to deflation of the chimney stent grafts to avoid inadvertent crushing of the renal/visceral stents.
- Once the entirety of the aortic endograft is deployed completion angiogram is done to ensure adequacy of repair and to look for any endoleaks, kinking, or crushing of the parallel stents. The initial run is done with the wires in place in case a type 1a endoleak is present or there is visceral/renal malperfusion. Evaluation for brisk filling of the distal renal, superior mesenteric, and celiac axis branch vessels should be performed without any stiff wires to insure adequate run off and evaluate for stent graft patency as they remodel and conform to the native anatomy. A high-resolution x-ray shot should be performed to evaluate satisfactory stent architecture and overlap (**FIGURE 7**). A cone-beam CT with or without contrast is a useful tool for 3D evaluation of the repair.
- Removal of the axillary and femoral sheaths with cinching of previously placed sutures allows for straight forward closure of the access sites. After removal of all sheaths, inspection for distal pulses is performed and documented.

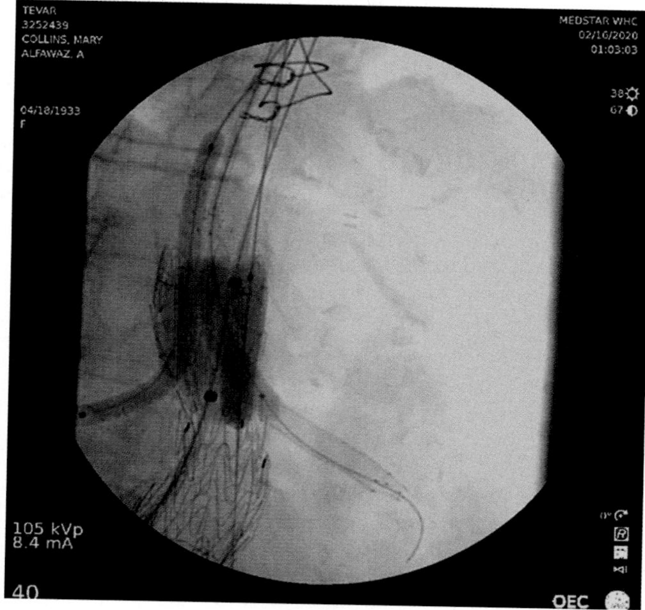

FIGURE 6 ● Inflation of CODA and parallel stents to allow for molding of stents.

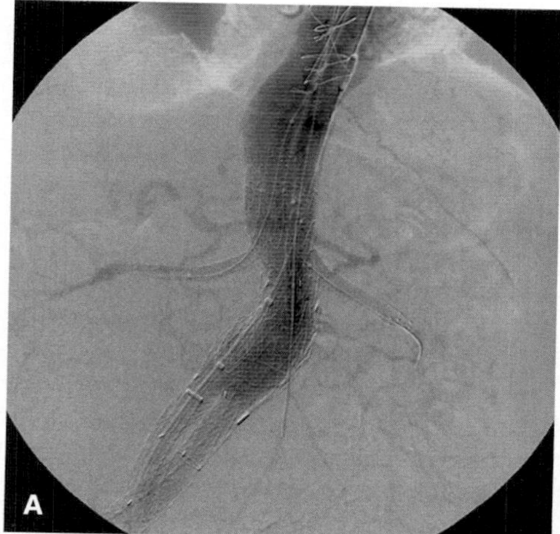

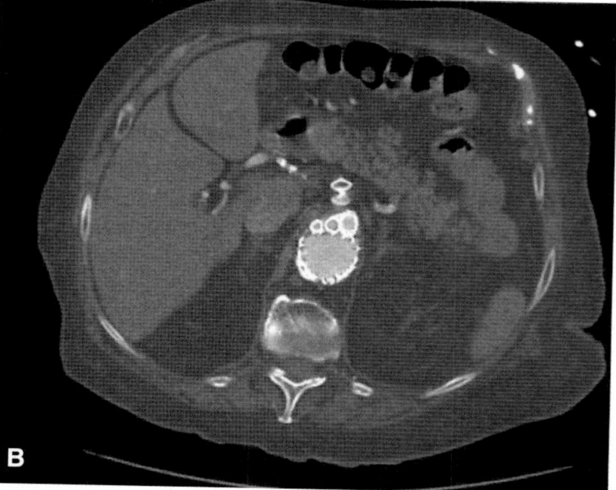

FIGURE 7 ● High resolution of completion angiogram demonstrating patency of all stent grafts and target vessels. **A,** Postoperative CT scan demonstrating celiac plug with 3 vessel snorkel repair **(B)**.

RETROGRADE PARALLEL STENTING IN EVAR

Femoral Access

- A periscope is a parallel stent positioned in a retrograde fashion alongside the aortic endograft. Femoral access is obtained under ultrasound guidance on the anterior surface of the common femoral artery. If there is concern for inadequate access or a significant underlying burden of disease, placement of an iliac conduit using 10-mm Dacron graft should be considered. After access is obtained, systemic anticoagulation is achieved with intravenous unfractionated heparin dosed to an ACT of at least 250 seconds.
- Access for cannulation is dependent on the size of the stents to be placed. Perclose sutures should be placed preemptively. A large bore sheath can be used to allow up to two or three smaller 6-Fr sheaths for cannulation of the branch vessels. If 7-Fr sheaths are required, placement of an external conduit with separate access of conduit for each sheath is preferred. Once adequate access is obtained, the branch vessels are cannulated as previously described. A hydrophilic Glidewire is exchanged for a stiffer wire and the sheath is advanced. Once branch sheaths are in place, stent grafts are advanced to their appropriate location as outlined above with same principles for positioning, and an adequate length of stent graft extended into the target vessel (minimum of 15 mm of apposition with the target vessel).
- The main endograft is advanced into the aorta, positioned at the appropriate level, and deployed with the sheaths still in place. The sheaths are slowly withdrawn, and the periscope stents are deployed. If the stents fall short of the end of the aortic graft, they should be extended with additional covered stents. With balloons inflated in all the parallel stents, a CODA balloon is inflated to mold the main endograft around the stents. Extension of the main body proximally to exclude the thoracic aneurysm or pathology is then completed. Finally, completion angiography is performed with similar principles as described above.

PEARLS AND PITFALLS

Chronic aortic dissection	■ A small true lumen diameter was initially considered a relative contraindication to parallel grafting, mostly due to concerns with possible stent-graft collapse, disruption of the septum, and difficulty to cannulate the vessels. This dogma has largely been debunked with increasing experience showing high technical success even in the presence of a compressed true lumen[11] (**FIGURE 8**).

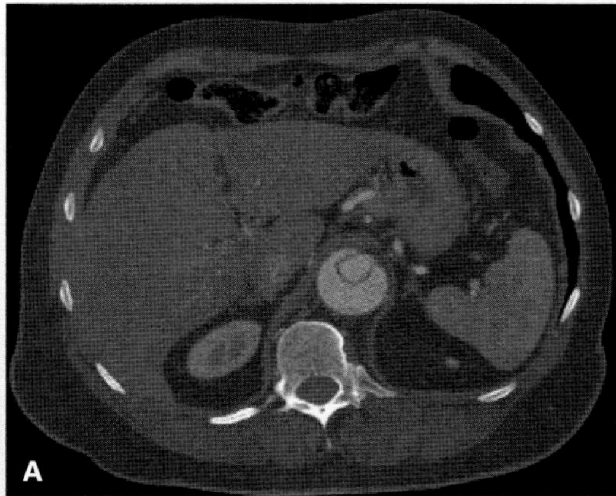

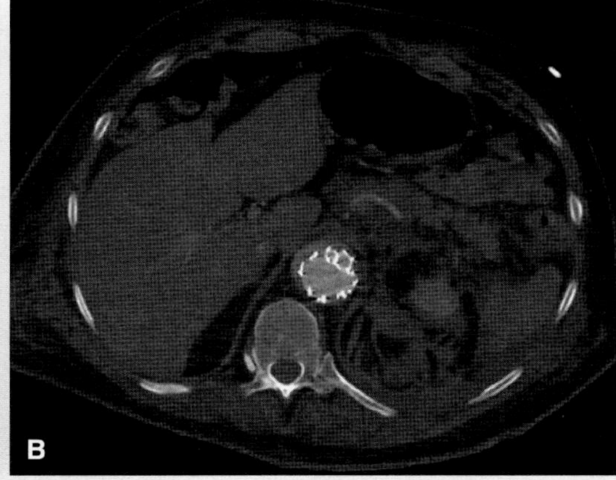

FIGURE 8 ● Chimney in aneurysms secondary to chronic aortic dissection; Initial preoperative CT scan demonstrating a compressed true lumen. **A,** Postoperative CT scan demonstrating a fully expanded true lumen with chimneys **(B)**.

Severely calcified or tortuous access vessels	▪ The limitations for standard TEVAR/EVAR are also applied to these endografts. Approximately 10%-20% of patients may require conduits. Most aortic devices require delivery systems with outer diameter of 20-25 Fr, requiring 7-9 mm of healthy external iliac artery diameter. In the setting of severe tortuosity, calcification, narrowing, or prior stents, a planned iliac conduit offers a suitable alternative to avoid inadvertent disruption of the iliac arteries. In addition to iliac artery access, brachial and axillary artery access should be assessed for dissection, narrowing or aneurysmal degeneration that can impact suitability as access vessels.
Short or early branching of the target branch artery	In cases of early branching or a solitary kidney with a short angulated renal artery, one may consider single vessel surgical debranching prior to endovascular repair of the aortic aneurysm.

POSTOPERATIVE CARE

- Almost all of our parallel stenting cases are admitted to the ICU postoperatively. This allows for hourly neurovascular and hemodynamic assessments for at least 24 hours. Our spinal cord protection protocol includes withholding of certain perioperative hypertensive medications (long-term beta blockers are continued), perioperative cerebrospinal fluid (CSF) drainage, perioperative mean arterial pressure maintenance ≥90 mm Hg, maintenance of hemoglobin to ≥10 g/dL intra- and postoperatively, as well as a steroid bolus in patients with any changes in intraoperative somatosensory and motor evoked potentials.
- Frequent laboratory checks are performed including troponin, lactate, CBC, and BMP. Close monitoring of urine output is continued with any sign of oliguria brought to the attention of the surgeon. When a patient has been neurologically intact for 24 hours, the spinal drain is clamped. After 6 to 24 hours of a stable neurologic exam depending on length of thoracic coverage, the drain is removed. The patient is discharged on aspirin and clopidogrel and a follow up CTA is performed within 1 month, followed by CTA or combination of noncontrast CT with duplex evaluation at 6 months, 1 year, and annually thereafter.

COMPLICATIONS

- Gutter leaks: Type I endoleaks that occur along the space between the main endograft and parallel stents are termed gutter leaks. These are best avoided by having an adequate length of overlap, at least 2 to 3 cm between the aortic wall, main endograft, and chimney grafts. Most gutter leaks resolve spontaneously within a year of implantation without evidence of sac expansion.[12]
- Kinked or crushed parallel stents: Kinked or crushed parallel stents can occur if the molding sequence is not followed. It is best to keep all wires in the branch vessels until after the completion angiogram to address this issue. This circumstance can occur if there is a long length of self-expanding stent as well. Typically, placement of a bare metal stent within the self-expanding stent can remediate this situation.

OUTCOMES

- The most comprehensive registry evaluating parallel stenting is the PERICLES registry.[13] Type IA endoleaks were noted in approximately 10% of patients intraoperatively. However, after intervention most are resolved prior to leaving the operating room. Ischemic stroke or TIA occurred in approximately 2% to 3% of patients in the PERICLES study. No patients suffered spinal cord ischemia. Two percent of patients suffered access complications requiring intervention. Two percent of patients suffered a postoperative myocardial infarction and 12% of patients suffered an AKI including 1.8% that required temporary or permanent dialysis. Of the 517 patients with parallel stenting, 2.5% required reintervention for an occluded chimney.[2,14]

CONCLUSION

- Parallel stenting has yielded acceptable short and midterm outcomes in carefully selected patients with complex aortic aneurysms that are not within the realm of repair using commercially available devices, or in urgent/emergent situations where access to a clinical trial device or a custom-made device is not an option.

REFERENCES

1. The UK EVAR Trial Investigators. Endovascular versus open repair of abdominal aortic aneurysm. *N Engl J Med*. 2010;362:1863-1871.
2. Donas K, Lee JT, LAchat M, Torsello G, Veith F. Collected world experience about the performance of the snorkel/chimney endovascular technique in the treatment of complex aortic pathologies: the PERICLES registry. *Ann Surg*. 2015;262(3):546-553.
3. Tanious A, Wooster M, Jung A, Nelson PR, Back M, Shames ML. Endovascular management of proximal fixation loss using parallel stent grafting techniques to preserve visceral flow. *Ann Vasc Surg*. 2017;42:169-175.
4. Kansagra K, Kang J, Taon M, et al. Advanced endografting techniques: snorkels, chimneys, periscopes, fenestrations, and branched endografts. *Cardiovasc Diagn Ther*. 2018;8(suppl 1):S175-S183.
5. Kölbel T, Carpenter SW, Taraz A, Taraz M, Larena-Avellaneda A, Debus ES. How to calculate the main aortic graft-diameter for a chimney-graft. *J Cardiovasc Surg*. 2016;57(1):66-71.
6. Doelare S, Smorenburg S, van Schaik T, et al. Image fusion during standard and complex endovascular aortic repair, to fuse or not to fuse? A meta-analysis and additional data from a single-center retrospective cohort. *J Endovasc Ther*. 2021;28(1):78-92. doi:10.1177/1526602820960444.
7. Scali S, Kim M, Kubilis P, et al. Implementation of a bundled protocol significantly reduces risk of spinal cord ischemia after branches or fenestrated endovascular aortic repair. *J Vasc Surg*. 2018;67(2):409-423.e4.
8. Sulzinski M; Rossi MJ; Alfawaz A, et al. Optimization of factors for the prevention of spinal cord ischemia in thoracic endovascular aortic repair. *Vascular*. 2022;30(2):199-205.
9. Meertens M, Lemmes C, Oderich G, Schurink G, Mees B. Cerebrovascular complications after upper extremity access for complex aortic interventions: a systematic review and meta-analysis. *Cardiovasc Intervent Radiol*. 2020;43:186-195.

10. Plotkin A, Ding L, Han S, et al. Association of upper extremity and neck access with stroke in endovascular aortic repair. *J Vasc Surg*. 2020;71(5):1602-1609.
11. Kitagawa A, Greenberg RK, Eagleton MJ, Mastracci TM, Roselli EE. Fenestrated and branched endovascular aortic repair for chronic type B aortic dissection with thoracoabdominal aneurysms. *J Vasc Surg*. 2013;58(3):625-634. doi:10.1016/j.jvs.2013.01.049
12. Ullery B, Tran K, Itoga N, Dalman RL, Lee JT. Natural history of gutter-related type Ia endoleaks after snorkel/chimney EVAR. *J Vasc Surg*. 2017;64(4):981-990.
13. Taneva GT, Lee JT, Tran K, et al. Long-term chimney/snorkel endovascular aortic aneurysm repair experience for complex abdominal aortic pathologies within the PERICLES registry. *J Vasc Surg*. 2021;73(6):1942-1949. doi:10.1016/j.jvs.2020.10.086
14. Li Y, Hu Z, Bai C, Liu J, Zhang T, Ge Y et al. Fenestrated and chimney technique for juxtarenal aortic aneurysm: a systematic review and pooled data analysis. *Sci Rep*. 2016;6:2.

Chapter **15**

Branched and Fenestrated Endovascular Stent Graft Techniques

Peter J. Rossi

- Endovascular repair of abdominal aortic aneurysms depends on specific anatomic constraints regarding infrarenal neck length and angulation in order to accommodate commercially available infrarenal devices. Fenestrated and branched endografts were introduced to enable minimally invasive repair of complex juxtarenal and suprarenal aortic aneurysms.[1] These devices incorporate reinforced fenestrations or directional branches, permitting incorporation of visceral and renal artery origins into the proximal endograft seal zone without compromising end-organ perfusion or aneurysm exclusion.[2] Devices can be manufactured to patient-specific specifications, or commercially available devices can by modified by the surgeon prior to being reconstrained and implanted. This chapter summarizes the technical features of endovascular aneurysm repair using fenestrated and branched stent grafts for pararenal and thoracoabdominal aortic aneurysms (TAAAs).

DEFINITION

- The term *fenestrated repair* refers to deployment of an endograft featuring custom orifices created and reinforced at precise locations around the aortic endograft to enable branch artery access, cannulation, and placement of a bridging stent graft during aneurysm exclusion. Fenestration sites are selected from analysis of patient-specific cross-sectional image data to enable exclusion of aneurysms with short or angled infrarenal necks. Graft design may be aided by three-dimensional reconstruction, and in some cases three-dimensional printing, of the aneurysm.[3] In general, the target arteries (renal or mesenteric) must arise from normal aorta to enable fenestrated repair. As a rule, fenestrations must be able to deploy flush with the aortic wall to ensure adequate aneurysm exclusion. "Alignment" stents (covered or uncovered, depending on individual patient circumstance) are deployed as needed to prevent target artery malperfusion as a consequence of misalignment between the fenestration and target artery orifice.
- *Branched repair* refers to endovascular aneurysm exclusion employing covered stents to directly connect the main lumen of the endograft to the target visceral artery. These devices enable repair of aneurysms involving or extending proximal to the origins of the renal or visceral vessels (eg, type IV TAAAs). Some distance must be present between the main body of the endograft at full deployment and the aortic wall at the target visceral artery orifice. Branched stent grafts are currently available in two distinct configurations:
  - *Fenestrated branches* arise from reinforced fenestrations bridged by balloon-expandable covered stents.
  - *Directional or cuffed branch* devices feature appended fabric cuffs, precisely located to enable straight, helical, down- or upgoing guidewire egress, target vessel cannulation, and deployment of bridging covered stents. Self-expanding flexible nitinol stents are usually employed for this purpose.
- Physician-modified endograft refers to back table modification of a commercially available endograft (thoracic or abdominal) which is subsequently reconstrained before being introduced into the patient. This technique is not approved for general use by the US Food and Drug Administration (FDA) and generally should be used within the confines of an ongoing clinical trial.

DIFFERENTIAL DIAGNOSIS

- Most aneurysms are degenerative (previously characterized as "atherosclerotic").
- Other etiologies include infection (eg, mycotic aneurysms), inflammation (eg, inflammatory aneurysm or aortitis), development of penetrating ulcers or asymmetric saccular enlargement, connective tissue disorders (eg, Marfan syndrome), and related aortic pathologies (dissection or intramural hematoma).

PATIENT HISTORY AND PHYSICAL FINDINGS

- Aortic aneurysms are asymptomatic prior to rupture and are diagnosed incidentally or during screening. The Society for Vascular Surgery (SVS) recommends elective aneurysm repair at a size greater than 5.5 cm for males and greater than 5 cm for females or enlargement greater than 5 mm in 6 months.[4]
- In up to 10% of patients, aneurysms may be accompanied by periaortic inflammation and resultant retroperitoneal fibrosis involving adjacent structures, including the duodenum and ureters.[5] These patients may present with abdominal or back pain, fatigue, malaise, or low-grade fever even at relatively small diameters. The SVS recommends repair of aneurysms where symptoms are attributable to the aneurysm regardless of size.[4]
- A comprehensive history should be obtained to fully appreciate the potential natural history of each patient's disease, including a full assessment of cardiovascular risk factors, current smoking habits, and a family history of aneurysm disease or connective tissue disorders.
- Evaluation of perioperative clinical risk emphasizes cardiac, pulmonary, and renal functional status and reserve, including baseline laboratory testing, noninvasive cardiac stress testing, pulmonary function assessment, and carotid duplex ultrasonography when indicated.

DIAGNOSTIC IMAGING

- Preprocedural aortic imaging studies provide fundamental and necessary guidance for endovascular repair strategies of all types. Aneurysm morphology is best analyzed through acquisition of high-resolution computed tomography angiography (CTA) datasets.[3] CTA with submillimeter slice acquisition is recommended for optimal acquisition, allowing three-dimensional reformatting techniques, maximum intensity projections, and volume rendering.

- Stent grafts are currently custom-made to conform to patient anatomy, based on estimates of longitudinal distance, axial clock position, arc lengths, and angles derived from centerline of flow measurements.
- Anatomic limitations to be considered include difficult iliac access, excessive aortic tortuosity or angulation,[6] visceral artery occlusive disease, and anatomic variants including multiple accessory renal arteries or early renal branch bifurcation.

STENT GRAFT DESIGN

- Device planning starts with selection of the proximal landing zone based on "healthy" aorta. The proximal landing zone should include at least a 2-cm length of "normal," noncalcified, parallel aortic wall and at least 25 to 30 mm of proximal seal for endovascular TAAA treatment.[7] The outer-to-outer aortic diameter should be more than 18 mm and less than 32 mm for pararenal aneurysms and more than 18 mm and less than 38 mm for TAAAs.[8] Landing zone diameter should be no larger than the diameter of the next most proximal aortic segment.
- Fenestrated stent grafts are currently manufactured with three fenestration options: small and large circles and more proximal scallops (**FIGURE 1A**). *Small fenestrations* are 6 × 6 mm or 6 × 8 mm, created without crossing struts and reinforced by circumferential nitinol rings. *Large fenestrations'* diameters are 8, 10, or 12 mm and may incorporate stent struts crossing the edge or middle of the circular defect, limiting space available for alignment stents. *Scallops* are contoured indentations along the upper edge of the main body endograft fabric, 10 mm wide and ranging in height from 6 to 12 mm, depending on individual patient anatomy.[9]
- Device designs vary with aneurysm extent. For pararenal aneurysms, 70% of patients are adequately treated with two small fenestrations for the renal arteries and a scallop for the superior mesenteric artery (SMA),[9] though increasing the number of fenestrations to 3 or 4 to increase the proximal seal has been shown to improve the proximal seal from an average of 26 mm up to an average of 48 mm.[7] Suprarenal and type IV TAAAs typically require four fenestrations (no scallops). Extensive TAAAs (types I to III) need directional branches, particularly if the aortic diameter is relatively large or aneurysmal at the level of the visceral arteries. The combination of directional branches for celiac and SMA management with fenestrations for the renal arteries is increasingly popular.

SURGICAL MANAGEMENT

Ancillary Tools

- These procedures require advanced endovascular skills and a comprehensive inventory of applicable catheters, balloons, and stents (**TABLE 1**). Dedicated training in fenestrated and branched techniques is highly recommended for physicians already experienced in endovascular disease management and ancillary procedures including renal and visceral artery disease management.

Perioperative Measures

- Patients with difficult aneurysm anatomy, chronic kidney disease, or advanced age are preadmitted for bowel preparation and intravenous hydration with bicarbonate infusion. Oral acetylcysteine is no longer routinely recommended to minimize risk of periprocedural renal dysfunction following administration of iodinated contrast and should be used on a case-by-case basis.[10]

A

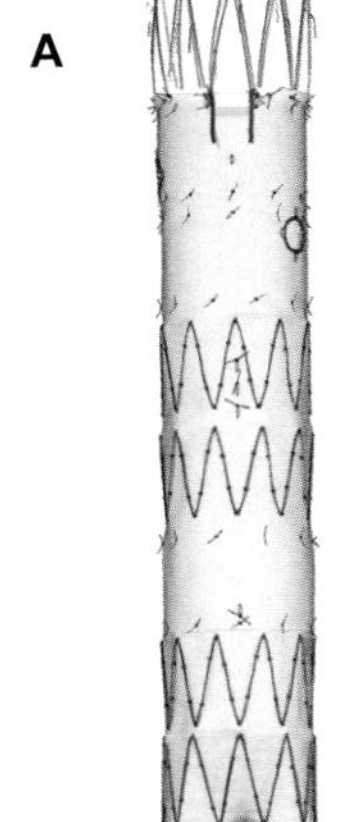

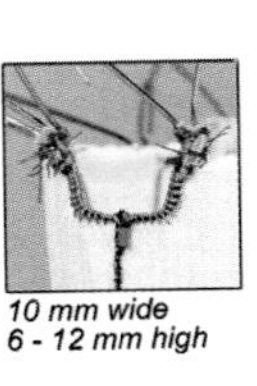

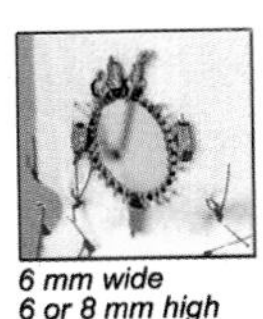

B

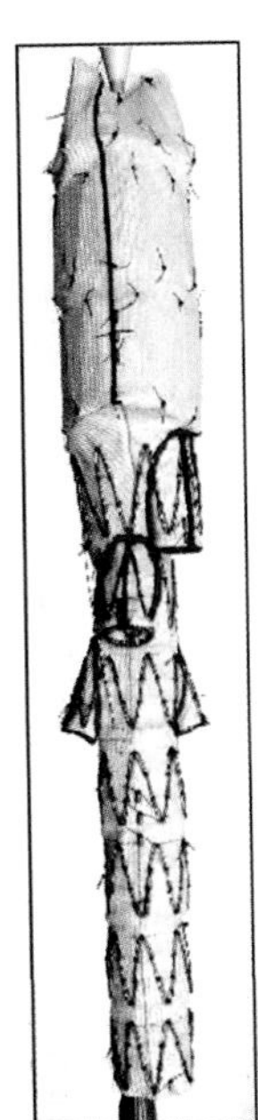

C

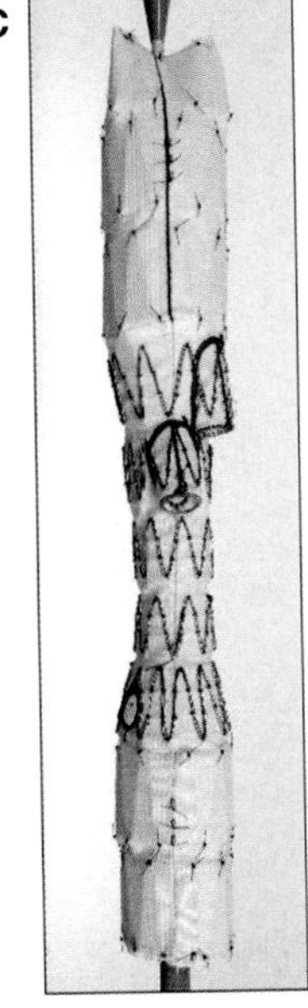

FIGURE 1 ● **A,** There are three types of fenestrations that can be manufactured: small, large, and scallop fenestrations. The fenestrated stent graft consists of a proximal fenestrated tubular component, a distal bifurcated universal component, and a contralateral iliac limb extension. **B,** The Cook Zenith stent graft lineage. **C,** Newer design with two straight downgoing branches and two fenestrations.

- Hybrid, fixed imaging platforms are essential for optimal results of these complex procedures. Most are performed using general endotracheal anesthesia; local or regional anesthesia may be sufficient in select cases.
- Intraoperative blood salvage systems ("cell saver") are recommended for difficult cases and all TAAAs. The creation of large, impermeable pockets within dependent portions of the surgical drapes will facilitate pooling and collection via the cell saver.
- The use of iodinated contrast is minimized by avoidance of power injector digital subtraction angiography runs during device implantation and side stent placement. Whenever possible, hand injections of dilute contrast are used to locate the side branches. Completion aortography is obtained only after all stents are positioned and post-dilated, again using diluted contrast (50%).
- To minimize contrast, use of onlay computed tomography (CT) images is recommended. In experienced hands, branch vessel precatheterization adds little to the overall procedure time.
- Spinal drainage should be strongly considered in high-risk patients including Crawford extent I-III aneurysms, previous open or endovascular infrarenal aortic repair, "shaggy" aorta, hypogastric artery occlusion, and left subclavian artery occlusion.[11]

Positioning

- Patients are positioned supine with the imaging unit oriented from the head of the table. Both arms are tucked for repair of pararenal aneurysms requiring up to three fenestrations.
- Brachial artery access is used in patients treated by directional branches or those who need four fenestrations.

Table 1: List of Ancillary Tools Recommended for Physicians Performing Fenestrated Stent Graft Procedures

Category	Manufacturer	Application
Sheaths		
20-Fr to 24-Fr Check-Flo sheath (30 cm)	Cook Medical, Bloomington, IN	Femoral access for multivessel catheterization
6-Fr or 7-Fr Ansel sheath (55 cm, flexible dilator)	Cook Medical, Bloomington, IN	Femoral access for branch artery stenting
6-Fr or 7-Fr TourGuide steerable sheath	Medtronic, Minneapolis, MN	Femoral access for branch artery stenting
7-Fr or 8-Fr Raabe sheath (90 cm long)	Cook Medical, Bloomington, IN	Brachial access for branch artery stenting
12-Fr Ansel sheath (55 cm, flexible dilator)	Cook Medical, Bloomington, IN	Brachial access for tortuous aortic arch to facilitate branch artery stenting
5-Fr Shuttle sheath (90 cm)	Cook Medical, Bloomington, IN	Branch artery access during difficult arch
Catheters		
Kumpe or Berenstein catheter 5-Fr (65 cm)	Multiple	Selective vessel catheterization
Kumpe or Berenstein catheter 5-Fr (100 cm)	Multiple	Selective vessel catheterization
C1 catheter 5-Fr (100 cm)	Multiple	Selective vessel catheterization
MPA catheter 5-Fr (125 cm)	Multiple	Selective vessel catheterization
MPB catheter 5-Fr (100 cm)	Multiple	Selective vessel catheterization
Van Schie 3 catheter 5-Fr (65 cm)	Cook Medical, Bloomington, IN	Selective vessel catheterization
Vertebral catheter 4-Fr (125 cm)	Multiple	Selective vessel catheterization
VS1 catheter 5-Fr (80 cm)	Multiple	Selective vessel catheterization
Simmons I catheter 5-Fr (100 cm)	Multiple	Selective vessel catheterization
Diagnostic flush catheter 5-Fr (100 cm)	Multiple	Diagnostic angiography
Diagnostic pigtail catheter 5-Fr (100 cm)	Multiple	Diagnostic angiography, selective vessel catheterization
Quick-cross catheter 0.014 in to 0.035 in (150 cm)	Phillips Medical	Selective vessel catheterization
Renegade catheter (150 cm)	Boston Scientific, Minneapolis, MN	Selective vessel catheterization
Guide catheters		
LIMA guide 7 Fr (55 cm)	Cordis Corporation, Bridgewater, NJ	Precatheterization
Internal mammary (IM) guide 7 Fr (100 cm)	Multiple	Selective vessel catheterization
MPA guide 7 Fr (100 cm)	Multiple	Selective vessel catheterization
Balloons		
10 mm × 2 cm angioplasty balloon	Multiple	Proximal stent flare
12 mm × 2 cm angioplasty balloon	Multiple	Proximal stent flare
5 mm × 2 cm angioplasty balloon	Multiple	Advance sheath over balloon
Wires		
Bentson wire 0.035 in (150 cm)	Multiple	Initial access
Soft glidewire 0.035 in (260 cm)	Multiple	Target vessel catheterization
Stiff glidewire 0.035 in (260 cm)	Multiple	Target vessel catheterization
Rosen wire 0.035 in (260 cm)	Multiple	Branch artery stenting
1-cm tip Amplatz wire 0.035 in (260 cm)	Multiple	Branch artery stenting
Lunderquist wire 0.035 in (260 cm)	Multiple	Aortic stent graft
Glidegold wire 0.018 in (180 cm)	Multiple	Target vessel catherization
Stents		
iCAST stent grafts 5-10 mm	Atrium, Hudson, NH	Branch artery stenting
Gore VBX balloon-expandable stent grafts, 6-8 mm	Gore Medical, Phoenix, AZ	Branch artery stenting
LifeStream balloon-expandable stent grafts, 5-10 mm	Becton-Dickinson, Franklin Lakes, NJ	Branch artery stenting
Balloon-expandable stents 0.035 in	Multiple	Branch artery stenting or reinforcement
Self-expandable stents 0.035 in	Multiple	Distal branch artery stenting
Self-expandable stents 0.014 in	Multiple	Distal branch artery stenting

LIMA, left internal mammary artery; MPA, main pulmonary artery; VS1, Van Schie 1.

The left arm is abducted and prepped in the surgical field up to the axilla. A working sterile side table is oriented in the same axis of the abducted arm for optimal support of necessary wires and catheters.

- Electrocardiogram (EKG) leads, urinary catheter, and other monitoring cables and lines should be taped or secured so that they are not in the path of the X-ray beam of the fluoroscopic unit and do not impede movement of the C-arm gantry.

Arterial Access

- Access is established in the femoral arteries. Patients with small, calcified, or stenotic iliac arteries may require creation of an iliac conduit for safe device delivery.
- Total percutaneous femoral access is the preferred approach in patients with noncalcified arteries or mild posterior plaque. Appropriately applied standard "preclosure" with suture-mediated closure devices allows hemostasis in 99% of femoral arteries with a 30-day complication rate of 3.1% per artery.[11] When femoral arteries are small, calcified, or bifurcate close to the inguinal ligament, standard surgical exposure and access is obtained. Proximal and distal control is obtained using vessel loops.
- The left brachial artery is surgically exposed via small longitudinal incision in the upper arm, just proximal to the origin of the deep brachial artery. Likewise, percutaneous axillary access with standard preclosure may be utilized when anatomically feasible.
- Intravenous heparin (80-100 U/kg) is administered immediately after femoral and brachial access is established. An activated clotting time longer than 250 seconds is maintained throughout the procedure with frequent rechecks every 30 minutes. Prior to deployment of the stent graft, diuresis is induced with intravenous mannitol and/or furosemide.

ENDOVASCULAR REPAIR USING FENESTRATED STENT GRAFTS

- Fenestrated–branched repair is currently performed using the Cook Zenith stent graft lineage. Newer designs by Medtronic (Valiant), Terumo (Anaconda), and Cook Medical (p-Branch) remain under clinical investigation. A four-branched device (Gore TAMBE) is under investigation as well.
- The Cook Zenith fenestrated stent graft consists of a proximal fenestrated tubular component, a distal bifurcated universal component, and a contralateral iliac limb extension (**FIGURE 1A**). The fenestrated tubular component is custom-made to fit the patient's anatomy. Four to 8 weeks are required for manufacturing and delivery in the United States.
- Bilateral percutaneous femoral access is established under ultrasound guidance; each femoral puncture is preclosed using two Perclose devices. Bilateral 8-Fr sheaths are introduced to the external iliac arteries over Benson guidewires (Cook Medical, Bloomington, IN). The guidewires are exchanged to 0.035-in soft glidewires and Kumpe catheters, which are advanced to the ascending aorta and exchanged for stiff 0.035-in Lunderquist guidewires (Cook Medical, Bloomington, IN).
- Choice of access site is dependent on tortuosity and vessel diameter. Provided there are no issues with both iliac arteries, the branches are performed via the right femoral approach, whereas the fenestrated and bifurcated devices are introduced via the left femoral approach. A 20-Fr (two fenestrations) or 22-Fr (three fenestrations) Check-Flo sheath (Cook Medical, Bloomington, IN) is introduced via the right femoral approach (**FIGURE 2A**). The valve of the Check-Flo sheath has four leaflets, which are accessed by two short 7-Fr sheaths at 2- and 7-o'clock positions.
- Precatheterization of the renal arteries is performed using 0.035-in soft glidewires and 5-Fr Kumpe or C1 catheters (Cook Medical, Bloomington, IN), which are supported by 7-Fr left internal mammary artery (LIMA) guide catheters (**FIGURE 2B**). Alternatively, onlay fusion CTA is recommended to minimize contrast use. Generally, for two-vessel fenestrated endograft, precatheterization is not necessary with the use of onlay fusion techniques.
- The fenestrated stent graft is oriented extracorporeally, introduced via the left femoral approach, and deployed with optimal apposition between the fenestrations and the target catheters.
- Proper device orientation, using the anterior and posterior markers, is essential. It is useful to deploy the first two or three stents and then rotate the imaging unit laterally, confirming alignment. The device should be deployed slightly higher than what is anticipated, with lowest of the four radiopaque markers in the fenestration at the upper edge of the renal artery. The diameter-reducing wire on the fenestrated component allows for some rotational and cranial–caudal movement to optimize alignment following initial deployment.
- After deployment of the fenestrated component, if precatheterization has been used, each catheter is removed from its target artery and used to sequentially regain target vessel access through the respective fenestration (**FIGURE 2C**). In most cases, when alignment is carefully confirmed prior to attempted cannulation, the target vessel is accessed without difficulty. When access is challenging, catheterization of the fenestration may be facilitated by the use of a steerable sheath (ie, 6-Fr Tour Guide [Medtronic, Minneapolis, MN]).
- After the target vessel is catheterized, soft glidewire is removed and hand injection is used to confirm location. The glidewire is exchanged for a 0.035-in Rosen guidewire (Cook Medical, Bloomington, IN). The Rosen guidewire has a floppy J tip, reducing the risk of branch renal artery perforations. When additional support is required, the Amplatz guidewire (Cook Medical, Bloomington, IN) with 1-cm soft tip can be used.
- After the Rosen or stiff guidewire of choice is positioned, a 7-Fr Ansel sheath with flexible dilator is advanced. If there is difficulty to advance the sheath, an undersized balloon may be used as a dilator to facilitate advancement.
- Once the sheath is in position, an alignment stent is positioned under protection of the sheath with the tip of the stent just beyond the tip of the sheath (**FIGURE 2D**).

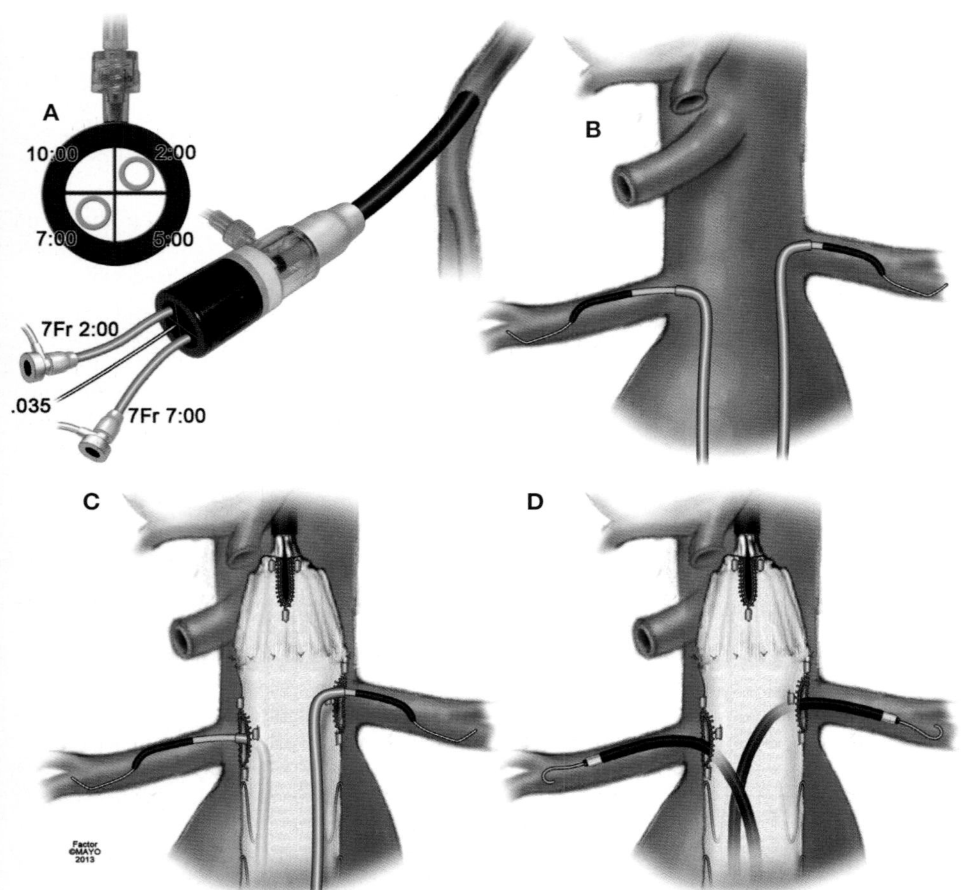

FIGURE 2 • **A,** A 20-Fr (two fenestrations) or 22-Fr (three fenestrations) Check-Flo sheath is introduced via the right femoral approach. **B,** Precatheterization of the renal arteries. **C,** Sequentially regain access into the fenestrated component, fenestration, and target vessel. **D,** An alignment stent is advanced under protection of the sheath. (A, Used with permission of Mayo Foundation for Medical Education and Research, all rights reserved.)

- For repairs requiring two or three vessel fenestrations, the target vessels are accessed sequentially using femoral approach. For those requiring four fenestrations, the celiac axis is accessed via brachial approach using a preloaded catheter, which is placed through the celiac fenestration and exits the stent graft via an access scallop at the top of the device.
- The diameter-reducing tie on the fenestrated segment is removed after all the target arteries are accessed and secured by 7-Fr hydrophilic sheaths.
- The top cap of the device is advanced forward to deploy the uncovered fixation stent (**FIGURE 3A**). The top cap is retrieved prior to deployment of the alignment stents.
- After the top cap and dilator are removed, the proximal landing zone is gently dilated using a compliable balloon such as the Coda balloon (Cook Medical, Bloomington IN, **FIGURE 3B**). It is critical that the balloon dilatation is performed prior to placement of alignment stents, or alternatively, each stent has to be protected by separate balloons.
- The alignment stents are sequentially deployed following removal of the diameter-reducing tie, retrieval of the top cap, and balloon dilatation of the neck. **The sequence of stent deployment is renal arteries followed by SMA and celiac axis**. Prior to each stent deployment, the position of the stent is confirmed by hand injection. The stent is deployed 3 to 5 mm into the aorta (**FIGURE 3C**) and flared using a 10 mm × 2 cm balloon (**FIGURE 3D**). A completion angiography of each branch is performed using hand injection after direct injection of 100 to 200 μg of nitroglycerin to minimize spasm.
- Following placement of the alignment stents, a distal bifurcated stent graft is oriented, advanced, and deployed with preservation of the ipsilateral internal iliac artery. The dilator of the bifurcated device may encroach the contralateral renal stent or the SMA stent. In these cases, it is useful to leave a 10-mm balloon ready to be inflated in the renal stent to prevent damage (**FIGURE 4A**, *inset*). The minimum overlap between the bifurcated and the fenestrated component is two full-length stents (17 mm each), but ideally, more than three full stents is recommended to minimize risk of component separation (**FIGURE 4B**).[12,13] After deployment of the bifurcated device, the dilator is removed with care to avoid damage or dislodgement of the renal stents.
- The contralateral gate is catheterized using a soft glidewire and 5-Fr catheter (**FIGURE 4B**). Access is confirmed by 360° catheter rotation. The glidewire is exchanged for a 0.035-in Lunderquist guidewire. Limited iliac angiography using contralateral oblique views with hand injection. The contralateral limb extension is deployed with preservation of the internal iliac artery (**FIGURE 4C**).
- A completion cone beam CT angiography of the aorta and iliac arteries is obtained using power injection to demonstrate patency of the visceral arteries, main body, iliac limbs, and iliac arteries.

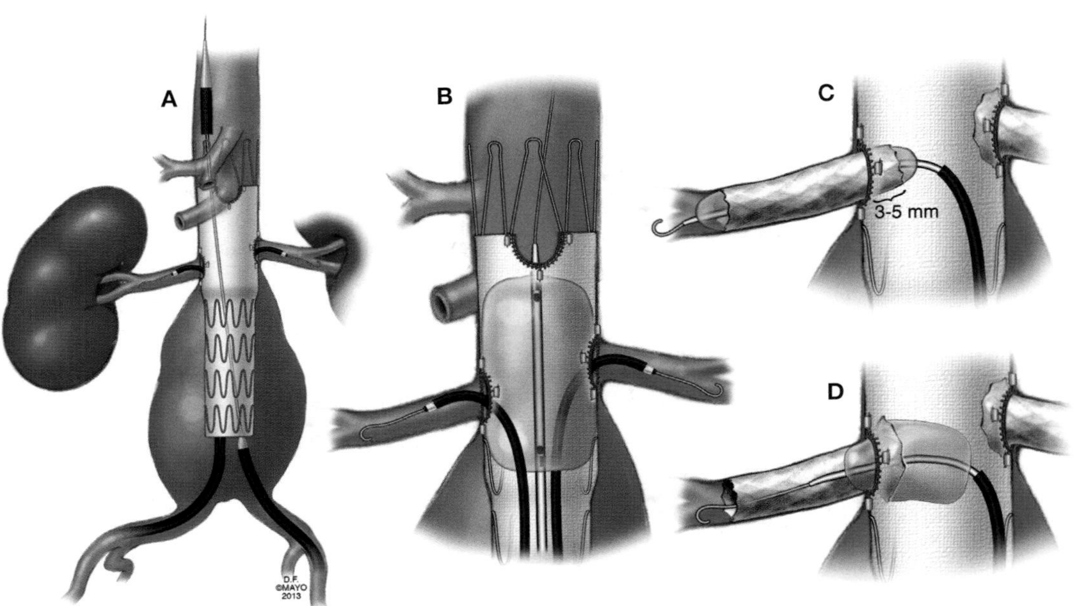

FIGURE 3 ● **A,** The top cap of the device is advancing forward allowing deployment of the uncovered fixation stent. **B,** The proximal landing zone is gently dilated using a compliable balloon. Stent deployed 3 to 5 mm into the aorta **(C)** and flared using a 10 mm × 2 cm balloon **(D)**.

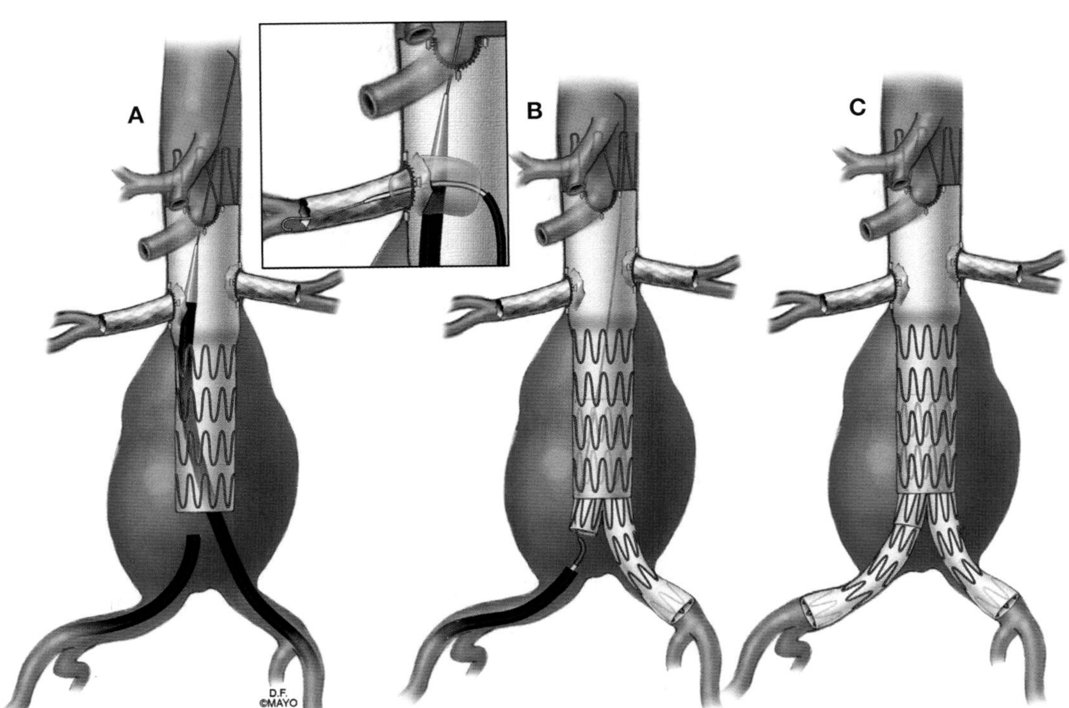

FIGURE 4 ● To avoid the dilator of the bifurcated device encroaching the contralateral renal stent or the superior mesenteric artery stent, leave a 10-mm balloon ready to be inflated in the renal stent (**A,** *inset*). **B,** The minimum overlap between the bifurcated and the fenestrated component is more than two full-length stents. **C,** The contralateral limb extension is deployed with preservation of the internal iliac artery.

ENDOVASCULAR REPAIR USING MULTIPLE DIRECTIONAL BRANCHES (MULTIBRANCH T-BRANCH STENT GRAFT)

- Directional branches created with presewn cuffs are currently available from Cook Zenith stent graft lineage on an investigational use basis (**FIGURE 1B**). A four-vessel multibranch stent graft design (T-branch) remains under investigation for treatment of TAAAs.
- The extent of repair varies depending on the proximal extension of aneurysm within the thoracic aorta. The procedure is performed using bilateral femoral and left brachial approach. In general, the repair starts with deployment of a proximal thoracic TX2 stent graft (Cook Medical, Bloomington, IN) followed by deployment of the T-branch stent graft (Cook Medical, Brisbane, Australia) and distal bifurcated component and contralateral limb extension. The self-expandable stents are placed into the four branches following deployment of all aortic components. The critical steps are reviewed as follows:
- Bilateral femoral and left brachial arterial access is obtained (**FIGURE 5A**). A proximal thoracic stent graft is deployed if needed depending on aneurysm extent.

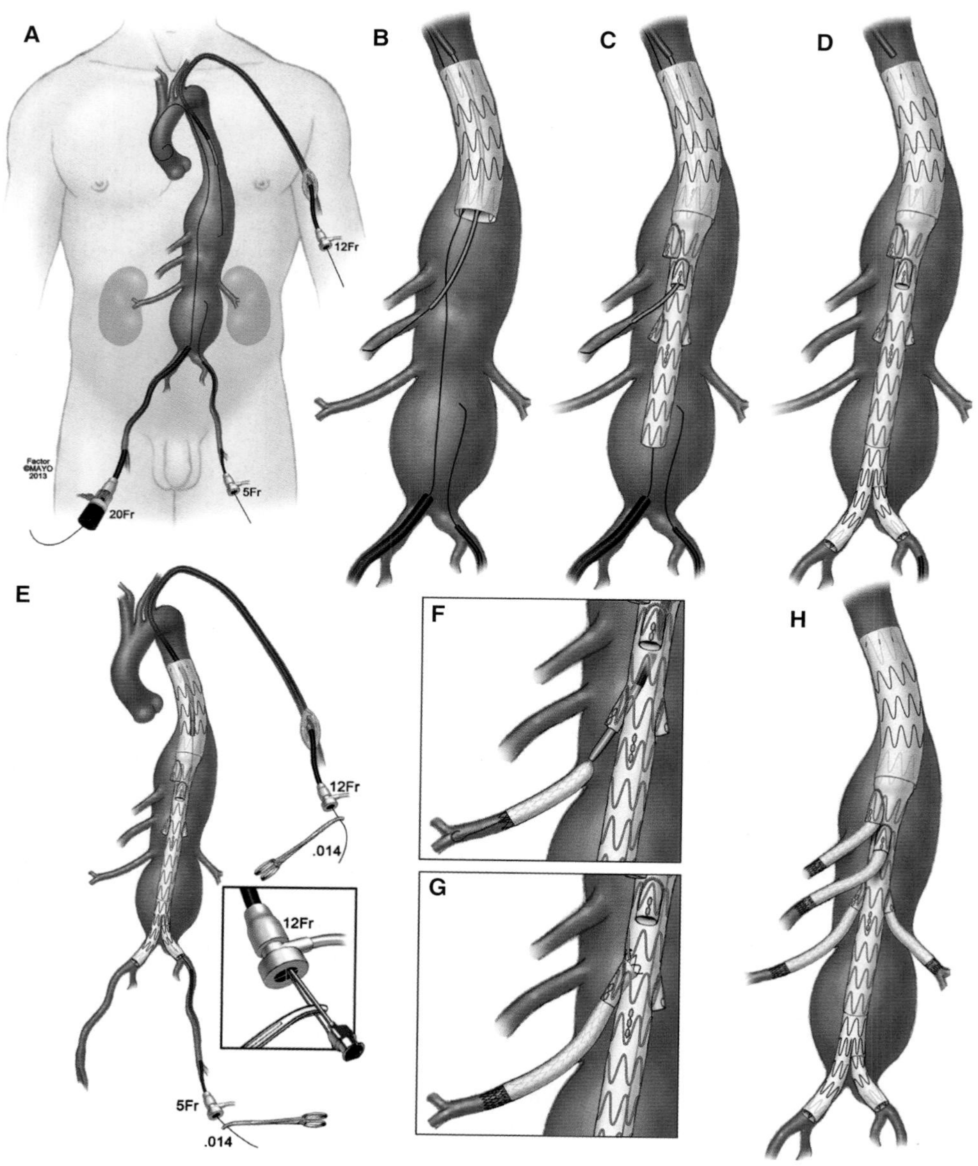

FIGURE 5 ● **A,** Endovascular repair using multiple directional branches is performed using bilateral femoral and left brachial approach. Deployment of proximal thoracic TX2 stent graft **(B)**, followed by deployment of the T-branch stent graft **(C)**, and distal bifurcated component and contralateral limb extension **(D)**. The femoral arteries may be closed, restoring flow into the lower extremities; maintain access into one of the femoral arteries using a 5-Fr sheath **(E,** *inset***)**. **F** and **G**. 9-Fr 80-cm flexor sheath is advanced into the target vessel, followed by placement of a self-expandable stent graft. **H,** Complete procedure. (A, B, F, and G Used with permission of Mayo Foundation for Medical Education and Research, all rights reserved.)

- Precatheterization of the renal arteries is not required, but it is critical that the distal edge of the directional branch is deployed above its intended target vessel. To guide deployment of the T-branch component, the SMA is precatheterized via the brachial approach (**FIGURE 5B**).
- The T-branch stent graft is oriented extracorporeally, introduced via the femoral approach, and deployed with the directional branches located proximal to its intended target vessel (**FIGURE 5C**).
- Deployment of the distal universal bifurcated stent graft and contralateral iliac extension are identical to what was described in the fenestrated technique (**FIGURE 5D**).
- The femoral arteries are closed at this point, restoring flow into the lower extremities. It is useful to maintain access into one of the femoral arteries with a 5-Fr sheath (**FIGURE 5E**, *inset*). This maneuver allows passage of a 0.014-in guidewire from the left brachial artery to femoral artery. The guidewire is clamped in both ends, which locks the 12-Fr sheath in place and provides support for deployment of the side branches.
- The 12-Fr Ansel I sheath (Cook Medical, Bloomington, IN) is advanced via the left brachial approach and positioned inside the T-branch component in the descending thoracic aorta (**FIGURE 5E**). At this point, a 0.014-in guidewire is advanced through and through from the left brachial to femoral artery, preventing movement of the 12-Fr sheath in the aortic arch.
- Each side branch is individually catheterized in a sequential fashion, starting with the renal arteries (**FIGURE 5F**) followed by the SMA and celiac axis. A 5-Fr main pulmonary artery (MPA) or Kumpe catheter (Cook Medical, Bloomington, IN) is used to access the directional branch and target vessel. Once the vessel is catheterized, the soft glidewire is exchanged for a stiff guidewire (Rosen or short-tip Amplatzer, Cook Medical, Bloomington, IN), which is positioned in the target vessel.
- A 9-Fr 80-cm flexor sheath (Cook Medical, Bloomington, IN) is advanced coaxially within the 12-Fr sheath into the target vessel.
- Each target vessel is stented with a self-expandable stent graft (**FIGURE 5F**). The stent graft should be oversized by 1 to 2 mm and should provide at least 2 cm of distal landing zone in the target vessel, extending 3 to 5 mm into the aortic lumen of the T-branch device.
- To prevent kinks in the transition of the stent graft to the target artery, each self-expandable stent graft is reinforced by a second self-expandable uncovered stent, which is deployed 1 cm beyond the distal edge of the stent graft (**FIGURE 5G**). Selective completion angiography is obtained for each sequential branch.
- A completion angiography of the arch and thoracoabdominal aorta is obtained after all matting stent grafts are deployed (**FIGURE 5H**).

ENDOVASCULAR REPAIR USING TWO DIRECTIONAL BRANCHES AND TWO FENESTRATIONS (TWO BRANCH–TWO FENESTRATED STENT GRAFT)

- A design with directional branches for the celiac and SMA and fenestrations for the renal arteries has been widely used at the Cleveland Clinic.[14] A design with two straight downgoing branches and two fenestrations has been used (**FIGURE 1C**). The advantage of the latter is the ability to provide short, transversely oriented branches for the renal arteries.
- The same principles already described for fenestrated stent grafts are applied with respect to device design, planning, and arterial access.
- Bilateral femoral access and left brachial artery access are needed (**FIGURE 6A**). The right femoral access is used for precatheterization of the renal arteries. The left brachial access is used for the celiac axis and SMA (**FIGURE 6B**).
- A proximal thoracic TX2 stent graft (Cook Medical, Bloomington, IN) is deployed first, depending on proximal extension of the aneurysm (**FIGURE 6A**).
- After the renal arteries and SMA are precatheterized, the fenestrated–branched stent graft is oriented extracorporeally, introduced via the femoral approach and deployed with perfect apposition between the renal fenestrations and the target renal arteries (**FIGURE 6B**).
- The celiac and SMA branch are accessed using preloaded catheters and glidewires, which are snared via the left brachial approach (**FIGURE 6B**).
- Each catheter is sequentially removed from the renal arteries and used to regain access into the fenestrated component, renal fenestration, and target renal artery (**FIGURE 6C**). Hydrophilic sheaths and alignment renal stents are advanced as previously described.
- The preloaded catheters in the SMA and celiac branch allow advancement of a 0.035-in soft glidewire, which is snared via the left brachial approach (**FIGURE 6B**). A sheath and catheter are advanced into the celiac branch. Following access into the celiac axis, a 0.035-in Amplatz guidewire is placed.
- The SMA is accessed using similar steps, and after access is established with Amplatz guidewire, a 9-Fr sheath is advanced to allow positioning of a self-expandable stent graft.
- Once all four vessels are catheterized and sheaths are positioned into the renal arteries and SMA, the diameter-reducing tie is removed, allowing complete expansion of the fenestrated–branched component (**FIGURE 6D**).
- Sequential target artery stenting is performed using balloon-expandable covered stents for the renal fenestrated branches (**FIGURE 6E**, *inset*) and self-expandable stent grafts for the SMA and celiac axis (**FIGURE 6E**, *inset*). Selective branch angiography is performed after each branch stent is placed.
- Deployment of distal bifurcated component and contralateral iliac limb extension is identical to what has been described for fenestrated stent grafts (**FIGURE 6F**).

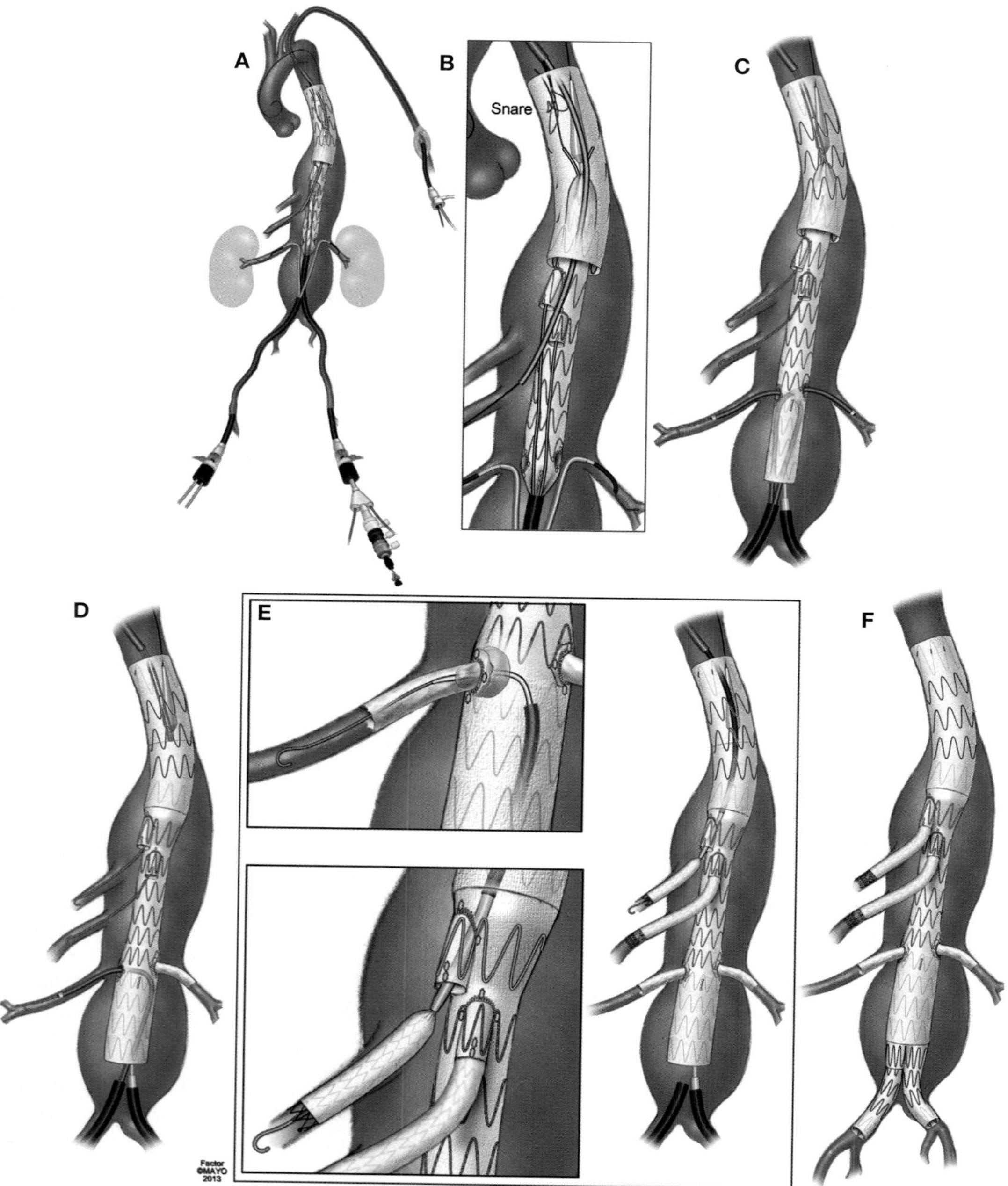

FIGURE 6 ● **A,** Bilateral femoral access and left brachial artery access is needed. **B,** After the renal arteries and superior mesenteric artery (SMA) are precatheterized, the fenestrated–branched stent graft is oriented extracorporeally, introduced via the femoral approach. The celiac and SMA branch are accessed using preloaded catheters and glidewires, which are snared via the left brachial approach. **C,** Regain access into the fenestrated component, renal fenestration, and target renal artery. **D,** Complete expansion of the fenestrated–branched component. Sequential target artery stenting is performed using balloon-expandable covered stents for the renal fenestrated branches and self-expandable stent grafts for the SMA and celiac axis (**E,** *inset*). **F,** Deployment of distal bifurcated component and contralateral iliac limb extension.

PEARLS AND PITFALLS

Preoperative evaluation	▪ Complete history and physical examination with emphasis on cardiovascular risk factors, family history of aneurysm disease, and connective tissue disorders. ▪ Preoperative medical evaluation focused on cardiac, pulmonary, and renal performance. ▪ Aortic imaging with CTA allows detailed analysis of aneurysm morphology for stent graft design and procedure planning.
Arterial access	▪ Iliac conduits are recommended in patients with small, diseased, or excessively tortuous iliac arteries. ▪ Pelvic perfusion with maintenance of internal iliac artery flow decreases risk of spinal cord injury.
Stent graft implantation	▪ Precise stent graft design and implantation are critical aspects of the procedure. ▪ Minimize use of iodinated contrast by avoiding contrast aortography during device implantation. ▪ Precatheterization and/or onlay CT allows precise device implantation with minimal need of angiography. ▪ Fenestrations are typically accessed via the femoral approach and stented using balloon-expandable covered stents. ▪ Directional branches are accessed via the brachial approach and stented using self-expandable stent grafts.
Misaligned fenestrations	▪ Excessive tortuosity in the iliac or visceral segment may cause misalignment of fenestrations and difficult target vessel catheterization. ▪ Rotation of the device, which is constrained by a diameter-reducing tie, and use of balloon displacement or curved catheters allow successful catheterization in most cases.
Branch perforation or dissection	▪ Small, diseased, and tortuous visceral arteries are prone to perforation or dissection, particularly if an Amplatz guidewire is needed to provide more support. ▪ Careful attention to detail and minimizing guidewire manipulation with close attention to the tip of the guidewire help prevent this complication.
Stent kinks	▪ Branch tortuosity may lead to kinks within the side stents. ▪ This should be immediately recognized and treated by placement of a second self-expandable stent to prevent branch occlusion.

POSTOPERATIVE CARE

- Length of stay averages 2 to 3 days for endovascular repair of pararenal aneurysms and 4 to 5 days for TAAAs.
- Cerebrospinal fluid drainage, if used, is discontinued on postoperative day 2, after a 6-hour clamp trial and documentation of normal coagulation profile.
- Oral diet is resumed the day after the operation for uncomplicated cases requiring two to three fenestrations, but it is typically withheld for 1 or 2 days for difficult cases or those requiring four fenestrations or branches.
- Cone beam CTA is obtained at the completion of stent graft deployment in the operating room, which may reveal a technical issue requiring intervention in up to 31% of patients.[15] Follow-up includes clinical examination and imaging (CTA and ultrasound) in 6 to 8 weeks, every 6 months during the first year, and yearly 1 year, and early thereafter.
- Patients are started on aspirin indefinitely. Clopidogrel is not recommended unless there is a specific concern with one of the side branches because of small size (<4 mm), occlusive disease, or dissection. Clopidogrel should be avoided early after extensive TAAA repair because of risk of delayed spinal cord injury and paraplegia, which may necessitate replacement of the spinal drain.

OUTCOMES

- Branched and fenestrated aortic repairs have become more common and devices continue to evolve. The European Society for Vascular and Endovascular Surgery has recommended B/FEVAR over open repair of pararenal and TAAAs in patients with appropriate anatomy.[16] Short-term and mid-term outcomes have been good for these devices, with perioperative death rates of 0.9%, 5-year freedom from aortic-related mortality of 98%, and 64% freedom from reintervention at 5 years.[17] Freedom from reintervention is lower in patients undergoing F/BEVAR to treat type Ia endoleak after failed infrarenal EVAR.[18]
- Technical success is high for endovascular repair using fenestrated stent grafts, with branch artery preservation successful in up to 99.2% of vessels for extent IV TAAA and pararenal AAA, and 98.5% in extent I-III TAAA.[17]
- Up to 20% of patients undergoing F/BEVAR may require a secondary intervention for endoleak (type I or type III), highlighting the need for life-long postoperative surveillance.[17]
- Likelihood of reintervention for branch artery instability (type Ic endoleak or loss of patency) becomes more likely with increasing extent of repair.[19] Mastracci and associates have reported a freedom from branch-related complications of 84% at 5 years.[20]

COMPLICATIONS

Intraprocedural Complications

- ***Fenestration misalignment***: Neck angulation, tortuosity, and errors of design or implantation can lead to misalignment between the fenestration and the target vessel. Several maneuvers can be used to overcome misalignment between the fenestration and the vessel. Initially, the catheter and guidewire are rotated to "probe" the aortic wall in search for the vessel. To maintain access into the fenestration, a 7-Fr Ansel sheath is advanced into the fenestration and secured by a 0.018-in guidewire, whereas a 5-Fr "buddy" catheter (eg, Van Schie [VS] 3) is used to locate the renal artery. In patients with downgoing or stenosed renal arteries, it may be difficult to advance the catheter over a soft glidewire. The catheter and glidewire may bounce up into the top cap, providing support for the catheter to be advanced deep into the renal artery.

- Diameter-reducing ties are located posteriorly, which may result in the fenestrations being pulled slightly more posterior than its intended location. A useful maneuver is to gently rotate each fenestration, usually anteriorly. Other maneuvers are rarely needed but included use of reverse-curved catheters (eg, Omni-Select or SOS) for downgoing vessels or vessels that are originating from the lower part of the fenestration, microcatheters, and balloon displacement of the main stent graft. The latter is rarely needed but may provide more room for catheter manipulations.
- ***Branch perforation or dissection***: Branch vessel perforation and/or dissection can be prevented by meticulous technique, visualization of the tip of the wire, and avoiding wire manipulations. The guidewire should not be positioned in small terminal branches, which are prone to perforate or dissect. It should be visualized and stabilized during exchanges manipulations, avoiding forward or retrograde movement. If perforation occurs, it should be immediately recognized and treated using a microcatheter and coil embolization. Dissections within the main renal artery can be treated by placement of a self-expandable stent.
- ***Endoleaks***: Type II and type IV endoleaks may occur and should be left untreated. Type I and type III endoleaks occur in up to 8% of patients with proper selection of a healthy landing zone and adequate planning.[21] In the event of a type Ia endoleak, the proximal neck may be redilated, but all the alignment stents need to be protected by separate balloons. Type III endoleaks may result from inadequate flare, lack of apposition, use of bare metal stent, or inadequate length into the aorta.
- ***Stent kinks or narrowing***: Kinks are preventable and can be anticipated from careful review of vessel anatomy by CTA. These remain a cause of reintervention or branch vessel loss if not recognized. Short stents (<2 cm) tend to avoid bends and the mid- or distal portion of the renal artery, which has greater respiratory motion. The right renal may have a posterior orientation from its course behind the inferior vena cava. If a kink is anticipated by CTA or is evident by completion angiography, a self-expandable stent should be placed. Kinks or narrowing may also result from inadequate flare, strut compression, and ostial disease. In these cases, angioplasty or stenting with a reinforcing balloon-expandable stent may be recommended.

Postoperative Complications

- Spinal cord injury
- Stroke
- Cardiac events (myocardial infarction, arrhythmias, congestive heart failure)
- Pulmonary complications (pneumonia, prolonged ventilation, tracheostomy)
- Gastrointestinal complications (ileus, pancreatitis, cholecystitis)
- Systemic inflammatory response (fever, leukocytosis, thrombocytopenia)
- Renal function deterioration
- Access-related problems (bleeding, thrombosis, pseudoaneurysm)

ACKNOWLEDGEMENT

We gratefully acknowledge the contributions of Gustavo S. Oderich and Karina S. Kanamori as portions of their chapter were retained in this revision.

REFERENCES

1. Park JH, Chung JW, Choo IW, et al. Fenestrated stent-grafts for preserving visceral arterial branches in the treatment of abdominal aortic aneurysms: preliminary experience. *J Vasc Interv Radiol*. 1996;7(6):819-823.
2. Nordon IM, Hinchliffe RJ, Holt PJ, et al. Modern treatment of juxtarenal abdominal aortic aneurysms with fenestrated endografting and open repair—a systematic review. *Eur J Vasc Endovasc Surg*. 2009;38(1):35-41.
3. Coles-Black J, Barber T, Bolton D, Chuen J. A systematic review of three-dimensional printed template-assisted physician-modified stent grafts for fenestrated endovascular aneurysm repair. *J Vasc Surg*. 2021;74:296-306.
4. Chaikof EL, Dalman RL, Eskandari MK, et al. The Society for Vascular Surgery practice guidelines on the care of patients with an abdominal aortic aneurysm. *J Vasc Surg*. 2018;67:2-77.
5. Ketha SS, Warrington KJ, McPhail IR. Inflammatory abdominal aortic aneurysm: a case report and review of the literature. *Vasc Endovasc Surg*. 2014;48:65-69.
6. Squizzato F, Oderich GS, Balachandran P, Tenorio ER, Mendes BC, De Martino RR. Effect of aortic angulation on the outcomes of fenestrated-branched endovascular aortic repair. *J Vasc Surg*. 2021;74:372-382.
7. Katsargyris A, Marques de Marino P, Verhoeven EL. Graft design and selection of fenestrations vs. branches for renal and mesenteric incorporation in endovascular treatment of pararenal and thoracoabdominal aortic aneurysms. *J Cardiovasc Surg*. 2019;60:35-40.
8. Mendes BC, Oderich GS, Correa MP, et al. Endovascular repair of complex aortic pathology. *Curr Surg Rep*. 2013;1(2):67-77.
9. Greenberg RK, Sternbergh III WC, Makaroun M, et al. Intermediate results of a United States multicenter trial of fenestrated endograft repair for juxtarenal abdominal aortic aneurysms. *J Vasc Surg*. 2009;50(4):730-737.
10. Aucoin VJ, Eagleton MJ, Farber MA, et al. Spinal cord protection practices used during endovascular repair of complex aortic aneurysms by the US Aortic Research Consortium. *J Vasc Surg*. 2021;73:323-330.
11. Bradley NA, Orawiec P, Bhat R, Pal S, Suttie SA, Flett MM, Guthrie GJK. Mid-term follow-up of percutaneous access for standard and complex EVAR using the ProGlide device. *Surgeon*. doi:10.1016/j.surge.2021.03.005
12. Dowdall JF, Greenberg RK, West K, et al. Separation of components in fenestrated and branched endovascular grafting—branch protection or a potentially new mode of failure? *Eur J Vasc Endovasc Surg*. 2008;36(1):2-9.
13. Wang SK, Lemmon GW, Gupta AK, et al. Aggressive surveillance is needed to detect endoleaks and junctional separation between device components after zenith fenestrated aortic reconstruction. *Ann Vasc Surg*. 2019;57:129-136.
14. Barrett T, Khwaja A, Carmona C, et al. Acute kidney injury: prevention, detection, and management. Summary of updated NICE guidance for adults receiving iodine-based contrast media. *Clin Radiol*. 2021;76:193-199.
15. Mezzetto L, Mastrorilli D, Abatucci G, et al. Impact of cone beam computed tomography in advanced endovascular aortic aneurysm repair using latest generation 3D c-arm. *Ann Vasc Surg*. 2021;78:132-140. doi:10.1016/j.avsg.2021.04.035

16. Wanhainen A, Verzini F, Van Herzeele I, et al. Editor's choice – European Society for Vascular Surgery (ESVS) 2019 clinical practice guidelines on the management of abdominal aorto-iliac artery aneurysms. *Eur J Vasc Endovasc Surg*. 2019;57:8-93.
17. Oderich GS, Tenorio ER, Mendes BC, et al. Midterm outcomes of a prospective, nonrandomized study to evaluate endovascular repair of complex aortic aneurysms using fenestrated-branched endografts. *Ann Surg*. 2021;274:491-499.
18. Hostralich A, Mesnard T, Soler R, et al. Prospective multicentre cohort study of fenestrated and branched endografts after failed endovascular infrarenal aortic aneurysm repair with type Ia endoleak. *Eur J Vasc Endovasc Surg*. 2021;62:540-548.
19. Diamond KR, Simons JP, Crawford AS, et al. Effect of thoracoabdominal aortic aneurysm extent on outcomes in patients undergoing fenestrated/branched endovascular aneurysm repair. *J Vasc Surg*. 2021;74:833-842.
20. Mastracci TM, Greenberg RK, Eagleton MJ, et al. Durability of branches in branched and fenestrated endografts. *J Vasc Surg*. 2013;57(4):926-933; discussion 933.
21. Edman NI, Schanzer A, Crawford A, et al. Sex-related outcomes after fenestrated-branched endovascular repair for thoracoabdominal aortic aneurysms in the US Fenestrated and Branched Aortic Research Consortium. *J Vasc Surg*. 2021;74:861-870.

SECTION IV: Visceral and Renal Artery Disease Management

Chapter **16**

Stenting, Endografting, and Embolization Techniques: Celiac, Mesenteric, Splenic, Hepatic, and Renal Artery Disease Management

Mohamed A. Zayed and Ronald L. Dalman

DEFINITION

- The content discussed in the following text presupposes familiarity with basic wire and catheter-based endovascular techniques. For a summary of such techniques, the reader may refer to excellent existing references.[1]
- Various occlusive and/or aneurysmal disease processes in renal and visceral arteries may necessitate endovascular interventions (**TABLE 1**).
- Progressive renal artery stenosis (RAS) or occlusion may predispose to renovascular hypertension (RVH; most common form of secondary hypertension) and ischemic nephropathy.[2] Aortic atherosclerosis at the ostia or proximal renal artery accounts for two-thirds of cases.[3] Fibromuscular dysplasia (FMD) also causes progressive serial stenoses throughout the renal arteries and may also predispose to RVH. FMD occurs most commonly in younger female patients.[4]
- Acute mesenteric ischemia (AMI) and chronic mesenteric ischemia (CMI) are life threatening but fortunately rate conditions (1 in 1000 and 1 in 100,000 hospital admissions, respectively).[5,6] The infrequent nature of symptomatic mesenteric ischemia may be due to the rich collateral supply derived from the celiac, superior, and inferior mesenteric arteries. CMI most commonly develops following progressive atherosclerotic occlusion of two or more mesenteric arteries, with the superior mesenteric artery (SMA) being the most critical of the three. Arterial embolization, leading to acute occlusion of the celiac artery or SMA, more commonly is associated with AMI.[6] In rare circumstances, in critically ill patients, impaired intestinal perfusion due to arterial vasospasm may occur in the absence of thromboembolic occlusion.
- Extra- and intraparenchymal renal artery branch aneurysms occur with a reported autopsy incidence between 0.01% and 0.7% and may arise from various disease etiologies.[7] Overall, the risk of acute clinical evolution (rupture or thrombosis) is low but may be increased during pregnancy, with high resultant maternal and fetal mortality. The risk of progression/rupture, as is the case in most visceral artery aneurysms, is presumed to decline significantly following menopause.
- Aneurysms of the celiac artery, SMA, and their branches are also infrequent and associated with varying etiologic entities. Splenic artery aneurysms are the most common (60%), followed by aneurysms in the hepatic (20%), superior mesenteric, and celiac arteries, in that order.[8,9] Syndromes such as polyarteritis nodosa or Kawasaki disease may be associated with aneurysms in various segments of the mesenteric arterial circulation. Guidelines for intervention vary,[10] depending on aneurysm location, rate of enlargement, symptom status, and demographic considerations: age, gender, and menstruation status.

Table 1: Renal/Visceral Arterial Disease

Causes of renal/visceral artery stenosis or occlusion	• Atherosclerosis • Fibromuscular dysplasia • Dissection • Coarctation syndromes • Extrinsic compression • Vasculitis • Hypercoagulable state
Causes of renal/visceral artery aneurysm	• Extension of aortic aneurysmal disease • Atherosclerotic degeneration • Blunt or penetrating trauma • Fibromuscular dysplasia • Connective tissue disorder • Iatrogenic injury

PATIENT HISTORY AND PHYSICAL FINDINGS

- RVH, with or without concurrent evidence of ischemic nephropathy, is seen in less than 50% of individuals manifesting severe RAS.[2,3] Hypertension in children, new onset hypertension in individuals younger than 30 or older than 55 years old, or accelerated hypertension should prompt suspicion for the presence of RAS. Older patients with RVH/RAS typically manifest other stigmata of systemic vascular disease, including coronary and cerebrovascular disease, in addition to peripheral vascular disease. In patients with severe bilateral RAS, renal failure may be exacerbated with recent initiation of an angiotensin-converting enzyme (ACE) inhibitor.[11] Acute exacerbations of poorly controlled RVH may manifest with "hypertensive crisis," flash pulmonary edema, or neurologic symptoms ranging from headache to seizure and stroke. Physical examination may reveal severe elevation of both systolic and diastolic blood pressures, abdominal bruits, and other manifestations of peripheral arterial occlusive disease.

- Patients with CMI are typically elderly and have a prior history of symptomatic vascular disease. Like RAS/RVH patients, CMI rarely is present without other signs and symptoms of advanced vascular disease, including aortic and mesenteric branch arterial calcification on plain x-ray films of the abdomen. Symptoms produced by CMI are frequently nonspecific and intermittent, leading to delayed diagnosis and disease progression. Classical symptoms usually include postprandial dull/crampy midepigastric abdominal pain, progressive weight loss, and "food fear" with decreased caloric intake.[12] Findings on physical examination are usually noncontributory, similar to those related to advanced peripheral arterial disease (eg, absent pedal pulses); patients frequently are malnourished and cachectic. Abdominal auscultation frequently reveals hyperactive bowel sounds, and a bruit may sometimes be auscultated.
- AMI presents more dramatically, with sudden onset of abdominal pain, often in patients suffering acute embolic occlusion of the SMA. Although pain may seem out of proportion to objective physical examination findings initially, progressive tenderness to palpation and ultimately peritoneal signs develop in parallel with diminishing bowel viability. Clinical status also rapidly deteriorates, with progressive metabolic acidosis, shock, and multisystem organ failure.[6]
- Patients with renal artery aneurysms (RAAs) may provide a history of trauma, arterial dissection, syndromic vascular conditions, connective tissue disorders, or RAS. The majority of RAAs are asymptomatic at the time of diagnosis, identified as incidental findings on cross-sectional imaging studies ordered for unrelated indications. Specific associated historical and physical findings are rare but may include acute onset hypertension, abdominal distension, flank pain, hematuria, syncope, and shock. Occasionally, an abdominal pulsatile mass is present on physical examination.[7] Although not always fatal, RAA rupture, particularly those in segmental branches, frequently predisposes to renal infarction and resultant decrease in glomerular filtration capacity.
- Patients with aneurysms of the celiac and SMAs and derived branches may manifest with a history of arterial dissection, trauma, pancreatitis, or other local inflammatory processes or infections. One-third of patients may also have aneurysmal disease in other segments of their arterial anatomy.[8] As is the case with RAAs, patients rarely present with symptoms other than rupture, which itself is also rare. Free rupture may result in hemoperitoneum, hematobilia, or life-threatening gastrointestinal hemorrhage. The risk of rupture is highest with hepatic (20%-44% of mesenteric arterial aneurysm ruptures) and splenic artery aneurysms, the latter notoriously at risk during the third trimester of pregnancy.[13,14] Presence of a splenic artery aneurysm recognized during pregnancy should prompt consideration of immediate repair, regardless of the status of the pregnancy.[15]

IMAGING AND OTHER DIAGNOSTIC STUDIES

- Renal artery disease assessment usually begins with duplex ultrasonography, which has a reported sensitivity of 86% to 93%, specificity of 98%, and overall accuracy of 96%.[16] Duplex criteria used to diagnose more than 60% RAS include an arterial peak systolic velocity of more than 180 to 200 cm per second, a ratio of renal artery to aortic peak systolic velocity of more than 3.5, or acceleration time between onset and peak of systole of more than 100 m per second. Kidney length and resistive indexes derived from parenchymal insonation may also provide important insight into the presence, nature, and severity of end-organ disease.
- Similarly, duplex ultrasound provides a useful, noninvasive method of assessing for the presence of chronic mesenteric occlusive disease.[17] In the celiac artery, peak systolic velocities of more than 200 cm per second provides a sensitivity and accuracy for detecting a greater than 70% stenosis of 87% and 82%, respectively. In the SMA, peak systolic velocities of more than 275 cm per second provides a sensitivity and accuracy for detecting a greater than 70% stenosis of 92% and 96%, respectively.
- Computed tomography angiography (CTA) is the current gold standard for confirming the presence, severity, and extent of occlusive mesenteric vascular disease. CTA-derived images also provide insights into the potential underlying mechanism of occlusion, including FMD, associated dissection, evidence of inflammation/infection, or thromboembolic occlusion. Moreover, three-dimensional reconstructions generated from CTA datasets also provide valuable guidance for preprocedural planning. In emergent circumstances, such as those associated with suspected AMI, CTA usually represents the "go-to" diagnostic test.
- For patients with contrast allergies or other contraindications to computed tomography (CT) scanning, magnetic resonance angiography (MRA) may provide a suitable alternative, particularly for initial diagnosis and screening purposes. Overall resolution of MRA is not equal to that of CTA, and in some circumstances may not provide sufficient detail for the precise surgical or interventional planning.

SURGICAL MANAGEMENT

Patient Selection

- Appropriate patient selection for endovascular intervention is paramount and dependent on therapeutic indication, anatomy, patient comorbidities, and acuity of the disease process. In the following text, we discuss considerations for patients with renal/mesenteric arterial occlusive disease, followed by considerations for patients with renal/mesenteric arterial aneurysmal disease.
- For RAS, the indication for endovascular intervention is contingent on severity of stenosis, the presence and severity of presumed resulting hypertension, and extent of residual glomerular filtration capacity. For RAS, there is no accepted indication currently for "prophylactic" intervention. Endovascular intervention is considered only in patients with severe hypertension, who have failed medical management with at least three concurrent antihypertensive medications or have demonstrated progressive loss of renal

function due to ischemic nephropathy in the setting of more than 60% RAS. The future role for endovascular intervention in treating RVH has been called into question by level I data demonstrating only modest reductions in blood pressure following renal artery stenting.[18]

- Patients with critical stenosis or occlusion of at least two mesenteric arteries, in the setting of signs and symptoms consistent with CMI, are also potential candidates for endovascular management. Patients with atypical symptoms who may meet anatomic criteria for mesenteric occlusive disease often experience disappointing results following endovascular intervention.
- Given the compromises inherent in management of AMI, often in the setting of uncertain bowel viability, hybrid open and endovascular approaches may represent the safest and most expeditious option. Particularly in regard to "acute-on-chronic" occlusion of the proximal SMA, with a patent distal segment preserved by collateral flow, surgical exposure at celiotomy enables distal SMA cannulation and sheath placement. Standard angiographic techniques are then employed to cross the occlusive proximal lesion in a retrograde fashion, with subsequent angioplasty and stenting performed to restore pulsatile antegrade flow.[19] We have employed this technique reliably under a variety of challenging clinical conditions with consistently good results.
- In patients with disease in multiple mesenteric arterial segments and symptoms concerning for mesenteric ischemia, SMA revascularization, either via endovascular or open surgical approaches, represents the most reliable and effective method for resolving critical mid- and distal gut ischemia. Decompressive laparotomy should always be considered as an essential adjunct in these circumstances, regardless of revascularization method used, to facilitate selective resection of nonviable bowel if needed and limit the noxious effects of abdominal compartment syndrome in these already compromised patients.
- In comparison, the safety and use of primary inferior mesenteric artery (IMA) endovascular intervention remains controversial in patients with disease in multiple mesenteric arteries. Recent series report relatively frequent procedure-related complications and poor outcomes following attempted IMA intervention.[20] These results may in part be due to the progressive nature of occlusive vascular disease in the most distal aortic segment at the level of the IMA and resulting difficulty in resolving significant ostial stenoses with even high-pressure angioplasty techniques.
- The criteria for elective repair of asymptomatic RAAs are controversial. Recommendations vary for intervention based on aneurysm diameter, also taking into account the size of the parent artery, extent of mural calcification, and rate of enlargement, if available. Consensus exists regarding treatment for all aneurysms larger than 3 cm in diameter.[21,22] Similarly, patients with intact but symptomatic true aneurysms, recent-onset false (pseudo-) aneurysms, and aneurysms resulting from associated FMD are also typically repaired promptly, given their presumed higher risk of rupture. RAAs in women of childbearing age with plans for future pregnancies are usually repaired, when recognized, at almost any size. Less agreement is present for RAAs larger than 2 cm but smaller than 3 cm in diameter, with treatment recommendations often customized based on individual circumstances.
- There are no set size criteria for visceral artery aneurysm repair. Although larger aneurysms are thought to have an increased potential risk of rupture, small visceral artery aneurysms are also known to rupture and manifest with life-threatening hemorrhage. Therefore, most visceral aneurysms larger than 2 cm should be repaired when identified. This recommendation does not necessarily apply to poststenotic arterial dilations (not true aneurysms) and distal SMA aneurysms. The latter are generally best managed by embolization and/or resection of the dependent loops of adjacent small intestine. In most circumstances, ruptured visceral artery aneurysms are best managed by open or hybrid approaches, allowing for assessment of bowel or end-organ ischemia in conjunction with restoration of arterial flow.

Preoperative Planning

- Prior to attempted repair or exclusion, aneurysm location and access issues should be precisely determined via cross-sectional imaging studies. Luminal plaque, thrombus burden, associated aneurysms, and pre-existing dissections should also be noted. Finally, target vessel diameter should be determined at several intervals before, within, and after the lesion of interest to optimize coil, stent, and graft selection.
- The preferred method of critical renal artery ostial lesion management is by balloon-expandable stent placement. In rare circumstance, angioplasty predilation may be required to advance the appropriate stent through the renal ostia and across the stenotic lesion. Renal artery stents range from 10 to 30 mm in length and 4 to 7 mm in diameter. Transfemoral approaches to the renal artery are generally preferred due to the shorter distance to target, smaller imaging fields, and abundant availability of purpose-specific instrumentation. However, cephalad angulation of the renal artery origins relative to the aorta, the presence of extensive infrarenal aortoiliofemoral arterial occlusive disease, or significant iliac artery tortuosity may favor consideration of the left brachial artery and descending thoracic aorta as the preferred route of access.
- For the treatment of mid- to distal RAS in the setting of FMD, angioplasty alone is generally the preferred treatment modality. Either transfemoral or transbrachial approaches may be considered, depending on the considerations noted earlier. Care must be taken to minimize procedural trauma with precise determination of target artery diameter and selection of appropriately sized instruments (sheaths, balloons, and stents). Poor planning or ill-considered procedural technique may precipitate arterial dissection, thrombosis, and renal infarction.
- Depending on the degree of lesional calcification, the extent of associated juxtaostial aortic occlusive disease, lesion length, and associated target vessel tortuosity, balloon- or self-expanding stent grafts may be chosen for luminal reconstitution and may provide improved long-term patency in the proximal SMA.[23] Cannulation of either the celiac or SMA may be achieved from both femoral and brachial approaches. However, in emergent or extenuating circumstances, left brachial access often proves more expeditious and effective. This is particularly true in the setting of high-grade ostial

stenosis or occlusion, where brachial access and antegrade aortic sheath placement may provide improved guidewire, sheath, and crossing catheter pushability and trackability.

- Successful wire cannulation of ostial SMA and celiac lesions may require "telescoping" techniques with different sheath and wire combinations (see in the following text). This is also true of attempts to deploy devices in the mid- and distal splenic artery, where a triaxial catheter and sheath combination extending into the target lesion is frequently most effective. Given the short and often tortuous nature of the celiac artery, stable sheath placement is challenging, often representing the most difficult aspect of the procedure.
- Similar principles are used when treating aneurysms of renal and visceral arteries, including precise catheter positioning and stable sheath support. Aneurysm size, location, neck anatomy, and extent of tortuosity of feeding target vessels impact the strategy of repair. For example, for large retropancreatic splenic artery aneurysms, coil embolization of the aneurysm sac (preferably with large-end-first or nesting coils) prior to covered stent placement across the ostium of the aneurysm is necessary to ensure long-term procedural success. For precise embolization of shallow or wide-necked aneurysms, adjuncts such as distal balloon occlusion with deployment of detachable coils may be necessary. For more accessible aneurysms with a wide-based aneurysm neck, bare metal stenting may be performed across the ostium of the aneurysm first, followed by placement of coils through the open interstices of the stent to keep the coils localized to the area of interest. Branch artery aneurysms usually occur at bifurcation points and are accompanied by small, well-defined necks and are ideally suited for embolization with microcoils (0.018–in catheter compatible) delivered through a triaxial delivery system.
- The preferred size/shape of embolization devices or covered stents may be either accurately estimated from a preprocedural CT arteriogram or determined at the time of angiographic imaging and sheath placement. Based on these measurements, coil and plug diameters may be oversized by 20% of the target vessel diameter. The length of coils selected is derived from the anticipated arterial lumen surface area that requires embolization. Similarly, the length of vascular plugs selected depends on the target artery to be embolized and the estimated luminal flow. For example, higher flow arteries, such as those proximal to arteriovenous fistulae, usually need more extensive coverage to ensure definitive occlusion. Both self-expanding and balloon-expandable stent grafts are available. The former are also typically oversized by 20%, and the latter are usually sized 1 mm greater than the target artery diameter. Attention should be given to the sheath selection to ensure adequate diameter and length. The device-specific instructions for use (IFU) should be consulted in all circumstances prior to use of occlusion devices, or more generally, any endovascular device with the potential risk for significant vascular injury.
- Depending on their specific location, some visceral artery aneurysms may be embolized without specific end-organ ischemic injury. However, embolization of distal aneurysms, such as those located within the splenic hilum, may result in splenic infarction, further bleeding, or abscess formation. Therefore, splenectomy remains a viable alternative method of splenic artery aneurysm management for many patients. Appropriate vaccinations should be administered with sufficient lead time to allow for an appropriate immunization response prior to elective splenic artery embolization procedures or planned splenectomy.

Operating Room Setup

- Procedures may be performed in an angiography suite, or in an operating room, equipped with a floating-point carbon fiber, radiolucent operating table; fluoroscopy platform; and monitor-viewing bank. However, for precise visceral artery interventions requiring steep oblique/lateral imaging and higher fluoroscopic kilovolt (kV), portable systems in the operating room setting may not provide sufficient image clarity and resolution. Under these circumstances, use of a fixed-imaging system, either in an angiography suite or hybrid operating room, will maximize the likelihood of success.
- For the majority of elective renal and visceral artery interventions, conscious sedation with a combination of short-acting analgesic and sedative agents will provide adequate patient comfort, immobility, and optimal imaging parameters. Standard patient safety measures for conscious sedation, including supplemental oxygen, standard monitoring, and availability of resuscitation equipment should be employed in compliance with local hospital policy. However, general anesthesia is clearly indicated to facilitate treatment of AMI, urgent/emergent management of aneurysm rupture, and/or hemorrhage potentially requiring bowel resection or open conversion.
- For the most part, all renal and visceral artery endovascular interventions can be performed with the patient in the supine position. The left arm may be positioned out at 90° to allow for transbrachial interventions. If a transfemoral intervention is planned, the patient's arms may be extended over the head to aid with image clarity; however, most patients can only tolerate this for certain time periods prior to fatigue. Placing the patient in a 30° rotation to the right, on bolsters placed behind the left flank, at the time of the procedure, will facilitate "true lateral" position to localize and cannulate the origin of the SMA without requiring the image intensifier and radiation source to be in full horizontal position and limiting operator access to the patient as a result.
- In addition to a full array of complementary wires, catheters, and sheaths, premounted balloon-expandable stents and stent grafts should be available, including in low-profile platforms (0.014 in or 0.018 in). Appropriate sizes of coils and plugs should also be identified and readily available.

RENAL ARTERY ANGIOPLASTY AND STENTING

First Step

- For arterial access, a retrograde transfemoral approach is usually selected; however, antegrade transbrachial access may improve accessibility and sheath stability in the presence of significant abdominal/pelvic girth, significantly down-sloping renal arteries, or tortuosity/obstruction of the distal aorta or iliac arteries.
- Arterial access is usually obtained percutaneously using standard Seldinger technique. Bedside ultrasound may facilitate precise placement. Once an interventional sheath access is placed, intravenous unfractionated heparin is administered to maintain an activated clotting time (ACT) of more than 250 seconds.

Second Step

- Wire access to the pararenal aorta may be achieved with 0.035-in guidewire. A 4- or 5-French (Fr) flush catheter is advanced over the guidewire to approximately the level of the first lumbar vertebral body.
- If renal function permits, a complete aortoiliac arteriogram in anterior–posterior image intensifier orientation should be performed to assess both the renal arteries and renal accessory arteries. A power injector should be used for the road map aortogram, using a high injection rate (eg, 15-20 mL per second) and low volume (eg, 10-15 mL). Breath-holding instructions should be given to the patient or the assisting anesthesiologist to allow for aortogram acquisition during end expiration. Glucagon (0.25-2 mg intravenous; approximately 10 minutes preprocedure) can also be administered to diminish intestinal motility and enhance arterial visualization.
- A magnified angiogram can be repeated in areas of interest and intended treatment. For better visualization of the renal artery, the image intensifier should be oriented with a few degrees in cranial and lateral obliquity ipsilateral to the renal artery of interest.
- Intraoperative angiographic measurements are obtained to confirm device selection. A marked flush catheter or radiopaque ruler may facilitate accurate angiographic measurements.

Third Step

- A stiff 0.035-in guidewire (ie, Amplatz, Rosen) is placed in the pararenal aorta to facilitate advancement of a 45-cm 8-Fr renal dilation guide catheter (RDC), or 6-Fr RDC sheath (ie, Terumo Pinnacle destination or Cook Ansel Flexor). The sheath dilator tip should not be advanced into the target vessel to avoid compromise of the residual vessel lumen.
- Wire cannulation of the renal artery is the essential first step. Depending on the angle of entry at the orifice, a number of different catheter tip shapes may facilitate successful renal cannulation (Sos 1 or 2, Cobra, Vanchi, etc.). Once cannulated, the sheath tip is advanced immediately adjacent to, but not across, the renal artery orifice (**FIGURE 1**). A 0.014-in or 0.018-in stiff guidewire with a floppy or hydrophilic tip is then employed to probe across areas of severe stenosis, through a reverse curve or angled catheter, depending on the optimal angle for access. Alternatively, a 0.035-in guidewire, with improved handling and radiopacity, may provide suitable trackability for less critical stenoses.
- Once access is achieved, the wire should be advanced to a secondary branch to optimize positional stability. Care should be taken to maintain wire tip visualization in the field of view, particularly when using hydrophilic guidewires, as they can easily perforate parenchymal arterioles when advanced too

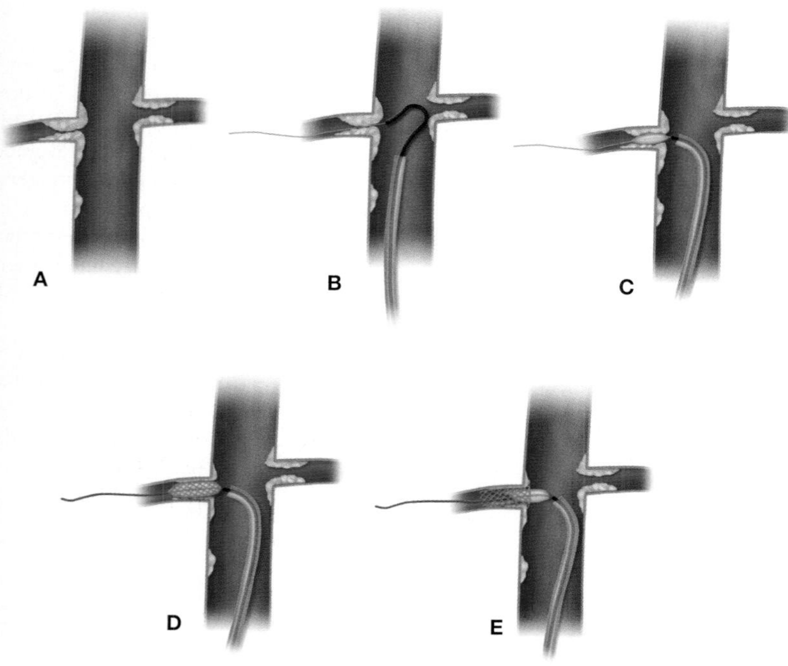

FIGURE 1 ● **A,** Pararenal aorta demonstrating high-grade stenosis at the right renal artery orifice. **B,** Cannulation of the right renal artery with a 0.014-in or 0.018-in Glidewire guided by a curved-tip catheter. Wire and catheter cannulation system are stabilized by a 6-Fr sheath. The cannulating wire is advanced into the distal right renal artery to provide additional stability to the system. **C,** The right renal artery orifice stenosis is predilated with a low-profile, small-diameter balloon. **D,** Using sheath support for stability, an appropriately sized balloon-expandable stent is deployed across the stenosis and is protruding 1 mm into the aortic lumen. **E,** While maintaining cannulation system, protruding edge of the stent is flared into the aortic lumen with an appropriate compliant angioplasty balloon.

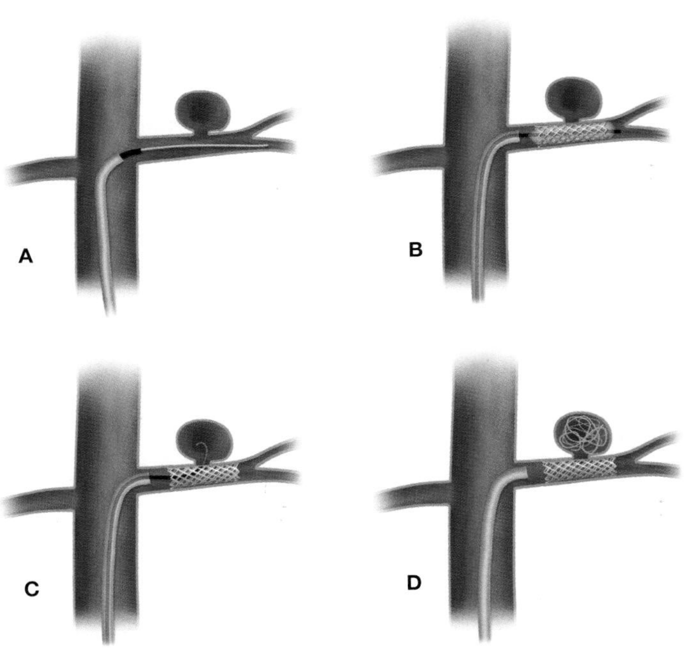

FIGURE 2 ● **A,** Left renal artery has an associated saccular aneurysm. Cannulation of the left renal artery is facilitated with an angled guidewire and curved-tip catheter. The cannulation system is stabilized by an appropriately sized sheath. **B,** A bare metal stent is deployed across the origin of the left RAA. **C,** A telescoping technique is used to cannulate the aneurysm sac through an interstice of the bare metal stent. Sheath tip is advanced to the renal artery orifice and catheter is advanced up to the inner luminal wall of the bare metal stent to stabilize and facilitate cannulation of the aneurysm sac. **D,** Appropriately sized coils are deployed into the aneurysm sac through the stent interstices.

far into the segmental renal circulation. Parenchymal perforation may precipitate intra- or extracapsular hematoma formation, renal hemorrhage, and circulatory collapse unless immediately recognized and corrected.

Fourth Step

- Prior to renal artery stenting, predilation may be necessary to provide sufficient luminal space for delivery of the crimped stent/delivery catheter (**FIGURE 1**). A 2- to 4-mm low-profile, semicompliant, or coronary balloon compatible with a 0.014-in or 0.018-in system can be used for this purpose. Care needs to be taken to maintain wire position during subsequent stent exchange; loss of wire position here can preclude stent delivery or precipitate luminal thrombosis if aortic and/or orificial atheroma is displaced by predilation.
- Using a low-profile 0.014-in or 0.018-in system (rapid exchange or over the wire [OTW]), a balloon-expandable stent (eg, Cordis Palmaz Blue, Boston Scientific Express SD, Cook Formula) is delivered across the lesion (**FIGURE 1**). The low-profile nature of these devices enables facile placement, as well as contrast delivery across the lesion to confirm appropriate position. Rapid exchange or monorail systems allow for shorter wire length, aiding procedural efficiency vis-à-vis catheter/wire/device exchanges. In contrast, OTW devices provide improved pushability and trackability across constricting lesions.
- For mid- or distal RAS, the shortest balloon-expandable stent length providing complete coverage should be selected. For mid- or distal RAAs, appropriate length self-expanding or balloon-expandable stent grafts should be selected to provide adequate pre- and postaneurysm renal artery sealing zones (**FIGURE 2**).
- Following stent placement under fluoroscopic guidance, the balloon should be deflated fully prior to its withdrawal to avoid movement or dislodging of the stent. Areas with substantial tortuosity may precipitate arterial kinking at the transition point between stented and nonstented segments. Excessive oversizing, or overinflation of stents mounted on semicompliant balloons, may promote renal artery injury, dissection, or thrombosis. Temptation to optimize the postprocedural angiographic image, potentially at the expense of vessel integrity or anticipated long-term patency, should also be avoided.
- For ostial renal artery lesions, the balloon-expandable stent should be positioned so that the aortic end is deployed approximately 1 mm into the aortic flow stream. The aortic edge of the stent can be "flared" outward with a repeat angioplasty using the distal edge of the same balloon (**FIGURE 1**).

Fifth Step

- After successful deployment, the sheath should only be withdrawn after the completion imaging encompassing the entire ipsilateral kidney is performed to confirm uniform perfusion and absence of parenchymal and/or capsular injury.
- Following withdrawal of the sheath from the renal orifice, while maintaining wire access, completion paraorificial aortography is performed to confirm stent positioning and target lumen diameter. Residual stenosis, kinking, or dissection should be confirmed to be absent prior to withdrawal of the wire.

VISCERAL ARTERY ANGIOPLASTY AND STENTING

First Step

- As previously noted, access considerations need to account for individual patient anatomy, operator experience and skill, available devices, potential complications, goals of treatment, and anticipated time of the procedure. Most internationalists prefer the transfemoral approach for visceral vascular access. However, proximal left brachial artery exposure and puncture often facilitates access to significantly down-sloping or tortuous mesenteric arteries.
- A 4- or 5-Fr sheath is placed in the arterial access site to facilitate advancement of a 4- or 5-Fr marked flush catheter to the paravisceral aorta.
- Intravenous unfractionated heparin is administered after sheath placement to achieve an ACT of more than 250 seconds.

Second Step

- After a standard aortogram, a magnified paravisceral aortogram can be performed with the image intensifier placed in a steep oblique or true lateral position to optimize localization and cannulation of the celiac artery and SMA origins.
- Care should also be taken here to visualize the major branches of the celiac artery and/or SMA. Attempts should be made to visualize the first significant branch of the SMA, usually the middle colic artery, to avoid inadvertent coverage and/or compromise of colonic arterial perfusion as a consequence of planned procedures.
- Visceral lesions of interest can be further characterized at this time by optimizing image intensifier obliquity. Accurate measurements are facilitated by marked flush catheter or radiopaque ruler placement.

Third Step

- After withdrawal of the flush catheter, a stiff guidewire and a long (90 cm), braided 6-Fr sheath (ie, Terumo Pinnacle destination, Cook Ansel Flexor) is advanced to the paravisceral aorta. Various angled sheath tips (ie, straight, angled hockey tip, curved) can be used depending on the degree of visceral artery angulation, aortic diameter, and access approach (femoral or brachial).
- Along with selected sheath, various guide catheter types (ie, angled, vertebral, cobra, RDC, or reverse curved SIM or Sos catheters) can be used to facilitate visceral artery cannulation.

Fourth Step

- An exchange-length, stiff 0.014-in or 0.018-in guidewire, with a floppy tip, is advanced through the preselected catheter and sheath combination. However, wire cannulation of a diseased visceral arteries orifice may be challenging. From the brachial approach, successful cannulation may be facilitated with sheath placement distal to the artery of interest, followed by gradual withdrawal of the sheath with the selected angled catheter inside the sheath protruding slightly outward. When the catheter "clicks" into place, an exploratory hydrophilic guidewire is then gently advanced to obtain luminal access. Once the lumen is cannulated, the guidewire is then advanced to a secondary visceral branch to facilitate catheter and sheath advancement, as indicated (**FIGURE 3**). Another cannulation strategy is to withdraw wire and catheter combinations from a stable sheath position across the anticipated vessel orifice area at various "clock" positions.
- For a "no-touch" technique, a shaped catheter or sheath tip is positioned luminally in direct proximity to the orifice of interest. A 0.014-in or 0.018-in hydrophilic guidewire is then

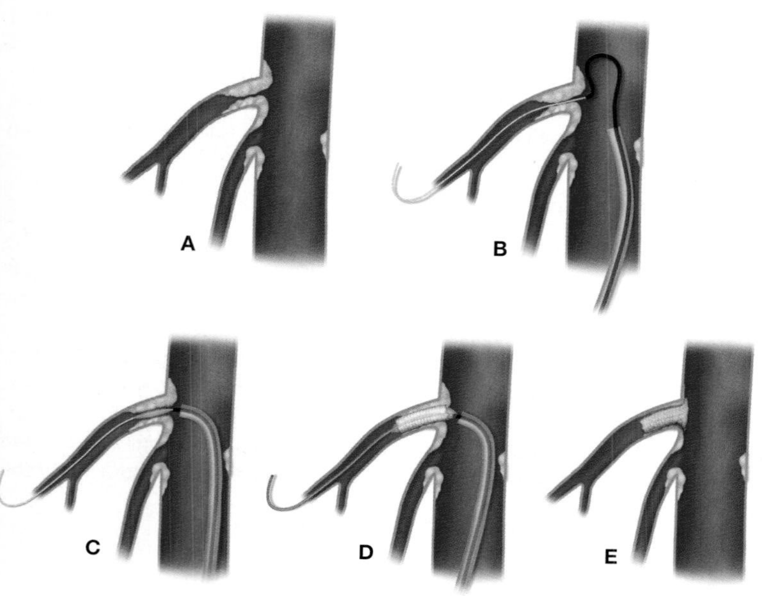

FIGURE 3 ● **A,** High-grade stenosis of the proximal celiac artery origin. **B,** A curved-tip guide catheter is used to facilitate celiac artery cannulated with a 0.014-in or 0.018-in guidewire. The cannulation system is stabilized with distal advancement of the guidewire into a celiac artery branch, as well as maintaining a sheath in the aortic lumen. **C,** A low-profile, compliant predilation balloon may be advanced over the guidewire to dilate the stenosis and provide a tract for future stenting. **D,** An appropriately sized balloon-expandable covered stent graft is deployed across the stenosis while slightly protruding into the aortic lumen. **E,** Full stent apposition following deployment and proximal flaring of the stent graft at the prior stenosis site.

used to localize and facilitate cannulation. To improve trackability and pushability of the system, a stabilizing "buddy" stiff guidewire may also be advanced, when necessary, to "pin" the cannulation sheath to the opposite wall.

- When single-wire cannulation proves inadequate to support catheter and sheath advancement into the target vessel, placement of a second, or even third 0.014-in or 0.018-in wire, across the area of stenosis may facilitate successful catheter/sheath advancement.

Fifth Step

- An appropriately sized self-expanding or balloon-expandable stent graft is preferred for the treatment of visceral artery stenoses. Predilation of the tract may be necessary with a small, low-profile balloon to facilitate advancement of the balloon-expandable stent (**FIGURE 3**).
- The aortic end of a balloon-expandable stent used for the treatment of ostial or proximal visceral artery lesions should be positioned 1 mm into aortic flow lumen, and the stent edge should be flared out with the edge of an angioplasty balloon.
- Accuracy of deployment of self-expanding stent grafts can be improved with partial deployment of the stent while maintaining the cannulation sheath in the orifice of the visceral artery. Once the distal portion of the stent graft is accurately deployed, the remainder of the proximal stent graft can be unsheathed to allow for full deployment. An appropriately sized compliant balloon may then be subsequently used to fully mold the self-expanding stent graft to profile and/or slightly flare the aortic edge.
- For friable lesions, or lesions that may include fresh thrombus, consideration should be given to advancing and deploying balloons and stents over a filter wire (0.014-in eV3 SpiderFX embolic protection system). Although placement of a distal filter may not preclude all embolic sequelae, it may reduce the severity or significance of associated potential complications. This option may be particularly valuable in SMA interventions.

HYBRID REPAIR OF PROXIMAL MESENTERIC ARTERY STENOSIS/OCCLUSION

First Step

- In the setting of acute or acute-on-chronic mesenteric ischemia, where exploratory laparotomy is otherwise indicated to assess bowel viability, a hybrid retrograde catheterization approach is generally preferred. At laparotomy, surgical exposure of the superior mesenteric or celiac artery is obtained. To expose the celiac artery, the left triangular ligament is incised, the left hepatic lobe is retracted to the right, and the gastroesophageal junction is retracted to the left. Further caudal dissection along the surface of the aorta may be used to expose the SMA origin.
- For purposes of both embolectomy and hybrid retrograde catheterization, exposure of the proximal section/midsection of the SMA is preferentially obtained at the superior root of the small bowel mesentery (**FIGURE 4**). This location generally provides access four or more centimeters distal to the SMA orifice, which allows stable sheath positioning to facilitate retrograde cannulation and stenting. Distal to the lower margin of the pancreas, the length of the SMA is limited by early branching of the ileocolic artery and intestinal cascade, so relatively proximal positioning should be achieved to minimize excessive dilation/trauma to the vessel by the sheath.[19]

Second Step

- When embolic occlusion is present, embolectomy is performed gently through an anterior arteriotomy. The tapering nature of the SMA in this area requires gentle catheter withdrawal with gradual balloon deflation in order to avoid iatrogenic arterial damage, dissection, or thrombosis.
- Retrograde cannulation of an exposed distal segment of the target vessel provides optimal access for definitive endovascular intervention. In emergent conditions with compromised intestine, this approach is preferential to open revascularization strategies, which may require prosthetic graft placement following prolonged, extensive dissection of the mesentery and aortic root.
- Retrograde mesenteric cannulation is facilitated by placement of a longitudinal arteriotomy in the exposed distal segment of the target vessel. To reduce the risk of injury to the exposed artery during cannulation, the arteriotomy site is closed with a prosthetic or autogenous patch. The patch itself is then cannulated to facilitate sheath placement, angiogram, stent placement as well as expedited puncture site closure at the end of the procedure (**FIGURE 4**).
- Relatively long sheaths (20 cm or more) should be used during retrograde cannulation to ensure that the operator's hands are clear from the fluoroscopy field and minimize operator radiation exposure during catheterization maneuvers.[19]

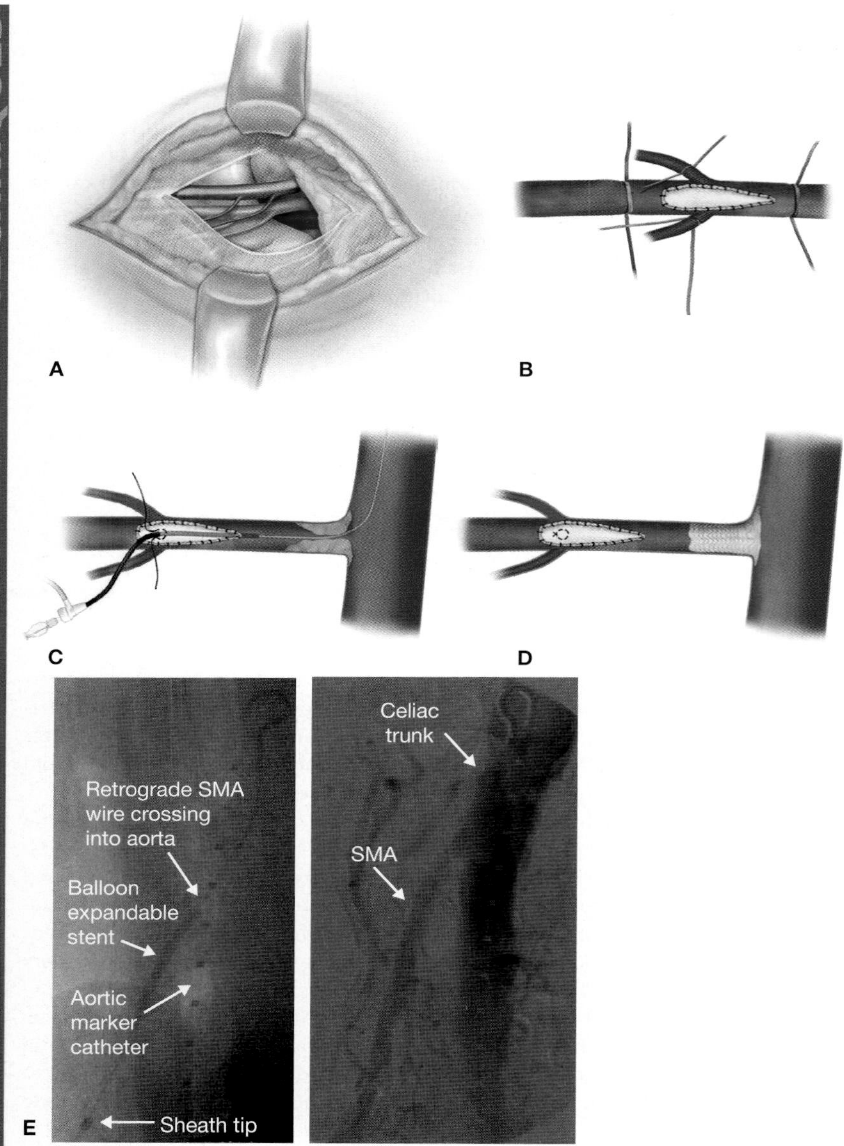

FIGURE 4 ● **A,** Open exposure of the proximal SMA at the caudal portion of the mesenteric root. **B,** The proximal SMA, ~3 to 4 cm from its aortic origin, is circumferentially exposed while preserving its side branches. A longitudinal arteriotomy is created and thrombectomy is performed with patch angioplasty. **C,** Sheath is placed through a puncture in the angioplasty patch and arteriogram is performed to evaluate stenosis in the proximal SMA origin. **D,** A stent is deployed using fluoroscopic guidance at the SMA origin across the identified hemodynamic stenosis. The patch puncture site is repaired to maintain hemostasis. Ei. Retrograde access to SMA, with inflation of balloon expandable stent extending into aorta proximally, spanning length of proximal occlusive lesion. Eii. Completion mesenteric arteriogram from aortic injection, showing complete restoration of mesenteric arterial lumen and normal distal arterial perfusion. Retrograde mesenteric wire has been removed, and arteriotomy closed at the patch site in distal SMA.

RENAL OR VISCERAL ARTERY EMBOLIZATION

First Step

- Arterial access can be secured via either a left brachial artery or transfemoral approach, depending on the intended target vessel and its angulation relative to the aorta.
- For standard coil embolization, a 5- or 6-Fr sheath access will be adequate. However, if an occlusion device will be used, a larger sheath size may be required depending on device specifications.
- Systemic anticoagulation with intravenous unfractionated heparin is also commonly used during these procedures.

Second Step

- Angiographic characterization may require angiograms in multiple different obliquities to fully appreciate size, extent, and angulation of the lesion of interest, particularly those affecting secondary visceral branches. In the angiographic parlance, regarding the extent, severity, and profile of a luminal obstruction, "one view is no view."
- One should note the extent of vascular collateralization associated with the vascular segment that will be embolized.

Third Step

- A telescoping cannulation technique is usually used to enhance the positioning and stability of the embolization system. To perform this, a sheath is advanced as close to the target lesion as possible. A catheter is then extended from beyond the tip of the sheath and used to protrude into target lesion (**FIGURE 5**).
- Embolization of remote target lesions may require higher orders of telescoping. Placing a sheath into another larger sheath, or a 0.018-in microcatheter (ie, Codman Prowler, Cook CXI, BSCI Renegade) into a standard 0.035-in

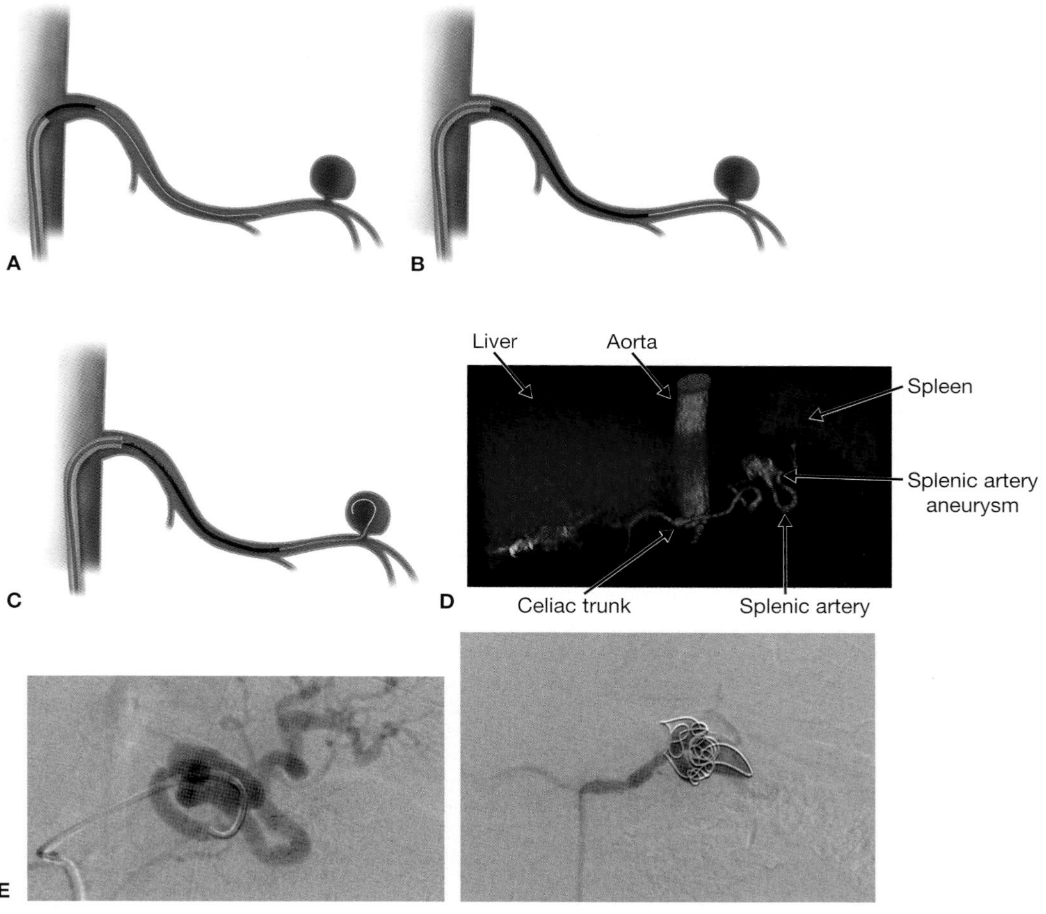

FIGURE 5 ● **A,** Cannulation is attempted of a saccular visceral artery aneurysm. A sheath and angled catheter facilitate cannulation of the visceral artery origin with a guidewire. **B,** A 0.035-In catheter and guidewire negotiate proximal arterial tortuosity. **C,** A microcatheter is telescoped through the 0.035-in catheter to facilitate wire cannulation of the aneurysm. **D,** Three-dimensional abdominal CTA of a female with a mid-splenic artery saccular aneurysm. **E,** Selective splenic artery aneurysm pre- and postselective coiling.

guide catheter, can help access more challenging lesions (**FIGURE 5**). Alternating wire and microcatheter advancements may facilitate cannulation of smaller and more tortuous arteries (such as the superior and inferior gastroduodenal arteries [**FIGURE 6**]) and distal/hilar splenic artery.

- If possible, the cannulation catheter/microcatheter should be advanced into the lesion slightly further than the intended embolization site, because the system can draw back during deployment of coils or plugs.

Fourth Step

- Once the cannulation catheter is positioned in the target lesion, 0.018-in or 0.035-in coils are delivered sequentially into the target area through their respective catheters. For detached coils, the metal tube housing the coil is attached to the back end of the cannulation catheter, and the stiff end of a guidewire is used to push the coil out of its housing unit and into the catheter shaft. The floppy tip of the guidewire is then replaced into the catheter to push the coil along the entire shaft of the catheter and into the lesion (**FIGURE 5**). The stiff end of the guidewire should not be used to push the coil into the lesion because it can change the cannulating catheter tip shape and lead to instability in the cannulation system and maldeployment.
- Alternatively, small aneurysm may be occluded with detachable or nondetachable microcoils or ethylene vinyl alcohol copolymer. IFU are variable and should be referred to for recommended deployment techniques.
- When coil deployment can be accurately localized, and precise coil positioning is critical to the success of the procedure, large-to-small tapered coils should be used. When arterial blood flow is needed/required to carry part of the coil into the preferred deployment location, small-to-large tapered coils are preferred in this situation. Newer "nesting" coils will reform immediately into larger, obstructing profiles. Older tubular coils need to be advanced as they are being deployed to avoid simply lining the target artery without sufficient luminal obstruction. Attention to understanding what coils are in inventory, and how respective coil choices are optimally deployed, is essential for procedural success.

- For larger aneurysms or planned occlusion of an entire vessel lumen, a vascular plug (ie, AGA Medical Amplatzer I or II vascular plug) may be preferable and a more effective means for target embolization. However, plug placement usually requires stable sheath target artery cannulation. Amplatzer I and II vascular plugs are produced in diameters ranging between 4 and 22 mm and lengths ranging between 6 and 18 mm. Recommended device IFU should be consulted to ensure proper device selection and deployment. When sheath access cannot be withdrawn to enable plug deployment, catheter-delivered coils should be deployed instead.
- Once a coil or plug is delivered into a lesion, its position may be modified slightly by catheter tip advancement. This maneuver, when performed properly, maximizes the obstructive surface area and resulting coil thrombogenicity.
- When multiple coils or plugs are used, deployment should also be strategized and deliberate. For example, the first coil should be placed in the deepest part of the lesion (base of an aneurysm), whereas the last coil should be placed in the entry point of the lesion (neck of an aneurysm).
- For acutely bleeding vessels (such as the gastroduodenal arteries in the setting of duodenal ulcerations), a "back-door"–"front-door" approach ensures hemostasis. This involves occluding the culprit vessel pre and post the area of bleeding (**FIGURE 6**). Coiling only one side of the bleeding artery may prevent further access attempts while not providing sufficient vessel occlusion and hemostasis. Small bleeding pelvic arteries may similarly be embolized using a Gelfoam slurry slush preparation.[24] Recommended IFU should be consulted to ensure proper preparation and administration of these slurries.

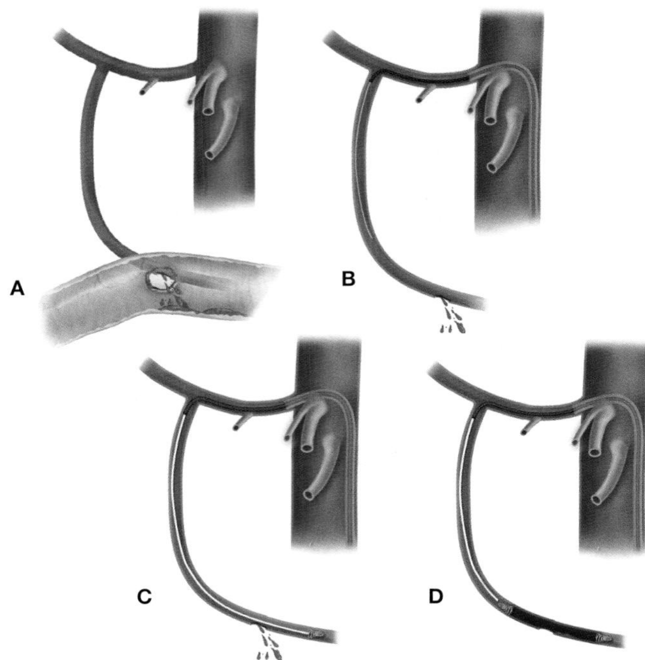

FIGURE 6 ● **A,** Bleeding gastroduodenal artery with an associated duodenal ulceration. **B,** Sheath cannulation of the common hepatic artery branch of the celiac artery, followed by catheter cannulation of the gastroduodenal artery. **C,** Back-door deployment of an embolization coil distal to the angiographically identified bleeding point in the gastroduodenal artery. **D,** Subsequent "front-door" embolization of the feeding segment of the gastroduodenal artery.

Fifth Step

- It is customary to perform postembolization arteriography to confirm final coil/plug positioning. Residual flow will still be evident in the recently embolized vessel segment, because the patient generally remains heparinized during this period of the procedure. If uncertainty persists as to the adequacy of embolization, arteriography may be repeated following reversal of anticoagulation, taking into account increased risks of thrombosis/embolization around the delivery sheaths and catheters proximal to the targeted lesion.

PEARLS AND PITFALLS

Indications	▪ Preoperative imaging (duplex and CTA) should be reviewed in detail to ensure patient suitability and help plan out appropriate intervention. ▪ Combining information gathered from duplex and CTA is beneficial, especially in situations when the stenosis is overestimated due to heavy luminal calcification.
Vessel cannulation	▪ One should note the angulation of the target vessel relative to the aorta. Because this angle may vary with respiration, angiograms should be obtained while the patient is apneic (if intubated) or at end expiration. ▪ Generally, renal arteries and up-sloping visceral vessels may be easier to cannulate from a transfemoral artery approach. Down-sloping renal and visceral vessels may be easier to cannulate from a proximal left brachial artery puncture. ▪ Using an angulated, flexible, low-profile sheath system also aids in the cannulation process.
Angioplasty balloon selection	▪ Care should be taken in selecting appropriate size and types of balloons. ▪ Generally, only low-profile compliant balloons should be used for angioplasty interventions in the renal and visceral arteries. In rare circumstances, a noncompliant balloon may be used to help mold a stent graft to full profile. ▪ Diameter of angioplasty balloon should be estimated relative to adjacent normal vessel lumen. Oversizing is generally not necessary, and a smaller diameter balloon may be preferred when performing angioplasty across highly calcified lesions.

(Continued)

Stent selection	■ Care should also be taken in selecting appropriately sized stents for desired interventions. ■ Stent diameter should be estimated relative to normal vessel lumen diameter adjacent to target lesion to be treated and is generally oversized by approximately 1 mm. ■ Stent length should be estimated relative to the length of the target lesion while providing enough coverage into the adjacent normal vessel lumen (area of needed coverage is variable depending on type of lesion and intervention). ■ Oversized stents are prone to kinking and may risk damaging the target vessel. Undersized stents may lead to maldeployment, migration, and ineffective seal with adjacent vessel lumen. ■ Sometimes, the angioplasty balloon of a balloon-expandable stent gets stuck in the stent during its removal. In this situation, pulling the balloon risks misplacing or dislodging the stent from its desired location. Instead, the operator should ensure complete deflation of the balloon and attempt slowly advancing the balloon while rotating its catheter.
Coil/plug selection	■ Size of coils and plugs should be selected relative to lesion dimensions. Undersized coils and plugs risk migration to unintended vascular beds. ■ Stability of the embolization delivery system should be selected relative to the size of the embolization device. Larger embolization devices may cause instability in low-profile delivery systems.
Renal/visceral artery dissection	■ Sheath and large catheter cannulation of renal and visceral arteries should be avoided to prevent damage or dissection. ■ If a dissection occurs, angiographic evaluation is required to determine whether it is flow limiting. All flow-limiting dissections should be stented with an appropriately sized balloon-expandable stent.
Renal/visceral arterial spasm	■ Arterial spasms may be induced with vessel cannulation, angioplasty, or stenting. Younger patients are typically more prone for this. Arterial vasodilators, such as nitroglycerin or papaverine, may be infused into the vessel lumen by way of cannulation sheath or catheter to help relieve this. ■ The operator should be aware that papaverine may precipitate out of solution if mixed with heparin.
Renal capsular perforation or hematoma	■ This may be caused by inadvertent advancement of cannulating wire into the renal parenchyma. To avoid this complication, always keep the end of the wire in sight during sheath and device advancements over the wire. Also, avoiding the use of straight or angled-tip stiff Glidewires in this circumstance can decrease the risk of this complication. ■ Symptoms of renal capsular hematoma or perforation include abdominal pain and nausea, accompanied by a vasovagal response, which frequently requires aggressive resuscitation and stabilization maneuvers by the interventional team. ■ If this complication is encountered, maintain wire access (do not remove the offending wire) to facilitate a catheter exchange to provide access to coil placement and occlusion of the perforation site. Loss of wire access can further complicate this situation; however, as long as sheath access remains in the renal artery, the relevant segmental branches can be reaccessed for coil delivery.
Removal of malpositioned/misplaced devices	■ All attempts should be made to safely reposition malpositioned/misplaced stents, endografts, coils, or plugs. This may involve secondary cannulations, larger sheath placement, and balloon angioplasty with gentle directional force. ■ If endovascular retrieval or repositioning is unsuccessful, angiographic flow across malpositioned/misplaced devices should be evaluated. If arterial flow is clearly obstructed to unintended vital structures or may become a significant nidus for thrombosis or hemodynamic stenosis, open surgical removal may be indicated or attempted repositioning of devices in areas of less critical hemodynamic significance (eg, iliac arterial system).

POSTOPERATIVE CARE

- At the conclusion of the procedure, hemostasis is achieved with manual compression or, in cases requiring larger than 6-Fr sheath size, closure devices. Heparin reversal with protamine administration is also helpful unless anticoagulation is to be continued following the procedure.
- As is the case with all patients undergoing peripheral arterial intervention in our practice, patients are observed for a 6- to 24-hour period following device placement. During this period, access site hemostasis and ipsilateral pedal perfusion status is monitored periodically, along with hydration status/urine output and signs of unintended end-organ malperfusion.
- Patients treated with renal/visceral artery angioplasty or stenting receive exaggerated antiplatelet therapy in the immediate perioperative period. In our practice, we load patients with 300 mg of Plavix following the procedure, therapy continuing at 75 mg daily for 6 additional weeks.
- Postoperative surveillance of patients with renal/visceral artery interventions is necessary. Duplex evaluation of renal/visceral artery stents 1 to 3 months following intervention is usually recommended, followed by repeat duplex evaluation every 6 months for at least 1 to 2 years. Afterward, stents with no evidence of in-stent restenosis or de novo disease progression may be imaged at yearly intervals. Evidence of restenosis, either by end-organ dysfunction or surveillance

imaging studies, should prompt reevaluation and reintervention as necessary to maintain luminal patency and long-term success.

OUTCOMES

- Endovascular treatment of RAS has a reported technical success rate of 88% to 100%. Treatment effects on hypertension alone are quantitatively modest and inconsistent between studies.[25,26] Improvement in renal function is reported in approximately 25% of patients.
- Treatment of mesenteric occlusive disease has a reported technical success rate of 96%. Postoperative symptom improvement/resolution is reported in approximately 88% of treated patients. Primary patency is estimated at 65% to 92%, with primary assisted patency at 92% to 100%, and secondary patency at 99%.[27,28]
- Embolization and stent graft techniques for repair of renal and visceral artery aneurysms are limited to variably sized retrospective series but with acceptable technical success rates in appropriately selected patients.

COMPLICATIONS

- For renal artery interventions, complications most commonly arise from access site complications, contrast-induced nephropathy, or atheroembolization. Renal artery restenosis is reported between 5% and 66%, depending on duration of follow-up and criteria used for continued surveillance. The perioperative 30-day mortality is estimated at 0% to 5% and survival at 3 years is estimated at 74%.[29] Other less frequent complications include iatrogenic renal parenchymal perforation, capsular hematoma, arterial dissection, thrombosis, or distal plaque embolization into branch or accessory arteries.
- For mesenteric artery interventions, restenosis or occlusion of treated visceral vessels is documented in 10% to 27% of patients,[30] emphasizing the need for continued postprocedural surveillance. Less common complications include mesenteric artery perforation, dissection, or distal parenchymal embolization due to wire/catheter manipulation of areas with fresh thrombus or friable plaque. While treating branch artery aneurysms of the spleen, occasionally, portions of the splenic parenchyma may be lost due to coiling and branch occlusion, with attendant symptoms consistent with segmental splenic infarction.

REFERENCES

1. Schneider PA. *Endovascular Skills, Guidewire and Catheter Skills for Endovascular Surgery*. 3rd ed. Informa Healthcare; 2009.
2. Garovic VD, Textor SC. Renovascular hypertension and ischemic nephropathy. *Circulation*. 2005;112:1362-1374.
3. Hansen KJ, Edwards MS, Craven TE, et al. Prevalence of renovascular disease in the elderly: a population-based study. *J Vasc Surg*. 2002;36:443-451.
4. Beregi JP, Louvegny S, Gautier C, et al. Fibromuscular dysplasia of the renal arteries: comparison of helical CT angiography and arteriography. *AJR Am J Roentgenol*. 1999;172:27-34.
5. McMillan WD, McCarthy WJ, Bresticker MR, et al. Mesenteric artery bypass: objective patency determination. *J Vasc Surg*. 1995;21:729-740.
6. Stoney RJ, Cunningham CG. Acute mesenteric ischemia. *Surgery*. 1993;114:489-490.
7. Tham G, Ekelund L, Herrlin K, et al. Renal artery aneurysms. Natural history and prognosis. *Ann Surg*. 1983;197:348-352.
8. Messina LM, Shanley CJ. Visceral artery aneurysms. *Surg Clin North Am*. 1997;77:425-442.
9. Tessier DJ, Abbas MA, Fowl RJ, et al. Management of rare mesenteric arterial branch aneurysms. *Ann Vasc Surg*. 2002;16:586-590.
10. Chaer RA, Abularrage CJ, Coleman DM, et al. The Society for Vascular Surgery clinical practice guidelines on the management of visceral aneurysms. *J Vasc Surg*. 2020;72:3s-39s.
11. Hobbs SD, Thomas ME, Bradbury AW. Manipulation of the renin angiotensin system in peripheral arterial disease. *Eur J Vasc Endovasc Surg*. 2004;28:573-582.
12. Chang JB, Stein TA. Mesenteric ischemia: acute and chronic. *Ann Vasc Surg*. 2003;17:323-328.
13. Carr SC, Mahvi DM, Hoch JR, et al. Visceral artery aneurysm rupture. *J Vasc Surg*. 2001;33:806-811.
14. Dave SP, Reis ED, Hossain A, et al. Splenic artery aneurysm in the 1990s. *Ann Vasc Surg*. 2000;14:223-229.
15. Selo-Ojeme DO, Welch CC. Review: spontaneous rupture of splenic artery aneurysm in pregnancy. *Eur J Obstet Gynecol Reprod Biol*. 2003;109:124-127.
16. House MK, Dowling RJ, King P, et al. Using Doppler sonography to reveal renal artery stenosis: an evaluation of optimal imaging parameters. *AJR Am J Roentgenol*. 1999;173:761-765.
17. Moneta GL, Lee RW, Yeager RA, et al. Mesenteric duplex scanning: a blinded prospective study. *J Vasc Surg*. 1993;17:79-84.
18. Wheatley K, Ives N, Gray R, et al. Revascularization versus medical therapy for renal-artery stenosis. *N Engl J Med*. 2009;361:1953-1962.
19. Wyers MC, Powell RJ, Nolan BW, et al. Retrograde mesenteric stenting during laparotomy for acute occlusive mesenteric ischemia. *J Vasc Surg*. 2007;45:269-275.
20. Oderich GS. Current concepts in the management of chronic mesenteric ischemia. *Curr Treat Options Cardiovasc Med*. 2010;12:117-130.
21. Pfeiffer T, Reiher L, Grabitz K, et al. Reconstruction for renal artery aneurysm: operative techniques and long-term results. *J Vasc Surg*. 2003;37:293-300.
22. Panayiotopoulos YP, Assadourian R, Taylor PR. Aneurysms of the visceral and renal arteries. *Ann R Coll Surg Engl*. 1996;78:412-419.
23. Tallarita T, Oderich GS, Macedo TA, et al. Reinterventions for stent restenosis in patients treated for atherosclerotic mesenteric artery disease. *J Vasc Surg*. 2011;54:1422-1429.
24. Bauer JR, Ray CE. Transcatheter arterial embolization in the trauma patient: a review. *Semin Intervent Radiol*. 2004;21:11-22.
25. Corriere MA, Pearce JD, Edwards MS, et al. Endovascular management of atherosclerotic renovascular disease: early results following primary intervention. *J Vasc Surg*. 2008;48:580-587.
26. Tuttle KR, Chouinard RF, Webber JT, et al. Treatment of atherosclerotic ostial renal artery stenosis with the intravascular stent. *Am J Kidney Dis*. 1998;32:611-622.
27. Sharafuddin MJ, Olson CH, Sun S, et al. Endovascular treatment of celiac and mesenteric arteries stenoses: applications and results. *J Vasc Surg*. 2003;38:692-698.
28. Sivamurthy N, Rhodes JM, Lee D, et al. Endovascular versus open mesenteric revascularization: immediate benefits do not equate with short-term functional outcomes. *J Am Coll Surg*. 2006;202:859-867.
29. Yutan E, Glickerman DJ, Caps MT, et al. Percutaneous transluminal revascularization for renal artery stenosis: Veterans Affairs Puget Sound Health Care System experience. *J Vasc Surg*. 2001;34:685-693.
30. Brown DJ, Schermerhorn ML, Powell RJ, et al. Mesenteric stenting for chronic mesenteric ischemia. *J Vasc Surg*. 2005;42:268-274.

Chapter 17

Visceral Reconstruction to Facilitate Cancer Management: Celiac, Mesenteric, Splenic, Hepatic, and Renal Artery Disease Management

Arash Fereydooni and E. John Harris Jr.

DEFINITION

- This chapter assumes basic knowledge of surgical oncology principles and the management of patients with intra-abdominal tumor pathology. For further review of these topics, please refer to relevant background sources.[1]
- Advanced primary and recurrent abdominal malignant tumors may frequently involve adjacent arterial and venous structures. Surgical management may require curative en bloc tumor resection, with the goal of achieving negative macroscopic and microscopic margins. Adjunct vascular reconstruction may be necessary to achieve complete tumor removal.
- A wide variety of malignancies may develop in the peritoneal space and retroperitoneum. A representative range of pathologies involving intra-abdominal arterial and venous structures is summarized in **TABLE 1**.
- Primary vascular tumors are exceedingly rare, frequently mimic other oncologic disease processes, and may evolve slowly—leading to delay in diagnosis and treatment. Although most commonly arising from large vessels such as the aorta and vena cava, primary vascular tumors may also originate from distal branches of the iliac, mesenteric, and renal arteries. Classification systems (Wright/Salm classification) have broadly categorized primary vascular tumors as intimal (majority, 70%) and mural.[2]

Table 1: Range of Intra-abdominal Oncological Pathologies That Can Potentially Involve Arterial and Venous Structures

Arterial	
Aorta	Angiosarcoma,[a] paraganglioma, pheochromocytoma, leiomyosarcoma, rhabdomyosarcoma
Superior mesenteric artery	Adenocarcinoma, neuroendocrine carcinoma, adenosquamous carcinoma, cystadenocarcinoma
Iliac artery	Adenocarcinoma, leiomyoma, endometrial stromal carcinoma, fibrosarcoma, fibroma
Venous	
Inferior vena cava	Angiosarcoma,[a] adrenocortical carcinoma, teratoma, Wilms tumor, pheochromocytoma, neuroendocrine carcinoma, intestinal carcinoma, hepatocellular carcinoma
Renal vein	Renal cell carcinoma, adrenocortical carcinoma, pheochromocytoma
Portal vein	Adenoma, adenocarcinoma, cholangiocarcinoma, neuroendocrine carcinoma, hepatocellular carcinoma
Iliac vein	Intestinal carcinoma, leiomyoma, endometrial stromal carcinoma, fibrosarcoma, fibroma, transitional cell carcinoma, liposarcoma. leiomyosarcoma

[a]*Primary vascular tumor.*

PATIENT HISTORY AND PHYSICAL FINDINGS

- Patients with complex intra-abdominal oncologic pathology are best managed by a multidisciplinary care team at a tertiary care center. If tumor extension to adjacent vascular structures is suspected, surgical planning should include evaluation of potential revascularization options by a vascular surgeon.
- The initial assessment should include a thorough evaluation of the patient's presenting symptoms. This may include focal or regional abdominal pain resulting in tumor parenchyma pressing against adjacent structures. Patients may also present with gastrointestinal symptoms such as early satiety, nausea, and vomiting. Erosive gastrointestinal lesions may manifest with hematochezia, melena, or hematemesis. Constitutional flu-like symptoms, fevers, malaise, fatigue, night sweats, and muscle aches may also rarely present in patients with certain patients with rapidly expanding tumors.
- Depending on the primary site and tissue of origin, tumor-associated physical findings may not be obvious until relatively late in the disease process. Abdominal distension can result from increasing tumor volume or from serous ascites due to portal venous compression. Tumor mass effect or infiltration of the inferior vena cava (IVC) or iliac venous system may lead to unilateral or bilateral lower extremity edema, dilated abdominal wall veins, evidence of deep venous thrombosis (DVT), biliary symptoms, and renal insufficiency. Accordingly, physical examination should not only include a thorough abdominal exam with palpation of all nodal basins but also a complete vascular exam with evaluation of limb pulses, Doppler signals, and assessment of extent/grade of limb edema.
- Patients with primary vascular tumors, particularly ones with intimal expansion and growth, can present with evidence of venous or arterial embolization. Manifestations of recurrent venous pulmonary emboli include shortness of breath, respiratory distress, and hemodynamic changes including tachycardia and right heart failure. Depending on the volume of arterial emboli, symptoms can range from lower extremity pain to digital discoloration.

IMAGING AND OTHER DIAGNOSTIC STUDIES

- Tumor staging and classification systems are beyond the scope of this chapter. Please refer to other excellent references for tumor-specific staging modalities and requirements.[1,3]

- Patients deemed candidates for surgical resection by a multidisciplinary team should receive a high-resolution, thin-slice (at least 1 mm), multidetector computed tomography (MDCT) scan with intravenous contrast injection to allow for imaging during arterial, and venous phases. Image acquisition should allow for multiplanar sagittal, coronal, and three-dimensional reconstructions. This type of detailed imaging provides valuable information regarding tumor margins, suspected histologic subtype, and grade and can also help determine the morphology, patency, and extent of involvement of adjacent vascular structures.
- In situations where mesenteric venous thrombosis is visualized on MDCT, specific postprocessing protocols may be further implemented to improve clarity regarding the extent of thrombus burden and associated and/or resultant venous congestion.
- Adjunct imaging studies may also include magnetic resonance imaging (MRI), ultrasonography, and rarely angiography/venography. Particularly, in patients with concern for osseous or neurogenic tumor involvement, MRI may be particularly useful in defining tissue planes and tumor parenchyma boundaries. MRI also has a nearly 100% sensitivity for detecting intracaval tumor thrombus.
- Autogenous vascular conduit may be necessary for adequate revascularization, particularly following bowel resection and reconstruction. When anticipated, preoperative venous duplex scanning of the lower extremities will help document the presence and usage of superficial femoral vein as potential graft conduit. The presence of deep venous obstruction, either acute or chronic, may preclude venous harvest from that particular extremity. Similarly, the bilateral lower extremity greater saphenous veins should be evaluated for patency, diameter, and adequate length.
- Occasionally, preoperative or intraoperative transesophageal echocardiography may be needed to confirm the proximal extent of intracaval tumor thrombus visualized using other cross-sectional imaging modalities and determine whether the tumor thrombus is encroaching into the right atrium.[4]

SURGICAL MANAGEMENT

Patient Selection

- Whenever possible, the goal of surgical extirpation of abdominal solid organ tumors should be oncologic cure. This assumption presupposes tumor localization to a distinct anatomic region that will allow for resection with negative macroscopic and microscopic margins. Thus, the goals of the procedure should be clearly defined by sufficient preoperative high-quality anatomic cross-sectional imaging, multidisciplinary consultation, and discussions with the patient regarding the operative risks, benefits, expectant outcomes, and overall prognosis.[1,5]
- Abdominal solid organ tumors are traditionally considered unresectable when they involve the arterial or venous vasculature, are diffusely metastatic throughout the peritoneum or at remote sites, or involve the root of the mesentery or spinal cord to a significant extent. Patients with extensive tumor burden precluding resection may still be offered incomplete removal or debulking operations to potentially prolong survival and improve symptom palliation.[5]
- Equally as important as the anatomic considerations, preoperative patient functional status is a significant determinant of surgical eligibility. Performance assessments, such as outlined by the Karnofsky or Eastern Cooperative Oncology Group (ECOG) score, help predict patient-specific postoperative quality of life.[1,6] At our institution, patients who are bedridden at the time of initial assessment, severely disabled, or unable to independently perform activities of self-care are often not offered curative resection.
- Candidacy for intra-abdominal vascular reconstruction is also contingent on the extent of potential or preexisting vascular compromise. As such, we have typically attempted arterial reconstruction when tumors involve critical arterial structures such as the aorta, celiac artery and its branches, proximal superior mesenteric artery (SMA), common/external iliac artery, and the internal iliac artery in the setting of an embolized, occluded, or resected contralateral internal iliac artery. Similarly, venous reconstruction is also anticipated when tumor margins appear to include the vena cava, portal, superior mesenteric, common, and external iliac veins.

Preoperative Planning

- Items to consider in preoperative multidisciplinary review include the extent of planned gross surgical resection margins, the need for preoperative arterial or venous embolization, the need for other prophylactic procedures such as placement of ureteral stents or nephrostomy tubes, and the likelihood for intestinal resection and/or reconstruction.
- Ureteral stent placement should be considered in all patients who demonstrate evidence of ureteral obstruction, renal hydronephrosis, or urinary obstructive signs or symptoms from either tumor mass effect or invasion of urologic structures. Moreover, ureteral stents should also be considered in patients with pelvic tumors where there is potential concern of ureteral injury during resection of the tumor or during vascular reconstruction.
- A thorough review of detailed preoperative imaging will greatly facilitate proper conduit selection and preparation and, ultimately, a successful outcome. Particular attention should be directed to the length of vascular segment involved by adjacent tumor, the branch points and bifurcations present along this length, and which segments, if any, are circumferentially encased by tumor parenchyma.
- Attention should be paid as to whether planned resection will include vessels which are already occluded with adequate collateral circulation already in place or whether adjacent or contralateral vascular structures are capable of supplying adequate inflow and outflow. Vascular segments to be reconstructed should be patent and preserved to the greatest extent possible during the planned tumor resection.
- Endovascular embolization is the preferred method of preoperative vascular occlusion prior to open surgical resection. This strategy is commonly used for preoperative splenic artery/vein embolization prior to planned surgical splenectomy, internal iliac artery embolization prior to planned pelvic tumor resection, and renal artery/vein embolization prior to planned nephrectomy with or without the need for further exposure of the retrohepatic IVC. Moreover, retroperitoneal liposarcoma encompassing the abdominal aorta may have

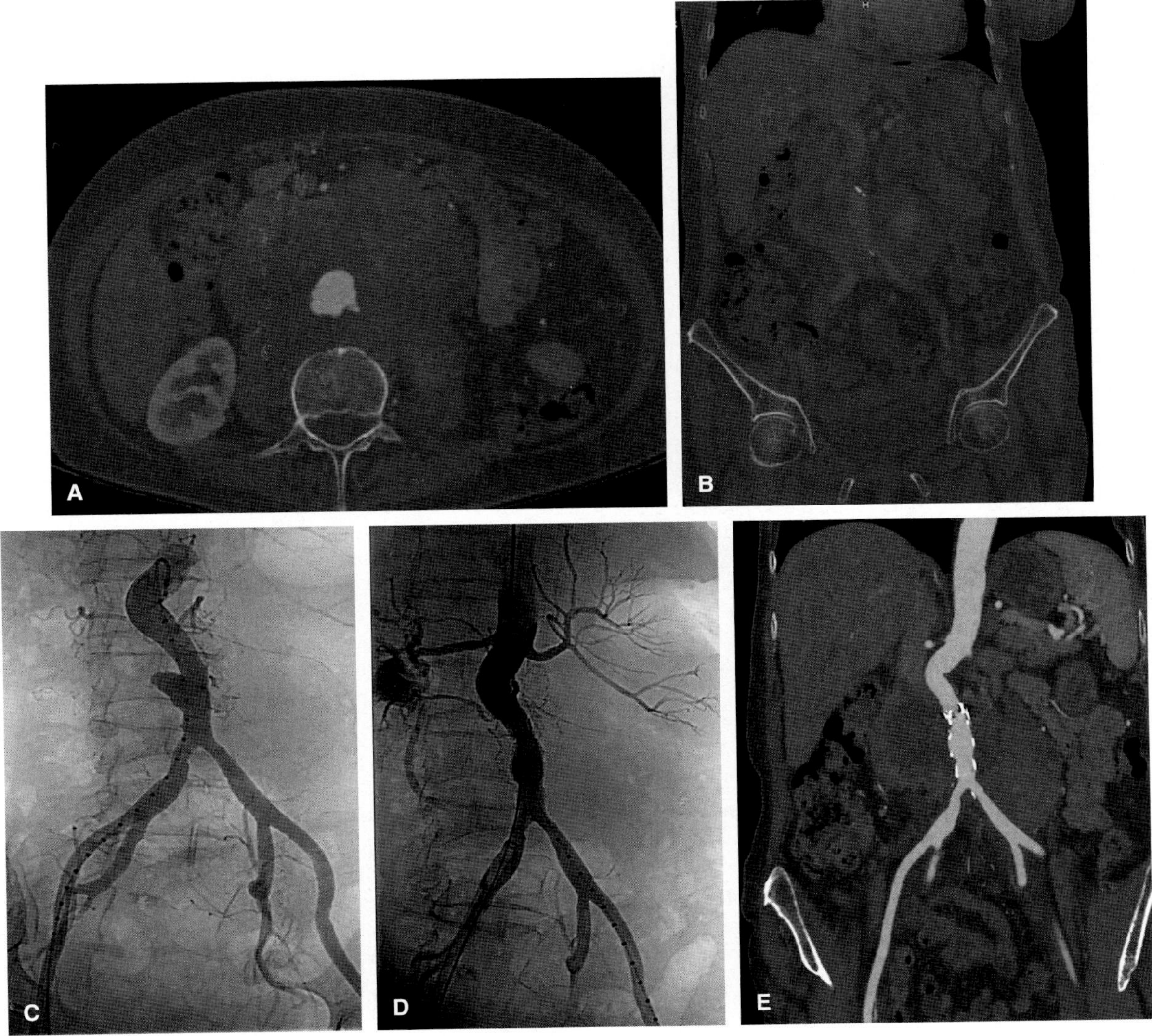

FIGURE 1 ● **A** and **B,** Circumferential encasement of the infrarenal abdominal aorta by a bulky, heterogeneously enhancing retroperitoneal liposarcoma. Much of the infrarenal segment of the abdominal aorta extending into the bifurcation is encased by a large heterogenous retroperitoneal mass. Associated with this tumor is a saccular infrarenal abdominal aortic aneurysm within the tumor, **(C)** well-demonstrated on the diagnostic angiogram. **D,** Endovascular repair of the infrarenal abdominal aortic intratumoral pseudoaneurysm with an aortic cuff extender covering the aneurysmal segment of the aorta prior to neoadjuvant chemotherapy and surgical resection. **E,** Computed tomographic angiography demonstrating complete exclusion of the pseudoaneurysm with an aortic cuff endograft, with no evidence of endoleak.

associated saccular aneurysms within the tumor. Given the risk of degradation of the tumor and subsequent rupture of the aneurysm with neoadjuvant chemotherapy or surgical resection, the degenerated segment of the artery may be preemptively excluded (**FIGURE 1**). For this purpose, the preferred size of coils/plugs or endograft are estimated based on the diameter and length measurements of the target vessel on preoperative cross-sectional imaging and is typically oversized by up to 20% of the target vessel diameter. For additional details regarding visceral embolization techniques, refer to Part 6, Chapter 16 (Stenting, Endografting, and Embolization Techniques). For additional details regarding endovascular abdominal aortic aneurysm repair, refer to Part 6, Chapter 21 (Advanced Aortic Aneurysm Management: Endovascular Aneurysm Repair—Standard and Emergency Management). For additional details regarding internal iliac artery embolization techniques, refer to Part 6, Chapter 22 (Advanced Aneurysm Management Techniques: Management of Internal Iliac Artery Aneurysm Disease).

- Aortoiliac arterial involvement often requires resection followed by reconstruction with patch angioplasty, interposition, or extra-anatomic bypass. Type of reconstruction and conduit type (autogenous venous allograft, cryopreserved homograft, or synthetic conduit) is contingent on the type of tumor, extent of vascular segment involvement, and degree to which intestinal reconstruction is also anticipated. In the latter case, when contamination by succus entericus is likely, autogenous femoral vein conduits for iliac artery reconstructions and IVC or spliced femoral vein conduits for aortic reconstructions are preferred. Alternatively, when not available, rifampin-soaked, gel-sealed knitted Dacron conduit may serve as a potential substitute with acceptable results.[7]

- Reconstruction of the celiac trunk, common hepatic artery, SMA, portal vein, and superior mesenteric vein (SMV) are similarly contingent on the extent of involvement of these structures with tumor pathology. Unless the artery in question is circumferentially involved, it is our preference to resect only the portion of vessel wall directly involved with tumor while preserving the remaining vessel architecture with patch repair. Autogenous venous conduit (using superficial femoral vein or greater saphenous vein or femoral vein) is preferred for vessel segments requiring interposition grafting.
- The mainstay of treatment of primary and secondary tumors of the IVC is surgical resection and reconstruction. The extent of reconstruction is contingent on the type of tumor, extent of caval involvement, and the anatomic segments involved. Adequate retrohepatic caval exposure is challenging and may require total vascular isolation of the liver to minimize blood loss during this maneuver. In circumstances where the IVC is chronically occluded with tolerable lower extremity edema and adequate renal function, ligation and resection without reconstruction should be considered. On the other hand, patients with recent occlusion of the IVC, few venous collaterals, notable lower extremity symptoms, or renal insufficiency should be considered for either interposition grafting or patch venoplasty.

Operating Room Setup

- Preoperative endovascular embolization procedures should be performed in an angiography suite or hybrid operating room. A full complement of compatible guidewires, catheters, sheaths, coils, and plugs should be available.
- Open tumor resection is best performed in an operating room setting with adequate space to facilitate the maneuvering of multiple surgical subspecialty teams and their necessary operative trays/equipment.
- Most intra-abdominal tumor resection and reconstruction procedures may be performed with the patient in the supine position. In the surgical field, the patient's lower extremities should be prepared for vein harvest if potentially necessary.
- In patients who require retrohepatic IVC exposure and reconstruction, the left lateral decubitus position should be employed to facilitate right thoracoabdominal exposure through the 8th or 9th rib interspace.
- Placement of ureteral stents will require initial positioning of the patient in lithotomy position and then subsequent repositioning of the patient to facilitate further planned surgical intervention.

AORTIC RECONSTRUCTION

- For a discussion of the technical exposure of the paravisceral, pararenal, and infrarenal aorta, please refer to Part 6, Chapter 18 (Advanced Aneurysm Management Techniques: Open Surgical Anatomy Repair).

First Step

- The surgical exposure of an intra-abdominal tumor either directly adjacent or involving the aorta should aim to not only provide adequate exposure of tumor resection but also facilitate adequate proximal and distal arterial control. A traditional midline abdominal incision, extending from the xiphoid process to the pubis, can facilitate this in the majority of patients.
- In patients with wide costal margins or an anticipated need for wide parahepatic or parasplenic exposure, a bilateral subcostal incision may also be useful.
- For large abdominal tumors, renal tumors, or tumors with cephalad intra-abdominal extension to the level of the diaphragm, a lateral decubitus thoracoabdominal approach to facilitate both adequate tumor exposure and vascular proximal control and reconstruction is advised.

Second Step

- Proximal aortic control can often be obtained directly above the anticipated cephalad margin of the tumor. In this circumstance, via either retroperitoneal or transperitoneal approaches, the medial and lateral aortic margins are cleared for 2 to 3 cm proximal to the tumor margin. The exposed segment is inspected for lumbar vessel branches, which may be externally ligated as necessary to aid in exposure and control. A large, slightly curved vascular aortic clamp (eg, DeBakey aortic occlusion clamp) is best suited to obtain proximal aortic control.
- Supraceliac or suprarenal aortic exposure may be necessary for optimal control (**FIGURE 2**).
- For control of the supraceliac aorta, the peritoneal cavity is entered below the level of the xiphoid process. With cephalad retraction of the left lobe of the liver, the left triangular ligament of the liver is divided and the lesser sac is entered via a longitudinal incision in the gastrohepatic ligament. Care should be taken here to avoid injury to the esophagus (identified by aid of orogastric/nasogastric tube placement) or a replaced left hepatic artery. For additional exposure, the median arcuate ligament and the right crus may be divided (**FIGURE 2**).
- Suprarenal aortic control is obtained following circumferential dissection and mobilization of the left renal vein off the ventral surface of the aorta. Left renal vein inferior lumbar branches should be ligated to facilitate mobilization. In rare circumstances, the left renal vein may need to be ligated during this maneuver. When this is anticipated, existing collateral veins such as the left gonadal, adrenal, or lumbar should be intentionally preserved prior to division of the left renal vein.
- Infrarenal aortic exposure can be achieved either via transperitoneal or retroperitoneal approaches. If the tumor has pelvic extensions or if exposure/control of the right iliac system is anticipated, a transperitoneal approach may be preferable.

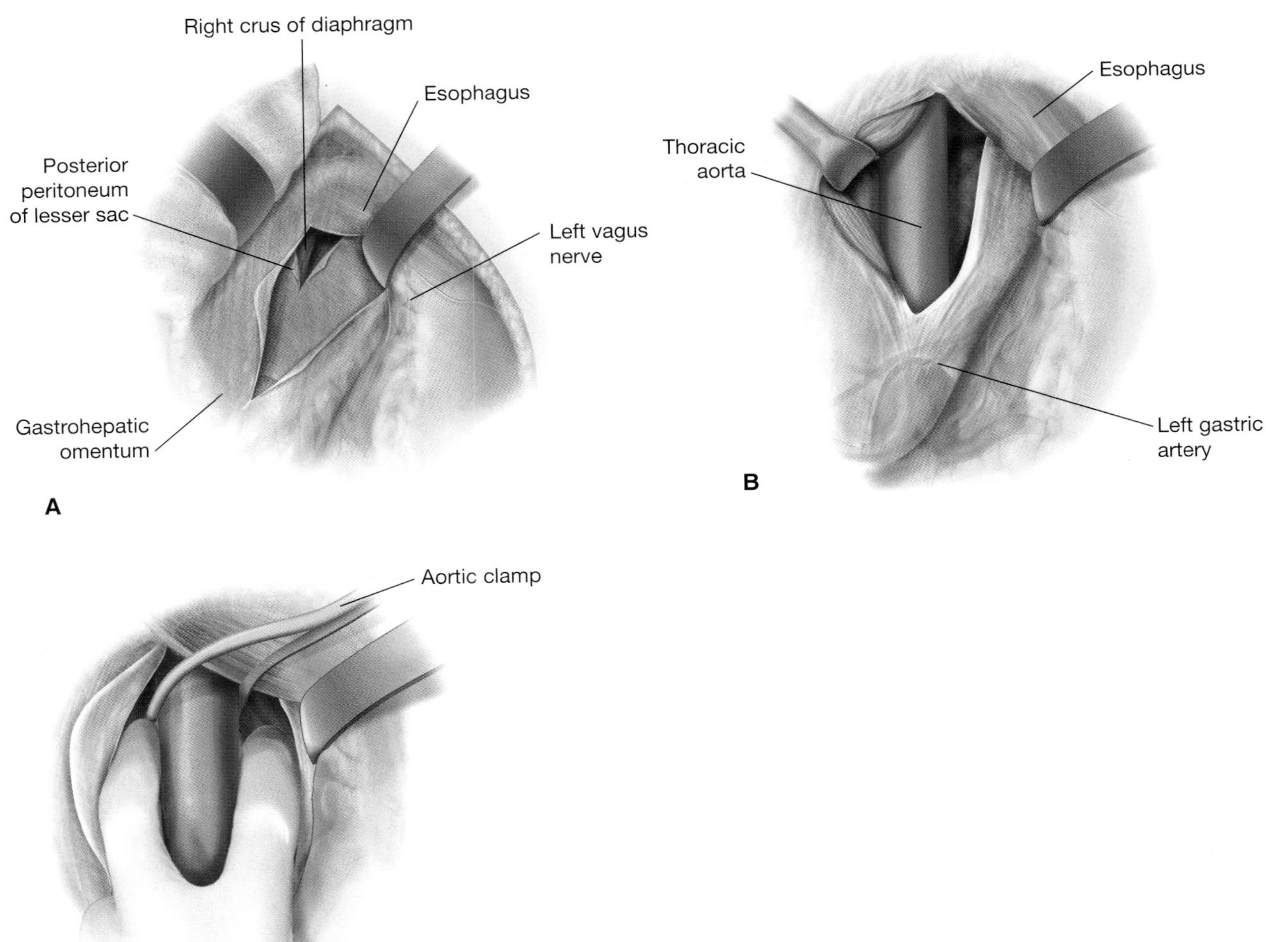

FIGURE 2 ● Transabdominal exposure of the supraceliac aorta for proximal aortic control. **A,** The left lobe of the liver is retracted superiorly and to the patient's right. The distal esophagus is identified and gently retracted to the patient's left. A longitudinal incision is made in between these structures through the gastrohepatic ligament to enter the lesser sac. **B,** The posterior peritoneum and the right crus of the diaphragm can then be incised to expose the supraceliac aorta. **C,** Blunt digital dissection can aid with circumferential exposure of this aortic segment to allow for proximal control with vascular clamping.

Third Step

- Depending on the extent of aortic tumor involvement, durable repair may be achieved using either patch angioplasty or interposition grafting.
- Patch repair is commonly performed with a woven Dacron, bovine pericardium, or autogenous femoral vein. The patch is fashioned in a manner to facilitate a wide repair without narrowing the residual the aortic lumen. The anastomosis is usually performed with 4-0 Prolene sutures, in a running fashion, with one suture starting from each end of the patch repair. Depending on the age of the patient, presence and extent of retroperitoneal soilage by intestinal contents, and amount of retroperitoneal inflammation present, polyester pledgets may be required to minimize suture-related aortic injury and needle hole bleeding (**FIGURE 3**).
- Alternatively, when more extensive aortic segments are involved or the tumor cannot be safely mobilized circumferentially around the aorta, interposition grafting may be more appropriate. After resection, the residual aorta should be inspected for any intimal defects, tumor infiltration, or intraluminal thrombus. Once clean endpoints are determined, the interposition graft of choice can be brought to the field. Conduit choices include autogenous vena cava or spliced femoral veins, cryopreserved homogenous arterial conduit, or knitted or woven polyester and expanded polytetrafluoroethylene (ePTFE). Once selected, the proximal end is fashioned in a way to minimize diameter differences between the aorta and graft. The anastomosis is usually performed with a running 3-0 or 4-0 polypropylene suture. Once completed, the proximal clamp is temporarily released to allow the conduit to be routed in such a way to avoid redundancy, kinking, or twisting. After reclamping the graft (to avoid repeated aortic clamping), the distal anastomosis is completed in a similar fashion after sufficient proximal and distal flushing maneuvers (**FIGURE 4**).

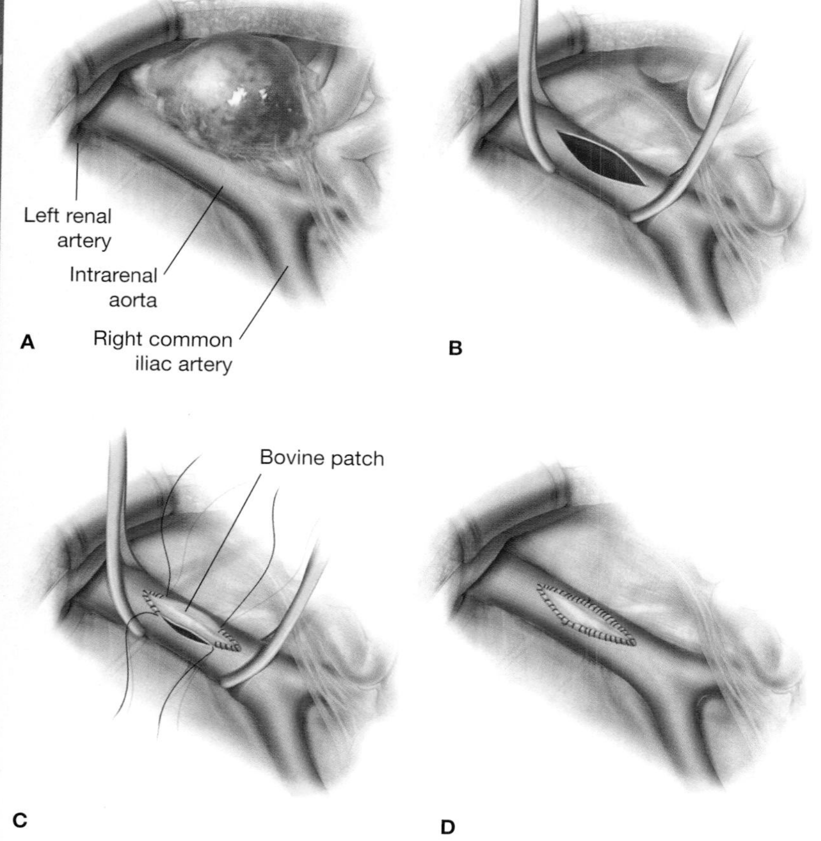

FIGURE 3 ● Patch angioplasty repair of infrarenal aorta. **A,** Transabdominal exposure of the infrarenal abdominal aorta and adjacent tumor mass. **B,** Following proximal and distal aortic control, mass is removed along with associated aortic wall. **C** and **D,** Aortotomy repaired with a bovine pericardial patch.

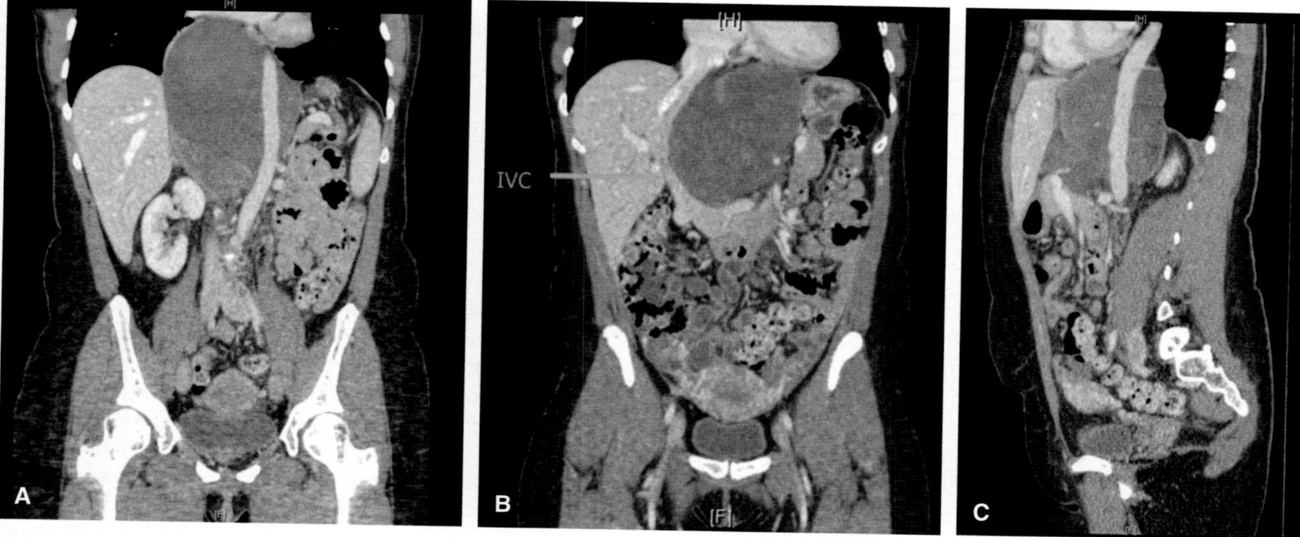

FIGURE 4 ● Branched aortovisceral repair following resection of a large retroperitoneal thoracoabdominal myxoid sarcoma mass. **A,** Coronal abdominal computed tomography (CT) demonstrates large thoracoabdominal and mediastinal mass directly adjacent to major organ structures and the paravisceral aorta. **B,** CT demonstrates retroperitoneal portion of tumor mass displacing inferior vena cava toward the patient's right. **C,** Sagittal CT demonstrates circumferential involvement of the paravisceral aorta with the tumor mass. **D,** Left thoracoabdominal exposure reveals a large retroperitoneal mass extending proximally directly underneath the diaphragm. The supradiaphragmatic aorta **(E)**, proximal left renal artery **(F)**, and proximal superior mesenteric artery (SMA) **(G)** were all exposed to facilitate tumor resection and aortic branched repair. **H,** Aortic branch graft was constructed on the operative back table by attaching a 14-mm bifurcated Dacron graft to the side of a 16-mm Dacron tube graft. Following en bloc resection of the mass along with associated aortic segment **(I** and **J)**, the resected aortic segment was then repaired with the constructed graft. Branches were used for end-to-end anastomosis to the left renal artery and SMA.

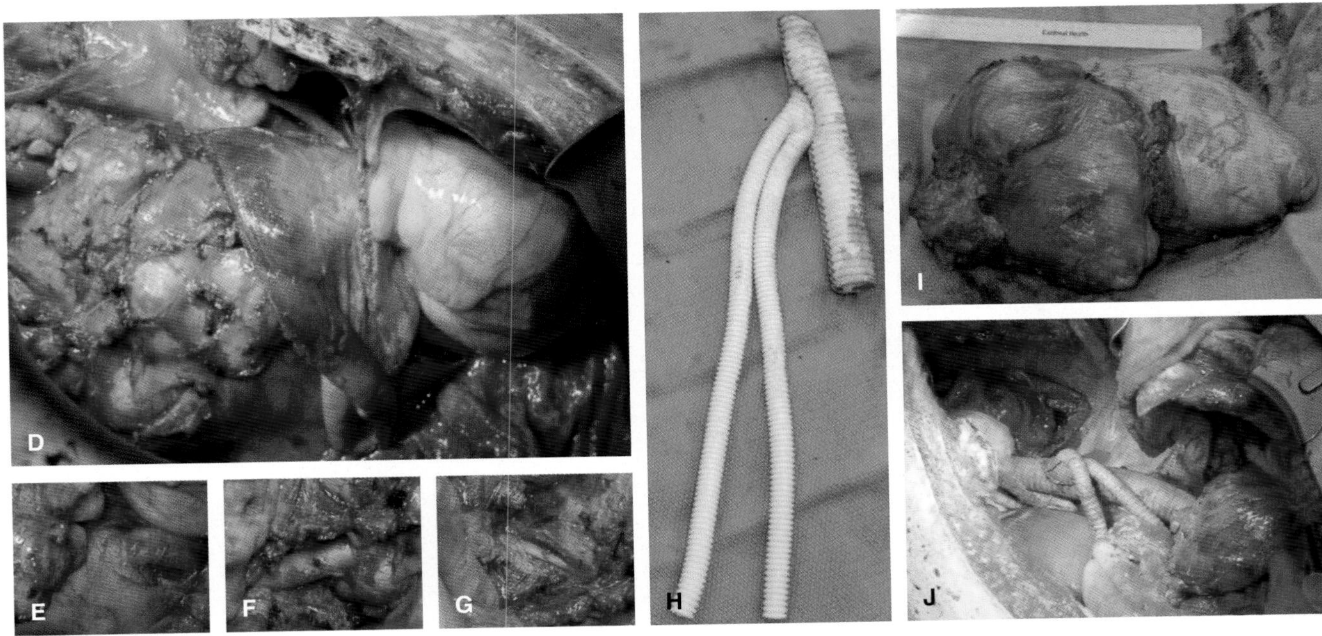

FIGURE 4 ● Continued

- Autogenous tissue repairs of the aorta are preferred in circumstances where intestinal continuity has been interrupted. However, if autogenous tissue is not available or not adequate for use, gel-impregnated woven polyester graft material immersed in rifampin solution is the prosthetic conduit of choice. To achieve adequate coverage, the graft is immersed in 50 mL of normal saline containing 600 mg of rifampin for at least 30 minutes.
- If the paravisceral or pararenal aorta reconstruction is required, visceral and renal vessels can be reimplanted to the interposition aortic graft. Alternatively, a premanufactured or surgeon-modified branched aortic graft can be used to facilitate end-to-end anastomoses to the visceral or renal vessels following aortic interposition graft repair, with side limbs typically 6 to 8 mm in diameter (**FIGURE 4**).

SUPERIOR MESENTERIC ARTERY RECONSTRUCTION

First Step

- Exposure of the SMA, in situations where it is involved with the tumor, may be performed jointly with the surgical oncology team. Particularly in situations where the SMA is extensively involved, sufficient vascular control should be obtained prior to significant debulking or resection maneuvers.
- To expose the SMA at the base of the mesentery, the transverse colon and omentum are elevated while packing the small bowel to the right. The peritoneum is then incised at the base of the transverse mesocolon, taking care to identify and preserve the middle colic and jejunal arterial branches. Judicious cephalad retraction of the inferior border of the pancreas may also improve exposure (**FIGURE 5**).
- Alternatively, proximal SMA exposure may be gained laterally, following division of the ligament of Treitz and mobilization of the fourth portion of the duodenum. Visualization of the underlying SMA can be further enhanced with gentle retraction of the inferior border of the pancreas to the level of the left renal vein (**FIGURE 5**).
- The splanchnic nerves must be sharply excised to effectively elevate the SMA off the anterior aortic wall.

Second Step

- Reconstruction approach is dictated by the extent of tumor ingrowth. SMA involvement may be tangential or require segmental resection to achieve appropriate tumor margins.
- Partial SMA involvement may only require resection and reconstruction of one of the SMA walls. With arterial control established, the tumor tissue and involved SMA can be sharply resected en bloc. Following inspection to ensure a disease-free patent lumen, the arteriotomy is repaired with a patch angioplasty technique. Autogenous vein is the preferred patch material when available, especially following interruption of intestinal continuity. When alimentary tract continuity is not disrupted, bovine pericardial tissue, polytetrafluoroethylene (PTFE), or polyester patch may be used for repair. 6-0 Polypropylene monofilament suture is a good choice for arteriotomy closure and repair.

Third Step

- More extensive tumor involvement with the SMA may require segmental resection and interposition grafting. Variables to consider include the length of the defect, whether the SMA

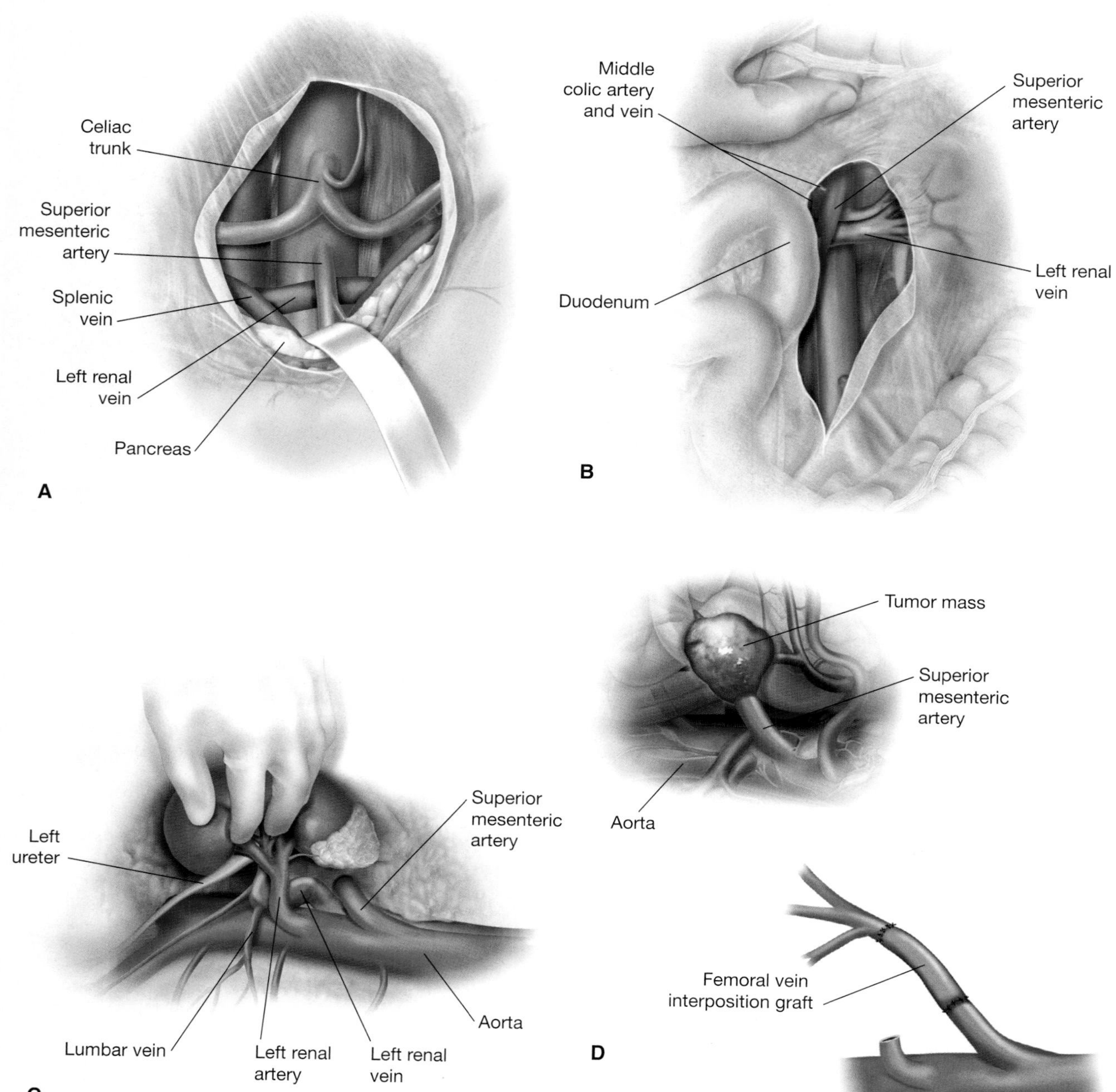

FIGURE 5 • Transabdominal exposure and reconstruction of the superior mesenteric artery (SMA). **A,** The origin of the SMA may be exposed with mobilization and gentle retraction of the superior border of the pancreas along with extended cephalad exposure of the aorta to the level of the celiac trunk. **B,** Alternatively, the SMA can be exposed from a lateral approach with division of the ligament of Treitz and right lateral mobilization of the fourth portion of the duodenum. **C,** Exposure can be enhanced with gentle cephalad retraction of the inferior border of the pancreas and ventral mobilization of the left kidney. Care should be taken to not avulse left renal vein lumbar, gonadal, or adrenal branches during mobilization of the left kidney. **D,** Tumor mass resection with associated segment of SMA. The arterial segment is repaired with an autogenous interposition greater saphenous vein graft.

origin is also involved, and conduit material available for repair.

- For short segment replacement, reversed greater saphenous vein is the preferred conduit for SMA grafting. Appropriately sized saphenous vein is usually harvested from the thigh, distended, and prepared for interposition. The tumor tissue is resected en bloc with the involved segment of SMA. Following confirmation of adequate margins, sequential end-to-end proximal anastomosis is performed. The graft is then brought to length while avoiding any twisting or kinking of the graft. The distal end-to-end anastomosis is then similarly performed. Spatulation of both the arterial endpoints and saphenous conduit may or may not be helpful, depending on size discrepancy.
- For long segment resections or resections involving the origin of the SMA, a long retrograde "question mark" graft, so named for its appearance on contrast arteriography following the procedure, is used to route arterial blood from the right iliac artery around the base of the mesentery to the distal SMA. Alternatively, an antegrade bypass from the supraceliac aorta may be tunneled posterior to the pancreas and brought out coaxially along the course of the distal SMA. Finally, when the SMA origin is involved but sufficient distal SMA is present to allow mobilization, the SMA may be reimplanted on the distal aorta if a disease-free segment can be identified by palpation or from assessment of preoperative imaging studies. For bypass options under these circumstances, cryopreserved arterial homograft or 6-mm polyester or externally supported PTFE are typically preferred conduits. Care is once again taken to avoid conduit twisting or kinking during placement or tunneling.
- Although a potential option, direct bypass from the region of the origin of the SMA to the distal mesenteric artery is problematic in that fashioning the bypass requires elevation of the mesentery, with the distal anastomosis positioned on the posterior aspect of the distal mesenteric artery. Although the graft may function well with the mesentery elevated, reduction of the intestines into the abdomen invariably causes graft conduit, autogenous or prosthetic, to kink and potentially thrombose. In this circumstance, it is almost impossible to fashion an interposition graft of appropriate length, so approaches such as retrograde grafting or reimplantation should be considered as preferred alternatives.

SUPERIOR MESENTERIC VEIN OR PORTAL VEIN RECONSTRUCTION

First Step

- Exposure of the portal vein is facilitated via entry of the peritoneal cavity and interruption of the umbilical vein and falciform ligament. The porta hepatis can be better visualized with cephalad retraction of the right lobe of the liver, downward retraction of the colonic hepatic flexure, and medial mobilization of the first and second portions of the duodenum. The portal vein is then easily identified in the right posterior border of the hepatoduodenal ligament. This exposure can be extended from the hilum of the liver to the head of the pancreas inferiorly. Inferiorly, care should be taken to identify and preserve the coronary vein and splenic vein (**FIGURE 6**).
- In most instances, the neck of the pancreas is divided as part of the tumor exposure and resection, which improves caudal exposure of the portal vein, splenic vein, and SMV.
- Exposure of the SMV can be achieved via exposure distal to the splenic vein confluence or via similar techniques used to expose the SMA. At the base of the transverse mesocolon, the SMV can be found lying to the right of the SMA near the midline. Multiple dense lymphatics overlying the vein often require careful dissection and meticulous control. Care should also be taken to identify and preserve the middle colic vein proximally and ventral venous tributaries distally (**FIGURE 6**).

Second Step

- The extent of tumor involvement with the SMV and portal vein is variable. Reconstruction is often required to preserve mesenteric outflow.
- Following establishment of vascular control, en bloc resection of the tumor and associated venous structures can be performed. Partial involvement is best managed via patch venoplasty. Preservation of an intact back wall of the splenic SMV confluence is often beneficial in maintaining the structural integrity of the bifurcation. SMV and portal vein patch venoplasty repairs can be performed using autogenous saphenous vein or bovine pericardium. A 6-0 polypropylene suture repair is used to close the vein, running or interrupted (**FIGURE 6**).
- Tumor involvement requiring complete resection of the portal vein or SMV will require interposition graft reconstruction. Interposition grafting with autogenous superficial femoral vein or cryopreserved venous homograft is preferred when intestinal resection and reconstruction is anticipated. Alternatively, 6- or 8-mm ringed PTFE when venous conduit is unavailable or inadequate. The distal end-to-end anastomosis is completed first, followed by the proximal end, with either interrupted or triangulated running sutures to prevent purse-stringing and anastomotic narrowing (**FIGURE 6**).

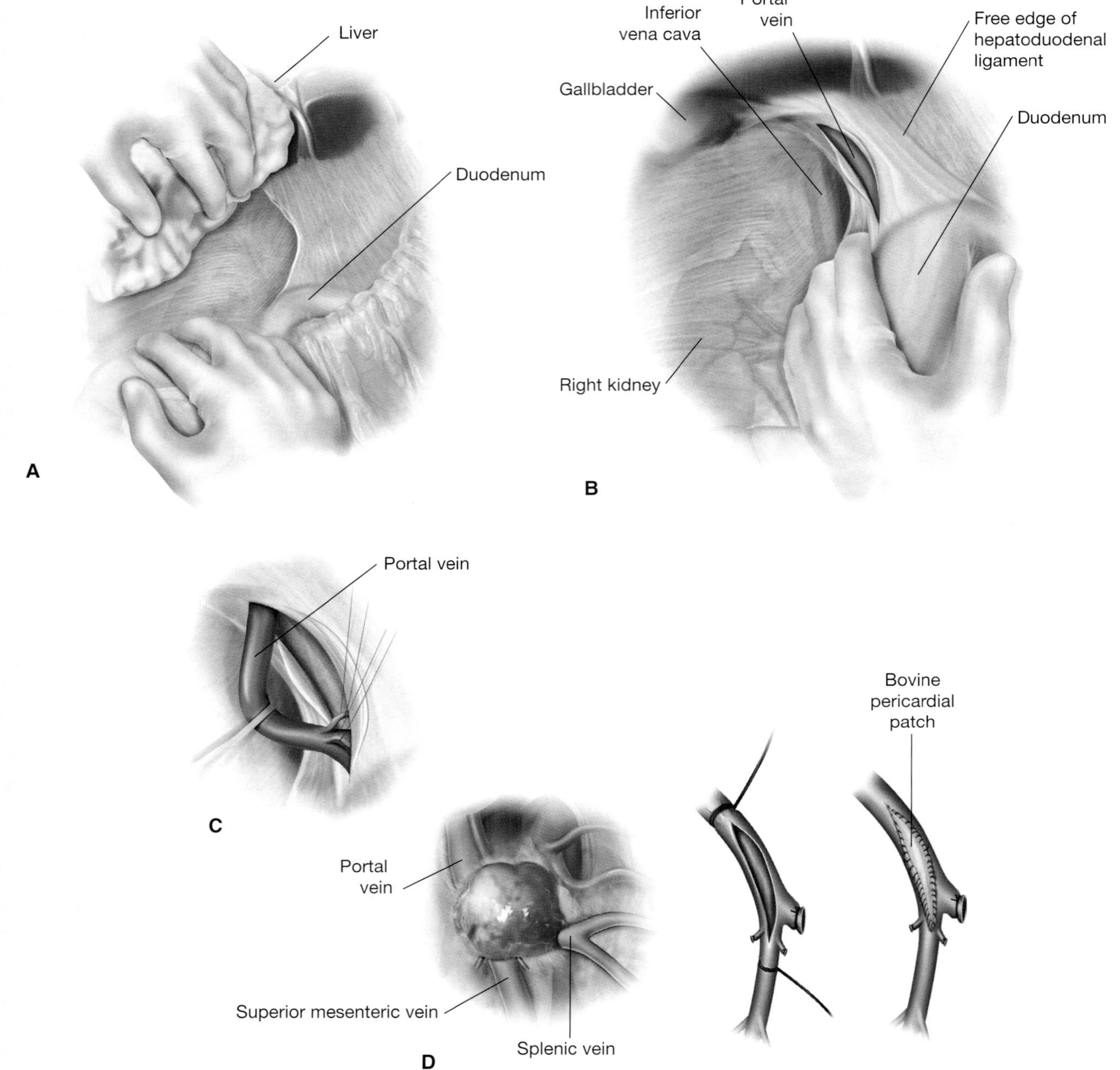

FIGURE 6 ● Transabdominal exposure and reconstruction of the portal vein and superior mesenteric vein (SMV) confluence. **A,** With cephalad retraction of the right lobe of the liver, the posterior peritoneal attachments of the first and second portions of the duodenum may be visualized. **B,** The portal vein and proximal SMV may be exposed through a longitudinal incision along the lateral free aspect of the hepatoduodenal ligament. **C,** Venous tributaries draining into the portal vein and SMV confluence may be ligated to facilitate exposure and reconstruction of this venous segment. **D,** Tumor mass resection with associated ventral segment of the portal vein and SMV confluence and repair with a patch venoplasty using a bovine pericardial patch.

INFERIOR VENA CAVA RECONSTRUCTION

First Step

- Infrahepatic IVC exposure can be facilitated either through right retroperitoneal or transperitoneal exposure. Exposure is typically dictated by the extent of other planned intra-abdominal procedures and anticipated tumor resection margins.
- For right retroperitoneal exposure, the flank is elevated to 15° to 20° with the patient positioned in the supine position. A transverse incision can then be made extending from the rectus abdominis to the tip of the 11th or 12th rib. The external oblique, internal oblique, transversus abdominis muscles, and transversalis fascia are divided to create the retroperitoneal plane via blunt dissection. With judiciously placed self-retaining retractors, a 6-cm segment of the right lateral aspect of the pararenal and infrarenal vena cava may be easily exposed (**FIGURE 7**).

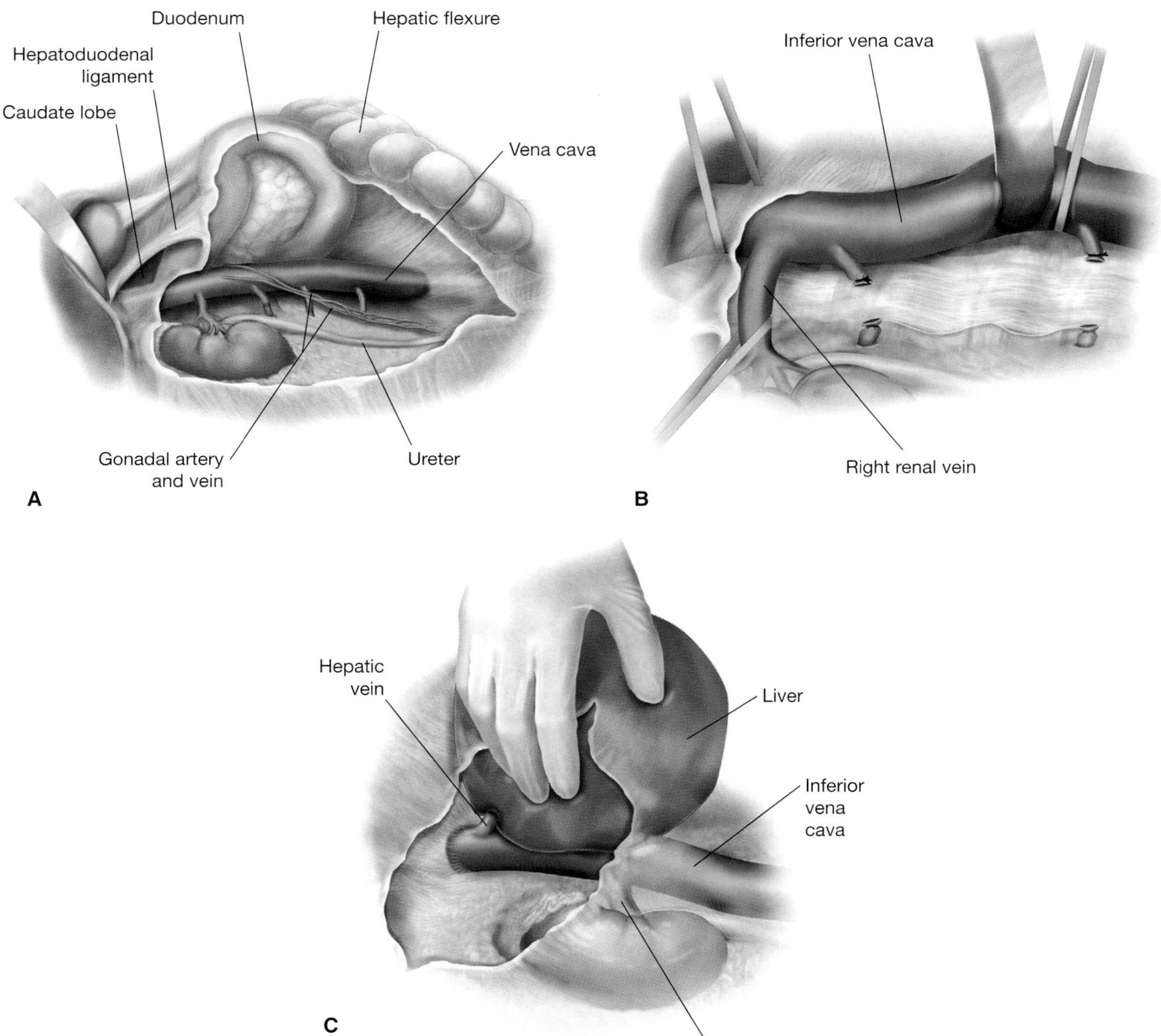

FIGURE 7 ● Transabdominal exposure of the inferior vena cava (IVC) to facilitate operative reconstruction. **A,** An extended right retroperitoneal exposure of the IVC can be achieved with mobilization of the small bowel to the patient's left, division of the lateral peritoneal attachments of the right colon to allow its medial reflection, and division of the retroperitoneal attachments of the second and third portions of the duodenum. **B,** Posterolateral lumbar veins can be ligated to allow for full anterior mobilization of the IVC and facilitate circumferential control. **C,** The retrohepatic vena cava is visualized with medial mobilization of the right hepatic lobe. Small hepatic vein branches enter the IVC at this level and will require careful dissection and division to facilitate this segment of the IVC.

- For a transperitoneal exposure, either a midline laparotomy or bilateral subcostal incision will facilitate adequate exposure. Once the peritoneal space is entered, the small bowel is retracted to the left and the lateral peritoneal attachments of the right colon are divided. This facilitates medial mobilization of the right colon and mesentery and provides access to the retroperitoneal attachments of the second and third portions of the duodenum. Once these attachments are divided, the underlying vena cava can then be adequately exposed from the suprarenal level to the common iliac veins. Ligation and division of the ventral pararenal lymphatics, right lateral lumbar veins, and anterior crossing left gonadal vein will aid in caval mobilization during proximal and distal circumferential dissection. Vascular tapes may be placed around the proximal and distal exposed segments of the vena cava to facilitate vascular control. Care should be taken to not avulse medial lumbar veins with overaggressive mobilization of the vena cava during these maneuvers (**FIGURE 7**).
- For extended retrohepatic IVC exposure, a right thoracoabdominal incision may be performed with the patient positioned in a left lateral decubitus position. Once the peritoneal cavity is entered, the right triangular ligament and lateral and posterior peritoneal attachments to the right hepatic lobe can be divided. Medial retraction of the right hepatic lobe can then be performed to facilitate visualization of the lateral surface of the retrohepatic IVC (**FIGURE 7**). Hepatic compression here, especially following placement of self-retaining retractors, can increase hepatic congestion and ischemia and should be minimized to the greatest extent possible. In situations where caval visualization is not adequate despite optimal hepatic retraction, proximal extension or even division of the sternum may be necessary to facilitate safe exposure. Once adequate exposure is achieved, circumferential control can be achieved following ligation and division of small hepatic venous branches that course between the caudate lobe of the liver and the IVC in this region.
- The suprahepatic IVC can be exposed following ligation and division of the round ligament and wide division of the falciform and coronary ligaments. Caudal retraction of the bare dome of the liver facilitates visualization of the suprahepatic vena cava and at least two of the three main hepatic veins. Careful dissection of the areolar tissue surrounding these veins allows for circumferential exposure of each of these veins as well as this segment of the vena cava.

Second Step

- Once the vena cava is controlled both proximally and distally, the tumor mass can be dissected off other pertinent structures to facilitate en bloc resection. Systemic anticoagulation is accomplished with unfractionated heparin sulfate (100 U/kg intravenous infusion) and reversed with protamine sulfate, 1 mg/100 units of heparin, when vascular reconstruction or retraction is complete.
- Prior to removal of the tumor mass, the patient is placed in Trendelenburg position and vascular clamps positioned proximal and distal to the anticipated margins of resection. If the involved segment of the IVC is limited to only a few centimeters or one side wall, a long Satinsky side-biting vascular clamp may be used for partial caval occlusion (**FIGURE 7**).
- Acute occlusion of the suprarenal or retrohepatic IVC may induce profound hypotension due to significant preload reduction. In these circumstances, preemptive aggressive fluid resuscitation, gradual clamping of the vena cava, or partial occlusion may be better tolerated. Alternatively, venovenous bypass or atriocaval shunt placement may be necessary. Please refer to prior references for further details regarding preparation and placement of atriocaval shunts.[8,9]
- Specific isolation of the retrohepatic vena cava requires control of both the hepatic inflow and outflow. Inflow control is achieved with cross-clamping of the infrahepatic vena cava as well as with a Pringle maneuver (clamping of the hepatic artery and portal vein). Outflow control is achieved with suprahepatic or infradiaphragmatic clamping of the IVC.

Third Step

- The strategy for reconstruction is dictated by the extent of the IVC defect and the concomitant need for other vascular reconstructions. Typically, the vena cava is repaired, when necessary, following arterial reconstructions to decrease end-organ ischemia. The duration of caval occlusion should be limited to less than 30 minutes to minimize venous congestion and resultant ischemia.
- For small caval defects, primary repair may suffice when the lumen diameter is reduced by less than 50%. Otherwise, autogenous internal jugular vein or bovine pericardial patch repair may be incorporated into the repair. Lower extremity vein harvest is not preferred for caval reconstruction due to increased risk for distal thrombotic complications.
- For replacement of the IVC, when necessary, interposition graft using externally supported ePTFE is the preferred conduit. Following resection of the involved segment, the transected ends of the vena cava are inspected for any residual disease within the lumen. Controlled sequential flushing of the transected ends also ensures patency. The graft diameter is chosen to be deliberately smaller than the caval segment being replaced to promote higher velocities within the graft segment following reconstruction. The proximal anastomosis is completed first using either a running 4-0 or 5-0 Prolene suture. The distal anastomosis is then similarly performed with the patient in Trendelenburg position. Prior to completion of the distal anastomosis, proximal and distal clamps are sequentially removed, a Valsalva maneuver is induced by the anesthesiologist, and the graft is filled with heparinized saline while flushing is performed to minimize retained air and the risk for air embolization.
- External support rings are maintained to the greatest extent possible to avoid compression of the graft, including at midgraft segments where end-to-side anastomoses are necessary for renal vein or common iliac vein reimplantation. For repair of the confluence of the common iliac veins, we have successfully modified this procedure by incorporating a short segment of nonsupported bifurcated ePTFE graft into the repair. Externally supported ePTFE grafts are then sutured to the nonringed segment with ePTFE suture. The suture lines are then covered with BioGlue or sterile Dermabond to prevent suture line bleeding and the graft is then placed in situ (**FIGURE 8**).

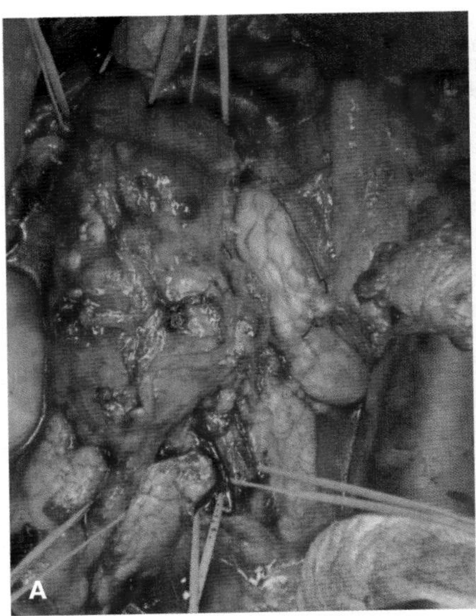

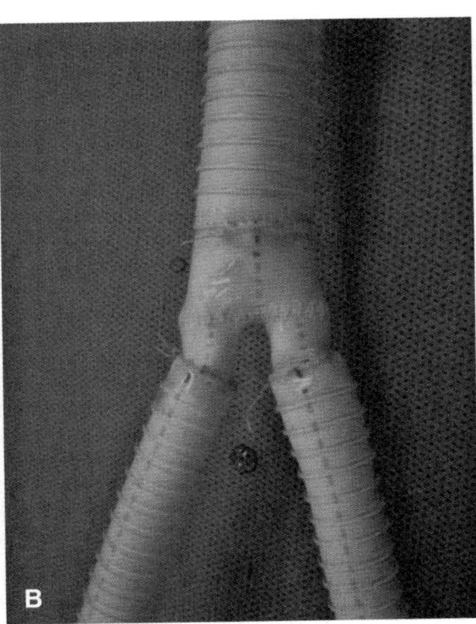

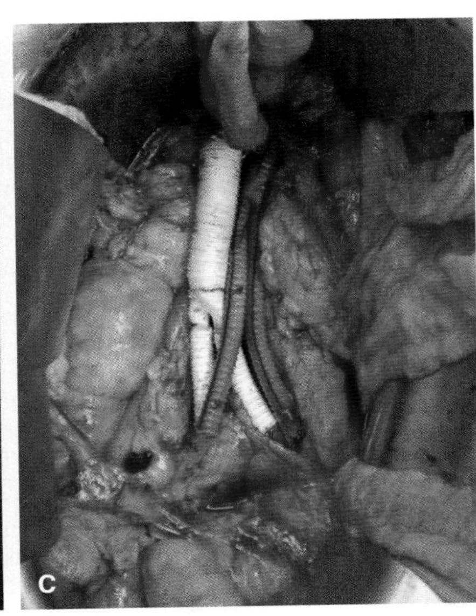

FIGURE 8 ● Inferior vena cava (IVC) and aortic reconstruction in the setting of intra-abdominal resection of a large retroperitoneal high-grade leiomyosarcoma. **A,** Operative exploration demonstrated a large retroperitoneal mass with circumferential involvement with the infrarenal aorta and IVC. Proximal infrarenal aorta and distal bilateral common iliac arteries were circumferentially exposed and controlled. The proximal infrarenal IVC and distal left common iliac vein were also controlled. **B,** Back-table construction of a custom polytetrafluoroethylene (PTFE) bifurcated graft for reconstruction of the IVC. This was performed by suturing a 16-mm ringed PTFE graft to two 10-mm ringed PTFE grafts using a 6-0 Gore-Tex suture. The anastomosis was reinforced with Dermabond. **C,** Following tumor mass resection along with associated IVC, infrarenal aorta, and proximal bilateral common iliac arteries, the vena cava is reconstructed using the custom-constructed bifurcated PTFE graft. The resected aortoiliac segment was reconstructed using traditional techniques using a bifurcated Dacron graft.

PEARLS AND PITFALLS

Preoperative workup	■ It is imperative that a comprehensive plan for resection and vascular reconstruction be developed and agreed upon by all participating surgical specialties well in advance of the procedure. ■ Adequate preoperative evaluation will facilitate discussion of planned vascular reconstructions as well as the risks and anticipated outcomes of the procedure.
Intraoperative anticoagulation	■ The presence of adequate systemic anticoagulation prior to vascular occlusion is essential to the optimal outcome of the procedure. Anticoagulation may be delayed to minimize tumor bed bleeding during resection but should be established well in advance of planned vascular reconstruction. ■ An activated clotting time of greater than 250 seconds is recommended during vascular repairs to avoid thrombotic complications. Reversal of anticoagulation following completion of arterial repairs is also standard practice.
Arterial repairs	■ If the aorta is known to be involved with tumor, it is imperative that proximal control be established well proximal to the anticipated margin of resection. ■ To optimize outcome, the presence and extent of underlying vascular arterial disease should be fully appreciated. For example, complete aortoiliac or aortofemoral reconstruction may be necessary when significant atherosclerotic disease is present in the distal aorta (as an alternative to segmental patching or replacement). Similarly, endarterectomy of residual SMA or celiac artery diseased lumens may be necessary to optimize patency of patch or interposition graft repairs. ■ Attempts should be made to preserve as many SMA and celiac artery branches as possible during vascular reconstruction to maintain adequate bowel perfusion. This is particularly important if concomitant bowel resection is anticipated.

Venous repairs	■ In the setting of complete compression or occlusion of the IVC, the indications for reconstruction following resection may be less compelling. Reconstruction of chronically occluded iliac veins is generally not indicated under any circumstances during oncologic resections—particularly when patients are free preoperatively of significant lower extremity edema. ■ Air embolus is a significant potential complication of extensive venous reconstruction. The risk of air embolization may be minimized when repairs are performed with the patient in Trendelenburg position and with timely Valsalva induction by the anesthesiologist during retrograde flushing maneuvers prior to completion. If a large air embolus is suspected, blood can be aspirated directly from the vena cava or right atrium while the patient is maintained in Trendelenburg and left lateral decubitus position.
Renal vascular repairs	■ Right renal vein reconstruction and/or reimplantation to the vena cava is necessary because there is no adequate collateral venous outflow from the right kidney. During right renal vein reimplantation, the right renal artery should also be controlled and clamped to avoid venous congestion injury to the kidney. ■ Left renal vein can be sacrificed and ligated if the left adrenal and gonadal veins are intact. However, if left kidney venous outflow collaterals were ligated during exposure and reconstruction, the left renal vein should be preserved or reconstructed whenever possible.
Postoperative bleeding	■ In the immediate postoperative period, sudden or acute anemia, abdominal pain, abdominal distension, or hemodynamic instability should be approached with heightened awareness for possible intra-abdominal bleeding. ■ Particularly in patients with recent pancreatic reconstructions, bowel-associated leaks may compromise arterial/venous repairs and can lead to acute catastrophic bleeding requiring urgent intervention.
Methods to avoid lower extremity edema	■ Patients are prone to increased lower extremity edema following lower extremity venous harvest or intra-abdominal vena cava reconstructions. For these patients, lower extremity elevation in the immediate postoperative period is recommended. ■ Early compression therapy of the lower extremity can also significantly minimize the extent of lower extremity edema in the perioperative period. Arterial insufficiency should be ruled out prior to initiation of compression therapy to avoid compromise of already limited arterial inflow.

POSTOPERATIVE CARE

- Patients are typically managed in a monitored setting where periodic vascular examination is available and vasoactive agents are administered as necessary to maintain homeostatic arterial perfusion pressure.
- Intravenous fluid resuscitation is maintained in the short-term perioperative period until the patient resolves an anticipated course of intestinal ileus.
- All patients should be initiated and maintained on an antiplatelet agent, typically 325 mg aspirin daily.
- In patients who preoperatively received therapeutic anticoagulation, this should slowly be restarted 1 to 2 days following the patient's operation to minimize perioperative bleeding complications.
- Patients with large PTFE interposition caval grafts are typically anticoagulated for at least 6 months postoperatively and potentially lifelong depending on risk factors, history of prior DVT, and extent of reconstruction required to restore caval continuity.
- Early mobilization and DVT mechanical and/or chemical prophylaxis should be initiated as soon as safely possible in the postoperative period.

OUTCOMES

- Abdominal tumor resection with vascular reconstruction is feasible for many malignancies previously deemed unresectable.
- In a series of 47 patients who underwent IVC reconstruction with en bloc tumor resection, there was an 80% 5-year patency rate of the vascular reconstruction and a 45% 5-year survival.[10]
- In a series of 17 patients with SMA and portal vein reconstructions with pancreatic mass resection, there was an 88% primary patency rate. Two patients returned to the operating room for vascular-related complications. Eighty-two percent of patients were reported alive over follow-up period (4-48 months).[11]
- In a series of 120 patients undergoing vein resection, 41.7% had primary repair or patch venoplasty, 29.2% had primary anastomosis, and 29.2% had interposition graft. Around 28% of patients developed portal vein thrombosis, 26.5% of which happened in the preoperative period. Late thrombosis was often detected concurrently with local recurrence.[12]
- In a series of 35 patients who underwent pancreatectomy with arterial reconstruction, including 18 hepatic, 8 celiac, 3 splenic, 3 middle colic, 2 superior mesenteric, and 1 left renal artery, had an overall patency of 97% at a mean follow-up of 510 ± 184 days with 1 hepatic artery thrombosis.
- In a series of 14 patients receiving retroperitoneal sarcoma resection and major arterial and venous reconstruction, primary arterial patency was 58% and primary-assisted patency was 83%. Venous patency was 78%. Local recurrence occurred in 21% of patients and 5-year disease-free survival was 52%.[13]
- In a series of 141 patients who underwent resection of retroperitoneal soft tissue sarcomas with either major arterial or venous structure involvement, arterial continuity was retained in all patients and venous continuity was retained in 80%. Perioperative morbidity was 36% and mortality was 4%. Midterm arterial patency was 88.9% and venous patency was 93.8%. The overall 5-year patient survival was 66.7%.[14]

COMPLICATIONS

- Intraoperative bleeding
- Perioperative infection
- Thrombosis or occlusion of repair or graft site
- Venous air embolism
- Wound complications due to poor nutrition or possible radiation to operative field
- DVT from hypercoagulable state

REFERENCES

1. Feig BW, Ching CD. *The M.D. Anderson Surgical Oncology Handbook*. University of Texas MD Anderson Cancer Center; 2012.
2. Wright EP, Glick AD, Virmani R, Page DL. Aortic intimal sarcoma with embolic metastases. *Am J Surg Pathol*. 1985;9(12):890-897.
3. Amin MB, Greene FL, Edge SB, et al. The Eighth Edition AJCC Cancer Staging Manual: continuing to build a bridge from a population-based to a more "personalized" approach to cancer staging. *CA Cancer J Clin*. 2017;67(2):93-99.
4. Sigman DB, Hasnain JU, Del Pizzo JJ, Sklar GN. Real-time transesophageal echocardiography for intraoperative surveillance of patients with renal cell carcinoma and vena caval extension undergoing radical nephrectomy. *J Urol*. 1999;161(1):36-38.
5. Swallow CJ, Strauss DC, Bonvalot S, et al. Management of primary retroperitoneal sarcoma (RPS) in the adult: an updated consensus approach from the transatlantic australasian RPS working group. *Ann Surg Oncol*. 2021;28(12):7873-7888.
6. Ghosh J, Bhowmick A, Baguneid M. Oncovascular surgery. *Eur J Surg Oncol*. 2011;37(12):1017-1024.
7. Bandyk DF, Novotney ML, Johnson BL, Back MR, Roth SR. Use of rifampin-soaked gelatin-sealed polyester grafts for in situ treatment of primary aortic and vascular prosthetic infections. *J Surg Res*. 2001;95(1):44-49.
8. Baumgartner F, Scudamore C, Nair C, Karusseit O, Hemming A. Venovenous bypass for major hepatic and caval trauma. *J Trauma*. 1995;39(4):671-673.
9. Klein SR, Baumgartner FJ, Bongard FS. Contemporary management strategy for major inferior vena caval injuries. *J Trauma*. 1994;37(1):35-41; discussion 41-42.
10. Quinones-Baldrich W, Alktaifi A, Eilber F, Eilber F. Inferior vena cava resection and reconstruction for retroperitoneal tumor excision. *J Vasc Surg*. 2012;55(5):1386-1393.
11. Song TK, Harris EJ Jr, Raghavan S, Norton JA. Major blood vessel reconstruction during sarcoma surgery. *Arch Surg*. 2009;144(9):817-822.
12. Snyder RA, Prakash LR, Nogueras-Gonzalez GM, et al. Vein resection during pancreaticoduodenectomy for pancreatic adenocarcinoma: patency rates and outcomes associated with thrombosis. *J Surg Oncol*. 2018;117(8):1648-1654.
13. Tedesco MM, Norton JA, Cisco RM, Song TK, Harris EJ Jr. Pancreatic mass resection and revascularization. *J Vasc Surg*. 2010;52(2):530.
14. Schwarzbach MH, Hormann Y, Hinz U, et al. Clinical results of surgery for retroperitoneal sarcoma with major blood vessel involvement. *J Vasc Surg*. 2006;44(1):46-55.

Chapter **18**

Open Renal Revascularization: Hepatorenal, Splenorenal, and Aortorenal Bypass

Fred Arthur Weaver and Gregory A. Magee

DEFINITION

- While the aorta is the most commonly used source of inflow for renal artery revascularization, the hepatic and splenic arteries can be used as an alternative inflow source when the aorta is severely diseased, occluded, or there is a hostile periaortic retroperitoneum. Patients with congestive heart failure may benefit from hepatic- or splenic-based revascularization as it minimizes the increase in cardiac afterload induced by aortic crossclamping, and these approaches have been shown to be durable alternatives to aorta-renal bypass. Alternative terms for hepatic- or splenic-based renal revascularization include hepatorenal, splenorenal bypass, splanchnorenal bypass, or extra-anatomic renal revascularization.

DIFFERENTIAL DIAGNOSIS

- Renal revascularization is most commonly performed to alleviate "resistant" renovascular hypertension. Resistant hypertension is defined as a systolic blood pressure greater than 140 mm Hg in patients on at least three antihypertensives, representing 5% to 10% of all hypertensives. A subset of these patients has secondary hypertension due to renal artery pathology or endocrine tumors. Alternative causes of resistant hypertension include:
  - Renal artery
    - Atherosclerosis
    - Aneurysm arteriovenous fistula
    - Fibromuscular dysplasia
    - Takayasu arteritis
    - Other vasculitidies involving the renal artery (eg, Behçet syndrome, polyarteritis nodosa)
    - Trauma
    - Aortic and/or renal artery dissection
  - Endocrine tumors associated with hypertension
    - Pheochromocytoma
    - Primary aldosteronism (Conn disease)
    - Cushing syndrome
    - Primary adrenal hyperplasia
    - Hyperthyroidism
    - Acromegaly

PATIENT HISTORY AND PHYSICAL FINDINGS

- Patient age: In younger patients, renovascular hypertension generally arises from nonatherosclerotic pathologies, such as Takayasu arteritis or fibromuscular dysplasia. In patients older than 50 years of age, atherosclerosis is the most common etiology.
- Associated risk factors are those typical for all occlusive arterial disease: tobacco use, diabetes, hyperlipidemia, and hypertension.
- Length of the hypertensive diathesis: Was the hypertension easily controlled for a period of time, with a recent increase in the difficulty of control? Is the hypertensive diathesis severe and recent in onset? If either is true, the patient is more likely to have secondary hypertension.
- Recognition of the systemic burden of the vascular disease present provides an important perspective on indications and treatment options. Many vascular maladies involve multiple vascular beds. Is there evidence of disease involving the carotid arteries, lower extremity arterial tree, and/or thoracic and abdominal aorta?
- A history of postprandial pain, significant unintentional weight loss, and food avoidance is suggestive of mesenteric occlusive disease.
- Prior pancreatitis may complicate attempts at splenic-based renal revascularization.
- Prior Hodgkin disease or other neoplasms requiring mantle or midline abdominal radiation.
- For general operative risk considerations, recognition and documentation of the presence of coronary artery disease, previous coronary stents, or surgical coronary revascularization as well as valvular disease and congestive heart failure are fundamental to surgical planning.
- Documentation of renal function as evidenced by increased serum creatinine, pedal edema, and recent requirement for renal replacement therapy.
- Recognition of prior aortic procedures, or intra-abdominal nonvascular procedures such as a retroperitoneal lymphadenectomy for testicular cancer, which would complicate retroperitoneal dissection and aortic exposure.
- Family history of syndromic aortic connective tissue disorders such as Marfan, Ehlers-Danlos, or Loeys-Dietz.
- The specific antihypertensive regimen in place prior to surgery needs to be verified and documented.
- To obtain the most accurate baseline measurement, the highest blood pressure obtained from either arm should be recorded and retained.
- A complete vascular examination must be performed, with particular attention paid to pulse deficits and bruits. In particular, diminished femoral pulses or an abdominal bruit may indicate significant aortic or branch vessel occlusive disease, potentially complicating revascularization plans. The presence of concomitant carotid bruits may suggest carotid occlusive disease that should be assessed prior to renal revascularization. The presence of an aortic aneurysm should be assessed by abdominal palpation.

IMAGING AND OTHER DIAGNOSTIC STUDIES

- Laboratory assessment of renal function should include, at a minimum, serum creatinine, blood urea nitrogen (BUN), and electrolytes. Baseline glomerular filtration rate can be estimated from creatinine level, age, sex, and race using the Modification of Diet in Renal Disease (MDRD) or the Chronic Kidney Disease Epidemiology Collaboration (CKD-EPI) equations.

- The co-occurrence of endocrine syndromes, such as pheochromocytoma or functional adrenal tumors that potentially contribute to resistant hypertension must be evaluated with appropriate serologic and/or urine studies prior to operative intervention.
- Renal artery duplex ultrasonography is performed to document existing renal artery disease, renal mass, and intraparenchymal renal blood flow indices. Hemodynamically significant renal artery stenosis (>60%) is determined by duplex-derived assessment of peak systolic velocity measurements across lesions. Baseline characteristics (ie, kidney size, velocity, spectral waveforms, and resistive indices) serve as reference points for future surveillance imaging following revascularization.
- Selective visceral and renal arteriograms are obtained to define normal and variant vascular anatomy, including lateral imaging of both the celiac and superior mesenteric arteries (**FIGURES 1** and **2**).
- Computed tomography (CT) angiography of the abdomen and pelvis, with arterial and venous phases, may provide additional useful information regarding the extent of existing aortic disease and other associated abdominal pathology (**FIGURES 3** and **4**). Catheter-based arteriography alone may not identify significant arterial wall disease or the presence of aneurysmal lesions. However, the expense, contrast load, and radiation associated with complementary arteriographic imaging modalities may not be justified or appropriate in every patient, so anatomic information obtained from these examinations should be integrated into the operative plan on an iterative basis. Preoperative, imaging-based planning is combined with direct intraoperative assessment to create the most effective and durable revascularization possible for each patient.
- Documentation of celiac, hepatic, splenic, and superior mesenteric artery patency is a mandatory prerequisite for hepatic- or splenic-based revascularization procedures. Significant stenosis of the celiac origin or hepatic or splenic artery occlusive disease will prevent successful renal revascularization from these arteries. Associated superior mesenteric artery disease also needs to be considered, particularly when the gastroduodenal artery provides significant collateral flow from the celiac artery to the mesenteric bed. Renal artery anatomy, including branch vessel involvement and the presence of multiple renal arteries must also be documented.
- Bilateral lower extremity vein mapping is also necessary to identify potential graft conduit. Standard vein mapping techniques, including imaging in a warm room with the patient

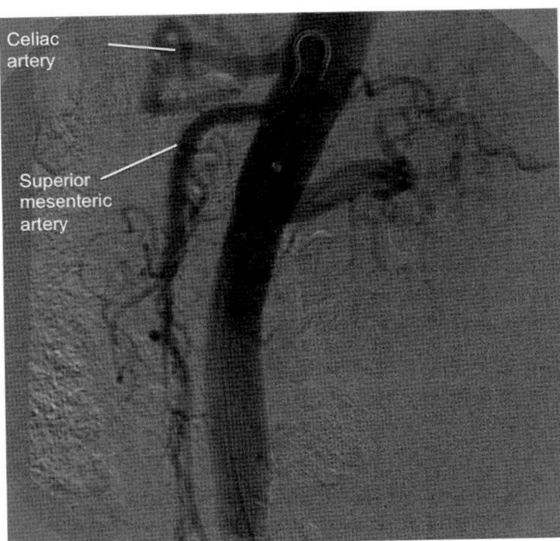

FIGURE 1 ● Abdominal angiogram with lateral view shows a normal celiac artery.

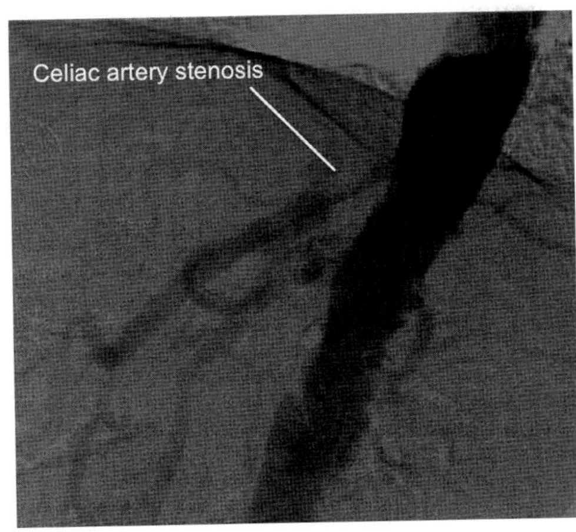

FIGURE 2 ● Abdominal angiogram with lateral view shows a stenotic celiac artery.

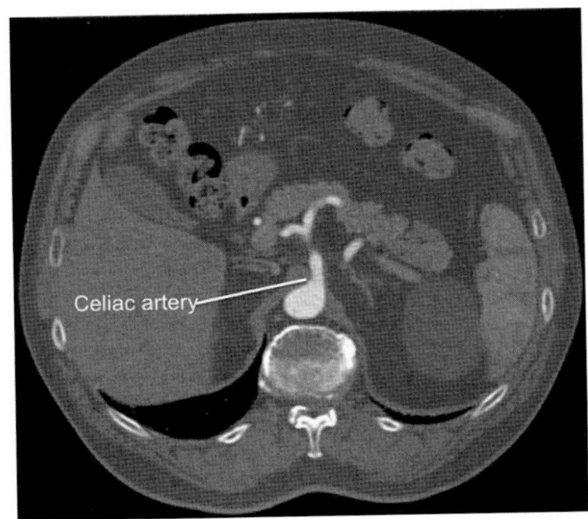

FIGURE 3 ● Axial CT scan image shows a normal celiac artery origin.

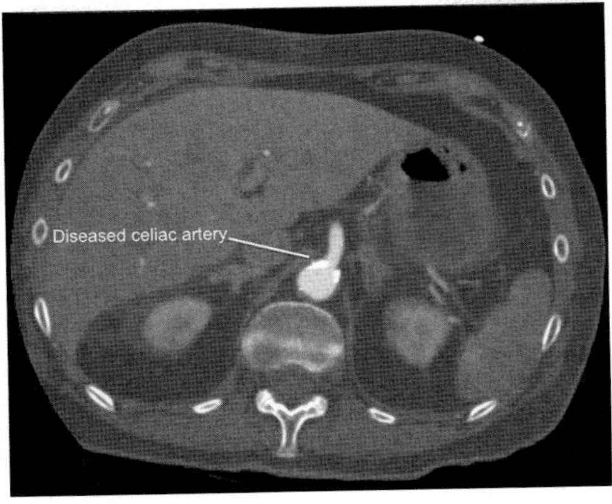

FIGURE 4 ● Axial CT scan image shows a diseased celiac artery origin.

in reverse Trendelenburg position, should be employed to ensure accuracy and reproducibility.

- For selected patients, a more extensive preoperative evaluation for coronary artery or valvular disease should be considered. This may include both a transthoracic echocardiogram and cardiac stress evaluation. Selective pulmonary evaluation may be required in patients with chronic obstructive pulmonary disease (COPD)-associated respiratory compromise. Additional vascular assessments should be performed as indicated, including carotid duplex ultrasonography to access the significance of carotid bruits identified on physical examination.

SURGICAL MANAGEMENT

Preoperative Planning

- Aorta-renal bypass is the most direct and generally most expeditious approach.[1,2] However, extra-anatomic renal artery revascularization may be preferable in selected circumstances as previously noted.
- Review of preoperative imaging is performed to determine variant vascular anatomy, if present. Anatomical extent of the existing renal artery disease is assessed.
- The aorto-renal and hepatic-right renal bypasses require a conduit, preferably autogenous vein.
- The splenic-left renal bypass may be performed with or without graft conduit. The native splenic artery has sufficient length, usually to extend directly to the left renal artery, when fully mobilized. When necessary due to variant anatomy, or prior scarring around the pancreas, a venous conduit can also be employed.
- Planning for availability of duplex ultrasonography in the operating room will facilitate intraoperative confirmation of adequate target revascularization and renal perfusion.

Positioning

- Patient is placed in supine position with both arms tucked.
- A small bump is placed under the respective flank.
- The operative field is prepped from the nipples to the knees.

TECHNIQUES

HEPATORENAL BYPASS

Placement of Incision

- Optimal access is gained through a right subcostal incision extending from the midline to the tip of the 12th rib. In large or obese patients, the medial extent of the incision can be extended across the midline as a chevron (**FIGURE 5**).
- When necessary, an upper midline incision may also provide sufficient exposure.

Hepatic Artery Exposure

- The hepatoduodenal ligament is exposed by retracting the right lobe of the liver cephalad.

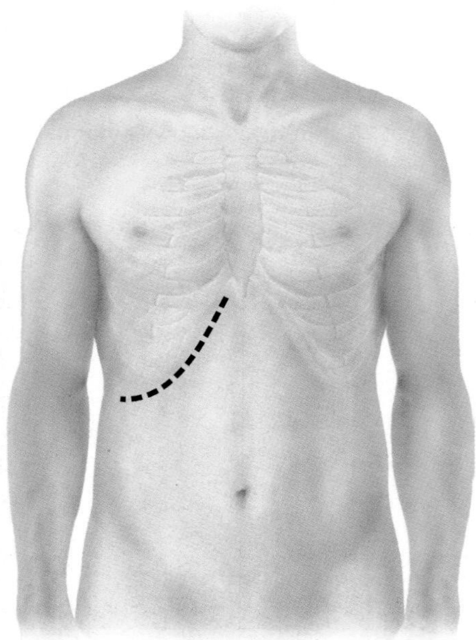

FIGURE 5 • Right subcostal incision extended to the tip of 12th rib.

- The right colon and duodenum are reflected anteriorly and to the left (Kocher maneuver). The small intestine is packed toward the pelvis with moist laparotomy pads.
- The hepatoduodenal ligament is incised longitudinally. The hepatic artery is located in the porta hepatis medial to the common bile duct (**FIGURE 6**).
- The gastroduodenal artery is identified as the first large branch coursing caudad and encircled with a silastic vessel loop. The gastroduodenal artery should be preserved in the presence of superior mesenteric artery occlusive disease as it provides important collateral circulation to the small intestines.
- The hepatic artery is controlled proximally and distally with silastic vessel loops (**FIGURE 7**).

Right Renal Artery Exposure

- The right colon and duodenum are reflected as detailed earlier to expose the inferior vena cava and right renal vein.
- The right renal artery is located posterior and superior to the main renal vein. Depending on its position, the renal vein is retracted either cephalad or caudad. To ensure the main renal artery is exposed, the dissection should be carried to its aortic origin. This requires medial retraction of the inferior vena cava and division of lumbar veins when necessary.
- The right renal artery is controlled using a silastic vessel loop.
- The main renal artery is exposed circumferentially and then distally to the three segmental renal artery branches. Each branch is identified and controlled with a silastic vessel loop. This is a critical operative maneuver that excludes the presence of branch disease and ensures a successful renal artery revascularization (**FIGURE 7**).

Distal Anastomosis

- The distal anastomosis is always performed first to take advantage of the additional degrees of freedom provided by the mobile graft.

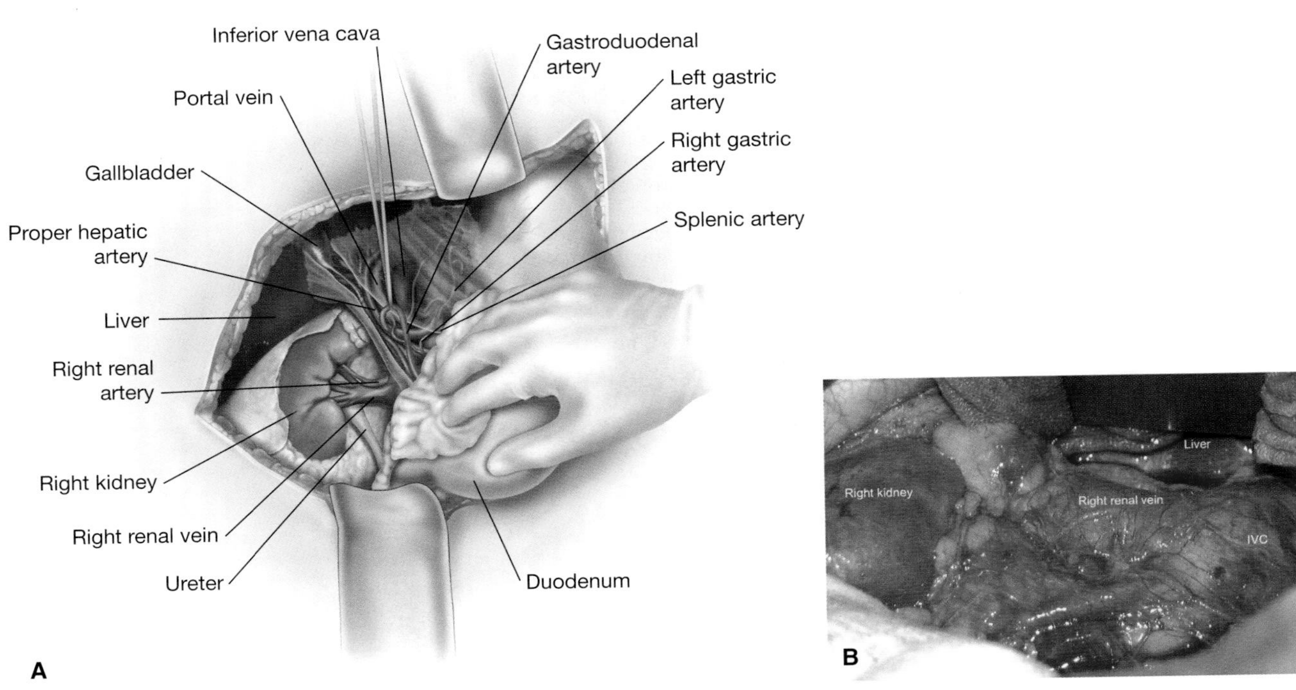

FIGURE 6 ● **A** and **B,** Kocher maneuver with porta hepatis dissected. IVC, inferior vena cava.

- An appropriate length of great saphenous vein is harvested from the thigh. The patient is then heparinized with 100 U/kg intravenously. The vein itself is reversed before placement.
- The proximal renal artery is mobilized following its division from the aorta, at its origin. The proximal stump is oversewn with 5-0 polypropylene suture.
- The redundant renal artery is trimmed distally from its origin until the disease-free segment is reached. The mobile renal artery is then transposed anterior to the inferior vena cava.
- The vein graft and renal artery are spatulated and an end-to-end anastomosis is created with 6-0 polypropylene suture, tied at opposite ends of the anastomosis to prevent purse-stringing. Alternatively, depending on renal artery diameter, eight interrupted sutures may be distributed circumferentially around the lumen. The smaller the renal artery diameter, the more advantageous the interrupted technique. Loupe magnification is necessary to ensure optimal results regardless of which suture technique is chosen (**FIGURE 7**).
- Once the distal anastomosis is completed, the vein graft is oriented longitudinally to prevent twisting or kinking prior to completion of the proximal anastomosis.

Proximal Anastomosis

Hepatic artery

- Small vascular clamps or removal clips are used to control the proximal and distal hepatic artery.
- A longitudinal arteriotomy is made on the hepatic artery and extended using Potts scissors.
- The vein is spatulated and an end-to-side anastomosis is performed using polypropylene (**FIGURE 8A**).

Gastroduodenal artery

- The gastroduodenal artery may be used as an alternative inflow vessel if sufficiently large size (4-6 mm in diameter). This anastomosis may be performed either end-to-end or end-to-side, but prior to division of the gastroduodenal artery, consideration should be given toward its contribution to the mesenteric circulation (**FIGURE 8B**).

Intraoperative Duplex Ultrasonography

- We recommend insonation of the graft and both anastomoses using an appropriately sized 7-MHz scan head to ensure technical proficiency following completion of the reconstruction. In recent years, our practice has come to rely on duplex ultrasonography for intraoperative assessment of all small and medium size autogenous reconstructions, especially in light of the reduced frequency of such procedures in the era of endovascular and hybrid reconstructions. Renal artery reconstruction is unforgiving. Less than a technically perfect anastomosis can result in bypass graft stenosis or occlusion leading to either recurrent hypertension and/or a decrease in renal function.
- Spectral waveforms, velocities, and B-mode are all employed to detect technical errors requiring immediate repair.

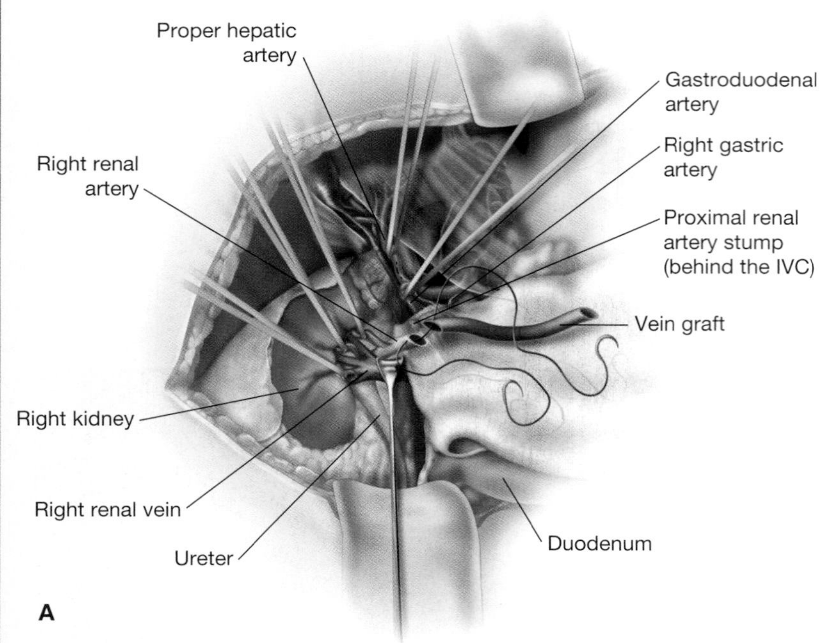

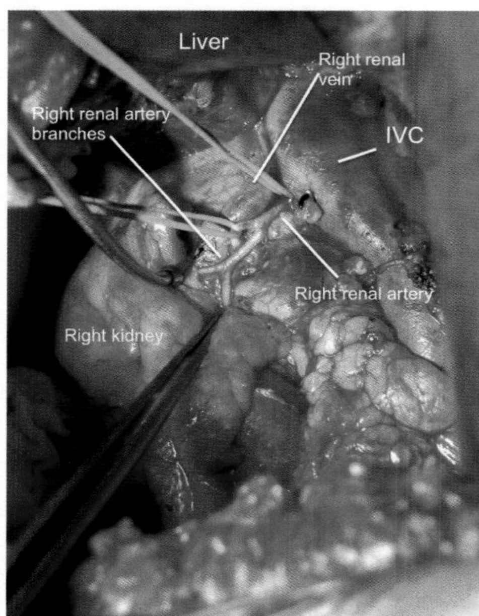

FIGURE 7 ● **A and B,** Right renal artery and distal branches encircled with silastic loops. Distal anastomosis is performed first. IVC, inferior vena cava.

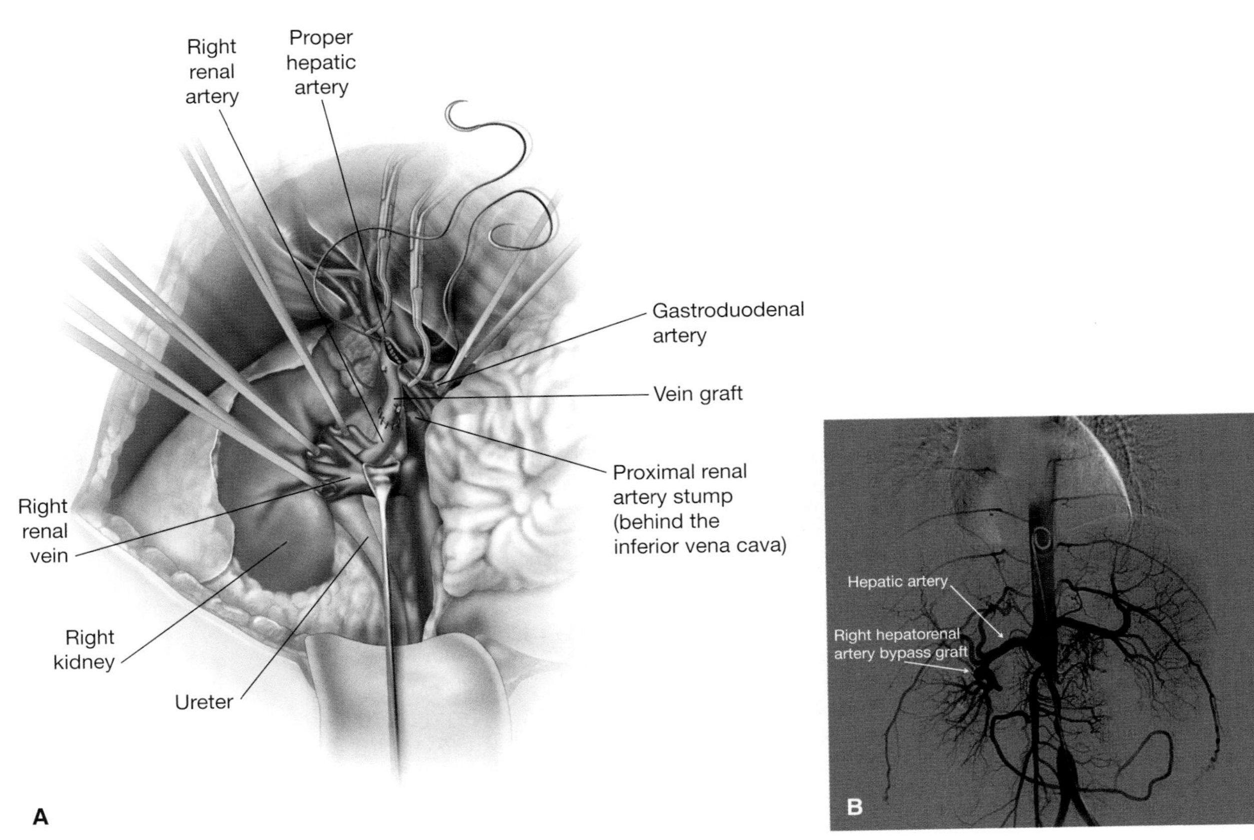

FIGURE 8 ● **A,** Proximal Anastomosis. **B,** Anterior-posterior angiographic image demonstrates a hepatorenal artery bypass.

SPLENORENAL BYPASS

Placement of Incision

- Exposure is obtained through a left subcostal incision extending from the midline to the tip of the 12th rib. In large or obese patients, the medial extent of the incision can be extended across the midline as a chevron (**FIGURE 9**).
- As was the case on the right side, the upper midline incision may also provide sufficient access depending on body habitus, prior operations, and operator experience.

Splenic Artery Exposure

- The greater omentum is elevated exposing the transverse mesocolon. The ligament of Treitz is taken down and the inferior mesenteric vein is ligated and divided. The plane between the pancreas and kidney is entered and the pancreas is elevated. The splenic vein is embedded in the body of the pancreas—avoid injury during mobilization of the distal pancreas. The splenic artery should be palpable along the cephalad border of the pancreas. It is mobilized medially and laterally until sufficient length is obtained to fashion either transposition or support an autogenous vein conduit bypass (**FIGURE 10**).

Left Renal Artery Exposure

- After mobilizing the distal pancreas, the left renal vein is located just posterior and caudad.

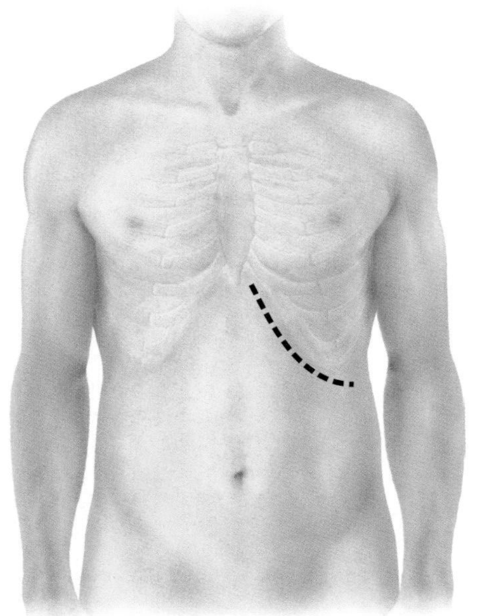

FIGURE 9 ● Left subcostal incision extended to the tip of 12th rib.

- The left renal vein is circumferentially mobilized. This requires division of its nonrenal tributaries: the gonadal, adrenal, and renolumbar veins. Dividing these veins greatly enhances renal vein mobility, facilitating renal artery exposure.
- As previously described on the right, the left renal artery is dissected to its aortic origin and controlled with a silastic vessel loop. The distal artery and its three segmental branches are identified and encircled with silastic vessel loops. The importance of mobilization of the segmental branches is again emphasized (**FIGURE 11**).

Splenorenal Anastomosis

- The patient is heparinized with 100 U/kg of unfractionated heparin intravenously. The left renal artery is clamped

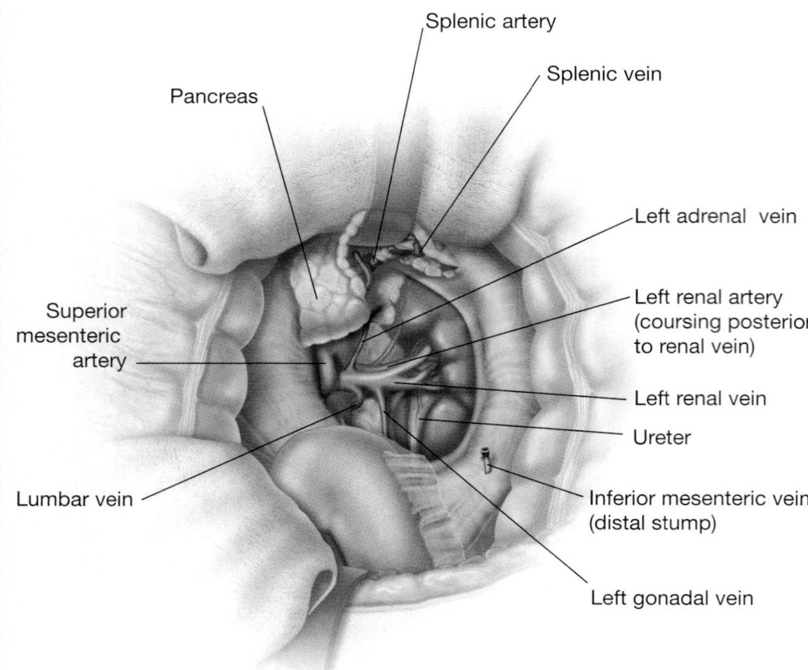

FIGURE 10 ● Left renal artery and vein exposure. Division of the inferior mesenteric vein allows cephalad retraction of the retropancreatic plane, which allows visualization of the splenic artery.

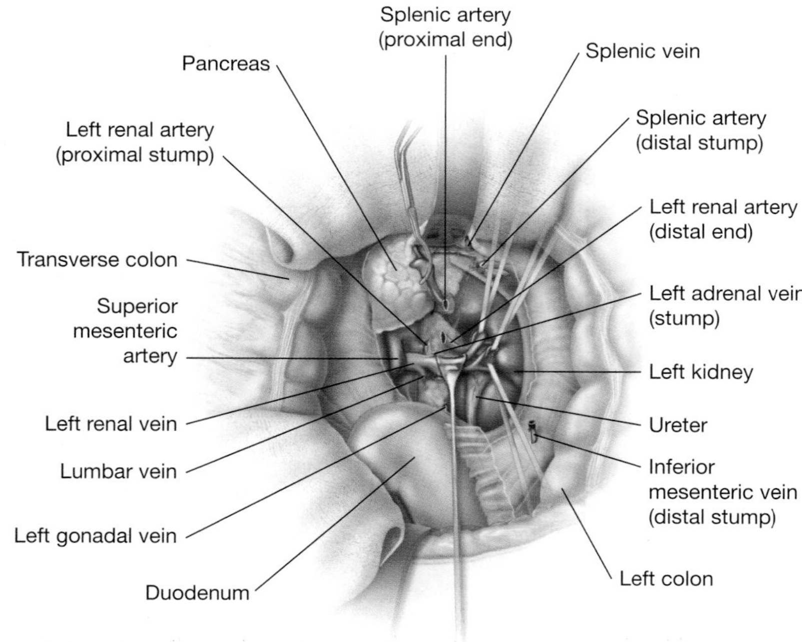

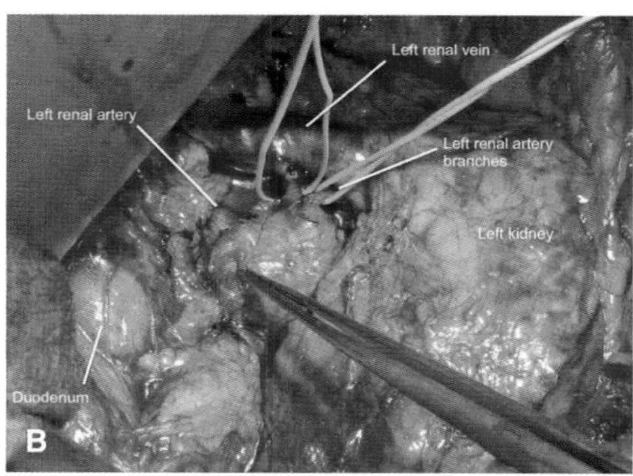

FIGURE 11 ● **A and B,** The splenic artery and left renal artery are divided. The gonadal, adrenal, and lumbar veins are ligated and divided, allowing complete mobilization of the left renal vein.

at the origin and divided. The proximal renal stump is oversewn with 5-0 polypropylene suture. The distal main renal artery is spatulated distal to the existing renal artery disease. The mobilized splenic artery is divided with sufficient length to extend behind the pancreas to the left renal artery without undue tension. The distal splenic artery is oversewn.

- The mobilized splenic artery is spatulated and transposed end to end to the left renal artery, again with either running or interrupted polypropylene suture depending on the respective arterial diameters (**FIGURE 12**).
- Alternatively, when splenic artery length is insufficient, reversed saphenous vein may be employed as a bridge graft. Again, to optimize the degrees of freedom, the distal anastomosis is performed first, followed by an end-to-end or end-to-side anastomosis to the splenic artery. The vein graft is positioned posterior and inferior to the body of the pancreas.

Intraoperative Duplex Ultrasonography

- As described earlier.

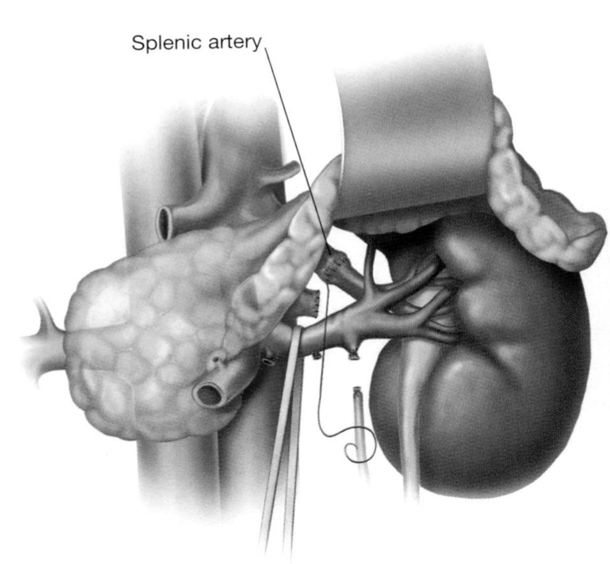

FIGURE 12 ● Completed anastomosis between the splenic artery and left renal artery.

AORTORENAL BYPASS

Placement of Incision

- A subcostal incision is performed on the appropriate side as described earlier.
- A midline incision may be used if bilateral aortorenal bypasses are planned.

Infrarenal Aortic Exposure

- The infrarenal aorta is exposed circumferentially from the renal artery origins to above the aortic bifurcation.
- Beware of lumbar arteries when placing the aortic clamps.

Renal Artery Exposure

- As described earlier.

Distal Anastomosis

- As described earlier.

Aortorenal Anastomosis

- The aorta is cross clamped below the contralateral renal artery and above the aortic bifurcation with sufficient length to easily perform the anastomosis.
- A small arteriotomy is performed on the lateral aspect of the aorta and an aortic punch is used to create a round arteriotomy appropriately sized to the vein graft.
- The vein graft is spatulated and an end-to-side anastomosis is performed using polypropylene suture.

Intraoperative Duplex Ultrasonography

- As described earlier.

FINAL INSPECTION

With completion of the revascularization procedure, all anastomoses and oversewn renal artery origins are inspected for hemostasis. Heparin anticoagulation is reversed with protamine, in a quantity sufficient to normalize the activated clotting time (ACT). Palpation of the superior mesenteric artery (SMA) at the base of the mesentery is performed to confirm a pulse. Operative traction and/or pre-existing disease may compromise SMA flow or precipitate an occult dissection. If the SMA pulse is absent, or the intestinal viability is uncertain, mesenteric artery revascularization may be necessary.

PEARLS AND PITFALLS

Preoperative imaging	▪ Surgical planning may require CT and catheter-based arteriography as complementary references. ▪ Celiac artery stenosis is an absolute contraindication for hepatic- and splenic-based renal revascularization.
Preoperative vein mapping	▪ Autogenous vein is the preferred conduit for renal revascularization. ▪ Lower extremity vein mapping allows assessment for suitable conduit.
Exposure of the renal artery	▪ Circumferential exposure of the entire main renal artery and the three segmental branches is imperative for placement of the renal anastomosis distal to existing disease.
Graft orientation	▪ Longitudinal orientation needs to be confirmed repeatedly during graft placement. Excessive reliance on graft marking or "striping" as the sole method of orientation may lead to inadvertent kinking or twisting.
Intraoperative duplex	▪ Completion duplex scanning is easy, quick, and invaluable in identifying technical errors, which may compromise graft patency and renal viability. ▪ Unlike lower extremity bypass procedures, perioperative graft occlusion cannot typically be identified expeditiously to prevent end-organ compromise.

POSTOPERATIVE CARE

- Postoperative care typically involves central venous and arterial pressure monitoring in the intensive care unit (ICU) for the first 24 to 48 hours.
- Serial monitoring of serum creatinine, urine output, and acid-base status is essential in the early postoperative period. Unexplained changes in acid-base status or elevation of serum creatinine could indicate occlusion of the revascularization or mesenteric ischemia.
- Blood pressure is maintained in a physiologic range with vasoactive medications as necessary. Oral antihypertensives are resumed on postoperative day one and adjusted depending on the response to renal revascularization.
- Diet is resumed as bowel function returns; nasogastric suction is usually not required.
- Blood pressure and antihypertensive medication requirements may decrease after renal revascularization and should be adjusted prior to discharge.
- Diet is resumed as bowel function returns; nasogastric suction is usually not required.
- Follow-up surveillance duplex ultrasonography is performed at 6 and 12 months, then annually thereafter. Detected abnormalities suggesting stenosis of the renal reconstruction may be addressed with remedial endovascular intervention or surgical revision when indicated.

OUTCOMES

- Large case series documenting the outcomes following isolated hepatorenal and splenorenal artery bypass are sparse. Published results are derived from two relatively large series, generally demonstrating acceptable perioperative morbidity and mortality with improved renal function and blood pressure and durable patency.
- Moncure et al. reported 77 patients who underwent 79 procedures (29 hepatorenal and 50 splenorenal bypasses) for the treatment of renovascular hypertension and renal preservation. The perioperative mortality was 6%. Deterioration in renal function occurred on three occasions but only in patients with bilateral simultaneous repair. Cure or improvement in hypertension was observed in 52 of 63 patients. Renal function was preserved or improved in 67 of 77 patients.[3]
- Another series by Geroulakos et al. document similar outcomes with extra-anatomic renal artery revascularization for atherosclerotic renal artery disease. Forty-five hepatorenal and/or splenorenal bypasses were performed in 38 patients for the treatment of renovascular hypertension, renal preservation, or both. There was one postoperative death from myocardial infarction and two cases of early graft thrombosis. There was a significant decrease in postoperative mean serum creatinine as well as the average number of antihypertensives. Over a median follow-up of 33 months, there were 10 deaths, all from cardiac issues.[4]

COMPLICATIONS

- Bypass graft thrombosis
- Intestinal ischemia due to pre-existing disease or traction injury to the SMA during operative exposure
- Bleeding from the renal, hepatic, splenic, aortic anastomoses, ligated renal artery stump, and portal or splenic vein if injured
- Acute renal failure requiring temporary or permanent renal replacement therapy
- Pancreatitis, splenic infarction, and common bile duct injury
- Incisional hernia

REFERENCES

1. Benjamin ME, Dean RH. Techniques in renal artery reconstruction: part II. *Ann Vasc Surg*. 1996;10(4):409-414.
2. Weaver FA, Kumar SR, Yellin AE, et al. Renal revascularization in Takayasu arteritis–induced renal artery stenosis. *J Vasc Surg*. 2004;39:749-757.
3. Moncure AC, Brewster DC, Darling RC, et al. Use of the splenic and hepatic arteries for renal revascularization. *J Vasc Surg*. 1986;3:196-203.
4. Geroulakos G, Wright JG, Tober JC, Anderson L, Smead WL. Use of the splenic and hepatic artery for renal revascularization in patients with atherosclerotic renal artery disease. *Ann Vasc Surg*. 1997;11:85-89.

Chapter **19**

Open Visceral Revascularizations for Ischemia: Superior Mesenteric Artery Embolectomy, SMA/Celiac Bypass/Endarterectomy

Robyn A. Macsata†, Benjamin Pomy, and Kellie R. Brown

DEFINITION

Acute/Subacute

- Acute mesenteric ischemia (AMI) is an uncommon, life-threatening, vascular and general surgical emergency effecting approximately 1 in 1000 patients annually. This disease is accompanied by significant morbidity and mortality following both endovascular and open surgical intervention.[1] The most common cause of AMI is secondary to an embolic event from a cardiac source, such as atrial fibrillation (**FIGURE 1**). Other causes include nonocclusive mesenteric ischemia (NOMI) and mesenteric venous thrombosis (MVT). NOMI is a result of a generalized low-flow state creating vasoconstriction to the mesenteric vessels in order to shunt blood to the more vital organs (heart and brain); treatment is of the underlying conditions and in some extreme circumstances catheter-directed vasodilatory agents. MVT is a result of a surrounding inflammatory event; treatment is directed at the involved organ, which may require removal (such as a cholecystectomy) and therapeutic anticoagulation. Both treatment of NOMI and MVT are outside the scope of this chapter.

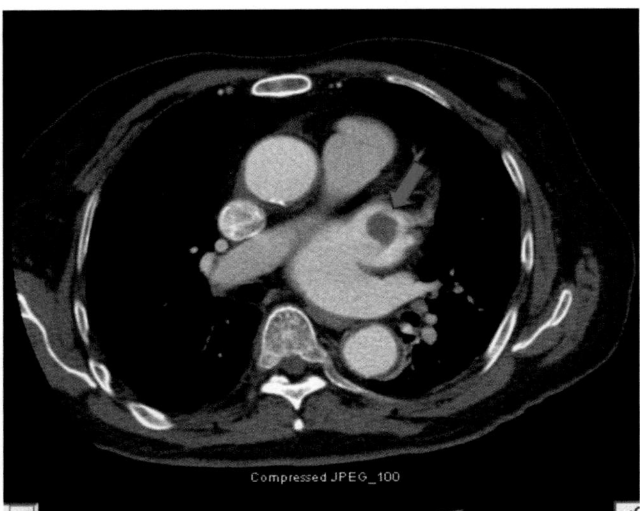

FIGURE 1 ● Left atrial appendage thrombus (*red arrow*) in a patient who presented with SMA occlusion. (Courtesy of Dr. Benjamin Pomy, George Washington University.)

†Deceased

- Subacute mesenteric ischemia is secondary to in situ thrombus of preexisting mesenteric artery occlusive disease (MAOD) in the proximal superior mesenteric artery (SMA). This occurs secondary to either plaque rupture or a generalized low-flow state with resulting in situ thrombus formation.

Chronic

- Chronic mesenteric ischemia (CMI) presents with chronic postprandial pain and weight loss and can be difficult to diagnose due to its nonspecific presentation. CMI is caused by the inability to maintain adequate postprandial blood flow to the visceral organs due to atherosclerotic severe stenosis or occlusion of multiple visceral vessels, resulting in oxygen and metabolite supply and demand mismatch. This is a result of MAOD; however, the presence of MAOD alone does not always correlate with CMI symptoms.[2]

DIFFERENTIAL DIAGNOSIS

Acute/Subacute

The differential diagnosis for AMI is broad and includes many abdominal pathologies, which may present with peritonitis, such as:

- Appendicitis
- Cholecystitis
- Pancreatitis
- Diverticulitis
- Bowel obstruction
- Perforated ulcer disease

Chronic

The differential diagnosis for CMI is even more broad than that of AMI due to the often-vague nature of presentation. The differential for CMI includes:

- Gallstones
- Peptic ulcer disease
- Various food intolerances (celiac disease, etc.)
- Chronic pancreatitis
- Occult malignancy
- Inflammatory bowel disease
- Irritable bowel syndrome
- Functional abdominal pain

PATIENT HISTORY AND PHYSICAL FINDINGS

Acute/Subacute

- Patients commonly present to the emergency department with acute onset of severe abdominal pain. In some patients this pain may be accompanied by bloody diarrhea, and it is not uncommon for patients to report a large bowel movement immediately following symptom onset. Patients often will have a diagnosis of cardiac dysrhythmias, most commonly atrial fibrillation, and may have reported a missed dose of their anticoagulation.
- "Pain out of proportion" to physical examination is a hallmark of AMI; however, this may be absent in 20% to 25% of cases. Patients may rapidly decline and exhibit profound metabolic acidosis, sepsis, and multisystem organ failure. Patients with preexisting MAOD may have a history of CMI symptoms with postprandial abdominal pain and weight loss that then develops into acute peritonitis. This presentation is very often difficult to diagnose given the nonspecific nature of the symptoms. Presentation is otherwise similar to AMI, but slightly more insidious with a history of vague abdominal symptoms.[1]

Chronic

- Chronic mesenteric ischemia is typically diagnosed in elderly, frail patients, with a classic triad of symptoms: vague abdominal pain, weight loss, and "food fear." These patients often have nonspecific symptoms for a prolonged period of time. They realize their pain is related to eating, which leads to anorexia, significant weight loss, and chronic malnutrition. Patients with CMI usually undergo an extensive workup for other abdominal pathologies including occult malignancies, ulcer disease, and functional abdominal pain prior to being diagnosed with CMI.[2]

IMAGING AND OTHER DIAGNOSTICS

Acute/Subacute

- Diagnosis of both acute and subacute mesenteric ischemia is best performed with computed tomography angiography (CTA) (**FIGURE 2**). CTA is both sensitive and specific for acute arterial embolism, thrombosis, and MAOD and can evaluate the bowel for ischemia and necrosis.[3] CTA can then be used for either endovascular or open surgical operative planning, including need for possible bowel resection. Arteriogram is generally reserved for when endovascular treatment is planned.

Chronic

- Given the noninvasive nature and low cost, screening is done with duplex ultrasound (DUS) in the noninvasive vascular laboratory. Patients should be fasting before this procedure for better visualization of the vessels, to decrease bowel gas, and to assure a resting state. Patients without any mesenteric stenosis will have high resistance waveforms preprandial that become low resistance postprandial, and velocities will all be below 200 cm/s^2 in the celiac and below 275 cm/s^2 in the SMA. Patients with a greater than 70% celiac and/or SMA stenosis will have high resistance waveforms both pre- and postprandial, and velocities will be above 200 cm/s^2 in the celiac and 275 cm/s^2 in the SMA. CTA can be used to confirm the diagnosis, but most often patients progress straight to arteriogram, which is the gold standard for diagnosis and most commonly therapeutic as well.[4]

SURGICAL MANAGEMENT

Endovascular Options

- While out of scope of this chapter, it should be noted that endovascular strategies for mesenteric revascularization have become increasingly popular and, specifically for

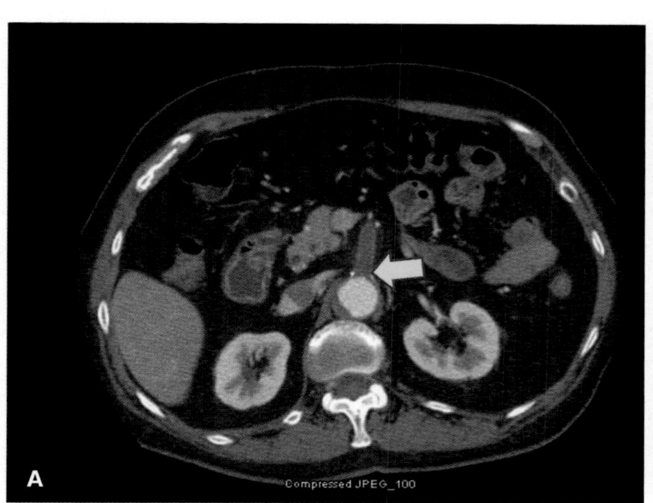

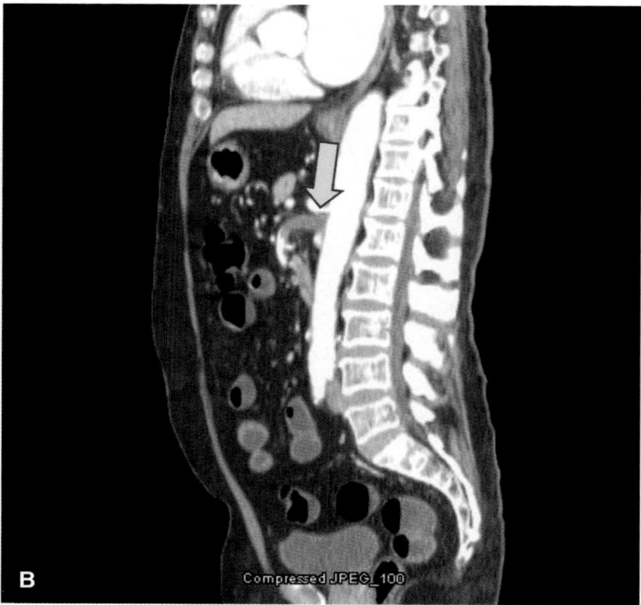

FIGURE 2 ● Acute SMA occlusion (*yellow arrows*) at the vessel origin. **A,** Axial view. **B,** Coronal view. (Courtesy of Dr. Benjamin Pomy, George Washington University.)

CMI, have become first-line therapy. This is due to the minimally invasive nature of these interventions resulting in improved perioperative morbidity with a relative trade-off for decreased long-term patency and freedom from symptom recurrence.[4] Obviously, endovascular options for AMI are limited to cases when bowel ischemia has not progressed to the point of requiring bowel resection. Endovascular strategies for mesenteric revascularization include catheter-directed mechanical thrombectomies and thrombolysis to treat acute thrombus followed by angioplasty and/or stenting to treat any underlying chronic occlusive disease. Mesenteric angioplasty and stenting can also be employed alone in the setting of symptomatic CMI (see Part 6, Chapter 13).

Acute/Subacute

Preoperative Planning

- Given the acute nature of their presentation and likelihood of underlying bowel ischemia, these patients are often septic and require ongoing aggressive resuscitation. This requires a full laboratory evaluation and type and cross for blood products. Once mesenteric thrombosis is identified by CTA, patients should be fully anticoagulated with full-dose intravenous (IV) heparin (70 U/kg) on the way to the operating room.

Positioning

- The patient should be placed on the operating table in supine position with at least one arm extended for anesthesia access for intravenous fluids and intra-arterial blood pressure monitoring. A nasogastric tube is placed for gastric decompression. A Foley catheter is placed for accurate urine monitoring. The patient is prepped and draped from the level of the nipples to the knees; this wide prep will allow harvesting of the greater saphenous vein (GSV) if needed for revascularization.

Chronic Mesenteric Ischemia

Preoperative Planning

- Given the prolonged nature of their presentation, these patients are often severely malnourished. Preoperative workup includes a full laboratory panel including liver enzymes and a full nutritional assessment. Improving preoperative nutrition via an oral route is often difficult given the underlying disease; preoperative total parenteral nutrition may be considered but has not been proven to show any benefit. Priority should be placed on revascularization, and the operation should not be delayed for nutritional optimization.
- In addition to nutritional concerns, patients with CMI should have undergone screening DUS (as described above) as well as either CTA or catheter-based angiography. These images are used to determine the optimal revascularization strategy (discussed in the sections that follow). If vein is to be used for bypass, patients should undergo vein mapping to ensure adequate length and caliber of GSV.

Positioning

- The patient is placed on the table in supine position with at least one arm extended to give the anesthesiologist access for intravenous fluids and intra-arterial pressure monitoring during the procedure. A nasogastric tube is placed for gastric decompression. A Foley catheter is placed to accurately measure urine output. A semi-lateral position with the patient's left side elevated with a shoulder roll to aid in accessing the retroperitoneum is an alternative option.

TECHNIQUES

EMBOLECTOMY (WITH OR WITHOUT ENDARTERECTOMY AND PATCH ANGIOPLASTY):

- ***FIRST STEP—laparotomy, control contamination:*** A midline laparotomy is performed extending from the xiphoid process to the public tubercle; this gives wide access to the abdomen to perform bowel evaluation and dissection of the aorta and mesenteric vessels as needed. The bowel is thoroughly evaluated upon opening the abdomen, any frankly necrotic or perforated bowel is resected, and any questionably ischemic bowel management is delayed until after revascularization.
- ***SECOND STEP—identify and expose the SMA (FIGURE 3):*** The SMA is reached by packing the small bowel to the patient's right side and the transverse colon along with its mesentery cephalad, similar to exposure of an infrarenal abdominal aortic aneurysm. Given the nature of the event, the SMA pulse usually cannot be felt at the base of the mesentery. Nevertheless, a longitudinal incision is made at the base of the mesentery followed by sharp dissection to identify the SMA. Of note, there are many crossing veins as well as lymphatics throughout the mesentery that should be identified, tied, and transected on the way to the SMA. Once identified, the SMA can be traced back to its origin at the aorta as well as forward to its first branches beyond the thrombus. The main trunk of the SMA as well as its branches are dissected free from the surrounding mesentery and controlled with vessel loops to maintain proximal and distal control (**FIGURE 4A** and **B**).
- ***THIRD STEP—heparinize and perform thrombectomy (optional endarterectomy):*** The patient is rebolused with heparin as needed depending on the preoperative emergency dosing. The SMA is inspected to determine the level of disease present. If it feels as if only acute thrombus is present, a transverse arteriotomy is made just proximal to any branch point (**FIGURE 3**). Proximal and distal embolectomy is performed using a range of #2 to 4 Fogarty balloons; when proximal embolectomy is completed pulsatile arterial flow from the aorta should be reestablished. Distal thrombectomy may

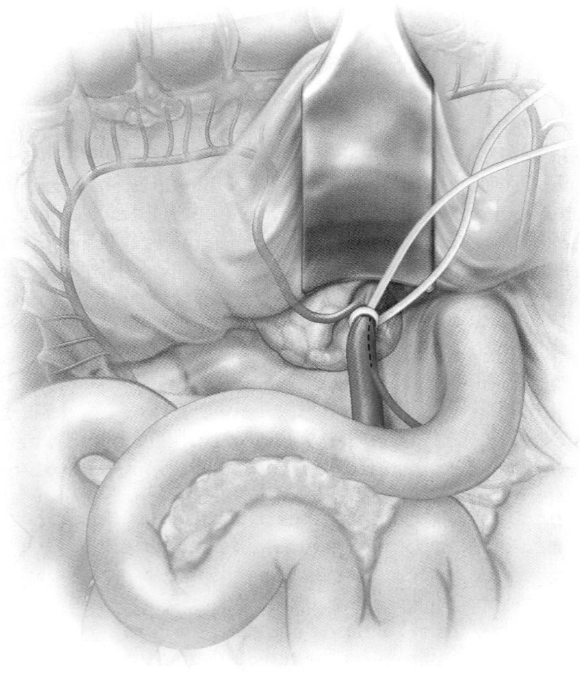

FIGURE 3 ● Exposure of the SMA: The colon is retracted cephalad, and small bowel to the right. The base of the mesentery is incised, and the SMA is identified at the base of the mesentery.

require embolectomy of multiple branches. When complete there should be back bleeding from all involved vessels. The arteriotomy is then closed using two 6-0 Prolene sutures running toward each other and tied together.

- If underlying plaque is identified upon palpation of the SMA, a longitudinal arteriotomy is performed as opposed to a transverse arteriotomy. Following thrombectomy, as described above, an endarterectomy is performed to remove bulky atherosclerotic plaque from the SMA. To perform the endarterectomy, the longitudinal arteriotomy should extend from the proximal aspect to the distal aspect of the atherosclerotic disease, a plaque elevator is then used to elevate the calcified thrombus off the vessel media. Following plaque removal, the artery is thoroughly irrigated with heparinized saline to prevent further embolization of atherosclerotic debris, and the arteriotomy is closed using a patch angioplasty, usually with a bovine pericardial patch, or if contamination is significant, a GSV vein patch.
- ***FOURTH STEP—manage ischemic bowel, determine closure strategy:*** Once the revascularization is complete, bowel viability is once again assessed. Any frankly necrotic or perforated bowel that was not identified or removed prior to revascularization is resected. At this time, the surgeon should use their best judgment of the strategy for abdominal closure, need for a second-look operation, bowel anastomosis, etc. In general, a second look operation is advocated, and bowel reanastomosis is deferred until this second look, when a full appraisal of viability can be undertaken.

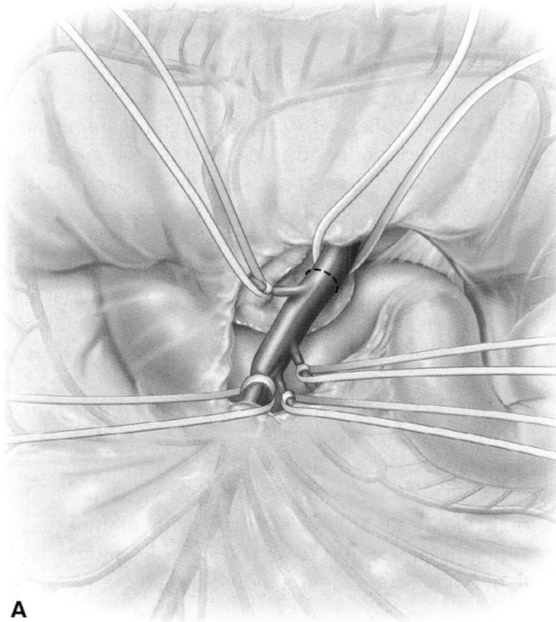

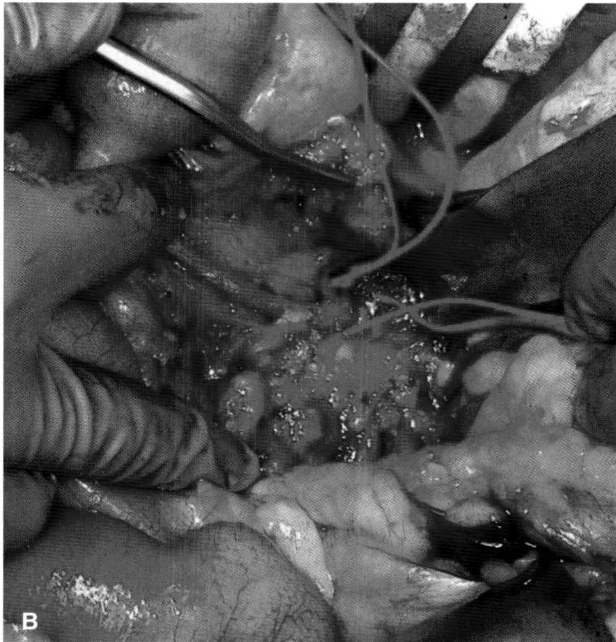

FIGURE 4 ● SMA dissection. **A,** The SMA is dissected free and vessel loops are used to control branches. Transverse incision is made to facilitate embolectomy. **B,** Intraoperative picture of SMA exposed and controlled. (Courtesy of Dr. Kellie R. Brown, The Medical College of Wisconsin.)

CHRONIC MESENTERIC ISCHEMIA

Surgical Decision Making

- Similar to bypasses in the lower extremity, mesenteric revascularization does require careful operative planning with knowledge of the patient's anatomy. As with all vascular bypasses, one needs:
  - Inflow
  - Outflow
  - Conduit

The section that follows provides a brief discussion of the surgical decision-making process for each of these considerations.

Inflow: Antegrade vs Retrograde Bypass

- An arterial bypass to the mesenteric vessels may be performed either antegrade, with the supraceliac aorta as the source of inflow, or retrograde, with either the infrarenal aorta or right common iliac artery as the source of inflow. Benefits of an antegrade approach are a less diseased (atherosclerosis/calcium) inflow vessel and a shorter straighter bypass to the outflow vessels. However, dissection of the supraceliac aorta may be difficult and cross clamping of the aorta is often required, which comes with hemodynamic consequences. Occasionally, a partially occluding clamp (such as a Satinsky clamp) may be used; however, this is not always possible. Benefits of a retrograde approach include an easier dissection and avoiding cross clamping of the aorta (if the right common iliac artery is used as inflow). However, often these more distal vessels have atherosclerotic disease and may be calcified; furthermore, the bypass requires retrograde flow and can be fraught with kinking on its way to the outflow vessels. Ultimately, no differences in outcomes have been reported between an antegrade or retrograde approach to inflow; therefore, this is left up to the surgeon's best judgment and usually based on the unique anatomy and pathophysiology of the patient.[4]

Outflow: One-Vessel vs Two-Vessel Revascularization

- The main two sources of outflow for a mesenteric bypass are the celiac (often extended to the common hepatic artery) and SMA. When patients present with clinically symptomatic CMI, the SMA nearly invariably has a high-grade stenosis while the celiac artery may or may not also be involved. There are little data available to support the number of vessels to revascularize, and, while the theoretical advantage to multivessel revascularization is better long-term patency, outcomes in the literature appear equivocal. Therefore, revascularization strategy is often based on surgeon preference along with patient anatomy and comorbidities. In younger patients with a longer life expectancy, two-vessel bypasses should be considered if the anatomy presents itself, while in patients with a lower life expectancy and more comorbidities, one-vessel bypass is a valid option.[4]

Conduit: Prosthetic vs Autogenous

- The main conduit choices for mesenteric reconstruction are autogenous (commonly GSV), polytetrafluorethylene (PTFE), and Dacron. In the acute setting, with bowel ischemia and necrosis, autogenous conduits are preferred even for vein patches. This is to reduce the risk of graft infection from bacterial translocation or frank contamination. When performing a retrograde bypass in a clean field, a ringed graft is preferred to reduce the chance of kinking. Ultimately, there is no solid evidence to support optimal conduit choice for long-term patency, and the conduit choice is largely left up to surgeon experience and patient factors.[5]

SMA/CELIAC BYPASS (WITH OR WITHOUT SMA ENDARTERECTOMY)

- ***FIRST STEP—laparotomy:*** A midline laparotomy is performed extending from the xiphoid process superiorly to the public tubercle inferiorly; this allows for wide access to the abdomen including the supraceliac and infrarenal aorta, as well as all mesenteric vessels.
- ***SECOND STEP—isolate and control the inflow vessel***
  - ***Antegrade bypass: supraceliac aorta and celiac artery (*FIGURE 5*)***: The supraceliac aorta is exposed by retracting the small bowel and colon inferiorly, dividing the left triangular ligament, followed by mobilization and retraction of the left lobe of the liver. The lesser sac is entered by dividing the gastrohepatic ligament, the stomach is retracted inferiorly, and the esophagus is retraced to the patient's left. Here, the diaphragmatic crura are overlying the aorta and must be divided to reach the supraceliac aorta. Enough distance must be cleared in order to place clamps and perform an anastomosis. This dissection can then be taken down inferiorly to the celiac artery and its branches that require exposure as well.
  - ***Retrograde bypass: isolate and control the infrarenal aorta/common iliac artery:*** The infrarenal aorta and the right common iliac are exposed by retracting the small bowel to the patient's right side and the colon superiorly followed by opening of the retroperitoneum. The retroperitoneum dissection is extended up the base of the colon mesentery to the SMA, as described earlier. The celiac artery may also be exposed in this direction by continuing this dissection further superior. The aorta/iliac artery is controlled with side biting clamps while the mesenteric vessels are controlled with vessel loops.
- ***THIRD STEP—Isolate outflow vessel:*** If the celiac artery is to be revascularized, it is exposed in the same manner as the supraceliac aorta, with slightly further distal dissection to identify and free the celiac artery (**FIGURE 6**). If the celiac artery has a long segment occlusion, the hepatic artery can be used for outflow. The hepatic artery is exposed through the lesser sac by retracting the stomach inferiorly and incising the gastrohepatic peritoneum. The celiac artery is identified and the common hepatic can be found extending to the left (**FIGURE 6**). In nearly every instance of mesenteric bypass the SMA is revascularized, with or without the celiac artery (or hepatic artery). The SMA is exposed in a similar manner as with acute mesenteric ischemia, described above.

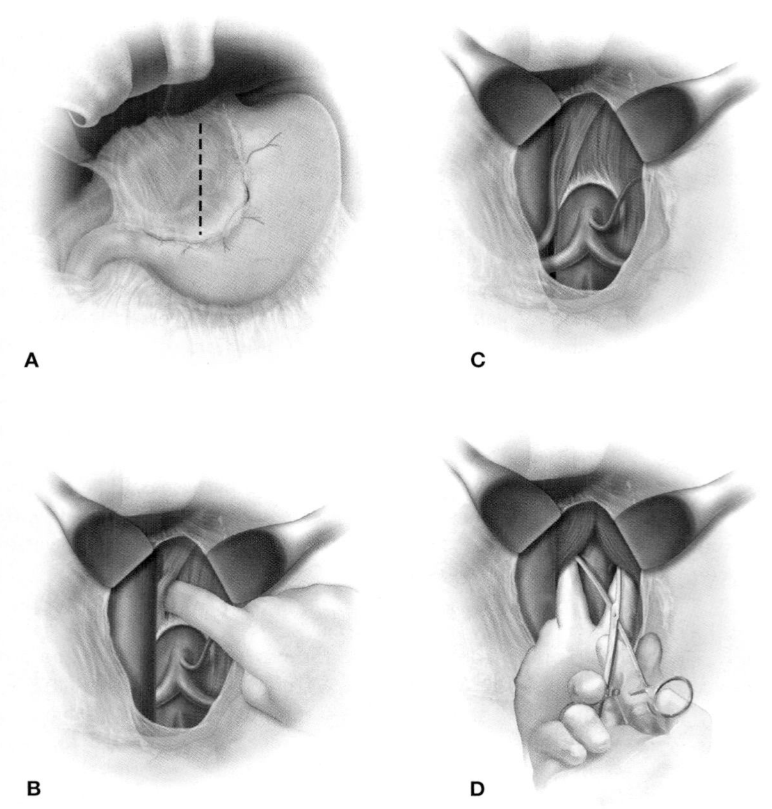

FIGURE 5 • Exposing the supraceliac aorta. **A,** Dotted line shows the location for division of the gastrohepatic ligament. **B,** Once the ligament is divided, the crus is encountered. **C,** Bluntly divide the fibers of the crus. **D,** Using fingers for retraction, control of the aorta can be gained with a clamp, although circumferential control is optimal.

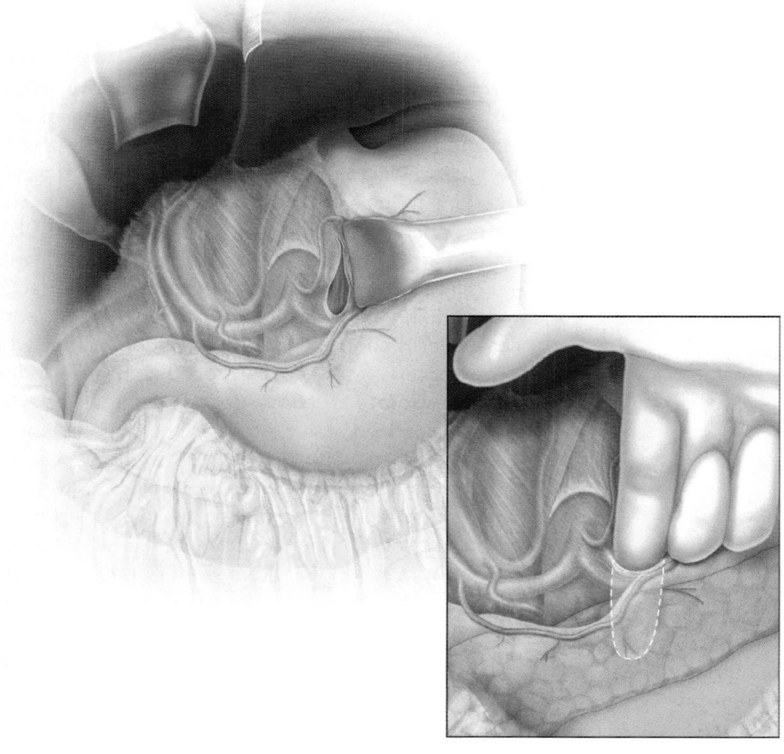

FIGURE 6 • Exposure of the hepatic artery is through the gastrohepatic peritoneum. The liver is retracted superiorly, and the stomach inferiorly. The peritoneum is incised to expose the celiac axis and the hepatic artery.

- ***FOURTH STEP—heparinize and perform revascularization:***
  - The patient is given an IV heparin bolus (70 mg/kg) for anticoagulation. If a one-vessel bypass is planned (most commonly to the SMA), a 6- or 8-mm Dacron tube graft is chosen, and if a two-vessel bypass is planned a 12 × 6 mm or 14 × 7 mm bifurcated Dacron graft is chosen (**FIGURE 7**). The proximal (inflow) anastomosis is sewn first to the aorta or iliac artery in an end-to-side fashion using running 5.0 Prolene sutures. Supraceliac inflow bypasses (antegrade) are tunneled under the pancreas to the SMA. The retropancreatic tunnel is created by careful blunt finger dissection posterior to the pancreas and anterior to the left renal vein. When tunneling care must be taken to assure there is no disruption of the underlying venous network. If a retropancreatic tunnel appears to be too dangerous then an anterior approach is also acceptable.
  - Infrarenal/common iliac bypasses (retrograde) are tunneled to the patient's left using a "lazy C" configuration passing a tunnel through the ligament of Treitz to the lateral aspect of the SMA and celiac arteries. This bypass can also be tunneled deep to the left renal pedicle in what is known as a "French bypass." At this time, the SMA is inspected to determine the need for endarterectomy prior to performing the anastomosis. If endarterectomy is required, this is performed as described above. If possible, the arteriotomy used for the endarterectomy can be used for the bypass anastomosis. The mesenteric (outflow) artery anastomosis is sewn in an end-to-side fashion using running 6.0 Prolene sutures. When performing a single-vessel bypass, priority should be placed on revascularizing the SMA unless the patient's anatomy dictates otherwise. In a two-vessel reconstruction, one limb of the graft is anastomosed to the SMA and the other to the celiac or hepatic artery. Prior to completing the anastomosis, the graft should be flushed and de-aired to prevent any distal embolization. It is of upmost importance to assure that there is no kinking of the conduit. This is especially critical in a retrograde bypass given the longer distance traveled and the "lazy C" configuration.

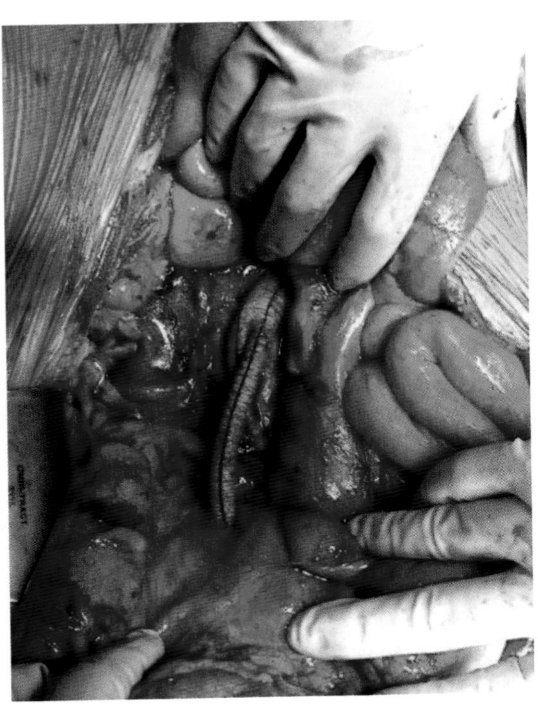

FIGURE 7 ● Orientation of bifurcated antegrade graft to celiac and SMA. (Courtesy of Dr. Benjamin Pomy, George Washington University.)

- ***FIFTH STEP—inspect bowel and close the abdomen:*** After completing the revascularization, the bowel should be inspected to note any areas of ischemia. In some cases, there is graft exposed in the retroperitoneum, and the tongue of the omentum may be used to cover the graft to avoid any contact with the bowel. The abdomen is then closed in usual fashion.

PEARLS AND PITFALLS

Inflow dissection	■ In order to gain access to the supraceliac aorta and successfully sew an anastomosis, appropriate exposure and retraction is imperative. This stresses the need for a full midline laparotomy extending to the xiphoid process superiorly. Given its mobile articulating arms and retractors, the Omni retractor system works best in this tight deep space.
■ Outflow dissection	■ When crossing the mesentery on the way to both the celiac and SMA, there are multiple crossing veins. Care should be taken to dissect carefully in this area to identify and ligate all crossing veins and prevent bleeding, which further disrupts visualization and will make dissection even harder. ■ The left gastric artery is typically the smallest of the celiac axis and may be divided in order to enhance retraction and space to perform the anastomosis and tunneling.

■ Embolectomy technique	■ Fogarty catheter sizes range from 2 to 7 Fr (4-14 mm inflated balloon diameter); given the size of mesenteric vessels are about 1 cm, 3-4 French Fogarty catheters usually work best. An embolectomy catheter should pass clean with residual back bleeding at least twice before it is felt to be successful. ■ When performing the proximal (aortic) embolectomy, it is imperative that the surgeon (or assistant) maintains proximal control on the SMA. As the thrombus is cleared there will be a torrential return of pulsatile flow from the aorta.
Endarterectomy technique	■ A full arterial incision beyond the plaque in both directions assures a complete endarterectomy. The distal flap is going against the direction of blood flow and should be tacked in order to prevent recurrent thrombosis of the vessel.
Bypass technique	■ When tunneling, consideration should always be made to the patient in different position, most importantly sitting up, when planning how to tunnel the bypass. ■ These patients are often very thin, and consideration of how to cover the prosthetic bypass with minimal mesenteric fat should also be made when planning how to tunnel the bypass. If needed, a tongue of omentum can be pulled beneath the small bowel mesentery to cover the bypass graft.

POSTOPERATIVE CARE

Acute/Subacute

- Given their emergent/urgent preoperative presentation, extensive nature of the surgery, and possibility of ongoing bowel ischemia and reperfusion, the aggressive resuscitation begun in the emergency department and continued in the operating room must be maintained in a surgical intensive care unit postoperatively. Often these patients will require open abdomens to facilitate planned return to the operating room to reevaluate bowel viability. The details of this intensive and general surgical care are beyond the scope of this chapter but are imperative to avoid the significant mortality and morbidity rates associated with these presentations and procedures. Therapeutic systemic anticoagulation with intravenous heparin should be maintained to avoid recurrent thrombosis of mesenteric vessels; this allows for easier surgical management of anticoagulation if repeated surgeries are necessary. Lastly, given the likely cardiac incitement of the event, a full cardiac workup looking for source of embolism should also be completed during this critical time.

Chronic

- Even in the elective setting, this is a large surgery on patients with multiple comorbidities; furthermore, bowel reperfusion may still occur creating electrolyte abnormalities. Therefore, these patients should be monitored in surgical intensive care unit postoperatively. Chronic poor nutrition will reverse over an extended time after the patient is able to tolerate greater oral intake; poor nutrition at the time of the procedure may lead to poor wound healing, gastritis, and bowel anastomosis failure, which should all be anticipated. Given the chronic nature of the atherosclerotic disease, systemic anticoagulation is not necessary; however, antiplatelets for treatment of generalized atherosclerosis, particularly coronary artery disease, should be started once oral intake is tolerated.

OUTCOMES

Acute/Subacute

- Acute mesenteric ischemia carries a very high risk of perioperative mortality. Most series estimate perioperative mortality as high as 70%. There are little long-term data available for mortality in these patients; however, 1-year survival has been reported to be around 70% in recent years. The complication rates following revascularization for AMI have been reported as high as 60%. The most common complications following these operations are cardiac and pulmonary complications.[6]

Chronic

- As discussed above, open revascularization for chronic mesenteric ischemia is increasingly reserved as a second-line option due to relatively higher perioperative morbidity and mortality compared with endovascular therapy. Perioperative mortality after revascularization for CMI is estimated at approximately 6%. In some high-volume centers, the mortality has been shown to be around 1% to 3% for good-risk patients, but it can be as high as 20% in low-volume settings. Perioperative morbidity is similarly high and is estimated to be about 30% overall. The most common complications after these operations are pulmonary are cardiac complications, including prolonged mechanical ventilation, myocardial infarction, and cardiac arrest. Long-term symptom relief is excellent after open revascularization, approximately 76% at 5 years. Patency for SMA bypass is also excellent, with primary patency rates estimated at 85% to 90% at 3 years.[2]

COMPLICATIONS

Acute/Subacute

Graft/Surgical-Related Complications

- SMA dissection/stenosis and resulting reocclusion
- Anastomosis failure with hemorrhage
- Other surgical bleeding requiring transfusion
- Limb ischemia secondary to showering emboli
- Enterotomy/missed intestinal ischemia with peritonitis

Hemodynamic Complications

- Myocardial infarction/cardiac arrest
- Prolonged mechanical ventilation
- Acute renal insufficiency/acute renal failure
- Refractory shock with multiorgan system failure
- Death

Chronic

Graft/Surgical-Related Complications

- Graft kinking with occlusion
- SMA/celiac dissection with occlusion
- Graft infection
- Anastomosis failure with hemorrhage
- Enterotomy
- Limb ischemia secondary to showering atherosclerotic emboli
- Surgical wound infection/breakdown (poor nutritional status)

Hemodynamic Complications

- Myocardial infarction/cardiac arrest
- Prolonged mechanical ventilation
- Acute kidney injury/acute renal failure
- Refeeding syndrome
- Death

ACKNOWLEDGMENT

The authors would like to acknowledge the guidance and input of Dr. Robyn Macsata who sadly passed away prior to publication of this text.

REFERENCES

1. Wyers MC, Martin MC. *Acute mesenteric arterial disease-clinicalKey. Rutherford's Textbook of Vascular Surgery and Endovascular Therapy*. 9th ed. Elsevier Inc; 2019. doi:10.1016/B978-0-323-42791-3.00133-X
2. Oderich GS, Ribeiro M. *Chronic mesenteric arterial disease: clinical evaluation, open surgical and endovascular treatment. Rutherford's Textbook of Vascular Surgery and Endovascular Therapy*. 9th ed. Elsevier Inc; 2019. doi:10.1016/B978-0-323-42791-3.00132-8
3. Ginsburg M, Obara P, Lambert DL, et al. ACR Appropriateness Criteria® imaging of mesenteric ischemia. *J Am Coll Radiol*. 2018;15(11):S332-S340. doi:10.1016/j.jacr.2018.09.018
4. Huber TS, Björck M, Chandra A, et al. Chronic mesenteric ischemia: clinical practice guidelines from the society for vascular surgery. *J Vasc Surg*. 2021;73(1):87S-115S. doi:10.1016/j.jvs.2020.10.029
5. Foley MI, Moneta GL, Abou-Zamzam AM, et al. Revascularization of the superior mesenteric artery alone for treatment of intestinal ischemia. *J Vasc Surg*. 2000;32(1):37-47. doi:10.1067/mva.2000.107314
6. Ryer EJ, Kalra M, Oderich GS, et al. Revascularization for acute mesenteric ischemia. *J Vasc Surg*. 2012;55(6):1682-1689. doi:10.1016/j.jvs.2011.12.017

Chapter 20

Advanced Aneurysm Management Techniques: Open Surgical Anatomy and Repair

Harold Davis Waller and Mark F. Conrad

DEFINITION

- An aneurysm is defined as a permanent, focal dilation of an artery to a size that is greater than 50% of the normal or expected transverse diameter of the vessel. Although dimensions differ slightly for men and women, practically speaking the normal diameter for the abdominal aorta is 2 cm; therefore, the abdominal aorta is considered aneurysmal when it reaches 3 cm in the transverse dimension.
- *A fusiform* aneurysm is the symmetric enlargement of the entire vessel and is the most common type of abdominal aortic aneurysm (AAA). A *saccular* aneurysm is a focal outpouching of the vessel wall to one side and is much less common.
- Aneurysms may occur in virtually any vessel in the body but are most commonly seen in the infrarenal AAA. The *neck* is the length of normal aorta between the ostium of the inferior-most renal artery and the beginning of the aneurysmal aorta. The term *juxtarenal* is used to describe AAAs that do not involve the renal arteries but, due to their proximity to the inferior-most renal artery (<1 cm neck), require clamping above the renal arteries to complete the proximal aortic anastomosis. For a *suprarenal* aneurysm, at least one of the renal arteries arises from aneurysmal aorta, which implies the need for both a proximal clamp and renal artery reconstruction at the time of the repair (**FIGURE 1**). This chapter will focus on the indications and techniques for open repair of infrarenal and juxtarenal AAAs.
- The dreaded complication of AAA is rupture. Size and expansion rate are the two most important predictors of rupture, such that they guide the indication for repair in asymptomatic patients.[1]
- Other factors that increase rupture risk include female gender, a family history of aneurysms, smoking status (higher risk for current smokers vs never and former smokers), hypertension, and chronic obstructive pulmonary disease (COPD).[2-5]

PATIENT HISTORY AND PHYSICAL FINDINGS

- A thorough history and physical exam is imperative in the evaluation of a patient being considered for aneurysm repair.
- History of present illness: Determine how the aneurysm was found. Often, AAAs are an incidental discovery on an imaging test performed for another purpose. It is critical to ask about abdominal or back pain as these symptoms may be caused by a "symptomatic" aneurysm that would require more urgent repair.
- Past medical history: Patients with concomitant cardiac, lung, and/or renal disease tend to have more complications perioperatively and should be medically optimized prior to proceeding with elective repair. Although there is no broad recommendation for preoperative cardiac revascularization in asymptomatic patients, those with known cardiac disease or risk factors should be evaluated by a cardiologist as there is some recent evidence that certain subgroups of these high-risk patients may benefit from preoperative revascularization.[6,7]
- Family history: Approximately 15% to 20% of patients with AAA will have a first-degree relative with aneurysmal disease. Patients with AAA should be counseled to alert their siblings and children to this condition, so they may be screened appropriately.[3,8]
- Social history: Smoking has been linked to an increased risk of aneurysm formation and rate of expansion. Patients should be counseled on smoking cessation.
- Review of systems: In addition to the generalized systems review appropriate for all patients undergoing major surgery, particular attention should be directed to other vascular comorbidities. In particular, query about previous cerebrovascular accident (CVA) or transient ischemic attack (TIA) symptoms, amaurosis fugax, mesenteric ischemia, and lower extremity ischemic symptoms (claudication, rest pain, ulcers). Work up positive symptoms as appropriate.

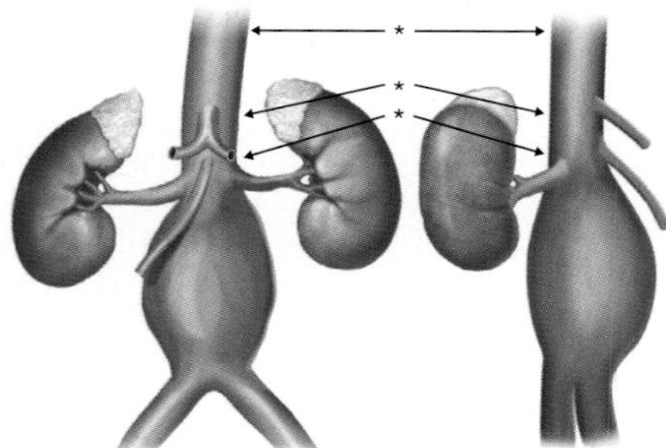

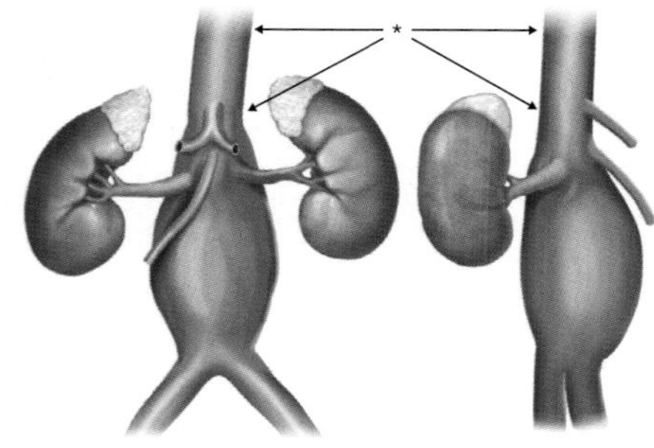

* Potential cross-clamp sites

FIGURE 1 • Anatomic differences between a juxtarenal AAA, where the neck of normal aortic diameter is less than 1 cm, and a suprarenal AAA, where the takeoff of at least one renal artery arises from the aneurysm.

- On physical exam, perform a thorough abdominal exam noting the location of surgical scars, and be aware that the positive predictive value for localizing a small- to moderate-sized AAA on exam is poor. A small proportion (1%-10%) of patients with AAA will have a concomitant aneurysm elsewhere, so be cognizant that those patients with known AAA and a prominent femoral or popliteal pulse may need further imaging to exclude an aneurysm in these locations.[9]
- Conversely, patients who initially present with peripheral aneurysms such as femoral (85%) or popliteal aneurysms (60%) have a much higher rate of concomitant AAA and aortic screening should be performed in these patients.[9,10]

IMAGING AND OTHER DIAGNOSTIC STUDIES

- Of all imaging techniques used for AAA screening and surveillance, B-mode ultrasonography is the least expensive and safest with regard to radiation exposure. Currently, the U.S. Preventative Services Task Force (USPSTF) recommends a one-time abdominal ultrasound as a AAA screening test for all males between the ages of 65 and 75 years who have ever smoked and selective abdominal ultrasound screening based on risk factors for all males in this age range who have never smoked. Women aged 65 to 75 years who have never smoked and have no family history of AAA should not undergo any routine ultrasound screening for AAA. It is generally accepted that a negative screening ultrasound exonerates the patient from further screening or surveillance imaging, as the likelihood of new aneurysm development of clinical significance after the age of screening is extremely low. If a screening ultrasound detects a small aneurysm, yearly ultrasounds are indicated until the sac approaches a size where repair may be indicated, at which time further imaging with computed tomography (CT) is recommended.[9,11,12]
- Computed tomography angiography (CTA) provides a more accurate assessment of aneurysm size, extent, branch vessel proximity, and involvement (which is used to determine if the aneurysm is amenable to endovascular or open repair, and if open repair is to be done, where the proximal clamp should be applied) and is the test that should be used for planning open AAA repair. A thorough exam should include thin (1.5 cm or smaller) cuts of the chest, abdomen, and pelvis with contrast administered in the arterial phase (**FIGURE 2**).

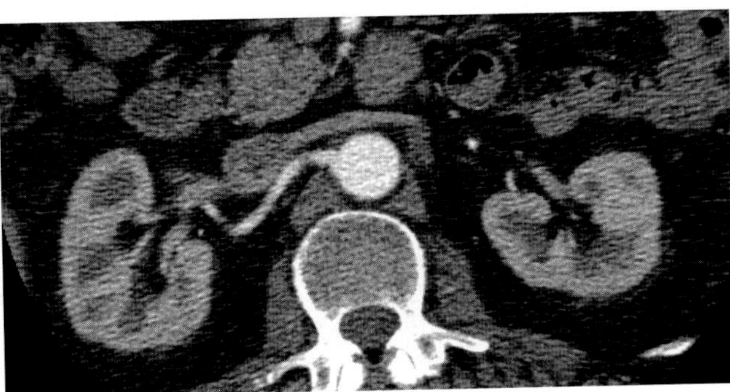

FIGURE 2 ● Axial cut of a CTA showing the takeoff or the right renal artery and the more commonly seen renal vein lying anterior to the aorta.

- It is important to note the location of the aneurysm and its relationship to the renal arteries. Renal anatomy should be noted as well, including any accessory renal arteries, renal vein course, and the presence of a pelvic or horseshoe kidney. The renal vein usually travels anterior to the aorta, but a retroaortic renal vein should be noted as it will influence the operative approach to the aorta. Other venous anatomy, such as a duplicated or left-sided inferior vena cava (IVC), should be noted as well.

SURGICAL MANAGEMENT

- The decision to operate on an asymptomatic patient is based on three primary factors: the risk of aneurysm rupture, the risk associated with aneurysm repair, and the patient's life expectancy. The operative risk and overall life expectancy should be assessed. Assuming that a patient is fit to proceed with repair, size is currently our best predictor of rupture. The UK Small Aneurysm Trial and ADAM VA Trial recommend treatment for all patients with an infrarenal AAA larger than 5.5 cm in size, with consideration for repair in women with AAA of 5.0 cm given their higher risk of rupture and likely smaller baseline aortic size. These studies also support repair for those patients who have an increase in diameter of greater than 0.5 cm over a 6-month period (**TABLE 1**).[13,14]
- Although there are no large trials looking specifically at iliac aneurysms, repair is generally recommended when they reach 4 cm or greater in size. Iliac aneurysms are more often seen in patients with a concomitant aortic aneurysm and only a quarter of patients with iliac aneurysms will have isolated disease.
- All open repairs should be performed under general anesthesia. It is preferable for the anesthesia team to evaluate the patient prior to the day of surgery so that appropriate time for developing an anesthetic plan, lines, and other means of hemodynamic monitoring are allowed. The use of an epidural for pain control in the postoperative period is useful as it limits narcotic use and improves pulmonary toilet during the early postoperative period. In addition, arrangements should be made for autotransfusion given the unavoidable amount of intraoperative blood loss, which is often measured in liters.
- Preoperative understanding of the patient's individual anatomy is of the utmost importance. The surgeon must know the proximity of the aneurysmal aorta to the renal and visceral vessels and whether these branch vessels arise from the aneurysm, as this will determine where the proximal cross clamp will be applied. If at all possible, clamps should only be applied to nonaneurysmal aorta with minimal thrombus

Table 1: Indications for Repair of Abdominal Aortic Aneurysm

- Leak or frank rupture
- Size (5.5 cm in men, 5 cm in women for aortic aneurysm, and 4 cm for iliac aneurysms)
- Increase in size of >0.5 cm over a 6-mo period
- Symptomatic (pain, compression on adjacent structures)
- Dissection within aneurysm

or calcification to minimize risk of clamp injury or distal embolization of debris, and all aneurysmal aorta should be resected even if this means involvement of the visceral or iliac segment. One exception to this rule is the case where the aneurysm arises directly below the renal artery but does not involve the artery. In this instance, a cuff of aneurysmal tissue can be plicated into the anastomosis to avoid the need for an aortorenal bypass, which can lead to increased operative times, length of stay, and a decline in renal function.[15] If the aorta contains a significant amount of debris or there is little space between branch vessels, a more proximal clamp site in the supraceliac aorta should be considered. It is important to discuss the proposed clamp site with anesthesia preoperatively, as this will affect their management of the patient. The choice of clamp site should be made during the preoperative planning stage, as the intraoperative need to move the clamp higher is associated with adverse outcomes.[16]

- Planning for the distal anastomosis requires review not only of the aortic bifurcation but of the iliac arteries as well. If there is aneurysmal or occlusive disease within the iliac arteries, concurrent repair with a bifurcated graft may be appropriate; otherwise, the majority of AAAs are repaired with a tube graft to the iliac bifurcation. The type of distal anastomosis may predicate the method of distal control, which can be obtained with a single clamp across the bifurcation or both iliac origins, or occlusion balloons (Foley catheters or Pruitt occlusion balloons) for heavily diseased vessels.
- Key preoperative planning concerns are summarized in **TABLE 2**.

Table 2: Operative Planning

- Is a retroperitoneal or transperitoneal approach better?
- Where is the best location for proximal control? What are the alternatives should intraoperative findings preclude using this site?
- Will clamping cause renal or visceral ischemia?
- Will the renal or visceral arteries need to be reconstructed as part of the repair? If so, what size grafts should be used for the bypass?
- Where is the renal vein? Does it pass anteriorly or posterior to the aorta? Will the kidney be taken up or left down?
- How will distal control be obtained? Will reconstruction involve the iliac arteries or can the distal anastomosis be to the bifurcation?
- What size/type graft should be used?

TECHNIQUES

- There are two approaches for the open repair of the infrarenal or juxtarenal aortic aneurysm: transperitoneal or retroperitoneal approach (**FIGURE 3**). The approach used for an infrarenal AAA is based on several factors: body habitus (obese patients are often best approached via retroperitoneal incision), prior abdominal surgery (concern for intraperitoneal adhesions), and clamp sites; above the renal arteries may favor a retroperitoneal approach, whereas planned intervention on the right renal or iliac artery would be easily performed from a transperitoneal approach.

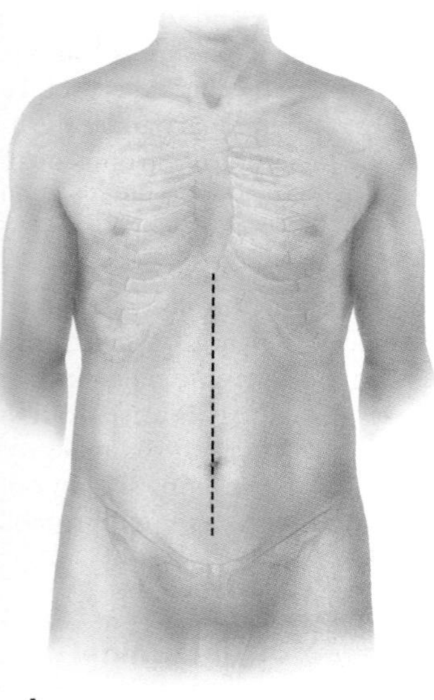

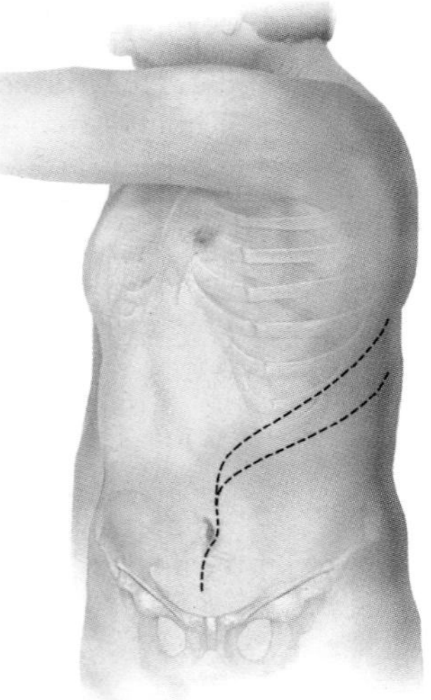

FIGURE 3 ● Incision for the two approaches to aneurysm repair. **A,** Transperitoneal and **B,** retroperitoneal. The retroperitoneal approach can be modified for higher exposure on the visceral aorta.

TRANSPERITONEAL APPROACH

- Positioning: The patient is positioned supine on a standard operating room (OR) table with both arms extended. The operative field should include the nipple line superiorly to midthighs inferiorly to allow exposure for a high incision as well as groin access should the femoral vessels be needed. The hair is clipped and a towel is placed over the perineum. Any previous incisions within the operative field are marked. A Steri-Drape or Ioban is used to secure the drapes in position. Once fully prepped, check pulse volume recording (PVRs) and/or distal pulses to establish a baseline for distal perfusion.
- Incision: A generous midline incision from the xiphoid to the pubis is made and dissection is carried through the underlying tissue until the peritoneal cavity is entered (**FIGURE 3**). It may be necessary to extend the incision cephalad lateral alongside the xiphoid if higher exposure is needed, or in emergent situations such as a rupture where immediate supraceliac control is needed. A self-retaining retractor system should then be positioned. Our preference is the Omni retractor as the open configuration of the system does not limit the width of exposure.
- Dissection: The greater omentum and transverse colon are retracted cephalad and packed away in a moistened towel or lap pad on top of the patient's chest. The small bowel is retracted to the right and packed within a separate moistened towel. The small bowel is gently placed behind a self-retaining retractor, taking care not to compromise the superior mesenteric artery (SMA). This exposes the ligament of Treitz (LOT), which can be divided along the jejunum to the level of the aorta (**FIGURE 4**). Reposition the retractor to displace as much small bowel as possible out of the field, and take down the LOT with electrocautery, taking care not to injure the bowel. The inferior mesenteric vein is usually ligated during this dissection. This allows access to the infrarenal aorta where the overlying retroperitoneal tissue can be dissected-free. Depending on the proximal extent of aorta needed for an adequate cuff of the proximal anastomosis, an anterior renal vein may need to be mobilized cephalad and surrounded with a red rubber catheter or Penrose drain for easy manipulation during creation of the proximal anastomosis. In order to gain the best mobility, the gonadal, adrenal, and renal lumbar branches are ligated if necessary (**FIGURE 5**).
- Exposure of the supraceliac aorta (**FIGURE 6**): This maneuver is only needed in cases where high abdominal aortic exposure is needed, such as in a rupture. The left lobe of the liver must be retracted laterally by taking down the triangular ligament. Next, identify and dissect-free the gastroesophageal junction after dividing the gastrohepatic ligament, which is most expeditiously done by palpating for

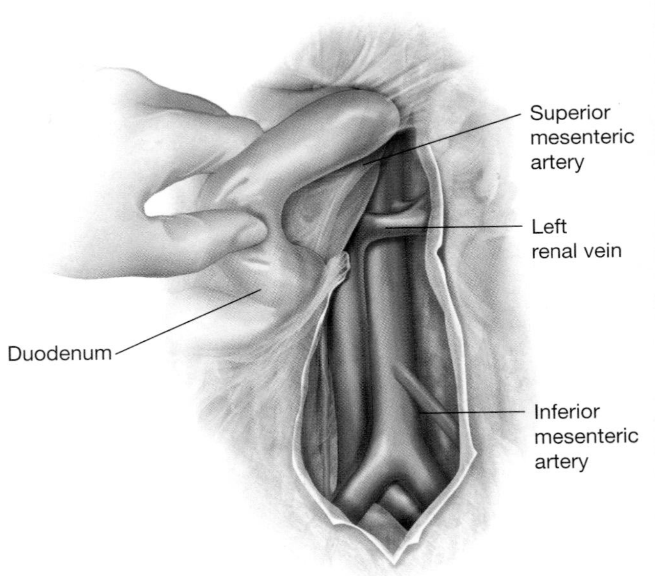

FIGURE 4 • Division of the ligament of Treitz (LOT). After reflecting the colon cephalad and the small bowel to the patient's right, the LOT can be divided to expose the infrarenal aorta.

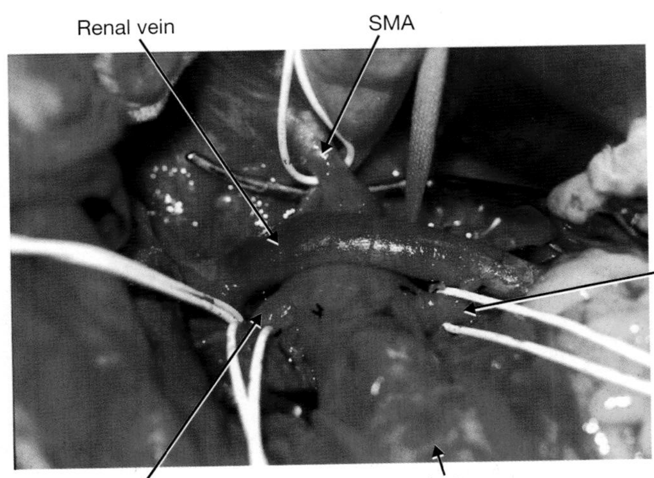

FIGURE 5 • (illustration and photo): Mobilization of the left renal vein. Cephalad or caudal mobilization of the left renal vein to expose the origin of the renal arteries. Ligation of several venous side branches may be needed for safe mobilization.

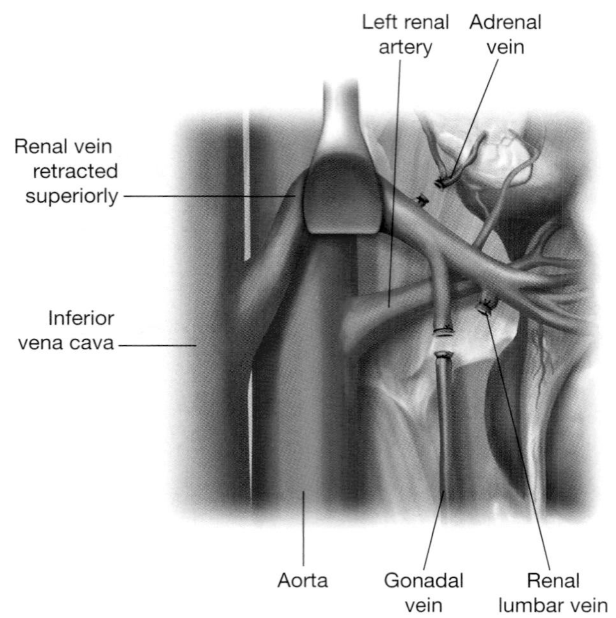

FIGURE 5 ● (*continued*)

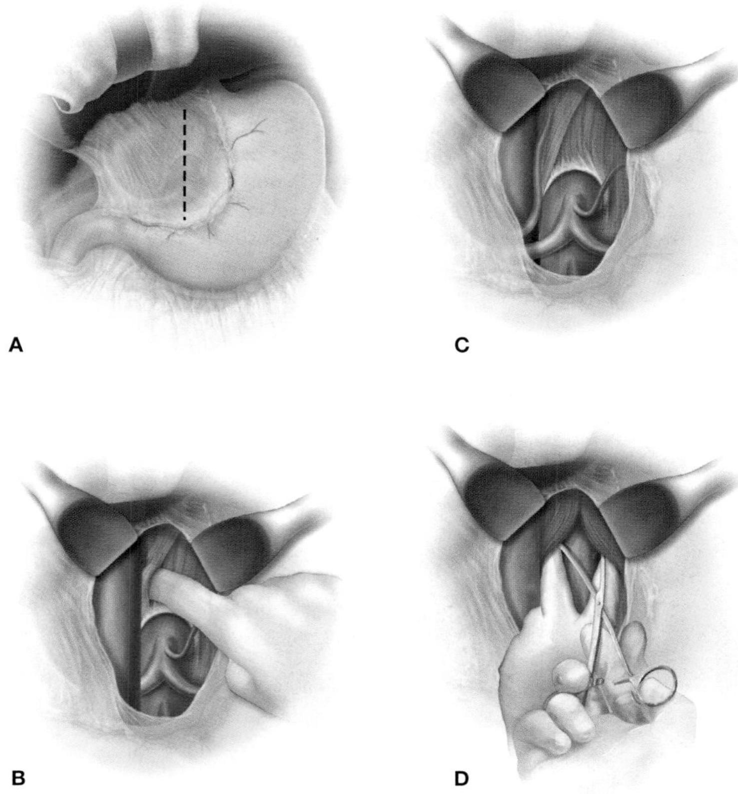

FIGURE 6 ● Gaining control of the supraceliac aorta. **A,** *Dotted line* shows the location for division of the gastrohepatic ligament. **B,** Once the ligament is divided, the crus is encountered. **C,** Bluntly divide the fibers of the crus. **D,** Using fingers for retraction, control of the aorta can be gained with a clamp, although circumferential control is optimal.

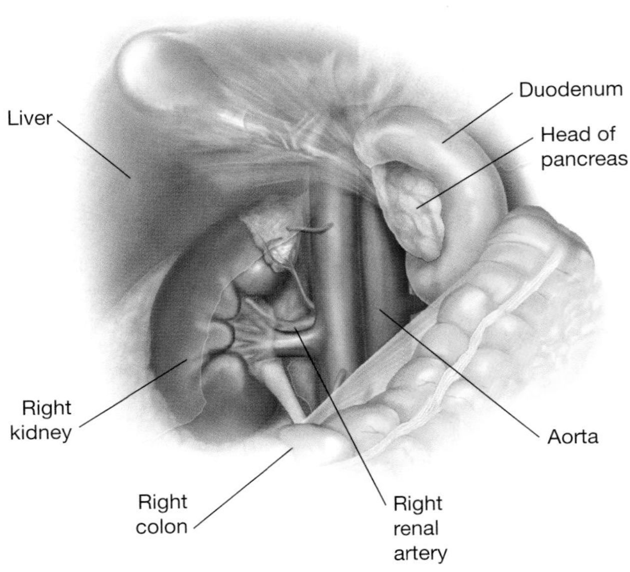

FIGURE 7 ● Exposure of the aorta and right renal artery via right medial visceral rotation.

the nasogastric tube and applying caudal traction. Division of the gastrohepatic ligament must be performed with the cautious consideration that a replaced left hepatic artery could be coursing beneath this structure. The esophagus can then be retracted to the patient's left, which exposes the aorta. To obtain control, an aortic compressor can be used in extreme circumstances; however, dissection of the aorta circumferentially and surrounding the aorta with a shoestring (if the patient's condition allows) is preferable. This exposure, although useful when urgent supraceliac control is needed, will not allow access to the visceral segment of the aorta. In order to gain visceral exposure, a right or left medial visceral rotation should be incorporated into the dissection. The use of a right medial visceral rotation will allow access to the right renal artery, as well as placing the SMA on 90° tension, and is useful for exposing a clamp site in those patients with a juxtarenal aneurysm with very little room between the renals and SMA (**FIGURE 7**). The use of a left medial visceral rotation also allows for exposure to the entire visceral segment of the aorta as well as the left renal artery. In this approach, care must be taken to avoid injury to the spleen and tail of the pancreas. In patients where a supra-SMA or supraceliac clamp is planned, the retroperitoneal approach is preferable.

RETROPERITONEAL APPROACH

- Positioning: Once asleep, the patient is placed in the lateral position with the left side up at an approximately 60° angle (**FIGURE 8**). The right arm is extended on an armboard, being sure to leave room for an Omni or other self-retaining retractor post. The upper left arm should be placed on another armboard and padded to prevent neural injury. The bed is flexed at the patient's flank to open up the area between the ribs and the left anterior superior iliac spine. Position the legs so that the lower leg is straight and the upper leg is flexed at the knee. Pillows are used as padding

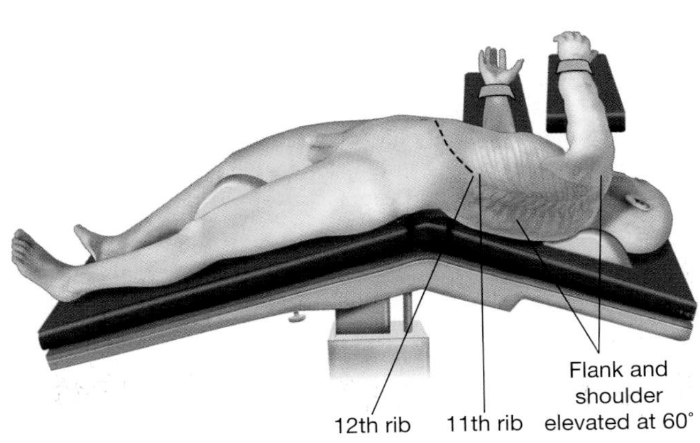

FIGURE 8 ● Positioning for retroperitoneal incision.

between legs. A beanbag can be inflated to keep the patient in place, and we secure thick cloth tape over the shoulder to keep the patient on their side with the shoulders at 90° and the hips rotated posteriorly. If a bean bag is not available, blanket rolls can be used anteriorly and posteriorly to further secure the patient. All bony prominences and pressure points should be well padded to avoid injury. Ultimately, positioning should allow access to prep an operative field from the spine posteriorly to the umbilicus anteriorly and from the nipple line to the groins. Use clippers to remove hair within the prep area. Prep from the axilla and nipple line to the upper thigh. Mark all previous incisions and use a Steri-Drape or Ioban over the entire prepped area to secure the drapes. Once fully prepped, check pulse volume recording (PVR) and/or distal pulses/signals to establish a baseline for distal perfusion.

- Incision: Unless clamping is planned at or above the level of the SMA, a standard retroperitoneal incision over the 11th rib (10th interspace) will provide adequate exposure (**FIGURE 3**). Some practitioners confirm this location by ultrasound. Carry the incision from the posterior axillary line to the anterior border of the rectus. Avoid entry into the pleural cavity if possible by being cognizant that the further posterior the incision is commenced, the higher likelihood this will occur.
- Dissection: Carry the dissection through the underlying tissue, dividing the transversalis fascia, and enter the retroperitoneal space down to but not violating Gerota's fascia. This space can be more easily identified by resecting a distal segment of the 11th rib, as the transversalis fascia and transversus abdominal musculature insert along the inferior border of this rib. It is possible to stay entirely within a retroperitoneal plane during this dissection; however, if the peritoneum is violated the abdominal contents can be packed away with retractors, or the peritoneum can be immediately repaired with a running 3-0 chromic suture and the dissection continued in the retroperitoneum. The aorta is approached via an anterorenal (colloquially referred to as "leaving the kidney down") or retrorenal plane ("taking the kidney up") (**FIGURE 9**). Generally, the aorta is approached via a retrorenal approach unless there is a retroaortic renal vein or a need to access the SMA beyond its origin. As the retroperitoneal dissection continues, the left ureter should be identified, swept toward the midline, and placed behind a retractor to avoid injury during the aortic dissection. The left renal artery is identified and dissected back to its aortic origin.
- The renal lumbar vein should be identified and ligated to avoid injury and excessive bleeding. Once the origin of the renal artery is identified, a right angle clamp can be placed along the surface of the aorta and the overlying retroperitoneal tissue divided with electrocautery. It is imperative to get on the aorta and stay on the aorta to avoid excessive bleeding from the retroperitoneal tissue. The aorta is exposed to the bifurcation and can be dissected circumferentially here if a clamp site is planned; however, note the left iliac vein can course posterior to the bifurcation and should be avoided. It is often easier to expose an area of the left common iliac artery for clamping and control the right common iliac artery with an occlusion balloon from within. It is unwise to gain distal circumferential control of the iliac arteries in this situation as the iliac veins are often adherent to the posterior aspect of the artery and are easily injured. Also, limiting dissection of the left common iliac artery will minimize the risk of retrograde ejaculation in men, which occurs when the surround nerve plexus is disrupted. Pay particular attention to identifying and not injuring the ureters, which eventually cross anterior to the iliac vessels. Identify and isolate the inferior mesenteric artery (IMA) with a vessel loop. If necessary, by commencing the incision along a higher rib space, the dissection can be carried caudal to expose the entire visceral segment (**FIGURE 10**).

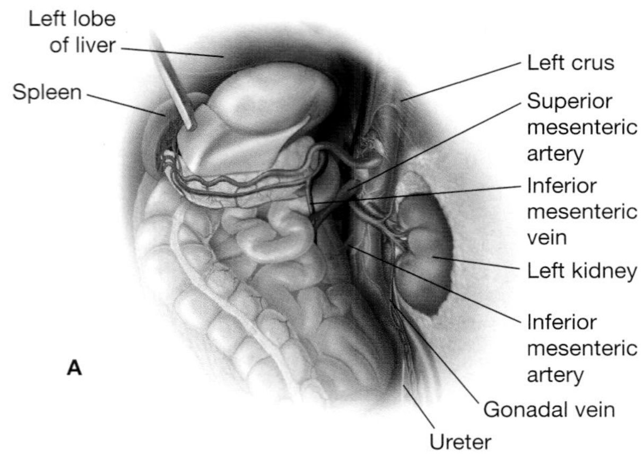

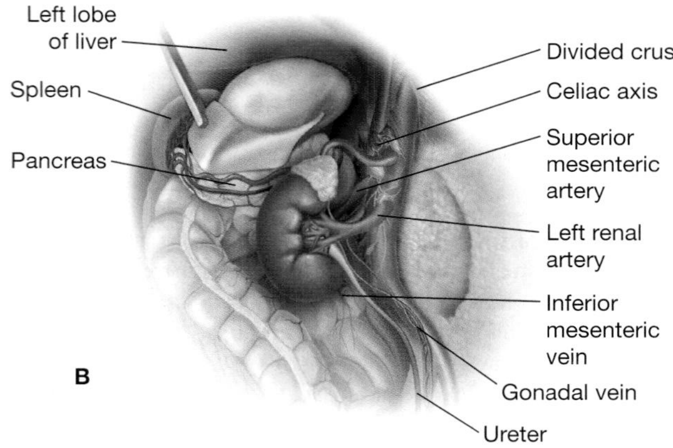

FIGURE 9 ● The aorta can be approached in an anterorenal plane **(A)** or a retrorenal plane **(B)**.

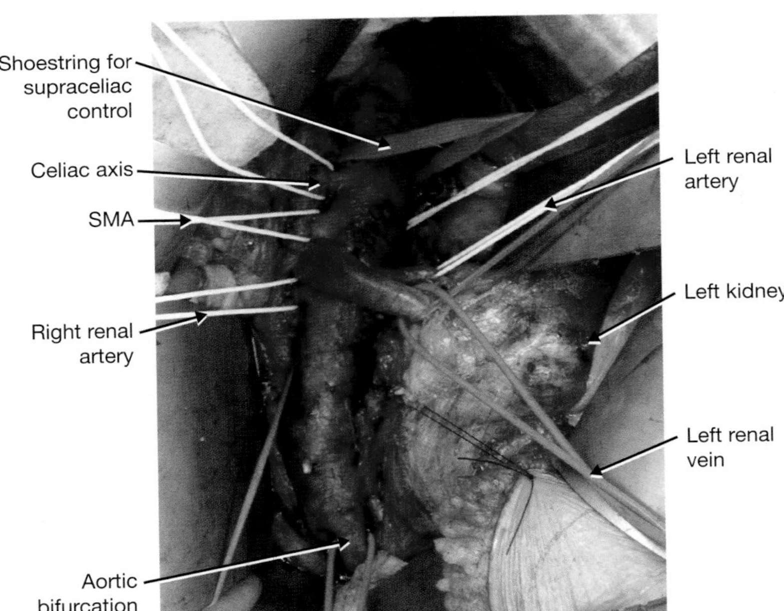

FIGURE 10 ● Exposure of the entire abdominal aorta from a retroperitoneal approach. Here, the kidney is "left down" in an anterorenal plane. All vessels are surrounded with vessels loops.

AORTIC CLAMPING AND REPAIR

- When dissecting on the aorta, care must be taken to minimize aggressive manipulation and subsequent atheroembolization, particularly if preoperative imaging shows extensive mural debris. Regardless of approach, it is important during circumferential dissection of the aorta to avoid injury to the posterior lumbar arteries, which are usually paired. The posterior aortic dissection is performed with a blunt sweeping motion of your finger. If the tissue does not pull away from the aorta easily, it is likely due to the presence of a branch vessel. In this instance, the aorta is gently retracted and the dissection is continued sharply under direct vision. If the lumbar vessels are encountered and require ligation, carefully circumferentially dissect out the artery, tie the proximal side of the vessel, and use another tie or apply a double clip to the distal end prior to dividing.
- Choice of graft: There are several choices for conduit during open AAA repair. Generally, a polytetrafluoroethylene (PTFE) or Dacron tube graft is sewn from the proximal aorta to the bifurcation. The aorta can be measured for the appropriate graft with aortic sizers, but often, an estimation of size can be made from the preoperative CTA. Regardless, the majority of patients can be repaired with an 18- to 22-mm graft. In patients with extensive bifurcation or iliac disease, a bifurcated graft may be used. If this is the case, the proximal single lumen portion of the graft should be as short as possible to prevent kinking. In contemporary practice, we make this portion 3 to 4 cm to provide a seal zone if future endografting is necessary. Tunneling the limb to the femoral level should be done only in special circumstances, and if so, care must be taken to position the graft posterior to the ureter (**FIGURE 11**).

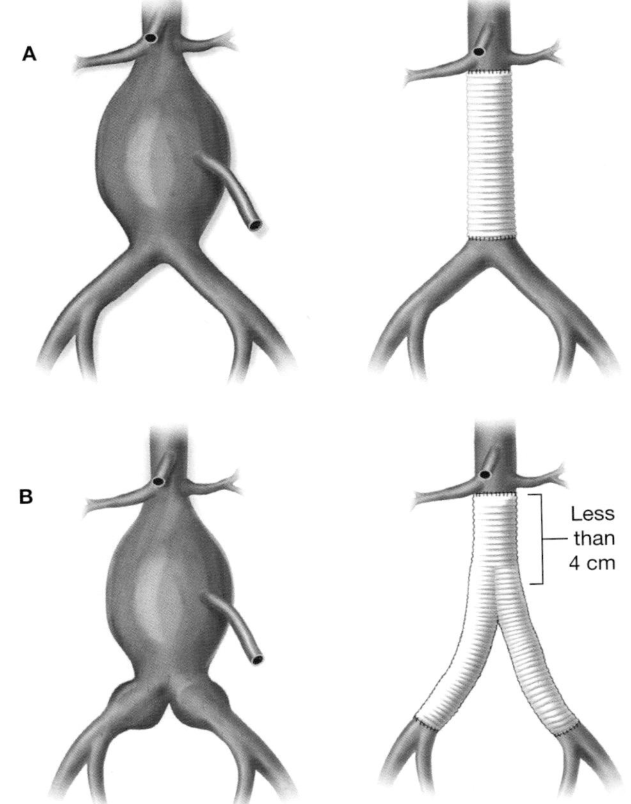

FIGURE 11 ● **A,** Tube graft from infrarenal aorta to bifurcation and **(B)** bifurcated graft from infrarenal aorta to iliac or femoral vessels.

- Choosing the site of the proximal anastomosis: This will depend on the quality of the proximal neck of the aneurysm and the vicinity of the visceral vessels. In the most straightforward scenario, an adequate cuff of normal aorta is present below the renal arteries to allow for infrarenal clamping and an end-to-end anastomosis. In the event of a short infrarenal cuff, a suprarenal clamp can be used to provide space to sew. If the aneurysmal tissue extends to the visceral branches, or if there is significant atherosclerotic disease of the branches, a beveled anastomosis may be required, possibly including an endarterectomy of the origin of a branch vessel or a bypass to the left renal artery (**FIGURE 12**). When there is aneurysmal tissue to the level of the renal arteries, whether one employs a suprarenal clamp and plication of the aneurysm cuff with the graft sewn below the renal arteries or a beveled anastomosis with left renal artery bypass, there is no difference in the 3-year incidence of aneurysmal degeneration of the proximal anastomosis, change in long-term renal function, or mortality (**FIGURE 13**).[15] Overall, these considerations should be apparent based on careful review of preoperative imaging and planned well before clamping of the aorta. From the retroperitoneal approach, every effort should be made to incorporate the right renal artery into the anastomosis.
- In preparation for clamping, the patient should be systemically heparinized at a dose of 70 U/kg and heparin is allowed to circulate for 3 to 5 minutes. It is important to communicate with anesthesia prior to clamping and unclamping so they may anticipate and address subsequent hemodynamic shifts. Generally, the systemic pressure should be reduced in preparation for the proximal clamping. If the visceral segment is involved, bulldog clamps should be applied to the visceral vessels prior to aortic clamping to avoid embolization. The proximal clamp is then carefully applied and secured with a shoestring around the clamp. The aortic sac is then opened with electrocautery and heavy scissors proximally and distally. Mural debris should be carefully removed to identify all patent lumbar arteries. Distal control can then be obtained by internal balloon occlusion of each iliac with Foley catheters if external control was not previously obtained. All back-bleeding lumbar vessels should be suture ligated with 2-0 silk in a figure-of-eight fashion. In heavily calcified aortas, focal endarterectomies may be necessary for effective ligation of each vessel.
- Sewing of the proximal anastomoses: There are several techniques to complete the anastomosis, and the choice is based on a combination of surgeon preference and tissue quality. Regardless of technique, however, the posterior row of sutures should be sewn first. Ensure that there is adequate exposure of the proximal aorta; this may require the use of a self-retaining retractor within the opened sac or stay sutures on the edges of the sac. Place the graft on the patient's chest upside down, so the posterior aspect of the graft lies anteriorly. If the posterior row is to be done in an interrupted fashion, the first mattress suture is placed in the middle of the graft from outside to inside, placing a snap on the needled ends of the sutures. Place four more mattress sutures, two on each side, working your way to the 3- and 9-o'clock positions on the graft. Care must be taken to ensure there are no gaps between sutures; all travel must be within a mattress stitch and not between stitches. Once all sutures are placed in the graft, begin placing the aortic sutures from inside to outside on the aorta. The proximal aorta is usually not completely transected and the posterior wall can be used to create a Creech bite that uses the aortic wall as a pledget. Once all sutures are placed, each individual stitch is pledgeted and tied down snugly. The anterior

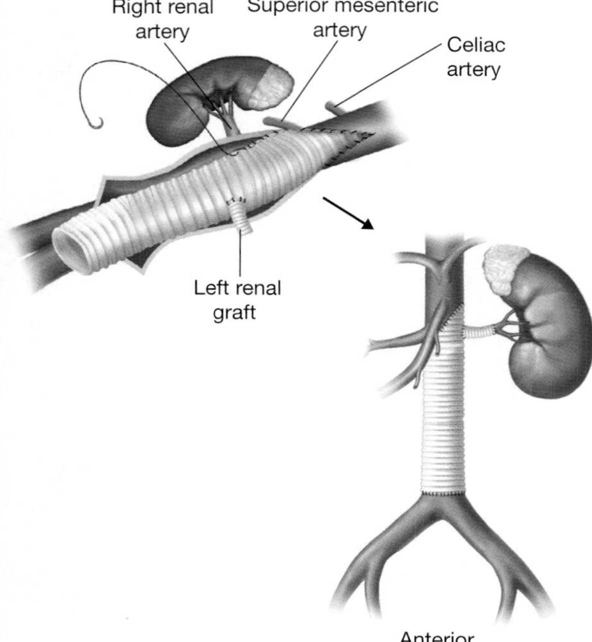

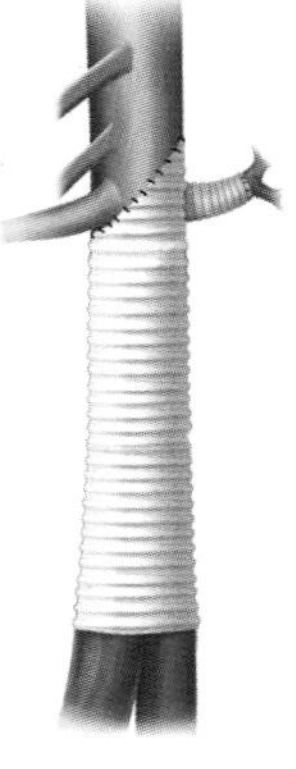

FIGURE 12 ● Beveled anastomosis with bypass to the left renal artery. The suture line runs just inferior to the right renal artery.

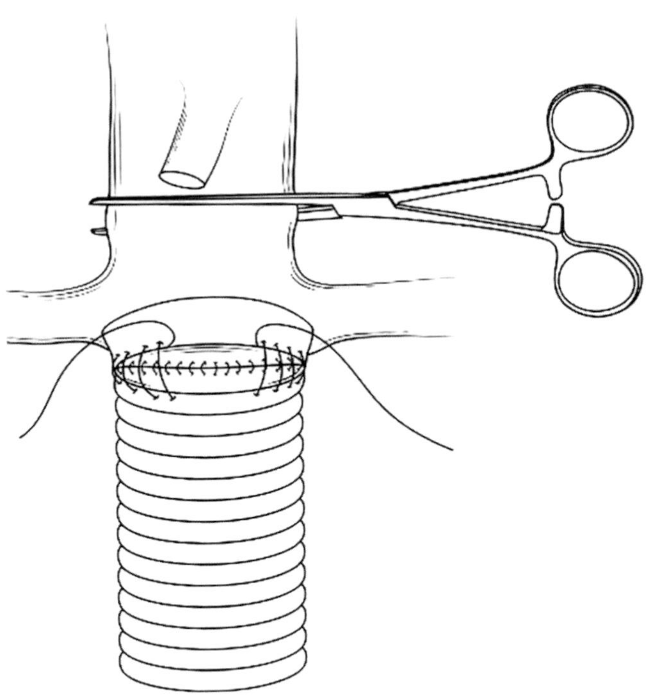

FIGURE 13 ● Plicated aneurysm cuff (PLI) technique, in which aneurysm cuff is plicated on itself and cuff is sewn to the graft up to the level of the renal arteries.

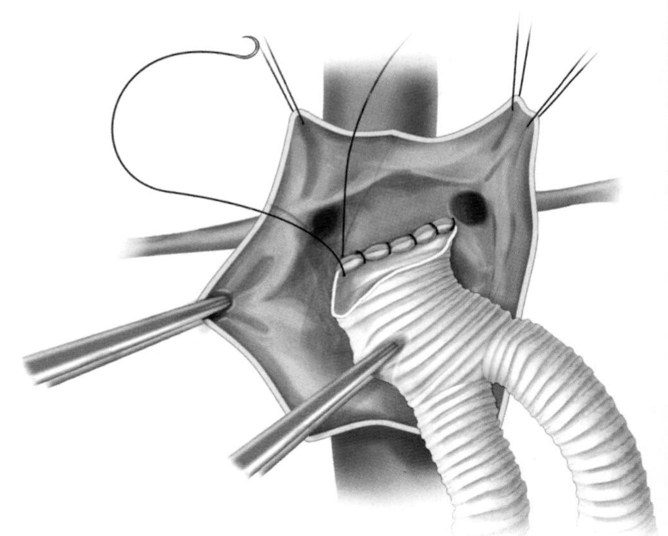

FIGURE 14 ● Construction of the posterior row of the proximal anastomosis. Note that the anterior and lateral aspects of the aorta are divided but the posterior wall is left intact in this figure, using "Creech" suturing technique.

row is then completed, starting from each side and working your way to the center, such that the anterior-most stitch is the final stitch placed. These are also pledgeted and tied into place. Once the proximal anastomosis is completed, an atraumatic clamp should be applied to the body of the graft, and the proximal aortic clamp is slowly released to test for integrity of the repair. Any leaks in the suture line should be addressed at this time, particularly along the posterior row, as this will be inaccessible once the distal anastomosis is in place. It is unwise to attempt to place stitches on a fully perfused aorta, and the proximal clamp should be reapplied if pledgeted repair stitches are necessary. A running anastomosis can also be performed with a 3-0 Prolene and an atraumatic needle. The back row is again begun in the middle of the graft with deep Creech bites on the aorta. The graft can be parachuted in to make the suture line taut. The back row should be inspected to ensure that it is snug and additional sutures are used at the 3- and 9-o'clock positions to secure the back row and run to the top of the aorta (**FIGURES 14** and **15**).

- IMA implantation: Although the IMA can generally be ligated without clinical consequence, there are certain situations where it may be beneficial to reimplant the vessel to avoid bowel ischemic complications. Reimplantation generally is associated with excellent long-term patency and a low risk of large bowel ischemia. Patients with altered pelvic blood flow, such as those with prior gastrointestinal surgery or occluded hypogastric arteries, should especially be considered for IMA reimplantation. Furthermore, visual inspection of the sigmoid colon prior to closure should be done, and IMA reimplantation is performed if there appears to be any questionable viability of the bowel. Additionally, prior to IMA ligation, an assessment of back-bleeding (and thus the collateral circulation to the IMA territory) should be performed and reimplantation is considered in cases where the back-bleeding is poor.[17]

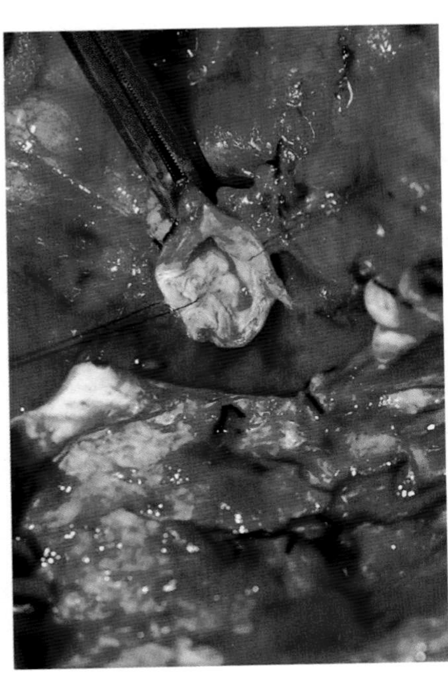

FIGURE 15 ● Aortic cuff. The aorta can be totally transected and stay sutures applied in preparation for the anastomosis.

- Creating the distal anastomosis: After the proximal anastomosis is completed and hemostasis is ensured, the graft should be pulled taut to the location of the distal anastomosis (or anastomoses if a bifurcated graft is to be used).

The graft should be measured to ensure no redundancy or kinking occurs but should not be so tight as to put undue strain on the proximal anastomosis. The distal anastomosis can be performed in a running or interrupted fashion, as described previously. While sewing, the assistant should use a forceps to pull the graft distally to relieve tension on the anastomosis, which decreases the incidence of loose sutures.

- Flushing and unclamping: Just prior to the completion of the distal anastomosis, the graft needs to be flushed proximally and distally to remove any clot, air, and/or debris. After flushing, irrigate the graft with heparinized saline and complete the anastomosis. Once both anastomoses are completed, communicate with the anesthesiologist that the clamps are ready to be removed as they need to prepare to react to a possibly substantial drop in systemic blood pressure when the lower extremities are reperfused. It is more appropriate to tolerate a slightly longer clamp time and allow the anesthesiologist to regulate the blood pressure accordingly than to unclamp a hypotensive patient. As the surgeon slowly unclamps, the assistant can exert manual pressure at the level of the femoral arteries to encourage any debris to flush into the pelvis, which may tolerate embolization better due to the extensive collateral network. Pressure is then released from the femoral vessels and systemic pressure is monitored. If there is substantial hypotension, partial or complete reclamping may need to be performed to allow the anesthesia team time to optimize hemodynamics. Once unclamped, inspect the anastomosis and sac for bleeding. There may be new lumbar bleeding as a result of pelvic reperfusion that was not apparent during the graft placement. Diffuse oozing can be treated with hemostatic agents. Check pulses and Doppler signals in the iliac arteries and any clamped branch vessels, as well as distal pulses and/or PVRs. If lower extremity PVRs are significantly worse than the preoperative assessment, this should heighten concern for embolization and may warrant groin exploration and distal thrombectomy.
- Sac closure: This is especially important for the transperitoneal approach, as an uncommon but equally disastrous late complication from open aortic surgery is an aortoenteric fistula, which occurs when graft and/or anastomosis erodes into the bowel. To help prevent this complication, the walls of the now decompressed aortic sac should be closed over the graft and sewn in a running fashion with a long 3-0 silk or chromic suture. If there is insufficient sac to cover the graft, an omental flap can be mobilized and placed over the graft prior to returning the viscera to its anatomic location. The sac of the aorta can be a significant source of bleeding, so the cut edge of the sac should be cauterized to ensure hemostasis and persistent bleeding should be suture ligated prior to sac closure.
- Drainage and closure: If the pleural cavity was violated, drainage can be achieved by a red rubber suction catheter, placed during diaphragmatic repair, or chest tube placement. Additional placement of a closed suction Jackson-Pratt (JP) or Blake drain in the peritoneal or retroperitoneal (RP) cavity can be done on a selective basis; we generally place a drain if there was excessive mobilization near the tail of the pancreas raising concern for a potential pancreatic leak, or in coagulopathic patients. The spleen should be carefully inspected for injury, and we have a low threshold for splenectomy if there is any injury. The abdominal wall should then be closed in layers.

PEARLS AND PITFALLS

- Ideally, proximal clamp time should be less than 30 min. It is therefore imperative to have all tools and grafts ready and all team members briefed on the operative plan prior to clamping. If the clamp is suprarenal, complications begin with more than 40 min of ischemia. However, for an infrarenal clamp, the operator will have several hours if necessary to complete the anastomosis.
- Injury to the common iliac vein or distal IVC during dissection is a potentially lethal complication. This is a complication that is much better to avoid than to treat. If necessary, it is important to completely mobilize the vein and perform a primary repair under direct vision. Blind suturing in a bleeding field will only lead to disaster. If exposure cannot be obtained, it is acceptable to transect the overlying artery (aorta or iliac) to allow access to the vein.
- The ureters can be injured during both the transperitoneal or retroperitoneal approach. The ureters should always be identified prior to repositioning retractors or beginning a new dissection plane.

POSTOPERATIVE CARE

- Patients should be monitored in an intensive care unit (ICU) postoperatively with systolic blood pressure goals of 100 to 140 mm Hg for a straightforward infrarenal or juxtarenal repair. Blood pressure goals should be higher for thoracoabdominal repairs to promote spinal cord perfusion.
- Suitable patients should be extubated as early as possible, even in the OR if appropriate as early extubation decreases complications.[18]
- A nasogastric tube (NGT) is kept in place given the bowel manipulation and likelihood of ileus. We keep the NGT in for the first full postoperative day and although it is not imperative to maintain it until full return of bowel function, we will keep it in place an additional day if outputs are unusually high. We generally start standing rectal suppositories on the first postoperative day.
- If a chest tube is placed, we leave this to suction until removal, which is done when output is less than 150 mL per 24 hours and the chest x-ray (CXR) shows no large effusion.

- Postoperative mobilization should be done as soon as possible. These patients will require physical therapy and many will ultimately require inpatient rehab.

OUTCOMES

- Mortality for an elective, open infrarenal AAA repair is less than 5%, and although the risk increases for those with a juxtarenal or suprarenal repair, our recent experience shows that 30-day mortality in patients with juxtarenal repair is 2.5%. Mortality increases in the instance of an urgent or rupture to as high as 70%.[1,5]
- Patient-specific predictors of postoperative complications and mortality include older age, higher modified frailty index (mFI) score, COPD, chronic renal disease (creatinine >1.8), or history of myocardial infarction (MI)/congestive heart failure (CHF).[1,19]
- Operative-specific predictors of postoperative complications include long OR or clamp times, hypothermia, high blood turnover, and a high perioperative fluid requirement.
- Open aneurysm repair cases are becoming more complex as EVAR and its fenestrated counterparts are increasingly employed for elective cases. When employed in urgent situations and for explantation, perioperative mortality and complications increase. However, elective repair of complex aneurysms (juxtarenal and suprarenal) showed no long-term survival difference when compared to elective open infrarenal AAA repair.[20,21]

COMPLICATIONS

- Bleeding
- Infection
- Splenic injury (consider adding splenectomy to operative consent)
- Renal failure
- MI
- CVA
- Spinal cord ischemia (increased risk with suprarenal and thoracoabdominal repairs)
- Anastomotic breakdown
- Aortoenteric fistula
- Pancreatitis

REFERENCES

1. Brewster DC, Cronenwett JL, Hallett JW Jr, et al. Guidelines for the treatment of abdominal aortic aneurysms. Report of a subcommittee of the Joint Council of the American association for vascular surgery and Society for vascular surgery. *J Vasc Surg*. 2003;37:1106-1117.
2. Cronenwett JL, Sargent SK, Wall MH, et al. Variables that affect the expansion rate and outcome of small abdominal aortic aneurysms. *J Vasc Surg*. 1990;11(2):260-269.
3. Darling RC III, Brewster DC, Darling RC, et al. Are familial abdominal aortic aneurysms different? *J Vasc Surg*. 1989;10(1):39-43.
4. Strachan DP. Predictors of death from aortic aneurysm among middle-aged men: the Whitehall study. *Br J Surg*. 1991;78(4):401-404.
5. Tsai S, Conrad MF, Patel VI, et al. Durability of open repair of juxtarenal abdominal aortic aneurysms. *J Vasc Surg*. 2012;56(1):2-7.
6. McFalls EO, Ward HB, Moritz TE, et al. Clinical factors associated with long-term mortality following vascular surgery: outcomes from the Coronary Artery Revascularization Prophylaxis (CARP) Trial. *J Vasc Surg*. 2007;46(4):694-700.
7. Garcia S, Rider JE, Moritz TE, et al. Preoperative coronary artery revascularization and long-term outcomes following abdominal aortic vascular surgery in patients with abnormal myocardial perfusion scans: a subgroup analysis of the coronary artery revascularization prophylaxis trial. *Catheter Cardiovasc Interv*. 2011;77(1):134-141.
8. Van de Luijtgaarden KM, Bastos Gonçalves F, Hoeks SE, Majoor-Krakauer D, et al. Familial abdominal aortic aneurysm is associated with more complications after endovascular aneurysm repair. *J Vasc Surg*. 2014;59(2):275-282.
9. Chaikof EL, Brewster DC, Dalman RL, et al. SVS practice guidelines for the care of patients with an abdominal aortic aneurysm: executive summary. *J Vasc Surg*. 2009;50(4):880-896.
10. Dawson I, Sie RB, van Bockel JH. Atherosclerotic popliteal aneurysm. *Br J Surg*. 1997;84(3):293.
11. Johnston KW, Rutherford RB, Tilson MD, et al. Suggested standards for reporting on arterial aneurysms. Subcommittee on Reporting standards for arterial aneurysms, Ad Hoc Committee on Reporting standards, Society for vascular surgery and North American chapter, International Society for Cardiovascular surgery. *J Vasc Surg*. 1991;13(3):452-458.
12. US Preventive Services Task Force; Owens DK, Davidson KW, Krist AH, et al. Screening for abdominal aortic aneurysm: US preventive Services Task Force recommendation Statement. *JAMA*. 2019;322(22):2211-2218.
13. Lederle FA, Johnson GR, Wilson SE, et al. The aneurysm detection and management study screening program: validation cohort and final results. Aneurysm Detection and Management Veterans Affairs Cooperative Study Investigators. *Arch Intern Med*. 2000;160:1425-1430.
14. Lederle FA, Wilson SE, Johnson GR, et al. Immediate repair compared with surveillance of small abdominal aortic aneurysms. *N Engl J Med*. 2002;346(19):1437-1444.
15. Wang LJ, Tsougranis GH, Tanious A, et al. The removal of all proximal aneurysmal aortic tissue does not affect anastomotic degeneration after open juxtarenal aortic aneurysm repair. *J Vasc Surg*. 2020;71(2):390-399.
16. Green RM, Ricotta JJ, Ouriel K, DeWeese JA. Results of supraceliac aortic clamping in the difficult elective resection of infrarenal abdominal aortic aneurysm. *J Vasc Surg*. 1989;9(1):124-134.
17. Jayaraj A, DeMartino RR, Bower TC, et al. Outcomes following inferior mesenteric artery reimplantation during elective aortic aneurysm surgery. *Ann Vasc Surg*. 2020;66:65-69.
18. Zettervall SL, Soden PA, Shean KE, et al. Early extubation reduces respiratory complications and hospital length of stay following repair of abdominal aortic aneurysms. *J Vasc Surg*. 2017;65(1):58-64.
19. Barbey SM, Scali ST, Kubilis P, et al. Interaction between frailty and sex on mortality after elective abdominal aortic aneurysm repair. *J Vasc Surg*. 2019;70(6):1831-1843.
20. Fairman AS, Chin AL, Jackson BM, et al. The evolution of open abdominal aortic aneurysm repair at a tertiary care center. *J Vasc Surg*. 2020;72(4):1367-1374.
21. Deery SE, Lancaster RT, Baril DT, et al. Contemporary outcomes of open complex abdominal aortic aneurysm repair. *J Vasc Surg*. 2016;63(5):1195-1200.

Chapter 21 Advanced Aortic Aneurysm Management: Endovascular Aneurysm Repair—Standard and Emergency Management

Oonagh H. Scallan and Audra A. Duncan

DEFINITION

- Abdominal aortic aneurysm (AAA) is defined as abnormal dilatation of the abdominal aorta greater than 50% of the normal proximal segment, typically greater than 3 cm.
- The most common etiology of AAAs is degenerative, often also referred to as atherosclerotic. Other etiologies include inflammatory, dissection, trauma, developmental or congenital, and infectious.

DIFFERENTIAL DIAGNOSIS

- Most AAAs are asymptomatic and are identified incidentally during an exam for an unrelated pathology. The classic triad of symptoms in a patient with a ruptured aneurysm includes acute-onset abdominal or back pain, hypotension, and a pulsatile abdominal mass.
- The differential diagnosis is broad and is dependent on the presentation of the patient. Possible alternative diagnoses include:
  - Renal colic
  - Diverticulitis
  - Perforated ulcer
  - Pancreatitis
  - Gastrointestinal bleed
  - Myocardial infarction
  - Pulmonary embolism

PATIENT HISTORY AND PHYSICAL FINDINGS

- Patients with AAA are typically asymptomatic and the aneurysm is diagnosed as an incidental finding. A patient of lower body habitus or with a large aneurysm may notice a palpable pulsatile mass.
- Rarely, patients may present with distal limb ischemia related to embolization of thrombus from within the aneurysm.
- Patients with a ruptured aneurysm may present with abdominal or back pain, or pain radiating to the testes, inguinal canal, rectum, or hip. A history of syncope or hypotension in a patient with a tender, pulsatile abdominal mass indicates a possible ruptured aneurysm. Rarely, patients may present with an aortocaval fistula secondary to the ruptured aneurysm and demonstrate symptoms of heart failure, a systolic bruit in the abdomen, and central venous hypertension.
- Risk factors for aneurysmal disease are similar to atherosclerotic disease and include advancing age, male gender, chronic obstructive pulmonary disease, smoking, family history of aneurysms, and connective tissue disorders. A thorough history should be taken from the patient to elicit risk factors for an aneurysm and medical comorbidities. The history and physical exam are important to determine the etiology of the aneurysm and overall health of the patient as this will influence the choice of operative approach.
- Risk factors for rupture include female gender, large initial aneurysm diameter, low forced expiration volume in 1 second, current smoking history, immunomodulation therapy after major organ transplantation, and elevated mean blood pressure.[1]
- An AAA may be identified on physical exam as a palpable pulsatile mass, typically supraumbilical and in the midline; however, the position may vary due to aortic tortuosity. The ability to palpate the aneurysm is affected by the aneurysm size and body habitus of the patient. Given the incidence of concomitant aneurysms, patients should be examined for other aneurysms such as femoral or popliteal aneurysms.

IMAGING AND OTHER DIAGNOSTIC STUDIES

- Multiple randomized controlled trials (RCTs) have demonstrated that a one-time screening for an AAA by ultrasound is effective at reducing aneurysm-related mortality and incidence of aneurysm rupture.[2] The Multicentre Aneurysm Screening Study (MASS) randomized over 67,000 men aged 65 to 74 to ultrasound AAA screening vs no screening, and found that screening led to a 40% reduction in aneurysm-related mortality, and this benefit persisted for over a decade.[3]
- Society for Vascular Surgery (SVS) guidelines recommend a one-time screening ultrasound for men and women aged 65 to 75, or over 75 in good health, with a history of tobacco use, and patients aged 65 to 75, or older than 75 years and in good health, with a first-degree relative with an AAA.[1]
- CT angiogram (CTA) is the current standard modality for operative planning and provides excellent imaging of AAAs, with increased accuracy of diameter measurements compared to ultrasound. CTA allows for three-dimensional reconstruction and includes essential anatomic information such as dimensions, neck angulation, thrombus, calcification, occlusive disease, and assessment of arterial access.

SURGICAL MANAGEMENT

Indications

- The goal of AAA repair is to prevent rupture; therefore the decision to treat is based on the risk of rupture, the risk of treatment, the patient's life expectancy, and patient preference.[2]
- The current recommendation for repair of AAA in low- and average-risk patients is aneurysms >5.5 cm in men and >5 cm in women. There is no long-term benefit of survival of open or endovascular repair in small aneurysms, 4 to 5.5 cm, as demonstrated by multiple RCTs.[4]

- Other indications include rupture, aneurysm growth rate of >1 cm in 1 year, and symptomatic aneurysms.

Preoperative Planning

- Successful EVAR excludes an aneurysm from blood flow through placement of the stent, typically through the common femoral arteries. A stent graft consisting of a metallic stent framework covered with a synthetic fabric material is used. The metal skeleton is made of nitinol or stainless steel. There are multiple aortic stent grafts currently available and the selection of the device should be tailored to the individual anatomic requirements, as each device has different parameters for the IFU.
- Anatomic measurements obtained from a high-quality CTA are essential for a successful EVAR. 3-D reconstruction software programs (eg, TeraRecon) provide precise diameter and path length measurements for operative planning. Graft oversizing of 10% to 20% is typically used in the aortic neck. Length measurements are obtained from the lowest renal artery to the iliac bifurcations and can be repeated intraoperatively with marking catheters.
- The IFU of the device and the patient's anatomy should be carefully scrutinized for suitability for EVAR and device selection. If the patient does not have good anatomy for standard EVAR, they should be considered for fenestrated or branched EVAR or open repair. Other patient characteristics to factor into the decision for operative repair include the age of the patient and durability of repair, and potential for the presence of a connective tissue disorder.
- When EVAR is performed within IFU criteria, the results are excellent, with <1% type 1a endoleaks. However, a large number of patients undergo standard EVAR with anatomy outside IFU. Reduced adherence to IFU is associated with higher rates of aneurysm sac expansion, which ultimately translates into treatment failure, costly reintervention, and possibly late aneurysm rupture.[5] The Ad Hoc Committee of Standardized Reporting Practices for the Society of Vascular Surgery defined a marginal neck as having length <15 mm, diameter >28 mm, angle >60, and presence of significant calcification or thrombus. These guidelines predominantly coincide with the instructions for use for the majority of EVAR devices.[6]
- With the increasing use of EVAR for patients with hostile or short necks, techniques to prevent or treat type 1a endoleaks have become important tools, such as the Heli-FX EndoAnchor System (Medtronic Vascular). This is an adjunctive sealing device that can be placed to treat or prevent type 1a endoleak. It delivers 3.0 × 4.5 mm helical screws to improve the seal between the endograft and the aortic wall (**FIGURE 1**).
- The decreasing profile of endovascular devices is beneficial in not only allowing navigation of tortuous, diseased, or small iliac arteries, it also makes totally percutaneous access for the procedure appealing. This technique uses suture-mediated closure devices, such as Perclose ProGlide or Prostar XL, in a "preclose" technique. The Prostar XL Percutaneous Vascular surgery device (Abbott Vascular) is a suture-mediated arterial closure device. It is a CE Mark-approved closure device for large size femoral artery punctures from 8 to 24 Fr; it is delivered over a 0.038 wire. The ProGlide (Abbott Vascular) is also a suture-mediated arterial closure device that will track over a standard 0.035 wire and accommodates 5- to 21-Fr arteriotomies. In arteriotomies >8 Fr, at least two devices are required to close the arteriotomy. Risk factors for failure include heavy arterial calcification, increased ratio of sheath size to common femoral artery diameter, increased patient age, and female sex.[7] In patients with inadequate access vessels for a percutaneous approach, open femoral exposure may be required. Adjunctive measures for inadequate access include the use of a conduit or endoconduit.

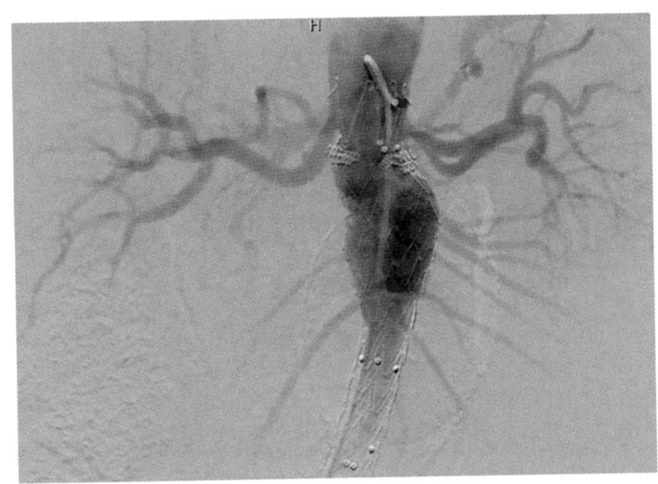

FIGURE 1 ● Seven endoanchors inserted in the infrarenal aorta using the Heli-FX EndoAnchor System in an EVAR treating an aneurysm with a short infrarenal neck.

- In patients who do not have ideal anatomy for a standard EVAR with a bifurcated device, an aortouni-iliac endograft may be more appropriate. Some relative indications for aortouni-iliac endograft configuration include a very small (<15 mm) terminal aorta, which would not accommodate a bifurcated device, severe unilateral iliac occlusive disease, or secondary treatment of migration of short body endograft.
- The SMA and celiac arteries should also be examined preoperatively for patency and evidence of severe stenosis or occlusion. If present, the patient should be carefully assessed for symptoms of chronic mesenteric ischemia. In the setting of severe visceral disease, revascularization should be considered prior to EVAR or open repair should be considered given the obligation of covering the IMA during EVAR.

ENDOVASCULAR ANEURYSM REPAIR STANDARD

Percutaneous Access

- After confirming the location of the inguinal ligament, femoral bifurcation, and appropriateness of the artery for percutaneous access, ultrasound guidance is used to puncture the common femoral artery with a 0.018-in micropuncture kit. A 0.035-in starter wire (eg, Bentson, Cook Medical, Bloomington, IN) is advanced into the abdominal aorta and the sheath is exchanged for a 7-Fr sheath.

Preclose Technique

- While the assistant maintains pressure, the 7-Fr sheath is exchanged for a Perclose Proglide (Abbott, Abbott Park, IL) device. This is advanced until the guidewire exit line on the device and the wire is temporarily removed. The device is advanced until pulsatile blood is seen through the pilot tube lumen. The device is turned to the 10-o'clock position and the footplate is activated. Holding back tension on the device, the suture is deployed. The footplate is lowered, and the device removed from the artery until the guidewire is reintroduced. The suture ends are clamped together to avoid premature cinching of the knots (**FIGURE 2**).
- A second Perclose Proglide (Abbott, Abbott Park, IL) device is loaded and deployed at the 2-o'clock position.

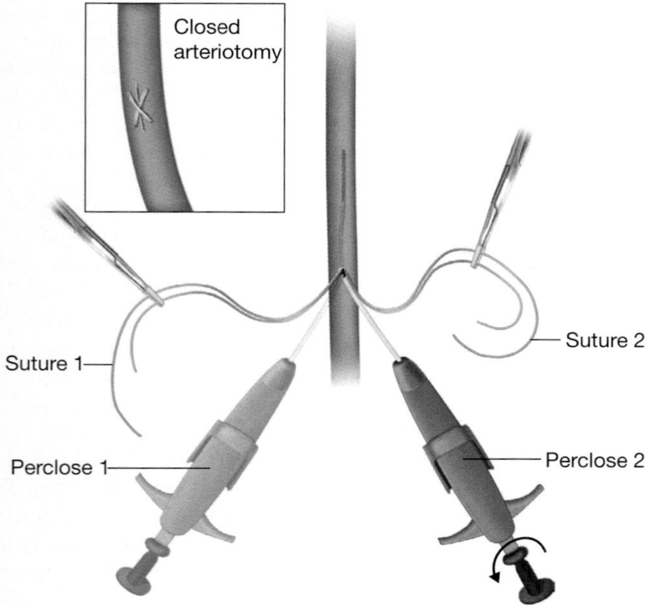

FIGURE 2 ● Preclose technique. Two ProGlides are deployed, one at the 10-o'clock position and the other at the 2-o'clock position before beginning serial dilation maneuvers and deployment of delivery catheters. Once the procedure is complete, and large diameter devices are removed, both knots are seated to close the arteriotomy (see inset). Until closure, the free sutures are controlled on suture boots. Once the procedure is complete, both knots are pushed down to close the arteriotomy.

- Once both devices are deployed and the sutures controlled, a 9-Fr sheath may be placed to continue dilation.

Delivery and Deployment of Endograft

- Bilateral straight stiff 260 cm Lunderquist (Cook Medical) or equivalent wires are placed in the proximal descending thoracic aorta. Serial dilation is then performed to place the sheaths required for the chosen device.
- Systemic anticoagulation is established with intravenous unfractionated heparin (100 units/kg) and confirmed with an activated clotting time (ACT) greater than 250 seconds.
- A flush catheter is advanced into the proximal abdominal aorta from the contralateral femoral artery. A catheter with 1 cm markers can be used to concomitantly confirm the length measurements obtained from preoperative imaging.
- The main body endograft is oriented to deploy the contralateral gate anterolaterally, and advanced over the ipsilateral Lunderquist wire (Cook Medical) (**FIGURE 3A**).
- The flush catheter is connected to a power injector and air is flushed from the system. The image intensifier is adjusted cranially to limit parallax in the setting of neck angulation to obtain an orthogonal view to the takeoff of the lowest renal artery, based on the preoperative CT. With the ventilator held to minimize motion artifact, an initial aortogram is obtained to identify the position of the renal arteries.
- The main body endograft is then deployed according to the IFU, with the proximal fabric margin positioned just below the lowest renal artery to obtain maximum seal. Deployment continues until the contralateral gate is open. The flush catheter should be pulled back before deployment of suprarenal fixation to avoid entrapment of the catheter. The suprarenal stents are then deployed (**FIGURE 3B**).

Gate Cannulation

- The flush catheter is retracted to below the contralateral gate, and a combination of hydrophilic wires (such as a Terumo Glidewire guidewire) and direction catheters can be used to cannulate the contralateral gate. Positioning the contralateral sheath within 1 to 2 cm of the gate may assist this (**FIGURE 3C**).
- Once the gate has been cannulated, the flush pigtail catheter is reformed within the limb and presence within the device is confirmed by visualizing the spinning catheter. Cannulation can also be confirmed by using a molding balloon and inflating it across the origin of the limb resulting in a mushroom appearance of the balloon.[8]
- Strategies to obtain gate cannulation include various guidewires, shaped catheters, adjusting the C-arm, or using a snare from the other side. Brachial access can also be used for this same purpose.

Limb extension

- Retrograde iliac angiography is performed through the sheath with the C-arm in the contralateral oblique position to identify the origin of the internal iliac artery. A marker catheter is used to measure the appropriate length limb. For three-piece bifurcated devices, this is completed on both sides. Adequate overlap between stent components and length of seal in the common iliac artery must be considered (**FIGURE 3D**).

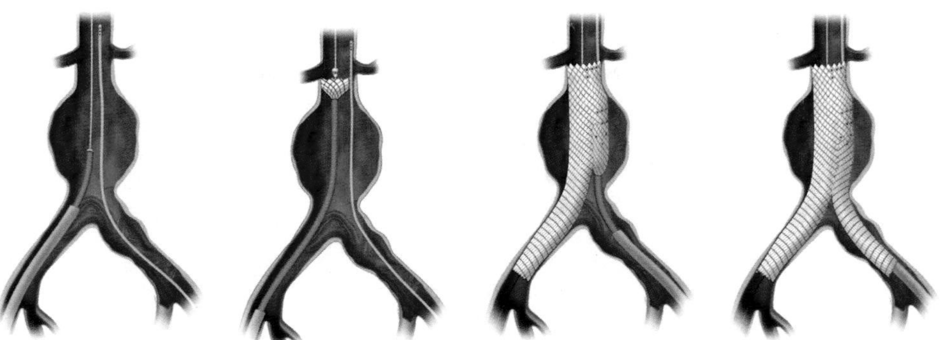

FIGURE 3 ● Delivery and deployment of endograft. **A,** The main body is brought up the ipsilateral iliac artery to the level of the renal arteries. An Omni Flush catheter is brought up the contralateral iliac artery and an angiogram is performed. **B,** The main body endograft is deployed under fluoroscopic guidance until the contralateral gate is opened. **C,** The contralateral gate is cannulated. **D,** An extension limb is placed proximal to the iliac bifurcation on the contralateral side and the ipsilateral endograft is finished being deployed (one docking limb systems) or an extension limb is placed (two docking limb systems) to the level of the ipsilateral iliac bifurcation.

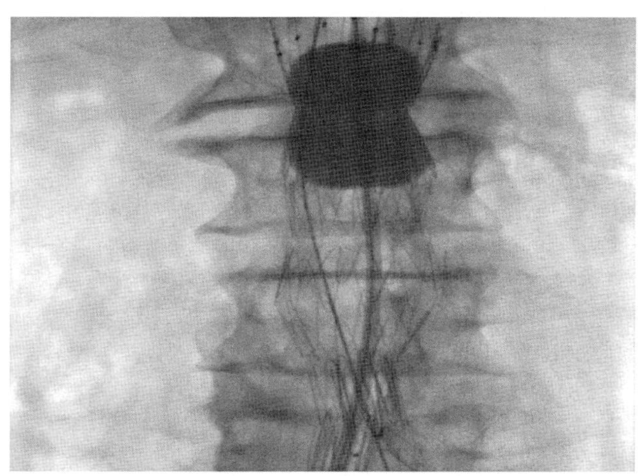

FIGURE 4 ● Balloon molding. A semicompliant balloon is inflated at proximal and distal landing zones as well as at all overlapping endografts.

Balloon Molding

- A semicompliant balloon is expanded with diluted contrast solution at all three landing zones, the neck and iliac arteries, areas of overlap, and areas within the gates as appropriate for the specific device. Kissing balloons may be used to treat the presence of a common iliac artery stenosis or narrowing at the aortic bifurcation. Self-expanding bare metal stents may be used in areas of stenosis or at the end of the distal limb into the external iliac artery to prevent kinking (**FIGURE 4**).

Completion Arteriography

- The flush catheter is reintroduced and a completion aortogram is performed with the end of the catheter superior to the stent graft to assess for positioning, stent patency, and the presence of endoleaks (**FIGURE 5A-D**).
- Type I and III endoleaks present as earlier, brisker antegrade filling of the aneurysm sac as opposed to type II endoleaks, which tend to be delayed, slower, retrograde filling of the aneurysm sac.
- All type I and III endoleaks should be addressed prior to completion of the procedure, whereas many type II endoleaks resolve on their own over the first year. If proximal aortic endoanchors are required, they are placed at this time.

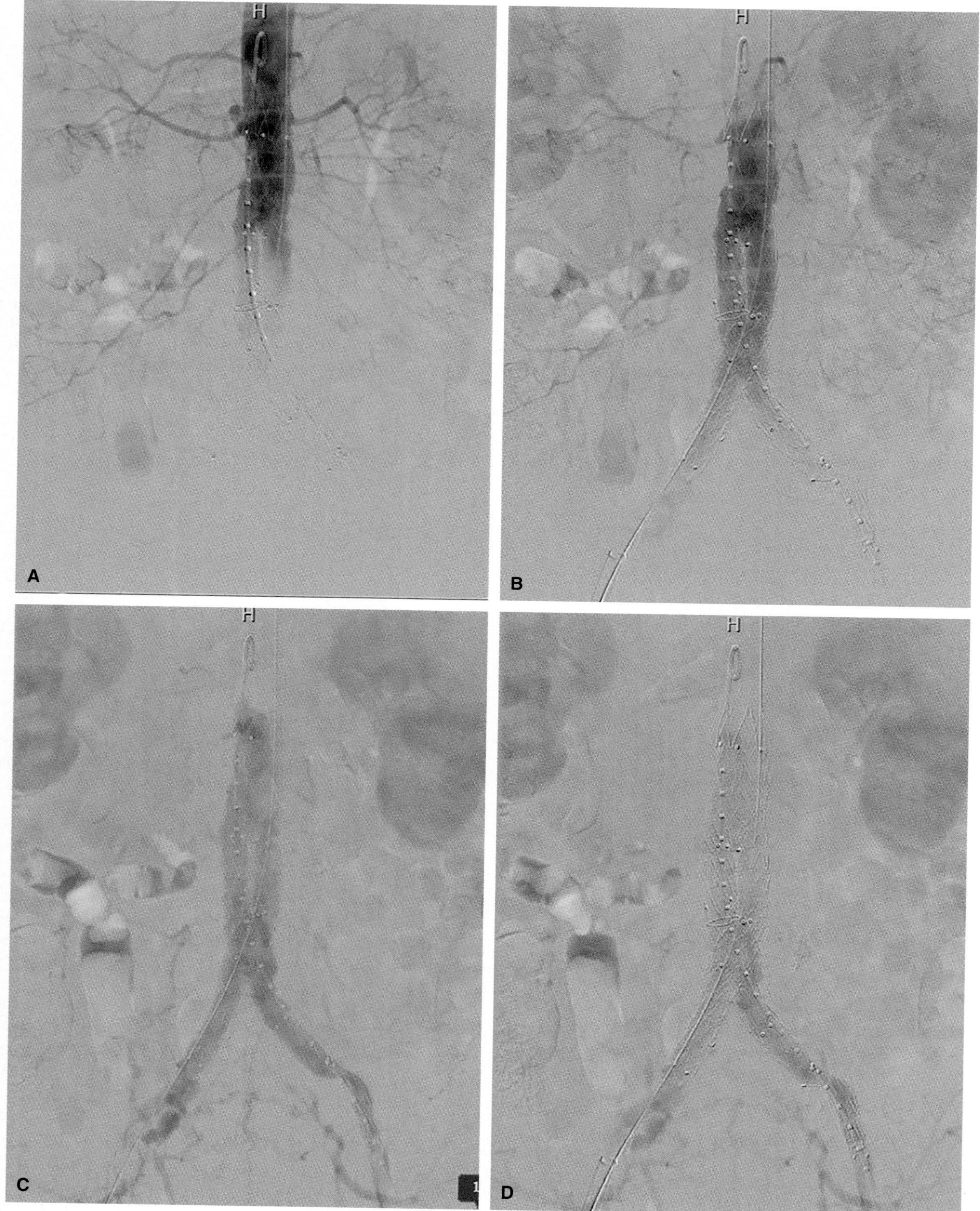

FIGURE 5 ● Completion arteriography. Special attention is paid to ensure the renal and iliac arteries are patent, as well as to identify if an endoleak is present. The endograft itself should be scrutinized for any evidence of limb kinking. **A,** Renal artery patency confirmed. **B,** No type 1A endoleak confirmed. **C,** The right external and internal iliac arteries are confirmed to be patient. The left iliac limb extends into the external iliac artery to exclude the left internal iliac aneurysm. The endograft itself should be scrutinized for any evidence of limb kinking. **D,** No type 1B, 2, 3, or 4 endoleak identified with delayed imaging.

ENDOVASCULAR ANEURYSM REPAIR FOR RUPTURED ANEURYSMS OR REVAR

Preoperative Considerations

- Successful treatment of a ruptured AAA with EVAR relies on early diagnosis, rapid completion of a CT scan, and timely transport to the operating room. A standardized protocol developed by the Albany Vascular Group to manage patients with ruptured AAA has shown significant improvements in patient survival.[9]
- In a hybrid OR, the patient is prepped and draped in supine position, including the abdomen for potential conversion to open repair if necessary.

Access

- Access to the common femoral arteries may be performed through a percutaneous approach or open exposure depending on the clinical circumstances, operator experience, and logistics. In hemodynamically unstable patients, access may be obtained under local anesthesia with conversion to general anesthesia once balloon control of the aorta has been obtained if necessary. If time does not permit for the preclose technique, conversion to open femoral closure after the endograft has been fully deployed may be completed.
- After placement of bilateral stiff wires (eg, Lunderquist, Cook Medical), the sheaths are upsized as outlined in the previous section. If an aortic occlusion balloon is to be used due to hemodynamic instability, the sheath on the contralateral side should be advanced into the supraceliac aorta to provide support for the balloon and prevent downward displacement into the aneurysm sac. This also allows for removal of the balloon through the sheath to avoid the balloon getting caught on the barbs of the endograft.
- The use of systemic anticoagulation in the setting of ruptured aortic aneurysm repair is controversial and dependent on the hemodynamic status of the patient, presence of active bleeding, and existing consumptive coagulopathy. Anticoagulation may be withheld until the main body and extension limbs are deployed.

Aortic Balloon Control

- A semicompliant balloon (Coda, Cook Medical) is advanced and positioned in the supraceliac aorta under fluoroscopic guidance (**FIGURE 6**). Once in position, the balloon can be inflated depending on the patient's hemodynamic status.

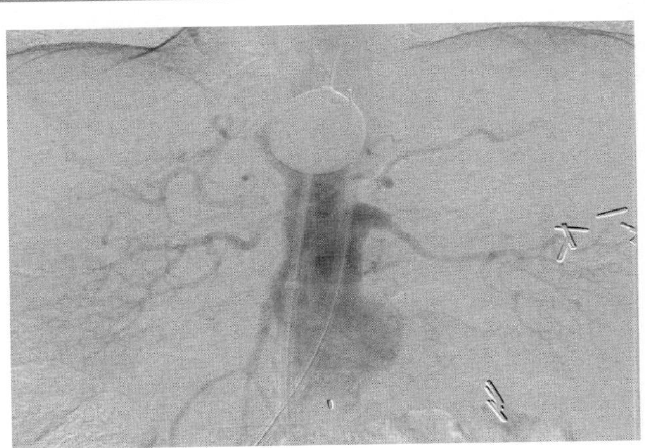

FIGURE 6 ● Aortic balloon control for REVAR. A semicompliant balloon is placed up the contralateral iliac artery proximal to the celiac trunk. It can be inflated depending on hemodynamic instability.

Endograft Delivery and Deployment

- Aortography is performed through the contralateral sheath below the balloon to localize the origins of the renal arteries.
- The main body endograft is oriented for anterolateral deployment of the contralateral gate, then placed through the ipsilateral sheath to the level of the renal arteries. A repeat angiogram after adjusting for parallax may be necessary if there is angulation of the aortic neck (**FIGURE 7**).
- If the aortic occlusion balloon is in place without the support of a sheath, it should be deflated and withdrawn to avoid trapping the balloon between the aortic neck and the stent graft. The main body is then deployed just distal to the lowest renal artery, according to the device IFU, and the entirety of the ipsilateral gate is deployed. This allows for a second semicompliant balloon to be advanced up the ipsilateral endograft limb and placed into the main body for inflation depending on hemodynamic instability (**FIGURE 8**).

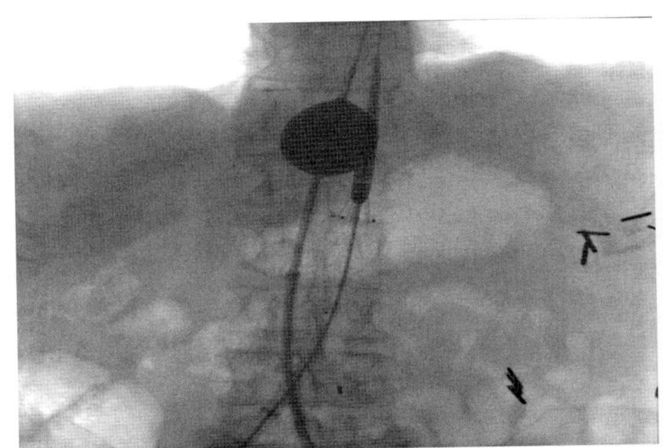

FIGURE 7 ● Main body deployment for REVAR. After an angiogram is performed to identify the renal arteries and aortic neck, the main body is deployed up the ipsilateral iliac artery. This can be done with the semicompliant balloon inflated.

Gate Cannulation

- Gate cannulation proceeds in a standard fashion during REVAR. Time awareness is critical to ensure that aneurysm sealing is accomplished in the most expeditious manner possible.

Limb Extension

- Limb extension proceeds in a standard fashion during REVAR.

Balloon Molding

- Balloon molding is performed at all seal zones to optimize hemostasis.

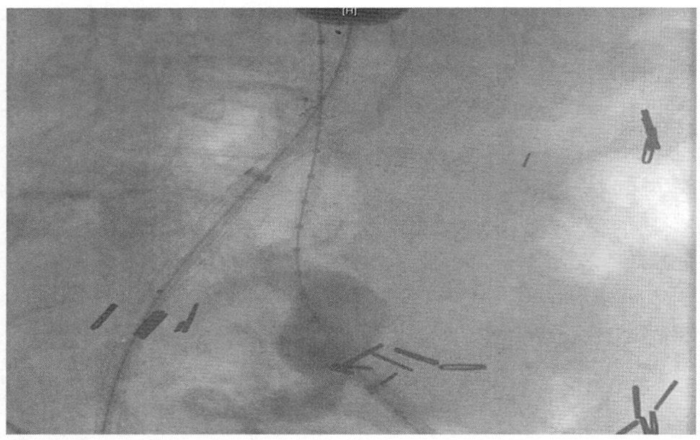

FIGURE 8 ● Balloon exchange and gate cannulation for REVAR. The entire ipsilateral gate is deployed prior to contralateral gate cannulation. A second semicompliant balloon is placed up the ipsilateral endograft limb (top of image) and placed into the main body of the endograft. It can be inflated depending on hemodynamic instability. The first semicompliant balloon is removed and the sheath is brought to distal to the contralateral gate to prepare for gate cannulation. Retrograde angiography with a marking catheter is performed through the contralateral sheath to identify the iliac bifurcation and desired limb extension length.

Completion Aortography

- Completion aortography is performed as previously described. Attention should be paid to all the general considerations of presence and nature of endoleaks, kinking of the limbs, and sufficient overlap in the landing zones to meet IFU.

Closure

- Closure proceeds as indicated for standard EVAR.

Abdominal compartment syndrome (ACS)

- Abdominal compartment syndrome occurs in up to 20% of patients after treatment of a ruptured AAA by EVAR, with a high rate of perioperative mortality of 50%.[10]
- The pathophysiology of ACS after EVAR for ruptured AAA is multifactorial and includes the presence of the retroperitoneal hematoma, ongoing bleeding from lumbar arteries and the IMA, and shock associated with rupture, which can induce alterations in microvascular permeability and lead to visceral and soft tissue edema.[9]
- Several variables have been identified as contributing factors to ACS including the use of an aortic occlusion balloon, need for massive blood transfusion, and coagulopathy at the com pletion of the case.

PEARLS AND PITFALLS

Patient selection and preoperative planning	Careful preoperative assessment of the patient and their anatomy is essential to obtaining a good, durable result from EVAR to ensure anatomic suitability and availability of equipment.
Access	Ultrasound guidance is essential to limiting access complications. The needle tip should be visualized entering the anterior artery wall, in an area deemed appropriate for access.
Gate cannulation	In general, the main body should be advanced through the more tortuous of the iliac arteries to all a more "straight shot" for the contralateral gate cannulation. However, in some scenarios this may not be practical if the tortuosity of the iliac precludes main body positioning and deployment altogether. Crossing the iliac limbs of the graft during placement of the main body graft may allow a straighter line for gate access.
Tortuous iliacs	Remove the stiff wires and leave catheters in place for the completion angiogram. This allows the vessels to take their native position and reveal any type 1a endoleak or kinking of the limbs that may not be evident when the graft is straightened out by the stiff wire.
Graft angioplasty	If using one smaller sheath (ie, 12 or 14 Fr) and one larger, place the compliant balloon through the smaller sheath first. Once the balloon is inflated, it is more difficult to pass through a 12-Fr sheath.
Closure	Tie down the sutures of the closure device with the wire in place. If there is still significant bleeding, deploy another closure device or place an occlusive sheath and proceed with open conversion of the femoral artery closure under more controlled circumstances.

POSTOPERATIVE CARE

- After percutaneous EVAR, patients should remain supine for 3 hours and are free to ambulate thereafter. Most elective EVARs are discharged on postoperative day 1, or in some cases as same-day surgery. Given the decreasing size of access sheaths, the preclose technique, and advanced anesthesia techniques, several centers have advocated for the safety and efficacy of outpatient EVAR, with nearly 40% of patients estimated to be candidates.
- As recommended by SVS guidelines, an initial postoperative contrast-enhanced CT is performed at 1 month to assess stability of the aneurysm sac, and for endoleaks and graft position. Patients are then reassessed with CT or color duplex ultrasound at 6 months if there is a type II endoleak or 1 year if there is no endoleak and no aneurysm sac enlargement[1] (**FIGURE 9**).
- EVAR has been shown to have lower perioperative morbidity and mortality compared to OSR. The early survival

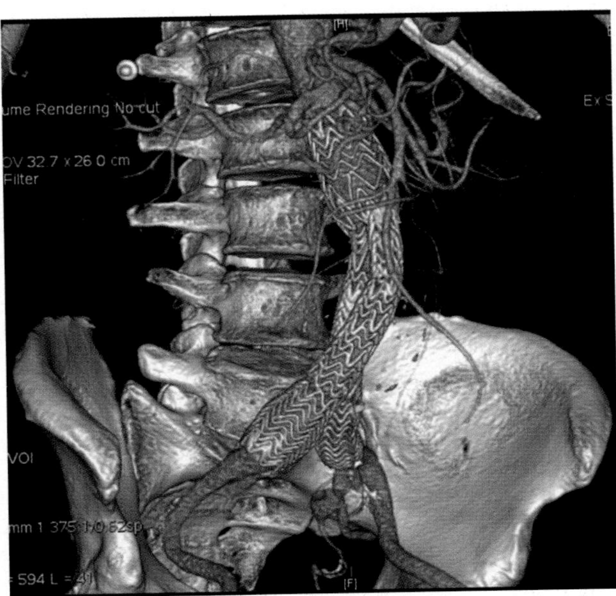

FIGURE 9 ● Postoperative imaging. 3-D reconstruction of a CT aortogram in a patient who have undergone successful EVAR at 1-month follow-up.

benefit of EVAR is lost over time; the 15-year results from EVAR-1 showed now difference in survival between EVAR vs OSR.[11] Beyond 8 years, EVAR has been found to have higher all-cause and aneurysm-related mortality, primarily due to aneurysm rupture in the EVAR group.[11]

COMPLICATIONS

- Endoleak and delayed rupture
- Graft limb occlusion
- Thromboembolism
- Migration
- Stent graft infection
- Renal dysfunction
- Renal artery occlusion
- Bowel ischemia
- Pelvic ischemia

REFERENCES

1. Chaikof EL, Dalman RL, Eskandari MK, et al. The Society for Vascular Surgery practice guidelines on the care of patients with an abdominal aortic aneurysm. *J Vasc Surg*. 2018;67(1):2-77.e2. doi:10.1016/j.jvs.2017.10.044
2. Swerdlow NJ, Wu WW, Schermerhorn ML. Open and endovascular management of aortic aneurysms. *Circ Res*. 2019;124(4):647-661. doi:10.1161/CIRCRESAHA.118.313186
3. Ashton HA, Buxton MJ, Day NE, et al. The Multicentre Aneurysm Screening Study (MASS) into the effect of abdominal aortic aneurysm screening on mortality in men: a randomised controlled trial. *Lancet*. 2002;360(9345):1531-1539. doi:10.1016/s0140-6736(02)11522-4
4. Filardo G, Powell JT, Martinez MA, Ballard DJ. Surgery for small asymptomatic abdominal aortic aneurysms. *Cochrane Database Syst Rev*. 2015;2015(2):CD001835. Published 2015 Feb 8. doi:10.1002/14651858.CD001835.pub4
5. Schanzer A, Greenberg RK, Hevelone N, et al. Predictors of abdominal aortic aneurysm sac enlargement after endovascular repair [published correction appears in Circulation. 2012 Jan 17;125(2):e266]. *Circulation*. 2011;123(24):2848-2855. doi:10.1161/CIRCULATIONAHA.110.014902
6. Chaikof EL, Blankensteijn JD, Harris PL, et al. Reporting standards for endovascular aortic aneurysm repair. *J Vasc Surg*. 2002;35(5):1048-1060. doi:10.1067/mva.2002.123763
7. Smeds MR, Charlton-Ouw KM. Infrarenal endovascular aneurysm repair: new developments and decision making in 2016. *Semin Vasc Surg*. 2016;29(1-2):27-34. doi:10.1053/j.semvascsurg.2016.06.001
8. Wilson WRW, Benveniste GL. Confirmation of contralateral limb gate cannulation using a moulding balloon. *Eur J Vasc Endovasc Surg Extra*. 2010;20:25-26.
9. Mehta M. Technical tips for EVAR for ruptured AAA. *Semin Vasc Surg*. 2009;22(3):181-186. doi:10.1053/j.semvascsurg.2009.07.010
10. SÁ P, Oliveira-Pinto J, Mansilha A. Abdominal compartment syndrome after r-EVAR: a systematic review with meta-analysis on incidence and mortality. *Int Angiol*. 2020;39(5):411-421. doi:10.23736/S0392-9590.20.04406-5
11. Patel R, Sweeting MJ, Powell JT, Greenhalgh RM. EVAR trial investigators. Endovascular versus open repair of abdominal aortic aneurysm in 15-years' follow-up of the UK endovascular aneurysm repair trial 1 (EVAR trial 1): a randomised controlled trial. *Lancet*. 2016;388(10058):2366-2374. doi:10.1016/S0140-6736(16)31135-7

Chapter 22

Advanced Aneurysm Management Techniques: Management of Internal Iliac Artery Aneurysm Disease

Olamide Alabi, Erica L. Mitchell, and Laura B. Pride

DEFINITION

- An internal iliac artery aneurysm (IIAA) is defined as a ≥50% increase in the expected diameter. Internal iliac arteries for both men and women measure 0.54 ± 0.15 cm,[1] therefore threshold diameter of 8 mm is used to define IIAA.
- IIAA are exceedingly rare, representing <0.5% of all aortoiliac aneurysms. Ninety percent are unilateral and not associated with abdominal aortic aneurysms (AAA)[2,3] (**FIGURE 1**).
- Patients with IIAA are typically males in their seventh and eighth decade of life in line with their association with atherosclerotic disease.[2,3]
- The natural history of IIAA is not well described as prospective studies are lacking. Retrospective data show that IIAAs are typically slow growing and aneurysms <4 cm rarely rupture.[4,5]

DIFFERENTIAL DIAGNOSIS

- The differential diagnosis of IIAA is primarily limited to atherosclerotic degenerative aneurysms.
- Aneurysmal degeneration of the internal iliac artery may result from infection, trauma, inflammatory or connective tissue disorders, and dissection.[6]

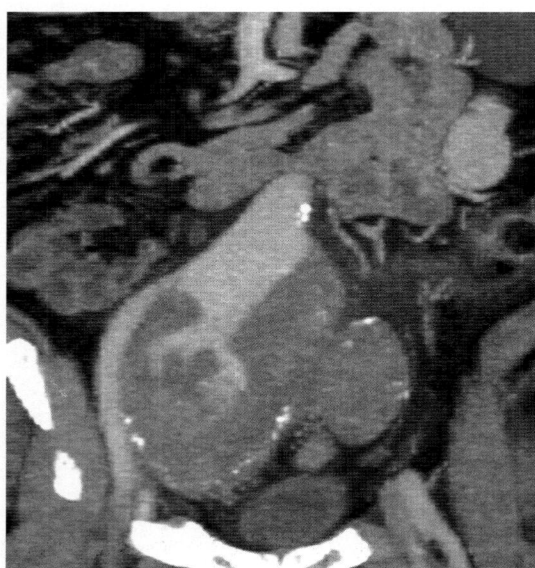

FIGURE 1 • Large right internal iliac artery aneurysm.

PATIENT HISTORY AND PHYSICAL FINDINGS

- IIAAs are difficult to detect on physical examination because they are situated deep in the posteromedial pelvis.
- Most IIAAs are asymptomatic and found incidentally on imaging.
- Symptoms may result from compression of adjacent structures including lumbosacral nerves, pelvic veins, and portions of the urinary or lower gastrointestinal tract and result in lower back, flank, or groin discomfort, as well as urinary changes. The nonspecific nature of these symptoms often delays diagnosis and treatment of IIAA. Less common presentations include renal failure, rectal bleeding from fistulization, constipation, lower extremity swelling, and deep vein thrombosis.[2,6]
- When IIAA present as rupture, mortality rates are high and reported at >30%.[6] Survival for ruptured IIAA is improving with endovascular treatment.[5]
- Data related to rupture risk and threshold for repair are limited to common iliac artery (CIA) aneurysms, with treatment indicated for aneurysms >3 to 3.5 cm in diameter.[4,5,7] This threshold can be extended to IIAA management as well.
- Repair is indicated for all symptomatic IIAA, regardless of size.

IMAGING AND OTHER DIAGNOSTIC STUDIES

- Although plain abdominal x-rays can detect heavily calcified aortoiliac aneurysms, the imaging modalities used to make the diagnosis include duplex ultrasound (DUS), computed tomography angiography (CTA), magnetic resonance imaging (MRI), and magnetic resonance angiography (MRA).
- DUS is an excellent screening and surveillance tool for asymptomatic aortoiliac disease; however, image quality can be limited by bowel gas and increased abdominal girth. Distinguishing common, internal, or external iliac artery (EIA) aneurysmal involvement may be challenging by DUS alone.[6,8,9]
- CTA, with 1-mm cuts, represents the "gold standard" for the diagnosis and anatomic evaluation of abdominal aneurysms and is essential for endovascular case planning. Contrast enhancement allows for comprehensive evaluation of luminal irregularities, relationship to other anatomic structures, and for the identification of impending or overt rupture.[9,10]
- MRI and MRA are highly sensitive and allow for detailed evaluation of aneurysmal disease without the use of ionizing radiation. Their use is limited for operative planning because they are less able to demonstrate aortic wall calcification.
- Digital subtraction angiography (DSA) is invasive and adds little to the identification and analysis of iliac aneurysms.

SURGICAL MANAGEMENT

- The goals of surgical management are to prevent death from rupture and maintain suitable pelvic perfusion.
- The majority of IIAAs are now repaired via endovascular methods[2] as traditional surgical repair can be challenging and fraught with pelvic venous bleeding complications.
- Endovascular repair is associated with lower operative morbidity and mortality rates and shorter inpatient length of stays compared with open repair.[3,4,11]
- Open surgical repair remains a reasonable option with excellent long-term durability for patients with aneurysm anatomy not suitable for endovascular repair, failed endovascular repair, aneurysmal compression of local structures, and/or the presence of an infected endovascular graft.

Preoperative Planning

- High-quality preoperative imaging is essential for precase planning.
- CTA, with multiple phases, is optimal for this purpose. Multiple phases allow for complete evaluation as precontrast phase provides information regarding vessel calcification, contrast images reveal luminal irregularities such as mural thrombus, dissections or ulcerations, and delayed phase images allow for endoleaks to be detected postprocedurally.[12]
- A combination of axial imaging and 3D postprocessing should allow for complete evaluation of the following:
  - IIAA diameter and length of proximal and distal landing zones
  - Iliac artery tortuosity and angulation
  - Presence and severity of associated occlusive disease
  - Ipsilateral and contralateral internal iliac artery patency
  - Status of the ipsilateral deep femoral artery
  - Concomitant CIA, abdominal or thoracic aortic pathology
- Determination of IIAA endovascular repair suitability needs to be answered at the start. Suitability is determined by pelvic perfusion, landing zone, vessel tortuosity, and access.
- The optimal method for endovascular repair of IIAA depends largely on the adequacy of pelvic perfusion. Preservation of at least one internal iliac artery, if feasible, is recommended to prevent future buttock claudication and erectile dysfunction.
- Spinal cord ischemia, colonic ischemia, and buttock necrosis can result from loss of flow to both internal iliac arteries.[2,13,14] If obliteration of perfusion to both internal iliac arteries is planned, a staged approach can minimize ischemic complications.[9]
- In general, landing zones are sited in nonaneurysmal arterial segments that manifest minimal angulation, tortuosity, and/or occlusive disease. The allowable diameter range for treatment may vary, depending on the device deployed. In all circumstances, reference should be made to the "Instructions for Use," or IFU, included in the package insert or available online.
- Device selection is based on the need for durable aneurysm exclusion and endograft fixation, accomplished with the fewest component pieces possible.
- If the patient is not an endovascular candidate, then a decision needs to be made on how best to manage the IIAA via open surgical techniques.
- Options for open repair include total internal iliac artery aneurysm inflow and outflow ligation, endoaneurysmorrhaphy, or aneurysmectomy with interposition grafting. Treatment option will drive operative exposure and extent of IIAA dissection.

Positioning

- Open surgical repair is typically performed under general or spinal anesthesia. The iliac artery can be accessed through a low midline/transperitoneal or a paramedian/retroperitoneal approach. Exposure will depend on the patient's body habitus, extent of the aneurysm, presence of concomitant AAA and/or CIA aneurysm, or if there are bilateral IIAAs.
- Endovascular repair can be performed under general, regional, spinal, or local anesthesia. For this approach, the patient is positioned supine, arms by their side, with both groins and the entire abdomen prepared and draped into the sterile field. The C-arm is typically positioned contralateral to the operative team.

OPEN SURGICAL REPAIR

- Exposure of the Internal Iliac Artery Aneurysm
  - Our preferred approach for open repair of a unilateral IIAA is an ipsilateral lower quadrant retroperitoneal approach.
  - A curvilinear, or "kidney transplant-type," incision is created with dissection through the skin, subcutaneous tissue, external and internal oblique muscles, and transversus abdominis musculature to the retroperitoneal space. Sweep the preperitoneal fat, peritoneum, and contents medially.
  - Note the psoas muscle, the iliac artery lies laterally. The iliac vein is posteromedial to the artery.
  - Utilize a Bookwalter or an OMNI-TRACT retractor system to aid in exposure.
  - Identify the ureter as it crosses over the iliac artery bifurcation. Avoid devascularizing the ureter.
  - Appropriately expose the common and external iliac arteries at the origin while avoiding injury to the underlying iliac veins.
  - If the operative plan includes total internal iliac artery aneurysm inflow and outflow ligation, endoaneurysmorrhaphy, or aneurysmectomy with interposition grafting, dissect medially and caudally to expose the outflow branches of the internal iliac artery.

Options

- Proximal Ligation: One of the simplest options for management of an IIAA is surgical ligation of proximal internal iliac artery. Unfortunately, this procedure is associated with a high recurrence rate with IIAA enlargement resulting from retrograde filling of the aneurysm sac.[15] Continued surveillance is needed for all IIAA treated in this manner.
- Distal Ligation: Distal ligation eliminates retrograde filling of a residual IIAA. The procedure can be technically difficult due to the depth of the dissection deep in the pelvis.
- Endoaneurysmorrhaphy: Involves proximal ligation of the internal iliac artery followed by opening of the aneurysm sac and ligation of the branch vessels from within. Endoaneurysmorrhaphy is used to treat proximal ligation failures.

TECHNIQUES

- Aneurysmectomy: Maintaining perfusion to the distal internal iliac artery can be achieved with aneurysmectomy and interposition bypass. This option is generally applied for concomitant treatment of EIA aneurysms. Jump grafts can arise off of this bypass for EIA perfusion.[14] Transposition of the internal iliac artery to the external iliac artery has also been described.[13]

ENDOVASCULAR REPAIR

- There are various methods to perform endovascular flow interruption or exclusion of the IIAA.
- Proximal Exclusion:
    - In the setting of normal bilateral pelvic perfusion, simple stent graft coverage of the arterial origin of the IIAA is an option. Continued aneurysm growth is inevitable with this approach since the IIAA is still perfused via distal branches. Further IIAA treatment, especially for an enlarging IIAA, can be a challenge with this treatment algorithm.[2] Continued surveillance is needed for all IIAA treated in this manner.
- Proximal Embolization:
    - Coil embolization of the IIAA ostium carries similar risk and outcome as proximal exclusion.
- Distal Embolization with Proximal Exclusion/Embolization:
    - The preferred IIAA obliterative endovascular treatment option involves coil embolization or plug occlusion of the internal iliac artery branch vessels and/or the aneurysm itself. A stent graft is then deployed across the origin of the internal iliac artery (**FIGURE 2**).
    - Outflow vessel embolization with proximal exclusion is chosen in the setting of no adequate proximal landing zone for embolic devices. Proximal embolization is selected for adequate proximal landing zone for embolic devices.
    - Some interventionalists choose to fill the aneurysm sac in addition to outflow vessel embolization to decrease the risk for future endoleak. There are no studies to determine how prevalent or effective this technique is.
- Internal iliac artery preservation: Given the risk of associated ischemic complications with the above-mentioned techniques, several methods have been employed in attempt to preserve pelvic perfusion.
    - Iliac branch endoprosthesis:
        - While outside of the manufacturer's IFU, an iliac branch endoprosthesis (IBE) can be used to treat IIAA while preserving internal iliac artery flow. In these cases, a large internal iliac artery branch vessel is used as the distal landing target[4,16,17] (**FIGURE 3**).
    - Parallel stent grafts
        - For IIAA lacking an adequate proximal landing zone for stent grafting, a "chimney" or "snorkel" type graft can be extended from the internal iliac artery into the EIA or CIA. Alternately, a "sandwich" technique can be used, via simultaneous release of parallel covered stent grafts, to create an iliac artery neo-bifurcation.[2]
    - Hybrid Stent and Embolization
        - In the absence of a distal landing zone, a stent graft can be placed into the largest of the branch vessels after coil embolization of smaller vessels draining the aneurysm.

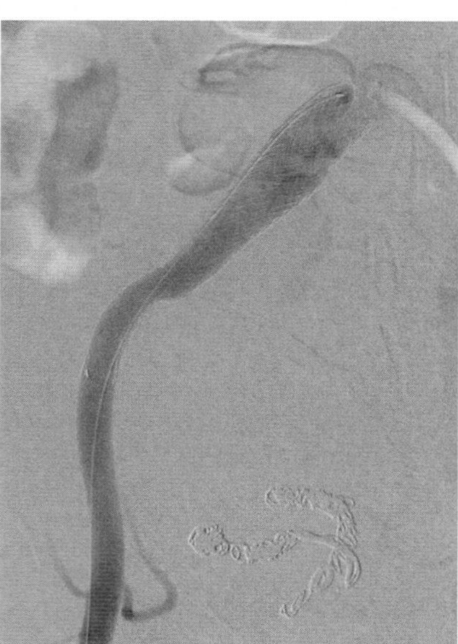

FIGURE 2 • Endovascular exclusion of large internal iliac artery aneurysm with distal coil embolization and proximal exclusion with stent graft.

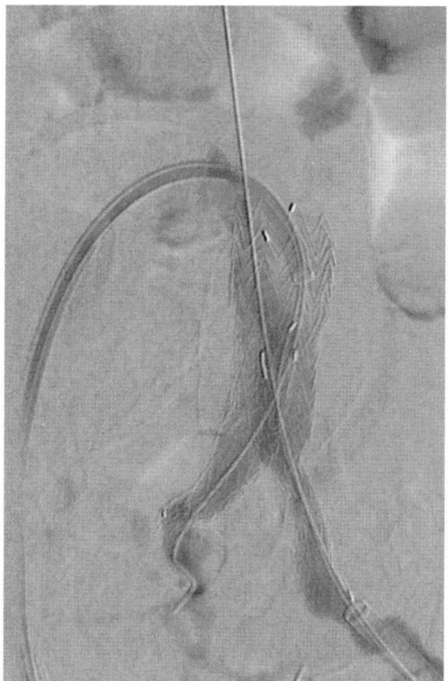

FIGURE 3 • Iliac branch endoprosthesis delivery for exclusion of left internal iliac artery aneurysm.

PEARLS AND PITFALLS

Open vs endovascular management	▪ The preferred treatment for IIAAs is endovascular over open repair because endovascular repair is associated with lower operative morbidity and mortality rates and shorter inpatient length of stays compared with open repair.[3,4,11]
Preoperative planning	▪ Determination of IIAA endovascular repair suitability needs to be answered at the start. ▪ Suitability is determined by pelvic perfusion, landing zone, vessel tortuosity, and access as described above. CTA, with multiple phases, is optimal for this purpose.
Adequate exposure (Open)	▪ The iliac artery can be accessed through a low midline/transperitoneal or a paramedian/retroperitoneal approach. Exposure will depend on the patient's body habitus, extent of the aneurysm, presence of concomitant AAA and/or CIA aneurysm, or if there are bilateral IIAAs.
Adequate access	▪ Endovascular access requires suitable arterial access. Arterial suitability is driven by arterial diameter, degree of atherosclerotic burden, and vessel tortuosity. These parameters are typically outlined and driven by the device IFU.

POSTOPERATIVE CARE

- For endovascular treatment of the IIAA, postoperative care is similar to a standard endovascular aneurysm repair. Complete blood count and basic metabolic panel may be checked the following morning.
- Groin access should be checked routinely immediately after the procedure, the following morning, and prior to discharge. The duration for strict immobilization is driven by the arterial closure technique of the interventionalist. Oral intake is started immediately, the Foley catheter is removed, and the patient is encouraged to ambulate and discharged on following postoperative day.
- For open surgical treatment, both trans- and retroperitoneal approaches, diet can be advanced, and labs drawn in alignment with institutional protocols. Patients can be discharged when ambulatory, pain is well managed, and bowel function resumes.

COMPLICATIONS

- In general, morbidity and mortality rates are higher for open surgical vs endovascular repair of IIAA.
- Thirty-day mortality rates for both urgent and elective open surgical repair is 4% to 6% compared to 1% to 2% for endovascular repair.
- Hospital length of stay (LOS) is greater for open (5-9 days) vs endovascular (2-3 days) IIAA repair.[11]
- The main complication associated with open IIAA repair is bleeding related to venous injury. Other less common complications include ureteral injury, bowel injury, ipsilateral leg ischemia, and early graft thrombosis.
- Complications related to endovascular treatment include access site injuries, early graft thrombosis, and ischemia related to iliac artery occlusion.
- Graft occlusions to both the external and internal iliac arteries occur at significantly higher frequency with endovascular preservation techniques than with open surgery.[13,16]
- Complications specifically related to internal iliac artery occlusion include buttock claudication (30% unilateral, 40% bilateral),[13,16,18] ischemic colitis or ischemic bowel requiring surgery (0.5% unilateral, 1% bilateral), gluteal necrosis and spinal ischemia (<1%),[18] and erectile dysfunction (10%-15% of cases).[13,18]
- IBE with preservation of at least one internal iliac artery for the management of aortoiliac disease is associated with a notably lower (2%) rate of buttock claudication with 97% technical success, 7% reintervention rate, and <1% 30-day mortality.[16]
- Embolization of the internal iliac artery with vascular plugs vs coil embolization is associated with lower procedural time, total fluoroscopy time, and radiation dose when applied to EVAR (**FIGURE 4**).[19] Unfortunately, in the management of IIAA, it may not be feasible to use plugs alone to sufficiently embolize the distal branch vessels.[18]

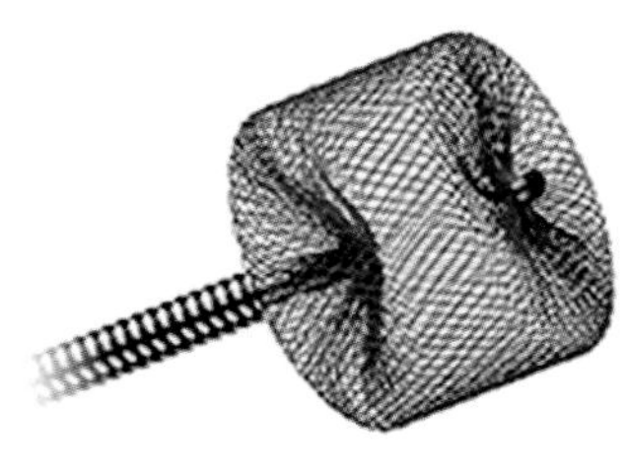

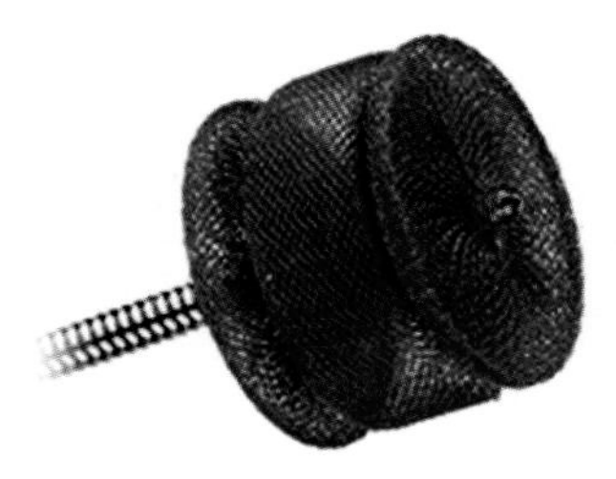

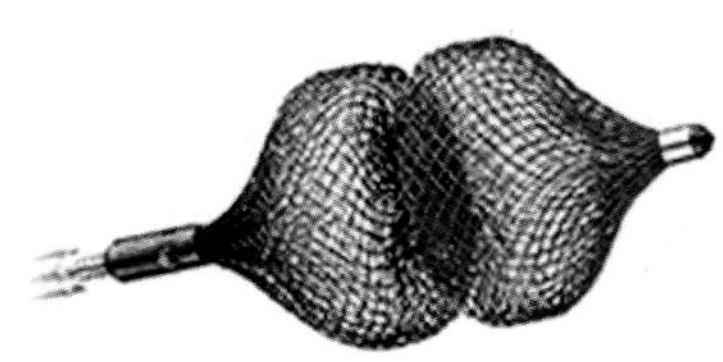

FIGURE 4 ● Variety of vascular plugs used for vessel embolization. (Amplatzer is a trademark of Abbott or its related companies. Reproduced with permission of Abbott, © 2022. All rights reserved.)

REFERENCES

1. Johnston KW, Rutherford RB, Tilson MD, Shah DM, Hollier L, Stanley JC. Suggested standards for reporting on arterial aneurysms. Subcommittee on reporting standards for arterial aneurysms, Ad Hoc Committee on reporting standards, Society for vascular surgery and North American Chapter, International Society for Cardiovascular surgery. *J Vasc Surg*. 1991;13(3):452-458.
2. Perini P, Mariani E, Fanelli M, et al. Surgical and endovascular management of isolated internal iliac artery aneurysms: a systematic review and meta-analysis. *Vasc Endovasc Surg*. 2021;55(3):254-264.
3. Antoniou GA, Nassef AH, Antoniou SA, Loh SYY, Turner DR, Beard JD. Endovascular treatment of isolated internal iliac artery aneurysms. *Vascular*. 2011;19(6):291-300.
4. Wanhainen A, Verzini F, Van Herzeele I, et al. Editor's Choice - European Society for Vascular Surgery (ESVS) 2019 Clinical practice guidelines on the management of abdominal Aorto-iliac artery aneurysms. *Eur J Vasc Endovasc Surg*. 2019;57(1):8-93.
5. Laine MT, Björck M, Beiles CB, et al. Few internal iliac artery aneurysms rupture under 4 cm. *J Vasc Surg*. 2017;65(1):76-81.
6. Dix FP, Titi M, Al-Khaffaf H. The isolated internal iliac artery aneurysm—a review. *Eur J Vasc Endovasc Surg*. 2005;30(2):119-129.
7. Santilli SM, Wernsing SE, Lee ES. Expansion rates and outcomes for iliac artery aneurysms. *J Vasc Surg*. 2000;31(1 pt 1):114-121.
8. Freel KA, Nutley WK. Internal iliac artery aneurysm detected by sonography. *J Diagn Med Sonogr*. 2013;29(5):234-237.
9. Chaikof EL, Dalman RL, Eskandari MK, et al. The Society for Vascular Surgery practice guidelines on the care of patients with an abdominal aortic aneurysm. *J Vasc Surg*. 2018;67(1):2-77 e2.
10. Biancari F, Paone R, Venermo M, D'Andrea V, PeräläJ. Diagnostic accuracy of computed tomography in patients with suspected abdominal aortic aneurysm rupture. *Eur J Vasc Endovasc Surg*. 2013;45(3):227-230.
11. Buck DB, Bensley RP, Darling J, et al. The effect of endovascular treatment on isolated iliac artery aneurysm treatment and mortality. *J Vasc Surg*. 2015;62(2):331-335.
12. Lau C, Feldman DN, Girardi LN, Kim LK. Imaging for surveillance and operative management for endovascular aortic aneurysm repairs. *J Thorac Dis*. 2017;9(suppl 4):S309-S316.
13. Kouvelos GN, Katsargyris A, Antoniou GA, Oikonomou K, Verhoeven ELG. Outcome after interruption or preservation of internal iliac artery flow during endovascular repair of abdominal aorto-iliac aneurysms. *Eur J Vasc Endovasc Surg*. 2016;52(5):621-634.
14. Bacharach JM, Slovut DP. State of the art: management of iliac artery aneurysmal disease. *Cathet Cardiovasc Interv*. 2008;71(5):708-714.
15. Wilhelm BJ, Sakharpe A, Ibrahim G, Baccaro LM, Fisher J. The 100-year evolution of the isolated internal iliac artery aneurysm. *Ann Vasc Surg*. 2014;28(4):1070-1077.
16. Giosdekos A, Antonopoulos CN, Sfyroeras GS, et al. The use of iliac branch devices for preservation of flow in internal iliac artery during endovascular aortic aneurysm repair. *J Vasc Surg*. 2020;71(6):2133-2144.
17. Noel-Lamy M, Jaskolka J, Lindsay TF, Oreopoulos GD, Tan KT. Internal iliac aneurysm repair outcomes using a modification of the iliac branch graft. *Eur J Vasc Endovasc Surg*. 2015;50(4):474-479.
18. Bosanquet DC, Wilcox C, Whitehurst L, et al. Systematic review and meta-analysis of the effect of internal iliac artery exclusion for patients undergoing EVAR. *Eur J Vasc Endovasc Surg*. 2017;53(4):534-548.
19. Abbott C *The Amplatzer Family of Vascular Plugs*. 2021 [cited January 9, 2021] https://www.cardiovascular.abbott/int/en/hcp/products/peripheral-intervention/amplatzer-family-vascular-plugs.html.

Chapter 23

Aortoiliac Occlusive Disease: Open Surgical Management

Ashley R. Gutwein and Raghu L. Motaganahalli

DEFINITIONS

- Peripheral artery disease (PAD) is a condition that, due to atherosclerosis and chronic plaque accumulation, leads to arterial occlusion that results in diminished blood supply to distal arterial beds. Patients experience a wide range of symptoms from claudication to rest pain, nonhealing wounds, and gangrene.
- PAD is then further subclassified depending on the anatomical location of the atherosclerotic burden. In general, PAD is classified as aortoiliac, femoral-popliteal, tibial, or multilevel disease.[1,2]
- The Trans-Atlantic Inter-Society Consensus Classification (TASC) historically was used to help classify the anatomic disease patterns and recommend open vs endovascular therapy.[3] TASC has made way for the Global Anatomic Staging System (GLASS).
- GLASS evaluates the arterial occlusive disease of the entire limb as well as the presence of wounds and infections to help determine the chances of success with endovascular vs open treatment[2] (**TABLE 1**).
- When patients have the multilevel disease, treatment is first focused on treating the aortoiliac and femoral occlusive disease (termed inflow disease), followed by the more distal (or outflow) arterial occlusive disease.[1]
- This chapter will focus on open surgical options for aortoiliac occlusive disease.

DIFFERENTIAL DIAGNOSIS

- Several conditions can mimic vascular claudication. It is important to differentiate if the lower extremity pain is due to vascular occlusive disease or due to neurogenic or musculoskeletal etiology. A thorough history, physical examination, x-rays, and continuous-wave Doppler can help differentiate between arterial, venous, neurogenic, or musculoskeletal causes for pain.[4,5]

Table 1: GLASS Classifications of Aortoiliac Occlusive Disease

I. Stenosis of the common and/or external iliac artery, chronic total occlusion of either common or external iliac artery (not both), stenosis of the infrarenal aorta: any combination of these
II. Chronic total occlusion of the aorta; chronic total occlusion of common and external iliac arteries; severe diffuse disease and/or small-caliber (<6 mm) common and external iliac arteries; concomitant aneurysm disease; severe diffuse in-stent restenosis in the AI system
A, no significant CFA disease; B, significant CFA disease (>50% stenosis)

AI, aortoiliac; CFA, common femoral artery.

A simplified staging system for inflow (AI and CFA) disease is suggested. Hemodynamically significant disease (>50% stenosis) of the CFA is considered a key modifier (A/B).

Adapted from Conte MS, Bradbury AW, Kolh P, et al. Global vascular guidelines on the management of chronic limb-threatening ischemia [published correction appears in J Vasc Surg. 2019 Aug; 70(2):662]. J Vasc Surg. 2019;69(6S):3S-125S.e40. Copyright © 2019 by the Society for Vascular Surgery and European Society for Vascular Surgery. With permission.

- Patients with aortoiliac occlusive disease may experience gluteal, thigh, or calf muscle pain. Symptoms are reproducible and occur with walking.
- Neurogenic claudication occurs with standing, does not require walking to bring it on, and can be relieved by positional changes. Use of spinal support while walking, such as a shopping cart or wheeled walker, may relieve the pain. Patients with neurogenic claudication may also have vasculogenic claudication complicating the diagnosis. Spinal imaging and ankle-brachial indices (ABIs) can help differentiate between neurogenic and arterial occlusive disease. It is important to understand the patient's symptoms and expectations before proceeding with any form of intervention.
- Venous claudication is described as a bursting type of pain that occurs after walking longer distances and requires a longer rest period with leg elevation. Physical examination findings of swelling and discoloration are often present. Once again, ABIs and duplex examinations can help distinguish the etiology.
- Pain secondary to osteoarthritis can mimic arterial claudication; however, the pain is localized to the joints, exacerbated by activity, and relieved by rest. X-rays and ABIs can help differentiate these two diagnoses.

PATIENT HISTORY AND PHYSICAL FINDINGS

- Patients with aortoiliac disease have up to a 50% risk of concomitant coronary artery disease with the same risk factors of smoking, hypertension, lipid abnormalities, diabetes mellitus, male gender, increased age, and family history.
- The disease burden in the internal and external iliac blood supply leads to a variety of clinical presentations, which is most notable for Leriche syndrome, which comprises the symptoms of buttock claudication, impotence in men, muscle atrophy, and absent or diminished femoral pulses.[6,7] Impotence as an isolated symptom in men should be evaluated for other possible causes. Impotence is only seen in 30% of men with decreased hypogastric perfusion as there are abundant collaterals from the mesenteric, profunda, and lumbar arteries.
- A physical examination will show a decrease or lack of femoral and distal pulses, although at rest the pulses may be present. More severe disease may present with extremity hair loss, coolness, decreased capillary refill, dependent rubor, as well as gangrene.
- ABIs are decreased but not generally below 0.5 to 0.6 unless the patient also has outflow disease.

IMAGING AND OTHER DIAGNOSTIC STUDIES

- Noninvasive vascular laboratories
  - Patients with aortoiliac disease will have decreased ABI with dampened waveforms of the common femoral artery indicating proximal stenosis or occlusion[7] (**FIGURE 1**).

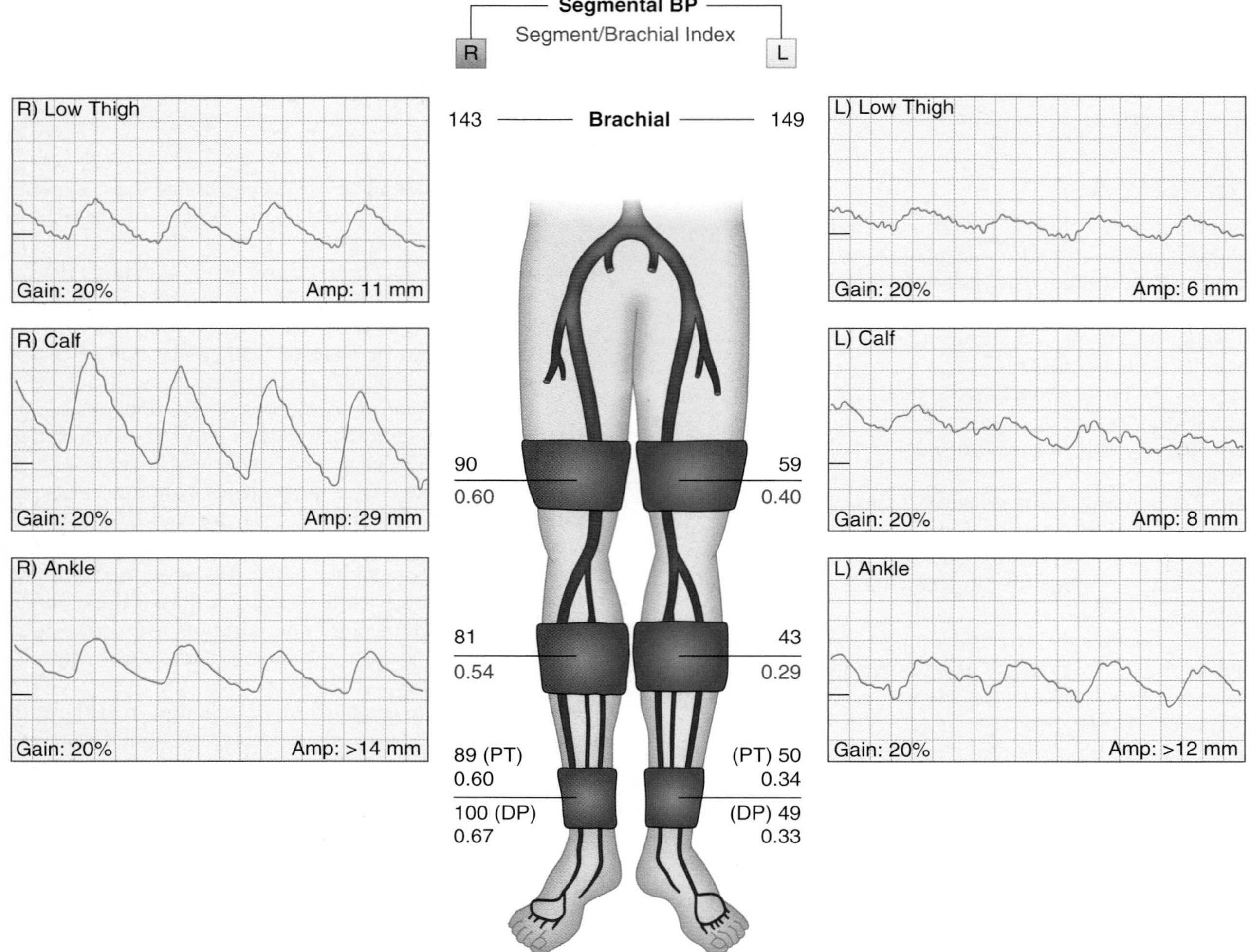

FIGURE 1 ● Arterial waveforms showing monophasic waveform in both lower extremities with decreased ABI suggestive of aortoiliac occlusive disease.

  - If the patient has a normal ABI at rest, exercise testing should be completed. A drop by 15% of the ABI from resting value is considered significant and leads to diminished blood flow distal to the point of stenosis or obstruction during exercise.
  - Duplex ultrasound for the aortoiliac system is limited by body habitus and bowel gas.
- Computed tomography angiography (CTA)
  - CTA is excellent at estimating the degree of stenosis as well as the degree of calcification. It is often considered the noninvasive imaging study of choice for preoperative planning. It is important to evaluate the aortoiliac, femoral, popliteal, and tibial vessels.
  - CTA can help in deciding graft size, location of cross-clamping, enlarged collateral pathways to preserve, and operative approach (open, endovascular, or hybrid)[8] (**FIGURE 2**).
- Magnetic resonance angiography (MRA)
  - MRA often can overestimate the degree of stenosis, and the presence of stents and other metallic objects can interfere with imaging. Motion artifacts may limit the quality of the study.
  - MRA can be considered if the patient has a contraindication to CTA, such as contrast allergy.
- Arteriography
  - Iliac occlusion and diseased femoral arteries can make diagnostic angiography complicated and may require using a radial or brachial artery approach.
  - Arteriography does not always show the degree of calcification, which is important in operative planning.
  - CO_2 angiography may be the best option in patients with severe renal insufficiency.

SURGICAL MANAGEMENT

- The decision to proceed with revascularization vs medical therapy is based on the patient's symptoms. Claudication is generally treated medically while rest pain or tissue loss require revascularization.[4]
- Patients should be advised to quit smoking and start statin therapy and aspirin if tolerated.

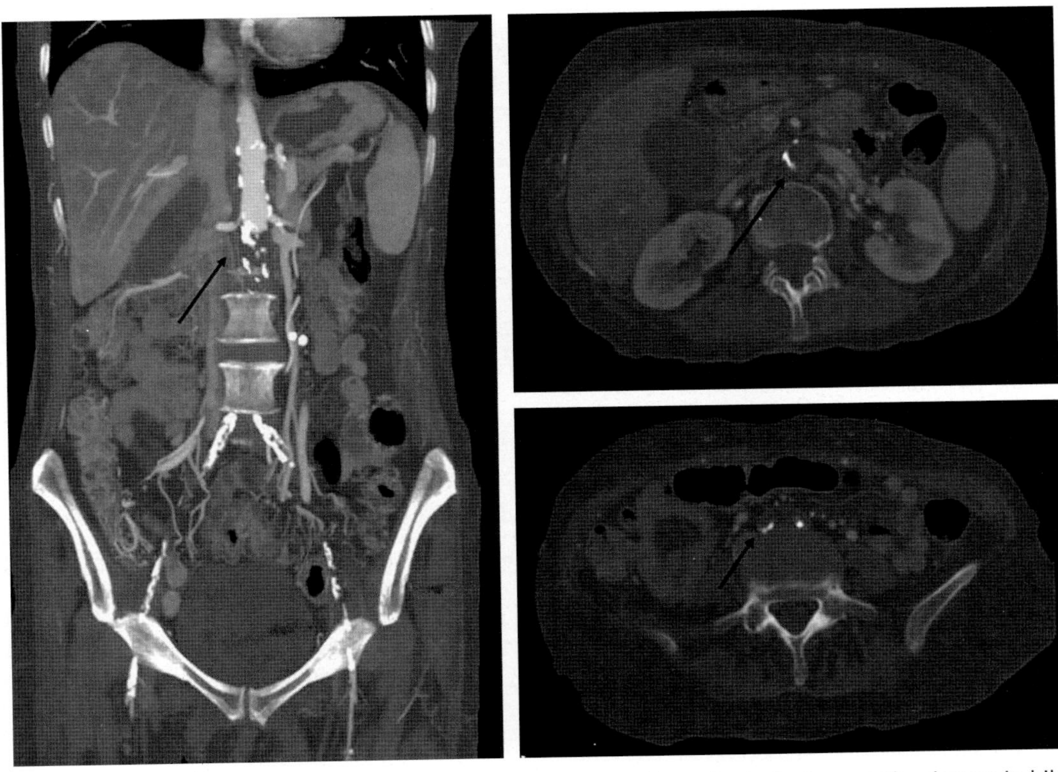

FIGURE 2 ● CTA showing juxtarenal aortic occlusion at the level of the renal arteries including calcific plaques in bilateral common iliac arteries (*black arrows*).

- Preoperative anesthesia visits should include inquiries into cardiac, lung, and renal systems to evaluate overall operative risk as patients with PAD are at high risk for coronary artery disease, chronic obstructive pulmonary disease, and chronic kidney disease.[6]
- The decision to proceed with open vs endovascular interventions is multifactorial and depends on the patient's anatomy, comorbidities, and age, as well as the surgeon's experience.
- Patients with aortoiliac occlusive disease can be treated with either an inline direct reconstruction such as aortobifemoral or thoracobifemoral bypass. Extra-anatomic options include an axillofemoral or femoral-to-femoral bypass. In general, aortobifemoral bypass (AFB) is durable with excellent long-term patency, but if the patient is not a candidate due to comorbidities, anatomy, or prior abdominal surgeries, extra-anatomic bypass is a good alternative.

AORTOBIFEMORAL BYPASS

- The patient is prepared from nipples to knees with chlorhexidine preparation and draped with a sterile technique using skin-protective barriers.

Exposure of Femoral Vessels

- Exposure of femoral outflow vessels is the initial step in AFB.
- The inguinal ligament marks the transition point from the external iliac artery to the common femoral artery and is identified by connecting the anterior superior iliac spine to the pubic tubercle. The common femoral artery is located over the medial third of the femoral head and two finger breaths lateral to pubic symphysis but may be difficult to palpate in aortoiliac occlusive disease. Ultrasound can be used to identify the common femoral artery and femoral bifurcation to allow for optimal incision placement.
- There are two options for groin incision: vertical and oblique. A vertical incision over the common femoral artery and bifurcation allows for greater access to the proximal and distal vessels in extensive femoral artery disease that requires common femoral endarterectomy and profundoplasty. These techniques are discussed in Part 6, Chapter 24. If the patient has no significant common femoral or deep femoral artery disease noted on imaging studies, then an oblique incision is better for cosmesis and wound healing. A transverse incision is made parallel and just caudal to the inguinal ligament.
- The subcutaneous tissue is then dissected with electrocautery with careful attention to ligate superficial crossing vessels to control bleeding and ligating lymphatics to prevent seroma formation. A self-retaining retractor is used to help expose the tissues and is repositioned as the dissection proceeds deeper.
- Once the fascia lata is divided vertically, the femoral sheath is identified. The femoral artery lies lateral to the femoral vein. Dissection is carried out cranially to identify the distal external iliac artery. Circumflex femoral veins cross the femoral artery just beneath the inguinal ligament. It is advisable to

ligate this venous branch to prevent inadvertent injury resulting in bleeding during the tunneling process. Circumferential control is also obtained of the inferior epigastric artery, circumflex femoral artery branches. These branches provide important collateral flow to the lower extremities and pelvis in case of aortoiliac occlusive disease. Progressing caudally, circumferential dissection of the profunda femoral and superficial femoral arteries is performed until a soft healthy portion of the artery is encountered and tagged with a vessel loop or moist umbilical tape using a right angle. All arterial side branches are identified and are controlled with vessel loops or temporary clips. The branches are rarely ligated to help preserve collaterals. The extent of femoral dissection depends on the patient's outflow, and if diseased adjunct endarterectomy may be required.

- Dissecting the femoral arteries before opening the abdomen minimizes the time that the abdomen is open. The groin incision is then packed with an antibacterial saline-soaked gauze to avoid desiccation.

Exposure of the Aorta

- A transperitoneal approach is routinely used to expose the infrarenal aorta, although a retroperitoneal approach may also be used depending on surgeons' preference and associated visceral arterial occlusive disease being addressed.
- For transabdominal exposure, a longitudinal midline incision is made from just below the xiphoid process to a few centimeters below the umbilicus or down to the symphysis pubis when iliac arterial exposure will be required. Subcutaneous tissue is dissected, and the abdomen is entered through linea alba between the rectus muscles.
- In a transabdominal approach, the transverse colon is retracted cephalad, and the small bowel is shifted to the patient's right side and packed in soft, moist lap sponges to the right. The ligament of Treitz is taken down and the duodenum is mobilized to the right. A self-retaining retractor is then placed to sweep the bowel to the right with a moist laparotomy pad. The retroperitoneal tissue overlying the aorta is dissected, and the aorta is exposed superiorly to at least the level of the left renal vein.
- Retroperitoneal aortic exposure offers the advantages of exposing the aorta at or above the level of the renal arteries. The benefits of retroperitoneal exposure include less postop morbidity and decreased pulmonary complications. The disadvantage of retroperitoneal exposure includes difficulty to expose the right femoral artery with difficulties experienced during the tunneling process. The risk of bleeding due to venous injuries also limits the use of this technique for AFB. These limitations could be overcome by limiting the extent to which the patient is positioned in the lateral decubitus position. The incision is made beginning at the tip of the 12th rib and extended toward the umbilicus. The Rectus muscle is not generally divided. Care is taken to prevent inadvertently entering the peritoneal cavity while entering the retroperitoneal space. Blunt dissection ensures that peritoneal contents are swept off the abdominal wall providing additional working space in the retroperitoneum.
- Preoperative CTA can help identify renal arteries anatomy, the position of the left renal vein, inferior mesenteric artery (IMA), and a portion of the aorta that is free of disease for clamping and sewing the proximal anastomosis. Manual palpation is also used to identify a portion of the artery amenable to clamping. Care should be taken to prevent circumferential dissection of the aortic neck in patients with a retro aortic renal vein.
- If there is a juxtarenal occlusion of the aorta, or if there is a need for an aortic endarterectomy at the level of the renal arteries or adjunct aortic endarterectomy is needed, then one should expose a segment of suprarenal aorta. The left renal vein is either ligated between sutures or mobilized by dividing the lumbar and adrenal veins. This will enable mobilization and control of the origins of the renal arteries, which are controlled with doubly passed silastic loops so that they may be occluded during endarterectomy to prevent atheroma embolization. Accessory renal arteries and the IMA should be identified and be evaluated if reimplantation is necessary.

Tunneling and Graft Selection

- Blunt finger dissection under the inguinal ligament and over the aortic bifurcation is used to make the tunnel. It is important to stay directly anterior to the external iliac artery and posterior to the ureter. The crossing vein off the femoral vein beneath the inguinal ligament must be ligated or carefully avoided. Moist umbilical tapes, Penrose drain, or red rubber catheters are fed through to the tunnels using a smooth aortic clamp to mark the tunnels.
- Aortic sizers and preoperative imaging are used to select the appropriately sized graft. Typically, a bifurcated polyester (Dacron) graft is used, although others prefer polytetrafluoroethylene (PTFE). Grafts range from 12 × 6 mm to 22 × 11 mm.

Proximal Anastomosis

- There are two options for proximal aortic anastomosis: end to end and end to side. Both are acceptable and have advantages depending on the patient's anatomy and surgeon preference. End-to-side anastomosis can preserve blood flow to the pelvis and is necessary when there is bilateral external iliac artery occlusion with patent hypogastric arteries and IMA. An end-to-end anastomosis allows an aortic endarterectomy of the proximal aorta as well as the renal arteries to be performed. This configuration has a decreased risk of aortoenteric fistula as it lies flat in the retroperitoneum; however, it does not preserve antegrade flow into the pelvis or IMA. Before aortic clamping, heparin is given intravenously. Typically, 100 units/kg is administered and allowed to circulate for 3 minutes with a goal activated clotting time (ACT) around 250. ACT is checked every 30 minutes and readministered as needed.
- If a patient has juxtarenal aortic occlusion (**FIGURE 3A**), both the renal artery vessel loops are placed on tension to prevent any embolic debris from embolizing into renal arteries at the time of clamping the proximal neck. Suprarenal clamps are placed followed by transecting the aorta leaving a stump to move the clamps down below the renal arteries soon after endarterectomy (**FIGURE 3B**). This will reduce the renal ischemia time and resultant postoperative acute kidney injury.
- If end-to-side anastomosis is planned a side-biting aortic clamp can be used. For the infrarenal aorta it may be difficult to perform an anastomosis using a side-biting clam without

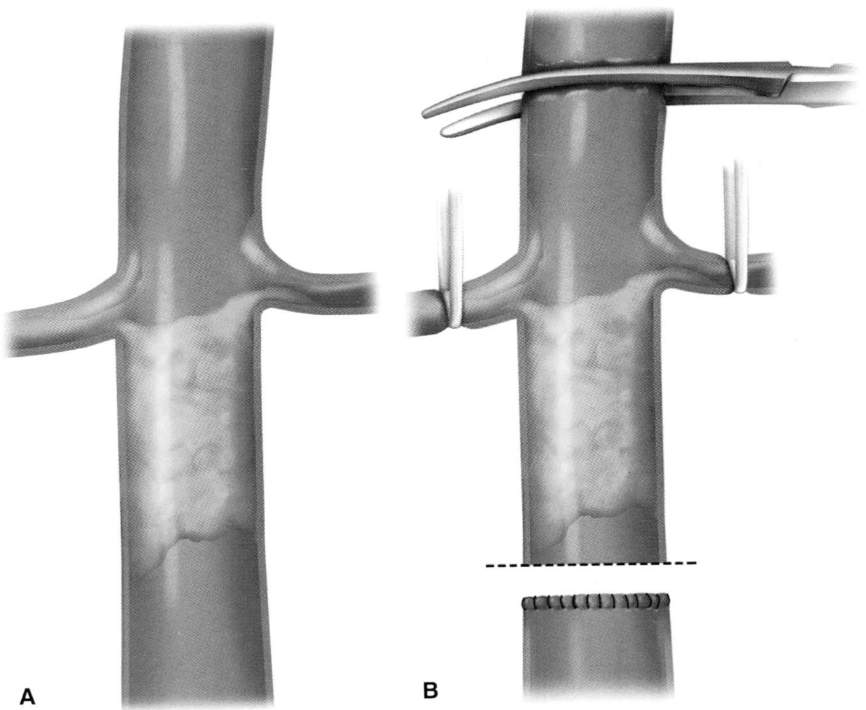

FIGURE 3 ● Image showing juxtarenal aortic occlusion with stenosis of both renal arteries **(A)**. Adjunct aortic endarterectomy, renal endarterectomy with brief suprarenal control would be necessary to complete the proximal anastomosis **(B)**.

risking bleeding from the suture line due to the caliber of the aorta and thickness of the aortic wall. Hence the authors prefer using two clamps to occlude the aorta before aortotomy below the level of renal arteries. An appropriately sized graft is chosen; the graft is then trimmed and beveled. The anastomosis is completed using a running 3.0 polypropylene (**FIGURE 4A**). When there is need to preserve the flow into the internal iliac artery, one can also consider doing the distal anastomosis to the common iliac artery or to the internal iliac artery with additional graft limbs to the femoral artery (**FIGURE 4B**).

- If an end-to-end anastomosis is planned: The aorta is transected just distal to the renal arteries leaving sufficient length for anastomosis. If the aorta is heavily calcified, an aortic endarterectomy can be done to facilitate the proximal anastomosis. The graft is trimmed to leave the main body length of 3 to 4 cm, and a running 3.0 polypropylene is used for anastomosis (**FIGURE 6C**). Felt pledged sutures can be used if the aortic wall is thinned due to endarterectomy. If the aortic wall is thin, authors prefer to use interrupted sutures using a 4-0 Prolene to complete the anastomosis. One can also reinforce the proximal suture line with a sleeve of the Dacron especially if the aorta is of poor quality at the suture line. The distal aorta then is oversewn with a 3-0 Prolene. The graft limbs are then clamped, and the proximal clamp is then released to check for suture line bleeding. Repair sutures can be used for any suture line bleeding with 4-0 or 5-0 sutures on a pledget as needed.
- The decision to reimplant the IMA depends on the status of pelvic perfusion and superior mesenteric arterial collaterals. Traditionally, if there is no pulsatile back bleeding from the ostium of the IMA, then a reimplantation is indicated. If the IMA is occluded, then reimplantation is not indicated. However, reimplantation itself cannot prevent colonic ischemia (**FIGURE 5A** and **B**).

Graft Tunneling

- Using the umbilical tape or Penrose drain as a guide, an aortic clamp is then used to tunnel each graft limb from the abdomen into the femoral incision. The graft is then pulled gently through the tunnel above the external iliac vessels and below the ureter. Care must be taken to minimize kinking, twisting, and redundancy in the graft tunnels. Once tunneled the graft limbs are flushed to confirm adequate inflow, reclamped in the abdomen, and flushed with heparinized saline solution.

Distal Anastomosis

- The common femoral, superficial femoral, and profunda arteries are clamped, using the surgeon's preferred clamp, on healthy portions of the artery. Side branches are controlled by placing the vessel loops on tension. A longitudinal arteriotomy is then made with a no. 11 blade followed by Potts scissors. If there is significant common femoral or profunda disease the arteriotomy should be carried onto the profunda, and common femoral endarterectomy or profundoplasty performed if needed as poor outflow is a common cause of late graft occlusion. The graft is then cut on a taper to allow a natural reimplantation angle into the common femoral artery with minimal tension. The anastomosis is then completed as an end-to-side fashion with 5-0 or 6-0 polypropylene sutures in a running fashion (**FIGURE 6**).

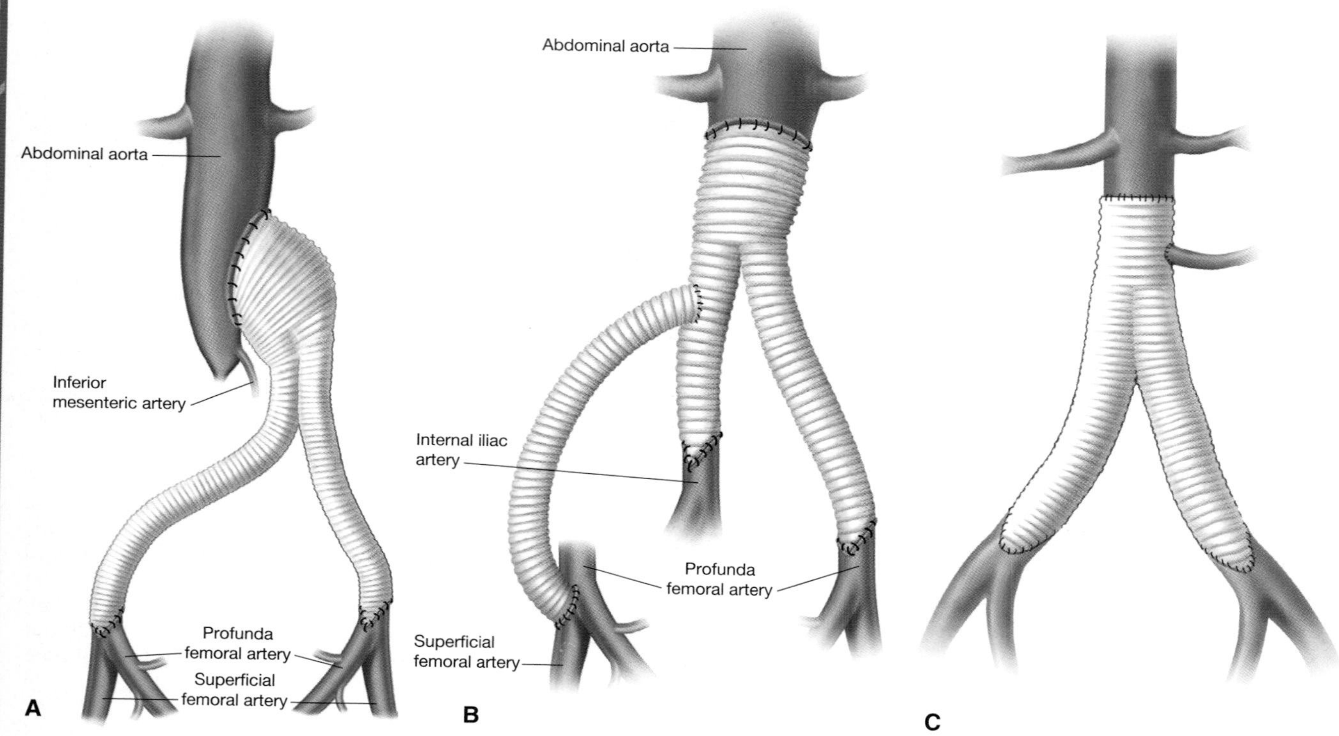

FIGURE 4 ● Configurations for aortobifemoral artery bypass. End-to-side aortobifemoral bypass for patients with occluded bilateral external iliac arteries **(A)**. Frame **(B)** shows aorta to common iliac or to internal iliac bypass with an additional graft limb to the femoral artery. Both **(A and B)** techniques are designed to preserve pelvic arterial flow. Frame **(C)** shows aorta to bifemoral bypass with reimplantation of the inferior mesenteric artery.

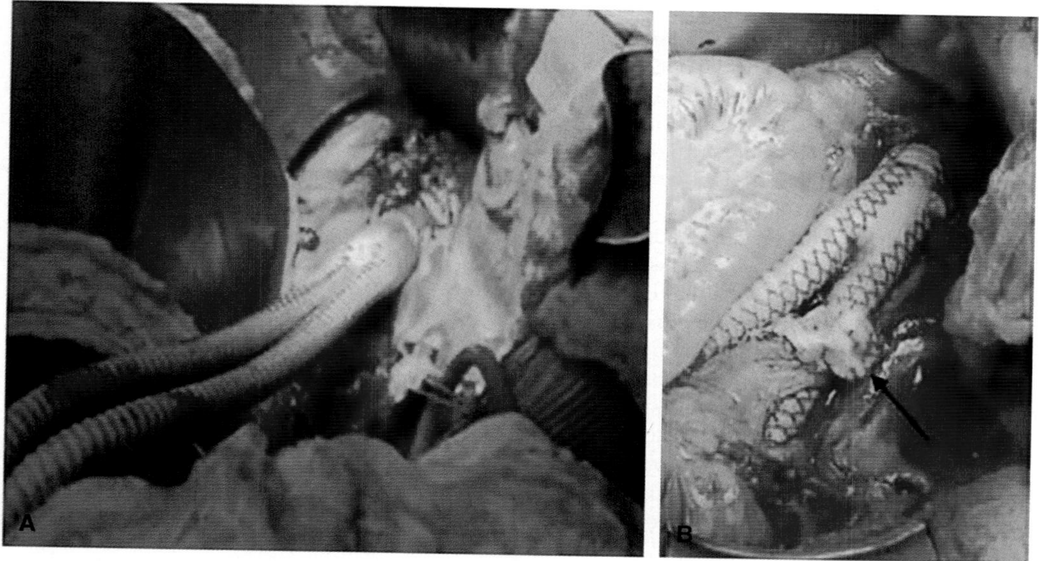

FIGURE 5 ● Intraoperative image shows completion of the proximal anastomosis to aorta with end-to-end technique **(A)**. Frame **(B)** shows completion of the aortobifemoral artery bypass. *Black arrow* shows the inferior mesenteric artery patch ready to be reimplanted to the graft limb.

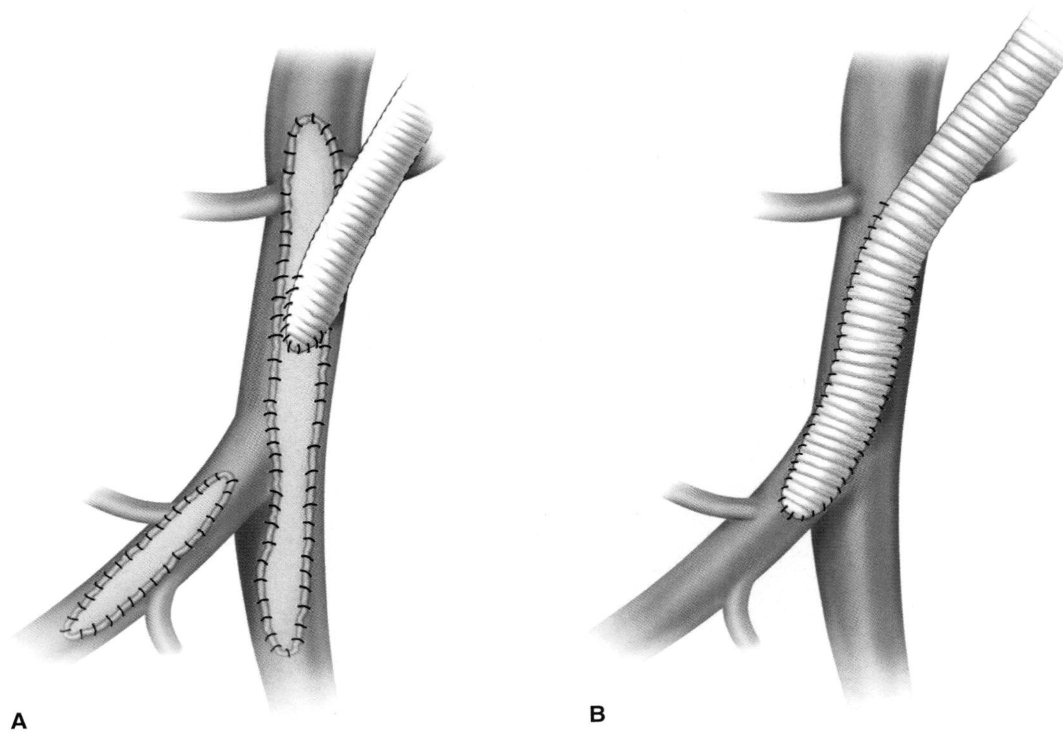

FIGURE 6 ● Femoral artery reconstruction configurations. Common femoral endarterectomy with deep femoral endarterectomy, patch angioplasty, and reimplantation of the aortofemoral graft limb onto the patch **(A)**. Femoral endarterectomy with profundoplasty extending the hood of the graft onto deep femoral artery **(B)**.

The same procedure is completed for the contralateral limb. Graft limbs and native vessels are flushed and back bled before completion of the arteriotomy closure.

Closure

- Protamine may be given, depending on the time of the last heparin bolus or according to the intraoperative ACT reading. Approximately 10 mg is given for every 1000 units of heparin given, adjusted for time decay and the heparin half-life or can be estimated of the last ACT measurement. After adequate hemostasis is achieved, the groins are closed in multiple layers and the dead space is closed to prevent seroma formation and minimize groin infections. In the case of redo groin incisions, if tissue is not adequate for closure, a prophylactic muscle flap should be strongly considered. Groin complications can be catastrophic as they can place the graft at risk for infection.
- In the abdomen, the retroperitoneum is closed over the graft to prevent aortoenteric fistulas and the abdominal fascia is closed according to surgeon preference. In situations where the retroperitoneum cannot be approximated with ease, a tongue of omentum is brought into the infracolic compartment through the transverse mesocolon and placed over the graft to keep the bowel and the graft separated.[5,6]

Thoracofemoral Bypass

- If the infrarenal aorta is not suitable for clamping due to heavy calcification, or if there is extensive disease burden in the paravisceral aorta (**FIGURE 7A**), thoracofemoral bypass may be considered. In addition, in a patient with a hostile abdomen, making it difficult to gain access to retroperitoneum without risking injury to peritoneal contents, thoracofemoral bypass may be preferred.
- In general, patients undergoing thoracobifemoral bypass will need a similar preprocedure evaluation as for an AFB. One anticipates that patients can withstand single lung ventilation and recover from a thoracotomy.
- Preparation will include chest wall, abdomen, pelvis, both lower extremities up to the knee with the patient in semidecubitus position to allow access to the right femoral artery. As described earlier for the retroperitoneal exposure, one would anticipate some difficulty with the tunneling process specifically for the right lower extremity if the patient is positioned in true lateral decubitus position.
- The procedure involves the following major components:
  - Bilateral femoral artery exposure as described above.
  - Thoracotomy through the 8th intercostal space to gain access into the left hemithorax. The inferior pulmonary ligament is divided to allow mobilization of the left lung. Single lung ventilation is required at this point to expose the descending thoracic aorta. Care should be taken to prevent injury to the thoracic duct for complications of chylothorax. Once the mediastinal pleura is divided, the distal descending thoracic aorta is exposed.
  - The thoracic aorta is partially occluded with a side biting Satinsky clamp of appropriate configuration.
  - As described above, an end-to-side anastomosis is performed with 3-0/4-0 Prolene sutures. The suture line is examined for any bleeding before proceeding to the infrainguinal reconstruction.

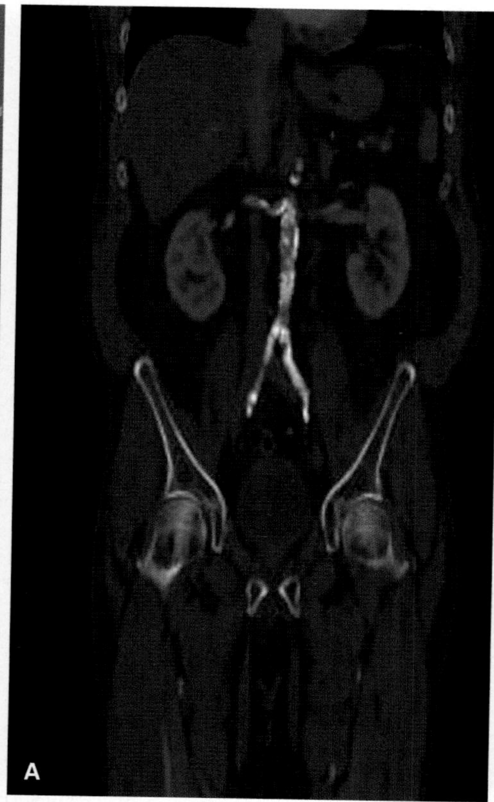

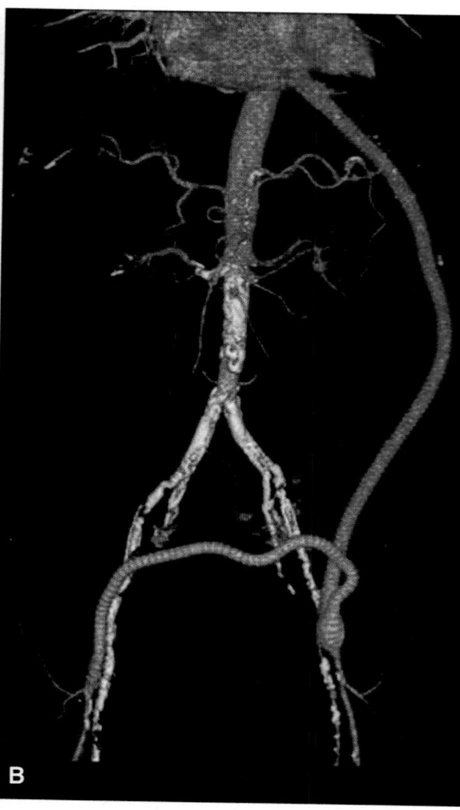

FIGURE 7 • CT Angiographic image shows heavily calcific juxtarenal aorta not suitable for placing a clamp **(A)**. Frame **(B)** shows a completed thoracic aorta to bifemoral bypass.

- The retroperitoneal tunnel lies behind the diaphragm along the posterolateral abdominal wall into the pelvis (**FIGURE 7B**).
- Typically, a 10- to 12-mm straight Dacron tube or an externally supported PTFE is chosen as the conduit. A femoral-to-femoral artery graft is then performed to revascularize the right lower extremity.
- A chest tube is placed in the left hemithorax to allow the drainage and removed at the earliest opportunity after ensuring adequate lung expansion. Wound closure is performed in multiple layers by approximating the anatomical layers with absorbable suture material.[8,9]

EXTRA-ANATOMIC BYPASS

Graft Configuration

- Depending on the extent of the aortoiliac occlusive disease and symptoms a variety of graft configurations may be used: axillofemoral bypass using commercially available PTFE grafts or axillounifemoral bypass using an 8-mm externally supported straight graft along with femoral-to-femoral bypass. **Femoral Exposure**: See section under Aortobifemoral Bypass-Exposure of Femoral Vessels.

Axillary Exposures

- Choosing the donor axillary artery: In general, patients will need an upper extremity arterial Doppler study including blood pressure in both upper extremities to look for pressure gradients before choosing the donor artery. The decision also depends on the presence of other prosthetic material, pacemaker, defibrillator, access port, prior radiation, dialysis access, presence of ostomies and fistulas, and coexisting conditions that would require thoracotomy in the future.
- The patient should be positioned with the arm abducted at 90° with a shoulder roll. The surgical field involves the upper arm, shoulder, chest wall, abdomen, as well as both lower extremities to the knees. A two-team approach is useful to limit the duration of the procedure in these critically ill patients.
- An oblique incision is made a couple of centimeters inferior to the middle third of the clavicle. The deep fascia is opened, and the pectoralis major muscles are split. Pectoralis minor tendon may have to be divided to obtain exposure of the axillary artery. The axillary artery is then dissected. There are often large venous branches that need to be ligated. Several branches of the axillary artery must be controlled to prevent back bleeding during the anastomosis.
- The anastomosis is performed to the first part of the axillary artery, which is medial to the tendon of the pectoralis major muscle. Anastomosis at this location generally prevents anastomotic disruption that may result from hyperabduction of the upper extremity.

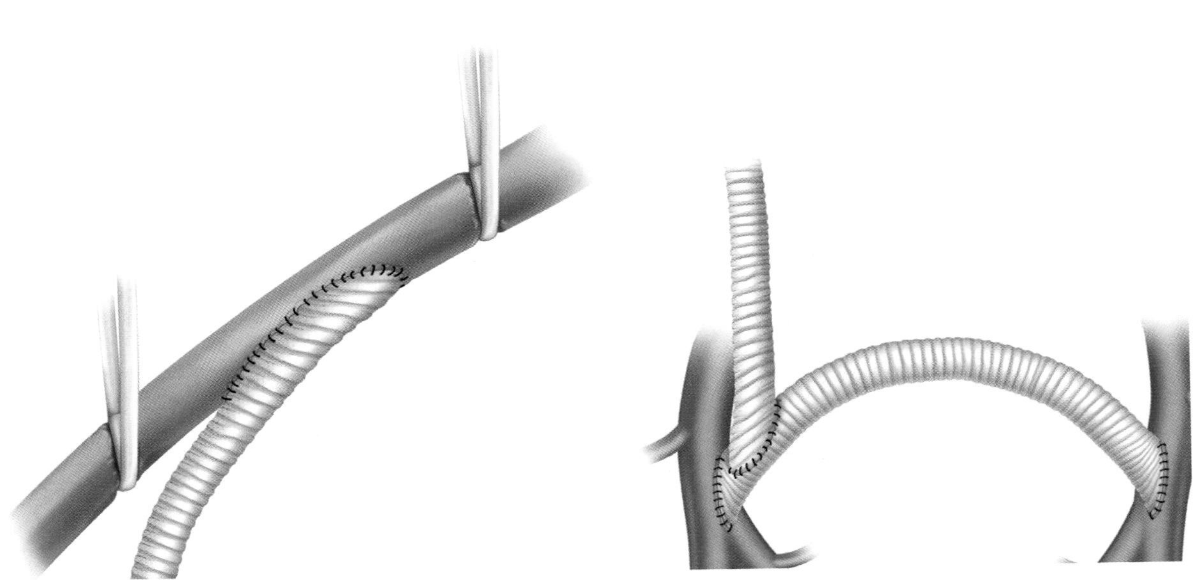

FIGURE 8 ● Axillary artery to externally supported PTFE graft. Note configuration of the inflow anastomosis to axially artery **(A)**, axillounifemoral bypass and femoral to femoral bypass **(B)**.

Tunneling and Graft Selection

- For the axillofemoral bypass an 8-mm externally supported PTFE graft is typically used, and 6- to 8-mm externally supported PTFE is used for the femoral-to-femoral bypass. If planning an axillobifemoral bypass, there is a bifurcated externally supported PTFE graft available.
- The tunneling process differs if an axillary unifemoral bypass is planned vs using an off the shelf axillobifemoral bypass graft.
- The axillofemoral tunnel is started using blunt dissection from the axillary incision medial and posterior to the pectoralis minor muscle and groin incision medial to the anterior superior iliac spine. A long metallic tunneler is then passed between the incisions on the anterior lateral aspect of the abdominal and chest wall, anterior to the external oblique aponeurosis. Occasionally one may need a counter incision over the lower chest wall to facilitate the tunneling process.
- The femoral-to-femoral artery bypass tunnel is completed by using blunt dissection just anterior to the inguinal ligament. The tunnel is then completed in the suprapubic region just anterior to the external oblique aponeurosis fascia with a gentle large arc using blunt dissection. A long aortic clamp can be used to pass the graft from one side to the other in the subcutaneous tissue, avoiding entry into the peritoneal cavity.

Axillary Anastomosis

- After heparinizing the patient as previously described, the axillary artery is clamped. The arteriotomy should be made as medial as safely possible to avoid tension on the graft that could result in an axillary artery anastomotic disruption. An 11 blade is used to make the arteriotomy along the inferior wall of the axillary artery and extended using Potts scissors. The graft is spatulated and an end-to-side anastomosis is completed with a running 5-0 or 6-0 polypropylene. A gentle curve is then allowed before the graft takes a vertical course inferiorly (**FIGURE 8A**).
- After completion, the anastomosis is inspected for hemostasis before feeding the graft through the tunnel. Some redundancy should be left in the graft to avoid tension on the axillary artery, which could cause anastomotic disruption.

Femoral Anastomosis

- Similar principles described in the aortobifemoral portion of this chapter are used in the femoral anastomosis of extra-anatomic reconstruction, ensuring adequate outflow with the adjunct endarterectomy or profundaplasty in patients with extensive femoral artery disease.
- If planning an axillobifemoral configuration, an oval graftotomy is made on the hood of the axillounifemoral bypass for the femoral-femoral graft (**FIGURE 8B**). This is an additional anastomosis that is required if one is not using a prefabricated axillobifemoral graft configuration.

Closure:

- Protamine can be administered as described earlier in this chapter. Continuous waveform Doppler is used to evaluate the outflow arteries with the graft open and clamped. The groin incisions are closed in the same fashion as described in the aortobifemoral portion of this chapter. The axillary incision is closed first by approximating the deep fascia followed by soft tissue and skin.[10,11]

PEARLS AND PITFALLS

Aortofemoral reconstruction	▪ Adequate exposure is critical to success. ▪ Localized endarterectomy at both proximal and distal anastomotic sites is generally required. ▪ Tunneling errors can lead to both early and late complications with graft failure. ▪ The hood of the distal anastomosis should be placed onto the deep femoral artery to improve graft patency.
Extra-anatomical reconstruction	▪ Adequate inflow and outflow must be assured for success. ▪ Concomitant femoral endarterectomy should be used freely. ▪ Tunneling and closure errors frequently cause early graft failure. ▪ Axillary anastomosis should be placed as medially as possible to prevent anastomotic disruption.

POSTOPERATIVE CARE

- Patients are admitted to a cardiac monitored floor postoperatively as patients are at high risk for cardiac and respiratory disease.
- High-frequency neurovascular checks are needed to assess early graft thrombosis requiring reintervention or initiation of anticoagulation.
- Patients are encouraged to ambulate at the earliest once they have no bleeding concerns and have adequate pain control.
- When the abdomen is entered, in the case of aortobifemoral grafting, patients are kept NPO until bowel function returns while enhanced recovery protocols suggest early return to feeding.
- The decision to place the patient on antiplatelet and anticoagulation is based on the patient's comorbidities, and prior vascular procedure history.
- Patients should be seen in clinic immediately postoperatively and then 3, 6, and 12 months and then every 6 to 12 months thereafter with an ABI and graft duplex.[12]

COMPLICATIONS

- Early
  - Hemorrhage
  - Early graft thrombosis
  - Infections
  - Colon ischemia
  - Femoral nerve injury
  - Venous thrombosis
  - Abdominal or lower extremity compartment syndrome
  - Postoperative pneumonia
  - Acute kidney injury
- Late
  - Aortoenteric fistula
  - Graft restenosis, thrombosis of graft
  - Anastomotic pseudoaneurysm
  - Graft infection

REFERENCES

1. Bismuth J, Duran C. Bypass surgery in limb salvage: inflow procedures. *Methodist Debakey Cardiovasc J*. 2013;9(2):66-68.
2. Conte MS, Bradbury AW, Kolh P, et al. Global vascular guidelines on the management of chronic limb-threatening ischemia. *J Vasc Surg*. 2019;69(6s):3S-125S.e140.
3. Norgren L, Hiatt WR, Dormandy JA, Nehler MR, Harris KA, Fowkes FG. Inter-Society Consensus for the management of peripheral arterial disease (TASC II). *Journal of vascular surgery*. 2007;45(suppl S):S5-S67.
4. Conte MS, Pomposelli FB, Clair DG, et al. Society for Vascular Surgery practice guidelines for atherosclerotic occlusive disease of the lower extremities: management of asymptomatic disease and claudication. *J Vasc Surg*. 2015;61(3 suppl):2s-41s.
5. Menard M, Shah SK, Belkin M. Aortoiliac disease: direct reconstruction. In: Sidway AN, ed. *Rutherfords Vascular Surgery and Endovascular Therapy*. Vol IV. Elesvier; 2019:1397-1415.
6. Crawford R, Brewster D. *Direct Surgical repair of aortoiliac disease*. In: *Atlas of Vascular Surgery and Endovascular Therapy*. Vol IV. Elsevier; 2014:350-361.
7. Mylankal KJ, Fitridge R. Assessment of chronic limb ischemia. In: Loftus I, Hinchliffe RJ, eds. *Vascular and Endovascular Surgery: A Companion to Specialist Surgical Practice*. Vol. VI. Elseiver; 2019:13-35.
8. Crawford JD, Scali ST, Giles KA, et al. Contemporary outcomes of thoracofemoral bypass. *Journal of vascular surgery*. 2019;69(4):1150-1159.e1151.
9. Kalman PG, Johnston KW, Walker PM. Descending thoracic aortofemoral bypass as an alternative for aortoiliac revascularization. *J Cardiovasc Surg*. 1991;32(4):443-446.
10. Schneide JR. Extraanatomic repair of aortoiliac occlusive disease. In: Chaikof EL, ed. *Atlas of Vascular Surgery and Endovasular Therapy*. Vol IV. Elsever; 2014:362-372.
11. Schneide JR. Aortoiliac disease: open extraanatomic bypass. In: Sidawy AN, ed. *Rutherfords Vascualr Surgery and Endovascular Therapy*. Vol. IV. Elsevier; 2019:1416-1422.
12. Zierler RE, Jordan WD, Lal BK, et al. The Society for Vascular Surgery practice guidelines on follow-up after vascular surgery arterial procedures. *J Vasc Surg*. 2018;68(1):256-284.

Chapter 24

Aortoiliac Occlusive Disease: Endovascular and Hybrid Management

Shernaz S. Dossabhoy and Venita Chandra

DEFINITION

- Multilevel atherosclerotic occlusive disease involving the distal aorta, iliac vessels, and common femoral arteries is a commonly occurring pathology seen often by vascular surgeons. Traditional approaches to this disease process involved open surgical reconstruction with an aortobifemoral bypass or iliofemoral bypass. Over the past 20 years, however, there has been a paradigm shift toward endovascular and hybrid approaches often as first-line therapy. Combining femoral endarterectomy with endovascular iliac stenting is now a common minimally invasive approach to this problem, providing an effective alternative to open strategies with the potential of shorter hospitalizations and decreased morbidity. Compared to iliac stenting alone, proper evaluation of femoral disease and, if indicated, a hybrid approach with concomitant femoral endarterectomy has been associated with increased durability of endovascular aortoiliac interventions.[1]

PATIENT HISTORY AND PHYSICAL FINDINGS

- Aortoiliac and femoral occlusive disease can present, as with all peripheral arterial diseases (PADs), in a variety of ways.
- The typical presentation of aortoiliac occlusive disease includes claudication of the buttock and upper thigh and erectile dysfunction. When multilevel vascular disease occurs, as in the case of combined aortoiliac and femoral occlusive disease, distal lower extremity symptoms such as calf claudication, rest pain, and tissue loss may ensue.
- Typical physical examination includes the absence or diminution of femoral pulses. Other than the peripheral pulse assessment, the physical examination can demonstrate other signs of PAD such as cool digits and active wounds or ulcers, including more subtle findings such as shiny skin and lack of hair over the shins.

IMAGING AND OTHER DIAGNOSTIC STUDIES

- The initial evaluation of a patient with PAD should involve noninvasive evaluation of peripheral blood flow with arterial waveforms and ankle–brachial indices (ABIs) (**FIGURE 1**). These studies provide objective data regarding the extent of occlusive disease; however, they do not provide adequate anatomic data for preoperative planning.
- Once the degree and physiologic impact of the disease are determined by noninvasive testing, high-resolution anatomic imaging via either computed tomographic angiography (CTA) or magnetic resonance angiography (MRA) should be obtained for surgical planning.
- CTAs are currently the gold standard for preoperative planning. They have the advantage of providing information regarding the degree and location of stenosis as well as the anatomy of the arterial wall (including degree of calcification and presence of aneurysms). Three-dimensional reformatting can provide additional valuable information (**FIGURE 2**). CTAs, however, are limited by the fact that they involve the use of contrast as well as radiation exposure. MRAs avoid radiation exposure and contrast often, however, at the risk

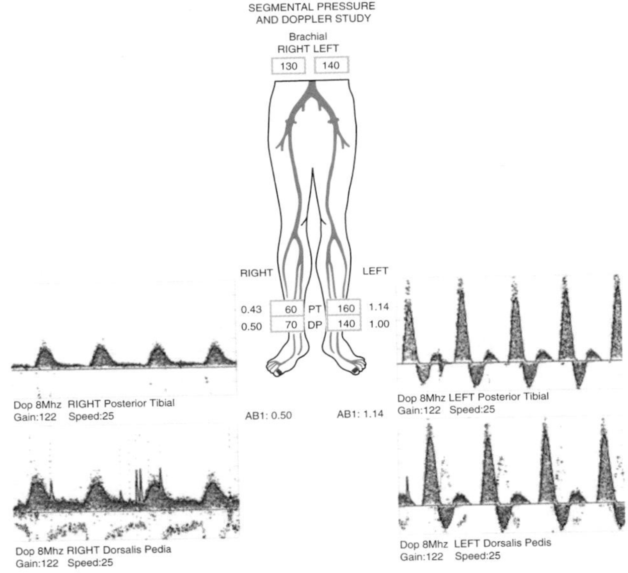

FIGURE 1 ● Arterial waveforms and ankle–brachial indices for a patient with aortoiliac disease. Note the monophasic waveforms on the right.

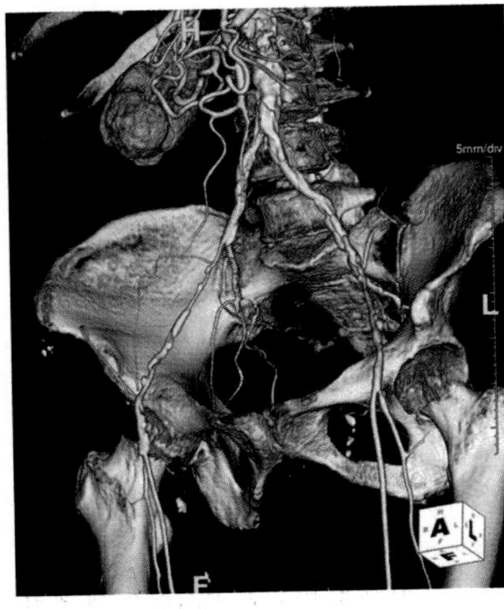

FIGURE 2 ● Computed tomographic angiography with 3D reconstruction demonstrating diffuse aortoiliac as well as femoral occlusive disease.

of reduced anatomic precision. Gadolinium magnetic resonance contrast also entails risk of long-term renal dysfunction and nephrogenic systemic fibrosis.

- Catheter-based diagnostic aortography also provides anatomic data; however, it is an invasive procedure with potential complications. In addition, arteriograms only provide an understanding of the luminal anatomy, occasionally obscuring features such as aneurysms, inclusion cysts, or periarterial inflammation. Particularly for aortoiliac-femoral disease, preprocedural CTA identifies significant common femoral disease that may benefit from concomitant open endarterectomy at the time of catheter-based intervention. Alternatively, relying on catheter-based arteriography as the primary diagnostic modality may reduce overall contrast burden, radiation exposure, and need for additional procedures if common femoral level intervention is not required. In general, careful preprocedural physical examination and duplex imaging may suffice to help determine whether the additional cost and potential risks of CTA are justified prior to catheter-based intervention for aortoiliac arterial occlusive disease.

SURGICAL MANAGEMENT

- As with all patients with PAD, initial treatment approach should include comprehensive assessment and management of concomitant cardiovascular disease risk factors. Details regarding maximal medical management of PAD are beyond the scope or purpose of this chapter; at a minimum, however, consideration should be given to beginning statin and antiplatelet therapy prior to intervention, along with consideration of beta blockade and angiotensin receptor blocker or converting enzyme inhibitor therapy in selected patients. Patients should be counseled on risk factor behavior modification including smoking cessation, exercise or walking program such as supervised exercise therapy, and diet modification.
- Regardless of medical or anesthetic risk, however, all patients with critical limb ischemia should be considered candidates for revascularization when faced with potential limb loss. Major limb amputation above or below the knee is not necessarily a "safer" surgical alternative to multilevel hybrid revascularization for these patients. Indications for intervention for intermittent claudication are somewhat more complicated and controversial, however. The risks of a procedure are weighed against the potential gain; typically, only patients with severe lifestyle-limiting claudication who have failed nonoperative strategies are offered surgical revascularization.

Preoperative Planning

- Determining the anatomic distribution of disease is essential to obtaining optimal results. The imperative for precision imaging cannot be emphasized enough—if you cannot appreciate the full extent of disease, you cannot expect to comprehensively address it. As in all aspects of vascular surgery, the biggest disappointments, both during and after the procedure, usually arise from underestimating the extent of underlying disease.
- Historically, the Trans-Atlantic Inter-Society Consensus (TASC) II guidelines have provided a classification scheme based on anatomic patterns of disease (**FIGURE 3**).[2] The recommendations of the TASC II guidelines is an endovascular management for TASC A and B iliac lesions, whereas open surgical reconstruction is recommended for TASC C and D lesions in good-risk patients. Frequently, however, patients with multilevel disease as seen in TASC C and D lesions have more virulent atherosclerotic processes that often make them poorer surgical candidates. In addition, the development of an increasingly sophisticated armamentarium of endovascular tools and strategies is leading more and more vascular surgeons to attempt endovascular revascularization first, even for patients with TASC C or D lesions.
- More recently, the 2019 Global Limb Anatomic Staging System (GLASS) for critical limb threatening ischemia (CLTI) provided a simplified staging system for inflow disease (both aortoiliac and common femoral artery) (**TABLE 1**).[3] These guidelines recommend an endovascular-first approach for the treatment of CLTI patients with moderate to severe (eg, GLASS stage IA) aortoiliac disease.[3]
- Targeted perioperative risk assessment should be undertaken in appropriate patients, particularly in those with reduced exercise tolerance, known or suspected congestive heart failure, clinically significant pulmonary disease, exercise-induced angina, arrhythmias, or recent history of myocardial infarction. The presence of additional relevant comorbidities, including diabetes, reduced glomerular filtration rate, iodinated contrast allergies, thrombophilia or coagulopathic disorders, concomitant bacterial infection, or liver disease, should also be identified and, when present, evaluated.

Positioning

- Patients are generally placed in the supine position, either in a hybrid operating suite with fixed imaging capabilities or on a radiolucent table with a mobile imaging unit (C-arm) in a traditional operating room environment.
- Positioning should be arranged in such a way as to ensure adequate exposure of the entire aortoiliac and femoral vasculature, with room on either side of the patient to rotate the imaging unit to various angles to obtain appropriate oblique images. In angiographic parlance, in many important circumstances (such as identifying and protecting the origin of the ipsilateral internal iliac artery), "one view is no view."

Type A Lesions

- Unilateral or bilateral stenosis of CIA
- Unilateral or bilateral single short (<3 cm) stenosis of EIA

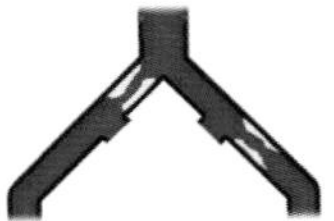

Type B Lesions

- Short (<3 cm) stenosis of infrarenal aorta
- Unilateral CIA occlusion
- Single or multiple stenoses totaling 3-10 cm involving the EIA not extending into the CFA
- Unilateral EIA occlusion not involving the origins of internal iliac of CFA

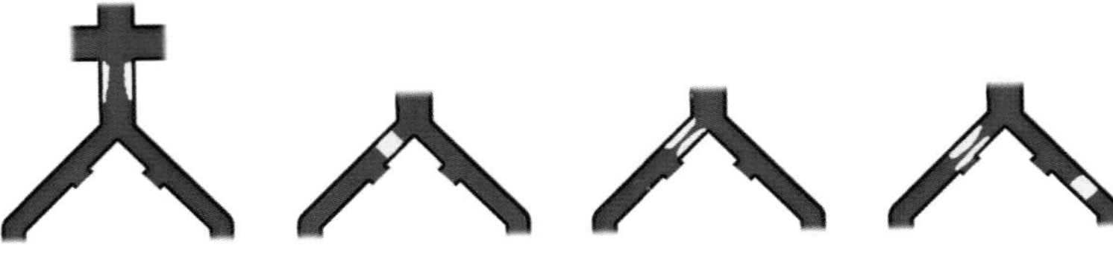

Type C Lesions

- Bilateral CIA occlusions
- Bilateral EIA stenoses 3-10 cm long not extending into the CFA
- Unilateral EIA stenosis extending into the CFA
- Unilateral EIA occlusion that involves the origins of internal iliac and/or CFA
- Heavily calcified unilateral EIA occlustion with or without involvement of origins of internal iliac and/or CFA

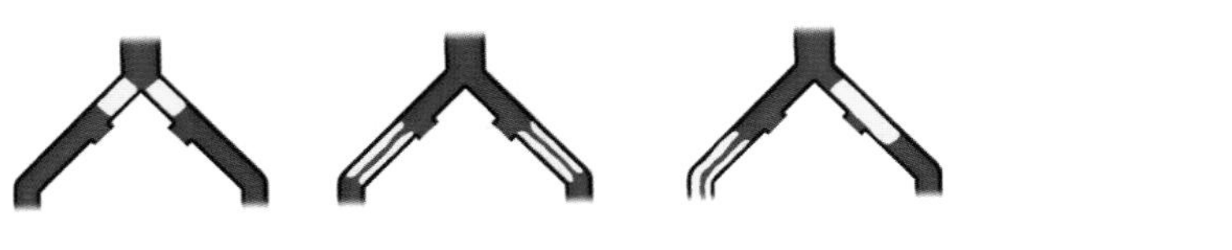

Type D Lesions

- Infrarenal aortoiliac occlusion
- Diffuse disease involving the aorta and both iliac arteries requiring treatment
- Diffuse multiple stenoses involving the unilateral CIA, EIA, and CFA
- Unilateral occlusions of both CIA and EIA
- Bilateral occlusions of EIA
- Iliac stenoses in patients with AAA requiring treatment and not amenable to endograft placement or other lesions requiring open aortic or iliac surgery

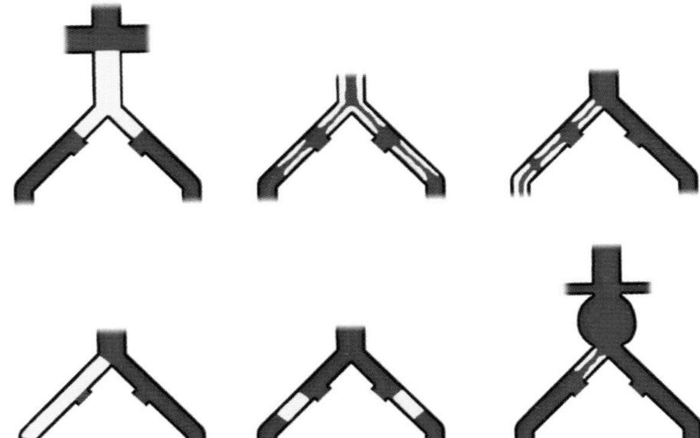

FIGURE 3 ● TASC II classification scheme for iliac disease. (Reprinted from Norgren L, Hiatt WR, Dormandy JA, et al. Inter-Society Consensus for the Management of Peripheral Arterial Disease [TASC II]. *J Vasc Surg*. 2007;45(suppl S):S5–S67. Copyright © 2007 The Society for Vascular Surgery. With permission.)

Table 1: Global Anatomic Staging System (GLASS) Simplified Staging System for Aortoiliac Inflow Disease

GLASS stage	Description
I	• Stenosis of common and/or external iliac artery • Chronic total occlusion of common or external iliac artery (not both) • Stenosis of infrarenal aorta, or • Any combination of the above
A	No significant CFA disease
B	Significant CFA disease (>50% stenosis)
II	• Chronic total occlusion of aorta • Chronic total occlusion of common and external iliac arteries • Severe diffuse disease and/or small-caliber (<6 mm) common and external iliac arteries • Concomitant aneurysmal disease • Severe diffuse in-stent restenosis of aortoiliac system
A	No significant CFA disease
B	Significant CFA disease (>50% stenosis)

CFA, common femoral artery.
Adapted from Conte MS, Bradbury AW, Kolh P, et al. Global vascular guidelines on the management of chronic limb-threatening ischemia. J Vasc Surg. 2019;69(6S):3S-125S. Copyright © 2019 by the Society for Vascular Surgery and European Society for Vascular Surgery. With permission.

FEMORAL ENDARTERECTOMY

First Step

- For extended femoral endarterectomy (often requiring exposure of the proximal deep femoral or "profunda" artery as well as the entire length of common femoral artery), optimal exposure is obtained via a longitudinal incision placed directly over the femoral artery (**FIGURE 4**). The inguinal ligament should be identified by palpation of the pubic tubercle and anterior superior iliac spine (an oblique line between these two structures is the typical course of the inguinal ligament) and used as a guide for femoral localization. Typically, the femoral artery is located approximately one-third the distance from the pubic tubercle to anterior superior iliac crest. Even when no pulse is palpable, a firm calcified linear mass can usually be palpated in this area. Alternatively, duplex ultrasound or fluoroscopic imaging may be used to ensure accurate placement of the incision. Failure to incise directly over the common femoral artery may increase risk for chronic lymphatic drainage, delayed or complicated wound healing, and femoral nerve or venous injury. Although oblique femoral incisions have gained in popularity, especially when used to obtain femoral access for proximal aneurysm repair, these often do not provide sufficient exposure as distal external iliac exposure is often required for a complete endarterectomy.
- The subcutaneous tissues are divided, ligating any lymphatic channels that are encountered. The inferior edge of the inguinal ligament is identified, and the common femoral artery is exposed through the femoral sheath as it exits underneath the inguinal ligament.

Second Step

- Full circumferential dissection of the distal external iliac artery (under the inguinal ligament), the common femoral artery, the superficial femoral artery, and the origin of the deep femoral artery and its initial branches are obtained sequentially (**FIGURE 4**).
- The individual arteries should be assessed for areas of calcification and extensive plaque burden. Soft sections with minimal calcification, or plaque limited to the posterior arterial wall, should be identified for consideration of clamp placement as appropriate for the planned procedure.
- The inguinal ligament may be divided for adequate exposure of the distal external iliac artery when necessary to ensure adequate endarterectomy. When considering the relative margin of distal endarterectomy vs proximal stent placement, it is important to avoid stent placement across the inguinal ligament, as this may greatly reduce long-term patency of the procedure as well as complicate stent delivery through an ipsilateral retrograde sheath. In general, operators should err of the side of more extensive proximal endarterectomies as opposed to distal extension of external iliac stents.
- Careful ligation of the circumflex iliac vein as it crosses over the external iliac artery under the inguinal ligament should be considered to prevent accidental tearing of the vessel during clamping.
- External iliac collaterals, like the epigastric artery or circumflex iliac artery, should be preserved during dissection and endarterectomy whenever possible to ensure optimal long-term outcome.

Third Step

- Once exposure is complete, the common femoral artery can be punctured under direct visualization with advancement of a wire under fluoroscopic guidance across the iliac lesion (**FIGURE 5**).

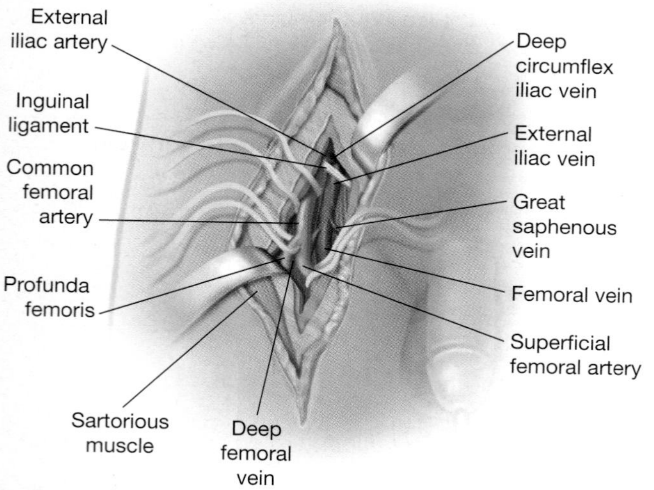

FIGURE 4 ● Typical longitudinal femoral artery exposure and anatomy. CFA, common femoral artery; DCIV, deep circumflex iliac vein; EIA, external iliac artery; EIV, external iliac vein; GSV, greater saphenous vein; SFA, superficial femoral artery.

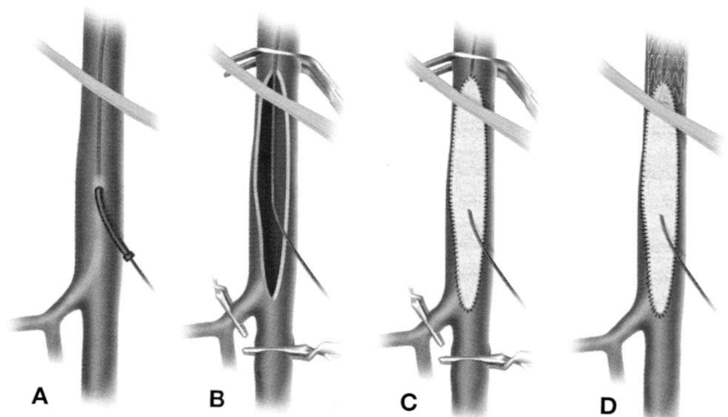

FIGURE 5 ● Technique for concurrent femoral endarterectomy and iliac stenting. **A,** Direct puncture of common femoral artery and advancement of wire under fluoroscopic guidance. **B,** With wire across iliac lesion, clamp proximal and distal end proceed with arteriotomy. **C,** After endarterectomy, patch is sewn in. Prior to completion of patch center, the distal portion of the patch is punctured with an 18-gauge needle and the wire is passed through the patch. **D,** After completion of the patch, flow is restored and a sheath can be advanced over the wire and iliac stenting can proceed. For patients with distal external iliac disease, the iliac stents can be carried down into the proximal portion of the endarterectomy and patch.

- This approach eliminates the possibility of creating a retrograde dissection when a wire is passed after the endarterectomy is performed, as well as the need to puncture the endarterectomy patch to gain access.
- If the disease burden is confined to the common iliac artery or only the proximal external iliac artery, then iliac stenting can proceed at this point, prior to proceeding with the endarterectomy. Occasionally, however, the amount of femoral disease burden is so great that the sheath will be occlusive or otherwise impair runoff, which may limit the ability to obtain digital subtraction angiography images during or after stent placement. Therefore, consideration should be given to initial endarterectomy depending on individual anatomic circumstances.
- When retrograde wire passage is not possible due to extensive proximal plaque burden, tortuosity, or other anatomic considerations, antegrade passage from the contralateral iliofemoral system (obtained via either percutaneous or open femoral access) or left axillary or brachial access may be attempted. Importantly, longer sheath/catheter/guidewire combinations will be needed for these procedures and positioning considerations will be affected as well (eg, arm will need to be exposed and prepped on a radiolucent surface). Once antegrade wire access is accomplished, this may be used to deliver treatment devices directly or snared and externalized through the ipsilateral femoral access for retrograde intervention as originally planned.

Fourth Step

- Leaving the wire in place, the patient is systemically heparinized, and proximal and distal femoral control is obtained with vascular clamps. Especially proximally, a padded clamp (eg, Fogarty Hydragrip) should be chosen to allow the external iliac artery to be clamped over the existing wire to prevent or minimize wire-related injury.
- A longitudinal common femoral arteriotomy is performed to expose the full extent of femoral disease that needs to be addressed to ensure adequate runoff from the iliac intervention. A single femoral incision for the femoral endarterectomy is often sufficient to achieve adequate outflow; however, additional distal femoral bypass procedures may be required if extensive forefoot gangrene is present, which is often a consequence of multilevel arterial occlusive disease. Extended deep femoral endarterectomy is highly effective in achieving suitable runoff when few other revascularization options may be available (**FIGURE 4**).
- The arteriotomy can extend onto either the superficial or deep femoral artery. Occasionally, an eversion endarterectomy of the deep femoral artery can be performed when the arteriotomy extends onto the superficial femoral artery. Alternatively, the arteriotomy may be extended down the deep femoral artery when the superficial femoral artery is chronically occluded. Selection of the reconstruction technique is influenced by the occlusive pathology, level of debility, indications for revascularization, and optimal revascularization strategy (**FIGURE 6**).

Fifth Step

- Carefully, an endarterectomy plane is developed between the plaque and remaining mural media or adventitia using a Penfield dissector or Beaver blade. The plane most typically is developed within or exterior to the media, leaving the adventitia intact. Failure to appreciate the appropriate endarterectomy plane may weaken the adventitia, leading to bleeding or postoperative hematoma or pseudoaneurysm formation. Care should be taken to dissect the plaque away from the remaining arterial wall, not vice versa. The endarterectomy plane is developed on each side of the vessel and advanced posteriorly until the planes meet in the midline. Following this maneuver, the plaque is transected flush with

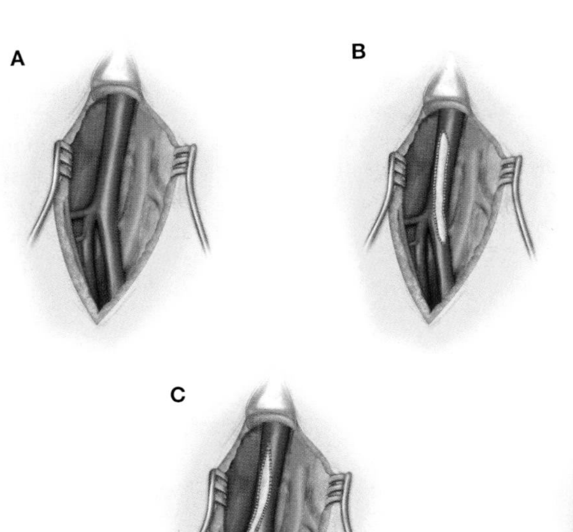

FIGURE 6 ● Various femoral endarterectomy closure strategies. **A,** Typical anatomy; occasionally, primary repair, can be considered if common femoral artery is of adequate size. **B,** Arteriotomy and patch extended onto superficial femoral artery; deep femoral artery endarterectomy can be performed using an eversion technique. **C,** Arteriotomy and patch extended onto deep femoral artery. Particularly useful in chronically occluded superficial femoral artery (SFA). **D,** Interposition repair of common femoral artery; can syndactylize deep femoral artery and SFA if needed.

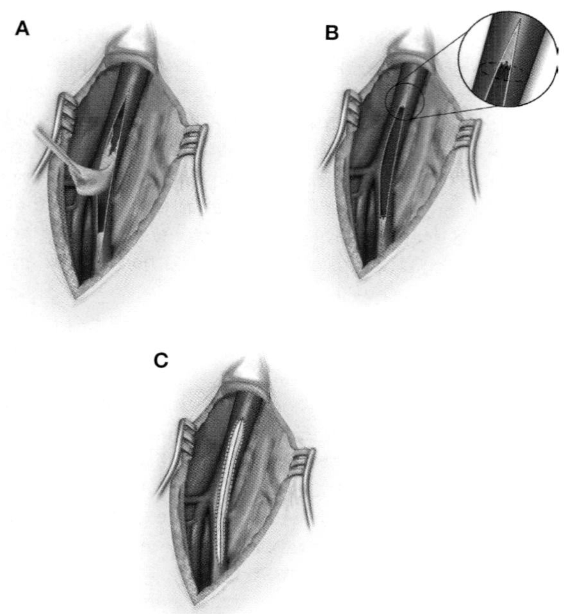

FIGURE 7 ● Femoral endarterectomy technique. **A,** Longitudinal arteriotomy and development of endarterectomy plane. **B,** Ensure adequate endpoints on either end. **C,** Patch closure.

the arterial wall. Care should be taken to achieve good quality and minimally diseased endpoints in both the superficial and deep femoral arteries as necessary (**FIGURE 7**). Tacking sutures, as commonly employed during carotid endarterectomy, may also be necessary in the femoral artery to ensure adequate endpoints. Particularly in the case of the deep femoral artery, care should be taken to extend the endarterectomy well past the mass of common femoral artery–related plaque. This may require exposing the deep femoral artery well beyond its initial branches, dividing crossing branches of the deep femoral vein, and avoiding excessively deep placement of self-retaining retractors to limit the possibility of traction injury to femoral nerve branches.

- Often, significant posterior plaque extends proximally into the external iliac arteries. As previously discussed, care should be taken in deciding at which point the endarterectomy should end vs distal extension of iliac stents (**FIGURE 5**).

Sixth Step

- Once the full extent of plaque has been removed and suitable irrigation performed to identify and eliminate remaining mobile fragments of residual media, patch angioplasty should be performed typically using running 5-0 polypropylene suture initiated at both the proximal and distal endpoints and tied in the middle. Bovine pericardium, extruded polytetrafluoroethylene (ePTFE), and polyester or autogenous vein segments all may represent reasonable patch options, depending on individual circumstances. In general, autogenous vein is more resistant to infection, whereas prosthetic patch options are available off the shelf in a variety of configurations. ePTFE patches tend to bleed more through their suture holes following placement, although this tendency may be tempered by use of ePTFE sutures. Currently, our preference is to use bovine pericardial patch as the default choice in the absence of infection or other contraindication (eg, patient objection due to religious reasons) (**FIGURE 6**).
- Rarely, when arterial wall integrity appears compromised following endarterectomy, femoral interposition grafting may be performed in lieu of patch angioplasty. Interposition grafting may also be a good choice when the femoral plaque burden is so great that endarterectomy is impractical; in this case, an interposition graft (ePTFE or knitted polyester) can be placed instead of a patch. This can be configured in any number of ways:
    - Distal anastomosis to distal common femoral artery
    - Distal anastomosis to syndactylized superficial and deep femoral arteries (**FIGURE 6**)
    - Distal anastomosis to superficial femoral artery with reimplantation of the deep femoral artery
    - Distal anastomosis to the deep femoral artery with reimplantation of superficial femoral artery
    - Distal anastomosis to the deep femoral artery only, when the superficial femoral artery is already occluded

Seventh Step

- Before completion of patch closure, the middle or distal portion of the patch is punctured with an 18-gauge needle and the back of the previously placed wire is routed through the needle. Patch closure is then completed and the clamps are removed; at this point, an appropriately sized sheath can be advanced over the wire, through the patch, in preparation for iliac stenting.

COMMON ILIAC STENTING

First Step

- Typically, a 6-Fr or 7-Fr sheath is adequate for iliac stenting. Once the sheath is placed after completion of the patch, appropriate arteriogram images are obtained.
- For distal aorta and proximal common iliac disease, often the best approach is passage of a flush catheter into the aorta and a power-injected aortogram.
- For primarily iliac disease, retrograde arteriography through the femoral sheath is usually sufficient to obtain adequate iliac opacification.
- Contralateral anterior oblique (15°-30°) projections are typically chosen for visualization of the respective iliac systems to ensure identification of the origin of the ipsilateral internal iliac arteries. Also, the full extent of disease burden may be most adequately addressed by multiple obliquities in any circumstance.
- A marking catheter may be used to assist in length measurements and "buddy" wires may also be placed from contralateral femoral access. Every effort should be made to maintain perfusion to the hypogastric arteries.

Second Step

- Selection of the appropriate balloon and stent diameter for the common iliac arteries is crucial. Slight oversizing of 5% to 10% is recommended, except in the case of heavily calcified lesions, where oversizing may increase the risk of arterial rupture.
- Optimal target vessel diameter can be estimated preoperatively from CTA measurements based on the diameter of adjacent or contralateral nondiseased arterial segments and confirmed intraoperatively during the hybrid procedure itself. Common iliac artery target diameters range from 7 to 10 mm while external iliac artery diameters range from 5 to 8 mm with both depending on patient gender, body habitus, and burden of disease.
- Balloon "predilation" may facilitate stent placement and assist with stent sizing.
- Mild pain during dilation is to be anticipated and indicates stretching of the adventitia; excessive or persistent pain, however, may indicate arterial compromise or rupture. In the latter circumstance, consideration should be given to additional placement of a covered stent when contrast extravasation is present on arteriography and not immediately controlled with extended balloon deployment. In the retroperitoneum, unlike the lower extremities, tamponade will not likely limit further bleeding and extended balloon deployment may not be advisable as definitive treatment. When general anesthesia is required for the concomitant endarterectomy, this warning sign may not be present and completion arteriography should be closely examined for indications of iliac artery disruption or contrast extravasation.
- There are numerous commercially available stents, with some specifically indicated for iliac arterial intervention (eg, "on label") (**TABLE 2**). Appropriate diameter and length stents generally fall into two categories, balloon-expandable or self-expanding, and can be covered or uncovered (eg, with adherent graft material).

Table 2: Various Stent Options for Treating Aortoiliac Disease[a]

	Balloon-expandable	Self-expanding
Covered	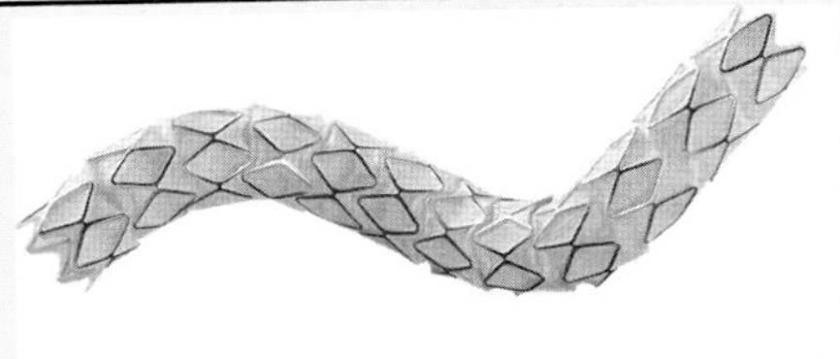 GORE® VIABAHN® VBX Balloon Expandable. See Instructions for Use for complete device information, including approved indications and safety information. (Copyright © 2014 W. L. Gore & Associates, Inc. Used with permission) Lifestream™ Balloon Expandable Vascular Covered Stent (Bard Peripheral Vascular Inc., Tempe, Ariz) iCAST (Atrium Medical, Hudson, NH)[a]	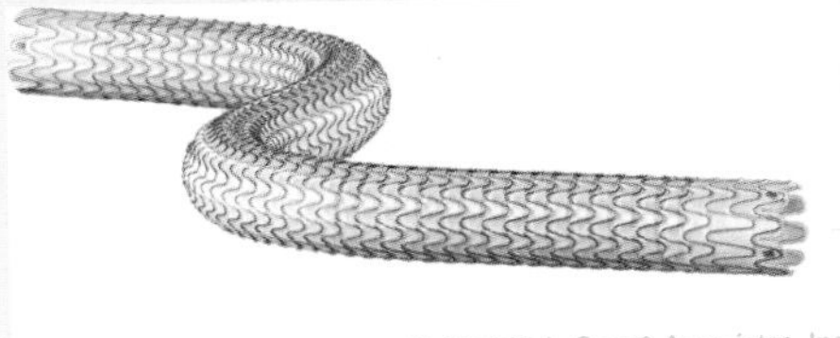 GORE® VIABAHN® Endoprosthesis. See Instructions for Use for complete device information, including approved indications and safety information. (Copyright © 2020 W. L. Gore & Associates, Inc. Used with permission.)

(Continued)

Table 2: Various Stent Options for Treating Aortoiliac Disease[a] (Continued)

	Balloon-expandable	Self-expanding
Uncovered (Bare metal)	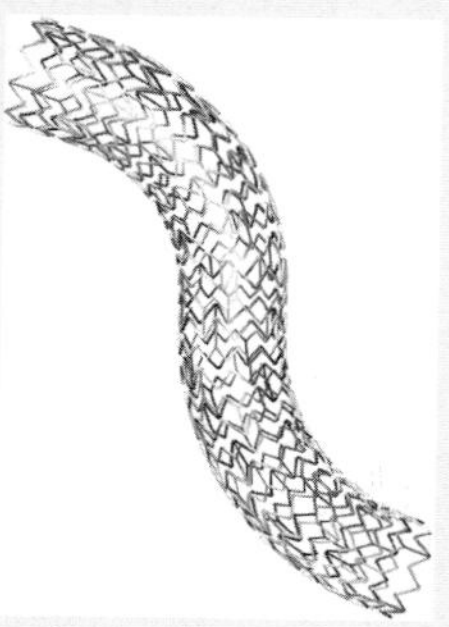 Image provided courtesy of Boston Scientific. Copyright © 2022 Boston Scientific Corporation or its affiliates. All rights reserved.	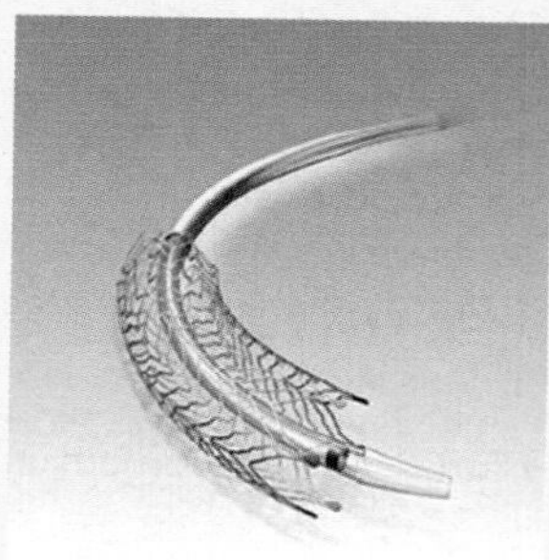 Absolute Pro and OmniLink Elite are trademarks of Abbott or its related companies. Reproduced with permission of Abbott, © 2022. All rights reserved.
	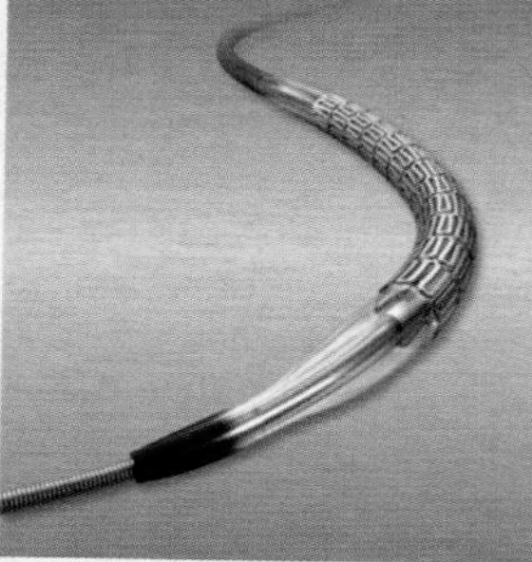 Absolute Pro and OmniLink Elite are trademarks of Abbott or its related companies. Reproduced with permission of Abbott, © 2022. All rights reserved.	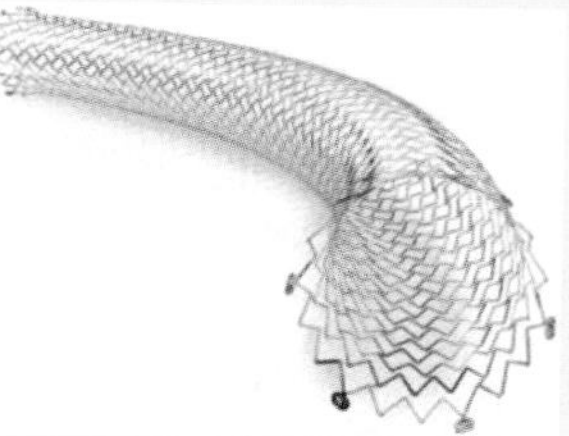 S.M.A.R.T Vascular Stent (Cordis, Miami Lakes, FL)
	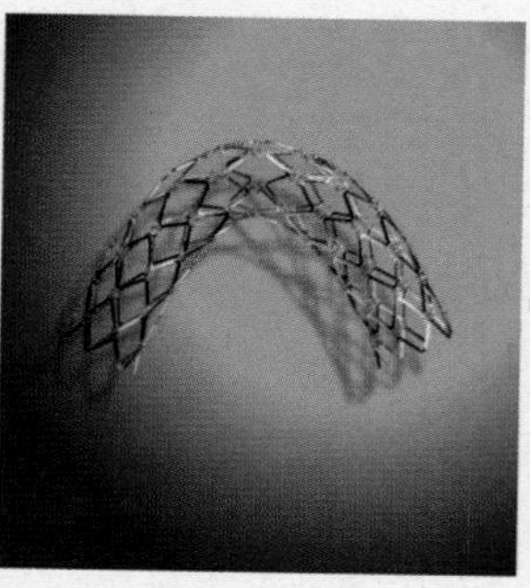 Palmaz Genesis Balloon Expandable Stent (Cordis, Miami Lakes, FL)	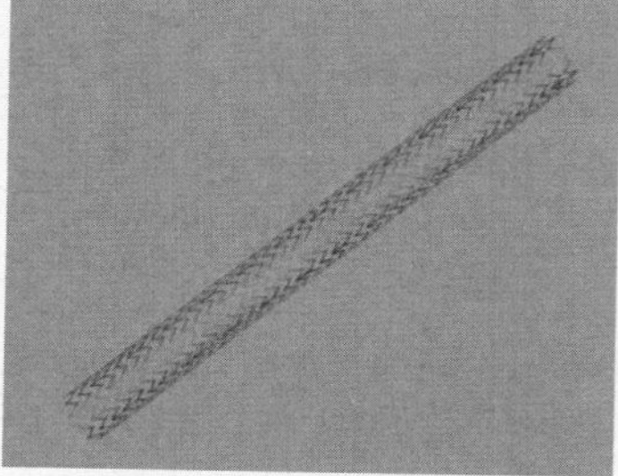 Zilver 635 Vascular Self-Expanding Stent (Courtesy of Cook Medical, Bloomington, Ind)
	Assurant Cobalt Iliac Stent System (Medtronic, Minneapolis, Minn)	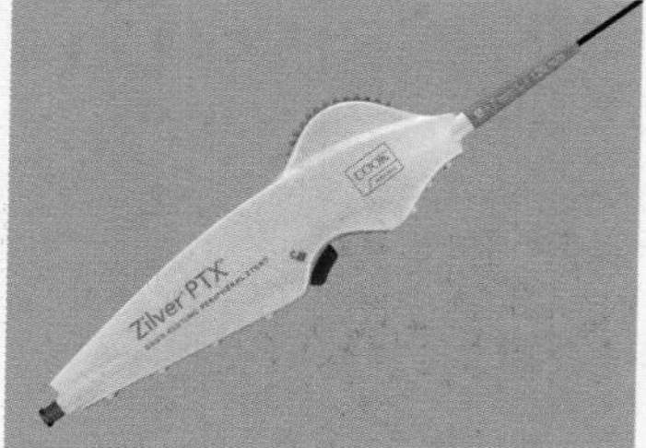 Zilver PTX Drug-Eluting Peripheral Stent (Courtesy of Cook Medical, Bloomington, Ind)[b]
		LifeStent™ and LifeStent™ XL Vascular Stent System (Bard Peripheral Vascular Inc., Tempe, Ariz)[b]

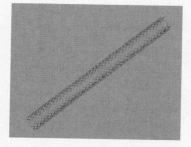

[a]*The devices listed are approved by the FDA for iliac disease, unless otherwise stated.*
[b]*Off-label use; not FDA-approved for iliac lesions.*

- The length of the balloon or stent should cover the entire length of the diseased area.
- Balloon-expandable stents have the advantage of higher precision of placement and greater radial strength; however, they are less flexible than self-expanding stents. In general, balloon-expandable stents are best suited for common iliac artery lesions where "kissing" stents in the contralateral iliac artery may be needed to deal with excessive plaque burden or calcification, or the aortic bifurcation may need to be "advanced" into the distal aorta to completely ensure adequate luminal recanalization. Alternatively, external iliac lesions are often best treated with self-expanding stents, which are more flexible and compliant with the radius of curvature present in this artery. Exceptions exist for both indications, however, and device placement should be individualized to specific anatomic and clinical requirements.
- In heavily calcified vessels, to better facilitate angioplasty and stenting, plaque modification with intravascular lithotripsy (eg, Shockwave, Shockwave Medical Inc., Santa Clara, CA) can be considered.

Third Step

- In the setting of bilateral or even unilateral proximal common iliac artery disease or distal aortic disease, bilateral aortic bifurcation balloon dilation and stenting should be completed simultaneously to protect the contralateral common iliac artery from dissection, plaque dislodgement, or subsequent embolization. This is generally referred to as "kissing" iliac stents.
- Alternatively, the Covered Endovascular Reconstruction of the Aortic Bifurcation (CERAB) technique can be used when the distal aortic wall is calcified. This involves placing two kissing iliac stents (usually covered) within a covered aortic stent graft to endovascularly reconstruct the aortic bifurcation in a more anatomic and physiologic fashion (**FIGURE 8**).[4]
- Balloon-expandable stents are typically used for these proximal common iliac lesions and may be deployed well into the distal aorta, essentially raising the level of the aortic bifurcation.

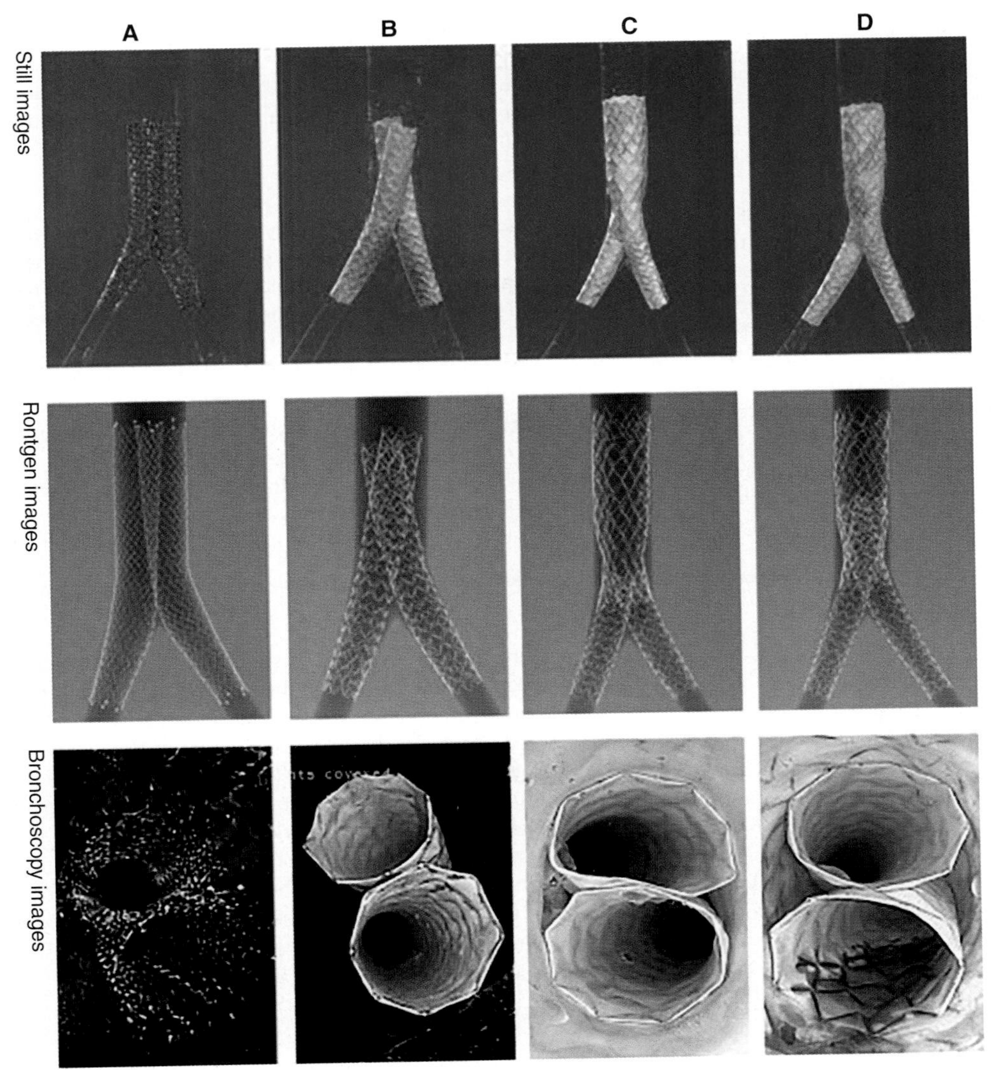

FIGURE 8 • Still, Rontgen, and bronchoscopic images of **(A)** self-expandable nitinol kissing bare metal stents; **(B)** balloon-expandable kissing covered stents; **(C)** Covered Endovascular Reconstruction of the Aortic Bifurcation (CERAB)-1 with limbs starting in the tapered portion of the aortic cuff; **(D)** CERAB-2 with the iliac limbs starting just above the tapered part of the aortic cuff. (Reprinted with permission from Groot Jebbink E, Grimme FA, Goverde PC, et al. Geometrical consequences of kissing stents and the Covered Endovascular Reconstruction of the Aortic Bifurcation configuration in an in vitro model for endovascular reconstruction of aortic bifurcation. *J Vasc Surg*. 2015;61(5):1306-1311.)

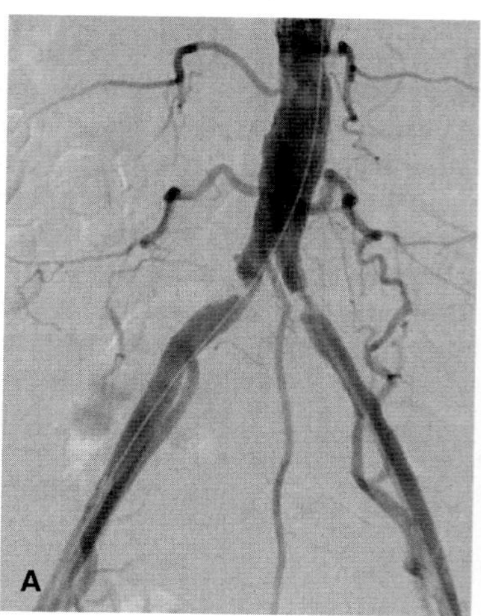

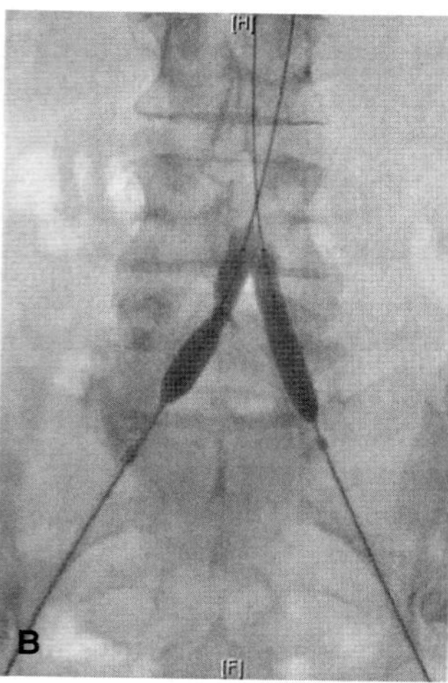

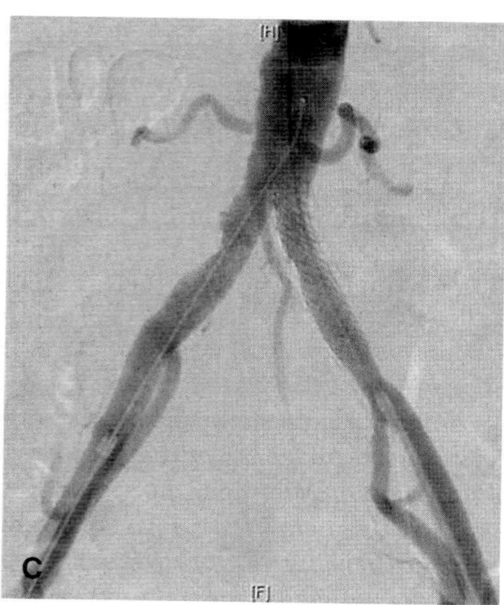

FIGURE 9 ● Bilateral common iliac artery stenosis treated with kissing stent technique. **A,** Initial aortogram demonstrating high-grade bilateral proximal common iliac stenosis. **B,** Balloon dilation demonstrating waist in balloon at location of stenosis. **C,** Completion aortogram with bilateral kissing iliac stents, raising the aortic bifurcation by a few centimeters.

Fourth Step

- For common iliac lesions immediately adjacent to the aortic bifurcation, after precise arteriographic localization of the aortic and iliac bifurcations and extent of plaque burden, appropriately sized stents are selected. Unilateral or bilateral sheaths of sufficient diameter for the selected stents are advanced into the distal aorta. When common iliac lesions are not strictly "orificial," concomitant contralateral stenting is generally not required. Again, careful angiographic assessment should be made to determine the extent of plaque burden present at the origin of the common iliac arteries to make this determination.
- Appropriately sized balloon-expandable stents are advanced within the sheaths and positioned across the respective lesions. The sheaths are then pulled back to expose the entire stent; this sequence prevents accidental dislodgement of the stent off the balloon, attempting to cross the lesion, and limits the risk of plaque embolization during stent passage.
- Once both stents are positioned appropriately, they are inflated simultaneously to achieve the kissing configuration (**FIGURE 9**).

Fifth Step

- Completion arteriography, typically through a pressure injection in the distal aorta through "side-hole" or flush catheters, is obtained to confirm stent placement, evaluate degree of residual stenosis, and rule out complications such as dissection or thrombus/embolization.
- When the clinical significance of plaque in the aorta or iliac arteries is unknown, pressure measurement may be required. Pull-back pressures are obtained with the goal of eliminating pressure gradients across the treated lesion at rest or limiting to less than 15 mm Hg following injection of a distal vasodilator such as papaverine.

EXTERNAL ILIAC ARTERY STENTING

First Step

- When the external iliac artery is diseased, particularly the distal segment, self-expanding stents are typically used due to the increased tortuosity of these vessels and the increased flexibility of self-expanding stents as opposed to balloon-expandable stents (as described in *Common Iliac Stenting, Second Step*).
- The same principles exist in terms of sizing, although for self-expanding stents, 10% to 20% oversizing is typically recommended in the respective instructions for use.

Second Step

- Deployment of self-expanding stents does not require advancement of the introducer sheath past the lesion. The self-expanding stents usually are mounted on a carrier and constrained. The stents should be positioned across the lesion and deployed.
- Close fluoroscopic monitoring should occur during deployment, as self-expanding stents tend to be far less precise in positioning in comparison to balloon-expandable stents and typically may advance across the lesion during deployment. Carefully applying negative tension and ensuring slow deployment can help increase accuracy of stent placement.

Third Step

- Predilation and postdilation may be performed as necessary with appropriately sized balloons before and after stent deployment.
- In the setting of very distal external iliac artery disease or incomplete distal external iliac endarterectomy (as described earlier), the distal end of the stent may be carried down to the level of the endarterectomy, again with care to avoid crossing the inguinal ligament as previously described (**FIGURE 5**).

Fourth Step

- Just as in common iliac stenting, completion arteriograms should be performed, and pressure gradients may be obtained as necessary to confirm sufficient resolution of the stenosis.

Fifth Step

- Usually, a single-repair stitch can be used to close the patch sheath access site, regardless of the diameter of the sheath used for stent deployment.
- Once hemostasis is achieved, the sheaths removed, and anticoagulation reversed with protamine injection, the femoral exposure should be closed with a multilayer, anatomic closure with absorbable suture.

PEARLS AND PITFALLS

Occluded iliac artery strategies

Reentry devices	■ When attempting to cross an occluded segment with catheter-guidewire combinations, a subintimal plane may be developed. This subintimal technique is appropriate as long as the true lumen can once again be regained prior to entering the aorta. In some circumstances, this reentry may be challenging. In these situations, reentry devices can be employed. These devices have nitinol cannula that can be advanced through the device and used to puncture into the true lumen; a 0.014-in wire is then advanced. Free passage of the wire indicates true lumen access, which is confirmed by contrast injection. The passage can then be dilated and stented in a conventional manner (**FIGURE 10**). Care should be taken to attempt reentry before the dissection plane is advanced too far proximally into the distal aorta, as this may compromise the ability to properly deploy balloon-expandable stents and/or compromise inferior mesenteric arterial flow. Similarly, reentry systems should be used with caution in the iliac arterial system to avoid perforation and retroperitoneal bleeding.

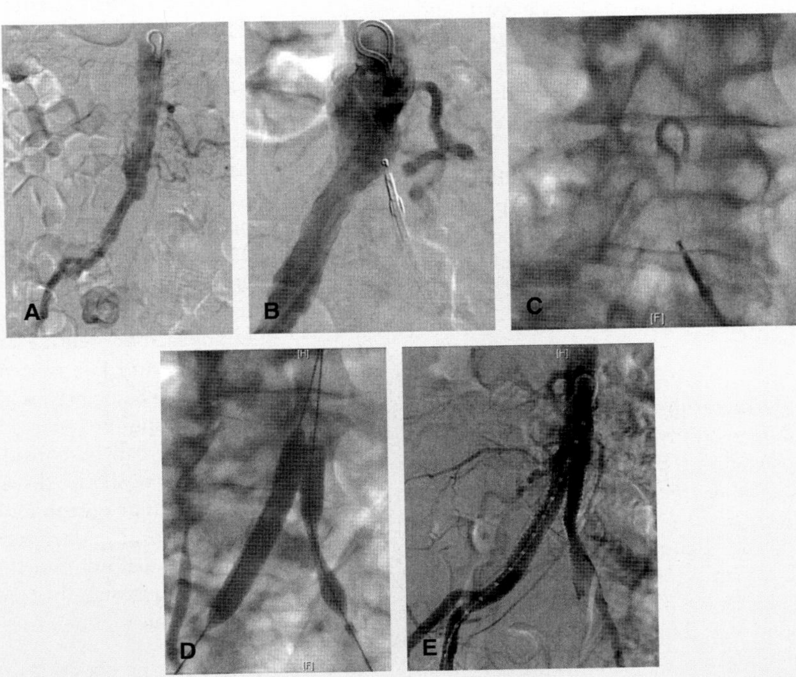

FIGURE 10 ● Use of an Outback reentry catheter in treatment of a chronic total iliac occlusion. **A,** Aortogram showing complete occlusion of the left iliac arterial system. **B,** The majority of the occlusion was crossed; however, reentry into the true aortic lumen was unsuccessful using traditional techniques. The Outback reentry catheter was advanced and positioned. **C,** After advancement of the reentry needle, a 0.014-in wire was able to be passed into the aorta. **D,** Retrograde kissing balloon-expandable stent placement into bilateral common iliac arteries. **E,** Completion aortogram demonstrating reconstitution of flow in left iliac system. (Cordis, Miami Lakes, FL.)

Alternative approach	■ Antegrade approach from either a brachial or contralateral femoral access sometimes provides more "pushability" across recalcitrant lesions and may be more successful at obtaining wire access. This is particularly true when a small invagination is apparent angiographically in the ipsilateral common iliac artery (when totally occluded). Once the occlusion or stenosis is traversed, the wire can be snared from the ipsilateral femoral and an ipsilateral sheath can still be advanced to complete the procedure as previously described from the ipsilateral femoral access. This is generally advisable as compared to attempted stent placement from left brachial access, due to proximity and control issues, as well as the availability of suitably sized stents on long delivery catheters.
Severe calcified disease strategies	■ In patients with significant atherosclerotic burden, care should be taken during the intervention to minimize atheroembolization. Use of covered stent grafts can be considered in these scenarios. Additionally, as an added benefit of the hybrid approach, flushing maneuvers of the patch angioplasty site may be performed to eliminate embolic debris. ■ Prior to angioplasty or stenting, plaque modification with intravascular lithotripsy (eg, Shockwave) can be considered. ■ If the distal aorta is diseased, the Covered Endovascular Reconstruction of the Aortic Bifurcation (CERAB) technique deploys two kissing iliac stents within a covered aortic stent graft to more anatomically and physiologically reconstruct the aortic bifurcation.
Arterial rupture	■ Cover with stent graft. Consider proximal balloon occlusion.
Arterial dissection	■ Extend stent if the dissection is flow limiting.

POSTOPERATIVE CARE

- Following femoral endarterectomy and iliac stenting, patients are usually monitored in the hospital for 1 to 2 days.
- Postoperative antithrombotic management is not well studied in this population; however, most surgeons treat patients with dual antiplatelet therapy such as aspirin and clopidogrel (Plavix), with a loading dose of clopidogrel (ie, 300 mg) followed by a daily dose (ie, 75 mg), for the first 6 weeks following the procedure. Long-term antiplatelet management is usually achieved with acetylsalicylic acid (ASA 81 mg) alone, except in circumstances of aspirin allergy.
- Routine follow-up with arterial duplex and ABIs is important to monitor for continued patency and potential need for secondary intervention. Typical postoperative surveillance includes 1 month, 3 month, 6 months, and annually thereafter. Patients with active wounds should be more closely monitored until healed.

OUTCOMES

- Early and long-term results of concomitant common femoral artery endarterectomy and iliac stenting have been excellent since their first reports in the early 2000s.[5,6] More recent studies continue to report excellent patency results. In a series of 108 patients (127 procedures), 2-year primary, primary-assisted, and secondary patency were 91%, 94%, and 98%, while 5-year patency rates were 87%, 92%, and 98%, respectively.[7]
- There is some evidence that covered stent grafts may have improved patency compared to bare metal stents, particularly in TASC C and D lesions.[6,8] In a study of 61 patients with TASC C and D iliac lesions all treated with the VIABAHN self-expanding PTFE-covered stent graft (W.L. Gore and Associates, Flagstaff, Ariz), primary patency at three years was 95%.[9]
- Iliac artery stenting combined with open femoral endarterectomy also appears to be equally effective as open surgical revascularization with aortobifemoral or iliofemoral bypass. Piazza and colleagues[10] found similar 30-day morbidity and mortality as well as primary patency at 3 years when comparing a 10-year cohort of patients treated in both manners. These similarities were maintained even after stratification for TASC group. In the long-term, endovascular repair with kissing iliac stents (with and without femoral endarterectomy) continues to have comparable outcomes with open aortobifemoral bypass. Dorigo and colleagues studied 210 patients (82 aortobifemoral, 128 iliac stenting) with TASC C and D lesions and found a significantly lower rate of postoperative complications in the stenting group (7% vs 21%, $P < .001$) but no significant difference in 6-year survival, patency (primary, primary-assisted, or secondary), or reintervention.[11]
- Endovascular stenting and/or hybrid therapy has comparable early and late outcomes to open surgical revascularization but is associated with shorter hospital length of stay and lower hospital expense.[12] Therefore, endovascular or hybrid treatment can be considered a first-line therapy option for aortoiliac occlusive disease in appropriate patients.
- Endovascular aortobifemoral bypass or hybrid iliac stenting with femoral endarterectomy is associated with complications (see below) and the need for reinterventions, ranging from approximately 6% to 11%.[9,11] Thus, routine surveillance, often lifelong, is critical for these patients.

COMPLICATIONS

- Contrast nephropathy
- Wound complications, including infection, dehiscence, seroma formation, and nerve entrapment
- Arterial rupture

- Arterial dissection
- Embolization
- Common or external iliac stent stenosis, thrombosis, or occlusion
- Common femoral artery stenosis
- Common femoral artery pseudoaneurysm

REFERENCES

1. Rzucidlo EM, Powell RJ, Zwolak RM, et al. Early results of stent-grafting to treat diffuse aortoiliac occlusive disease. *J Vasc Surg*. 2003;37(6):1175-1180.
2. Norgren L, Hiatt WR, Dormandy JA, Nehler MR, Harris KA, Fowkes FGR. Inter-society Consensus for the management of peripheral arterial disease (TASC II). *J Vasc Surg*. 2007;45:S5-67.
3. Conte MS, Bradbury AW, Kolh P, et al. Global vascular guidelines on the management of chronic limb-threatening ischemia. *J Vasc Surg*. 2019;69(6):3S-125S.e40.
4. Groot Jebbink E, Grimme F, Goverde P, van Oostayen J, Slump C, Reijnen M. Geometrical consequences of kissing stents and the covered endovascular reconstruction of the aortic bifurcation configuration in an in vitro model for endovascular reconstruction of aortic bifurcation. *J Vasc Surg*. 2015;61(5):1306-1311.
5. Nelson PR, Powell RJ, Schermerhorn ML, et al. Early results of external iliac artery stenting combined with common femoral artery endarterectomy. *J Vasc Surg*. 2002;35(6):1107-1113.
6. Chang RW, Goodney PP, Baek JH, Nolan BW, Rzucidlo EM, Powell RJ. Long-term results of combined common femoral endarterectomy and iliac stenting/stent grafting for occlusive disease. *J Vasc Surg*. 2008;48(2):362-367.
7. Maitrias P, Deltombe G, Molin V, Reix T. Iliofemoral endarterectomy associated with systematic iliac stent grafting for the treatment of severe iliofemoral occlusive disease. *J Vasc Surg*. 2017;65(2):406-413.
8. Mwipatayi BP, Thomas S, Wong J, et al. A comparison of covered vs bare expandable stents for the treatment of aortoiliac occlusive disease. *J Vasc Surg*. 2011;54(6):1561-1570.
9. Bracale UM, Giribono AM, Spinelli D, et al. Long-term results of endovascular treatment of TASC C and D aortoiliac occlusive disease with expanded polytetrafluoroethylene stent graft. *Ann Vasc Surg*. 2019;56:254-260.
10. Piazza M, Ricotta JJ, Bower TC, et al. Iliac artery stenting combined with open femoral endarterectomy is as effective as open surgical reconstruction for severe iliac and common femoral occlusive disease. *J Vasc Surg*. 2011;54(2):402-411.
11. Dorigo W, Piffaretti G, Benedetto F, et al. A comparison between aortobifemoral bypass and aortoiliac kissing stents in patients with complex aortoiliac obstructive disease. *J Vasc Surg*. 2017;65(1):99-107.
12. Rocha-Neves J, Ferreira A, Sousa J, et al. Endovascular approach versus aortobifemoral bypass grafting: outcomes in extensive aortoiliac occlusive disease. *Vasc Endovasc Surg*. 2020;54(2):102-110.

Chapter 25 Surgical Exposure of the Lower Extremity Arteries

Young Kim and Anahita Dua

DEFINITION

- The primary etiology of chronic lower extremity ischemia is atherosclerosis, although other, rare causes may exist. These include embolic disease, adventitial cystic disease, popliteal artery entrapment, radiation arteritis, and other disease processes. The symptomatic manifestation of chronic lower extremity ischemia is termed peripheral arterial disease (PAD). Atherosclerotic stenosis or occlusion of the peripheral arterial tree results in arterial insufficiency and limb ischemia. PAD is a major contributor to reduced quality of life (QOL) and increased morbidity and mortality among an increasing elderly patient population.

DIFFERENTIAL DIAGNOSIS

- The challenge for the vascular specialist is to determine whether the nature and severity of presenting symptoms correlate with the degree of chronic arterial insufficiency present. Many alternative diagnoses must be considered, including neuropathy (eg, spinal stenosis), inflammation, infection, lymphatic or venous disease, repetitive trauma (eg, diabetic foot ulcers), or peripheral embolism. Definitive diagnosis is derived from a detailed history and physical examination correlated with appropriately directed noninvasive vascular laboratory and adjunctive imaging studies. The vascular specialist must also differentiate chronic limb ischemia from acute limb ischemia, which is quicker-onset (within 14 days) and more likely to require an urgent intervention.

PATIENT HISTORY AND PHYSICAL FINDINGS

- Approximately half of patients with PAD are asymptomatic. Symptoms related to PAD can range from intermittent claudication to chronic limb-threatening ischemia (CLTI), where CLTI includes ischemic rest pain, ulceration, and gangrene. Pulse examination is an integral component of the vascular-focused physical examination. Femoral, popliteal, posterior tibial, and dorsalis pedis pulses should be noted and graded (0 = absent; 1+ = diminished; 2+ = normal; 3+ = enlarged/aneurysmal). If pulses are absent, a handheld Doppler probe may be utilized to localize signals. Additionally, the femoral pulses may be auscultated to listen for bruits, indicating aortoiliac occlusive disease (as opposed to an infrainguinal process). Femoral bruits may be further exacerbated by having the patient perform several squats prior to auscultation.
- Claudication is defined as muscular pain, cramping, aching, or discomfort in the lower limb, reproducibly elicited by exercise and relieved within 10 minutes of cessation. Classically, the muscle group impacted by claudication is one level inferior to the atherosclerotic lesion. For example, aortoiliac lesions present with buttock claudication, and femoropopliteal lesions present with calf claudication. Lesions at multiple levels are responsible for the development of CLTI. CLTI has traditionally been defined as (1) persistent, recurring ischemic rest pain requiring opiate analgesia for longer than 2 weeks and (2) ankle systolic blood pressure (SBP) less than 50 mm Hg or toe pressures less than 30 mm Hg (or absent pedal pulse in patients with diabetes).[1] Ischemic rest pain worsens with leg elevation and is relieved by dependency. In addition to absent pulses, dependent rubor, elevation pallor, and calf muscle atrophy are frequently present among patients with CLTI. CLTI also includes ischemic foot ulceration and gangrene in the setting of ankle SBP less than 50 mm Hg or toe pressures less than 40 mm Hg in patients without diabetes (<50 mm Hg in diabetics).
- Patients with PAD often have multiple medical comorbidities. These include coronary artery disease (CAD), diabetes mellitus, hypertension, hyperlipidemia, chronic kidney disease, chronic obstructive pulmonary disease, and a prolonged smoking history. Frailty is also common among patients with PAD due to older age and limited ambulation. Therefore, all patients with PAD require comprehensive medical management and risk factor modification. Additionally, given that PAD often manifests through pain, patients with PAD should also be questioned regarding use of narcotic and non-narcotic analgesics.
- For patients with intermittent claudication, revascularization is indicated for those with persistent, lifestyle-limiting symptoms, despite adequate risk factor modification, exercise, and optimal medical management. For patients with lifestyle-limiting claudication, the primary goal of intervention is to improve exercise tolerance and thereby QOL. All patients with CLTI, on the other hand, are indicated for surgical revascularization to prevent limb loss. Therefore, revascularization among the CLTI cohort is focused on wound healing and functional limb salvage, in addition to symptomatic relief and QOL improvements.[2,3]

IMAGING AND OTHER DIAGNOSTIC STUDIES

- Adequate preoperative planning depends on a thorough history and detailed physical examination. The vascular specialist must determine the severity of ischemic symptoms, along with any infectious complications, functional status, and anticipated longevity. Once it is decided that revascularization will improve the patient's functional status and QOL, imaging and other diagnostic studies can be utilized to determine the location, extent, and severity of occlusive arterial lesions. These studies can also help determine whether endovascular, open, or hybrid revascularization procedures are indicated.
- The delineation of the relevant arterial anatomy on the index limb is facilitated by high-quality, noninvasive vascular laboratory studies (ankle-brachial index and toe pressure measurements). These are supplemented by arterial color duplex ultrasound imaging. Arterial duplex is extremely accurate in the assessment of iliofemoral and femoropopliteal arterial occlusive disease but less so for infrageniculate lesions. Duplex enables differentiation of stenosis from occlusion and determination of lesion length and degree of calcification.
- Cross-sectional imaging studies, such as computed tomography angiography (CTA) or magnetic resonance arteriography, can also help define arterial anatomy when defining disease extent and severity. CTA is better suited for assessing aortoiliac and femoral disease and suboptimal for infrageniculate arteries. Catheter-based angiography is better suited for assessing infrageniculate disease. Both CTA and conventional angiography utilize intravenous contrast, and the practitioner should be cognizant of contrast-induced nephropathy.

SURGICAL MANAGEMENT

Preoperative Planning

- In terms of cardiovascular health, PAD is considered equivalent to CAD. Therefore, preoperative risk evaluation for overall cardiovascular-related mortality represents an integral component of preoperative planning. For patients with stable or minimally symptomatic CAD, preoperative evaluation is focused on risk-reduction efforts. Frequently, this includes antiplatelet therapy, plaque stabilization via statin therapy, β-blockade, and optimization of hypertension management.
- For an open bypass, the goals of preoperative planning include identification of diseased arterial segment(s), selection of the most appropriate arterial inflow source, selection of the optimal bypass target for maximal outflow and target bed perfusion, and selection of the best available conduit. Conduit availability is almost always the rate-limiting factor because the best quality conduit is a single-segment great saphenous vein (GSV). Alternatives to GSV grafts include prosthetic conduits (eg, polytetrafluoroethylene, Dacron), arm veins, and spliced vein segments.
- The surgical plan should be individualized based on patient's functional status, medical comorbidities, extent of arterial disease, and conduit availability. Infrainguinal bypass may originate from the common femoral artery (CFA), superficial femoral artery (SFA), profunda femoris artery (PFA), or popliteal artery, with a bypass target of the popliteal, tibial, or pedal/plantar arteries. Patient positioning, selection of incisions, and surgical techniques are all dictated by the type of bypass procedure deemed most appropriate under the circumstances.

EXPOSURE OF THE FEMORAL VESSELS

Positioning

- The patient is placed in supine position. Foley catheter should be inserted, as long as the patient is not anuric at baseline. Arms may be tucked to facilitate intraoperative and completion angiography.

Placement of Incision

- The inguinal ligament can be identified as a line between the pubic tubercle and anterior superior iliac spine. The CFA is located along this imaginary line, two fingerbreadths lateral to pubic tubercle. Palpation of the inguinal ligament and femoral pulse, or direct visualization with duplex ultrasound, can localize the CFA bifurcation and help to guide optimal incision placement. Even when pulseless due to excessive calcification or occlusive disease, the CFA may be localized by reliance on anatomic landmarks and direct palpation, recognized as a firm tubular structure positioned within the femoral sheath.
- The vertical groin incision is most commonly employed to provide optimal access to the entire length of the CFA. This should be created coaxially along the artery itself, continued from the inguinal ligament distally, and aimed at the medial aspect of the knee. This incision may be extended cephalad or caudad to increase arterial exposure as necessary (**FIGURE 1**, *incision A*).
- Alternatively, a transverse incision can be placed 1 cm below and parallel to the inguinal ligament to avoid potential skin maceration and wound complications that may accompany vertical incisions in this situation (**FIGURE 1**, *incision B*). This incision is particularly useful in obese patients with substantial abdominal pannus. Although the proximal SFA and PFA may be exposed through a transverse incision, further proximal or distal exposure is prohibited by the incision itself. Therefore, if an extensive common and deep femoral endarterectomy is anticipated to optimize inflow, a vertical incision should be planned.

Dissection and Control of the Common, Superficial, and Proximal Deep Femoral Arteries

- The incision is carried through the subcutaneous tissue and superficial fascia using electrocautery. A self-retaining retractor, such as a Weitlaner or Beckmann, may be placed at this time. Deep to the subcutaneous tissue and superficial fascia, the dissection is extended longitudinally, even when using an oblique incision, to optimize the length of femoral exposure. Self-retaining retractors are carefully repositioned to

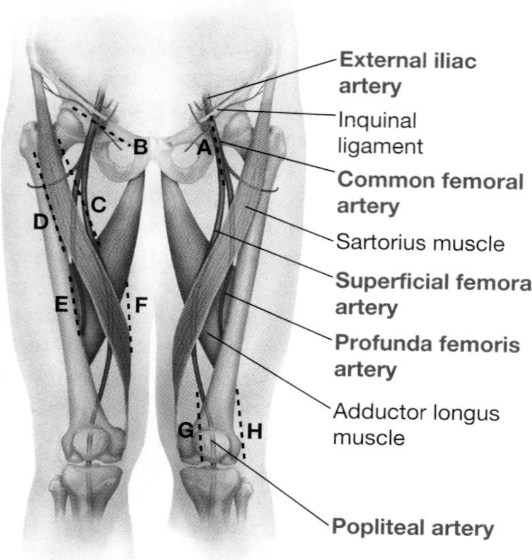

FIGURE 1 ● Exposure of the femoral vessels. The proximal femoral vessels may be exposed through a *(A)* longitudinal or *(B)* transverse incision. The mid- and distal superficial femoral and profunda femoris arteries may be exposed through a number of incisions *(C-F)*. The suprageniculate popliteal artery may be exposed through a *(G)* medial or *(H)* lateral approach.

optimize exposure, while avoiding traction injury to femoral nerve branches or the common femoral vein. Sharp dissection through the femoral sheath exposes the anterior surface of the CFA.

- The dissection plane should remain centered directly over the CFA, which can be identified by digital palpation. Encountering venous structures indicates medial deviation from the optimal plane; whereas the iliopsoas muscle, femoral nerve fibers, or lymphatic vessels are indicative of lateral deviation. Incorrectly placed femoral incisions are associated with an increased risk of wound complications, including wound necrosis and separation, lymphatic leaks, femoral neuropraxia, and venous injury.
- Sharp dissection should proceed along the CFA both proximally and distally. The CFA and its branches are circumferentially dissected and individually isolated. Placement of a red rubber catheter or silastic vessel loops around the CFA and its branches aid in retraction, dissection, and mobilization.
- Proximal dissection is continued along the CFA to the inguinal ligament. At this point, the inguinal ligament may be divided if exposure of the external iliac artery is necessary. Caution is necessary in this area, as a prominent femoral vein tributary crosses anteriorly over the CFA in this area, underneath the inguinal ligament, and is prone to injury if not identified, ligated, and divided early in the dissection. Inadvertent injury to this so-called "vein of pain" results in retraction and troublesome bleeding. If the inguinal ligament is divided, it should be repaired prior to the end of the procedure to prevent hernia formation.
- The medial and lateral femoral circumflex arteries, important collaterals in iliofemoral arterial occlusive disease, are identified at level of the inguinal ligament and individually controlled with removable clips or silastic vessel loops. Use of the former reduces clutter in the wound during endarterectomy or creation of the proximal anastomosis. If removable clips are placed, then they should be removed prior to the end of the procedure.
- As the dissection proceeds distally, an abrupt caliber change marks the femoral bifurcation and the origins of the PFA (Latin for *deep femoral artery*) and SFA. The SFA continues distally in the same plane, while the PFA usually courses posteriorly and laterally away from the femoral bifurcation. Occasionally, multiple PFAs may be encountered. The lateral circumflex iliac vein is encountered crossing the anterior surface of the PFA and should preclude any blind dissection in this area. After silastic loops are placed on each vessel, gentle upward traction on the CFA and SFA may help bring the PFA into view (**FIGURE 2A**).
- Medial and distal dissection provides extended exposure of the proximal SFA (**FIGURE 1**, *incision F*). This vessel only occasionally has small branches in its proximal segment. A sensory branch of the femoral nerve may be present crossing the SFA from lateral to medial. Transection may result in pain, numbness, and paresthesia along the medial thigh distribution. Even extended femoral bifurcation dissections rarely require division of femoral nerve branches, which should be avoided to minimize postoperative discomfort.

Exposure of the Profunda Femoris Artery—Middle and Distal Segments

- Exposure of the distal portions of the PFA often enables use of shorter vein conduit in distal leg bypass or may improve outflow from proximal revascularization procedures (eg, iliac angioplasty and stenting, aortobifemoral bypass). These segments can be exposed through either posteromedial or anteromedial approaches (**FIGURE 1**, *incisions C–F*). The approach should be dictated by the surgical indication (inflow sources or outflow target), with additional consideration for native vs reoperative field.
- Incisions are placed along either the medial (**FIGURE 1**, *incisions C and F*) or lateral borders of the sartorius muscle (**FIGURE 1**, *incisions D and E*). The dissection plane is deepened through the subcutaneous tissue and fascia using electrocautery, passing lateral or medial to the sartorius, respectively. The sartorius muscle is then mobilized and retracted laterally or medially, depending on the approach. Dissection is carried posteriorly, passing lateral to the superficial femoral vessels and accompanying nerve, to the space between the adductor longus muscle (medially) and vastus medialis (laterally) (**FIGURE 2B**, *incisions C–E*). The PFA and profunda vein pass directly underneath.
- Dissection between adductor longus and vastus medialis muscle exposes the middle segments of the PFA. Crossing venous tributaries should be ligated and divided as necessary to provide optimal exposure. Distal segments of PFA begin to course posterior to the femur beyond this point and are therefore less useful for bypass planning.
- Alternatively, dissection between the adductor longus (anteriorly) and gracilis muscle (posteriorly) allows for medial exposure of the PFA in the distal thigh (**FIGURE 1**, *incision F*; **FIGURE 2B**, *incision F*).

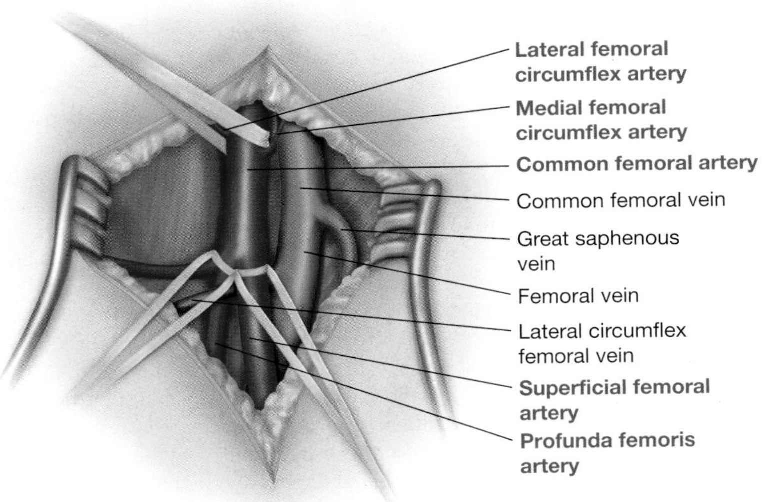

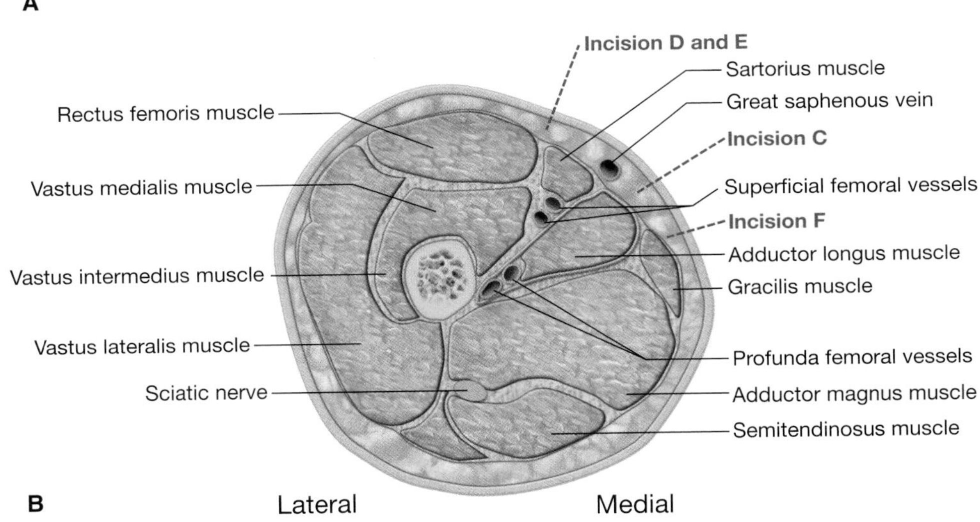

FIGURE 2 ● **A,** Exposure of femoral vessels at groin through a longitudinal incision. **B,** Anteromedial and posterolateral approaches to expose middle and distal segments of the superficial and deep femoral arteries. Incisions *(C-F)* correspond to **FIGURE 1**.

EXPOSURE OF THE POPLITEAL ARTERY

Medial Exposure of the Above-Knee Popliteal Artery

- The patient is placed in a supine position. The operative leg is then flexed and rotated laterally. A bump may be placed underneath the knee for stabilization; however, this may hinder the use of gravity to aid in exposure.
- A longitudinal incision is made along the groove formed by the vastus medialis (anteriorly) and the sartorius muscles (posteromedially), measuring approximately 10 to 12 cm (**FIGURE 3A**, *incision A*). The incision is carried through the subcutaneous tissue and fascia using electrocautery. A self-retaining retractor is carefully placed without undue tension, taking care not to injure the GSV or saphenous nerve. At this location, the GSV is likely to be encountered more posteromedially in the subcutaneous tissue. The saphenous nerve may be encountered at distal end of the incision as it joins the GSV near the medial aspect of the knee.
- The deep fascia is then longitudinally incised above the sartorius muscle to enter the above-knee popliteal fossa. The popliteal artery can be palpated against the posterior surface of the femur (**FIGURE 3B**).
- Multiple veins are encountered in the popliteal fossa. The popliteal artery is often surrounded by venae comitantes (Latin for *accompanying veins*), and the popliteal vein is posterolateral to the artery in this location. The popliteal and/or superficial femoral veins may be duplicated throughout the popliteal fossa and distal thigh. Isolation and control of the artery usually requires ligation and division of surrounding collateral veins. A sclerotic popliteal vein can easily be mistaken for the popliteal artery, and care must be taken to distinguish the two vessels.

Lateral Exposure of the Above-Knee Popliteal Artery

- Lateral exposure of the above-knee popliteal artery is useful in select clinical scenarios. For instance, axillopopliteal bypass is logistically easier through a lateral approach. Another instance is when the medial approach has previously been dissected or is complicated by infection or injury.
- The patient is placed in a supine position. The operative leg is then flexed and rotated medially. A bump may be placed underneath the knee for stabilization.
- A longitudinal incision is made between the vastus lateralis and the biceps femoris muscles, measuring approximately 10 to 12 cm (**FIGURE 4A**, *incision A*). The incision is carried through the subcutaneous tissue and fascia using electrocautery. A self-retaining retractor is carefully placed without undue tension. Once the fascia lata has been exposed, a generous cruciate incision ("T-ed") is created at both ends to prevent bypass graft impingement by its dense fibers.
- After self-retaining retractors are placed, the popliteal space is entered. The sciatic nerve and popliteal vein will be encountered first, as they are lateral to the popliteal artery. The sciatic nerve is gently retracted downward. The popliteal vein is then circumferentially dissected and mobilized to expose the above-knee popliteal artery.

Posterior Exposure of the Popliteal Vessels

- Although direct and relatively uncomplicated, posterior access is limited by the medial and lateral heads of the gastrocnemius muscle distally and the hamstrings proximally. Therefore, only limited popliteal artery access is achievable through this incision. Despite its limitations, posterior exposure may be the preferred approach for management of popliteal artery entrapment syndrome, popliteal adventitial cystic disease, focal popliteal artery aneurysms, or arterial injury following traumatic posterior knee dislocation.
- The patient is placed in a prone position, using a pillow to prop up the lower leg and foot.

An S-shaped incision is made, starting medially at the distal thigh. The incision is carried across the posterior crease of the knee joint, ending laterally at the proximal leg. Dissection is then carried anteriorly through the subcutaneous tissue and superficial fascia, entering the popliteal fossa. After placing self-retaining retractors, exposure is maximized by mobilizing the popliteal artery between the two heads of the gastrocnemius muscle inferiorly and between the hamstring muscles (semimembranosus and biceps femoris) superiorly.

- The muscles are gently retracted to expose the entire popliteal fossa. The tibial and common peroneal nerves are

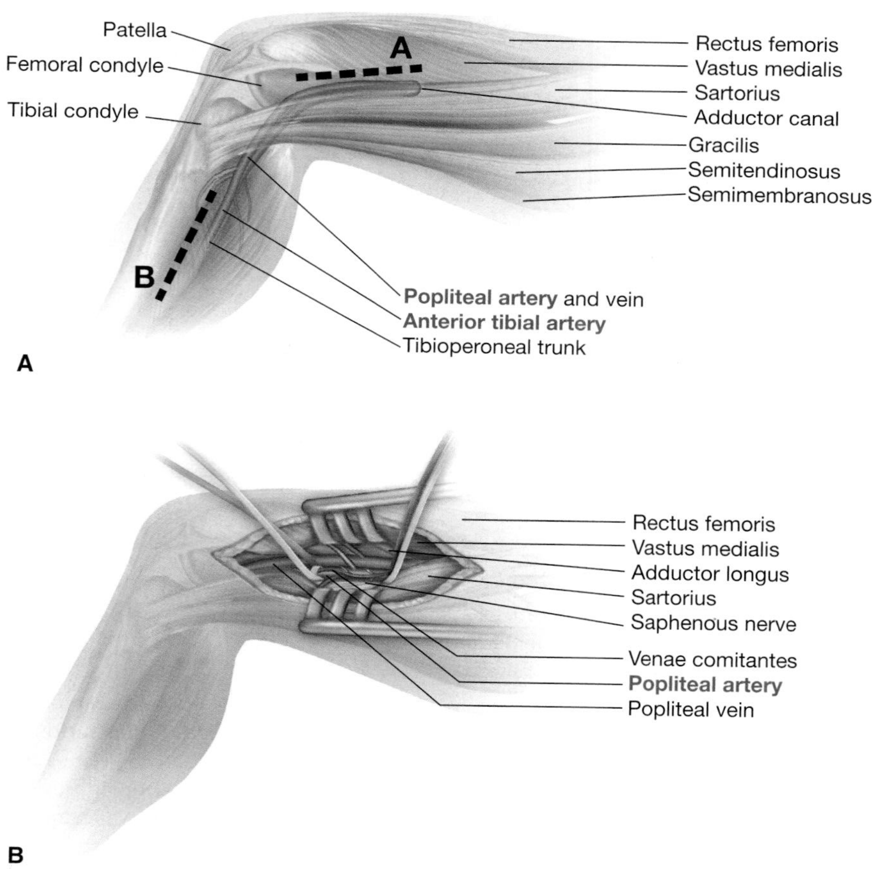

FIGURE 3 ● **A,** Medial exposure of the *(A)* suprageniculate and *(B)* infrageniculate popliteal artery. **B,** Exposure of the suprageniculate popliteal artery. **C,** Exposure of the infrageniculate popliteal artery and its trifurcation. **D,** Exposure of the popliteal artery through a posterior approach.

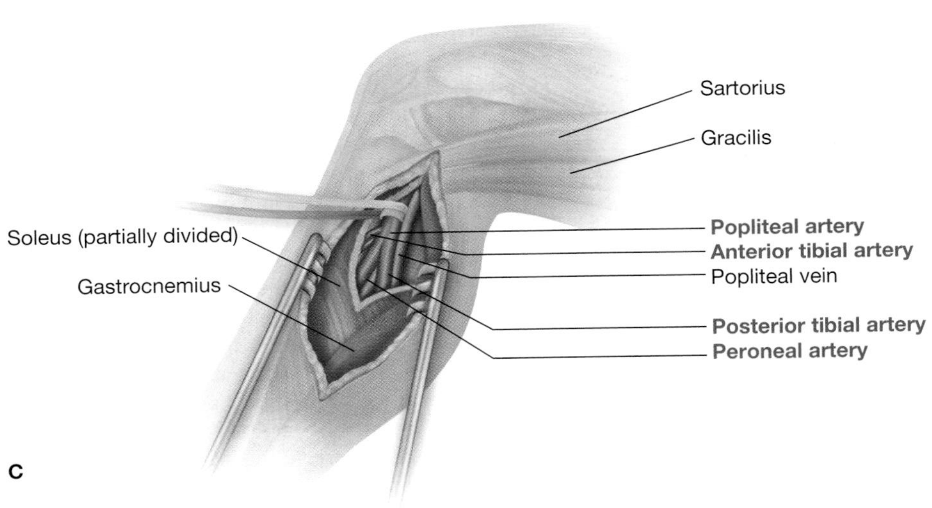

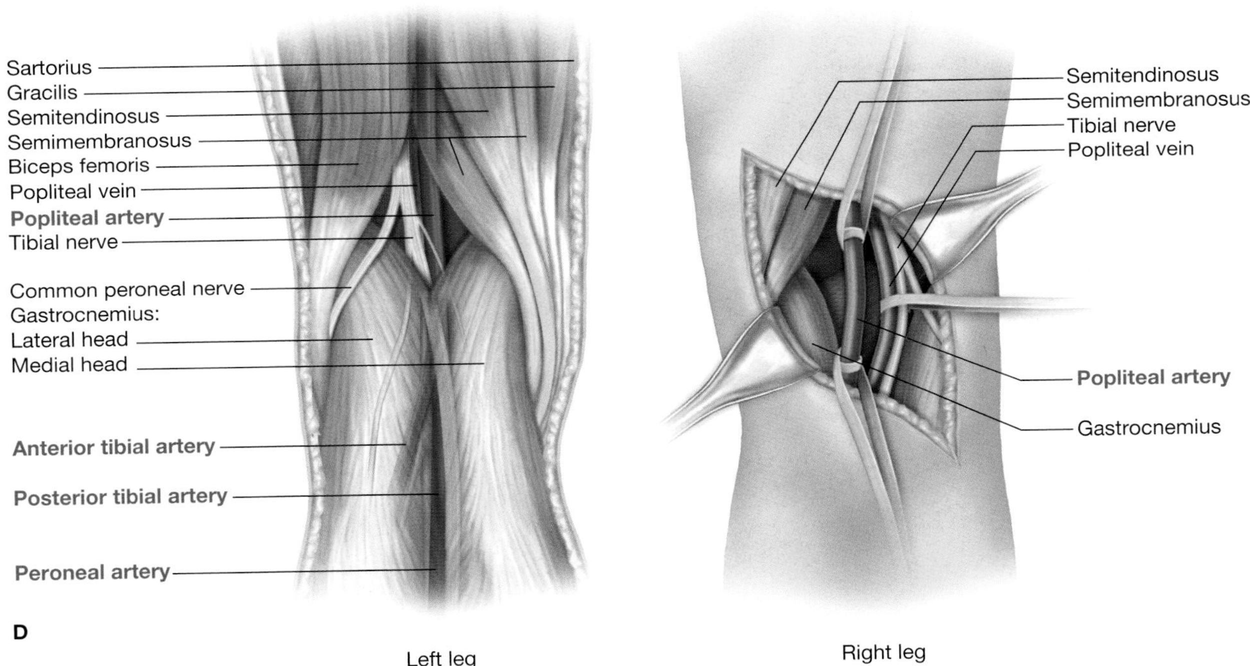

FIGURE 3 ● Cont'd

encountered superficially in this exposure. The popliteal artery is anterior (deep) to the popliteal vein in the popliteal fossa.

- It may be necessary to mobilize the popliteal vein with ligation and division of popliteal venous tributaries to fully expose the artery. Once the appropriate segment is circumferentially dissected, silastic vessel loops are placed proximally and distally.

Medial Exposure of the Infrageniculate Popliteal Artery

- The medial approach to the below-knee popliteal artery is the most common approach (**FIGURE 3A**).
- The patient is placed in a supine position. The operative leg is then flexed and rotated laterally. A bump may be placed underneath the knee for stabilization; however, this may hinder the use of gravity to aid in exposure.
- A longitudinal incision is made one fingerbreadth below the edge of the tibia, along the course of the GSV (**FIGURE 3A**, *incision B*). The dissection is carried through subcutaneous tissue and fascia into the deep posterior compartment. The infrageniculate popliteal vessels reside in the deep posterior compartment and are partially covered by the origin of the soleus muscle.
- Division of the soleus muscle fibers (**FIGURE 3C**) will facilitate exposure of the tibioperoneal trunk and takeoff of the anterior tibial artery; however, it is not entirely necessary for exposure of the below-knee popliteal artery itself. As previously described, the popliteal artery lies

in close proximity to the popliteal vein and tibial nerve. Mobilization of the popliteal vein from the adjacent artery is imperative to provide adequate exposure of all relevant structures, including the anterior tibial artery, tibioperoneal trunk, and its two branches (posterior tibial and peroneal arteries). It may be necessary to ligate and divide the anterior tibial vein at its confluence with the (often paired) popliteal vein to expose the tibial vessels. Dissection and retraction must proceed deliberately in this location to avoid injury to the neighboring tibial nerve and its distal branches.

Lateral Exposure of the Infrageniculate Popliteal Artery

- The lateral approach to the below-knee popliteal artery is rarely performed, given the need for fibulectomy, but may be beneficial in the setting of active infection or a reoperative surgical field.
- A longitudinal incision is made a fingerbreadth anterior to the fibula, starting 2 cm inferior to the fibular head and extending caudally. Dissection is carried directly onto fibula (**FIGURE 4A**, *incision B*). Note the location of the common peroneal nerve, which courses from posterior to anterior around the neck of the upper fibula just below its head, before it branches into the superficial and deep peroneal nerves. Injury to the common peroneal nerve can result in foot drop and sensory deficits.
- After exposure of the fibula, the periosteum of the fibula is circumferentially dissected. A bone saw is then used to excise the exposed segment of the fibula, while protecting the underlying structures. The popliteal vessels and branches are found directly underneath the fibular periosteum, with the popliteal artery usually located anterior to the popliteal vein and posterior tibial nerve. By extending the dissection distally, the anterior tibial artery takeoff and the tibioperoneal trunk can also be exposed.

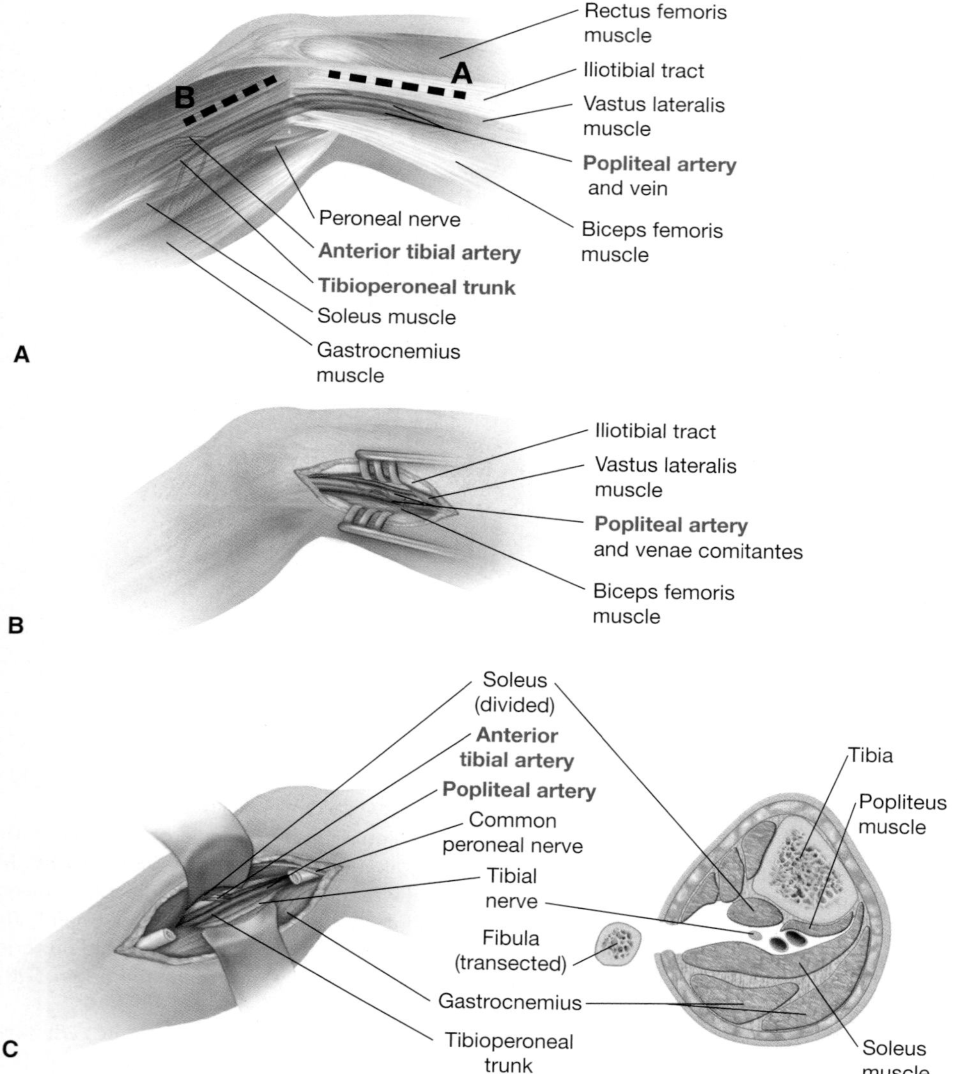

FIGURE 4 ● **A,** Lateral exposure of *(A)* suprageniculate and *(B)* infrageniculate popliteal artery. **B,** Exposure of suprageniculate popliteal artery. **C,** Exposure of infrageniculate popliteal artery and its trifurcation.

EXPOSURE OF THE TIBIAL VESSELS

Exposure of the Anterior Tibial Artery—Proximal Segment

- Exposure of the origin of the anterior tibial artery is similar to the technique for medial exposure for the infrageniculate popliteal artery.

Exposure of the Anterior Tibial Artery—Middle Segment

- Exposure of the middle segment of the anterior tibial artery is useful for situations in which there is limited length of autogenous vein graft.
- An axial incision is made in a vertical plane about two fingerbreadths lateral to the anterior edge of the tibia (**FIGURE 5A**). The incision is then deepened between the tibialis anterior and the extensor hallucis longus muscles. The anterior tibial artery is found superficial to the interosseus membrane between the cleft formed by these two muscles.
- Dissecting away the overlying collateral veins allows for exposure and control of the middle segment of the anterior tibial artery. Use of a proximal sterile tourniquet during exposure of all the crural arteries may significantly accelerate the dissection while limiting bleeding from the numerous and redundant collateral veins. Prior to placing the sterile tourniquet, an Esmarch bandage should be used to drain the leg of its venous blood, otherwise venous congestion may result in persistent bleeding from any venous structures.

Exposure of the Posterior Tibial Artery—Proximal Segment

- Exposure of the proximal segment of the posterior tibial artery is similar to the technique for medial exposure for the infrageniculate popliteal artery. The soleus muscle must be dissected free from its tibial attachments for adequate exposure.

Exposure of the Posterior Tibial Artery—Middle Segment

- Exposure of the middle segment of the posterior tibial artery is useful for situations in which there is limited length of autogenous vein graft.
- A longitudinal incision is made just anterior to the soleus muscle. The overlying soleus muscle must be divided to expose the underlying vessels (**FIGURE 5B**). The posterior tibial artery lies anterior to soleus muscle with the peroneal artery located laterally, in the same plane, between the soleus and tibialis posterior muscles.
- Careful dissection is necessary to avoid injury to the tibial nerve, which commonly runs between the posterior tibial and peroneal vessels.

Exposure of the Peroneal Artery—Proximal Segment

- Exposure of the proximal segment of the peroneal artery is similar to the technique for medial exposure for the infrageniculate popliteal artery, extended caudally to expose the tibioperoneal trunk and its branches.

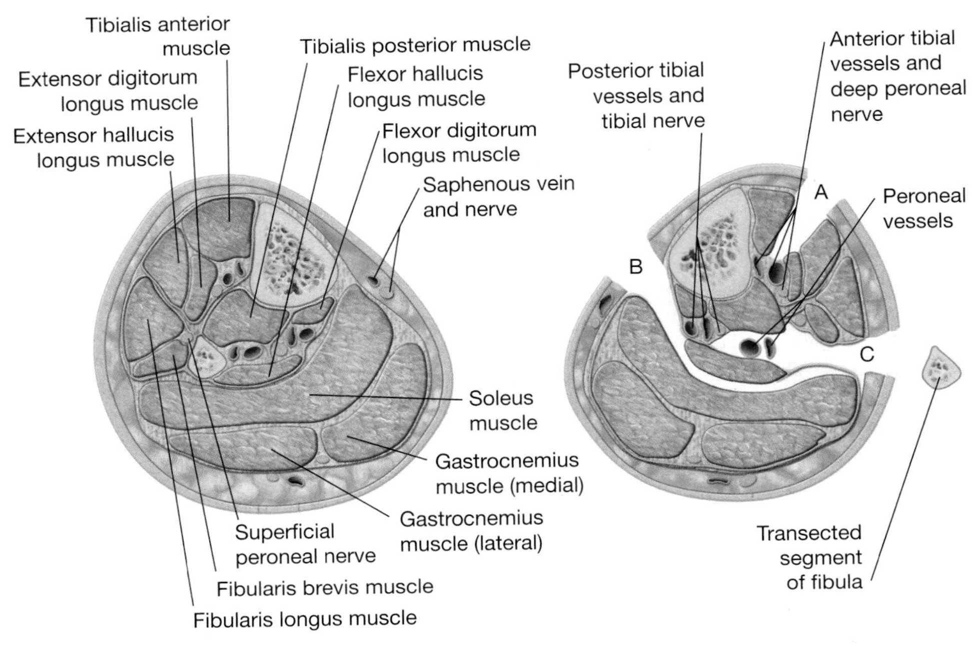

FIGURE 5 ● Exposure of anterior tibial, posterior tibial, and peroneal arteries at mid-lower leg.

Exposure of the Peroneal Artery—Middle Segment

- Exposure of the middle segment of the peroneal artery may also be performed from an anterolateral approach. This is rarely performed, given the need for fibulectomy.
- A vertical incision is made over the fibula at the desired level of exposure (**FIGURE 5C**). Dissection is then carried down through the overlying muscle using electrocautery, eventually exposing the fibula. The fibular periosteum is dissected circumferentially. A bone saw is then used to excise the exposed segment of the fibula, while protecting the underlying structures. After incising the inner periosteal membrane, the peroneal vessels are found immediately beneath this structure. The artery usually is anterior to flexor hallucis longus and posterior to the tibialis posterior muscles.
- The peroneal artery is exposed and controlled after mobilization from circumferential collateral veins and the main peroneal vein. Use of a proximal sterile tourniquet and Esmarch bandage is prudent.

EXPOSURE OF PEDAL VESSELS

Exposure of the Inframalleolar Posterior Tibial Artery

- Exposure of the distal segment of the posterior tibial artery enables pedal bypass, which may be useful in patients with tibial disease (eg, diabetic macroangiopathy).
- Intraoperative ultrasound may be used to locate the trajectory of the posterior tibial artery. A longitudinal incision is made through skin and fascia at the midpoint between the medial malleolus and the Achilles tendon. If this exposure is used for an *in situ* bypass procedure, the incision should be deviated anteriorly to accommodate the anterior course of the GSV, as it crosses the medial malleolus.
- The flexor retinaculum is identified as a thick tendon sheath and divided sharply to provide optimal exposure. The posterior tibial vessels are located between the flexor digitorum longus and flexor hallucis longus muscles/tendons. A small Weitlaner self-retaining retractor is placed for exposure. The neurovascular bundle is usually enveloped by fatty tissue underneath the fascia. Within the neurovascular bundle, the posterior tibial artery is usually found anterior to the tibial nerve. There is typically a rich network of venous collaterals present. These may either be mobilized or (more commonly) divided to facilitate distal posterior tibial artery exposure.
- When more distal bypass targets are needed (eg, prohibitive burden of disease in the posterior tibial artery itself), the dissection may be continued distally along the posterior tibial artery to its bifurcation into the medial and lateral plantar arteries. In these cases, however, preoperative angiogram is paramount to immediate and long-term surgical success and only in rare circumstances should the operative plan be changed by unexpected findings at the time of surgery. The presence of luminal calcification alone, without substantial compromise to the target lumen diameter, is not a contraindication to bypass reconstruction. If there is any uncertainty regarding the optimal bypass target, consideration should be given to intraoperative arteriography to guide surgical decision-making. To this end, we perform all open bypass procedures in a hybrid operating room environment with high-quality imaging capabilities to ensure the optimal outcome of all procedures, regardless of the initial operative plan.

Exposure of the Supramalleolar Anterior Tibial Artery

- Exposure of the supramalleolar anterior tibial artery is useful as a distal bypass target, especially in the presence of substantial tibial atherosclerosis. It may also be preferable to bypass to this segment in the presence of a dorsal foot wound.
- Ultrasound may help to localize this artery intraoperatively. A longitudinal incision is placed made between the tibialis anterior (medially) and extensor hallucis longus and the extensor digitorum longus (laterally) (**FIGURE 6A**). The anterior tibial artery and peroneal nerve usually course through the groove between these structures. Dissection and retraction of these tendons will expose the supramalleolar segment of the anterior tibial artery.

Exposure of the Dorsalis Pedis Artery

- The dorsalis pedis artery (Latin for *dorsal artery of foot*) is the extension of the anterior tibial artery as it passes beneath the extensor retinaculum. It can serve as a suitable distal bypass target, especially in patients with diabetes.
- Ultrasound may help to localize this artery intraoperatively, as the location and course of this artery can vary widely between patients. The artery is best exposed beyond the inferior extensor retinaculum. A longitudinal incision is made on the dorsum of the foot, between the first and second metatarsal shafts and distal to the extensor retinaculum (**FIGURE 6B**).
- The dorsalis pedis artery typically resides in the groove between the first and second metatarsal heads, lateral to the extensor hallucis longus tendon, which is readily identified by dorsiflexion of the great toe, and medial to extensor hallucis brevis. Dissection is carried through subcutaneous tissue and the fascial layer must be divided to expose the artery. The dorsalis pedis artery is surrounded by two venous structures which must be carefully identified prior to placement of a sterile tourniquet. Methylene blue dye is useful for marking the artery at this point. After placement of the tourniquet, it can be quite difficult to differentiate the artery from the surrounding veins.

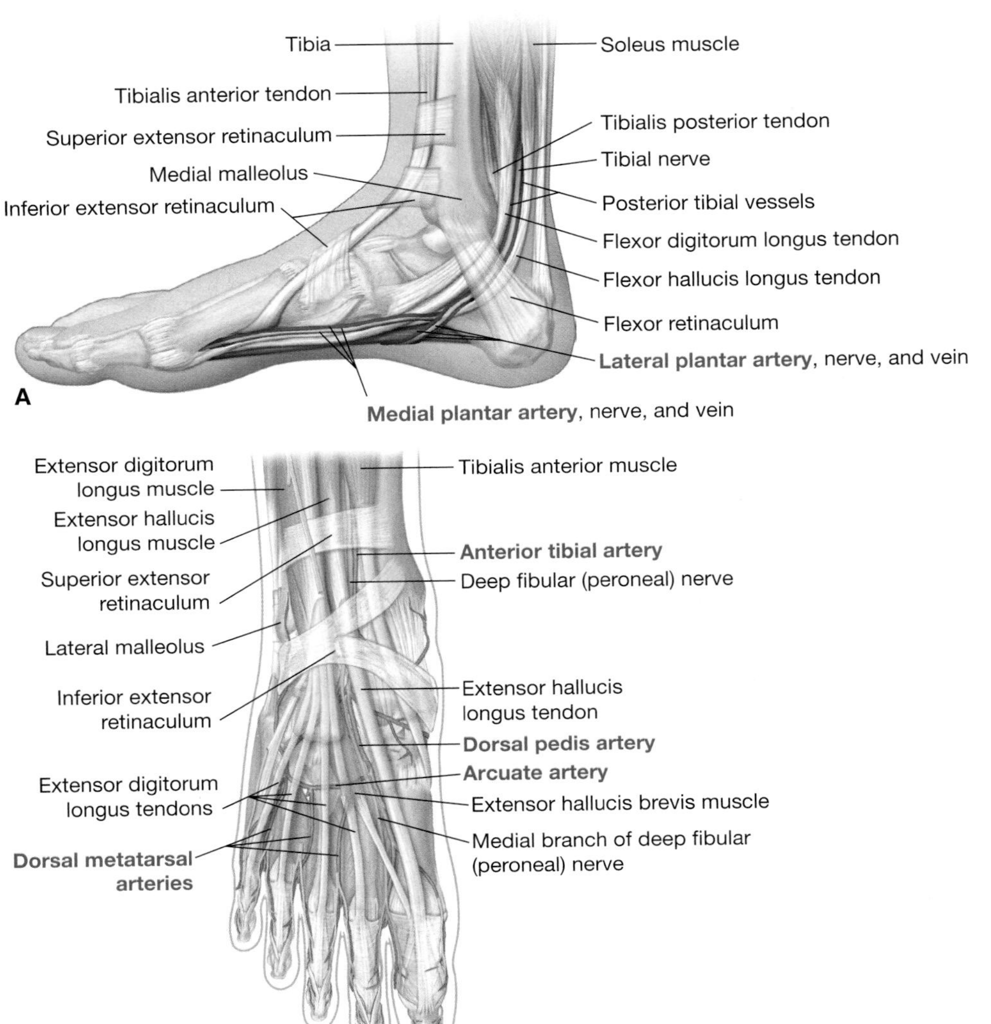

FIGURE 6 ● **A,** Exposure of posterior tibial artery. **B,** Exposure of anterior tibial and dorsalis pedis arteries.

PEARLS AND PITFALLS

- Preoperative and intraoperative ultrasound aids the selection and placement of the incision. Dissection can be guided by palpation of the underlying arterial pulse. In many cases, given the burden of atherosclerotic disease, distal pulses are frequently absent or difficult to palpate. Use of an intraoperative Doppler probe can aid in the localization and dissection of target vessel. Nonetheless, knowledge of appropriate anatomic landmarks will greatly facilitate careful and expeditious exposure and avoid inadvertent injury to surrounding structures. In all circumstances, dissection should be directly targeted on and around the artery. This principle is similar in many ways to the orthopedic axiom to "stay on the bone" during dissection—keeping exposure centered on the target artery minimizes venous bleeding and damage to surrounding structures. Placement of an encircling silastic vessel loop will aid in vascular control and further mobilization.
- In the exposures of the thigh arteries, the sartorius muscle serves as an important landmark for the exposure of the common, superficial, and profunda femoris arteries.
- In the setting of reoperation, alternative surgical exposures allow operation in a virgin field that is unscarred by previous operation. Active infection may also preclude certain approaches to a target vessel, and alternative access is prudent in these situations.
- At the end of the procedure, if the inguinal ligament was divided for proximal exposure, it should be reapproximated. Any removable clips placed on the femoral circumflex arteries should be removed. Completion angiography is not always necessary, but may be useful if there is any question regarding the quality of the bypass.

POSTOPERATIVE CARE

- Following bypass, patients should be maintained on a comprehensive medical regimen to optimize their cardiopulmonary status. Lower extremity bypass operations are often performed on patients with diabetes and debilitating symptoms of claudication or CLTI. Postoperative care should also aim to optimize nutritional status, functional status, and maintenance of euglycemia. If the indication for bypass was tissue loss, the patient may develop a worsening infection secondary to increased distal perfusion.
- Most surgeons routinely employ routine antiplatelet and selective anticoagulation therapy to improve graft patency in lower extremity bypass patients. The Dutch Bypass Oral Anticoagulants or Aspirin (BOA) trial suggested that oral anticoagulation improved vein graft patency compared with aspirin, whereas aspirin improved prosthetic graft patency compared with anticoagulation.[10] The antiplatelet and/or anticoagulation regimen must be tailored to each individual patient following bypass with consideration of risk for graft failure vs risk of bleeding.
- We routinely administer aspirin to bypass patients and reserve anticoagulation (warfarin) for high-risk situations (redo bypass, marginal or alternative vein conduits, spliced vein grafts, poor outflow, prior graft thrombosis) due to the increased bleeding risk associated with anticoagulation. If anticoagulation is initiated, we begin with a low-dose heparin infusion after a routine postoperative check and then titrate accordingly if there is no evidence of hematoma or bleeding. The patient is transitioned to an oral anticoagulant following dietary intake and ambulation.
- Considerable efforts on wound care are required to achieve wound healing after lower extremity revascularization in patients with CLTI and tissue loss. Meticulous nursing care and early ambulation are also crucial to prevent decubitus ulcer in the lower extremities and the sacrum, creating new wounds in patients with lower extremity ischemia. Physical therapy consultation is advisable following bypass procedures. We routinely use *Prevalon* boots to protect the affected extremity from developing pressure ulcers against the bedpost.

OUTCOMES

- Outcomes of revascularization should be reported and interpreted through the reporting standards created and updated by the Society for Vascular Surgery.
- In general, autogenous vein conduits are superior to all others for infrainguinal bypass, even for the suprageniculate popliteal insertion site, where vein has proven superior to PTFE beyond 2 to 3 years. Ipsilateral and contralateral GSV conduits exhibit patency rates superior to alternative vein grafts, such as small saphenous vein, arm vein, and spliced veins. Vein graft primary patency rates for femoral-to-infrageniculate popliteal bypasses are approximately 70% to 75% at 5 years, and assisted primary patency can be improved even further by a duplex vein graft surveillance protocol. Infrapopliteal vein graft primary patency rates range from 60% to 70% at 5 years. Multiple randomized trials have shown no benefit of reversed vs in situ vein configurations.
- PTFE grafts have acceptable short-term and intermediate-term patency rates only in the suprageniculate popliteal position and therefore should only be used in limb salvage situations if autologous vein is truly unavailable. When PTFE must be used, an adjunctive venous Miller cuff or Taylor patch may improve results. The primary factors influencing graft patency are indication, conduit type, conduit quality (diameter), and arterial runoff. Poor runoff adversely impacts prosthetic graft patency.
- The reader is further referred to standard textbook sources such as *Rutherford's Vascular Surgery*, 7th edition, Chapter 109, for a more detailed discussion of the expected outcomes after surgical revascularization for infrainguinal disease.[2]

COMPLICATIONS

- Incomplete hemostasis: Satisfactory hemostasis should be achieved prior to skin closure. Full anticoagulation from heparin can be reversed with protamine to reduce the risk of postoperative bleeding. Channel drains may be placed in extensively dissected wounds. Hypertension is also a strong risk factor for postoperative hemorrhage and blood pressure should be strictly controlled during the postoperative phase.
- Vascular injury: Vascular clamps or silastic loops can lift atherosclerotic plaques and create inadvertent dissection planes and arterial injury in the presence of calcified plaques. Vascular clamps should therefore be placed at relatively soft, disease-free segments. Occasionally, this requires lateral positioning of a clamp to provide anterior/posterior rather than lateral compression of a vessel. In the CFA, the accumulation of significant posterior plaque often mandates modification of "atraumatic" clamp placement. In the tibial vessels, care should be taken to obtain control in the least traumatic fashion possible to limit compression of inelastic runoff vessels and the potential for clamp injury and restenosis. Alternative devices (eg, *Pruitt* occlusion catheters, *Fogarty* embolectomy catheters) may provide sufficient control to maintain a hemostatic field during completion of the distal anastomosis without exerting undue tension on the target vessel. As previously mentioned, strategic use of proximal thigh tourniquets and Esmarch bandage, deployed following creation of the proximal anastomosis and graft tunneling, may also be useful in minimizing bleeding and the risk of clamp injury in diseased tibial vessels.
- Distal embolization: Most frequently, periprocedural embolization is due to fragmentation of atherosclerotic plaque fragments or thrombus during dissection or clamping. Full systemic anticoagulation with intravenous heparin prior to clamping the vessel and intraoperative monitoring of activated clotting time will minimize the risk of graft or native vessel thrombosis. Prior to closure of arteriotomy and clamp release, all involved arteries must be meticulously back-bled and flushed to remove residual thrombus or loosen plaque fragments. Attention to this portion of the procedure, as well as to the precise course of graft tunneling, will optimize outcome and eliminate the need for revisions at the end of a long procedure.
- Nerve injury: Nerves and vessels are often intimately associated. Nerve injury can be caused by surgical dissection, a poorly placed self-retaining retractor, aggressive

spreading and clamp placement, and thermal energy from diathermy. These injuries can be prevented via intimate knowledge of appropriate anatomic landmarks, accurate incision placement, and meticulous sharp dissection. Importantly, excessively deep placement of self-retaining retractors during CFA/PFA exposure can result in substantial traction injuries to motor branches of the femoral nerve, significantly limiting the ability of patients to stand or bear weight for weeks following the procedure. As a general rule, retractors should be placed in the most superficial plane possible to obtain sufficient exposure of target vessels. All retractors should be removed as soon as they are no longer needed, or if attention is turned to alternative sites or other portions of the procedure that do not require continuous exposure.

- Lymphatic injury: Lymphatic vessels usually course close to the arteries and veins. Any visible lymphatic vessels should be suture ligated. Cautery may be used to the divided end of lymphatic channels. Careful dissection respecting tissue planes allows layered closure to eliminate dead space and lymphatic accumulation, formation of seroma, or hematoma. Lymph nodes should not be transected. When lymph nodes are inadvertently injured, extra time should be taken to control, ligate, and divide afferent and efferent vessels and remove the node completely.

REFERENCES

1. Norgren L, Hiatt WR, Dormandy JA, et al. Inter-society consensus for the management of peripheral arterial disease (TASC II). *J Vasc Surg*. 2007;45(suppl S):S5-S67.
2. Mills JL. Infrainguinal bypass. In: Cronenwett JL, Johnston KW, Rutherford RB, eds. *Rutherford's Vascular Surgery*. 7th ed. Saunders/Elsevier; 2010:1682-1703.
3. London NJM. Surgical intervention for lower extremity arterial occlusive disease: femoropopliteal and tibial interventions. In: Hallett JW, Mills JL, Earnshaw J, et al, eds. *Comprehensive Vascular and Endovascular Surgery*. 2nd ed. Mosby, Inc; 2009:192-214.
4. Netter FH. *Atlas of Human Anatomy*. 5th ed. Saunders/Elsevier; 2010.
5. Ouriel K, Rutherford RB. *Atlas of Vascular Surgery: Operative Procedures*. Saunders; 1998.
6. Rohen JW, Yokochi C, Lutjen-Drecoli E. *Color Atlas of Anatomy: A Photographic Study of the Human Body*. 7th ed. Lippincott Williams & Wilkins; 2011.
7. Zarins CK, Gewertz BL. *Atlas of Vascular Surgery*. Churchill Livingstone; 1989.
8. Mills JL, ed. *Management of Chronic Lower Limb Ischemia*. Arnold Publishing Inc and Oxford University Press; 2000.
9. Mills JL, Lucas LC. Reversed vein bypass grafts to popliteal, tibial and peroneal arteries. In: Fischer JE, ed. *Mastery of Surgery*. 6th ed. Lippincott Williams & Wilkins; 2012.
10. Efficacy of oral anticoagulants compared with aspirin after infrainguinal bypass surgery (The Dutch Bypass Oral Anticoagulants or Aspirin Study): a randomised trial. *Lancet*. 2000;355(9201):346-351.

Chapter 26

Management of the Infected Femoral Graft

Alyssa Jaesun Pyun and Vincent Lopez Rowe

DEFINITION

- Early prosthetic graft infection: <4 months, often hospital acquired, more virulent, associated with more severe presentation
- Late prosthetic graft infection: >4 months, often low virulence (eg, *Staphylococcus epidermidis*)
- Szilagyi Classification (postoperative wound infection)
  - Grade I: cellulitis
  - Grade II: extend into subcutaneous tissue
  - Grade III: involving vascular prosthesis

PATIENT HISTORY AND PHYSICAL FINDINGS

- The symptoms of an infected femoral graft can vary widely, from a chronically draining wound to sepsis and hemodynamic collapse.
- Symptoms may have been present from hours to weeks.
- Infections are more likely to occur when bypass grafts are implanted emergently or required prolonged operative times.
- Physical examination should include inspection of the surgical wounds and graft tunnels for induration, erythema, tenderness, open wounds, aneurysmal degeneration of the graft or anastomosis, or drainage.

IMAGING AND OTHER DIAGNOSTIC STUDIES

- When possible, causative organisms should be identified prior to surgery to aid in choosing appropriate systemic antibiotics and the optimal surgical approach. Surface culture swabs may result in false negatives, especially for low-virulent organisms with low numbers and slow growth not penetrating the perigraft tissue.
- Positive blood cultures are uncommon and laboratory testing may be normal, especially in late appearing low-virulent perigraft infections.
- Duplex ultrasonography is often the first imaging study obtained as it can be performed quickly, can demonstrate graft patency, and can differentiate anastomotic pseudoaneurysms, hematomas, seromas/fluid collections, and solid tissue masses. Duplex ultrasonography can also help define the tissue planes involved and proximity to the underlying bypass graft.
- Prior to surgery, detailed imaging with computed tomographic angiography (CTA) can provide critical information for developing a cohesive plan for surgical exploration with graft removal and replacement.
- CT can accurately identify anatomic signs of infection including loss of normal tissue planes, soft tissue gas, and presence of fluid collections/abscesses or anastomotic pseudoaneurysms.
- CTA provides high-resolution imaging of the aorta and run-off vessels, which will aid in determining revascularization options, including in situ reconstruction, obturator bypass, or ilioprofunda bypass.
- Radionuclide scans may provide evidence for graft infection when other imaging studies are nondiagnostic; however, this may result in false positives in the early postoperative period due to nonspecific uptake of healing perigraft tissue.

SURGICAL MANAGEMENT

- Aggressive and wide debridement of devitalized or infected tissue must accompany graft excision and replacement in the setting of infection. This may require multiple/staged debridements.
- Partial or complete excision of infected prosthetic grafts is generally required to eliminate the infection.
- Excision of infected autogenous graft infections may be necessary when associated with sepsis caused by *Escherichia coli*, *Pseudomonas*, or *Proteus* spp.
- Graft preservation with local debridement may be considered when low-virulent infections of shorter graft segments do not include the anastomoses and are limited to the immediate perigraft area. We recommend against graft preservation with virulent organisms such as *Pseudomonas*, *Serratia*, *methicillin-resistant Staphylococcus aureus*, and *E. coli*.
- Thrombosed grafts with adequate collateral circulation may tolerate excision without reconstruction.
- Graft excision and extra-anatomic bypass is preferred in the presence of severe sepsis and/or hemorrhage. Examples of extra-anatomic bypasses include axillary-to-femoral bypass (**FIGURE 1**), obturator bypass, or cross-femoral bypass.

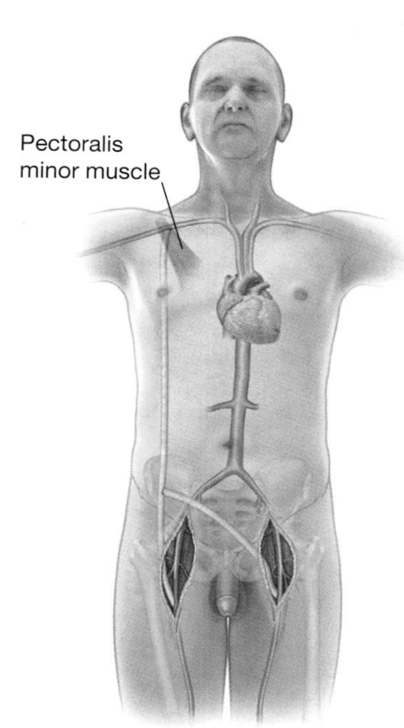

FIGURE 1 ● Axillofemoral bypass. Note that the proximal graft is placed behind the pectoralis minor muscle.

- In situ replacement is generally preferred in low-virulent infections without sepsis or invasive infection and in those with distal occlusive disease.
- There continues to be a limited role for endovascular therapy in the setting of femoral graft infections; however, it has been described in rare circumstances.[1]
- Potential options for replacement graft material include autogenous vein (saphenous, cephalic, basilic, or superficial femoral vein [SFV]), cryopreserved tissue (aorto-iliac-femoral artery, femoral vein, saphenous vein),[2] or antibiotic-impregnated prosthetic graft (rifampin-soaked Dacron or polytetrafluoroethylene [PTFE]).
- Debridement of an infected groin wound may result in a large defect that either cannot be covered or closed. Muscle flaps can provide coverage of healthy well-vascularized tissue to protect the repair.
- Small to medium defects can be covered with a sartorius muscle flap, which is divided from its attachment to the anterior superior iliac spine and mobilized medially to cover the wound.
- A pedicled flap from the leg or abdominal wall may be required for larger wounds. These flaps may utilize the rectus femoris, rectus abdominis, tensor fasciae latae, or gracilis.[3-5]
- Negative pressure wound therapy can be considered with adequate tissue coverage over the bypass graft.

GENERAL CONSIDERATIONS

- It is preferable when considering an extra-anatomic reconstruction to revascularize before excising the infected graft. This can be accomplished with a bypass and tunnel performed across clean tissue planes. Once the bypass is completed and wounds closed, the groin can be explored and the infected graft removed. With this approach, the continuity between the superficial femoral and deep femoral arteries should be maintained by either oversewing the distal common femoral artery or anastomosing the profunda femoris artery (PFA) to the superficial femoral artery with proximal ligation (**FIGURE 2**).
- Debridement of the infected site should include removal of infected or necrotic tissue and complete excision of the anastomosis. Dissection may be aided by lack of incorporation of the infected graft but also may prove challenging due to the extensive scarring in the reoperative field. Sharp dissection techniques are critical for minimizing the risk of inadvertent injury to vessels or adjacent structures.
- Other measures such as the use of antibiotic-loaded beads and pulse lavage irrigation can be used as adjunctive measures for wound sterilization.[6,7]
- It is important to send cultures of the perigraft fluid, tissue, and graft.[8] Instructions can be given to the microbiology lab to perform sonication of the graft to separate biofilm from graft and maximize the bacteriology yield.

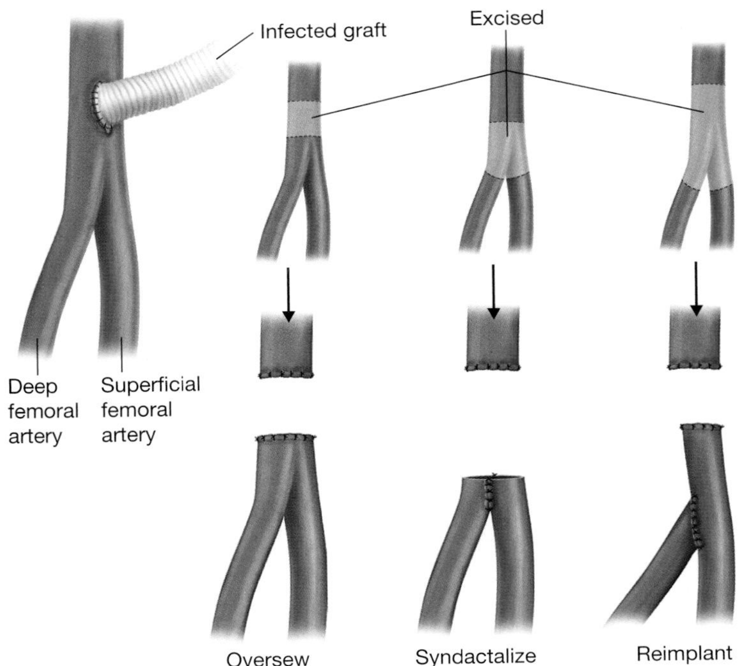

FIGURE 2 ● Surgical options for maintaining continuity of arterial flow to the profunda femoris artery after obturator bypass and common femoral artery ligation.

OBTURATOR BYPASS

- Using the obturator foramen may be a useful approach for bypassing an infected groin through a sterile field.[9-11] A reinforced PTFE graft is preferred and can be used if sepsis has been controlled and the bypass can be performed without violating the infected field.
- The proximal anastomosis can be performed to the common iliac artery, external iliac artery (ipsilateral or contralateral), or previous graft if not infected (**FIGURE 3**). Exposure can be obtained through a standard retroperitoneal incision, by dividing the external and internal oblique and transversus abdominis muscles, identifying the preperitoneal space, and retracting the peritoneum medially with blunt dissection techniques. The obturator foramen is just posterior to the anterior ramus of the pelvis, although it may not be easily palpated due to the overlying obturator membrane.
- The distal anastomosis can be performed to the distal superficial femoral artery, the midportion of the PFA (see the following section, lateral approach to the Lateral Profunda Femoris Artery Exposure), or the popliteal artery. During this dissection, the adductor longus and magnus can be identified with the leg abducted and externally rotated. The tunnel will be placed deep to these muscles, which insert on the external surface of the obturator foramen.
- The tunnel should be performed in a cranial direction with a long aortic clamp or tunneling instrument (**FIGURE 4**). The instrument is passed deep to the adductor magnus while a hand is placed over the obturator foramen from the retroperitoneal incision. The instrument can be directed through the obturator foramen. The tunnel should be made through the anteriomedial portion of the obturator foramen to avoid injury to the obturator artery and nerve, which traverses laterally.
- Once the tunnel is made, the graft can be placed and the bypass performed. Once completed, the incisions should be closed and protected before proceeding with excision of the infected graft.

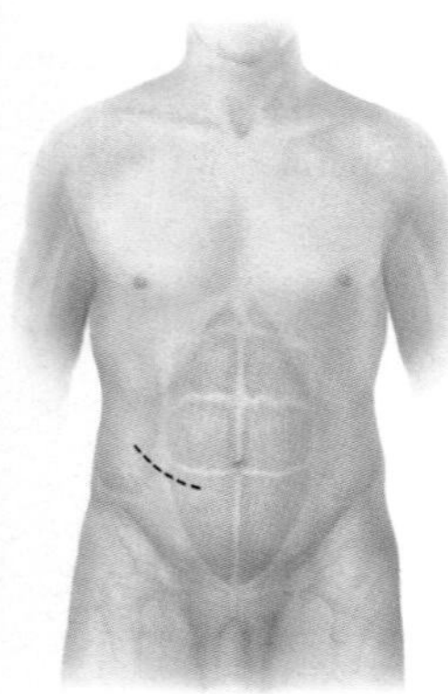

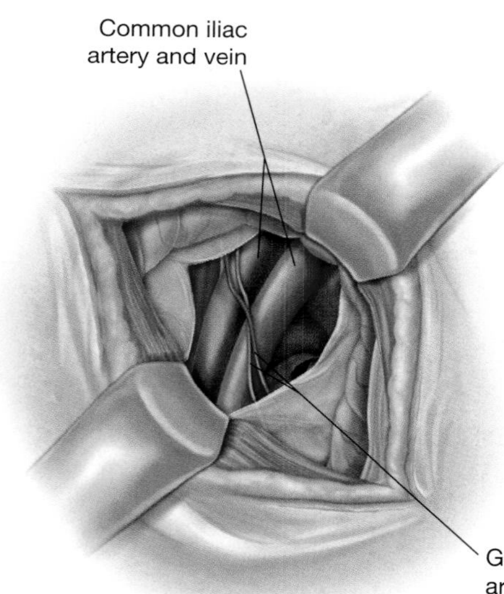

FIGURE 3 ● Operative incision for retroperitoneal exposure of the iliac artery. Peritoneum and its contents are retracted medially to aid in exposure.

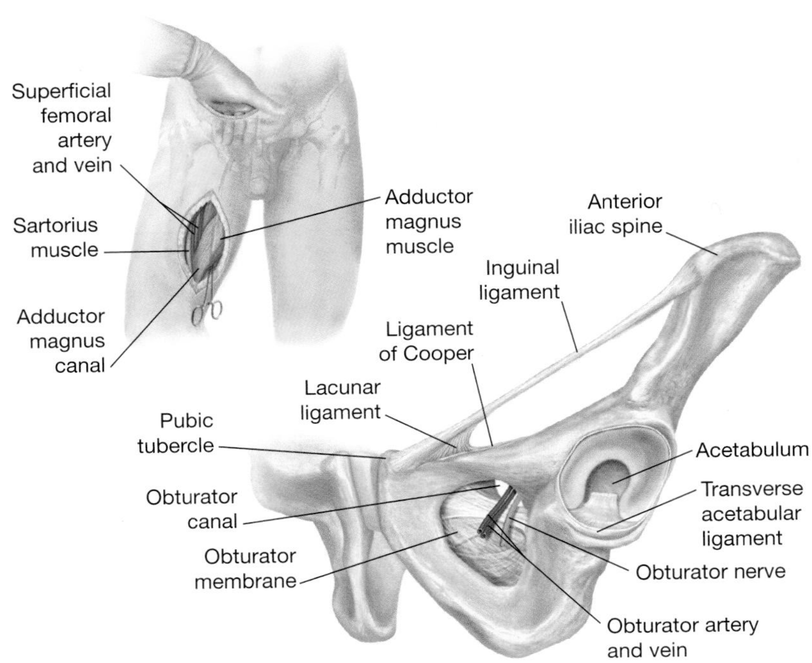

FIGURE 4 • Exposure of the superficial femoral artery and tunneling for an obturator bypass. **Left:** creating the tunnel behind the adductor magnus muscle. **Right:** placement of the tunnel through the obturator membrane.

LATERAL FEMORAL BYPASS

- The lateral femoral bypass allows for tunneling lateral to the infected field.
- A retroperitoneal approach allows for inflow vessel exposure and anastomosis. The graft is then tunneled medial to the anterior iliac spine and under the inguinal ligament through the psoas canal before continuing anterolaterally, coursing lateral to the femoral nerve subcutaneously to the outflow vessel for distal anastomosis.[12]

LATERAL PROFUNDA FEMORIS ARTERY EXPOSURE

- Another option for remote revascularization is to use the second portion of the PFA, exposed through a lateral incision.[13] This approach may be useful if the superficial femoral artery is occluded and the goal is to establish flow from the axillary artery via a tunnel medial to the anterior iliac spine and lateral to the femoral infection.
- The PFA is exposed through an incision placed along the lateral border of the sartorius muscle 4 to 6 cm below the anterior superior iliac spine (**FIGURE 5**). The sartorius and superficial femoral vessels can be retracted medially to expose the adductor longus. Its overlying fascia is divided, and with medial retraction, the PFA is exposed.

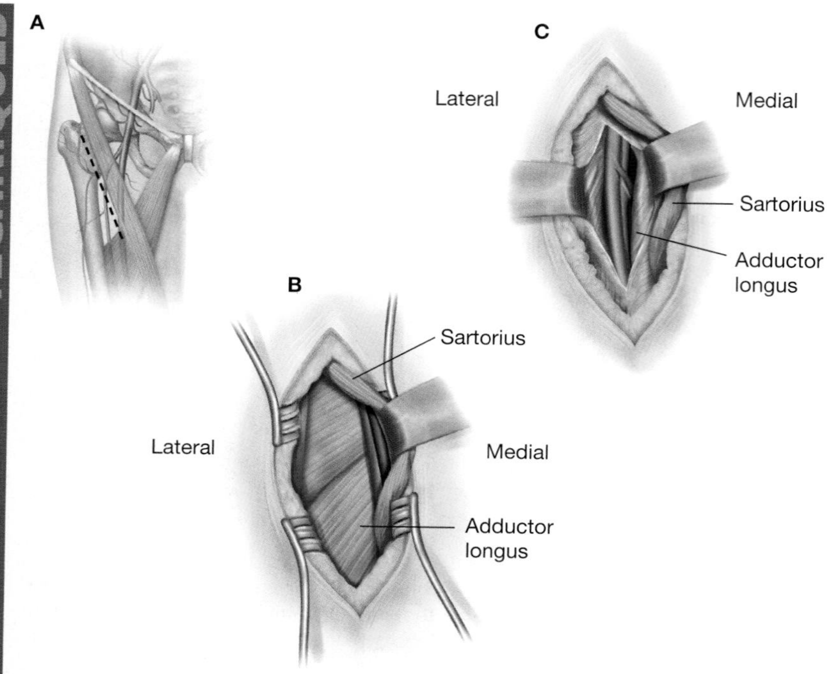

FIGURE 5 ● Lateral exposure of the profunda femoris artery. **A,** Incision along the lateral border of the sartorius muscle. **B,** Medial retraction of the superficial femoral artery and vein to expose the adductor longus. **C,** Fascial incision and medial retraction of the adductor longus to expose the profunda femoris vessels.

SUPERFICIAL FEMORAL VEIN HARVEST

- SFV can be a suitable graft for reconstruction, with a low incidence of recurrent or uncontrolled infection.[14] Preoperative evaluation should include duplex imaging of the SFV to exclude deep venous thrombosis and to determine the vessel diameter.
- Dissection can be performed through a standard anteromedial leg incision or placed over the lateral border of the sartorius (**FIGURE 6**). The vein should be dissected from its confluence with the profunda femoris vein distally to obtain sufficient length for reconstruction. Care should be taken to preserve the profunda femoris vein and the common femoral vein. The dissection can be continued distally through the adductor canal if an extensive segment of vein is required for reconstruction.
- Once harvested, branches of the SFV should be doubly ligated or suture ligated a distance 2 mm from their junction with the SFV to prevent slippage of the ligature once the conduit is pressurized.

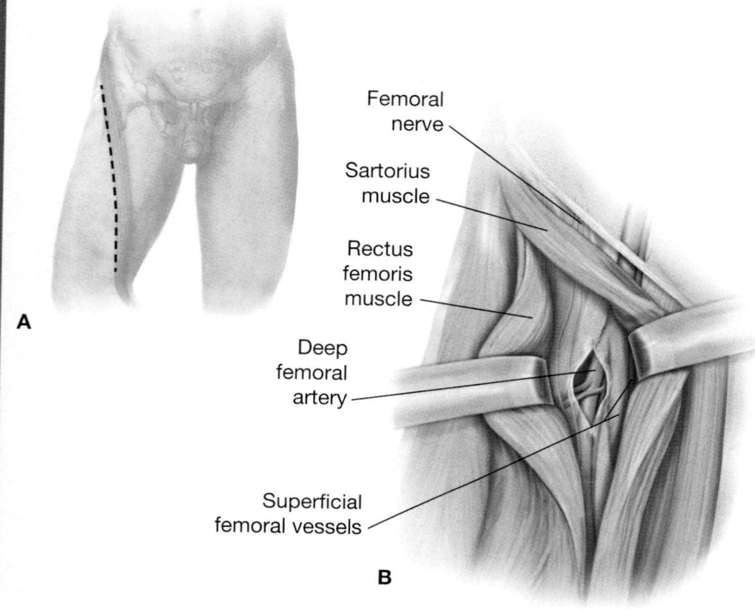

FIGURE 6 ● Exposure of the superficial femoral vein. **A,** Incision along the sartorius muscle. **B,** medial retraction of the sartorius to expose the superficial femoral vein.

CRYOPRESERVED GRAFTS

- Some studies have shown favorable results for cryopreserved allografts with regard to limb loss, recurrent infection, and survival compared with other in situ replacements.[15]
- When considering an allograft, greater than 24 hours may be required to locate suitable graft material and length if there is no on-site inventory.
- Grafts should be prepared immediately before implantation. The thaw-and-rinse process takes approximately 45 minutes.
- Ligated branches should be tested for hemostasis and suture ligatures placed if necessary. Antibiotic-impregnated fibrin glue may be considered at suture lines. If using an aortoiliac homograft, it is easier to confirm hemostasis if the graft is placed with the lumbar branches facing anterior.
- Graft length should allow for a tension-free anastomosis. When possible, avoid allograft-to-allograft anastomoses.

PROFUNDA TO SUPERFICIAL FEMORAL ARTERY TRANSPOSITION

- Alternatively, in scenarios of significant common femoral artery interruption with gross infection and no suitable conduits available, a profunda to superficial femoral artery transposition can be done.
- Femoral artery exposure with common femoral, profunda, and superficial femoral artery control should be obtained, followed by sufficient profunda and superficial femoral artery mobilization to minimize tension while avoiding redundancy/kinking. After suture ligation of the common femoral artery, an end-to-side or end-to-end anastomosis of the profunda and superficial femoral artery can be done to maintain distal perfusion (**FIGURE 2**). In theory, by maintaining the continuity of the femoral bifurcation, the collaterals from the profunda femoral artery are allowed back into the axial circulation earlier, as opposed to through the small collateral networks around the knee.

PEARLS AND PITFALLS

Preoperative considerations	■ When possible, consideration should be made prior to surgery for the best option(s) of graft material, allowing time to obtain it if required. For autogenous vein, preoperative duplex is essential to determine the size and quality of the proposed conduit.
Proximal and distal vessel control	■ When possible, proximal and distal vessel control should be obtained through extension of the original incision or through separate incisions before dissecting the infected vessels. Remote bypass with subsequent removal of infected material may be preferable to in situ repair.
Intraoperative cultures	■ It is important to obtain Gram stain, aerobic, and anaerobic cultures of the perigraft fluid, perigraft tissue, and graft. The yield of the graft will be increased if sonication of the graft is performed in the microbiology lab prior to incubation.
Tunnels	■ Tunnels, when possible, should be placed in sterile fields.
Systemic antibiotic treatment	■ Broad-spectrum antibiotics should be initially considered for patients with severe sepsis. For those without sepsis, blood and wound cultures should be performed prior to starting antibiotics. Initial antibiotics should include coverage for methicillin-resistant *Staphylococcus aureus* (MRSA). After surgery, parenteral antibiotics should be considered for 2-6 weeks, especially for invasive infections or in situ repair.

POSTOPERATIVE CARE

- Antibiotics should be continued for at least 2 to 6 weeks, depending on the type of organism, and should be chosen based on antimicrobial sensitivity when available.
- Patients should be inspected daily for signs of infection, which may include fever, leukocytosis, erythema or drainage from the wound, or wound breakdown. Persistent infection should trigger consideration of wound exploration and reevaluation of the antibiotic regimen.
- Drains, if placed, should be removed as soon as possible, based on quantity and appearance of fluid. Ongoing purulent drainage or continued fever and leukocytosis may indicate lack of source control, which may require wound exploration and washout.
- Arterial surveillance should be performed prior to discharge to confirm the integrity of the repair and establish a baseline for future surveillance examinations.

COMPLICATIONS

- Bleeding from the wound should raise immediate concern for arterial disruption from persistent infection leading to tissue destruction. If present, patients should undergo arterial duplex and be considered for re-exploration. Under these circumstances, complete evaluation of the arterial reconstruction (even if remote) is advisable as vascular resection and reconstruction may be required. At times, arterial ligation may be the only option for local control of sepsis.

- If not already performed, patients requiring re-exploration and debridement for persistent infection will most often benefit from muscle flap coverage of the defect.

REFERENCES

1. Naddaf A, Hasanadka R, Hood D, Hodgson K. Repair of an anastomotic pseudoaneurysm with a novel hybrid technique. *Ann Vasc Surg*. 2020;63:439-442.
2. Furlough CL, Jain AK, Ho KJ, Rodriguez HE, Tomita TM, Eskandari MK. Peripheral artery reconstructions using cryopreserved arterial allografts in infected fields. *J Vasc Surg*. 2019;70(2):562-568.
3. Ryer EJ, Garvin RP, Kapadia RN, et al. Outcome of rectus femoris muscle flaps performed by vascular surgeons for the management of complex groin wounds after femoral artery reconstructions. *J Vasc Surg*. 2020;71(3):905-911.
4. Ali AT, Rueda M, Desikan S, et al. Outcomes after retroflexed gracilis muscle flap for vascular infections in the groin. *J Vasc Surg*. 2016;64(2):452-457.
5. Dua A, Rothenberg KA, Lavingia K, Ho VT, Rao C, Desai SS. Outcomes of gracilis muscle flaps in the management of groin complications after arterial bypass with prosthetic graft. *Ann Vasc Surg*. 2018;51:113-118.
6. Stone PA, Armstrong PA, Bandyk DF, et al. Use of antibiotic-loaded polymethylmethacrylate beads for the treatment of extracavitary prosthetic vascular graft infections. *J Vasc Surg*. 2006;44(4):757-761.
7. Mote GA, Malay DS. Efficacy of power-pulsed lavage in lower extremity wound infections: a prospective observational study. *J Foot Ankle Surg*. 2010;49(2):135-142.
8. Bandyk DF, Bergamini TM, Kinney EV, et al. In situ replacement of vascular prostheses infected by bacterial biofilms. *J Vasc Surg*. 1991;13(5):575-583.
9. Pearce WH, Ricco JB, Yao JS, et al. Modified technique of obturator bypass in failed or infected grafts. *Ann Surg*. 1983;197(3):344-347.
10. Bath J, Rahimi M, Long B, Avgerinos E, Giglia J. Clinical outcomes of obturator canal bypass. *J Vasc Surg*. 2017;66(1):160-166.
11. Dunphy KM, Hassey J, Vallabjaneni R, et al. Results of obturator foramen bypass in patients with groin infection and arterial involvement. *Ann Vasc Surg*. 2021;S0890-5096(21):00202-00208.
12. Madden NJ, Calligaro KD, Dougherty MJ, Zheng H, Troutman DA. Lateral femoral bypass for prosthetic arterial graft infections in the groin. *J Vasc Surg*. 2019;69(4):1129-1136.
13. Bridges R, Gewertz BL. Lateral incision for exposure of femoral vessels. *Surg Gynecol Obstet*. 1980;150(5):732-733.
14. Smith ST, Clagett GP. Femoral vein harvest for vascular reconstructions: pitfalls and tips for success. *Semin Vasc Surg*. 2008;21(1):35-40.
15. Kieffer E, Gomes D, Chiche L, et al. Allograft replacement for infrarenal aortic graft infection: early and late results in 179 patients. *J Vasc Surg*. 2004;39(5):1009-1017.

Chapter 27

Femoral Pseudoaneurysm Management: Open and Endovascular

Joseph Patrick Hart

DEFINITION

- Common femoral aneurysms are either true aneurysms or pseudoaneurysms and are usually chronic. True aneurysms are typically either degenerative or due to familial or genetic disease. Pseudoaneurysms differ in that not all the arterial wall layers are typically involved, and they are most often acute. The name pseudoaneurysm indicates an aneurysm wall consisting only of connective tissue histologically similar to the adventitia.
- Femoral pseudoaneurysms are a common reason for urgent or emergent vascular surgery inpatient consultation that usually arise from transfemoral vascular access with or without iatrogenic procedural and periprocedural mishaps. Active pseudoaneurysms contain a nonthrombosed or partially thrombosed area of extravascular flow. This chapter focuses on the treatment of pseudoaneurysms of the femoral artery and bifurcation.
- Consultation for femoral pseudoaneurysms (PSAs) remains common due to increasing utilization of endovascular access as well as the use of larger devices. Closure devices have become routine and have led to earlier discharge and mobilization times; however, closure devices can cause their own set of possible complications, including concomitant dissection, back wall to front wall closure, vessel occlusion, distal embolization, and infection. These concerns should inform the approach to any patient with PSA after closure device use.

DIFFERENTIAL DIAGNOSIS

- If concern for femoral PSA arises, a mass may be present anterior to the femoral artery, which may or may not be pulsatile. It is generally considered most appropriate to obtain an early directed vascular ultrasound whenever suspicion arises.
- The differential diagnosis includes:
  - Periprocedural hematoma without pseudoaneurysm
  - Femoral arterial to venous fistula
  - Lymphadenopathy
  - Seroma
  - Abscess
- An isolated iatrogenic arteriovenous fistula (AVF) will often have a palpable thrill or audible bruit and may present with limb swelling. This can coexist with a femoral PSA. A firm groin mass can be either a hematoma or thrombosed pseudoaneurysm or could represent groin lymphadenopathy from a variety of causes. An abscess or seroma typically presents with a softer mass in the groin, with or without overlying cellulitis. Simple duplex ultrasound can often confirm the diagnosis when a groin mass is discovered on physical examination.

PATIENT HISTORY AND PHYSICAL FINDINGS

- Patients with femoral PSA often present with history of recent cardiac catheterization, peripheral angiography or intervention, endovascular graft placement, intracardiac device placement, extracorporeal life support (ECMO) use, or any other procedure via a transfemoral arterial access.
- Closure device use is an essential historical point to elucidate as the presence of a closure device may change the spectrum of anticipated concomitant findings and proposed repair.
- Many patients who develop PSA after arterial access are on aggressive perioperative antiplatelet and anticoagulation regimens, which increase their risk for PSA formation. These may not be able to be discontinued, depending on the procedure performed or devices placed (eg, drug-eluting devices).
- Multiple femoral accesses, previous open common femoral surgery, prosthetic patch graft or adjacent stent deployments, radiation, or other historical factors are important details to determine in the patient's history.
- Morbid obesity is an important risk factor, history element, and potentially complicating perioperative/-interventional factor.
- Some patients report a sudden popping sensation preceding groin mass formation. Not infrequently, an episode of straining or lifting just precedes complaints of PSA formation.
- Physical examination of PSA can vary from obvious and quite striking to relatively benign and occult. Tenderness anterior to the common femoral artery on the side of access is common, and concomitant ecchymosis and hematoma is often noted. A pulsatile mass on the side of the access is often appreciated if the femoral artery pseudoaneurysm is patent. A bruit may be audible and may be due to PSA, or concomitant AVF, stenosis, or dissection.
- The ipsilateral limb should be examined carefully for distal perfusion, and pulse examination should be documented. The contralateral limb distal vascular examination is also important as the status of distal perfusion is critical. If pulses are not palpable, the status of Doppler signals should be assessed and documented bilaterally.
- Skin viability over the PSA should be assessed. If the pseudoaneurysm or pseudoaneurysm and hematoma in combination have led to so-called shiny skin or otherwise evident compromised skin perfusion, expeditious and most likely open surgical management will be necessary.
- Hemoglobin concentration may be decreased, especially if there is a concomitant large groin or retroperitoneal hematoma.
- Patients with hemodynamic instability or requiring ongoing transfusion should undergo rapid assessment with stabilization and may then require expedited treatment.

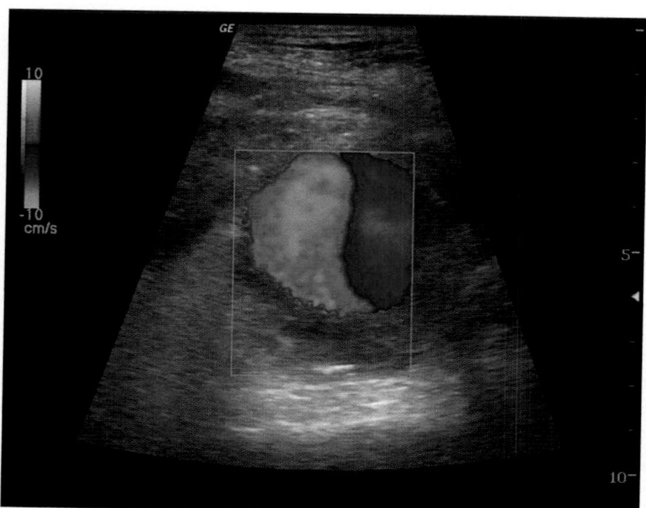

FIGURE 1 ● Duplex ultrasound of CFA with pathognomonic finding of arterial pseudoaneurysm.

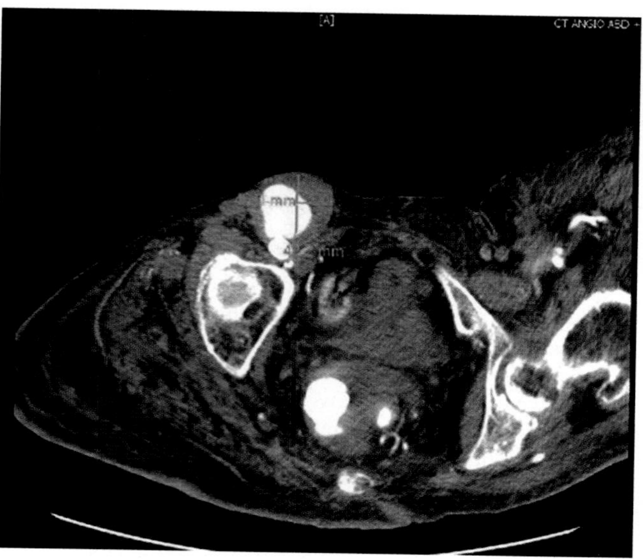

FIGURE 2 ● CT angiography of pelvis with finding of arterial pseudoaneurysm.

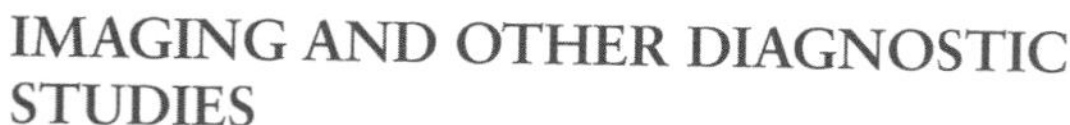

IMAGING AND OTHER DIAGNOSTIC STUDIES

- Imaging to confirm or exclude groin PSA is usually initiated by a screening duplex ultrasound (**FIGURE 1**). This will often confirm the diagnosis and may be all the imaging necessary prior to attempting repair. Typical and pathognomonic bicolor signal within the pseudoaneurysm cavity makes the diagnosis. In addition, ultrasound can provide confirmation of the length and dimensions of the pseudoaneurysm neck, which is critical to confirming suitability for thrombin injection to treat noninvasively.
- Other potential findings on ultrasound can include AVF, femoral or common femoral deep venous thrombosis, additional technical problems within the common femoral artery (CFA) lumen, existing occlusive disease, arterial thrombosis, hematoma, seroma, or other problems.
- CT angiography (CTA), contrasted or even noncontrast CT, magnetic resonance angiography all may detect a groin pseudoaneurysm in various clinical scenarios. If malperfusion is detected on physical examination, CTA is indicated to confirm or exclude distal embolization, femoral artery bifurcation or other related vessel thromboses, chronic occlusive disease, and/or steal (**FIGURE 2**).
- While CTA can be omitted from the workup in many cases, it may be helpful to establish the runoff status below the pseudoaneurysm, as well provide information regarding inflow and surrounding anatomy.
- Catheter angiography may be a useful adjunct to either thrombin injection or, in some cases, even operative repair.

NONOPERATIVE MANAGEMENT

- Importantly, under a certain threshold size, PSAs are likely to thrombose spontaneously. Observation with serial weekly ultrasound follow-up is indicated in those patients with PSAs under 2 cm, with no associated skin compromise or infection.[1] Repeat ultrasound often will demonstrate occlusion of the PSA after 1 to 2 weeks, obviating any need for intervention. If the patient is maintained on anticoagulation the PSA is less likely to occlude without assistance.
- Ultrasound-guided compression is a potentially successful, although tedious, approach that accelerates otherwise spontaneous closure in some patients. This approach is undertaken by the ultrasound tech. The femoral vessels and the PSA neck is visualized. Ultrasound-guided compression is held to occlude flow through the neck but allow flow through the femoral vessels. This is held for 15 to 30 minutes, and the flow in the PSA is evaluated. Repeat pressure can be applied if partial occlusion is observed. This technique can be very uncomfortable for the patient and may require sedation. If the patient is maintained on anticoagulation, this technique is not likely to be successful, and this technique is generally reserved for those PSAs that are smaller. We typically reserve ultrasound-guided compression for those PSAs that are less than 2 cm but are not candidates for observation only.[1]

ENDOVASCULAR APPROACH

- Endovascular management is the most common approach to femoral PSA today. With its less invasive approach without the need for a formal open incision, thrombin injection remains the workhorse of femoral PSA treatment.
- After a femoral PSA is identified by duplex ultrasound, neck length and width must be evaluated carefully and confirmed to be greater than or equal to 10 mm long and less than 5 mm wide.[2]
- In PSAs that do not have otherwise acceptable necks, some can still be salvaged for endovascular management by use of endoluminal angioplasty balloon protection, usually from a contralateral approach to protect against distal embolization of thrombin, when a neck of more conventional dimensions for unprotected thrombin injection is not present.

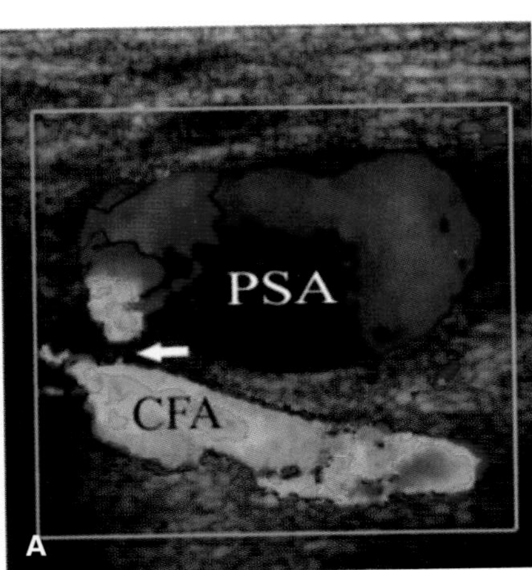

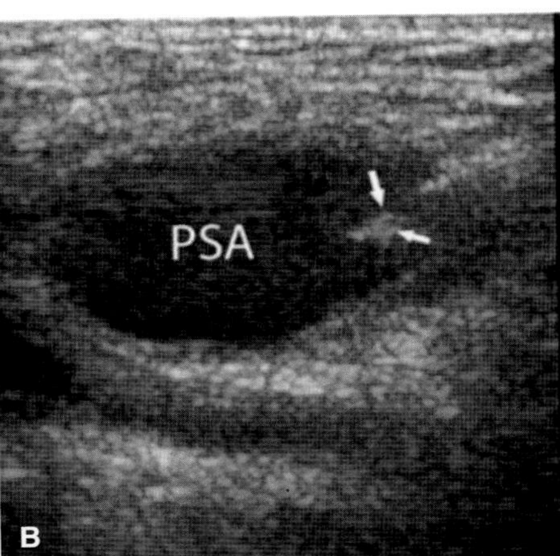

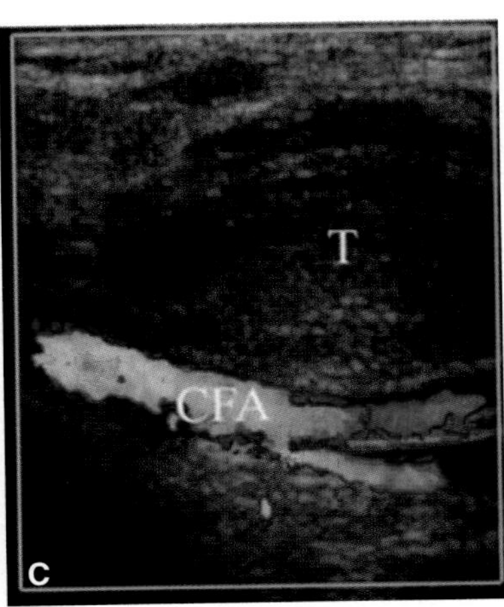

FIGURE 3 ● Duplex ultrasound of CFA with **(A)** arterial pseudoaneurysm (arrow indicates PSA neck), **(B)** needle tip for thrombin injection (arrow indicates needle tip), and **(C)** thrombotic pseudoaneurysm occlusion with preservation of native vessel luminal flow.

- Following prep and drape and a time out, an appropriately prepped and draped ultrasound probe is used to confirm the presence of the pseudoaneurysm again and that spontaneous thrombosis has not occurred. Neck length and width are quickly generally confirmed.
- A micropuncture needle on an injection system using extension tubing and a three-way stopcock is placed under ultrasound guidance into the PSA sac. Agitated saline without thrombin is then injected to confirm luminal access to the PSA (**FIGURE 3**). (Alternatively, an etched EchoTip micropuncture needle can also provide direct evidence of correct needle position.)
- After this is confirmed by a swirling pattern on grayscale duplex (or etched tip needle use), thrombin can be injected while maintaining meticulous attention to awareness of needle tip position. An initial injection of as little as 0.1 mL of a 1000 U/mL thrombin solution is used, and ultrasound visualization of the PSA is maintained.[3] Use of a total dose greater than 1.0 mL of such a solution should not be necessary in most moderate-sized PSAs. Thrombosis of the PSA is visualized, usually almost immediately, upon thrombin injection. Continuous duplex monitoring is used during extremely slow and measured injection to look for increased echogenicity and/or loss of color flow indicating PSA thrombosis.
- Avoiding overinjection and treatment beyond the PSA or its neck into the CFA is most critical and necessitates excellent on-field ultrasound imaging guidance and highly coordinated, stable injection technique.
- Ultrasound is then used to confirm complete thrombosis during the index procedure. Visualization of appropriate thrombosis of the pseudoaneurysm lumen by grayscale as well as elimination of color flow within the pseudoaneurysm with preservation of flow within the arterial lumen are confirmed and documented.
- Critically, those attempting thrombin injection should be prepared to perform rescue thrombus aspiration or other catheter-directed intervention should there be distal thrombin embolization.
- Most vascular surgeons perform a follow-up duplex ultrasound to confirm pseudoaneurysm thrombosis and exclude the need for retreatment or further observation at 24 to 48 hours post procedure.

SURGICAL MANAGEMENT

- Surgical management first mandates orderly control of inflow and outflow. PSA having surgical repair will usually be larger, present with one of the other complications outlined above, and occur in patients who have failed, or were not a candidate for, ultrasound-guided compression or thrombin injection.
- The first step is to obtain proximal control. Given the common femoral PSA proximity to the inguinal ligament in many cases, this raises specific challenges with regards to proximal control. In patients with adequate distance above the pseudoaneurysm, relatively high exposure of the common femoral from the groin can be accomplished. In this case, a longitudinal incision is made over the femoral vessels and, in the most proximal aspect, carried down to the femoral artery at the level of the inguinal ligament. Care must be taken to avoid entrance into the pseudoaneurysm itself. Circumferential control is obtained, and a vessel loop is placed around the vessel. Extensive mobilization of the inguinal ligament to allow high external iliac control through the groin is critical if working to do the whole repair from the groin only.
- If there is not enough room proximal to the pseudoaneurysm to facilitate operative exposure of the common femoral artery, there are two choices. A separate curvilinear incision can be made above the inguinal ligament, and the retroperitoneal space can be entered after dividing the abdominal musculature and dissecting the retroperitoneal space. The distal external iliac artery can be circumferentially controlled above the inguinal ligament via this approach, which provides excellent proximal control.
- Alternatively, endovascular balloon control can be obtained from the contralateral groin or, if necessary, the arm or the ipsilateral superficial femoral artery (SFA). However, this provides another arterial access site at risk for PSA or other

complication; therefore, careful planning and execution of this access must be taken (**FIGURE 4**).

- The second step is to obtain distal control of the femoral bifurcation. This is generally done by dissecting distal from the PSA sac and getting circumferential control of both the SFA and the profunda.
- Once proximal control is obtained, distal control of the femoral bifurcation is also required.
- The third step is then to clamp both proximally and distally, typically after heparin is administered, and then directly enter the PSA sac. Further dissection of the common femoral artery is done at this point, and the arterial defect should be clearly seen. Often, the defect is small and can be repaired with one or two interrupted Prolene sutures. If the defect is large, or the edges require resection due to friable tissue, a patch angioplasty should be undertaken. In our practice, this is typically completed with bovine pericardium (**FIGURE 5**).
- However, in the setting of infection, a section of saphenous vein should be used. In the presence of a known chronically occluded SFA (and absent chronic limb threatening ischemia), the occluded SFA may be harvested (caudally away from the bifurcation) and endarterectomized to create autologous conduit with which to form a patch.
- Occasionally, despite all intentions, the PSA sac is entered directly prior to control being obtained. While clearly a secondary strategy, in this situation more formal proximal control can be obtained by one operator while another operator applies direct digital hemostasis at the femoral arteriotomy site.
- Once the arterial repair is complete, evacuation of large communicating hematomas either within the groin and thigh or retroperitoneum should be completed as necessary. Any necrotic skin should be resected. Wide drainage, careful and meticulous incision

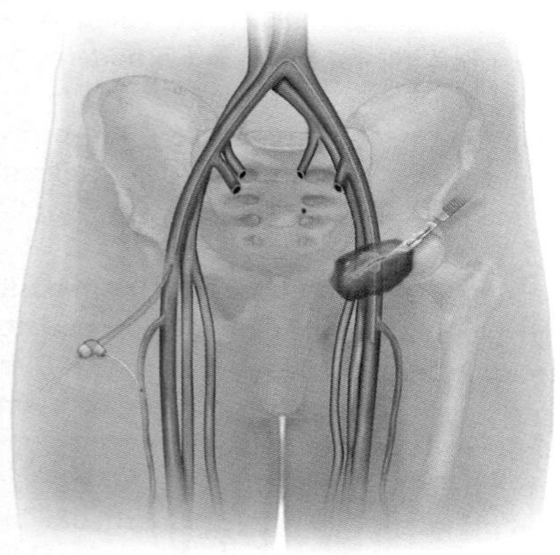

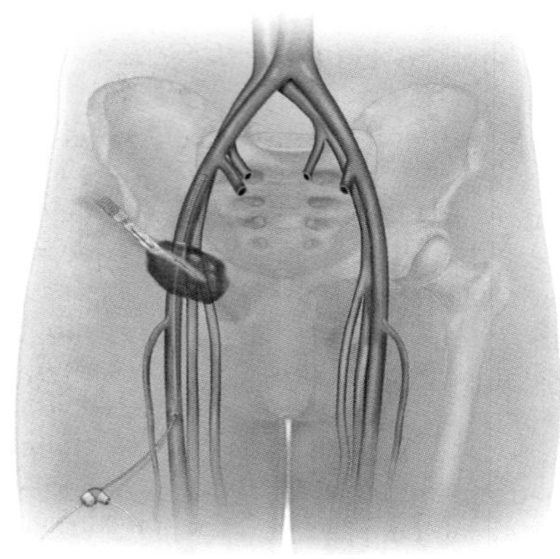

FIGURE 4 ● Strategies (contralateral CFA and ipsilateral SFA) for endovascular external iliac artery control to facilitate dissection.

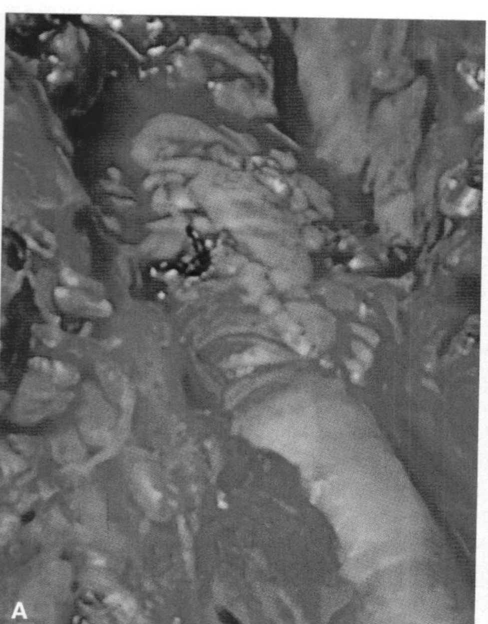

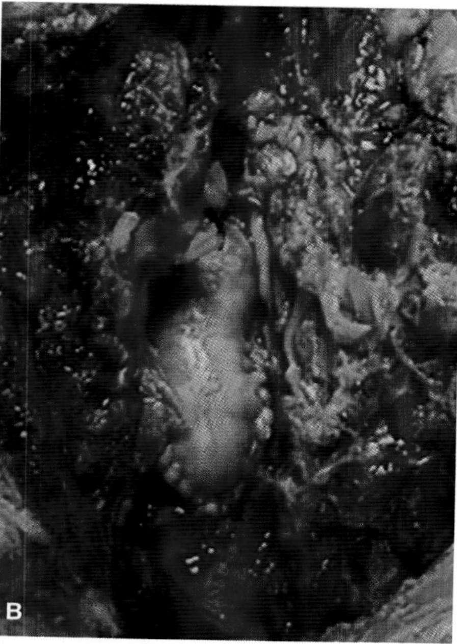

FIGURE 5 ● If primary repair is not an option, **(A)** bovine patch angioplasty and **(B)** vein patch angioplasty are options. Dacron (with Rifampin) or PTFE interposition grafting can also be considered in more severe cases.

management, delayed primary closure techniques (with a planned return to the operating room for definitive closure once infection clearance is achieved), vacuum assisted closure dressings with specialized sponges for atraumatic dressing near or directly on vascular structures, temporary antibiotic bone cement bead placement, and other steps may be considered.

- It is usually feasible to do a multilayer primary closure. However, in the event of a large soft tissue defect, it may be necessary to perform a sartorial or other muscle flap, and plastic surgery assistance for formal muscle flap or other composite closure may be necessary to achieve a satisfactory outcome.
- If primary closure is feasible, it is our practice to place drains into these wounds to prevent seroma formation. Often it is necessary to get some tissue closure over the vessels and use the vacuum-assisted closure device for the skin, when there is a skin defect due to necrosis.

PEARLS AND PITFALLS

Duplex ultrasound	■ The workhorse of femoral artery PSA diagnosis is color duplex ultrasound with a stereotypical two-color flow pattern within the PSA.
Management	■ The mainstay of active management of the iatrogenic common femoral PSA, beyond observation or ultrasound-guided compression, is thrombin injection. ■ Clinicians performing thrombin injection must be familiar with limits regarding the neck geometry, balloon protection techniques, and operative or endovascular techniques to treat luminal displacement of thrombin as needed or should distal thrombosis occur.
Operative approach	■ In the case of operative approaches, the extent of proximal control concomitant with the overall clinical situation balancing patient body habitus, adjacent disease, previous procedures, and comorbidities vs security of proximal artery inflow control is critical.
Endovascular adjuncts	■ Endovascular adjuncts to inflow control may be critical as a hybrid approach to open repair. Likewise, definitive open control of the external iliac artery either by extensive mobilization of the inguinal ligament for more proximal control or formal counter incision to access the iliac arteries in the pelvis will be needed in a subset of cases.
Open repair	■ In the case of open repair, successful operative management or even staged operative management with delayed closure is only the beginning of successful treatment. Careful management of this incision with close monitoring of skin closure both prior to discharge and follow-up as an outpatient is critical. Reoperation, management of seromas, and a need for secondary plastics coverage will be frequent in the open management group.

POSTOPERATIVE CARE

- Operative repairs, especially those in the case of infection or extensive hematoma creating dead space and or increasing risk of seroma, will require meticulous postoperative care and frequent reintervention. Re-exploration, seroma evacuation, adjuncts to achieve primary closure, and early plastic surgery consultation will be the cornerstone of successful management of wound problems.
- Finding a way to at once be both hopeful and reassuring—yet clear—with patients and families that these are risks in these cases is important from a patient satisfaction and medical-legal standpoint in this author's estimate.
- Duplex follow-up even of operative repairs is helpful to exclude seroma, technical defects, thrombosis, and other problems. If an occlusive process component was of concern, follow-up ankle brachial indexes may also be valuable.
- In most cases anticoagulation regimen will not be impacted by a successful minimal direct primary pseudoaneurysm repair. In the event of a more complex repair, antiplatelet or other medication recommendations may need tailoring to the specific patient scenario.
- Patients treated with thrombin injection or ultrasound-guided compression should be kept on strict bed rest for a minimum of 6 hours with close observation immediately following the procedure and then general bed rest with minimal necessary activity overnight. Duplex ultrasound confirmation of satisfactory thrombosis without local complication should be performed at 24 to 48 hours post injection.

COMPLICATIONS

- Complications of open repair of femoral pseudoaneurysm align closely with those of any open procedure involving the common femoral artery or its bifurcation.
- Groin wound infection, incisional dehiscence, seroma, infection, anastomotic suture line or patch dehiscence, neuropathic pain or injury, venous thrombosis or bleeding, postoperative

thrombosis or hemorrhage, chronic wound formation, biologic or prosthetic implant infection with need for removal, and other typical perioperative problems may arise.

- Multiple complicating comorbid conditions may combine to leave a given patient at significant risk of extensive and complex local wound problems.
- In complex cardiac patients, volume overload, renal failure, pulmonary compromise, further cardiac issues, or related problems may serve to undermine an otherwise technically successful operative repair.
- For local wound complications, prolonged serial washouts and VAC dressing placements to support delayed reclosure or formal plastic surgery operative coverage with muscle flap or other pedicled coverage for ultimate definitive closure may be necessary.
- Thrombin injection has potential complications of immune reaction, incomplete thrombosis, failure, distal embolization of thrombin with distal leg ischemia, recurrence, or other similar problems.
- Recurrent or persistent pseudoaneurysms can be treated with further thrombin injection if it is felt a safe neck still exists or (if small) with expectant management and observation/reimaging for further complete pseudoaneurysm thrombosis and resolution.

REFERENCES

1. Fellmeth BD, Roberts AC, Bookstein JJ, et al. Postangiographic femoral artery injuries: nonsurgical repair with US-guided compression. *Radiology*. 1991;178(3):671-675. doi:10.1148/radiology.178.3.1994400
2. Saad NE, Saad WE, Davies MG, Waldman DL, Fultz PJ, Rubens DJ. Pseudoaneurysms and the role of minimally invasive techniques in their management. *Radiographics*. 2005;25(suppl 1):S173-S189. doi:10.1148/rg.25si055503
3. Stone PA, Campbell JE, AbuRahma AF. Femoral pseudoaneurysms after percutaneous access. *J Vasc Surg*. 2014;60(5):1359-1366. doi:10.1016/j.jvs.2014.07.035

SUGGESTED READINGS

1. Altin RS, Flicker S, Naidech HJ. Pseudoaneurysm and arteriovenous fistula after femoral artery catheterization: association with low femoral punctures. *AJR Am J Roentgenol*. 1989;152(3):629-631. doi:10.2214/ajr.152.3.629
2. Dzijan-Horn M, Langwieser N, Groha P, et al. Safety and efficacy of a potential treatment algorithm by using manual compression repair and ultrasound-guided thrombin injection for the management of iatrogenic femoral artery pseudoaneurysm in a large patient cohort. *Circ Cardiovasc Interv*. 2014;7(2):207-215. doi:10.1161/CIRCINTERVENTIONS.113.000836
3. Gorecka J, Chen JF, Shah S, Dardik A, Guzman RJ, Nassiri N. A hybrid approach for vascular control and repair of an expanding iatrogenic femoral artery pseudoaneurysm. *J Vasc Surg Cases Innov Tech*. 2020;6(3):460-463. doi:10.1016/j.jvscit.2020.07.010
4. Hayakawa N, Kodera S, Miyauchi A, et al. Effective treatment of iatrogenic femoral pseudoaneurysms by combined endovascular balloon inflation and percutaneous thrombin injection. *Cardiovasc Interv Ther*. 2021;37(1):158-166. doi:10.1007/s12928-021-00764-9
5. Kalapatapu VR, Shelton KR, Ali AT, Moursi MM, Eidt JF. Pseudoaneurysm: a review. *Curr Treat Options Cardiovasc Med*. 2008;10(2):173-183. doi:10.1007/s11936-008-0019-8
6. Kang SS, Labropoulos N, Mansour MA, et al. Expanded indications for ultrasound-guided thrombin injection of pseudoaneurysms. *J Vasc Surg*. 2000;31(2):289-298. doi:10.1016/s0741-5214(00)90160-5
7. La Perna L, Olin JW, Goines D, Childs MB, Ouriel K. Ultrasound-guided thrombin injection for the treatment of postcatheterization pseudoaneurysms. *Circulation*. 2000;102(19):2391-2395. doi:10.1161/01.cir.102.19.2391
8. Liau CS, Ho FM, Chen MF, Lee YT. Treatment of iatrogenic femoral artery pseudoaneurysm with percutaneous thrombin injection. *J Vasc Surg*. 1997;26(1):18-23. doi:10.1016/s0741-5214(97)70141-1
9. Madia C. Management trends for postcatheterization femoral artery pseudoaneurysms. *JAAPA*. 2019;32(6):15-18. doi:10.1097/01.JAA.0000558236.60240.02
10. Schahab N, Kavsur R, Mahn T, et al. Endovascular management of femoral access-site and access-related vascular complications following percutaneous coronary interventions (PCI). *PLoS One*. 2020;15(3):e0230535. doi:10.1371/journal.pone.0230535
11. Stone PA, AbuRahma AF, Flaherty SK, Bates MC. Femoral pseudoaneurysms. *Vasc Endovasc Surg*. 2006;40(2):109-117. doi:10.1177/153857440604000204
12. Yang EY, Tabbara MM, Sanchez PG, et al. Comparison of ultrasound-guided thrombin injection of iatrogenic pseudoaneurysms based on neck dimension. *Ann Vasc Surg*. 2018;47:121-127. doi:10.1016/j.avsg.2017.07.029

Chapter 28

Infrainguinal Embolectomy Techniques

Kathryn Marie Swanson and Malachi G. Sheahan

DEFINITION

- Acute limb ischemia is defined as the sudden loss of blood flow to an extremity resulting in acute ischemia. If the ischemia persists untreated, it can lead to muscle death, limb loss, and possibly death. To be considered acute limb ischemia, the onset must be within 2 weeks of presentation. The condition is often associated with embolic events secondary to atrial fibrillation or aortic mural thrombus. In addition, acute limb ischemia can be thrombotic in nature secondary to preexisting atherosclerotic disease or trauma. Occlusions can occur at the aortic, iliac, femoral, popliteal or tibial levels. Based on the anatomy and etiology of ischemia, a broad range of techniques exist, both open and endovascular, which can be used to restore blood flow to an acutely ischemic extremity. In this chapter, we will focus on the technique for infrainguinal embolectomy.

DIFFERENTIAL DIAGNOSIS

- The diagnosis of acute limb ischemia can be attributed to an embolic source or a thrombotic state (**TABLE 1**). Sources of embolism can be cardiac or noncardiac. Examples of a thrombotic state include atherosclerotic obstruction, arterial bypass thrombosis, hypercoagulable state, vasospasm, and aortic dissection.

PATIENT HISTORY AND PHYSICAL FINDINGS

- Acute limb ischemia can occur secondary to an embolic or thrombotic event.
- Embolic events can be cardiac or noncardiac in origin. Cardiogenic embolism usually arises from a thrombus that forms in the heart due to an arrhythmia or from wall motion abnormality after a myocardial infarction. Noncardiac sources of emboli are usually due to aortic mural thrombus secondary to trauma or underlying atherosclerotic lesions.
- Thrombotic events can be precipitated by vessel dissection, hypercoagulable state, lower extremity bypass thrombosis, or trauma.
- Acute limb ischemia usually presents with severe pain to the affected extremity. This can progress to motor and/or sensory loss depending on the duration of ischemia time.
- Acute limb ischemia can be classified according to the Rutherford classification (**TABLE 2**).
- In the setting of acute on chronic limb ischemia, the sudden onset of worsening pain with motor/sensory loss is usually preceded by a history of claudication and/or rest pain.
- The presentation of acute limb ischemia differs from chronic limb ischemia due to the development of collateral vessels surrounding the chronic occlusion. Chronic occlusions can lead to progressive claudication symptoms and occasionally pain at rest. This progression happens over months to years, rather than hours, as is seen in acute limb ischemia.
- Physical examination findings include tenderness to palpation in the affected limb, pallor, decreased or absent pulses, and motor and sensory loss. If the acute limb ischemia is advanced, the extremity will appear mottled with absent pulses and total loss of motor and sensory function.
- In the setting of acute on chronic limb ischemia, the presence of chronic limb ischemia signs may be present as well. These signs include hair loss, hypertrophic toenails, dependent rubor, and chronic wounds.

IMAGING AND OTHER DIAGNOSTIC STUDIES

- Historically, catheter-based angiography is the gold standard for evaluating acute limb ischemia as it allows simultaneous diagnosis and treatment of the occlusion. In addition, contralateral femoral or brachial access will allow you to obtain inflow images of the aortoiliac segments. Angiography is limited, however, by the availability of an angiography suite, potentially poor visualization of the outflow vessels, and the

Table 1: Etiology of Acute Limb Ischemia

Embolic	Thrombotic	Miscellaneous
Cardiac embolism secondary to atrial fibrillation or myocardial infarction, cardiac mural thrombus, aortic mural thrombus, thrombus from more proximal aneurysm	Acute thrombosis of preexisting atherosclerotic lesion, trauma with resulting vessel thrombosis, aneurysm thrombosis, hypercoagulable states, dissection	Dynamic flap from aortic dissection, access site complication

Table 2: Rutherford Classification of Acute Limb Ischemia

Rutherford class	Prognosis	Arterial signal	Venous signal	Sensory loss	Motor loss
I	Viable	+	+	–	–
IIa	Threatened	–	+	+	–
IIb	Threatened	–	+	+	+
III	Nonviable	–	–	+	+

calcium burden in the affected vessels, which might inhibit imaging.

- Computed tomography angiogram (CTA) has become the test of choice due to widespread availability and high speed when diagnosing acute limb ischemia. However, the use of CTA is limited by the risk of contrast-induced nephropathy, especially in patients with preexisting renal dysfunction. CTAs allow the physician to view relevant anatomy and pathology, including aortoiliac disease, as well as calcification along the vessels in the affected extremity. In addition, CTA may allow for better visualization of distal runoff when compared with catheter-based angiography.
- Duplex ultrasonography is also available to evaluate blood flow in an ischemic extremity. This modality has the advantage of being low cost and easy to access. However, it is operator dependent and can be limited by body habitus. In addition, duplex ultrasonography does not provide images of the aortoiliac segment.

SURGICAL MANAGEMENT

Preoperative Planning

- Surgical management of acute limb ischemia is largely guided by the Rutherford ischemia classification (**TABLE 2**). All patients with acute limb ischemia should be placed on a heparin drip upon presentation to prevent thrombus propagation unless a contraindication exists. In the setting of Rutherford class 1 ischemia, the patient may be managed conservatively with anticoagulation alone. Rutherford class IIa or IIb warrants revascularization. Endovascular revascularization can be attempted with Rutherford class IIa ischemia. Rutherford class IIb ischemia requires immediate open surgical revascularization such as open embolectomy. Rutherford class III ischemia is nonviable, and primary amputation should be considered to avoid sequelae of systemic reperfusion injury. In the event that there is a role for endovascular or hybrid intervention or a completion angiogram, most cases should be performed in a hybrid suite with both operative and angiographic capabilities.

Positioning

- The patient should be positioned supine on the table. The sterile prep should include the abdomen along with the affected lower extremity and the contralateral groin and thigh. In certain circumstances, the antecubital fossa should be prepared for brachial access and the entire contralateral lower extremity may be prepped for saphenous vein harvest. The entire involved extremity should always be included in the sterile field in case an embolectomy is not possible and a bypass procedure is required. In addition, depending on ischemia time, concurrent four-compartment fasciotomy may be necessary.

TECHNIQUES

- Prior to revascularization, four-compartment fasciotomies should be performed in the lower extremity if the ischemic time is greater than 6 hours or if any concern for compartment syndrome exists. For further information, please see the corresponding chapter in this text.
- A longitudinal skin incision is made overlying the femoral artery in the groin of the affected limb. The landmark halfway between the pubic symphysis and the anterior superior iliac spine can be used to guide incision placement as the femoral pulse will frequently be absent (**FIGURE 1**).

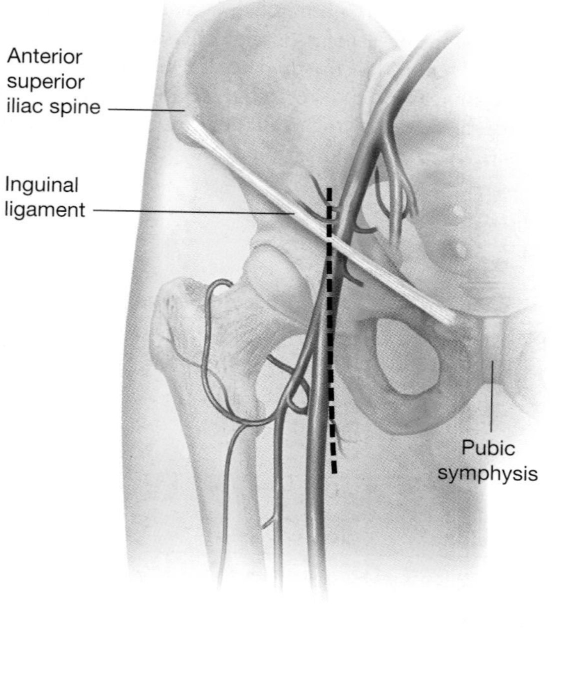

Anterior superior iliac spine

Inguinal ligament

Pubic symphysis

FIGURE 1 ● The halfway point between the anterior superior iliac spine and public symphysis is the anatomic landmark used to guide incision placement for common femoral artery exposure.

- Dissection is then carried down to the level of the common femoral artery with Bovie electrocautery and Metzenbaum scissors, taking care to ligate or cauterize any exposed lymphatics to avoid postoperative groin seroma. Care should be taken not to injure any of the other contents of the femoral triangle including the femoral nerve and femoral vein (**FIGURE 2**).
- As there are rarely anterior branches of the femoral artery, the vessel is safely approached from this direction.
- The distal external iliac artery and proximal profunda femoris and superficial femoral arteries are encircled with Silastic vessel loops. Any side branches are controlled with vessel loops or ligated with silk suture or surgical clips (**FIGURE 3**).

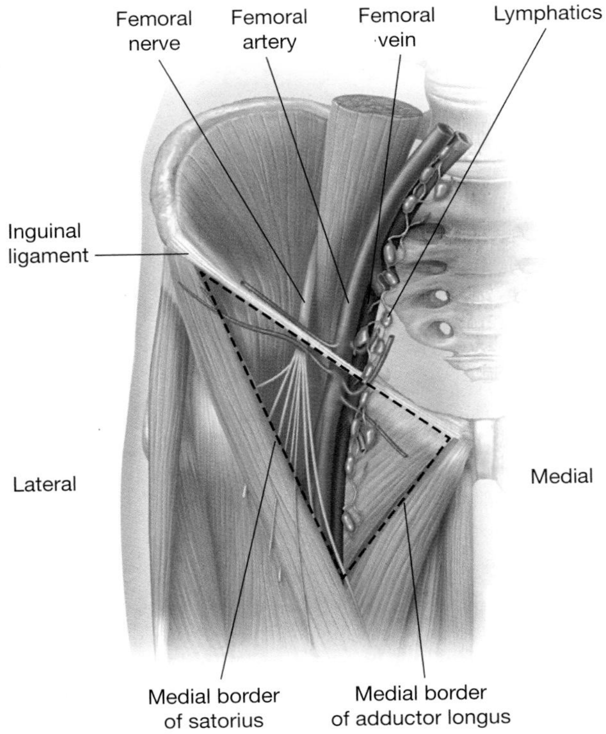

FIGURE 2 ● The femoral triangle is bound by the inguinal ligament, medial border of the sartorius muscle, and border of the adductor longus muscle. The femoral triangle contains, from lateral to medial, the femoral nerve, femoral artery, femoral vein, and inguinal lymphatics.

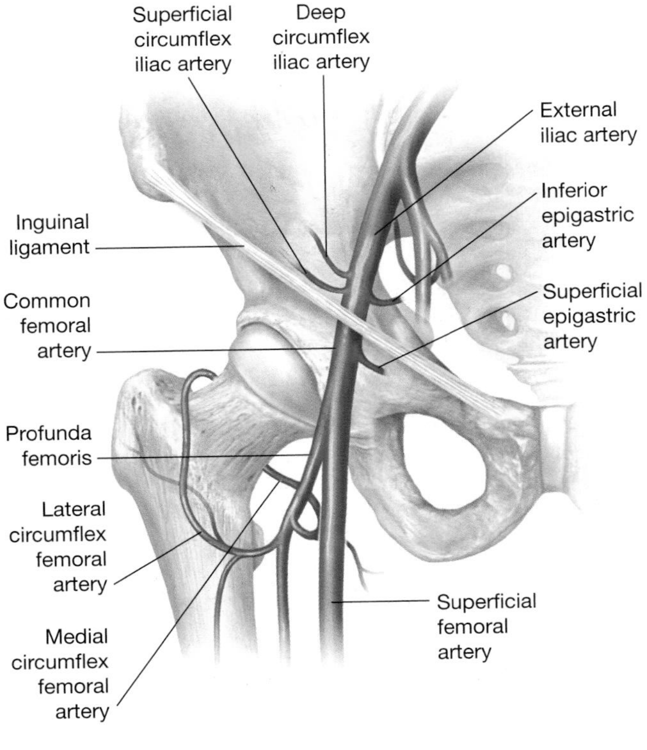

FIGURE 3 ● Branches of the common femoral artery.

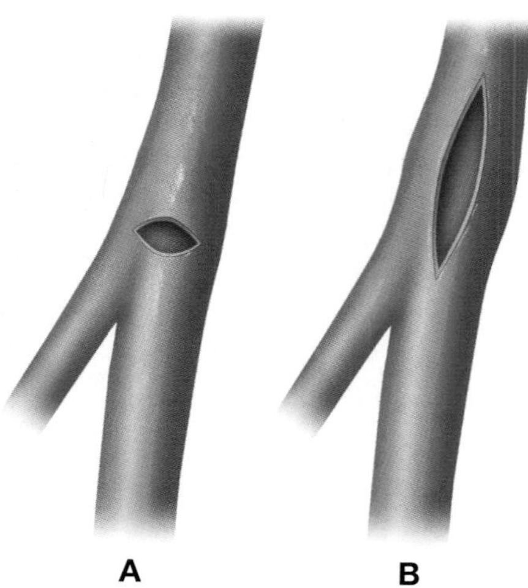

FIGURE 4 • Transverse **(A)** vs longitudinal **(B)** arteriotomy.

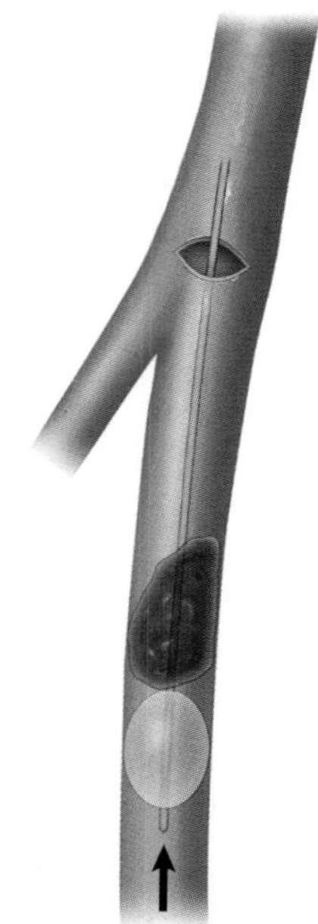

FIGURE 6 • The Fogarty embolectomy catheter is advanced down the artery past the point of thrombus. The balloon is gently inflated and then pulled back so as to remove any thrombus in the artery.

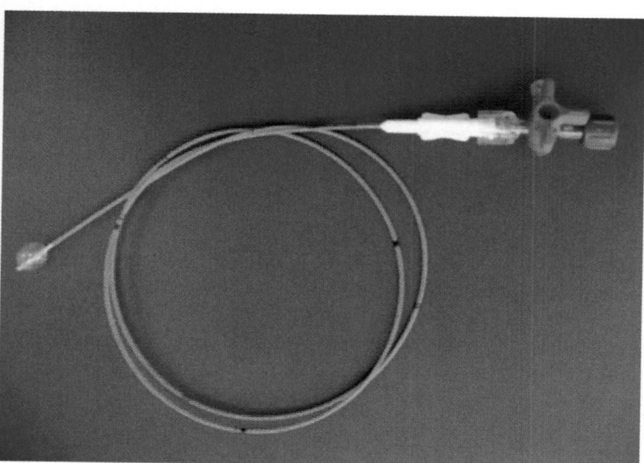

FIGURE 5 • Fogarty embolectomy catheter.

- If they are not already on a heparin drip, the patient is systemically heparinized to obtain an activated clotting time (ACT) greater than 250 seconds. The heparin should be redosed as needed every 30 minutes throughout the case to maintain an ACT >250 seconds.
- If thrombus is suspected in the common femoral artery, clamping in this region should be avoided so as not to transect any preexisting clot.
- An arteriotomy is made in the common femoral artery with a #11 blade scalpel and extended with Potts scissors. A transverse vs longitudinal arteriotomy is chosen based on the presence or absence of chronic disease in the femoral artery (**FIGURE 4**) (see pearls and pitfalls for more information).
- Any thrombus initially encountered can be removed with DeBakey forceps and sent to pathology as a specimen.
- A Fogarty balloon embolectomy catheter (**FIGURE 5**) is then advanced down the superficial artery into the popliteal artery. The authors usually start with a 3 French catheter. The balloon is inflated with saline as indicated and withdrawn from the artery in order to remove any thrombus from the vessel (**FIGURE 6**). As the balloon is withdrawn the control of the superficial femoral artery is released to allow concurrent back-bleeding. Multiple passes are made with the Fogarty catheter until there is adequate back-bleeding and no return of thrombus. If there is concern for thrombus in the profunda femoris artery, Fogarty embolectomy is again performed down the profunda until good back-bleeding is encountered and there is no further return of thrombus.
- Distal control is then obtained by placing tension on the Silastic vessel loops.
- Attention is then turned toward the inflow. Fogarty embolectomy is performed of the inflow until there is strong pulsatile inflow bleeding and no return of thrombus. Proximal control is then reestablished with a vascular clamp or a Silastic vessel loop.
- At this point, the foot should be checked for pulses or Doppler signals. If signals are present and adequate in the ipsilateral foot, the arteriotomy can be closed. If the arteriotomy was made in transverse fashion, arterial closure is performed by primary repair of the arteriotomy using 5-0 Prolene suture with a C1 needle in an interrupted fashion. If a longitudinal arteriotomy was performed, it is prudent

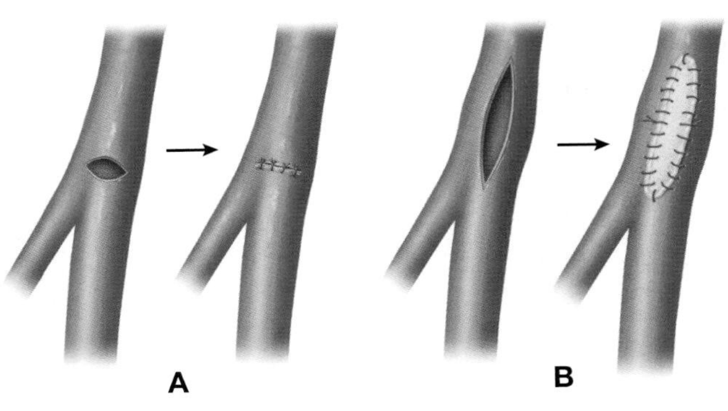

FIGURE 7 ● Arterial closure techniques. Transverse arteriotomy should be closed primarily with interrupted Prolene suture **(A)**. Longitudinal arteriotomy should be closed with bovine pericardial or autologous vein patch angioplasty **(B)**.

to proceed with patch angioplasty with bovine pericardial patch vs autologous vein so as not to cause stenosis of the vessel (**FIGURE 7**).

- If palpable pulses are not obtained in the foot, an angiogram should be performed. This will help guide further decision making. If there are no fluoroscopic capabilities, the above-knee vs below-knee popliteal artery should be exposed.
- The above-knee popliteal artery is exposed through a distal medial thigh incision. With the leg externally rotated and knee flexed, an incision is made along the anterior border of the sartorius muscle in the distal third of the thigh (**FIGURE 8**). The sartorius muscle is then retracted posteriorly, and the vastus medialis muscle is identified and retracted anteriorly. This will expose the popliteal vessels. The sheath enveloping the popliteal artery and vein is incised. The artery should immediately be encountered as it lies medial to the vein (**FIGURE 9**).
- Proximal and distal control of the artery should be obtained with Silastic vessel loops. A longitudinal arteriotomy is made with a #11 blade scalpel and Fogarty embolectomy is again performed both distally and proximally.
- At this point, if there are adequate distal signals or pulses, the arteriotomy should be closed as described above.
- If there are not adequate signals or pulses in the foot at this point, the below-knee popliteal artery should be exposed. This is usually performed via a medial calf incision with the leg externally rotated and flexed at the knee. The incision is made 1 cm posterior to the tibial border in the proximal third of the calf (**FIGURE 10**). Care should be taken not to injure the great saphenous vein.
- Dissection is carried down to the level of the gastrocnemius, which is retracted posteriorly to expose the neurovascular sheath (**FIGURE 11**). The popliteal vein will be encountered first in the neurovascular bundle. This should be encircled with a Silastic vessel loop and retracted to expose the popliteal artery laterally. The tibial nerve lies posterior to the artery. Care should be taken not to injure the tibial nerve during this dissection.

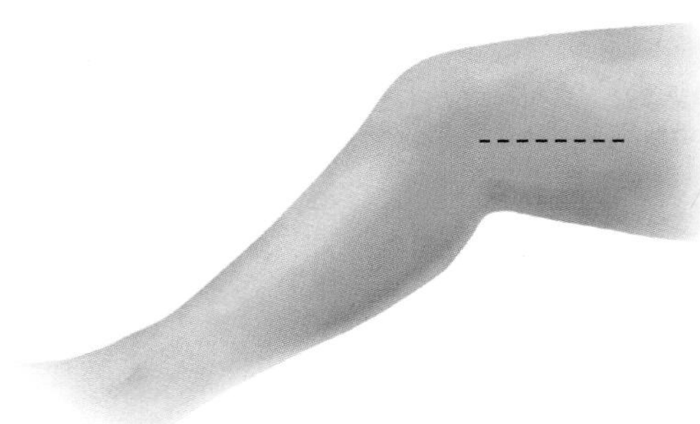

FIGURE 8 ● The skin incision for suprageniculate popliteal exposure is made along the anterior border of the sartorius in the distal third of the thigh.

- For more distal exposure, the soleus can be divided and retracted posteriorly (**FIGURE 11**). This will allow further dissection of the popliteal artery to identify the tibioperoneal trunk as well as anterior tibial arteries. These should be encircled with Silastic vessel loops, so as to allow for selective Fogarty catheterization of each tibial vessel.
- For more proximal exposure, the tendons of the semitendinosus, gracilus, and sartorius can be divided (**FIGURE 11**). These should be reapproximated at the time of closure.

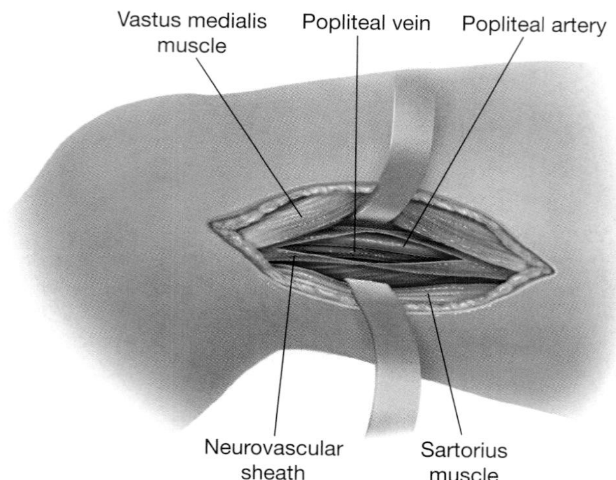

FIGURE 9 • The suprageniculate popliteal artery is exposed by retracting the sartorius muscle posteriorly and the vastus medialis muscle anteriorly. This will expose the neurovascular bundle containing the popliteal artery.

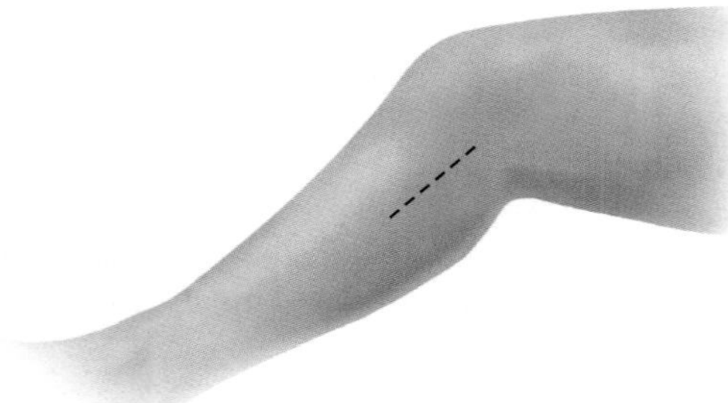

FIGURE 10 • Skin incision for infrageniculate popliteal exposure is made 1 cm posterior to the tibial border in the proximal third of the calf.

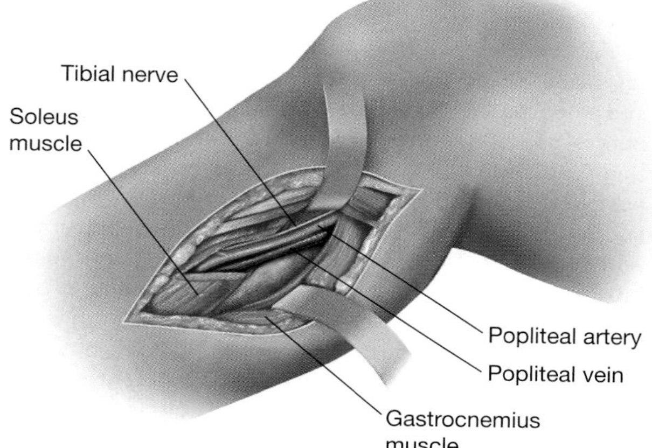

FIGURE 11 • The infrageniculate popliteal artery is exposed by retracting the gastrocnemius posteriorly. Division of the soleus may be necessary to further expose the distal infrageniculate popliteal artery and tibial arteries.

- A longitudinal arteriotomy is then made with a #11 blade scalpel and extended with Potts scissors. Fogarty embolectomy is then performed of all three tibial vessels. For Fogarty embolectomy technique, see above.
- At this point, the below-knee popliteal artery should be closed with bovine pericardial patch angioplasty or autologous vein patch angioplasty.
- The groin incision is closed in *multiple* layers including the femoral sheath, deep dermal layer, and skin. If incisions from distal arterial exposures were made, a layered closure of these should be performed as well.

PEARLS AND PITFALLS

Common femoral embolectomy	■ For common femoral embolectomy, transverse arteriotomy is sufficient as long as the artery is free of significant atherosclerosis. In the setting of moderate to substantial calcium and plaque burden, it is prudent to perform a longitudinal arteriotomy with endarterectomy and patch angioplasty. ■ In the event of a common femoral embolectomy, it is important to make the arteriotomy sufficiently close to the bifurcation of the superficial femoral and profunda femoris arteries. This will allow the catheter to be directed into either lumen for embolectomy.
Popliteal embolectomy	■ For above-knee popliteal embolectomy, it is advised to perform a longitudinal arteriotomy with patch angioplasty with bovine pericardium or autologous vein patch. ■ Below-knee popliteal embolectomy should always be performed with longitudinal arteriotomy and patch angioplasty closure so as not to narrow the lumen of the vessel significantly.
Complications	■ In the event that the embolectomy catheter cannot be passed due to chronic disease or a dissection, a bypass may be necessary to reestablish inline flow.
Fasciotomy	■ Concurrent fasciotomy should be performed for ischemia time greater than 6 hours, or if the patient develops signs of compartment syndrome. The threshold for fasciotomy should be low as a missed compartment syndrome has devastating long-term effects.

POSTOPERATIVE CARE

- Postoperatively, the patient should be admitted to a hospital unit capable of performing cardiac monitoring and hourly neurovascular checks.
- The patient will require embolic workup including CTA chest/abdomen/pelvis with runoff and echocardiogram. If those studies do not reveal an embolic source, the patient will need a hypercoagulability workup. This can be done as an outpatient.
- In most cases, the patient should be anticoagulated postoperatively on a heparin drip with transition to an appropriate oral agent upon discharge.

COMPLICATIONS

- Postoperative cardiac events: As is true of most vascular surgery procedures, myocardial infarction remains a leading cause of morbidity and mortality after this procedure secondary to the prevalence of preexisting cardiac vascular disease and the increased stress on the body caused by acute limb ischemia. In addition, arrhythmias are a common cause of emboli and may be encountered postoperatively. All patients should be monitored on telemetry in the postoperative period.
- Renal failure: Circulating myoglobin, a by-product of muscle death, is associated with prolonged periods of limb ischemia. Elevated myoglobinemia can lead to toxic nephropathy. This, combined with contrast load from preoperative imaging or on-table angiography, puts the patient at risk for acute renal failure.
- Infection: Groin wounds should be closely monitored for signs of infection. Suspected infections should be treated promptly with antibiotics to avoid involvement of any underlying prosthetic material, such as bovine pericardial patch used for angioplasty. Groin wounds have high rates of infections.
- Lymphocele: Groin lymphoceles are a possible sequela of inadequately ligated lymphatic channels. These can be observed if they are small. However, if they persist or cause compressive symptoms, the lymphocele should be surgically excised and closed in multiple layers. Groin muscle flaps can also prove helpful in preventing lymphocele recurrence.
- Arterial complications: Dissection can occur during Fogarty embolectomy if the catheter is advanced into a subintimal plane. If the entry flap is easy to identify, the intimal flap should be tacked down with interrupted Prolene suture. If the dissection flap occurs proximally or distally in the artery, endovascular intervention with balloon or stent placement may be required. In addition, postoperative pseudoaneurysm can develop at the arteriotomy site if there is not an adequate seal on the arteriotomy after repair. This will usually require reexploration and open repair.
- Distal embolization: Distal embolization may occur following angiography or after advancing the Fogarty catheter through the thrombus in the artery.
- Compartment syndrome: Compartment syndrome can develop secondary to ischemia-reperfusion phenomenon. This results in muscle death and worsening interstitial edema. It is associated with ischemia times greater than 6 hours. Generally speaking, the threshold to perform fasciotomy at the time of reperfusion is low as missed compartment syndrome has devastating consequences including permanent motor/sensory deficits and limb loss.
- Limb loss: Rates of limb loss despite revascularization remain high as many patients have underlying vascular disease prior to their acute ischemic event. In addition, patients who present with higher Rutherford acute limb ischemia scores are found to have decreased rates of limb salvage.

SUGGESTED READING

1. Creager M, Kaufman J, Conte M. Acute limb ischemia. *N Engl J Med.* 2012;366:2198-2206.
2. Hemingway J, Emanuels D, Aarabi S, et al. Safety of transfer, type of procedure, and factors predictive of limb salvage in a modern series of acute limb ischemia. *J Vasc Surg.* 2019;69(4):1174-1179.
3. Kempe K, Starr B, Stafford J, et al. Results of surgical management of acute thromboembolic lower extremity ischemia. *J Vasc Surg.* 2014;60(3):702-707.
4. Suggested standards for reports dealing with lower extremity ischemia. Prepared by the Ad Hoc Committee on Reporting Standards, Society for Vascular Surgery/North American Chapter, International Society for Cardiovascular Surgery. [published correction appears in J Vasc Surg. 1986;4(4):350]. *J Vasc Surg.* 1986;4(1):80-94.
5. Tawes R, Harris E, Brown W, et al. Acute limb ischemia: thromboembolism. Symposium: Nontraumatic Vascular Emergencies. *J Vasc Surg.* 1987;5(6):901-903.
6. Wang J, Kim A, Kashyap V. Open Surgical or endovascular revascularization for acute limb ischemia. *J Vasc Surg.* 2016;63(1):270-278.

Chapter 29 Percutaneous Femoral-Popliteal Reconstruction Techniques: Antegrade Approaches

Kellie R. Brown

DEFINITION

- Femoral-popliteal revascularization for indications of limb salvage or claudication is performed using open, endovascular, or hybrid approaches. Advanced open surgical techniques are detailed elsewhere.
- Basic procedural goals: Improve functional status, quality of life, and, in the setting of ischemic tissue loss, augment wound healing and limb preservation.
- Challenges influencing long-term clinical success: (1) superficial femoral and popliteal artery movement during activities of daily living, including flexion, compression, torsion, and stretching; (2) compromised runoff; (3) the generally diffuse nature of femoral-popliteal disease, requiring angioplasty of long segments of diseased and stiffened artery; and (4) complex pathology, including ostial lesions, luminal thrombus accumulation, and mural calcification.
- Indications for intervention:
  - Rutherford class 1, 2, and 3 ischemia—exercise therapy and medical management are pursued as primary intervention.[1]
  - Rutherford class 4, 5, and 6 ischemia—rest pain, ischemic ulcer, and gangrene warrant revascularization as initial therapy.
- Guidewire-catheter combinations are particularly effective and widely used to cross femoral-popliteal stenoses or occlusions. Once across, reconstructions are performed with any combination of angioplasty, stenting, stent grafting, or atherectomy.
- Reentry devices facilitate true lumen reentry after subintimal recanalization for endovascular treatment of complex lesion morphologies and occlusions in the femoral-popliteal segment.
- Subintimal recanalization and reconstruction of the femoral and popliteal arteries have diminished reliance upon femoral-popliteal bypass. Reentry into the true lumen can be challenging and is often the rate-limiting factor for the success of this procedure. Improved wires, support catheters, and reentry devices have been developed for crossing chronic total occlusions (CTOs).
- Tools for managing CTOs are listed in **TABLE 1** CTO support catheters may be used to support the guidewire that is being used to cross the occlusion. These typically have lubricious surface and a stiff tip. Distal access may be used to recanalize infrainguinal occlusions from a retrograde direction. Reentry catheters may be used to reenter the true lumen.

Table 1: Tools for Managing Chronic Total Occlusions in the Lower Extremity

Tool for managing CTO	Purpose	Examples
CTO support catheters	Support during wire crossing	CXI (Cook Medical) Quick-Cross (Spectranetics) TrailBlazer (Covidien) Gopher (Vascular Solutions) Seeker (BD)
Distal access	Access for bidirectional approach	Retrograde puncture of SFA–popliteal Tibial-pedal
Reentry catheters	Enter true lumen from subintimal space	Outback (Cordis) Pioneer (Medtronic) Enteer (Covidien) OffRoad (Boston Scientific)
CTO crossing devices	True lumen crossing	Crosser (Bard) Frontrunner (Cordis) Laser (Spectranetics) TruePath (Boston Scientific) Wildcat (Avinger) Viance (Covidien)

CTO, chronic total occlusion; SFA, superficial femoral artery.

PATIENT HISTORY AND PHYSICAL FINDINGS

- History includes a detailed description of ischemic symptoms pertaining to claudication, rest pain, or tissue loss. The progression of symptoms and timeframe are helpful in determining the urgency of therapy.
- The presence and severity of cardiovascular disease risk factors should be assessed and managed to ensure optimal perioperative and long-term clinical results, including tobacco use, diabetes, hypertension, hyperlipidemia, renal dysfunction, and sedentary lifestyle.
- Previous vascular or endovascular procedures should be reviewed in detail, including obtaining operative notes, prior imaging and surveillance studies, and prior physiologic testing results whenever possible.
- For claudicants, the potential presence and contribution of nonvascular causes of leg pain with exercise should be considered; for example, neurologic claudication secondary to lumbar radiculopathy and other degenerative spine diseases.[2]
- Physical examination should document peripheral pulses at all levels, both lower extremities, including the strength and quality of femoral pulses and skin integrity at potential access sites.
- The severity and extent of ischemia, degree of existing tissue damage, and presence of infection are documented prior to initiating intervention.

IMAGING AND OTHER DIAGNOSTIC STUDIES

- Physiologic vascular testing provides objective determination of the location and severity of disease, assists in procedural planning, and provides documentation of baseline conditions.
  - Ankle-brachial index (ABI): ratio of the continuous wave Doppler–determined blood pressure in the anterior or posterior tibial arteries (whichever is higher) to the

blood pressure in the brachial artery (>0.9 = normal; 0.5-0.9 = usually consistent with mild to severe claudication; <0.5 = present in patients with very short distance claudication, rest pain, or tissue loss).

- Toe pressures: The ABI may be artifactually elevated in diabetic patients with calcified tibial arteries. Toe pressures may provide more reliable assessment of pedal and forefoot perfusion when the ABI is greater than 1.2. Hallux pressure less than 50 mm Hg may predict delayed or inadequate wound resolution, 50 to 80 mm Hg is indeterminant, and greater than 80 mm Hg is generally sufficient to promote healing.
- Duplex arterial imaging: Direct insonation provides insight into the location and severity of disease. The ratio of the peak systolic velocities (PSV) obtained from the most compromised location divided by PSV from the most adjacent, proximal noninvolved segment provides additional guidance regarding the severity of disease; greater than or equal to 2.5:1 usually identifies a stenosis greater than 50% (**FIGURE 1**).
- Computed tomographic arteriography (CTA): CTA has assumed an increasing role in guiding peripheral vascular intervention, particularly in regard to choosing appropriate devices and optimal interventional approach (eg, ipsilateral antegrade vs contralateral retrograde). Patients who might benefit from subintimal recanalization and reentry typically have complex lesion morphology, such as arterial occlusion, that may be managed by creating a new channel outside of the potential space offered by the subintimal area. Imaging studies that define the anatomy and lesion morphology are

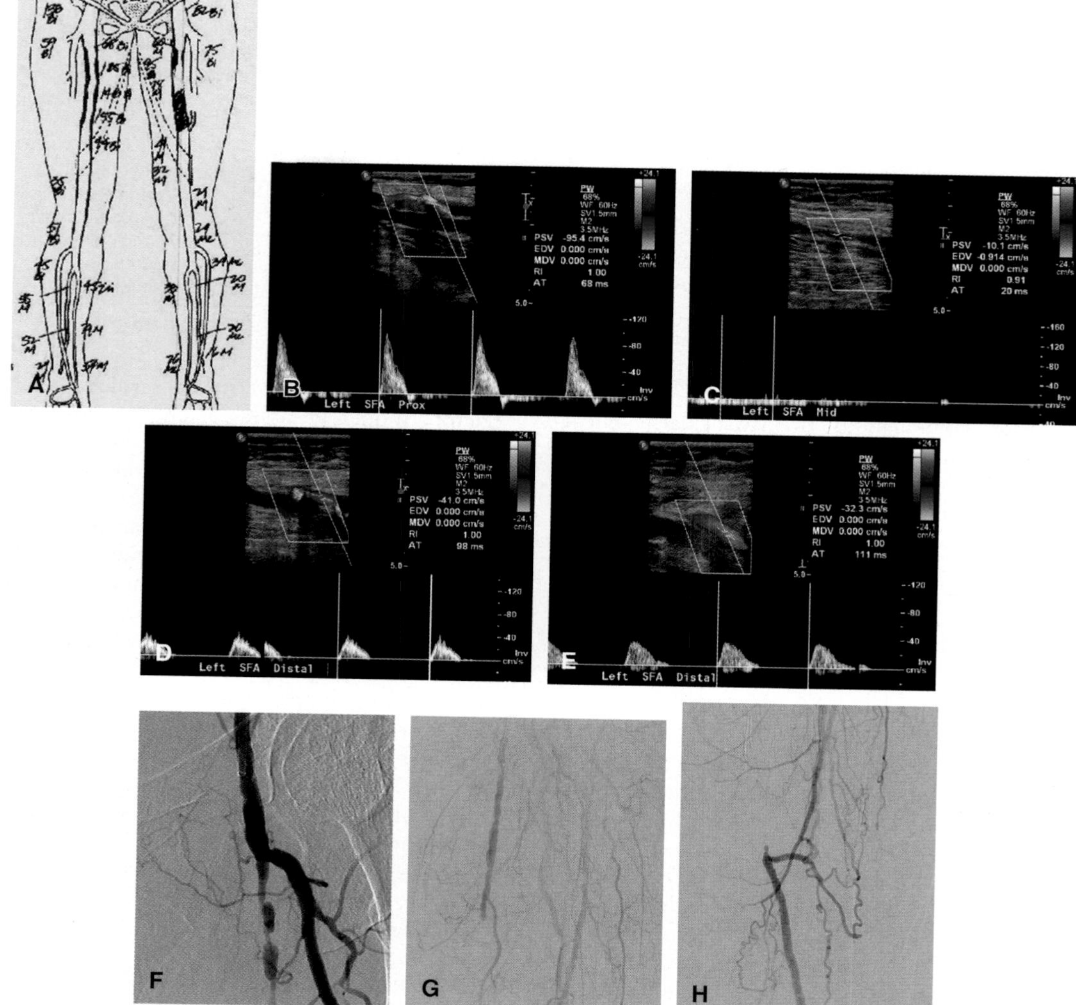

FIGURE 1 ● Duplex evaluation of lower extremity arteries. **A,** Duplex mapping was performed on a patient with very severe left lower extremity claudication. There is a left SFA occlusion with reconstitution of the distal SFA. **B,** Duplex image of proximal left SFA shows some plaque formation and a peak velocity of 95 cm per second. **C,** This duplex image demonstrates no flow in the occluded segment of the SFA. **D,** The left distal SFA duplex image shows the point of reconstitution of the artery with a patent distal artery and low velocity flow. **E,** The more distal SFA is a healthier artery with a reasonable lumen, but it has a low peak velocity of 32 cm per second. **F,** The arteriogram performed on the left lower extremity of this patient at the time of intervention showed a patent but diseased proximal SFA. The CFA and profunda femoris artery do not have significant occlusive disease. **G,** There is a mid-SFA occlusion as demonstrated by duplex evaluation. **H,** There is reconstitution of the left distal SFA as indicated by duplex mapping.

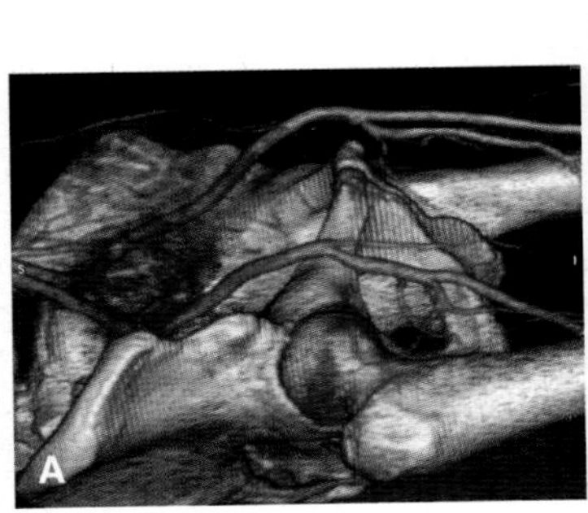

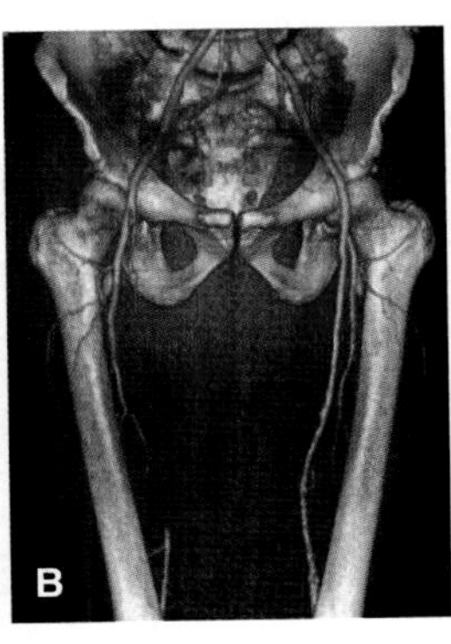

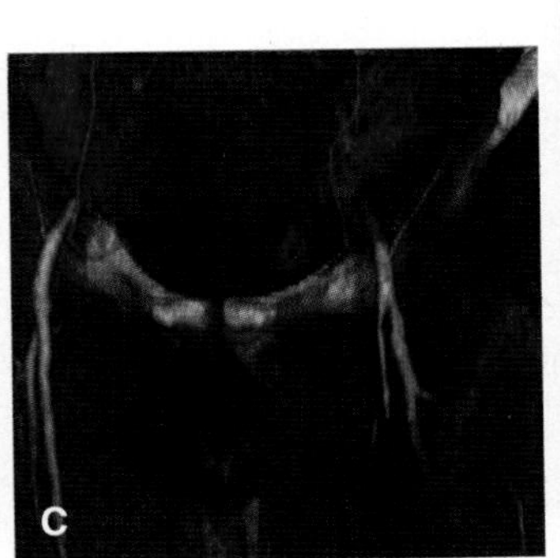

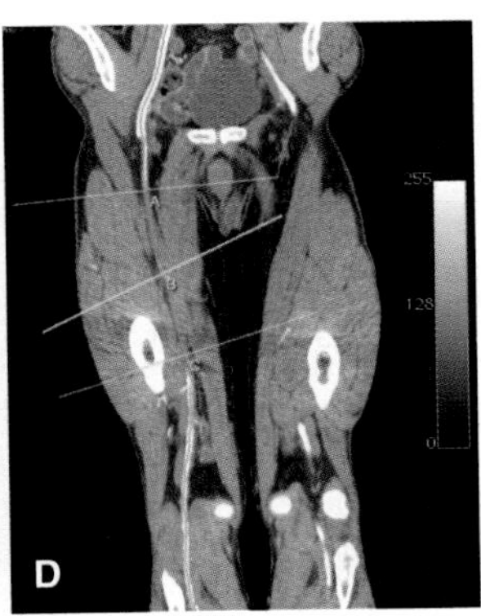

FIGURE 2 ● CT angiography for infrainguinal occlusive disease. Volume rendering technique. Preoperative study of puncture zones in the CFA in a patient with a long right SFA occlusion. **A,** Evaluation of iliac artery inflow. **B,** Long right SFA occlusion with reconstitution of the above-the-knee popliteal artery. **C,** CT evaluation of the CFAs and femoral bifurcations prior to access. **D,** Centerline measurements performed to measure diameters and plan for stent graft placement in the right SFA.

useful prior to revascularization. This additional guidance, however, comes at the cost of substantially more iodinated contrast and radiation exposure than that provided by catheter-directed, intra-arterial contrast arteriography, augmented by direct ultrasonic visualization and physiologic testing (**FIGURE 2**).

- Magnetic resonance arteriography (MRA): MRA may also assist preoperative planning. Although MRA does not expose patients to ionizing radiation, artifactual overestimation of disease severity is common in low-flow conditions. Also, gadolinium contrast administration is contraindicated in patients with a glomerular filtration rate of less than 30 mL per minute due to risk of contrast-associated glomerulosclerosis (**FIGURE 3**).

SURGICAL MANAGEMENT

- Overview—Success in percutaneous management of femoral-popliteal occlusive disease requires detailed preoperative planning, thoughtful choice of access site and closure techniques, and familiarity and facility with a wide range of complementary intraluminal wire-guided devices.

Preoperative Planning

- The operative plan includes access site selection, planned method of crossing, and options for arterial reconstruction.
- Endovascular inventory: An essential element of endovascular success is a robust and redundant device inventory. In contrast to open reconstruction techniques, where similar instruments will suffice for all lower extremity bypass configurations regardless of routing, a unique and task-specific repertoire is required for almost every endovascular approach. Procedural success requires that the necessary devices, including guidewires, sheaths, catheters, angioplasty balloons, stents, reentry devices, stent grafts, and atherectomy catheters are identified and available before intervention is attempted.
- Appropriate radiation protection must be available for all individuals involved in interventional procedures. All team members must conscientiously wear a radiation dosimeter, submitted monthly for aggregate exposure documentation. Leadership ensures that all team members adhere to basic radiation safety tenants, including limiting the length and intensity of exposure to the minimum required for precision imaging and intervention (the "as low as reasonably achievable" [ALARA] principle). Safety principles, including distance from the radiation source, appropriate shielding and optimal table height, and source-image intensifier distance, must be understood and applied during every procedure.

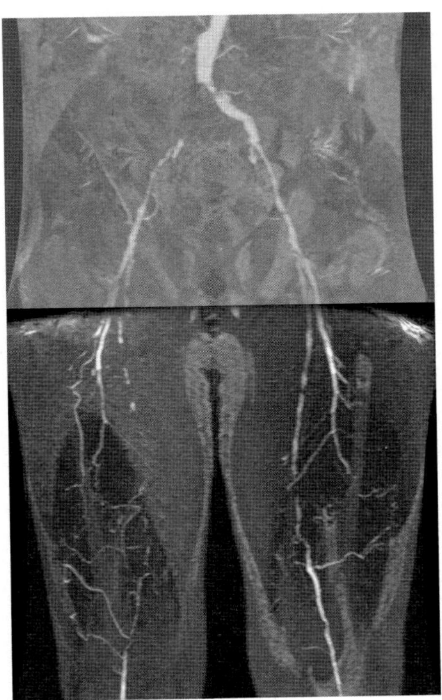

FIGURE 3 ● Magnetic resonance angiography as preoperative assessment of lesion location and severity. This patient has extensive iliac and femoral artery occlusive disease. Both femoral artery puncture sites are compromised. There are long lesions in both superficial femoral arteries.

- Antibiotic prophylaxis is administered prior to the initiation of the procedure, whenever permanent implants are considered.
- Percutaneous procedures are performed under local anesthesia with appropriate sedation. Care should be taken to avoid

oversedation to ensure that patients can cooperate with instructions and imaging requirements during the procedure. When hybrid open endovascular procedures are contemplated, general anesthesia may facilitate more rapid and accurate device deployment, with reciprocally less radiation exposure for the patient, catheterization laboratory team, and operator.

- An important initial consideration is the approach and optimal puncture site. The common femoral artery (CFA) is the most frequent access site. The approach is typically either up and over the aortic bifurcation from the contralateral femoral artery or ipsilateral antegrade femoral puncture. The transbrachial, transthoracic approach may also provide optimal antegrade access under certain circumstances.
- Subintimal recanalization of the femoral-popliteal segment may be performed using an up and over approach from the contralateral common femoral artery or using an antegrade approach from the ipsilateral common femoral artery. A reentry catheter may be used through either of these access choices. Preoperative noninvasive imaging is very helpful in making this plan for approach.
- The location of lesion helps determine access site and approach. Many patients with superficial femoral artery (SFA) and/or popliteal artery disease are treated with an up and over approach. If the patient has inflow iliac artery disease or has an SFA lesion that begins near the origin of the SFA, an up and over approach is warranted. Reentry devices require placement of a 6-French (Fr) sheath. If an up and over approach is anticipated, the aortic bifurcation should also be assessed to make sure that the reentry device can be passed.
- Patients with extensive disease below the knee and without iliac or proximal SFA disease and who are not obese can be treated using an antegrade approach.

Positioning

- Surgeon position should provide forehand access, whenever possible (**FIGURE 4**).
- Retrograde femoral puncture: This is the most common type of access for all endovascular procedures, including femoral-popliteal revascularization (**FIGURE 5**). The needle is placed in the CFA and the guidewire is advanced retrograde into the iliac artery.

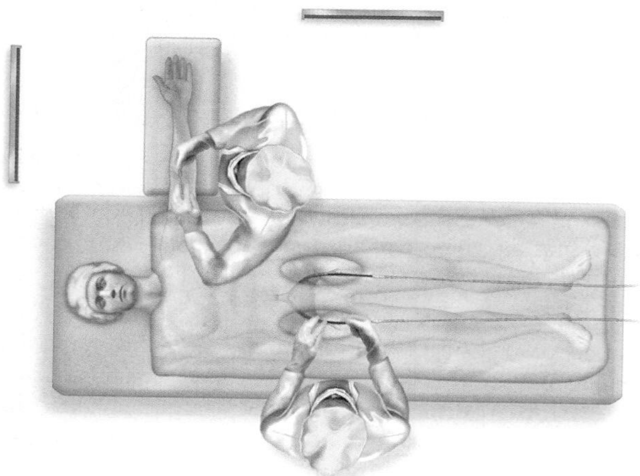

FIGURE 4 • Patient positioning. The operator works forehand when possible. The right-handed operator stands on the patient's right side for a retrograde femoral puncture of either groin. The right-handed operator stands at the inferior aspect of the left arm when performing a left brachial puncture. The monitors are placed so that they can be comfortably observed by the operator.

- The femoral area is examined prior to puncture of the artery. The inguinal ligament extends from the anterior superior iliac spine to the pubic tubercle. The best puncture site is inferior to the inguinal ligament and at least a centimeter superior to the femoral bifurcation. Ultrasound provides useful guidance for arterial puncture and is used routinely in the authors practice (**FIGURE 6**). Following needle insertion, spot fluoroscopy from an ipsilateral oblique angle is obtained to confirm position. If arterial insertion is determined to be proximal to the femoral head, the access attempt is aborted before larger devices are inserted to minimize the risk of retroperitoneal hematoma formation due to inadequate compression or control following the procedure. Common femoral access also enables closure devices to be employed with confidence when necessary.
- Closure devices: recommended for retrograde femoral access site management following insertion of greater than or equal to 6-Fr sheaths. Sheath puncture less than 6 Fr is best managed by compression for 10 to 15 minutes, with or without adjuncts such as a thrombin-impregnated dressing (eg, D-stat patch).
- When pulses are not palpable at the desired access site, ultrasound or fluoroscopic guidance (assisted by mural femoral artery calcification) may provide valuable assistance. Under these circumstances, bilateral femoral access and ipsilateral iliac intervention may be required for procedural success. Ideally, this eventuality is anticipated based on the results of preprocedural examination and physiologic testing. Fortunately, the pulseless femoral artery is often palpable based on mural calcification alone. Patience and spot fluoroscopic images to confirm needle and artery position following failed needle passes often ensures ultimate success.
- Secondary puncture of the postoperative groin presents special challenges. Whenever possible, scar tissue and anastomoses should be avoided. Access in native artery is preferable to prosthetic or autogenous grafts. Considerable force may be required for needle and micropuncture set access; consideration should be given to using "stiff" 0.018-in wires and micropuncture sets specifically manufactured to facilitate difficult groin access.
- Antegrade femoral puncture: The femoral pulse and inguinal ligament are carefully marked (**FIGURE 7**). Needle placement is directed proximal to the femoral artery bifurcation under real-time ultrasound guidance.
- Guidewire placement into the superficial femoral artery (SFA) requires patience and practice. Ultrasound imaging in a longitudinal view may facilitate SFA wire intubation. When using a micropuncture set with a "steerable" 0.018-in wire (eg, one with a slight curve placed at the tip), fluoroscopic control may also be employed. If repeated attempts result in deep femoral artery placement, the micropuncture set should be exchanged for an 11-cm 4- or 5-Fr sheath over a standard multipurpose (eg, Bentsen) wire. Once safe antegrade deep femoral access is obtained, the 5-Fr sheath may be gradually withdrawn with sequential fluoroscopic contrast "puffs" of 1 mL or less performed until the femoral bifurcation is imaged (but while the sheath tip is still in the CFA). At this juncture, roadmapping or last-image-hold digital subtraction

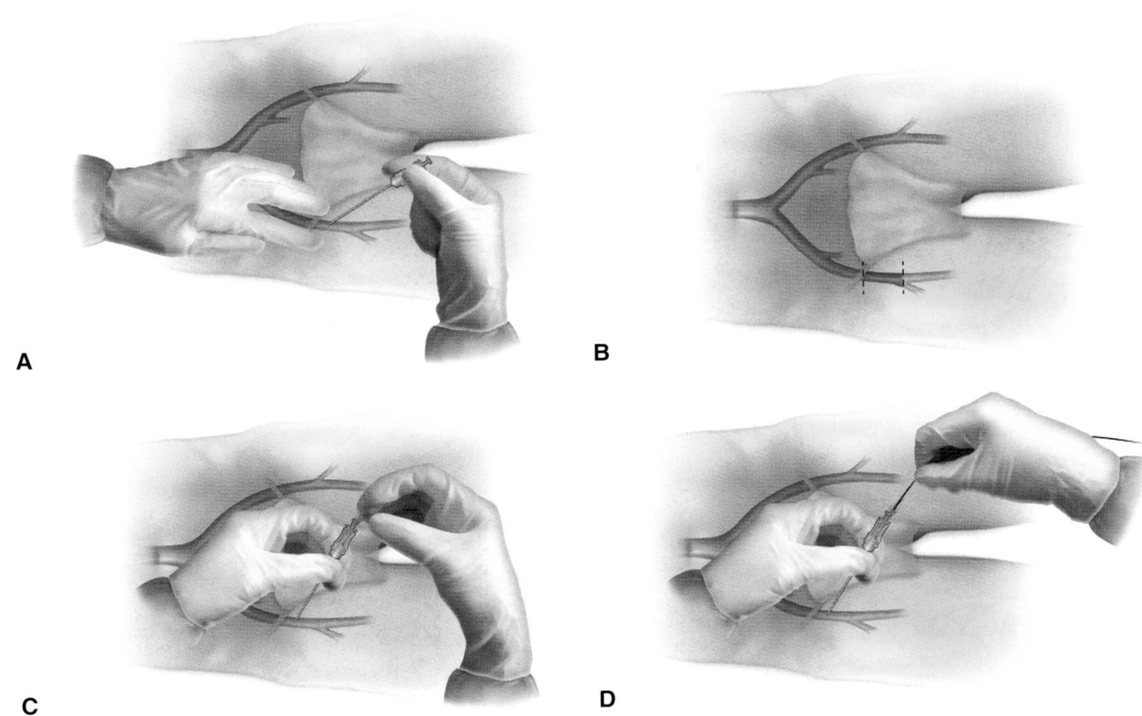

FIGURE 5 ● Retrograde femoral puncture. **A,** The anatomic relationships are evaluated. The left hand may be used to help guide the needle. **B,** The access needle is placed in the CFA inferior to the inguinal ligament and superior to the femoral bifurcation. **C,** The needle is advanced into the CFA until arterial blood return is apparent. **D,** In the image a prolongation of the guide inside the retrograde femoral should be included, in order to understand that with this approach and these needle angulation the guide should never go to the SFA, or profunda artery.

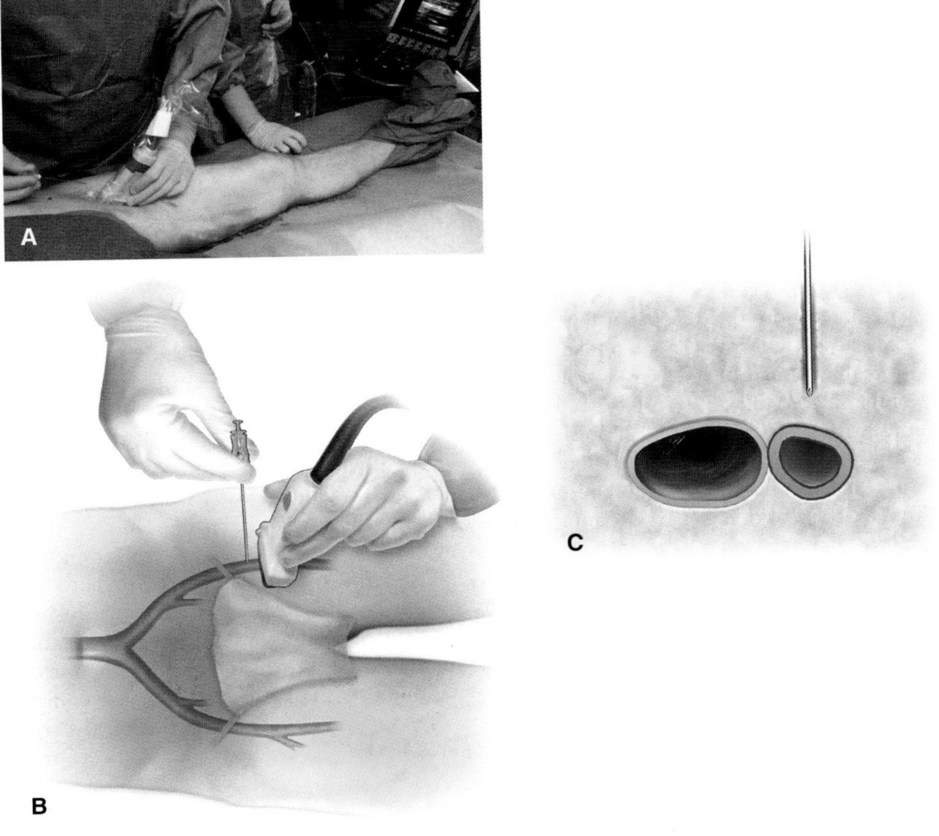

FIGURE 6 ● Ultrasound-guided puncture. **A,** In this case, the operator is evaluating the left CFA using the ultrasound probe with a longitudinal orientation. The monitor is placed in a location where the operator can visualize the arterial puncture real time. **B,** In the drawing, the operator is preparing for an antegrade femoral puncture with ultrasound guidance. **C,** In this rendering of an ultrasound image that is seen during common femoral arterial puncture, the common femoral vein is typically much larger in diameter, lies side by side to the artery, and the vein is typically easily compressible. The entry needle can be visualized as it enters the artery to ensure the correct location of the puncture.

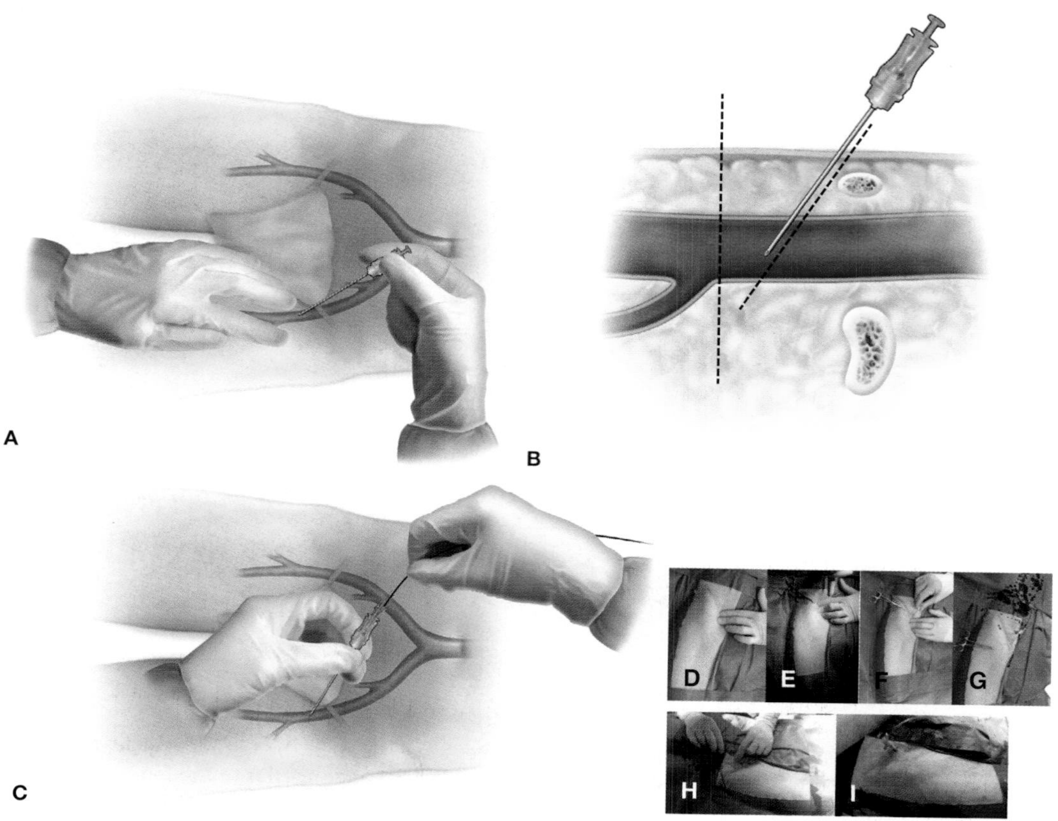

FIGURE 7 ● Antegrade puncture. **A,** The needle punctures the skin at the level of the inguinal ligament or just superior to that level. The angle of trajectory of the needle will permit the artery puncture to be proximal to the femoral bifurcation. **B,** The further proximal to the femoral bifurcation the artery puncture is located, the easier it is to steer the wire into the SFA. The best location for needle placement is inferior to the inguinal ligament but well proximal to the femoral bifurcation. **C,** The needle enters the CFA, and when arterial return is achieved, the floppy-tip guidewire is advanced into the artery. **D,** The artery and the anatomic boundaries are palpated. **E,** A clamp is used to assist with fluoroscopic identification of the desired puncture location. **F,** The needle is placed. **G,** Arterial return is achieved. **H,** A guidewire is placed. **I,** A sheath is advanced.

angiography from an ipsilateral oblique angle is performed to outline femoral bifurcation anatomy, after which a steerable hydrophilic guidewire and, ultimately, the 5-Fr sheath is directed under fluoroscopic imaging into the SFA.

- Antegrade femoral access should be avoided in the obese, in patients with a short CFA, or in patients with extreme proximal or orificial SFA disease. Although antegrade access improves "pushability" across total occlusions and enables usage of a wider inventory of guidewire-catheter combinations, there is no option for inflow disease management using this approach.
- Brachial puncture and transaortic sheath placement may provide an alternative option for "antegrade" femoral access. Upper extremity arteries are smaller, less forgiving, more prone to spasm, and less predictably managed with compression following access. Notoriously, small amounts of arterial extravasation may catalyze debilitating and permanent neurapraxia, even when brachial access is obtained well distal to the axillary fossa. Debilitating nerve injury from "axillary" sheath hematomas may occur at any location proximal to the antecubitum. Open exposure effectively minimizes this risk, and exposure is easily obtained with local anesthetic in most patients.
- The longer guidewires and catheters required to access the femoral and popliteal arteries are less responsive to surgeon manipulation from a brachial approach and also limit the available inventory of appropriate devices for femoral or popliteal intervention.
- When brachial access is required, the level of access is determined by the diameter of the largest sheath required to complete the procedure. For 6- or 7-Fr sheaths, the segment immediately proximal to the antecubital fossa is sufficient. For larger sheaths, access should be obtained in the distal axillary artery, proximal to the bifurcation of the deep brachial artery. The left arm should be used whenever possible to minimize risk for embolic iatrogenic stroke. During micropuncture access, even under direct vision, back-bleeding may not be pulsatile due to the smaller caliber of the brachial artery. Sheaths should be managed with frequent flushing with 100 U/mL heparin, as well as systemic anticoagulation once definitive interventional sheaths (6-7 Fr, 55-90 cm from the arm) are positioned in the target artery, or whenever sheaths appear to be occlusive. Intra-arterial nitroglycerine injection may reduce arterial vasospasm to the distal extremity when necessary.

- Percutaneous femoral-popliteal revascularization techniques include balloon angioplasty alone, or self-expanding stent graft implantation as an adjunct to angioplasty. These techniques require placement of interventional-grade sheaths, braided when required to cross the aortic arch or bifurcation to prevent kinking as well as sufficient length to reach the treatment site without limiting device selection. Sheath access also permits serial angiographic imaging to guide device positioning, deployment, and confirm procedural success.

SHEATH PLACEMENT

- Ensure that the appropriate sheath is selected and that alternatives are available should plans or needs change.
- Decide on optimal sheath positioning. Usually, placement immediately adjacent to the target lesion maximizes the ability to cross the lesion, control the procedure, and minimize contrast usage. In many circumstances, it may not be possible or practical to advance the sheath past the femoral bifurcation when approaching from the contralateral femoral artery.
- Heparin is typically administered, 50 to 100 U/kg, following sheath placement and prior to intervention.

Up and Over Approach

- Crossing the aortic bifurcation (**FIGURE 8**): Through a contralateral retrograde puncture, an infrarenal aortogram is performed to evaluate aortic bifurcation anatomy and location. Usually located at the level of the iliac crest, vascular calcifications may outline the bifurcation and guide positioning. The aortic bifurcation must be free of occlusive or aneurysmal disease to ensure safe sheath passage. Occasionally, iliac artery lesions must be treated prior to femoral intervention to ensure optimal outcome.
- Selective catheterization of the aortic bifurcation is performed, followed by antegrade catheterization of the contralateral iliac artery system, either with the flush or pigtail catheter used for the aortogram or an exchange catheter advanced at least to the femoral bifurcation.
- The sheath tip is placed somewhere between mid-iliac artery and the mid- to distal SFA, depending on lesion location and interventional intention. A 6-Fr sheath may be adequate for this purpose, but 7 Fr may be required for many devices (read the package insert). The angioplasty catheter length for proximal SFA lesions is 75 to 80 cm; for more distal lesions, 90 to 110 cm.
- Access to the deep femoral artery may be required to safely advance the "up and over" sheath over a stiff exchange wire (eg, Rosen). After flushing and dilator placement, ensure that the sheath sidearm stopcock is turned to the "off" position. The skin incision may need to be enlarged to facilitate placement. Consider serial dilator exchanges when upsizing a sheath by two or more French sizes. Occasionally, depending on the angle of the aortic bifurcation, sheath placement may be facilitated by passage over a stiff, exchange length hydrophilic wire. When using hydrophilic wires for this purpose, care should always be taken to keep the tip of the wire in the image screen field to prevent inadvertent arterial puncture and extravasation from wire injury. Similarly, when confronted by extreme tortuosity in the iliac arterial system, interval advancement of the sheath into the internal iliac artery may be required to gain access to the contralateral iliac artery with a second or "buddy" wire, following which, standard catheter and guidewire techniques may be used to advance the sheath to its ultimate desired location.
- Regardless of procedure or access approach, it is always advisable to keep the wire tip in the imaging field whenever sheaths are exchanged or advanced—arterial perforation and extravasation may limit procedural options, or the ability to initiate systemic anticoagulation, and may increase compartment pressures to the point of requiring surgical release if not recognized and managed promptly.

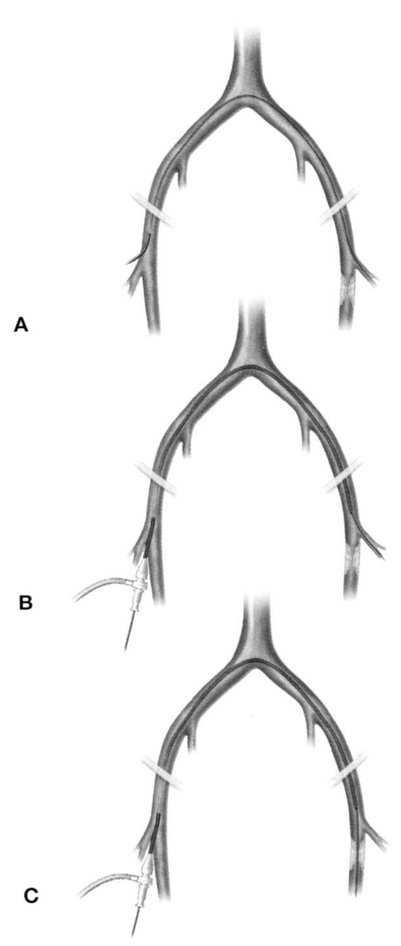

FIGURE 8 ● Sheath access. **A,** An exchange guidewire is placed over the aortic bifurcation. The tip of the guidewire is placed in a large, safe branch. In this example, the profunda femoris artery is used to anchor the wire. **B,** The sheath is advanced over the stiff guidewire. The advancement of the sheath is observed under fluoroscopic control to ensure that it is being passed safely. **C,** After sheath placement over the aortic bifurcation, the stiff wire is removed and the directional wire is advanced across the lesion in preparation for treatment.

Table 2: Approach: Up and Over or Ipsilateral Antegrade

Approach	Antegrade	Up and over	Brachial
Puncture	More challenging	Simple retrograde femoral	Retrograde brachial
Catheterization	Proximal femoral puncture and selective catheters	Challenging with tortuous arteries, diseased bifurcation	Challenging, long distance, diseased aorta
		Easy to catheterize SFA	
Catheter control	Excellent	Fair	Fair
Catheter inventory	Minimal	More supplies, long catheters	Specific material, long sheaths, catheters
		Up and over sheaths	
Indications	Infrapopliteal, femoropopliteal disease	Proximal SFA disease	Proximal SFA, femoropopliteal disease
Limitations	Obesity, CFA disease, proximal SFA disease	Contralateral disease, bifurcation disease	Aortic disease, infrapopliteal disease

CFA, common femoral artery; SFA, superficial femoral artery.

Ipsilateral Approach

- See prior recommendations for securing access (**TABLE 2**). Obesity and excessive abdominal pannus may significantly limit the use of this approach. Before initiating treatment, obtain angiographic documentation of existing ipsilateral anatomy, including infrapopliteal runoff.
- Shorter guidewires and devices improve the efficiency of the ipsilateral antegrade approach.
- If balloon angioplasty alone is planned, 4- or 5-Fr sheath can be used to treat ipsilateral SFA lesions. More complex reconstructions require 6-Fr and occasionally 7-Fr sheaths.

CROSSING OCCLUSIVE LESIONS

- Guidewire-catheter skills form the basis of all endovascular procedures. Successful guidewire positioning requires familiarity with a range of devices and guidewire-catheter pairings. The guidewire required for crossing the lesion could not be adequate for working or deploying a stent or a stent graft. Familiarity with and access to a wide selection of wires (depending on length, diameter, tip pressure, and hydrophilic qualities) is essential for success (**FIGURE 9**).
- Guidewire features to be considered:
  - Length: Must be adequate to cover the cumulative distance, both inside and outside the patient, to perform the procedure and support the catheter.

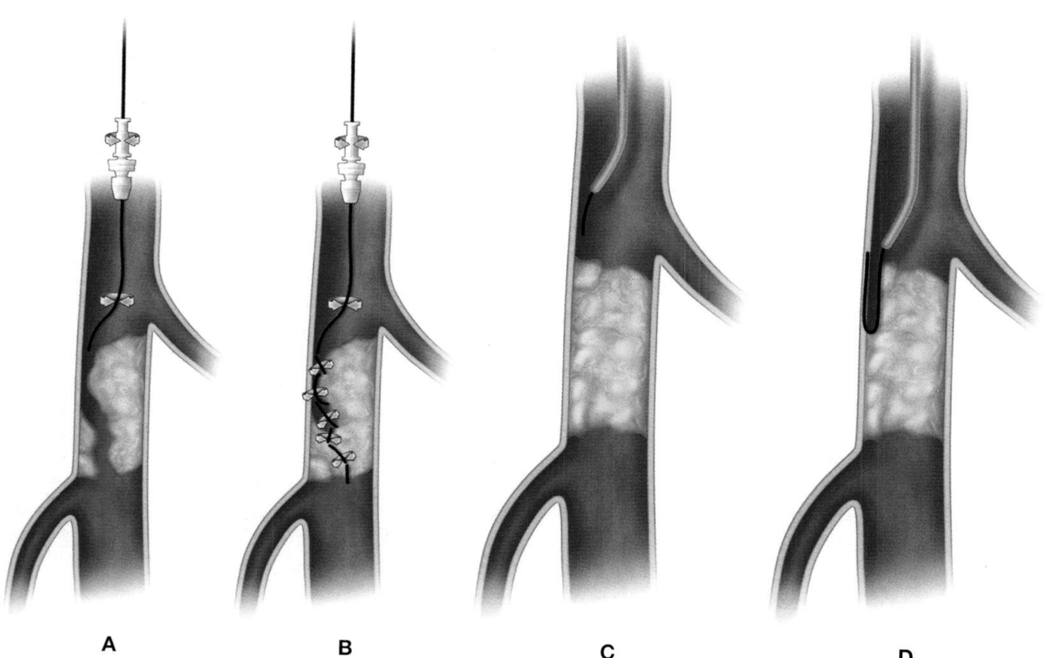

FIGURE 9 ● Crossing the lesion. **A,** In this case, a critical stenosis is crossed. The image intensifier is angulated to get the best view of the pathway through the lesion. **B,** Typically, a hydrophilic wire with a directional tip is used and the wire tip is steered through the lesion. **C,** In this case, an occlusion is crossed using subintimal technique. The guidewire is advanced and is supported by a catheter with an angled tip. **D,** The guidewire is pointed toward the arterial wall at the beginning of the lesion and is pointed away from the collateral that fills the segment and is near the location where the lesion begins. The wire is pushed until an elbow forms and enters the subintimal space. **E,** The loop is advanced. The loop is maintained in a narrow configuration by supporting it closely with the catheter. **F,** After the loop pops into the patent distal segment, the catheter is advanced. The wire is removed and contrast is administered to confirm the location of the catheter tip in the true lumen.

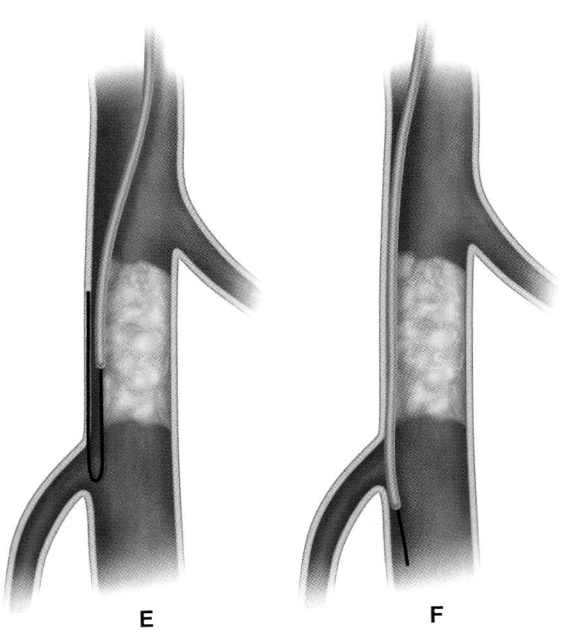

FIGURE 9 ● Continued

Guidewire lengths vary from 145 to 300 cm. For an ipsilateral antegrade approach, 145- to 180-cm guidewires are adequate, but for contralateral or brachial access 260- to 300-cm lengths are necessary.

As a general rule of thumb, guidewire length must be at least twice that of the coaxial device to be positioned over the wire.

- Diameter: Most femoral-popliteal procedures are performed with 0.035-in guidewires, but smaller-caliber angioplasty is generally performed with 0.018-in or 0.014-in guidewires.
- Stiffness: An inner steel core confers different magnitudes of stiffness on the shaft of the wire. A stiffer wire may help to cross a calcified lesion, but it is also easier to injure the vessels. In wires specifically designed to cross femoral-popliteal lesions, tip pressure may also vary across wires with similar stiffness along the majority of their length.
- Coating: Hydrophilic guidewires may reduce the coefficient of friction. Typically, they are passed in conjunction with purpose-specific crossing catheters.

- Crossing catheters support guidewire passage and, depending on design, confer varying degrees of support and directionality. After the guidewire is used to cross the lesion, the catheter may be advanced so that the choice working wire may be placed. Crossing catheter technology has advanced considerably in the last 5 to 10 years. Options abound for torsionality (braided or unbraided), tip taper, tip shape, length, and diameter. Examples include the Quick-Cross and CTX catheter families. Some experience is required to learn how to use these catheters optimally in most situations.

RECANALIZATION STRATEGY IN CHRONIC TOTAL OCCLUSIONS

- With most complex lesions of the femoral and popliteal arteries, it is quite common to recanalize the true lumen. Stenosis can almost always be crossed transluminally using a wire supported by a catheter. A steerable, hydrophilic, low-profile wire is best. Long lesions, particularly if completely occluded, may not be able to be crossed in the true lumen. In this case, subintimal recanalization and reentry is the best option.
- Strategy is based on selection of a reentry site where the artery has an acceptable lumen, collaterals can be preserved, calcification is avoided, and potential bypass sites remain intact. Staying in the true lumen offers the shortest reconstruction and preservation of the most collaterals. When subintimal passage is required, reentry should be accomplished as close to the distal true lumen reconstitution as possible. The most common method of subintimal recanalization is using a loop of hydrophilic wire to dissect the subintimal space reenter the true lumen.
- There is typically a large incoming collateral feeding the reconstituted segment. If the reentry site is calcified, the success rate for loop passage is lower and use of a reentry catheter is more likely to be needed.
- If there is a substantial plaque at the intended reentry site, consider a site more distal than the initial reconstitution site. If there is another lesion distal to but near the reentry site, this can pose a challenge for passing the guidewire distally after it has popped into the true lumen.
- The operator must decide in this case whether to reenter distal to all the lesions, given that it might negatively affect bypass options. If reentry fails and the patient needs a bypass, target sites for distal anastomosis should be anticipated, although failed reentry usually does not result in thrombosis of that segment.

TREATMENT PLATFORM

Sheath Placement

- Place the sheath tip close to the origin of the occlusion. Contrast administered through the sheath fills the distal reconstitution site through collaterals. For an SFA occlusion, the tip of the sheath is usually positioned near the femoral bifurcation and the distal artery is visualized with contrast flowing through profunda collaterals. Use a sheath that is one size larger than that used for angioplasty and stenting, usually 7 Fr. This permits contrast administration even if a reentry device is being positioned (**FIGURE 10**).

- Heparin is typically administered, 50 to 100 U/kg following sheath placement and prior to intervention.

Entering the Subintimal Space

- Place an angled-tip catheter pointing toward the artery wall at the origin of the occlusion. Point it opposite the location where the largest runoff collateral is located. Advance a Glidewire into the wall. Push it and the tip will catch and a loop will form (**FIGURE 11**).

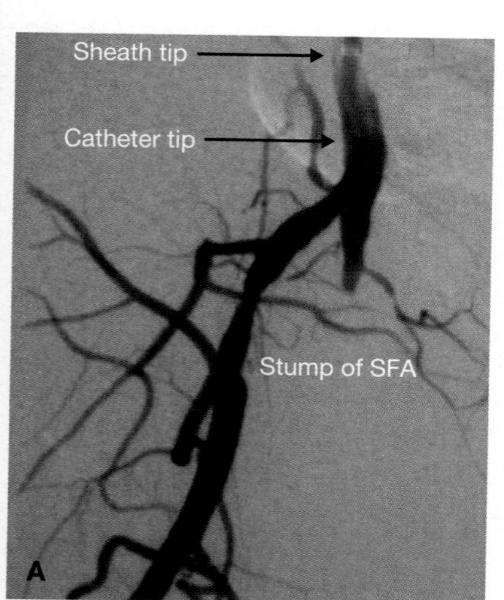

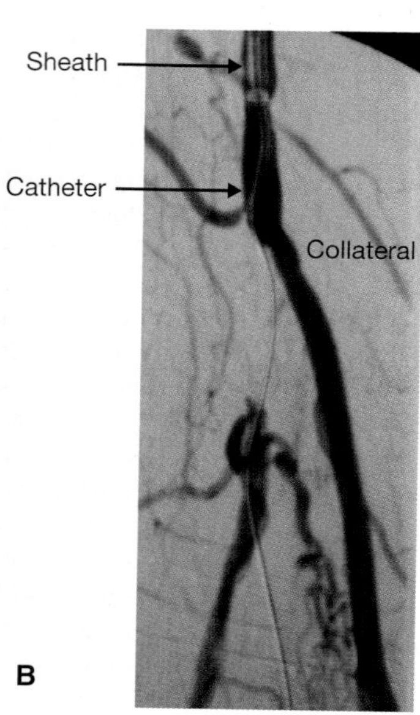

FIGURE 10 ● Sheath placement. **A,** There is a stump of proximal SFA that is patent. The sheath was placed up and over the aortic bifurcation. The tip of the sheath is in the common femoral artery and can be recognized by a radiopaque tip. The catheter is used to direct the guidewire into the blind sac of the occluded proximal SFA. **B,** This arteriogram shows a short popliteal artery occlusion. The tip of the sheath is placed directly into the proximal popliteal artery to support the recanalization. There is a large perigenicular collateral that originates from the popliteal artery at the location where the artery occludes. Typically, the subintimal space is entered by directing the catheter tip and the guidewire to the arterial wall on the side opposite the origin of the large collateral.

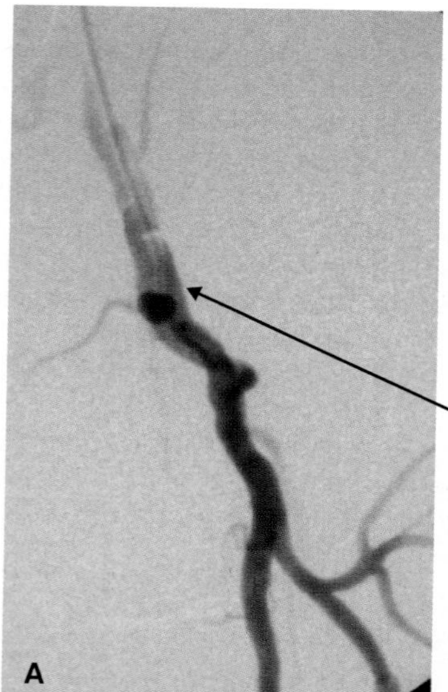

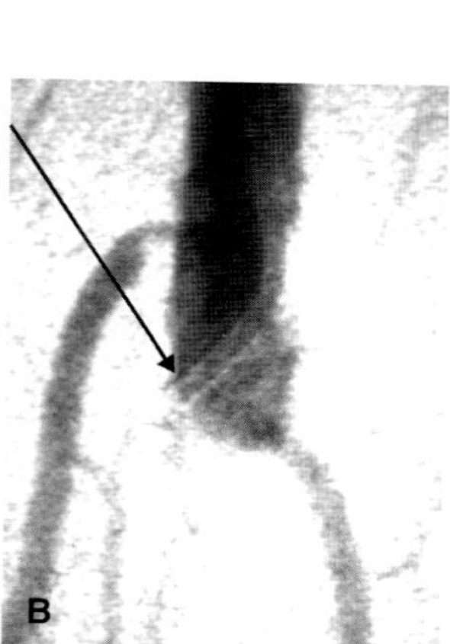

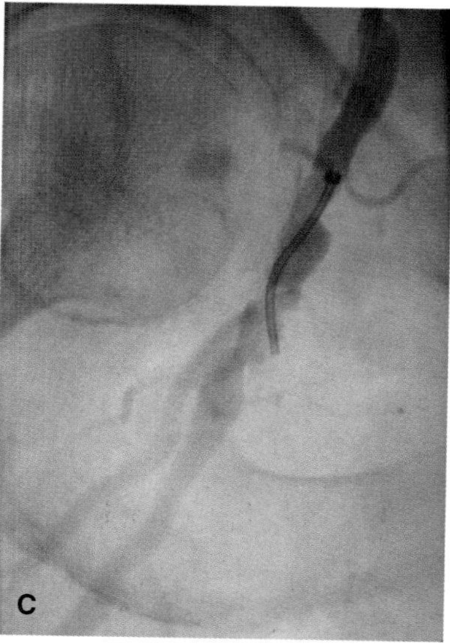

FIGURE 11 ● Enter the subintimal space. **A,** After sheath tip placement near the origin of the occlusion and where the administered contrast will opacify the location where the artery reconstitutes. An angled-tip catheter is used (*arrow*) to direct the wire toward the superficial femoral artery origin. **B,** In the popliteal artery, the catheter is pointed to the interface between the artery and the occlusion on the side opposite the largest exiting collateral (*arrow*). **C,** The tip of the catheter is pointed against the artery wall at the location where the occlusion starts. **D,** The hydrophilic guidewire is pushed into the wall until the tip of the wire catches and a loop forms. The loop usually forms at the transition zone along the wire between the soft, floppy tip of the hydrophilic wire and the stiffer shaft of the wire. **E,** After the wire loop is embedded within the occlusion, the supporting catheter is advanced.

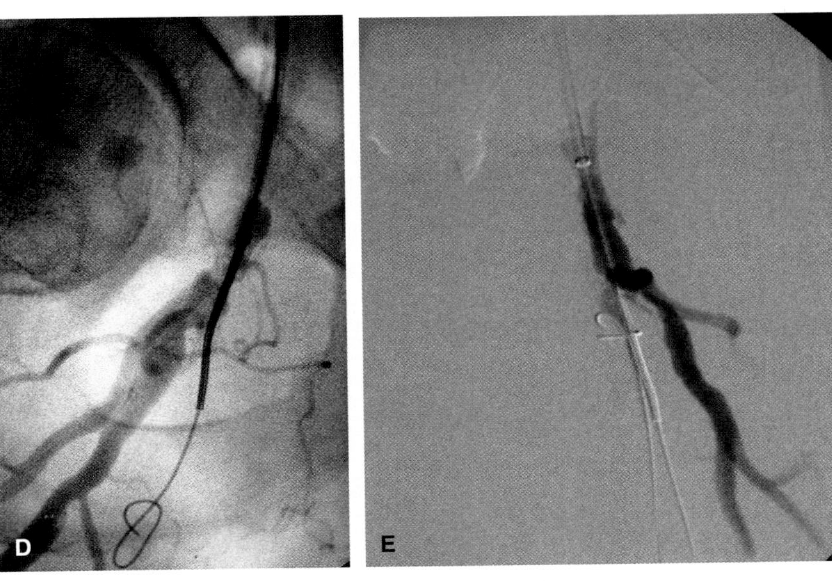

FIGURE 11 ● Continued

LOOP MANAGEMENT

Loop Advancement

- Visualization, loop management, and assessment of the reentry site are the maneuvers that enhance success. The looped hydrophilic wire is advanced past the lesion (**FIGURE 12**). The loop is kept narrow and is optimal if less than the diameter of the artery lumen. This is done by closely following the loop with a supporting catheter. Because the loop is in the subintimal space, keeping the loop narrow keeps the subintimal space tight. This helps to direct the wire in a straighter trajectory toward its target and makes the knuckle of the wire loop a more effective tool for piercing tissue to get into the true lumen.
- The standard Glidewire (Terumo) has a directional tip with a soft shaft. If subintimal passage is being performed past a heavily calcified lesion, the artery wall may be more adherent to the calcified segment, making wire passage alone more difficult. Catheter support is required, and sometimes a low-profile balloon must be used to create space in the

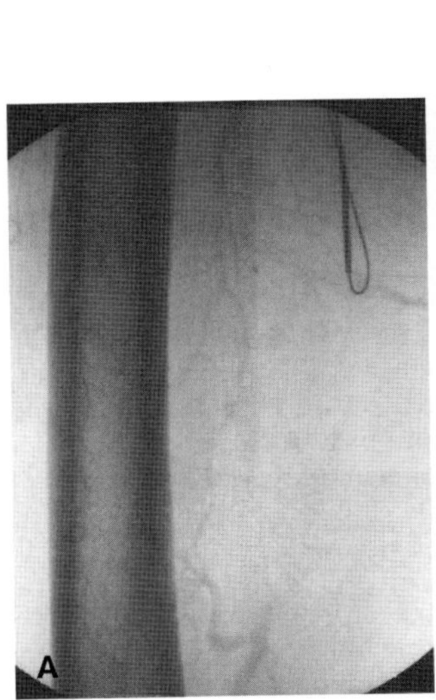

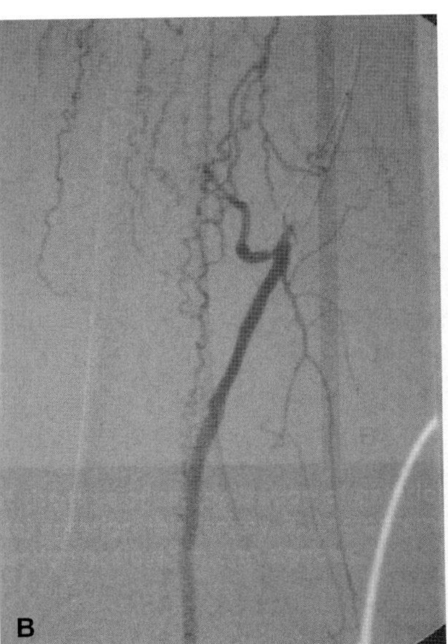

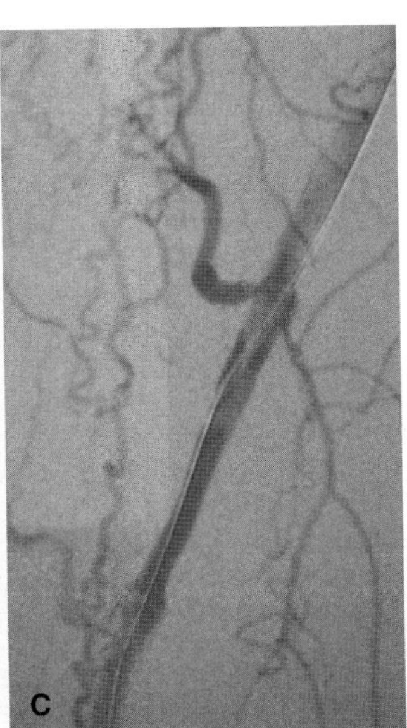

FIGURE 12 ● Loop advancement. **A,** After entering the subintimal space, the loop is advanced with the support of the catheter. The loop works best when it is maintained in a narrow configuration. This is enhanced by closely following the loop with the supporting catheter. If the loop encounters a heavily calcified segment, it tends to widen or to spiral around the calcific segment. **B,** The loop is advanced to the arterial segment where the true lumen is reconstituted. Quite commonly, the loop of wire will pass into the true lumen. The location where the artery reconstitutes is visualized by administering contrast into the sheath. **C,** After the loop passes into the true lumen, advance the catheter into the true lumen. Always confirm location in the true lumen before starting reconstruction. This is usually done by removing the wire and administering contrast into the catheter. The guidewire of choice for use during treatment can then be placed.

subintimal plane. Typically, a standard Glidewire is used, but when passing a very calcified lesion, a stiff Glidewire should be considered. A nylon catheter, 4 or 5 Fr, with an angled tip and a hydrophilic coating is best.

- CTO support catheters, such as the Quick-Cross (Spectranetics) or the CXI (Cook Medical), offer more support and low profile than a standard catheter and are generally helpful in crossing CTOs. The loop usually seeks the weakest point in the tissue and breaks across the membrane from subintimal potential space to true lumen more than 70% of the time in our experience. Orthogonal views are helpful in assessing the trajectory of the loop and whether it is progressing toward the reentry site.
- Even if the reentry site is calcified, a wire loop or a stiff wire with catheter support may reenter the true lumen, and it is worth an attempt. If this approach is unsuccessful, a reentry catheter is used as the next step, both to save time and to maintain the integrity of the reentry before too much manipulation has taken place.

REENTRY DEVICE

Reentry Device Placement

- The subintimal wire is exchanged for a stiff 0.014-in guidewire.
- The reentry device is advanced.
  - If the proximal part of the subintimal space is too tight to allow passage of a 6-Fr reentry catheter (approximately 2 mm), a long, low-caliber balloon may be used to slightly enlarge the subintimal space. Do not dilate the area intended for reentry. If the subintimal space at the reentry site is enlarged, it prevents the reentry needle from having adequate support to puncture the true lumen.

REENTRY INTO TRUE LUMEN

- After the catheter is in place, a needle in the tip of the catheter is advanced into the true lumen.
- A 0.014-in guidewire is advanced from the reentry catheter into the true lumen.
  - The direction of the needle is oriented using fluoroscopy.
  - Orthogonal views are obtained to locate the juxtaposition of the true and false lumens.
  - The image intensifier is positioned so that the catheter and an acceptable target vessel segment are viewed side by side.
- Rotate the catheter until the "L" shape appears at the tip.
- Advance the needle into the true lumen.
  - Multiple needle passes may be required. The risk of a needle pass is low.
  - The needle may only require a partial advancement to get into the true lumen. A full advancement may go through the true lumen and into the wall on the opposite side.
  - Multiple small adjustments are often required before the true lumen is reentered, especially if the reentry site is diseased.
- The needle throw is oriented with intravascular ultrasound (IVUS) when using the Pioneer catheter (Medtronic). The needle is at the 12-o'clock position on the IVUS image, and the catheter is rotated to face the true lumen. Using color ultrasound, the true and false lumens can be distinguished and the wire passed into the true lumen.
- After passing the wire, the needle is retracted and the reentry catheter is removed over the wire.
- Some commercially available reentry catheters are listed in **TABLE 1**. Reentry catheters may be guided by fluoroscopy or IVUS, and reentry is achieved by passage of a needle, stiff wire tip, or drill. Orthogonal views are obtained to locate the juxtaposition of the true and false lumens, and the image intensifier is positioned so that the catheter and an acceptable target vessel segment are viewed side by side (**FIGURE 13**).

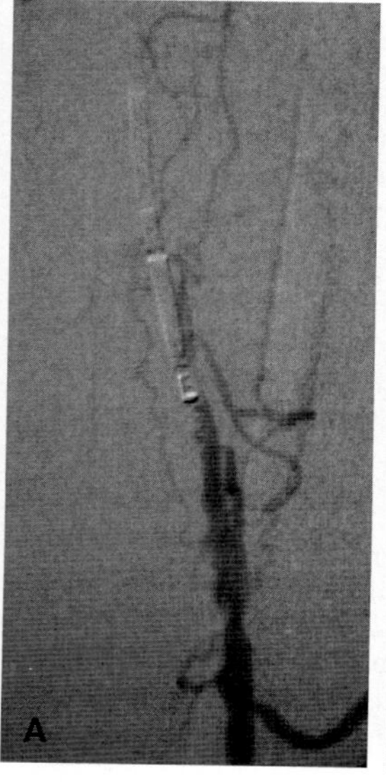

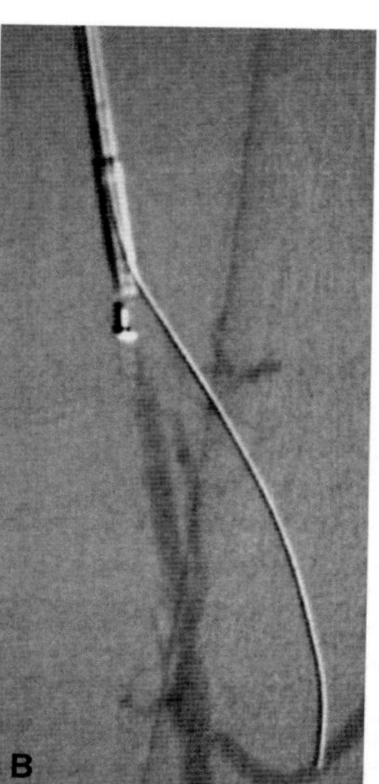

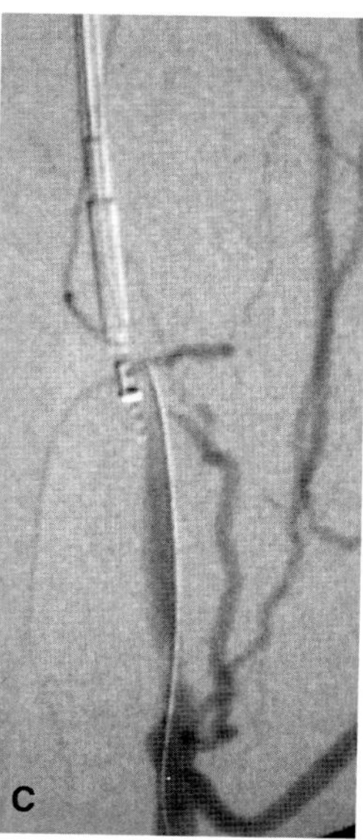

FIGURE 13 ● Use of a reentry catheter. **A,** If the wire loop does not pass into the true lumen, consider a reentry device. In this example, the Outback (Cordis) device is used. This is a 6-Fr catheter that is advanced in the subintimal space, along the same course where the channel was created by the catheter and guidewire. The reentry catheter is oriented side by side with the true lumen. The catheter is rotated so that the "L" shape at the tip of the reentry catheter is pointing toward the true lumen. **B,** The needle is advanced. In this case, the tip of the needle had passed beyond the true lumen and the wire is outside the artery. **C,** The needle is passed again, this time not quite so deeply, and the wire passes into the true lumen. After each throw of the needle, if it appears to be going in the correct direction into the true lumen, the wire is passed to explore and see if the tip progresses into the correct location in the true lumen.

ALTERNATIVE REENTRY OPTIONS

Reentry Device Cannot Be Used

- Use a catheter with a stiff tip to bluntly push on the reentry site or use a low-profile balloon angioplasty to break up the tissue membrane in hopes of achieving a fenestration as shown by active blood return.
- This approach is sometimes successful, but it enlarges and occasionally perforates the subintimal space at the reentry site and will render the reentry catheters less efficacious because they rely on a tight subintimal space to provide leverage for the needle passage into the true lumen.
- Another option is to consider a straight 0.035-in Glidewire or a straight 0.014-in or 0.018-in CTO wire to push on the reentry site to see if it can be drilled into place.

Retrograde Approach

- Retrograde puncture can be performed on a distal artery, such as a tibial or pedal artery. Retrograde passage of a wire is often possible, even when antegrade passage across the same lesion was not. This is especially the case for occlusions of the popliteal and proximal tibial level where there are collaterals that an antegrade wire tends to follow blindly along and where reentry devices are not as applicable.
  - Contrast is administered through the proximal access to obtain a roadmap of the distal puncture site, or ultrasound is used to guide the access.
  - A 4-cm 21-gauge micropuncture needle is used.
- A V18 wire (Boston Scientific) is introduced.
  - Sheath placement is avoided if possible to keep the arteriotomy small.
  - If the retrograde wire cannot break into the true lumen, a coronary balloon catheter is passed over it.
- A balloon introduced from the antegrade direction and the balloon introduced retrograde are juxtaposed and inflated and are usually able to split the dissection flap to open the true lumen (**FIGURE 14**).

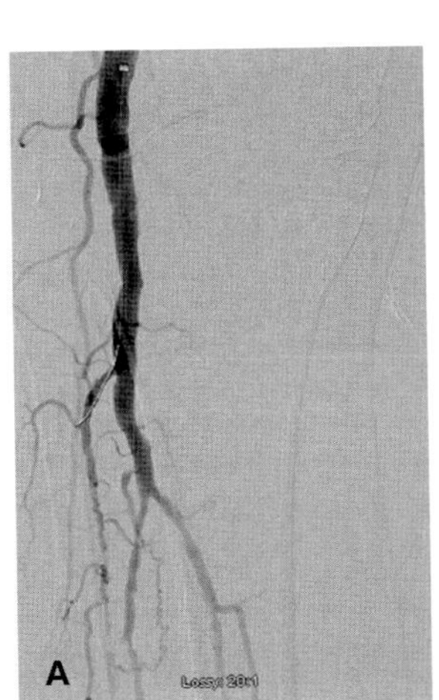

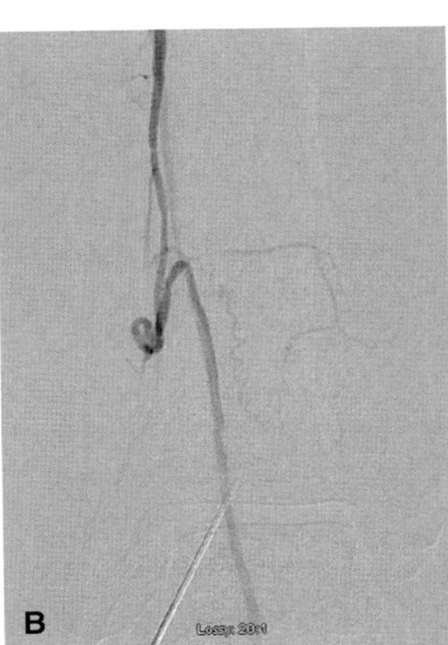

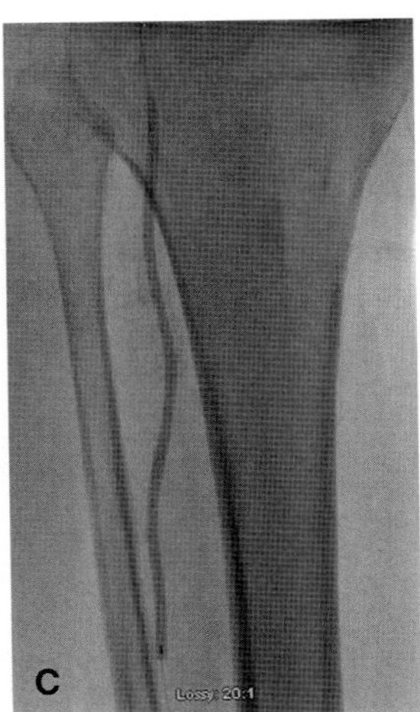

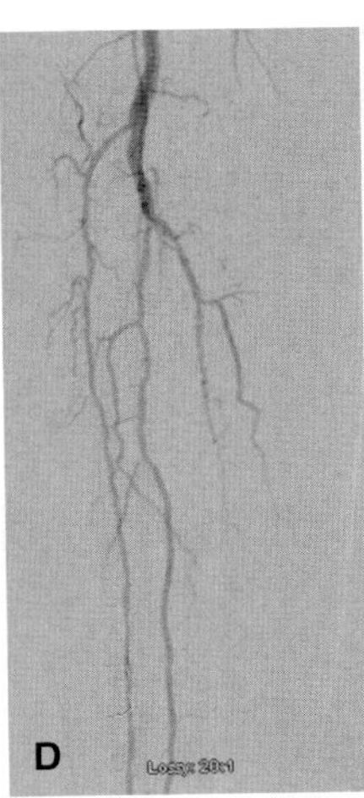

FIGURE 14 ● Retrograde puncture using pedal access. **A,** This patient has a pedal gangrene in an angiosome that is perfused by the anterior tibial artery. Revascularization of the anterior tibial artery using a traditional antegrade approach was not successful. **B,** A roadmap of the distal anterior tibial artery was performed. The arterial access needle is advanced into the distal anterior tibial artery under roadmapping. **C,** After retrograde access, the guidewire is passed into the antegrade sheath. The angioplasty balloon is then introduced through the antegrade sheath. **D,** After angioplasty, the anterior tibial artery is patent.

BALLOON ANGIOPLASTY

- Once wire access is obtained across the lesion, angioplasty is undertaken. The angioplasty process enlarges the lumen by compressing and rupturing the plaque, as well as stretching and, in some cases, damaging the media and adventitia (**FIGURE 15**).
- The balloon length and diameter are typically selected to treat the entire lesion, with minimal proximal or distal overlap, to restore the original diameter as determined by proximal or distal measurement. The balloon catheter is positioned over the guidewire and inflated to nominal pressure to achieve the specified diameter. Occasionally, higher pressures may be required to reduce lesion "waisting."
- Inflate slowly. Balloon inflation is maintained for 2 minutes.
- Deflate slowly, and ensure full deflation fluoroscopically before withdrawal.
- The balloon angioplasty catheter may be used repeatedly during the same procedure; however, its capacity to recover the predeployment diameter following deflation degrades with sequential use.
- Balloon diameters range from 4 to 7 mm for the SFA and 3 to 6 mm in the popliteal artery.
- Conventional angioplasty is limited somewhat by target artery dissection. Not all dissections need further treatment. In general, only flow-limiting dissections as judged by sequential contrast injections through the interventional sheath need additional treatment. Dissections may be managed by prolonged periods of inflation followed by gradual deflation to "tack" the plaque up to the arterial wall. Persistent flow obstruction following angioplasty is the most common indication for subsequent secondary stenting.

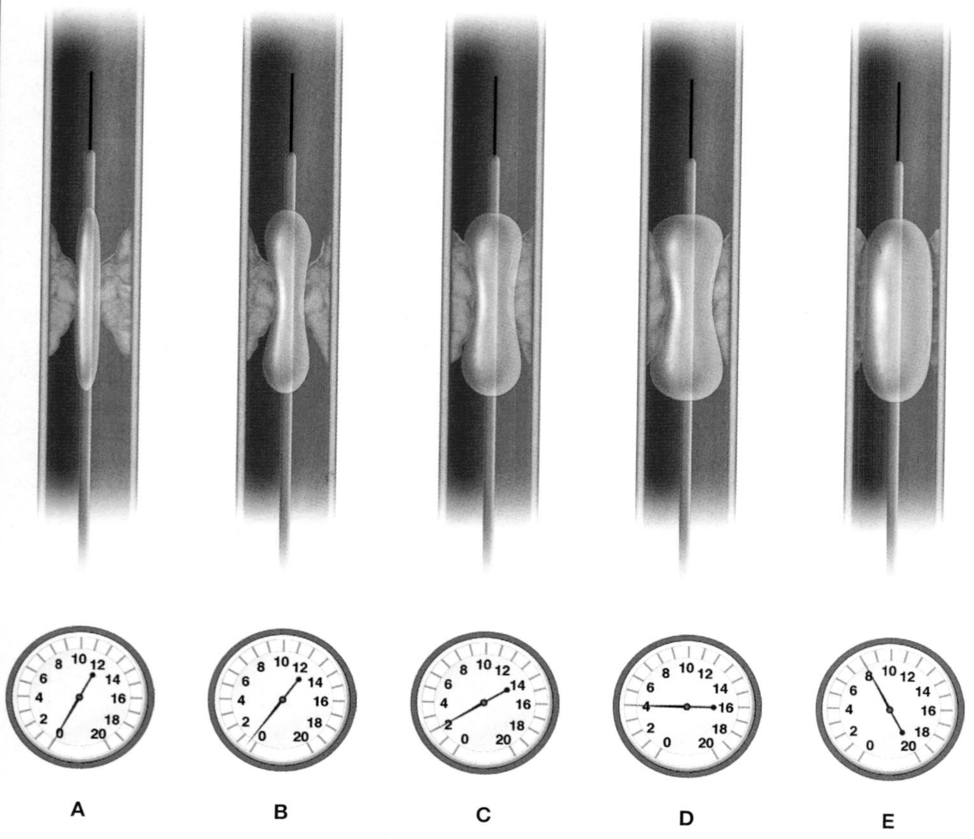

FIGURE 15 ● Balloon angioplasty. **A,** The balloon catheter is advanced over the guidewire and into the lesion. If possible, an angioplasty balloon is selected that is able to treat the whole lesion length with a single inflation. **B,** The balloon is inflated, and this is observed using fluoroscopy. At very low pressure, the balloon will inflate freely in the locations where there is minimal or no impingement of the lesion on the balloon. **C,** Usually with 2 atm of pressure, the waist on the balloon becomes apparent and the lesion begins to yield to the outward force exerted by the balloon. **D,** The balloon is inflated gradually. This helps to avoid delivering more pressure to the artery than is required. This also allows the lesion to gradually give way. At higher pressure, the waist becomes smaller. **E,** Pressure in the balloon is gradually increased until the balloon reaches its full diameter. The balloon is typically inflated for 2 to 3 minutes in situations where the operator is hoping to use angioplasty as stand-alone therapy.

STENTS

- Although all vascular-compatible, size-appropriate, self-expanding (nitinol) stents may be deployed in the superficial femoral or popliteal arteries as clinically indicated, select devices have obtained specific indications for this application from the US Food and Drug Administration. The operator is encouraged to familiarize themselves with this designation and to use application-approved devices whenever appropriate to ensure optimal outcome.
- Material and characteristics of peripheral stents have evolved in recent years. Self-expanding nitinol stents are most appropriate for SFA and popliteal applications. The ideal stent should have the ability to adapt to the vessel with a precise deployment and without kinking, collapsing, or fracturing as well as limit long-term arterial injury and restenosis. More recently, drug-eluting stents have been developed and are approved for use in the United States to limit chronic restenosis of the stent arterial segment following deployment. The potential clinical benefits derived from these devices are offset to a significant degree by their substantial increase in cost over "bare metal" stents.
- Femoral-popliteal stents may be placed routinely or selectively. Selective stent placement may be considered for significant postangioplasty dissection, long lesions (>15 cm), residual stenosis postangioplasty, pressure gradient (>10 mm Hg) after angioplasty, recurrent stenosis, occlusion, or to prevent or limit postangioplasty embolization of plaque.
- Localization: A stent is typically deployed to span the distance between the relatively healthy artery proximal and distal to the target lesion. "Healthy" is a relative term in this sense, and care should be taken to limit stent coverage to the minimal distance required to achieve an optimal result. Long lesions in the SFA are most commonly stented, but be aware that stents in the distal superficial femoral and popliteal arteries may be damaged by stress from knee flexion (**FIGURE 16**). Excessive stent coverage may accelerate long-term restenosis and luminal compromise, regardless of the degree of initial success or the type or size of deployed stent.
- Sheath size: Most stents for infrainguinal deployment require a 6- or 7-Fr sheath. Refer to the individual instructions for use for each individual device.
- Deployment: Most infrainguinal nitinol stents are deployed using a pin and pull maneuver that retracts the cover from the constrained stent and the underlying mandrel. A ratcheting mechanism may also be integrated into the deployment process. Typically, these may be removed for basic pin/pull deployment if the ratchet becomes jammed or disabled. After deployment, completion angioplasty is performed to bring the stent to profile.
- Complications of stent deployment:
  - Acute: arterial dissection, occlusion, rupture, stent migration or embolization, embolization of atherosclerotic material, thrombosis
  - Chronic: intimal hyperplasia, recurrent stenosis, infection, stent damage, thrombosis

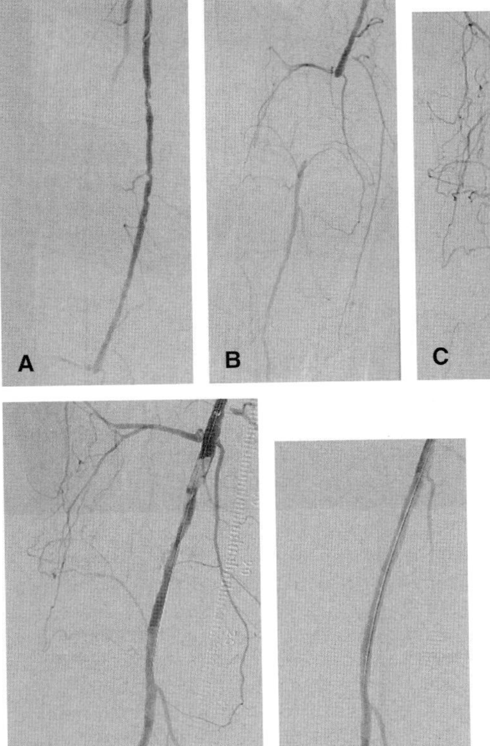

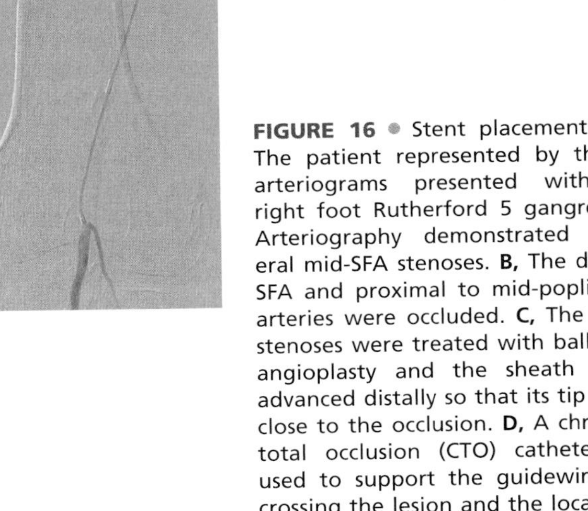

FIGURE 16 ● Stent placement. **A,** The patient represented by these arteriograms presented with a right foot Rutherford 5 gangrene. Arteriography demonstrated several mid-SFA stenoses. **B,** The distal SFA and proximal to mid-popliteal arteries were occluded. **C,** The SFA stenoses were treated with balloon angioplasty and the sheath was advanced distally so that its tip was close to the occlusion. **D,** A chronic total occlusion (CTO) catheter is used to support the guidewire in crossing the lesion and the location in the true lumen is confirmed. **E,** After balloon angioplasty, there was a significant dissection and residual stenosis. **F,** A self-expanding nitinol stent was placed for mechanical support of the arterial wall and to enhance immediate patency of the reconstruction.

STENT GRAFTS

- Nitinol-based, flexible stent grafts may be deployed over long and calcified SFA lesions as an alternative to bare metal or drug-eluting stents. In general, the longer and more complex the target lesion(s) and length of required coverage, the more suitable the indication for covered stent placement.
- Stent grafting may require exchange of a 0.035-in wire system for smaller guidewires (eg, 0.025 in or 0.018 in); the operator is again cautioned to refer to the instructions for use for each device considered for placement. Stent grafts must be deployed over the specific guidewire adequate for the stent graft. Sheath upsizing may also be required, depending on the diameter selected. Choosing a larger sheath at the outset will minimize the need for awkward or inefficient sheath exchange after the procedure is well underway. Aggressive predilatation is also often necessary in order to create sufficient space for bulkier covered stent to pass the lesion prior to deployment. Similar to bare metal stents, covered stent deployment is usually followed by completion angioplasty to bring the covered lumen to profile (**FIGURE 17**).
- Relative advantages of stent grafts compared with bare metal stents include the ability to create an entirely new lining for a disease arterial segment. This coverage obviates the possibility of in-stent stenosis within the graft. However, experience has shown that unlike surgically placed prosthetic bypass grafts, covered stents in the superficial femoral and popliteal arteries tend to incite restenosis at the proximal end. Thus, placement usually requires coverage up to the origin of the SFA. Any uncovered artery in this region is likely to develop critical restenosis. Disadvantages include the necessary coverage of all collateral vessels encompassed in the covered segment, as well as the increased risk for graft infection inherent in fabric-covered metal stents. Also, although some stent grafts are heparin bonded, the thrombogenicity of covered stents varies directly with the length of segment covered, such that complete SFA coverage from the origin to the adductor canal necessitates long-term oral anticoagulation therapy in patients treated in our practice. Anticoagulation in this circumstance is designed to limit thrombus extension following future graft occlusion rather than increasing long-term graft patency. Anticoagulation does not typically extend prosthetic graft patency in the lower extremity, regardless of open or endovascular placement.

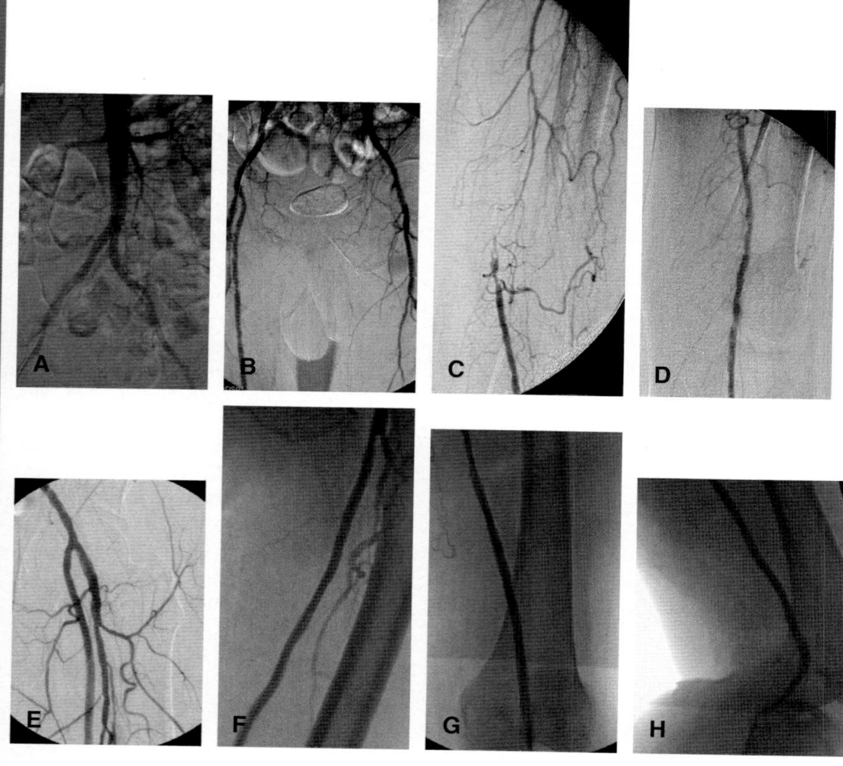

FIGURE 17 ● Stent graft. **A,** This patient has a long SFA occlusion that was relined with Viabahn stent graft. An aortoiliac arteriogram was performed using contralateral access. **B,** The left SFA is occluded. There is a patent proximal stump of SFA. **C,** The point of reconstitution is the above-the-knee popliteal artery. **D,** The proximal popliteal artery, extending to the knee, is diffusely diseased. **E and F,** After recanalization and aggressive balloon angioplasty, the artery is reconstructed with Viabahn stent graft placement. **G and H,** The distal end of the graft is fully dilated and without flow limitation in the straight leg and bent knee positions.

PEARLS AND PITFALLS

Artery puncture	▪ The puncture is planned prior to the procedure. Access site issues are the most common type of complication. A well-performed access will set the procedure up for success.
Specific material	▪ In planning the procedure, check to make sure that all the necessary inventory is available prior to the procedure.
Crossing the lesion	▪ Do not force the wire across the lesion. If staying within the true lumen is not successful, utilize subintimal passage or try a retrograde approach.
Subintimal passage	▪ The subintimal space often can be converted to a smooth, large-diameter conduit. ▪ Entry and reentry sites usually require extra angioplasty or mechanical support from implants.
Optimal reentry site	▪ Minimal calcifications. ▪ Healthy true lumen. ▪ Shortest subintimal channel.
Collaterals	▪ Reenter as close to distal reconstitution as possible. ▪ Typically, a large incoming collateral feeds the reconstituted segment. ▪ The subintimal space has collaterals and can fail suddenly. Consider anticoagulation or dual antiplatelet therapy post procedure to maintain patency.
Follow-up	▪ The patient is evaluated after the procedure at 1 week and 1 month and then 6-month intervals after that. We typically obtain some assessment of perfusion (ABI). Duplex mapping may also be performed for surveillance.

POSTOPERATIVE CARE

- The patient should remain at bedrest for at least 6 hours after the procedure. After use of a closure device, usually 2 hours of bedrest is required.
- Puncture site management: Obtaining hemostasis is made safer and simpler when the arteriotomy site is carefully managed during the procedure. Ensure the patient is comfortable prior to removing the sheath.
- Holding pressure: After ipsilateral antegrade puncture, use two hands to hold pressure. One is placed proximal to the inguinal ligament to apply pressure over distal external iliac artery to decrease the pressure flowing through the puncture. The other hand applies pressure over the area of arterial puncture just distal to the inguinal ligament. There are no approved closure devices for antegrade puncture. Following a retrograde puncture, digital pressure is held at the location of arteriotomy, proximal to the skin puncture site.
- Closure devices: Closure devices are used whenever possible to reduce risk of access site complications and limit patient immobility following the procedure.
- The patient is seen in clinic 1 week post procedure for an access site check and at 1 month where a new baseline ABI and duplex ultrasound of the treated segment is obtained. In our practice we then follow these patients with ABI and duplex every 6 months. This surveillance program is modified as necessary for high-risk patients, who are sometimes seen at closer intervals.
- True lumen recanalizations have collaterals, whereas subintimal passages do not. Patients with subintimal recanalization should be monitored with duplex because they may fail suddenly in a manner similar to a bypass. We typically perform duplex surveillance every 6 months.
- The patient should be encouraged to:
  - Avoid smoking
  - Walk daily
  - Follow best medical treatment
  - Follow-up with the vascular clinic

OUTCOMES

- Patients with peripheral artery disease and critical limb ischemia (CLI) have a shorter life expectancy than the general population. The most effective method of revascularization with the shortest recovery time and the least amount of surgical risk is considered ideal. In this regard, most centers have adopted a percutaneous-first approach to lower extremity revascularization, when intervention is indicated.[3]
- Successful percutaneous revascularization is considered equivalent to traditional open bypass surgery in providing freedom from major and minor amputation in patients with severe limb ischemia up to 2 years following revascularization. To date, the Bypass vs Angioplasty in Severe Ischemia of the Leg (BASIL) trial remains the only randomized prospective trial comparing the success of open surgical bypass vs endovascular therapy for CLI. When life expectancy extends beyond 2 years, bypass patency is superior.[4] With recent advances in technology, the patency of the endovascular procedures may approach that which can be achieved with autogenous vein bypass.[5]
- Others studies have reported that, despite the reduced primary patency, limb salvage rates remain comparable with surgical bypass and range from 74% at 5 years to 84.7% at 8 years.[6]
- On a population level, an endovascular approach has been shown to be associated with improved amputation-free survival as compared with open bypass in a study of propensity matched Medicare beneficiaries. Patients undergoing endovascular repair had improved amputation-free survival compared with open repair at 30 days (92.6 vs 91.1%, $P = .002$) and at 4 years (51 vs 46%, $P < .001$).[7]
- Lower limb revascularization of diabetic patients affected by intermittent claudication, in addition to improved walking performance, is associated with a reduction in the incidence of future major cardiovascular events when accompanied by increased physical exercise and improved glucose management and weight control.[8]
- Loop reentry using standard technique is successful in about 70% to 80% of cases.[9]
- In patients who failed loop reentry, reentry catheters are successful approximately 80% of the time.[9]
- Reentry success was 90% successful in a study using the Outback (Cordis) reentry catheter for all-comers.[10]

COMPLICATIONS

- Artery puncture: hematoma, occlusion, dissection, pseudoaneurysm, arteriovenous fistula
- Failure of recanalization: intimal dissection, branch occlusion, thrombosis, embolization, vessel rupture, remote hemorrhage
- Stent/stent graft complications: stent embolization, stent will not expand lesion, stent kink, stent thrombosis
- Infection

ACKNOWLEDGMENT

We gratefully acknowledge the contributions of F. Gallardo Pedrajas and Peter A. Schneider as portions of their chapter were retained in this revision.

REFERENCES

1. Hirsch AT, Haskal ZJ, Hertzer NR, et al. ACC/AHA 2005 guidelines for the management of patients with peripheral arterial disease (lower extremity, renal, mesenteric, and abdominal aortic): executive summary a collaborative report from the American Association for Vascular Surgery/Society for Vascular Surgery, Society for Cardiovascular Angiography and Interventions, Society for Vascular Medicine and Biology, Society of Interventional Radiology, and the ACC/AHA Task Force on Practice Guidelines (Writing Committee to Develop Guidelines for the Management of Patients With Peripheral Arterial Disease) endorsed by the American Association of Cardiovascular and Pulmonary Rehabilitation; National Heart, Lung, and Blood Institute; Society for Vascular Nursing; TransAtlantic Inter-Society Consensus; and Vascular Disease Foundation. *J Am Coll Cardiol*. 2006;47:1239-1312.
2. Issack PS, Cunningham ME, Pumberger M, et al. Degenerative lumbar spinal stenosis: evaluation and management. *J Am Acad Orthop Surg*. 2012;20(8):527-535.
3. Giugliano G, Perrino C, Schiano V, et al. Endovascular treatment of lower extremity arteries is associated with an improved outcome in diabetic patients affected by intermittent claudication. *BMC Surg*. 2012;12(suppl 1):S19.
4. Adam DJ, Beard JD, Cleveland T. Bypass versus angioplasty in severe ischaemia of the leg (BASIL): multicentre, randomised controlled trial. *Lancet*. 2005;366:1925-1934.

5. Almasri J, Adusumalli J, Asi N, et al. A systematic review and meta-analysis of revascularization outcomes of infrainguinal chronic limb-threatening ischemia. *J Vasc Surg*. 2018;68:624-633. doi:10.1016/j.jvs.2018.01.066
6. Houbballah R, Raux M, LaMuraglia G. Trans-Atlantic debate: lower extremity bypass versus endovascular therapy for young patients with symptomatic peripheral arterial disease. Part two—against the motion. Endovascular therapy is the preferred treatment for patients <65 years old with symptomatic infrainguinal arterial disease. *Eur J Vasc Endovasc Surg*. 2012;44:116-119.
7. Wiseman JT, Fernandes-Taylor S, Saha S, et al. Endovascular versus open revascularization for peripheral arterial disease. *Ann Surg*. 2017;265(2):424-430. doi:10.1097/SLA.0000000000001676 PMID: 28059972; PMCID: PMC6174695.
8. Conrad MF, Crawford RS, Hackney LA, et al. Endovascular management of patients with critical limb ischemia. *J Vasc Surg*. 2011;53:1020-1025.
9. Setacci C, Chisci E, de Donato G, et al. Subintimal angioplasty with the aid of a re-entry device for TASC C and D lesions of the SFA. *Eur J Vasc Endovasc Surg*. 2009;38(1):76-87.
10. Bausback Y, Botsios S, Flux J, et al. Outback catheter for femoropopliteal occlusions: immediate and long-term results. *J Endovasc Ther*. 2011;18(1):13-21.

Chapter 30

Tibial Interventions: Tibial-Specific Angioplasty Considerations and Retrograde Approaches

Georges E. Al Khoury, Adham N. Abou Ali, and Rabih A. Chaer

DEFINITION

- Endovascular tibial intervention is a minimally invasive, endoluminal revascularization of the infrapopliteal vessels. It is an accepted treatment of critical limb ischemia (CLI) in patients with tibial occlusive disease. It is usually performed from a transfemoral access (antegrade approach) and, in selected cases, from transpedal or tibial access (retrograde approach).
- Therapeutic interventions performed in tibial arteries include plain or drug-eluting balloon angioplasty, atherectomy, or bare metal or drug-eluting stents.
- Procedures are typically performed under local anesthesia with moderate conscious sedation in a fixed-imaging hybrid operating room or in the interventional angiography suite. Portable imaging systems may also provide sufficient resolution for precise, image-guided intervention depending on circumstances.

DIFFERENTIAL DIAGNOSIS

The differential diagnosis for peripheral arterial disease includes, and is not limited to, the following:

- Diabetic neuropathy pain is described as a burning or aching sensation that commonly occurs at night associated with numbness or hypoesthesia. The symptom complex of diabetic neuropathy may be confused with ischemic rest pain or metatarsalgia, given the similar dermatomal distribution and overlapping risk factors.
- Venous ulcers are associated with skin pigmentation, induration from chronic venous hypertension, and inflammation. They develop primarily in the perimalleolar region of the ankle and usually do not involve the forefoot.
- Musculoskeletal pain resulting from mechanical etiology, stress fracture, arthritis, and plantar fasciitis.
- Soft tissue infection and malperforans ulcers in diabetic patients with advanced sensory neuropathy and/or Charcot deformity of the foot.
- Chronic, nondiabetic peripheral neuropathies such as dorsal foot paresthesias and dysesthesias following long saphenous vein harvest.

PATIENT HISTORY AND PHYSICAL FINDINGS

- Patients with infrainguinal occlusive disease present with symptoms of claudication (Rutherford ischemia classification categories 1, 2, and 3), ischemic rest pain, or tissue loss (Rutherford ischemia categories 4, 5, and 6). When the atherosclerotic disease is limited to the infrapopliteal arterial segments, pain is mainly located in the forefoot. Advanced arterial insufficiency can also lead to ischemic ulceration, gangrenous changes, and nonhealing wounds. This constellation of symptoms represents chronic limb-threatening ischemia and typically occurs when the ankle pressure is less than 50 mm Hg, the ankle-brachial index is less than 0.4, and the great toe pressure is less than 30 mm Hg (**FIGURE 1A** and **B**).

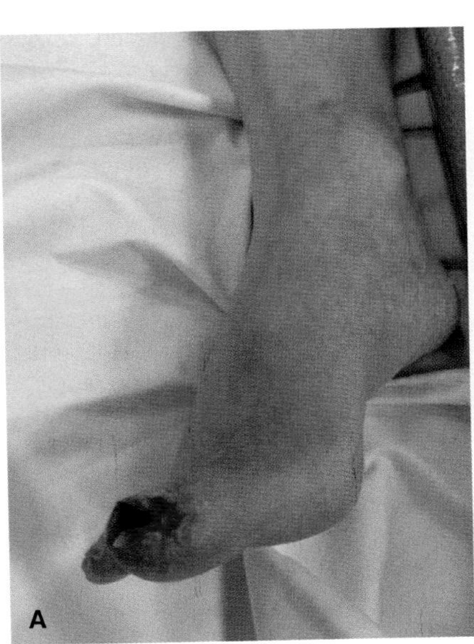

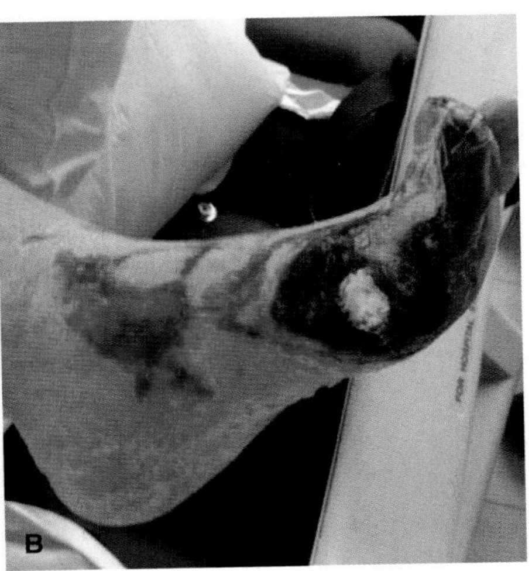

FIGURE 1 ● **A,** Patient with tibial occlusive disease and ischemic right first toe ulceration. Rutherford class 5. **B,** Patient with severe multilevel occlusive disease with gangrene of the left first toe and ulcerations on the dorsum of the foot. Rutherford class 6.

- CLI with tissue loss often occurs not only in the setting of multilevel arterial occlusive disease but also with isolated diabetic tibial occlusive disease. In that setting, femoral, and frequently popliteal, pulses remain palpable. In either circumstance, limb-threatening ischemia may ensue. In the latter circumstance, multilevel approaches to complete revascularization, either staged or simultaneous, should be pursued.
- Neurovascular examination, with particular focus on the wound location and the extent of tissue loss, should be evaluated and documented. Probably, the most deterministic variable is the extent of tissue loss—Wagner wound classification, the presence and severity of osteomyelitis, exposure or involvement of the calcaneus bone, residual intact skin on either the dorsal or plantar foot.
- The Society of Vascular Surgery Lower Extremity Threatened Limb (SVS WIfI) classification system categorizes critical limb ischemia based on wound, ischemia, and foot infection grades. The resulting score and clinical stage correlate with the amputation risk for each limb.[1] Wound grading depends on the size, depth, and severity of the wound. Ischemia grading depends on the ankle-brachial index, ankle pressures, and transcutaneous oxygen pressure levels. Foot infection grading depends on local and/or systemic signs of infection.
- These conditions all impact decision making and clinical outcomes. Patient's functional capacity also plays an important role in the intensity of the therapeutic strategy. Options and outcome goals vary substantially between ambulatory and nonambulatory patients.

IMAGING AND OTHER DIAGNOSTIC STUDIES

- Pulse volume recordings (PVRs) and toe pressure measurements when possible (**FIGURE 2**).
- Duplex (**FIGURE 3**).
- Computed tomography and magnetic resonance angiograms have limited diagnostic utility in the infrapopliteal vessels. This is usually due to inaccurate contrast bolus timing with distal extremity cross-sectional imaging techniques, heavy vessel wall calcification, and the diminutive size of reconstituted target arteries.
- Intra-arterial angiography remains the gold standard imaging study for tibial occlusive disease for both diagnostic and therapeutic purposes (**FIGURE 4**).

SURGICAL MANAGEMENT

- Technical skills, careful planning, and knowledge of the relevant arterial anatomy determine tibial revascularization strategies for limb salvage. Current controversies include the potential value of restoring patency in more than one tibial vessel to optimize blood flow and maximize the chances of wound healing. Proponents of this approach reference the "angiosome" concept of the foot or the idea that specific skin regions derive primary perfusion from end arterioles arising primarily from either the dorsal pedal or posterior tibial arteries as they cross the ankle. This practice is pursued in marked contradistinction to the open surgical imperative to restore in-line flow to the foot in the single largest, most continuous crural artery. The many advantages of endovascular reconstruction techniques in tibial reconstruction include restoring partial flow in multiple target arteries as compared with a single artery following surgical bypass, as well as opportunities to repeat procedures with relatively simple outpatient interventions as needed, to maintain patency and skin integrity. Treatment decisions regarding revascularization strategy in individual circumstances should be guided by patient-specific comorbidities and anatomic considerations, arterial runoff into the foot, patient habitus and ambulatory status as well as patency and feasibility considerations related to either open or endovascular options.
- Currently available endovascular technology facilitates successful treatment of complex occlusive lesions at and below the malleolar level. Limitations remain and include limited durability and patency, as well as technical limitations highlighted by risks of arterial perforation (**FIGURE 5**), difficulty in true lumen reentry in complete occlusions (**FIGURE 6**), procedure-related distal arterial embolization, and limited pedal vessel outflow in certain circumstances.

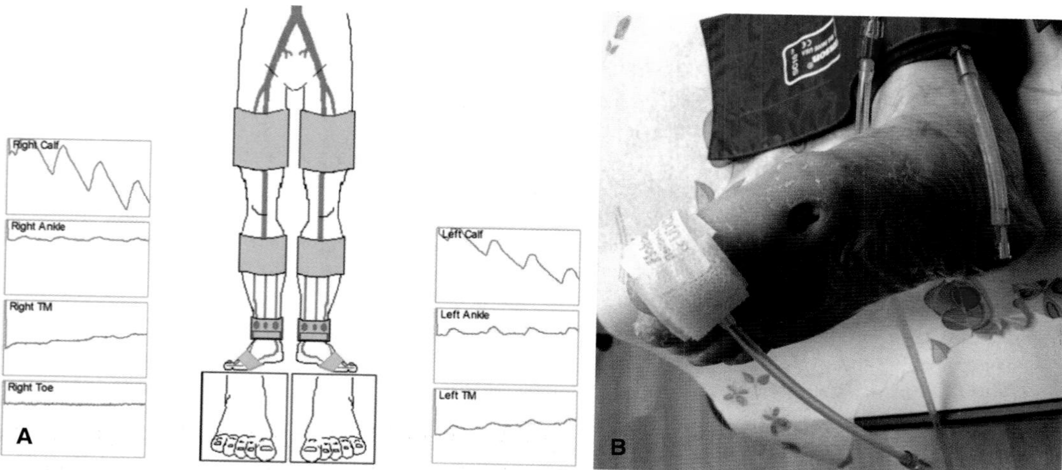

FIGURE 2 • PVR on a patient with severe right tibial occlusive disease and nonhealing toe ulcer. The tracings are pulsatile at the calf level consistent with adequate femoropopliteal flow; however, the waveforms are flat, distally suggestive of tibial occlusive disease.

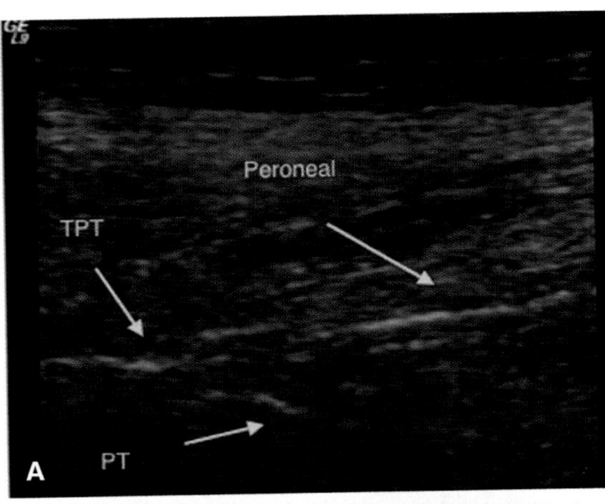

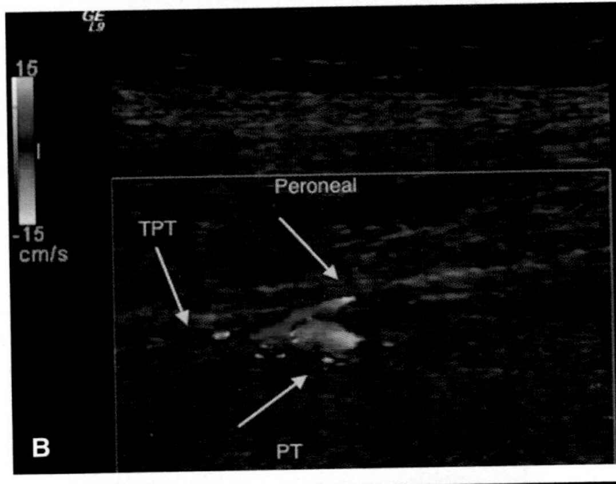

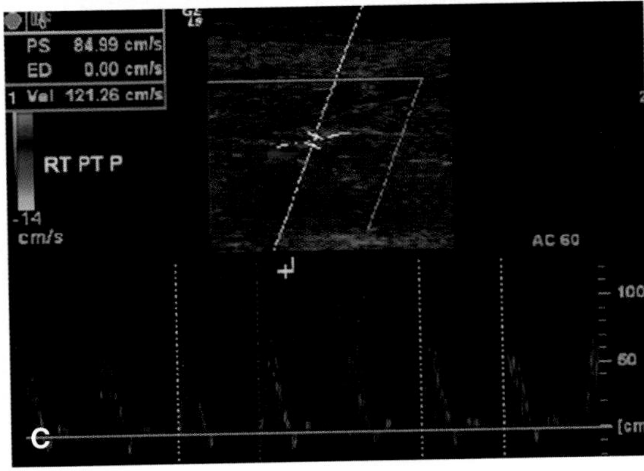

FIGURE 3 ● **A,** Duplex B-mode image shows the calcified tibioperoneal trunk bifurcation into the posterior tibial artery and peroneal artery. **B,** Duplex of the tibioperoneal trunk bifurcation shows flow into the posterior tibial artery. **C,** Duplex of the proximal posterior tibial artery shows normal triphasic Doppler waveform.

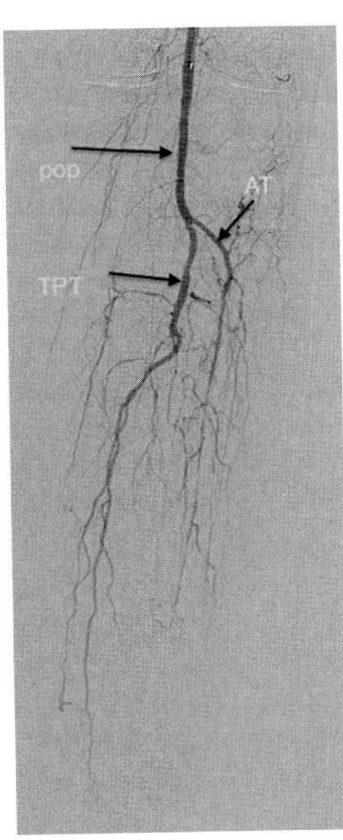

FIGURE 4 ● Selective left leg angiogram shows patent popliteal artery, patent tibioperoneal trunk, complete occlusion of the anterior tibial artery, and complete occlusion of the peroneal artery.

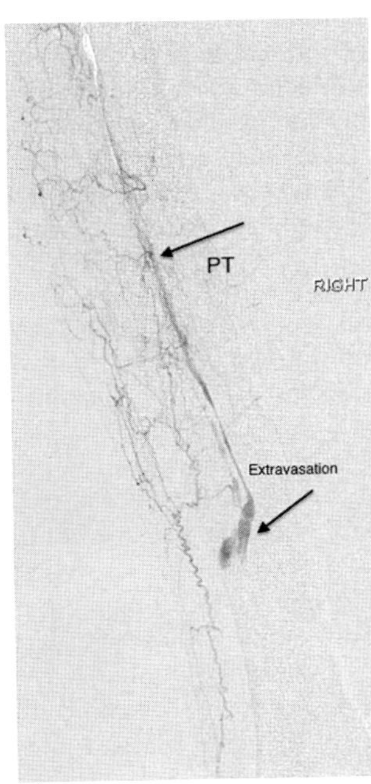

FIGURE 5 ● Angiogram shows extravasation from distal posterior tibial artery in an attempt to cross a total occlusion with a catheter and wire.

- The retrograde or SAFARI (Subintimal Flossing with Antegrade-Retrograde Intervention) tibial intervention technique may improve technical results in challenging lesions, particularly those resistant to ipsilateral antegrade access, including flush occlusions at the origin of the target artery or with large collateral arteries adjacent to the occluded origin. In nearly every circumstance, even chronic and recalcitrant occlusions may be crossed more easily from the retrograde rather than antegrade approach; this is true regardless of the chronicity of the lesion in question, degree of calcification, or length of occlusion.
- The pedal loop technique has been proposed in certain clinical situations requiring significant improvement in blood flow via the restoration of flow through both the anterior tibial and posterior tibial arteries (through the plantar arteries and their

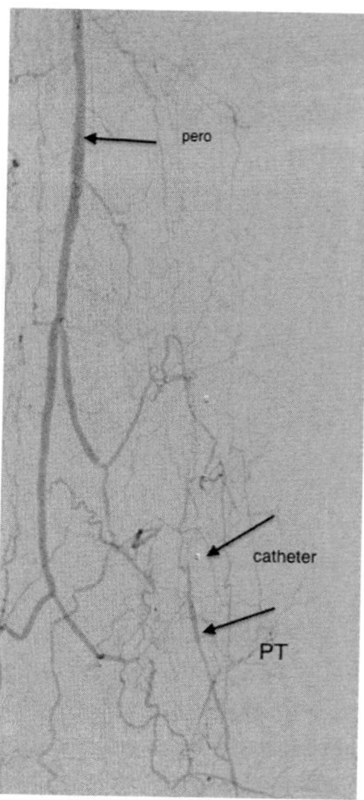

FIGURE 6 ● Angiogram from sheath shows the catheter in the subintimal plane after recanalization of posterior tibial (PT) with reconstitution of distal PT away from the catheter.

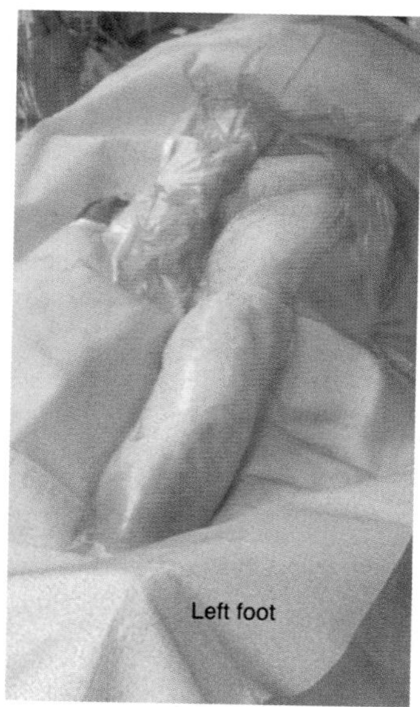

FIGURE 7 ● Patient is placed in the supine position on the angiographic table; the groins and lower extremity are prepped and draped in anticipation of antegrade and retrograde approaches.

anatomical anastomoses). It entails one of two approaches: A. Antegrade recanalization of the anterior tibial artery (ATA) and the dorsalis pedis (DP) and then retrograde recanalization of the plantar artery and then the posterior tibial artery. B. Antegrade recanalization of the posterior tibial artery and the plantar artery and then retrograde recanalization of the DP and then the ATA. Very low-profile balloon catheters are recommended particularly while navigating the tortuous vessels of the foot.

Preoperative Planning

- Preoperative vein mapping prior to the diagnostic angiogram is helpful in handicapping potential surgical alternatives and determining the extent to which interventional alternatives are to be pursued.
- Patients should be medically optimized prior to their procedure: preventive strategies are advised to reduce the risk of kidney injury in patients at risk for contrast nephropathy; smoking cessation is encouraged as well as antiplatelet and statin therapy. Carbon dioxide angiography is a useful tool in aortoiliac and femoral (inflow) evaluation; however, its utility in tibial angiography is limited.
- Tibial interventions can entail significant radiation exposure. Protective shields, lead glasses, and judicious use of fluoroscopy are recommended to protect all participants in the procedure. Ultrasound-guided access can minimize radiation exposure, particularly for pedal access; needle extenders allow the operator to puncture remotely and minimize hand exposure.
- Micropuncture and pedal access kits are useful access tools.
- Sheaths: 5- and 6-Fr, braided, 90 cm or 110 cm from contralateral femoral access; 45- to 55-cm sheath from the ipsilateral transfemoral access; 4- and 5-Fr Slender Glidesheaths (Terumo) with the ultrathin wall technology have been suggested for diagnostic angiograms from the transradial access; 120- to 150-cm (Sublime) length sheaths are currently available for intervention.
- Wires: 300-cm, 0.014-in, or 0.018-in wires; 260-cm, 0.035-in floppy Glidewire.
- Catheters: 150- to 170-cm catheters and balloons.
- Medications: heparin (or other anticoagulant), clopidogrel, nitroglycerin, papaverine, alteplase, and calcium channel blockers.

Positioning

- The patient is placed supine on the angiographic table with both groins prepped and draped. Consider preparing the foot and the leg in anticipation for retrograde approach if needed (**FIGURE 7**).

ANTEGRADE TIBIAL REVASCULARIZATION

First Step: A. Femoral Access and Anticoagulation

- Contralateral femoral access with standard up and over technique is our routine approach for diagnostic arteriograms and most tibial interventions.
- Antegrade femoral approach has distinct advantages for tibial or pedal interventions, especially in the setting of a hostile and narrow aortic bifurcation. Antegrade access generally provides easier pushability and reduced radiation to the patient and procedural team. Therefore, it is our preferred approach in the treatment of recurrent disease or known distal disease.
- Ultrasound-guided access may minimize risk for access site complications.
- Diagnostic arteriogram to image the inflow is performed.

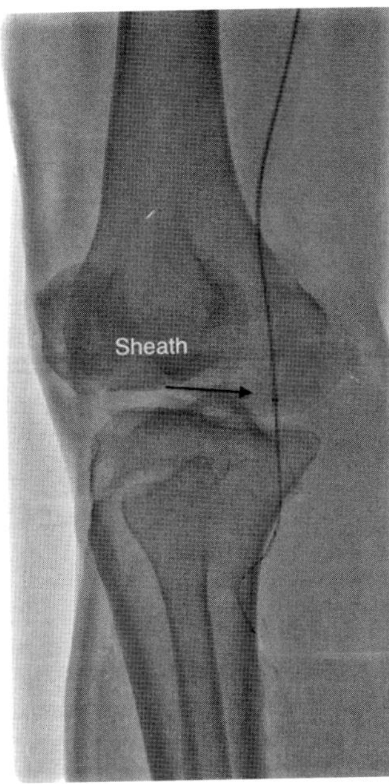

FIGURE 8 ● After obtaining femoral access, the sheath is advanced to the popliteal artery for the intervention. It allows better visualization of the tibial vessels and facilitates the pushability and the ability to cross total occlusions.

- A 5- or 6-Fr sheath is advanced over a stiff wire to the popliteal artery, positioned as close as possible to the tibial trifurcation (Sheath: 90-110 cm from the contralateral femoral access and 45 to 55 cm from the ipsilateral femoral access) (**FIGURE 8**).
- Sheath tip positioning close to the target vessel maximizes pushability across total occlusions. Also, improved visualization of tibial vessels is achieved with reduced contrast volumes.
- Anticoagulation is established using unfractionated heparin or other alternatives to achieve an activated clotting time (ACT) of more than 250 seconds.

B. Transradial Access

- The improved safety and patient convenience profile for transradial compared with transfemoral access has made this approach attractive to interventionalists with lower access site complication rates and shorter ambulation times.
- Patient selection is of paramount importance given the greater distance that needs to be traversed compared with transfemoral access. Typical distances to tibial arteries are 200 to 250 cm.
- Left radial access is typically preferred (to right radial access) given the shorter working distance and avoiding the need to cross the aortic arch and compromising the cerebral vessels.
- It is helpful to have the working table parallel to the abducted left arm and to have the imaging monitor to the left of the patient's head (if accessing from the left radial artery) for improved working flow.
- Ultrasound-guided access is also encouraged to minimize access site complications.
- Slender Glidesheaths (Terumo), 4 and 5 Fr, with the ultrathin wall technology have been suggested for diagnostic angiograms through the transradial access.
- An antispasmodic cocktail of vasodilators (a calcium channel blocker and nitroglycerin with a heparinized saline solution) is subsequently administered.
- An angled catheter (Kumpe, Angled Glidecath) can be used to traverse the arch into the descending thoracic aorta with the image intensifier in a left anterior oblique view. An upper extremity angiogram may be helpful if the operator encounters difficulties crossing the subclavian artery.
- Selective lower extremity diagnostic angiograms can be performed utilizing a 5-Fr 125-cm-long pigtail catheter.
- The relatively recent Terumo R2P Destination Slender sheath available in 149 cm lengths allows for placing the sheath tip as close as possible to the target lesion to allow for better pushability.
- Similarly, anticoagulation is established using unfractionated heparin to achieve an ACT of more than 250 seconds.

Second Step: Selective Angiogram

- Imaging of the tibial outflow is obtained from sheath injections or through diagnostic catheters (5- to 10-mL power or hand injection). To reduce contrast load, contrast may be diluted 50% for all but the most distal arterial beds.
- Anteroposterior or ipsilateral anterior oblique projections are obtained to visualize the popliteal "trifurcation" and separate the tibia and fibula. True lateral oblique projections are obtained to visualize pedal outflow.
- Arteriographic images must be carefully examined to optimize outcome; multiple projections may be required to sufficiently opacify tibial and pedal vascular anatomy, especially distal to extended or serial occlusions. Delayed views (prolonged digital subtraction angiography [DSA] time) may improve opacification of patent tibial or pedal vessels distal to occluded segments (**FIGURE 9**). Withdrawing the sheath to the femoral bifurcation may uncover reconstitution of distal tibial artery segments through extended deep femoral artery collateral pathways.

Third Step: Crossing the Occlusion

- Angled catheters and guidewires are typically used to select the respective tibial arteries.
- The catheter/guidewire combination is advanced into the target tibial artery proximal to the occlusion or stenosis.
- Anatomy is confirmed with magnified arteriographic views.
- "Road mapping" may improve guidance across occlusions. The wire leads through the occlusion, followed by the crossing catheter (eg, Quick-Cross or Cook CXI or TrailBlazer, 0.014 in or 0.018 in) (**FIGURE 10**).
- Transluminal passage is preferred to subintimal access because reentry into the true lumen may be unpredictable and challenging.
- Soft-tipped hydrophilic guidewires are used to negotiate and traverse tibial stenosis with the support of crossing catheters under magnified road map guidance.
- Heavier weighted tip, chronic total occlusion (CTO) guidewires (either 0.014-in or 0.018-in platforms) are designed to provide improved performance and penetration across total occlusions.
- For longer occlusions, leading with a 2-mm percutaneous transluminal angioplasty (PTA) balloon as an alternative to low-profile crossing catheters (eg, Quick-Cross or CXI) can

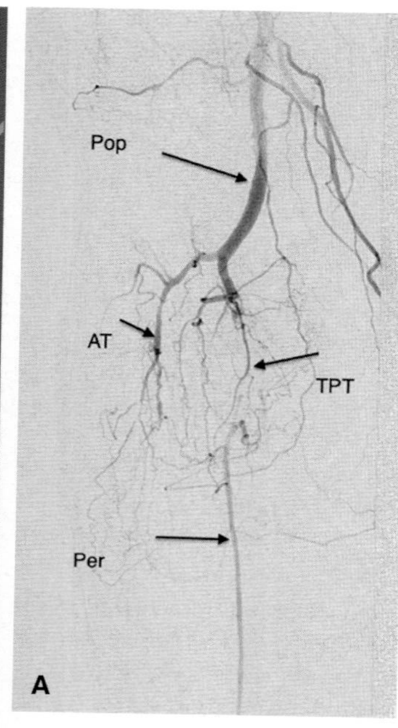

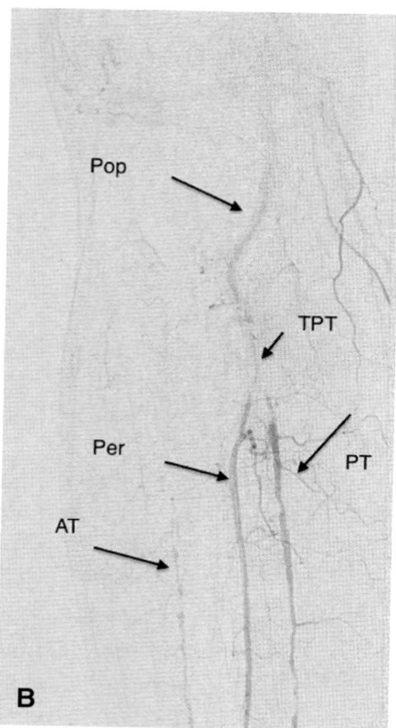

FIGURE 9 ● **A,** Diagnostic angiogram from the popliteal sheath demonstrates patent right popliteal artery, occluded anterior tibial artery, and occluded distal tibioperoneal trunk with reconstitution of peroneal artery. The posterior tibial artery appears to be occluded. **B,** Angiogram with delayed DSA time identifies a patent diseased posterior tibial artery distal to the occluded tibioperoneal trunk and patent peroneal artery.

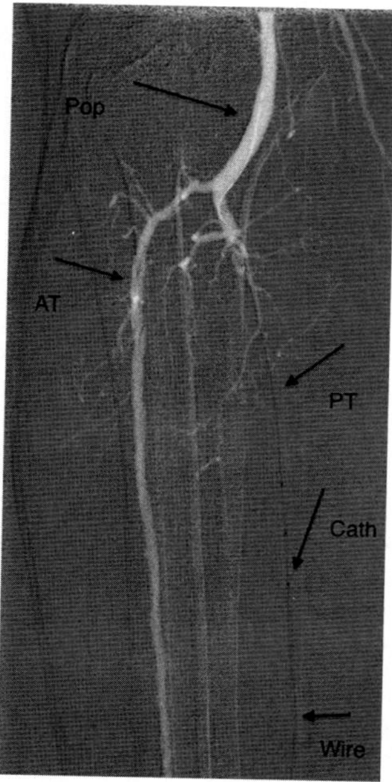

FIGURE 10 ● Recanalization of occluded PT. Under road map guidance, the PT was selected, and using a wire and support catheter, the occlusion was crossed.

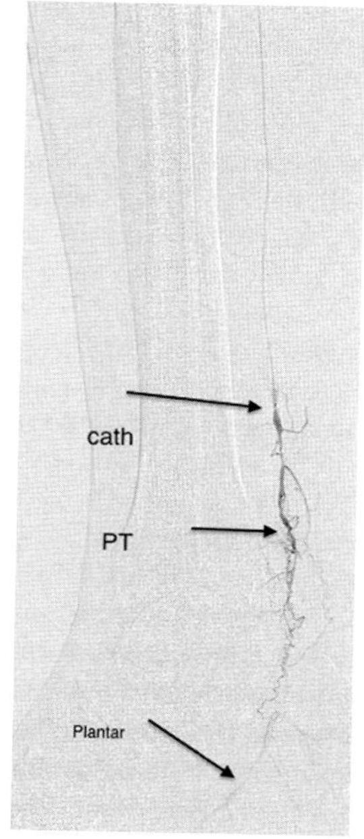

FIGURE 11 ● Angiogram from catheter in PT during recanalization of occluded PT.

improve access by extending or reestablishing the recanalization plane during transit.

Fourth Step: Reentry Into the True Lumen

- Reenter into the true lumen under road map guidance (**FIGURE 11**).
- Advance the catheter over the wire into the true lumen beyond the target lesion and remove the wire.
- Check for back-bleeding and subsequently perform a selective angiogram through the catheter to confirm the proper intraluminal position (**FIGURE 12**).
- Advance a stiff wire with long, soft tip into the target vessel as distal as possible (**FIGURE 13**).
- Remove the catheter carefully under fluoroscopic guidance while maintaining wire access into the distal patent artery.
- Reentry devices can be used to select the true lumen from a dissection plane. Alternatively, if failure to reenter the true lumen persists despite the use of reentry devices or balloon angioplasty to disrupt the dissection membrane, retrograde access into the distal true lumen can be attempted at the time or in a staged future setting.

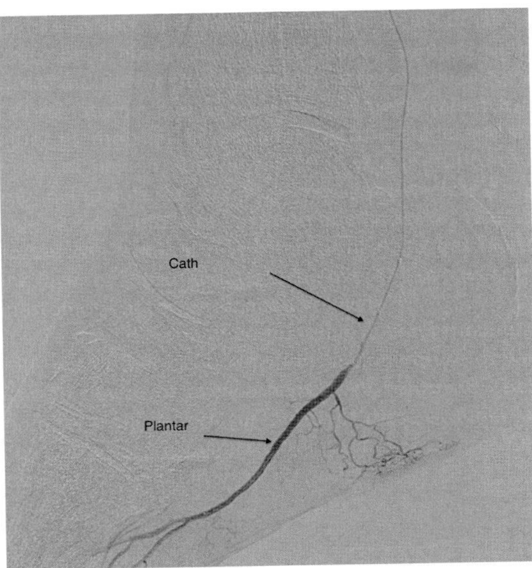

FIGURE 12 ● Angiogram from catheter in the plantar artery to confirm the proper intraluminal position after recanalization of PT.

Fifth Step: Treatment With Balloon Angioplasty

- The proximal and distal ends of the lesion are demarcated by a repeat contrast injection through the sheath. The use of radiopaque adhesive rulers applied on the affected leg may help with measurement and device selection.
- Deliver the appropriate size balloon (typically 2-3.5 mm in diameter) to the target lesion and perform the balloon angioplasty for 2- to 3-minute inflation time (**FIGURE 14**).
- Single inflation using a long balloon decreases the procedural time and reduces the risk of postangioplasty dissection requiring reintervention (**FIGURE 15**). Tapered balloons can help treat lesions across vessels of variable size.

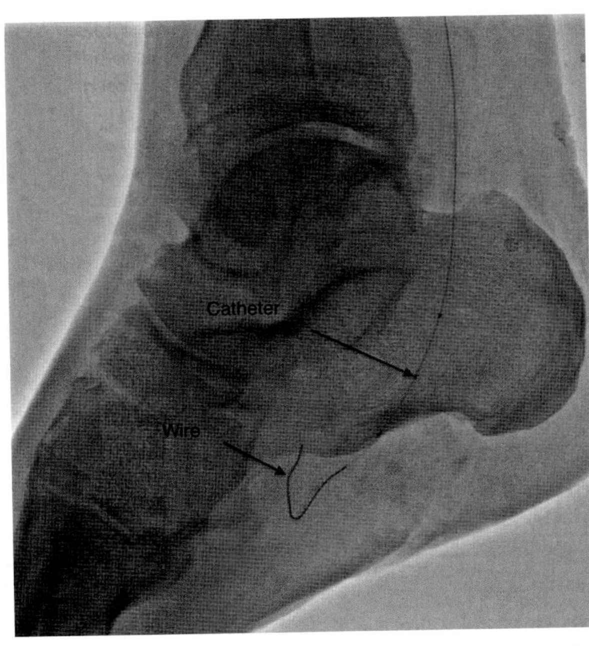

FIGURE 13 ● Placement of wire into the plantar artery prior to angioplasty of the occluded PT.

- Heparin flush, continuous or intermittent, through the sheath is recommended during balloon inflation and throughout the procedure.
- Selective injection of intra-arterial nitroglycerin through the sheath will minimize the effects of spasm at or distal to the intervention.

Sixth Step: Angiogram Post Balloon Angioplasty

- The treatment balloon is retracted back over the wire to the popliteal artery level.
- The completion arteriogram is performed from a sheath injection to assess the angioplasty outcome and pedal runoff (**FIGURE 16**).

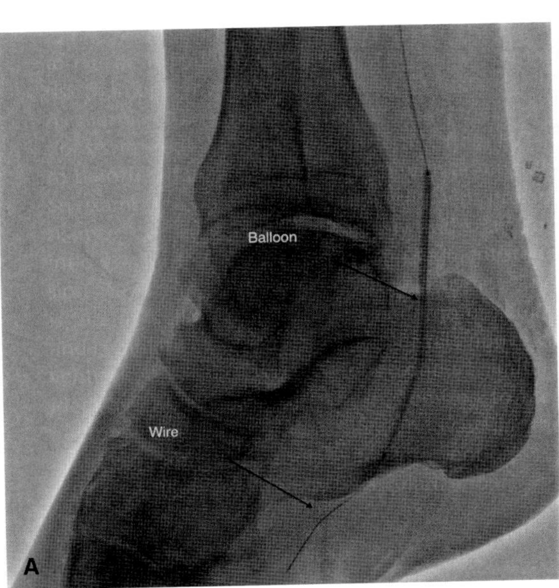

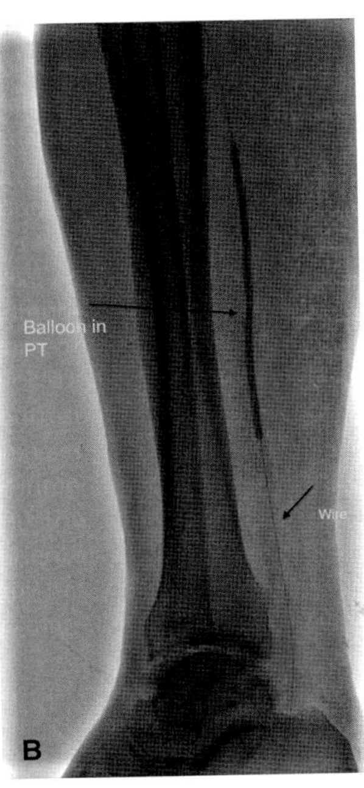

FIGURE 14 ● **A,** Balloon angioplasty of distal PT with 2-mm balloon for 2-minute inflation time. **B,** Balloon angioplasty of PT with 3-mm balloon for 2-minute inflation time.

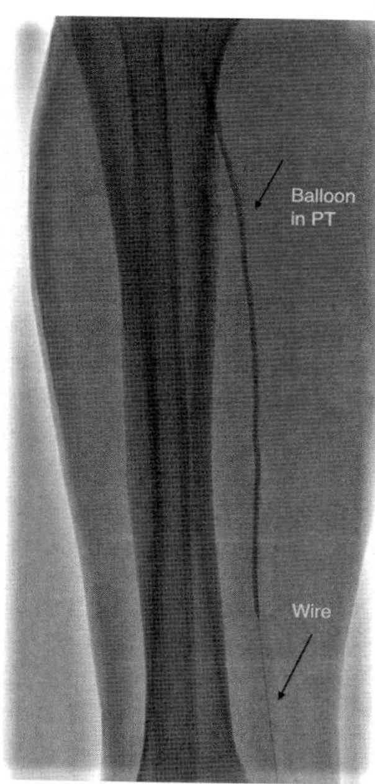

FIGURE 15 ● Angioplasty of PT with long balloon.

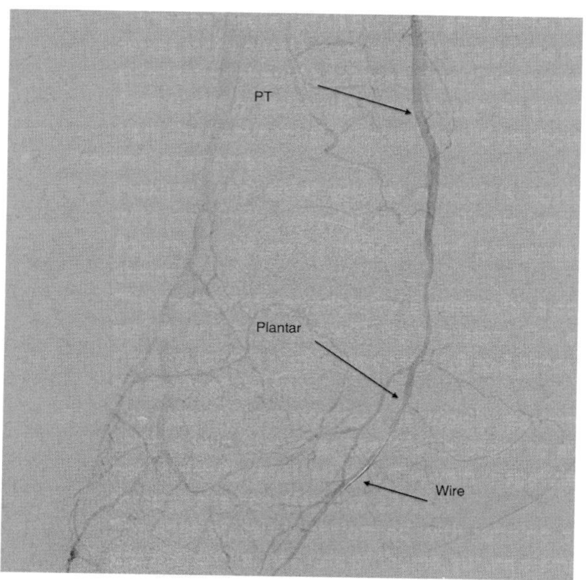

FIGURE 16 ● Angiogram from sheath postrecanalization and angioplasty of PT shows good flow without any flow-limiting dissection.

- Recoil or dissections are treated with sustained reinflation of the balloon for 3 to 5 minutes or by upsizing the balloon, followed by more gradual deflation.
- Flow-limiting dissections in the proximal tibioperoneal trunk and proximal tibial arteries may be resolved with stent or tack placement when necessary.
- Distal embolization can be managed by aspiration through the existing catheter or aspiration with a purpose-specific catheter such as the Export. Catheter-directed thrombolysis may be attempted in select cases.
- Other modalities may be useful in restoring patency, such as atherectomy devices and can be used as stand-alone therapy or as adjuncts to balloon angioplasty.
- The routine use of tibial stenting is not advocated at this stage. Although there is some evidence to suggest that drug-eluting stents may result in improved durability, these are subject to cost restrictions, regulatory approvals, and availability depending on the country of practice. Ongoing trials on bioabsorbable drug eluting tibial scaffolds may add to the device armamentarium.

Seventh Step: Treatment With Atherectomy

- Treatment with atherectomy devices necessitates crossing the occlusive lesion with a wire prior to device use. In our practice it is reserved to heavily calcified lesions that cannot be crossed with a catheter or a balloon over the wire (**FIGURE 17**).
- Different atherectomy devices have different technical considerations. Operator familiarity with the respective device is important for the technical success of the procedure.
- After crossing the lesion as described in step 3 above, the existing wire is exchanged for a 0.014-in wire.
- The atherectomy device is typically introduced over its respective 0.014-in wire. Atherectomy is performed following device-specific instructions for use.
- Postatherectomy balloon angioplasty is subsequently performed as mentioned in the fifth step above (**FIGURE 17**).
- Distal embolic protection devices are frequently employed during atherectomy of femoropopliteal lesions due to the concern for embolization. These devices are rarely employed with atherectomy of tibial vessels.

Eighth Step: Revascularization of Another Tibial Vessel

- The ultimate goal is to reestablish direct, in-line arterial flow to the ischemic part of the foot. A secondary goal is to optimize flow by reconstructing more than one occluded tibial artery, when possible.
- The wire is redirected into another tibial vessel, and recanalization is performed as described earlier (**FIGURE 18**).
- When the peroneal artery is the sole outflow vessel, revascularization to the level of the peroneal collaterals at ankle is needed.
- Ostial lesions at the bifurcation of anterior tibial artery and tibioperoneal trunk can be treated with kissing balloon technique to prevent plaque shifting.

Ninth Step: Completion Angiogram and Hemostasis

- If the completion angiography is satisfactory (**FIGURE 19**), the sheath is pulled back to the common femoral artery and injection from that level is recommended to rule out any complications in the femoropopliteal segment related to sheath position.
- The sheath is removed, and hemostasis is obtained at the access site either by using closure device or manual compression without heparin reversal unless necessary.

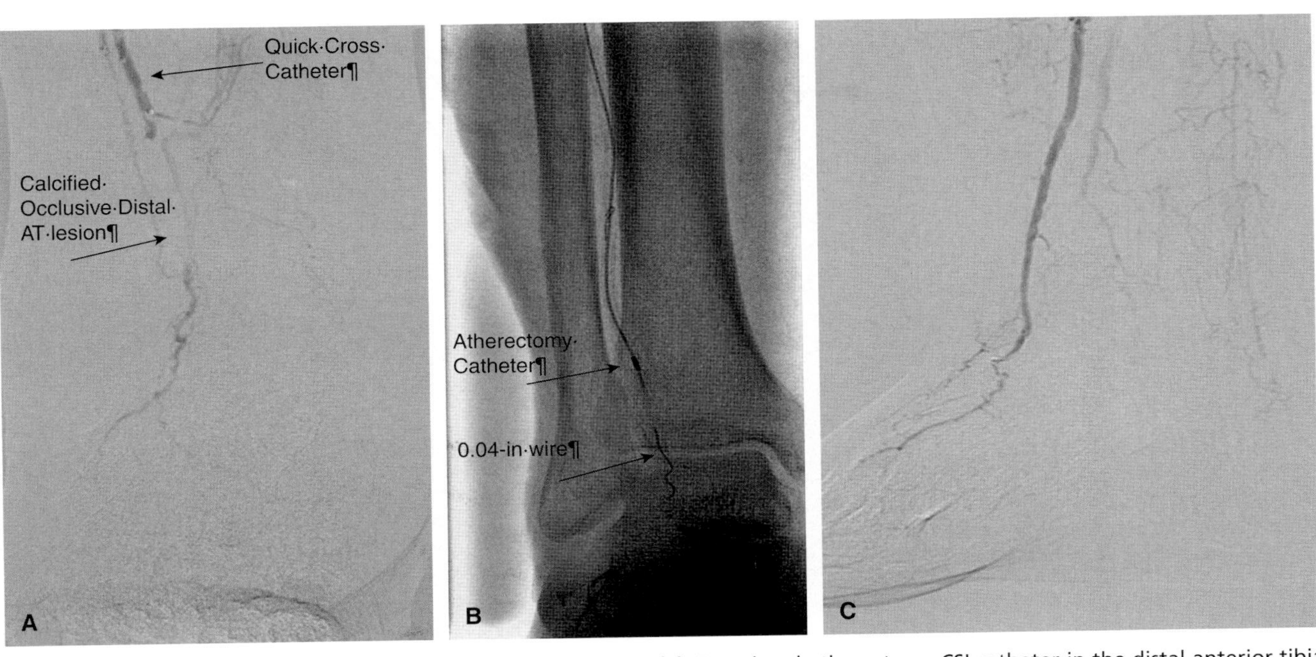

FIGURE 17 ● **A,** Occluded distal anterior tibial (AT) artery lesion **(B)**. Rotational atherectomy CSI catheter in the distal anterior tibial artery over a 0.014-in wire. **C,** Postatherectomy and standard balloon angioplasty completion angiogram.

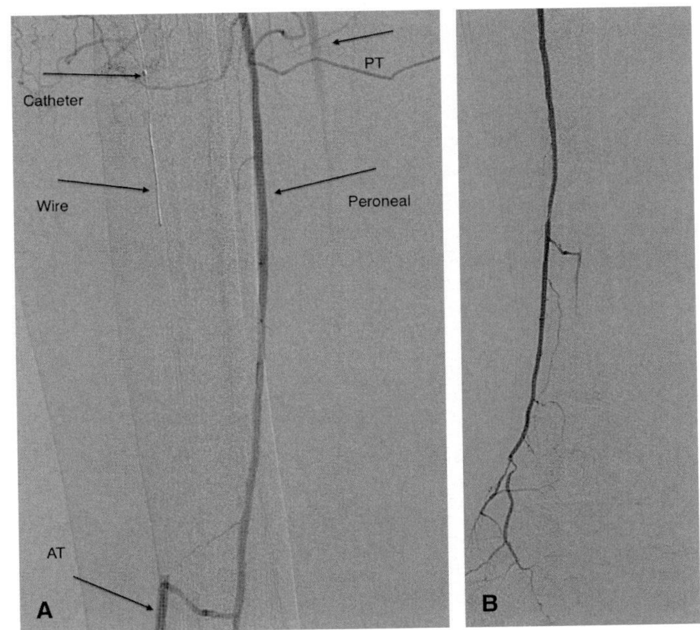

FIGURE 18 ● **A,** Angiogram from the sheath at the time of recanalization of anterior tibial (AT) artery with a wire and catheter. The peroneal artery is patent and reconstitutes a distal anterior tibial artery. **B,** Angiogram from the sheath postangioplasty of the AT with 3-mm balloon shows patent AT without any dissection or flow-limiting stenosis.

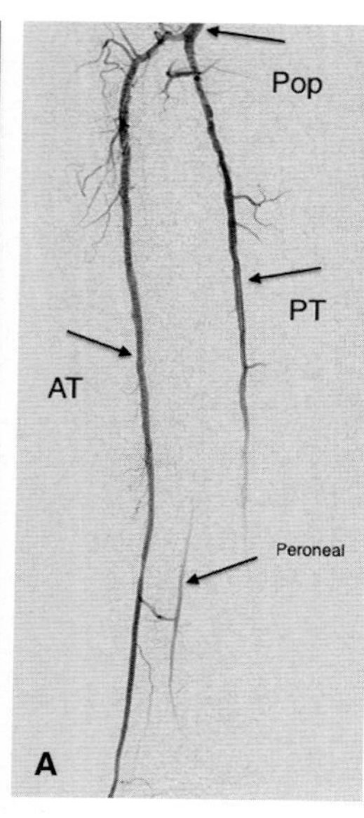

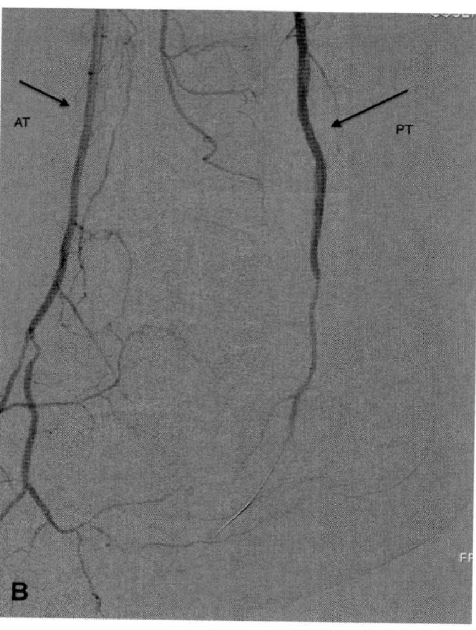

FIGURE 19 ● **A,** Completion angiogram from the sheath postrecanalization of occluded AT and PT shows patent vessels with good flow mainly in the AT without any significant dissection. The peroneal artery reconstituted in a retrograde fashion from the AT. **B,** Patent distal AT and PT runoff into the foot.

RETROGRADE TIBIAL RECANALIZATION

First Step: Retrograde Access

- Antegrade access is obtained first as described earlier. This is used for initial imaging and delivery of treatment devices.
- Administration of vasodilators through the antegrade sheath can facilitate tibial access and minimize vasospasm.
- Retrograde tibial arterial access is performed under ultrasound or fluoroscopic guidance using a micropuncture 21-gauge needle; a 300-cm, 0.018-in or 0.014-in wire; and balloon or support catheter. An introducer dilator, although potentially useful, is not essential.
- Sedation should be managed to minimize movement when road mapping is used to identify target arteries; excess sedation will worsen patient cooperation as they will not be able to follow the physician's instructions.
- Local anesthesia is infiltrated at the intended puncture site; excess anesthetic volume may deepen the vessel and make cannulation more difficult.
- Access to the posterior tibial artery is obtained in the region of the medial malleolus. Dorsiflexion and/or eversion of the foot may facilitate access.
- Access to the anterior tibial artery is obtained on the dorsum of the foot or the distal aspect of the leg anteriorly, where the target artery may be larger. Dorsalis pedis access is facilitated by plantar flexion of the foot.
- The peroneal artery should be approached laterally through the interosseous membrane.
- More proximal access to the posterior or anterior tibial arteries may be obtained with road map guidance when necessary. The use of intra-arterial vasodilators will help with vessel visualization and subsequent access.
- Inadvertent venous puncture may occur during attempts at retrograde access, and when it does, consider leaving the wire in place to help guide further attempts at arterial access.
- Ultrasound-assisted retrograde access, as an adjunct to road map guidance alone, may help to define the three-dimensional orientation of the needle in relation to the target artery (**FIGURE 20**).
- Image quality is optimized by incorporating a sufficient delay following contrast injection to maximize opacification of the target artery. Selective use of intra-arterial vasodilators through the antegrade sheath may reduce the severity of access-related vasospasm, when present, distally.
- The C-arm is adjusted to best align the needle to the target vessel, typically using an ipsilateral oblique projection.
- Surgical exposure may become necessary to ensure adequate access for retrograde tibial reconstruction. Retrograde access may also be obtained concomitant with planned

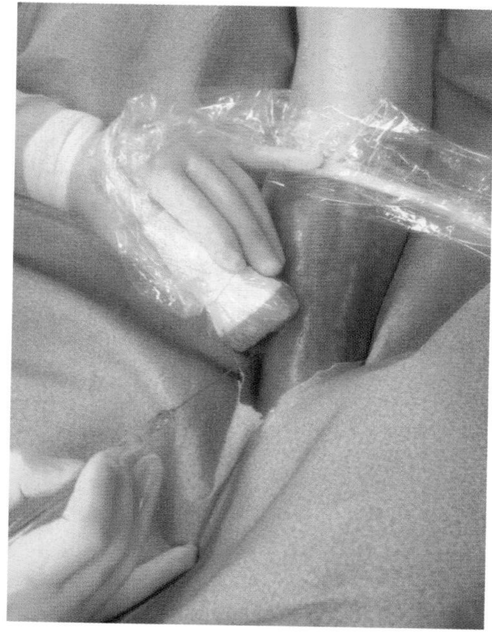

FIGURE 20 ● Retrograde approach: access to PT under ultrasound guidance.

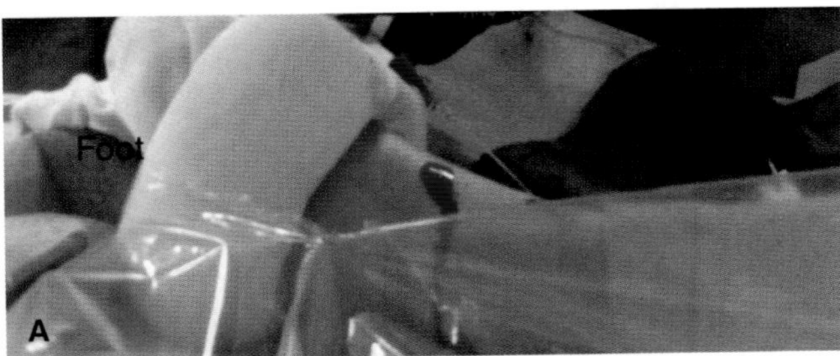

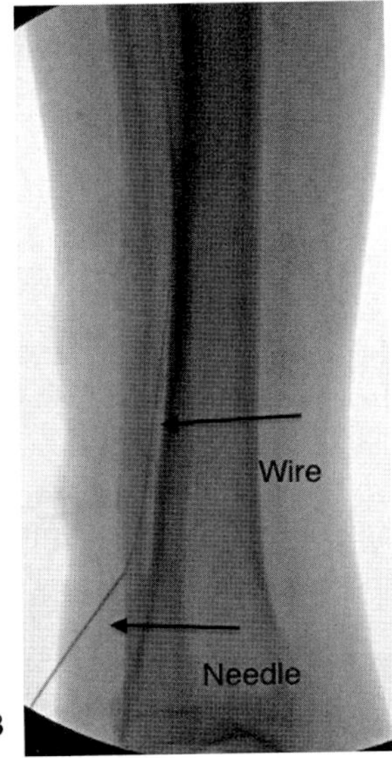

FIGURE 21 ● A, Retrograde access to AT with adequate arterial back-bleeding from the micropuncture needle. B, Needle in AT and wire advanced proximally under fluoroscopic guidance.

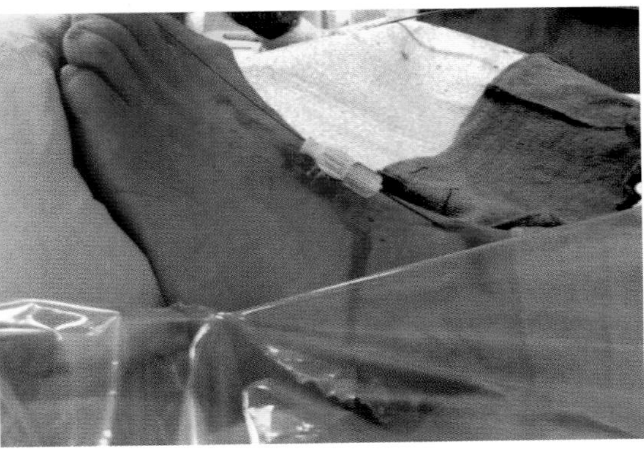

FIGURE 22 ● Retrograde access: wire and inner dilator of the microsheath.

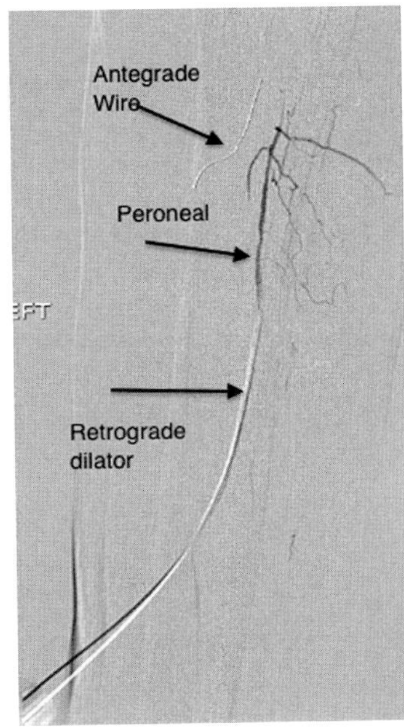

FIGURE 23 ● Retrograde access of the peroneal artery angiogram from the introducer confirms the intraluminal position.

transmetatarsal amputation by identifying and cannulating the open end of transected distal dorsal pedal artery.

Second Step: Retrograde Angiogram

- Once back-bleeding is seen, the micropuncture 0.018-in access wire is advanced under fluoroscopic guidance (FIGURE 21), followed by an appropriately sized support catheter, balloon, or the inner dilator of the 4-Fr microsheath.
- In most cases, retrograde sheaths are generally *not* deployed to minimize trauma to the puncture site and distal target artery (FIGURE 22). When sheaths are required, use of a radial access sheath will facilitate atraumatic access.
- Intraluminal position is confirmed by retrograde angiography through the catheter or dilator (FIGURE 23).

Third Step: Recanalization of Tibial Occlusion

- Antegrade sheath arteriography is used to delineate the extent of the target lesion.
- The occlusion is crossed using 0.018-in or 0.014-in wires, supported by a crossing catheter or low-profile angioplasty balloon (FIGURE 24). The 0.014-in wire may lack the necessary support to allow retrograde crossing of tibial lesions, and therefore, the 0.018-in wire can be utilized.
- The wire and crossing catheter combination is advanced from distal to proximal and into the popliteal artery if possible. The wire is removed.
- Following aspiration to confirm luminal position, a selective arteriogram is performed from the retrograde catheter.

Fourth Step: Exteriorization of the Wire From the Femoral Access Site

- Next, an attempt is made to advance the guidewire into the antegrade sheath or catheter (FIGURE 25).
- When this proves difficult on its own, a snare is deployed through the antegrade sheath to capture and externalize the distal retrograde wire (FIGURE 26).
- Following successful externalization of the retrograde wire, through and through "wire access" is available from both ends.
- A crossing catheter is then advanced from the antegrade access site over the wire to the patent tibial vessel distal to the occlusion.
- Distal intraluminal position is confirmed with arteriography through the crossing catheter.

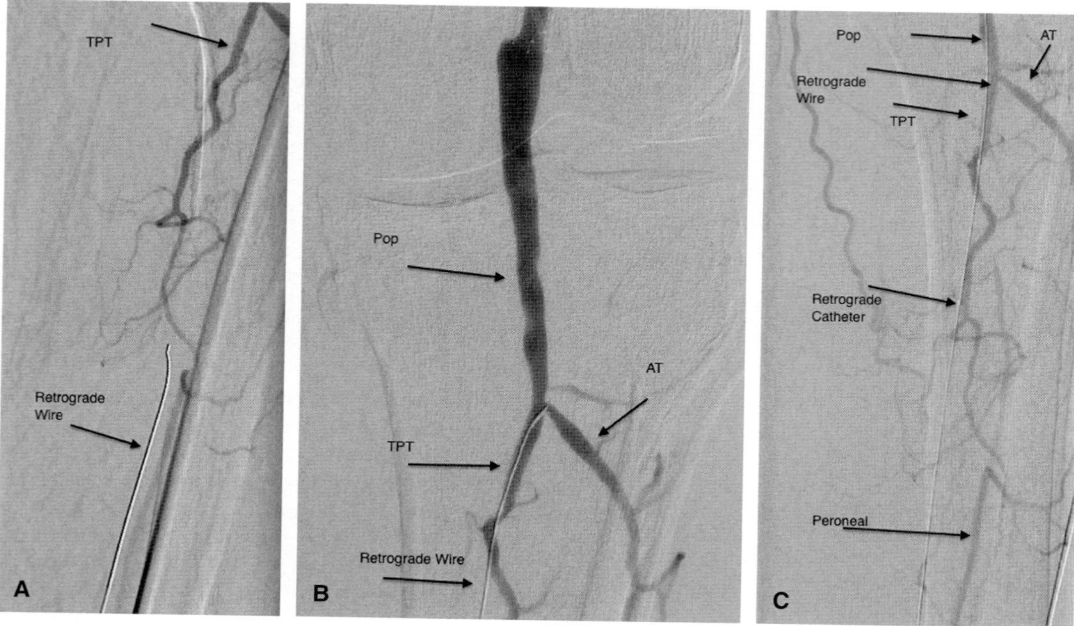

FIGURE 24 ● **A,** Angiogram from antegrade sheath. Wire crossing the occluded PT. **B,** Angiogram confirming entry of the wire into the tibioperoneal trunk (TPT). **C,** Angiogram shows the retrograde wire and catheter across the occlusion into the popliteal artery proximally.

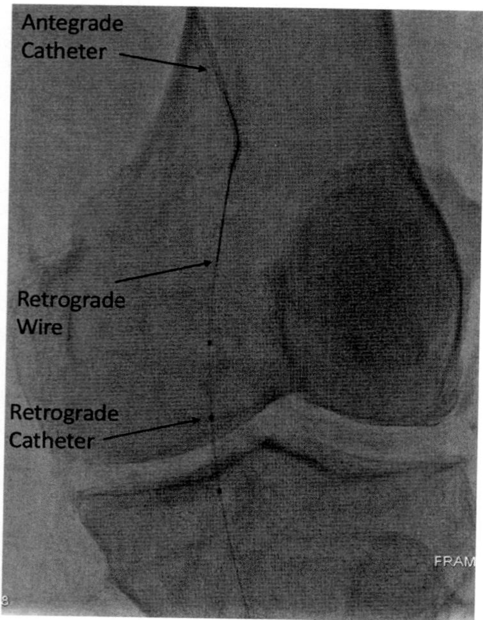

FIGURE 25 ● Retrograde wire is advanced into the antegrade catheter to establish "wire access" from both antegrade and retrograde access sites.

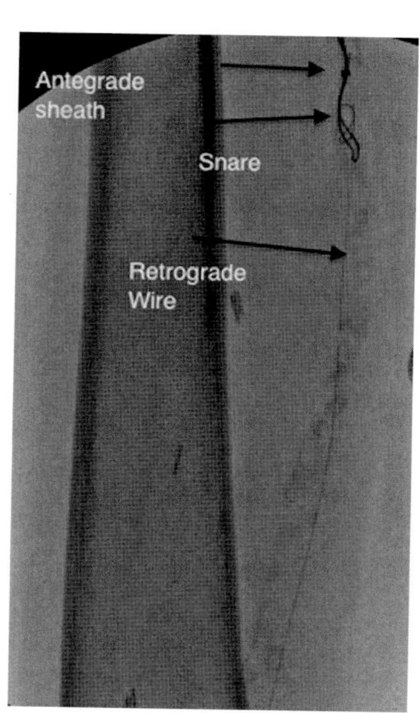

FIGURE 26 ● Snaring the retrograde wire into the proximal sheath.

- Next, the through and through wire is removed from the antegrade sheath, leaving the crossing catheter across the lesion. The wire is exchanged for a 300-cm 0.014-in working wire, advanced distally through the antegrade crossing catheter.
- The retrograde access catheter or micropuncture 4-Fr access dilator is subsequently removed from the distal target artery.

Hemostasis is obtained and maintained by manual pressure at the access site (**FIGURE 27**), the application of a blood pressure cuff across the site (**FIGURE 28**), or a radial compression device (Dstat Radial Hemostat Band). Vasospasm at the retrograde access sites can be addressed with intra-arterial vasodilator administration.

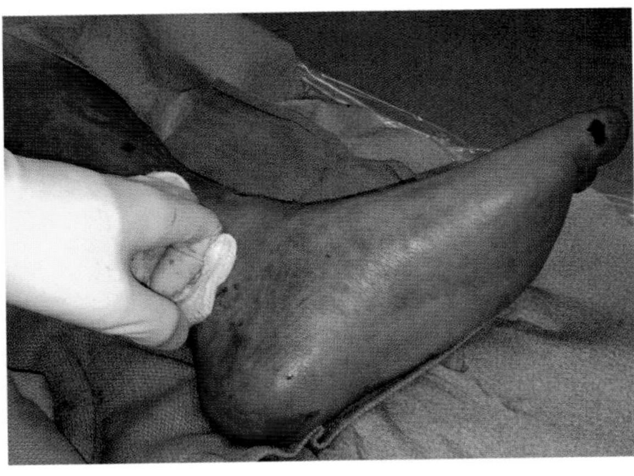

FIGURE 27 ● Hemostasis with manual compression postretrograde PT access.

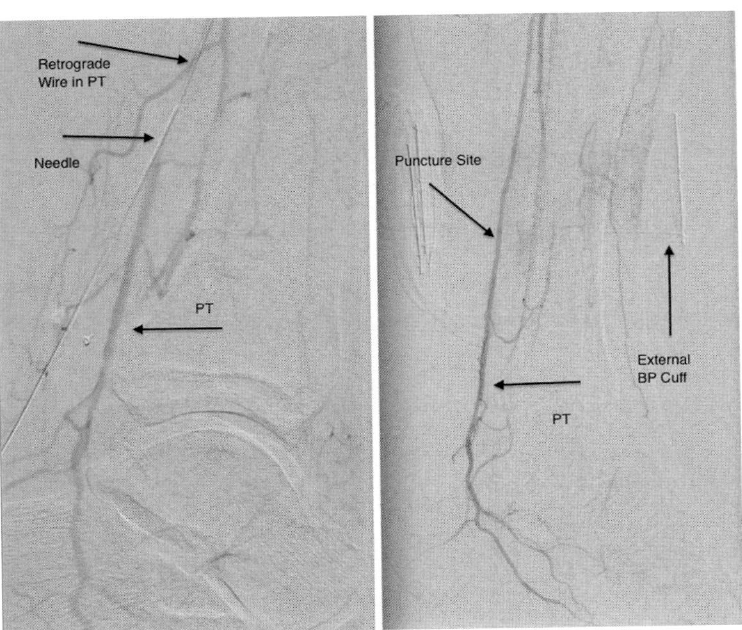

FIGURE 28 ● Angiogram of PT access site with blood pressure cuff used for hemostasis (image on the right of the screen).

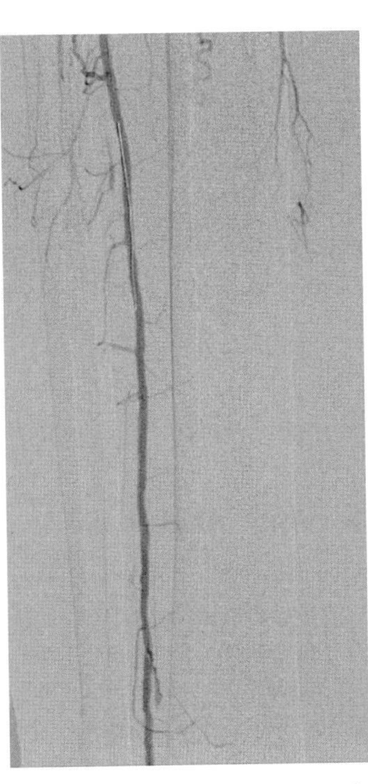

FIGURE 29 ● Angiogram shows extravasation from retrograde peroneal access site postrecanalization of TPT.

- Removing all devices from the retrograde access site as quickly as possible reduces instrumentation time and potential for arterial injury and distal thrombosis.
- Inflating a balloon advanced from the antegrade access sheath across the retrograde access site (**FIGURE 29**) not only may affect hemostasis but can also increase traumatic injury and access site bleeding and is rarely needed.

Fifth Step: Treatment With Balloon Angioplasty

- The intervention is then performed in the standard fashion from the antegrade approach (**FIGURE 30**).

Antegrade-Retrograde Approach

- If the retrograde wire is not able to cross the lesion and regain access to the true lumen, an antegrade-retrograde approach may be used to create adjacent subintimal planes in opposing directions (CART technique or controlled antegrade and retrograde subintimal tracking) (**FIGURE 31**).
- The dissection flap separating the adjacent subintimal spaces may be disrupted by simultaneous inflation in both directions.
- This allows visualization and recanalization of true lumen from either or both directions. The two PTA balloons selected for this maneuver should be sized appropriately to minimize risk for target arterial rupture.

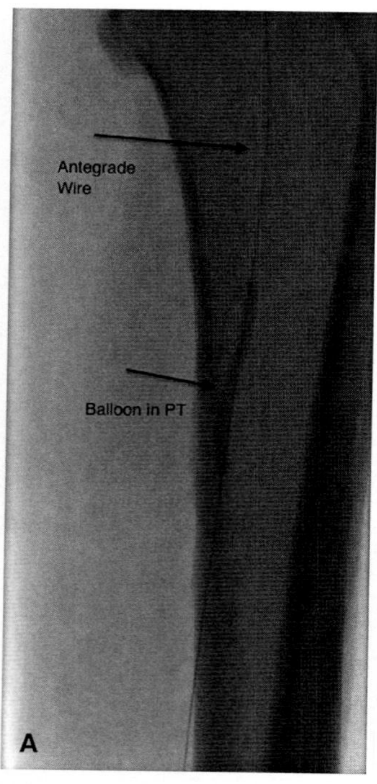

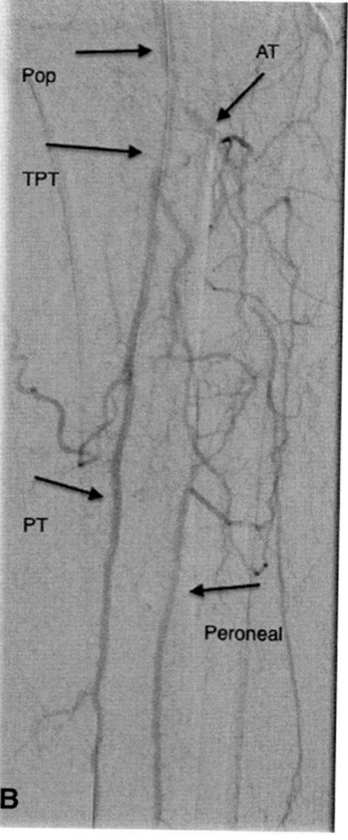

FIGURE 30 ● **A,** Balloon angioplasty of the occluded PT postretrograde recanalization and exteriorization of the wire from the antegrade sheath. **B,** Completion angiogram shows good flow into the PT without any dissection.

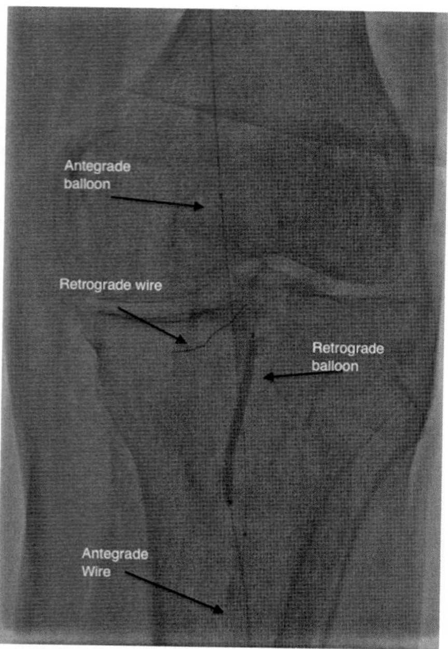

FIGURE 31 ● Retrograde/antegrade PTA to disrupt the membrane between two subintimal planes.

PEARLS AND PITFALLS

Goals for percutaneous tibial revascularization	■ Achieve direct in-line flow to the ischemic foot and, when possible, optimize pedal perfusion by recanalizing more than one occluded tibial artery.
Contralateral or antegrade femoral access	■ Choice based on inflow anatomy and target lesion. Advancement of the antegrade sheath tip into the popliteal artery is key for support and successful tibial revascularization.
Ultrasound-guided access	■ Can help access the anterior wall of the vessel in a relatively disease-free spot and minimize access site complications. It is recommended in antegrade femoral access and retrograde pedal access.
Retrograde approach	■ Should not be regarded as the first option for tibial interventions. It is selectively considered after failed attempts at antegrade access and in the setting of flush occlusions of the antegrade artery with large, adjacent collaterals.
Sheathless retrograde technique	■ Is preferred to minimize tibial artery access complications such as dissection and thrombosis. Recanalization is achieved with a wire and support catheter. Hemostasis with manual compression is usually sufficient.
Crossing total occlusions	■ The intraluminal plane is attempted first with a stiff wire and crossing catheter. The proper catheter position should be confirmed with a selective arteriography prior to definitive angioplasty.
Balloon-assisted recanalization	■ Inflation of a 2-mm balloon may assist with the recanalization of long calcified occlusions.
Kissing balloon technique	■ Is sometimes needed to treat the ostial lesions at the origin of the anterior tibial or posterior tibial artery, depending on the amount of plaque in the adjacent peroneal artery or tibioperoneal trunk.
Anticoagulation	■ Maintain an ACT of greater than 250 seconds throughout the intervention. Continuous or intermittent flushing of the popliteal sheath with heparinized solution is recommended.
Vasodilators	■ Are used from the antegrade sheath and at the pedal access site to prevent vasospasm and to allow better visualization of tibial vessels distal to the occlusion. Heparin, verapamil, and nitroglycerin is a frequently used "cocktail" through the pedal access to address vasospasm.

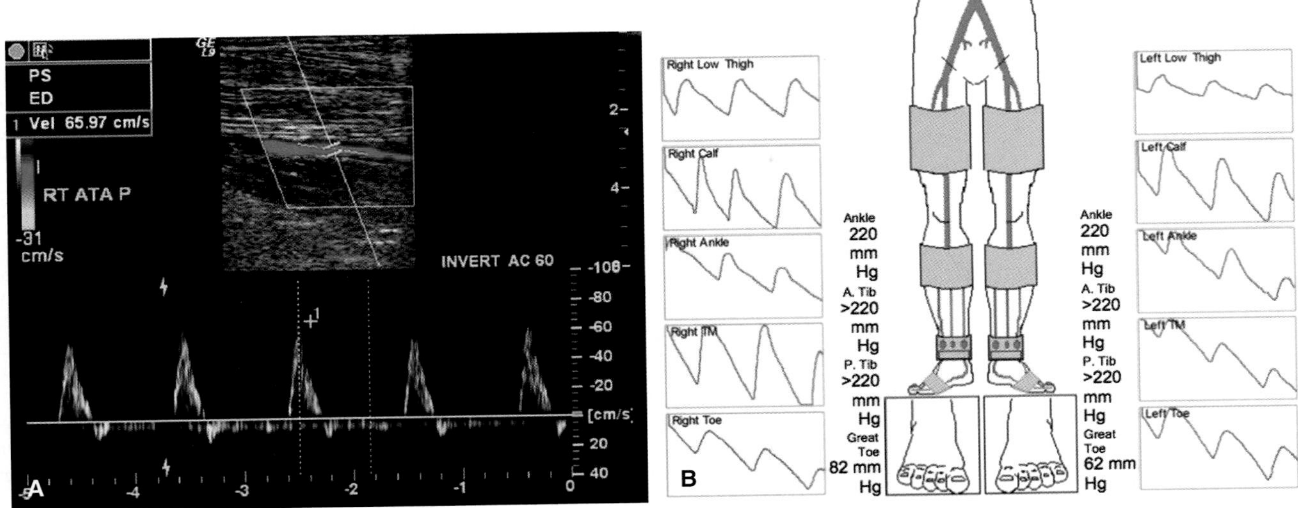

FIGURE 32 ● **A,** Duplex of the anterior tibial artery postrecanalization and angioplasty shows patent vessel with relatively normal Doppler flow. **B,** Follow-up PVRs postrecanalization and angioplasty of the right anterior tibial artery and right posterior tibial artery demonstrate normal PVR waveforms in the foot with adequate toe pressure.

POSTOPERATIVE CARE

- Following the procedure, the patient is observed in the recovery unit with serial neurovascular examinations and intravenous and oral hydration.
- A clopidogrel loading dose (usually 300 mg) is administered when the patient is not already on dual antiplatelet therapy. Dual antiplatelet therapy is recommended for at least 3 months, longer when stents are used.
- Clinical follow-up is obtained 2 to 4 weeks after the procedure is performed, including vascular laboratory studies (usually PVRs, segmental pressures, and Duplex arterial insonation) (**FIGURE 32**).
- Close follow-up is essential to ensure optimal symptom resolution and limb salvage.

OUTCOMES

- Tibial balloon angioplasty carries a relatively low primary patency rate but can greatly augment long-term limb salvage rates. The minimally invasive nature of the procedure is especially advantageous in high-medical-risk patients. One-year primary patency rates in experienced hands range from 30% to 40%; secondary patency rates approach 60%, with ultimate limb salvage greater than 70%.[2,3]
- Retrograde interventions do not impact the patency rates of tibial interventions compared with antegrade transfemoral access. Access site thrombosis appears to be an uncommon complication.[4,5]
- Literature results remain inconsistent regarding drug-eluting balloons for tibial lesions. Results from the randomized IN.PACT DEEP trial comparing drug-coated balloons vs standard angioplasty for the treatment of infrapopliteal lesions revealed no significant differences in amputation rates between the two groups.[6]
- Primary stenting does not appear to offer any advantage over tibial angioplasty alone. A Cochrane review of randomized clinical trials revealed no differences in primary patency, secondary patency, or major amputations between angioplasty alone vs angioplasty and stenting.[7,8] There may be some patency advantage associated with drug eluting, as compared with bare metal stents.[9] Nonetheless, stenting under all circumstances should be considered as a "bailout," used to improve suboptimal results of angioplasty alone.[10]
- Tibial atherectomy does not offer an added benefit compared with plain balloon angioplasty with comparable patency and limb salvage rates.[11]
- Patients with significant tissue loss and gangrene should be followed very closely after successful tibial angioplasty. Lesion restenosis rates trend higher in patients at increased risk for limb loss.[12]
- Multilevel interventions, when necessary, are associated with improved limb salvage rate and wound healing compared with isolated tibial interventions.[3]
- Postangioplasty arterial restenosis may portend less clinical significance once healing is achieved in the distal limb or forefoot. The temporary increase in blood flow following angioplasty is often sufficient to heal small ulcerations.[13]
- There is some evidence of improved patency with drug-eluting stents and drug-eluting balloons.[9,14]
- The LIFE BTK trial is currently enrolling patients in the prospective trial evaluating the safety and effectiveness of the new Everolimus Eluting Resorbable Scaffold system in the tibial vessels.

COMPLICATIONS

- Access site complications (hematoma, bleeding, pseudoaneurysm) are more common with the ipsilateral antegrade femoral approach.
- Contrast-induced nephropathy can be avoided by sufficient preoperative, intraoperative, and postoperative hydration as well as judicious use of contrast.
- Vessel thrombosis can be avoided by maintaining a therapeutic anticoagulation level throughout the procedure. The use of nitroglycerin can help prevent vasospasm and a

low-flow state. Dual antiplatelet therapy is recommended to avoid early postprocedural target artery thrombosis.

- Outflow embolization may be successfully treated with catheter aspiration or thrombolysis if needed.
- Retrograde access site bleeding, dissection, and vessel thrombosis are described after the retrograde pedal access. Using ultrasound-guided access, sheathless technique and the use of local vasodilators may minimize the risk of retrograde access site complications.
- Compartment syndrome may develop either from reperfusion injury following successful intervention or, more commonly, perforation of tibial arteries in the deep compartments of the leg.
- Limb loss may result from failed intervention, iatrogenic vessel thrombosis, distal arterial occlusion following embolization, and compartment syndrome.

REFERENCES

1. Mills JL, Sr., Conte MS, Armstrong DG, et al. The Society for Vascular Surgery Lower Extremity Threatened Limb Classification System: risk stratification based on wound, ischemia, and foot infection (WIfI). *J Vasc Surg* 2014;59:220-234.e1-2.
2. Fernandez N, McEnaney R, Marone LK, et al. Predictors of failure and success of tibial interventions for critical limb ischemia. *J Vasc Surg*. 2010;52:834-842.
3. Fernandez N, McEnaney R, Marone LK, et al. Multilevel versus isolated endovascular tibial interventions for critical limb ischemia. *J Vasc Surg*. 2011;54:722-729.
4. Taha AG, Abou Ali AN, Al-Khoury G, et al. Outcomes of infrageniculate retrograde versus transfemoral access for endovascular intervention for chronic lower extremity ischemia. *J Vasc Surg*. 2018;68:1088-1095.
5. Lai SH, Fenlon J, Roush BB, et al. Analysis of the retrograde tibial artery approach in lower extremity revascularization in an office endovascular center. *J Vasc Surg*. 2019;70:157-165.
6. Zeller T, Micari A, Scheinert D, et al. The IN.PACT DEEP clinical drug-coated balloon trial: 5-year outcomes. *JACC Cardiovasc Interv*. 2020;13:431-443.
7. Hsu CC, Kwan GN, Singh D, Rophael JA, Anthony C, van Driel ML. Angioplasty versus stenting for infrapopliteal arterial lesions in chronic limb-threatening ischaemia. *Cochrane Database Syst Rev*. 2018;12:Cd009195.
8. Randon C, Jacobs B, De Ryck F, Vermassen F. Angioplasty or primary stenting for infrapopliteal lesions: results of a prospective randomized trial. *Cardiovasc Intervent Radiol*. 2010;33:260-269.
9. Bosiers M, Scheinert D, Peeters P, et al. Randomized comparison of everolimus-eluting versus bare-metal stents in patients with critical limb ischemia and infrapopliteal arterial occlusive disease. *J Vasc Surg*. 2012;55:390-398.
10. Donas KP, Torsello G, Schwindt A, Schönefeld E, Boldt O, Pitoulias GA. Below knee bare nitinol stent placement in high-risk patients with critical limb ischemia is still durable after 24 months of follow-up. *J Vasc Surg*. 2010;52:356-361.
11. Todd KE Jr, Ahanchi SS, Maurer CA, Kim JH, Chipman CR, Panneton JM. Atherectomy offers no benefits over balloon angioplasty in tibial interventions for critical limb ischemia. *J Vasc Surg*. 2013;58:941-948.
12. Saqib NU, Domenick N, Cho JS, et al. Predictors and outcomes of restenosis following tibial artery endovascular interventions for critical limb ischemia. *J Vasc Surg*. 2013;57:692-699.
13. Schmidt A, Ulrich M, Winkler B, et al. Angiographic patency and clinical outcome after balloon-angioplasty for extensive infrapopliteal arterial disease. *Cathet Cardiovasc Interv*. 2010;76:1047-1054.
14. Schmidt A, Piorkowski M, Werner M, et al. First experience with drug-eluting balloons in infrapopliteal arteries: restenosis rate and clinical outcome. *J Am Coll Cardiol*. 2011;58:1105-1109.

Chapter 31 Open Infrainguinal Reconstruction Techniques

Gregory J. Landry

DEFINITION

- Lower extremity bypasses are named by the corresponding inflow and outflow arteries. The most common inflow source is the femoral artery (common, superficial, profunda). For disease that is more distal the popliteal or tibial arteries can also be used for inflow. Common sources of outflow include the popliteal (above and below knee), tibial (anterior tibial, posterior tibial, peroneal), and pedal (dorsalis pedis, posterior tibial, medial and lateral plantar) arteries.
- Autogenous conduit is preferred for all lower extremity bypasses when available. The greater saphenous vein (GSV) is the most frequently used conduit. Other options for native conduit include the short saphenous vein, arm vein (basilic, cephalic, brachial), and femoral vein.
- If suitable autogenous conduit is not available, alternate conduit options include prosthetic (polytetrafluoroethylene, polyester) or cryopreserved cadaver grafts.

DIFFERENTIAL DIAGNOSIS

- The majority of patients for whom lower extremity bypass is necessary will have atherosclerotic peripheral arterial disease (PAD).
- Other conditions for which lower extremity bypass may be necessary include aneurysms (eg, femoral, popliteal), trauma, and vasculitis.

PATIENT HISTORY AND PHYSICAL FINDINGS

- PAD can be asymptomatic; however, revascularization is rarely performed in the absence of symptoms. The most frequent symptomatic presentation of PAD is intermittent claudication (leg pain with walking relieved by rest). More severe PAD presents with chronic limb threatening ischemia (CLTI), including rest pain, ulcers, and gangrene.
- A history of cardiovascular risk factors should be elicited in all patients undergoing lower extremity bypass, including history of smoking, cardiac disease, cerebrovascular disease, diabetes, chronic kidney disease, hyperlipidemia, and chronic obstructive pulmonary disease.
- Upper and lower extremity pulse examination should be performed. Because atherosclerosis is a systemic disorder, the following pulses should be assessed bilaterally: carotid, brachial, radial, femoral, popliteal, dorsalis pedis, and posterior tibial. Both the presence and strength of pulses should be recorded.
- If lower extremity pulses are absent, which is usually the case in patients undergoing surgery for peripheral arterial disease, ankle-brachial indices (ABIs) should be measured. The highest ankle pressure is divided by the highest brachial pressure.
- A history of prior vein use or removal should be elicited. Veins may have previously been used for prior lower extremity or coronary artery bypass. Patients with varicose veins may have undergone prior vein stripping or ablation. Patients with chronic kidney disease may have had prior upper extremity arteriovenous fistula placement. In dialysis-dependent patients, upper extremity veins should be used judiciously as they may be necessary for future arteriovenous access.

IMAGING AND OTHER DIAGNOSTIC STUDIES

- ABIs should be calculated in all patients considered for lower extremity bypass. A normal ABI is between 0.9 and 1.3. While there is some overlap, in general, an ABI 0.5 to 0.9 is consistent with intermittent claudication and <0.5 is consistent with CLTI. An ABI >1.3 is likely falsely elevated due to arterial calcification and may or may not be associated with significant arterial occlusive disease.
- Arterial duplex ultrasonography can be performed to determine sites of arterial stenosis and occlusion. In some centers, ultrasonography is the only diagnostic test performed before revascularization; however, in most centers, additional imaging is performed.
- Patients considered for lower extremity bypass should undergo arteriography to define the proximal (inflow) and distal (outflow) targets.
  - Digital subtraction angiography remains the gold standard and provides the greatest anatomic detail for operative planning.
  - Alternative imaging modalities include computed tomography and magnetic resonance angiography or duplex ultrasonography.
- Duplex ultrasonography should be used for preoperative vein mapping to identify suitable autogenous conduit (**FIGURE 1**). If the patient has good-quality GSV, no further

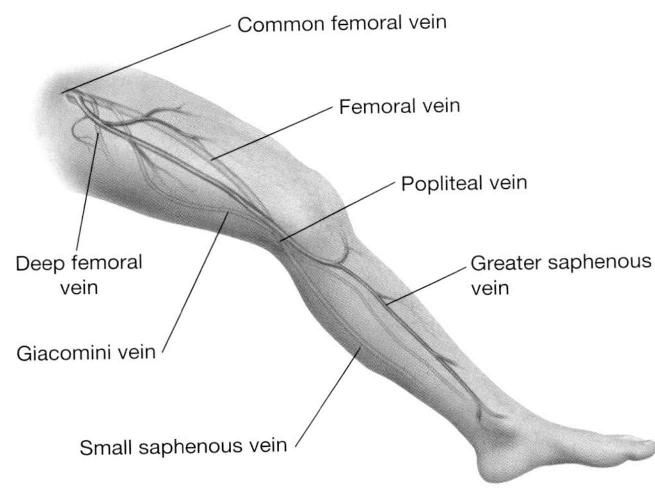

FIGURE 1 • Lower extremity venous anatomy.

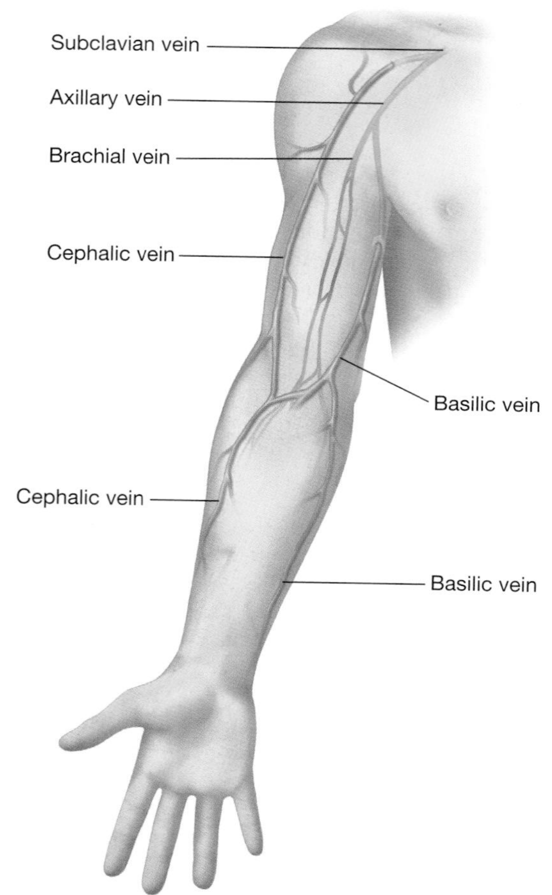

FIGURE 2 ● Upper extremity venous anatomy.

vein mapping is typically necessary. If the GSV is of poor quality or absent, small saphenous vein and arm vein should be mapped (**FIGURE 2**).

- Ideal conduit diameter is 3.5 mm or greater.
- The vein should be easily compressible. A thick-walled or noncompressible vein may indicate prior superficial venous thrombosis, and the vein is likely not suitable for bypass.
- Mapping should ideally immediately precede surgery with vein course marked with an indelible marker on the skin.

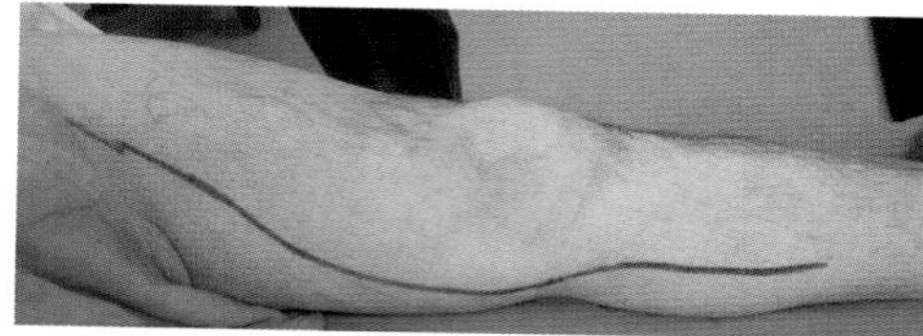

FIGURE 3 ● Lower extremity vein mapping with marking of GSV.

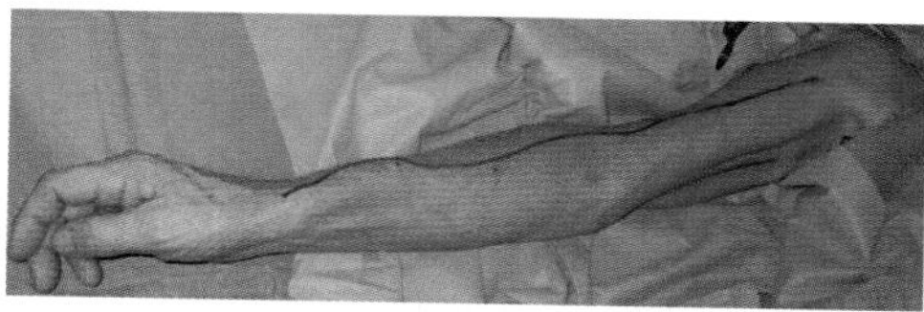

FIGURE 4 ● Upper extremity vein mapping with marking of the cephalic and basilic veins.

This allows precise placement of incisions, which avoids the creation of skin and tissue flaps that might impede wound healing.

SURGICAL MANAGEMENT

- Preoperative planning
  - If not previously marked or if marks have faded, it is useful to re-mark the intended venous conduit with ultrasound guidance prior to surgery (**FIGURES 3** and **4**).
  - Open foot lesions or gangrene should be covered with sterile adhesive to prevent contamination of sterile incisions.
  - Prophylactic intravenous antibiotics should be administered to reduce risk of perioperative infection.
  - If arm vein is to be harvested, it is important to avoid blood draws or intravenous lines in the intended arm(s). If veins from both arms are necessary, central venous access may be necessary.
- Positioning
  - The majority of the procedures are performed with the patient supine. If small saphenous vein is the intended conduit, it is often easier to perform this part of the procedure with the patient prone and then to reprepare and drape with the patient supine.
  - If arm vein is to be harvested, the arms should be abducted and placed on arm boards.

TECHNIQUES

- Arterial exposure (for additional details see Part 6, Chapter 25):
  - The common, superficial, and profunda femoral arteries are exposed through a proximal groin incision. This incision can be either longitudinal or oblique per surgeon preference. The femoral vessels are located in the femoral triangle bordered medially by the adductor longus muscle, laterally by the sartorius muscle, and superiorly by the inguinal ligament.
  - The above-knee popliteal artery is exposed through a medial above-knee incision. The sartorius muscle is reflected posteriorly and the popliteal space entered. The popliteal artery and vein are closely apposed and dissected free from each other.
  - The below-knee popliteal artery is exposed through a medial below-knee incision. The fascia is opened and the popliteal space entered. The gastrocnemius muscle is reflected posteriorly and the popliteal artery identified cephalad to the soleus muscle.
  - Division of the proximal soleus muscle allows dissection of the proximal anterior tibial artery, tibioperoneal trunk, and proximal posterior tibial and peroneal arteries.
  - The mid and distal anterior tibial artery is exposed through a lateral calf incision. The anterior compartment is entered and the tibialis anterior and extensor hallucis longus muscle are separated, with the artery found at the base of the compartment between these two muscles.

- The mid and distal posterior tibial and peroneal arteries are exposed through a medial calf incision. The fascia is opened to enter the superficial posterior compartment. The soleus muscle is divided to enter the deep posterior compartment. Upon entering the deep posterior compartment, the first vessels encountered are the posterior tibial artery and veins. Tibial veins are often paired with branches over the artery. In the same plane, further lateral dissection is needed to expose the peroneal artery, which is adjacent to the fibula.
- This distal peroneal artery can be exposed through a lateral calf incision with removal of the distal fibula. The common peroneal nerve should be protected. The lateral malleolus should be preserved to maintain joint stability. Muscle attachments to the fibula should be disconnected with a periosteal elevator or similar device and the fibular segment resected using a saw or bone cutters. Great care should be taken on the medial aspect of the fibula as the peroneal vessels lie immediately underneath.
- Inframalleolar arteries can be exposed on the foot for pedal bypass. The dorsalis pedis artery is typically located between the first and second metatarsal. The distal posterior tibial and proximal medial and lateral plantar arteries are posterior to the medial malleolus and extend onto the plantar surface of the foot.

- Open vein harvest: GSV
  - A longitudinal incision is made directly over the marked vein. Either a single incision or multiple skip incisions can be used, with some evidence of fewer wound infections with the latter approach (**FIGURE 5**).
  - The necessary length of vein is unroofed. Using blunt and sharp dissection with Metzenbaum scissors, the vein is freed from surrounding structures. Side branches are ligated and divided with silk ligatures and hemoclips.
  - The GSV is divided proximally at the saphenofemoral junction (**FIGURE 6**), distally according to the length of vein needed, once both proximal and distal anastomosis sites have been dissected.
  - It is helpful distally to identify a branch point in the vein that can subsequently be used for the proximal anastomosis if the graft is placed in reversed configuration (**FIGURE 7A** and **B**).
- Open vein harvest: small saphenous vein
  - The same technique is used as for the GSV, except typically with the patient prone.
  - Proximally, the vein is typically divided at the saphenopopliteal junction. Some patients will have continuation of the small saphenous vein in the thigh (Giacomini vein), which allows harvesting additional length of vein in the thigh.
- Open vein harvest: arm vein
  - Both the cephalic and basilic veins can be harvested through longitudinal arm incisions. The same technique is used as for leg vein; however, care must be taken, as the arm veins tend to be more thin walled and fragile than leg vein.
  - The cephalic vein can frequently be harvested as a single conduit from the wrist to the deltopectoral groove (**FIGURE 8A-C**). A single segment is frequently adequate for a femoral-popliteal or femoral to proximal tibial bypass.
  - The basilic vein tends to be larger in diameter than the cephalic vein, although often, only a short segment in the upper arm is available. The basilic vein is well suited for use as an extension graft when revision of a previously placed bypass is necessary. When used as a new bypass, a composite graft composed of two or more vein segments is frequently necessary.
  - The basilic vein often has large branches that communicate medially with the brachial vein. These branches are often broad based and are better ligated with a running monofilament suture than simple ligation.
  - The median antebrachial cutaneous nerve frequently interdigitates with the basilic vein. With meticulous dissection, this nerve can be preserved (**FIGURE 9**).
  - The brachial vein is intimately associated with both the brachial artery and median nerve. This vein can also be

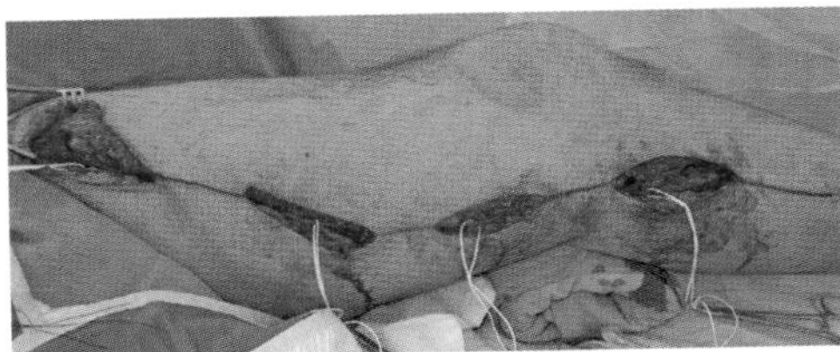

FIGURE 5 ● Open GSV harvest through skip incisions. The vein is encircled with silastic vessel loops.

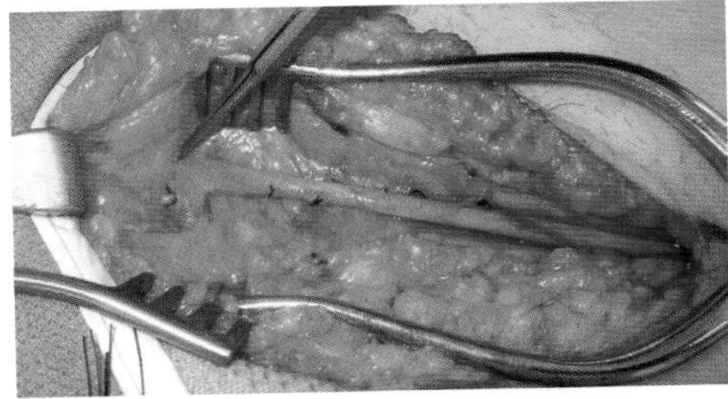

FIGURE 6 ● GSV mobilized proximally to saphenofemoral junction. Side branches ligated with silk ligatures.

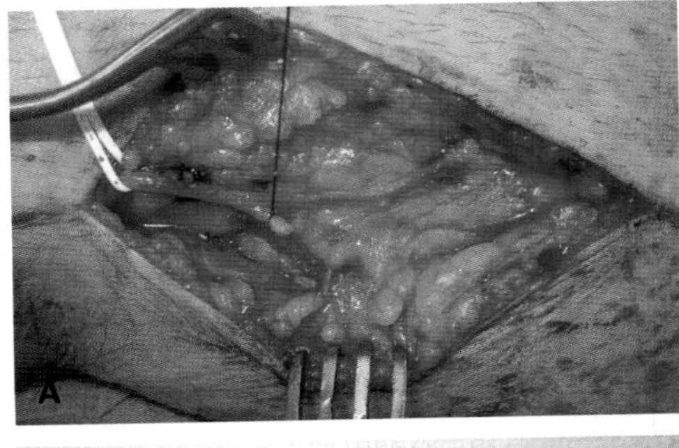

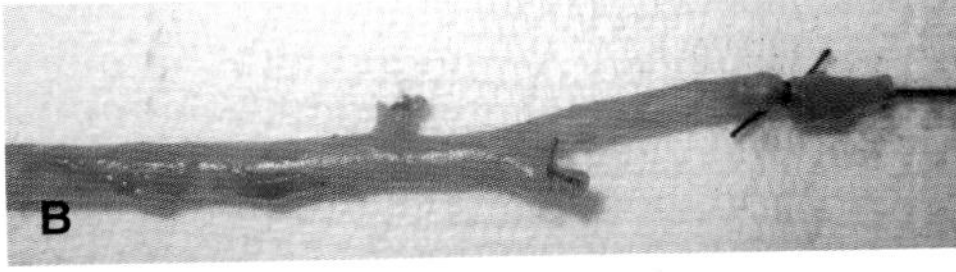

FIGURE 7 ● **A and B,** Distal GSV divided at branch point to provide starting spot for proximal anastomosis of reversed vein graft.

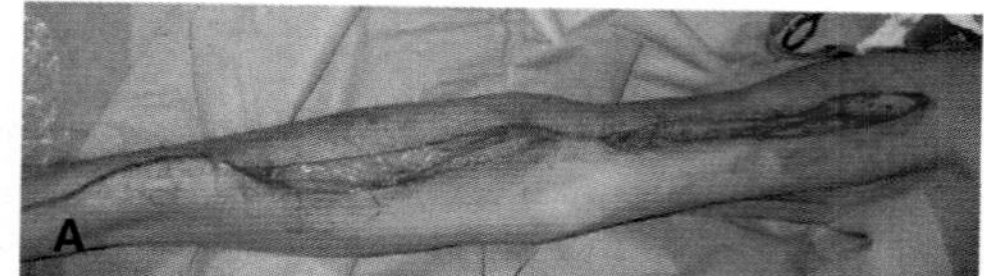

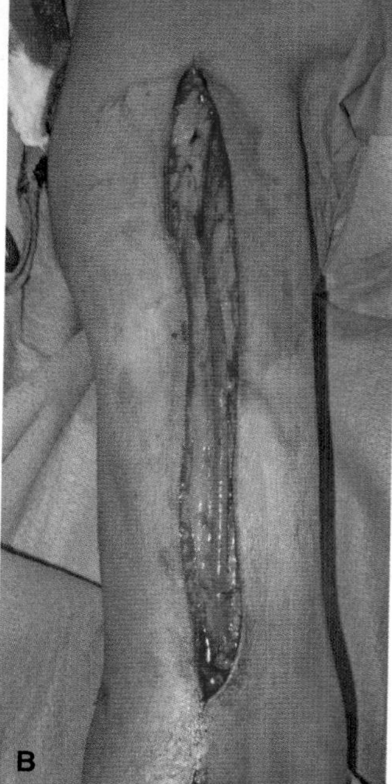

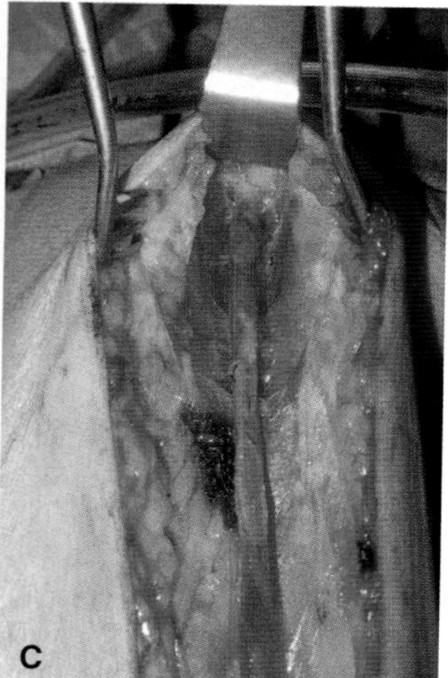

FIGURE 8 ● **A,** Cephalic vein harvested the full length of the arm with skin bridge at antecubital fossa. **B,** Upper arm cephalic vein. **C,** Cephalic vein harvested medially to deltopectoral groove.

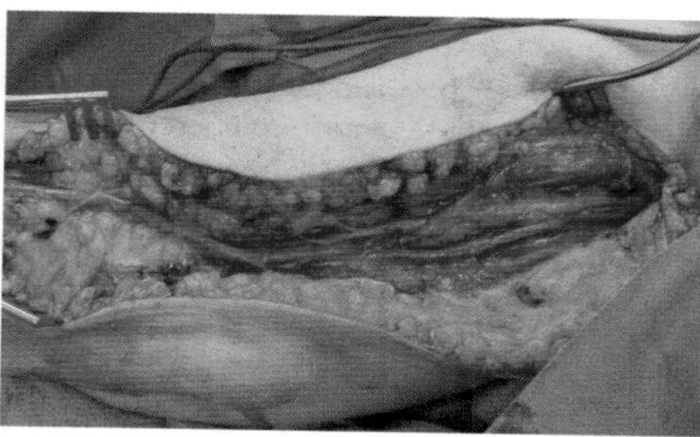

FIGURE 9 ● Basilic vein harvested in upper arm. Median antebrachial cutaneous nerve adjacent to and interdigitating with vein.

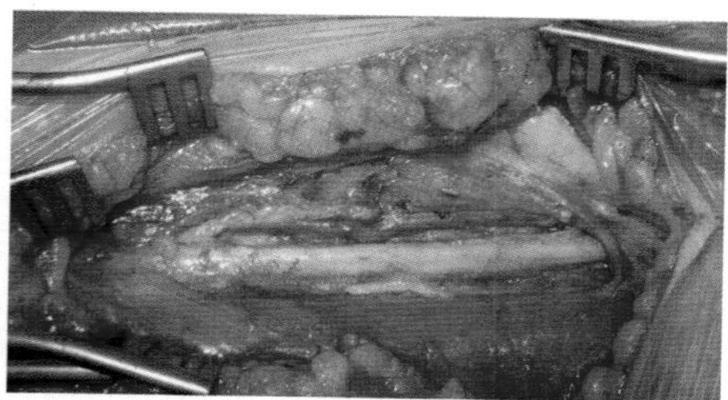

FIGURE 10 ● Brachial vein harvest with vein adjacent to median nerve. Brachial artery deep to nerve.

harvested as conduit, but great care needs to be taken to avoid injury to adjacent structures (**FIGURE 10**).

- Open harvest: femoral vein
  - Although typically used for larger vessel reconstruction, the femoral vein can be used for autogenous lower extremity bypass if necessary.
  - The proximal femoral vein is harvested medial to sartorius muscle. The vein is adjacent to the superficial femoral artery. The vein can be harvested proximally up to the profunda femoral vein.
  - Distally, the femoral vein is easier to harvest with the sartorius muscle reflected posteriorly. The vein can easily be harvested as far as the adductor canal.
  - If a longer segment is needed, the vein can be further harvested caudal to the adductor tendon into the popliteal fossa.
- Endoscopic harvest: GSV
  - Endoscopic harvest works best for veins within the saphenous fascial envelope (**FIGURE 11A**). It is technically more difficult in cases where the vein leaves this fascial envelope and is situated more superficially or in the subcutaneous fatty tissue (**FIGURE 11B**).
  - Available harvesting systems are described in **TABLE 1**.
  - A 2-cm incision is made at the level of the knee and the GSV dissected free at this site and encircled with a silastic vessel loop (**FIGURE 12**).
  - The vein is dissected from the knee to the saphenofemoral junction using a conical dissecting tip (**FIGURE 13**). CO_2 insufflation is performed through an inflatable trocar.
  - The vein is held in place with the C-ring or V-lock mechanism, and side branches are divided with bipolar electrocautery or harmonic scissors depending on the manufacturer (**FIGURE 14**).
  - Harvesting can also be performed in the calf; however, this is more technically challenging due to multiple geniculate venous branches, subcutaneous position of vein, and close approximation with saphenous nerve.
  - If an incision in the groin is going to be made for the proximal anastomosis of the graft, the incision can be

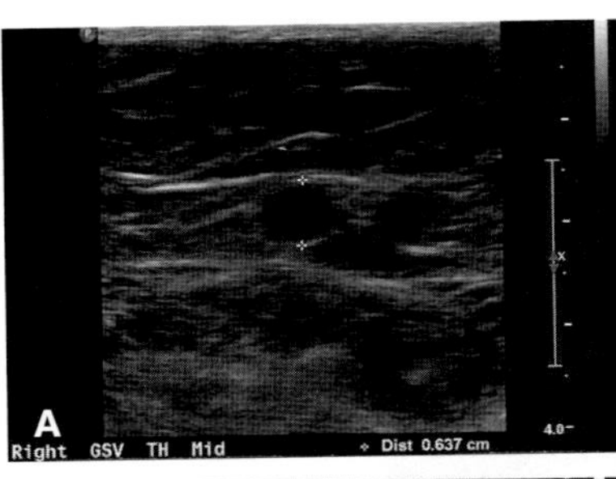

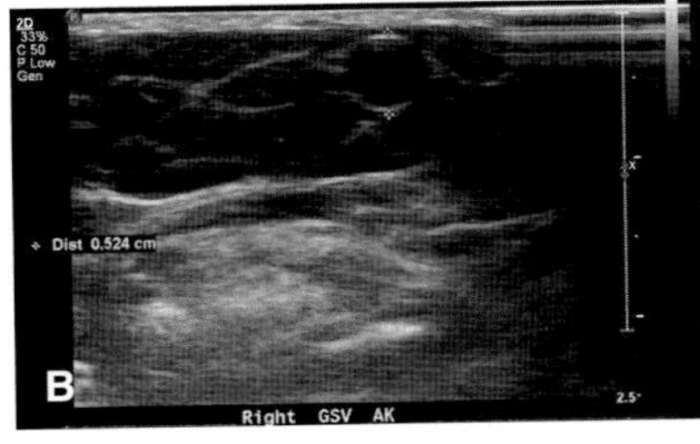

FIGURE 11 ● **A,** GSV (marked by *cursors*) within the saphenous fascial envelope suitable for endoscopic vein harvest. **B,** Subcutaneous GSV outside of saphenous fascial envelope, less suitable for endoscopic harvest.

Table 1: Endoscopic Vein Harvesting Systems

Manufacturer	Device	Dissecting tool	Vein securing	Side branch ligation
Maquet	Vasoview	Conical tip	C-ring	Bipolar ligating forceps
Maquet	Vasoview Hemopro	Conical tip	C-ring	Thermostatic cut and seal
Terumo	VirtuoSaph	Conical tip	V-lock	Bipolar cut and coagulation

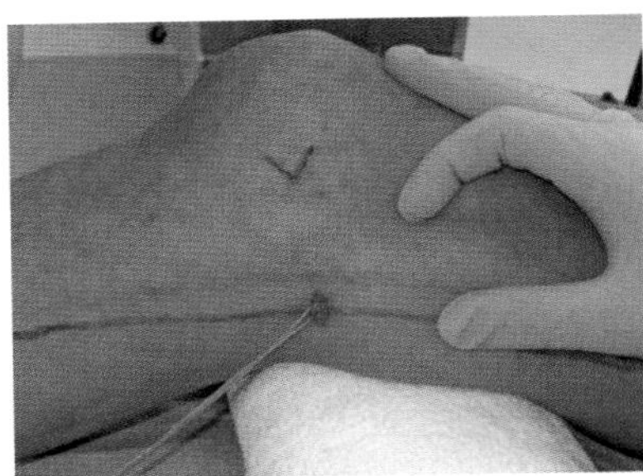

FIGURE 12 ● A 2-cm incision at the level of the knee through which GSV (encircled with silastic loop) dissected for endoscopic harvest.

made at this point to complete the proximal harvest. If an incision is not going to be made in the groin, a stab incision is made in the groin and the vein grasped under direct vision with a tonsil clamp. The vein is then pulled through the incision and ligated and divided with silk ligatures.

- After proximal division, the vein can be pulled out of the tunnel through the knee incision.

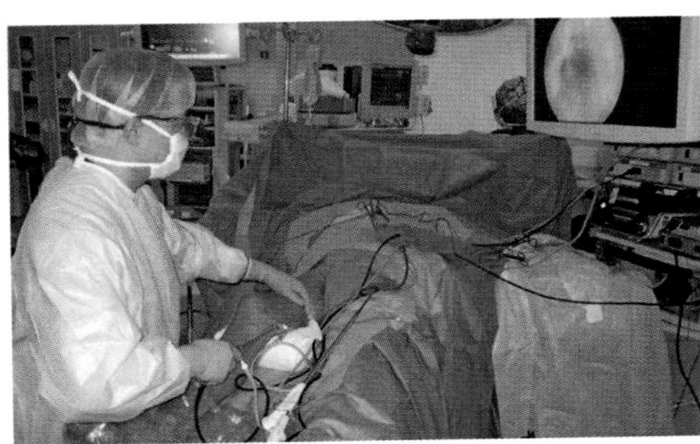

FIGURE 13 ● Conical dissecting tool mounted on camera used to isolate GSV. Operator standing opposite screen depicting endoscopic image.

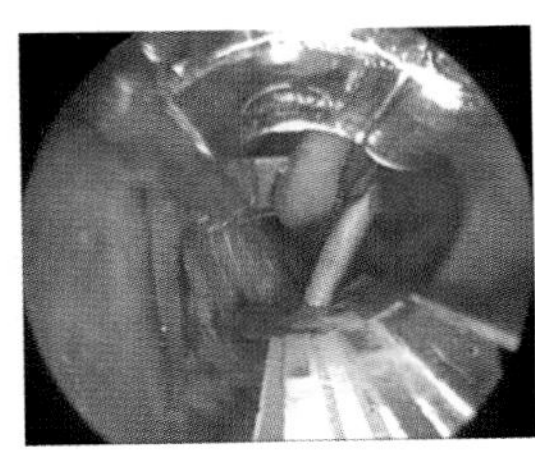

FIGURE 14 ● GSV held in plastic cradle while side branch ligated and divided with bipolar electrocautery.

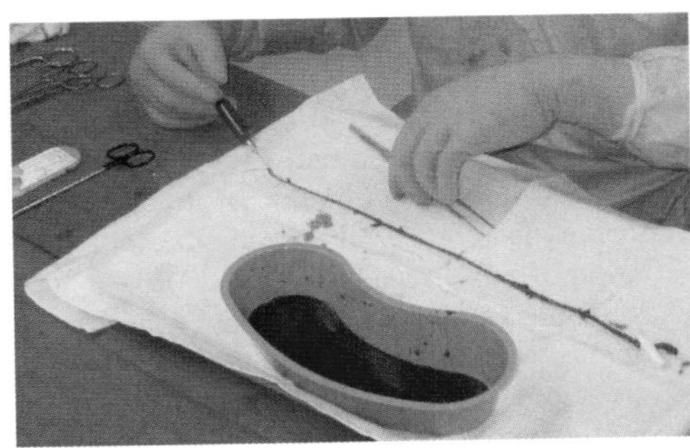

FIGURE 15 ● Back-table preparation of harvested vein.

  - A below-knee incision can be made to harvest the distal vein if this incision is already intended for the distal anastomotic site.
- Back-table vein preparation
  - Harvested veins are prepared on a back table (**FIGURE 15**). Veins are distended with the surgeon's solution of choice. The author prefers using chilled, heparinized autologous blood, although heparinized saline is also sufficient.
  - Any side branches not ligated during the initial harvest are ligated with silk ligatures or, if too small or short, with 7-0 polypropylene suture.
  - For endoscopically harvested veins, because the side branches are not ligated during the initial harvest, they are ligated at a back table with silk ligatures or 7-0 polypropylene suture after vein removal.
- Composite graft creation
  - A venovenostomy can be performed with two (or more) venous segments to create a single conduit of adequate length. The vein of larger diameter should be

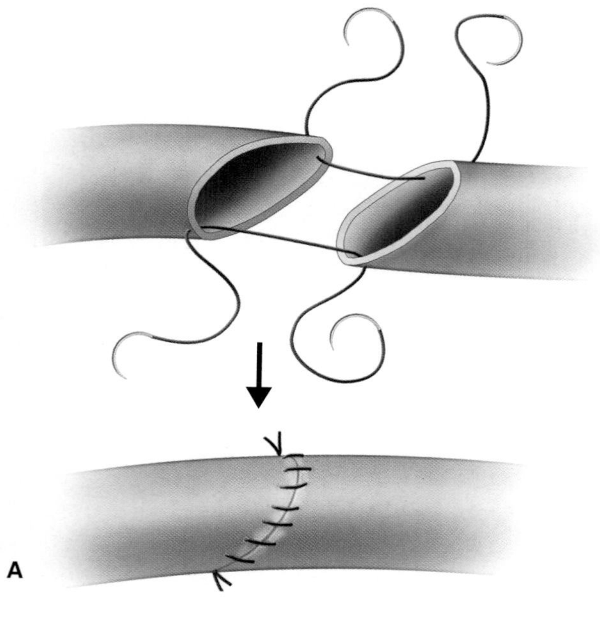

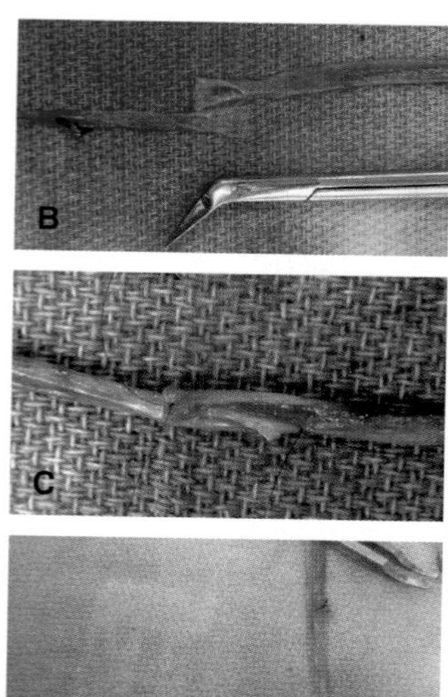

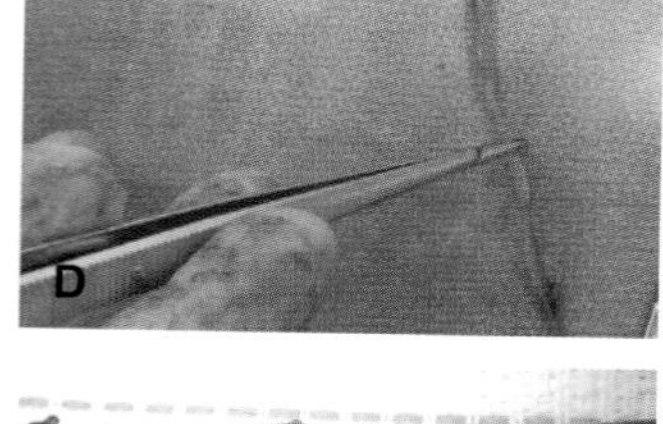

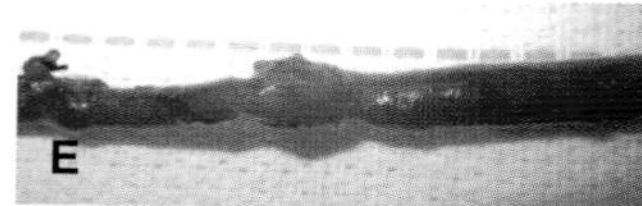

FIGURE 16 ● **A,** Diagram depicting vein splicing. **B,** Splicing of arm veins to create single conduit. Veins spatulated with Potts scissors. **C,** A 7-0 polypropylene suture placed to approximate the heel and toe of the two veins. **D,** Venovenostomy performed with running suture. **E,** Final spatulated venovenostomy.

placed proximally. The veins are spatulated and sewn end to end with running 7-0 polypropylene suture (**FIGURE 16A-E**). Additional vein segments can be added as necessary with the same technique to create a conduit of adequate length.

- Nonautogenous conduit
  - The most commonly used prosthetic bypasses are externally supported polytetrafluoroethylene or polyester. Typical diameters are 6 or 8 mm depending on the size of the arteries. No special preparation for these grafts is required.
  - Cryopreserved greater saphenous vein is the most frequently used cryopreserved conduit. Cryopreserved femoral artery and vein can also be used. These conduits are frozen and must be thawed and prepared according to manufacturer specifications.
- Graft tunneling
  - Grafts are best tunneled using a hollow tube tunneler, such as a Scanlan tunneler, in order to avoid unnecessary tension on the vein as it is pulled through the subcutaneous tissue. This is particularly important in a composite graft where suture line disruption can potentially occur. The same tunnelers can be used for prosthetic conduits.
  - Tunneling performed after the proximal anastomosis allows the graft to be passed under pressure, which lessens the likelihood of twisting or kinking during tunneling.
  - In a first-time bypass, tunneling anatomically through the popliteal fossa for below-knee targets provides the most direct route to minimize vein length (**FIGURE 17**). In redo procedures in which previous grafts were tunneled

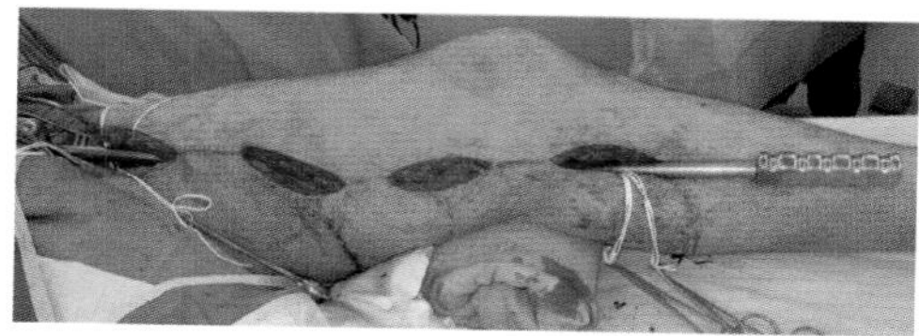

FIGURE 17 ● Anatomic tunnel through popliteal fossa for femoral to below-knee popliteal artery bypass.

through the popliteal fossa, a subcutaneously tunneled graft may be necessary.
  - Two options exist for grafts tunneled to the anterior tibial artery. For grafts based on the common femoral artery, a lateral, subcutaneously tunneled graft is the most straightforward. For grafts based further distally on the superficial femoral or profunda femoral arteries, an anatomic tunnel through the popliteal fossa and interosseous membrane is more direct and minimizes vein length. The interosseous membrane should be directly visualized and a cruciate incision made to prevent graft stricture. Grafts to the posterior tibial or peroneal artery are tunneled either through the popliteal fossa or medially and subcutaneously (**FIGURE 18**).
  - Vein grafts can either be placed reversed or nonreversed depending on the size match at the proximal and distal anastomotic site. Reversed grafts require no further treatment. Nonreversed grafts require valve lysis with a valvulotome. This is best performed with the vein pressurized, so is typically performed after placement of the proximal anastomosis prior to tunneling so that lysis occurs under direct vision.

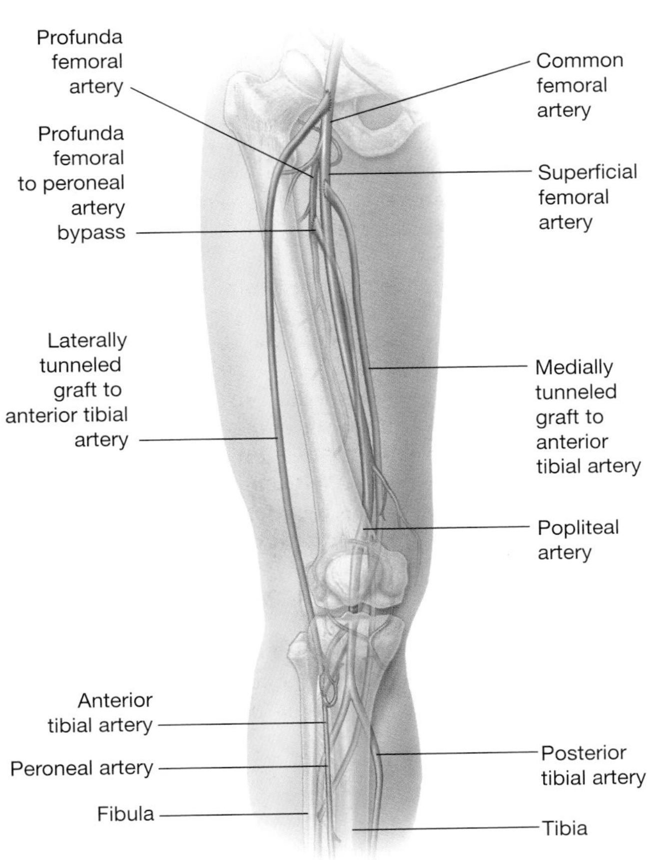

FIGURE 18 ● Diagram depicting tunneling options for tibial grafts.

- Choice of proximal anastomotic site
  - The choice of proximal anastomotic site depends on the anatomy, available vein length, and quality.
    - If adequate vein length is present, an anastomosis to the common femoral artery is generally preferred.
    - If vein length is insufficient, the graft can be based on either the superficial or the profunda femoral artery. For patients with atherosclerotic lower extremity arterial occlusive disease, the profunda femoral artery is more likely to be better preserved than the superficial femoral artery, which is more likely to be affected by atherosclerosis (**FIGURE 19A** and **B**).
    - In the presence of common femoral or proximal profunda femoral artery stenosis, a common and/or profunda femoral endarterectomy with placement of a vein or prosthetic patch (Linton patch) can provide adequate inflow for the graft, with the proximal anastomosis to the distal end of the patch (**FIGURE 20**).
    - In patients with patent superficial femoral arteries and more distal tibial artery disease, as is often seen in patients with diabetes, grafts may be based on either the above- or below-knee popliteal artery.
    - For patients requiring tibial or pedal bypasses with insufficient vein length, the superficial femoral

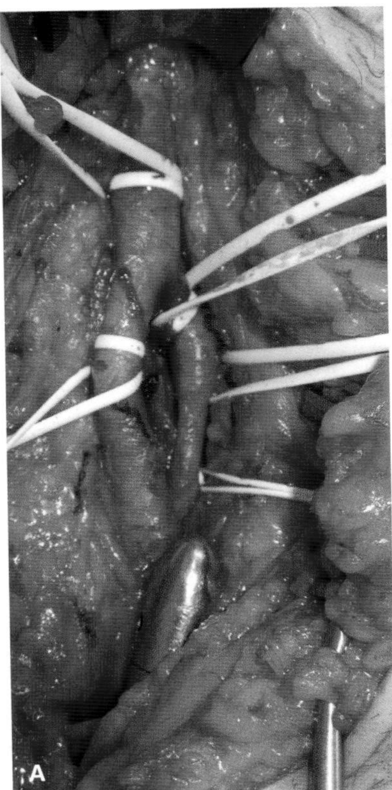

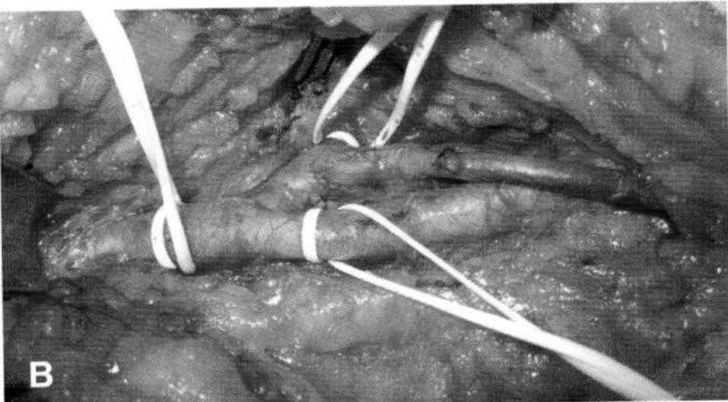

FIGURE 19 ● **A,** Common, superficial, and profunda femoral arteries dissected for proximal anastomosis. Vessels encircled with silastic loops. **B,** Proximal anastomosis to profunda femoral artery in patient with inadequate vein length to base graft on common femoral artery. Note tunneling device in subsartorial position.

artery can be treated with angioplasty with or without stenting to provide inflow for a graft based on the above- or below-knee popliteal artery. This is ideally performed either in a hybrid operating room (OR) suite or in a standard OR with C-arm fluoroscopy.

- Choice of distal anastomotic site
  - In general, the shortest bypass configuration that provides adequate distal flow is chosen.
    - If direct runoff to the foot can be achieved through a bypass to the popliteal artery, this is preferred.

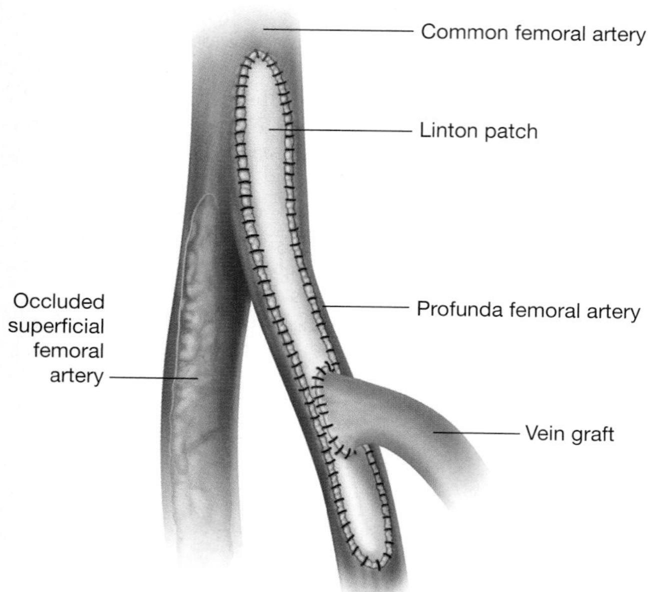

FIGURE 20 ● Diagram of Linton patch on common and profunda femoral arteries from which proximal anastomosis of bypass is based.

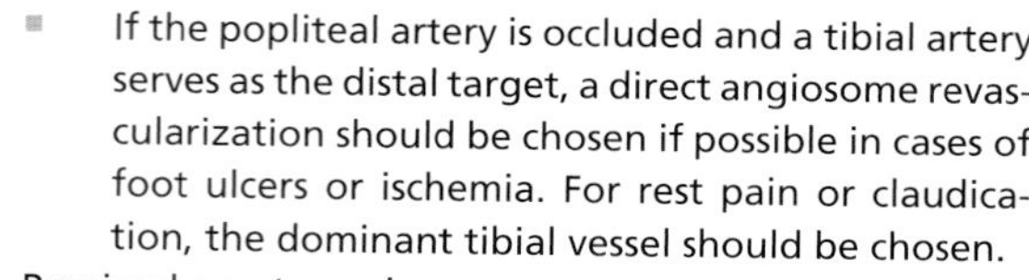

    - If the popliteal artery is occluded and a tibial artery serves as the distal target, a direct angiosome revascularization should be chosen if possible in cases of foot ulcers or ischemia. For rest pain or claudication, the dominant tibial vessel should be chosen.
- Proximal anastomosis
  - Proximal and distal arterial control is obtained with atraumatic vascular clamps, silastic loops, or Fogarty catheters as needed and per surgeon's choice.
  - The anastomotic arteriotomy is made with a no. 11 scalpel and extended with Potts scissors. The arteriotomy length should be about 1.5 to 2 times the diameter of the vein.
  - The proximal anastomosis is ideally performed using a vein branch as the heel in order to avoid heel stricture (**FIGURE 21**). The vein is spatulated through the heel (**FIGURE 22A-C**).
  - The anastomosis is performed with running polypropylene rule. As a rule of thumb, suture diameter is 4-0 in the iliac artery, 5-0 femoral, 6-0 popliteal, and 7-0 tibial (**FIGURE 23**).
- Distal anastomosis
  - This is performed in similar fashion to the proximal anastomosis, although spatulation through a side branch is generally not possible and less necessary as for the proximal anastomosis, because the graft toe geometry is more important for patency than the heel geometry in the outflow (**FIGURE 24**).
  - Some surgeons prefer using a tourniquet inflated to 250 mm Hg for distal control below the knee. This requires less dissection than control with vascular clamps or silastic loops. In patients with extensive arterial calcification, however, tourniquet control may not be adequate.
  - When prosthetic grafts are used, especially if placed in an infrageniculate position, it is common to use a vein patch or cuff at the distal anastomosis. Since most stenoses occur at the distal outflow

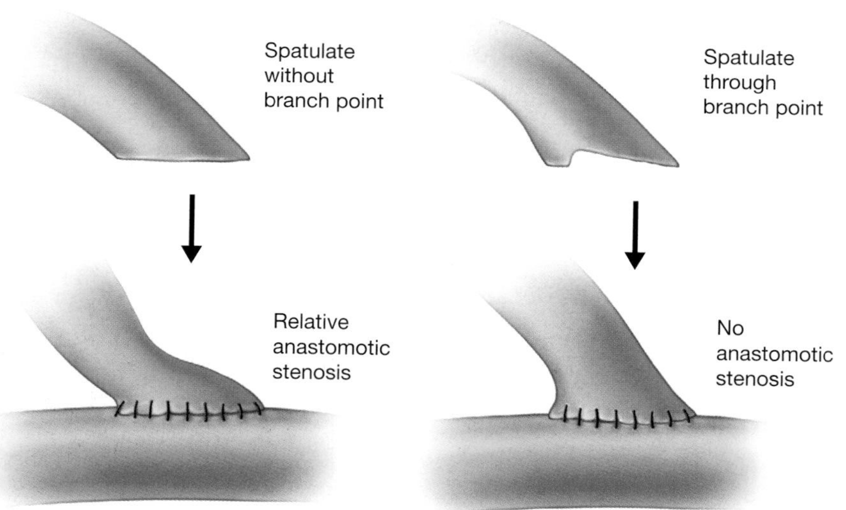

FIGURE 21 ● The vein is spatulated through a branch point to avoid a stricture at the heel of the proximal anastomosis, which can occur if a side branch is not used.

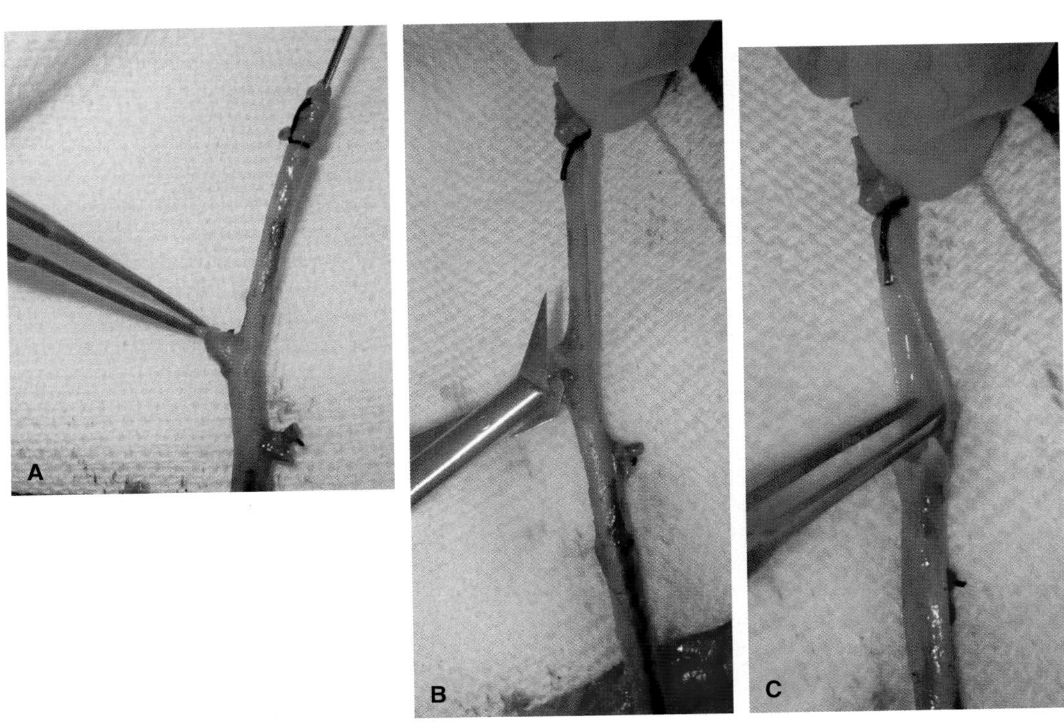

FIGURE 22 ● **A,** Preparation of vein for proximal anastomosis. If possible, side branch is chosen for heel of proximal anastomosis to prevent anastomotic stricture. **B,** Vein spatulated with Potts scissors through branch point. **C,** Spatulated vein prepared for proximal anastomosis.

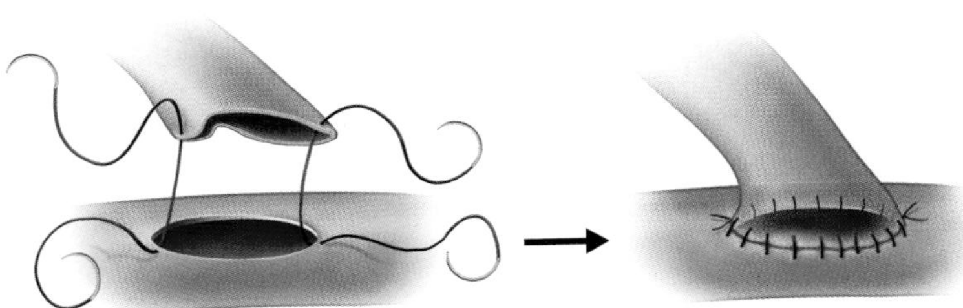

FIGURE 23 ● Diagram demonstrating proximal graft anastomosis.

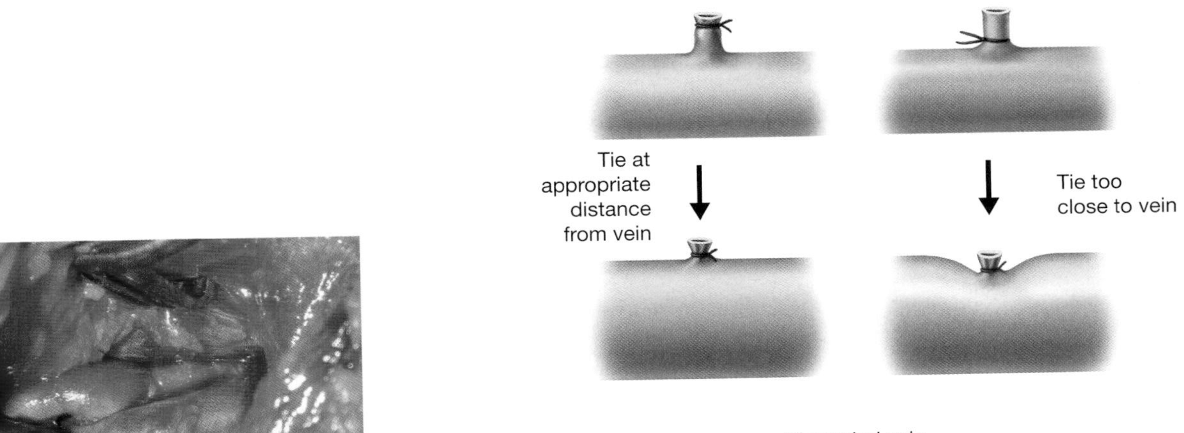

FIGURE 24 ● Distal anastomosis to below-knee popliteal artery.

FIGURE 25 ● "Dimpling" can occur with graft distention if side branch tie is too close to vein.

due to the formation of intimal hyperplasia, a vein patch or cuff can help to mitigate intimal hyperplasia formation. Commonly used techniques include the Taylor patch, Linton patch, or Miller cuff.

- In situ bypass:
  - An alternative bypass method utilizing the greater saphenous vein is an in situ bypass. In these bypasses the greater saphenous vein is not harvested, rather, it is left in place. The same graft configurations as a reversed or nonreversed saphenous vein graft can be performed, with the proximal greater saphenous vein and inflow artery exposed in the proximal incision and the distal greater saphenous vein and outflow artery exposed in the distal incision. The greater saphenous vein is ligated and divided at the saphenofemoral junction and the most cephalad vein valve manually lysed. The vein is then anastomosed to the inflow artery in standard fashion. The saphenous vein is then ligated and divided distally, and the valves are lysed with a valvulotome. This is best accomplished with the vein pressurized and can typically be achieved with one or two passages of the valvulotome. The distal anastomosis is then performed in standard fashion.
  - After completing the proximal and distal anastomosis, greater saphenous vein branches must be ligated. This can be done through a continuous or staggered incision. Branches can be identified with intraoperative duplex ultrasound or angiography.
- Adjunctive techniques:
  - In distal tibial or pedal bypasses, if the arterial outflow is deemed suboptimal, an adjunctive arteriovenous fistula can be created. An adjacent tibial or pedal vein is mobilized and the proximal end anastomosed to the bypass graft. This creates a low resistance outflow bed for the graft that may assist in maintaining graft patency in situations where the arterial outflow has high resistance.
- Intraoperative assessment:
  - Augmentation of Doppler signals at the ankle with the graft open compared with the graft occluded generally indicates graft patency with improved arterial perfusion. Intraoperative duplex or arteriography should also be considered to rule out technical problems with the graft.

PEARLS AND PITFALLS

Open vein harvest	■ Preoperative vein mapping is important to localize the site of the incision to avoid tissue flaps that can lead to poor wound healing. ■ Vein branches should not be ligated flush with the vein as "dimpling" can occur when the vein is distended. It is good to ligate the vein branch at least 1 mm away from the vein to allow proper vein expansion (**FIGURE 25**). ■ Arm veins tend to be more fragile than leg veins, requiring gentler handling during harvest.
Endoscopic vein harvest	■ Avoid harvesting veins that are subcutaneous or not enclosed within a fascial envelope as these are technically more difficult to harvest and therefore more prone to injury.
Vein preparation	■ Avoid overdistending the vein during preparation. A good technique is to inject a small amount of fluid into the vein and then manually distending the vein in segments rather than trying to inflate the vein with the syringe.
Graft tunneling	■ Passing the graft while distended reduces the risk of twisting or kinking. ■ Using a sterile marking pen, a line can be drawn on the anterior surface of the vein to help orient the graft distally and prevent twisting.
Anastomotic placement	■ Severely diseased vessels tend to delaminate when handled. Great care must be taken to include all layers in the anastomosis to prevent dissection. ■ In severely calcified vessels, vessel loops may not provide adequate control and vascular clamps may cause a crush injury. In these cases, Fogarty balloons may be needed for arterial control. A thigh tourniquet can also be used to facilitate arterial control.

POSTOPERATIVE CARE

- Patients should be monitored postoperatively in either an intensive care unit or a surgical ward. Hourly vascular checks should be performed with continuous wave Doppler.
- Early ambulation, generally on the first postoperative day, is encouraged, particularly in patients with claudication or rest pain. Patients with ulcers or gangrene may require a longer period of non–weight-bearing if lesions are on a weight-bearing surface.

OUTCOMES

- Anticipated 3-year primary patency rates for reversed saphenous vein grafts are 70% to 80% for femoral-popliteal and 60% to 75% for femoral-tibial. Comparable patency rates for arm vein bypasses are 60% to 70% and 50% to 60%, respectively, and for prosthetic grafts, 45% to 65% and 20% to 30%, respectively. Anticipated 5-year limb salvage in patients with critical limb ischemia is 80% to 90%, with 5-year survival in 40% to 70%.[1-5]

- Reversed and in situ vein grafts have been shown to have comparable patency rates in multiple studies.[6]
- Ambulatory function and independent living status is preserved in the majority of patients who undergo successful revascularization.
- Quality of life measures are improved in the majority of patients who undergo successful revascularization.[7]
- About 20% to 30% of patients will develop vein graft stenoses requiring either open or endovascular revision during follow-up.[8,9]
- Data on patency rates of open vs endoscopically harvested vein grafts are mixed, making definitive recommendations on the preferred approach difficult.[10,11]

COMPLICATIONS

- Wound infection
- Seroma
- Hematoma
- Graft occlusion
- Myocardial infarction

REFERENCES

1. Chew DK, Owens CD, Belkin M, et al. Bypass in the absence of ipsilateral greater saphenous vein: safety and superiority of the contralateral greater saphenous vein. *J Vasc Surg*. 2002;35(6):1085-1092.
2. Curi MA, Skelly CL, Woo DH, et al. Long-term results of infrageniculate bypass grafting using all-autogenous composite vein. *Ann Vasc Surg*. 2002;16(5):618-623.
3. Faries PL, Arora S, Pomposelli FB, et al. The use of arm vein in lower-extremity revascularization: results of 520 procedures performed in eight years. *J Vasc Surg*. 2000;31(1):50-59.
4. Gentile AT, Lee RW, Moneta GL, et al. Results of bypass to the popliteal and tibial arteries with alternative sources of autogenous vein. *J Vasc Surg*. 1996;23(2):272-279.
5. Taylor LM Jr, Edwards JM, Porter JM. Present status of reversed vein bypass: five-year results of a modern series. *J Vasc Surg*. 1990;11(2):193-206.
6. Harris PL, Veith FJ, Shanik GD, et al. Prospective randomized comparison of in situ and reversed infrapopliteal vein grafts. *Br J Surg*. 1993;80(2):173-176.
7. Nguyen LL, Moneta GL, Conte MS, et al. Prospective multicenter study of quality of life before and after lower extremity vein bypass in 1404 patients with critical limb ischemia. *J Vasc Surg*. 2006;44(5):977-983.
8. Idu MM, Buth J, Hop WCJ, et al. Factors influencing the development of vein-graft stenosis and their significance for clinical management. *Eur J Vasc Endovasc Surg*. 1999;17:15-21.
9. Conte MS, Bandyk DF, Clowes AW, et al. Results of PREVENT III: a multicenter randomized trial of edifoligide for the prevention of vein graft failure in lower extremity bypass surgery. *J Vasc Surg*. 2006;43(4):742-751.
10. Kronick M, Liem TK, Jung E, et al. Experienced operators achieve superior patency and wound complication rates with endoscopic great saphenous vein bypass compared with open harvest in lower extremity bypass. *J Vasc Surg*. 2019;70:1534-1542.
11. Guo Q, Huang B, Zhao J. Systematic review and meta-analysis of saphenous vein harvesting and grafting for lower extremity arterial bypass. *J Vasc Surg*. 2021;73(3):1075-1086.

Chapter 32 Perimalleolar Bypass and Hybrid Techniques

Robin B. Osofsky and Erika R. Ketteler

DEFINITION

- Perimalleolar bypasses are defined by the anatomic location of the distal target outflow vessel and refer to any revascularization in which the distal target vessel is the posterior tibialis, anterior tibialis, or peroneal arteries in the distal lower leg and usually referring to the level just above the ankle malleoli. The pedal vessels (dorsalis pedis, posterior tibialis, and lateral or medial plantar artery) can also be target vessels, but by definition these bypasses should be identified as pedal as there are different patency expectations as compared with perimalleolar targets.
- Infrapopliteal (perimalleolar and pedal) bypasses are generally performed in patients with advanced critical limb threatening ischemia (CLTI), which includes tissue loss and/or ischemic rest pain. Surgical management of distal tibial disease can be performed with open surgical bypass, endovascular therapy (EVT), or a hybrid approach. To the date of this chapter publication, no randomized control trials exist that clarify whether EVT or surgical bypass is better in patients with distal tibial disease. Regardless of technique, the specific therapy is tailored to an individual's clinical picture, functional status, and correlating anatomic limitations.

DIFFERENTIAL DIAGNOSIS

- The three major etiologies of lower extremity ulceration include ischemic, neuropathic, and venous stasis disease. Although all of these can have poor perfusion as a primary contributing factor, the diagnostic workup and management is different. Arterial ulcerations typically have a punched-out dry appearance and occur on the distal forefoot and toes, whereas neuropathic ulcerations often occur due to pressure at callus points. Venous stasis ulcerations are typically located on the medial malleolus ("gaiter") location and have associated edema, skin changes, and brawny induration and possible serous drainage.

PATIENT HISTORY AND PHYSICAL FINDINGS

- Peripheral arterial occlusive disease (PAOD) is the chronic atherosclerotic disease of the lower extremities. It is a spectrum of disease that ranges from asymptomatic to intermittent claudication (IC) and finally critical limb threatening ischemia (CLTI). Patients with CLTI will present with one or both of the following factors: rest pain or tissue necrosis (gangrene or nonhealing ulceration). Ischemic rest pain is characterized specifically by burning pain localized primarily to the distal forefoot and is associated with dependent rubor and elevation pallor.
- It should be noted that the natural history of PAOD and IC differ drastically from that of patients with CLTI. Rates of limb loss for patients with IC is <1% per year of life, whereas patients with CLTI have rates of 22% (2%-42%) at 1 year.[1]
- In general, the demographics for patients with PAOD, IC, and CLTI are similar and can differentiate into modifiable and nonmodifiable risk factors. Modifiable risks factors include smoking, hypertension, hyperlipemia, and diabetes, with smoking being the risk offering most opportunities for physician input. Nonmodifiable risk factors include age, gender, African American ethnicity, and family history of atherosclerosis. Of note, patients with CLTI have a higher prevalence of renal disease and diabetes. In addition, many of such patients do have the classic history of IC but rather present initially with tissue loss (embolic or caused by minor trauma). This fact is especially pertinent in diabetic patients who may not have any pain as a symptom of the critical limb ischemia.
- Due to significant comorbid conditions, it is critical to perform risk stratification when deciding between different revascularization modalities. In addition, managing and optimizing risk factors are keys to a successful outcome following lower extremity revascularization, regardless of the technique used. As such, optimizing lipid profile, glycemic control, smoking cessation, minimizing renal dysfunction, and managing hypercoagulable states are all essential components to the perioperative medical management, in addition to managing any concomitant coronary disease. Many patients may already be followed by a team of physicians for their co-morbidities and it is imperative that consultants remain actively involved in the perioperative period to optimize both the short-term quality of life and long-term limb salvage and overall survival.
- Included in surgical decision making is understanding that, although operative procedures may be technically and anatomically feasible, palliative expectant wound care may be more appropriate. This is important especially if the patient has small, limited wounds without pain or infection in a high-risk surgical patient who may be nonambulatory.
- Primary amputation may sometimes best meet patient expectations and goals of care rather than revascularization, especially if there is limited life-expectancy, nonambulatory status, or an imminent dying trajectory.
- Physical examination should include a thorough peripheral vascular examination, including assessment of the potential presence of a palpable aortic aneurysm on abdominal examination as a source of emboli causing the limb ischemic changes. The quality and symmetry of pulses and/or handheld Doppler signals at the femoral, popliteal, and pedal levels will assist in determining the anatomic level of disease. Wound documentation, when present, should note location, depth, presence of infection, bone exposure, and extent of soft tissue defects. Neuropathic deformities of the foot should also be taken into careful consideration for offloading purposes. If there is gross purulence or systemic signs of infection, a debridement of the affected area is usually required prior to revascularization for sepsis control.

- Classically, scoring systems for CLTI such as the Fontaine and Rutherford systems have been utilized to determine the likelihood of amputation and need for revascularization. However, in the past decade, such systems have been replaced with the Society for Vascular Surgery Lower Extremity Threatened Limb Classification System. The system stratifies limb risk by three factors: Wound, Ischemia, and foot Infection (WIFI) score. This system is similar to the "TMN" score for malignancy and grades each of the three main criteria on a four-point severity scale (0,1,2,3), which altogether yield a total of 64 distinct combinations. These 64 combinations are then assigned to one of four stages of clinical severity that are expected to correlate with amputation risk at 1 year. Clinical stage 1 is "very low risk" with 1 year rate of major amputations 0.75%, whereas stage 5 corresponds to an unsalvageable limb (**FIGURE 1**).[2]

IMAGING AND DIAGNOSTIC STUDIES

- The initial diagnostic workup of patients with ischemic ulcerations, rest pain, or significant claudication involves noninvasive vascular testing. This involves calculation of ankle-brachial indices (ABIs) and pulsed volume recordings in addition to duplex imaging of the extremity. An ABI of less than 0.4 is typically seen in patients with CLTI (**FIGURE 2**). Toe pressures of less than 40 mm Hg suggest inadequate microvascular perfusion for wound healing even with normal macrovascular arterial perfusion (eg, palpable dorsalis pedis [DP] and posterior tibial [PT] pulses). In cases of severely calcified vessels, it is important to obtain associated pulsed volume recordings or segmental waveforms along with toe pressures because ABIs can be falsely elevated due to vessel incompressibility generating an ABI >1.4. Transcutaneous oxygen tension ($TcPO_2$) measurement can also be used to determine the severity of ischemia and probability of wound healing (**FIGURE 3**).
- Computed tomography arteriography (CTA) is the preferred imaging modality for aortoiliac and femoropopliteal disease. However, CTA is limited in assessment of the tibial vessels often due to calcification or concomitant proximal stenosis, which ultimately limits distal contrast opacification. Magnetic resonance angiography has some use in CLTI but in general infrapopliteal disease tends to be overestimated by this modality and the injection of heavy metal gadolinium is not without concern for patients with concomitant renal insufficiency. Thus, digital subtraction angiography (DSA) remains the gold standard for diagnosis of infrapopliteal disease especially as the treatment of arterial stenoses/occlusions could occur in the same setting in an endovascular approach. Prior to obtaining either CTA or DSA, the surgeon must consider to optimize renal function to decrease the risk for contrast-induced nephropathy.

TREATMENT STRATEGY

- The goal of therapy in patients with CLTI should be to relieve pain, heal wounds, preserve functional status, and avoid major amputation. Pulsatile flow at the level of the tissue loss is the general goal; however, sometimes a pulse is not achievable and global improvement of perfusion to the

Assessment of the risk of amputation: the WIFI classification (for further details see Mills et al[317])

Component	Score	Description		
W (Wound)	0	No ulcer (Ischaemic rest pain)		
	1	Small, shallow ulcer on distal leg or foot without gangrene		
	2	Deeper ulcer with exposed bone, joint or tendon ± gangrenous changes limited to toes		
	3	Extensive deep ulcer, full thickness heel ulcer ± calcaneal involvement ± extensive gangrene		
I (Ischaemia)		ABI	Ankle pressure (mmHg)	Toe pressure or $TcPO_2$
	0	≥0.80	> 100	≥60
	1	0.60–0.79	70–100	40–59
	2	0.40–0.59	50–70	30–39
	3	<0.40	<50	<30
fI (foot infection)	0	No symptoms/signs of infection		
	1	Local infection involving only skin and subcutaneous tissue		
	2	Local infection involving deeper than skin/subcutaneous tissue		
	3	Systemic inflammatory response syndrome		

Example: A 65-year-old male diabetic patient with gangrene of the big toe and a <2 cm rim of cellulitis at the base of the toe, without any clinical/biological sign of general infection/inflammation, whose toe pressure is at 30 mmHg would be classified as Wound 2, Ischaemia 2, foot infection 1 (WIfI 2-2-1). The clinical stage would be 4 (high risk of amputation). The benefit of revascularization (if feasible) is high, also depending on infection control.

ABI = ankle-brachial index, $TcPO_2$ = transcutaneous oxygen pressure.

FIGURE 1 ● Society for Vascular Surgery Lower Extremity Threatened Limb Classification. (System: Risk stratification based on Wound, Ischemia, and foot Infection [WifI].) (Reprinted from Mills JL, Conte MS, Armstrong DG, et al. The Society for Vascular Surgery Lower Extremity Threatened Limb Classification System: risk stratification based on wound, ischemia, and foot infection (WIfI). *J Vasc Surg*. 2014;59(1):220-234.e1-2. Copyright © 2014 The Authors. With permission.)

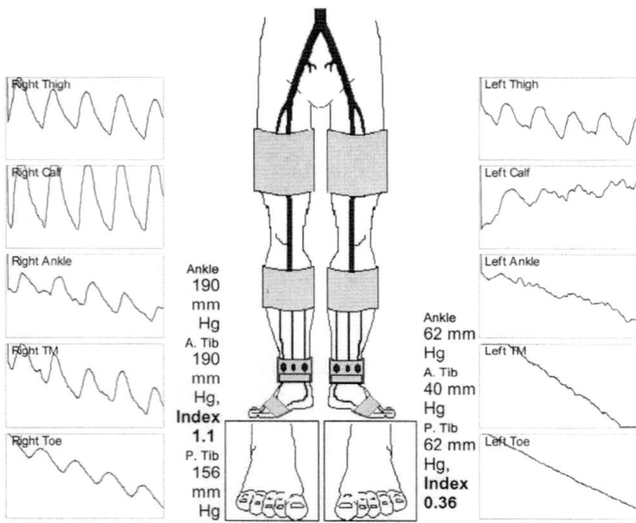

FIGURE 2 ● Severely reduced ABI and flattened distal pulsed volume recordings.

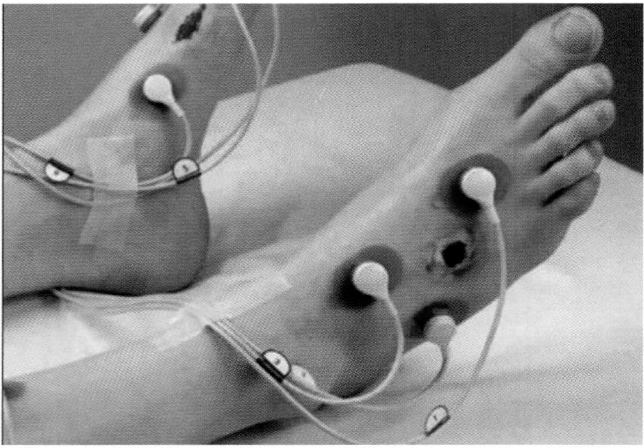

FIGURE 3 ● Transcutaneous oxygen tension ($TcPO_2$).

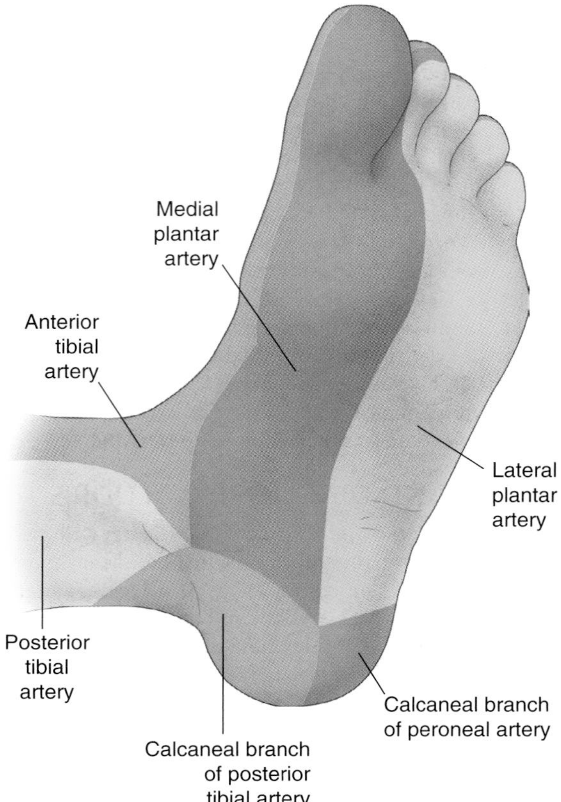

FIGURE 4 ● Angiosome concept.

ischemic area is the objective. Historically, angiosome revascularization (**FIGURE 4**) was implemented to guide the choice of distal anastomosis, based on the feeding vessel for the vascular territory of interest.[3] Attempts at distal revascularization should only proceed when adequate arterial inflow is present. Hence, proximal revascularization of the aorta and iliac and femoral arteries may need to be performed prior to or concomitantly with perimalleolar revascularization.

- Treatment strategy regarding choice of EVT vs open surgical bypass remains complex. The Trans-Atlantic Inter-Society Consensus (TASC) classification system does assist in such decision-making. In 2007, the TASC II classifications were published, which classified disease pattern involvement from types A through D for both aortoiliac and femoropopliteal segments. The group advocated for endovascular treatment for TASC type A and open surgical treatment for TASC type D. For TASC type B and C lesions, the authors stated there was insufficient evidence for recommending one modality over another (**FIGURE 5**). As mentioned in the introduction, there are no trials that ideally compare tibial EVT to surgical bypass and at the time of this publication, the ongoing BEST CLI and BASIL2 trials remain open to try to answer such questions.
- The decision to proceed with open perimalleolar bypass is made in the context of the patient's overall clinical functional status, cardiopulmonary and renal comorbidities, presence of autogenous saphenous vein conduit, and options for endovascular revascularization. Preoperative autogenous conduit assessment is best performed by detailed duplex imaging along the length of the vein. Preference is always given to a single segment of the great saphenous vein (GSV) from the ipsilateral leg that is at least 2.5 to 3 mm in diameter, compressible, and free of thrombus throughout. Assessment of the contralateral GSV is useful in cases that ipsilateral vein is found to be of poor quality during operative exploration. Small saphenous vein or arm vein is rarely used, but both are options realizing that the quality and frequency of valves is less ideal for long conduits. Combining multiple segments of veins may be necessary for adequate length with each anastomosis being a future site of stenosis impacting long-term patency. Composite bypass with vein and prosthetic, or full prosthetic bypass, is least ideal due to patency and infection risks but may be necessary if autogenous vein is not available. Composite bypasses do have limited long-term patency but may be appropriate if patency is only needed for wound healing and/or pain control in unique patient scenarios.
- Inflow artery selection for perimalleolar bypass is usually based on the length of available conduit and extent of proximal disease. The common, superficial, or deep femoral arteries or the popliteal artery may all serve as suitable inflow. Pulse by examination of such vessels is usually adequate

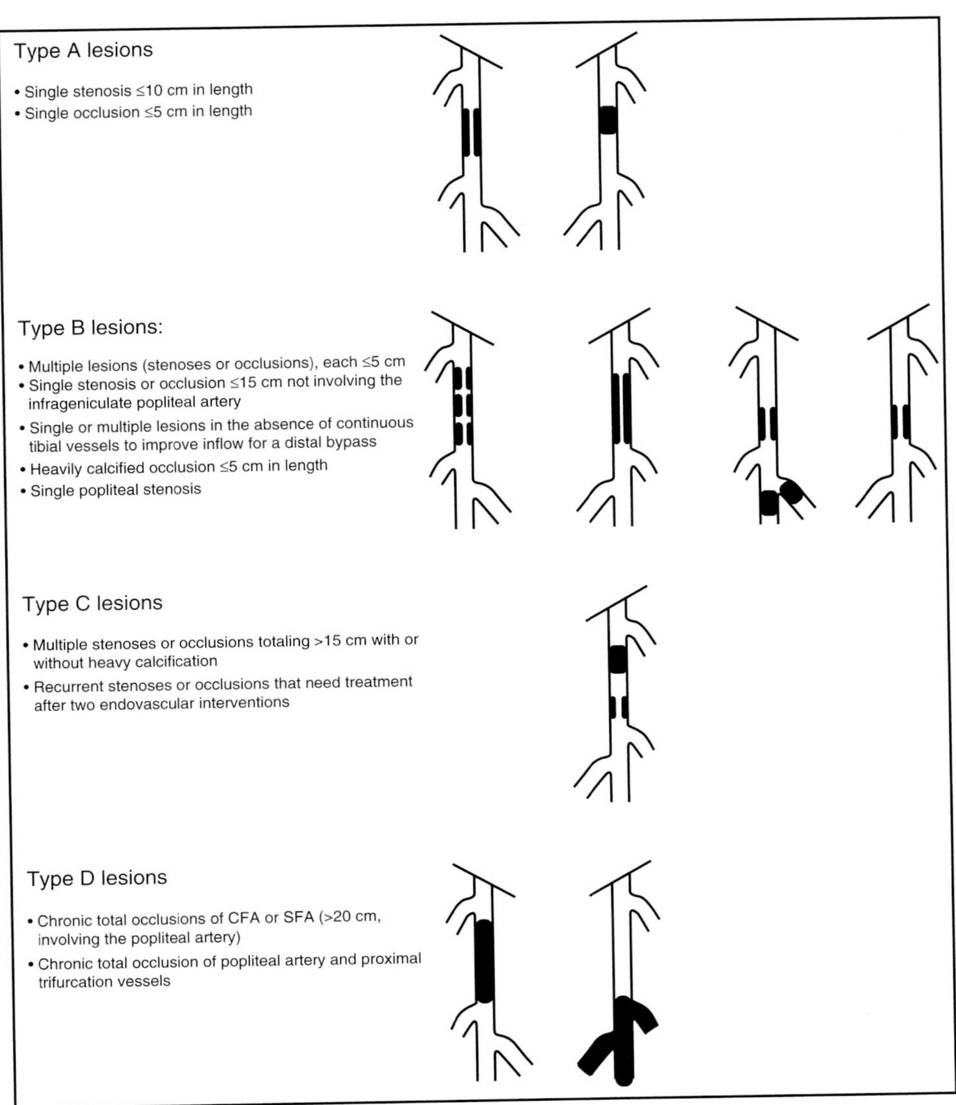

Type A lesions
• Single stenosis ≤10 cm in length
• Single occlusion ≤5 cm in length
Type B lesions:
• Multiple lesions (stenoses or occlusions), each ≤5 cm
• Single stenosis or occlusion ≤15 cm not involving the infrageniculate popliteal artery
• Single or multiple lesions in the absence of continuous tibial vessels to improve inflow for a distal bypass
• Heavily calcified occlusion ≤5 cm in length
• Single popliteal stenosis
Type C lesions
• Multiple stenoses or occlusions totaling >15 cm with or without heavy calcification
• Recurrent stenoses or occlusions that need treatment after two endovascular interventions
Type D lesions
• Chronic total occlusions of CFA or SFA (>20 cm, involving the popliteal artery)
• Chronic total occlusion of popliteal artery and proximal trifurcation vessels

FIGURE 5 ● Trans-Atlantic Inter-Society Consensus (TASC) classification for femoropopliteal disease. (Reprinted from Kukkonen T, Korhonen M, Halmesmäki K, Lehti L, Tiitola M, Aho P, Lepäntalo M, Venermo M. Poor inter-observer agreement on the TASC II classification of femoropopliteal lesions. *Eur J Vasc Endovasc Surg*. 2010;39(2):220-224. Copyright © 2010 European Society for Vascular Surgery. With permission.)

but can be supplemented by duplex imaging or even with diagnostic angiography. The need for concomitant endarterectomy should also be evaluated at this time and may be needed to ensure inflow is adequate to service the revascularization method by vein, prosthetic, or endovascular recanalization.

SURGICAL MANAGEMENT

Preoperative Planning

- The type of anesthesia is determined by the type of cardiopulmonary comorbidities and the anatomic level of arterial occlusive disease. Preoperative consultation with anesthesiology and cardiology can be utilized in the CLTI patient population to gauge the appropriate amount of surgical risk vs a nonoperative approach. Generally, limb threat with tissue loss does not require preoperative cardiac testing as time to allow cardiac revascularization is not appropriate. Cardiac disease optimization with medical management should be continued or initiated with antiplatelet, anti-inflammatory statin therapy and blood pressure and diabetic control to assist in prevention of perioperative complications. General anesthesia, peripheral nerve block, and spinal anesthesia are all potential options for bypass procedures. Intraoperative fluid administration should be used judiciously, and preoperative preparation should include blood type determination and crossmatching as necessary. Therapeutic anticoagulation may be held prior to the revascularization procedure, but most patients remain on antiplatelet agents without cessation.

Positioning

- Any lower extremity bypass might require intraoperative angiography and, as such, procedures should be performed on a fluoroscopy-appropriate table. The patient is positioned supine, with the leg slightly abducted and externally rotated to provide optimal exposure of the ipsilateral GSV harvest site. It is our practice to localize the GSV by ultrasound to assist in incision planning and try to access the conduit vein in discontinuous incisions to provide for better healing with less disruption of the lymphatics to avoid excessive edema. Intraoperative vein mapping also helps determine whether the contralateral leg should also be prepped as an alternative site for vein harvesting.

- Other items that should be available in the room include a sterile pneumatic tourniquet and a surgical bump constructed of towels to allow elevation of the knee for best anatomic exposure and dissection. A sterile on-table tourniquet can be useful to avoid clamp injury to target distal artery. Open forefoot wounds should be excluded from the operative field with adhesive drapes prior to limb preparation.

OPEN BYPASS

Perimalleolar Bypass to the Distal Posterior Tibialis Artery

First Step: Exposure of the Posterior Tibialis Artery at the Ankle

- The distal incision is marked by palpating posterior to the medial malleolus, taking care to avoid injury to adjacent GSV (**FIGURE 6**). Dissection is carried sharply through skin and subcutaneous tissues and through the flexor retinaculum. The tendons of the flexor digitorum longus muscle and flexor hallucis longus pass anteriorly and posteriorly, respectively, to the neurovascular bundle at this level. Careful attention to finding perforating collaterals can guide the dissection to the main artery of interest especially as a pulse is generally not present to assist. The paired tibial veins are often seen first as overlying the artery. The tibial nerve travels posterior to the artery and may not be seen clearly during this exposure. The tibial artery does not need to be dissected circumferentially if a pneumatic tourniquet is deployed for proximal control. For plantar bypass/exposure of the medial and lateral plantar arteries, the same incision can be carried further distally onto the medial aspect of the foot. Avoidance of circumferential occlusion of the target artery is recommended, and often only single vessel loop retraction can occlude any arterial flow to allow visualization for anastomosis creation.

Second Step: Exposure of the Inflow Artery

- Concurrent dissection of the arterial inflow can be performed with a second surgical team if available while the tibial target is being exposed to assist in limiting operative time in high-risk patients with CLTI. If the common femoral artery is chosen, then a longitudinal vertical incision just below the inguinal ligament will allow for simultaneous exposure of both the femoral bifurcation and the saphenofemoral confluence for dissection of the GSV. If femoral bifurcation disease is not suspected by prior imaging, then a transverse groin incision localized over the femoral artery erring medially toward the GSV is also a useful exposure as it is more anatomic with less tension to provide for decreased risks of wound separation and lymph leak (**FIGURE 7**). If the deep femoral artery is to be used as inflow, then division of the lateral femoral circumflex vein may be helpful in controlling the first-order branches past the origin. If the deep femoral origin is more posterior, the muscle bellies of the adductor longus and vastus medialis can be divided to limit the angle from which the graft originates from the arterial anastomosis. Another approach to the deep femoral artery for inflow is a lateral sartorius approach (**FIGURE 8**).
- If the below-knee popliteal artery is to be used as the inflow, which might be the case in diabetic patients with severe tibial disease not amenable to endovascular revascularization, this exposure is best obtained through a medial calf incision 1 cm posterior to the tibia (**FIGURE 9**). Utilizing the surgical bump under the distal thigh to allow the calf muscles to be tension-free, the infrageniculate popliteal artery is found by dividing the skin and avoiding the GSV. The crural fascia is incised again 1 cm posterior to the tibia with the incision extended to the border of the semitendinosus tendon to allow retraction of the gastrocnemius muscle (and sometimes also the deeper soleus muscle) posterior to enter the

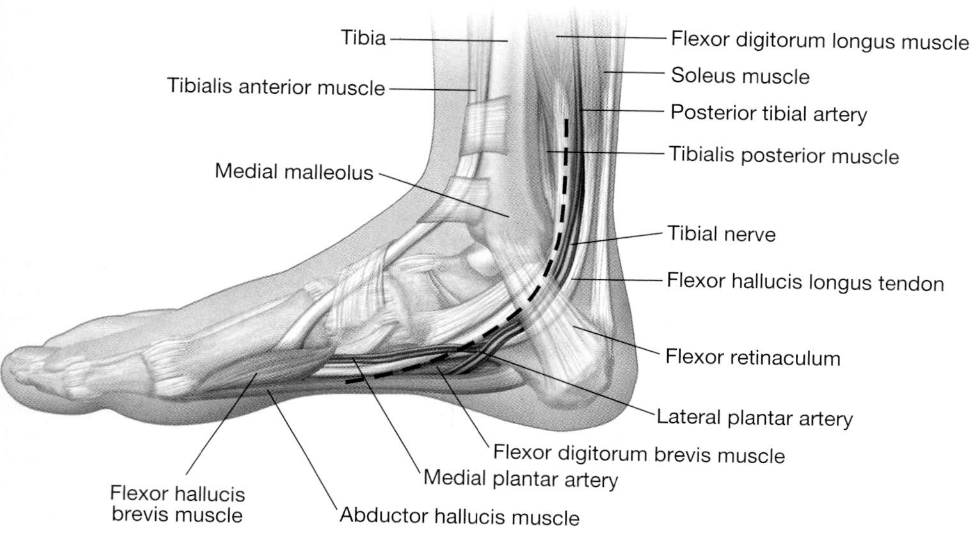

FIGURE 6 ● Incision for exposure of the posterior tibialis artery at the medial malleolus.

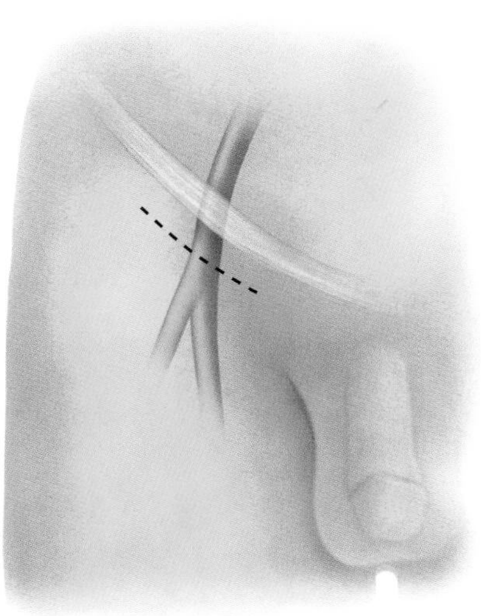

FIGURE 7 ● Transverse groin incision for femoral artery exposure.

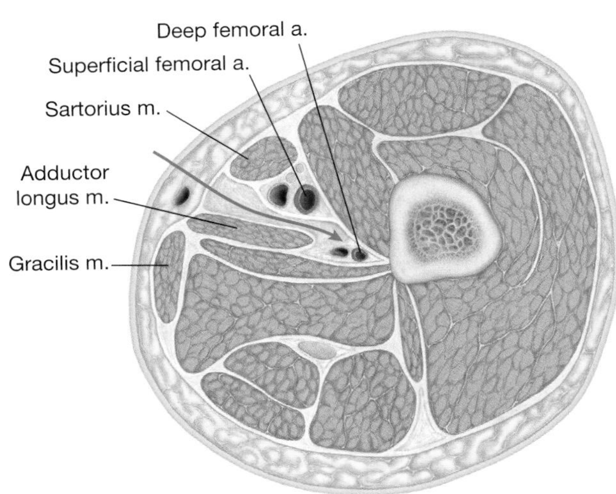

FIGURE 8 ● Deep femoral artery exposure via lateral sartorius approach (*solid blue arrow*).

fascia of an avascular plane to find the neurovascular popliteal bundle proximal and deep along the tibia (**FIGURE 10**).

Third Step: Harvest and Preparation of Autogenous Vein

- The course of the GSV is marked on the skin prior to prepping. The shortest segment of suitable caliber and quality GSV is harvested. Incision placement is partially determined by the location of the arterial access incisions. Care should be taken to avoid creating skin flaps during vein exposure. Harvesting vein through skip incisions may help to minimize wound complications but is not necessary for a good result. Minimal vein manipulations, with care being taken to accurately ligate side branches with permanent suture without crimping the main vein lumen is important. Minimal dissection of the vein is typically required when in situ bypass is planned, as the vein can be left in its bed with only limited dissection of the anastomotic segments. Skip incisions provide access to ligate larger side venous branches.

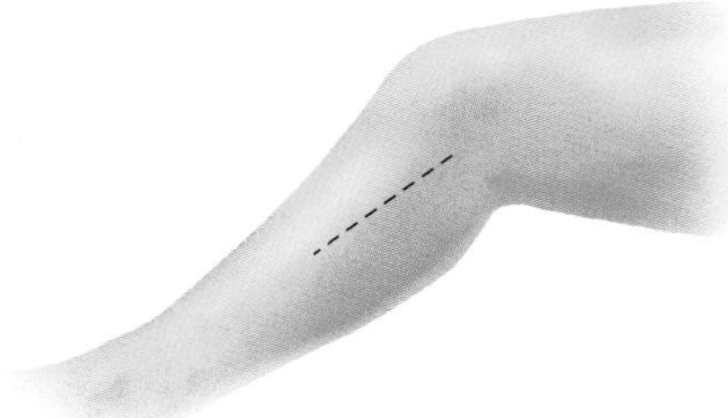

FIGURE 9 ● Incision for below-knee popliteal exposure.

- After an adequate length of saphenous is exposed, it is prepared for use. If a reversed bypass is being planned, the vein is removed from its bed and reversed for bypass placement. The saphenofemoral confluence is oversewn or suture ligated. If an in situ bypass is planned, the saphenous vein is transected at the saphenofemoral confluence, and the proximal vein is transposed to the femoral bifurcation and the anastomosis is constructed. Value lysis is performed after proximal anastomosis creation to allow dilation of the vein for ease in using the valvulotome. A third option, nonreversed translocated, is used when the size mismatch is too great to use the reversed technique but the vein needs to be tunneled under the muscle or across the leg (as in a distal anterior tibial bypass). In situ and translocated vein conduits are useful, but there is a technical learning curve with needed ability to troubleshoot patent branches especially if skip incisions were created (**FIGURE 11**).
- When using reversed vein, we generally try to use the largest overall diameter segment for the bypass conduit. The vein is distended gently with heparinized saline, any branches that are not ligated well are repaired using 7-0 polypropylene suture, and small holes are oversewn in a longitudinal fashion taking care not to narrow the vein. Depending on institutional expertise, endoscopic vein harvest is an alternative method to minimize incisional length and potential wound complications, but it has a steep learning curve. There is evidence to suggest that endoscopic vein harvest may decrease the infection risks but this benefit may be outweighed by long-term patency concerns.[4]
- After systemic anticoagulation is achieved with intravenous heparin, the proximal anastomosis is performed after controlling the inflow artery with vessel loops or vascular clamps. The loops or clamps are released, and the anastomosis is confirmed to be hemostatic. If significant atherosclerotic disease in the inflow artery is present, a separate arterial patch repair may be needed with our preference in using bovine pericardium on the host artery with the vein conduit anastomosed to such. Other patch options can be a separate segment of vein or even prosthetic such as Dacron or PTFE (**FIGURE 12**).
- If valve lysis is required, it is done after proximal anastomosis creation. Once complete, the vein is distended with blood. The vein is then marked for orientation with marker to avoid twisting and it is passed through the tunneler to exit the distal incision and clamped proximally with an atraumatic bulldog clamp or Yasargil clip. The length of vein needed is determined after the vein has already been tunneled and distended, with the leg in a maximally extended position.

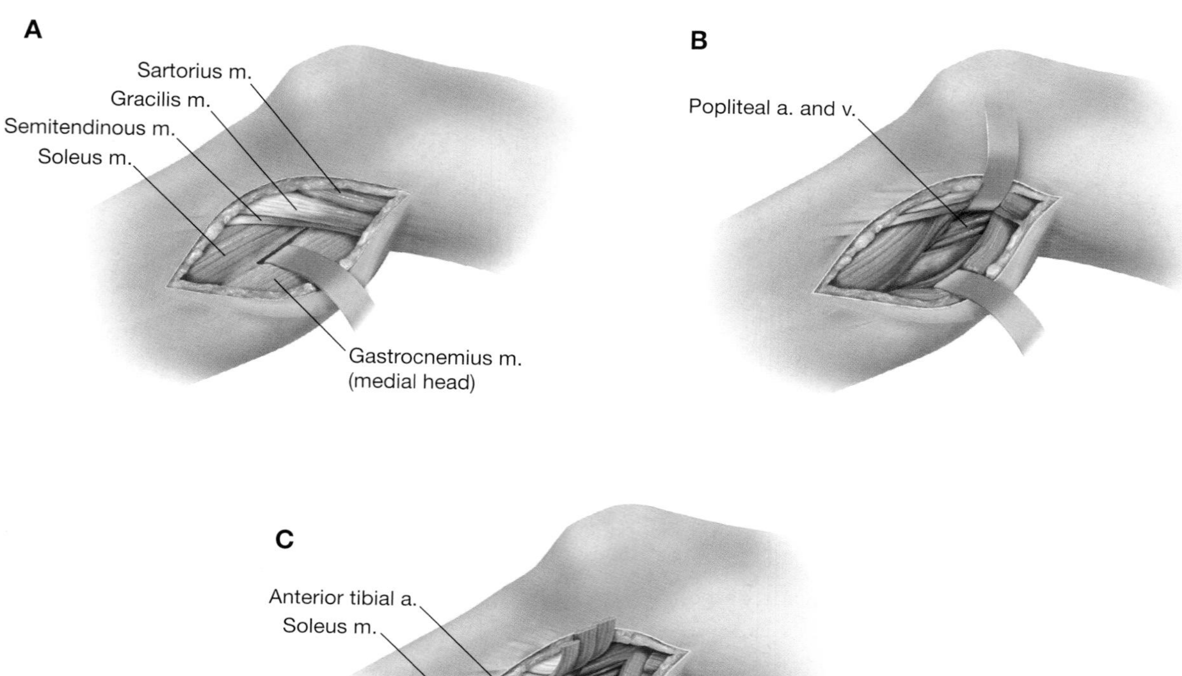

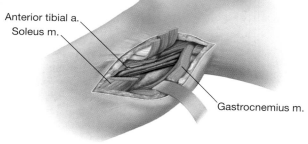

FIGURE 10 ● **A-C,** Dissection for below-knee popliteal exposure.

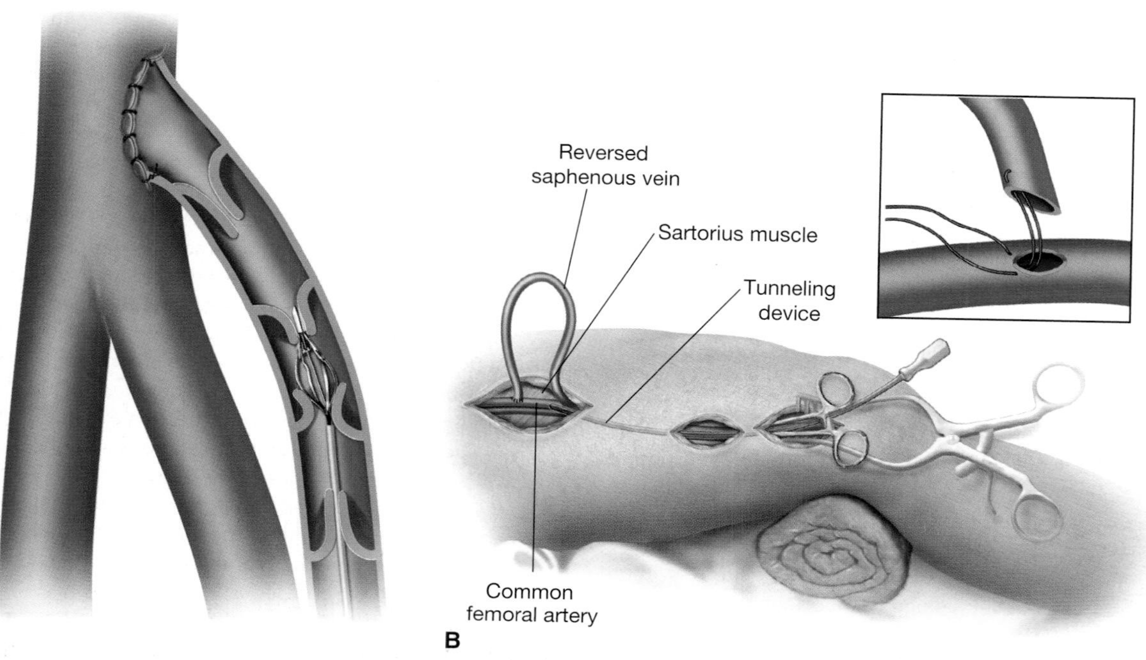

FIGURE 11 ● **A,** A valvulotome being used to lyse valves in a nonreversed vein under distension. **B,** Tunneling with hollow tunneling device through the subcutaneous tissues away from saphenectomy site.

The leg can be manipulated in various positions with knee flexion to make sure any excess or redundant vein is appropriately trimmed prior to embarking on the distal anastomosis.

- Tunneling is generally performed using a hollow tunneler (eg, Gore, Scanlan, Jenkner) with a blunt appropriately sized tip (6 mm at least) in a subcutaneous plane away from the saphenectomy incision, if possible, to avoid wound complications. The vein is carefully inspected at the entry and exit site of the tunnel to ensure it is not constrained by fascial or muscular bands. Of note, unique vein tunneling may be required as situations arise in a more anatomic approach (such as through the tibial/fibular space when going from medial inflow artery to ATA).

Fourth Step: Distal Anastomosis Creation

- If a tourniquet is to be used for distal control, then the lower leg is exsanguinated using an Esmarch bandage. The tourniquet is placed around the thigh if the inflow is at the level of the common femoral, profunda femoris, or proximal superficial femoral arteries. It is inflated to 250 to 300 mm Hg. The target is then identified. Care is taken to identify the artery instead of the vein because they can appear deceptively similar when exsanguinated under tourniquet hemostasis. The distal anastomosis is created using a 6-0, 7-0, or 8-0 polypropylene suture depending on the size of the target artery. Loupe magnification is helpful and generally mandatory in this setting. The first assistant should sit beside the operating surgeon to maintain suture tension around the anastomosis and suction away blood and debris from the operative field.
- Tourniquet, intra-arterial balloon occlusion, occlusion without circumferential occlusion, or cautious atraumatic clamps are all options for hemostatic control. If the tourniquet fails to maintain sufficient hemostasis due to medial calcification in the larger proximal arteries, other options for hemostasis include vessel loops and vascular clamps for tibial control, use of vessel stoppers, or use of a carbon dioxide (CO_2) blower suction device. Circumferential tibial artery dissection must be done with care to avoid injury to the adjacent paired tibial veins, or venae comitantes, that give off several crossing branches above and below the target artery.
- Prior to completion of the anastomosis, the tourniquet is deflated and flushed. The proximal graft clamp or bulldog is released, and the anastomosis is thoroughly flushed prior to tying down and completing the anastomosis. Cautious limited probing of the outflow artery with coronary dilators can ensure no concerns of the anastomosis but should be judiciously utilized as dissection or injury to the artery can occur even with proper technique. Topical agents such as thrombin/Gelfoam, Surgicel, or Floseal may be helpful in obtaining hemostasis following reversal of anticoagulation with protamine. Wound closure is covered later in the chapter.

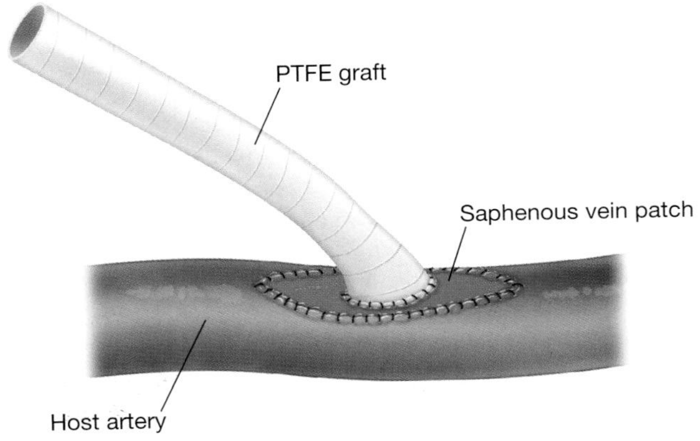

FIGURE 12 ● Schematic for Linton patch anastomosis.

Perimalleolar Bypass to the Distal Anterior Tibialis Artery

First Step: Exposure of the Anterior Tibialis Artery at the Ankle

- Simultaneous dissection of the vein and proximal inflow artery should occur while the distal bypass target is identified and controlled as described earlier. The distal exposure of the anterior tibial above the ankle is performed by identifying the tendon of the extensor hallucis longus and creating an incision just lateral to this and medial to the tibialis anterior tendon. Plantar flexing the ankle and palpating the space that opens between the two tendons often easily identify this groove in which the artery runs. The extensor retinaculum is divided at the malleolus and the vascular bundle should be easily identified at this level lying along the anterior surface of the tibia (**FIGURE 13**).

Second Step: Tunneling the Vein to the Anterior Tibialis Artery

- The GSV is harvested and either reversed or used in a nonreversed fashion depending on factors described earlier. The tunnel from the inflow artery to the anterior tibial can be maintained in a subcutaneous plane across the anterior surface of the tibia medial to the exposure site, but this is difficult due to thin skin and limited subcutaneous tissue in most patients. A counterincision may be needed at the ankle to allow for a gentler curvature of the vein graft toward the dorsum of the foot. If there is concern about potential compression of the vein graft in this region because of its superficial nature, the alternative is to tunnel through the interosseus membrane. This tunnel is created higher in the calf between the deep posterior and anterior compartments (**FIGURE 14**). Because the GSV harvest incision is already on the medial calf, the dissection can be extended deeper by retracting the gastrocnemius muscles posteriorly and partially dividing the soleus to reach the posterior tibial vessels. These are protected and gently retracted posteriorly while the fibers of the tibialis posterior muscle are separated and the tunneler is bluntly passed through the interosseus membrane here. Once the vein graft is in the anterior compartment, it can be tunneled in a subcutaneous or subfascial plane to reach the exposed anterior tibialis artery just above the ankle. Another path for the vein conduit if there is enough length is to tunnel across the anterior thigh to the lateral calf, taking care in the subcutaneous space of the lateral knee, which should be kept lateral/posterior to avoid the fibular head where nerve injury can occur.

Third Step: Exposure of the Dorsalis Pedis Artery

- If the dorsal pedal artery is the target vessel, then the exposure distally is on the dorsum of the foot and the tunneling

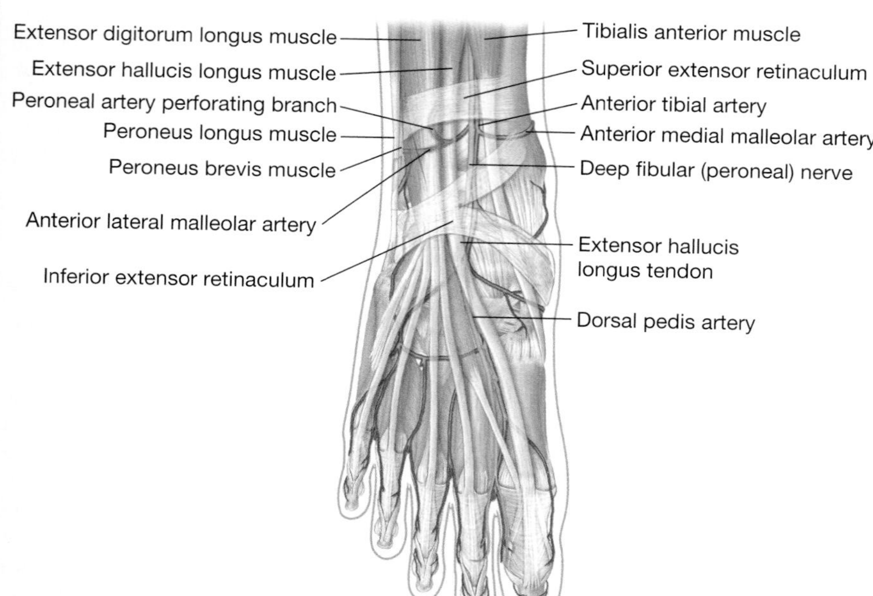

FIGURE 13 ● Exposing the anterior tibialis artery at the ankle.

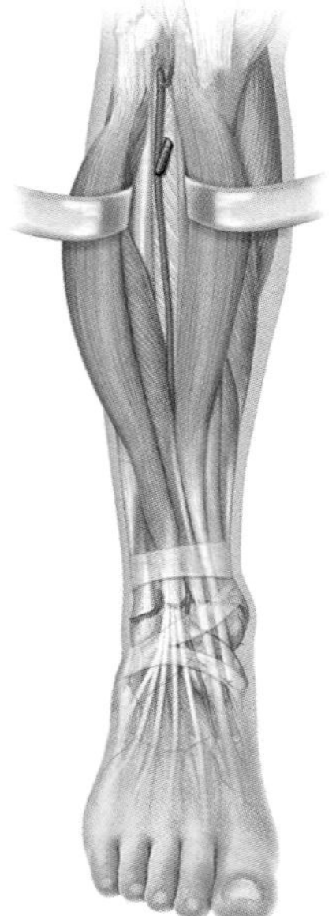

FIGURE 14 ● Tunneling through the interosseous membrane at the midcalf.

techniques remain similar to what is outlined earlier for the anterior tibial artery at the ankle. An incision is created on the dorsum of the foot just lateral to the extensor hallucis longus tendon and carried down through the fascia. The dorsal pedal artery lies lateral to the deep peroneal nerve here (**FIGURE 15**).

- Care should be taken to not leave self-retaining retractors in for too long in these smaller distal incisions to avoid tension on the wound edges and potential skin necrosis.

Exposure of the Peroneal Artery at the Ankle

First Step: Peroneal Artery Anatomy

- The peroneal artery comes off the tibioperoneal trunk at the upper calf and then distally branches into two perforating branches at the ankle joint, termed anterior and posterior perforating peroneal arteries, which supply the anterior and lateral compartments and communicate with the anterior tibial artery and some tarsal branches.

Second Step: Exposure of the Distal Third of the Peroneal Artery

- The proximal segment of the peroneal artery can be accessed easily from a medial approach similar to the posterior tibial artery exposure just dissection more laterally toward the fibula. Using Doppler signal can ensure proper trajectory. The perimalleolar or distal third of the peroneal artery needs to be approached laterally and requires resection of a portion of the fibula. An incision is created along the lateral border of the fibula, and dissection is carried down through the fascia to the fibula after which the periosteum is cleared proximally and distally (**FIGURE 16**). The peroneal artery is near the fibula medially, and care should be taken to avoid injury to the vascular bundle when clearing the bone (**FIGURE 17**). The bone can then be excised, and the peroneal artery is identified behind the interosseus membrane. The bone can be transected using a Gigli saw or oscillating power saw. The advantage of either a traditional bone cutter or power saw is that the bone does not necessarily have to be circumferentially dissected.
- The peroneal artery can also be exposed posteriorly, but this is somewhat challenging to do when the patient is supine. An incision just above the ankle posterolaterally between the tendons of the flexor hallucis longus and the flexor digitorum longus reveals the artery in its most distal segment

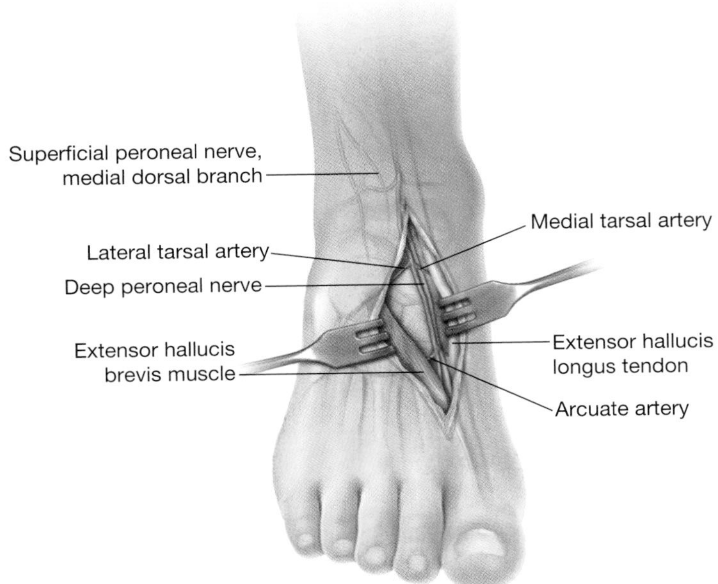

FIGURE 15 ● Exposure of the dorsalis pedis artery.

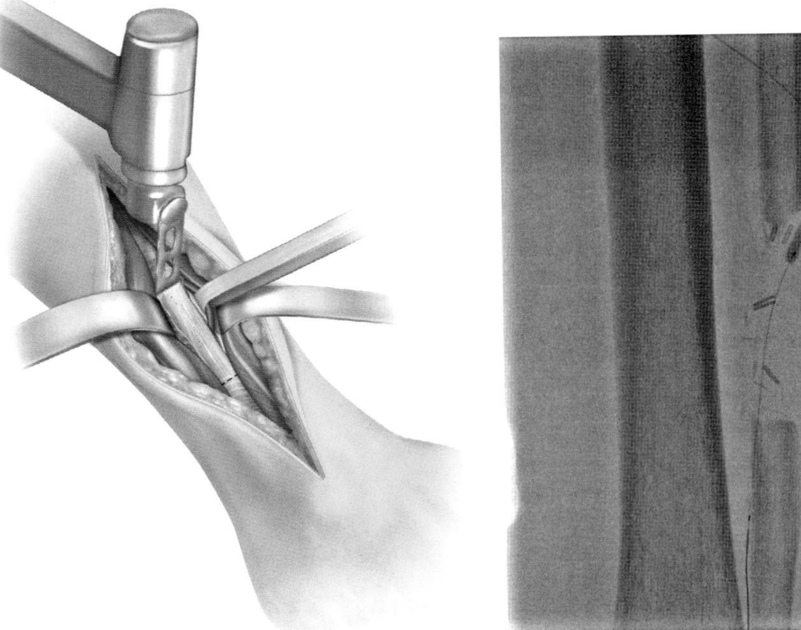

FIGURE 16 ● Clearing the fibula and resection for exposure of the distal peroneal artery.

(**FIGURE 18**). This approach is favored when the small saphenous vein will also be harvested for the graft conduit.

Additional Considerations

Alternative Conduits

- Despite careful preoperative planning and efforts to fully interrogate adequate conduit, the great saphenous vein may prove to be unsuitable for the intended purpose once exposed. If length of vein is a concern, then careful consideration should be given to either moving the inflow anastomosis more distally or moving the target artery more proximally. An additional alternative is to create a shorter tunnel, harvest the great saphenous vein from the contralateral leg, or harvest arm vein when other options are not available or advisable.
- Occasionally, if no suitable autogenous vein conduit exists (especially in the case of redo bypasses), consideration may

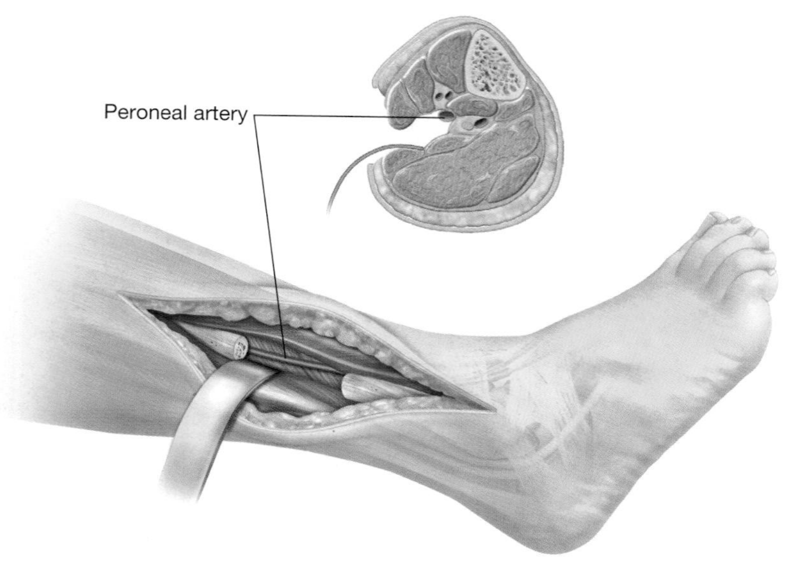

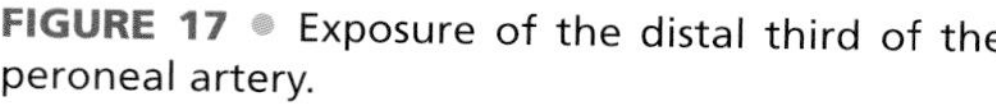
FIGURE 17 ● Exposure of the distal third of the peroneal artery.

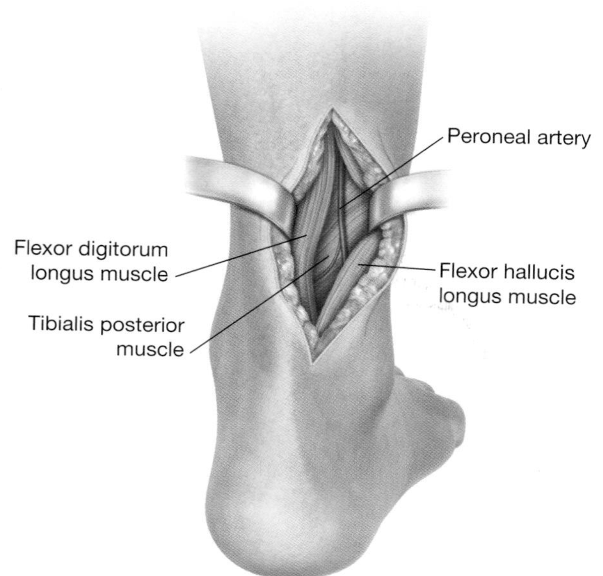

FIGURE 18 ● Posterior approach to the distal third of the peroneal artery.

be given to cadaveric cryopreserved vein or prosthetic bypass with vein cuffs or patches or creation of arteriovenous fistulae distally. The limitations of these nonautogenous options must be weighed against the known patency limitations of spliced vein or arm vein grafts. In addition, composite vein/PTFE remains a viable option, but patency and infection limitations must also be considered.

Bypass Evaluation

- Following open, endovascular, or hybrid procedures the authors advocate for thorough evaluation of the intervention performed. The patency of the bypass is assessed intraoperatively by multiple potential methods. Feeling a strong bypass pulse in the tunnel and in the target vessel distal to the anastomosis is reassuring but could suggest nonideal outflow (obstructive at or distal to anastomosis). Listening with a handheld Doppler to assess the quality of the Doppler signal of the artery distal to the distal anastomosis is also helpful. A multiphasic strong Doppler signal that augments significantly when the graft is first compressed and then released is suggestive of a patent bypass. In the absence of strong clinical signs of graft patency (eg, palpable distal pulse), an intraoperative color flow duplex scan may be used to identify potential flow limiting defects, such as retained valves in the bypass if in situ or transposed or focal velocity elevations or low flow in the graft itself due to twisting or vein injury.
- Completion arteriography provides useful detail regarding potential technical problems, including the status of the anastomoses, tunneling issues, and the presence of retained valves, if any. Angiography is performed using a small-caliber needle in the most proximal artery or vein bypass with runoff views through the venous conduit into the outflow arterial tree. Some degree of spasm may be seen at the site of clamp placement or vessel loop manipulation but should be considered thrombus or stenosis until proven otherwise. Reimaging, treatment of spasm with intra-arterial papaverine, or exploration of the concerning area of vein or artery is required if angiography reveals concerns. When tunneling concerns arise, dynamic arteriography with the leg flexed and extended in various positions can be helpful to prevent kinking of the bypass in the early postoperative period.

Wound Closure

- Wound closure is a key component of the operation and should not be minimized or relegated to inexperienced team members as much of the morbidity from bypass procedures arises from wound complications. These patients have significant postoperative edema related to vein harvesting as well as the arterial reperfusion of the ischemic limb. The vein harvest bed should be irrigated, inspected for hemostasis, and closed in multiple layers of running or interrupted absorbable suture and/or staples. Generally, suture multilayer closure is preferably for any areas where a nonanatomic bypass is present. Care is taken to avoid injury to the saphenous nerve. At the ankle and around points of flexion, such as the knee, it is useful to use mattress nylon sutures. It is also important to close the ankle incision first before reperfusion edema makes tension-free closure challenging. It is often difficult to get more than one layer of subcutaneous tissue over the bypass and distal anastomosis at the perimalleolar level (**FIGURE 19**). Wound closure should be planned for while making the initial incisions with other closure options including use of vacuum-assisted device or even a bedside or return to operating room for secondary closure; both of these closure management options are generally rare events but are useful to consider if needed in some scenarios.

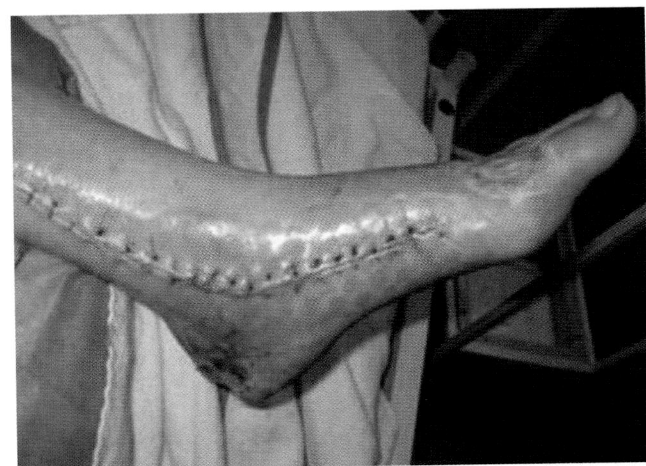

FIGURE 19 ● Perimalleolar wound closure.

ENDOVASCULAR TECHNIQUES

Endovascular and Hybrid Approaches

- For completeness in presentation of the perimalleolar revascularization topic, a discussion must occur regarding endovascular interventions. In the past few decades, there have been numerous advances in endovascular techniques pertaining to lower extremity arterial disease. These endovascular approaches provide many advantages and generally are associated with less morbidity in the patient with CLTI with many comorbidities because endovascular interventions can be performed under local sedation without needing general or regional anesthesia as is needed for open bypass. Nonetheless endovascular revascularization techniques have their own limitations and disadvantages. Hence, it is of paramount importance to first identify appropriate anatomic stenoses and/or occlusions amenable to EVT as discussed above in TASC II guidelines. In addition, it is essential to identify the patient is an appropriate candidate for EVT from the clinical presentation, functional status and comorbidities, and anatomic pattern of disease. Surgical calculators can be helpful to decide if endovascular approaches offer the patient less risk than open bypass revascularization.
- As mentioned, PAOD can present in a variety of permutations with regards to disease pattern. Often, EVT may need to be offered in a hybrid approach with an open bypass. As an example, a patient with a short segment proximal stenosis may be treated with angioplasty and stent to augment inflow while the patient's distal long segment stenosis/occlusion may be managed with open vein bypass. The contrast is true as well, as many patients undergo proximal bypasses and completion management with distal endovascular interventions especially with venous conduit limitations. The ideal hybrid approach must be customized to the patient's anatomy and disease distribution. Endovascular therapy has greatly expanded the toolbox for interventions in the management of lower extremity revascularization.

Endovascular Arterial Access

Endovascular access approaches and outcomes are topics that need to be discussed in greater detail than this chapter covers. In general, the percutaneous Seldinger technique is utilized to gain arterial access via a retrograde or anterograde approach. Once access is obtained with a micropuncture (4Fr) system, an appropriately sized working sheath is inserted to guide wires and catheters to cross and treat the angiographic stenoses and occlusions that are imaged (**FIGURE 20**).

- Retrograde access via the contralateral common femoral artery is commonly utilized for lower extremity revascularization. Once a working sheath is situated, the treatment limb is accessed by fluoroscopical guidance of wires and catheters up and over the aortic bifurcation. The retrograde technique offers advantages given ease of access and less risk of the development of dissection flaps.
- Alternatively, retrograde access can be accomplished in the ipsilateral limb distal to the target lesion for intervention. For example, the dorsalis pedis artery can be used allowing for direct access below a tibial arterial target lesion. Nonetheless, this technique is limited by sheath size as well as the quality of distal access and is technically challenging with a learning curve.
- Finally, anterograde access via the ipsilateral common femoral and superficial femoral with the patient supine or the popliteal artery with the patient prone. Each technique has advantages and disadvantages based on target vessel intervention goals, but in general an antegrade approach provides shorter distance for maneuvers and allows for greater ease in push ability and maneuverability of wires and catheters. With that said, anterograde access carries a risk for the development of anterograde dissection flap, which can result in acute limb ischemia and need for emergent open repair. Furthermore, anterograde access can be technically difficult in obese patients especially for common femoral artery access through a large pannus.

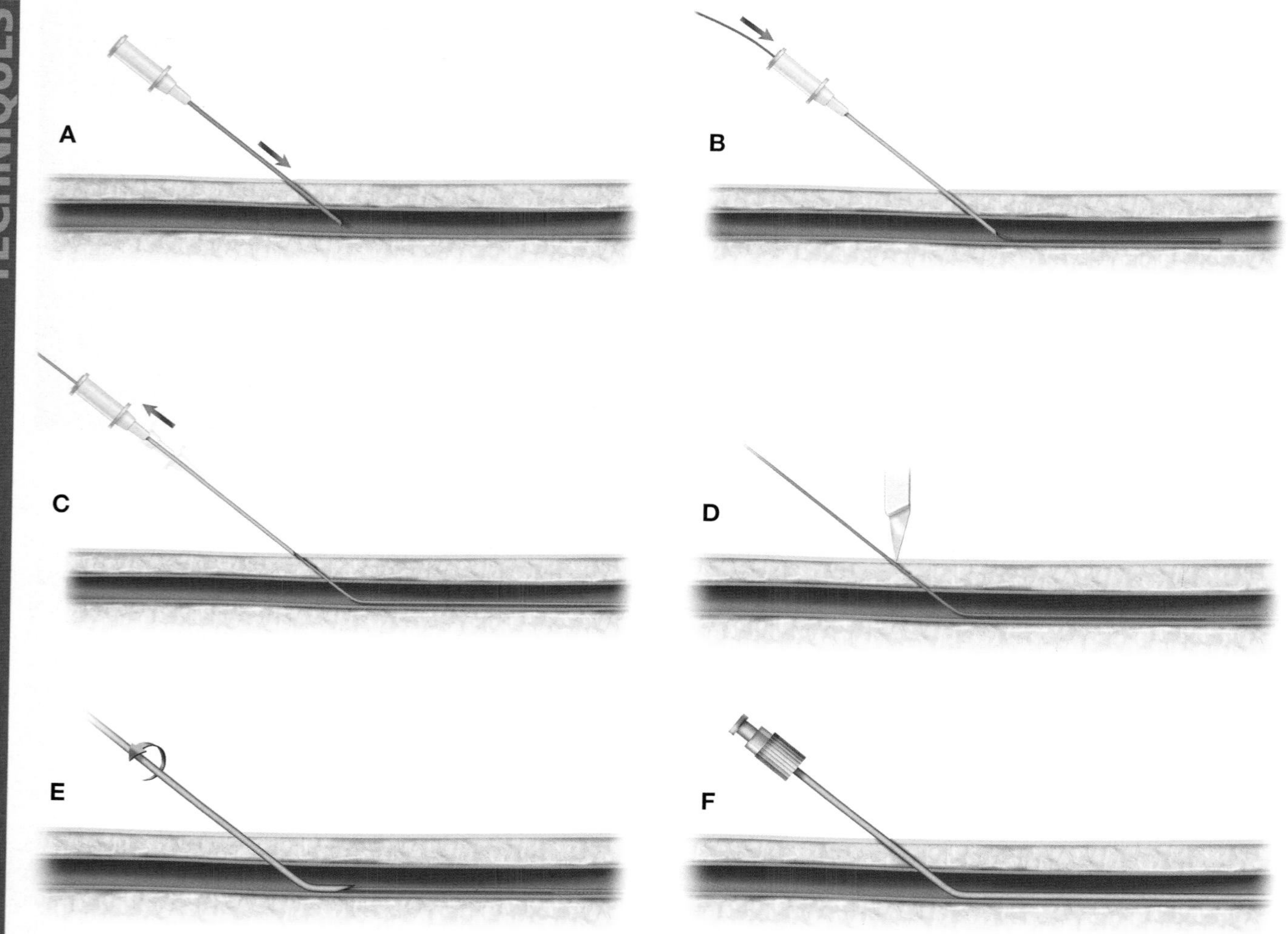

FIGURE 20 ● Seldinger technique. **A,** Hollow needle introduction into artery. **B,** Passage of guidewire into artery via hollow needle. **C,** Removal of needle over the wire. **D,** Incision of skin along wire. **E,** Placement of dilator over the wire into the artery and then removal of dilator. **F,** Placement of the sheath over the wire into the artery and removal of the wire.

Image Acquisition

- Equipment and room setup are essential components for successful endovascular revascularization procedures. The surgeon must ensure they have access to a procedure room with fluoroscopy imaging on an appropriate table. Preoperatively the patient's renal function should be assessed, and if needed, preoperative hydration should be provided. In addition, surgeons should have appropriate radiation safety equipment available. Contrast agents can ultimately be injected via syringe or with power injector. Finally, digital subtraction angiography should be utilized to optimally interpret the fluoroscopic images.

Treatment

- The rate-limiting step of endovascular revascularization procedures is the ability to cross or traverse the target lesion or lesions. This process often requires an ability to modify the operative plan based on the patient's anatomy, therapeutic goals, and comorbidities. The intervention performed will ultimately be determined by the quality of the lesion (eg, calcific) and total length of the stenosis or occlusion. Various treatment modalities available include percutaneous balloon angioplasty (PTA) with or without stent placement, cryotherapy, and atherectomy. The rationale and details of such techniques is complex and beyond the scope of this chapter, but each endovascular technique is deployed based on the goal of the procedure related to the desired clinical outcome and the time for patency of the intervention. These outcomes are weighed with the expense of both the endovascular supplies and the degree of patient and staff radiation and the contrast dye requirements for a patient especially if there is underlying renal insufficiency. Perimalleolar endovascular revascularization procedures should be performed by providers with experience and training to allow appropriate technical skills combined with clinical judgments to obtain optimal outcomes with least risk and most benefit.

Closure

- Access site closure is a broad topic with goal to avoid hematomas or arterial injury. In general, manual pressure can be employed for sheath sizes less than 8 French, but this method requires movement restrictions for a period to prevent pseudoaneurysm or bleeding. Thus, to expedite time and patient comfort, numerous percutaneous closure devices exist on the market that include a variety of physical, chemical, and combination of such to close the percutaneous access site without complications of bleeding, thrombosis, or arterial injury and stenosis. Postoperative anticoagulation also is a consideration when selecting a closure method. If hemostasis is not satisfactorily achieved following removal of access sheath and appropriate manual pressure, a deferral to an open repair is required with resultant risks and benefits.

PEARLS AND PITFALLS

	Open bypass perimalleolar procedures
Preoperative planning	▪ The bypass target is chosen to provide the best option for direct in-line perfusion to area of tissue loss on the forefoot. Autogenous vein bypass is preferred over prosthetic for both patency and limb-salvage outcomes.
Placement of incision	▪ Using ultrasound in the operating room to identify the GSV in relation to the proximal and distal incisions can help avoid raising flaps or creating postoperative wound complications. ▪ Use of a tourniquet above the knee can assist in avoiding unnecessary manipulation and potential injury to distal tibial vessels.
Tunneling	▪ Tunneling the bypass away from the vein harvest incision can help protect the bypass from exposure and infection in case of wound complications and wound dehiscence postoperatively.
Intraoperative assessment of bypass	▪ Manipulating the leg in slightly different positions can assist with evaluating the course of the vein bypass in the tunnel during intraoperative assessment with on-table angiography.
Wound closure	▪ Avoid leaving self-retaining retractors in distal incisions for prolonged periods to avoid skin edge necrosis. ▪ Closure of distal wounds is best accomplished with nylon suture in a mattress fashion to avoid tension on the wound. Wounds over the dorsum of the foot can be closed with mattress sutures. Alternatively, deep-dermal Vicryl sutures and subcuticular Monocryl sutures can be employed and dressed with Dermabond. Occasionally, a counter incision may be necessary to provide adequate coverage over the exposed artery at the ankle. Rare cases may need secondary wound closure after reperfusion edema and/or utilization of vacuum-assisted devices.
Postoperative care	▪ A gently placed soft cast can prevent significant lower leg edema and subsequent wound breakdown in the immediate postoperative period. ▪ Predischarge duplex assessment of the graft is important if intraoperative assessment of the bypass was not performed with angiography or duplex.

POSTOPERATIVE CARE

Open Bypass

- Because of the length and location of the vein harvested for conduit, the patient will undoubtedly have significant edema postoperatively throughout the affected leg. Drains (eg, flat 10Fr Jackson-Pratt to bulb) can be placed in the vein harvest sites especially with deep harvest sites and if the patient requires postoperative anticoagulation; key is to exit the drain proximal to the drain placement in a separate skin incision to avoid creating any more distal wounds that could leak or weep. Tape should be avoided on all skin in the lower leg especially as postoperative edema can cause blisters and infection in compromised skin. The authors do not routinely wrap the leg for at least 48 hours to prevent conduit compression and thrombosis. Limb elevation must be employed in the postoperative setting such that the ankle is above the knee and the knee is above the hip. When the patient is ready for compression wrappings, the foot, ankle, and lower leg may be wrapped in a soft cast consisting of an inner layer of Webril and outer layer of gently compressive Ace wrap or Coban. Care needs to be taken to minimize external compression on the vein graft itself, especially in the areas around the ankle. The patient can ambulate starting on postoperative day 1, but the leg should be elevated when the patient is sitting or in bed.
- The authors will universally put the bypass patient on single or dual antiplatelet therapy in the perioperative setting. Depending on the clinical scenario and the surgeon's assessment of the conduit and runoff quality, a short course of

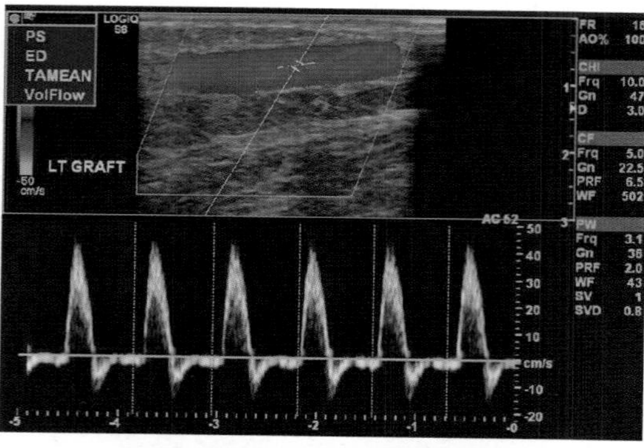

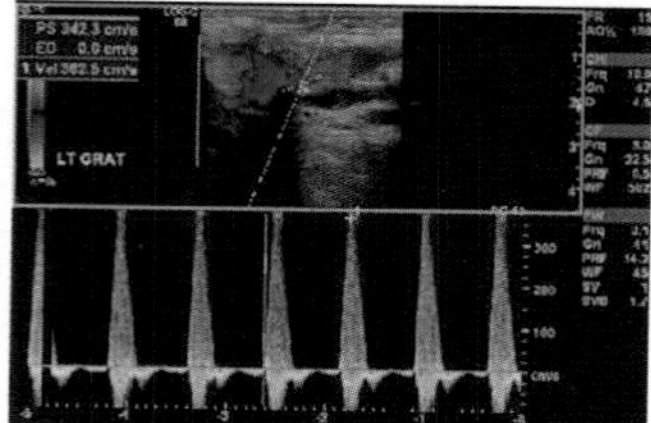

FIGURE 21 ● Surveillance duplex of vein bypass.

therapeutic anticoagulation may be employed; however, this must be balanced against the risk of bleeding in individual patients. In addition, the patient should remain on a statin, ensure adequate glucose control, and remain normotensive.

- For perimalleolar bypass patients who did not get an intraoperative assessment of their bypass with an on-table angiography, a predischarge duplex is performed to document patency and pedal perfusion. If a significant abnormality is identified on duplex (significantly low flows in the bypass or focally high velocities), then this should be addressed prior to discharge with angiography or exploration of the area with appropriate intervention.
- Once discharged, patients either return weekly for a change of their soft cast until their edema has sufficiently resolved or follow up at the 1-month interval for formal duplex interrogation of the bypass. Certainly, more frequent visits may be warranted in patients with wound concerns.
- Surveillance duplex of vein bypasses is obtained at the 3-month, 6-month, and 12-month postoperative time points and then every 6 or 12 months with both ABI and graft duplex (**FIGURE 21**). After the 1-year time point with no previous abnormalities on postoperative imaging, the surveillance can be moved to once a year. Occasionally, the surveillance interval is shortened for high-risk bypasses or prosthetic tibial bypasses and especially if the patient is still using tobacco.

COMPLICATIONS

- Early complications of distal bypasses include bleeding, wound infection/breakdown, and graft occlusion. Early graft occlusion in the first 24 to 48 hours must be considered technical errors and require urgent operative re-exploration.

Late complications include graft stenosis, limb swelling, graft occlusion, and aneurysmal degeneration of the vein bypass. Most patients with CLTI have concomitant coronary disease, and the rate of perioperative myocardial infarction can be as high as 5%. It is very important to maintain patients on their cardiac medications in the perioperative period and manage fluids judiciously to avoid precipitating coronary events.

OUTCOMES

Perimalleolar Bypass Revascularization

- In a systemic review and meta-analysis in 2018 for bypass surgery to any infrainguinal target, the incidence rate of major amputation within 1 year was 0.11 with great saphenous vein graft, 0.24 with nonautogenous graft, and 0.16 with ectopic vein or spliced arm vein graft. Primary patency of the bypass at 1 year was 0.77 in nonautogenous grafts, 0.64 in great saphenous vein grafts, and 0.45 in ectopic vein or spliced arm vein graft. At 2 years and beyond, superior patency (primary and secondary) and limb salvage rates for great saphenous vein over nonautogenous and ectopic vein conduits were evident and increasingly amplified. Mortality was similar for the three types of bypass grafts. Data for major adverse cardiovascular events, reintervention/readmission, amputation-free survival, reintervention and amputation-free survival, quality of life, and wound healing were limited.[5]

Perimalleolar Endovascular Revascularization

- In a systemic review and meta-analysis in 2018, in patients with infrapopliteal artery lesions, primary patency at 1 year was as follows: bare-metal stent (BMS): 0.50, drug-eluting stent (DES): 0.73, atherectomy 0.78, and balloon angioplasty 0.66. At 3 years, in patients with infrapopliteal artery lesions, primary patency of DES was 0.49 and that of BMS was 0.10 with no data available for PTA. Data on major amputation and mortality in patients with infrapopliteal disease were not significantly different for various endovascular techniques at 1 and 3 years of follow-up.[5]

REFERENCES

1. Anton N. Sidawy BAP. *Rutherford's Vascular Surgery and Endovascular Therapy*. 9th ed. Russell Gabbedy; 2014.
2. Aboyans V, Ricco JB, Bartelink MLEL, et al. 2017 ESC Guidelines on the Diagnosis and Treatment of Peripheral Arterial Diseases, in collaboration with the European Society for Vascular Surgery (ESVS): document covering atherosclerotic disease of extracranial carotid and vertebral, mesenteric, renal. *Eur Heart J*. 2018;39(9):763-816. doi:10.1093/eurheartj/ehx095
3. Fujii M, Terashi H. Angiosome and tissue healing. *Ann Vasc Dis*. 2019;12(2):147-150. doi:10.3400/avd.ra.19-00036
4. Zhao AH, Kwok CHR, Jansen SJ. How to prevent surgical site infection in vascular surgery: a review of the evidence. *Ann Vasc Surg*. 2022;78:336-361. doi:10.1016/j.avsg.2021.06.0455
5. Almasri J, Adusumalli J, Asi N, et al. A systematic review and meta-analysis of revascularization outcomes of infrainguinal chronic limb-threatening ischemia. *J Vasc Surg*. 2018;68:2 PMID: 29804736 doi:10.1016/j.jvs.2018.01.066

Chapter 33 Popliteal Aneurysm Management: Open and Endovascular Repair

Lindsey Marie Korepta and Bernadette Aulivola

DEFINITION

- Popliteal artery aneurysms (PAAs) are the most frequently encountered peripheral arterial aneurysm, accounting for 70% of aneurysms in the peripheral vasculature. In general, an artery is considered aneurysmal when it measures 1.5 times the diameter of the normal adjacent segment. Normal popliteal artery diameter varies depending on body habitus but is typically between 5 and 9 mm and can be up to 1 to 2 mm larger in men than in women.[1,2]
- In characterizing PAAs for indications for repair, not only the maximal diameter but also the presence or absence of intraluminal thrombus and the symptomatic status are important.
- Clinical practice guidelines advocate for repair of any PAA measuring greater than 2 cm in diameter, although smaller aneurysms may have an indication for repair if they are symptomatic or if there is evidence of thromboembolism. The diameter of the popliteal artery is typically larger proximally, at its transition from the superficial femoral artery as it emerges from the adductor hiatus, than in the more distal portion. Aneurysms are more common in the proximal or mid portions of the popliteal artery and may extend to involve the superficial femoral artery proximally or tibial vessels distally.[3]

DIFFERENTIAL DIAGNOSIS

- The asymptomatic PAA may present with a palpable pulsatile mass or fullness in the popliteal fossa on physical examination. The differential diagnosis for a popliteal fossa mass includes PAA, Baker cyst, deep venous thrombosis, and neoplasms such as rhabdomyosarcoma. In the symptomatic patient with ischemia, the differential diagnosis includes other etiologies of acute or chronic ischemia, including popliteal entrapment syndrome, cystic adventitial disease, atherosclerotic peripheral artery disease (PAD), and thromboembolism.

PATIENT HISTORY AND PHYSICAL FINDINGS

- When evaluating any patient, it is important to consider risk factors for aneurysm disease in general, including advanced age, male sex, smoking history, personal history of PAD or atherosclerosis in other vascular beds, and family history of aneurysm disease or connective tissue disorder. Most patients with PAAs are male, accounting for approximately 95% of those affected.[1] Additional risk factors for atherosclerotic disease include hypertension and hyperlipidemia. Diabetes, while a risk factor for atherosclerotic peripheral artery disease, is protective against the development of aneurysm disease.
- In patients with a diagnosis of abdominal aortic aneurysm (AAA), a thorough physical examination should be performed to rule out the presence of concomitant peripheral aneurysms including PAAs, which are present in over 10% of these patients. Palpation of the popliteal pulse is best performed using a technique where the examiner encircles both hands around the knee with thumbs positioned anteriorly over the patella and all other fingertips of both hands pressed against the popliteal fossa. If palpation reveals evidence of a widened popliteal pulse or pulsatile mass, or if the examination is equivocal, duplex ultrasound should be performed to evaluate further for the presence of a popliteal artery aneurysm.
- In patients with PAA, bilateral involvement is present in over 60%, emphasizing the importance of evaluating the contralateral extremity in patients diagnosed with PAA. In addition, approximately 40% of patients with PAA will also have an AAA; therefore, aortic imaging is indicated in all patients with PAA.[4] While femoral artery aneurysms are less common, they may be seen with increased frequency in patients with other extremity aneurysms or AAA; therefore, femoral pulse palpation and/or imaging is recommended as well.
- While PAAs may be diagnosed when small and asymptomatic, patients may present with symptoms of acute or chronic ischemia due to thromboembolism, mass effect on surrounding structures, or rupture, the latter of which is quite rare. Popliteal artery aneurysms, in contrast to AAAs, more commonly present with ischemic symptoms when symptomatic rather than rupture. PAAs can develop intraluminal thrombus, which may embolize to distal vessels. Distal embolization may, in fact, be asymptomatic. Most patients presenting with acute limb ischemia (ALI) related to PAA do so given popliteal artery thrombosis; therefore, PAA should be in the differential diagnosis of any patient presenting with ALI.
- It is important to remember that digital subtraction angiography (DSA) alone may not identify PAA in the patient presenting with ALI; therefore, duplex ultrasound or axial imaging such as computed tomography angiography (CTA) or magnetic resonance angiography (MRA) is essential to identify the presence of PAA and characterize the maximal diameter of the artery.
- Distal embolization due to intraluminal thrombus may present in the asymptomatic state or with intermittent claudication, ischemic rest pain, or tissue loss with distal ulceration or gangrene.
- While uncommon, patients with large PAAs may present with compressive symptoms related to mass effect on the surrounding structures. This may result in complaints of popliteal fossa fullness, discomfort or pain, or lower extremity swelling from popliteal vein compression, which may result in deep venous thrombosis. Compression of the common peroneal nerve by the PAA may present with neurologic symptoms such as foot drop.[5]
- Significant risk of limb loss exists in the patient presenting with signs and symptoms of ALI associated with PAA thromboembolism (36%).[4] This emphasizes the importance of diagnosis of the PAA at an early stage such that proper surveillance

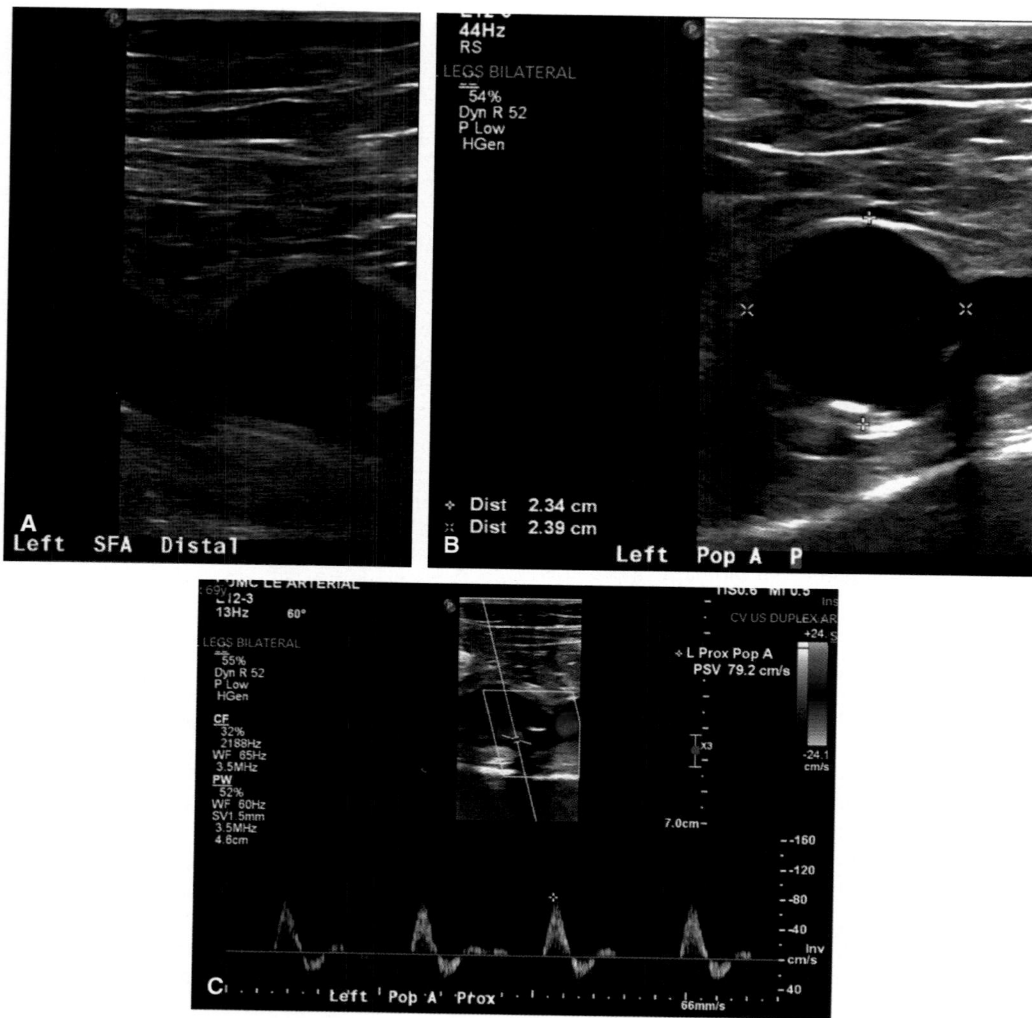

FIGURE 1 ● Popliteal artery aneurysm imaging using duplex ultrasound, depicted in **(A)** b-mode longitudinal view, **(B)** b-mode transverse view and **(C)** color flow longitudinal view.

and elective intervention may be performed when indicated. Of PAAs that are identified when asymptomatic, 14% to 24% will become symptomatic within 1 to 2 years and 31% to 68% will become symptomatic within their lifetime.[4,6]

IMAGING AND OTHER DIAGNOSTIC STUDIES

- As previously mentioned, given the high rate of bilateral PAAs and concomitant AAA, bilateral lower extremity arterial duplex ultrasound (US) and abdominal aortic US should be performed whenever a popliteal artery aneurysm is identified. Screening duplex US has been demonstrated to have a nearly 100% accuracy in detection of PAAs and thus is recommended by the Society for Vascular Surgery clinical practice guidelines to be the first step in diagnosis.[1] As demonstrated in **FIGURE 1**, duplex US is able to determine PAA diameter and can detect color Doppler flow through the aneurysm lumen and presence of intraluminal thrombus.
- When repair is indicated for a PAA, CTA (**FIGURE 2**), MRA, or DSA can be used to further characterize the size and extent of the PAA and the runoff vasculature beyond the aneurysm.

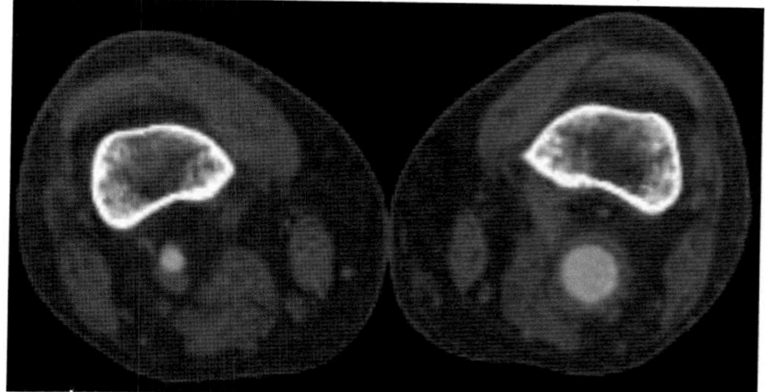

FIGURE 2 ● Axial slices of computed tomography angiogram (CTA) imaging demonstrating a left popliteal aneurysm with contrast enhancement of the lumen and presence of a rim of intraluminal thrombus.

It is important to note that DSA demonstrates only the flow lumen and therefore is not an accurate technique to determine aneurysm diameter and may not detect aneurysm at all in cases of PAA thrombosis.

SURGICAL MANAGEMENT

Preoperative Planning

- Workup may vary significantly in the asymptomatic vs the acutely symptomatic patient. Ideally, if the PAA is identified in the asymptomatic state, surveillance may be performed with duplex US and elective repair may be planned once the aneurysm meets size criteria for repair. Asymptomatic PAAs should be considered for elective repair if they measure >2 cm in maximal diameter, or smaller if there is evidence of intraluminal thrombus and runoff vessel occlusion, a possible result of distal embolization. In all cases of elective aneurysm repair, the risk–benefit ratio is assessed prior to recommending intervention. The size of the aneurysm, evidence of distal embolization, and the patient's overall health and medical comorbidities should be taken into consideration. Risks of intervention vary based upon whether the aneurysm is repaired using open surgical or endovascular means. Planning prior to operative repair typically includes venous mapping to identify the suitability of autogenous conduit. Cardiac risk stratification and optimization is essential, as in all elective vascular procedures.
- In the elective setting, lower extremity runoff CTA is the ideal imaging study to provide anatomic detail for intervention planning. This imaging modality provides an adequate assessment of thrombus burden within the aneurysm and runoff to the foot. If the aneurysm is large, contrast enhancement of the aneurysm sac and runoff may be slow, requiring a delayed phase of imaging to properly assess the distal runoff vessels (**FIGURE 3**). During an on-table angiogram, the catheter can be advanced into and beyond the aneurysm to better identify the runoff vessels. Either technique will be able to identify the anatomy of the patent arteries including any large geniculate arteries in the vicinity of the aneurysm, which can be helpful when determining appropriate operative management. Both endovascular and open techniques are used to treat PAAs.
- Endovascular stent placement is a reasonable treatment option for PAA, but patency outcomes are improved in patients with better distal runoff. In our practice, to be considered a candidate for endovascular therapy the patient must have more than one tibial artery vessel runoff to the foot and an adequate sealing zone proximal and distal to the aneurysmal segment. The proximal and distal landing zones must measure between 4 and 12 mm in diameter, as currently available self-expanding covered stents for use in the peripheral vasculature range between 5 and 13 mm in diameter (Viabahn, W. L. Gore & Associates, Flagstaff, AZ). Geniculate vessel anatomy should be assessed preoperatively, as there is potential for retrograde flow via these vessels into the aneurysm sac after stent graft placement (type 2 endoleak), which may lead to progressive aneurysm growth. Preoperative side branch embolization with coils or plugs may be considered if such branches are present and the patient is not a candidate for open repair.
- In general, open repair of PAAs is preferred if the patient is deemed to be reasonable operative risk with life expectancy >2 years, especially if the patient is at a young age at intervention, if compressive symptoms are present, or if the aneurysm crosses the knee joint, which is often the case. Techniques for open repair include posterior approach to the popliteal artery with interposition grafting or medial approach with ligation of the artery proximal and distal to the aneurysm and surgical bypass around the aneurysmal segment. Infrequently in the patient presenting with ALI due to acute PAA thrombosis, primary amputation may be considered if the limb is deemed to be nonviable or if the patient is nonambulatory.

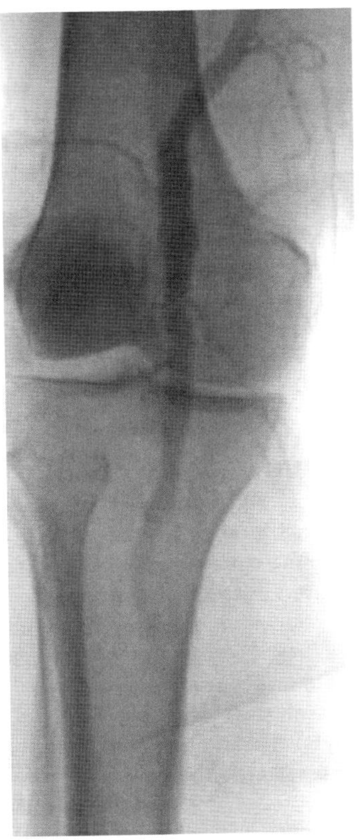

FIGURE 3 ● Preintervention angiography with catheter positioned in the distal superficial femoral artery.

POSITIONING AND TECHNIQUE

Endovascular Technique

First Step: Thrombolytic Therapy

- If the patient presents with acute thrombosis of a PAA and endovascular PAA repair is being considered, a patent flow lumen must be restored and runoff artery flow must be optimized prior to stent graft deployment. Typically, on initial diagnosis with ALI, a therapeutic heparin bolus (80 U/kg intravenous [IV]) is given and IV infusion (18 U/kg/h) is instituted.
- Restoration of flow of the occluded popliteal artery is performed typically via a contralateral retrograde femoral artery ultrasound-guided access. The access site must be assessed for the presence of an aneurysm, and it is helpful to know if AAA is also present since puncture site and catheter navigation may be affected by this knowledge. A sheath is placed

up and over the aortic bifurcation with its tip positioned within the external iliac or femoral artery of the affected lower extremity.

- If ischemic symptoms are mild, thrombolytic agent may be infused over a course of hours to dissolve thrombus in the artery. This typically commits the patient to a 12- to 24-hour course of thrombolysis, sometimes longer. For catheter-directed thrombolysis, a multi-side hole catheter is positioned through the thrombosed segment over a guidewire. The location of the tip of the catheter must be confirmed within a patent artery distally prior to infusion. Tissue plasminogen activator (TPA) is then infused at a rate of 1 mg/h through the catheter, which instills the medication throughout the length of the thrombus through multiple side-holes of the catheter. The sheath side-arm is flushed continuously with a low-dose heparin infusion, typically 500 U/h. This is intended to assure patency of the sheath, rather than as a therapeutic dose of anticoagulation. The patient undergoing drip thrombolytic therapy requires close observation, often in the intensive care unit, with Q1 hour neurovascular checks and access site inspection for bleeding complications. Laboratory values including CBC, PT, PTT, and fibrinogen should be checked every 6 hours looking for signs of bleeding or coagulopathy that may alter plans for ongoing thrombolytic therapy. The administration of thrombolytic agents is associated with a risk of bleeding, so patients should be appropriately screened for bleeding risks prior to instituting therapy.
- Often, the degree of ischemia in the patient presenting with a thrombosed PAA does not lend itself to pharmacologic thrombolysis, as described above, given the risk of ongoing nerve, muscle and soft tissue damage from prolonged ischemia during the treatment time. In that case, more rapid thrombolysis results may be seen with the use of pharmacomechanical thrombectomy techniques. There are several commercially available mechanical thrombectomy devices available. In our practice, we pulse-spray 10 mg of TPA (diluted in 100 mL of normal saline) into the thrombus, let it dwell within the thrombus for 20 minutes, then perform thrombus removal using suction thrombectomy. If persistent residual thrombus is seen, a lytic catheter may be left in place for 12 to 24 hours as described above for more complete thrombolysis. After lysis, the patient can be considered for endovascular or open repair. The use of thrombolytic therapy in general requires that the degree of ischemia present would allow for time for thrombolysis, which is generally faster when using mechanical adjunctions to pharmacologic therapy. Open operative thrombectomy should always be a consideration if the degree of ischemia is advanced and rapid flow resolution is warranted.

Second Step: Endovascular Stent Graft Repair

- If endovascular PAA repair is planned, whether in the setting of elective PAA repair or in the symptomatic patient after thrombolysis, the patient is placed on a radiolucent table in the supine position. The sheaths required for delivery of large covered self-expanding stents can be as large as 10 French. In our practice, an up and over technique is used from a contralateral groin approach if there is a favorable access site and aortic bifurcation anatomy. Otherwise an open cut-down on the ipsilateral groin with antegrade access of the common femoral artery may be performed.
- A preintervention DSA run is performed, and the proximal and distal landing zones are identified. A marker catheter can be used to guide stent graft length selection (**FIGURE 4**). Large geniculate branches may be coil embolized prior to stent graft placement. The patient is systemically heparinized (80 U/kg), with a goal activated clotting time (ACT) >200 seconds. The stent is selected based upon seal zone vessel diameter, typically upsizing the stent graft 1 mm from the size of the artery.
- The stent graft is then deployed across the aneurysm, and postdeployment angioplasty may be performed with the appropriate-sized balloon at the seal zones to assure adequate graft expansion and seal. Completion DSA is performed to evaluate the stented segment and runoff arteries. This will assess for artery patency as well as presence of endoleaks (**FIGURES 5** and **6**). Runoff DSA images to the foot are then obtained to document outflow to the foot.

Third Step: Closure of Access

- If endovascular access from the contralateral groin has been carried out, we use PerClose ProGlide closure (Abbot Laboratories, Abbott Park, IL). If open arterial exposure has been performed, the sheath is removed and the artery is closed in a transverse arteriotomy technique with running 6-0 Prolene suture, flushing the artery antegrade and retrograde before completion of the closure down. The femoral exposure is then closed in a standard layered technique.

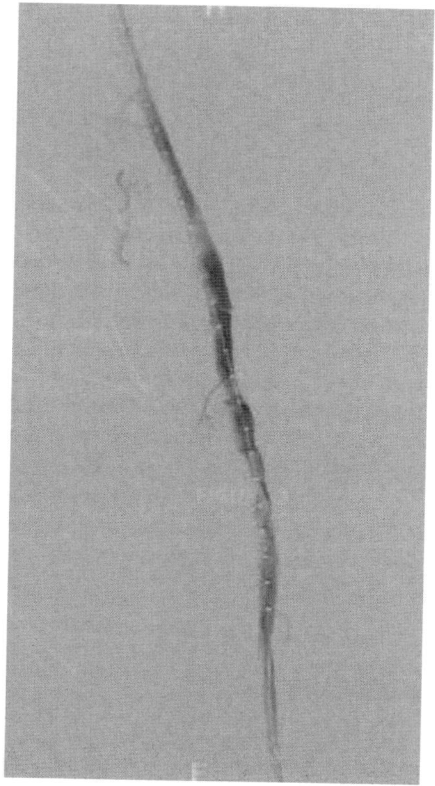

FIGURE 4 ● Marker catheter in place to assist with choosing stent length during endovascular repair of PAA.

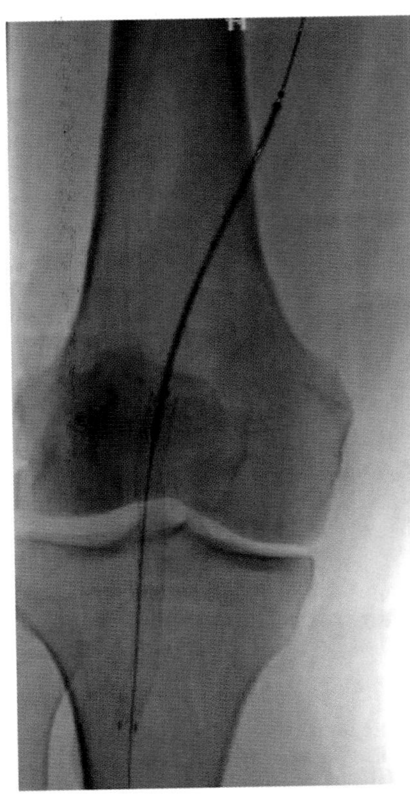

FIGURE 5 ● Intraoperative angiogram depicting two covered stent deployment with one stent deployed and adequate overlap with second stent about to be deployed.

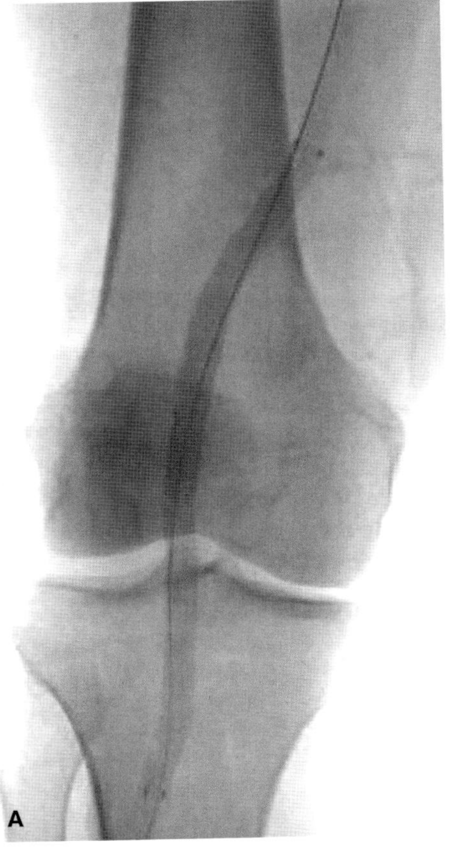

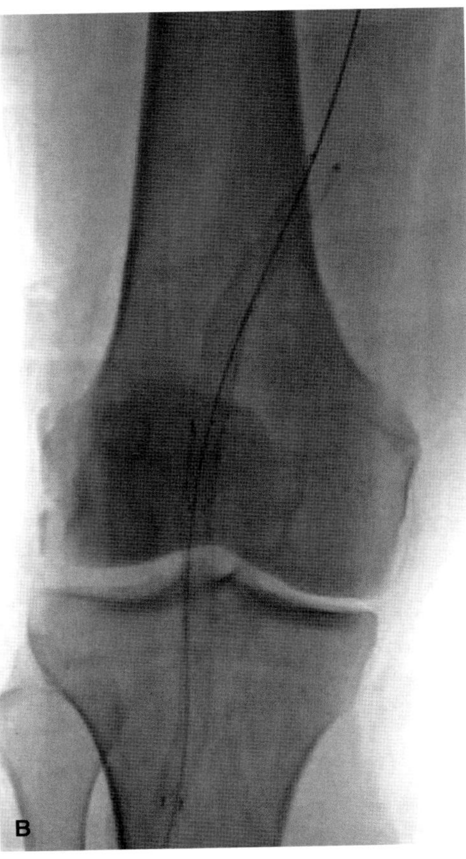

FIGURE 6 ● Completion angiogram after covered stent deployment in endovascular repair technique with **(A)** and without **(B)** contrast.

OPEN OPERATIVE TECHNIQUE

- Depending on the size and location of the aneurysm, there are two standard approaches to open popliteal artery aneurysm repair.

Medial Approach (Ligation and Bypass)

First Step: Harvest of Autogenous Conduit

- Preoperatively, the patient should undergo venous mapping with ultrasound. Ipsilateral great saphenous vein (GSV) is the conduit of choice. Before prepping and draping the patient, ultrasound may be performed, marking the course of the GSV with a skin marker on the surface. If autogenous vein is not available, prosthetic graft may be used, typically 6 mm or 8 mm ringed polytetrafluoroethylene (PTFE). The patient is positioned supine, and the extremity is then prepped and draped in the standard sterile fashion. Before or after proximal and distal arterial exposure, the GSV is harvested from one incision to the other, assuming that the size of the vein at this location is adequate. If better conduit quality is present more proximally, then separate GSV harvest incisions may be made. The goal is to use the highest-quality segment of the GSV for bypass.

Second step: Exposure of the Proximal Popliteal Artery

- Assuming the PAA does not extend proximally into the distal superficial femoral artery, proximal exposure is achieved with a longitudinal incision above the knee, taking care to identify and preserve the GSV. A bump is placed just below the knee, facilitating exposure of the above-knee popliteal artery. The artery is exposed by retracting the sartorius muscle posteriorly and entering the popliteal space. The popliteal vein is usually encountered first, and the popliteal artery is located just lateral to this. The artery is dissected free of the neighboring veins and surrounding tissue sufficiently to allow for passage of a vessel loop proximal and distal to the planned proximal anastomosis site. There should be enough space distal to this to ligate the popliteal artery proximal to the aneurysm.

Third Step: Exposure of the Distal Popliteal Artery

- Depending on the extent of the aneurysm, the distal anastomosis of the bypass graft may be the above-knee popliteal artery for very focal aneurysms, but more commonly is located at the distal popliteal artery and approached from a medial incision below the knee. The bump is repositioned under the distal thigh. A longitudinal incision is made below the knee on the medial aspect of the proximal calf. Again, care is taken to avoid injury to the GSV. The fascia of the superficial posterior compartment of the calf is opened longitudinally and the popliteal space is entered. As with the proximal exposure, the vein is encountered first and retracted posteriorly to dissect the artery and place a proximal and distal vessel loop for control. Care should be taken to avoid traction on the nearby tibial nerve. Since the inflow and the outflow to the PAA will be ligated during the operation, one may choose to place a 0-silk tie around the popliteal artery at the proximal aspect of the exposed artery here for ligation rather than a vessel loop in order to tie off the vessel later. If the popliteal artery is aneurysmal throughout its length, the exposure may be extended distally to identify and control a tibial artery target for bypass. The posterior tibial or peroneal arteries can be easily accessed from a medial approach. If the anterior tibial artery or mid to distal peroneal arteries are chosen as the distal bypass target, a separate lateral incision is needed.

Fourth Step: Tunneling

- The bypass conduit can be tunneled anatomically between the heads of the gastrocnemius along the course of the native popliteal artery; however, if the aneurysm is large this may not be feasible due to risk of compression of the bypass graft or risk of rupture/bleeding during tunneling. In this case a "bucket handle" bypass may be performed with subcutaneous tunneling of the bypass instead. Once the tunnel is created with a vascular clamp or tunneling device, the patient is systemically heparinized with 80 U/kg of IV heparin and an ACT is checked to assure therapeutic anticoagulation with a goal ACT of 200 to 250 s.

Fifth Step: Conduit Preparation

- Assuming adequate GSV conduit is available for use, it is harvested assuring adequate length, ligating all branches with 3-0 or 4-0 silk ties and tying it off proximally and distally using 2-0 silk ties. The GSV is stored in an isotonic solution (500 cc of Plasmalyte or Normosol with 60 mg papaverine and 5000 U heparin) in an effort to reduce vasospasm. The GSV conduit may be used in the reversed or nonreversed orientation. This is typically based on surgeon preference as there is no significant impact of vein orientation on bypass patency rates. If the plan is to position it nonreversed, then standard preparation with valve lysis should be performed. If GSV is not available, the bypass may be performed with ringed PTFE, and if so, a distal target artery vein or bovine pericardium patch may be performed prior distal anastomosis at the target site.

Sixth Step: Arterial Bypass

- Arterial bypass is performed in standard fashion with either proximal end-to-side or end-to-end anastomosis. End to side is usually easier from a technical standpoint given size discrepancy with the artery larger than the conduit. The proximal anastomosis is performed first, then the bypass conduit is allowed to inflate with pulsatile inflow and inspected for hemostasis prior to tunneling to the distal anastomosis site. The distal anastomosis is then performed. The inflow and outflow arteries to the aneurysm sac should be ligated as close to the aneurysm sac as possible to ensure aneurysm thrombosis and to decrease the risk of further growth. Completion arteriography can be performed if there is a question about the status of the bypass based on Doppler signal and pulse examination at the end of the case, but it is not our routine to perform completion arteriography.

- When possible, the medial approach is our preferred method of bypass given the ability to harvest the entire length of the GSV, the familiarity of the exposure, and the ability to reach the tibial vessels, if needed for the distal bypass target.

Posterior Approach (Interposition Grafting)

First Step: Harvest of Autogenous Conduit

- If the aneurysm is located directly behind the knee or demonstrates significant compressive symptoms requiring decompression, the posterior approach is preferable. If GSV is to be harvested from the groin of proximal thigh, this is performed supine, then the patient is turned prone. The distal GSV may be harvested in the prone position. The patient is then placed in prone position, assuring proper padding with axillary rolls, a pillow beneath the hips, soft padding underneath the knees, and a roll beneath the ankles. If the small saphenous vein is of adequate size, it can be used as the bypass conduit and harvested via the same incision as outlined below. The popliteal artery is exposed from a posterior approach and aneurysmorrhapy with aneurysm sac decompression can be performed at the same time.

Second step: Exposure of the Proximal Popliteal Artery

- A lazy S-shaped incision is used with the proximal incision positioned on the medial aspect of the posterior distal thigh and the distal part of the incision on the lateral aspect of the posterior calf (**FIGURE 7**). The proximal popliteal artery is identified distal to the adductor canal and exposed by separating the semimembranous and semitendinosus muscles medially from the long head of the biceps femoris, which lies laterally.

Third Step: Exposure of the Distal Popliteal Artery

- Dissection is then carried along the course of the popliteal artery distally to gain distal control of the artery beyond the aneurysm. Care should be taken to gently retract the tibial nerve to gain visualization of the popliteal artery along its course if needed. As there is no tunneling required, the patient is then systemically anticoagulated with heparin as previously described.

Fourth Step: Arterial Bypass

- Vascular clamps are placed distally and proximally for arterial control. The aneurysm sac is opened longitudinally and any intraluminal thrombus is removed. Back bleeding geniculate arteries are oversewn with silk figure-of-eight sutures. End-to-end interposition bypass is then performed in a method similar to that used for open repair of aortic aneurysms (**FIGURE 8**). Alternatively, an end-to-side proximal and distal anastomosis can be carried out, which may be preferable if there is a significant size discrepancy between the bypass conduit and the native artery. An alternative is to use appropriately sized prosthetic conduit, either Dacron or PTFE, to assure a better size match. Often, posterior approach repair may be performed with a short interposition graft. Wound closure is performed with two deep layers and a subcuticular stitch.

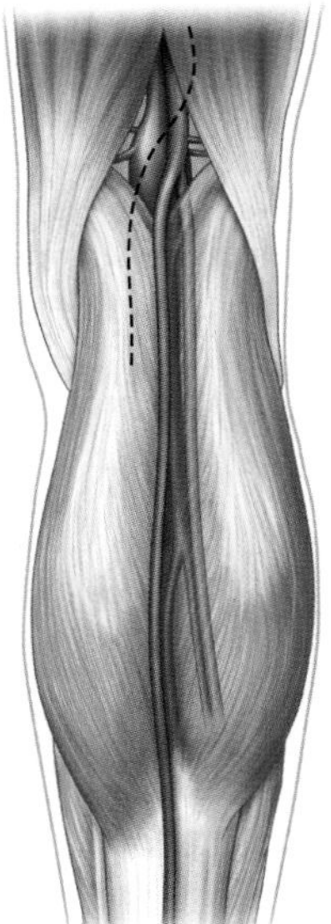

FIGURE 7 Posterior approach to the popliteal artery depicting the lazy-S incision with the incision medial on the thigh and lateral on the calf.

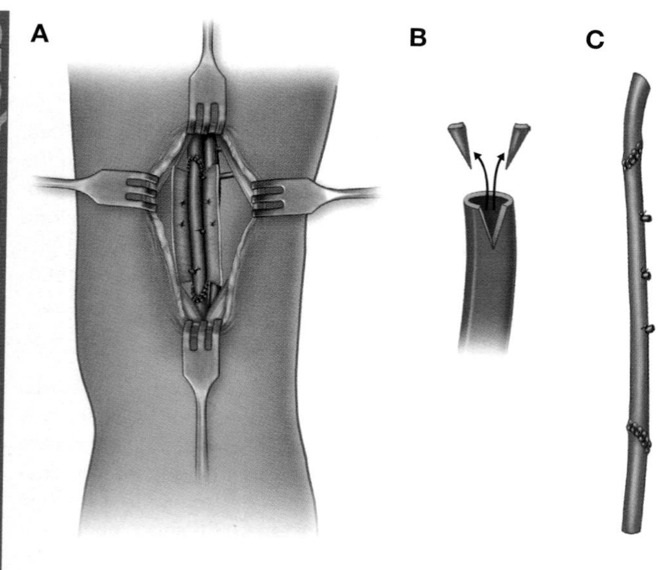

FIGURE 8 • End-to-end bypass technique with saphenous vein conduit using a splicing technique of the proximal and distal arteries and veins to prevent stenosis at the anastomoses.

PEARLS AND PITFALLS

Popliteal artery aneurysm thrombosis	■ As with any acute limb ischemia case, the potential to develop compartment syndrome after revascularization should be taken into consideration and calf four-compartment fasciotomies should be performed when the risk of this is deemed to be significant. If calf fasciotomies are required, we often apply a vessel loop with staples in a "Roman sandal" configuration across the fasciotomy site. This allows for the vessel loop to be tightened at the bedside day by day, and eventually bedside wound closure may be performed without a return trip to the operating room. ■ If open intervention is planned in a patient with PAA thrombosis and there is an adequate runoff artery, bypass may and should be performed without efforts at thrombolysis as long as the runoff artery is deemed to be adequate.
Endovascular technique considerations	■ When planning an endovascular approach to repair of a PAA, we try to use as few stents as possible to decrease the risk of stent migration or thrombosis. We ensure adequate proximal and distal seal into healthy artery to prevent the development of endoleaks in the future. We often perform an open cutdown onto the proximal superficial femoral artery (SFA) or distal common femoral for safe delivery of larger sheaths (typically greater than 8 French in diameter or a steep aortic bifurcation).
Open surgery technique considerations	■ Size mismatch between the artery and the bypass conduit can be considerable. For larger arteries or arteriomegaly, a PTFE bypass conduit that can be chosen closer to the size of the artery should be considered. Studies have demonstrated acceptable patency rates with prosthetic conduit.[7]

POSTOPERATIVE CARE

- With either technique, the popliteal aneurysm can continue to grow if patent geniculate arteries are left unaddressed. Careful postoperative duplex ultrasound (DUS) surveillance should be carried out to assure the best chance of long-term patency. Clinical practice guidelines recommend DUS surveillance be performed at 30 days, 3 months, 6 months, 12 months, and then yearly if the aneurysm does not grow during this interval.[1]
- We place all patients treated with endovascular repair on dual antiplatelet therapy with aspirin 81 mg/d and clopidogrel 75 mg/d for at least 90 days. For vein bypasses, we place

all patients on aspirin 81 mg daily indefinitely. For patients with prosthetic bypass conduits or compromised tibial runoff, we consider dual antiplatelet therapy. For patients presenting with ALI and PAA thrombosis, we often treat with therapeutic anticoagulation in addition to antiplatelet therapy for at least 1 to 3 months.

- The posterior approach incision may be compromised if significant edema is present, therefore we apply compression wraps to the lower extremity for at least a few weeks or until edema is under control.

COMPLICATIONS

- Stent thrombosis has been noted with single vessel runoff, stent coverage below the knee, and large aneurysm size.[1] Stent thrombosis can be detected on DUS surveillance (**FIGURE 9**), CT angiography, or digital subtraction angiography. These stents can often be reopened with pharmacomechanical thrombolysis using the same technique as referenced above. If an underlying lesion is noted as a cause of the stent thrombosis, it may undergo angioplasty or stenting as needed (**FIGURE 10**). In patients with only single vessel runoff, open bypass should be considered given the elevated risk of stent graft thrombosis.
- In order to prevent stent and bypass thrombosis, initiation of postoperative anticoagulation and/or antiplatelet therapy is very important.
- Poor tibial artery runoff is associated with worse outcomes for both open and endovascular interventions.[8] In a patient with poor tibial runoff after open bypass we often will add low-dose rivaroxaban 2.5 mg BID to aspirin 81 mg. We ensure that all stented patients are on dual antiplatelet therapy for at least 90 days and occasionally lifelong if they are noted to have poor tibial runoff.
- Wound complications are increased in open repair over endovascular repair.[1,8] We make every effort to ensure that our patients are medically optimized before surgery. This includes initiation of antihypertensive and statin medications as indicated as well as nutritional support.

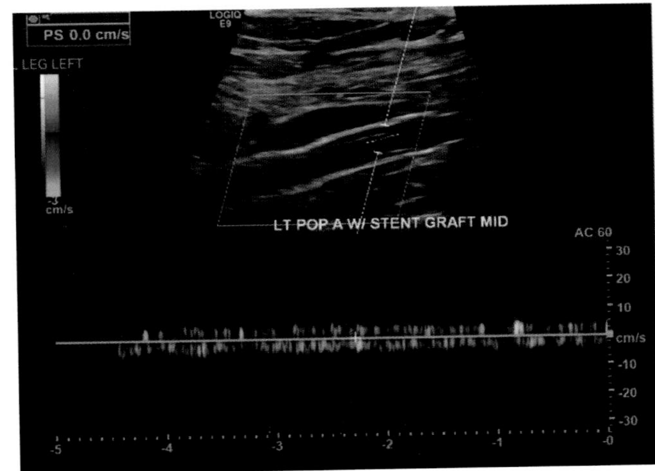

FIGURE 9 • Duplex US demonstrated stent occlusion.

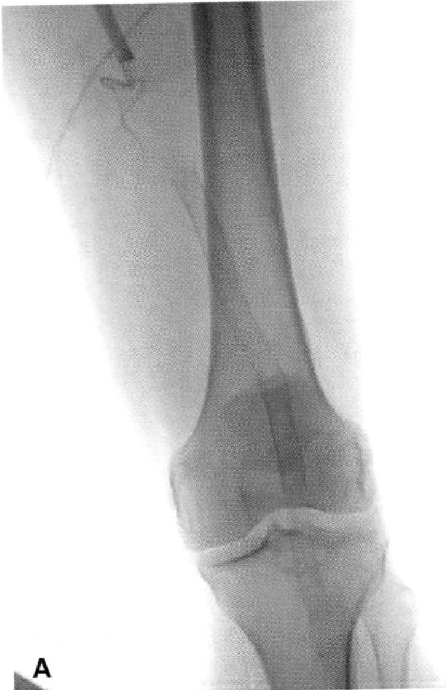

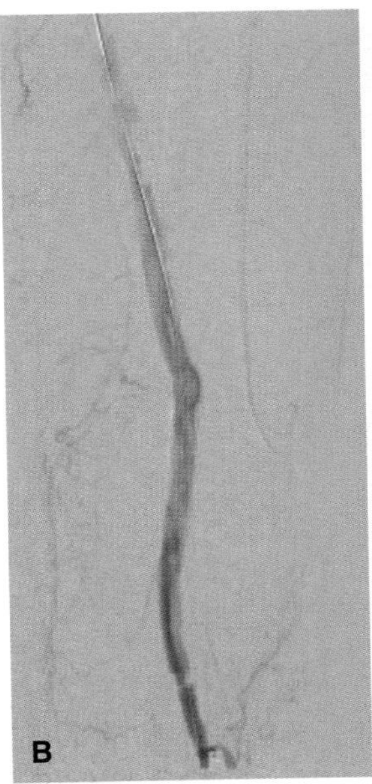

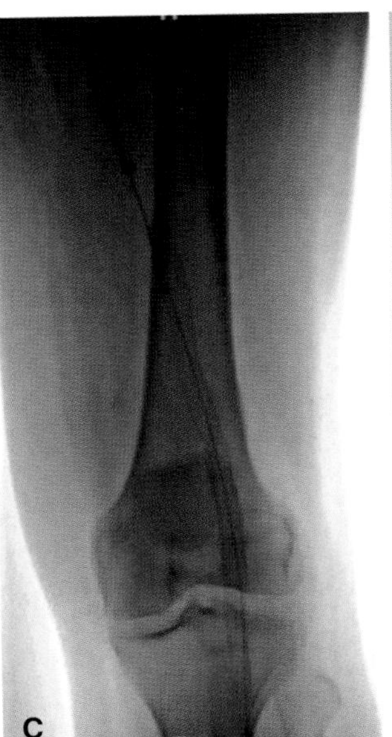

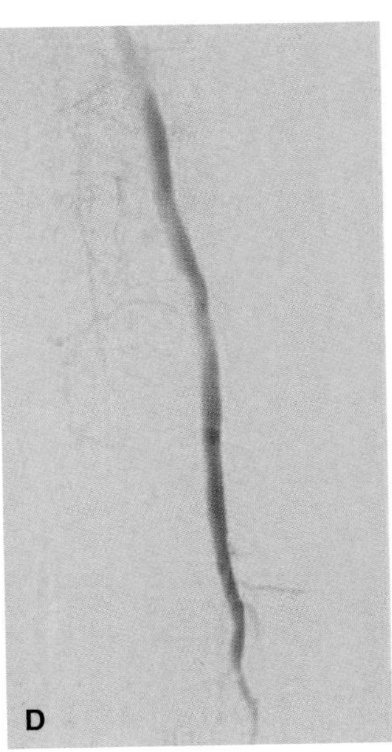

FIGURE 10 • Digital subtraction angiography depicting an occluded stent **(A)**, which was able to be reopened with AngioJet thrombectomy **(B)**, and an area of stenosis just distal to the existing stents **(C)** was treated with an additional stent **(C)** with good result **(D)**.

REFERENCES

1. Farber A, Angle N, Averginos E, et al. The Society for Vascular Surgery clinical practice guidelines on popliteal artery aneurysms. *J Vasc Surg*. 2022;75(1S):109S-120S.
2. Johnston KW, Rutherford RB, Tilson MD, et al. Suggested standards for reporting on arterial aneurysms, Ad Hoc Committee on Reporting Standards, Society of Vascular Surgery and North American chapter, International Society for Cardiovascular Surgery. *J Vasc Surg*. 1991;13(3):452-458.
3. Pomposelli F, Hamdan A. Rutherford's vascular surgery, chapter 136: Lower extremity aneurysms. In: Cronenwett JL, Johnston KW, Rutherford BS, eds. *Rutherford's Vascular Surgery*. 7th ed. Saunders/Elsevier; 2010.
4. Vermilion BD, Kimmins SA, Pace WG, Evans WE. A review of one hundred forty-seven popliteal aneurysms with long-term follow-up. *Surgery*. 1981;90(6):1009-1014.
5. Dawson I, Sie R, van Baalen JM, et al. Asymptomatic popliteal aneurysm: elective operation versus conservative follow-up. *Br J Surg*. 1994;81(10):1504-1507.
6. Dawson I, Sie RB, van Bockel JH. Atherosclerotic popliteal aneurysm. *Br J Surg*. 1997;84(3):293-299.
7. Beseth BD, Moore WS. The posterior approach for repair of popliteal artery aneurysms. *J Vasc Surg*. 2006;43(5):940-944; discussion 944-5.
8. Leake AE, Segal MA, Chaer RA, et al. Meta-analysis of open and endovascular repair of popliteal artery aneurysms. *J Vasc Surg*. 2017;65:246-256.

SECTION VI: Surgical Management of Venous Disease

Chapter 34

Acute Iliofemoral Deep Vein Thrombosis and May-Thurner Syndrome: Surgical and Interventional Management

Sharon C. Kiang and Brian G. DeRubertis

DEFINITION

- Acute iliofemoral occlusion is defined as complete or partial thrombosis of any part of the iliac vein and/or the common femoral vein (CFV), with or without associated femoropopliteal thrombosis, in which symptoms have been present for 14 days or less or for which imaging indicates that thrombosis has occurred within the past 14 days or less.[1] Acute iliofemoral occlusion may occur de novo following unprovoked deep vein thrombosis (DVT) or may occur (or reoccur) in the setting of prior ipsilateral DVT or external compression (May-Thurner syndrome or neoplasia). Treatment options include (1) systemic anticoagulation alone, (2) open surgical venous thrombectomy, or (3) percutaneous intervention, including catheter-directed thrombolysis, pharmacomechanical thrombectomy, and stenting of intrinsic or extrinsic obstructive lesions or masses.

DIFFERENTIAL DIAGNOSIS

- Iliofemoral DVT most commonly presents with unilateral leg swelling and pain. Although patient history and simple diagnostic testing can generally distinguish from other causes, differential diagnoses include cellulitis or worsening of chronic conditions such as venous insufficiency or lymphedema.

PATIENT HISTORY AND PHYSICAL FINDINGS

- There are three objectives in the treatment of iliofemoral thrombotic occlusion: (1) prevent propagation of DVT and subsequent pulmonary embolism (PE), (2) provide symptomatic relief for the patient, and (3) prevent the development of postthrombotic syndrome (PTS).
- A thorough history must be obtained prior to treatment because decisions regarding choice of treatment modality are impacted by severity of symptoms as well as the patient's overall functional status.
- Specific risk factors that merit individualized questioning include history of trauma, current or past episodes of DVT or PE, history of thrombophilia, history or current diagnosis of cancer, and a history of tobacco or substance use. Family history of DVT or PE is important to ascertain. A thorough investigation of current medications should be undertaken, making note of any contraceptive therapy, hormone replacement therapy, or use of anticoagulation (ie, warfarin, enoxaparin).
- Symptoms of iliofemoral occlusion can range from nondescript mild symptoms to severe disabling symptoms, and manifestations of symptoms can vary widely. Commonly reported symptoms of iliofemoral occlusion include limb edema, heaviness, pain, lifestyle-limiting venous claudication, stasis dermatitis, and, in advanced cases, venous ulcerations.[2] Duration of symptoms and consideration of inciting events at the time of symptom development will help differentiate acute occlusion from exacerbation of chronic disease.
- Symptom severity is an important differentiating variable in the management rubric of acute iliofemoral occlusion; severe and persistent symptoms, especially those continuing following the initiation of therapeutic anticoagulation, increase the likelihood of long-term disabling sequelae. The more severe and persistent the symptoms, the more justified the indication for aggressive thrombus removal.
- A detailed physical examination is essential. Conditions that produce symptoms mimicking those associated with iliofemoral occlusion should be excluded. A thorough abdominal and lower extremity pulse examination, with noninvasive physiologic testing, if necessary, will exclude possibility of arterial insufficiency. Comprehensive assessment of peripheral motor and sensory nerve function and of the spine and lower limb joints can rule out these confounding etiologies.
- The affected limb(s) should be examined for evidence of chronic venous insufficiency and/or stasis dermatitis, as well as signs and symptoms of acute DVT. Signs of acute iliofemoral occlusion may include pain, swelling, and bluish discoloration. Extensive thrombus propagation throughout the ipsilateral venous system may lead to phlegmasia alba dolens, characterized by profound painful swelling and a pale, milk-like skin hue. Further thrombus propagation from the deep to the superficial venous system increases outflow obstruction to the point of impeding arterial inflow, precipitating phlegmasia cerulea dolens, limb threat, and tissue loss.
- In patients with either acute or chronic venous disease, objective evaluation and prognostic stratification is best accomplished by using the CEAP (Clinical, Etiology, Anatomy, Pathophysiology) system and venous clinical severity score (VCSS).[3,4]
- Because multiple interventions may be required to optimize outcome in acute iliofemoral disease, patients' expectations

should be managed accordingly. In addition, iliac and femoral venous intervention commonly requires extended periods of postoperative anticoagulation (warfarin and/or low-molecular-weight heparin) to ensure long-term procedural success. The likelihood of patient compliance thus represents an additional important prognostic indicator.

- Long-term functional outcomes are discouraging for patients who refuse interventional management of acute iliofemoral occlusive disease. Forty-four percent of patients treated with medical therapy alone will experience venous claudication, and up to 60% will develop PTS within 2 years.[5-7]

IMAGING AND OTHER DIAGNOSTIC STUDIES

- Imaging provides important prognostic and interventional guidance to surgical management of acute iliofemoral occlusive disease. Current modalities include duplex ultrasonography; catheter-based contrast phlebography; and reconstructed, cross-sectional, contrast-based whole body (computed tomography [CT] and magnetic resonance [MR]) imaging.

Duplex Ultrasonography

- In experienced hands, duplex ultrasonography (US) provides extremely sensitive and specific information regarding the chronicity and extent of infrainguinal venous obstruction. Diagnostic accuracy in the iliocaval venous system is less predictable due to the presence of overlying bowel gas and abdominal adiposity.
- Duplex-derived criteria for acute venous occlusion include incompressibility under direct vision, partial luminal obstruction within the normally echo-free lumen, and absent or abnormal venous flow characteristics with respiration or following a Valsalva maneuver or distal compression.[8]
- The primary advantages of duplex imaging include its noninvasive nature, avoidance of ionizing radiation or nephrotoxic contrast agents, easy reproducibility, portability, and accessibility in the outpatient setting. In addition, substantial cost savings are realized compared with other imaging modalities. Other advantages include the ability of duplex scanning to differentiate hematomas, lymphatic system obstruction, superficial thrombophlebitis, and other soft tissue abnormalities from deep venous obstruction. Thus, duplex scanning is the initial imaging modality of choice in all patients with suspected iliofemoral DVT. When sufficient imaging parameters are met, definitive therapeutic intervention may be safely performed based on duplex-derived anatomic and diagnostic imaging alone.

Computed Tomography Venography

- CT phlebography is frequently ordered for assessment of limb swelling in the inpatient setting. Advantages of this modality include nearly universal availability day or night, less reliance on skill and experience of the technical staff performing the procedure, outstanding spatial resolution, reproducibility and sensitivity throughout the entire venous system, the simultaneous ability to image pulmonary arterial flow and lung perfusion, freedom from limb pain induced by direct probe compression during ultrasound examinations, and the ability to incidentally diagnose concurrent conditions (such as solid organ neoplasia) that may influence thrombogenicity or suitability for treatment with open vs endovascular techniques.
- The modern helical CT phlebogram provides a diagnostic sensitivity and a specificity of nearly 100% per year and was found to detect previously unsuspected venous thrombosis at a prevalence of 1.1%.[9,10]
- CT phlebography also provides useful information regarding thrombus density (and thus chronicity), the presence of residual luminal patency in obstructed veins, and the nature and severity of extrinsic iliac vein compression when present.
- The applicability of CT phlebography to the diagnosis of venous obstruction is limited by the volume of iodinated intravenous contrast required to obtain optimal spatial resolution in target vessels, as well as considerable whole-body radiation exposure inherent in CT imaging. On average, the radiation dosage delivered by diagnostic CT phlebography is equivalent to that of over 1200 chest x-rays or over 10 years environmental exposure at sea level (dosage equivalents courtesy of Radiation Physics Department, Stanford Hospital & Clinics). This is particularly true in patients with reduced creatinine clearance, women of childbearing age who may be pregnant, or in children. For many reasons, including the considerable expense associated with the study, CT phlebography should not be considered a first-line study but rather reserved for patients in whom duplex scanning does not provide sufficient anatomic guidance or where additional diagnoses (eg, pulmonary embolization, solid organ malignancy, or external iliac vein compression) merit evaluation or exclusion.

Magnetic Resonance Venography

- MR phlebography shares many of the advantages and disadvantages of CT-derived cross-sectional imaging, including the ability to obtain high-quality, high-resolution images of surrounding soft tissues and delineate the extent of accompanying lymphadenopathy, soft tissue sarcomas, venous aneurysms, malformations, and compression syndromes that may influence treatment and long-term management considerations. MR phlebography also provides a sensitivity and specificity of nearly 100%, respectively, in the diagnosis of acute iliofemoral venous occlusion.[11]
- However, unlike computed tomography venography, magnetic resonance venography can be used during pregnancy and provide reduced risk of nephrotoxicity in patients with reduced creatinine clearance (although gadolinium is contraindicated in patients with an estimated glomerular filtration rate [eGFR] of more than 60 mL/min).
- Contraindications for MR-based venous imaging include the presence of implantable pacemakers/defibrillators/infusion systems or other ferromagnetic devices and surgical clips/endografts, as well as claustrophobia in affected patients. MR studies are also expensive compared with duplex US, and dedicated personnel and equipment are less widely available than are modern, multirow-detector CT imaging capabilities. Thus, MR phlebography is considered most appropriate as a secondary examination in the absence of suitable duplex imaging or in the presence of contraindications to CT phlebography. MR phlebography may be particularly useful in the evaluation of coexisting or complicating ipsilateral or central venous vascular malformations.

Catheter-Based Contrast Phlebography

- Despite continuing improvements in the quality and widespread availability of noninvasive imaging, catheter-based contrast phlebography remains the gold standard for iliofemoral venous evaluation. Sensitivity and specificity are also nearly 100%, and in addition to anatomic information, physiologic venous pressure and flow information are also provided throughout the iliocaval system when accessed in a retrograde fashion from the CFV.
- Typical fluoroscopic findings include abrupt vessel cutoff in the case of total occlusion or visualization of a filling defect with residual luminal flow around the margins, a phenomenon known as "tram tracking."
- An obvious limitation is the relatively high degree of operator dependency, both in terms of physician and facility capabilities. Catheter-based contrast phlebography may be nondiagnostic in up to 18% of cases due to misinterpretations, artifacts, or superimposition of overlying structures.[12] Thus, experience and suitable infrastructure are necessary to ensure accuracy and precision.
- Other major drawbacks include the inherent invasiveness of the procedure and attendant procedural risk, radiation and contrast exposure (although significantly less than that required for CT imaging), and cost. Thus, contrast phlebography is also inappropriate as the initial diagnostic modality for most patients and best employed in conjunction with planned interventions directed at active thrombus removal.

Intravascular Ultrasound

- Intravascular ultrasound (IVUS) with the 9F Volcano IVUS catheter (Volcano Corporation, San Diego, CA) provides direct intraluminal visualization during catheter-based phlebographic assessment and intervention.
- IVUS-based imaging allows for precise measurement of cross-sectional area and maximum and minimum lumen diameter. Flow within the residual lumen may be determined, as well as precise analysis of residual luminal irregularities. The superior two-dimensional imaging characteristics of IVUS compared with contrast phlebography make this modality the measurement instrument of choice when assessing extrinsic iliac vein compression from tumors or overlying iliac arteries (eg, May-Thurner syndrome).

INTERVENTIONAL AND SURGICAL MANAGEMENT

Preoperative Planning

- Serologic and hematologic evaluation should include the basic metabolic panel (to assess renal function and concomitant electrolyte abnormalities), complete blood count, and a coagulation profile. It is also important to ascertain the status of antiplatelet or anticoagulation therapies when present (eg, dose, dosing frequency, prior complications).
- Prior to operative intervention, the index treatment limb should be marked as required for World Health Organization's preoperative checklist and "time-out" requirements and extent and severity of edema "baselined" for future comparison.
- When appropriate access requires multiple sites (eg, bilateral femoral and/or internal jugular vein approaches), those should be marked and initialed as well.

Positioning

- Patients can be placed supine or prone depending on the site necessary for access. On the operating table, the patient should be placed supine, with their arms secured at the side to facilitate ancillary access from the groin or neck. When popliteal access is required, prone positioning is required.

TECHNIQUES

PERCUTANEOUS MANAGEMENT OF ILIOFEMORAL DEEP VEIN THROMBOSIS (± VENOUS COMPRESSION SYNDROMES)

Duplex-Guided Femoral Vein Access

- Access site is chosen based on duplex US findings, proximal (peripheral) to the site of thrombotic occlusion. This may be the CFV in patients with isolated iliac DVT or the popliteal or tibial veins in patients with iliofemoral DVT.
- Under ultrasound guidance, a 0.018-in micropuncture set is used to access the target vein. In the setting of proximal obstruction, the vein is typically large and easily identified. Wire and catheter exchange is performed to upsize to a 5-Fr interventional sheath.

Baseline Phlebography

- The initial phlebogram is performed either through the interventional sheath or through a diagnostic catheter advanced to the suspected site of occlusion. When using digital subtraction angiography, a mixture of 50% Visipaque and 50% saline provides adequate volume and visualization while minimizing contrast load.
- The ease with which guidewire passage is accomplished, as well as historical information regarding duration of symptoms, informs interventional decision making. Patients with symptoms of less than 7 days duration are frequently conclusively treated with single-session pharmacomechanical thrombectomy, whereas patients with longer duration will more frequently require pretreatment with multiday courses of catheter-directed thrombolytic therapy. The initial phlebogram is instrumental in determining the course of therapy in this regard. Regardless of approach, the goal of therapy is to achieve rapid thrombus removal, minimize venous obstruction, reduce the likelihood of venous valvular damage, uncover underlying venous compression syndromes, and at least theoretically, reduce the likelihood of symptomatic recurrence.

Catheter-Directed Thrombolysis

- Until recently, catheter-directed thrombolysis has been the mainstay of interventional management for iliofemoral

DVT. Following guidewire traversal of thrombus, treatment length is determined via insertion of a marker catheter. Subsequently, an appropriately sized side-hole infusion catheter is positioned over the occluding thrombus. Infusion catheters come with infusion (perforated segment lengths) ranging from 5 to 50 cm or longer, and infusion segment length should be selected to direct infusate specifically into luminal thrombus only—for example, not into patent luminal segments where it will be rapidly dissipated into the venous and systemic circulation. Prior to initiating infusion, the multipurpose guidewire used to position the catheter is exchanged for a purpose and catheter-specific end-occlusion wire, which typically forces the infusate to exit through the side holes rather than leak out coaxially along the guidewire lumen.

- Once proper positioning is obtained, a continuous infusion of tissue plasminogen activator (tPA or alteplase, Genentech, San Francisco, CA) is initiated at the rate of 0.25 to 1.0 mg/h, depending on the extent of thrombus burden and perceived chronicity. A concurrent, coaxial heparin infusion (400-700 U/h) is administered through the sheath to prevent thrombus accumulation around the infusion system.
- Monitoring in a step-down or intensive care environment is an essential safety requirement during extended periods of catheter-directed intravenous thrombolysis outside of the catheterization laboratory. Fibrinogen levels, coagulation profile, and hematocrit are assessed every 4 to 6 hours. Typically, tPA infusion is halted if/when fibrinogen levels drop below 200 mg/dL or evidence of bleeding is present. Repeat phlebography is performed every 12 to 24 hours to assess therapeutic progress and residual thrombus load. As thrombus burden recedes, replacement catheters with shorter infusion segments are typically chosen to concentrate drug delivery within the remaining clot. Infusion rarely continues beyond 48 hours regardless of progress, as experience has demonstrated that complication rates vary directly with total tPA dosage and length of infusion. Also, infusion rates may be reduced when significant progress is noted during periodic phlebographic assessment, again to reduce risks of dosage-related bleeding complications while still pursuing complete dissolution of clot.
- Ultrasound-assisted thrombolysis using the EKOS infusion catheter (EKOS Corporation, Bothell, WA) may reduce the duration of infusion and total tPA dose. This 6-Fr catheter is also available in multiple infusion lengths and contains a core wire producing ultrasound energy that may disrupt fibrin bonds and increase tPA diffusion within thrombus. Clinical studies have demonstrated equivalent clinical outcomes with reduced infusion times using the EKOS system.

Pharmacomechanical Thrombectomy

- Pharmacomechanical thrombectomy (PMT) uses mechanical forces to assist tPA dispersion within the thrombus, typically during a single treatment session. Concurrent aspiration capabilities help remove thrombus fragments during treatment sessions. Devices currently used for this purpose in the venous system include the AngioJet catheter (MEDRAD, Warrendale, PA) and Trellis (Covidien, Mansfield, MA) infusion systems.
- The AngioJet systems comprise an infusion catheter and dedicated reusable drive unit. Radially oriented infusion ports generate high-pressure jets to disperse heparinized saline, with or without tPA, into the thrombus and an adjacent aspiration port to export fragments and debris.
- The AngioJet catheter is most commonly used in acute iliofemoral occlusion in the "power pulse" mode; in this setting, the aspiration function of the catheter is temporarily disabled, whereas tPA pulsation is delivered directly into the thrombus. Typically, 6 to 8 mg of tPA is delivered in this fashion at the beginning of a treatment session. With power pulse activated, the catheter is repeatedly advanced and withdrawn through the thrombus over the guidewire (**FIGURE 1**). After allowing the tPA to dwell for 10 to 15 minutes, the aspiration function is activated and thrombus removed to the greatest extent possible.

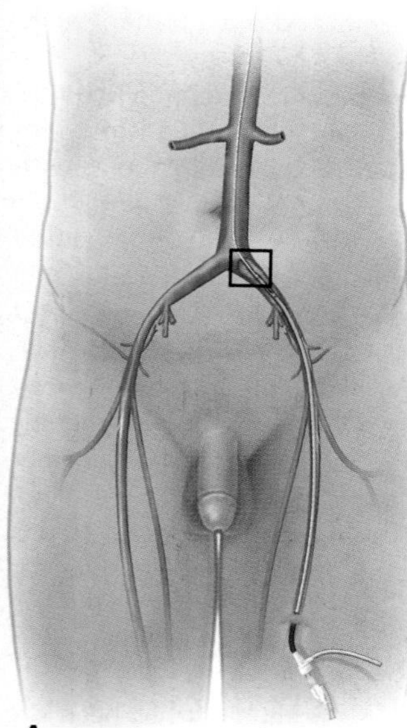

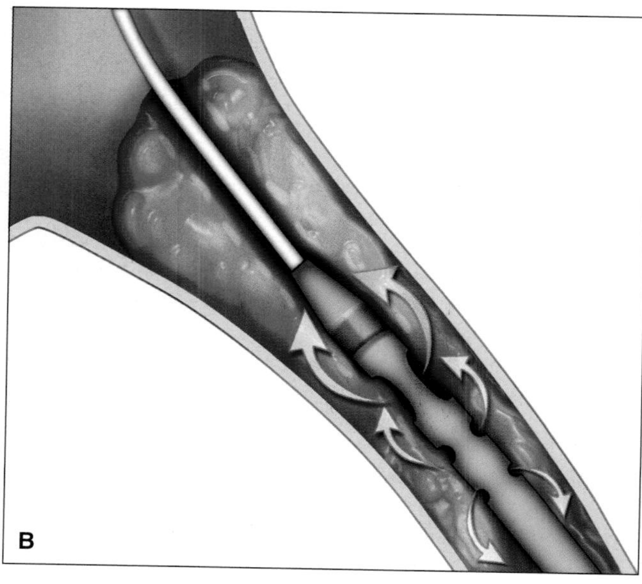

FIGURE 1 ● **A,** The 6-Fr AngioJet thrombectomy catheter is useful in the treatment of DVT. This catheter is advanced through a sheath situated in the popliteal or femoral vein over a 0.035-in guidewire. The catheter has radially oriented infusion side holes that deliver saline and tPA directly into the thrombus **B,** and aspiration ports that remove dissolved thrombus and debris.

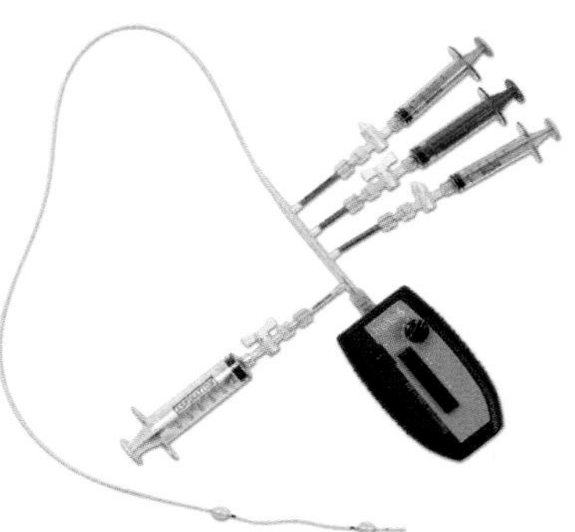

FIGURE 2 ● The Trellis peripheral infusion system is an 8-Fr catheter with a single-use disposable drive unit. The catheter has compliant occlusion balloons that are inflated on either side of the treatment zone after advancing the catheter over the guidewire through the thrombus. The treatment zone of the catheter (either 15 or 30 cm length) contains both infusion side holes and aspiration ports. (©2022 Medtronic. All rights reserved. Used with the permission of Medtronic.)

- The Trellis system is composed of an infusion catheter of either 15- or 30-cm infusion length, with compliant occlusion balloons at either end of the infusion ports (**FIGURE 2**). Following placement over the guidewire, the end occlusion balloons are inflated in order to isolate the area of planned pharmacomechanical thrombolysis (**FIGURE 3**). A sinusoidal dispersion wire is then advanced through the core of the catheter and attached to a disposable drive unit, which when activated uses mechanical forces to disperse the tPA through the thrombus. After an infusion of 6 mg of tPA over the span of 10 minutes, aspiration of thrombus and debris is performed from the treated segment. The occlusion balloons concentrate tPA within the treatment segment, enabling multiple infusion and dispersal sessions during the same procedure with minimal systemic delivery of thrombolytic agent (**FIGURE 4**).

Stenting of Underlying Venous Stenoses or Venous Compression Syndromes

- Following clearance of acute thrombus from the iliofemoral system, underlying venous lesions that provoked DVT formation or focal external compression may become apparent on completion phlebography. These lesions should be addressed during the same treatment session to minimize the risk of recurrence. IVUS may be particularly useful in this regard.

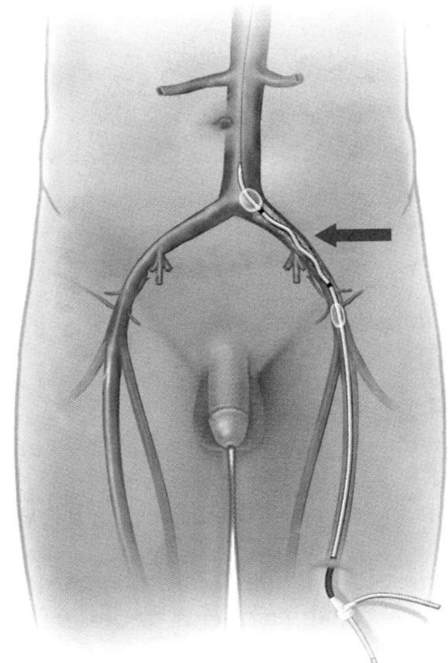

FIGURE 3 ● Once the Trellis catheter is in position, the guidewire is replaced by the mechanical dispersion wire, which is attached to the drive unit and enables the treatment portion of the catheter to oscillate back and forth (*arrow*) to facilitate tPA dispersion. During the 10-minute treatment time, tPA is infused through the infusion port at a rate of 1 mg (1 mL) per minute, and following treatment, the dissolved thrombus and remaining tPA is aspirated through the aspiration port.

- Although fixed stenoses may occur throughout the venous system, the most common location for extrinsic compression occurs at the point where the left common iliac vein passes beneath the overlying right common iliac artery (RCIA) (**FIGURE 5**). After recognizing this compression and successful removal of thrombus proximal or distal to this lesion, the stenosis may be safely resolved with stenting (**FIGURE 6**). This is best performed by upsizing the interventional sheath to at least 10 Fr followed by deployment of a self-expanding, braided, stainless steel Wallstent (Boston Scientific, Watertown, MA). In conjunction with completion venography, IVUS is then used to quantify the extent of residual compression.

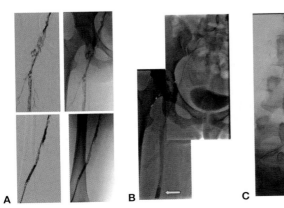

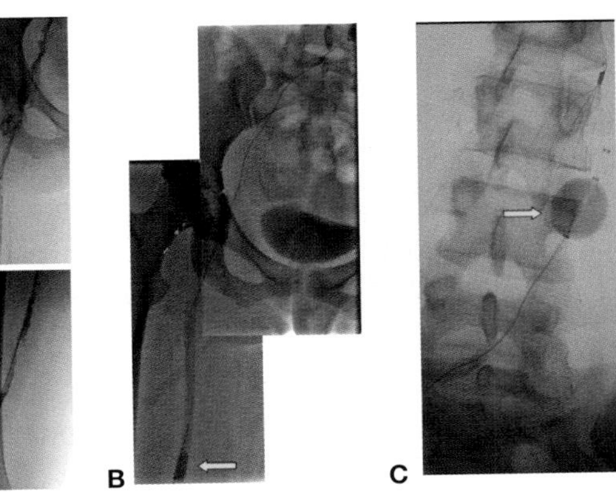

FIGURE 4 ● Patient with left iliofemoral venous thrombosis secondary to May-Thurner syndrome. Note the extensive thrombus within the iliac and femoral veins **(A)**. **B and C,** The patient is being treated in the prone position through popliteal vein access. The Trellis catheter has been inserted and advanced through the thrombus, and the occlusion balloons are inflated on either side of the treatment zone (*arrows*). Note the oscillating dispersion wire that improves tPA delivery during infusion.

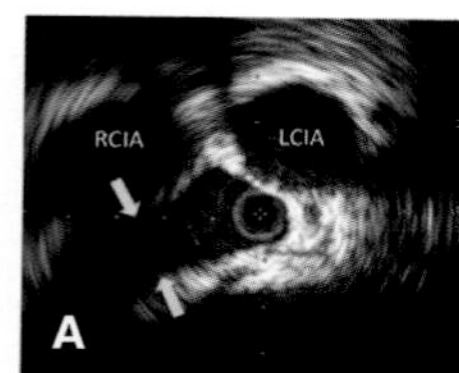

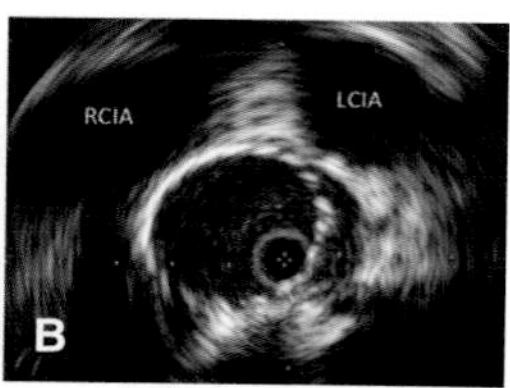

FIGURE 5 ● Intravascular ultrasound is the most sensitive assessment tool for detecting May-Thurner compression of the left common iliac vein. **A,** The RCIA is lying directly over and compressing the left common iliac vein (between *yellow arrows*). **B,** Following stenting of the left common iliac vein, there is complete resolution of the compression by the RCIA.

- Stent diameter is chosen based on IVUS-obtained measurements, but diameters commonly chosen for common iliac vein placement in May-Thurner patients range from 16 to 20 mm. In this application, it is important to choose longer stents that provide additional surface apposition in the common or even external iliac veins to present stent dislodgement and migration. Wallstents are particularly appropriate in this regard as they will shorten or extend in proportion to the ultimate treatment diameter and feature exposed wires at either end to optimize vein wall engagement.
- Once appropriately sited and deployed, poststent dilation is necessary to ensure optimal deployment and migration resistance. Some discomfort will be experienced by the "awake" patient during these procedures, and stenting molding should be guided by patient tolerance under these circumstances.

Completion Imaging

- Completion phlebography documents resolution of target stenosis and reciprocal reduction in collateral venous flow.

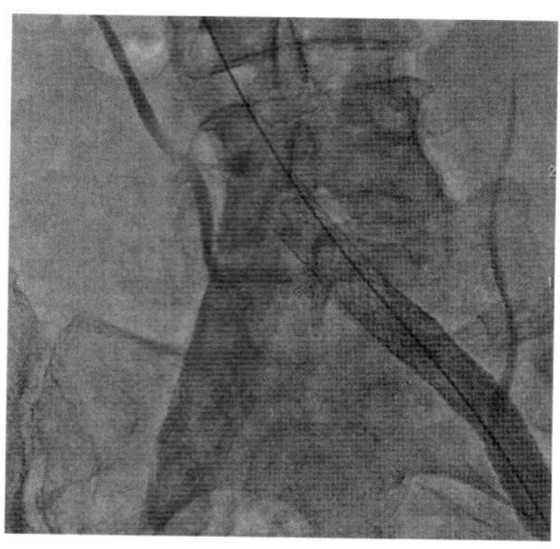

FIGURE 6 ● Stenting of the left common iliac vein for May-Thurner syndrome is performed with a braided self-expanding stainless steel stent, usually in diameters ranging from 16 to 20 mm.

- The presence of persistent collaterals suggests residual venous stenosis or compression; IVUS should be reperformed in this circumstance to confirm wall apposition and stent expansion. Repeat balloon dilation may be necessary in these circumstances until sufficient expansion is achieved.

Closure of the Femoral Vein Access

- Following sheath removal, manual pressure is held over the venous puncture site. Closure devices are not appropriate or indicated for management of venous access.
- Patients need to remain supine for at least 1 hour following sheath removal.
- Therapeutic intravenous anticoagulation with unfractionated heparin is initiated at the completion of the procedure. Maintenance of full anticoagulation without interruption throughout the early postoperative period is imperative to procedural success.

OPERATIVE MANAGEMENT OF ILIOFEMORAL DEEP VEIN THROMBOSIS

Iliac Venous Thrombectomy

- For most clinical scenarios, open venous thrombectomy has largely been supplanted by the interventional, image-guided techniques described in the preceding sections. In patients with limb-threatening phlegmasia cerulean dolens or those with contraindications to lytic therapy or contrast administration, open surgical thrombectomy remains an effective and necessary treatment modality.
- Whenever possible, surgical thrombectomy is performed under general anesthesia with positive pressure ventilation to reduce the risk of intraoperative PE.
- A vertical inguinal incision is made to allow exposure and control of the CFV, femoral vein, saphenofemoral junction, and the profunda femoris vein. Once these venous structures have been exposed, the patient is systemically anticoagulated with 100 U/kg of intravenous heparin.
- A longitudinal venotomy is made in the CFV, and a no. 8 or no. 10 venous thrombectomy catheter is then passed up to the level of the common iliac vein and thrombectomy is performed. Attempts are made to clear the majority of the iliac thrombus before passing the thrombectomy catheter into the vena cava in order to reduce the likelihood of pulmonary embolization.
- Back-bleeding may not be present due to competent iliac vein valves, or back-bleeding can occur from the hypogastric vein even without clearance of the thrombus within the common iliac vein. Therefore, back-bleeding should not be used as an indicator of effective thrombus clearance and venography should be performed as a routine after completion of iliac and infrainguinal thrombectomy.

Infrainguinal Femoral Venous Thrombectomy

- Following iliac venous thrombectomy, heparinized saline should be used to flush the iliac vein, the proximal external iliac vein (or distal CFV) should be clamped, and then any thrombus at the proximal (peripheral) aspect of the venotomy should be extracted with forceps.
- Infrainguinal thrombus can then be removed by manual massage or by exsanguinating the leg with an Esmarch bandage, sequentially applied from the foot to the groin, with sufficient overlap to provide continuous compression (**FIGURE 7**). Clot is delivered through the venotomy at the groin.
- Balloon thrombectomy can be performed using a no. 3 thrombectomy catheter passed from the venotomy in the CFV in a retrograde fashion down toward the popliteal

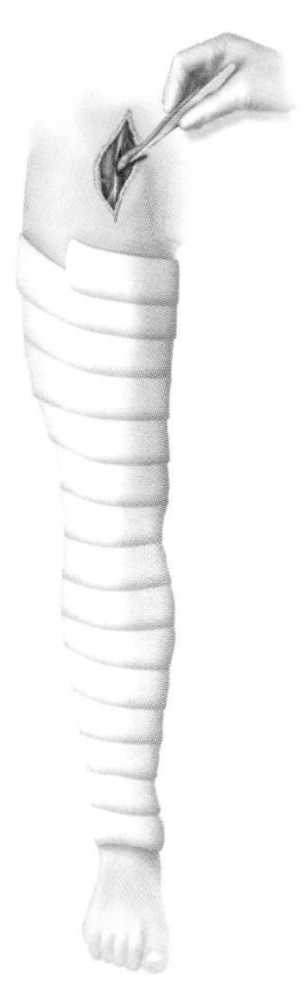

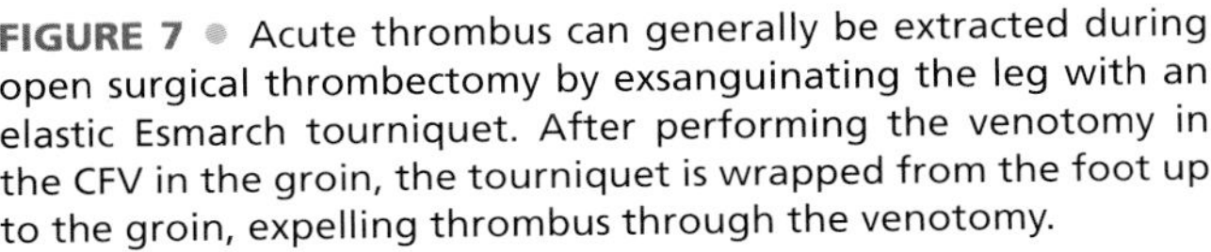

FIGURE 7 ● Acute thrombus can generally be extracted during open surgical thrombectomy by exsanguinating the leg with an elastic Esmarch tourniquet. After performing the venotomy in the CFV in the groin, the tourniquet is wrapped from the foot up to the groin, expelling thrombus through the venotomy.

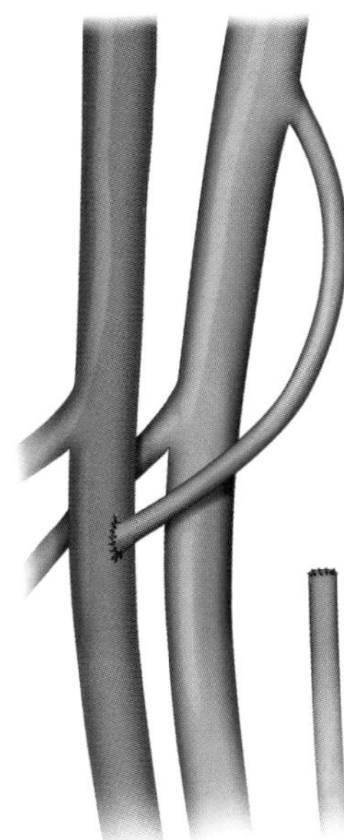

FIGURE 8 ● Patency rate following open surgical thrombectomy is significantly improved by creation of an AVF. Following thrombectomy of the iliac and femoral veins, the venotomy is closed with running monofilament suture and an end-to-side anastomosis is created between the saphenous vein and superficial femoral artery.

and tibial veins. Following thrombectomy, the infrainguinal venous circulation should be flushed vigorously with heparinized saline before closure of the venotomy.

- If infrainguinal thrombus persists after thrombectomy, additional techniques for thrombus removal include on-table tPA administration. For on-table tPA administration, 6 mg of alteplase in 200 mL saline is infused retrograde into the femoral vein through the venotomy in the CFV, then the vein is clamped and the solution is allowed to dwell for 10 to 30 minutes.
- If the infrainguinal venous thrombectomy is not successful due to chronic thrombus in the femoral vein, the femoral vein is then ligated below the profunda, and balloon thrombectomy is then performed on the profunda vein and its branches.
- After open thrombectomy is complete, the venotomy is closed with running continuous monofilament suture, avoiding postclosure stricture of the CFV by precision suture placement. If narrowing is apparent, vein or bovine pericardial patch angioplasty may be performed as necessary to restore luminal diameter.

Adjunct Arteriovenous Fistula Creation

- Rates of rethrombosis following surgical thrombectomy can be as high as 80%. Creation of an arteriovenous fistula (AVF) may significantly reduce this risk and is incorporated in the procedure by most surgeons.
- The same groin incision may be employed for AVF creation, transposing the proximal segment of the ipsilateral greater saphenous vein to the superficial femoral artery (**FIGURE 8**).
- Surgical ligation or interventional occlusion of the AVF is ultimately required for optimal long-term outcome, usually employed within 6 weeks following the procedure. Documented patency of the venous system should be demonstrated on follow-up duplex imaging. Failure to close this fistula may result in significant long-term limb and cardiovascular complications, and follow-up is essential to ensure that this part of the procedure is completed.
- Open thrombectomy procedures by their nature are associated with significant blood loss from the central venous system, and preparations should be made both to crossmatch and bank sufficient packed red blood cells, as well as employ operative scavenging systems to recycle and reinfuse lost blood to ensure that appropriate hemodynamic conditions may be maintained throughout the procedure.

Completion Imaging

- Completion venography of the iliac venous system should be performed following open surgical thrombectomy to assess the adequacy of the thrombectomy.
- Following closure of the venotomy and reestablishment of venous flow through the iliofemoral venous system, an 18-gauge access needle and guidewire can be used to puncture the CFV and place a 5-Fr sheath. Contrast injection directly through this sheath is performed to evaluate the iliac veins and assess for residual thrombus. Following venography, the sheath is removed, and a single monofilament stitch can be used to close the puncture site.

Wound Closure

- A careful search for any transected lymphatics should be conducted prior to wound closure.
- A closed suction drain should be placed in the groin wound to prevent seroma formation.
- The wound is then closed with multilayered running absorbable sutures for hemostatic and lymphostatic closure.

POSTOPERATIVE CARE

- Following open surgical thrombectomy, full therapeutic anticoagulation is imperative to prevent rethrombosis. An intravenous heparin infusion is immediately initiated and maintained for 24 to 48 hours before the patient is transitioned to oral anticoagulation with a low-molecular-weight heparin bridge prior to discharge.
- Ambulation should begin on the first postoperative day. Patients may usually be discharged within 48 to 72 hours following thrombectomy.
- On discharge, the patient should be placed in elastic compression stockings (30- to 40-mm Hg ankle gradient), and the importance of compression should be stressed to the patient in the discharge instructions.

OUTCOMES

Endovascular Intervention

- Pharmacomechanical venous thrombectomy provides clinical success rates of 70% to 100% and may reduce the incidence of the PTS, although this latter conclusion remains controversial.
- Following successful procedures, long-term venous patency is reported at 84% in 5 years.
- Valvular competence is preserved at 80% in 5 years and 56% in 10 years in recent series.

Surgical Thrombectomy

- Surgical thrombectomy provides long-term iliac venous patency, with rates approaching 80% when combined with inclusion of a temporary AVF.
- At 5 years, over one-third of patients can be expected to be symptom free and have retained valvular competence.

REFERENCES

1. Vedantham S, Grassi CJ, Ferral H, et al. Reporting standards for endovascular treatment of lower extremity deep vein thrombosis. *J Vasc Intervent Radiol.* 2005;17:417-434.
2. Kahn SR, Ginsberg JS. Relationship between deep venous thrombosis and the postthrombotic syndrome. *Arch Intern Med.* 2004;164:17-26.
3. Porter JM, Moneta GL. Reporting standards in venous disease: an update. International consensus committee on chronic venous disease. *J Vasc Surg.* 1995;21:635-645.
4. Rutherford RB, Padberg FT, Comerota AJ, et al. Venous severity scoring: an adjunct to venous outcome assessment. *J Vasc Surg.* 2000;31:1307-1312.
5. Prandoni P, Lensing AW, Prins MH, et al. Below-knee elastic compression stockings to prevent the postthrombotic syndrome. *Ann Intern Med.* 2004;141:249-256.
6. Brandjes DP, Buller HR, Heijboer H, et al. Randomized trial of effect of compression stockings in patients with symptomatic proximal-vein thrombosis. *Lancet.* 1997;349:759-762.
7. Delis KT, Bountouroglou D, Mansfield AO. Venous claudication in iliofemoral thrombosis: long-term effects on venous hemodynamics, clinical status, and quality of life. *Ann Surg.* 2004;239:118-126.
8. Kearon C, Ginsberg JS, Hirsh J. The role of venous ultrasonography in the diagnosis of suspected deep venous thrombosis and pulmonary embolism. *Ann Intern Med.* 1998;129:1044-1049.
9. Weinmann EE, Salzman EW. Deep-vein thrombosis. *N Engl J Med.* 1994;15:1630-1641.
10. Zontsich T, Turetschek K, Baldt M. CT-phlebography. A new method for the diagnosis of venous thrombosis of the upper and lower extremities. *Radiology.* 1998;38:586-590.
11. Burke B, Sostman HD, Carroll BA, et al. The diagnostic approach to deep venous thrombosis. Which technique? *Clin Chest Med.* 1995;16:253-268.
12. Allie DE, Hebert CJ, Lirtzman MD, et al. Novel simultaneous combination chemical thrombolysis/rheolytic thrombectomy therapy for acute limb ischemia: the power pulse spray technique. *Catheter Cardiovasc Interv.* 2004;63(4):512-522.

Chapter 35 Vena Cava Filter Placement and Removal

Courtney M. Morgan and John E. Rectenwald

DEFINITION

- An inferior vena cava (IVC) filter is a device designed to filter venous blood returning to the right-sided heart and prevent large venous thrombi from the lower extremities and vena cava below the IVC filter from reaching the pulmonary arteries. Venous thrombus reaching the pulmonary arteries (pulmonary embolus, PE) can inhibit oxygenation of blood in the pulmonary capillaries and venous return to the left-sided heart resulting in a decreased arterial oxygen saturation. In addition, pulmonary emboli increase pulmonary artery pressures resulting in pulmonary hypertension and right heart strain or failure. The combination of these two phenomena may result in significant morbidity and mortality in those in which it occurs.
- Inferior vena cava filters are made from various metal alloys including iron, chromium and nickel (stainless steel), nickel and titanium (Nitinol), or cobalt chromium alloy (Elgiloy). They are generally designed in a classic conical design (**FIGURE 1**) although alternative variations exist. The conical design is very efficient and allows up to 70% of the cone volume to be occupied with thrombus with only a 50% obstruction of cross-sectional area of the IVC. In addition, it allows captured thrombus to be centered within the vena cava, thus allowing venous flow around the clot to facilitate thrombolysis.[1] IVC filters are all designed to be placed within the vena cava through a transvenous route primarily by the internal jugular or common femoral venous route. IVC filters are generally designed to be oversized compared to the IVC at rest and are therefore held in place in the IVC by a combination of the radial force and the presence of hooks at the ends of the filter struts that penetrate the wall of the vena cava.

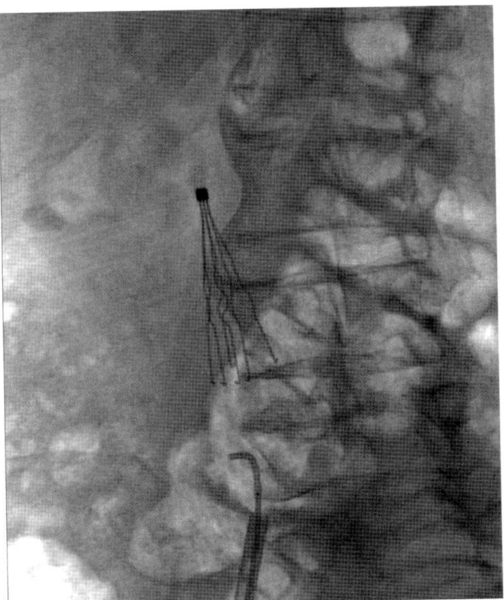

FIGURE 1 ● A Greenfield Stainless Steel over-the-wire inferior vena cava filter demonstrating the classic conical design structure. This design allows maximal capture of thrombus while retaining IVC patency as well as promoting venous blood flow around the thrombus to facilitate thrombolysis.

Types of IVC Filters

- Permanent filters, as the name implies, originally developed in the 1960s to 1970s, are intended to be placed in patients indefinitely and are designed to provide life-long filtration, with features that allow maximal fixation to the vena cava intimal surface and promote tissue ingrowth. Permanent IVC filters include the Greenfield Stainless Steel filter (Boston Scientific, MA. USA), the VenaTech LP filter (B. Braun, PA, USA), the TrapEase filter (Cordis, FL, USA), the Simon Nitinol filter (B. Braun, PA, USA), and the Bird's Nest filter (Cook Medical, IN, USA) (**FIGURE 2**).
- Retrievable IVC filters, developed in the early 2000s, are filters that are intentionally designed for removal once the patient no longer needs IVC filtration for the prevention of PE. They are specifically designed to be reconstrained and removed and frequently have hooks incorporated into their designs to facilitate loop ensnarement of the filter and subsequent retrieval. As detailed below, these design features are thought to contribute to the increased complication rates associated with retrievable filters. Examples of currently available retrievable IVC filters include the Günther Tulip and Celect filters (Cook Medical, IN, USA), OptEase filter (Cordis FL, USA), the Option ELITE filter (Argon Medical, TX, USA), the Denali Filter (Bard Medical, NJ, USA) (**FIGURE 3**), and ALN filter (KM Medical, MA, USA).
- Convertible IVC filters are a relatively new concept the first of which only being released in the last few years. This category of IVC filters are intended to be placed permanently but only provide temporary IVC filtration. They convert from an IVC filter to what is essentially a caval stent by means of an absorbable suture or cap that can be removed percutaneously. Examples of this category of IVC filters includes the Sentry Bioconvertible filter (Boston Scientific, MA, USA) and the VenaTech Convertible filter (B. Braun, PA, USA) (**FIGURE 4**). All retrievable and convertible IVC filters are approved by the US Food and Drug Administration for permanent use.

IVC Filter Retrieval

- The rationale for removal of IVC filters has evolved over time. In 1998, PREPIC, a prospective, randomized study that compared patients with IVC filters in place to anticoagulation concluded that patients with filters were at lower risk for symptomatic PE but elevated risk of recurrent deep

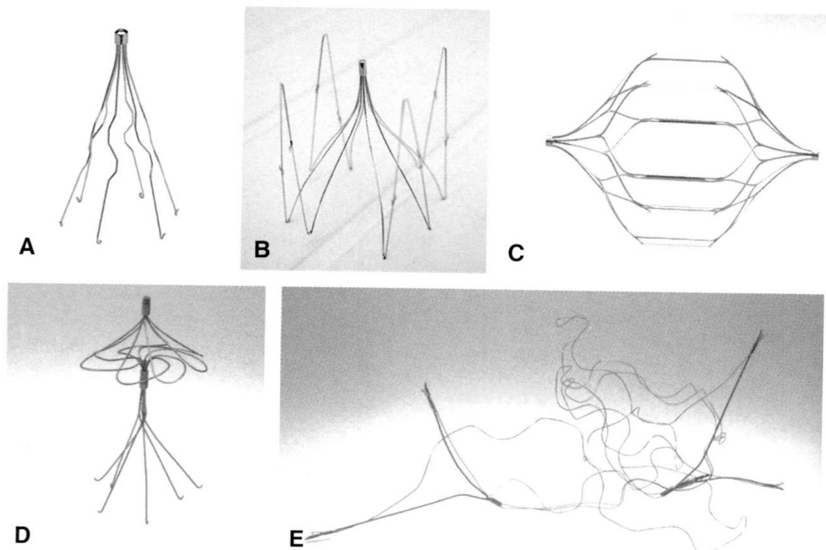

FIGURE 2 ● FDA-approved Permanent IVC filters. From left to right: **A,** Boston Scientific Greenfield Stainless Steel over-the-wire filter **B,** B. Braun Vena Tech LP filter; **C,** Cordis Trapease Filter; **D,** BD Interventional Systems, Simon Nitinol Filter; and **E,** Cook Medical Cook Medical Gianturco-Roehm Bird Nest filter. (A, Image provided courtesy of Boston Scientific. Copyright © 2022 Boston Scientific Corporation or its affiliates. All rights reserved. B, © B. Braun SE. C, Cordis, Miami Lakes, FL. D and E, Courtesy of Cook Medical, Bloomington, Ind.)

vein thrombosis (DVT).[2] This finding, combined with the data suggesting that risk of death from venous thromboembolism (VTE) is highest in the first 2 weeks after occurrence,[3] spurred the development of IVC filters that could be retrieved to allow for protection from PE when at risk early in the course of VTE and then removed to decrease the risk of recurrent DVT. While this was the intent of retrievable IVC filter, in practicality very few (as low as 5%) of these retrievable filters were actually retrieved.[4-6]

- Recently, the FDA published two safety communications regarding retrievable IVC filters based on analysis of the poor long-term performance of retrievable filters observed in the FDA's Manufacturer and User Facility Device Experience database.[7] Retrievable filters appeared to have significantly higher rates of complications when compared to traditional, permanent IVC filters. The first of these communications, published in August of 2010, recommended that "implanting physicians and clinicians responsible for the ongoing care of

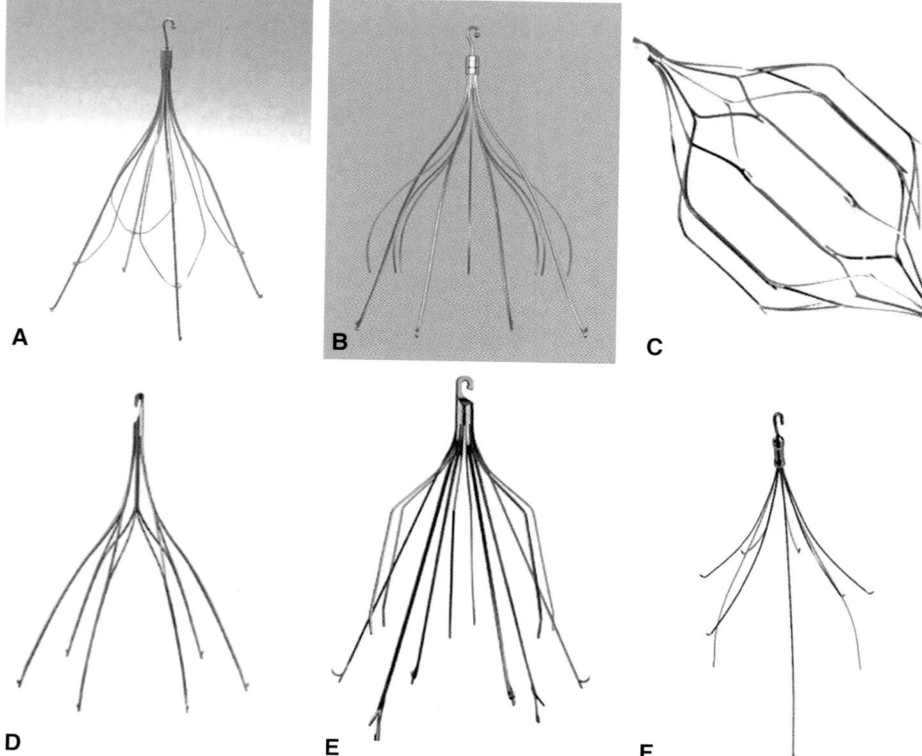

FIGURE 3 ● FDA-approved Retrievable IVC filters. From left to right. **A,** Cook Medical Günther Tulip filter; **B,** Cook Medical Celect Platinum filter; **C,** Cordis Optease Filter; **D,** Argon Medical Devices Option ELITE filter; **E,** BD Interventional Systems Denali filter; and **F,** ALN Optional Filter with hook. (A and B, Courtesy of Cook Medical, Bloomington, Ind. C, Cordis, Miami Lakes, FL. D, Argon Medical. E, Courtesy and © Becton, Dickinson and Company. F, Used with permission from ALN.)

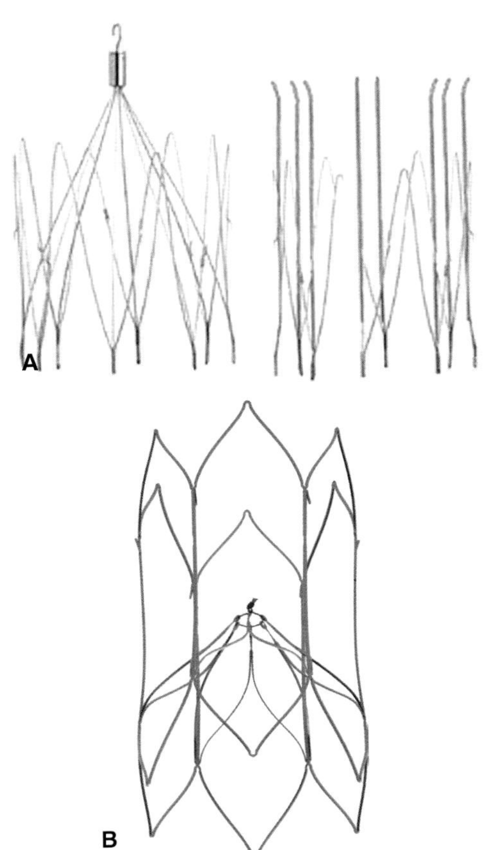

FIGURE 4 ● FDA-approved Convertible IVC filters. **A,** B. Braun Vena Tech Convertible filter, and **B,** Boston Scientific Sentry Bioconvertible filter. (A, © B. Braun SE. B, Image provided courtesy of Boston Scientific. Copyright © 2022 Boston Scientific Corporation or its affiliates. All rights reserved.)

patients with retrievable IVC filters consider removing the filter as soon as protection from PE is no longer needed." In May of 2014, the second FDA safety alert letter was published regarding its own decision-analysis regarding IVC filter removal in patients without pulmonary embolism. Based on this analysis, this alert recommends that if the retrievable filter is no longer needed it should be removed between 29 and 54 days after implantation. Based on the FDA's model, the risks of the presence of an IVC filter outweigh the benefits after this time interval.[8]

DIFFERENTIAL DIAGNOSIS

- Patients who are candidates for IVC filters generally present with the signs and symptoms of VTE. These may include unilateral extremity swelling and pain or bilateral lower extremity edema in the case of extensive iliofemoral DVT.
- Patients who suffer PE frequently experience sudden pleuritic chest pain associated with shortness of breath, hypoxia, and signs of right-sided heart failure.
- The diagnosis of VTE can be readily established by assessing for risk factors of VTE and ruling out other potential causes such as lymphedema, chronic venous insufficiency, or cellulitis in the case of extremity DVT and pneumonia, myocardial infarction, pericarditis, and others in the case of pulmonary embolus.

PATIENT HISTORY AND PHYSICAL FINDINGS

- In the United States, DVT occurs in approximately 1 per 1000 people each year. Nearly one-third of patients with symptomatic untreated DVT present with PE.[9] Anticoagulation is the treatment of choice for most cases of VTE, with evidence-based guidelines supporting the use of a vena cava filter when anticoagulation is not possible due to contraindications to anticoagulation or hemorrhagic complications, recurrent PE despite therapeutic anticoagulation, or an inability to achieve therapeutic anticoagulation.[10]
- Expanded indications for prophylactic use of IVC filters are based on clinical factors that place a patient at high risk for both PE and bleeding, making the use of prophylactic anticoagulation for prevention of VTE prohibitive.[11]
- Likewise, relative indications for filter placement include poor compliance with anticoagulation, free-floating iliocaval thrombus, renal cell carcinoma with extension into the renal vein and vena cava, thrombolysis or thromboembolectomy of the iliofemoral veins or IVC, and risk of recurrent PE with pre-existing pulmonary hypertension or limited cardiopulmonary reserve.
- Filter placement may also be considered after DVT in patients with cancer, burns, and pregnancy or for prophylaxis in multitrauma patients, including those with severe closed head injury (Glasgow Coma Scale score <8), spinal cord injury, complex pelvic or multiple long-bone fractures, intra-abdominal injury, pelvic or retroperitoneal hematoma, and ocular trauma.
- Contraindications to vena cava filter placement are few and include chronic occlusion or significant compression of the vena cava and agenesis of the vena cava.
- Upper extremity DVT is becoming more common with the increasing use of central venous lines (particularly peripherally inserted central catheters or P.I.C.C. lines), pacemakers, and implantable defibrillators, with an estimated risk of PE approaching 9% in some series.[12] Standard treatment involves anticoagulation, but with contraindications or complications arising from anticoagulation, superior vena cava (SVC) filter placement can be considered.
    - Since there are no filters specifically designed for placement in the SVC, an adaptation of current IVC filter and available techniques is required. A conical filter with a filter leg hook attachment is most appropriate that these are placed at the confluence of the innominate veins. Filter length should be considered to prevent protrusion into the right atrium. Filter placement is not recommended within an SVC with a diameter >28 to 30 mm.

IMAGING AND OTHER DIAGNOSTIC STUDIES

- In general, there are no required imaging studies prior to placing an IVC filter. This is due to the fact that an IVC venogram is performed at the time of IVC filter placement.

Despite this, the vast majority of patients in which IVC filters are being considered have already had computed tomography (CT) scans or other imaging previously. These studies can be reviewed with special attention paid to the appearance of the common femoral and iliac veins as well as that of the inferior vena cava. Noting the location of the lowest renal vein in relation to the adjacent vertebral bodies can also be a helpful maneuver.

- In patients with renal insufficiency or severe iodinated contrast allergy, alternative contrast agents such as carbon dioxide (CO_2)[13-15] and even gadolinium[13,16] can be used to define and evaluate the IVC and other structures immediately prior to IVC filter placement (**FIGURE 5**). These alternatives to iodinate contrast agents allow for evaluation of IVC patency, presence and location of thrombus, caval anatomy, and location of the renal veins.
- The use of both intravenous[17,18] and transabdominal ultrasound[19,20] for IVC filter placement has become more mainstream. These techniques allow for filter placement without the use of x-ray or contrast agents and are especially well suited for intensive care patients who cannot be easily transported to the fluoroscopy suite for the procedure.[18,21]

SURGICAL MANAGEMENT

Preoperative Planning

- The patient is examined and a thorough history is completed. A review of the indications for filter placement should be conducted prior to filter placement. Based on the clinical scenario, either a permanent or a retrievable filter should be selected for use.

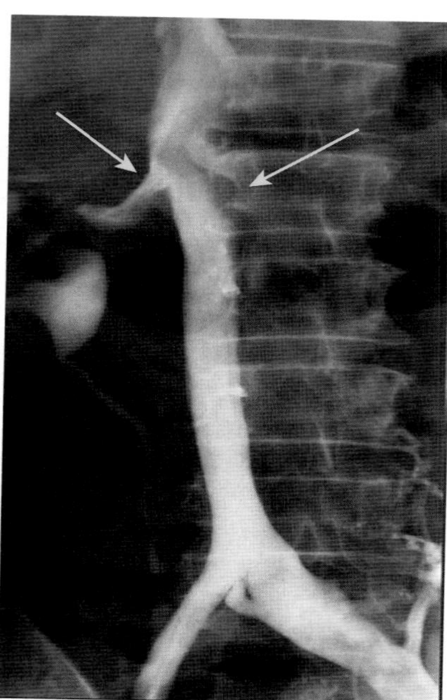

FIGURE 5 ● An example of the use of alternative contrast agent for real-time imaging of the vena cava for IVC filter placement. This carbon dioxide (CO_2) inferior vena cavagram well demonstrates the bilateral iliac veins, the inferior vena cava, and the bilateral renal veins (*yellow arrows*).

- Central venous catheters that may be present at the proposed site of access or that extend across the intended location for filter deployment should be removed.
- Coagulopathy or other hematologic issues should be assessed. Discontinuation of anticoagulation before the procedure should be considered based on clinical indication and hemorrhagic risk profile.
- Preoperative imaging studies such as duplex ultrasound or available computed tomography (CT) images, if available, should be reviewed to identify anatomic vena cava variants or other venous anomalies that could potentially alter the treatment plan. During filter placement, selective venography may also help to identify venous anomalies. In this regard, accessory renal veins, retroaortic, and circumferential left renal vein anomalies (5%-7%) are the most common anatomic variation but do not affect filter position. Transposition of the vena cava to the left side with drainage into the left renal vein is rare (0.2%-0.5%) but necessitates accurate anatomic definition. Duplication of the vena cava is also rare (0.2%-0.3%), with the right-sided IVC draining the right iliac vein and right renal vein, whereas the left-sided IVC drains the left iliac veins and joins the left renal vein where it crosses over into the right-sided vena cava. Undiagnosed duplication of the IVC may leave the duplicated vena cava unprotected against PE and would require either separate filters in each vena cava or a suprarenal filter placed above the junction of the left renal vein and the right-sided vena cava. Agenesis of the vena cava is extremely rare, but when present, filter insertion should be avoided, although filter placement into an enlarged azygous segment has been described.[22]
- A preprocedure duplex ultrasound should be obtained to evaluate the presence of venous thrombosis at the intended percutaneous access site or extending into iliofemoral or vena cava. Jugular venous access may be needed if femoral vein access is not possible. A vena cavagram should be performed just before positioning and deployment of a filter to assess the presence and location of any thrombus within the vena cava. The presence of thrombus in the infrarenal IVC may necessitate suprarenal filter placement.
- Ultrasound-guided percutaneous access is generally recommended to allow for direct visualization of the access vein and real-time image guidance for venous cannulation, as well as to avoid concomitant arterial injury.
- The diameter of the IVC, including major and minor axes, should be measured either from venography, transabdominal duplex ultrasound, intravascular ultrasound (IVUS), or a preprocedure CT scan to assist in appropriate filter selection. Vena cava diameter measurements can vary depending on intravascular fluid status and respiratory variation. Vena cava geometry can also range from circular to elliptical.[18] Major and minor axes both should be measured. Nearly all current FDA-approved filters are indicated for vena cava diameters of less than 28 to 30 mm. In patients with a "megacava" defined as a vena cava with diameters larger than 30 mm, a Bird Nest IVC filter can be used within the enlarged IVC. If a Bird Nest IVC filter is not immediately available, either bilateral iliac vein IVC filters or placement for a filter within the suprarenal vena cava (if <30 mm in diameter) can be considered.

- Accurate identification of both renal and common iliac veins is important before filter deployment. The tip of the filter should be positioned at, or below, the lowest renal vein after confirmation of adequate clearance of the filter base above the iliac vein confluence.

Positioning

- The patient is brought to the endovascular suite and placed supine on a radiolucent table.
- If the procedure is being done in the operating room, the patient should be positioned on the radiolucent operating table such that the portable C-arm can be maneuvered over the patient's groin and abdomen for sufficient fluoroscopic visualization of the femoral and iliac vessels as well as the inferior vena cava.
- The patient's arms are placed at their sides and secured to facilitate imaging of the upper abdomen for filter placement.
- If the IVC filter is being delivered via the internal jugular vein, a shoulder roll should be placed beneath the patient's scapulae and the neck extended. In addition, the patient's head should be rotated to the contralateral side. These manipulations better position the internal jugular vein for access.
- In an obese patient, retraction of the abdominal pannus from the groin onto the abdomen can facilitate access of the common femoral vein.

INFERIOR VENA CAVA FILTER PLACEMENT FROM THE GROIN

- The site of puncture is first surveyed with duplex ultrasound to identify the access vessel, nearby structures and assure patency of the vein. The site is then prepped and surgically draped appropriately.
- Local anesthesia is obtained with 1% lidocaine injection over the site of puncture and into the subcutaneous tissues. Conscious sedation can also be utilized if appropriate.
- The right common femoral vein is access with either a 21-gauge micropuncture set or a 19-gauge single-wall puncture needle. The left common femoral vein can also be used for filter placement, however, this approach is less of a straight shot to the IVC and can result in a deployed IVC filter with significantly more tilt.
- After successful access of the common femoral vein, a 0.035 inch "J" or Bentson wire is then advanced through the micropuncture sheath or single-wall puncture needle into the vein and advanced into the inferior vena cava.
- Once the guidewire is in position, a 6-Fr sheath is placed over the wire to secure hemostatic venous access. A 5-Fr marker flush catheter is then advanced over the wire and positioned in the cephalad portion right iliac vein just below the confluence of the inferior vena cava. Many IVC filter manufacturers have designed their IVC filter delivery catheters/sheaths such that the inner dilator functions as a flush catheter and recommend placement of the sheath directly thus skipping this step. The authors choose not to do this as the use of a 6-Fr sheath and flush catheter avoids the risk of unnecessarily opening the IVC filter packaging in the event that an IVC filter cannot be placed such as an occluded IVC for thrombus in the vena cava where the filter is to be positioned.
- An initial contrast venography is performed through a flush catheter or filter delivery sheath to define anatomy and confirm absence of thrombus. A marker or calibrated catheter is positioned at or just below the confluence of the IVC and iliac veins, and a power injection of 20 mL/sec of contrast for 2 seconds for a total of 40 mL ("20 for 40") should confirm normal vena cava and iliac vein relationships. Performance of a breath hold or vagal maneuver will augment filling of the cava. The marker flush catheter facilitates accurate measurement of the diameter of the IVC.
- The inferior vena cava venogram is then carefully reviewed. Special note is made of any thrombus within the vena cava and its location. The contralateral common iliac vein is visualized to confirm normal caval anatomy. The diameter of the IVC is measured with the marker flush catheter to assure that the diameter is not greater than 28 to 30 mm. Finally, the renal veins are identified either directly by contrast refluxed into the vessels or indirectly but the mixing of uncontrasted blood from the renal veins with contrasted blood from the blood within the IVC. The level of the lowest renal vein is then related to a bony anatomic landmark, usually an endplate of a lumbar vertebral body or a vertebral disc space.
- Selection of an IVC filter oriented to the specific approach is essential. In this case, a *femoral*-oriented IVC filter should be selected. Use of a *jugular*-oriented IVC filter from the femoral approach will result in a maldeployed or "up-side down" filter. Review of the device instructions for use is essential. Depending on the specific filter device used, the deployment sequence and technique can vary. Understanding sheath and delivery catheter interactions is essential for successful and accurate deployment of each filter type.
- In general, however, once the IVC filter package is opened and the IVC filter and delivery catheter is flushed, the 5-Fr flush catheter is removed over a stiff 0.035 wire (such as an Amplatz). The skin incision and venotomy are then serially dilated to the size of the delivery sheath. This ranges from 7 to 9 Fr for most devices. The IVC filter delivery sheath is advanced over the wire and positioned appropriately.
- The wire and inner dilator for the filter delivery sheath is removed and the IVC filter with its delivery catheter is advanced into and secured to the filter delivery sheath.
- The authors prefer to have the filter delivery sheath advanced above the level of filter deployment so that the filter can be advanced to the level of deployment within the delivery sheath. The delivery sheath can then be retracted exposing the filter for deployment. This method avoids retracting or worse advancing the exposed IVC filter. Advancing the exposed IVC filter without the benefit of wire guidance risks perforation of the IVC and maldeployment of the IVC filter (**FIGURE 6**).

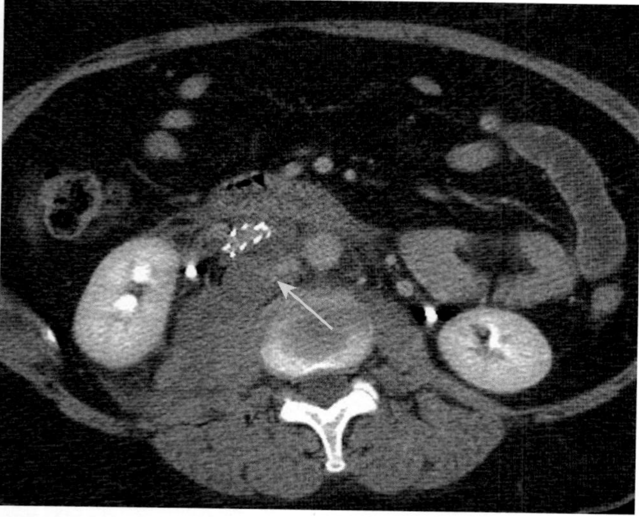

FIGURE 6 ● A computed tomographic venogram demonstrating inferior vena cava perforation and surrounding hematoma (*yellow arrow*) after infrarenal IVC filter placement. The filter and IVC are patent but compressed by the resulting retroperitoneal hematoma.

- Once the filter is in the correct position based upon landmarks established on review of the IVC venogram, the filter is deployed according to the manufacturer's instruction for use. Actual deployment of the filter can be accomplished by simple retraction of the deployment sheath over the IVC filter or exposure of the IVC filter and then deployment via a "pin and pull" technique.
- Once the IVC filter has been successfully deployed and is in position, the delivery sheath and catheter are retracted caudally and magnified anterior-posterior and orthogonal single shot x-ray images are obtained. These images are carefully reviewed to assure that the IVC filter has been fully and correctly deployed without crossing of the filter tines or significant tilting with in the vena cava.
- Following successful deployment of an IVC filter, all wires and catheters are removed and pressure is held at the femoral venotomy site until hemostasis is achieved. A sterile dressing is placed and the patient is taken back to the postoperative care unit and remains flat for 4 hours. The patient is then taken back to their inpatient unit or allowed to ambulate and then discharged home.

INFERIOR VENA CAVA FILTER PLACEMENT FROM THE NECK

For the sake of brevity, identical steps in placement of an IVC filter from the internal jugular vein that are identical to placement from the common femoral vein are omitted or truncated.

- As previously mentioned, a shoulder roll is placed beneath the patient scapulae and the neck extended. The patient's head is then rotated toward the opposite side of the site of access.
- The site of puncture is first surveyed with duplex ultrasound to identify the access vessel, nearby structures and assure patency of the vein. The site is then prepped and surgically draped appropriately.
- The right jugular vein is access with either a 21-gauge micropuncture set or a 19 gauge single-wall puncture needle after the area is anesthetized. A 0.035 inch "J" or Bentson wire is then advanced through the micropuncture sheath or needle into the vein and advanced into the inferior vena cava. This may require fluoroscopic guidance and the use of an angled catheter to guide the wire and traverse the right atrium, avoid the right-heart and gain access to the IVC. If catheter guidance is require for traversal of the right heart, then the 6 Fr. sheath is placed at this time with the guide wire within the right atrium or ventricle. Care is taken to monitor the patient's cardiac telemetry and retract the guide wire or catheter if cardiac arrhythmias are observed.
- Once the guidewire is in position and a sheath is in place, the marker flush catheter is advanced into the right or left iliac vein just below the confluence of the inferior vena cava. Again, the IVC filter delivery sheath with the specially designed flush inner dilator can be used instead.
- A power injection of 20 mL/sec of contrast for 2 seconds for a total of 40 mL ("20 for 40") is injected for the vena cavagram prior to IVC filter placement.
- The inferior vena cava venogram is then carefully reviewed as previously detailed and the level of the lowest renal vein is identified and referenced to a boney anatomic landmark.
- Again, selection of a correctly oriented IVC filter delivery device is essential. In this case, a *jugular*-oriented IVC filter should be selected. Use of a *femoral*-oriented IVC filter from the femoral approach will result in a maldeployed filter. Review of the devices instruction for use is essential.
- The IVC filter package is opened and the IVC filter and delivery catheter is flushed, the 5-Fr flush catheter is removed over a stiff 0.035 wire. The skin incision and venotomy are serially dilated. The IVC filter delivery sheath is advanced over the wire and positioned appropriately.
- The wire and inner dilator for the filter delivery sheath is removed and the IVC filter with its delivery catheter is advanced into and secured to the filter delivery sheath.
- Once the filter is in the correct position based upon landmarks established on review of the IVC venogram, the filter is deployed according to the manufacturer's instruction for use. Actual deployment of the filter can be accomplished by simple retraction of the deployment sheath via a "pin and pull" technique.
- Once the IVC filter has been successfully deployed and is in position, the delivery sheath and catheter is retracted cranially and AP and orthogonal single-shot x-rays are obtained to confirm proper filter deployment.
- All wires and catheters are removed and pressure is held at the femoral venotomy site until hemostasis is achieved. For the internal jugular approach, the authors make a point of always placing an occlusive sterile dressing in order to decrease the risk of potential air embolus. The patient allowed to sit upright and is taken back to the postoperative unit. Unlike the femoral approach, there is no need for the patient to remain flat for any period of time. The patient is then taken back to their inpatient unit or allowed to ambulate and then discharged home.

SUPERIOR VENA CAVA FILTER PLACEMENT

Practitioners should consult the applicable Instructions For Use for device indications and contraindications.

A SVC filter can be placed from the common femoral, the internal jugular, and even the subclavian veins depending on circumstances. The femoral approach to placement may be limited by the length of IVC filter delivery devices and patient height. In general, the internal jugular approach is preferred.

- The patient is positioned as previously described for an IVC filter placement placed from the right internal jugular vein approach with the head extended and the neck rotated to the patient's left.
- The skin in anesthetized and the internal jugular vein is punctured and cannulated with a wire under real-time ultrasound guidance.
- A 0.035 guidewire is advanced into and ideally through the right heart and into the perihepatic IVC. A 6-Fr sheath is placed over the wire to secure access.
- A marker pigtail catheter is placed and a venogram is obtained to identify the innominate vein and SVC confluence and unexpected anatomic venous anomalies. Duplication of the SVC occurs in 0.1% to 0.3%. The presence of occlusion, stenosis, or thrombus in the SVC precludes filter placement.
- The IVC filter is then deployed within the SVC using the previously described methods.
- Correct orientation of the filter requires use of a *jugular* filter kit from the *femoral* position or a *femoral* filter set deployed from the *jugular* or *subclavian* position. The filter is deployed so that leg hooks attach at the confluence of the innominate veins and the tip extends into the SVC (see **FIGURE 7**). Care must be taken to avoid filter intrusion in to the right atrium as this may predispose the patient to cardiac arrhythmias and filter migration.
- A chest radiograph is obtained to confirm filter position following placement.

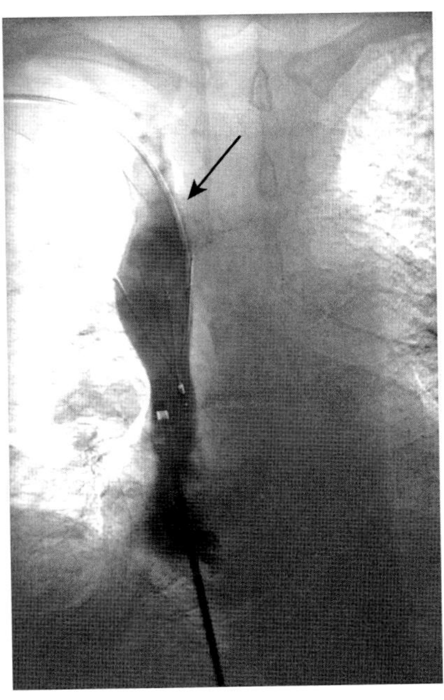

FIGURE 7 • A superior vena cavagram with SVC filter in place. The superior vena cava filter is positioned with the filter base just central to the confluence of the innominate veins (*black arrow*) and the tip proximal to the right atrium.

INFERIOR VENA CAVA FILTER RETRIEVAL

- Prior to an attempt at IVC filter retrieval, the filter should be evaluated radiologically to detect potential technical problems that may complicate or prohibit removal.
- Removal is contraindicated if conventional or CT venography or duplex ultrasound demonstrates thrombus in the filter (**FIGURE 8**).
- Imaging that suggests filter migration, severe tilt, fracture, or other mechanical failure may suggest the need for use of more advanced techniques for IVC filter retrieval.
- Nearly all current retrievable IVC filters require removal from a neck approach due to the conical design of most filters at present.
- For IVC filter retrieval, the patient is positioned and prepped as if undergoing IVC filter from the right internal jugular approach. The skin is anesthetized and the internal jugular vein accessed using real-time ultrasound guidance. Conscious sedation is frequently employed.
- A straight 0.035 guide wire is advanced through the SVC, right atrium of the heart, and into the IVC and a 6-Fr sheath is placed. A 5-Fr straight flush catheter is advanced over the wire. It is the author's preference to avoid recurved wire and catheters for retrieval to avoid the possibility of ensnarement of these instruments with the IVC filter.

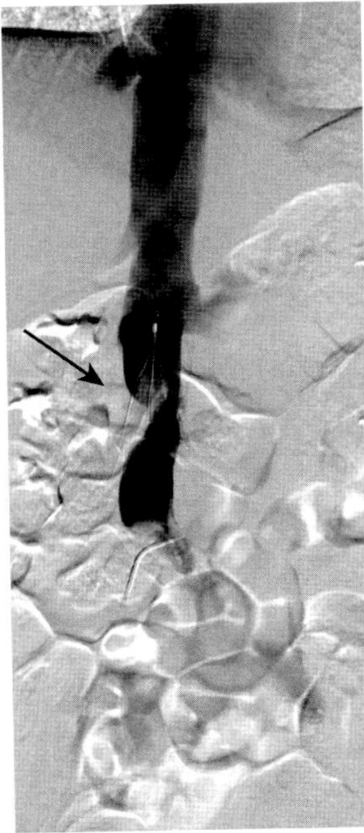

FIGURE 8 • Visualized thrombus (*black arrow*) within an IVC filter on vena cavagram obtained prior to a planned retrieval attempt.

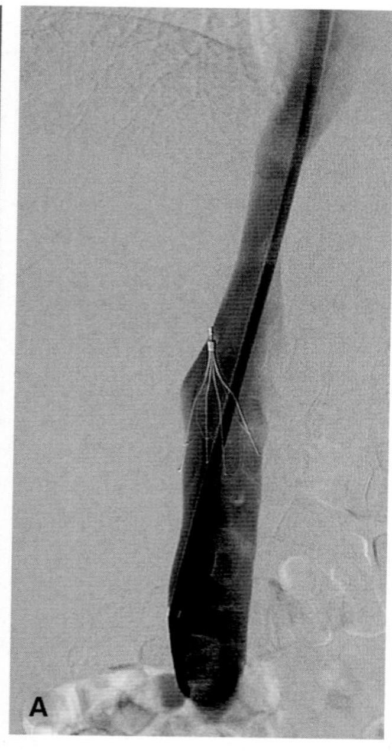

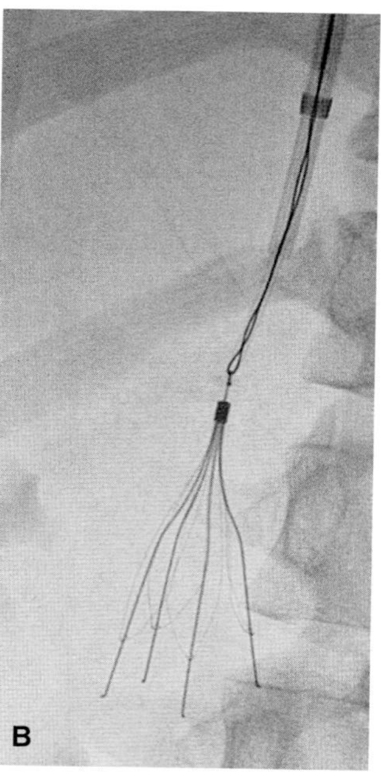

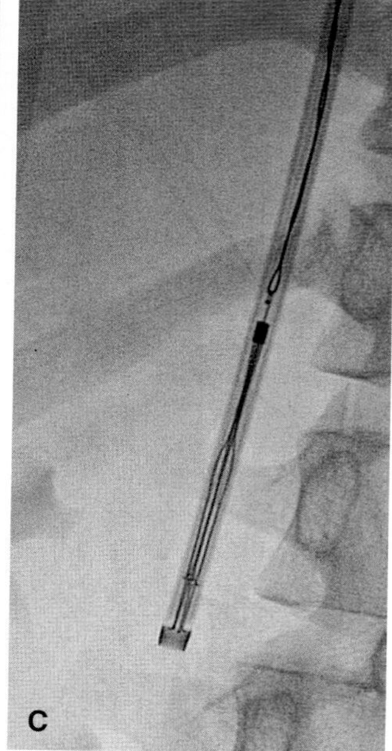

FIGURE 9 ● Steps involved in the uncomplicated removal of a Günther tulip retrievable IVC filter. An IVC venogram is first obtained demonstrating patency of the IVC and the absence of thrombus within the filter and visualized cava **(A)**. The tip of the retrieval IVC is then ensnared with snare or conical grappling device **(B)**. The 12-Fr sheath is then advanced over the hooks of IVC filter fully disengaging it from the caval wall and the filter is removed **(C)**.

- The flush catheter is positioned proximally into one of the common iliac veins and an inferior vena cavagram is performed by power injection of 20 mL/sec of contrast over 2 seconds. The venogram is carefully reviewed for the presence of thrombus within the visualized iliac veins, vena cava, and IVC filter (**FIGURE 9A**). If there is significant thrombus present within the filter, the retrieval should be aborted and the filter left in place. The patient can be restudied in 4 to 8 weeks and the IVC filter is removed at that time if imaging demonstrates resolution of the filter thrombus.
- Many manufacturers of IVC filter offer packaged retrieval systems that contain dilators, coaxial retrieval sheaths, and snares that can be used for removal. These are convenient but not necessary.
- The 5-Fr flush catheter is removed over a stiff 0.035 straight-tip Amplatz wire. The 6-Fr sheath is removed and the venotomy site serially dilated to 12 Fr. and a 55 cm 12-Fr sheath is placed over the wire and positioned just at or above the IVC filter.
- A 20 to 30 mm goose neck for multiloop endovascular snare catheter is advanced over the Amplatz wire and the wire is removed and replaced with the snare itself. The snare is used to capture the apex of the filter or apical hook if present (**FIGURE 9B**).
- Once the filter is engaged, the 12-Fr sheath is advanced over the snared filter. The filter legs should release from the vena cava wall allowing the ensnared filter to be retracted into the sheath and removed from the patient (**FIGURE 9C**). It is important to maintain tension on the filter with the snare, but not to retract it into the sheath, rather advance the sheath over the filter.
- If significant resistance is met while attempting to remove the IVC filter, retrieval should be aborted with a plan to consider an additional retrieval attempt utilizing advanced retrieval techniques.
- Once the IVC filter is removed from the patient, it should be carefully inspected to assure that it is intact and without unexpected missing component. Given the current medico-legal environment around IVC filters, the authors routinely photograph the removed IVC filters and upload the images into the patient's medical record.
- A guidewire is replaced into the vena cava and the flush catheter is replaced in the proximal iliac vein. A completion cavagram is performed and carefully reviewed for possible contrast extravasation that might indicate a caval injury or vena cava thrombosis.
- All instruments are removed and the venotomy managed as previously described.

TROUBLESHOOTING IVC/SVC FILTER PLACEMENT AND RETRIEVALS

- A filter deployed with crossed tines can frequently be corrected with simple IVC filter manipulation. This can be as simple as placement of a stiff wire within the vena cava and across the IVC filter or manipulation of the filter with a catheter.
- If the filter is retrievable, then crossed limbs or significant filter tilt can be dealt with by capture, reconstraint, and redeployment of the IVC filter. Complete removal of the filter and replacement should be considered if attempts at correction are not successful.
- A filter that is deployed and exhibits significant tilt >15° can frequently be adjusted and tilt improved by use of stiff wires

and catheters from below the IVC filter. If this should fail, the removable filters can be captured, reconstrained and redeployed to correct tilt.

- IVC filters that are significantly tilted and whose apices abut the wall of the vena cava can make standard retrieval extremely difficult. A simple maneuver such as placement of a stiff wire across the filter to displace it can be used to center the apex and facilitate ensnarement. If this is unsuccessful, after establishing additional venous access, an 8 to 12 mm angioplasty balloon can placed across the filter and inflated. This maneuver frequently displaces the apex of the filter and allows ensnarement and removal. Both of these techniques are simple, frequently successful,[23] and generally within the capabilities of most surgeons placing IVC filters.

PEARLS AND PITFALLS

Vena cava anatomy	■ Before filter placement, it is best to define the vena cava diameter, the location of the iliac vein confluence and renal veins, as well as the presence of vena cava and renal vein anomalies or thrombus in the vena cava.
Access site complications	■ Ultrasonography-guided access can evaluate whether there is thrombus at the access site before puncture and also help to avoid concomitant arterial and/or venous injury.
Limitations of imaging	■ Although the third lumbar vertebral body (or L1/L2 disc space) has been used as a landmark for filter deployment, bony lumbar vertebral anatomy alone is not adequate for proper filter placement as the renal veins and the iliac vein confluence may be found at this level in 5% to 10% of patients.[24] Whether venography, transabdominal duplex ultrasound, or IVUS is used for placement, understanding the limitations of each modality is critical for accurate filter placement.
Filter deployment problems	■ Filter tilt, crossing of filter legs, entrapment of the filter device inside the filter delivery catheter, filter migration, maldeployment, and vena cava perforation can occur during filter deployment. A thorough understanding of catheter-based techniques, imaging, and *specific filter delivery systems* is required.
The pregnant patient	■ Indications for filter placement in the pregnant patient include DVT with contraindication to anticoagulation. A suprarenal filter is preferred because of compression of the infrarenal portion of the IVC by the gravid uterus. Jugular access should be considered as well as limiting radiation exposure through use of IVUS if possible. Imaging at the time of placement should confirm the level of the renal veins and the hepatic vein confluence as distal and proximal landmarks. Measurements of the suprarenal IVC should confirm a diameter less than 28 to 30 mm. The filter should be deployed so that the leg attachment point is just above the highest renal vein and below the hepatic vein confluence. This usually positions the filter between the T11 and the L1 vertebral bodies.

Practitioners should consult the applicable Instructions For Use for device indications and contraindications.

POSTOPERATIVE CARE

- *Access site*: Initial postoperative care dictates removal of the sheath from the accessed vein and manual pressure over the puncture site for approximately 15 minutes. A pressure dressing is applied for a few hours, and then the access site is reinspected. If a femoral access is used for filter placement, the patient is keep flat and immobile for 2 to 4 hours. Swelling, hematoma, or bruit would indicate the need for a groin ultrasound to rule out a pseudoaneurysm or arteriovenous fistula.
- *Postprocedural imaging*: An abdominal radiograph is obtained after filter placement to document the position of the filter. The tip should reside between the L1 and the L2 vertebral bodies, but bony vertebral level can vary in relation to renal vein position. Filter tilt should be less than 15°. Tilt greater than 15° suggests filter malpositioning in the iliac vein or migration of the filter tip into a renal or gonadal vein.

COMPLICATIONS

- **Overview on IVC filter-related complications.** Reported technical success rates for a properly positioned filter range between 98% and 100%. Early complications involve access site hematoma, ecchymosis, arteriovenous fistulae, or maldeployment of the filter. Late complications include vena cava thrombosis, pulmonary embolus, access site thrombosis, migration, tilt, and leg penetration through the wall of the vena cava.[25,26] Although most filter types are roughly equivalent in prevention of PE, there is some variation in complication rates among devices.[27-29]
- **Vena cava thrombosis.** Filter design and shape may have some impact on propensity for vena cava thrombosis and rates of vena cava thrombosis varies between 6% and 30%.[30] Conical filter designs seem to have less flow impedance compared with nonconical designs. In a conical design, filling of the filter with thrombus occurs centrally while blood flows peripherally, which may help to maintain vena cava patency.
- **Venous access site thrombosis.** Complications from vascular access for IVC filter placement is reported at a rate of 4% to 11%[31] and similar to that of central line catheter insertion. The two most common access site complications are bleeding at the site of access (6%-15%)[32] and insertion site thrombosis (2%-35%)[33] more common in patient with hypercoagulable states. Factors contributing to access site thrombosis may include larger filter delivery catheter and

sheath size, multiple venous access attempts, extended post-procedure puncture site pressure, and clotting tendency.

- **Filter malpositioning and misplacement.** Filter tilt exceeding 15° may decrease filtration efficiency and lead to pulmonary emboli or vena cava occlusion. Rates of significant tilt vary in the literature between 0% to 39% and may be dependent on the particular filter being used.[34] Filter malpositioning and misplacement occurs at a rate of approximately 1% to 10%.[31] Inadvertent misplacement of the filter in the suprarenal vena cava can lead to renal vein thrombosis, and deployment in the iliac vein can contribute to iliofemoral venous thrombosis. Special care should be taken to delineate vena cava anatomy when using internal jugular access for IVC filter placement. The jugular approach to IVC filter is associated with a higher incidence of nontarget vessel malposition with misdeployment of the IVC filter in the gonadal, paraspinal, and renal veins.[35]
- **Filter leg or hook penetration.** Filter leg or hook penetration through the vena cava wall is fairly common (9%-24%)[36] and is usually asymptomatic. Filter design features such as recurved hooks, thickened J-hooks, and longitudinal filter struts have decreased but not eliminated the risk of penetration. Occasional erosion into the aorta, duodenum, small bowel, colon, ureter, and adjacent vertebral body has been described and, if associated with pseudoaneurysm or infection, may necessitate operative filter removal.
- **Filter migration.** Filters can migrate to a more central vena cava segment or to the heart and can be associated with severe cardiopulmonary compromise and death. Migration occurs in approximately 2% to 5% of cases[37] and is usually the result of inappropriate sizing, deployment over a thrombus with inadequate attachment to the wall of the vena cava, or dislodgement when catheters or guidewires becoming entangled within the filter struts.
- **Filter fracture.** Rates of IVC filter fracture are directly related to design, with variable fracture rates for each individual filter. Retrievable IVC filter fracture rates appear to increase over time and can reach rates of up to 16%.[30,38] Fortunately, overall filter fracture is a relatively rare event occurring in less than 1% of all IVC filters. Filters made from nitinol tend to be more prone to material fatigue and fracture, with an attendant risk of migration.
- **Guidewire entrapment.** Entrapment of guidewires, central venous catheters, or other intravascular devices has been reported and is less than 1%.[39]
- **PE and death.** Nonfatal PE (2%-5%), fatal PE (0.7%), and deaths linked to filter insertion (0.12%) are rare.[32]

REFERENCES

1. Greenfield LJ, Proctor MC. Suprarenal filter placement. *J Vasc Surg*. 1998;28(3):432-438; discussion 438. doi:10.1016/s0741-5214(98)70128-4
2. Decousus H, Leizorovicz A, Parent F, et al. A clinical trial of vena caval filters in the prevention of pulmonary embolism in patients with proximal deep-vein thrombosis. Prévention du Risque d'Embolie Pulmonaire par Interruption Cave Study Group. *N Engl J Med*. 1998;338(7):409-415. doi:10.1056/NEJM199802123380701
3. Carson JL, Kelley MA, Duff A, et al. The clinical course of pulmonary embolism. *N Engl J Med*. 1992;326(19):1240-1245. doi:10.1056/NEJM199205073261902
4. Duszak R, Parker L, Levin DC, Rao VM. Placement and removal of inferior vena cava filters: national trends in the medicare population. *J Am Coll Radiol JACR*. 2011;8(7):483-489. doi:10.1016/j.jacr.2010.12.021
5. Dixon A, Stavropoulos SW. Improving retrieval rates for retrievable inferior vena cava filters. *Expet Rev Med Dev*. 2013;10(1):135-141. doi:10.1586/erd.12.65
6. Guez D, Hansberry DR, Eschelman DJ, et al. Inferior vena cava filter placement and retrieval rates among radiologists and nonradiologists. *J Vasc Interv Radiol JVIR*. 2018;29(4):482-485. doi:10.1016/j.jvir.2017.11.008
7. Andreoli JM, Lewandowski RJ, Vogelzang RL, Ryu RK. Comparison of complication rates associated with permanent and retrievable inferior vena cava filters: a review of the MAUDE database. *J Vasc Interv Radiol JVIR*. 2014;25(8):1181-1185. doi:10.1016/j.jvir.2014.04.016
8. Morales JP, Li X, Irony TZ, Ibrahim NG, Moynahan M, Cavanaugh KJ. Decision analysis of retrievable inferior vena cava filters in patients without pulmonary embolism. *J Vasc Surg Venous Lymphat Disord*. 2013;1(4):376-384. doi:10.1016/j.jvsv.2013.04.005
9. Office of the Surgeon General (US), National Heart, Lung, and Blood Institute (US). *The Surgeon General's Call to Action to Prevent Deep Vein Thrombosis and Pulmonary Embolism*. Office of the Surgeon General (US); 2008. Accessed February 27, 2022. http://www.ncbi.nlm.nih.gov/books/NBK44178/
10. Kearon C, Kahn SR, Agnelli G, Goldhaber S, Raskob GE, Comerota AJ. Antithrombotic therapy for venous thromboembolic disease: American College of Chest Physicians Evidence-Based Clinical Practice Guidelines (8th Edition). *Chest*. 2008;133(6 Suppl):454S-545S. doi:10.1378/chest.08-0658.
11. Rogers FB, Cipolle MD, Velmahos G, Rozycki G, Luchette FA. Practice management guidelines for the prevention of venous thromboembolism in trauma patients: the EAST practice management guidelines work group. *J Trauma*. 2002;53(1):142-164. doi:10.1097/00005373-200207000-00032
12. Muñoz FJ, Mismetti P, Poggio R, et al. Clinical outcome of patients with upper-extremity deep vein thrombosis: results from the RIETE Registry. *Chest*. 2008;133(1):143-148. doi:10.1378/chest.07-1432
13. Brown DB, Pappas JA, Vedantham S, Pilgram TK, Olsen RV, Duncan JR. Gadolinium, carbon dioxide, and iodinated contrast material for planning inferior vena cava filter placement: a prospective trial. *J Vasc Interv Radiol JVIR*. 2003;14(8):1017-1022. doi:10.1097/01.rvi.0000082865.05622.ad
14. Boyd-Kranis R, Sullivan KL, Eschelman DJ, Bonn J, Gardiner GA. Accuracy and safety of carbon dioxide inferior vena cavography. *J Vasc Interv Radiol JVIR*. 1999;10(9):1183-1189. doi:10.1016/s1051-0443(99)70218-6
15. Dewald CL, Jensen CC, Park YH, et al. Vena cavography with CO(2) versus with iodinated contrast material for inferior vena cava filter placement: a prospective evaluation. *Radiology*. 2000;216(3):752-757. doi:10.1148/radiology.216.3.r00au15752
16. Spinosa DJ, Angle JF, Hartwell GD, Hagspiel KD, Leung DA, Matsumoto AH. Gadolinium-based contrast agents in angiography and interventional radiology. *Radiol Clin North Am*. 2002;40(4):693-710. doi:10.1016/s0033-8389(02)00022-2
17. Gunn AJ, Iqbal SI, Kalva SP, et al. Intravascular ultrasound-guided inferior vena cava filter placement using a single-puncture technique in 99 patients. *Vasc Endovascular Surg*. 2013;47(2):97-101. doi:10.1177/1538574412473186
18. Killingsworth CD, Taylor SM, Patterson MA, et al. Prospective implementation of an algorithm for bedside intravascular ultrasound-guided filter placement in critically ill patients. *J Vasc Surg*. 2010;51(5):1215-1221. doi:10.1016/j.jvs.2009.12.041
19. Corriere MA, Passman MA, Guzman RJ, Dattilo JB, Naslund TC. Comparison of bedside transabdominal duplex ultrasound versus contrast venography for inferior vena cava filter placement: what is the best imaging modality?. *Ann Vasc Surg*. 2005;19(2):229-234. doi:10.1007/s10016-004-0163-x
20. Garrett JV, Passman MA, Guzman RJ, Dattilo JB, Naslund TC. Expanding options for bedside placement of inferior vena cava filters with intravascular ultrasound when transabdominal duplex ultrasound imaging is inadequate. *Ann Vasc Surg*. 2004;18(3):329-334. doi:10.1007/s10016-004-0029-2

21. Wellons ED, Matsuura JH, Shuler FW, Franklin JS, Rosenthal D. Bedside intravascular ultrasound-guided vena cava filter placement. *J Vasc Surg*. 2003;38(3):455-457; discussion 457-458. doi:10.1016/s0741-5214(03)00471-3
22. Tanju S, Düşünceli E, Sancak T. Placement of an inferior vena cava filter in a patient with azygos continuation complicated by pulmonary embolism. *Cardiovasc Intervent Radiol*. 2006;29(4):681-684. doi:10.1007/s00270-005-0112-2
23. Brahmandam A, Skrip L, Mojibian H, et al. Costs and complications of endovascular inferior vena cava filter retrieval. *J Vasc Surg Venous Lymphat Disord*. 2019;7(5):653-659.e1. doi:10.1016/j.jvsv.2019.02.017
24. Danetz JS, McLafferty RB, Ayerdi J, Gruneiro LA, Ramsey DE, Hodgson KJ. Selective venography versus nonselective venography before vena cava filter placement: evidence for more, not less. *J Vasc Surg*. 2003;38(5):928-934. doi:10.1016/s0741-5214(03)00911-x
25. Ballew KA, Philbrick JT, Becker DM. Vena cava filter devices. *Clin Chest Med*. 1995;16(2):295-305.
26. Ray CE, Kaufman JA. Complications of inferior vena cava filters. *Abdom Imaging*. 1996;21(4):368-374. doi:10.1007/s002619900084
27. Vena Caval Filter Consensus Conference. Recommended reporting standards for vena caval filter placement and patient follow-up. *J Vasc Surg*. 1999;30(3):573-579.
28. Streiff MB. Vena caval filters: a comprehensive review. *Blood*. 2000;95(12):3669-3677.
29. Hann CL, Streiff MB. The role of vena caval filters in the management of venous thromboembolism. *Blood Rev*. 2005;19(4):179-202. doi:10.1016/j.blre.2004.08.002
30. Wang SL, Siddiqui A, Rosenthal E. Long-term complications of inferior vena cava filters. *J Vasc Surg Venous Lymphat Disord*. 2017;5(1):33-41. doi:10.1016/j.jvsv.2016.07.002
31. Kinney TB. Update on inferior vena cava filters. *J Vasc Interv Radiol JVIR*. 2003;14(4):425-440. doi:10.1097/01.rvi.0000064860.87207.77
32. Joels CS, Sing RF, Heniford BT. Complications of inferior vena cava filters. *Am Surg*. 2003;69(8):654-659.
33. Martin MJ, Blair KS, Curry TK, Singh N. Vena cava filters: current concepts and controversies for the surgeon. *Curr Probl Surg*. 2010;47(7):524-618. doi:10.1067/j.cpsurg.2010.03.004
34. Bae JH, Lee SY. Filter tilting and retrievability of the Celect and Denali inferior vena cava filters using propensity score-matching analysis. *Eur J Radiol Open*. 2018;5:153-158. doi:10.1016/j.ejro.2018.09.001
35. Yun JH, Khanna V, Ahuja RS, Natarajan B. Not so fast with the filter! Is it really in the inferior vena cava? *Am J Interv Radiol*. 2020;4:20. doi:10.25259/AJIR_29_2020
36. Kesselman A, Oo TH, Johnson M, Stecker MS, Kaufman J, Trost D. Current controversies in inferior vena cava filter placement: AJR expert panel narrative review. *AJR Am J Roentgenol*. 2021;216(3):563-569. doi:10.2214/AJR.20.24817
37. Bélénotti P, Sarlon-Bartoli G, Bartoli MA, et al. Vena cava filter migration: an unappreciated complication. About four cases and review of the literature. *Ann Vasc Surg*. 2011;25(8):1141.e9-14. doi:10.1016/j.avsg.2011.03.016
38. Geerts W, Selby R. Inferior vena cava filter use and patient safety: legacy or science?. *Hematol Am Soc Hematol Educ Program*. 2017;2017(1):686-692. doi:10.1182/asheducation-2017.1.686
39. Almestady R, Spain J, Bayona-Molano MDP, Wang W. Iatrogenic migration of VenaTech LP IVC filter to superior vena cava secondary to guidewire entrapment: case report and review of literature. *Vasc Endovascular Surg*. 2013;47(1):48-50. doi:10.1177/1538574412467861

Chapter 36 Superficial Venous Disease Management: Ablation, Phlebectomy, and Sclerotherapy

Meryl Simon Logan and Ruth L. Bush

DEFINITION

- Many consider varicose veins to be a cosmetic concern, yet they can often be a source of pain, distress, and debility.
- Varicose vein symptomatology ranges from asymptomatic to a contributor of nonhealing venous ulcers.
- The diagnosis and management of superficial venous disease has rapidly expanded in recent years, making what was once a surgery performed in the operating room with significant blood loss, now an outpatient in-office procedure with minimal down time.
- In the USA, superficial venous disease, including varicose veins, are common conditions affecting 30% of women and 15% of men. Up to 25% of the Western population is affected by lower extremity venous disease.[1]

Basic Anatomy of the Superficial Venous System

- Superficial veins are located between the skin and deep fascia.
- The main lower limb superficial veins are the great saphenous vein (GSV) and small saphenous vein (SSV).
- The GSV runs from the dorsum of the foot to the proximal thigh, where it empties into the common femoral vein at the saphenofemoral junction. The GSV lies within its own fascial compartment, the "saphenous fascia," and is accompanied by the saphenous nerve, which typically joins at or just below the knee.
- There are *anterior and posterior accessory saphenous veins* throughout the leg. These tributaries lie within the same tissue plane as the GSV.[2]
- There can also be a *duplicated saphenous vein*: a second vein that lies in the same plane as the GSV, has a similar diameter, and drains common cutaneous territories. A duplicated GSV can also be a source of recurrent varicosities after main GSV ablation.[3]
- Varicose veins are dilated subcutaneous veins measuring >3 mm in diameter in the standing position.[4] Of note, most insurance companies will not cover ablation of a GSV measuring <5 mm diameter.
- Pathophysiologic reflux of the superficial veins is defined as reflux lasting >500 ms.

DIFFERENTIAL DIAGNOSIS

- Not all visible veins are varicosities or due to reflux. Leg edema itself has a wide differential, including systemic causes which often lead to bilateral leg swelling (cardiac, renal, liver diseases), lymphedema (which can be primary or secondary), lipedema, as well as rare congenital syndromes such as Klippel-Trenaunay.
- Klippel-Trenaunay is a disorder classically described by a triad of varicosities, cutaneous vascular malformations, and soft tissue or bone overgrowth. This disorder can be associated with absence of the deep venous system. Ablation of superficial veins in a patient with an absent deep system could be catastrophic, highlighting the critical importance of both an appropriate H&P and venous imaging studies preoperatively.[5]
- Symptoms of deep venous disease are similar to those of superficial disease. One must evaluate both deep and superficial venous systems prior to any superficial venous intervention.

PATIENT HISTORY AND PHYSICAL FINDINGS

- Symptoms of venous insufficiency include heaviness, swelling, pain, itching, cramping, and throbbing. Patients can have bleeding from varicosities, or the varicosities can thrombose resulting in thrombophlebitis. Venous ulcer formation can be a result of longstanding venous hypertension due to superficial venous insufficiency.
- Important aspects of the history include prior deep vein thromboses (DVTs), prior venous treatment, hypercoagulable state, smoking, prior surgeries, prior trauma, family history, pregnancy history, and compression use.
- Physical exam should be done in the standing position. The presence/absence of varicosities, palpable cords, tenderness, pulsatility, thrills, or bruits should be noted. Skin changes, including brown discoloration due to hemosiderin staining, fibrotic changes, and thinning of the skin in the distal calf are evidence of more advanced disease and should be noted.
- A full pulse exam should be obtained, including femoral, popliteal, and pedal pulses.
- A standard way of documenting disease severity is using the CEAP classification, which stands for class, etiology, anatomy, pathophysiology. This is an internationally accepted standard for describing chronic venous disease.[6]
- Use of the Venous Clinical Severity Score (VCSS)[7] or other validated scoring tool to document the severity of chronic venous insufficiency is also recommended.

IMAGING AND OTHER DIAGNOSTIC STUDIES

- Venous duplex is the imaging test of choice. This allows DVT to be ruled out, and can evaluate for reflux in both the deep and superficial venous systems. Reflux in the deep system is defined as reflux lasting >1000 milliseconds (ms). Reflux in the superficial system is defined as lasting >500 ms. Perforator reflux is pathologic when it is >500 ms and the perforator measures >3.5 mm in diameter or more.
- A complete venous duplex is typically all that is needed to plan treatment for superficial varicosities. However, abnormal waveforms in the common femoral vein may hint at iliac venous disease, necessitating either CT venogram or catheter-based venogram to evaluate.

SURGICAL MANAGEMENT

General Considerations

- It is important to note that first-line treatment is conservative management, which includes compression therapy, leg elevation, weight loss, and over-the-counter pain medications.
- Compression stockings come in a variety of options (grade, size, length), and are useful in reducing swelling and thus providing symptomatic relief.[1]
- It is important to know the contraindications to surgery, which can include the absence or occlusion of the deep venous system, pregnancy, and the presence of an arteriovenous fistula.

Ablation

- Minimally invasive treatment options have generally supplanted the now mostly historical high ligation and stripping.
- There are multiple options for endovenous ablation including the use of radiofrequency, laser, and glues or sclerosants. All have the common goal of addressing the venous reflux by eliminating the veins that have reflux (**TABLE 1**).

Table 1: Various Endovenous Ablation Options for Axial Vein Reflux

Closure treatment	Thermal?	Tumescent use?	FDA-approved medication
Radiofrequency ablation (RFA)	yes	Yes	N/A
Laser	yes	Yes	N/A
Tissue adhesive "glue"	no	No	VenaSeal
Sclerosant	no	No	ClariVein
Polidocanol Injectable foam	no	No	Varithena

Preoperative Planning

- Most GSV/SSV incompetence can be considered for treatment. The 2020 Appropriate Use Criteria for Chronic Lower Extremity Venous Disease can give further guidance on when to treat.[8]
- These procedures are usually performed in the clinic or minor procedure room. Rarely is an operating room necessary.
- The patient can take an oral benzodiazepine 1 hour preoperatively to handle anxiety, if necessary.
- It is useful to keep the room warm to reduce vasospasm. In addition, the environment should be calming, and often music is chosen to assist in patient relaxation and comfort.

TECHNIQUES

STEP 1. POSITIONING

- The veins are marked in the preoperative area in the *standing position* (**FIGURE 1**).
- The patient is placed supine for GSV treatment and prone for SSV treatment (**FIGURE 2**). If both veins are to be treated at the same setting, we typically start with the GSV and have the patient turn on their side or stomach once this is complete to facilitate access to the SSV.
- The leg is prepped circumferentially and externally rotated into a frog-leg position. The table can be placed into reverse Trendelenburg to increase venous pressure and distend the vein to facilitate access.

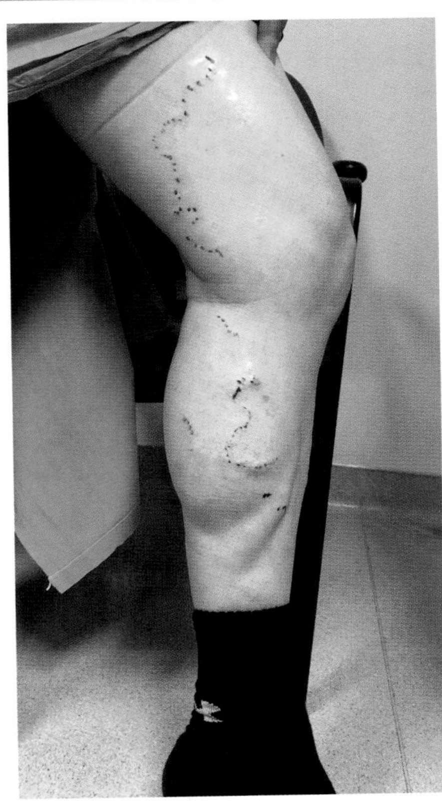

FIGURE 1 ● The great saphenous vein and varicosities have been marked in the standing position.

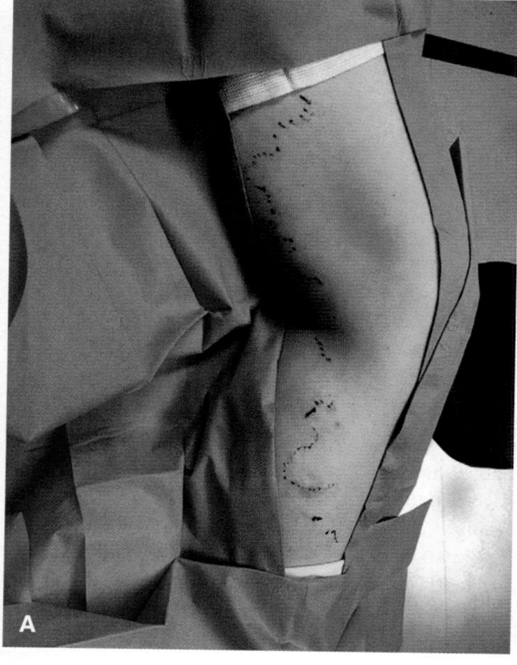

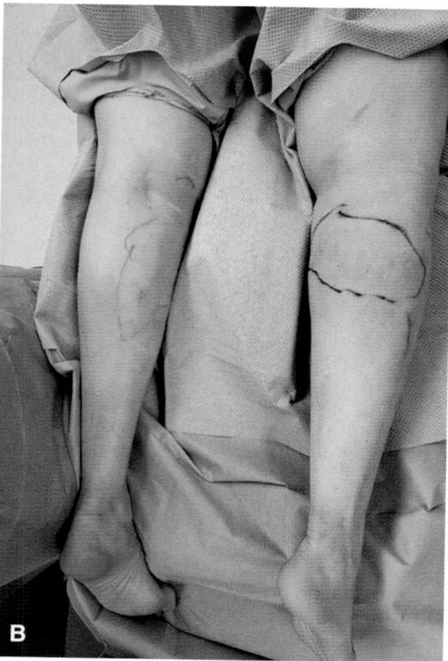

FIGURE 2 ● **A,** supine frog-leg position for GSV treatment. **B,** Prone positioning for SSV treatment.

STEP 2. REPEAT THE ULTRASOUND AND CHOOSE AN ACCESS SITE LOCATION

- The ideal access site is as distal on the leg as possible; however, below the knee ablation risks injury to the accompanying saphenous nerve (**FIGURE 3**).

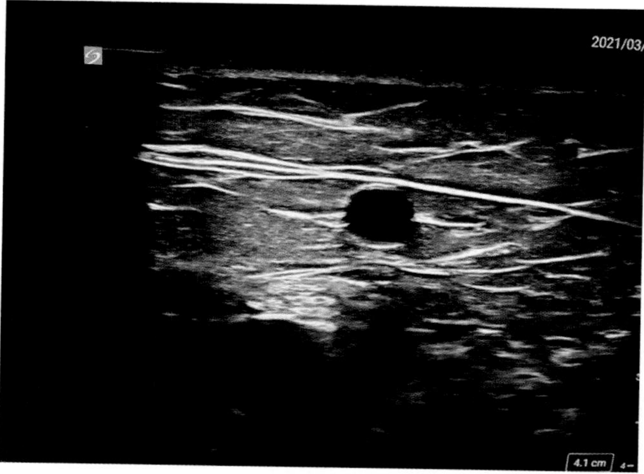

FIGURE 3 ● The GSV is seen on B mode ultrasound within the saphenous fascia.

STEP 3 ULTRASOUND-GUIDED ACCESS

- After local anesthetic is placed at the intended access site, using ultrasound guidance a micropuncture needle is placed into the vein, followed by advancement of a .018-inch wire (**FIGURE 4**). The wire is advanced to the SJF (or SPJ) under ultrasound guidance (**FIGURE 5**).
- The micropuncture sheath is exchanged for an appropriately sized sheath for the ablative device.

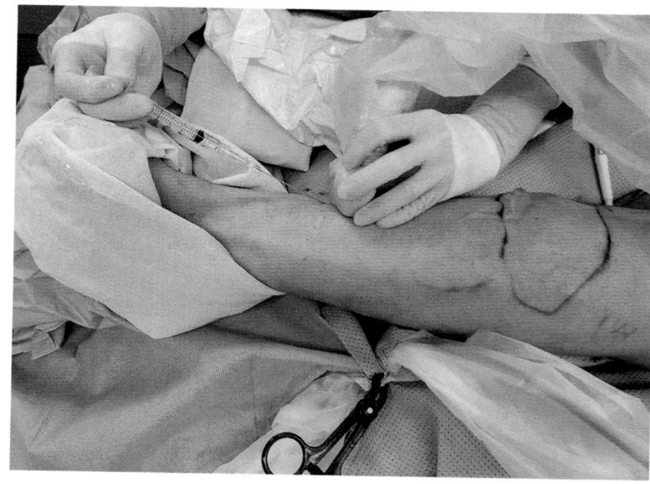

FIGURE 4 ● The vein (SSV in this image) is accessed under ultrasound guidance.

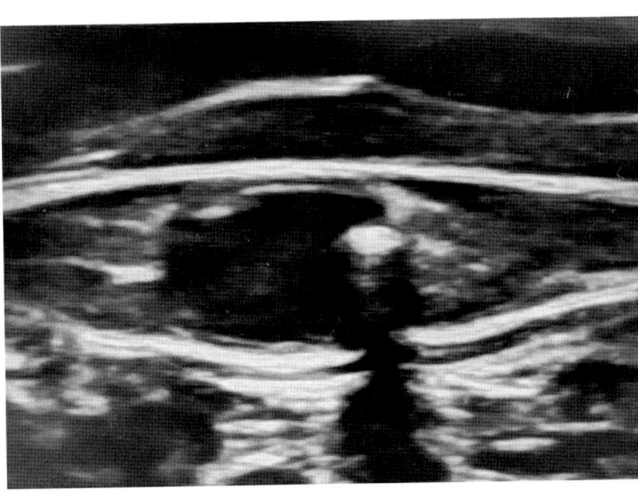

FIGURE 5 ● This B mode ultrasound image shows the radiopaque wire within the GSV lumen. Again, note the saphenous fascia surrounding the vein.

STEP 4

Thermal Ablation

- The tip of the laser or RFA catheter should be 2 to 2.5 cm distal to the SFJ or SPJ or distal to superficial epigastric veins.
- Administer tumescent fluid (approximately 10 mL/cm vein): saline, lidocaine, epinephrine mixture (**FIGURE 6**) to circumferentially surround the vein.
- Treat the vein per device instruction.

Nonthermal Ablation

Includes VenaSeal (n-butyl cyanoacrylate glue) or ultrasound-guided foam sclerotherapy.

- Inject cyanoacrylate glue per instructions for use; Screen patients for adhesive allergic reaction.
- Important to have constant compression at SFJ or SPJ to avoid embolism of glue or sclerosing agent.

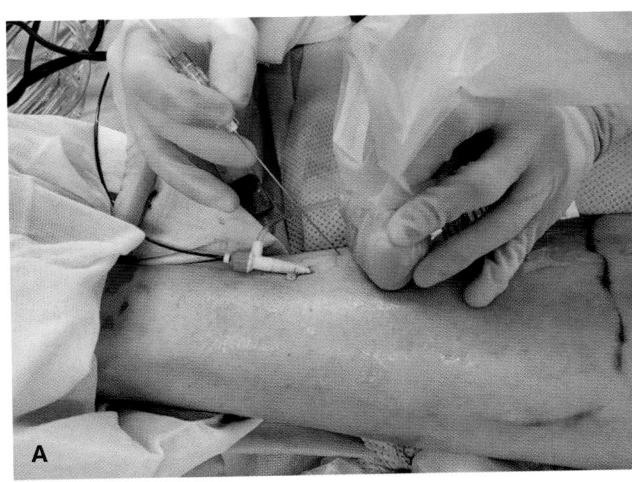

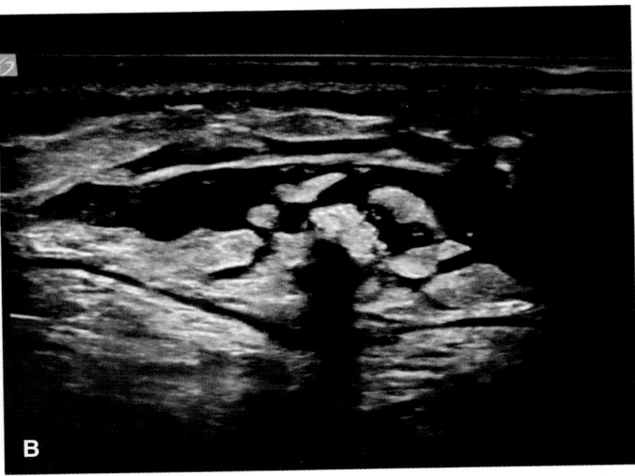

FIGURE 6 ● **A,** The ablation device sheath is in place. The tumescent anesthetic is placed with ultrasound guidance. **B,** Tumescent is seen on B mode ultrasound surrounding the vein, separating the soft tissue off the vein.

STEP 5. REMOVE SHEATH

- Remove sheath, hold light pressure × 5 minutes.

STEP 6. ELEVATE AND WRAP THE LEG

- We use bandage rolls (ie, Kerlix) and elastic wraps (ie, ACE) from foot to proximal thigh. If using cyanoacrylate glue, compression/wraps are not necessary.

PHLEBECTOMY AND SCLEROTHERAPY

- Phlebectomy and sclerotherapy are adjunctive procedures that can be utilized for additional varicosities and spider veins.
- This can be done simultaneously with ablation, or at a later date.
- Preoperative assessment and positioning are as noted in the *Surgical Management* section.

Phlebectomy

- Small "stabs" are made over the varicosities to be excised.
- This is often performed with an 11 blade, followed by a phlebectomy hooks or small hemostats to find, and grab the vein—this is a blind procedure!
- Once grasped, the vein is then gently pulled in a back and forth motion to remove as much vein as possible without tearing (**FIGURE 7**).
- Closure of the stabs can be accomplished with Dermabond or Steri-Strips.
- Compression is then applied as above.

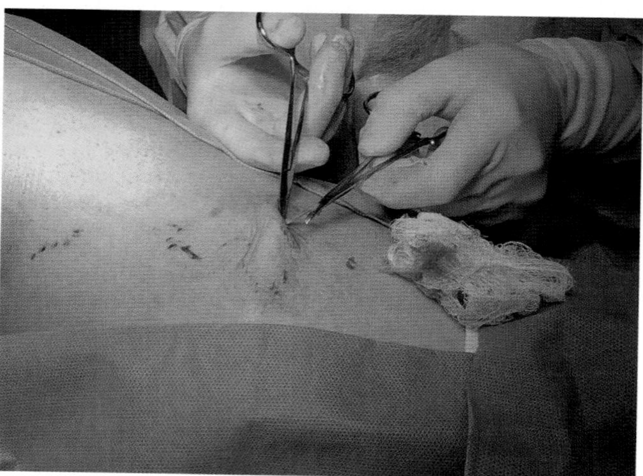

FIGURE 7 ● Through a stab incision, a varicose vein has been grasped and is being gently pulled during phlebectomy.

Sclerotherapy

- FDA-approved agents include sodium tetradecyl sulfate (Sotradecol) & polidocanol (Asclera)
- Tools needed-small syringes ideally 3 mL, small needle sizes (such as a 27 or 32 gauge)
    - Use of loupes or a vein light is an option to assist with small vein visualization, but is an added expense
    - It is important to let patients know that the treated areas will initially disappear, but then immediately return and may look red or "angry"—this is temporary
- Compression therapy is applied after sclerotherapy as well to improve outcomes[9]

PEARLS AND PITFALLS

Appropriate patient selection is key	■ Make sure you under promise and over deliver on expectations. No treatment will be perfect in relieving symptoms or providing cosmesis.
Venous insufficiency is a chronic disease	■ Recurrence is the rule rather than the exception. ■ Repeated procedures are often necessary in the patient's lifetime.
Pearl	■ Make sure there is appropriate distance between the end of the catheter and the SFJ or SPJ. Maintaining 2 cm distance for thermal ablation and 5 cm for cyanoacrylate is critical to avoiding femoral vein thrombus.
Postoperative care	■ Make sure patient is up and ambulating immediately after the procedure, if possible. This will decrease the incidence of post procedure DVT.

POSTOPERATIVE CARE

- Patients are instructed to remove compression wrapping after 48 hours, then transition to their compression stockings.
    - 2 weeks minimum use, recommend continued routine wear
- Acetaminophen or ibuprofen for post-procedure discomfort.
- Ambulation is encouraged immediately.
- Patients are brought back to clinic for a follow-up duplex in 3 to 7 days to confirm saphenous vein ablation and rule out endothermal heat-induced thrombosis (EHIT).

COMPLICATIONS

- Bruising/hematoma
- Superficial thrombophlebitis
- EHIT
    - Classification and treatment recommendations can be found elsewhere. We recommend those provided by the American Venous Forum and Society for Vascular Surgery (https://www.jvsvenous.org/article/S2213-333X(20)30343-7/fulltext)
- Skin reactions/thermal injury/pigmentation

- Saphenous nerve injury and paresthesia
- Recanalization/incomplete ablation
- Neovascularization (less common with ablation then seen with open ligation)

REFERENCES

1. Zhan HT, Bush RL. A review of the current management and treatment options for superficial venous insufficiency. *World J Surg*. 2014;38:2580-2588.
2. Schul MW, Vauvegula S. The clinical relevance of anterior accessory great saphenous vein reflux. *J Vasc Surg Venous Lymphat Disord*. 2020;8:1014-1020.
3. Kockaert M, De Ross KP, Dijk LV, Nijsten T, Neumann M. Duplication of the great saphenous vein: a definition problem and implications for therapy. *Dermatol Surg*. 2012;38:77-82.
4. Gloviczki P, Comerota AJ, Dalsing MC, et al. The care of patients with varicose veins and associated chronic venous diseases: clinical practice guidelines of the Society for Vascular Surgery and the American Venous Forum. *J Vasc Surg*. 2011;53:2S-48S.
5. Wang SK, Drucker NA, Gupta AK, Mashalleck FE, Dalsing MC. Diagnosis and management of the venous malformations of Klippel-Trénaunay syndrome. *J Vasc Surg Venous Lymphat Disord*. 2017;5:587-595.
6. Lurie F, Passman M, Meisner M, et al. The 2020 update of the CEAP classification system reporting standards. *J Vasc Surg Venous Lymphat Disord*. 2020;8:342-352.
7. Passman MA, McLafferty RB, Lentz MF, et al. Validation of Venous Clinical Severity Score (VCSS) with other venous severity assessment tools from the American Venous Forum, National Venous Screening Program. *J Vasc Surg*. 2011;54(6 Suppl):2s-9s.
8. Masuda E, Ozsvath K, Vossler J, et al. The 2020 appropriate use criteria for chronic lower extremity Venous disease of the American Venous Forum, the Society for Vascular Surgery, the American Vein and Lymphatic Society, and the Society of Interventional Radiology. *J Vasc Surg Venous Lymphat Disord*. 2020;8:505-525.
9. Lurie F, Lal BK, Antignani PL, et al. Compression therapy after invasive treatment of superficial veins of the lower extremities: clinical practice guidelines of the American Venous Forum, Society for Vascular Surgery, American College of Phlebology, Society for Vascular Medicine, and International Union of Phlebology. *J Vasc Surg Venous Lymphat Disord*. 2019;7:17-28.

Chapter 37 Hemodialysis: Open Access Construction

Thomas S. Huber and Salvatore T. Scali

DEFINITION

- The simplistic concept of hemodialysis is that blood is removed from the circulation, filtered through the dialysis machine and then returned. Effective hemodialysis requires a high-flow, low-resistance circuit such that a sufficient quantity of blood can be withdrawn for filtration and then returned. Therefore, the ideal hemodialysis access would be easy to cannulate, sustain sufficient blood flow, maintain patency, have minimal long-term complications, and be cost-effective while remaining acceptable to patients from both an ease of cannulation and cosmetic appearance standpoint.
- The currently available hemodialysis access options include nontunneled and tunneled dialysis catheters (TDCs), usually for more temporary use, and autogenous arteriovenous fistulas (AVFs) and prosthetic arteriovenous grafts (AVGs) for more permanent use. Unfortunately, none of the currently available access options fulfill all criteria for an ideal access and, therefore, they should be viewed as complementary.
- It is generally accepted that a *mature* AVF is the optimal access, although it has been recognized that AVFs are not universally appropriate and that the increased emphasis on their creation has resulted in a higher rate of nonmaturation.[1] In contrast, the potential advantages of AVGs include an unlimited supply of conduit, greater ease of cannulation, a larger surface area for cannulation, and the potential for immediate use.
- The recommendations for permanent hemodialysis access have evolved from a strong emphasis on AVFs, stemming from the original Dialysis Outcome Quality Initiative Guidelines (DOQI)[1] and the Fistula First Breakthrough Initiative (FFBI)[2] to the concept of a "functional access," as summarized by the concept of the "right access, right time, right patient, right reason," that is advocated in the most recent KDOQI Guidelines.[3] The guidelines recommend that each patient should have an ESKD (end-stage kidney disease) Life Plan that is updated on a regular basis and identifies the next dialysis access alternative in the event of failure. Furthermore, the guidelines make recommendations about the role of TDCs for both short-and long-term use (Guideline 2) along with permanent vascular access type and location (Guideline 3). Notably, the guidelines state that AVFs and AVGs are preferred over TDCs, although the choice between AVFs and AVGs should be deferred to the provider, emphasizing that a *usable* AVF is preferred over an AVG if possible.

DIFFERENTIAL DIAGNOSIS

- Patients with ESKD need some type of renal replacement therapy to survive. Although the focus of the chapter is on the open surgical techniques for hemodialysis access, it is important to emphasize that transplantation and peritoneal dialysis are both excellent renal replacement therapies that should be addressed with patients as part of the discussion about their ongoing ESKD Life Plan.
- The traditional choices for permanent upper extremity hemodialysis access are listed in **TABLE 1**. The generic recommendations about the access choice includes AVF > AVG, upper extremity > lower extremity, nondominant extremity > dominant extremity, and forearm > proximal upper arm. However, the optimal choice should be individualized understanding that most access configurations will inevitably fail, further underscoring the importance of the ESKD Life Plan and the need for a remedial access solution. The key determinants that inform the hemodialysis access choice include comorbidities, anatomy, life expectancy, anticipated duration of dialysis, and patient preference.

PATIENT HISTORY AND PHYSICAL FINDINGS

- All patients undergoing evaluation for a permanent hemodialysis access should receive a complete history and physical examination, similar to any major surgical procedure. The physical examination should include assessment of the arterial inflow/venous outflow to the extremity with a focus on any findings such as arm edema, facial swelling, or prominent veins on the chest or shoulder that would suggest central venous obstruction.

Table 1: Traditional Upper Extremity Hemodialysis Access Configurations

Arteriovenous fistula (AVF)
Radial-cephalic (radial artery—wrist)
Radial-basilic (radial artery—wrist)
Radial-cephalic (radial artery—proximal forearm)
Brachial-cephalic (brachial artery—antecubital fossa)
Brachial-basilic (brachial artery—antecubital fossa, distal upper arm)
Arteriovenous graft (AVG)
Brachial-antecubital vein (forearm loop, brachial artery—antecubital fossa, antecubital vein—cephalic, basilic, median antecubital, brachial)
Brachial-axillary (brachial artery—distal upper arm)
Brachial-axillary (brachial artery—proximal upper arm)

- It is important to document all prior access procedures, including any central venous catheters, along with any access-related complications (eg, hand ischemia).
- Notably, pacer and defibrillators with central venous wires are particularly problematic since they can induce an intense fibrotic response that can result in central stenoses or occlusions.

IMAGING AND OTHER DIAGNOSTIC STUDIES

- The noninvasive imaging in the vascular laboratory complements the physical examination.[4] The goals of the duplex ultrasound imaging are to identify all possible artery and vein combinations that can be used for a permanent access. The preoperative imaging includes measurement of the brachial and radial artery diameters, pressures, and velocity waveforms. In addition, an Allen test is performed to determine the dominant blood flow to the hand. The basilic and cephalic vein patency and diameters are measured, and any sign of thickening, scarring, or previous thrombosis is noted. Visualization of the central veins is attempted, although this is limited given the bony thoracic cavity. The potential access configurations can then be determined based upon the history, physical examination, and the noninvasive studies.
- The criteria for a suitable artery include a diameter of ≥2 mm, no evidence of an inflow stenosis, and the ability to vasodilate such that the inflow circuit can sustain adequate blood flow for dialysis. Assessment of vasodilation ability is difficult, but caution should be exercised in patients with severely calcified arteries, as commonly observed in older diabetic patients. The criteria for a suitable vein include a diameter of ≥3 mm, an adequate length for cannulation (in the case of AVFs), and no evidence of venous outflow obstruction.
- Additional imaging with either computed tomography– or catheter-based arteriography/venography can be obtained if necessary. This additional imaging is helpful in patients with presumed arterial inflow problems based upon a history of diabetes mellitus, peripheral artery disease, access-related hand ischemia (ie, steal), abnormal arterial segmental pressures, and/or those individuals undergoing complex access procedures. Similarly, it can be helpful for patients with presumed venous outflow lesions based upon a history of central venous catheters, pacer/defibrillators, arm edema, and/or those undergoing complex procedures.

SURGICAL MANAGEMENT

- The KDOQI Guidelines recommend that the choice of access procedure be dictated by the planned duration of dialysis, after consideration of their ESKD Life Plan (Guideline 3). Specifically, they recommend a forearm AVF, followed by a forearm AVG or a brachial-cephalic AVF, followed by an upper arm AVG or brachial-basilic AVF in patients who are anticipated to be on long-term hemodialysis. In contrast, they recommend a forearm AVG or brachial-cephalic AVF, followed by an upper arm AVG for those with predicted short-term dialysis duration. The Guidelines endorse consideration of early cannulation AVGs for individuals starting dialysis urgently (eg, renal failure without predialysis care) and provide recommendations for patients with complex access needs related to multiple prior failures, although the latter is outside the scope of the current chapter.
- The timing of access creation is dictated by the patient's renal function (ie, chronic kidney disease [CKD] vs ESKD) and the proposed access configuration (ie, AVF vs AVG). The KDOQI Guidelines recommend that patients with CKD with an estimated glomerular filtration rate (eGFR) ≤ 30 mL/min/1.73 m^2 be educated about the various renal replacement therapies while those with an eGFR 15 to 20 mL/min/1.73 m^2 should be referred for access creation. Given the requisite period for AVF maturation, it is ideal to operate on patients with CKD well in advance of their projected dialysis start date, hoping that their access will be suitable for cannulation when needed and obviate the need for TDC placement. Unfortunately, this scenario occurs less than 20% of the time and most individuals start dialysis with a catheter. If an AVG is the only permanent access option for patients with CKD, we prefer to wait until they initiate dialysis before access construction given the uncertainty of predicting when individuals will actually start dialysis, attempting to avoid the scenario that some of the usable lifespan of the AVG is expended before it is actually needed.
- It is imperative that strategies to preserve all potential access options are implemented preoperatively. Central venous catheters should be avoided to prevent the development of stenoses and/or occlusions, particularly subclavian vein catheters and percutaneously inserted central catheters. Similarly, leadless pacers should be used to prevent any fibrotic response from the leads in the central venous system. The cephalic and basilic veins should be spared from blood draws, intravenous catheters, and use as arterial conduits (for example, for lower extremity bypass with arm vein).

Preoperative Preparation

- The preoperative preparation for patients undergoing permanent access should be comparable with any major surgical procedure. It is important to emphasize that patients with CKD and ESKD typically have multiple active medical problems and that these should be optimized, despite that fact that access procedures are generally considered "minor." All infections should be completely treated (ie, catheter-related infection), particularly for those patients in which an AVG is planned. It may be helpful to consult the patient's nephrologist and dialysis center to optimize their preparation. In addition, we prefer to operate on individuals between their dialysis days when possible.

Choice of Anesthesia

- The intraoperative conduct of the various upper extremity permanent access procedures is similar, regardless of whether an AVF or AVG is being created. The options for anesthesia include local, regional, or general with the choice contingent upon the proposed configuration, as well as patient and provider preference. Although regional anesthesia has been purported to provide beneficial vasodilatory effects, the KDOQI Guidelines defer the choice to the provider's discretion (Guideline 8). It is our preference to use regional anesthesia for access procedures based in the antecubital fossa and distally on the forearm while general anesthesia is used for more proximal procedures that extend to the axilla. Importantly, we request that the anesthesiologist use shorter-acting regional agents so that it is possible to perform a neurologic examination of the hand in the recovery room. Intraoperative ultrasound, particularly after the induction of anesthesia, can be particularly helpful to identify the location and size of the outflow veins.

Positioning

- The selected upper extremity is positioned on an arm board or hand table with the shoulder abducted at 90°. The extent of the operative field and skin preparation is dictated by the procedure, typically extending from the hand to the axilla and shoulder. The KDOQI Guidelines failed to identify any intraoperative adjuncts (ie, anastomotic technique, suture type, topical agents) that improved outcome (Guideline 8). Similarly, they did not support the use of one specific graft material, deferring the choice to the operator's discretion (Guideline 4). Although not specifically addressed in the Guidelines, we prefer a fixed dose of heparin (ie, 5000 U intravenously) prior to arterial cross-clamp application in contrast to our more conventional dose for nondialysis-based arterial reconstructions (ie, 100 U/kg), given the intrinsic platelet dysfunction associated with renal failure. It has been our anecdotal impression that there is wide variation in the dosing of heparin across the country with a large percentage of surgeons not using it at all during hemodialysis access procedures.

FOREARM AVF

Radial-Cephalic AVF (FIGURE 1)

- A 3-cm longitudinal incision is made at the midpoint between the radial artery and the cephalic vein and extended distally to the wrist crease. Skin flaps are elevated both medially and laterally to facilitate exposure of the underlying vein and artery, and this can be facilitated with small spring retractors.
- The cephalic vein is dissected and a sufficient length is mobilized to facilitate transposing it to the adjacent artery; this may require ligating any small branches that tether the main vein.
- The vein is then transected proximally (ie, proximal on the vein, distal on the wrist) and the residual segment is suture ligated.
- The mobilized vein is then gently dilated with sterile heparinized saline and marked to prevent any inadvertent twisting during transposition.
- The radial artery is mobilized for approximately 2 to 3 cm, a sufficient length to allow placement of the vascular clamps and create the arteriotomy.
- Patients are administered a fixed heparin dose, the vessels are clamped, and a 1-cm longitudinal arteriotomy is created using an 11-blade scalpel and fine scissors.
- The vein is spatulated and an end of vein to side of artery anastomosis is completed using a running 6-0 monofilament suture under loupe magnification.

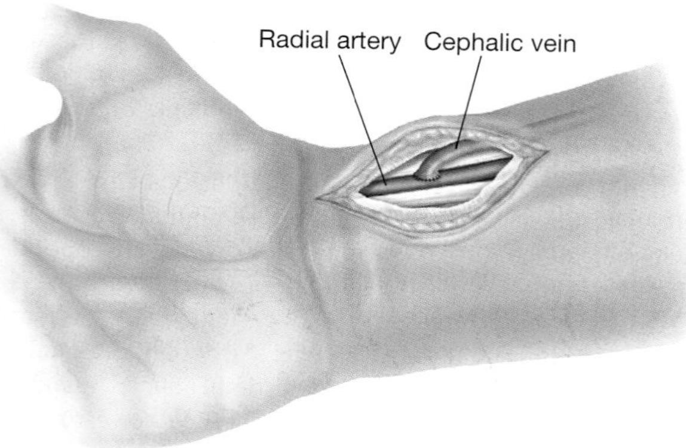

FIGURE 1 ● A distal radial artery–cephalic vein AVF at the wrist. A longitudinal incision is made between the radial artery and cephalic vein at the wrist. The cephalic vein is mobilized and anastomosed to the radial artery in an end-to-side fashion.

- There should be a thrill in the proximal cephalic vein upon completion of the anastomosis, although this is not always detected intraoperatively due to the small caliber of the radial artery and any residual spasm resulting from the dissection and clamp placement. Regardless, a bruit should be detected using continuous wave Doppler.
- A pulsatile signal in the cephalic veins suggests an outflow stenosis that mandates further investigation, potentially a twist in the vein or stenosis resulting from inadequate mobilization.
- The patient's heparin effect is not usually reversed given the small caliber of the vessels. The skin is reapproximated with interrupted, absorbable sutures, and the skin is closed with a monofilament, absorbable suture.

Radial-Basilic AVF (FIGURE 2)

- A 3-cm longitudinal incision is made over the distal radial artery proximal to the wrist crease and the vessel is dissected free, similar to the approach for the radial-cephalic AVF.[5]
- An incision is made over the course of the basilic vein in the forearm from the antecubital fossa to the wrist. This vein is easily identifiable in thin patients, but its location can be facilitated by an intraoperative ultrasound if necessary.
- The basilic vein is completely dissected and the branches are ligated.
- The vein is transected at the wrist, gently distended with heparinized saline, and then passed across the volar aspect of the forearm immediately deep to the skin. This can be facilitated using an aortic clamp or a hollow tunneling device.

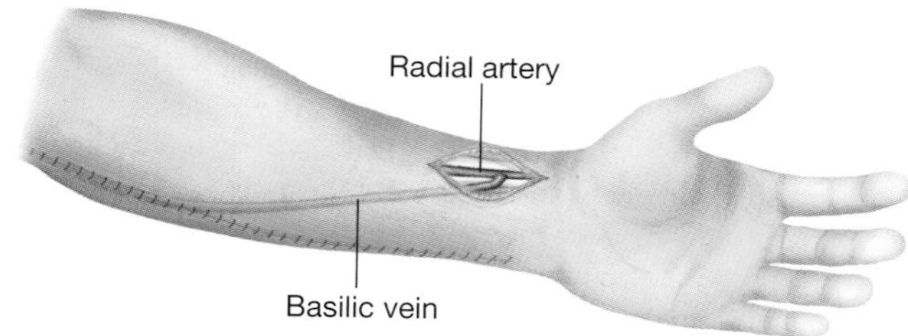

FIGURE 2 ● A radial artery–basilic vein AVF. A longitudinal incision is made over the distal radial artery near the wrist. An incision is made over the basilic vein from the antecubital crease to the wrist, and the vein is dissected free. The vein is transposed over the volar aspect of the forearm in a subcutaneous plane, and an end-to-side anastomosis is performed.

Caution should be exercised to assure a gentle curve of the vein at the antecubital fossa to prevent compressing it on the adjacent soft tissue.

- The remaining components of the procedure including the anastomosis, completion assessment and closure are identical to the radial-cephalic AVF.

Alternatives

- The radial-cephalic AVF can be created distal to the wrist in the anatomic snuffbox located between the extensor pollicis brevis and the extensor pollicis longus tendons.[6] Although the radial artery and cephalic vein are somewhat smaller in this location, the reported outcomes are comparable with the more traditional configuration at the wrist.
- The distal radial artery at the wrist can be transected and anastomosed to the cephalic vein in an end artery–side vein configuration, termed the RADAR AVF (radial artery deviation and reimplantation).[7] This configuration may have better patency and a lower rate of anastomotic hyperplasia but concerns remain about the potential for hand edema resulting from the end artery–side vein configuration.
- The ulnar artery can be used for both cephalic- or basilic-based AVFs, although caution should be exercised given the fact that most individuals are ulnar dominant.

UPPER ARM AVF

Brachial-Cephalic AVF (FIGURE 3)

- A transverse incision is made across the antecubital crease and the cephalic vein (or median antecubital vein) is exposed. Care should be exercised when making the skin incision since the target vein runs very superficial and can be inadvertently injured.
- Alternatively, a sigmoidal incision over the distal cephalic vein in the upper arm extending across the antecubital crease and then longitudinally over the brachial artery can be used if additional mobilization of the cephalic vein is required (or if the proximal radial artery will be used for the anastomosis).
- The vein is dissected free and its branches are suture ligated. This may require mobilizing the vein more proximal on the upper arm by elevating the skin flap if the vein and brachial artery are somewhat far apart.
- We will occasionally use the median antecubital vein, preserving both the cephalic and basilic outflow, if the outflow veins are somewhat diminutive. This affords both the opportunity to dilate and mature, conceding that the basilic vein will need to be transposed in the future if it emerges as the dominant outflow and that the dual outflow configuration may be associated with a higher incidence of hand ischemia.
- The brachial artery is exposed by incising the overlying bicipital aponeurosis and a sufficient length is mobilized to facilitate applying the vascular clamps and creating the anastomosis.
- Approximately 20% of individuals will have an "early take-off" of the radial artery proximal to the antecubital fossa.[8] In this scenario, the radial artery courses superficial to the larger ulnar artery in the antecubital fossa and can be mistaken for the brachial artery. Concern for a high takeoff of the radial artery should be raised if the vessel seems smaller than anticipated.
- A 1-cm longitudinal arteriotomy is created after vascular control. The cephalic (or median antecubital) vein is spatulated and distended and the anastomosis performed using a 6-0 monofilament vascular suture. The deeper tributary branches of the cephalic vein may be partially preserved to create a more patulous anastomosis.
- A robust bruit and thrill should be detected upon completion of the anastomosis. The cephalic vein may occasionally be compressed by the adjacent soft tissue or tethered by one of its branches, which can be remediated by incising any concerning soft tissue and raising a larger skin flap or transecting the offending branch and further mobilizing the vein.
- The wound is reapproximated with interrupted, absorbable sutures, and the final layer of skin is closed using a subcutaneous monofilament suture. It is helpful to mark the skin using lines perpendicular to the planned transverse component of the skin incision to assure correct alignment of the skin flaps.

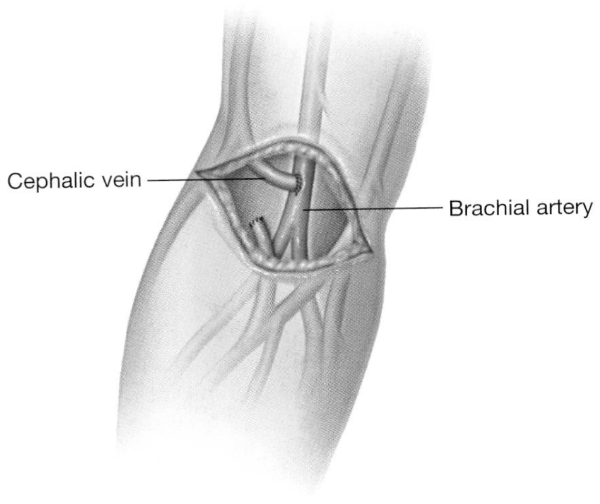

FIGURE 3 ● A brachial artery–cephalic vein AVF. A transverse incision is made across the antecubital fossa, and the cephalic vein and brachial artery are dissected. The anastomosis is performed in an end-to-side fashion.

Brachial-Basilic AVF (FIGURE 4)

- The brachial-basilic AVF can be created as a single- or two-stage procedure. The available evidence is somewhat equivocal, but it suggests that the two-stage procedure may allow smaller veins to mature and ultimately be suitable for dialysis.[9] We prefer the two-stage procedure since it avoids a larger surgical procedure unless the vein has dilated sufficiently. Given the need to transpose the vein and elevate it from its deeper position compared with the skin, it is relatively contraindicated in obese patients.

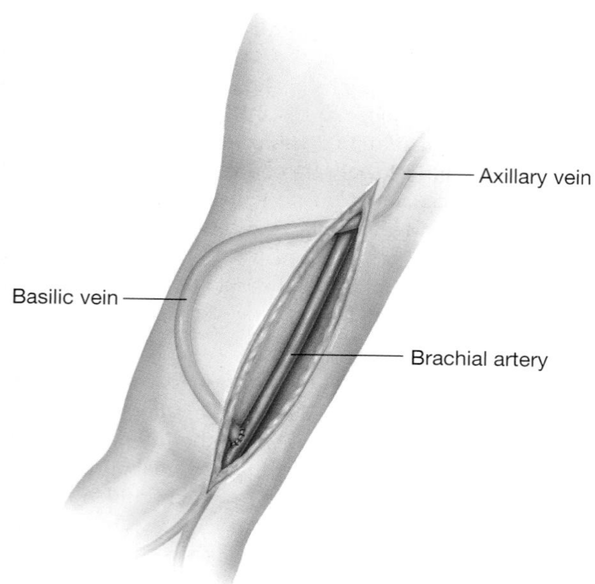

FIGURE 4 ● A brachial artery–basilic vein AVF. Note that the image could represent a single- or the two-stage procedure. An incision is made from the antecubital fossa to the axilla, and the basilic vein is dissected free. The vein is transposed through a lateral, subcutaneous tunnel and anastomosed in an end-to-side fashion.

- A 3-cm incision is made halfway between the basilic vein and brachial artery in the distal upper arm, immediately proximal to the antecubital fossa, as the initial step of the two-stage procedure. The exposure of the basilic vein may be simplified by marking its course with duplex. The vein is identified, confirmed by the overlying median antecubital cutaneous nerve that bifurcates in the distal upper arm, and then circumferentially dissected. The adjacent brachial artery is dissected free by incising the brachial sheath and approximately 2 to 3 cm is exposed. The basilic vein is transected and its proximal portion (ie, distal extent) is suture ligated. The vein is spatulated and mobilized to create the end vein to side brachial artery anastomosis using a standard technique.
- The second stage procedure is performed when the outflow basilic vein has dilated sufficiently for cannulation, typically >5 mm in diameter. A longitudinal incision is made from the antecubital crease to the axilla, incorporating the incision from the first-stage operation. We will typically make a series of smaller, subtotal incisions (rather than one continuous initial incision) to make sure that the incision overlies the basilic vein, minimizing the extent of the skin flaps. The basilic vein is then circumferentially exposed from the anastomosis to the axilla and completely dissected free. The vein may elongate as well as dilate after the first stage thereby increasing the available length for transposition. The broader-based branches of the basilic vein should be suture ligated to reduce the likelihood of the tie inadvertently falling off. The dissection is continued to the anastomosis to optimize the available length despite the surrounding scar tissue, although we do not typically dissect out the brachial artery at the anastomosis.
- The vein can be elevated and/or transposed with several different techniques including simple mobilization and elevation, mobilization and elevation beneath a subcutaneous flap, or transection of the anastomosis and transposition through a new subcutaneous tunnel with re-siting the anastomosis more proximally. We prefer the later technique since it facilitates rerouting the vein more lateral on the upper arm, which is more anatomically favorable for cannulation, although it mandates redoing the anastomosis. Furthermore, this approach does not mandate transecting the cutaneous nerve.
- The initial anastomosis is dissembled by transecting the vein at the anastomosis and oversewing its hood. The vein is then distended and marked to prevent twisting. It is imperative to fully mobilize the vein in the axilla to avoid creating any tension at the swing segment (ie, "hinge point"), a common site of neointimal hyperplasia formation. The distended vein is then gently draped over the skin, and its proposed course is marked on the skin. A tunnel is created as lateral as possible, immediately deep to the skin, using a curved, hollow tunneller, and the vein is passed through the tunnel.
- The brachial artery adjacent to the exit site of the basilic vein tunnel is then exposed by incision of the overlying brachial sheath. The anastomosis is completed using standard technique.
- A #10 Jackson-Pratt drain is placed throughout the basilic vein harvest site, and the overlying soft tissue is closed, exercising care not to somehow crimp or narrow the AVF. The deep dermal and skin layers are closed using a continuous braided and monofilament absorbable suture, respectively.

Alternatives

- The distal radial artery can be used as an alternative to the brachial artery at the antecubital fossa as the inflow source for both the cephalic- and basilic-based upper extremity AVFs.[10] The potential advantage includes a lower access flow rate that can result in a lower incidence hand ischemia, venous hypertension, arm edema, and central vein stenoses.
- One of the deeper, perforating vessels off the antecubital vein can be used with the proximal radial or brachial radial arteries in a configuration traditionally referred to as the Gracz AVF.[11]
- The brachial vein may be used as an alternative to the basilic vein with either a single- or two-stage procedure as outlined above.[12] The brachial veins are paired structures that course along the brachial artery, and they tend to be fairly thin walled and friable. It is our preference to perform a two-stage procedure, selecting the largest of the two branches during the first stage.

FOREARM AVG (FIGURE 5)

- A 3-cm incision is made across the antecubital crease, and the median antecubital vein and brachial artery are exposed. Alternatively, a horizontal incision can be made approximately 1 to 1.5 cm distal to the antecubital crease and skin flaps can be raised to expose the vessels. The cephalic, basilic, brachial, or median antecubital veins can be used as the venous outflow, and we traditionally just use the largest vein with the best outflow. Exposure of the brachial artery requires incising the overlying biceps aponeurosis. The course of the proposed prosthetic loop over the forearm is marked, extending approximately 2 to 3 cm from the wrist crease in a nice gentle curve. A separate longitudinal skin incision is made over this course near the wrist and a 6-mm nonringed graft, typically PTFE, is passed along the identified path using a hollow tunneller.
- The arterial and venous anastomoses are performed in sequence using a 6-0 monofilament vascular suture. We prefer to do the venous anastomosis first to minimize the amount of bleeding from the needle holes at the arterial anastomoses. A nice thrill should be detected at the venous anastomosis upon completion.
- The skin flaps are reapproximated with interrupted, absorbable sutures, and the final layer of the skin is closed with a monofilament, absorbable suture. The use of an early cannulation graft may avoid the use of a TDC in some settings.

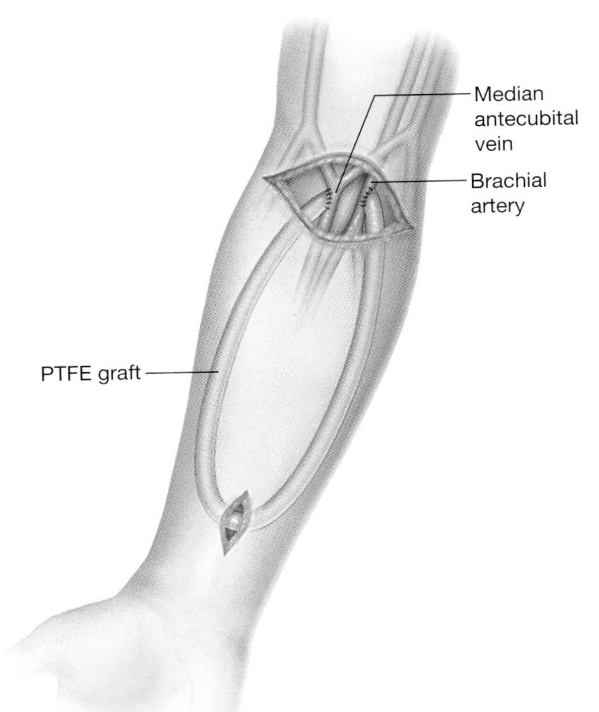

FIGURE 5 ● A forearm brachial artery–median antecubital vein AVG. A transverse incision is made across the antecubital fossa, and the median antecubital vein and brachial artery are dissected free. A 6-mm polytetrafluoroethylene (PTFE) graft is tunneled in a looped configuration with the aid of a second counter incision. Both anastomoses are completed in an end-to-side fashion.

UPPER ARM AVG

- The upper arm AVG can be created in two configurations: a gentle, semicircle from the brachial artery immediately proximal to the antecubital fossa to the axillary vein in the axilla (**FIGURE 6A**) or a complete loop from the brachial artery in the axilla to the adjacent axillary vein (**FIGURE 6B**). Our preference is to use the brachial artery in the axilla for individuals at a higher risk of developing access-related hand ischemia given the higher incidence associated with the brachial artery near the antecubital fossa, typically women and older individuals. We favor using the more distal brachial artery for those at lower risk for ischemia (eg, younger men) because the tunnel is a bit easier to make, particularly for some of the early cannulation grafts that require removing an investing plastic sheath.
- The distal brachial artery is exposed through a 3-cm incision over its course proximal to the antecubital crease. This requires incising the overlying brachial sheath and dissecting 2 to 3 cm of the vessel. The axillary vein (and proximal brachial artery for the other looped configuration) is exposed using a 3- to 4-cm longitudinal incision over the course of the vessels that extends to the axillary skin fold. Adequate exposure may require proximal extension of the incision and retracting the pectoralis major muscle and adjacent soft tissue. Two deep Weitlander retractors oriented at about 60° from the longitudinal axis of the vessels provides adequate exposure.
- The venous anatomy in the axilla can be somewhat confusing. The paired brachial and basilic vein drain into the axillary vein, although these configurations are not universal and there can be paired outflow veins. Additional proximal dissection should be performed if the initially identified veins appear to be too small.
- The proximal brachial artery can be exposed by incising its overlying sheath, typically distal to the takeoff of the profunda brachial artery.
- The course of the graft is marked on the skin (ie, gentle curve for distal brachial artery and complete "tear drop" loop for proximal brachial artery). A separate incision sited at the mid portion of the tunnel in the distal, lateral upper arm is required to tunnel the complete loop for the proximal brachial artery configuration. The hollow tunneller is passed from the axillary incision to the separate arm incision in such a fashion that its course is relatively deep to the skin near the axilla but immediately below the dermis for the portion of the graft that will be used for cannulation, roughly all but the 3 to 4 cm length near the axilla.
- The anastomoses are completed using standard technique. We prefer to construct the venous anastomosis first since it is more challenging given its proximal location. The soft tissue of the axilla is closed in multiple layers using interrupted, absorbable sutures, and the final later of skin is closed in a subcuticular fashion.

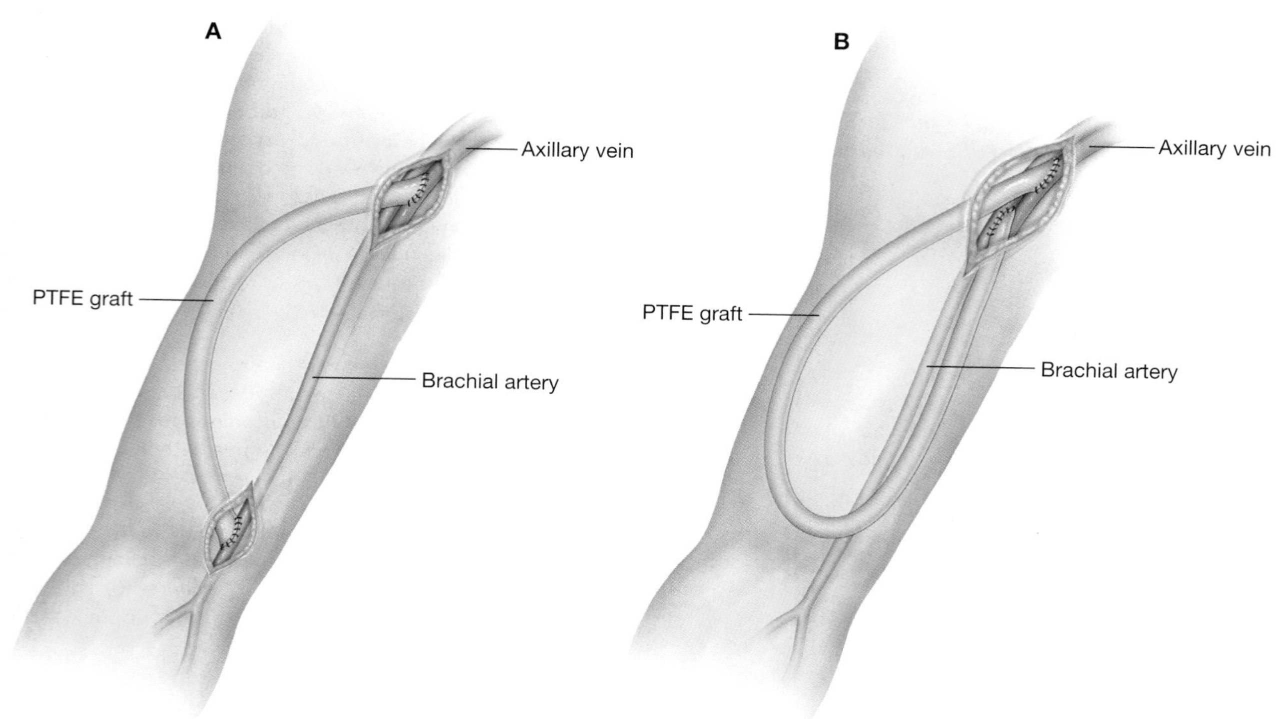

FIGURE 6 ● **A,** An upper arm brachial artery–axillary vein AVG is shown with the brachial artery exposed near the antecubital fossa. The 6-mm PTFE graft is tunneled through a lateral, subcutaneous plane, and both anastomoses are completed in an end-to-side fashion. **B,** An upper arm brachial artery–axillary vein AVG is shown with both anastomoses located in the axilla. A separate counter incision is made to facilitate the tunnel.

PEARLS AND PITFALLS

Access choice	▪ The choice of access procedure should be based upon anatomy, life expectancy, anticipated duration of dialysis, and patient preference within the context of the patient's ESKD Life Plan.
Access preservation	▪ Strategies should be implemented to preserve all potential access configurations and salvage all failing or thrombosed accesses.
Anastomosis	▪ The venous anastomosis should be constructed first when creating an AVG to minimize arterial bleeding from the needle holes.
Access Tunnel	▪ The course of the tunnel should extend laterally over the upper arm when creating an AVG to facilitate a comfortable position for cannulation while the patient's arm rests on the table during dialysis. Flexing the elbow to 90° prior to marking the tunnel to ensure that the graft is tunneled sufficiently lateral is helpful.
Complication prevention	▪ Strategies should be implemented preoperatively in patients deemed higher risk for ARHI including excluding any arterial inflow stenosis, avoiding the brachial artery at the antecubital fossa as the inflow source, and avoiding the use of large conduits (ie., transposed femoral vein). Furthermore, a potential remedial strategy should be generated *preoperatively* in the event that they develop ischemia. These higher-risk patients include the elderly, diabetic patients, those with peripheral vascular disease, and those with prior episodes of hand ischemia.

POSTOPERATIVE CARE

- A set of serum electrolytes should be obtained in the recovery room to determine the need for urgent hemodialysis. The new access and upper extremity pulses should be interrogated using a combination of physical examination and/or Doppler ultrasound. A brief neurological examination should be performed on the ipsilateral hand to assess both motor and sensory function.
- Patients undergoing second-stage brachial-basilic AVFs are routinely admitted overnight, and their drains are removed the following day at the time of discharge; all other patients are admitted selectively with the determinants being pain control, comorbidities, and urgent need for dialysis.
- Patients are seen in the outpatient clinic 2 weeks postoperatively and then monthly thereafter. The appearance of the wound and patency of the access are assessed along with the presence of any complications.
- Standard AVGs are cleared for use at 3 to 6 weeks postoperatively after the surgical incisions have healed, while early cannulation AVGs can be released almost immediately provided that the patient can tolerate graft cannulation through the surgical tunnel.
- An ultrasound of AVFs is obtained at 6 weeks to assess the outflow vein diameter and the access flow rates. AVFs are cleared for cannulation when the vein diameter exceeds 5 mm and the flow rates exceed 500 mL/min, typically in 3 to 4 months.[13]
- AVFs that fail to mature are evaluated further by AVF duplex. The etiology of this failure to mature includes inflow lesions, anastomotic stenosis, venous outflow stenosis, central vein lesions, accessory veins, excessive depth (ie, obesity), and diffuse narrowing.[4,14] Additional imaging with a catheter-based fistulagram or arteriogram is obtained with the choice dictated by the presumed problem and the need to image from the AVF anastomosis to the central veins or the whole access circuit including the arterial inflow. Remedial treatment with balloon angioplasty and/or an intraluminal stent can be performed as dictated by the findings. Unfortunately, up to one-third of AVFs require some type of remedial intervention to facilitate maturation.[4,14]

COMPLICATIONS

Access-Related Hand Ischemia

- The presence of any access-related hand ischemia (ARHI) or "steal" in the recovery room is particularly concerning. The symptoms of hand ischemia may range from mild (Grade 1—cool extremity, minimal symptoms) to moderate (Grade 2—pain during dialysis) to severe (Grade 3—rest pain, tissue loss).[15] Most of these complaints are more chronic, but the presence and any sensory or motor deficit in the immediate postoperative period merits further intervention. A small subset of patients, typically diabetic patients with peripheral arterial disease undergoing an AVG, can present with intense pain, paresthesia, and motor weakness in the early postoperative period despite normal wrist pulses. This condition, often termed ischemic monomelic neuropathy, is likely a variant of ARHI that primarily affects the nerves and is best treated with emergent access ligation, although some of the neurologic symptoms may not be reversible.[16,17]
- The management of ARHI or the steal syndrome remains an ongoing problem beyond the immediate postoperative period, and up to 20% of individuals receiving a brachial artery–based access at the antecubital fossa will develop some type of steal symptoms with roughly half of these requiring intervention.[18] The timing of the symptoms and ultimate need for intervention are somewhat variable with roughly one-third of the remedial interventions occurring within a week, one-third within a month, and the final one-third beyond a month.[18,19]
- The treatments for ARHI include correction of an arterial inflow stenosis, access flow restriction or "banding," proximalization of the arterial inflow (PAI), revision using distal inflow (RUDI), distal revascularization with interval ligation (DRIL), or ligation. The optimal choice is contingent access type (ie, AVF vs AVG), location (ie, brachial vs radial artery), comorbidities, patient life expectancy, available conduit, future access options, and anticipated dialysis access success. However, the practical choices for a brachial-axillary AVG with the anastomosis near the antecubital fossa include a PAI or ligation, while those for a brachial-based AVF include a RUDI, DRIL, or ligation.
- All patients with any motor compromise merit intervention to reduce the symptoms while, ideally, saving the access. The remedial treatment should include an arteriogram to exclude any inflow stenoses. Notably, the various treatment options (eg, DRIL, RUDI, banding) should be viewed as complementary rather than competitive strategies, with the DRIL and PAI potentially most beneficial for "low-flow" accesses (AVFs < 800 mL/min, AVG < 1200 mL/min) and the RUDI and banding techniques most beneficial for "high-flow" accesses.[20] We do not perform a DRIL or RUDI for steal symptoms associated with an AVG given their more limited patency but will correct the arterial inflow or perform a PAI.

Other Complications

- Patients undergoing permanent access procedures are prone to both systemic and access-specific complications. Owing to their comorbidities, these patients are prone to the typical cardiac and pulmonary complications.
- The access-specific complications commonly include ARHI, failing/thrombosed access, infection, arm edema, neuropathy, high-output congestive heart failure, and seroma. Although most of these complications are chronic, they can occur in the early postoperative period.
- Both AVFs and AVGs can thrombose in the early postoperative period with the incidence being around <10%.[21,22] Early access thromboses are typically attributed to technical issues or a hypercoagulable condition. We have taken an aggressive approach in this setting and have attempted access thrombectomy and surgical revision as dictated by the intraoperative findings and imaging.
- Surgical site infection can occur, and the spectrum of infection ranges from mild cellulitis to more extensive soft tissue infections. Minor wound infections can be treated with antibiotics targeted against the typical microorganisms. More extensive infections are less common and may mandate removal of all prosthetic material. These more extensive infections do not usually occur with autogenous AVFs.

- Postoperative edema is common. This usually resolves within the first couple of weeks. Persistent swelling merits further investigation with duplex ultrasound to exclude a hematoma or a venous outflow stenosis or occlusion. A catheter-based fistulagram may be necessary to evaluate for central venous stenosis. We typically wait 4 weeks after the access creation to obtain a fistulagram to allow the access to be incorporated in the surrounding soft tissue in an attempt to minimize cannulation complications at the time of the fistulagram.
- A seroma can develop in any of the surgical incisions from persistent lymph leak. These are usually self-limited and resolve with expectant management. Persistent leaks merit surgical exploration with ligation of all potential sources, although they can mandate access excision if they persist.

REFERENCES

1. NKF-DOQI clinical practice guidelines for vascular access. National Kidney Foundation-Dialysis Outcomes Quality Initiative. *Am J Kidney Dis*. 1997;30(4 suppl 3):S150-S191. http://www.ncbi.nlm.nih.gov/pubmed/9339150
2. Gold JA, Hoffman K. Fistula first: the National Vascular Access Improvement Initiative. *WMJ*. 2006;105(3):71-73.
3. Lok CE, Huber TS, Lee T, et al. KDOQI clinical practice guideline for vascular access: 2019 update. *Am J Kidney Dis*. 2020;75(4 suppl 2): S1-s164. (In Eng). doi:10.1053/j.ajkd.2019.12.001
4. Huber TS, Ozaki CK, Flynn TC, et al. Prospective validation of an algorithm to maximize native arteriovenous fistulae for chronic hemodialysis access. *J Vasc Surg*. 2002;36(3):452-459.
5. Silva MB, Jr., Hobson RW, Pappas PJ, et al. Vein transposition in the forearm for autogenous hemodialysis access. *J Vasc Surg*. 1997;26(6):981-986. http://www.ncbi.nlm.nih.gov/pubmed/9423713
6. Heindel P, Dieffenbach BV, Sharma G, Belkin M, Ozaki CK, Hentschel DM. Contemporary outcomes of a "snuffbox first" hemodialysis access approach in the United States. *J Vasc Surg* 2021;74(3):947-956. (In Eng). doi:10.1016/j.jvs.2021.01.069
7. Sadaghianloo N, Declemy S, Jean-Baptiste E, et al. Radial artery deviation and reimplantation inhibits venous juxta-anastomotic stenosis and increases primary patency of radial-cephalic fistulas for hemodialysis. *J Vasc Surg*. 2016;64(3):698-706.e1. (In Eng). doi:10.1016/j.jvs.2016.04.023
8. Kirksey L. Unrecognized high brachial artery bifurcation is associated with higher rate of dialysis access failure. *Semin Dial*. 2011;24(6):698-702.
9. Cooper J, Power AH, DeRose G, Forbes TL, Dubois L. Similar failure and patency rates when comparing one- and two-stage basilic vein transposition. *J Vasc Surg*. 2015;61(3):809-816.
10. Arnaoutakis DJ, Deroo EP, McGlynn P, et al. Improved outcomes with proximal radial-cephalic arteriovenous fistulas compared with brachial-cephalic arteriovenous fistulas. *J Vasc Surg*. 2017;66(5):1497-1503. (In Eng). doi:10.1016/j.jvs.2017.04.075
11. Gracz KC, Ing TS, Soung LS, Armbruster KF, Seim SK, Merkel FK. Proximal forearm fistula for maintenance hemodialysis. *Kidney Int*. 1977;11(1):71-75. http://www.ncbi.nlm.nih.gov/pubmed/839655
12. Jennings WC, Sideman MJ, Taubman KE, Broughan TA. Brachial vein transposition arteriovenous fistulas for hemodialysis access. *J Vasc Surg*. 2009;50(5):1121-1125.
13. Beathard GA, Lok CE, Glickman MH, et al. Definitions and end points for interventional studies for arteriovenous dialysis access. *Clin J Am Soc Nephrol*. 2018;13(3):501-512. (In Eng). doi:10.2215/cjn.11531116
14. Huber TS, Berceli SA, Scali ST, et al. Arteriovenous fistula maturation, functional patency, and intervention rates. *JAMA Surg*. 2021;156(12):1111-1118. (In Eng). doi:10.1001/jamasurg.2021.4527
15. Sidawy AN, Gray R, Besarab A, et al. Recommended standards for reports dealing with arteriovenous hemodialysis accesses. *J Vasc Surg*. 2002;35(3):603-610. http://www.ncbi.nlm.nih.gov/pubmed/11877717
16. Wilbourn AJ, Furlan AJ, Hulley W, Ruschhaupt W. Ischemic monomelic neuropathy. *Neurology*. 1983;33(4):447-451.
17. Thimmisetty RK, Pedavally S, Rossi NF, Fernandes JAM, Fixley J. Ischemic monomelic neuropathy: diagnosis, pathophysiology, and management. *Kidney Int Rep*. 2017;2(1):76-79. (In Eng). doi:10.1016/j.ekir.2016.08.013
18. Huber TS, Brown MP, Seeger JM, Lee WA. Midterm outcome after the distal revascularization and interval ligation (DRIL) procedure. *J Vasc Surg*. 2008;48(4):926-932.
19. Scali ST, Chang CK, Raghinaru D, et al. Prediction of graft patency and mortality after distal revascularization and interval ligation for hemodialysis access-related hand ischemia. *J Vasc Surg*. 2013;57(2):451-458.
20. Zanow J, Petzold K, Petzold M, Krueger U, Scholz H. Flow reduction in high-flow arteriovenous access using intraoperative flow monitoring. *J Vasc Surg*. 2006;44(6):1273-1278.
21. Farber A, Imrey PB, Huber TS, et al. Multiple preoperative and intraoperative factors predict early fistula thrombosis in the Hemodialysis Fistula Maturation Study. *J Vasc Surg*. 2016;63(1):163-170.e6. (In Eng). doi:10.1016/j.jvs.2015.07.086
22. Huber TS, Carter JW, Carter RL, Seeger JM. Patency of autogenous and PTFE upper extremity arteriovenous hemodialysis accesses: a systematic review. *J Vasc Surg*. 2003;38(5):1005-1011.

Chapter **38**

Hemodialysis Catheter Placement and Maintenance

Nathan W. Kugler and Kellie R. Brown

DEFINITION

- Hemodialysis is defined as the direct mechanical alteration of both blood volume and composition through filtering of blood. This differs from other forms of dialysis, such as peritoneal dialysis, in which volume and composition are indirectly altered.
- Hemodialysis catheters are central venous catheters placed for the purpose of and to facilitate administration of hemodialysis, either in a continuous or intermittent fashion. Typically, these are large-bore (up to 16Fr) dual-lumen catheters designed to facilitate exchange of large volumes of blood at rates (up to 500 mL/min) required for dialysis. Based on the most recent KDOQI guidelines the recommended catheter blood flow rates should be >350 mL/min.[1]
- Catheters can be either tunneled or nontunneled. Tunneled catheters often have a cuffed portion positioned subcutaneously near the skin exit site designed to prevent catheter migration and to decrease the risk of infection.
- A multitude of different hemodialysis catheter tip configurations are on the market, all of which have their own benefits and drawbacks (**FIGURE 1**).
- Hemodialysis catheter placement is typically defined by the vessel of venous access:
  - Internal jugular vein
  - Subclavian vein
  - Femoral vein

PATIENT HISTORY AND PHYSICAL FINDINGS

- A detailed history and physical examination are crucial when evaluating patients in need of a hemodialysis catheter for access.
- History:
  - Special attention to previous central venous line (CVL), peripherally inserted central catheter (PICC), and pacemaker placement is key to understanding risk for central venous stenosis.
  - History of previous upper extremity or neck vein deep venous thrombosis (DVT) provides insight to potential access site difficulties. History of previous lower extremity DVT is important when planning femoral vein access.
- Physical examination:
  - Face and chest wall swelling, with or without chest wall collaterals, can indicate significant central venous stenosis, possibly within the superior vena cava.
  - Chest wall scars can be indicative of previous tunneled lines or implantable port. In addition, palpation of chest wall can aid with evaluation of an underlying pacemaker.
  - Evaluation of the bilateral upper and lower extremities should include investigation of scars consistent with previous hemodialysis access attempts.
  - Unilateral upper extremity swelling can be indicative of either deep venous thrombus or more central venous stenosis.
- Bedside ultrasound evaluation is an important adjunct available in many provider offices. Such technology is becoming more readily available and is now often taught in conjunction with physical examination skills.

IMAGING AND OTHER DIAGNOSTIC STUDIES

- Any available previous imaging should be reviewed in detail. Prior chest x-ray and computed tomography (CT) imaging may demonstrate the presence of a pacemaker, previous central venous lines, peripherally inserted central catheters, or venous stents.

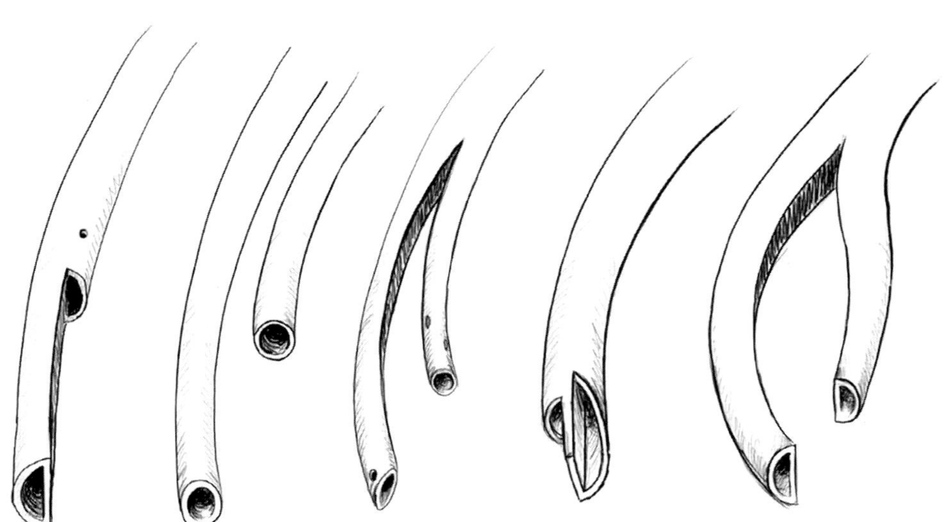

FIGURE 1 ● Diagram outlining the different tip designs of tunneled hemodialysis catheters. (Courtesy of Jacob C. Wood, MD.)

- Imaging review can help clinicians understand anatomic challenges to central catheter placement. In addition, it may aid in the understanding of and predict potential issues that may result in catheter dysfunction following placement.
- Ultrasound evaluation of the venous system is helpful in establishing the presence of thrombus and evidence of central obstruction and determining technical feasibility.
- In the situation of numerous previous central venous lines and no previous imaging, a reasonable start to evaluation is a dedicated CT venogram of the chest. Such imaging will help assess central venous anatomy and patency.

SURGICAL MANAGEMENT

Preprocedural Planning

- Determining whether the hemodialysis catheter will be tunneled or temporary is key to procedural planning. Absolute contraindications to placement of tunneled dialysis catheters include ongoing bacteremia and uncorrected coagulopathy, and overlying skin infection or breakdown. Relative contraindications include severe metabolic abnormalities, chest wall neoplasms, anticipated site of radiation therapy, ongoing cellulitis, chest wall burns, and those requiring ongoing chest physiotherapy.
- Tunneled dialysis catheters are available in different calibers and appropriate lengths. Choice of the appropriate length is critical as the anticipated duration of these catheters is significantly longer.
- Temporary nontunneled catheters are preferred for short-term (less than 2 weeks) dialysis access, or in the case of ongoing bacteremia or when multiple line exchanges are anticipated. Nontunneled catheters are available in different calibers, configurations (straight vs curved), and lengths. Differences in configuration lend advantages and disadvantages based on the venous access location.
- Appropriate preprocedural laboratory studies should include a basic metabolic panel to assess potassium and uremia along with an international normalized ratio for all patients. Those receiving heparin products should have a recent activated partial thromboplastin time. Patients with a history of or risk factors for thrombocytopenia should have a recent platelet count.
- Preprocedural antibiotic administration should be used in accordance with your institutional policy.
- Venous access location
  - The preferred location for venous access is the right internal jugular vein.
  - Catheters should not be placed on the side of a maturing fistula or anticipated hemodialysis fistula or graft as ipsilateral placement puts the patient at risk for central stenosis and potential for failure to mature.

Patient Positioning

- Patient positioning for catheter placement is dependent upon planned location of venous access and whether tunneled or nontunneled catheter is being placed.
- When utilizing internal jugular or subclavian vein access, the head should be rotated to the contralateral side. This technique will open the jugular triangle facilitating the most direct venous access. Restrictions such as associated cervical spine injury or previous spinal fusion may preclude this maneuver and may play a role in choice of venous access location.
- Trendelenburg positioning is an important aspect of safe venous access when utilizing either an internal jugular or a subclavian venous approach.
- When placing a tunneled hemodialysis catheter, the operator must ensure patient positioning allows sufficient exposure of the venous access site, skin tunnel, and catheter exit site.
- Overall room setup is a consideration with the understanding that alternative venous access sites might be required. Patient and bed positioning if planned fluoroscopy with a C-arm ensures adequate working room with minimal movement. Planning of optimal room setup and patient position can minimize unnecessary movements that may compromise sterile technique.
- Supplies:
  - It is critical to ensure all needed supplies for catheter placement are gathered and present prior to beginning the procedure. This ensures the most efficient means of placement while lessening risk of breaks in your sterile field.
  - Typical setups include a central venous access kit including the necessary wires, dilators, and catheters. Local anesthetic, skin knife, and dressings are necessary for all line placements. When planning for tunneled line placement, a tunneler is essential along with suture and dressing to close with the counter incision at the venous access site.

TECHNIQUES

GENERAL CONSIDERATIONS

- Ensuring adequate sterile technique is essential to reducing catheter-associated infections. Chlorhexidine and alcohol-based skin preparation products are best suited for prevention of infection,[2] and utilization of full body sterile draping minimizes potential exposure and equipment contamination.
- Utilization of a central line dressing kit, which typically includes an antimicrobial dressing such as BIOPATCH (Ethicon Inc., Cincinnati, OH) or Tegaderm CHG (3M Health Care, St. Paul, MN) dressing. There is some evidence that utilization of chlorhexidine dressings can reduce early catheter-associated blood stream infections.[3]
- Ultrasound should be utilized for both preprocedural assessment of the venous access site and for direct visualization of the needle and wire within the venous lumen. Use of ultrasound has been shown to improve first access attempt success while decreasing access site complications.[4]

GENERAL SELDINGER VENOUS ACCESS TECHNIQUE

- Step 1: Access site is chosen after ultrasound identification of the vessel. Local anesthesia is administered to the site. Ultrasound-guided needle access into the vein is performed with direct visualization of the needle tip within the lumen. This can be performed with an open needle technique or with negative aspiration utilizing a partially saline-filled syringe.
- Step 2: Evaluation of back bleeding can aid in confirmation of venous access. Back bleeding evaluation is often limited with micropuncture needle use. Back bleeding assessment can be confounded in severely hypotensive and/or hypoxic patients. If necessary, an arterial line transducer can be used to confirm that the access is within a vein, rather than an artery.
- Step 3: A wire is advanced through the needle to facilitate durable venous access. Ultrasound images of the wire within the venous lumen should be obtained and saved to the medical record. Wire position can then be manipulated under fluoroscopic guidance to ensure positioning within the inferior vena cava.

INTERNAL JUGULAR AND SUBCLAVIAN VEIN APPROACH

- Following Seldinger access of the appropriate vein the optimal position of the catheter must be determined with fluoroscopy. The wire can be positioned at the desired tip location and removed from the venous access sheath to measure the intravascular length for the catheter.
- Under fluoroscopy a 0.038-in wire is positioned within the inferior vena cava. In a subclavian vein approach or left internal jugular approach, directional catheters can be utilized to achieve proper wire position.
- A series of dilators are passed over the wire prior to introduction of the peel-away introducer sheath through which the dialysis catheter will be introduced and positioned under fluoroscopy. Trendelenburg positioning and a breath hold maneuver during removal of the dilator can minimize the risk of air embolism.
- The wire is removed from the peel-away introducer sheath prior to passing the hemodialysis catheter. Sheaths with a hemostatic valve will prevent significant back bleeding prior to advancing the catheter. If the peel-away sheath does not have a hemostatic valve, finger occlusion of the ostium can prevent significant back bleeding and minimize risk for air embolism.
- The hemodialysis catheter is advanced through the peel-away sheath into the venous system. Utilizing finger manipulation or small nontoothed forceps, the catheter is stabilized at the level of the venous access site as the peel-away sheath is removed.
- Following complete removal of the sheath the catheter should be evaluated with fluoroscopy to ensure no major kinks are identified and the appropriate tip position has been achieved (**FIGURE 2**).

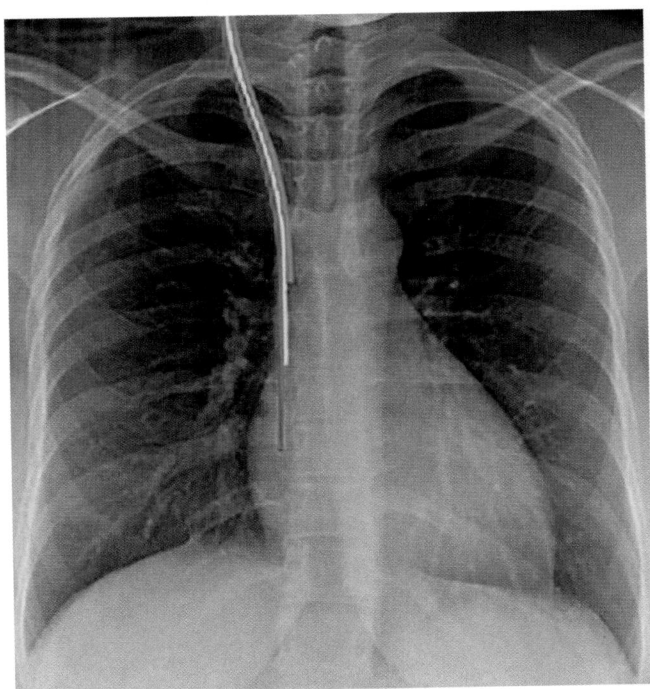

FIGURE 2 ● Chest x-ray or fluoroscopy aids in determination of the hemodialysis catheter as too shallow (blue), appropriately positioned (yellow), or too deep (pink). (Courtesy of Jacob C Wood, MD.)

FEMORAL VEIN APPROACH

- The general Seldinger technique is utilized to achieve femoral vein access with confirmation of venous access as detailed above.
- Catheter length is typically less of a consideration as often the longest available catheter is chosen. If concern for central stenosis exists, a venogram can help identify any areas of stenosis. The appropriate position of a femoral catheter is within the inferior vena cava, central to any significant stenosis if one exists. Placement central to any stenosis minimizes the risk for recirculation during hemodialysis sessions.
- If tunneled catheter placement is performed, tunnels should be positioned to ensure changes in patient position do not result in kinks in the catheter.

TUNNELED DIALYSIS CATHETER PLACEMENT

- The traditional Seldinger technique is utilized to gain venous access with a small skin incision made at the venous access site. Compared with nontunneled line placement, a more lateral venous access approach is utilized to minimize the impact of the catheter course of the vein.
- Utilization of a small Kelly forceps can release the surrounding soft tissues. It is important to establish venous sheath access prior to removal of the wire, which will facilitate catheter measurement.
- The wire is positioned at the location of the desired catheter tip using fluoroscopic guidance. Removal of the wire facilitates measurement of the intravascular length of the catheter. The intravascular length of the catheter is subtracted from the overall catheter length to determine the external catheter length. This external catheter length determines the length of the tunnel and thus the position of the skin exit site on the chest wall.
- After determination of the skin exit site and tunnel course, local anesthesia is instilled along the tract to facilitate comfortable passage of the tunneler.
- All tunneled dialysis catheter kits include a tunneler that is attached to the catheter. This is utilized to pass the catheter in a subcutaneous fashion from the skin exit site to the venous access site. The cuff should be positioned approximately 1-2 cm from the skin exit site within the tunnel (**FIGURE 3**). After tunneling, all lumens of the catheter should be flushed and capped.
- After tunneling to the venous access site, a stiff 0.038-in guidewire is positioned through the venous sheath into the inferior vena cava with the aid of fluoroscopy.
- A series of dilators are advanced at the venous access site prior to placement of the peel-away introducer sheath. The tip of the dilators only needs to be advanced 2 to 3 cm into the vein as they aid primarily in subcutaneous tissue dilation. The peel-away introducer sheath should be advanced under fluoroscopy to ensure smooth placement without kinking or concern for a more central obstruction.
- The dilator is removed from the peel-away sheath after which the dialysis catheter is inserted. Expeditious placement of the catheter within the sheath after dilator removal minimizes the chances of an air entry. In addition, Trendelenburg positioning and breath holding techniques help minimize risk for air embolism.
- The dialysis catheter should be firmly held at the level of the venous access site while the split peel-away introducer sheath is carefully removed.

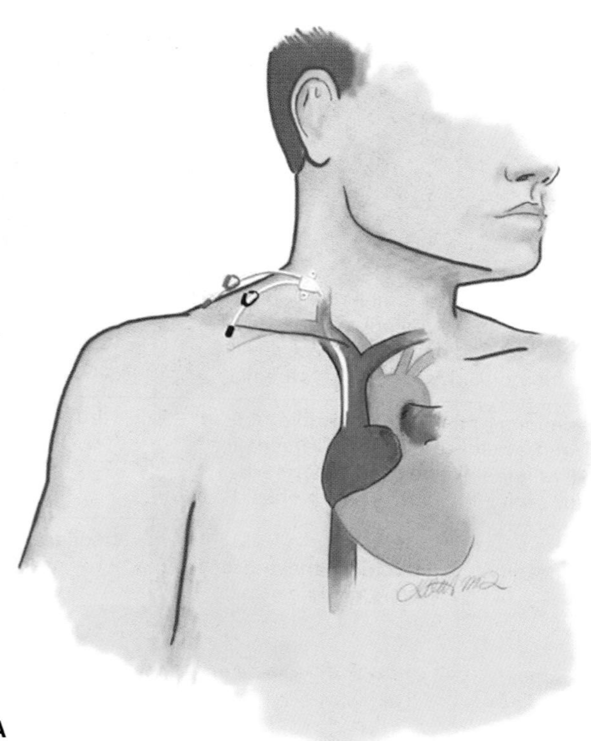

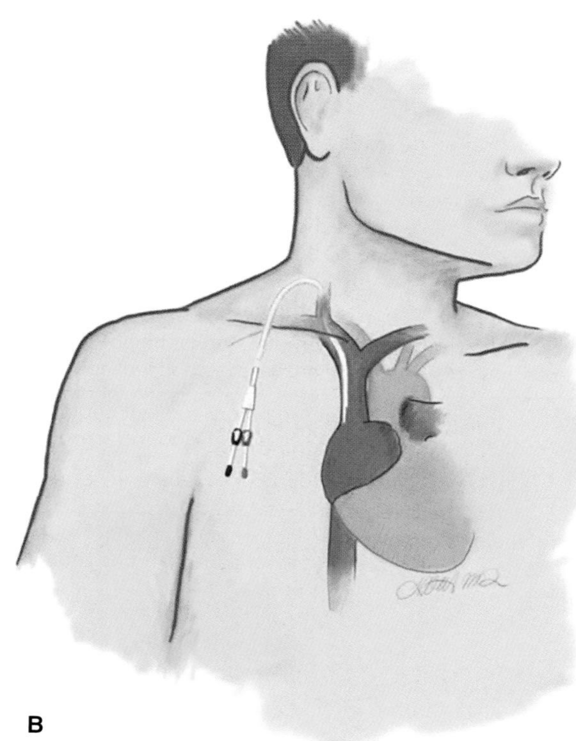

FIGURE 3 ● Nontunneled **(A)** and tunneled lines **(B)** with appropriate subcutaneous cuff position. (Courtesy Jacob C. Wood, MD.)

FINISHING CONSIDERATIONS

- All dialysis catheters, tunneled or not, should be flushed and aspirated prior to completion of the procedure to ensure appropriate line function.
- Prior to completion, all lines should be capped with the appropriate solution based on institutional protocols.
- For tunneled dialysis catheters the venous access site should be closed with both subcutaneous suture and a sterile dressing, often a sterile surgical adhesive.
- All catheters should be secured in place to ensure limited movement. Multiple different techniques and devices are available to proceduralists to accomplish this task.
- Sterile dressings in compliance with institution protocol should be placed prior to breaking down the sterile field. Antibiotic ointment can be applied at the catheter exit site during the initial healing period.[5]

HEMODIALYSIS CATHETER EXCHANGE

- Passage of a 0.035-in guidewire through the catheter port under fluoroscopy allows the operator to remove the dialysis catheter while maintaining venous access. The catheter should be inspected to ensure the tip is intact following removal.
- The guidewire should ideally be positioned into the inferior vena cava (IVC) prior to removal of the hemodialysis catheter. If having difficulty navigating to the IVC, use of an angled hydrophilic wire and torque device can facilitate IVC selection prior to catheter removal. A catheter can then be advanced over the hydrophilic wire to facilitate exchange for a stiffer 0.035-in wire. After removal of the catheter, pressure at the venous access site can help minimize bleeding.
- If bacteremia is present, wiping the wire with either Betadine or an alcohol-based solution can minimize risk of reinfection. When bacteremia exists and venous access options make it feasible, transition to a nontunneled catheter until bacteremia has completely resolved is best.
- When exchanging a nontunneled hemodialysis catheter, a new peel-away sheath can be advanced over the wire to facilitate placement of the new catheter.
- When exchanging a tunneled catheter, prior to passage of the guide wire, the catheter exit site is infiltrated with local anesthetic to allow adequate dissection of the subcutaneous cuff. Infiltration directly around the cuff can aid in dissection of the surrounding tissues. Adequate dissection of the cuff from the surrounding soft tissue is key to a smooth successful exchange.
- The guidewire is positioned within the IVC as noted above, and the replacement catheter is loaded onto the guidewire, and under fluoroscopic guidance the catheter is advanced to ensure passage without loss of wire position.

PEARLS AND PITFALLS

Patient selection	■ Thorough evaluation of all previous central venous lines and pacemakers is incredibly important when assessing for potential placement challenges.
Imaging evaluation	■ Optimal positioning of a nontunneled hemodialysis catheter is within the central superior vena cava. Nontunneled catheters are stiffer, and thus, atrium placement should be avoided. ■ Optimal positioning of the tunneled hemodialysis catheter tip is within the right atrium as catheters will retract several centimeters with upright positioning.[6] ■ Careful consideration of catheter length is crucial to the long-term function. Catheters terminating in the superior vena cava (SVC) risk dysfunction due to dislodging into the brachiocephalic or jugular veins. In addition, catheters terminating within the ventricle can be a source of ongoing arrhythmias.

Technique	■ In a tunneled dialysis catheter, the cuff of the catheter should not be placed more than 3 cm into the tract as it may complicate future removal. ■ For internal jugular venous access, entry into the jugular vein higher on the neck will create an unfavorable catheter course for tunneled lines leading to increased risk of kinking and dysfunction. ■ If unable to achieve stable wire access in the IVC, utilization of an angled catheter and glide wire under fluoroscopic guidance can facilitate IVC selection. ■ If positioning of the catheter is not ideal or if a kink exists within the catheter, placement of a stiff wire via one of the infusion ports can facilitate repositioning. ■ With tunneled dialysis catheter exchange, placement of an exchange length stiff glide wire in each catheter port facilitates a more stable platform over which to advance and position the replacement catheter (**FIGURE 4**).

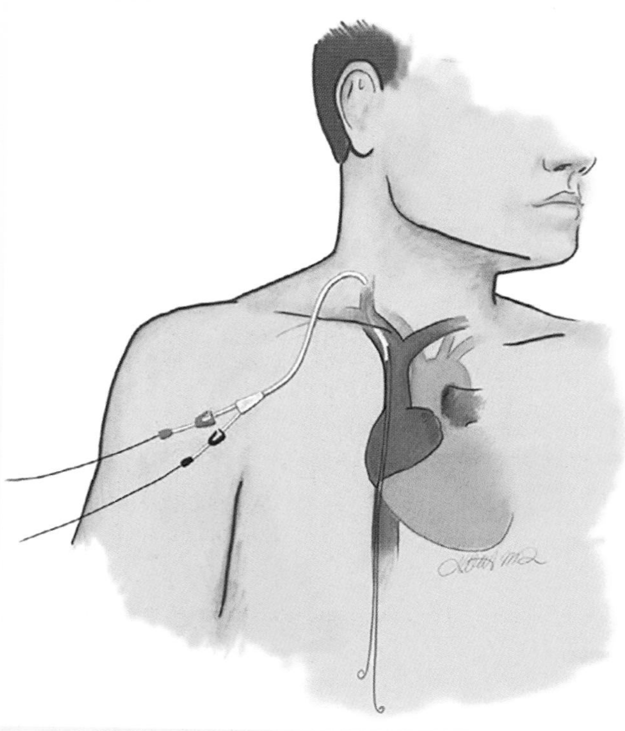

FIGURE 4 ● Illustration showing stiff glide wire access through each port of the tunneled dialysis catheter and into the infrarenal aorta. (Courtesy of Jacob C. Wood, MD.)

POSTOPERATIVE CARE

- Hemodialysis catheter maintenance:
  - When initiating dialysis, the catheter hub should be sani- with a chlorhexidine-based solution. The locking solution should be withdrawn till blood is visualized prior to connecting to the dialysis circuit.
  - After hemodialysis is complete, the catheter should be flushed with a locking solution based on institutional policy. Flushing all blood from the catheter minimizes the risk of thrombus formation. The most common catheter locking solutions include saline or heparin-saline (variable concentrations). Alternative options include antibiotic locks, tissue plasminogen activator, sodium citrate, and sodium bicarbonate.
  - The catheter hubs and skin entry site should be cleaned with a chlorhexidine-based solution and new sterile dressings applied.
- Any catheter should be removed when no longer clinically necessary. Removal of a nontunneled temporary hemodialysis line is easily performed at the bedside. Appropriate positioning and adequate manual pressure reduce risks of air embolism and hematoma formation. Removal of a tunneled catheter is typically performed in a procedural suite due to need for dissection of the subcutaneous cuff, which requires local anesthesia along with a scalpel and a small hemostat to aid with the dissection.
- All nonfunctional catheters that fail conservative techniques aimed at restoring function will need to be exchanged. Preservation of the venous access site should be of the utmost importance unless it is thought this factor is the reason for dysfunction.
- In patients with bacteremia, based on the most recent guidelines, antibiotic treatment with delayed line exchange over a nonbraided wire is encouraged. In cases with persistent exit site infection, other venous access sites should be explored.[1]
- Trouble shooting
  - Most issues related to a malfunctioning hemodialysis catheter are related to positioning. Repositioning of the

catheter over a wire to preventing kinking, particularly in the situation of a recently place tunneled catheter, may resolve the issue.

- Power aspiration and flushing of hemodialysis catheters can aid with clearing potential thrombus debris in a line resulting in improved function. If such techniques are required frequently then line exchange should be considered.
- When pressure for urgent dialysis exists, maneuvers such as flipping the inflow and outflow ports may help improve flow rates if mechanical catheter issues exist. This is not a long-term solution but can alleviate the need for urgent line exchanges.

COMPLICATIONS

- Iatrogenic arterial injury is a well-documented complication of percutaneous venous access. While inadvertent arterial needle access has been estimated up to 10%, use of ultrasound guidance has significantly lessened this event.[7,8] The true incidence is hard to calculate as fortunately the majority are detected prior to cannulation. Intra-arterial catheter placement rates are reported in less than 1%.[8]
- Removal of an inadvertent central line placed in the arterial system utilizing manual pressure alone for hemostasis has high rates of bleeding complications.[9]
- Pneumothorax can occur after internal jugular or subclavian venous access. The incidence of pneumothorax varies greatly by location of access, failed previous attempts, underlying lung disease, and operator experience but remains highest with a subclavian approach in up to 2% of cases.[10] While the majority of these will require simple observation, routine postprocedural chest x-ray imaging should be obtained.
- Access site hematoma is a complication seen with both tunneled and nontunneled lines.
- SVC and/or myocardial perforation is a rare but potentially fatal complication of either hemodialysis catheter placement or delayed complication of inappropriate catheter length. Hemothorax can occur, and if discovered should prompt contrast-enhanced CT imaging to better define potential site of injury.
- Infection is a significant complication after catheter placement, which can be catheter-related blood stream infections, catheter colonization, or exit site infections. Not all catheter-associated bloodstream infections require line removal or exchange, and based on the most recent guidelines there are very few instances where abandoning venous access for a line holiday is necessary.[1]
- Exit site infections are typically defined by hyperemia, induration, or tenderness less than 2 cm from the catheter exit site, and if associated with drainage this should be cultured. These infections can be treated with a 7- to 14-day course of appropriate antibiotic therapy. If unable to clear the associated infection, then line removal and/or exchange will be necessary.
- Catheter-associated thrombus is a common complication of any indwelling central catheter. Determination of ongoing need for the associated hemodialysis catheter is important when considering treatment options. Anticoagulation should be initiated per CHEST guidelines with line removal only if no longer clinically necessary.[11]
- Catheter-associated thrombus can affect catheter performance. Late catheter dysfunction is most commonly the result of thrombus formation either within or around the catheter. Anticoagulation remains the mainstay of external thrombus management with potential line removal if it is no longer necessary. Treatment should be continued based on the most recent CHEST guidelines. Internal thrombus can be managed with intraluminal lysis therapy or forceful saline flush techniques. Mixed results of the efficacy of these techniques have been reported. Ultimately, if unsuccessful in resolving the associated dysfunction, catheter exchange is necessary.
- Central venous stenosis is a well-documented complication of long-standing indwelling hemodialysis catheters and can affect longevity of future permanent dialysis access in that extremity.

OUTCOMES

- The general life expectancy of a hemodialysis catheter is highly variable, with tunneled catheters typically having a longer lifespan due to a decreased risk of infection.[12,13]
- Previous work has shown venous access location does significantly affect longevity of hemodialysis catheters, with right internal jugular (median 633 days) longer than either left internal jugular (430 days) or femoral (116 days).[14] Other studies have failed to replicate these results between right and left internal jugular approaches while femoral catheters universally have been shown to have the shortest life expectancy.
- Studies have demonstrated differences in longevity of hemodialysis catheters based upon distal tip design, with better catheter survival seen with split tips and/or split catheters.[14]
- While variability in institutional protocols for removal or exchange make long-term data difficult, no studies have shown that scheduled catheter exchanges improve long-term catheter-based hemodialysis success.
- Infection rates are often one of the greatest quality measures of catheter care following placement. The Centers for Disease Control and Prevention previously issued recommendations for interventions aimed at reducing catheter-associated infections including hand washing, full barrier precautions during insertion, chlorhexidine skin disinfection, avoidance of femoral cannulation, and removal when clinically indicated.[15] A study published in the *NEJM* evaluated the rate of catheter-related blood stream infections in ICU patients with indwelling central venous catheters following implementation of a safety bundle. They demonstrated a significant improvement in the mean number of infections per 1000 catheter days from 7.7 to 1.4 over an 18-month period.[16]

REFERENCES

1. Lok CE, Huber TS, Lee T, et al. KDOQI clinical practice guideline for vascular access: 2019 update. *Am J Kidney Dis*. 2020;75(4):S1-S164.
2. Yasuda H, Sanui M, Abe T, et al. Comparison of the efficacy of three topical antiseptic solutions for the prevention of catheter colonization: a multicenter randomized controlled study. *Crit Care*. 2017;21(1):320.
3. Puig-Asensio M, Marra AR, Childs CA, Kukla ME, Perencevich EN, Schweizer ML. Effectiveness of chlorhexidine dressings to prevent catheter-related bloodstream infections. Does one size fit all? A systematic literature review and meta-analysis. *Infect Control Hosp Epidemiol*. 2020;41(12):1388-1395.

4. Rabindranath KS, Kumar E, Shail R, Vaux EC. Ultrasound use for the placement of haemodialysis catheters. *Cochrane Database Syst Rev.* 2011(11):CD005279.
5. O'Grady NP, Alexander M, Burns LA, et al. Summary of recommendations: guidelines for the prevention of intravascular catheter-related infections. *Clin Infect Dis.* 2011;52(9):1087-1099.
6. Engstrom BI, Horvath JJ, Stewart JK, et al. Tunneled internal jugular hemodialysis catheters: impact of laterality and tip position on catheter dysfunction and infection rates. *J Vasc Intervent Radiol.* 2013;24(9):1295-1302.
7. Farrell J, Walshe J, Gellens M, Martin KJ. Complications associated with insertion of jugular venous catheters for hemodialysis: the value of postprocedural radiograph. *Am J Kidney Dis.* 1997;30(5):690-692.
8. Bowdle A. Vascular complications of central venous catheter placement: evidence-based methods for prevention and treatment. *J Cardiothorac Vasc Anesth.* 2014;28(2):358-368.
9. Dixon OGB, Smith GE, Carradice D, Chetter IC. A systematic review of management of inadvertent arterial injury during central venous catheterisation. *J Vasc Access.* 2017;18(2):97-102.
10. Vinson DR, Ballard DW, Hance LG, et al. Pneumothorax is a rare complication of thoracic central venous catheterization in community EDs. *Am J Emerg Med.* 2015;33(1):60-66.
11. Stevens SM, Woller SC, Kreuziger LB, et al. Antithrombotic therapy for VTE disease. *Chest.* 2021;160(6):e545-e608.
12. Dryden MS, Samson A, Ludlam HA, Wing AJ, Phillips I. Infective complications associated with the use of the Quinton "Permcath" for long-term central vascular access in haemodialysis. *J Hosp Infect.* 1991;19(4):257-262.
13. Mandolfo S, Acconcia P, Bucci R, et al. Hemodialysis tunneled central venous catheters: five-year outcome analysis. *J Vasc Access.* 2014;15(6):461-465.
14. Fry AC, Stratton J, Farrington K, et al. Factors affecting long-term survival of tunnelled haemodialysis catheters a prospective audit of 812 tunnelled catheters. *Nephrol Dial Transplant.* 2008;23(1):275-281.
15. O'Grady NP, Alexander M, Burns LA, et al. Guidelines for the prevention of intravascular catheter-related infections. *Clin Infect Dis.* 2011;52(9):e162-e93.
16. Pronovost P, Needham D, Berenholtz S, et al. An intervention to decrease catheter-related bloodstream infections in the ICU. *N Engl J Med.* 2006;355(26):2725-2732.

Chapter 39

Insertion of a Peritoneal Dialysis Catheter

An Alternative to Creating Vascular Access in the Treatment of Renal Failure

Ashley Nicole Krepline and Dean Edward Klinger

DEFINITION

- Peritoneal dialysis (PD) is a means of treating patients with end-stage renal disease. A catheter is placed within the peritoneal cavity to allow installation of a dextrose-based dialysate. PD uses the concept of diffusion gradients across a membrane. In PD, the membrane is all of the peritoneal surfaces within the abdomen.
- The diffusion gradient is created by the dialysate fluid instilled in the abdomen. Toxins, electrolytes, and water can diffuse across the membrane as dictated by the concentration gradients, the exposed surface area of peritoneum, and the length of time the dialysate is in the abdomen.

Alternatives to Peritoneal Dialysis

- The treatment options for patients with significant renal failure include kidney transplantation, hemodialysis, and PD. If possible, a kidney transplant is the preferred treatment. Renal replacement therapy with PD and hemodialysis offer comparable survival outcomes. PD, for the appropriate patient, offers several advantages to hemodialysis. Compared to hemodialysis, PD is associated with a slower decline in residual renal function. While hemodialysis is primarily performed in dialysis centers, PD is performed in the home allowing for more independence. Additionally, PD is associated with a lower cost per year as it does not require a dialysis center, requires fewer support staff, and patients require less erythropoietin stimulating agents when undergoing peritoneal dialysis.
- The rates of peritoneal dialysis vary widely across the world. Worldwide, approximately 11% of patients on dialysis undergo peritoneal dialysis; however, the rate of peritoneal dialysis is increasing at a faster rate than the utilization of hemodialysis (8% vs 6%-7%). Rates of peritoneal dialysis are highest in Hong Kong, Thailand, New Zealand, and Australia. Conversely, hemodialysis is utilized more frequently in Africa, North America, and Europe. In this chapter, we will focus on PD.

PATIENT HISTORY AND PHYSICAL FINDINGS

- A good history and physical exam will help ensure that you have a good candidate for PD. Hemodialysis is also an option for the treatment of renal failure and may be the better choice of dialysis for some patients.
- PD is a very good option for those patients that want to be independent as it is done at home. PD is less stressful on the heart and therefore is a good option in patients with heart failure. It is also a good option for patients with ascites from right sided heart failure and liver disease as PD provides treatment for both the renal failure and ascites.
- Patients with hernias should have them repaired at the time of insertion of the catheter unless the hernias are too large or complicated, in which case hemodialysis should be considered. Individuals that tell you of prior abdominal operations and having a lot of adhesions may not be able to have PD. Operations may leave the patient with too many adhesions such that a catheter cannot be inserted or there is insufficient surface area for adequate dialysis. Patients with ostomies and feeding tubes are also considered to be poor candidates for PD.

IMAGING AND OTHER DIAGNOSTIC STUDIES

- There is no preoperative imaging required prior to placement of a PD catheter. There is no imaging modality that quantifies the degree of adhesions that would prevent insertion of a catheter or predict adequate surface area and function of PD.

SURGICAL MANAGEMENT

Preoperative Planning

- Patients are required to meet with the home PD staff prior to insertion of the catheter. Assessments are made to ensure that the patient will be able to care for the catheter as well as do the dialysis. This requires adequate mental and physical abilities. An example of a patient where there could be problems might be in someone who has had a stroke. It is also advisable that the patient have a safe home environment that is clean and there is a live-in caregiver who can assist with the PD should the need arise. The PD staff make a home visit to assess the physical layout to assess the ability to store all the supplies and dispose of the waste.
- Care must be taken to keep in mind the patient's body habitus and disabilities when planning the location of the exit site of the PD catheter. The exit site should not be in a skin fold or at the beltline and when possible in a location that the patient can see.
- Chlorhexidine wipes or soap are given to the patient to use the day before and day of the operation. Prior to the operation, the patient is given preoperative antibiotics.

Positioning

- The patient is placed supine with arms out on the operating room table with appropriate padding of dependent areas. If the PD catheter is being inserted laparoscopically, a monitor is placed at the foot of the bed for visualization.

INSERTION OF A PD CATHETER

- The three means by which a PD catheter can be inserted are percutaneous, open, and laparoscopic. There are advantages and disadvantages to each (**TABLE 1**).
- The advantage of percutaneous and open insertion is that the procedure can be done under local anesthesia, with less cost as the procedure is shorter, and there is no requirement for use of the postanesthesia recovery unit. The advantage of laparoscopic insertion is that there is about 10% reduction in the patient having problems with the catheter being obstructed by the omentum.
- It is unknown if there is an increased risk of complications with insertion of the PD catheter using the laparoscopic technique compared to the open technique. This remains a controversy as some studies have demonstrated laparoscopic placement of PD catheters is associated with a higher rate of intraoperative complications; however, not all studies have demonstrated this.

Table 1: Advantages and Disadvantages of Each Method of PD Catheter Insertion

	Anesthesia	Cost	Catheter obstruction	Complications
Percutaneous	+	+	–	–
Open	+	+	–	+
Laparoscopic	–	–	+	+/–

PERCUTANEOUS PLACEMENT

- PD catheters can be placed using ultrasound and a percutaneous technique in a Seldigner fashion. Our practice does not utilize this technique and is beyond the scope of this chapter.

OPEN TECHNIQUE

- The operation begins with determining where to make the incision for insertion of the PD catheter. Markings are placed on the patient to indicate skin folds and where the patient's beltline is located. The surgeon's PD catheter of choice is used to help locate the position of the incision. The intra-abdominal portion of the catheter is positioned about 2 cm above the symphysis pubis. The first Dacron cuff on the catheter should be positioned in the rectus muscle through a paramedian incision. A mark is placed on the skin where the cuff will be positioned and marks can be placed on the skin to delineate the incision (**FIGURE 1**). At this time, assessment is made as to where the exit site will be located. The exit site of the catheter should not be in the skin folds or under the beltline. It is also preferred to have the exit site in a position where the patient is able to see it so as to make it easier to care for the catheter. The location of the incision can be shifted to accommodate the best position of the intra-abdominal portion of the catheter and exit site.
- The incision is carried through the skin and subcutaneous tissue down to the anterior rectus fascia (**FIGURE 2**). The fascia is incised in a craniocaudal direction to expose the rectus muscle. The rectus muscle is spread between its fibers to expose the posterior rectus fascia (**FIGURE 3**). A purse-string suture is placed in the posterior rectus fascia with care not to go too deep and catch underlying bowel (**FIGURE 4**). An opening is made in the posterior rectus and peritoneum. Care needs to be taken not to misinterpret bowel wall for the peritoneum.
- The PD catheter is thread onto a long stylet used to introduce the catheter. Initially, the catheter is thread on all

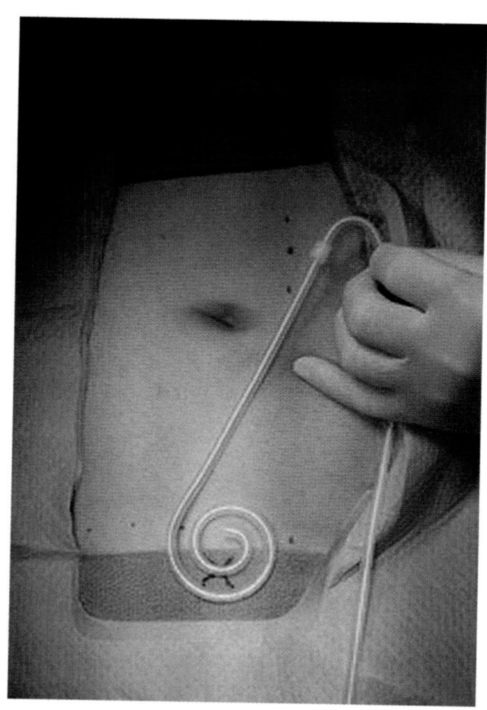

FIGURE 1 ● Prior to making an incision, preoperative landmarks are identified. The pubic symphysis is marked and skin folds and the beltline are noted. The end of the PD catheter is placed 2 cm cranially to the pubic symphysis and the location of the paramedian incision is marked at the level where the deep cuff lands.

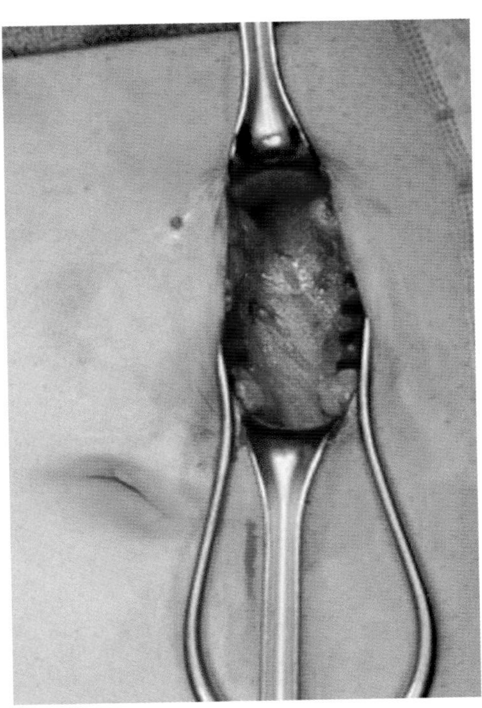

FIGURE 2 ● The incision is made and dissection through the subcutaneous tissues is done to expose the anterior rectus fascia.

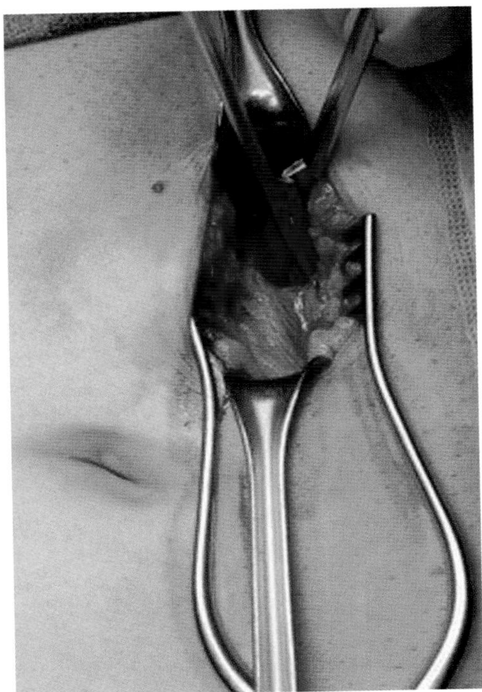

FIGURE 3 ● The anterior rectus fascia is incised. A Metzenbaum scissors is placed between rectus muscle fibers and spread perpendicular to the muscle fibers to expose the posterior rectus sheath.

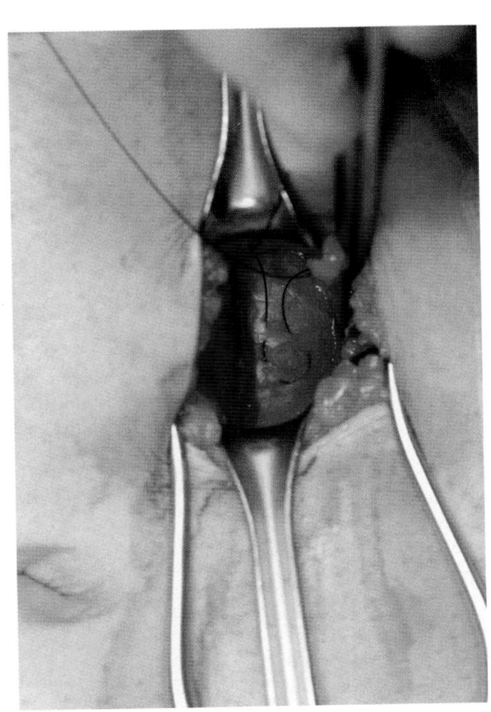

FIGURE 4 ● A purse-string suture is placed in the posterior rectus sheath.

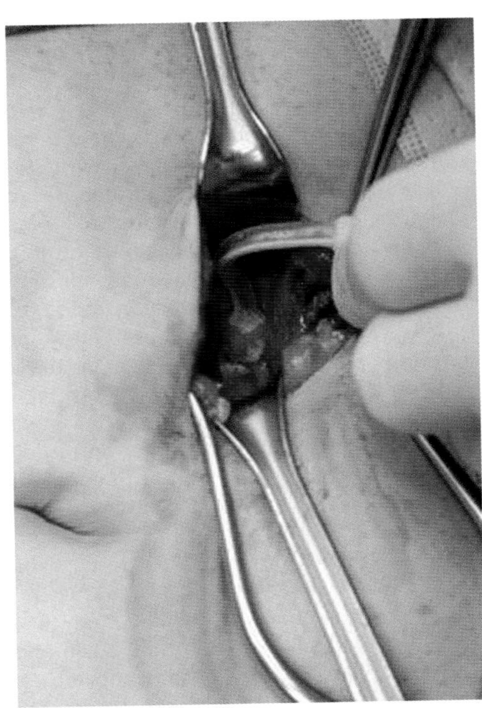

FIGURE 5 ● Once the PD catheter is inserted, the purse-string suture is tied.

the way to the end of the stylet to aid in easier insertion, but once the catheter is in the abdomen, the catheter is advanced over the stylet by several centimeters so that the end is not rigid. The catheter is gently directed toward the symphysis pubis. Once the stylet is in the correct position, the remainder of the catheter is introduced into the pelvis. The first Dacron cuff should come to lie in the rectus muscle and the purse-string suture is tied down about the catheter (**FIGURE 5**).

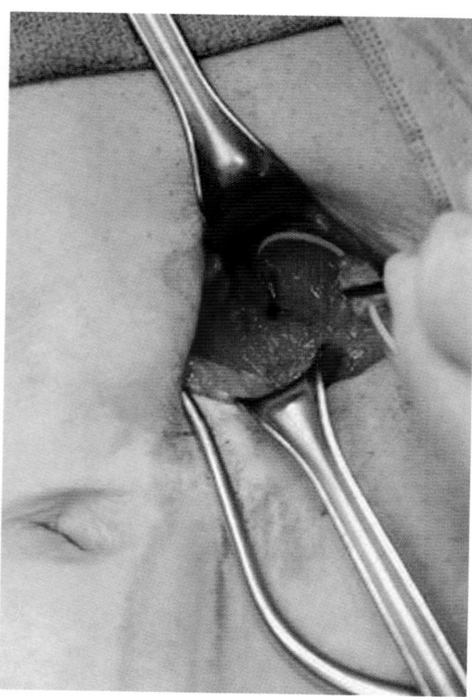

FIGURE 6 ● The catheter is flushed with saline solution and fluctuations of the meniscus in the catheter is observed during respiration or changes in the intra-abdominal pressure indicating a patent catheter.

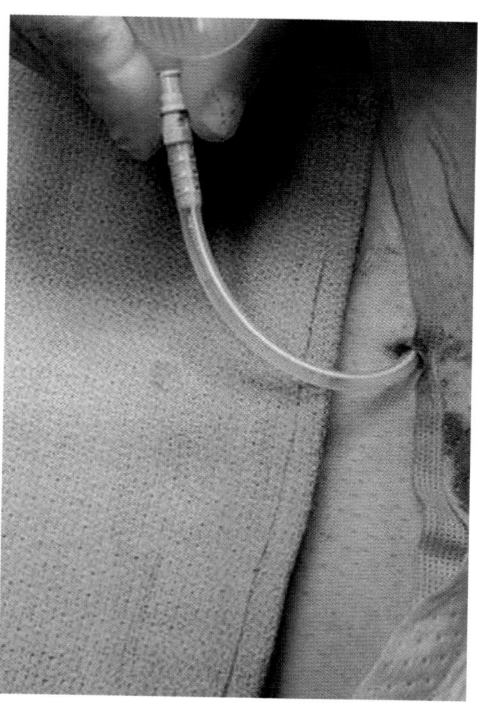

FIGURE 7 ● After insertion of the PD catheter, suture is used to close the anterior rectus sheath in a running fashion. The anterior sheath is closed from caudal to cranial to allow for the creation of a tunnel.

- The function of the catheter can now be tested. Approximately 20 to 30 mL of saline is instilled through the catheter. Ease of introduction is noted. Gentle aspiration can be attempted and the color of the fluid returned noted. It should be clear saline. A bit more saline is introduced and then the syringe is disconnected from the catheter. The meniscus of fluid in the catheter is observed. The meniscus should freely move up and down in the catheter, moving with changes of intra-abdominal pressure changes. Most often, variations can be seen just with respiration. If the meniscus freely fluctuates in the catheter, the catheter is in a good position (**FIGURE 6**).
- The anterior rectus fascia is closed from the caudal to cranial direction. The thought of closing it in this direction is to angle the catheter and get a bit of torque on the catheter to lever up the intra-abdominal end toward the anterior abdominal wall (**FIGURE 7**).
- The catheter is then tunneled to the exit site, avoiding skin folds and the beltline, and in a position where the second Dacron cuff is about 2 centimeters from the skin. The function of the catheter can be tested again and capped. The incision is closed and dressings applied (**FIGURE 8**, **Video 1**).

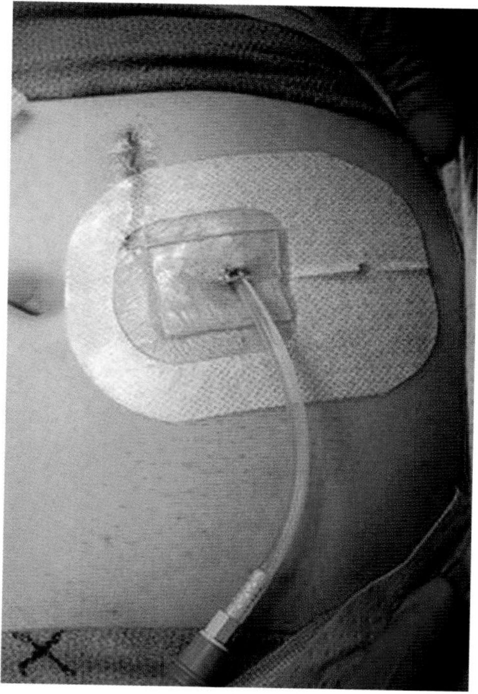

FIGURE 8 ● The PD catheter exit site is dressed with a chlorhexidine-impregnated Tegaderm and the incisions are dressed with Dermabond.

TECHNIQUES

LAPAROSCOPIC TECHNIQUE

- When inserting the PD catheter using the laparoscopic technique, considerations for the insertion site and exit site are the same as for the open technique. Pneumoperitoneum is obtained by placing a Veres needle at Palmer point in the left upper quadrant. A 5-mm radially dilating trocar is inserted in the left upper quadrant. A small incision is then made where the PD catheter is to be inserted and a second 5-mm trocar is inserted. A third 5-mm trocar is inserted in the opposite side of the abdomen from where the catheter is inserted.
- Using the three trocars, the omentum is pulled into the upper abdomen and sutured to the anterior abdominal wall in the right, middle, and left upper quadrants to prevent its migration back into the pelvis. A suture passing needle is used to place a stitch through the anterior abdominal wall. The suture is passed around a portion of the omentum, taking care to avoid vessels, and then taken back out the abdominal wall and secured. The purpose this maneuver is to prevent it from encasing and obstructing flow through the PD catheter.
- An alternative to suturing the omentum to the upper abdomen is to remove it. If this is to be done, we recommend placing a 12-mm Hasson cannula in the subxiphoid area. The insertion of the larger trocar is to help facilitate removal of the omentum from the abdomen. A harmonic scissors or LigaSure is used to remove the omentum following along the caudal border of the transverse colon.
- Attention is then directed toward inserting the PD catheter. The trocar at the PD catheter insertion site is removed. A peel away sheath and dilator is inserted at this site with the catheter going through the anterior rectus fascia, tunneling through the rectus muscle on an angle toward the pelvis, and exiting the posterior rectus fascia and peritoneum several inches caudal to the insertion site. The dilator is removed and the PD catheter is inserted through the sheath and directed toward the pelvis. The sheath is removed and the first Dacron cuff comes to lie in the rectus muscle. By tunneling the catheter at an angle through the rectus muscle, there is a torque on the catheter such that it will want to come to lie up against the anterior pelvic wall. The catheter is then tunneled to the exit site as described in the open technique, trocars removed, incisions closed, and dressings applied (**FIGURE 9**, **Video 2**).

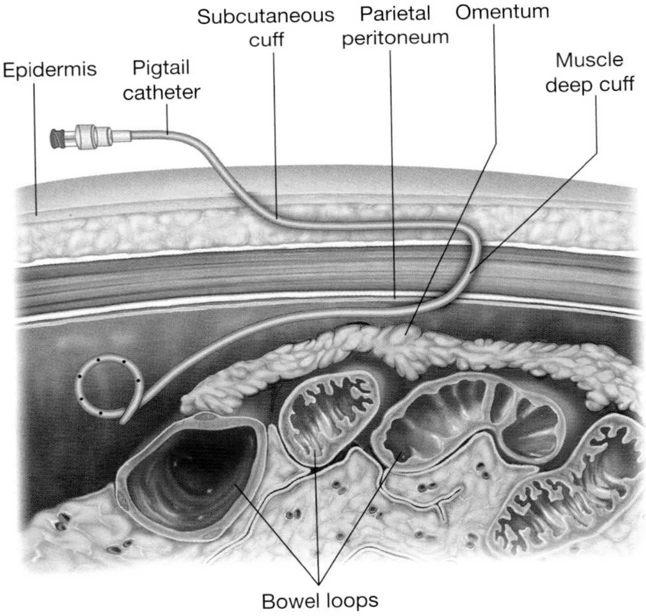

FIGURE 9 • A depiction of the tunnel created within the rectus muscle to allow the catheter to sit along the anterior abdominal wall.

PEARLS AND PITFALLS

Surgical management	■ When determining the position of the catheter in the pelvis, we aim to insert the catheter so the end of the catheter lays approximately 2 cm cephalad to the pubic symphysis so as to be just a bit further from the rectum and bladder. It has been our observation that patients may experience fewer symptoms of pressure in the pelvis during dialysis. ■ If the catheter is inserted laparoscopically, we recommend doing a concurrent omentectomy or pexy of the omentum to the upper abdomen. This is done to reduce the risk of the catheter being encased in the omentum, causing obstruction to drainage.

Technique

- Once the PD catheter is inserted, prior to leaving the operating room, it is important to flush the catheter to ensure patency. A syringe is used to inject approximately 20 to 30 mL of saline through the catheter. The saline should freely flow indicating the catheter is not kinked or obstructed. Once the saline is injected, the meniscus of the saline within the catheter tubing is observed and should vary with respiration or applying pressure to the abdominal wall.
- When suturing about the catheter, care must be taken not to puncture the catheter with the needle as this would result in leakage from the catheter during use.

POSTOPERATIVE CARE

- Traditional teachings suggest application of a nonocclusive gauze dressing over the PD catheter exit site to prevent contamination and to secure the PD catheter to prevent tugging on the catheter. Our practice has been to apply a chlorhexidine-impregnated Tegaderm to the PD catheter exit site. Regardless of the type of dressing applied, it is suggested the dressing be changed by experienced PD nurses in the perioperative period to prevent contamination.
- PD catheter flushing is performed weekly to assess the functionality of the PD catheter and closely monitor the patient in the postoperative period. It is recommended to wait 3 weeks following insertion of the PD catheter prior to initiating PD. The risk of leakage about the catheter decreases from 28% at 1 week postoperatively to just 2.4% at 3 weeks.

COMPLICATIONS

- Complications occur in approximately 20% to 35% of peritoneal dialysis catheter placement.

Bladder and Rectal Discomfort

- Patients may experience bladder and rectal discomfort following placement of a PD catheter. This is thought to be associated with the PD catheter resting against the rectum or bladder. Anecdotally, patients less frequently experience this discomfort if the PD catheter is placed so the catheter terminates approximately 2 cm cephalad from the pubic symphysis.

Leakage

- Leakage of dialysate from around the exit site most commonly occurs within 30 days of placement of the PD catheter and is usually a result of initiating PD too early, a technical error when placing the PD catheter, or poor tissue integrity and healing leading to inadequate incorporation of the Dacron cuff. Cessation of PD and transition to hemodialysis for several weeks will allow the exit site to heal and will typically stop the leakage of dialysate from the exit site.

Hernia

- As with all abdominal operations, hernias may occur. The risk of developing a hernia following insertion of a PD catheter is approximately 8.3%. A hernia may develop at the PD catheter exit site, most commonly this will only contain dialysate and will manifest as a bulge under the skin at the tract site. Hernias may also develop at port sites when PD catheters are placed laparoscopically, as is the risk with all laparoscopic abdominal surgery.
- Additionally, the increased intra-abdominal pressure associated with installation of the dialysate may result in hernias that were not detected on preoperative physical exam apparent. If a hernia develops, the patient may undergo either open or laparoscopic repair and eventual resumption of PD.

Catheter Malfunction

- A catheter malfunction can occur as a result in obstruction of the catheter side holes or kinking of the catheter. If a catheter is obstructed by bowel or omentum, the catheter will flush; however, the omentum or bowel will cover the side holes when dialysate is being removed. If the PD catheter is kinked or if there is fibrinous debris or clot within the catheter, the catheter will not flush or allow for drainage of the dialysate.
- Approximately 10% of patients develop catheter dysfunction due to omentum wrapping around the catheter, whether the catheter was placed with an open or laparoscopic technique, unless omentectomy or pexy of the omentum was performed at the time of laparoscopic PD catheter insertion.
- If the catheter malfunctions, laparoscopic intervention should be entertained. There is a 97% success rate of catheter function with laparoscopic intervention when combined with omentectomy or pexy of the omentum.

Infection

- An exit site infection may be present if the exit site is erythematous, indurated, or purulent drainage is observed from the exit site. If the exit site symptoms do not improve with antibiotics or recur after cessation of antibiotics, it is likely the cuff is involved. If this is the case, antibiotics should be given to suppress the infection. A new PD catheter can be inserted on the opposite side of the abdomen and dressings are applied. Following this, the old catheter is removed.
- The PD catheter cuff can extrude through the skin if tunneled too superficially and will act as a reservoir for bacteria. If the PD catheter cuff is completely exteriorized, it can be excised with a scalpel or pulled off with a forceps. If the cuff is incompletely exteriorized, it should be removed from the PD catheter tract and removed from the catheter.
- If there is concern for peritonitis, a peritoneal fluid sample should be obtained. A peritoneal fluid white blood cell count greater than 100/μL or bacteria identified on culture are indicative of peritonitis. Peritonitis can frequently be treated with appropriate antibiotics instilled via the PD catheter. If the pathogen causing peritonitis is yeast or mycobacterium, if the patient does not improve with antibiotic therapy, or if the patient develops recurrent peritonitis, the catheter will

need to be removed and replaced after successful treatment of peritonitis with an interval transition to hemodialysis while undergoing treatment for peritonitis.

SUGGESTED READING

1. Crabtree JH, Shrestha BM, Chow KM, et al. Creating and maintaining optimal peritoneal dialysis access in the adult patient: 2019 update. *Perit Dial Int*. 2019;39(5):414-436. doi:10.3747/pdi.2018.00232
2. Hagen SM, Lafranca JA, IJzermans JN, Dor FJ. A systematic review and meta-analysis of the influence of peritoneal dialysis catheter type on complication rate and catheter survival. *Kidney Int*. 2014;85(4):920-932. doi:10.1038/ki.2013.365
3. Krezalek MA, Bonamici N, Lapin B, et al. Laparoscopic peritoneal dialysis catheter insertion using rectus sheath tunnel and selective omentopexy significantly reduces catheter dysfunction and increases peritoneal dialysis longevity. *Surgery*. 2016;160(4):924-935. doi:10.1016/j.surg.2016.06.005
4. Li PK, Chow KM, Van de Luijtgaarden MW, et al. Changes in the worldwide epidemiology of peritoneal dialysis. *Nat Rev Nephrol*. 2017;13(2):90-103. doi:10.1038/nrneph.2016.181
5. Mehrotra R, Devuyst O, Davies SJ, Johnson DW. The current state of peritoneal dialysis. *J Am Soc Nephrol*. 2016;27(11):3238-3252. doi:10.1681/ASN.2016010112
6. Sodo M, Bracale U, Argentino G, et al. Simultaneous abdominal wall defect repair and Tenckhoff catheter placement in candidates for peritoneal dialysis. *J Nephrol*. 2016;29(5):699-702. doi:10.1007/s40620-015-0251-8

Chapter 40 Toe and Foot Amputations: Ray/Transmetatarsal/Symes*

Jacob C. Wood and Stephen Heisler

DEFINITION

- In the pursuit of limb preservation, it unfortunately is frequent that a patient may need a foot amputation to avoid compromising the entire extremity or even the individual. The development of nonviable tissue in one's foot may be due to the rapid onset of disease, poor comorbidity management, or delay in seeking medical attention. Diabetic patients suffer from a unique propensity for developing foot wounds secondary to the presence of macro- and microvascular disease and neuropathy—foot wounds can develop and spiral out of control without the patient even being aware.
- In this chapter we will be discussing several levels of foot amputations. A toe amputation is transecting a digit at the level of the phalanges. A ray amputation is transecting a digit at the level of the metatarsal bone. A transmetatarsal amputation (TMA) is transecting all digits at the metatarsal level. A Symes amputation is amputation of the foot through the distal tibia and fibula above the level of the malleoli.

DIFFERENTIAL DIAGNOSIS

- Diabetes mellitus with ulceration or gangrene
- Osteomyelitis
- Pressure-induced wounds
- Frostbite
- Vasculitis
- Vasospasm
- Peripheral arterial disease
- Thromboembolism
- Venous insufficiency
- Trauma
- Malignancy

PATIENT HISTORY AND PHYSICAL FINDINGS

- There are many things to take into consideration when evaluating a patient presenting with a foot wound. A careful history and physical should be sufficient to discover the etiology, extent, and acuity of a foot wound.
- A patient presenting with tachycardia, hypotension, leukocytosis, or other signs concerning for onset of sepsis warrants more urgent intervention.
- Foot wounds, particularly in the diabetic patient, can be much more extensive than they externally appear. There should be a low threshold to further interrogate a wound with purulent drainage or if the patient has systemic symptoms.
- The chronicity of a wound may be difficult to determine for diabetic patients. Not infrequently, patients present who have been completely unaware of the wound of concern until discovered by another person.
- To ensure healing potential and to prevent wound recurrence one maximizes medical optimization of comorbid conditions. This often requires a multidisciplinary approach. At our institution we regularly refer diabetic patients with marginal blood glucose control who present with foot wounds to endocrinology for optimization.
- Healing a wound requires an adequate blood supply to the affected area. A full pulse examination should be undertaken to evaluate for concomitant arterial insufficiency.
- Ischemic wounds can occur for several reasons, including atherosclerotic disease and digital ischemia in the setting of vasopressor use. After a revascularization procedure or after resolution of the offending condition, it is prudent to allow the ischemic wound to equilibrate prior to performing an amputation. Often what appears to be ischemic may prove to be viable if given time to declare itself.
- The more proximal an amputation the more it will affect the mechanics of ambulation. This will not affect a younger patient with excellent rehabilitation potential as much as an elderly patient who already has difficulty ambulating.

IMAGING AND OTHER DIAGNOSTIC STUDIES

- General laboratory data can help glean a patient's physiologic status on presentation including a basic metabolic panel and a complete blood count.
- C-reactive protein and erythrocyte sedimentation rate are general markers for inflammation and can suggest presence of osteomyelitis.
- The status of a diabetic patient's blood glucose control should be assessed with a hemoglobin A1c. The blood glucose level alone should not be used for this purpose as hyperglycemia may be a reflection of inflammation rather than poor glycemic control.
- When concerned for presence of osteomyelitis, foot X-ray with multiple views is a good initial imaging modality given a relatively low cost and the speed at which it can be performed. If the X-ray is inconclusive, or if more information is required to determine the extent of disease, magnetic resonance imaging may be necessary.

*Illustrations by Jacob C. Wood.

- If tibial pulses are not palpable an ankle-brachial index (ABI) with toe pressure is obtained to assess the vascular status of the foot. Values that are favorable for healing include an ABI greater than 0.8 (between 0.5 and 0.8 are marginal values) and a toe pressure greater than 50 mm Hg.
- Additional information can be obtained with segmental blood pressures, transcutaneous oxygen measurement, arterial duplex, and arteriography.

SURGICAL MANAGEMENT

Preoperative Planning

- The operation performed is dictated by the extent of disease, the vascular supply, and the rehabilitation potential of the patient. Minimizing the extent of the foot that is taken will maximize postoperative function; however, enough tissue should be taken to allow enough healthy skin and soft tissue to create a tension-free flap coverage for the amputation.
- Proximal amputations may cause tendon and ligamentous alterations that will cause unopposed plantarflexion or other deformity. Additional operations may be necessary to help the remaining foot reside in a maximally functional position, such a calcaneal (Achilles) tendon lengthening procedure.
- Foot amputations are well suited for nerve block with sedation, which most patients should tolerate.

Positioning

- Supine position is ideal for most foot amputations.
- The foot and distal leg are prepped and draped in circumferential fashion.

DIGIT AND RAY AMPUTATION

- When amputating a digit, the extent of the amputation dictates the incision that is made. A circumferential incision is sufficient for amputations at the phalangeal level or the distal aspect of a metatarsal bone. If the amputation must extend more proximally on the metatarsal bone a wedge-shaped incision or a racket-shaped incision is used. The incision should incorporate the ulcer if one is present with the goal of leaving behind only healthy and viable tissue. An incision should always be made with careful planning due to the unpredictable extent of underlying necrosis from infection. Making the incision about 1 cm or greater distal to the intended level of bone transection should allow for a tension-free closure (**FIGURES 1** and **2**).
- Electrocautery is used to divide the subcutaneous and soft tissues until the phalanx or metatarsal bone is encountered. Care is taken to not encroach on tissues in the territories of other digits so as to prevent unintentional devascularization of the adjoining digit. Electrocautery is usually sufficient to achieve hemostasis.
- If there is concern for vascular insufficiency, tissues should be handled as atraumatically as possible with sparing use of electrocautery, favoring suture ligation. Utilizing full-thickness flaps can lead to improved outcomes as these can protect vital vascular structures.
- Tendons are transected proximal to the incision. This is accomplished by grasping the tendons at the incision, putting tension on the tendons, and dividing them sharply at the incision. The remaining tendon should recoil within the foot proximal to the incision.
- The bone is isolated from the surrounding tissues using a periosteal elevator or other device. The bone should be transected along the diaphysis of the phalanx or metatarsal bone using bone shears or an oscillating saw. As mentioned above, the bone should be transected about 1 cm or greater proximal to the incision to allow a tension-free closure. Cartilage should not be left exposed at the wound surface. If any cartilage is exposed, it should be removed using a rongeur.
- If the amputation was done for osteomyelitis, a sample of the distal aspect of the remaining bone is sent for culture and pathology. This can be done using a rongeur. The specimen will guide further antibiotic needs and help dictate the length of antibiotic requirements.
- Any sesamoid bones within the affected area should be removed. This can be done using a combination of electrocautery and blunt dissection to divide the tissue surrounding the sesamoid bone(s). When enough of the bone is exposed

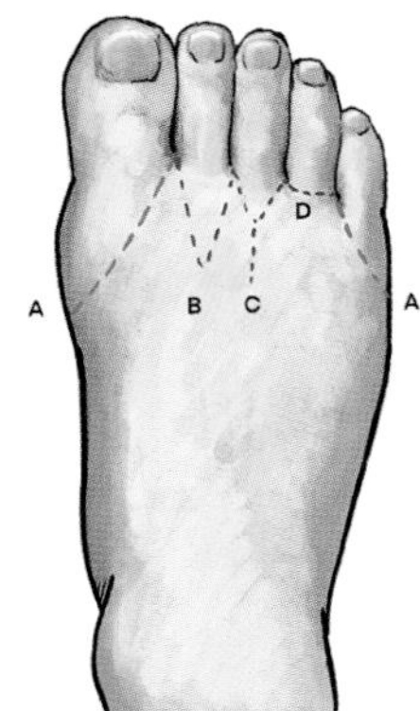

FIGURE 1 ● Incisions for toe/ray amputation. **A,** Beveled incisions are made for digits 1 and 5. Incisions for digits 2 to 4 require a **(B)** wedge-shaped or **(C)** racket-shaped incision. **D,** A circumferential incision at the base of the digit can be performed on any digit if the pathology is confined to the digit. (Illustration by Jacob C. Wood.)

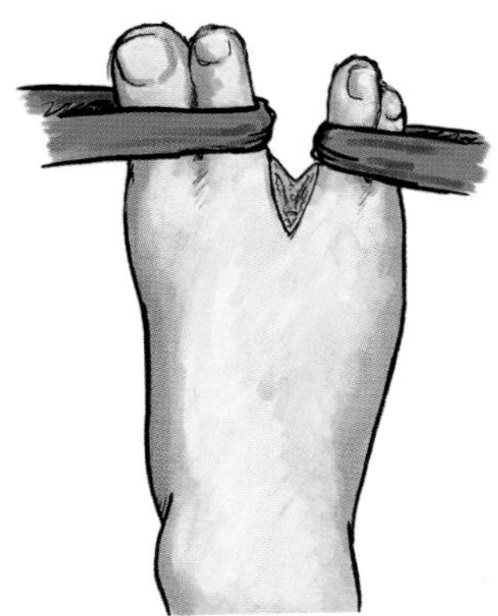

FIGURE 2 ● A wedge-shaped incision is made to perform a 3rd digit ray amputation. Loops from a lap pad are used to retract the medial and lateral toes away from the operative field. (Illustration by Jacob C. Wood.)

as can be grasped by toothed forceps (such as Kocher forceps), tension can be applied to the bone, which will facilitate circumferential dissection and removal.

- After infected and/or devitalized tissue is removed and hemostasis is obtained, the wound is closed in two layers with deep absorbable sutures in buried fashion and the skin approximated with permanent, monofilament sutures, usually in vertical mattress fashion.
- One may choose to leave the incision open or partially open if there is concern for retained infected tissue, which may worsen if the wound is closed. The wound may then be closed in a staged fashion or by secondary intention (**FIGURE 3**).
- When the offending pathology is focal to the distal digit, leaving the proximal one-third of the proximal phalanx of the toe has been found to reduce toe deviation of adjacent toes leading to ulcerations after the patient recovers.

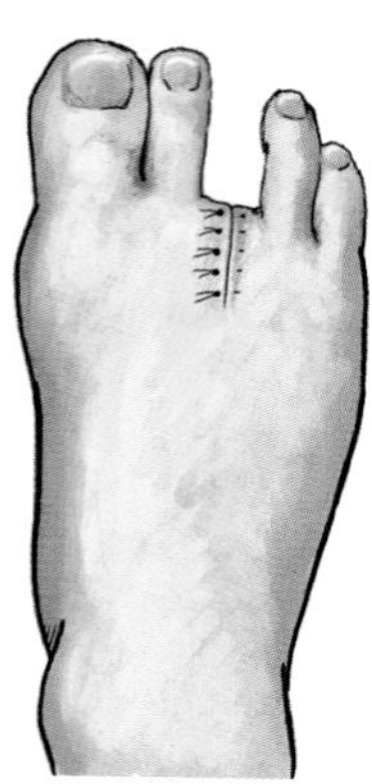

FIGURE 3 ● A 3rd digit ray amputation is completed with a multilayered closure. (Illustration by Jacob C. Wood.)

TRANSMETATARSAL AMPUTATION

- TMA is performed when all digits of a foot must be removed. The level of amputation is dictated by how much viable tissue the surgeon has to work with. Ideally, the metatarsal bones are transected at the distal aspects of the diaphyses just proximal to the flaring of the metaphyses and the parabolic relationship of metatarsal bone lengths is maintained.
- A modified fish-mouth incision is made, with the plantar flap longer than the dorsal flap (**FIGURE 4**).
- The dorsal incision is made 1 to 2 cm distal to the intended location of the metatarsal bone resection. The incision is sharply carried to the level of the metatarsal bones in a plane perpendicular to the surface of the skin. The medial and lateral apices of the incisions are placed midway between the dorsal and plantar aspects of the foot. The dorsal flap is retracted from the metatarsal bones (**FIGURE 5**).
- Each bone is individually isolated from the periosteum and surrounding tissue at the intended location of transection, then divided using either oscillating saw or bone shears. A power saw is preferred over the bone shears due to fragility of the metatarsal bones that can occur with advanced age or infection leading to longitudinal fractures. The tissue between each metatarsal bone is preserved to maintain the intermetatarsal vessels.

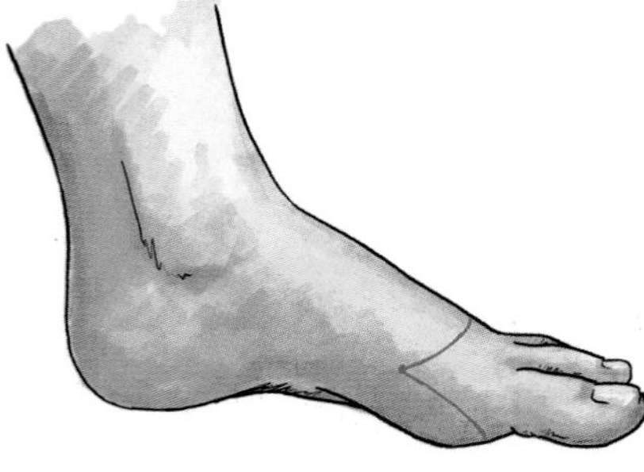

FIGURE 4 ● A fish-mouthed incision for a TMA. The plantar flap is longer than the dorsal flap. (Illustration by Jacob C. Wood.)

- The first and second metatarsal bones are cut at approximately the same length. The subsequent metatarsal bones are divided in a gently tapered fashion, aiming to maintain the curvature of the native metatarsal configuration.
- The metatarsal bones are cut at a 45° angle in the dorsoplantar projection. Beveling the bones at this angle reduces prominences on the plantar surface, thereby lowering focal pressure during propulsion that can otherwise lead to additional ulcerations after resuming ambulation.
- Proximal bone fragments can be sent for culture and pathology to ensure complete resection of osteomyelitic bone or to help guide antibiotic therapy for retained osteomyelitis.
- The plantar incision is made distal to the level of the metatarsal heads. The metatarsal bones and the toes are detached as the unit from the plantar flap. Care is taken to retain the intermetatarsal tissue.

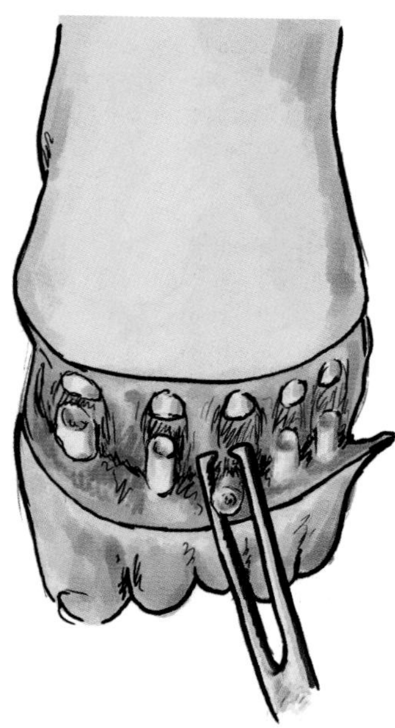

FIGURE 5 ● During a TMA, the metatarsal bones are transected at lengths that maintain the parabolic shape of the forefoot. The intermetatarsal tissue is preserved as the plantar flap is created. (Illustration by Jacob C. Wood.)

- Sesamoid bones and joint tissue are removed from the plantar flap to avoid development of heterotopic ossification and to decrease unnecessary bulk.
- After all compromised tissue has been removed and after hemostasis has been achieved, the flaps are brought together and closed. This is done using absorbable, braided suture in buried, interrupted fashion to approximate the deep tissues. The skin is brought together using either permanent, nonabsorbable suture in interrupted, vertical mattress fashion or with staples (**FIGURE 6**).
- When approximating tissue layers it is important to eliminate the amount of dead space as this can lead to wound dehiscence and reinfection of the amputation due to large flap remodeling and bone resection.
- If there is not enough tissue to accomplish complete closure or if there is concern for retained infected tissue that will not resolve with antibiotics, the surgeon may elect to perform partial closure or to leave the incision open.
- With good wound care, the wound may be able to be closed in delayed fashion if there is enough tissue, or closure can be obtained by secondary intention.

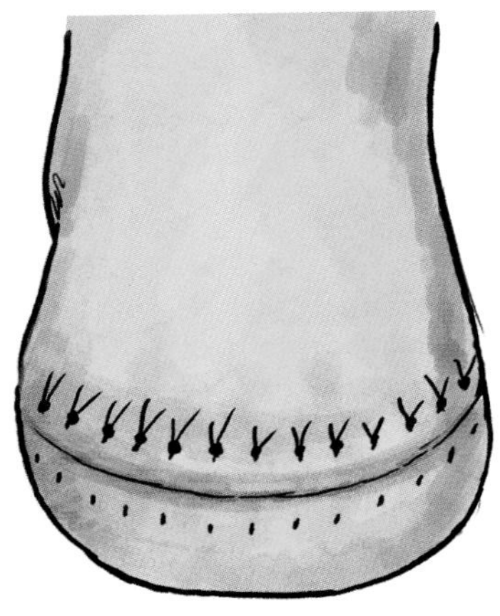

FIGURE 6 ● A TMA is completed with a multilayered closure. (Illustration by Jacob C. Wood.)

- Negative pressure wound therapy can facilitate wound closure or can bridge the gap for and maximize the wound bed for skin graft attempts.

SYMES AMPUTATION

- A Syme level amputation is a tibiotalar disarticulation with division of the tibia and fibula at the level of the malleoli. The flap is based on the heel fat pad (**FIGURE 7**).
- This operation can be done in one or two stages. The two-stage method involves ankle disarticulation followed by transection of the tibia and fibula approximately 6 weeks later. This is done when there is concern for retained infection or nonviable tissue.
- A fish-mouth incision is made based on the anatomic landmarks of the malleoli. The apices of the incision are placed 1 cm inferior and 1 cm anterior to the lateral malleolus and 1 cm inferior and 1 cm anterior to the medial malleolus. These points are connected extending anteriorly across the dorsal aspect of the ankle and in a plantar-ward direction.
- Planning of the medial incision must take the location of the posterior tibial artery into consideration, which must be preserved.

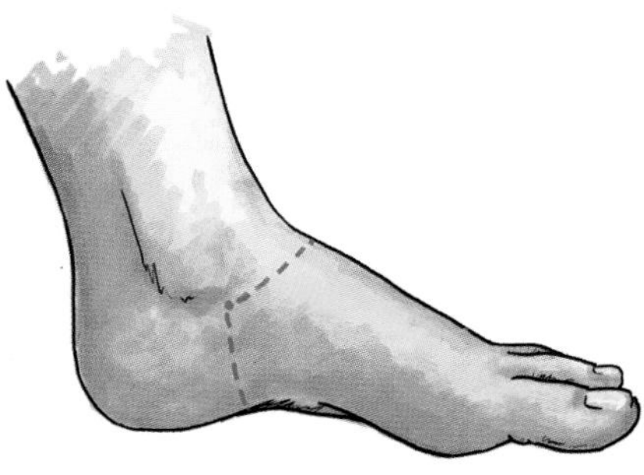

FIGURE 7 ● Syme amputation is done with a fish-mouthed incision with the apices about 1 cm inferior and 1 cm anterior to the medial and lateral malleoli. (Illustration by Jacob C. Wood.)

- The anterior/dorsal incision is made and carried directly to bone in a plane perpendicular to the skin surface. The extensor tendons encountered are stretched and divided to allow them to retract into the remaining tissue. The anterior tibial artery is ligated and divided.
- The talus bone is encountered. The talus bone is retracted with a bone hook, allowing dissection to and through the tibiotalar joint capsule and disarticulation of the ankle joint. Care is taken to preserve the posterior tibial artery with its branches, which will be encountered posterior to the medial malleolus thereby maintaining perfusion to the myocutaneous flap (**FIGURE 8**).
- The calcaneus is dissected free in a subperiosteal plane moving posteriorly to the calcaneal tuberosity where the tendocalcaneus (Achilles tendon) is encountered and dissected free from its insertion.

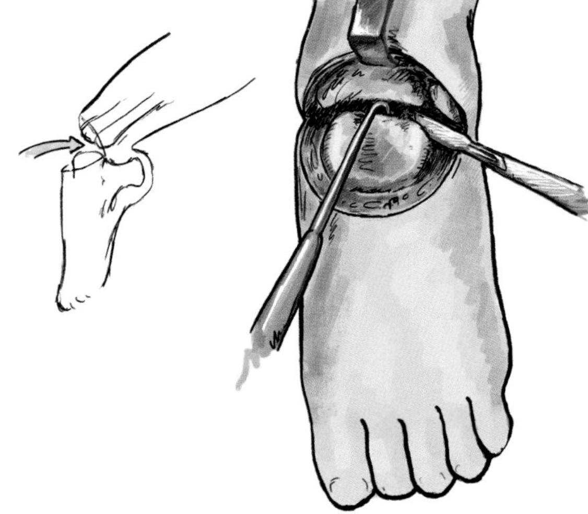

FIGURE 8 ● The tibiotalar joint is separated. Dissection is carried posteriorly around the calcaneus in a subperiosteal plane. (Illustration by Jacob C. Wood.)

- The calcaneus is further dissected in a subperiosteal plan until encountering the inferiorly directed incision. The calcaneus and foot are removed in one piece.
- The periosteum will assist with the weight-bearing potential of the flap and tends to heal to the tibia and fibula quite well.
- The heel fat pad has a unique aptitude for weight bearing and should be preserved at all costs—if it cannot be preserved, a different amputation should be considered.
- The tibia and the fibula are divided using an oscillating bone saw at a level proximal to the articular cartilage segments and distal to the diaphyses. Retaining the flaring segments of the tibia and fibula will assist with prosthesis fitting. Also, transecting in a point with a large amount of cortical bone will maximize the weight-bearing potential of the limb (**FIGURE 9**).
- The medial and lateral aspects of the malleoli are beveled to minimize pressure points while still maintaining a bulbous distal aspect of the amputation for prosthetic fitting.
- All synovial tissue and articular cartilage should be removed.
- A misplaced heel flap is an important complication after this amputation. It can be avoided by careful placement of the plantar surface of the flap directly beneath the center of the tibia. Removal of dog-ears, which will resolve with time, is thought to be a cause of flap migration.
- The peroneal tendons are anchored to the anterior flap fascia and retinaculum.

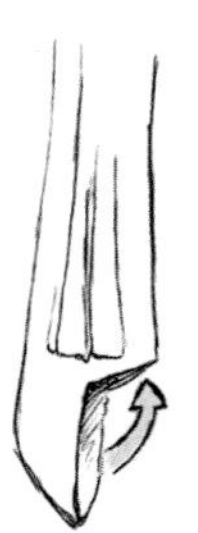
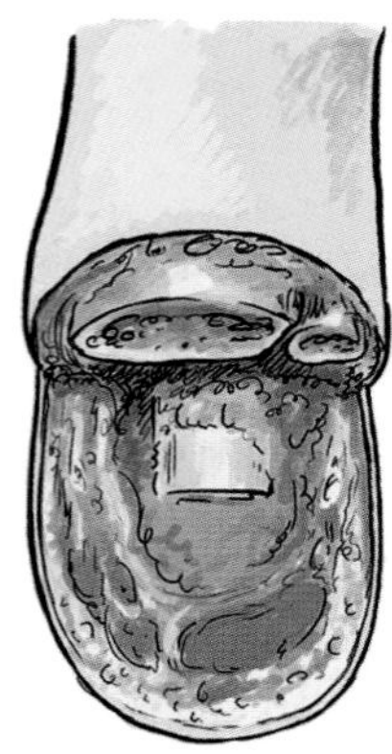
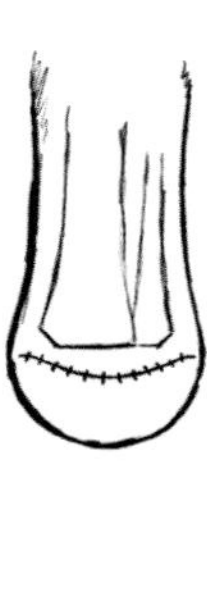

FIGURE 9 • The tibia and the fibula are transected. The medial and lateral aspects are beveled to avoid pressure points. The flap is made up of the Achilles tendon, the calcaneus periosteum, and the superficial tissues in this area including the plantar fat pad. The flap is rotated anteriorly to complete the amputation with a multilayered closure. Drains are often placed to eliminate the dead space under the flap—not pictured. (Illustration by Jacob C. Wood.)

- The wound is closed over drains to obliterate the dead space. Closure is performed in multiple layers using absorbable braided suture in deep interrupted fashion. The skin is closed using permanent monofilament suture in interrupted, vertical mattress fashion or with staples.

PEARLS AND PITFALLS

Closure	■ Striving for a tension-free skin closure while minimizing the trauma to the myocutaneous flaps during the operation will maximize success of the amputation. ■ Dog-ears from closure will resolve with time and healing.
Wound management and source control	■ Removing all infected tissue may not be possible. Microscopic disease will likely resolve with antibiotics with the wound being able to be closed. A grossly infected wound should be left open as closure will likely result in wound breakdown or worsening of the infection, potentially requiring a more proximal amputation. Counter incisions may be necessary for source control in the setting of severe infections.
Tourniquet use	■ Tourniquet can be used to minimize operative blood loss but should not be used in patients with severe ischemia or incompressible vessels. Tourniquet use is not only ineffective in patients with noncompressible arteries but is detrimental as it also causes venous hypertension resulting in more bleeding and bleeding that can be difficult to control.
Multidisciplinary approach	■ Most amputation patients benefit from a multidisciplinary approach to their preoperative and postoperative care to optimize their comorbid conditions and their functional rehabilitation.

POSTOPERATIVE CARE

- The postoperative hospital stay is largely dedicated to coordinating the patient's rehabilitation needs, antibiotic needs, medical management needs, and preparing the patient for ultimately living at home.
- Weight bearing of distal individual toe amputations and metatarsal amputations is variable based on patient needs and functional status prior to amputation. The preferable option is to be non–weight-bearing or heel weight bearing. For transmetatarsal amputations it is preferable to maintain a non–weight-bearing status for 4 weeks in a 90° splint or a tall boot to prevent dehiscence.
- Foot amputations require pressure offloading, which can be accomplished using specialized orthotic shoes. Offloading measures should be continued until the amputation is healed.
- Rehabilitation: becoming accustomed to a new configuration to one's foot may be quite challenging. The rehabilitation needs of a patient depend on the level of amputation and the

degree of deconditioning prior to the amputation. Physical and occupational therapy are useful for assessing a patient's rehabilitation needs as well as teaching patients how to ambulate while offloading the affected segment of the foot.

- Infection is a common reason for needing an amputation. The antibiotic requirements after an operation may range from none if the operation completely eradicates the infection to requiring a lengthy course of intravenous antibiotics if treating ongoing osteomyelitis.
- If the bone culture is positive then there is osteomyelitis that should be treated. The antibiotic of choice can be dictated by the speciation and sensitivities. We routinely seek Infectious Disease consultation for these patients. A peripherally inserted central catheter or equivalent will often need to be placed.
- If the bone culture is negative but there is concern for residual infected tissue, a short course of oral antibiotics may be desired. The wound should be monitored closely for evidence of recurrence of infection.
- Postoperative care should be coordinated in a multidisciplinary fashion to optimize the patient's comorbid conditions.

COMPLICATIONS

- Wound infection
- Wound breakdown
- Neuroma
- Pressure wounds
- Phantom limb pain
- Foot malformation

SUGGESTED READING

1. Bibbo C. Modification of the Syme amputation to prevent postoperative heel pad migration. *J Foot Ankle Surg*. 2013;52(6):766-770. doi:10.1053/j.jfas.2013.07.006
2. Boffeli TJ, Waverly BJ. Transmetatarsal and Lisfranc amputation. In: Boffeli T, ed. *Osteomyelitis of the Foot and Ankle*. Springer; 2015. doi:10.1007/978-3-319-18926-0_19
3. Eliassen A, Coleman DM. Transmetatarsal amputation. In: Upchurch GR, Henke PK, eds. *Clinical Scenarios in Vascular Surgery*. 2nd ed. Wolters Kluwer; 2015:468-471.
4. Harris RI. Syme's amputation. *J Bone Joint Surg*. 1956:38 B(3):614-632. doi:10.1302/0301-620X.38B3.614
5. Jimenez JC. Lower extremity amputation. In: Moore WS, Lawrence PF, Oderich GS, eds. *Vascular and Endovascular Surgery: A Comprehensive Review*. 9th ed. Saunders Elsevier; 2019:956-992.
6. Lavery LA, Ahn J, Ryan EC, et al. What are the optimal cutoff values for ESR and CRP to diagnose osteomyelitis in patients with diabetes-related foot infections?. *Clin Orthop Relat Res*, 2019;477(7):1594-1602. doi:10.1097/CORR.0000000000000718
7. Rios AL, Eidt JF. Lower extremity amputation: operative techniques and results. In: Sidawy AN, Rutherford RB, Perler BA, eds. *Rutherford's Vascular Surgery and Endovascular Therapy*. 9th ed. Saunders Elsevier; 2019:1496-1513.

Chapter 41 Lower Extremity Amputation: BKA/AKA/Hip Disarticulation

Shernaz S. Dossabhoy and Shipra Arya

DEFINITION

- Lower extremity amputations are a necessary set of procedures for vascular, orthopedic, plastic, and general surgeons to employ in various situations, including trauma, infection, ischemia/atherosclerotic disease, diabetic complications, malignancy, congenital or acquired deformities, and intractable pain (neuropathic, ischemic).
- The goals of lower extremity amputation are to remove ischemic, infected, or devitalized tissue and allow for eventual wound closure and healing. Amputation can also treat pain and improve mobility and function with the aid of rehabilitation and prosthetic limbs.
- Major amputations are proximal to the tarsometatarsal joint (Chopart, Boyd, Syme, Below Knee, and Above Knee). Minor amputations are distal or through the tarsometatarsal joint (Forefoot, Transmetatarsal, and Lisfranc). This chapter will focus on three types of major amputation, including: below-the-knee amputation (BKA), above-the-knee amputation (AKA), and hip disarticulations.
- Key terms: below-the-knee amputation (BKA) is a transtibial amputation, above-the-knee amputation (AKA) is a transfemoral amputation, and hip disarticulation is dislocation at the hip joint to allow for removal of the lower limb.

DIFFERENTIAL DIAGNOSIS

- Most amputations can be categorized as traumatic or nontraumatic. In this section, we discuss the differential diagnoses that lead to amputation and how the decision is made to proceed with limb salvage (secondary amputation) vs primary amputation. Primary amputation is defined as amputation occurring without prior attempt at limb salvage (eg, revascularization, bone repair, soft tissue/muscle flap coverage). On the other hand, secondary amputation includes amputations occurring after a failed attempt at revascularization and tissue reconstruction. This section will primarily focus on nontraumatic amputations. The operative techniques for BKA, AKA, and hip disarticulation, however, remain the same for both traumatic and nontraumatic amputations.
- Indications for primary amputation include "wet gangrene" (**FIGURE 1A**), nonsalvageable limb with loss of sensorimotor function (traumatic mangled extremity or acute limb ischemia), end-stage peripheral arterial disease (PAD), or critical limb threatening ischemia (CLTI) that is unable to be revascularized, comorbidities that preclude revascularization (ie, endovascular or open-bypass surgery), severe tissue loss or infection that precludes attempts at limb-salvage, intractable pain of the lower limb, refractory to management by pain specialist (ischemic, traumatic, neuropathic, or mechanical instability), and malignant tumors.
- Wet gangrene is a limb- and life-threatening event, presenting with swelling, purulence, blistering, erythema, and drainage in the setting of ischemic/under-perfused tissue with superimposed infection. Immediate guillotine amputation followed by definitive closure is advised (**FIGURE 2**).
- If primary amputation is not immediately indicated, patients will likely fall into one of the following categories: diabetic or other foot ulcer, dry gangrene, osteomyelitis, traumatic injury, peripheral arterial disease, or malignant tumor. Each should be closely monitored for signs of worsening ischemia, infection, or pain, which may necessitate future amputation.
- Diabetic foot ulcer (DFU): Diabetes is a major risk factor for lower extremity amputations worldwide. Approximately 25% to 90% of amputations within studied populations are associated with diabetes mellitus.[1] In Medicare patients, the incidence of DFU was 6.0% and lower extremity amputation 0.5% with 11% and 22% associated annual mortality, respectively.[2] Complications from diabetes mellitus are responsible for 60% to 80% of amputations.[2] Of patients with DFU, nearly 50% have concomitant PAD, which increases the risk of overall complications and amputation.[3]
- Other foot ulcers (neuropathic, pressure, arterial, venous): Amputations may be recommended for nonhealing nondiabetic ulcers, including neuropathic, pressure-related, or arterial. It is rare for amputation to be necessary for venous ulcers unless there is an association with intractable osteomyelitis.
- "Dry gangrene" (**FIGURE 1B**): In contrast to "wet gangrene," "dry gangrene" occurs in an extremity where the tissue "mummifies" and becomes discolored and ischemic, appearing dark or black. If there is no evidence of overt infection, dry gangrene does not require immediate amputation. The affected extremity can be conservatively managed or undergo revascularization with debridement. Amputation may often be avoided as an ischemic extremity will not heal properly. Dry gangrene or mummified tissue does not pass macrobacteria into the circulation.[2]
- Osteomyelitis: Especially in patients with diabetes, osteomyelitis of the forefoot, foot, and ankle may necessitate amputation. Often these infections are comanaged with podiatry and specific foot amputations are beyond the scope of this chapter (Part 6, Chapter 40). However, care must be taken to exclude osteomyelitis of the tibia or femur prior to transtibial or transfemoral amputation, respectively, to ensure adequate healing postoperatively.
- Traumatic injury: A mangled lower extremity in the setting of trauma may require amputation. Often, these injuries involve bone, muscle, and neurovascular structures, and it is helpful to involve specialists from orthopedic, vascular, and plastic surgery. Neurovascular structures should be assessed first as this will determine what portion of the limb may be salvageable as well as dictate level of amputation. Patient's age and functional status should be taken into consideration.
- PAD and nonsalvageable limb: Lower extremity ischemia is often due to chronic atherosclerotic disease, also known as PAD. Between 2000 and 2015, PAD was estimated to affect between 8.5 and 12 million Americans[4,5]—a 25% increase in prevalence over the prior decade. Risk factors for PAD

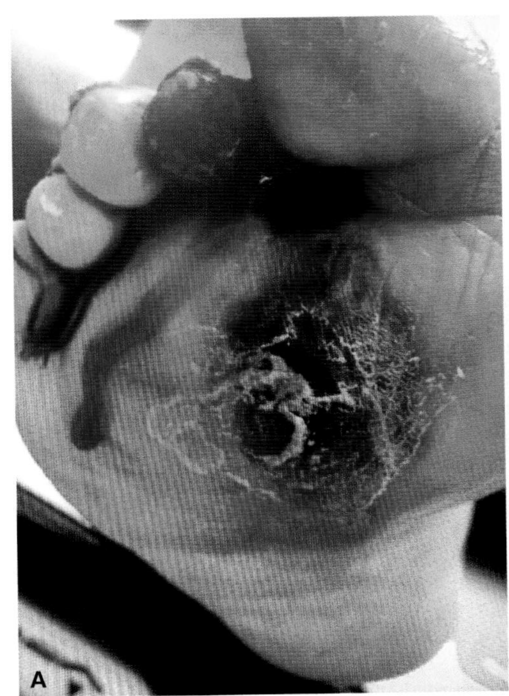

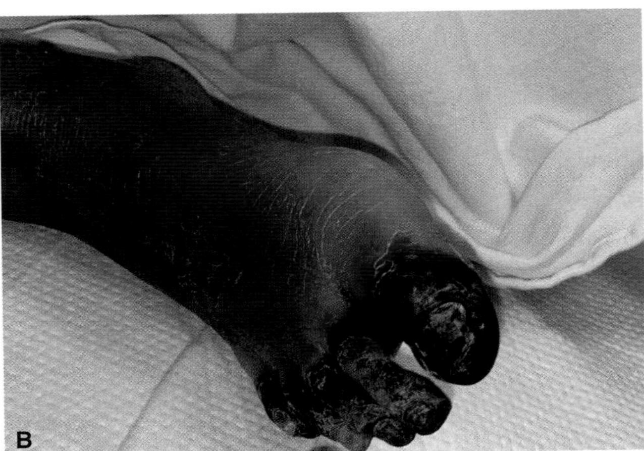

FIGURE 1 ● Gangrenous changes of foot with **(A)** wet gangrene with presence of infection and purulence on top of ischemic gangrenous changes and **(B)** dry gangrene with ischemia and necrosis of entire forefoot.

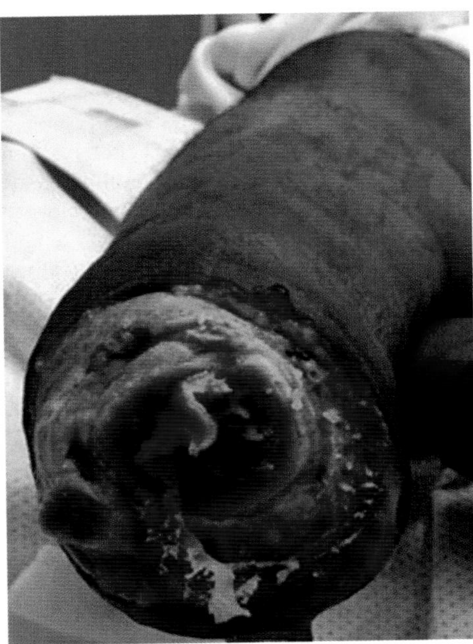

FIGURE 2 ● Staged amputation of lower extremity, also called "guillotine" amputation.

include age, cigarette smoking, dyslipidemia, and diabetes mellitus.[6] Late-stage, severe PAD is referred to as chronic critical limb threatening ischemia (CLTI) in the vascular surgery literature. Approximately 11% of patients with PAD will go on to develop CLTI,[7] which carries an associated 1-year amputation rate of 15% to 20% and 1-year mortality of 15% to 40%.[8] Once a limb is deemed "nonsalvageable" either due to failed prior revascularizations or inability to further revascularize, the patient should be evaluated for amputation. Urgency of amputation depends on degree of pain, presence of wound and/or infection, and often patient's desire or willingness to proceed with amputation.

- Malignant tumors of the proximal lower extremity: Malignant bony or soft tissue tumors with extensive involvement of the femur and soft tissues, not amenable to lesser resections, are treated with hip disarticulation. Hip disarticulation is reserved "for tumors more distal than those requiring a hemipelvectomy and more proximal than those that can be treated with a high thigh amputation."[9]

PATIENT HISTORY AND PHYSICAL FINDINGS

- Evaluation and planning for lower extremity amputation includes a thorough history and physical exam to optimize patient risk factors and assess for appropriateness of amputation.
- History should include risk factor assessment, extent of wound, infection, and ischemia that would guide efforts at limb salvage and functional status assessment. Risk factor assessment and modification to decrease perioperative morbidity and mortality includes smoking cessation, optimization of diabetes, hypertension, and hyperlipidemia, and consideration of perioperative beta-blockers in certain patients.
- Severe infections may require a two-stage approach, that is, "*guillotine*" amputation (see in "Surgical Management" section) followed by amputation formalization.
- Perioperative DVT prophylaxis and blood glucose control is important to minimize postoperative complications.

- Overall rehabilitation potential is based on individual patient's ability to ambulate, functional status, mental state, and overall life expectancy.
- Physical exam should include full vascular exam, including bilateral lower extremity femoral, popliteal, dorsalis pedis, and posterior tibial pulses. Additionally, one should assess for signs of infection, wounds, tissue loss, and any anatomic variations.
- The extent of amputation is determined by degree of tissue loss, ischemia, and infection as determined by physical exam. Ideally, there should be a palpable pulse proximal to the level of planned amputation as this is highly associated with stump healing. However, a nonpalpable pulse does not preclude amputation or mean the planned amputation will not heal; in these cases, further imaging and diagnostic studies are required, as described below (see in "Imaging and Other Diagnostic Studies" section).
- The Society for Vascular Surgery (SVS) Wound, Ischemia, and Foot Infection (WIfI) classification system can be used to assess threatened lower extremities by assigning a grade from 0-3 for each component (**TABLE 1**).[10] Based on this grading, a WIfI class is assigned. For example, a patient who presents with ischemic rest pain with ankle brachial index (ABI) 0.3, no wound, and no signs or symptoms of infection would be classified as Wound-0, Ischemia-3, Foot Infection-0, thus WIfI 030. This clinical stage can then be used to estimate the (a) risk of 1-year amputation and (b) likely need for/benefit of revascularization (assumes infection is controlled) (**FIGURE 3**). It should be noted that these estimates have been prospectively validated by numerous studies in select patient groups.[11]

Table 1: SVS Wound, Ischemia, and Foot Infection (WIfI) Classification System

Grade	(W) wound	(I) ischemia	(fI) foot infection
0	No ulcer; no gangrene	ABI ≥0.80 Ankle SBP > 100 mm Hg TP/$TcPO_2$ ≥ 60 mm Hg	No s/sx of infection
1	Small, shallow ulcer; no exposed bone; no gangrene	ABI 0.6-0.79 Ankle SBP 70-100 mm Hg TP/$TcPO_2$ 40-59 mm Hg	Local infection with at least 2 s/sx: • Local swelling or induration • Erythema 0.5-2 cm around ulcer • Local tenderness or pain • Local warmth • Purulent drainage
2	Deeper ulcer with exposed bone; gangrene on digits	ABI 0.4-0.59 Ankle SBP 50-70 mm Hg TP/$TcPO_2$ 30-39 mm Hg	Local infection (as above) with • Erythema >2 cm, or • Involving deeper structures (eg, abscess, osteomyelitis, septic arthritis, fasciitis)
3	Extensive, deep ulcer; extensive gangrene	ABI ≤0.39 Ankle SBP <50 mm Hg TP/$TcPO_2$ <30 mm Hg	Local infection (as above) with s/sx of SIRS: • Temp >38 °C or <36 °C • HR >90 beats/min • RR >20 breaths/min or $PaCO_2$ <32 mm Hg • WBC >12,000 or <4000 cu/mm or 10% bands

ABI, Ankle-brachial index; s/sx, signs/symptoms; $TcPO_2$, transcutaneous oximetry; TP, toe pressure.

IMAGING AND OTHER DIAGNOSTIC STUDIES

- The initial evaluation of a patient who may undergo lower extremity amputation should include noninvasive evaluation of peripheral circulation with arterial waveforms, ABIs, toe pressures or toe-brachial indices (TBIs), segmental pressures with pulse volume recordings (PVRs), and transcutaneous oxygen tensions ($TcPO_2$).
- ABIs >0.5 are associated with 90% healing of BKAs, while ABIs <0.35 correlate with poor wound healing of toe amputations.
- TBIs (also called "toe pressures") are a more reliable indicator of peripheral vascular disease and limb perfusion in diabetic patients. TBIs > 0.3 and absolute toe pressures >30 mm Hg are acceptable for wound healing in nondiabetic patients. In patients with diabetes, toe pressures >45 to 55 mm Hg may be required for healing.
- Segmental pressures with plethysmography, or pulse volume recordings (PVRs), are obtained by measuring blood pressure at successive levels along the length of the extremity combined with Doppler, which allows the examiner to localize the specific level of arterial disease. PVRs measure volume changes within the limb and are most useful in identifying disease in calcified vessels, which tend to yield falsely elevated pressure measurements (and thus falsely elevated ABIs). Regarding amputation prognosis, a calf Doppler systolic pressure of 50 to 70 mm Hg and a Doppler systolic thigh pressure of 80 mm Hg predict high success rate for wound healing after BKA.
- Transcutaneous oxygen tensions ($TcPO_2$s) of the lower extremity are obtained through platinum oxygen electrodes with patients positioned supine and with elevation of the limb. A $TcPO_2$ >40 torr predicts healing in 98% of amputations while $TcPO_2$ <20 torr has been historically associated with failure. Moreover, Columbo et al found that patients with $TcPO_2$ <40 torr had a two-fold increase of conversion to AKA or death.[12] Thus, $TcPO_2$ is a strong predictor of wound healing and may be more reliable than skin perfusion or segmental pressures.
- Duplex ultrasound (DUS) has recently been suggested to predict the best level of lower extremity amputation in patients with CLTI, as examination of lower extremity pulses may be unreliable. For example, in one study, all patients with aortoiliac or deep femoral arterial occlusion who initially received a BKA required reoperation with AKA due to poor wound healing, suggesting that performing a primary AKA for these patients could significantly reduce reoperation rates.[13]
- Often, if there has been concern for infection or osteomyelitis, X-ray (XR) or magnetic resonance imaging (MRI) of the foot and lower leg has been obtained. Both XR and/or MRI should be reviewed to ensure the tibial and fibular bones are free from infection prior to proceeding with amputation.
- While dedicated lower extremity imaging with computed tomographic angiography (CTA) or magnetic resonance angiography (MRA) is typically not required before amputation, they can provide an overall assessment for the degree of atherosclerotic vascular disease if noninvasive imaging is

A Estimate risk of amputation at 1 year for each combination

	Ischemia – 0				Ischemia – 1				Ischemia – 2				Ischemia – 3			
W-0	VI	VI	L	M	VI	L	M	H	L	L	M	H	L	M	M	H
W-1	VI	VI	L	M	VI	L	M	H	L	M	H	H	M	M	H	H
W-2	L	L	M	H	M	M	H	H	M	H	H	H	H	H	H	H
W-3	M	M	H	H	H	H	H	H	H	H	H	H	H	H	H	H
	fI-0	fI-1	fI-2	fI-3	fI-0	fI-1	fI-2	fI-3	fI-0	fI-1	fI-2	fI-3	fI-0	fI-1	fI-2	fI-3

B Estimate likelihood of benefit of/requirement for revascularization (assuming infection can be controlled first)

	Ischemia – 0				Ischemia – 1				Ischemia – 2				Ischemia – 3			
W-0	VI	VI	VI	VI	VI	L	L	M	L	L	M	M	M	H	H	H
W-1	VI	VI	VI	M	L	M	M	M	M	H	H	H	H	H	H	H
W-2	VI	VI	VI	VI	M	M	H	H	H	H	H	H	H	H	H	H
W-3	VI	VI	VI	VI	M	M	M	H	H	H	H	H	H	H	H	H
	f-0	fI-1	fI-2	fI-3	fI-0	fI-1	fI-2	fI-3	fI-0	fI-1	fI-2	fI-3	fI-0	fI-1	fI-2	fI-3

fI. foot Infection; I, Ischemia; W, Wound.

Premises:

1. Increase in wound class increases risk of amputation (based on PEDIS, UT, and other wound classification systems)
2. PAD and infection are synergistic (Eurodiale): infected wound + PAD increases likelihood revascularization will be needed to heal wound
3. Infection 3 category (systemic/metabolic instability): moderate to high-risk of amputation regardless of other factors (validated IDSA guidelines)

Four classes: for each box, group combination into one of these four classes

Very low = VL = clinical stage 1
Low = L = clinical stage 2
Moderate = M = clinical stage 3
High = H = clinical stage 4

Clinical stage 5 would signify an unsalvageable foot

FIGURE 3 ● Clinical staging of wound based on the SVS Wound, Ischemia, and Foot Infection (WIfI) classification system. (Reprinted from Mills JL Sr, Conte MS, Armstrong DG, et al. The Society for Vascular Surgery Lower Extremity Threatened Limb Classification System: Risk stratification based on Wound, Ischemia, and foot Infection (WIfI). *J Vasc Surg*. 2014;59(1):220-234.e2. Copyright © 2014 The Authors. With permission.)

inconclusive and demonstrate any anatomic variations not assessed by physical exam.

- An important note for DFU with infection: If there is tarsal and/or calcaneal bone involvement, then patient may require a BKA. If the infection is limited to only the forefoot, then can consider transmetatarsal amputation (TMA); however, further discussion is beyond the scope of this current chapter (Part 6, Chapter 40).

SURGICAL MANAGEMENT

Algorithm for Approach to Amputation

- The approach to lower extremity amputation must first consider if the limb is salvageable or not, followed by consideration of the patient's clinical status (septic or not), and potential for postoperative ambulation (see **FIGURE 4**, Management Algorithm).
- Throughout this process, shared decision-making between the multidisciplinary care team (including vascular surgeons, plastic surgery, orthopedic surgery, podiatry, wound care, physical medicine and rehabilitation (PM&R), nutrition, and palliative care, etc.) and the patient is of highest importance.[14] Patients must consider what is important for their quality of life, as some would rather proceed with terminal wound care and defer amputation until their clinical status changes, while others prefer to undergo primary amputation with the goal of increased rehab potential and ambulation with a prosthetic. It is helpful to engage PM&R physicians, who can often provide a more realistic assessment to patients and surgeons regarding ambulatory potential.

Preoperative Planning

- For patient preoperative management, see in "Preoperative Preparation." In addition, standard preoperative workup including anesthesia preassessment, ECG, echo, and chest x-ray if indicated, should be considered.
- Determining the appropriate level of amputation is essential for successful would healing and rehabilitation potential. Various objective criteria have been described to determine the level of amputation according to the degree of vascular perfusion (see in "Imaging and Other Diagnostic Studies"). Surgeon clinical judgment and experience complement the use of these adjunctive measures.

Positioning

- For any lower extremity amputation, the patient should be positioned supine on standard operating room table. A tourniquet of appropriate size should be available but kept sterile and only placed on the patient after prep and draping. A "bump" can be fashioned out of folded blue towels on the back table and is helpful for elevation of the limb during the procedure.

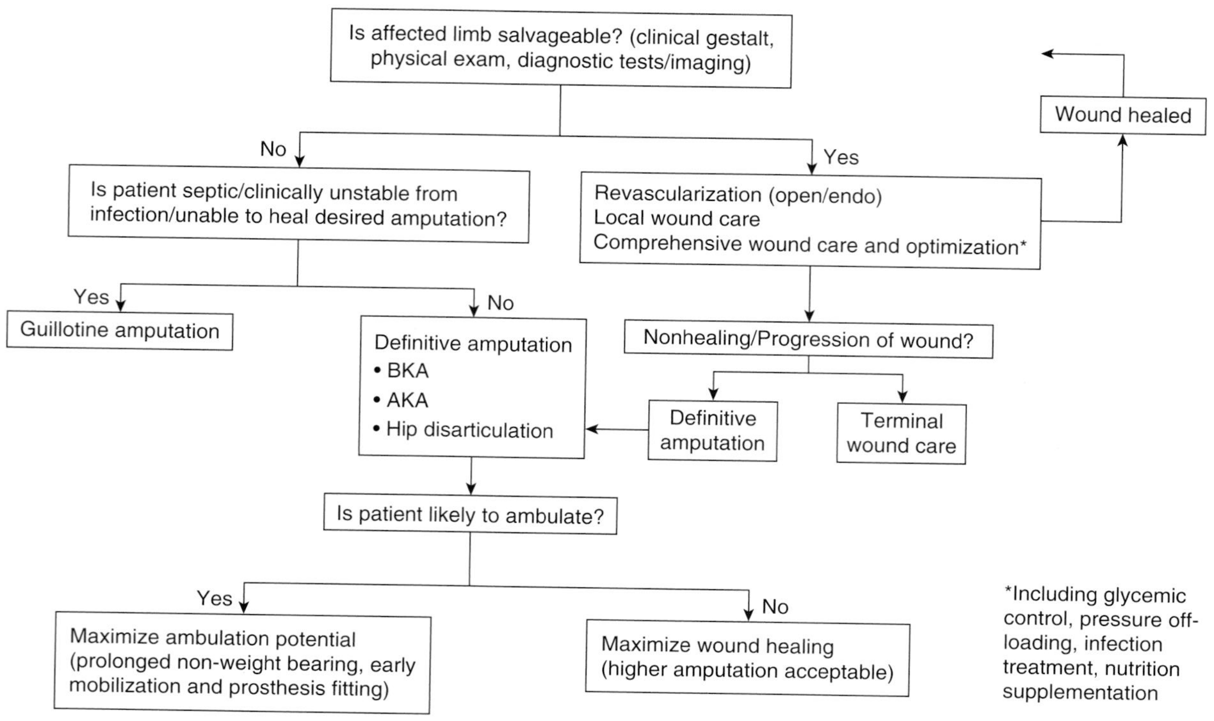

FIGURE 4 ● Algorithm for approach to limb salvage and amputation.

GENERAL PRINCIPLES

- Certain surgical principles can be applied to all amputation types. Selecting the appropriate amputation level is the first step and based on clinical and diagnostic factors (see in "Imaging and Other Diagnostic Studies") to assess vascular perfusion and structural bone integrity.
- Routine antibiotic and venous thromboembolism prophylaxis are administered. A tourniquet should be avoided in an ischemic limb unless the diseased arterial segment is located distally to the level of amputation only.
- Any dead or devitalized skin, muscle, and tissue is debrided and removed. Unnecessary trauma to healthy marginal tissue is minimized by careful dissection and avoiding excessive tissue handling with forceps or electrocautery.
- Skin and subcutaneous tissue should be kept intact with the fascia. Muscles are divided with electrocautery or sharply with scissors.
- Bone is divided with an electric or Gigli saw. Any bone dust is irrigated from the residual bone with saline. Bone edges are smoothed with a rasp. The anterior edge of larger bones (eg, femur or tibia) is beveled with an electric saw to minimize potential trauma with a future prosthesis.
- Large vessels are suture ligated.
- Nerves are tied off under stretch, divided sharply using scissors (not electrocautery), and allowed to retract into the residual limb. This prevents potential neuroma formation in the future. Injecting local anesthetic or neurolytic to the nerve stump prior to dividing has been proposed to ameliorate postoperative or phantom limb pain but is not in our routine practice.
- In patients who are at risk of having negative reactions to narcotic pain medications such as the elderly, the authors have had excellent results partnering with anesthesia to place preoperative nerve block catheters, which supply a continuous infusion of local anesthetic to the surgical limb and reduces postoperative opiate use.
- To keep the inferior muscle pad in place over the new residual limb in BKAs or AKAs, *myodesis* can be performed. The distal muscle is sutured to the bone through a predrilled hole, thereby securing the muscle to the bone. This prevents stump deformity and shifting of muscles during contraction, which can lead to progressive atrophy.
- In closing, the external fascia is reapproximated over the muscle and bone in a tension-free manner. Skin is approximated using staples, interrupted nonabsorbable sutures, or continuous suture (absorbable or nonabsorbable).
- No benefit has been shown to leaving drains in the wound and may increase the risk of infection. If drains are used, they should be removed by postoperative day 1 to 2 and placed away from the suture line.

TRANSTIBIAL OR BELOW KNEE AMPUTATION

- Transtibial amputation or BKA is the most common amputation used for lower extremity infection or ischemia (**FIGURE 5**). Typical BKA uses a long posterior flap that is well-vascularized, though other techniques have been described (eg, sagittal, skew, medial, or fish mouth flaps).
- An anterior skin incision is made 1 cm distal to the intended transection of the tibia, which is typically measured as one handbreadth (10-12 cm) below the tibial tuberosity. The incision is extended about one half to two thirds around the leg's circumference. The posterior flap includes the gastrocnemius and is 3 cm more than the transverse diameter of the calf to be eventually folded anteriorly and cover the tibia to cushion the bone for prosthesis.
- Muscles of the anterior and lateral compartments are divided with electrocautery.
- The tibia is divided 10 to 12 cm distal to the tibial tuberosity using a power saw perpendicular to the long axis of the bone. The anterior edge of the tibia is beveled to minimize prosthetic trauma. The fibula is next divided 1 to 2 cm proximal to the tibia, typically with Horsley bone cutters.
- Major vascular bundles are suture ligated. The tibial and peroneal nerves are divided sharply under stretch.
- The posterior flap is completed by dividing the residual posterior compartment musculature and soft tissue with a long amputation knife. To reduce bulk of the posterior flap, the soleus muscle can be excised at the level of the tibial osteotomy, preserving the gastrocnemius muscle and fascia.
- The deep fascia and skin are closed without tension.

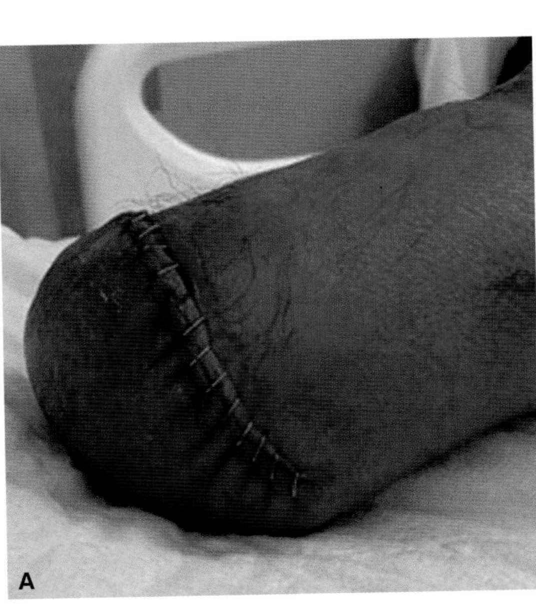

A

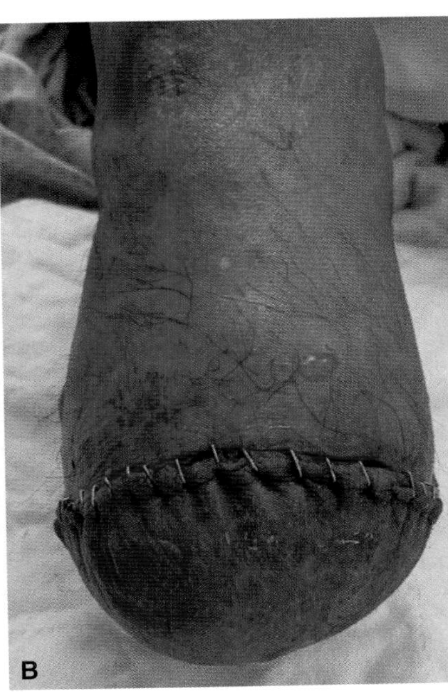

B

FIGURE 5 ● Transtibial or below-knee-amputation (BKA).

TRANSFEMORAL OR ABOVE KNEE AMPUTATION

- Transfemoral amputations or AKA can be performed at one of three levels (high, mid, or low) depending on the patient's expected postoperative function status and/or the extent of ischemia or infection.
- A circular (fish mouth) or sagittal incision is made 2 to 3 cm below the expected level of dividing the femur, followed by carrying the dissection down through the skin, fascia, and muscles. The femoral artery and vein are suture ligated in Hunter's canal. The femur is divided using an electric saw, proximal to the level of the divided muscles. The sciatic nerve is divided under stretch as described in "General Principles."
- Myodesis can be performed, whereby distal tendons of muscles are attached directly to bone via predrilled holes in the bone to maintain function and provide distal padding (**FIGURE 6**). While more common in tumor surgery, myodesis can be performed during both below-knee or above-knee amputations. In BKA, myodesis of the major leg muscle groups to the distal tibia provides soft-tissue coverage to the stump.[15] In AKA, a two-layer myodesis can be performed over the end of the femur, which provides added muscle stabilization of the bone.[16] Typically, the quadriceps and hamstrings muscles are myodesed to one another covering the distal bony femur edge. These muscles and the adductors are then secured to the femur using drill holes. Both absorbable and nonabsorbable suture have been described for this use.
- Myodesis, if performed, is followed by fascial closure with interrupted sutures.
- Skin is closed using sutures or staples.

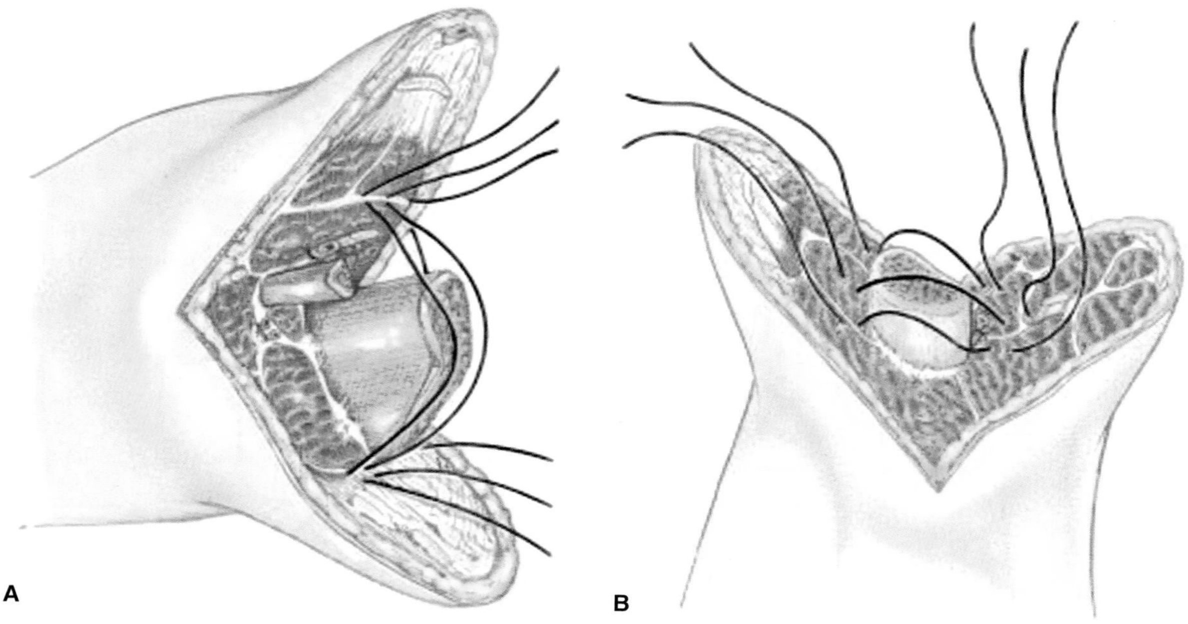

FIGURE 6 ● **A,** Myodesis over the distal tibia in below-knee-amputation. **B,** Two-layer myodesis over the femur stump in above-knee-amputation. (Reprinted by permission from Springer: Sugarbaker P, Bickels J, Malawer M. Above-knee amputation. In: Malawer MM, Sugarbaker PH, eds. *Musculoskeletal Cancer Surgery. Springer*; Reprinted by permission from Springer: Malawer M, Bickels J, Sugarbaker P. Below-knee amputation. In: Malawer MM, Sugarbaker PH, eds. *Musculoskeletal Cancer Surgery*. Springer; 2004:366.)

HIP DISARTICULATION

- Disarticulation of the femur at the hip joint is a rare procedure, performed for nonhealing amputations at a lower level, life-threatening infection/gangrene, tumors, or trauma. Patients commonly have impaired arterial inflow at the level of the iliac arteries, and so are at high risk of decubitus pressure ulcers and nonhealing wounds. Wound complication (60%) and mortality (21%) rates are high, even more so in the context of ischemia or urgent/emergent surgery.
- The patient is positioned in the lateral decubitus position to facilitate both a posterolateral and anterior approach to the hip (**FIGURE 7**).[17] For the first stage, the surgeon stands in an anterior position to the patient to perform the neurovascular bundle exposure and ligation. After an anterior oblique skin incision is made along and below the level of the inguinal ligament, the femoral vessels and nerve are divided, and the muscles of the anterior thigh are transected off the pelvic bone from lateral to medial, beginning with the sartorius and ending with the adductor magnus.
- The iliopsoas and obturator externus muscles are divided at their insertion on the lesser trochanter of the femur; all other muscles are divided at their origin. The quadratus femoris muscle is identified and preserved. The hip flexor muscles are transected from the ischial tuberosity at their origin.
- In the next phase, the surgeon moves to the contralateral side in a posterior position to the patient to facilitate gluteal muscular dissection and joint disarticulation. The pelvis is rotated from posterolateral to anterolateral position. The posterior skin incision is made. The gluteal fascia, tensor fascia lata, and gluteus maximus muscles are divided at their posterior attachments to reveal the muscles inserting onto the greater trochanter (via a common tendon). These muscles are transected at their insertion on the bone. The posterior joint capsule is exposed and transected. The sciatic nerve is identified and divided and then retracts below the piriformis muscle.
- The wound is closed with preserved muscles reapproximated over the joint capsule. Suction drains are placed, and over these, the gluteal fascia is secured to the inguinal ligament. Skin is closed with interrupted sutures.

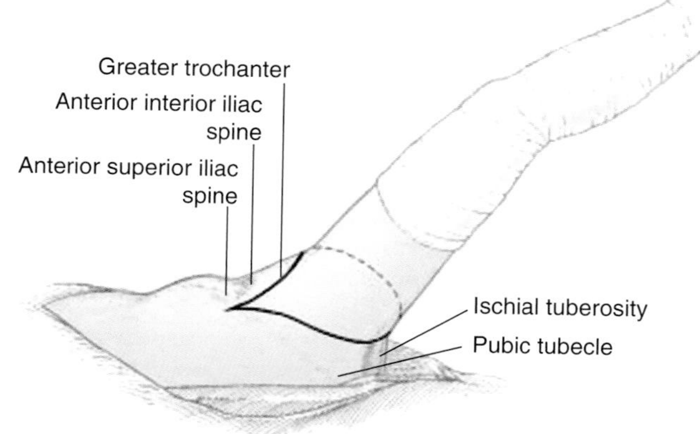

FIGURE 7 ● Hip disarticulation patient positioning and surgical incision. (Reprinted by permission from Springer: Sugarbaker P, Malawer M. Hip disarticulation. In: Malawer MM, Sugarbaker PH, eds. *Musculoskeletal Cancer Surgery*. Springer; 2004:340.)

PEARLS AND PITFALLS

BKA	■ For BKA, a long posterior flap is crucial to allow for successful padding and closure of the stump. The tibia should be resected 10-12 cm below the tuberosity with the fibula 1-2 cm above the level of the tibia. If the tibia is transected too proximally, the bony stump can erode through the anterior portion of the stump. If the fibula is left too long, then the patient will be unable to properly bear weight with a prosthesis.
AKA	■ For AKA, the length of the femur should be considered for either high or low AKA. High AKA is recommended if there is occlusion of the external iliac artery or profunda femoris for healing of the surgical incision site or if the extent of infection is extensive (ie, infected prosthesis or bone).
Hip disarticulations	■ For hip disarticulations, the lower extremity should be prepped and draped to allow for free manipulation of the hip joint, including hip flexion. Flexion at the knee joint is also important for developing the posterior amputation flap, which includes skin, subcutaneous tissue, fascia, and the gluteus maximus muscle maintaining its attachment at the deep surface to ensure adequate vascular supply for the flap. It is important to remember that the vascular supply to the posterior flap is dependent on leaving the gluteus maximus muscle attached to this flap.[9]

POSTOPERATIVE CARE

- Prior to leaving the operating room, the wound is commonly dressed in sterile fashion with vaseline gauze (Xeroform), layers of 4 × 4 cm gauze ("fluffs"), then wrapped with a Kerlix gauze bandage followed by an Ace compression bandage. This soft dressing with mild compression protects the wound and decreases edema. A knee immobilizer may be placed to keep the lower extremity extended at the knee joint to prevent contracture after BKA. The dressings are typically taken down on postoperative day 3 and further dressings with mild compression or shrinker stocking are continued until the wound is well healed (**FIGURE 8**). Compression over the patella should be avoided if possible as this can cause skin necrosis if placed too tightly.
- Instead, some surgeons have advocated for a rigid protective dressing. A rigid plaster of Paris stump dressing is applied immediately postoperatively and left on for 14 days. This dressing can be split longitudinally to allow for easy opening and closing (like a clamshell) for comfort and easier removal. This rigid dressing may reduce swelling and protect the stump from trauma and contracture. Disadvantages include its increased weight, inability to inspect the wound postoperatively, and possible compromise of blood flow to a stump with borderline perfusion.
- A recent Cochrane systematic review found no significant difference in benefits or harms when comparing rigid and soft dressings for patients undergoing transtibial amputations (BKAs).[18] Clinical judgment should be used after assessing the potential benefits and harms for each patient (ie, a high-fall risk patient may benefit more from a rigid protective dressing, while a patient with poor baseline skin integrity may benefit more from a soft dressing to decrease the risk of wound breakdown). While some studies favor rigid dressings immediately postoperatively for achieving faster stump healing[19] and reduction of stump volume, there is no apparent advantage in functional outcomes.
- Rigid removable dressings (RRDs) have also been utilized. These consist of sport tube socks to provide compression followed by a rigid plaster cast that is suspended by a stockinette to a supracondylar suspension cuff. Similar to a rigid

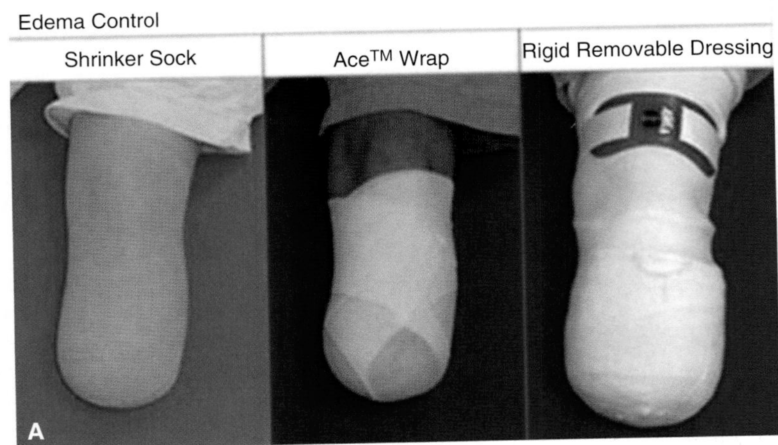

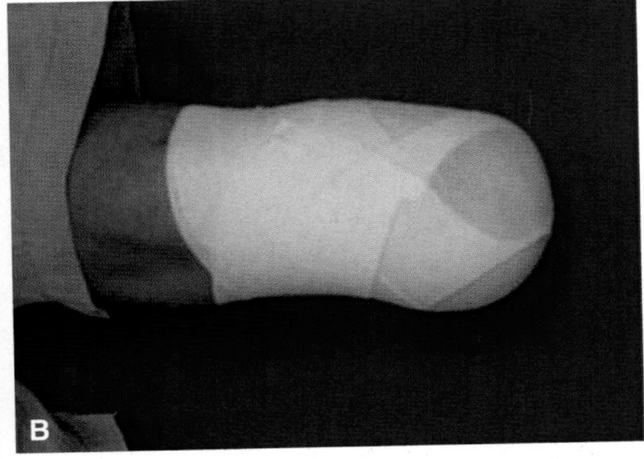

FIGURE 8 ● **A,** Types of postoperative dressings for compression and controlling edema after amputation. **B,** Ace wrap in figure-of-8 pattern. (Republished with permission of Springer, from Spires M. Lower extremity amputation: postamputation and residual limb care. In: Spires MC, Kelly BM, Davis AJ, eds. *Prosthetic Restoration and Rehabilitation of the Upper and Lower Extremity*. Demos Medical Publishing; 2014:26, Chapter 3; permission conveyed through Copyright Clearance Center, Inc.)

dressing, these reduce edema formation, but unlike the rigid protective dressing described above, their removability allows for more frequent wound inspections. Compression of the limb can be carefully controlled by adding more tube socks under the rigid cast.

- Regardless of dressing used, patients are made non-weight-bearing on the affected limb until the wounds are healed. An accidental traumatic injury to a fresh amputation site is a common cause of wound breakdown and complications.
- Other postoperative management should include standard postsurgical management including advancement of diet, adequate pain control, bowel regimen, and management of other medical conditions.

Rehabilitation and Prosthesis Preparation

- When patients have the time and opportunity to prepare for life with an amputation, consultation with PM&R specialists should be arranged prior to the surgery.
- With an adequate postoperative pain control regimen, rehabilitation begins as early as postoperative day 1 with joint exercises, bed and transfer mobility, and strengthening exercises for the contralateral leg and upper body.
- Inpatient consultation with PM&R service is made early to guide physical and occupational therapy, educate the patient about prosthetics, assist with rehabilitation placement, and help patients regain independence. Physical and occupational therapy should be prescribed early to facilitate mobility and training for activities of daily living (ADLs).
- The residual limb is fitted with an elastic compression stocking or "shrinker sock" to decrease edema and help shape and mold the limb to fit into the socket of a prosthesis. The shrinker sock is worn 24 hours a day to maximize edema reduction and optimize the shape of the residual limb for prosthesis fitting. Once the wound has healed, usually after 1 to 2 months, slow progression of weight-bearing is allowed.
- Long-term rehabilitation begins once the surgical incision is healed, which can take up to several weeks or longer depending on if there are any wound healing complications. Once healed, the patient can be fitted with a temporary prosthesis for gait training. Later, usually a minimum of 6 months postoperatively, a definitive prosthesis is prescribed, once the residual limb has stabilized in size and the patient has shown adequate ambulatory skill and training.

COMPLICATIONS AND OUTCOMES

- Multiple postoperative complications may arise after lower extremity amputations (**TABLE 2**), often due in large part to underlying comorbidities. In a large, retrospective review from 1990 to 2001, Aulivola et al identified 959 major lower extremity amputations (704 BKA = 73%, 255 AKA = 27%) in 788 patients.[20] The most commonly occurring complications included cardiac (10.2%), wound infection (5.5%), and pneumonia (4.5%). Amputation stump wound breakdown and failure for the residual limb to heal occur more commonly after BKA (13%) as compared to AKA (4%) (**FIGURE 9**).
- Outcomes on healing and revisions after amputations have been well studied. Nehler et al reported outcomes of 154 patients undergoing 172 major lower extremity amputations (94 BKA, 78 AKA) from 1997 to 2002.[21] Healing rates were lower for BKA vs AKA (55% BKA vs 76% AKA at 100 days; 83% BKA vs 85% AKA at 200 days). Thirty-nine patients (25%) required revision (23 BKA, 16 AKA) with 18 BKAs (19%) converted to AKA. In a more recent single-institution review from Columbo et al, 130 limbs undergoing BKA in 120 patients were examined. Thirty-eight percent of all BKAs achieved healing and ultimately ambulation. One-quarter of BKAs required reintervention with 9 limbs (7%) requiring BKA revision and 24 limbs (18%) converted to AKA.[12] In the series from Aulivola et al, 5% of AKA and 18% of BKA limbs required additional operation with 10% of BKAs requiring conversion to AKA at average time of 77 days postoperatively.[20]
- Ability to ambulate or wear a prosthesis is dependent on patient characteristics and amputation extent. In one study, 83% of BKA patients were ambulatory as compared to 45% of AKA patients; at 6-month follow up, these declined to 58% and 25%, respectively.[22] Of the patients who were ambulatory preoperatively, 74% of BKA and 63% of AKA

Table 2: Complications Following Major Lower Extremity Amputation With Relative Incidence

Complication	Reported incidence (%)
Deep vein thrombosis (DVT)	50% (without prophylaxis, AKA 38% vs BKA 21%)
Stump bleeding or hematoma	3%-9%
Infection	13%-40%
Need for reamputation	10%-20%
Phantom limb pain	50%-85%
Flexion contracture	3%-5%

Adapted with permission of Springer, from Arya S, Escobar GA. Principles of Lower Extremity Amputation: Etiology, Goals, Limb Length Decisions and Impact on Prosthetic Management. In: Spires MC, Kelly BM, Davis AJ, eds. Prosthetic Restoration and Rehabilitation of the Upper and Lower Extremity. Demos Medical Publishing; 2014:9-20; permission conveyed through Copyright Clearance Center, Inc..

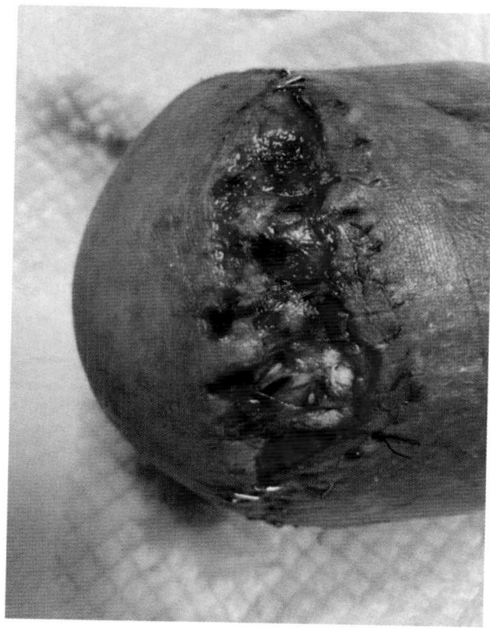

FIGURE 9 • Postoperative wound complication demonstrating below-knee-amputation (BKA) stump dehiscence.

remained so postamputation with similar rates observed at >1 year follow-up. Of all comorbidities studied (diabetes, renal insufficiency, PAD, or obesity), only age >70 years and female sex were independently associated with nonambulation postoperatively.

- Regarding mortality after amputation, in the large series from Aulivola et al, 30-day mortality was nearly 9% overall and significantly higher for AKA vs BKA (17% vs 6% $P < .001$) and for guillotine vs closed amputation (14% vs 8%, $P = .03$). Overall survival was 70% at 1 year and 35% at 5 years and significantly worse for AKA vs BKA (51% vs 75% at 1 year; 23% vs 38% at 5 years; $P < .001$). Gabel et al reviewed the Vascular Quality Initiative data registry for major lower extremity amputations (both BKA and AKA) from 2013 to 2015 and found an overall perioperative complication rate of 15% with 30-day mortality of 5%.[23] Patients undergoing AKA vs BKA were more likely to be female, >70 years old, underweight, nonambulatory, have ABI < 0.6, and have nonprivate insurance (all $P < .001$). AKA patients had a lower rate of 30-day postoperative complications (12% vs 18%) but a higher 30-day mortality (7% vs 3%) than BKA patients (all $P <.001$).
- Aspirin and statin therapy play an important role in risk prevention in PAD and nontraumatic amputations. In a population-based study from Arya et al, 155,647 patients with incident PAD were shown to have a significant reduction in both amputation and mortality with high-intensity statin therapy as compared to antiplatelet therapy only (HR 0.67; 95% CI 0.61-0.74 and HR 0.74; 95% CI 0.70-0.77, respectively).[24]

REFERENCES

1. Unwin N. Epidemiology of lower extremity amputation in centres in Europe, North America and East Asia. *Br J Surg*. 2000;87(3):328-337. doi:10.1046/j.1365-2168.2000.01344.x
2. Arya S, Escobar GA. Principles of lower extremity amputation: Etiology, goals, limb length decisions and Impact on prosthetic management. In: Spires MC, Kelly BM, Davis AJ, eds. *Prosthetic Restoration and Rehabilitation of the Upper and Lower Extremity*. Demos Medical Publishing; 2014:9-20.
3. Prompers L, Huijberts M, Apelqvist J, et al. High prevalence of ischaemia, infection and serious comorbidity in patients with diabetic foot disease in Europe. Baseline results from the Eurodiale study. *Diabetologia*. 2007;50(1):18-25. doi:10.1007/s00125-006-0491-1
4. Allison MA, Ho E, Denenberg JO, et al. Ethnic-specific prevalence of peripheral arterial disease in the United States. *Am J Prev Med*. 2007;32(4):328-333. doi:10.1016/j.amepre.2006.12.010
5. Thiruvoipati T, Kielhorn CE, Armstrong EJ. Peripheral artery disease in patients with diabetes: Epidemiology, mechanisms, and outcomes. *World J Diabetes*. 2015;6(7):961. doi:10.4239/wjd.v6.i7.961
6. Barnes JA, Eid MA, Creager MA, Goodney PP. Epidemiology and risk of amputation in patients with diabetes mellitus and peripheral artery disease. *Arterioscler Thromb Vasc Biol*. 2020;40(8):1808-1817. doi:10.1161/ATVBAHA.120.314595
7. Nehler MR, Duval S, Diao L, et al. Epidemiology of peripheral arterial disease and critical limb ischemia in an insured national population. *J Vasc Surg*. 2014;60(3):686-95.e2. doi:10.1016/j.jvs.2014.03.290
8. Duff S, Mafilios MS, Bhounsule P, Hasegawa JT. The burden of critical limb ischemia: a review of recent literature. *Vasc Health Risk Manag*. 2019;15:187-208. doi:10.2147/VHRM.S209241
9. Karakousis C. *Hip disarticulation*. In: *Operative Techniques in Orthopaedic Surgical Oncology*. Springer New York; 2014:217-222. doi:10.1177/0003134820923341
10. Mills JL, Conte MS, Armstrong DG, et al. The Society for vascular surgery lower extremity threatened limb classification system: risk stratification based on wound, ischemia, and foot infection (WIfI). *J Vasc Surg*. 2014;59(1):220-234.e2. doi:10.1016/J.JVS.2013.08.003
11. Darling JD, McCallum JC, Soden PA, et al. Predictive ability of the Society for Vascular Surgery Wound, Ischemia, and foot Infection (WIfI) classification system following infrapopliteal endovascular interventions for critical limb ischemia. *J Vasc Surg*. 2016;64:616-622. doi:10.1016/j.jvs.2016.03.417
12. Columbo JA, Nolan BW, Stucke RS, et al. Below-knee amputation failure and poor functional outcomes are higher than predicted in contemporary practice. *Vasc Endovasc Surg*. 2016;50(8):554-558. doi:10.1177/1538574416682159
13. Wagner WH, Keagy BA, Kotb MM, Burnham SJ, Johnson G. Noninvasive determination of healing of major lower extremity amputation: the continued role of clinical judgment. *J Vasc Surg*. 1988;8(6):703-710. doi:10.1016/0741-5214(88)90078-X
14. Gerhard-Herman MD, Gornik HL, Barrett C, et al. AHA/ACC guideline on the management of patients with lower extremity peripheral artery disease—Executive summary: a report of the American College of Cardiology/American Heart association task force on clinical practice guidelines. *J Am Coll Cardiol*. 2017;69(11):1465-1508. doi:10.1016/J.JACC.2016.11.008
15. Malawer M, Bickels J, Sugarbaker P. *Below-knee amputation*. In: *Musculoskeletal Cancer Surgery*. Springer; 2004:363-369. doi:10.1007/0-306-48407-2_23
16. Sugarbaker P, Bickels J, Malawer M. *Above-knee amputation*. In: *Musculoskeletal Cancer Surgery*. Springer; 2004:351-362. doi:10.1007/0-306-48407-2_22
17. Sugarbaker P, Malawer M. Hip disarticulation. In: *Musculoskeletal Cancer Surgery*. Springer; 2004:337-349. doi:10.1007/0-306-48407-2_21
18. Kwah LK, Webb MT, Goh L, Harvey LA. Rigid dressings versus soft dressings for transtibial amputations. *Cochrane Database Syst Rev*. 2019;6(6):CD012427. doi:10.1002/14651858.CD012427.pub2
19. Sumpio B, Shine SR, Mahler D, Sumpio BE. A comparison of immediate postoperative rigid and soft dressings for below-knee amputations. *Ann Vasc Surg*. 2013;27(6):774-780. doi:10.1016/j.avsg.2013.03.007
20. Aulivola B, Hile CN, Hamdan AD, et al. Major lower extremity amputation: outcome of a modern series. *Arch Surg*. 2004;139(4):395-399. doi:10.1001/archsurg.139.4.395
21. Nehler MR, Coll JR, Hiatt WR, et al. Functional outcome in a contemporary series of major lower extremity amputations. *J Vasc Surg*. 2003;38(1):7-14. doi:10.1016/S0741-5214(03)00092-2
22. MacCallum KP, Yau P, Phair J, Lipsitz EC, Scher LA, Garg K. Ambulatory status following major lower extremity amputation. *Ann Vasc Surg*. 2021;71:331-337. doi:10.1016/j.avsg.2020.07.038
23. Gabel J, Jabo B, Patel S, et al. Analysis of patients undergoing major lower extremity amputation in the Vascular Quality Initiative. *Ann Vasc Surg*. 2018;46:75-82. doi:10.1016/j.avsg.2017.07.034
24. Arya S, Khakharia A, Binney ZO, et al. Association of statin dose with amputation and survival in patients with peripheral artery disease. *Circulation*. 2018;137(14):1435-1446. doi:10.1161/CIRCULATIONAHA.117.032361

Part 7

Operative Techniques in Trauma and Critical Care

SECTION IV: THORACIC TRAUMATIC INJURIES

SECTION V: INJURY TO THE NECK

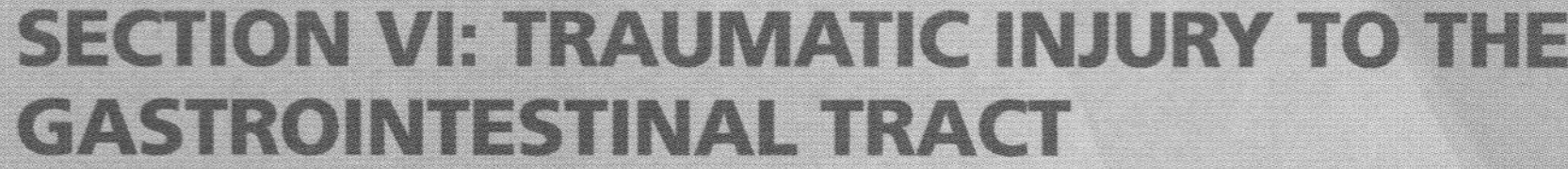

SECTION VI: TRAUMATIC INJURY TO THE GASTROINTESTINAL TRACT

SECTION VII: TRAUMATIC INJURY TO THE DUODENUM AND PANCREAS

SECTION VIII: TRAUMATIC INJURY TO THE SPLEEN AND LIVER

SECTION IX: TRAUMATIC INJURY TO THE GENITOURINARY TRACT

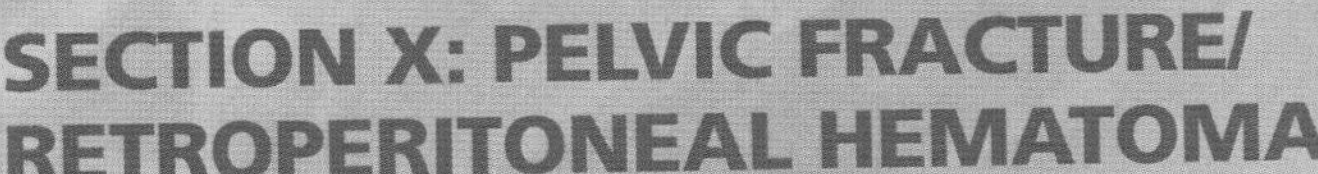

SECTION X: PELVIC FRACTURE/ RETROPERITONEAL HEMATOMA

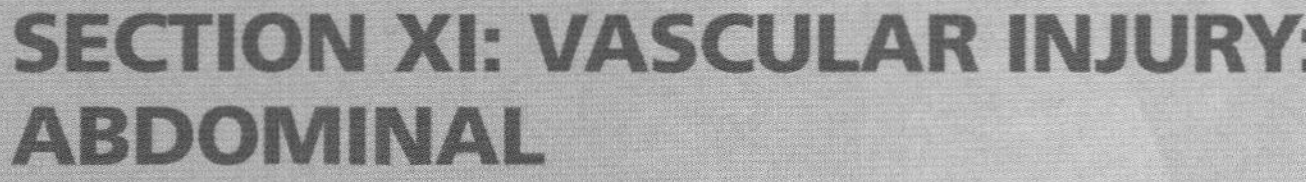

SECTION XI: VASCULAR INJURY: ABDOMINAL

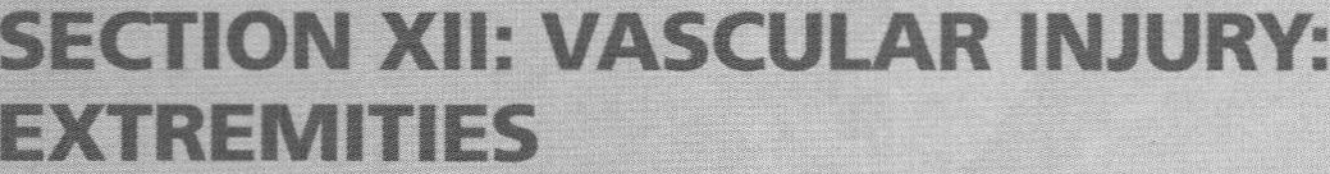

SECTION XII: VASCULAR INJURY: EXTREMITIES

SECTION XIII: TRAUMA IN PREGNANCY

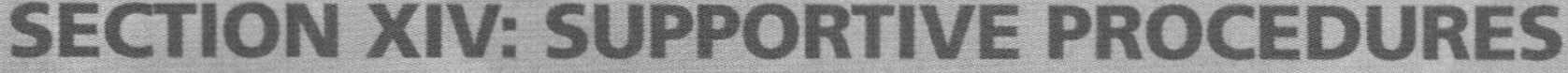

SECTION XIV: SUPPORTIVE PROCEDURES

Chapter 1 Burn Surgery: Escharotomy, Excision, and Split-Thickness Skin Grafting

Natalie J. Hodges and Sharmila Dissanaike

DEFINITION

- Burns are defined as injury to skin and subcutaneous structures from thermal energy, usually in the form of flame, scald, or steam. Chemicals, extremes of cold, and friction can result in injuries that require similar treatment, and they are often grouped alongside thermal burns.
- Classically, burns are categorized by depth: first degree are superficial burns, second degree are indeterminate, and third degree are considered full-thickness burns. Many burn centers further delineate second-degree burns into superficial partial thickness and deep partial thickness.
- A broad range of clinical strategies exist for the resuscitation, surgical management, and reconstruction of burn injuries.

DIFFERENTIAL DIAGNOSIS

- Certain desquamating skin conditions such as bullous pemphigoid, staphylococcal scalded skin syndrome, and toxic epidermal necrolysis can mimic the appearance of burns, although these are usually easily distinguished from the patient's clinical history.

PATIENT HISTORY AND PHYSICAL FINDINGS

- The incidence of burns has declined over the past century, with the implementation of improved fire safety measures in residences and workplaces.
- Burns can occur following exposure to both dry (eg, flame, explosion, heating element) and wet heat (eg, hot liquids), electricity, chemicals, and radiation.
- Physical examination is critically important to the identification and management of burn injuries. Large burns requiring resuscitation may have significant changes in vital signs or laboratory studies; however, smaller burns that still require clinical and possibly operative management most commonly have no noticeable physiologic changes.
- Classification and management of burn injuries is determined by clinical examination. Burn injuries can be classified as first degree when only the superficial epidermis is injured; these wounds are typically painful to touch, erythematous, and may be mildly edematous. Superficial partial-thickness burns typically are painful to touch with sloughing of the epidermis; they are erythematous and blanch and have a moist appearance. Deep partial-thickness burns exist closer on the spectrum to full-thickness burns but are still sensate and painful. They are either deep red or pale in color, without blanching, and tend to have a drier appearance than superficial partial-thickness burns. Full-thickness burns are not painful, are typically white in color, may have a dark leathery eschar and sloughing of skin, and are generally dry in appearance.
- Magnitude of injury is estimated by calculating the total body surface area (TBSA) involved in the burn. There are several methods to accomplish this; most commonly used are the rule of 9s, or the palmar method (**FIGURES 1** and **2**).
- For larger burns (in adults, >10% TBSA; in pediatrics, >1% TBSA; ideally managed at verified burn centers), the Lund-Browder chart is used to perform a more precise calculation of burn size, since this impacts resuscitation as well as surgical planning.
- It is important to note that burns may progress to become deeper over time, so ongoing clinical evaluation and expert reassessment is paramount.

IMAGING AND OTHER DIAGNOSTIC STUDIES

- Most burn injuries do not require imaging or diagnostic studies, unless associated with traumatic injury; management is based solely upon clinical examination. Concomitant inhalation injury is often diagnosed using fiberoptic flexible bronchoscopy.
- Chest radiography is performed broadly as an initial study in traumatically injured patients. Intubated burned patients require chest x-rays to confirm endotracheal tube placement, and in patients with suspected inhalation injury or large body surface area burns, plain films can establish a baseline prior to resuscitation. In patients with other associated traumatic chest injuries (eg, rib fractures or pneumothoraces), radiographs can be useful in determining need for further interventions (eg, thoracostomy, bronchoscopy). Burns sustained in significant blunt trauma (eg, motor vehicle collision, explosions) warrant standard trauma imaging via computed tomography scan to evaluate for internal organ injury.
- In the case of flash burns, chemical splash burns, or any injury where the face may be involved, it is appropriate to perform a Wood lamp examination to evaluate for corneal abrasions. This acts as a screening tool to identify burns requiring more formal ophthalmologic evaluation and treatment.
- Young children with burn injuries present a unique challenge, and a thorough assessment should include consideration of the possibility of nonaccidental trauma. If there is potential for abusive injury, then a full skeletal survey is usually performed.

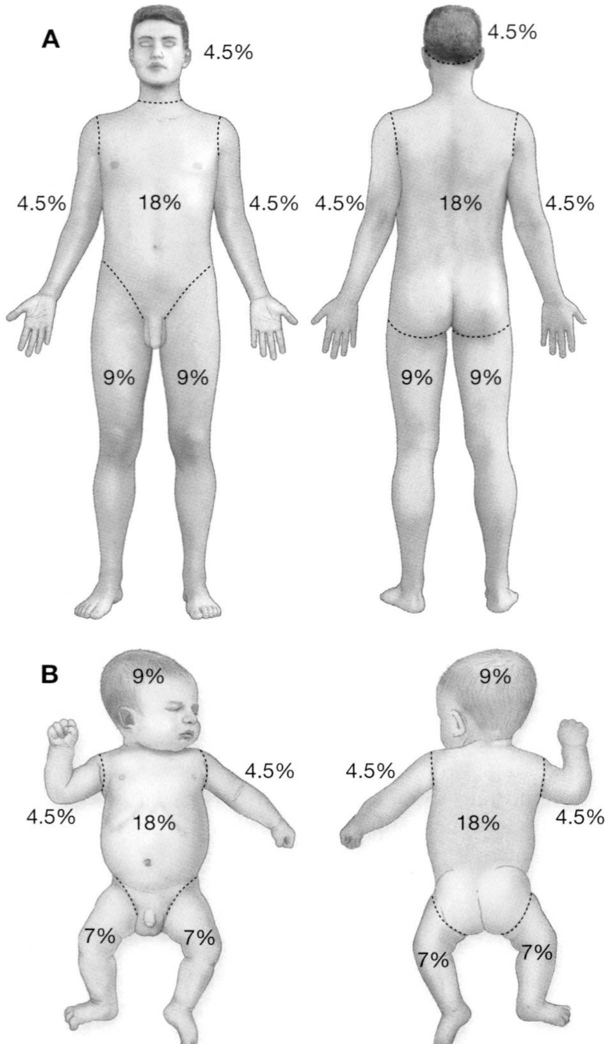

FIGURE 1 • Rule of 9's for estimation of burn size in children and adults.

SURGICAL MANAGEMENT

- Full-thickness burns will nearly all require surgical management. Nonoperative management by allowing natural scarring may be an option in burns smaller than a few centimeters in noncosmetic, nonfunctional areas of the body such as the back and buttocks. There are also reports of successful management of full-thickness small burns with enzymatic debridement; however, operative excision remains the standard of care. Staged closure, where a biologic or synthetic scaffold is used after excision, prior to closure with split-thickness skin graft, is often used in reconstructing deep full-thickness burns and may provide improved function and cosmesis over immediate skin grafting.
- Indeterminate-thickness burns (second degree), as their name suggests, may be managed using topical agents, enzymatic debridement, or a variety of surgical options. Often an initial trial of nonoperative management with topical wound care may be performed, to determine whether operative excision will be necessary.

Preoperative Planning

- Depending on patient stability, surgeon preference, and institutional resources, complete excision of the entire burn with immediate skin grafting may be performed in one operation in the immediate post-burn period, even in large burns; more commonly, however, different areas may be operated on in sequence over a number of operations spread over days and weeks.
- Where possible, tourniquets should be used to minimize blood loss.
- Hypothermia is a major challenge in burn surgery, and ambient room temperature, external warming devices, fluid

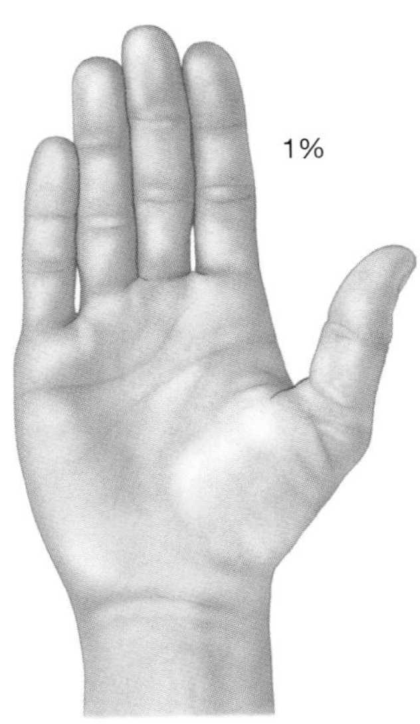

FIGURE 2 ● Palmar method of burn estimation, where the surface area of the patient's palm = 1% TBSA.

warmers, and internal warming catheters should all be considered to prevent hypothermia, which in turn can help prevent coagulopathy from developing during the operation, which may lead to increase blood loss.

- Proposed excision site and donor site(s) must be planned and marked prior to proceeding to the operating room, as well as proposed mesh ratio. Mesh ratio is influenced by burn size, donor site availability, and graft site, with the aim being to reduce time to closure of all affected skin areas while maximizing long-term cosmesis and functional outcome.
- As many burned patients requiring operative intervention are critically ill, hemodynamic and respiratory status should be optimized prior to surgery.

Positioning

- The goal of positioning in burn surgery should be to provide access to all planned operative sites without excessive strain on the patient or operating team. To this end, specially designed operating rooms with lifts and harnesses to safely elevate limbs are very helpful, although not essential.

ESCHAROTOMY

- Circumferential extremity burns can cause constriction and restrict perfusion, requiring escharotomy. Deeper burns may even cause compartment syndrome, requiring fasciotomy. It is crucial that these conditions are identified early, and surgical release performed immediately, in order to preserve function of the extremity.
- In similar fashion, deep circumferential burns of the thorax and abdomen can restrict ventilation, requiring escharotomy release.
- Since large burns require large-volume resuscitation, abdominal compartment syndrome can also result, leading to severe morbidity if untreated. With newer resuscitation protocols this complication has become less common; however, it should remain a consideration in any patient who has a tense, distended abdomen, elevated peak pressures on the ventilator, reduced urine output, and low blood pressure.
- Escharotomy is classically performed using two incisions along medial and lateral aspects of the injured limb, or torso. However, since these are usually only performed on full-thickness burns, which will require complete excision anyway, the exact location of the incision becomes less important. Therefore, it is wise to avoid areas directly over blood vessels (medial and lateral aspects of the fingers, for example, or directly over the saphenous vein in the leg) and instead perform the releasing incision in the area of maximal skin tension (**FIGURE 3**).

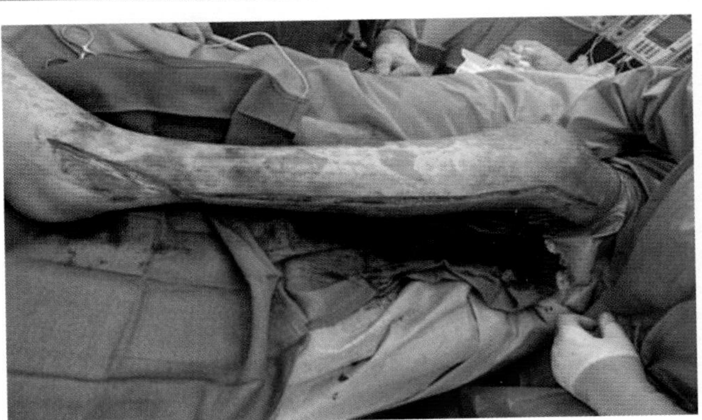

FIGURE 3 ● Escharotomies performed on a deep circumferential lower extremity burn.

EXCISION AND GRAFTING

- In order to achieve the best outcomes, excision and grafting should be performed as soon as possible after injury. While traditional practice has been to perform the first excision and grafting after resuscitation is completed yet within 5 to 7 days of injury, superior results can be obtained by performing excision during the resuscitative period. Since peripheral vasoconstriction is maximal in the first 24 hours after injury, this allows for less blood loss during operation.
- The most common form of excision is tangential excision, which is performed with a flat, sharp blade (eg, Weck or Watson). All burned tissue should be excised, including any areas of subcutaneous fat with thrombosed blood vessels (**FIGURES 4** and **5**).
- For deeper burns, it may be necessary to excise tissue down to fascia, termed fascial excision. This can be performed sharply with regular scalpels or electrocautery.
- Hemostasis should be achieved with nonadherent dressings soaked in epinephrine solution, and then covered with soaked laparotomy pads. Bleeding not controlled by this

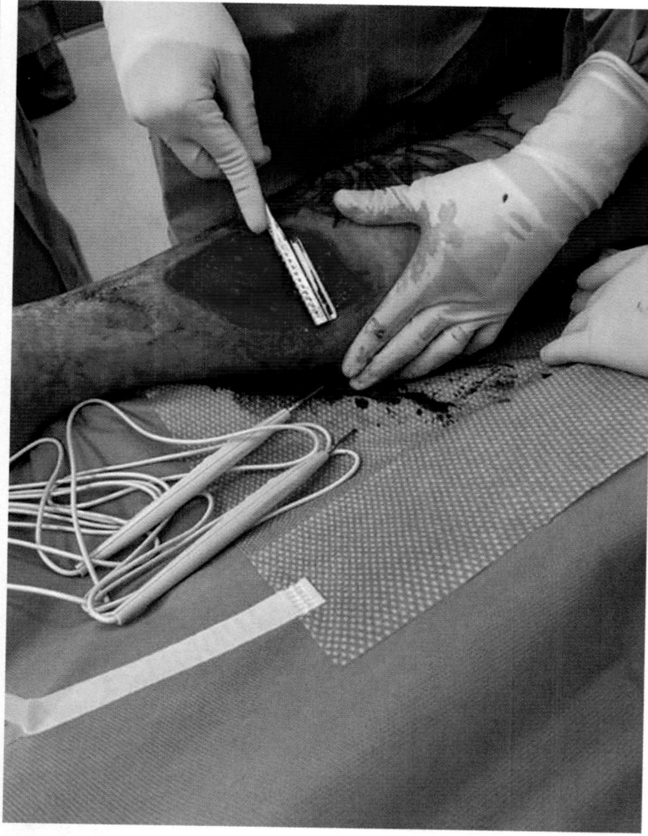

FIGURE 4 ● Sharp excision of burned tissue using a Weck Blade to reveal healthy bleeding tissue.

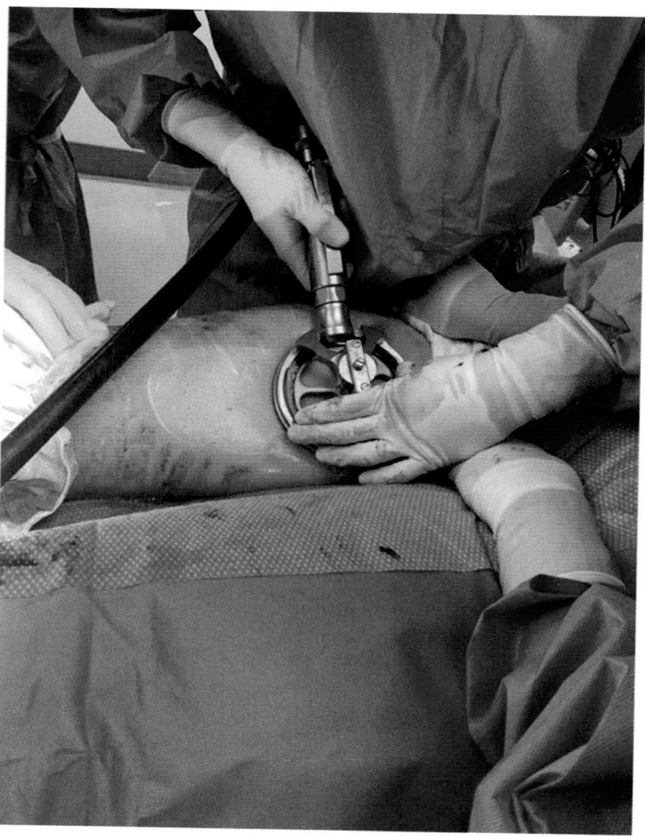

FIGURE 6 ● Use of the Amalgatome to harvest donor skin for split-thickness skin grafting.

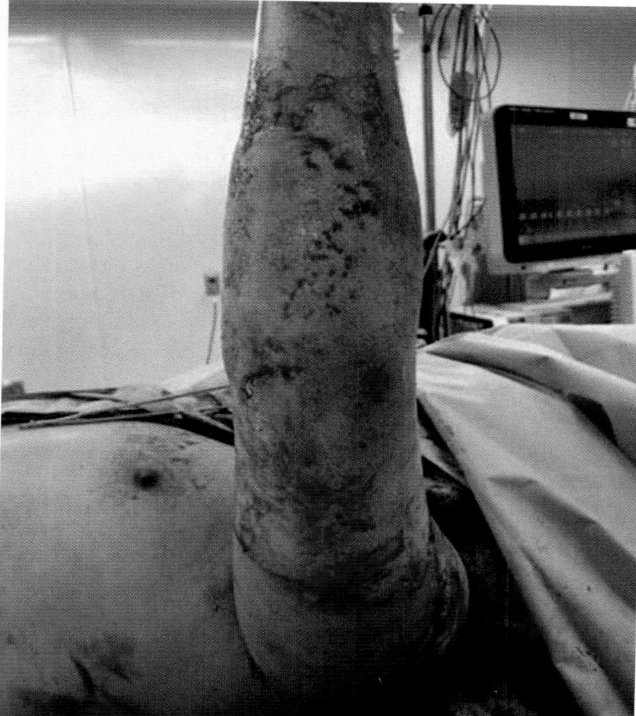

FIGURE 5 ● Arm after tangential excision; note the white appearance of the dermis with pinpoint bleeding.

dressing should be managed with electrocautery or suture ligation as required. Hemostasis is critically important to successful skin grafting, since the development of a hematoma will prevent imbibition and adherence of the skin graft, a common cause of early graft failure.

- The skin graft is harvested using a dermatome (**FIGURE 6**). Split-thickness skin grafts are usually taken at a depth between 8 and 18/1000 of an inch, with thinner grafts providing superior cosmetic outcomes, while thicker grafts are easier to handle and tend to be more durable.
- Harvested skin is then meshed in an appropriate ratio (**FIGURES 7** and **8**). Smaller ratios (1:1) provide superior cosmetic outcome; however, larger ratios (2:1, 3:1, and greater) allow coverage of a larger surface area using less donor skin. In addition to expanding the coverage area, meshing allows for evacuation of blood and serous fluid that may accumulate in the postoperative period, preventing graft imbibition and inosculation.
- Hemostasis is obtained at the graft site, and a fibrin glue solution is applied prior to the skin graft application. The skin graft is then sutured or stapled in place (**FIGURE 9**) prior to application of a nonadherent dressing (eg, petroleum or antibiotic-impregnated gauze) followed by a gauze wrap and compression bandage. Vacuum-assisted closure may also be used as a dressing.
- Staged closure may be used for several reasons. In larger burns, lack of availability of donor sites may require temporary coverage be performed. For deeper burns, the addition

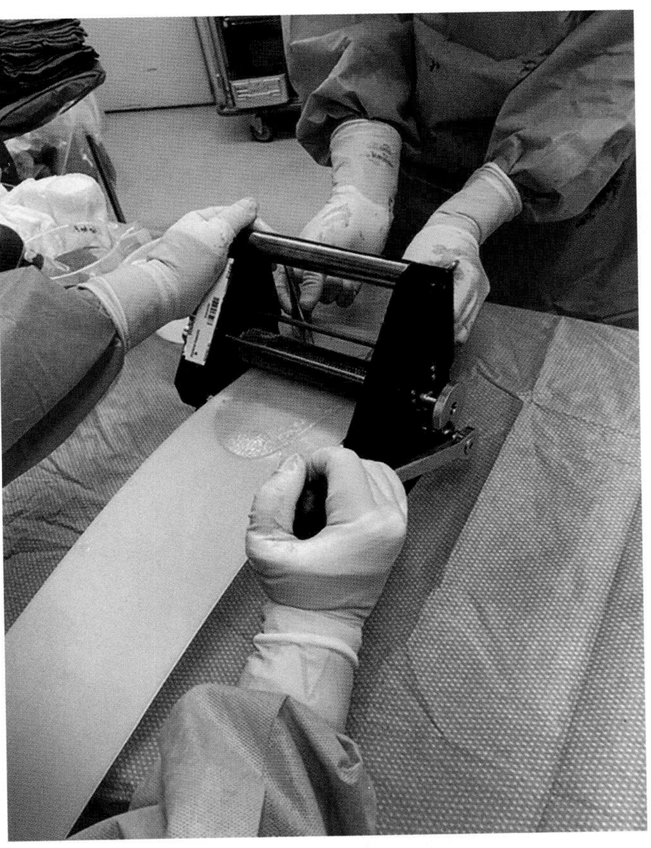

FIGURE 7 • Skin being placed through the mesher.

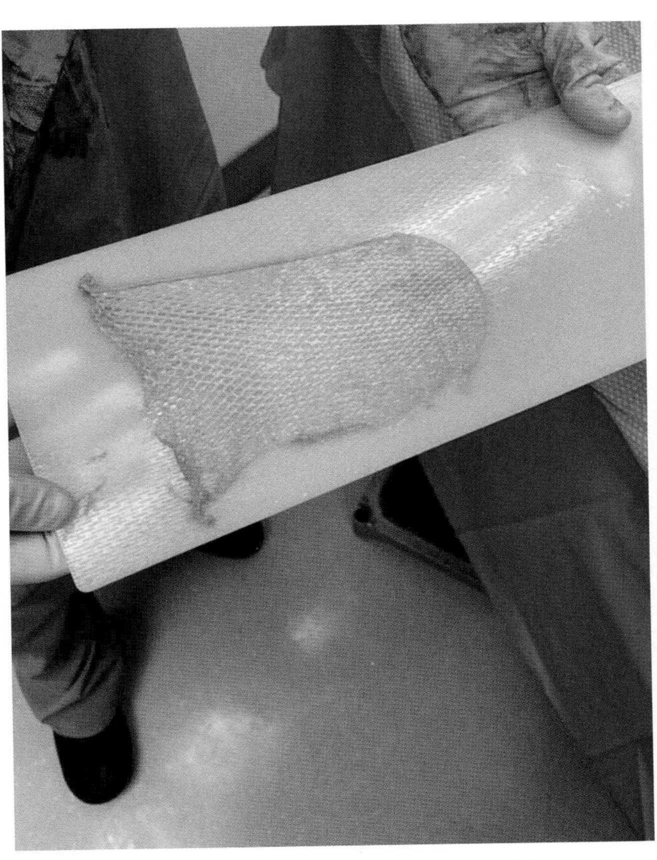

FIGURE 8 • Skin meshed in 2:1 ratio with dermal side exposed; this will be placed directly upon the wound bed.

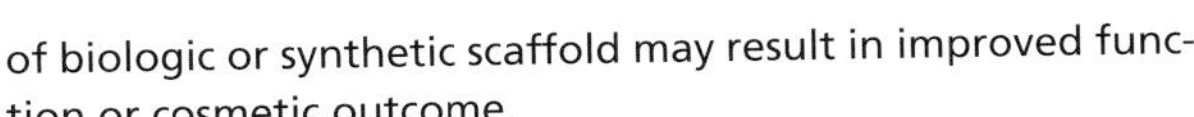

of biologic or synthetic scaffold may result in improved function or cosmetic outcome.

- There are several temporary coverage options for the wound bed of burns that have been excised, yet may not be ready for permanent closure, for a variety of reasons. Traditional options include xenograft, historically harvested porcine skin, and more recently tilapia skin, or allograft from donated cadaveric excision. These provide temporary biologic coverage of the wound bed without long-term integration.
- Biologic, synthetic, and hybrid products have been commercially developed (Acell, Primatrix, Integra, Novasorb BTM) to provide coverage for burns and wounds, while also integrating into the wound bed, providing a scaffolding for future skin grafts, and promoting faster wound healing. Typically, skin grafting is performed 2 to 3 weeks after application of these matrices, with timing and dressings individualized to each product.
- Cultured autograft, where a patient's own skin cells are grown in a laboratory and made available for subsequent grafting (Epicel) is an option in very large burns without adequate donor skin. Cultured cells are applied to excised wound beds in conjunction with widely meshed autograft (typically 1:4) to provide the best results.

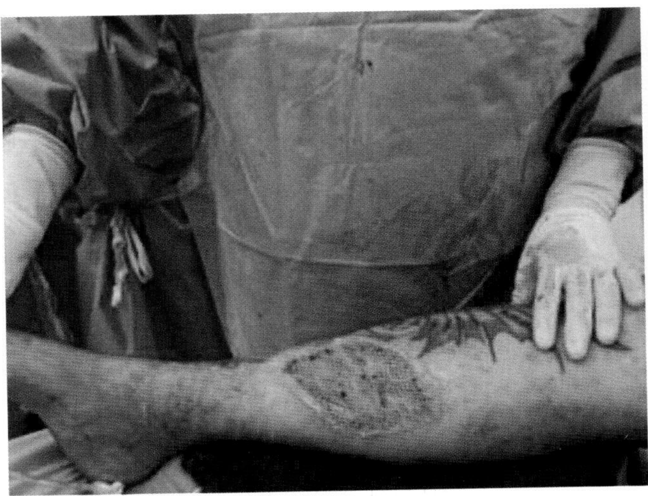

FIGURE 9 • Stapled skin graft in place on wound bed.

- RECELL is a commercially available platform that allows isolation of skin cells from a small skin sample, which is immersed in an enzyme solution to produce Spray-On Skin Cells. This technique is gaining popularity in burn centers and can reduce donor site burden by as much as 30%.

PEARLS AND PITFALLS

- Early excision and grafting of burns, along with adequate resuscitation, are the most important factors for successful short- and long-term outcome after burn injury.
- Inadequate hemostasis and dressings that allow shear forces on the graft in the early perioperative period are common reasons for graft failure.
- Incomplete debridement of all burned tissue, resulting in inadequate excision of the graft bed, is probably the most common reason for lack of successful graft take.

POSTOPERATIVE CARE

- Autologous split-thickness skin grafts are usually evaluated with takedown of dressings on postoperative day 3 to 5. Successful graft take is defined as viable, living skin tightly adhered to the underlying wound bed (**FIGURE 10**).
- Traditionally patients were immobilized during the immediate postoperative period; however, with use of adhesive glues, staples, and securely applied dressings to prevent graft shear, early mobility after surgery is now encouraged.
- Burn care is a multidisciplinary specialty, requiring active participation from surgeons, nurses, therapists, pharmacists, dieticians, psychologists, and others to assure the best outcome.

Complications

- Hemorrhage
  - Excision of large areas of skin rapidly often results in significant bleeding from capillaries and small vessels. The use of tourniquets over extremities during the excision phase is crucial to minimize unnecessary blood loss. The application of epinephrine-soaked gauze to the raw wound surface immediately after excision can also significantly reduce blood loss. For excisions of large areas, especially torso burns that cannot be controlled with tourniquet, preparations for blood transfusion during the operation should be made. In addition to hemorrhage resulting in shock and transfusion requirement from the initial debridement, later hematoma formation under the newly applied skin graft, as a result of inadequate hemostasis prior to graft application, will result in failure of graft take in that region.
- Infection
  - As burn patients have lost their primary immunologic barrier due to violation of the integument, they are at high risk of infectious complications. Infection can occur in the donor or recipient site.
- Graft failure
  - Early sources of graft failure include seroma or hematoma formation ("floated graft"), shear (caused by movement of the graft site causing dissociation), failure of neovascularization due to inadequate excision of all devitalized tissue, and infection.

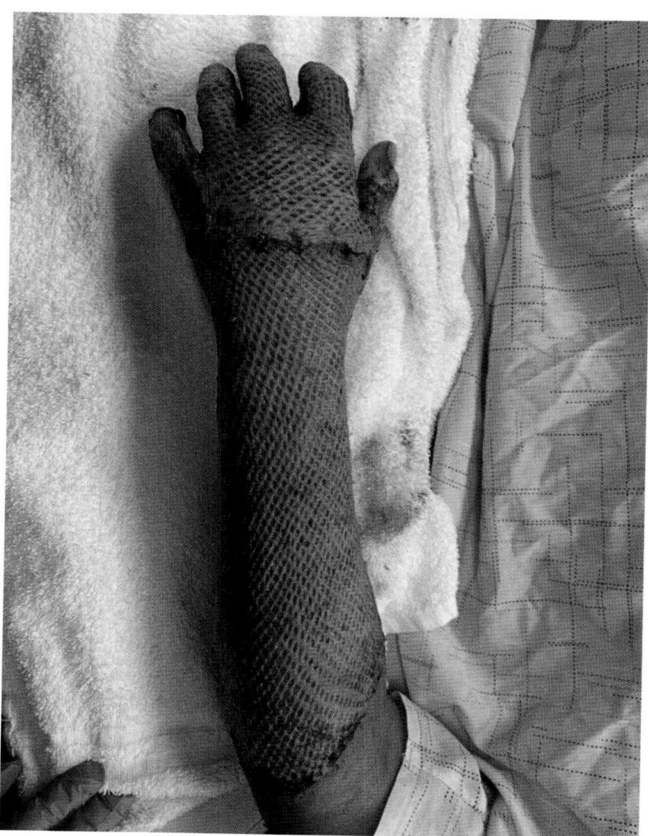

FIGURE 10 ● Split-thickness skin graft after dressing takedown on postoperative day 3, showing excellent take.

SUGGESTED READINGS

1. American Burn Association. *Burn Incidence Fact Sheet*. American Burn Association; 2017 https://ameriburn.org/who-we-are/media/burn-incidence-fact-sheet/
2. Engrav LH, Heimbach DM, Reus JL, Harnar TJ, Marvin JA. Early excision and grafting vs. nonoperative treatment of burns of indeterminant depth: a randomized prospective study. *J Trauma*. 1983;23(11):1001-1004.
3. Herndon DN. *Total Burn Care*. Elsevier; 2018.
4. Prohaska J, Cook C. *Skin grafting*. [Updated 2020 Sep 11]. In: *StatPearls* [Internet]. StatPearls Publishing; 2021. Available from: https://www.ncbi.nlm.nih.gov/books/NBK532874/

Chapter 2 Frostbite and Hypothermia: Surgical Management

Natalie J. Hodges and Sharmila Dissanaike

DEFINITION

- Frostbite is defined as an integument injury secondary to exposure to cold elements, typically lower than freezing, and can be delineated into first through fourth degree dependent upon depth and degree of tissue destruction.
- Hypothermia is defined as body temperature below normal, typically due to exposure to cold elements or environment.

DIFFERENTIAL DIAGNOSIS

- Frostnip refers to injuries secondary to exposure to cold elements related to vasoconstriction, which resolves completely without tissue destruction, following rewarming.
- Pernio is an inflammatory skin injury related to cold exposure above the freezing point that may be idiopathic or secondary to underlying cryoglobulinemia or connective tissue disease.
- Raynaud phenomenon causes vasoconstriction that can be triggered by cold temperature exposure, among other factors.
- Peripheral vascular disease can cause vasoconstriction and poor blood flow distally in extremities, mimicking frostbite.
- Cold-related tissue injury exists on a spectrum, like all thermal integument injuries. It can be graded as first through fourth degree depending on the degree of tissue injury. First-degree injuries have mild erythema and edema and may desquamate late in the injury course. Second-degree frostbite displays more erythema, significant edema, and vesicles in the acute phase, with desquamation and eschar in the late phase. Third-degree frostbite has hemorrhagic blisters in the early phase, progressing to blue/gray discoloration in the late phase (**FIGURE 1**). Finally, fourth-degree frostbite starts with a mottled initial appearance that progresses to dry, black mummified appearance, similar to dry gangrene (**FIGURE 2**).

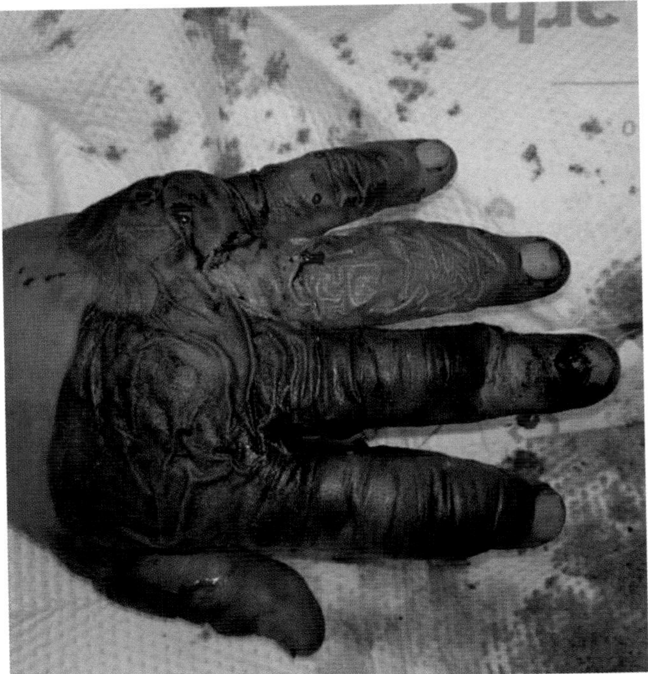

FIGURE 1 ● An example of early third-degree frostbite, prior to eventual desquamation and unroofing of blisters. This wound ultimately required split thickness skin grafting for coverage.

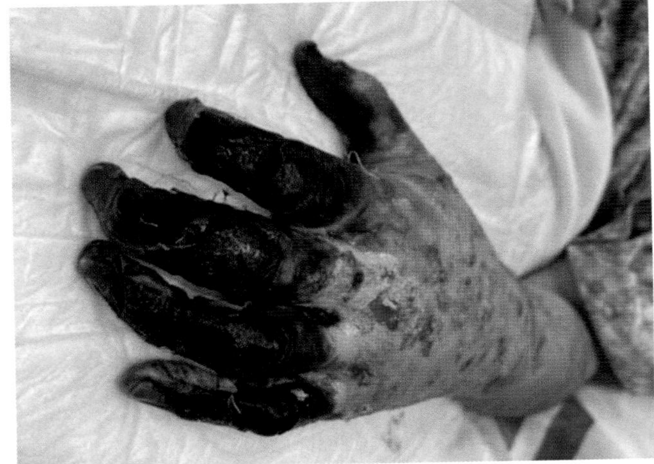

FIGURE 2 ● An example of fourth-degree frostbite, several weeks post injury. Note that while the distal tissue is clearly nonviable, it is not grossly infected and so not debrided.

PATIENT HISTORY AND PHYSICAL FINDINGS

- Prolonged exposure to cold environments, or brief exposure to extreme cold.
- Cold injuries can occur in concert with trauma or physiologic derangements related to the exposure (eg, dehydration and metabolic derangements in stranded hikers).

IMAGING AND OTHER DIAGNOSTIC STUDIES

- Diagnosis of cold-related tissue injuries is largely clinical. Diagnostic radiology in patients with unclear or confirmed history of trauma can be helpful.
- Imaging can guide therapy in deep injuries, for which multiple modalities have been investigated. Angiography and technecium-99 (99Tc) triple-phase bone scanning give the best prognostic information related to amputation and limb viability.
- Magnetic resonance angiography (MRA) may be superior to 99Tc as it allows finer delineation between viable and nonviable tissues and is more easily accessible in most hospitals.

- Either intravenous prostacyclin or tissue plasminogen activator (TPA), or a combination of the two should be considered for use in patients with severe frostbite and high risk of tissue loss; if used, it should be administered within 24 hours of injury.

SURGICAL MANAGEMENT

- It is important that rewarmed tissue is not reexposed to cold, since this can worsen injury. Therefore, active rewarming should only be initiated once the patient has arrived at the site of definitive care. Thawing should not be attempted until the victim can be kept warm and dry throughout the duration of their treatment.
- Rewarming of the affected extremity is critically important to stop the process of frostbite. This is ideally done in a 38-40 °C water bath, to quickly restore blood flow to tissues synergistically with rising metabolic rate.
- Within 24 hours of injury, administration of intravenous TPA) may be useful in salvaging vascular flow and maximizing retained tissue.
- Contrary to management of other thermal injuries, frostbite mandates delayed management. Optimally, cold-related injuries should be managed with supportive care—acutely with rewarming and resuscitation and chronically with pain control and wound care. Delayed surgical intervention allows for maximal post injury healing, neoinnervation, and neovascularization, therefore maximizing salvaged tissue. Amputation or excision should therefore be delayed as long as possible, as ongoing neovascularization can maximize retained tissue and function.
- Debridement of frostbite wounds is not typically indicated unless wounds become infected, in which only infected tissue should be debrided.

Preoperative Planning

Positioning

- Access to affected extremity, including circumferential preparation up to the level of the joint above what is affected by injury, is required for positioning. This may require adjuncts in the operating room such as foam supplements to provide adequate access to extremities needing excision or amputation.

TECHNIQUES

EXCISION

- Sharp excision to the most distal viable area should be undertaken at the latest possible time. This allows for maximal tissue salvage and neovascularization (**FIGURE 3**).
- Vascular supply to the remaining extremity or excised area should be ensured, and adequate coverage should be planned, whether by flap coverage, biologic coverage, skin graft, or other means.

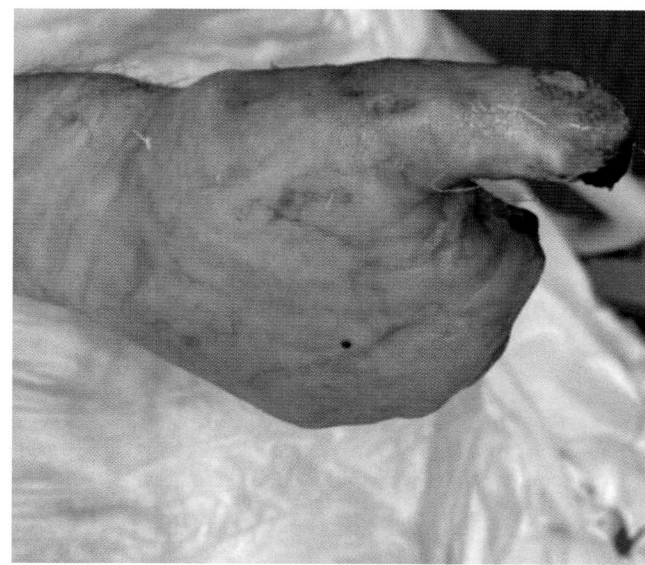

FIGURE 3 ● The same extremity after amputation with maximized tissue retention and satisfactory wound healing.

PEARLS AND PITFALLS

- Early excision or amputation of cold-related injuries is associated with unnecessary tissue loss. Surgical intervention should be delayed until clear demarcation of viable and nonviable tissue has occurred.
- Preoperative vascular evaluation by way of clinical examination and either CT angiogram or formal angiography should be performed to ensure wound healing and minimize tissue excision.
- Infection in cold-injured tissue mandates excision or amputation of the injured tissue, but this should be limited as much as possible to only grossly infected tissue.

POSTOPERATIVE CARE

- Wounds should be dressed in warm moist gauze initially to promote neovascularization and limit tissue dehydration. Infected wounds should be dressed in a debriding dressing such as a wet to dry dressing. Enzymatic or biologic dressings have not been shown to improve cold injury outcomes.
- Similar themes exist to burn injuries to cold injuries—early involvement of a multidisciplinary team to optimize wound care, therapy, and nutrition is critical to overall outcomes.

COMPLICATIONS

- Infection of cold injury wounds is highly prevalent secondary to compromised lymph and vascular flow. Infection of cold injury wounds is a challenging scenario, as it may force excision of otherwise viable tissue.
- Both acutely and chronically, pain is a significant cause of morbidity in the cold-injured patient population. Management with a multimodal regimen is critically important.
- Overaggressive attempts to rewarm cold-injured extremities (that have reduced sensation) can result in secondary burns, from too close/prolonged exposure to a heater, or scalding water. This increases tissue damage and often results in need for more extensive operation.

SUGGESTED READINGS

1. McIntosh SE, Freer L, Grissom CK, et al. Wilderness medical society clinical practice guidelines for the prevention and treatment of frostbite: 2019 update. *Wilderness Environ Med*. 2019;30(4S):S19-S32. doi: 10.1016/j.wem.2019.05.002. Epub 2019 Jul 17. PMID: 31326282.
2. Millet JD, Brown RK, Levi B, et al. Frostbite: spectrum of imaging findings and guidelines for management. *Radiographics*. 2016;36(7):2154-2169. doi: 10.1148/rg.2016160045. Epub 2016 Aug 5. PMID: 27494386; PMCID: PMC5131839.
3. Petrone P, Kuncir EJ, Asensio JA. Surgical management and strategies in the treatment of hypothermia and cold injury. *Emerg Med Clin North Am*. 2003;21(4):1165-1178. doi: 10.1016/s0733-8627(03)00074-9. PMID: 14708823.
4. Valnicek SM, Chasmar LR, Clapson JB. Frostbite in the prairies: a 12-year review. *Plast Reconstr Surg*. 1993;92(4):633-641. doi: 10.1097/00006534-199309001-00012. PMID: 8356126.
5. Verma P. Topical nitroglycerine in perniosis/chilblains. *Skinmed*. 2015;13(3):176-177. PMID: 26380502.

Chapter 3 Electrical Burns

Natalie J. Hodges and Sharmila Dissanaike

DEFINITION

- Injuries sustained to the skin, integument, and underlying tissues due to the transmission of electric current across a voltage differential.

DIFFERENTIAL DIAGNOSIS

- Electric current can spark fire, resulting in thermal injury rather than true electric injury. Since the timing of treatment, and potential for deep tissue injury, varies significantly between these two mechanisms, they are important to distinguish. They can also occur concurrently.

PATIENT HISTORY AND PHYSICAL FINDINGS

- It is important to determine whether current traveled through the body simply sparked at the source of contact or caused a thermal fire and the patient was exposed to flame.
- Distinguishing between high-voltage (>400 V) and low-voltage injury is crucial. The former is usually limited to workplace injuries, while the latter is common in household exposure. The potential for cardiac arrhythmia, spinal fracture, deep tissue, and ophthalmic injury is usually limited to high-voltage injury.
- Children may present with injury to the mouth from chewing on electric cords; this is typically a small, deep burn at the oral commissure.
- Electric burns commonly cause small, deep burns on the surface (**FIGURE 1**).

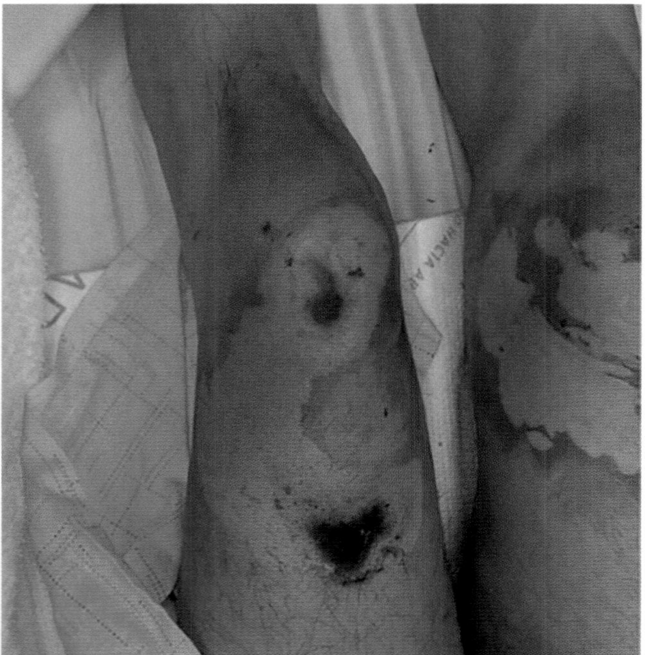

FIGURE 1 ● Deep partial and full-thickness electrical burns to the lower extremities.

- Electrical injuries are unique to burn injuries in that actual injury burden is far greater than what can be visually examined, due to current running through deeper tissues with relatively little surface changes.
- Nerves are particularly susceptible to electric current, so patients may present with weakness, paresthesia, and paralysis as a result. A thorough neurologic examination of all affected areas is essential. Entry and exit wounds can help ascertain the direction of current flow, which in turn can guide the areas to focus on most closely.
- High-ampere current can cause severe muscle edema and necrosis, resulting in compartment syndrome. This is a surgical emergency, so it is imperative that it is recognized quickly. A tense, tight, and swollen muscle compartment with pain on passive stretch is the hallmark of a compartment syndrome, and physical examination should be directed to search for these findings. Compartment syndrome of the arm, leg, hand, or foot may occur, based on the body part that was in closest contact with the electric current. If diagnosed, immediate fasciotomy is required. Abdominal compartment syndrome can also occur in major electric injuries; however, it is usually a result of large volume fluid resuscitation rather than the electricity itself.
- If compartment syndrome is not recognized, or with very high-voltage current (>10,000 V), instant necrosis and death of muscles, nerves, and vessels can occur, resulting in fixed contractures—a "claw hand," for example. Unfortunately, this is an indication that the limb is no longer viable, and immediate amputation can help reduce the systemic effects.
- Laboratory investigations for markers of muscle breakdown, such as serum potassium, creatinine kinase, and myoglobin should be measured, as well as markers of renal function such as serum creatinine. If elevated, these should be followed over time as significant rhabdomyolysis can occur in the days following electric injury.

IMAGING AND OTHER DIAGNOSTIC STUDIES

- Electrocardiogram should be obtained on all electric injuries. Patients who sustain high-voltage injuries should be placed on continuous telemetry for the first 24 hours.
- High-voltage injuries may cause fractures of the spine, so a physical examination for tenderness along the bony spine should be performed, and radiographs obtained.
- High-voltage injuries may cause premature development of cataracts; therefore, a formal ophthalmologic examination should be performed soon after injury to obtain a baseline assessment. This is particularly important for work-related injuries, to ensure patients are eligible for coverage of subsequent costs of medical treatment should this occur.
- High-voltage injuries can also cause cognitive impairment, both obvious and subtle. Baseline cognitive assessment is recommended, as cognitive therapy may be beneficial. Cognitive deficits may take up to a year to resolve, even with initial brain rest and subsequent cognitive therapy with trained speech and language pathologists.

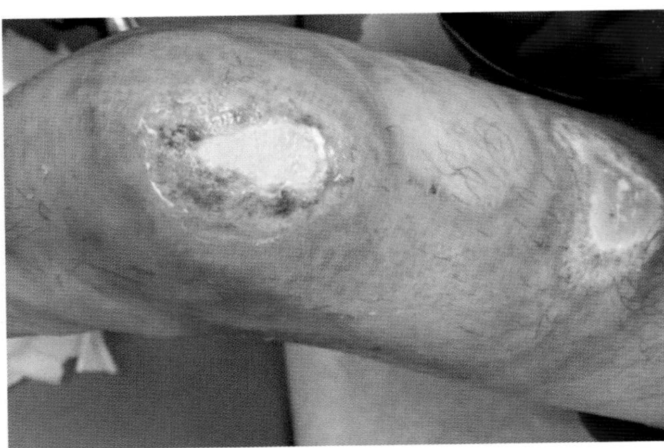

FIGURE 2 ● The same electric burns as in Figure 1, after resuscitation, and a period of wound care. Clear progression of the electric injury can be seen. The deeper areas in the center (white) required excision and split thickness skin graft, while the more superficial burns surrounding them (pink) healed with wound care alone.

SURGICAL MANAGEMENT

- Electric injuries may take up to 2 weeks to fully evolve; therefore, surgery is usually deferred until that time (**FIGURE 2**). However, in cases of acute compartment syndrome, or complete tissue necrosis, immediate decompression and excision, including amputation, may be necessary to save the patient's life or preserve as much function as possible.

PREOPERATIVE PLANNING

- Fluid resuscitation is critically important and typically requires larger volumes in electrically injured patients. While traditional resuscitation protocols relied on crystalloids such as lactated Ringer, many burn centers now use colloid resuscitation such as 5% albumin or even fresh frozen plasma relatively early in the resuscitation of larger burns, including electric injuries.
- Electric injuries often occur in people employed in occupations that require significant manual labor and dexterity, so functional outcome should be carefully considered in electrical burns. Operative technique used will depend on the type and location of the electric injury and can often require complex reconstructive measures and prolonged postoperative occupational and physical therapy. This is particularly true of burns to the oral commissures and hands (**FIGURE 3**).
- Patients requiring fasciotomy for compartment syndrome will often require multiple operations for re-evaluation of tissue viability, and debridement of necrotic tissue as the injury progresses, prior to final reconstruction.
- When amputation is required, it should be performed as distal as possible in order to preserve maximal function. Damage to nerves that typically occurs with electric injury can unfortunately reduce the opportunity for nerve reimplantation and advanced bioprosthetics.
- Since electric injuries are often deeper than thermal burn injuries, it is common to perform staged closure. This consists of initial excision, followed by placement of a dermal template or scaffolding matrix. A vacuum-assisted dressing is often placed over the matrix and continued for 2 to 3 weeks to allow tissue granulation and ingrowth. The scaffold is then delaminated and a split thickness skin graft placed.
- Deep electric injuries may also require rotational or free flaps to provide optimal coverage and function.

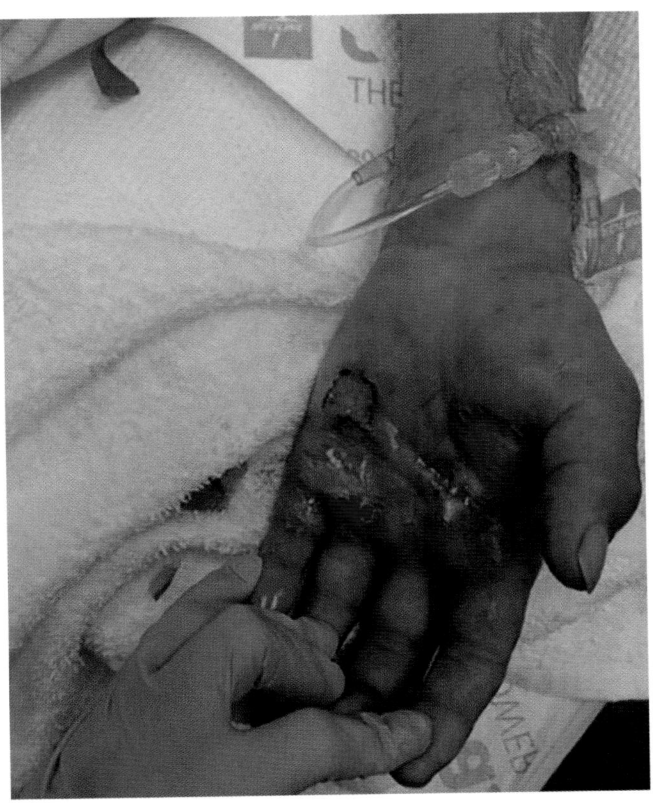

FIGURE 3 ● Deep partial thickness electrical burn to the hand. Full assessment of neurologic function is essential in this type of burn, and signs of compartment syndrome may require urgent carpal tunnel release.

PEARLS AND PITFALLS

- Underestimating burn burden based on exterior wounds alone.
- Performing surgery too early, when the burn is still evolving, will result in graft failure, infection of remaining necrotic tissue, and need for repeat operations.
- Failure to immediately decompress compartment syndrome, or perform amputation where needed, or lack of adequate fluid resuscitation may all result in worsening rhabdomyolysis, renal failure, and need for dialysis.

POSTOPERATIVE CARE

Postoperative care will be individualized based on the type of operation required.

COMPLICATIONS

- Since electric injuries cause a higher volume of tissue necrosis, especially in the deep soft tissues, infection is more common than with standard thermal burns.
- Rhabdomyolysis is a unique challenge in electric burns due to higher incidence of tetanic contractions.
- Cardiac arrhythmias can also be a significant complication in electrical burns secondary to current passing through the myocardium. Antiarrhythmics including calcium channel blockers and beta blockers may be necessary to convert or control these arrhythmias.

SUGGESTED READINGS

1. Aghakhani K, Heidari M, Tabatabaee SM, Abdolkarimi L. Effect of current pathway on mortality and morbidity in electrical burn patients. *Burns*. 2015;41(1):172-176. doi: 10.1016/j.burns.2014.06.008. Epub 2014 Jul 8. PMID: 25015707.
2. Ding H, Huang M, Li D, Lin Y, Qian W. Epidemiology of electrical burns: a 10-year retrospective analysis of 376 cases at a burn centre in South China. *J Int Med Res*. 2020;48(3):300060519891325. doi: 10.1177/0300060519891325. Epub 2019 Dec 19. PMID: 31854209; PMCID: PMC7782948.
3. Friedstat J, Brown DA, Levi B. Chemical, electrical, and radiation injuries. *Clin Plast Surg*. 2017;44(3):657-669. doi: 10.1016/j.cps.2017.02.021. Epub 2017 Apr 21. PMID: 28576255; PMCID: PMC5488710.
4. Hedawoo JB, Ali A. Electric burns and disability. *J Indian Med Assoc*. 2010;108(2):84-87. PMID: 20839563.
5. Winfree J, Barillo DJ. Burn management. Nonthermal injuries. *Nurs Clin North Am*. 1997;32(2):275-296. PMID: 9115477.

Chapter 4 Decision-Making and Operative Management of Necrotizing Soft Tissue Infections

Lisa Rae and Jeffery H. Anderson

DEFINITION

- Necrotizing soft tissue infection (NSTI) is defined as a rapidly progressive infection of the dermis, subcutaneous tissue, fascia, and/or muscle that is associated with significant local tissue destruction and results in systemic signs of toxicity and sepsis. NSTIs are classified by the type of infection (**TABLE 1**). Early diagnosis and urgent surgical treatment are needed for survival. NSTI can be categorized into three types.[1] Examples of NSTI include necrotizing fasciitis, Fournier gangrene, and gas gangrene.

DIFFERENTIAL DIAGNOSIS

- Cellulitis
- Myositis
- Erysipelas
- Stevens Johnson syndrome
- Bullous pemphigoid
- Skin manifestations of gram-negative sepsis: Erythema gangrenosum, thrombophlebitis, cutaneous bullae
- Note: Cellulitis with pain out of proportion to physical examination or signs of severe sepsis should be concerning for underlying NSTI.

PATIENT HISTORY AND PHYSICAL FINDINGS

- The history of the patient can vary greatly. Oftentimes, patients will report a prior history of a "boil" or "pimple" that progresses. Other times, patients will describe a preceding trauma with a small cutaneous injury or insect bite. Rarely, there will be no preceding cutaneous insult or the patient may report a muscle strain or bruise.
- NSTIs are often marked by rapid progression from the inciting source. The extent of the tissue involvement may not be determined by looking at the skin involvement. Often the necrotic tissue extends far beyond the overlying skin changes seen.[1]
- High-risk patient features include:
  - Injection drug use
  - Diabetes
  - Obesity
  - Peripheral vascular disease
  - Immunosuppression
- Physical examination
  - Cellulitis with skin blistering or sloughing (**FIGURES 1** and **2**)
  - Marked induration of overlying skin
  - Tenderness out of proportion to skin findings
  - Crepitus on examination (very poor sensitivity)
- Concerning features include:
  - White blood cell (WBC) > 20,000
  - Hyponatremia (Na < 135)
  - Acute kidney injury
  - Altered mental status
  - Septic physiology (tachycardia, hypotension, high fluid requirements)

Table 1: Types of Necrotizing Soft Tissue Infection

Necrotizing soft tissue infection classification[1]	
Type 1	Polymicrobial
Type 2	Monomicrobial (clostridial, Group A strep, etc.)
Type 3	Marine organism

IMAGING AND OTHER DIAGNOSTIC STUDIES

- NSTI is a clinical diagnosis; imaging is NOT indicated unless there is a concern regarding the accuracy of the diagnosis or concern for an underlying fluid collection. Computed tomography (CT) scan should not delay surgical treatment.

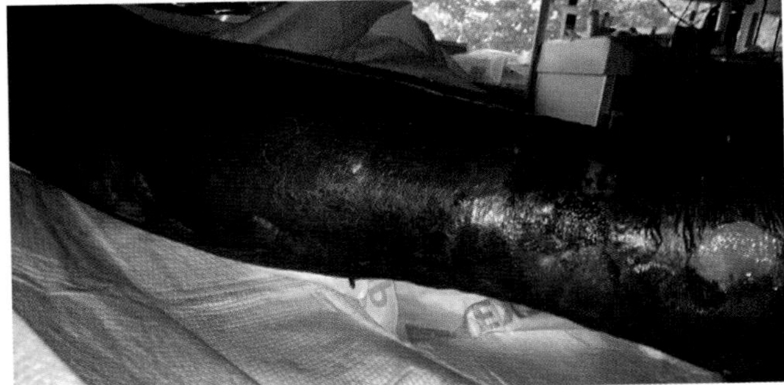

FIGURE 1 ● Bullae seen with necrotizing soft tissue infection.

- Pertinent laboratory values include basic metabolic panel (BMP), complete blood count (CBC), prothrombin time/partial thromboplastin time (PT/PTT), lactate, C-reactive protein (CRP), liver function tests (LFTs).
- X-rays of the affected area may demonstrate gas, although this finding is not sensitive.
- CT scan of the affected area may demonstrate gas and/or edema (**FIGURE 3**).
  - If performing a CT scan, we recommend that it be performed with contrast to rule out an underlying abscess or to differentiate between NSTI and myositis.

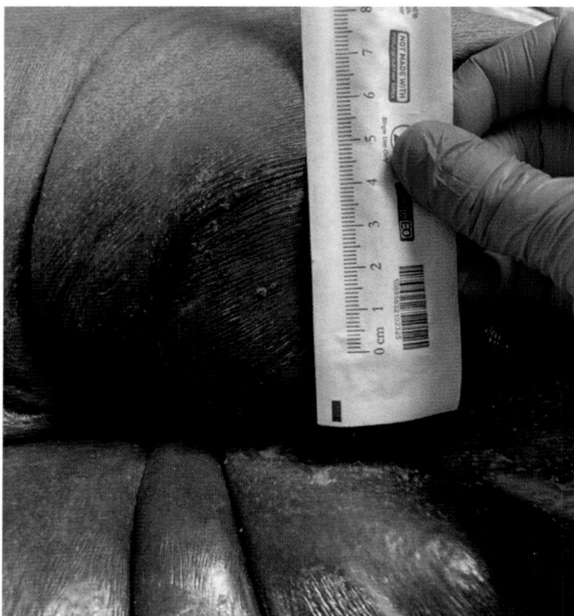

FIGURE 2 • Perianal and perineal physical examination of necrotizing soft tissue infection with skin changes and bullae.

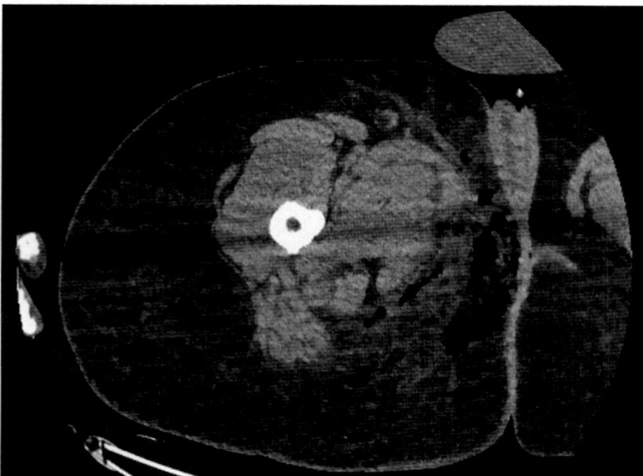

FIGURE 3 • Computed tomography scan demonstrating necrotizing soft tissue infection within deep pelvic tissues.

- The LRINEC score (**TABLE 2**) has been suggested to help distinguish NSTI from cellulitis when evaluating CRP, WBC count, hemoglobin (Hgb), serum Na^+ (sodium), serum creatinine, and blood glucose levels.[2]
  - LRINEC score ≥ 8 is a high risk of NSTI with a probability of 75% or greater. A score ≥ 6 is a moderate risk of NSTI, with a probability greater than 50%. This scoring system has not been validated and should only be used as an adjunct in decision-making.
  - Other studies have also shown that Na^+ ≥ 135 and WBC < 15,000 have a negative predictive value for NSTI[3] which correlates with LRINEC score.
  - Fernando et al note that the LRINEC score, presence of gas on X-ray, fever, hypotension, and bullae have poor sensitivity with regard to NSTI, thus emphasizing that this is a clinical diagnosis in which adjuncts can be used to aid in that diagnosis only when it is unclear.[4]
- Definitive diagnosis is made in the operating room (OR). The presence of necrotic fascia, dishwater fluid along fascial planes, and nonadherent tissue ultimately marks the diagnosis. A low threshold should exist to incise an area of cellulitic or necrotic overlying tissue to evaluate the fascia and underlying tissues in patients with clinical features concerning for NSTI.

SURGICAL MANAGEMENT

Preoperative Planning

- NSTI is a surgical emergency and once suspected the patient should be taken emergently to the OR.
- Obtain laboratory values including BMP, CBC, LFTs, PT/PTT, lactate, and CRP.
- Broad initial antimicrobial therapy should be initiated once NSTI is suspected in the emergency department.
  - At our institution, we use vancomycin, cefepime, clindamycin, and metronidazole.
    - Vancomycin covers methicillin-resistant *Staphylococcus aureus* (MRSA).
    - Cefepime covers gram-negative organisms and Group A strep.
    - Clindamycin covers both clostridial species and Group A strep and is used for toxin suppression.
    - Metronidazole covers anaerobes.

Table 2: Laboratory Risk Indicators for Necrotizing Fasciitis

Lab	Value	Score
C-reactive protein (mg/dL)	<15	0
	≥15	4
White blood cell (per cc)	<15	0
	15-25	1
	>25	2
Hemoglobin (g/dL)	>13.5	0
	11-13.5	1
	<11	2
Sodium (mEq/L)	≥135	0
	<135	2
Creatinine (mg/dL)	≤1.6	0
	>1.6	2
Glucose (mg/dL)	≤180	0
	>180	1

- Antibiotics should be tailored based on local cultures and sensitivities.
  - The timing of de-escalation of antibiotics per cultures and sensitivities is still poorly defined.[5]
  - At our institution de-escalation occurs once cultures are finalized and sepsis physiology has resolved.
- Treatment of sepsis as outlined by most recent Surviving Sepsis Guidelines include fluid resuscitation, vasopressors, and central access.[6]
- If the location of the NSTI includes the genitalia, neck, mediastinum, or forearm/hand, we recommend consultation of urology, otolaryngology, thoracic surgery, and hand surgery, respectively.

Positioning

- Positioning the patient depends on the area affected.
- A large area is recommended since the underlying tissues affected may be much larger than what is seen at the level of skin.
- Surgical management includes adequate debridement of all affected tissue; thus position should allow access to all potentially affected areas. If this is not possible, then the patient may need to be repositioned intraoperatively to obtain adequate exposure to all affected tissues.
  - For instance, a perineal NSTI should be positioned in lithotomy as many of these also progress into the abdominal wall, but the patient may also need to be positioned prone to obtain access to the back.

STEPS

- Effective management of NSTIs includes early, radical, sharp surgical debridement of ALL affected tissue, including the skin, subcutaneous fat, fascia, and muscle (**FIGURE 4**).
  - NSTI is often characterized by the presence of dishwater fluid once an incision over the affected area is made.
  - A positive "finger sign"—a finger placed in the fascial plane slides easily along the course of the infection—is often indicative of an NSTI.
  - Affected muscle often times will not respond to stimulation with electrocautery.
  - Affected tissue will often have visibly thrombosed vessels.
  - Unaffected tissue will appear healthy without signs of malperfusion.
  - Hemosiderin laden tissue should be excised even with evidence of bleeding.
  - Not uncommonly the amount of tissue affected will necessitate guillotine amputation.
- An adequate amount of tissue should be sent for culture rather than a swab to aid in identification of multiple potential organisms. Tissue culture should be obtained to allow for appropriate microbial coverage and eventual narrowing of antibiotics.
- Frequent re-evaluation of the tissues and laboratory values should be performed with a low threshold for return to OR for redebridement of any progression of infection.[7]
- For NSTIs not involving skin and subcutaneous tissue, a skin sparing technique (**FIGURES 5-8**) can be used to allow for easier postoperative reconstruction.[8]

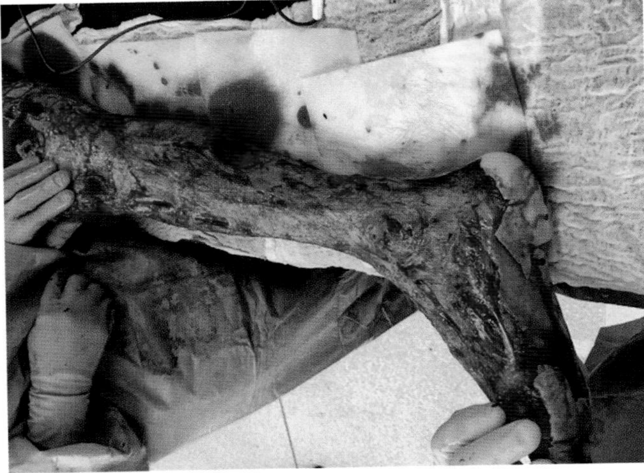

FIGURE 4 ● Adequate debridement of all affected tissue including skin and fascia.

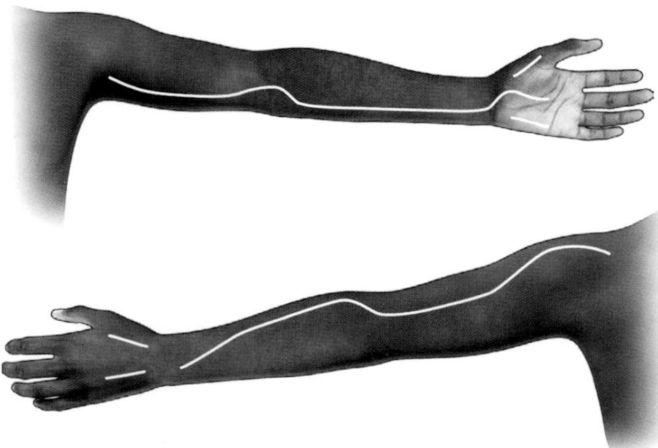

FIGURE 5 ● Skin sparing incision to upper extremities.

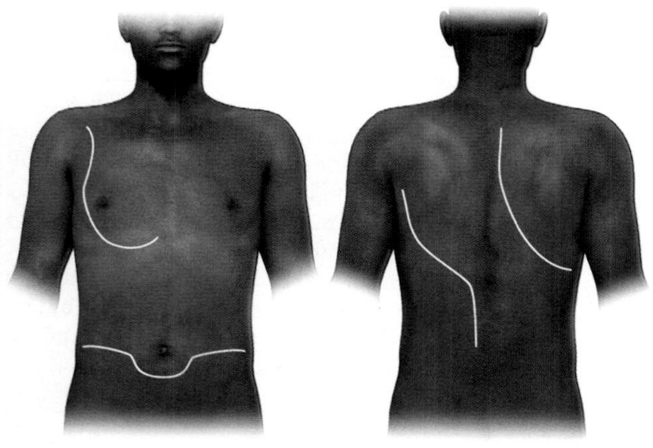

FIGURE 6 ● Skin sparring incision to trunk.

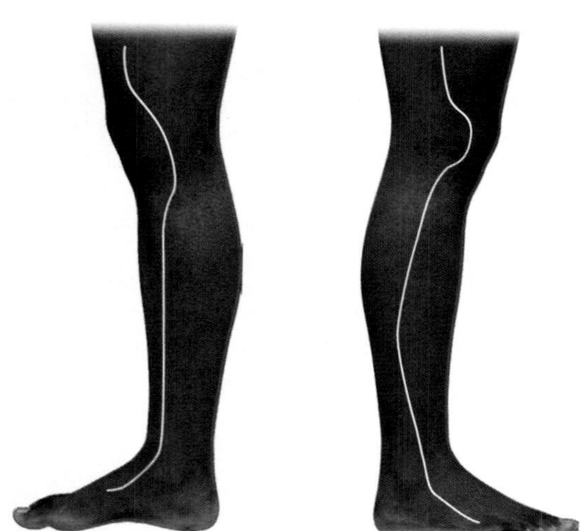

FIGURE 7 ● Skin sparring incision to lower legs.

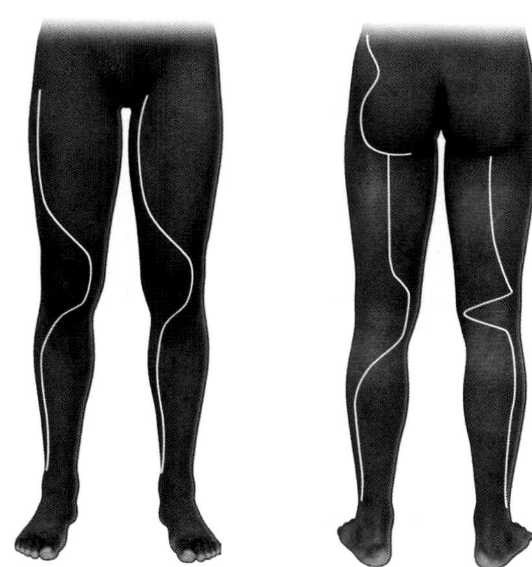

FIGURE 8 ● Skin sparring incision to lower extremities.

PEARLS AND PITFALLS

- When the diagnosis is in question, we recommend emergent surgical exploration as delays in surgical debridement (for instance to obtain a CT scan) can be life threatening. Mortality increases with delay in debridement greater than 24 hours.[4]
- Failure of wide and adequate surgical debridement often results in rapid progression of the disease and further morbidity and mortality (**FIGURE 9**).
- The appearance of healthy tissue (without hemosiderin) is the goal of excision rather than the presence of bleeding tissue.
- Amputation may be indicated and necessary when involving the extremities.

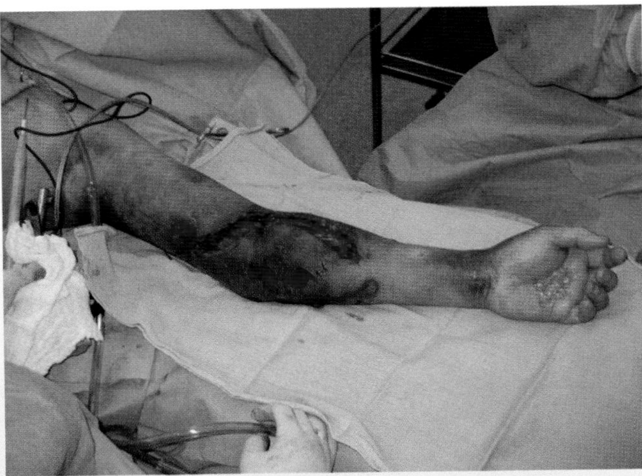

FIGURE 9 • Inadequate initial debridement leading to further spread of necrotizing soft tissue infection.

POSTOPERATIVE CARE

- Admission to surgical intensive care unit
- Leave wounds open to air to allow frequent reassessment for disease progression by nurses and surgical staff[7]
- Continuation of broad-spectrum antibiotics
  - These authors recommend narrowing antibiotics when septic physiology is resolving, WBC count is downtrending, and the wound appears healthy. Timing for de-escalation is variable in the literature.
- Tight blood glucose control with insulin drips is preferred
- Early enteral nutrition
- Frequent laboratory checks
  - A rising WBC after debridement may indicate inadequate debridement or progression of infection and should trigger prompt re-evaluation of the tissues and return the patient to the OR for further exploration and debridement.
- Consider transfer to a verified burn center as data have demonstrated improved outcomes of patients with NSTI at burn centers.[3] Burn centers are well versed in daily, painful, complex wound care that may be of benefit to recovery.
- Reconstruction may require skin grafting, use of dermal substitutes to cover exposed tendon and bone and/or flap coverage. Consider consulting burn and/or plastic surgeon for assistance if not already involved in the patient's care.
- Note: These authors do not recommend hyperbaric oxygen or intravenous immunoglobulin for the treatment of NSTI given the current evidence.

Rehabilitation is needed for optimal outcomes due to limb loss, prolonged critical illness, large tissue defects, contractures, pain, and distress.

COMPLICATIONS

- Failure to recognize an NSTI in a timely fashion, resulting in worsening infection and multiorgan failure, leading to greater morbidity and mortality.

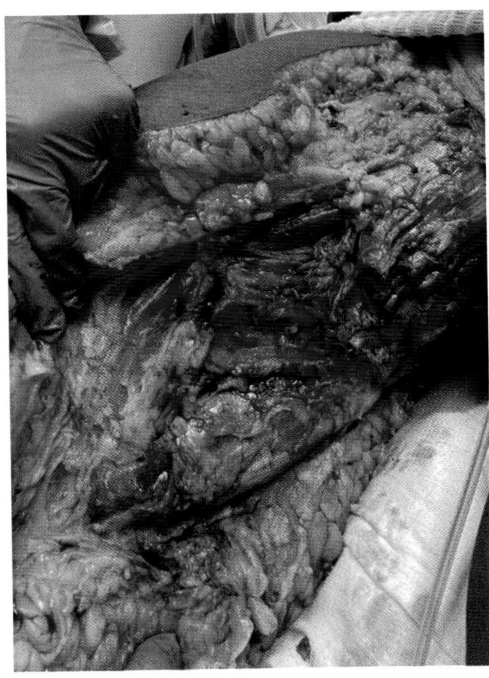

FIGURE 10 • Progression of infection seen at bedside with frequent assessment.

- Inadequate debridement or delayed return to OR for further debridement leading to progression of disease, further morbidity, and mortality (**FIGURE 10**).
- Bleeding, disseminated intravascular coagulopathy.

REFERENCES

1. Stevens DL, Bryant AE. Necrotizing soft-tissue infections. *N Engl J Med*. 2017;377(23):2253-2265. doi:10.1056/NEJMra1600673
2. Wong CH, Khin LW, Heng KS, Tan KC, Low CO. The LRINEC (Laboratory Risk Indicator for Necrotizing Fasciitis) score: a tool for distinguishing necrotizing fasciitis from other soft tissue

infections. *Crit Care Med*. 2004;32(7):1535-1541. doi:10.1097/01.ccm.0000129486.35458.7d

3. Hakkarainen TW, Kopari NM, Pham TN, Evans HL. Necrotizing soft tissue infections: review and current concepts in treatment, systems of care, and outcomes. *Curr Probl Surg*. 2014;51(8):344-362. doi:10.1067/j.cpsurg.2014.06.001
4. Fernando SM, Tran A, Cheng W, et al. Necrotizing soft tissue infection: diagnostic accuracy of physical examination, imaging, and LRINEC score—a systematic review and meta-analysis. *Ann Surg*. 2019;269(1):58-65. doi:10.1097/SLA.0000000000002774
5. Faraklas I, Yang D, Eggerstedt M, et al. A multi-center review of care patterns and outcomes in necrotizing soft tissue infections. *Surg Infect*. 2016;17(6):773-778. doi:10.1089/sur.2015.238
6. Rhodes A, Evans LE, Alhazzani W, et al. Surviving sepsis campaign—international Guidelines for management of sepsis and septic shock: 2016. *Intensive Care Med*. 2017;43(3):304-377. doi:10.1007/s00134-017-4683-6
7. Yang D, Davies A, Burge B, Watkins P, Dissanaike S. Open-to-Air is a viable option for initial wound care in necrotizing soft tissue infection that allows early detection of recurrence without need for painful dressing changes or return to operating room. *Surg Infect*. 2018;19(1):65-70. doi:10.1089/sur.2017.080
8. Tom LK, Wright TJ, Horn DL, Bulger EM, Pham TN, Keys KA. A skin-sparing approach to the treatment of necrotizing soft-tissue infections: thinking reconstruction at initial debridement. *J Am Coll Surg*. 2016;222(5):e47-e60. doi:10.1016/j.jamcollsurg.2016.01.008

SECTION III: Traumatic Injury to the Chest Wall, Pleura, and Diaphragm

Chapter 5 Rib Plating

Mitchell D. Gorman, Sagar S. Kadakia, and Joshua A. Marks

DEFINITION

- Rib fractures occur when an applied force exceeds the strength of the thoracic cage. They account for the majority of blunt chest trauma injuries.
- There are several different surgical techniques to stabilize these fractures including intramedullary rods, Kirschner wires, Judet struts, and plates with screws. The approach also varies: intrathoracic, percutaneous, and external. The technique of open external fixation using plates with screws has become one of the more popular approaches, and the one that will be discussed in this chapter.

CLASSIFICATION

- There are several chest wall scoring systems and most focus on the number of fractured ribs and whether they are unilateral or bilateral. The Chest Wall Injury Society proposed a standard nomenclature for multiple rib fracture classifications.[1] This provides a common language for communication regarding the degree of anatomic injury. Regarding displacement, characterization, and associated fractures, the society proposed three categories of individual fracture displacement, three characterizations of individual fractures, and a description of associated fractures on neighboring ribs.
  - Displacement (**FIGURE 1**)
    - **Undisplaced:** >90% contact between cortical surfaces
    - **Offset:** some cortical contact, but <90%
    - **Displaced:** no cortical contact due to either overlap of the ends or distraction
  - Fractures (**FIGURE 2**)
    - **Simple:** single fracture line across rib without fragmentation or comminution
    - **Wedge:** second fracture line not spanning the whole width of the rib, also known as a butterfly fragment

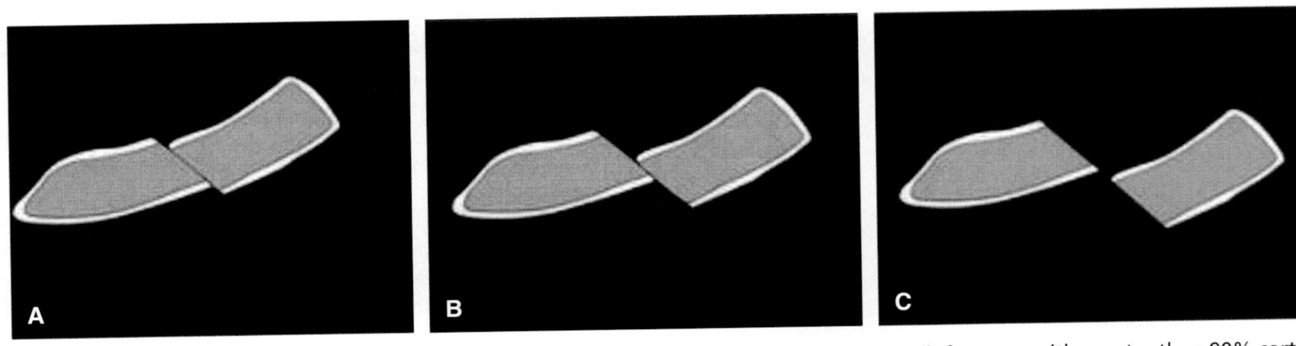

FIGURE 1 ● Diagrammatic representation of the CT axial images of **(A)** an undisplaced simple rib fracture, with greater than 90% cortical contact; **(B)** an offset simple rib fracture, with cortical contact but less than 90%; **(C)** a displaced simple rib fracture, with no cortical contact.

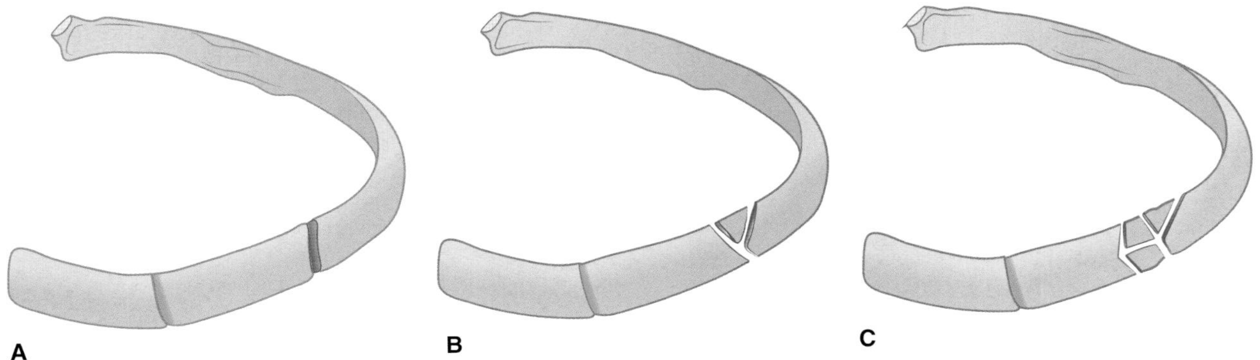

FIGURE 2 ● Diagrammatic representation of **(A)** an undisplaced simple rib fracture; **(B)** an undisplaced wedge rib fracture; **(C)** an undisplaced complex rib fracture.

      - **Complex:** At least two fracture lines with one or more fragments spanning the width of the rib
    - Associated fractures on neighboring ribs termed a "Series of Fractures"
- The Society also made recommendations regarding the anatomical sectors around the chest wall
    - Three anatomical sectors were delineated: anterior, lateral, and posterior. However, there is no consensus on the definition of anatomic boundaries.
        - In this chapter, the anatomic sectors are designated as follows:
            - Anterior: anterior to the anterior axillary line
            - Lateral: between the anterior and posterior axillary lines
            - Posterior: posterior to the posterior axillary line
    - Defining Flail Chest
        - The term "Flail Segment" should describe radiologic findings and "Flail Chest" describes the paradoxical motion seen on clinical exam.
        - Flail Segment is defined as three or more contiguous ribs fractured in two or more places.

PATIENT HISTORY AND PHYSICAL FINDINGS

- Ribs 1 to 3 are relatively protected, but when fractured, can be associated with severe intrathoracic injury.
- Ribs 9 to 12 are more mobile and have a higher association with intra-abdominal injury.
- Associated injuries
    - Pneumothorax/hemothorax
    - Lung herniation
    - Spleen, liver, and kidney injuries
    - Pulmonary contusions
    - Pulmonary lacerations
    - Brachial plexus compression/stretch/laceration

IMAGING AND OTHER DIAGNOSTIC STUDIES

- Plain Radiograph (**FIGURE 3**)
    - Rules out life-threatening injuries requiring immediate attention such as pneumothorax and hemothorax

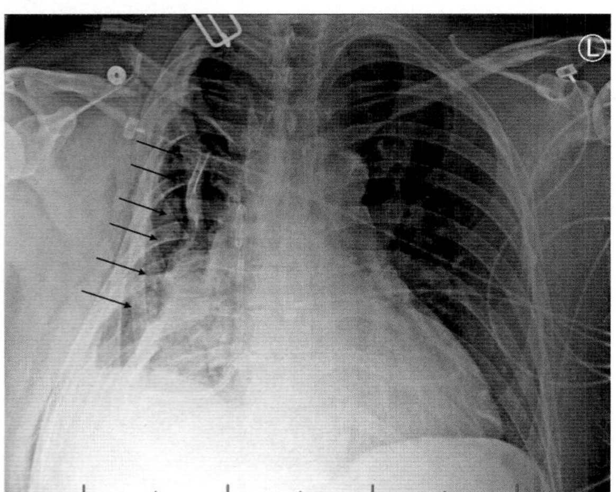

FIGURE 3 ● Anteroposterior chest x-ray of a patient showing multiple severely displaced segmental fractures involving the right ribs extending from ribs 1 to 9.

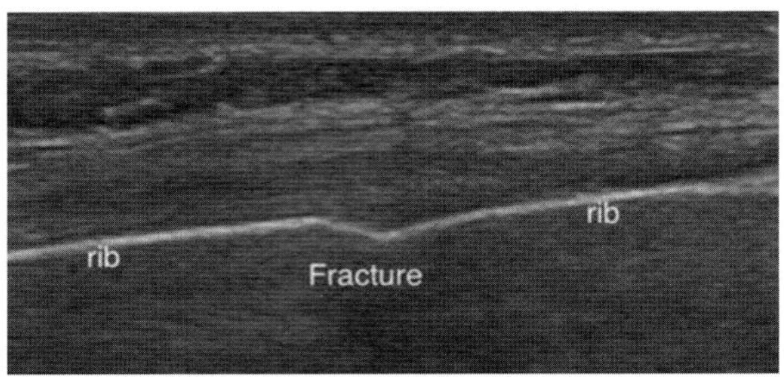

FIGURE 4 ● Ultrasound showing discontinuity of the rib cortex, indicating a fracture.[3]

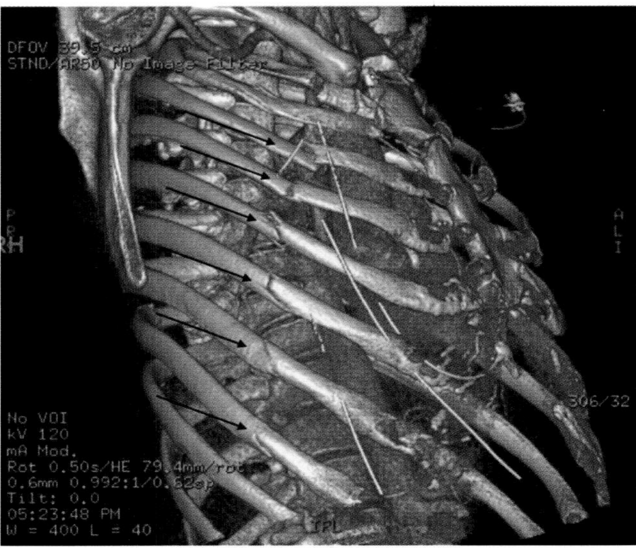

FIGURE 5 ● 3D reconstruction of a patient with multiple displaced right sided rib fractures.

    - Sensitivity is low compared to CT for detecting rib and sternal fractures.
    - Over half of patients with rib fractures on chest x-ray can have at least three additional fractures on CT.[2]
- Ultrasound (**FIGURE 4**)
    - More sensitive than chest x-ray.
    - Find the cortex of the rib and follow it to the point of discontinuity.
    - Discontinuity in the rib cortex represents the fracture.
    - Not recommended in the alert patient, as rib fractures are very tender to palpation. Can be used after induction of anesthesia to help locate rib fractures prior to incision.
- CT Scan (**FIGURE 5**)
    - In addition to traditional views (axial, coronal, and sagittal), 3D reconstructions allow for complete definition of all rib fractures and extent of displacement, as well as operative planning. Some rib fixation systems will print 3D models that are precontoured for each rib.

SURGICAL MANAGEMENT

- From the initial injury to the postoperative period, multimodal analgesia and pulmonary toilet remain key components of rib fracture management.
    - This consists of different classes of analgesics used simultaneously to manage pain.

- It is a tiered approach with standardized, sequentially escalated potency and objective measurements of response (vital capacity, incentive spirometry).
- Various classes include nonsteroidal anti-inflammatory drugs (NSAIDs), acetaminophen, opioids, epidural infusions of local anesthetics and/or opioids, and peripheral nerve blocks.

Goals

- Minimize the need for mechanical ventilation and tracheostomy
- Decrease ICU and hospital length of stay
- Diminish complication rates
- Decrease hospital costs
- Reduce pain
- Promote sooner return to activities of daily living (ADLs)/work
- As surgical stabilization of rib fractures becomes more routine, there remains ambiguity regarding its absolute indications.
  - Flail chest: Consensus from the Eastern Association for the Surgery of Trauma conditionally recommends consideration in all patients with flail chest after blunt trauma.[4]
  - Multiple displaced fractures, in the absence of flail chest: may be beneficial as these patients tend to express many of the same pathophysiologic symptoms as those with flail chest.[5]
  - Undisplaced fractures:
    - Currently, there is limited evidence to support surgical stabilization.
    - Interval displacement of the rib fractures is possible due to patient motion and changes in intrathoracic pressure.
    - Consider repeating a CT 48 to 72 hours after the initial injury to assess interval displacement for those patients with multiple undisplaced fractures or those who develop a worsening clinical status.
- Various algorithms have been developed by institutions; none having been externally validated. Notwithstanding, these can provide guidance in selecting patients who may benefit most from surgical stabilization. An example of one such algorithm comes from the Chest Wall Injury Society that has been adopted by many groups (**FIGURE 6**).[6]
- The Chest Wall Injury Society categorizes the indications by nonventilated and ventilated groups. Chest wall instability, rib fractures, and pulmonary derangement are evaluated.
  - Nonventilated
    - Chest wall instability
      - Three-rib flail chest
      - Three bicortically displaced/offset ribs
      - Clinical finding of paradoxical motion
      - Instability or "clicking" on palpation or as reported by the patient
    - Three or more displaced rib fractures (≥50% of the rib width) with two or more pulmonary physiologic derangements
      - Respiratory rate ≥20
      - Measured volumes on incentive spirometry <50% of predicted
      - Numerical pain score >5/10
      - Poor cough
  - Ventilated
    - Chest wall instability
      - Three-rib flail chest
      - Three bicortically displaced/offset ribs
      - Clinical finding of paradoxical motion
      - Instability or "clicking" on palpation or as reported by the patient

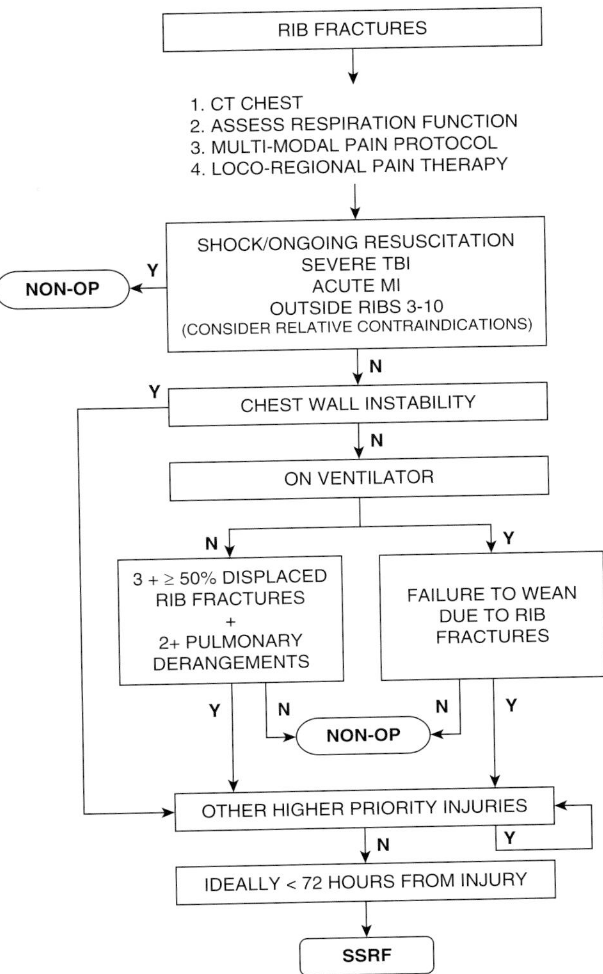

FIGURE 6 ● Chest Wall Injury Society algorithm for surgical stabilization of rib fractures.

      - Failure to wean from the ventilator that is clinically determined to be related to the rib fractures.

Contraindications

- Sepsis/infection
- Severe TBI (GCS < 8 or intracranial hypertension)
- Acute MI
- Unstable spine or pelvis fractures
- Hemodynamic instability/ongoing resuscitation
- Anticipated prolonged immobilization and/or ventilation
- Contaminated field

Relative Contraindications

- Less than three rib fractures
- Fractures <3 cm from the transverse process
- Moderate/mild traumatic brain injury (TBI)
- No fracture displacement
- Severe pulmonary contusion of the contralateral lung making single lung ventilation challenging
- Significant comorbidities
- Age < 18

Preoperative Planning

- Ideally fixation should be performed within 24 to 72 hours of injury.

- The goal of this timing is to stabilize the rib before peak tissue inflammation, which is typically between postinjury days 3 to 5.
- This timing can prove difficult in the polytrauma patient. Patients must be hemodynamically stable, and the correction of rib fractures may remain a low priority in the overall acute management of the patient. Injuries that are considered higher priority for intervention include, but are not limited to, preoperative spinal injuries, open abdomen, significant vascular trauma, and pelvic external fixation.
- In select patients, it may be beneficial to perform fixation as a "piggyback" to another operative procedure.

- Evaluate need for simultaneous thoracoscopy
  - May be needed for hemothorax evacuation or evaluation of the lung and/or diaphragm. May also be considered for post fixation evaluation of reduction as well as to perform nerve block.
  - It is not necessary, however, to enter the chest cavity in all cases, particularly if there is no hemothorax and the pleura is not violated during the fixation.
  - Single lung ventilation via double lumen tube or bronchial blocker should be considered in cases if the thoracic cavity is planned to be entered.
- Selecting ribs for plating
  - Ribs 1, 2, 11, and 12 are not plated. Ribs 11 and 12 are excised in cases of fracture with severe displacement.
- Sequence of plating
  - Preferred to approach fixation starting with the most displaced fracture and continuing outward.
  - Ideally the maximal number of ribs should be plated to help avoid any risks of subsequent displacement, deformity, or nonunion.

Positioning

- For anterior fractures, the patient is placed supine with arms abducted.
- For lateral and posterior fractures, the patient is placed in the lateral decubitus position with the affected side up, ensuring adequate padding. Flexing the table and raising the arm above the head allows for increased expansion of the thoracic cage. Prepping the hand and arm on the affected side assists with manipulation of the scapula and can help increase exposure.
  - Patients with bilateral fractures can be flipped to the contralateral side when complete or return to the OR for a separate procedure.

TECHNIQUES

- The incisions made are traditional for external reduction fixation and involve a muscle sparing technique. In regard to the components and fixation of plates, many proprietary systems exist that differ in the type of plates, malleability of the plates, amount of recommended fracture overlap, type, length and number of screws needed, and the instruments available to reduce and fixate the ribs. A description of all the diverse company systems is beyond the scope of this chapter. While it is necessary to learn the variances of the system available at one's own institution, the basic tenets of exposure and stabilization remain the same.

EXPOSURE

- Inframammary
  - This approach is preferred for anterior rib fractures and costochondral dislocations.
  - An incision is made horizontally, following the contour of the pectoralis major using the inframammary crease as a guide (**FIGURE 7**).
  - Dissection is carried down and superiorly below the pectoralis major to expose the serratus anterior and pectoralis minor (**FIGURE 8**).
- Axillary
  - This approach is preferred for anterior lateral and posterior lateral rib fractures.
  - Mark the location of the rib fractures on the patient. Plan an incision site that best allows for exposure of the most fractured ribs possible (**FIGURE 9**).
  - The incision is carried down and the fascia is elevated and freed from the latissimus muscle using sharp and blunt dissection (**FIGURE 10**). Take care to identify and avoid the long thoracic nerve that lies over the serratus anterior.

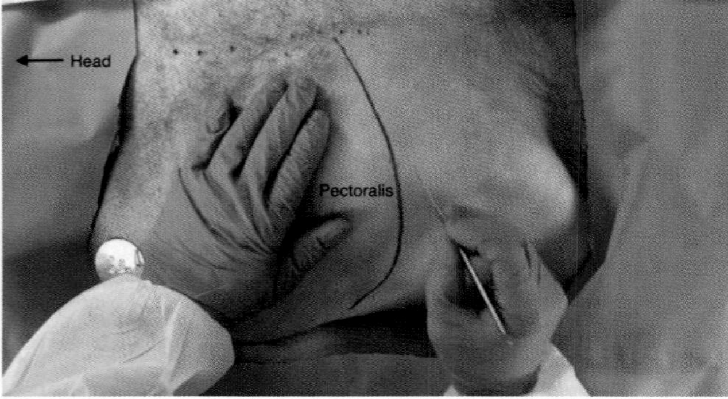

FIGURE 7 ● Planned incision for inframammary exposure. (Courtesy of Zimmer Biomet © 2021, Warsaw, IN.)

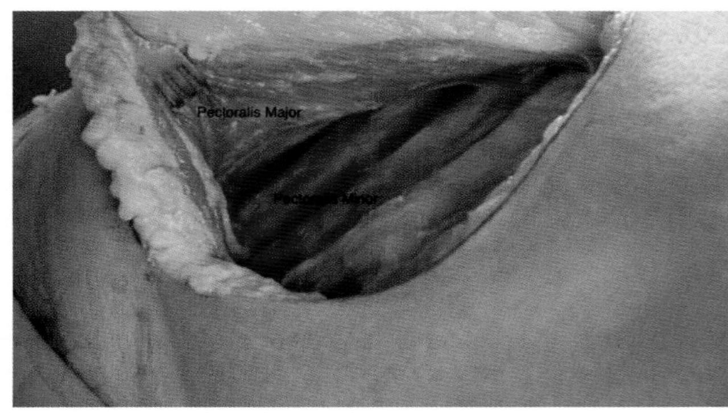

FIGURE 8 ● Inframammary exposure showing the pectoralis major and the pectoralis minor muscles. (Courtesy of Zimmer Biomet © 2021, Warsaw, IN.)

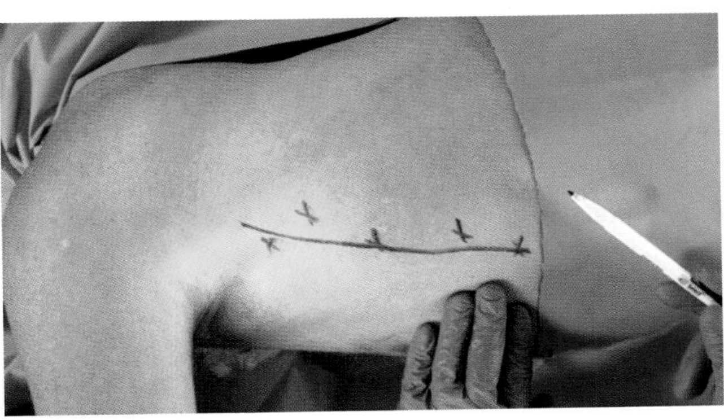

FIGURE 9 • Planned incision for axillary exposure. (Courtesy of Zimmer Biomet © 2021, Warsaw, IN.)

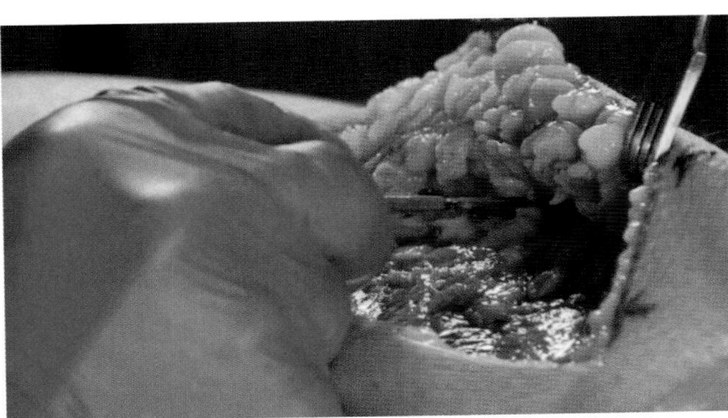

FIGURE 10 • The latissimus dorsi is dissected from the subcutaneous fat. (Courtesy of Zimmer Biomet © 2021, Warsaw, IN.)

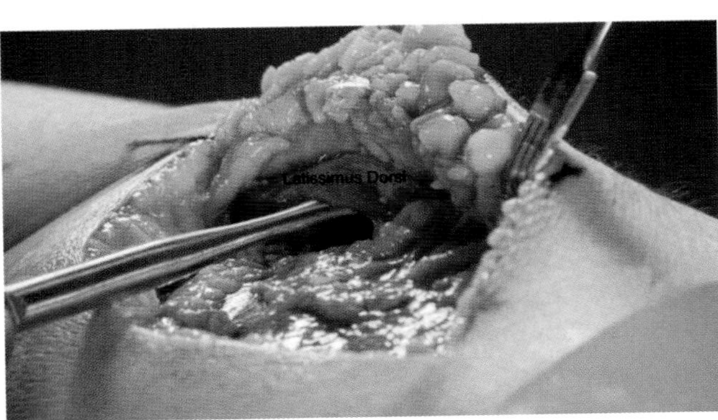

FIGURE 11 • The latissimus dorsi is lifted exposing posterior ribs. (Courtesy of Zimmer Biomet © 2021, Warsaw, IN.)

- Continue blunt dissection under the latissimus dorsi if needed to access rib fractures that lie more posteriorly (**FIGURE 11**).
- The serratus fibers are then split longitudinally, and the ribs are exposed (**FIGURE 12**). Avoid dissecting the intercostal muscles.

- Posterior Rib Fractures, subscapular
  - Make a posterolateral incision that extends below the tip of the scapula (**FIGURES 13** and **14**).
  - Continue the dissection down to the "triangle of auscultation" (latissimus, trapezius, and scapula) and elevate the fascia (**FIGURE 15**). Dissect below the latissimus dorsi and into the subscapular bursa with blunt and sharp dissection.

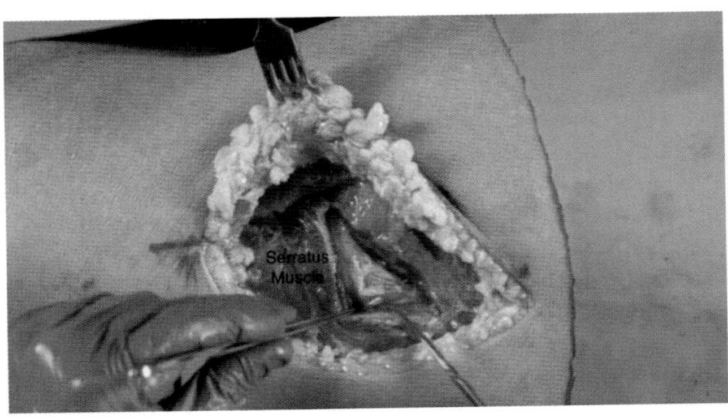

FIGURE 12 • The serratus muscle is split in a muscle sparing technique. (Courtesy of Zimmer Biomet © 2021, Warsaw, IN.)

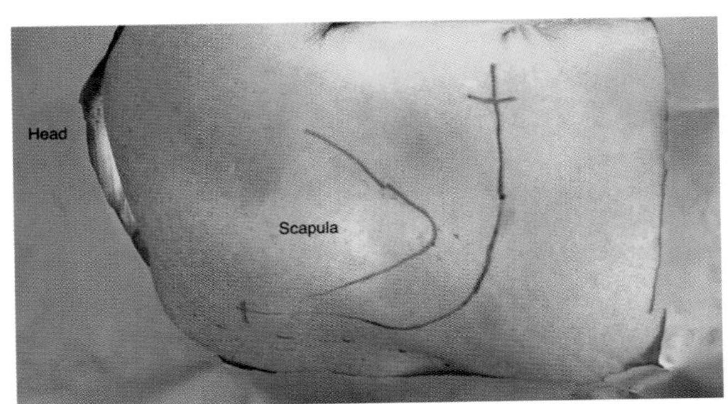

FIGURE 13 • Planned incision for subscapular exposure. (Courtesy of Zimmer Biomet © 2021, Warsaw, IN.)

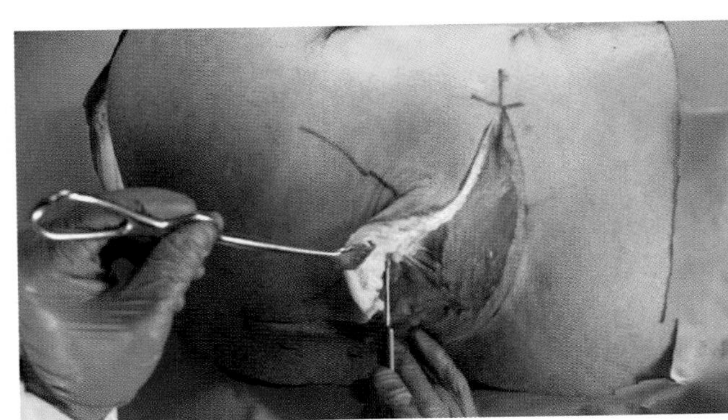

FIGURE 14 • Dissection through the subcutaneous fat. (Courtesy of Zimmer Biomet © 2021, Warsaw, IN.)

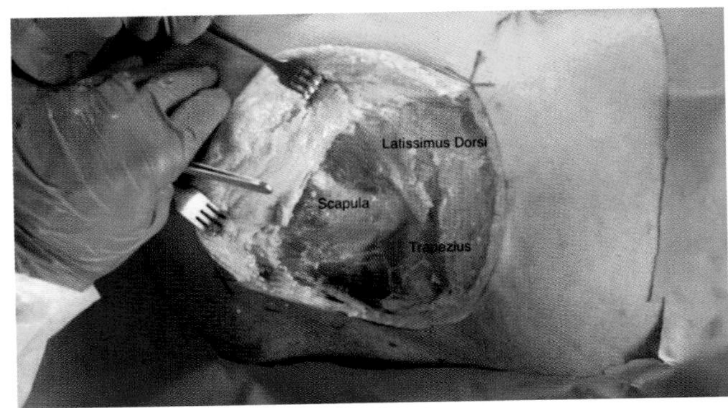

FIGURE 15 • Exposure of the "triangle of auscultation." (Courtesy of Zimmer Biomet © 2021, Warsaw, IN.)

PLATE PLACEMENT

- Going above the rib to avoid injury to the neurovascular bundle, measure the rib thickness using a caliper (**FIGURE 16**) and choose screw length based on the number in the view window. This is done on the medial and lateral aspects of the rib.
- Reduce the fracture using rib elevators or bone reducing forceps (**FIGURE 17**). If using a rib elevator, place it through so it lays under the posterior surface of the rib and not the inferior aspect to avoid injury to the neurovascular bundle. The goal of reduction is to align and fix the rib to restore the chest wall contour as closely as possible.
- Using a template, measure and cut the plate to allow an adequate landing zone on either side of the fracture (ie, a minimum of three screws on each side depending on the system). The template can be contoured by hand to match the rib anatomy.
- Select a plate and then cut to the length. If necessary, deburr the edges. The plate is then contoured to match the template using plate benders for in-plane and out-of-plane contouring (**FIGURE 18**). Threaded plate benders can also be used for minor bends.
- Position the plate over the fracture in the midbody of the rib using temporary fixation screws or plate holding forceps on the medial and lateral aspects of the rib fractures (**FIGURE 19**).
  - The plate should rest evenly over the rib without any tension. If tension is noted, remove the plate and use the plate benders to adjust the contour.
  - The clamps can also be adjusted medially and laterally as needed to help maintain plate contact with the rib.
- Select the appropriate screw length and fixate the plate to the rib (**FIGURE 20**). Systems vary as far as unicortical vs bicortical fixation, with the latter thought to be the more secure and a screw that is too long preferred over one that is short. Ensure adequate fixation on either side of the fracture (generally a minimum of three screws). If replacing a temporary fixation screw, a larger screw will be used to secure the plate.
- Repeat with ribs above and below as indicated.
- Consider performing a nerve block via injection of local anesthetic at the completion of the case.
- If the chest cavity is entered, a chest tube is placed.
- Dissected muscle and fascial plans are reapproximated and closed in layers, followed by skin closure.

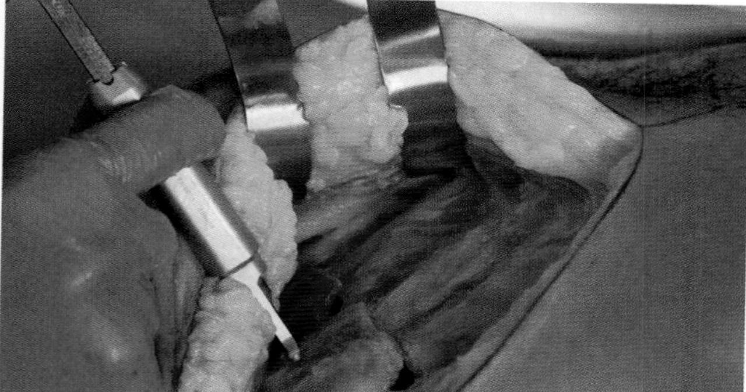

FIGURE 16 • Measuring the rib thickness with a caliper. (Courtesy of Zimmer Biomet © 2021, Warsaw, IN.)

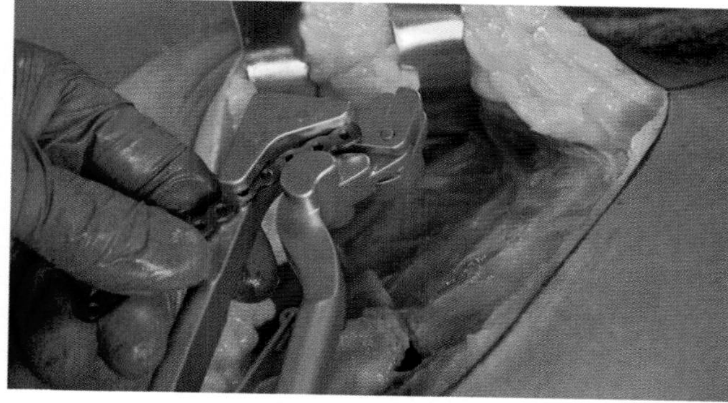

FIGURE 18 • Using plate benders to shape the plate to contour the rib. (Courtesy of Zimmer Biomet © 2021, Warsaw, IN.)

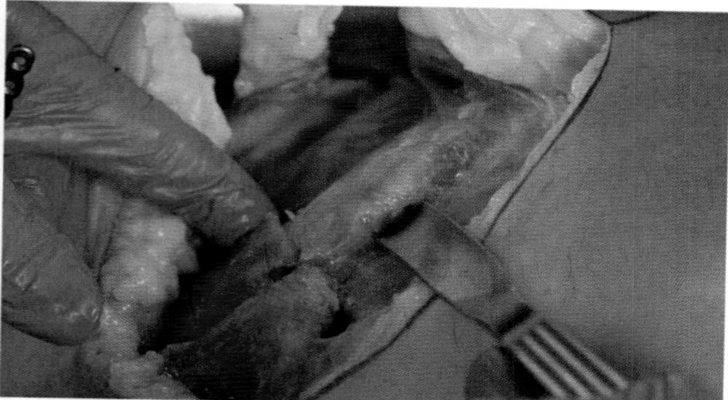

FIGURE 17 • The ribs are reduced as close to their anatomic position as possible. (Courtesy of Zimmer Biomet © 2021, Warsaw, IN.)

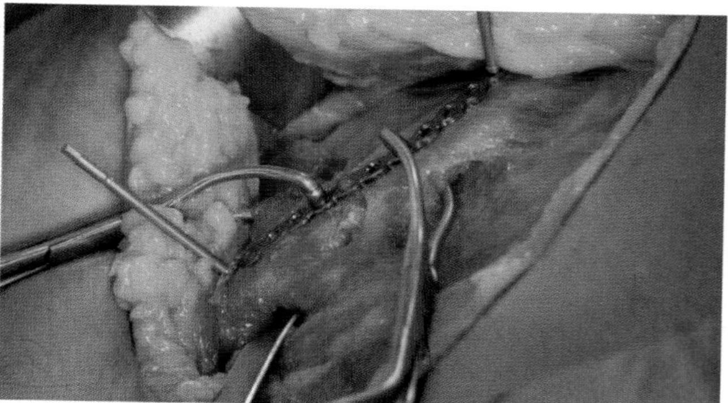

FIGURE 19 • Plate fixated to rib with temporary fixation screws and plate holding forceps. (Courtesy of Zimmer Biomet © 2021, Warsaw, IN.)

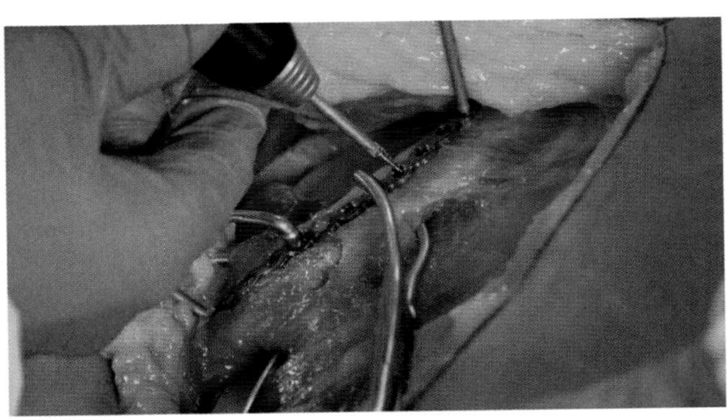

FIGURE 20 ● Placing screws on either side of the rib fracture. (Courtesy of Zimmer Biomet © 2021, Warsaw, IN.)

PEARLS AND PITFALLS

- Paravertebral rib fractures rarely need fixation.
- Do not strip the periosteum during the dissection. This can cause devascularization of the rib.
- Avoid excessive force when reducing fractures to avoid causing a synchronous fracture elsewhere along the rib.
- Take care to avoid injuring the neurovascular bundle along the inferior and posterior aspects of the rib during dissection or reduction of the fracture.
- If the rib is misaligned after all screws are placed, it may be necessary to loosen 1 or 2 screws and then clamp the plate to the bone. Once the clamp is in place with the plate and rib reapproximated, tighten the screws again and recheck the plate and rib position.
- In patients with severely comminuted fractures yielding large bone gaps (≥2 cm) between fracture segments, a bone graft or bone matrix may be necessary to support the plate and promote rib segment fixation healing.
- Thoracoscopic evaluation postplating allows for inspection of the diaphragm, lung parenchyma, lung expansion, and complete evacuation of hemothorax

POSTOPERATIVE CARE

- Obtain a postoperative chest x-ray (**FIGURE 21**) to evaluate for reduction of ribs and for residual or new hemothorax/pneumothorax.

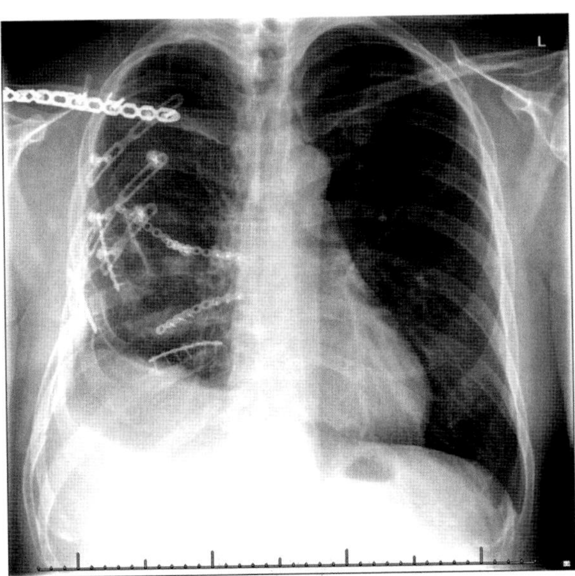

FIGURE 21 ● Completed fixation of patient's rib fractures from **FIGURE 3**. Fractures were stabilized using both extrathoracic and intrathoracic techniques.

- Continue multimodal pain management with aggressive pulmonary toilet.
- Venous thromboembolism (VTE) prophylaxis remains individualized to patient mobility and bleeding risk.
- Chest tube(s), if present and if there is no air leak and output is minimal, should be removed quickly, ideally within 24 hours postoperatively.

COMPLICATIONS

- Incidence less than 5%
  - Long-term follow up not reported in most series
- Intraoperative
  - Nerve, vascular, and lung parenchyma injury
- Immediate postoperative
  - Bleeding
  - Infection—wound or lung (atelectasis/pneumonia)
  - Retained hemothorax
  - Persistent air leak
- Late
  - Dislodgement and migration of hardware
    - Most common location: posteriorly due to rib angulation and shear forces
    - Most asymptomatic as ribs long since healed

REFERENCES

1. Edwards JG, Clarke P, Pieracci FM, et al. "Taxonomy of multiple rib fractures: results of the chest wall injury society international consensus survey." *J Trauma Acute Care Surg*. 2019;88(2):e40-e45. doi:10.1097/ta.0000000000002282

2. Chapman BC, Overbey DM, Tesfalidet F, et al. "Clinical utility of chest computed tomography in patients with rib fractures CT chest and rib fractures." *Arch Trauma Res*. 2016;5(4):e37070. doi:10.5812/atr.37070
3. Chen KC, Lin ACM, Chong CF, Wang TL. "An overview of point-of-care Ultrasound for soft tissue and musculoskeletal applications in the emergency department." *J Intensive Care*. 2016;4(1):55. doi:10.1186/s40560-016-0173-0
4. Kasotakis G, Hasenboehler EA, Streib EW, et al. "Operative fixation of rib fractures after blunt trauma." *J Trauma Acute Care Surg*. 2017;82(3):618-626. doi:10.1097/ta.0000000000001350
5. Pieracci FM, Leasia K, Bauman Z, et al. "A multicenter, prospective, controlled clinical trial of surgical stabilization of rib fractures in patients with severe, nonflail fracture patterns (Chest Wall Injury Society NONFLAIL)." *J Trauma Acute Care Surg*. 2020;88(2):249-257. doi: 10.1097/TA.0000000000002559
6. Delaplain PT, Schubl SD, Pieracci FM, et al. "*Chest Wall Injury Society Guideline for SSRF: Indications, Contraindications and Timing*." The Chest Wall Injury Society website; 2020. Accessed June 13, 2021. https://cwisociety.org/wp-content/uploads/2020/05/CWIS-SSRF-Guideline-01102020.pdf

Chapter 6

Needle Decompression, Tube Thoracostomy, Thoracentesis

Jennifer T. Cone and Selwyn O. Rogers Jr.

DEFINITION

- Needle decompression is the act of emergently placing a needle into the thoracic cavity in order to evacuate air that is causing a tension pneumothorax or hemothorax. Tube thoracostomy is the placement of a tube into the chest in order to evacuate air, fluid, or blood. It can be performed with tubes of multiple sizes depending on the indication for placement. Thoracentesis is defined as drainage of fluid from the thoracic cavity. A drainage catheter may be left in place after a thoracentesis procedure.

DIFFERENTIAL DIAGNOSIS

- Patients who require a needle decompression, tube thoracostomy, or thoracentesis may present with a variety of diagnoses. In the setting of trauma, both traumatic pneumothorax and hemothorax must be considered. In nontrauma patients, the differential diagnoses are broad. Patients with bullous lung disease may develop a spontaneous pneumothorax. Patients with cancer may develop malignant pleural effusions. Intra-abdominal inflammatory processes can lead to reactive pleural effusions. Finally, there are numerous potential iatrogenic reasons such as central line placement, chest wall procedures, or lung biopsy that may cause a pneumothorax or hemothorax requiring needle decompression or tube thoracostomy.

PATIENT HISTORY AND PHYSICAL FINDINGS

- In stable patients, a patient's history will help elicit the cause of the pneumothorax, pleural effusion, or hemothorax.
- In emergent situations where the patient is unstable or in distress, a history may not be possible. In these situations, it is important to rely on physical examination findings.
- In trauma patients, it is vital to assess the patient systematically using the ABCDE approach of a primary survey. The airway should be assessed first, followed by assessing breath sounds, then central pulses, then Glasgow Coma Scale score, and finally by exposing the patient. After adjuncts like a chest x-ray or FAST (Focused Assessment with Sonography in Trauma) examination, a secondary survey, which is a complete head-to-toe physical assessment, can take place.
- A pneumothorax may present with decreased or absent breath sounds, hyperresonance on percussion, tachypnea, and dyspnea. If a pneumothorax is loculated from previous chest surgery or infection, none of these findings may be present (**FIGURE 1**).
- A hemothorax may also present with decreased or absent breath sounds. Generally, one will find dullness on percussion of the chest. The patient may have tachypnea or dyspnea (**FIGURE 2**).
- Pleural effusions present similarly with decreased or absent breath sounds, tachypnea, and dyspnea. Chest wall percussion will generally reveal hyporesonance.

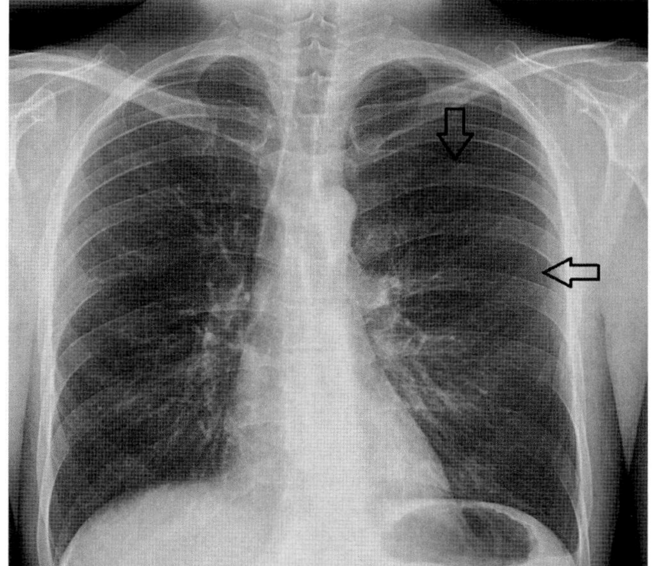

FIGURE 1 ● *Black arrows* point to left-sided pneumothorax. (Reprinted with permission from Daffner RH, Hartman M. *Clinical Radiology*. 4th ed. Wolters Kluwer; 2014. Figure 4.11a.)

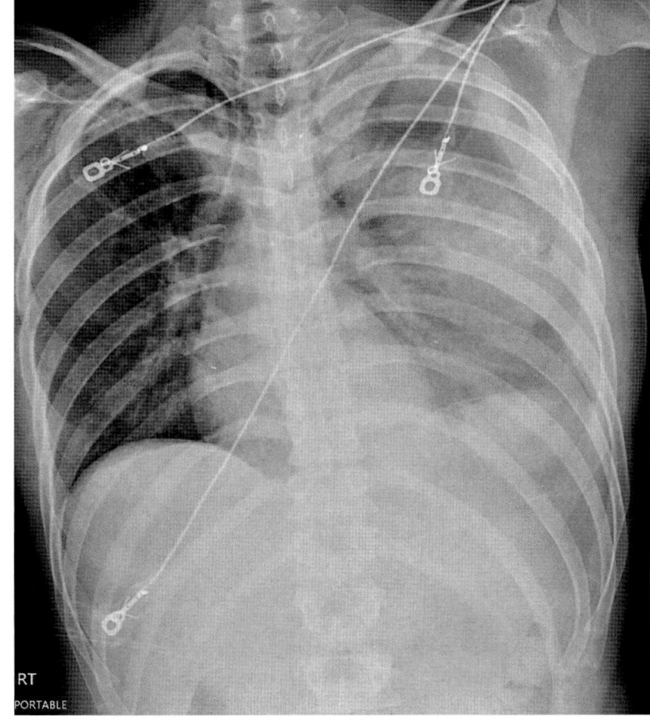

FIGURE 2 ● Chest x-ray showing left-sided hemothorax after gunshot wound of the left chest.

- Tension physiology presents with absent breath sounds on the affected side, tachycardia, hypotension, and distended neck veins. It is critical to be able to recognize tension physiology immediately and to not delay treatment, which is immediate decompression of the chest.

IMAGING AND OTHER DIAGNOSTIC STUDIES

- Imaging should only be employed in patients without tension physiology.
- A chest x-ray will often reveal a pneumothorax, pleural effusion, or hemothorax. Because of its speed and ease, it is generally the diagnostic procedure of choice. In the traumatic or urgent situation, a portable chest film should be obtained. However, supine or semireclined films can miss anterior pneumothoraces or small volumes of fluid or blood in the chest. Formal posterior-anterior and lateral chest films can be obtained in stable, elective patients.
- The extended FAST or eFAST examination, a point-of-care ultrasound of the chest, is becoming a more popular diagnostic modality and is being used as an adjunct to the primary trauma survey. The chest is examined with an ultrasound in both a coronal view over both diaphragms and a sagittal view over the 2nd intercostal space, midclavicular line to assess for lung sliding movement across the pleura, which correlates with no pneumothorax. Anechoic areas correlate with fluid in the chest. While the sensitivity of eFAST is varied in the published data, a recent meta-analysis has shown that the sensitivity of eFAST is higher than that of chest x-ray (91% vs 47%, respectively). The specificity of eFAST is similar to that of chest x-ray (99% vs 100%, respectively).[1]
- Chest computed tomography is the gold standard for diagnosing chest pathology. Venous or arterial contrast is used in cases of trauma and certain cancers, although this is not necessary to diagnose air or fluid in the chest. Simple fluid vs blood may be differentiated based on its density, with blood having higher Houndsfield units than simple fluid.

SURGICAL MANAGEMENT

Preoperative Planning

- In nonemergent situations, consent should be obtained and the surgeon should discuss the diagnosis, procedure, and potential complications with the patient.
- Needle decompression, tube thoracostomy, and thoracentesis all can be done at the bedside, whether on the floor, in the intensive care unit, or in the emergency department.
- In general, antibiotics are not needed as long as sterile technique is maintained. For procedures in which sterile technique is broken, a one-time dose of cefazolin (2 g) should suffice as antibiotic prophylaxis.[2]
- Prior to starting the procedure, the surgeon or practitioner should confirm the correct side is being addressed and ensure that all necessary materials are available at the bedside. When performing a thoracentesis, it is prudent to ensure quick access to the instruments necessary to perform a tube or finger thoracostomy in case of inadvertent tension pneumothorax or hemothorax.
- If a massive hemothorax is suspected, an autotransfuser collection chamber may be used to collect blood and transfuse back to the patient. The autotransfuser should be primed with 1 mL sterile sodium citrate per 10 mL of blood. There is controversy regarding the clinical benefit and utility of autotransfusing blood, as it is coagulopathic.
- If patient stability permits, a standard preprocedure time out should be performed prior to tube thoracostomy or thoracentesis. In addition, IV analgesia or local anesthesia should be used. Procedural moderate sedation can be considered in the stable patient to aid in patient comfort.
- Full sterile technique should be maintained for any nonemergent procedure. Sterile gloves, gown, and draping should be used in addition to provider masking, hair coverage, and eye protection.

Positioning

- Needle decompression
  - Patients may be positioned either supine or upright for a needle decompression.
- Tube thoracostomy
  - In the emergent trauma scenario, the patient should be positioned supine with the arm positioned over the head to open up the intercostal spaces.
  - In a nonemergent situation, the patient can be positioned either supine with the arm abducted at 90° or slightly propped in a lateral decubitus position.
- Thoracentesis
  - Positioning for a thoracentesis will depend somewhat on the volume of fluid, indication for the procedure, and experience of the practitioner.
  - Traditionally, a thoracentesis is performed with the patient upright and arms resting anteriorly.
  - A more common and applicable approach is often with the patient supine, slightly in reverse Trendelenburg position, with the arm abducted at 90°. This positioning allows a weak or less stable patient to rest in bed while also allowing the dependent collection of fluid in the base of the thoracic cavity.
  - Ultrasound of the chest prior to the procedure to ensure proper positioning increases the accuracy and decreases the chance of complications.

NEEDLE DECOMPRESSION

- A large-bore, size 10 to 14 gauge, angiocath needle is optimal for performing a needle decompression. The angiocath should not be less than 3.25 in in length. Alternatively, a similarly gauged spinal needle may be used and can be preferred for its increased length. Angiocath sheaths are prone to kinking if there is undue tension on the chest wall or skin.
- Needle decompression may be performed in the second intercostal space, midclavicular line, or the 4th or 5th intercostal space midaxillary line. Data show that providers are more comfortable, more confident, and more successful with the midaxillary line approach[3] (**FIGURE 3**).
- If there is time, which there is often not, the skin is quickly swiped with Betadine or chlorhexidine.
- The intercostal space is palpated and the needle is inserted at 90° over the rib directly into the thoracic cavity until air release is heard. Angling of the needle may result in inadvertent injury to the intercostal bundle.
- If an angiocath is used, the needle should be removed, leaving the catheter in place.

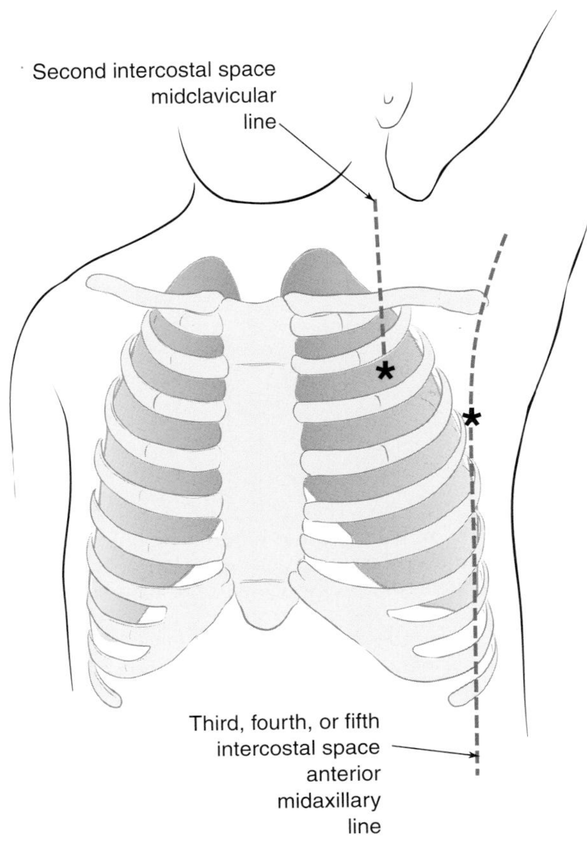

- The catheter or needle should be left open to the atmosphere to allow for continued release of air from the thoracic cavity.
- Needle decompression is a temporizing procedure and should be followed by a tube thoracostomy.

FIGURE 3 ● Needle decompression may occur at either the 2nd intercostal space in the midclavicular line or in the 3rd-5th intercostal space, midaxillary line. Asterisk marks the site of needle decompression. (Reprinted with permission from Connors KM, Terndrup TE. Tube thoracostomy and needle decompression of the chest. In: Henretig FM, King C, eds. *Textbook of Pediatric Emergency Procedures*. Lippincott Williams & Wilkins; 1997:399.)

TUBE THORACOSTOMY

- A 28 or 32 Fr straight chest tube is sufficient for most clinical applications, including traumatic hemothorax. No benefit has been found to using a larger-size chest tube for traumatic hemothorax.[4]
- With the arm positioned over the head to open up the intercostal spaces, the chest is prepped with Betadine or chlorhexidine from the axilla to the costal margin, and from medial to the nipple line to the bed. The chest should be draped with sterile blue towels and ideally surgical drapes.
- The 4th or 5th intercostal space is palpated in the midaxillary line.
- Local anesthetic, commonly 1% or 2% lidocaine with or without epinephrine, can be used to create a skin wheal in the planned incision site. Local anesthetic is then injected at a 90° angle to the ribs into the intercostal muscle and pleura.
- A 2-cm incision is made with a 15-blade scalpel in the direction of the ribs overlying the intercostal space or rib immediately beneath it.
- The subcutaneous tissue, including fat and muscle, is spread with a clamp, creating a tunnel wide enough for a finger or chest tube to pass easily. Alternatively, for emergent procedures, the subcutaneous tissue is cut with the scalpel down to the level of the rib. This facilitates quicker access to the chest cavity.
- There is no benefit to tunneling rib space above the incision site. This technique is often fraught with difficulty, increasing the chance of complications and making it more difficult to find the tunnel to insert the tube.
- A curved clamp is used to enter the thoracic cavity by pushing just over the superior surface of the rib (inferior surface of the intercostal space) until a pop into the pleura is felt. The dominant hand should control the clamp while the nondominant hand should be used to brace the clamp and ensure it does not continue to travel once the pleura has been entered (**FIGURE 4A**).
- The clamp is then spread open. It is prudent to use two hands to generate enough force to create a tract large enough to pass a finger or tube. As the clamp is slowly backed out of the chest wall, it is successively opened and spread.
- A finger is inserted through the tract into the thoracic cavity. The finger is swept along the internal pleural border to ensure proper entrance into the thoracic cavity and to ensure that there are no prohibitive adhesions from the lung or heart to the pleura (**FIGURE 4B**).
- The chest tube is clamped on its distal end to prevent unnecessary spillage of blood. A clamp is also placed on its proximal end in order to guide the chest tube (**FIGURE 4C**).
- The chest tube is then guided through the tract into the thoracic cavity. The clamp on the proximal end of the tube is removed. The chest tube should usually be directed in a posterior and apical position. The chest tube is further advanced into the chest (**FIGURE 5**).
- On an average-sized adult, the chest tube may be positioned at 12 cm at the level of the skin. Large adults may require chest tubes to be placed at deeper positions.
- The tube should be rotated 360° after insertion to confirm that it is not kinked or in the fissure of the lung.

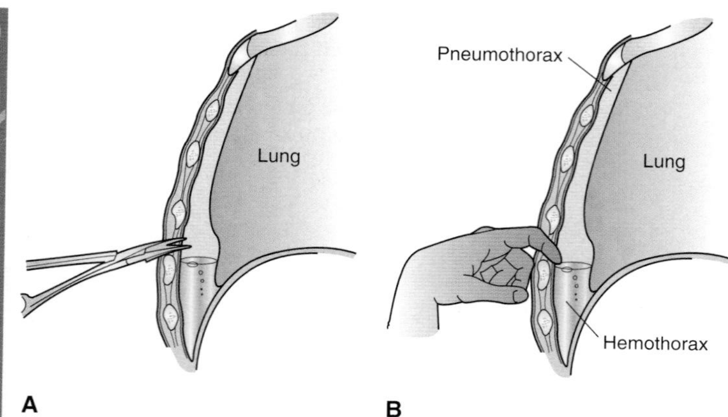

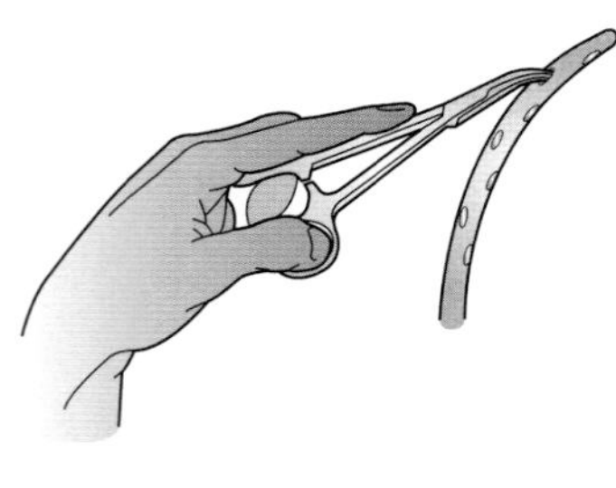

FIGURE 4 • **A,** Pleural space entered by blunt spreading of the clamp over the top of the adjacent rib. **B,** A finger is introduced to ensure position within the pleural space and to lyse adhesions. **C,** The thoracostomy tube is placed into the tunnel and directed with the help of a Kelly clamp. The tube is directed posterior and caudal for an effusion or hemothorax and cephalad for a pneumothorax. (Reprinted with permission from Klingensmith ME. *The Washington Manual of Surgery*. 7th ed. Wolters Kluwer; 2016. Figure 14.4.)

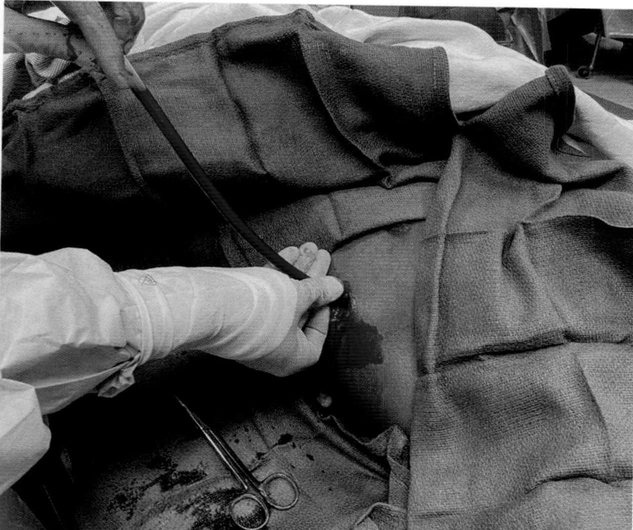

FIGURE 5 • The chest tube is advanced superiorly and posteriorly in the thoracic cavity.

- The chest tube should be secured to the skin with a heavy, nonabsorbable suture like a 0-silk.
- A "U-stitch" may be placed around the tube at time of insertion to facilitate airtight closure upon chest tube removal. This suture is not necessary, however, and is placed at the discretion of the provider. If placed, it should not be tied down until the chest tube is removed.
- The chest tube should be connected to a Pleur-evac at −20 mm H_2O suction.
- A sterile, occlusive dressing should be placed. Xeroform or Vaseline gauze is wrapped around the tube at its juncture with the skin. A 4 × 4 gauze is used to pad and cover the tube. The gauze is then covered with nonperforated tape.
- A portable chest x-ray should be obtained as soon as possible after insertion to confirm correct positioning (**FIGURE 6**).

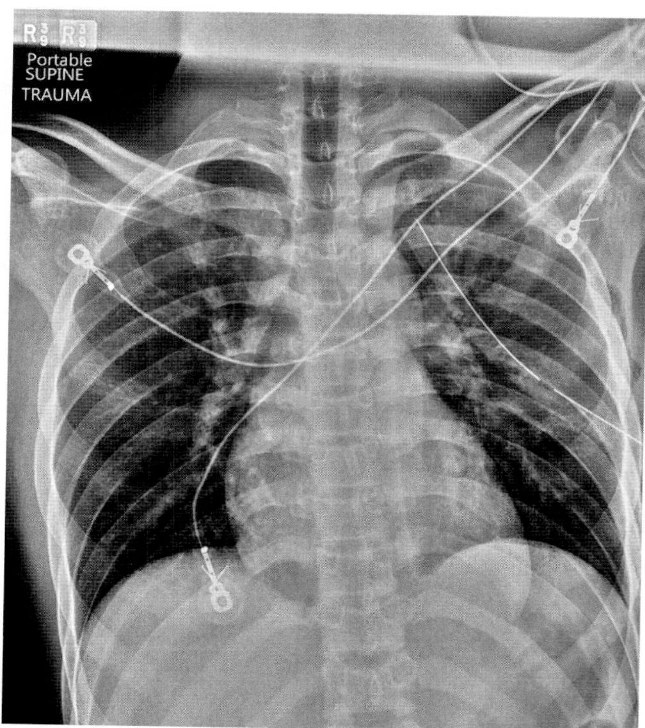

FIGURE 6 • A well-positioned left thoracostomy tube.

THORACENTESIS

- A thoracentesis may be performed posteriorly in an upright patient or in the mid- to posterior axillary line in a supine patient. In either case, the procedure should be performed in the 5th to 7th intercostal space. Lower drainage sites risk damage to the diaphragm or intra-abdominal organs while higher drainage sites risk missing the fluid collection and damaging the lung. Ultrasound will help to define these anatomic landmarks.
- After ultrasound localization, the site of thoracentesis is chosen. The skin is prepped with Betadine or chlorhexidine in a wide margin and draped with sterile blue towels and surgical drapes. The provider should be dressed in a sterile gown and gloves, with cap, mask, and eye protection.
- Similarly to a tube thoracostomy, local anesthetic should be used to create a skin wheal in the planned incision site. Local anesthetic is then injected at a 90° angle to the ribs into the intercostal muscle and pleura.
- The introducer needle with syringe attached is advanced at 90° to the ribs or chest wall on the superior border of the rib (inferior border of the intercostal space) through the incision, subcutaneous tissue and muscle and into the thoracic cavity. Negative pressure should be applied to the syringe as it is advanced forward (**FIGURE 7**).
- Needle advancement should stop when there is fluid return in the syringe.
- If a simple thoracentesis is planned, the needle is then connected to catheter tubing and a collection bag or negative pressure vacuum container until the desired amount of fluid is removed (**FIGURE 8**).
- If a temporary pigtail catheter is desired, while the needle is held steadily in place, the syringe is removed and the guidewire is inserted through the introducer needle. The needle is then removed, leaving the guidewire in place. A small, subcentimeter incision is made around the guidewire with an 11- or a 15-blade scalpel. Tissue dilators are then advanced over the guidewire with increasing succession in size, maintaining control of the guidewire at all times. A pigtail catheter with catheter stiffener inserted is then advanced over the guidewire into the thoracic cavity. The catheter stiffener and guidewire are then simultaneously removed, leaving the pigtail catheter in place. The pigtail can be secured with a large, nonabsorbable suture, such as a 0-silk. The pigtail catheter is then connected via tubing to a Pleur-evac system set to −20 mm H_2O (**FIGURE 9**)
- A chest x-ray should be obtained after the procedure to ensure proper drainage or catheter positioning.

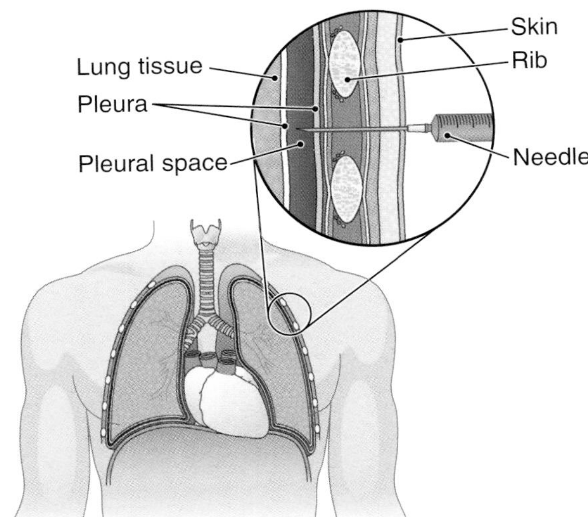

FIGURE 7 • The needle is directed at 90° into the fluid collection. (Reprinted with permission from: Cohen BJ, DePetris A. *Medical Terminology*. 8th ed. Wolters Kluwer; 2017. Figure 11.13.)

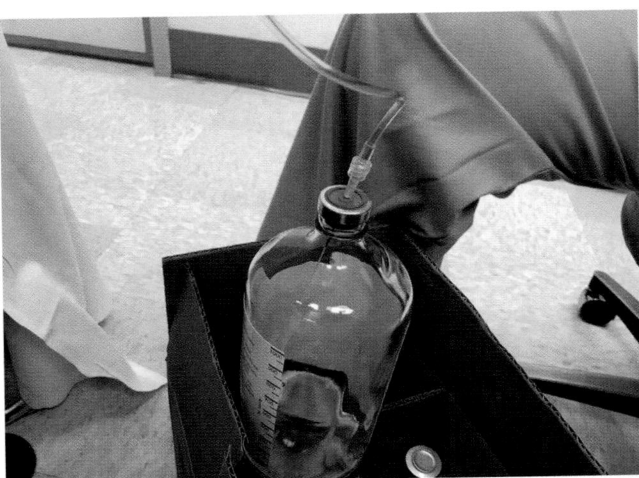

FIGURE 8 • Vacuum container for collecting effusion. (Reprinted with permission from Bornemann P. *Ultrasound for Primary Care*. Wolters Kluwer; 2021. Figure 54.15.)

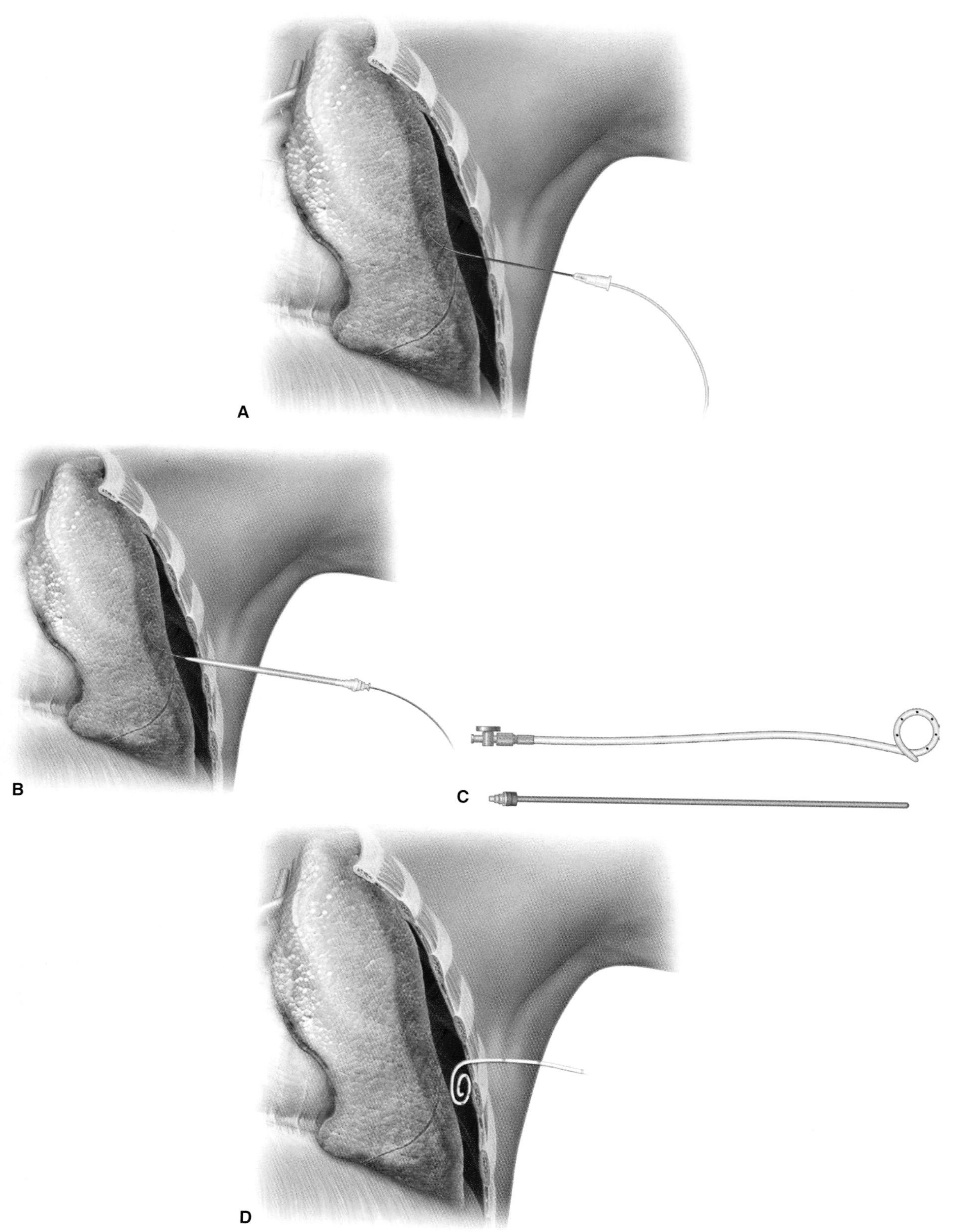

FIGURE 9 ● **A,** Syringe is removed and the guidewire is inserted through the introducer needle. **B,** Tissue dilators are then advanced over the guidewire with increasing succession in size, maintaining control of the guidewire at all times. **C,** A pigtail catheter with catheter stiffener inserted is then advanced over the guidewire into the thoracic cavity. **D,** The catheter stiffener and guidewire are then simultaneously removed, leaving the pigtail catheter in place.

PEARLS AND PITFALLS

Technique	▪ Care must be taken to avoid injury to the intercostal artery or vein by using an incorrect needle or clamp angle. The needle or clamp should be inserted straight into the chest over the ribs at 90° to minimize the chance of intercostal bundle damage. ▪ Air leaks in the Pleur-evac system should be investigated by first ensuring that all tubing is properly connected and the chest tube is in proper position in the chest, with the sentinel hole within the thoracic cavity. Air leaks from pulmonary parenchymal trauma are not uncommon and usually resolve in a matter of days. A persistent or large air leak should be worked up with a flexible bronchoscopy to check for tracheo- or bronchopulmonary fistula. ▪ Drainage of greater than 2 L at one time during a thoracentesis will increase the risk of re-expansion pulmonary edema. ▪ Maintaining control of the needle during a needle decompression or thoracentesis will decrease the risk of iatrogenic damage to intrathoracic structures.
Surgical management	▪ Adequate patient pain control, whether through local anesthesia or with sedation, will ensure a smoother and more comfortable operation.
Postoperative care	▪ Encouraging the patient to cough promotes lung re-expansion and drainage of blood and fluid.

POSTOPERATIVE CARE

- Needle decompression
  - A tube thoracostomy should be placed as soon as possible after a needle decompression.
- Tube thoracostomy
  - Chest tubes are normally maintained on wall suction with the Pleur-evac set to −20 cm H_2O suction. With resolution of the pneumothorax or hemothorax, the Pleur-evac may be placed on water seal.
  - Daily chest x-rays should be obtained to assess the patient and the chest tube system.
  - A malpositioned or nonfunctional tube should never be repositioned further into the chest after the sterile field of the index procedure is broken. If needed, an existing chest tube should be removed and a new chest tube should be inserted through a different incision.
  - Chest tubes should not be clamped except when treating retained hemothorax or loculations with intrathoracic tissue plasminogen activator (tPA).
  - Chest tubes may be considered for removal when the drainage is less than 100 to 200 mL/24 h and pneumothorax is absent or minimal and stable. The chest tube is placed on a trial of water seal for at least 4 hours prior to chest tube removal. A chest x-ray is obtained after this time to ensure there has not been the development of a pneumothorax.
  - Chest tubes may be removed at end inspiration, during expiration, or while the patient performs a Valsalva maneuver.
  - There are two methods of chest tube removal. In a two-provider scenario, one provider quickly pulls the chest tube while the second provider ties down the U-stitch skin suture. An occlusive dressing is then placed. A U-stitch closure should not generally be used if only one provider is present. In this case, after the securing sutures are cut, the tube is pulled while an occlusive dressing with Xeroform or Vaseline gauze covered with 4 × 4 gauze is simultaneously held against the insertion site.
  - Portable chest x-ray should be obtained within 4 hours after chest tube removal.
- Thoracentesis
  - After the desired amount of fluid is removed or the output is less than 50 to 100 mL/d, the needle or catheter is pulled from the chest and an occlusive dressing with Xeroform or Vaseline gauze covered with 4 × 4 gauze is immediately placed.
  - A chest x-ray should be obtained following catheter or needle removal.

COMPLICATIONS

- Injury to the intercostal bundle on the inferior surface of the rib can happen with incorrect needle or clamp angling. An injury to the intercostal vein will often stop on its own. An intercostal artery injury may require interventional radiology embolization or even thoracotomy to control.
- Chest tubes are often malpositioned in the fissure of the lung or basally. These tubes are usually not salvageable if the complication is not recognized immediately on placement (**FIGURE 10**).
- A chest tube that is placed too far into the chest may abut the mediastinum including heart and mediastinal vessels or apically abutting the subclavian vessels. These tubes should be pulled back to appropriate position based on chest x-ray to ensure no damage to the vessels (**FIGURE 11**).
- When not placed carefully, chest tubes can perforate thoracic organs and vascular structures. A chest tube placed through the parenchyma of the lung should be left in place for 24 to 48 hours to allow for tamponade through the tract.

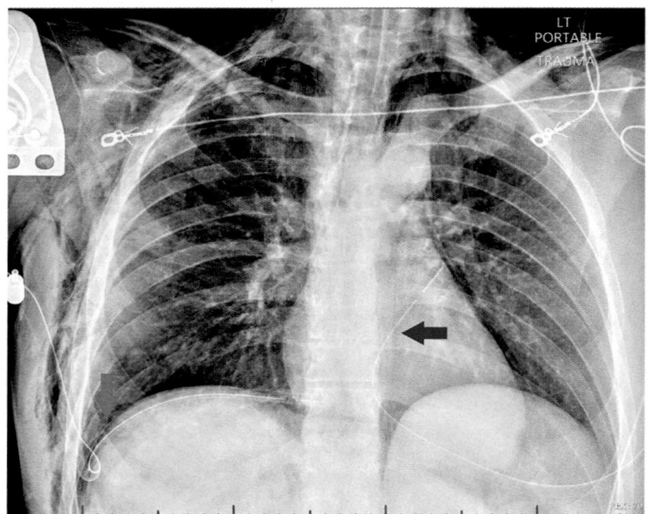

FIGURE 10 ● Bilateral malpositioned chest tubes. *Red arrow* points to basally directed chest tube. *Blue arrow* points to chest tube abutting the mediastinum.

Perforation of other mediastinal or thoracic structures may require immediate thoracotomy.

- A needle decompression, tube thoracostomy, or thoracentesis performed too inferior in the chest may cause iatrogenic damage to the diaphragm or intra-abdominal organs.
- Retained hemothorax is a frequent complication of tube thoracostomy placement for trauma to the chest. There are various management strategies depending on the preference of the surgeon and institution. A second chest tube may be placed to attempt to drain the residual blood. Administration of intrapleural thrombolytics (tPA) is also appropriate. Our protocol for tPA administration is to inject 50 mg tPA in 100 mL NS (tPA concentration 0.5 mg/mL) through chest tube daily × 3 days using sterile technique. The chest tube is clamped for 1 to 2 hours while the patient is rolled or allowed to ambulate to distribute the thrombolytics throughout the chest. The tube is then unclamped and the lytics are drained. Finally, VATS (Video Assisted Thoracoscopic Surgery) is an increasingly popular method of managing retained hemothorax. If chosen, it should be employed early, within 3 to 7 days of presentation, to reduce the chance of need for conversion to thoracotomy.

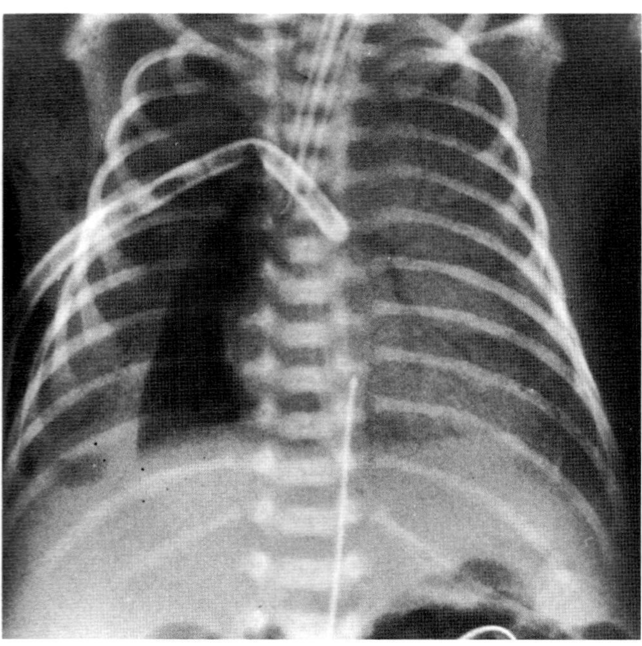

FIGURE 11 ● The tip of the thoracostomy tube has been advanced too far medially and is kinked against the mediastinum. Withdrawing the tube 1 or 2 cm would improve drainage at the medial thorax. Note the endotracheal tube tip in the right mainstem bronchus. (Reprinted with permission from MacDonald MG, Ramasethu J, Rais-Bahrami K. *Atlas of Procedures in Neonatology*. 5th ed. Wolters Kluwer; 2013. Figure 38.22.)

REFERENCES

1. Chan KK, Joo DA, McRae AD, et al. Chest ultrasonography versus supine chest radiography for diagnosis of pneumothorax in trauma patients in the emergency department. *Cochrane Database Syst Rev*. 2020;7(7):CD013031.
2. Cook A, Hu C, Ward J, et al. Presumptive antibiotics in tube thoracostomy for traumatic hemopneumothorax: a prospective, Multicenter American Association for the Surgery of Trauma Study. *Trauma Surg Acute Care Open*. 2019;4(1):e000356.
3. Inaba K, Karamanos E, Skiada D, et al. Cadaveric comparison of the optimal site for needle decompression of tension pneumothorax by prehospital care providers. *J Trauma Acute Care Surg*. 2015;79(6):1044-1048.
4. Inaba K, Lustenberger T, Recinos G, et al. Does size matter? A prospective analysis of 28-32 versus 36-40 French chest tube size in trauma. *J Trauma Acute Care Surg*. 2012;72(2):422-427.

Chapter 7 Pleurodesis

Jennifer T. Cone and Selwyn O. Rogers Jr.

DEFINITION

- Pleurodesis is defined as a procedure performed to adhere the visceral pleura of the lung to the parietal pleura of the chest wall to prevent the reaccumulation of fluid or air. It may be employed with various different techniques, including mechanical or chemical means. All methods of pleurodesis rely on an inflammatory process to create fibrinous adhesions between the visceral and parietal pleura, eliminating any potential space in the thoracic cavity.

Differential Diagnosis

- Pleurodesis can be used for a variety of clinical situations. Patients who have recurrent spontaneous pneumothoraces or malignant pleural effusions will benefit most from pleurodesis. Less commonly, pleurodesis can be used for persistent air leaks and recurrent chylothorax as an adjunct to more definitive surgical management.

Patient History and Physical Findings

- Patient history will vary based on diagnosis.
- Patients with recurrent spontaneous pneumothorax often have a diagnosis of bleb disease of the lung. Patients present with abrupt shortness of breath, decreased breath sounds, and hyperresonance on percussion. Management of this disease will vary based on surgeon and institution preference; however, pleurodesis can be indicated for the second episode of ipsilateral spontaneous pneumothorax.
- Patients with malignant pleural effusions generally have a pre-existing diagnosis of cancer. They present with worsening shortness of breath and cough. Exam findings include decreased breath sounds and dullness to percussion on the affected side. There is a high percentage of reaccumulation of fluid in the chest following a simple drainage procedure.[1] Patients with malignant pleural effusions have multifactorial causes of dyspnea. Pleurodesis should only be considered when drainage of fluid has shown symptom relief (**FIGURE 1**).

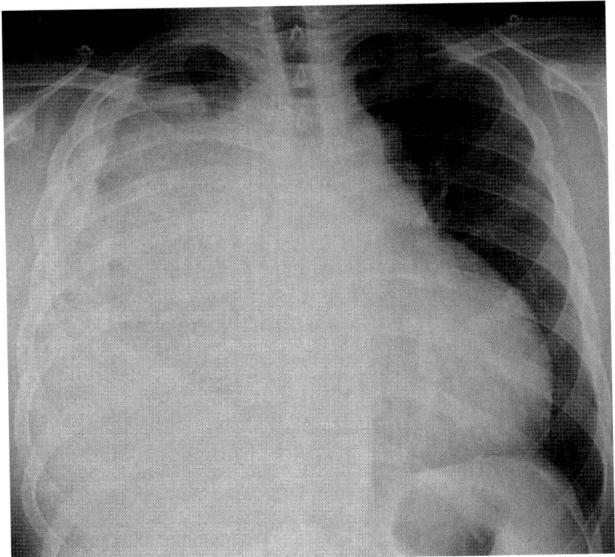

FIGURE 1 • Right sided malignant pleural effusion. (Reprinted with permission from Lee E. *Pediatric Radiology: Practical Imaging Evaluation of Infants and Children*. Wolters Kluwer; 2018. Figure 7.28A.)

IMAGING AND OTHER DIAGNOSTIC STUDIES

- A chest X-ray is usually sufficient for diagnosis of both recurrent pneumothorax and pleural effusion; however, chest computed tomography remains the gold standard diagnostic study.

SURGICAL MANAGEMENT

Preoperative Planning

- Consent should be obtained and the practitioner should discuss the diagnosis, procedure, and potential complications with the patient.
- Full sterile technique should be maintained if a new thoracostomy tube is placed for any operative intervention. For bedside chemical pleurodesis, it is acceptable to simply prep the insertion port on the tube and for the practitioner to use sterile gloves and a mask.
- Adequate analgesia should be provided as chemical pleurodesis can be painful. If performed at the bedside, IV pain medication can be used, but it may be more comfortable for the patient to receive moderate sedation during installation of chemicals into the chest.
- Local anesthetic, such as 1% or 2% lidocaine, should be directly applied to the pleura by infusing the anesthetic through the chest tube. There is no consensus on the volume of anesthetic to infuse, but volumes of up to 250 mg have been described. Clamp the tube for at least 10 minutes and rotate the patient to ensure even distribution.
- If performed at the bedside, continuous heart rate, blood pressure, and pulse oximetry monitoring should be used.
- Operative management for recurrent pneumothorax from bleb disease usually involves simultaneous blebectomy, which is described elsewhere.
- In general, a video-assisted thoracoscopic surgical (VATS) approach is preferred and better tolerated than an open thoracotomy.

Positioning

- For a bedside pleurodesis, the patient can be positioned supine with the arm abducted at 90° or in a lateral decubitus position with the arm overhead or resting anteriorly.
- Full positioning for VATS and thoracotomy is described elsewhere in this textbook.

STEPS

Chemical

- There are multiple methods of chemical pleurodesis. Talc, bleomycin, and tetracycline (and other cyclines) have all been described in the literature, with talc being more effective than bleomycin or tetracycline.[2]
- Chemical pleurodesis is most successful when there is already reasonable contact between the visceral and parietal pleura. If a large pneumothorax or pleural effusion is present, a chemical pleurodesis is not likely to be successful.
- A bedside procedure is possible if no decortication or lung exploration is required. However, this can be painful and adequate analgesia should be provided as described above.
- If no thoracostomy tube is present, one is placed as described in a previous chapter. A small bore chest tube, 14 to 16 Fr is acceptable in this clinical scenario.
- The sclerosing medication is instilled through the port site on an existing thoracostomy tube. The tube is then clamped with a heavy clamp while the medication is allowed to spread throughout the thoracic cavity. The patient can ambulate or be rolled to facilitate distribution throughout the thorax.
  - Talc slurry is used at a ratio of 4 g talc in 30 mL sterile saline. Flushing the thoracostomy tube with 10 to 20 mL saline will help ensure that the entire amount of slurry reaches the thoracic cavity. The infusion should be left in place for 60 minutes.
  - Talc may also be applied surgically as a powder (poudrage) during a thoracoscopy or a thoracotomy.
  - There is sparse evidence directly comparing a talc slurry to a talc powder application. One study does point to decreased recurrence rates in patients with secondary spontaneous pneumothorax with surgically placed talc powder during thoracostomy.[3] In patients with malignant pleural effusions, there appears to be no difference in outcomes between slurry and powder.[4]
    - Bleomycin is dosed at 1 U/kg.
    - Tetracycline is dosed at 10 to 20 mg/kg. It may be difficult to acquire in parenteral form.
  - The thoracostomy tube is then unclamped and the sclerosing agent is allowed to drain out of the chest.
  - A daily follow-up chest X-ray should be ordered.

Blood

- Blood pleurodesis has been described most commonly for patients with persistent air leaks that are unable to tolerate surgery. It is successful in up to 91% of patients.[5]
- Blood pleurodesis may be used in a manner similar to chemical pleurodesis described above. The patient's own blood is drawn and injected through a thoracostomy tube. There is no consensus regarding the volume of blood instilled through the chest tube. Described volumes range from 50 mL total up to 3 mL/kg.
- Blood pleurodesis has been shown to be superior to conservative management in patients with secondary spontaneous pneumothorax who cannot undergo surgery.[6]

Mechanical

- Mechanical pleurodesis can be achieved with pleural abrasion or with a formal pleurectomy. In patients undergoing decortication after retained hemothorax or empyema, pleural abrasions are created naturally as part of the debridement process.
- Pleurectomy has been found to be slightly more successful than creating pleural abrasions but is associated with a higher complication rate.[7,8]
- Both VATS and thoracotomy are described in other chapters.
  - During a VATS procedure, a 5- or 10-mm camera is inserted into the thoracic cavity. Additional ports are placed for retraction and surgical manipulation (**FIGURE 2**).
  - During a thoracotomy, a posterolateral incision is made in the chest, generally in the 5th-7th intercostal spaces. The chest is open to facilitate direct surgical access to the thoracic cavity (**FIGURE 3**).
  - Mechanical pleurodesis can occur naturally during a decortication procedure where adhesions and pleural rind are manually stripped off the lung and parietal pleura. It can also occur intentionally by creating abrasions with gauze or a dedicated pleural abrasion device.
  - Pleurectomy should be approached with caution. It is a major surgical procedure with the potential for complications. If follow-up thoracotomy will be needed for any indication, adhesions from prior pleurectomy make the procedure much more difficult. For this reason, most surgeons will perform a partial pleurectomy. Specifically, an apical pleurectomy will generally allow future thoracotomies. However, this is only applicable in cases of apical pneumothoraces.
  - In a parietal pleurectomy, the pleural lining of the thoracic cavity is surgically removed. This may be done sharply, but is often done with a combination of electrocautery and blunt dissection (**FIGURES 4** and **5**).

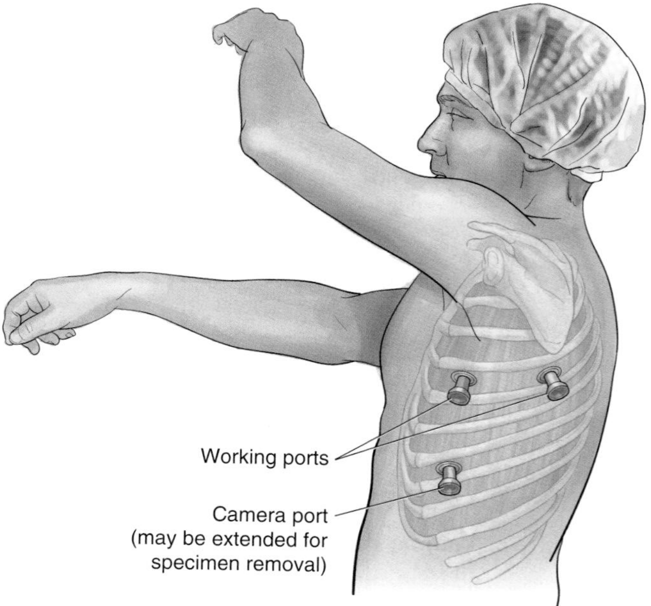

FIGURE 2 ● The standard patient and port positioning for a VATS procedure. (Reprinted with permission from LoCicero J. *Shields' General Thoracic Surgery*. 8th ed. Wolters Kluwer; 2019. Figure 27.6.)

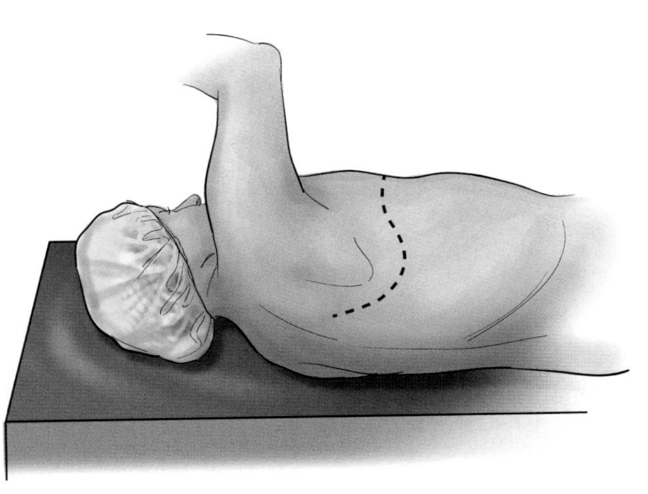

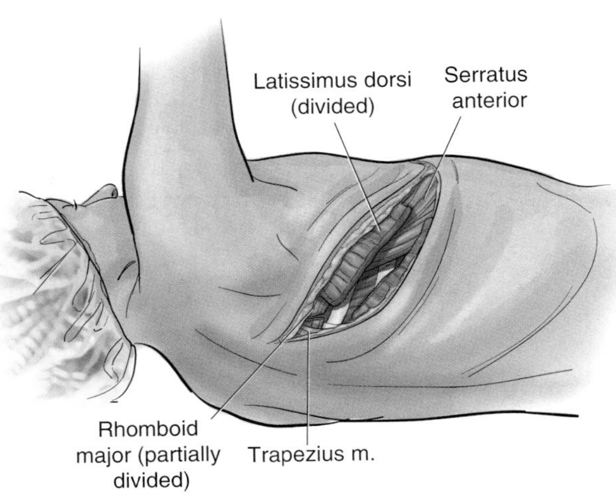

FIGURE 3 ● The patient is positioned in a lateral decubitus position and a curvilinear incision is made in the 5-7th intercostal spaces to best facilitate access to the thoracic cavity. (Reprinted with permission from LoCicero J. *Shields' General Thoracic Surgery*. 8th ed. Wolters Kluwer; 2019. Figure 27.9.)

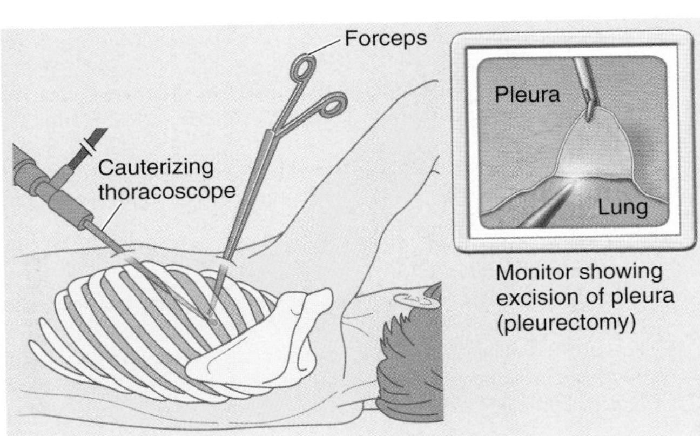

FIGURE 4 ● The pleura is stripped off the lung and pleural cavity. (Reprinted with permission from Agur AMR, Dalley AF II *Moore's Essential Clinical Anatomy*. 6th ed. Wolters Kluwer; 2020. UnFigure 4.9.)

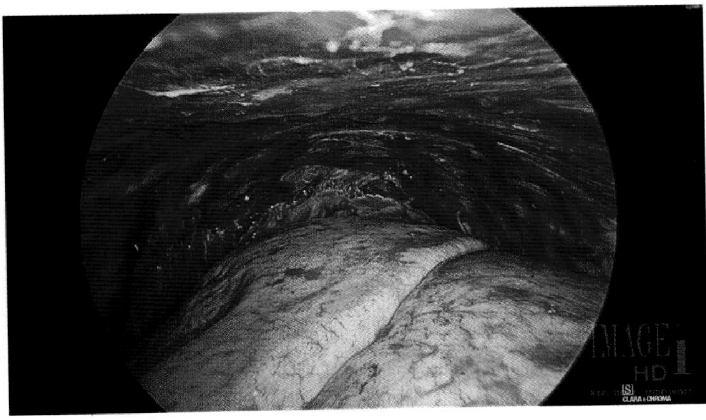

FIGURE 5 ● The appearance of the chest following a partial pleurectomy. (Reprinted with permission from DeVita VT, Rosenberg SA, Lawrence TS. *DeVita, Hellman, and Rosenberg's Cancer: Principles & Practice of Oncology*. 11th ed. Wolters Kluwer; 2019. Figure 120.4.)

PEARLS AND PITFALLS

Steroids	▪ The concurrent use of systemic steroids will decrease the success of pleurodesis, as the steroids will decrease the inflammation necessary for the sclerosing reaction to take place. If possible, stop use of steroids prior to pleurodesis.
Patient history and physical findings	▪ In patients with persistent air leaks, bedside clamping of a chest tube after chemical or blood pleurodesis should not be performed. Instead, gravity can be used to instill the pleurodesis material into the thorax while simultaneously allowing air to escape and preventing development of a tension pneumothorax.

POSTOPERATIVE CARE

- Following pleurodesis, a chest tube is maintained on suction at −20 mm H_2O to allow the best juxtaposition of the visceral and parietal pleura.
- The chest tube should remain in place until there is less than 100 mL/d.
- Chest tube removal is described in detail in previous chapters.

COMPLICATIONS

- The most common complications following pleurodesis are pain and fever.
- ARDS following talc infusion has been reported in multiple instances in the literature.[9,10] It has been reported with both high and low doses of talc and both powder and slurry installation. Small particle talc preparations, which are used predominantly in the United States, are associated with greater lung and systemic inflammatory response.[11]
- There is a higher rate of postoperative hemothorax with pleurectomy, as it is a more involved procedure than either chemical pleurodesis or the creation of pleural abrasions.

REFERENCES

1. Anderson CB, Philpott GW, Ferguson TB. The treatment of malignant pleural effusions. *Cancer*. 1974;33(4):916-922.
2. Dipper A, Jones HE, Bhatnagar R, Preston NJ, Maskell N, Clive AO. Interventions for the management of malignant pleural effusions: a network meta-analysis. *Cochrane Database Syst Rev*. 2020;4(4):CD010529.
3. Kim SJ, Lee HS, Kim HS et al. Outcome of video-assisted thoracoscopic surgery for spontaneous secondary pneumothorax. *Korean J Thorac Cardiovasc Surg*. 2011;44:225–228.
4. Bhatnagar R, Piotrowska HEG, Laskawiec-Szkonter M, et al. Effect of thoracoscopic talc poudrage vs talc slurry via chest tube on pleurodesis failure rate among patients with malignant pleural effusions: a randomized clinical trial. *JAMA*. 2020;323(1):60-69.
5. Chambers A, Routledge T, Billè A, Scarci M. Is blood pleurodesis effective for determining the cessation of persistent air leak? *Interact Cardiovasc Thorac Surg*. 2010;11(4):468-472. 6.
6. Ibrahim IM, Elaziz MEA, El-Hag-Aly MA. Early autologous blood-patch pleurodesis versus conservative management for treatment of secondary spontaneous pneumothorax. *Thorac Cardiovasc Surg*. 2019;67(3):222-226.
7. Weeden D, Smith GH. Surgical experience in the management of spontaneous pneumothorax, 1972–82. *Thorax*. 1983;38(10):737-743. 35.
8. Thomas P, Le Mee F, Le Hors H et al. Results of surgical treatment of persistent or recurrent pneumothorax. *Ann Chir*. 1993;47(2):136-140.
9. Campos JR, Werebe EC, Vargas FS et al. Respiratory failure due to insufflated talc. *Lancet*. 1997;349(9047):251-252. 150.
10. Rehse DH, Aye RW, Florence MG. Respiratory failure following talc pleurodesis. *Am J Surg*. 1999;177(5):437-440. 154.
11. Janssen JP, Collier G, Astoul P, et al. Safety of pleurodesis with talc poudrage in malignant pleural effusion: a prospective cohort study. *Lancet*. 2007;369(9572):1535-1539.

Chapter 8 Video-Assisted Thoracoscopic Surgery for Retained Hemothorax and Empyema

Morgan Schellenberg and Kenji Inaba

DEFINITION

- A retained hemothorax is defined as a hemothorax that is partially or completely undrained after chest tube insertion.
- The potential consequences of a retained hemothorax, if left in situ, include empyema, entrapped lung, and fibrothorax.
- Most retained hemothoraces occur in the setting of chest trauma, with larger initial hemothoraces predicting the development of retained hemothorax.[1]
- The optimal therapy for retained hemothorax remains controversial and depends largely on timing, volume of retained hemothorax, and institutional practices. Options include intrapleural fibrinolytics, additional chest tube or pigtail catheter placement, and video-assisted thoracoscopic surgery (VATS) for evacuation.
- VATS is a minimally invasive approach to thoracic surgery in which ports are placed percutaneously into the pleural space. Through these, instruments are passed into the pleural space to perform a variety of thoracic procedures. VATS for retained hemothorax or empyema typically involves, at a minimum, insertion of a camera port and one additional port to pass a suction catheter into the chest for removal of retained blood or pus, respectively.

DIFFERENTIAL DIAGNOSIS

- Initial diagnosis of a retained hemothorax is typically accomplished with a chest X-ray (CXR) (**FIGURE 1**). With this imaging modality, it may be challenging to distinguish a retained hemothorax from atelectasis or other lung consolidation of the lower lobes.[2] Therefore, if CXR suggests a retained hemothorax, a computed tomography (CT) scan of the chest with intravenous contrast is the next step to distinguish between these diagnoses.

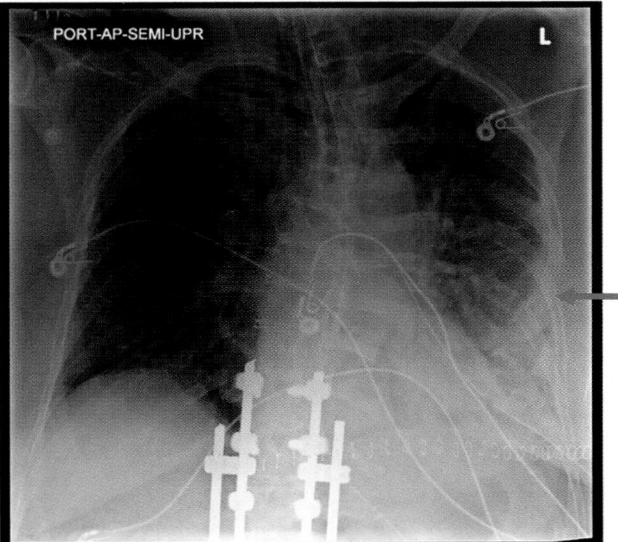

FIGURE 1 • Upright chest X-ray demonstrating left hemothorax following blunt trauma. Loss of the costodiaphragmatic recess and a meniscus sign against the chest wall (*arrow*) are demonstrated.

PATIENT HISTORY AND PHYSICAL FINDINGS

- Retained hemothoraces are typically the result of chest trauma but can also occur following thoracic surgery or procedures, such as lung biopsy. Empyemas occur from a variety of etiologies, including retained hemothoraces,[3] pneumonia, and as a complication of chest procedures. The patient history should elicit the presence or absence of these risk factors.
- In many patients, retained hemothoraces are asymptomatic. However, shortness of breath and chest pain may be present.
- Physical examination may be normal or reveal hypoxia, increased work of breathing, and dullness to percussion or diminished breath sounds over the lower lung fields.
- Signs and symptoms of empyema are similar to those of retained hemothorax but may additionally include infectious signs and symptoms, including fever.

IMAGING AND OTHER DIAGNOSTIC STUDIES

- Chest radiographs and CT scans are the most common imaging studies used to diagnose hemothoraces.
- An upright CXR will reveal loss of the costodiaphragmatic recess and sometimes a meniscus sign against the chest wall (**FIGURE 1**). If the CXR is taken supine, it may appear normal or demonstrate layering of the hemothorax throughout the ipsilateral chest cavity (**FIGURE 2**).
- CT scan will demonstrate the presence of pleural fluid (**FIGURE 3**). Measurement of the fluid's density in Houndsfield units can distinguish between simple effusion and blood or pus.
- The pleural fluid can also be sampled to assist in the diagnosis of retained hemothorax and empyema if necessary. Aspiration or drainage of blood from the pleural space is consistent with retained hemothorax. Pus evacuation from the pleural space is consistent with empyema. In milder cases, the fluid may appear cloudy instead of frankly purulent. In those cases, pleural fluid analysis can help to make the diagnosis of empyema, in which pleural fluid pH will be <7.20, glucose < 60, and/or lactate dehydrogenase level $>3\times$ serum.[4]

SURGICAL MANAGEMENT

Preoperative Planning

- After confirming the diagnosis of retained hemothorax or empyema as outlined earlier, there are a few additional considerations prior to VATS. First, VATS for retained hemothorax is most effective and associated with improved outcomes if undertaken within the first 5 days from injury. In terms of intervention timing, earlier is better and maximizes potential benefits to the patient.

- Secondly, because VATS is a nonemergent procedure, careful consideration of any associated traumatic injuries should occur prior to surgery. For example, vertebral fractures and necessary spinal precautions may preclude optimal positioning for VATS which is ideally performed with the patient extended at the hip to widen the intercostal spaces and facilitate port placement. The hip extension also results in the head positioned below the heart, which may increase intracranial pressure and should be avoided in patients with severe traumatic brain injuries.
- A third preoperative consideration is the fact that VATS requires placement of a double-lumen endotracheal tube for intraoperative mechanical ventilation. Therefore, the patient must be able to tolerate single-lung ventilation for the duration of the surgery.
- The necessary equipment should be gathered in advance of the procedure. Typically, this includes, at a minimum, thoracoscopic instruments including ports, camera, suction catheters, graspers, scissors, and electrocautery; a scalpel, open needle drivers, suture material, and chest tubes; and an open ring forceps if decortication is planned. A thoracotomy tray should be held on standby in case conversion to an open procedure is required.

Patient Positioning

- The patient is first positioned supine on a beanbag positioner for intubation with a double-lumen endotracheal tube and induction of general anesthesia. After intubation, VATS is best accomplished with the patient in lateral decubitus with the nonoperative hemithorax positioned down against the table (**FIGURE 4**). Extension at the hip is ideal to allow for enlargement of the intercostal spaces to ease port placement.

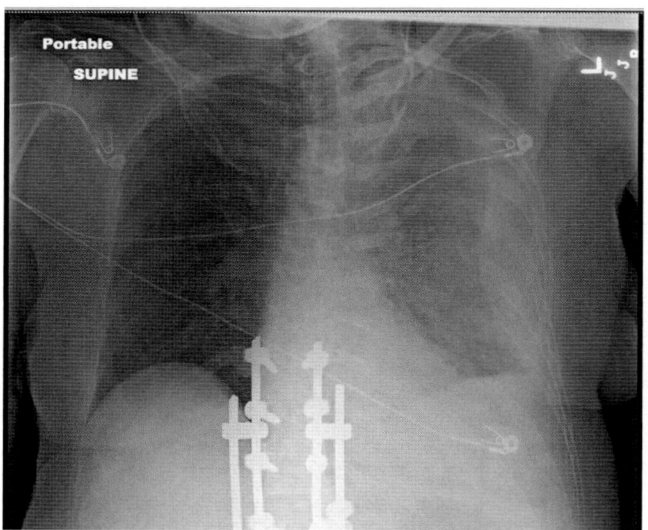

FIGURE 2 ● **Supine chest X-ray demonstrating left hemothorax following blunt trauma**. Opacity of the left hemithorax as a result of layering of the large left hemothorax.

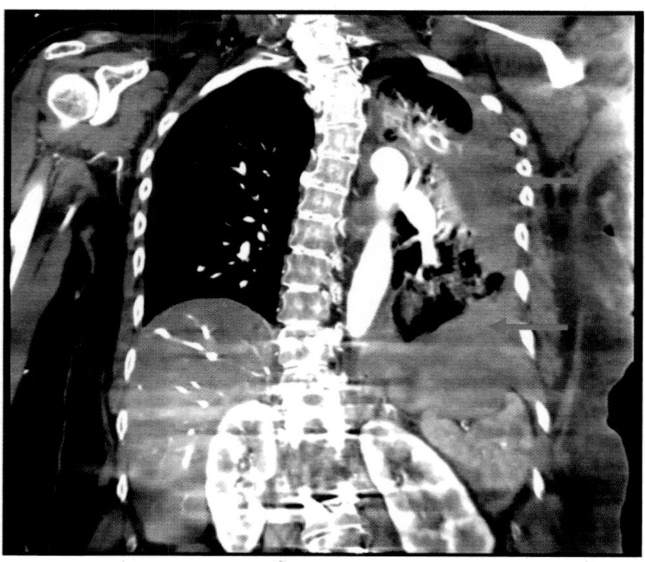

FIGURE 3 ● **Computed tomography (CT) scan of the chest demonstrating left hemothorax following blunt trauma.** After plain radiographs suggested the presence of a left retained hemothorax, CT scan was performed to distinguish retained hemothorax from consolidation. Hemothorax (*arrows*) is demonstrated.

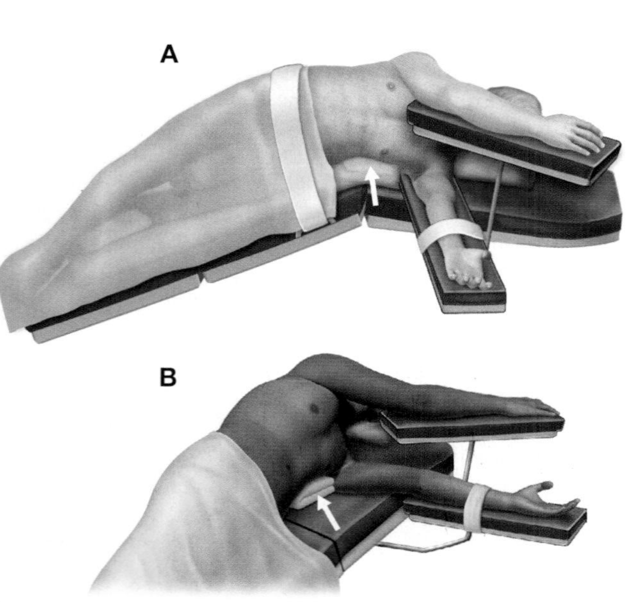

FIGURE 4 **Patient positioning for video-assisted thoracoscopic surgery.** The patient is placed in lateral decubitus with the nonoperative hemithorax positioned down against the operating table. All pressure points must be carefully padded. Hip extension allows for widening of the intercostal spaces to ease port placement.

- Next, careful attention must occur to pad all pressure points and avoid unnecessary strain on the joints of the body, particularly the shoulders, hips, and knees. For the upper body, an axillary roll placed under the dependent shoulder as well as gentle extension of the nondependent shoulder and placement of the arm onto an arm board will help avoid excessive tension on the respective brachial plexuses. As for the lower body, the hips and knees are slightly flexed with a pillow placed between the knees to avoid strain.

SKIN INCISIONS AND PORT PLACEMENT (VIDEO 1)

- After appropriate patient selection and careful positioning, the next step is to identify key surface landmarks in order to place the skin incisions for port placement in the optimal locations. We typically map out three port sites but begin by inserting only two: one working port and one camera port. A second working port is added if necessary.
- In general, the operator stands at the anterior aspect of the patient's torso and the camera assistant stands at the posterior aspect. Prior to port insertion, the patient should be placed on one-lung ventilation via the double-lumen tube, with respirations halted in the operative hemithorax to prevent injury to the lung parenchyma during port site placement or instrument insertion.
- The key surface landmarks to assist with port placement are the tip of the scapula; the fifth, sixth, and seventh ribs; and the anterior, mid, and posterior axillary lines (**FIGURE 5**). Most retained hemothoraces are located basolaterally or basoposteriorly, and the ports should be placed in locations that triangulate around the area of interest.
- In the typical positions for retained hemothorax evacuation, we begin by placing the camera port into the 6th-7th intercostal space in the mid axillary line (**FIGURE 6A** and **B**). The first working port is typically placed in the 5th-6th intercostal space in the anterior axillary line, through which the suction catheter can easily be based toward the basolateral aspect of the hemithorax. If needed, a second working port can be placed one or two intercostal spaces below the tip of the scapula, ie at the 7th-8th intercostal space in the posterior axillary line (**FIGURE 7**).

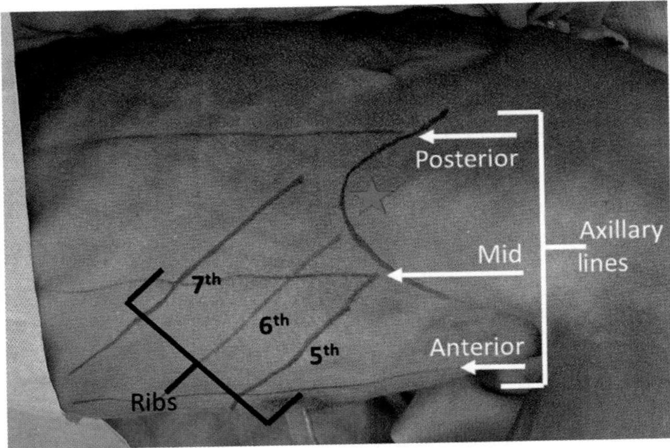

FIGURE 5 ● Surface landmarks for video-assisted thoracoscopic surgery. The key surface landmarks to assist with port placement are the tip of the scapula (*star*); the fifth, sixth, and seventh ribs; and the anterior, mid, and posterior axillary lines.

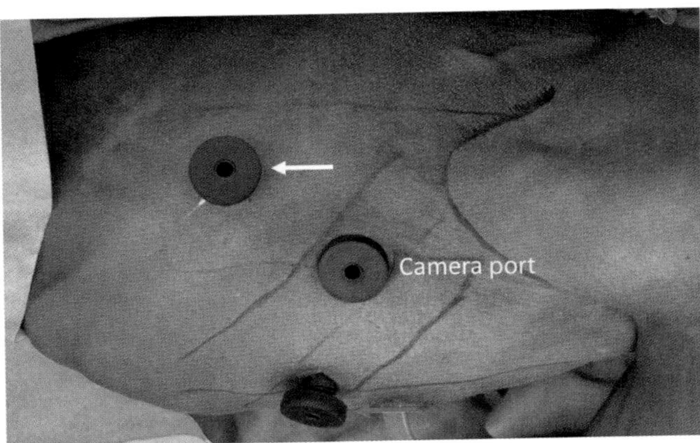

FIGURE 7 ● Port placement for video-assisted thoracoscopic surgery. In addition to the camera port (**FIGURE 6**), two additional working ports may be placed. These are inserted in the 5th-6th intercostal space in the anterior axillary line (*red arrow*) and, if a second working port is needed, to the 7th-8th intercostal space below the tip of the scapula in the posterior axillary line (*white arrow*). This triangulates the ports.

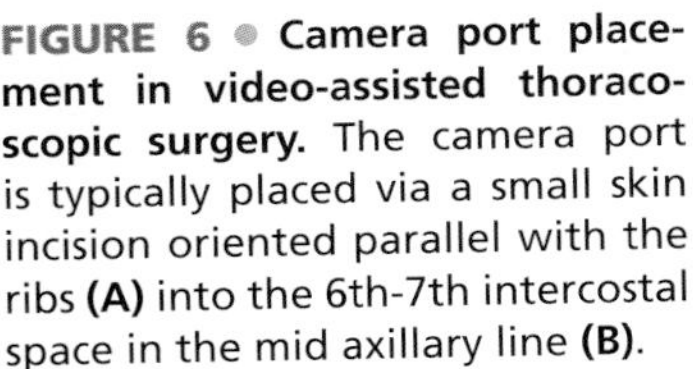
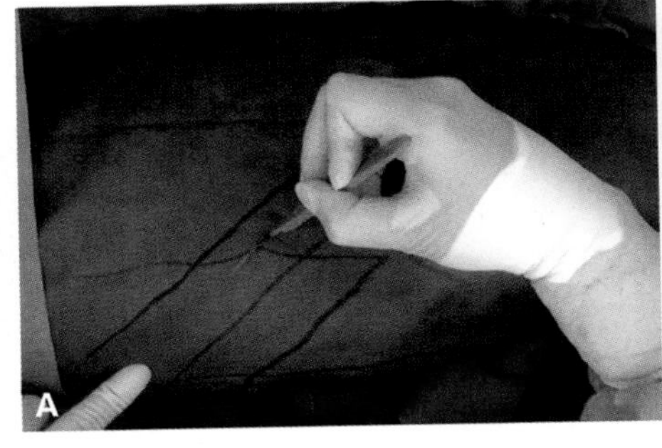

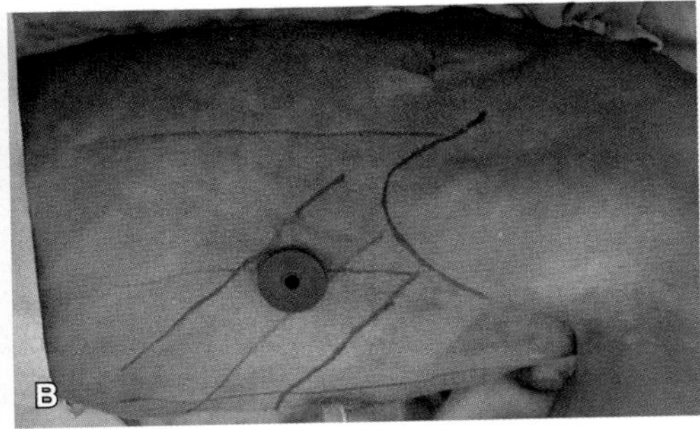

FIGURE 6 ● Camera port placement in video-assisted thoracoscopic surgery. The camera port is typically placed via a small skin incision oriented parallel with the ribs **(A)** into the 6th-7th intercostal space in the mid axillary line **(B)**.

EXPOSURE

- After establishing port site access into the hemithorax, there may be adhesions between the visceral and parietal pleurae. If these impede access to the retained hemothorax or empyema, or if they appear likely to tear during dissection or retraction, they should be carefully taken down with either sharp dissection or electrocautery as appropriate (**FIGURE 8**).

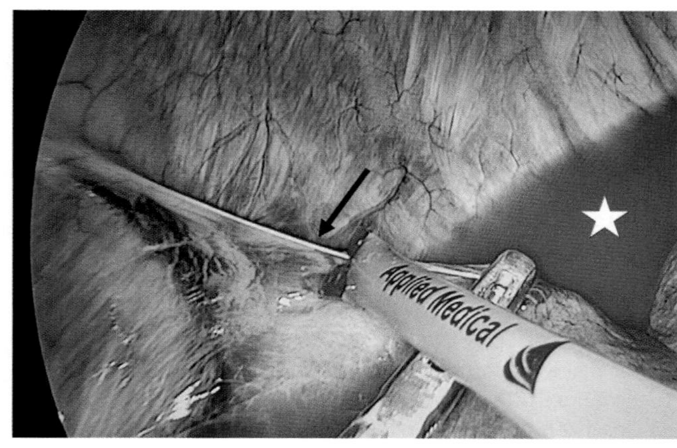

FIGURE 8 ● **Pleural Adhesions.** After entry into the hemithorax, the retained hemothorax is noted (*star*). If adhesions (*arrow*) between the visceral and parietal pleurae impede access to the retained hemothorax, they can be taken down with sharp or blunt dissection.

RETAINED HEMOTHORAX OR EMPYEMA EVACUATION

- Once unfettered access to the fluid collection of either blood or pus is achieved, the next step is to evacuate the fluid. Sometimes, this can be accomplished by simply passing a suction catheter, particularly one of 10 mm diameter, into the fluid collection (**FIGURE 9**).
- If the clotted blood cannot be removed in this manner, a grasper can be passed into the collection to disrupt the clot and evacuate it manually. Irrigation of the chest cavity can also help to disrupt clot and render it more accessible to evacuation, particularly with the suction catheter.
- If pus is encountered, sampling the fluid for culture prior to evacuation is prudent in order to allow for tailored antibiotic therapy.

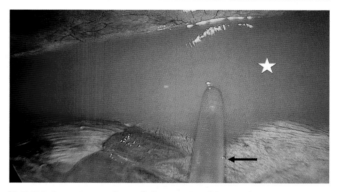

FIGURE 9 ● **Evacuation of the retained hemothorax.** Once the retained hemothorax (*star*) is accessible, the blood is evacuated via suction catheter (*arrow*).

DECORTICATION

- Although decortication is rarely needed during VATS for retained hemothorax, it is often a consideration after empyema evacuation in order to fully clear the infection and thereby help prevent recurrence.
- After the blood or pus has been removed from the hemithorax, the lung surface is inspected. Any purulence or clot coating the parenchymal surface of the lung is then removed (**FIGURE 10A**). A ring forceps can be helpful to accomplish this (**FIGURE 10B**).

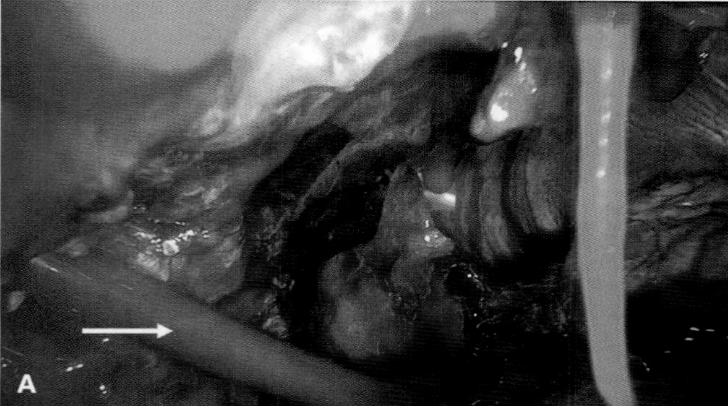

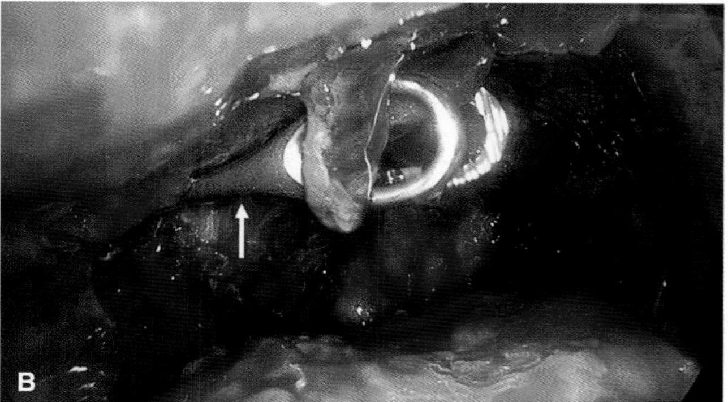

FIGURE 10 ● **Video-assisted thoracoscopic surgery decortication for retained hemothorax. A,** Any liquid blood is first evacuated via suction catheter (*arrow*). Clotted retained hemothorax is seen throughout, coating the parietal and visceral pleurae. **B,** The clotted retained hemothorax coating the parietal and visceral pleurae is removed with the assistance of a ring forceps (*arrow*).

FINAL STEPS

- Next, the pleural space is irrigated extensively until the effluent returns clear.
- One or two chest tubes are typically placed through the port sites: a single straight chest tube through the port at the mid axillary line, directed toward the apex of the lung, is often sufficient. If desired, a second angled chest tube can be placed through the port at the anterior axillary line and positioned to lie along the diaphragm and into the costodiaphragmatic recess.
- Port sites left without a chest tube should have the fascia closed with absorbable suture and the skin closed with staples.
- Lastly, the patient is returned to double-lung ventilation and then extubated if physiologically appropriate.

PEARLS AND PITFALLS

Analgesia	■ Postoperative pain control can be greatly assisted by performance of intercostal nerve blocks at the time of surgery.
Diagnosis	■ Cross-sectional imaging of the chest should generally be obtained prior to proceeding with VATS for retained hemothorax. ■ Associated pulmonary contusions, atelectasis, or other consolidations can appear isodense with any residual hemothorax on CXR and therefore CT scan of the chest is useful to distinguish a retained hemothorax from other etiologies of opacification of the costodiaphragmatic recess on CXR before proceeding with VATS.
Timing of surgery	■ The importance of timing cannot be overemphasized in the consideration of VATS for retained hemothorax evacuation. ■ VATS offers the most benefit in patient outcomes when pursued as early as feasible, ideally within 5 d of injury.
Conversion to open	■ Active bleeding from either the chest wall or the surface of the lung can be challenging to control from a thoracoscopic approach. ■ If there is concern for hemorrhage that is not easily accessible or controlled, the surgeon should not hesitate to convert to an open thoracotomy. ■ Particularly during decortication, if required, significant bleeding can occur from the lung's surface.

POSTOPERATIVE CARE

- A postoperative CXR is useful to verify chest tube placement and lung reexpansion. The chest tube(s) should remain in situ and connected to −20 cm H_2O suction until the lung is fully reexpanded, any air leak has resolved, and there is no residual pneumothorax on upright CXR. The chest tube(s) can then be transitioned to water seal and removed once the output is low, generally <200 cc/d, as long as the CXR is favorable and does not show residual pneumothorax or hemothorax.

COMPLICATIONS

Bleeding

- Intraoperative bleeding can be challenging to control from a minimally invasive approach, even for experienced surgeons. Care is taken during VATS to avoid injury to the intercostal vessels during port placement by inserting the ports directly above the superior border of the rib below. Injury to the intercostal vessels may not manifest with bleeding until after port removal, with the port tamponading the bleeding while it is in place. The non-camera ports should be removed under direct visualization for this reason. Injury to intercostal vessels may require conversion to open thoracotomy for management.
- Bleeding can also occur from the lung surface during decortication for empyema, a procedure that is notorious for its potential for significant blood loss. If significant blood loss is encountered, conversion to an open thoracotomy may be necessary to control hemorrhage.
- Lastly, bleeding can occur from injury to the pulmonary vasculature. Care must be taken during VATS for retained hemothorax or empyema evacuation to keep the dissection safely away from the pulmonary hilum.

Conversion to Open

- Conversion to a thoracotomy may be required to completely evacuate the retained hemothorax or empyema[5] or for control of bleeding as delineated above. The focus during the surgical care of these patients should be centered on resolving the retained hemothorax or empyema in a safe and careful manner. If the anatomy is unclear or the pathology is inaccessible, for example due to adhesions in the pleural space that cannot be carefully taken down, the surgeon should not hesitate to convert to an open procedure in order to proceed safely.

Persistent Air Leak

- Injury to the underlying lung parenchyma, either iatrogenically during the VATS or from the underlying etiology itself, may produce a persistent air leak via the chest tube. As long as this leak does not produce a large pneumothorax and patient physiology is not compromised, initial management should consist of close clinical observation with minimization of intrapleural suction to the extent possible while avoiding pneumothorax accumulation. The vast majority of persistent air leaks are self-limited.

Other Complications

- A small risk of other complications, including surgical site infection, pneumonia, and atelectasis, has also been reported after VATS.

REFERENCES

1. Prakash PS, Moore SA, Rezende-Neto JB, et al. Predictors of retained hemothorax in trauma: results of an eastern association for the surgery of trauma multi-institutional trial. *J Trauma*. 2020;89(4):679-685.
2. Velmahos GC, Demetriades D, Chan L, Tatevossian R, Cornwell EEIII, Yassa N, Murray JA, Asensio JA, Berne TV. Predicting the need for thoracoscopic evacuation of residual traumatic hemothorax: chest radiograph is insufficient. *J Trauma*. 1999;46(1):65-70.
3. DuBose J, Inaba K, Okoye O, et al. Development of posttraumatic empyema in patients with retained hemothorax: results of a prospective, observational AAST study. *J Trauma*. 2012;73(3):752-757.
4. Light RW. Parapneumonic effusions and empyema. *Proc Am Thorac Soc*. 2006;3(1):75-80.
5. DuBose J, Inaba K, Demetriades D, et al. Management of post-traumatic retained hemothorax: a prospective, observational, multicenter AAST study. *J Trauma*. 2012;72(1):11-22.

Chapter 9

Repair of Diaphragmatic Injury (Primary and Mesh)

Noelle N. Saillant and George C. Velmahos

DEFINITION

- The diaphragm is a dome-shaped muscular septum that separates the thoracic cavity from the abdomen.
- Superiorly the diaphragm is bounded by the bilateral hemithoraces and the mediastinum. Inferiorly the diaphragm bounds the abdominal viscera, namely, the stomach, small bowel, colon, omentum, liver, and spleen. The diaphragm is an essential muscle of respiration.
- Disruption of the diaphragm or its neural innervation, the phrenic nerve, can lead to ventilatory dysfunction and loss of the ability to manifest a "tidal volume," with each breath.
- In addition to its mechanical role in respiratory function, the diaphragm physically maintains the domain between the negative pressure of the intrathoracic cavity and the positive pressure of the abdominal cavity. Thus, when the muscle is traumatically breached, herniation of intra-abdominal structures into the chest occurs.
- Such herniation risks incarceration of the abdominal viscera and subsequently may lead to compression of the lung.

DIFFERENTIAL DIAGNOSIS

- The two major patterns of traumatic injury, blunt and penetrating, produce different patterns of destruction to the diaphragm. Blunt trauma transmits a high-energy, compressive or shearing force to the diaphragm that tends to cause large rents. Such defects are usually detected on the chest x-ray or computed tomography (CT) imaging as elevation of the hemidiaphragm, a supradiaphragmatic gastric or intestinal gas pattern, or a nasogastric tube in the intrathoracic position. This is in stark contrast to the insidious presentation of a penetrating diaphragmatic injury. Penetrating trauma often produces small defects at the direct site of the missile or object puncture. The resultant defect tends to be a small-caliber aperture that may, in time, provide a location for herniation and subsequent visceral incarceration or strangulation. Maintaining a high index of suspicion for diaphragmatic injury particularly in those patients who have sustained a penetrating trauma to the thoracoabdominal region is essential to the diagnosis.
- Congenital disruptions of the diaphragm can occasionally be diagnosed in the adult trauma patient. These are longstanding hernias that have a well-described appearance and anatomic location. A Bochdalek hernia is posterior and lateral to the left lateral arcuate ligament. The hernia may involve the intra-abdominal organs and is often associated with a hypoplastic ipsilateral lung. The Morgagni defect is a parasternal congenital defect that occurs in a muscular gap behind the xiphoid.[1] Hiatal hernias are easily distinguished from traumatic injuries as they involve the esophageal hiatus. Finally, the Chilaiditi sign, the radiographic appearance of the colon lying superiorly to the liver, can occasionally be misconstrued as a diaphragmatic disruption. This radiographic sign is present in under 0.3% of the population.[2]
- Finally, the radiographic findings of atelectasis, effusions, gastric dilatation, or pulmonary injury may mimic diaphragmatic injury on initial evaluation and should enter in the differential diagnosis.

PATIENT HISTORY AND PHYSICAL FINDINGS

- Patient history is essential to the diagnosis of a diaphragmatic injury. Patients may present in extremis or, alternatively, be hemodynamically normal with no physical examination findings.
- As with all trauma surveys, the initial evaluation requires assessment of the Airway, Breathing and Circulation portion of the ABCDEs of Advanced Trauma Life Support (ATLS).

By virtue of its anatomic position, the diaphragm is rarely injured in isolation, and the initial workup should be directed at identifying all life-threatening injuries. Airway and breathing may be compromised by concomitant injuries such as a hemothorax or pneumothorax or tension physiology. Large diaphragmatic injuries may also lead to compression of the lung from the herniated contents. Bleeding should be assessed and may occur in the chest, abdomen, or both cavities. Physical signs of diaphragmatic injury are generally secondary to a constellation of injuries above and below the diaphragm. Cardiac injuries, both blunt and penetrating, should be ruled out. The patient should be adequately examined for the evidence of peritonitis on examination suggestive of a hollow viscus injury within the abdomen. Posterior penetrating wounds may be associated with renal injuries, frequently manifesting with hematuria. Even in the absence of physical examination findings, all penetrating injuries of the thoracoabdominal region that overlie the rib cage at or below the 4th thoracic vertebral line should be strongly considered for a diaphragmatic injury. Similarly, any thoracic or abdominal gunshot wound may pass through the diaphragm, and thus, evaluating potential trajectories is essential to suspecting the diagnosis. High-energy mechanisms of injury, such as a high-velocity motor vehicle collision or fall from height, should also lead the trauma surgeon to suspect injury to the diaphragm.

Delayed presentations of diaphragmatic injuries have been described. Missed injuries may be diagnosed in the setting of subsequent radiographic inquiry or if hernias become symptomatic. Incarceration of abdominal contents may present with obstruction or obstipation, ischemia, and perforation. In the most severe forms, septic shock from such complications or cardiovascular collapse from tension physiology due to large-volume herniation may occur (**TABLE 1**).

IMAGING AND OTHER DIAGNOSTIC STUDIES

- Chest radiograph is an essential first tool for the diagnosis of diaphragm injury.
- Overt signs of injury include disruption of the diaphragmatic contour, evidence of herniation of intestinal contents

Table 1: Grading of Diaphragm Injuries

Grade	Findings
I	Contusion
II	Laceration <2 cm
III	Laceration 2-10 cm
IV	Laceration >10 cm with tissue loss ≤25 cm^2
V	Laceration with tissue loss ≥25 cm^2

Reprinted with permission from Moore EE, Malangoni MA, Cogbill TH, et al. Organ injury scaling. IV: Thoracic vascular, lung, cardiac, and diaphragm. J Trauma. 1994;36(3):299-300.

or naso/orogastric tubes within the thoracic cavity. New hemi-elevation of the diaphragms may be due to direct muscular injury or nerve dysfunction. Plain chest radiographs may be normal in up to 40% to 50% of patients and thus does not sufficiently rule out an injury.[3]

- Ultrasound, and specifically the focused assessment with sonography in trauma (FAST examination), is an important diagnostic tool during the initial trauma bay workup that may suggest the presence of a diaphragmatic injury. For instance, if a thoracoabdominal stab wound showed evidence of free fluid in the abdomen and in the chest, an injury should be considered. Furthermore, ultrasound is essential in the triage of "double jeopardy." Evidence suggests that 85% of bleeding from thoracoabdominal injuries is sourced from the abdomen, whereas 15% of injuries require primary thoracic exploration. Incorrect sequencing of thoracotomy and laparotomy, however frequent it may be, leads to high morbidity and mortality. The decision to first explore the chest vs abdomen is often predicated on the presence of fluid on the pericardial ultrasound. If there is a pericardial effusion, the chest is to be explored first. If there is no evidence of hemopericardium or massive hemothorax then the abdomen is prioritized.[4]
- CT imaging also lacks enough sensitivity and specificity to rule out a diaphragmatic injury. The pooled sensitivity and specificity are 0.77 and 0.91, respectively.[5] Side specificity is important to the discussion of diaphragm injuries. It has been reported that left-sided diaphragmatic injuries outnumber right-sided muscular injuries in a 3:1 ratio, due to the protection afforded to the right side by the liver and due to the predominance of right-handed assailants. However, left-sided injuries are more often diagnosed by surgical intervention and imaging findings, and therefore may lead to bias in this reporting. Owing to the position and association of the liver with the right hemidiaphragm, the sensitivity of diagnostic modalities also favors left-sided injury diagnosis over right-sided injuries in trauma patients.
- In hemodynamically normal patients, laparoscopy, or video-assisted thoracoscopy (VATS) is the definitive diagnostic method for occult diaphragm injuries and warranted when appropriate suspicion remains. Owing to inadequate sensitivity of other imaging modalities and the potential for catastrophic consequences of a delayed diagnosis, laparoscopic evaluation is conditionally recommended over CT for left-sided injury diagnosis.[5] Right-sided injuries may be managed nonoperatively in appropriate circumstances, based on the limited evidence supporting this practice. Again, risk of missed injury and incarceration must be weighed against the risk of operation and perioperative recovery. Patients who benefit from surgical exploration of the diaphragm are those suspected to have a transdiaphragmatic trajetory.[5-7]

SURGICAL MANAGEMENT

- Considerations to the technique are focused on stability and additional injuries.

Preoperative Planning

- If a preoperative chest tube is indicated, one should proceed with care as the tube is placed into the chest to avoid iatrogenic injury to any incarcerated viscera.
- Preoperative insertion of a nasogastric tube or orogastric tube will decompress the stomach and facilitate exposure.

TECHNIQUES

UNSTABLE PATIENTS

- The patient is brought to the operating room. Sterile prep and draping should expose the neck to the knees in accordance with basic trauma operative care. In the presence of other injuries, or hemodynamic instability, the diaphragm is typically of secondary consideration. The cavity with the compelling source of hemorrhage or injury should be explored first, as the diaphragm can be repaired through both cavities. The surgeon performs a meticulous evaluation of the injured cavities and attends to hemorrhage and contamination accordingly. Occasionally, an expeditious repair of a diaphragm laceration can help isolate the thorax from the abdomen in order to detect the source of bleeding or to prevent transcavitary contamination.

Simple Open Repair

- Simple diaphragm disruptions on the left may have visceral contents incarcerated into the "sucking chest wound" created by the laceration and the pressure differential between the abdominal and chest cavities. Careful reduction of the herniated contents should be performed to avoid iatrogenic injury of the involved viscera, particularly the spleen (see **FIGURE 1**).
- Once the contents are reduced, Allis clamps may be used to approximate the lacerated diaphragmatic edges and facilitate repair (see **FIGURE 2**).
- Interrupted or running sutures should be used to create an airtight and everted closure (see **FIGURE 3**).
- The authors prefer to use slowly absorbing sutures such as PDS (author GCV) or permanent sutures such as Ethibond (author NNS). A tension-free repair is essential to prevent recurrence of the rupture. A chest drain or chest tube should be considered to evacuate any chest soilage or residual hemothorax or pneumothorax. In the case of significant contamination of the chest or mediastinum, a washout of that cavity should be performed and drained with chest tubes (see **FIGURE 4**).

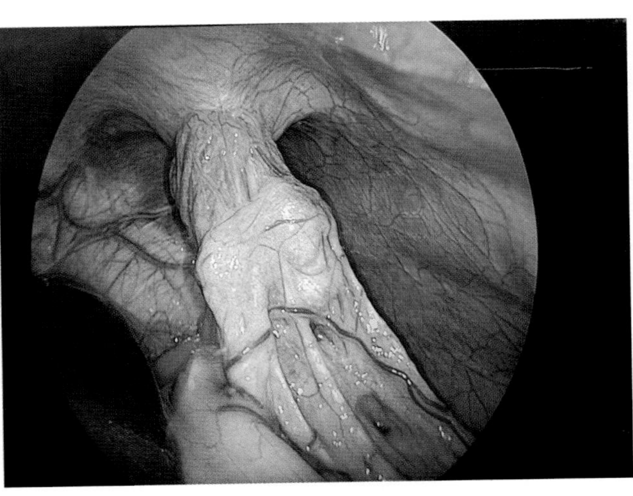

FIGURE 1 ● Herniated fat into diaphragm hernia.

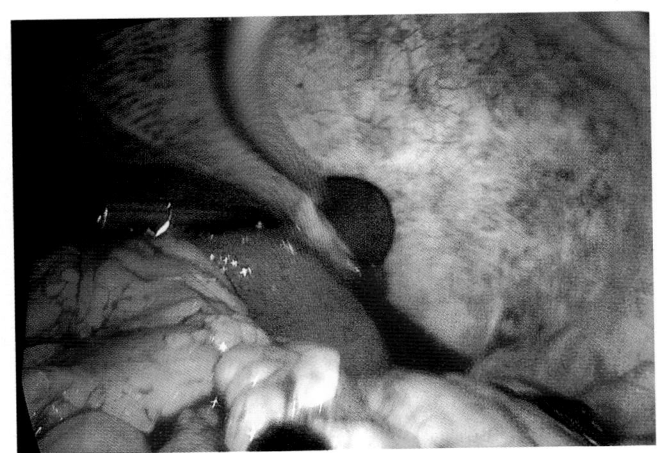

FIGURE 3 ● Use of red rubber to decompress chest/pneumothorax.

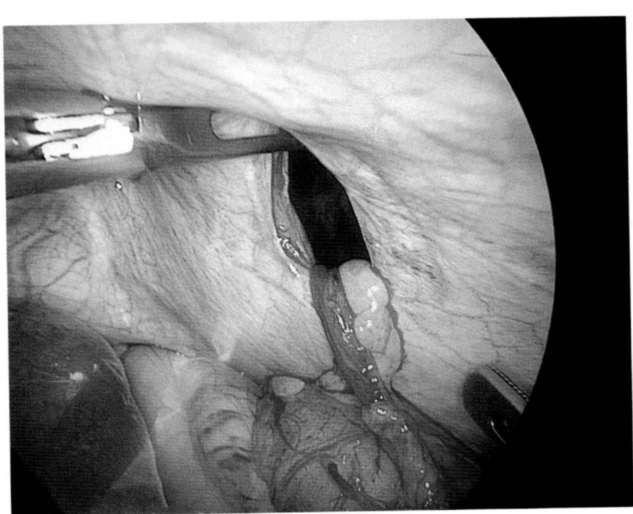

FIGURE 2 ● Status post reduction of contents.

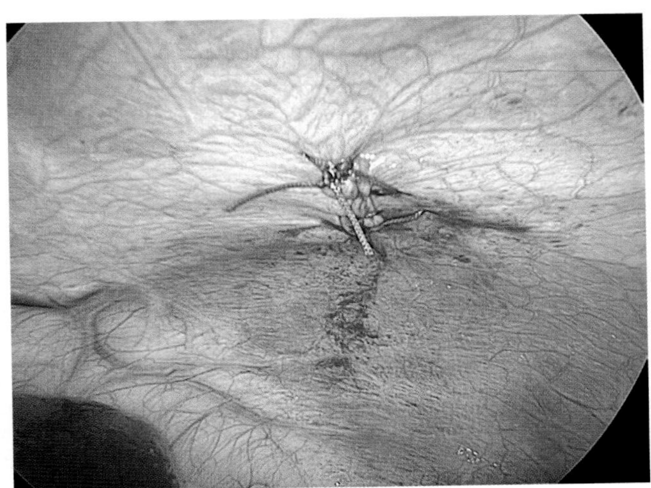

FIGURE 4 ● Airtight repair with sutures.

STABLE PATIENTS

Simple Laparoscopic Repair

- In the absence of other injuries, stable patients benefit from the minimally invasive approach of laparoscopy. A foot board is placed to facilitate positioning of the patient in anticipation of steep reverse Trendelenburg. This positioning helps gravitate the viscera caudally and away from the diaphragm to promote exposure. The patient is secured to the table and prepped and draped in the usual sterile fashion. Access to the abdomen may be via a Veress or cutdown technique; however, prior to insufflation, the anesthesia team should be alerted to the risk of creating a pneumothorax and subsequent tension with insufflation, especially if a preoperative chest tube is not in place. We insufflate slowly and then evaluate for potential injury by a 5-mm camera. Additional ports are placed if the diaphragm is truly injured and requires repair.
- When the likelihood of injury is high or preoperatively diagnosed, we often begin with a 12-mm Hasson port at the umbilicus, which can be easily extended to a laparotomy if needed. The exact location may be altered depending on the site of the wounds. Access is preferentially away from the wound site. Wounds may need temporary closure to prevent the escape of pneumoperitoneum. Pneumoperitoneum is carefully established at 15 mm Hg. A 30° scope is placed inside to compete the abdominal survey. Evaluation for blood or enteric contents is performed. Upon diagnosis of an injury a second 5-mm port is placed under direct visualization usually in the midclavicular line and a hand's breadth away from any causative wound. Atraumatic instruments are used to evaluate the abdomen. The stomach, spleen, and liver are inspected. The small bowel is run from the ligament of Treitz to terminal ileum. The colon is inspected with attention to the flexures. If no other injury is noted, the diaphragm laceration is repaired.

- Intracorporeal sutures cut to 15 cm are placed in an interrupted fashion and tied sequentially. As the final sutures are placed, a red rubber catheter is placed into the chest and the final sutures are secured around it. The red rubber is then placed to suction and pulled from the abdomen as the final suture is tied down to evacuate the pneumothorax. Alternatively, if there is concern for a residual pneumothorax/hemothorax or soiling of the chest cavity, the chest should be irrigated and suctioned prior to closure and a chest tube placed.
- You do not always have to close the fascia of every penetrating wound. Surgical wounds should be sutured closed. We typically leave the skin open on the penetrating soft tissue injury.

Complex Repairs

- Most diaphragmatic injuries can be repaired primarily. Occasionally, high-grade injuries (grade IV [10 cm laceration with tissue loss <25 cm^2] or grade V [laceration with tissue loss >25 cm^2]) may need additional techniques to address the tissue discrepancy. Injuries that are close to the pericardium or esophageal hiatus can also be challenging to repair. A transabdominal or transthoracic approach may be utilized. While most general surgeons prefer abdominal approaches, the thoracic approach may have some advantages in large defects that are difficult to access due to the liver, and in some chronic hernias, as it may represent a virgin surgical territory with less associated adhesiolysis.
- Reconstruction of the diaphragm with mesh requires full-thickness approximation to the surrounding tissue. Depending on the defect, the mesh can be fixed to the remaining muscular tissue. Lateral avulsions may require that the prothesis be secured with permanent sutures around the ribs. Medially, the mesh may need to be secured carefully to the pericardium. Posteriorly, the crus of the diaphragm is a good anchoring point. The repair should rest at about the 9th intercostal space at a lower position to facilitate lung expansion and minimize eventration. Care should be paid to avoid a high degree of tension at the repair site as this may result in rupture. The choice of prosthesis is at the discretion of the operator. In noncontaminated cases we prefer to use Parietex variety, with a dual surface to avoid visceral adhesions and incorporation. Biologics work reasonably well in the diaphragm as well even in noncontaminated cases.
- In contaminated cases, biologic mesh is utilized to bridge the tissue loss. Given the contamination that often necessitates this type of repair, excellent chest drainage is needed. In addition, the biologic meshes may stretch with time, which leads to eventration even when they are tensioned in a flat position at the initial placement. Finally, in cases of combined diaphragm loss and chest wall destruction, additional tissue coverage may be provided by the latissimus as a pedicled flap in severe cases.

PEARLS AND PITFALLS

Diagnosis	■ Occult diaphragm injures often occur in thoracoabdominal penetrating injuries. A high index of suspicion should be maintained and, when indicated, a diagnostic laparoscopy should be performed.
Preoperative decision making	■ When the patient has significant injury in the chest and abdomen, the sequencing of the abdominal and thoracic explorations is of paramount importance. The FAST examination may help guide this decision.
Operative pearls	■ During insufflation of the abdomen a pneumothorax can occur. Preoperative preparation for this complication is necessary by having a pleural tube in place or immediately available. In addition, communication with the OR team and anesthesia staff about this potential complication will allow prompt diagnosis and treatment should this occur. ■ In the patient with severe hemorrhage, closing the diaphragm defect can help isolate chest sources of bleeding from intra-abdominal sources of bleeding and stop the free flow of blood across the field. ■ In laparoscopic evaluations the optimal positioning is in a steep upright position Securing the patient and the presence of a foot board are essential to optimal exposure.

POSTOPERATIVE CARE

- Postoperatively the patient can usually be extubated in absence of other injuries.
- A chest x-ray should be performed to assess for pneumothorax.
- Most of the postoperative care is dictated by the supportive care of concomitant traumatic injuries.

COMPLICATIONS

- Atelectasis
- Pneumonia: 6% to 15% of patients
- Empyema and other associated deep space infections: 1% to 4%
- Severe sepsis is noted in 2%[8]

REFERENCES

1. Chandrasekharan PK, Rawat M, Madappa R, Rothstein DH, Lakshminrusimha S. Congenital diaphragmatic hernia—a review. *Matern Health Neonatol Perinatol.* 2016;3:6.
2. Moaven O, Hodin R. Chilaiditi syndrome. *Gastroenterol Hepatol.* 2012;8(4):276-278.
3. Lochum S, Ludig T, Walter F, Sebbag H, Grosdidier G, Blum AG. Imaging of diaphragmatic injury: a diagnostic challenge? *Radiographics.* 2002:22(suppl l_1):S103-S116.

4. Matsushima K, Khor D, Berona K, Antoku D, Dollbaum R, Khan M, Demetriades D. Double jeopardy in penetrating trauma: get FAST, get it right. *World J Surg*. 2018;42(1):99-106.
5. McDonald A, Robinson B, Alarcon L, et al. Evaluation and management of traumatic diaphragmatic injuries: a Practice Management Guideline from the Eastern Association for the Surgery of Trauma. *J Trauma*. 2018;85(1):198-207. (East guidelines).
6. Murray JA, Demetriades D, Asensio JA, et al. Occult injuries to the diaphragm: prospective evaluation of laparoscopy in penetrating injuries to the left lower chest. *J Am Coll Surg*. 1998;187(6):626-630.
7. Berg R, Karamanos E, Inaba K, Okoye O, Teixeira P, Demetriades D. The persistent diagnostic challenge of thoracoabdominal stab wounds. *J Trauma Acute Care Surg*. 2014;76(2):418-423.
8. Fair KA, Gordeon NT, Barbosa R, Rosell SE, Watter JM, Schreiber MA. Traumatic diaphragmatic injury in the American college of surgeons national trauma data bank: a new examination of a rare diagnosis. *Am J Surg*. 2105;209:864-869.

Chapter 10

Thoracic Incisions: Median Sternotomy, Anterolateral Thoracotomy, Bilateral Thoracotomy, Posterolateral Thoracotomy

Christina L. Jacovides and Mark J. Seamon

DEFINITION

- In trauma, the patient's physiology and suspected injury dictate the appropriate incision used to access the thorax and achieve operative exposure for repair.
- The thorax may be accessed via one of several standard incisions:
  - *Anterolateral thoracotomy and bilateral thoracotomy (clamshell)* are indicated for pulseless patients.
  - Patients in shock may require brief additional workup to determine the source of injury and proper thoracic incision.
    - Based on this focused workup, likely injuries may necessitate *median sternotomy*; *anterolateral thoracotomy; supraclavicular, infraclavicular,* or *cervical/anterior sternocleidomastoid extension* incisions.
  - Hemodynamically normal patients will tolerate a more extensive workup to determine precise anatomic injury and thus optimal thoracic incisions if required.
    - Depending on the injuries identified, *median sternotomy; anterolateral thoracotomy; supraclavicular, infraclavicular,* or *cervical/anterior sternocleidomastoid extension* incisions may be utilized. In rare circumstances, only after complete examination and imaging workup, a *posterolateral thoracotomy* may be considered.
- Thoracic exposure may be required to resuscitate a patient without signs of life, to repair injuries within the thoracic cavity, or to gain proximal control of vascular injuries of the neck, upper extremities, or abdomen.

DIFFERENTIAL DIAGNOSIS

- **Pulseless patient**[1]:
  - Tension pneumothorax
  - Open pneumothorax
  - Massive hemothorax
  - Cardiac tamponade
  - Airway disruption
  - Tracheobronchial injury
  - In addition, consider:
    - Exsanguination from nonthoracic source
- **Patient in shock:**
  - Clinically significant hemorrhage from thoracic source
    - Heart
    - Great vessels
    - Pulmonary hilum
    - Lung parenchyma
    - Chest wall
  - Clinically significant hemorrhage from nonthoracic source
    - Abdomen
    - Pelvis
    - Extremities
- **Hemodynamically normal patient:**
  - Lung injury
    - Contusion
    - Laceration
    - Pneumothorax
    - Hemothorax
  - Minor cardiac injury
  - Chest wall injuries
    - Rib fractures
    - Sternal fractures
    - Clavicle fractures
    - Scapular fractures
    - Shoulder injuries (bony, ligamentous)

PATIENT HISTORY AND PHYSICAL FINDINGS

- **Pulseless patient:**
  - Survival from resuscitative thoracotomy depends on a variety of factors including mechanism of injury, site of injury, presence or absence of signs of life, presence of vital signs, presenting cardiac rhythm, and need for cardiopulmonary resuscitation (CPR) (**FIGURE 1**).
  - Resuscitative thoracotomy is recommended in pulseless patients in the following situations (**TABLE 1**)[2]:
    - Patients with penetrating thoracic trauma with signs of life (strong recommendation)
    - Patients with penetrating thoracic trauma without signs of life (conditional recommendation)

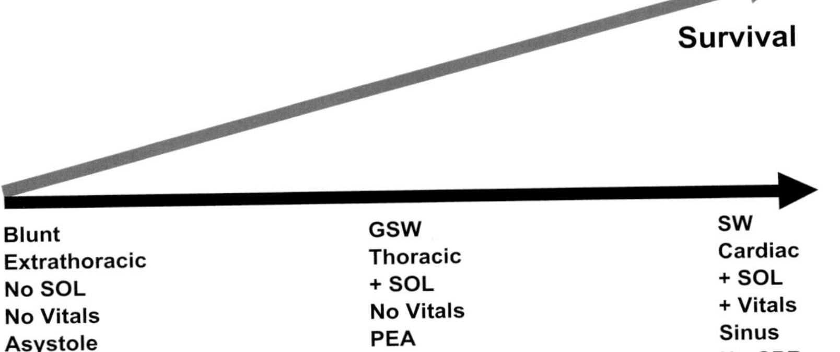

FIGURE 1 ● Resuscitative thoracotomy: The importance of survival predictors. Rates of survival after resuscitative thoracotomy vary by mechanism of injury, location of injury, whether the patient presents with signs of life or vital signs, the presenting cardiac rhythm, and whether the patient required cardiopulmonary resuscitation (CPR) before arrival to the trauma bay.

Table 1: EAST (Eastern Association for the Surgery of Trauma) Emergency Department Resuscitative Thoracotomy Recommendations

Question	Recommendation
PICO #1	In patients who present pulseless to the Emergency Department with signs of life after penetrating thoracic injury, we **strongly recommend** resuscitative Emergency Department thoracotomy. **Strong Recommendation**
PICO #2	In patients who present pulseless to the Emergency Department without signs of life after penetrating thoracic injury, we **conditionally recommend** resuscitative Emergency Department thoracotomy. **Conditional Recommendation**
PICO #3	In patients who present pulseless to the Emergency Department with signs of life after penetrating extrathoracic injury, we **conditionally recommend** resuscitative Emergency Department thoracotomy. **Conditional Recommendation**
PICO #4	In patients who present pulseless to the Emergency Department without signs of life after penetrating extrathoracic injury, we **conditionally recommend** resuscitative Emergency Department thoracotomy.[1] **Conditional Recommendation**
PICO #5	In patients who present pulseless to the Emergency Department with signs of life after blunt injury, we **conditionally recommend** resuscitative Emergency Department thoracotomy. **Conditional Recommendation**
PICO #6	In patients who present pulseless to the Emergency Department without signs of life after blunt injury, we **conditionally recommend against** resuscitative Emergency Department thoracotomy.[2] **Conditional Recommendation**

[1]Group voting for a recommendation was mixed. While all voted for a "conditional" recommendation, 11 members voted in favor of Emergency Department Thoracotomy and 4 voted against the procedure based on the PICO #4 Evidence Profile.
[2]Group voting for a recommendation was mixed. While all voted against the performance of Emergency Department Thoracotomy based on the PICO #6 Evidence Profile, 10 members voted for a "strong" recommendation and 5 voted for a "conditional" recommendation.
Recognizing the significant variability in outcomes after resuscitative thoracotomy based on mechanism of injury and patient presentation, the 2015 Eastern Association for the Surgery of Trauma (EAST) guidelines for use of resuscitative thoracotomy in patients who present pulseless to the Emergency Department differ based on whether the patient suffered penetrating thoracic, penetrating extrathoracic, or blunt trauma, as well as whether the patient presented with or without signs of life to the trauma bay.
Reprinted with permission from Seamon MJ, Haut ER, Van Arendonk K, et al. An evidence-based approach to patient selection for emergency department thoracotomy: a practice management guideline from the Eastern Association for the Surgery of Trauma. J Trauma Acute Care Surg. 2015;79(1):159-173.

    - Patients with penetrating extrathoracic trauma with or without signs of life (conditional recommendations)
    - Patients with blunt trauma with signs of life (conditional recommendation)
- Resuscitative thoracotomy is not recommended in pulseless patients with blunt trauma who present without signs of life.[2]
- Signs of life include:
    - Palpable pulse
    - Measurable blood pressure
    - Pupillary response
    - Spontaneous movement
    - Spontaneous respirations
    - Cardiac electrical activity
    - Cardiac motion or the presence of pericardial effusion on ultrasound
- In penetrating trauma, it is helpful to perform a quick roll to evaluate the patient for external injuries prior to resuscitative thoracotomy. This facilitates the decision to perform (or not perform) the thoracotomy (eg, transcranial gunshot wounds) and also facilitates the decision to proceed with an immediate "clamshell" thoracotomy (bilateral thoracic wounds) rather than left anterolateral thoracotomy and right chest triage with finger or tube thoracostomy.
- **Patient in shock:**
    - Primary and secondary survey according to Advanced Trauma Life Support (ATLS) protocols.
    - Establish a definitive airway only if necessary (based on oxygenation and ventilation) in the trauma bay. Endotracheal intubation may lead to further decrease in preload in hemorrhagic shock patients, precipitating cardiopulmonary arrest.[3,4]
    - Determine if bilateral breath sounds are present.
        - If diminished breath sounds are present, finger or immediate tube thoracostomy is performed. Ultrasound or chest x-ray (CXR) is not required for diagnosis.
    - Assess peripheral pulses to determine effectiveness of circulation. Establish intravenous access. Consider giving whole blood or blood products early in the resuscitation.
    - Assess Glasgow Coma Scale and disability.
    - Fully expose the patient and roll the patient both ways to ensure all injuries have been identified.
    - Perform focused secondary survey:
        - Consider external wounds in the chest, evidence of penetrating trauma, abrasions, bruising, bleeding, hematoma.

If there is a concern for open pneumothorax, place an occlusive flap dressing (open on one of four sides).
        - Consider chest wall instability and presence of flail segment—rib fractures may be associated with hemothorax, pneumothorax, or a combination. Sharp rib fragments may injure the lung and cause tension physiology, air leaks, and subcutaneous emphysema.
    - Obtain adjunctive studies including CXR and focused assessment with sonography for trauma (FAST) examination or extended FAST (eFAST) examination.
        - If CXR or eFAST suggests hemothorax or pneumothorax in the presence of shock, tube thoracostomy is indicated.
        - If pericardial FAST demonstrates pericardial effusion, consider pericardial window or emergent median sternotomy based on hemodynamics, injury mechanism, and patient age/comorbidities (renal failure is a common cause of chronic pericardial effusions).
- **Hemodynamically normal patient:**
    - Primary and secondary survey according to ATLS protocols.
    - Evaluate the patient for external signs of injury—ecchymosis, instability, crepitus, tenderness, bleeding, open wounds, etc.
    - Certain patterns of external injury are associated with specific injuries:
        - Sternal fractures (tenderness, ecchymosis, instability over sternum) are associated with high-velocity injuries and may be associated with blunt aortic or cardiac injuries.
        - Flail chest, crepitus, and chest wall instability may be associated with significant hemothorax, pneumothorax, or lung injury.
        - Shoulder dislocations may be associated with vascular injuries and loss of distal pulses in the upper extremities.
        - Penetrating neck or thoracic inlet injuries may be associated with aerodigestive and vascular injuries.
    - Note that patterns of observed injury differ in penetrating vs blunt trauma:
        - Penetrating trauma—trajectory and weapon determine injury.
        - Blunt trauma—a rough estimate of the amount of force exerted on the patient at the time of injury may guide differential and workup for injuries.

IMAGING AND OTHER DIAGNOSTIC STUDIES

- **Pulseless patient:**
    - Quickly roll and assess patient for all sites of injury.
    - If anterolateral or bilateral thoracotomy is indicated based on patient physiology, forego any imaging studies.
    - Consider immediate bilateral or clamshell thoracotomy for patient with bilateral thoracic wounds or begin with a left anterolateral thoracotomy and right-sided chest tube or finger thoracostomy to evaluate the right chest. Convert to bilateral thoracotomy if there is evidence of blood in the right chest.[5-7]
- **Patient in shock:**
    - Prior to imaging
        - For penetrating trauma patients, mark the sites of any penetrating injuries before obtaining imaging to assist in the assessment of trajectory. Consider using different markers on anterior and posterior wounds (eg, open and closed paper clips taped to the wounds).
- Adjunctive studies in the trauma bay
    - CXR
        - Use a systematic approach to read CXR to avoid missing injuries.
            - Airway
                - Is airway midline? If not, consider tension physiology or mediastinal hematoma.
                - If intubated, is the endotracheal tube (ETT) in correct position? If not, reposition.
            - Breathing
                - Is there hemothorax/pneumothorax present? If so, tube thoracostomy is indicated.
                - Is there evidence of pulmonary contusion? If so, monitor closely for respiratory deterioration (NB: contusions may not be evident on early CXR).
            - Circulation
                - Is there mediastinal widening? If so, consider computed tomography (CT) angiography of the chest to evaluate for great vessel injury if patient's hemodynamics improve enough to tolerate CT.
                - Is the cardiac silhouette unusually large or small? Although not diagnostic, an unusually large (hemopericardium) or small (hemorrhagic shock/hypovolemia) cardiac silhouette may give a hint at underlying pathology.
            - Diaphragm
                - Are the hemidiaphragms elevated? If so, consider diaphragmatic rupture or phrenic nerve injury.
                - Is there a deep sulcus sign? If so, consider pneumothorax.
                - Do there appear to be hollow viscous organs in the chest? If so, consider diaphragmatic rupture.
                - Are the costophrenic angles blunted? Consider hemothorax.
            - Everything else
                - Is there evidence of mediastinal air or subcutaneous emphysema? If so, consider pneumothorax or aerodigestive injuries.
                - Are rib, clavicle, or shoulder fractures present? If so, how unstable is the chest wall (consider intubation)? How is the patient's pain (consider pain control)?
                - Are there foreign bodies (eg, bullets)? Compare location and external wounds to determine trajectories and likely underlying injuries.
    - FAST examination—pericardial view
        - Evaluate for pericardial fluid on FAST examination in the trauma bay. The presence of pericardial fluid should raise suspicion for cardiac injury.
        - Be wary of a negative pericardial FAST examination with a corresponding pleural effusion or hemothorax—a cardiac injury may be decompressing itself into the pleural space and FAST examination has very limited sensitivity in this particular clinical scenario (**FIGURE 2**). An operative pericardial window should be strongly considered in this setting.

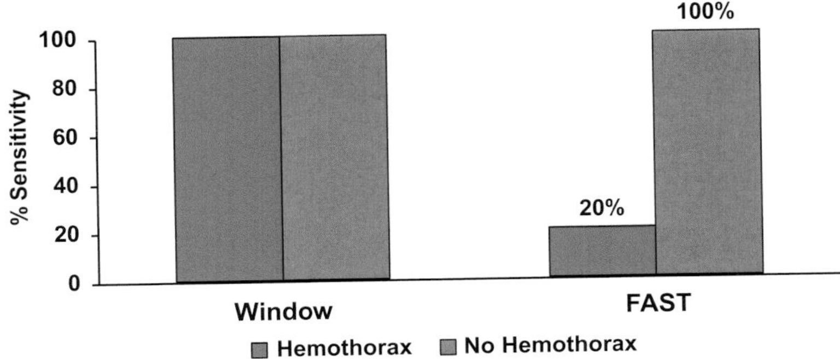

FIGURE 2 ● Cardiac injury detection. Subxiphoid pericardial window vs focused assessment with sonography for trauma (FAST) examination. In the presence of hemothorax, FAST has a decreased sensitivity for detection of cardiac injury. (Reprinted with permission from Meyer DM, Jessen ME, Grayburn PA. Use of echocardiography to detect occult cardiac injury after penetrating thoracic trauma: a prospective study. *J Trauma*. 1995;39(5):902-907; discussion 907-909.)

- Based on wound sites in penetrating trauma victims, consider additional plain films such as abdominal x-ray or head/neck x-rays to help rule out injury to extrathoracic body cavities.
- Utilize assessments and adjuncts to quickly and carefully plan the initial surgical incision in the operating room.

- **Hemodynamically normal patient:**
  - Diagnostic adjuncts (plain films, FAST) as above with additional imaging or workup considered.
  - Consider CT angiography if there is a concern for vascular injury (eg, mediastinal widening on CXR, pericardial fluid on FAST, periclavicular wounds).
  - Consider tube thoracostomy for diagnosis/therapeutic effect in:
    - Patients with respiratory instability and diminished breath sounds.
    - Patients with hemothorax or pneumothorax noted on CXR.
    - Note initial and ongoing output from chest tube once placed.
      - Operative exploration of the thoracic cavity has traditionally been indicated if the initial chest tube output is greater than 1500 cc or if ongoing output remains above 200 cc per hour for 4 hours, but patient physiology should dictate the need for operative intervention.[1,6]
      - If hemothorax does not resolve after initial chest tube placement, consider a second tube thoracostomy or operative exploration (**FIGURE 3**).
  - Despite favorable hemodynamics, consider subxiphoid pericardial window in the operating room (OR) for:
    - Positive pericardial FAST
    - Trajectory of penetrating trauma near the heart when operating for other indications such as abdominal injury. Clinically occult cardiac injuries are surprisingly common and should be "ruled out" in appropriate patients.
  - Mediastinal or transmediastinal injuries require special consideration[8]:
    - Thoracic CT angiography imaging both provides an effective initial roadmap to guide further management and detects clinically occult great vessel injuries.
    - In patients with posterior mediastinal injuries, esophageal injuries can be diagnosed with the aid of upper gastrointestinal (UGI) swallow study and esophagogastroduodenoscopy (EGD). Occult injury may present with delayed sepsis and adverse outcomes making repair options more limited and difficult.
    - Bronchoscopy is effective in diagnosing injuries of the proximal airways.
  - Also consider bronchoscopy for significant and/or persistent air leak despite a properly functioning chest tube. Bronchoscopy may demonstrate tracheal or bronchial injury.

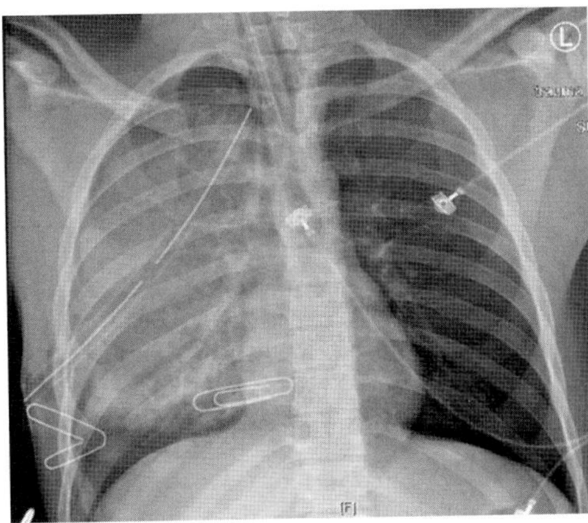

FIGURE 3 ● Massive hemothorax: shock. Young male patient presents in shock after multiple GSWs (closed paper clip marks anterior wound, open paper clip marks posterior). Chest x-ray confirms massive retained hemothorax after placement of right thoracostomy tube.

SURGICAL MANAGEMENT

Preoperative Planning

- **Pulseless patient:**
  - Prepare for left anterolateral or bilateral thoracotomy in the trauma bay.
  - Perform endotracheal intubation or establish a definitive airway.
  - Obtain intravenous or intraosseous access and begin blood product transfusion.
  - Transport immediately to OR for definitive repair if a perfusing rhythm is obtained.
- **Patient in shock:**
  - Immediate OR following initial resuscitation as above.
  - Choose incision based on site of suspected injury (**TABLE 2**) following primary/secondary survey, plain films, FAST examination.
  - Prep to allow maximal versatility, extension of incisions, or concurrent incisions when necessary. Specifically, include

Table 2: Summary: Initial Surgical Approaches

	Normal hemodynamics	Shock
Cardiac	Median sternotomy	Median sternotomy or "clamshell" thoracotomy for crossing transmediastinal injuries
Innominate	Median sternotomy	Median sternotomy
Right subclavian	Median sternotomy ± R supraclavicular extension ± clavicle resection	Median sternotomy ± R supraclavicular extension ± clavicle resection
Left subclavian	L anterolateral thoracotomy vs L supraclavicular incision ± clavicle resection	L anterolateral thoracotomy ± L supraclavicular incision ± clavicle resection
Proximal carotid	Median sternotomy with cervical extension	Median sternotomy with cervical extension
SVC	Median sternotomy	Median sternotomy
IVC	Median sternotomy	Median sternotomy
Pulmonary hilum	Anterolateral thoracotomy	Anterolateral thoracotomy
Lung parenchyma	Anterolateral thoracotomy	Anterolateral thoracotomy
Descending aorta	L anterolateral thoracotomy	L anterolateral thoracotomy
Esophagus	Proximal: R anterolateral thoracotomy Distal: L anterolateral thoracotomy	Proximal: R anterolateral thoracotomy Distal: L anterolateral thoracotomy
Trachea/airways	Proximal: median sternotomy Carina: R thoracotomy Main bronchus: R/L thoracotomy	Proximal: median sternotomy Carina: R thoracotomy Main bronchus: R/L thoracotomy

The incision of choice varies based on location of suspected injury and patient hemodynamics.

in prepped area the common vein harvest sites (eg, internal jugular, great saphenous vein) if vascular injury is suspected and interposition graft or bypass may be needed.

- **Hemodynamically normal patient:**
  - The specific injury pattern and initial workup determines the necessary interventions. Choose incision based on site of suspected injury (**TABLE 2**).
  - Consider endovascular repair options for aortic, subclavian, and proximal axillary artery injuries without evidence of free bleeding. Early contact to specialists and use of hybrid operative suites may facilitate endovascular repair in these select patients.

Positioning

- Median sternotomy
  - Supine with arms out
- Anterolateral and bilateral thoracotomy
  - Supine with arm abducted above the head
- Posterolateral thoracotomy
  - Lateral decubitus position if contralateral injuries have been ruled out.
  - Have a low threshold for chest tube placement on the side that will be down if there is a concern for injury to that side—placement of an emergent chest tube intraoperatively once the patient is positioned will be challenging.

TECHNIQUES

LEFT ANTEROLATERAL THORACOTOMY

- Positioning: supine with left arm abducted above the patient's head.
- Identify the fourth intercostal space. In men this will be in line with or just inferior to the nipple. In women it will be at or above the inframammary fold.
- Make an incision directly onto the rib from sternum to posterior axillary line, curving the incision toward the posterior axilla to follow the rib.
- Divide the intercostal muscles with a scalpel or with Mayo scissors.
- Divide the pleura with heavy curved Mayo scissors the entire length of incision.
- Place a Finochietto retractor and spread widely. Make sure that the bar for the retractor is toward the axilla to facilitate conversion to bilateral thoracotomy if necessary.
- Identify the pericardium and the phrenic nerves running cranially to caudally at the 3- and 9-o'clock positions on the pericardial sac.
- After grasping the pericardium with toothed forceps, open the pericardium with an anterior cranial-to-caudal incision to avoid injuring the lateral-lying phrenic nerve.
- Deliver the heart from the opened pericardial sac and inspect for any evidence of injury. Temporize any injuries with an occluding finger, atraumatic vascular clamp, skin staples, or suture. Of note, this left anterolateral thoracotomy incision may be utilized to achieve proximal control of left subclavian artery injuries (**FIGURE 4**).
- Cross-clamp the aorta by opening the pleura overlying the posterior mediastinum and identifying the aorta, which is visualized directly overlying the thoracic vertebrae (**FIGURE 5**). Once the aorta is identified, place an aortic Crawford clamp across the aorta at the level of the vertebral disc to avoid injuring segmental aortic branches to the spine. This maneuver shunts blood from "nonessential" organs to essential coronary and cerebral vasculature while limiting infradiaphragmatic exsanguination.
- Quickly assess for other injuries to temporize within the thoracic cavity.
- Open cardiac massage, or open chest CPR, is performed by rhythmically compressing the heat to augment blood flow until a perfusing rhythm is regained. This is much more effective than closed chest, standard CPR in hypovolemic, critically injured patients. Consider intracardiac injection of epinephrine and internal defibrillation depending on the visualized cardiac activity.

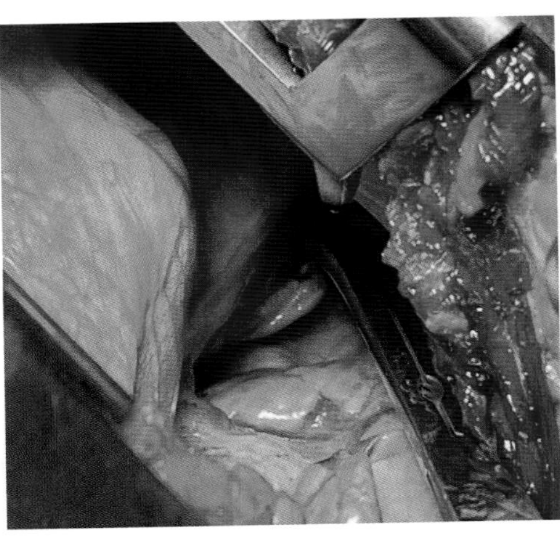

FIGURE 4 ● Proximal control of left subclavian artery via left anterolateral thoracotomy. The proximal left subclavian artery may be controlled via left anterolateral thoracotomy.

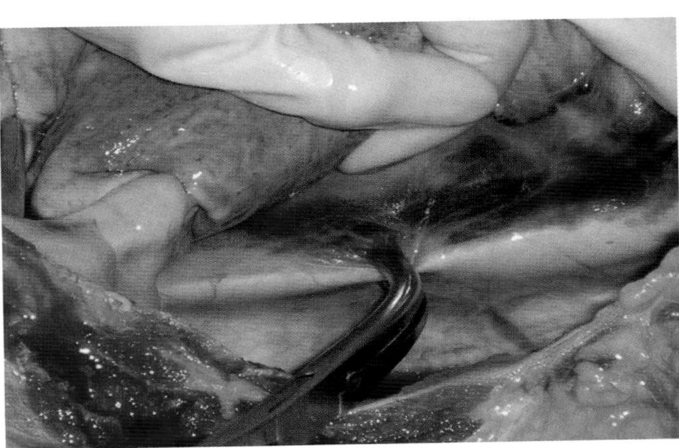

FIGURE 5 ● Resuscitative thoracotomy: placement of descending thoracic aortic cross-clamp. The aorta is clamped in the posterior mediastinum. In a pulseless patient, it may be difficult to distinguish the aorta from the esophagus.

- Ensure that intravenous access above and below the diaphragm has been established and resuscitate the patient with whole blood or blood components.
- Emergent transport to the OR for definitive management is indicated if a perfusing rhythm is achieved.
- Although less emergent and time sensitive, an anterolateral thoracotomy performed in the OR is performed in a similar fashion with greater initial attention paid to hemostasis (eg, use of electrocautery) and may not require pericardotomy, open cardiac massage, or placement of descending thoracic aortic cross-clamp depending on the clinical scenario.

BILATERAL THORACOTOMY

- If indicated based on wound pattern (eg, bilateral hemithoraces) or evidence of injury of the right thorax based on finger or tube thoracostomy, consider converting to a bilateral or clamshell thoracotomy.
- Begin by performing a left anterolateral thoracotomy, as detailed above.
- Extend the anterolateral thoracotomy incision over the sternum angling slightly up and to the right shoulder, and then across the chest above the right nipple, near the third intercostal space. This will ensure crossing the sternum in the bony portion and facilitate exposure of superior mediastinal structures.
- Divide soft tissue down to bone in the midline.
- Divide the sternum with a Lebsche knife or sternal saw.
- Continue across midline and open the third intercostal space of the right hemithorax.
- Place a second Finochietto retractor or replace a single retractor to spread the sternum.
- Follow other technical aspects of the left anterolateral thoracotomy as described above.

MEDIAN STERNOTOMY

- Identify the suprasternal notch and the xiphoid process.
- Make an incision in the midline overlying the sternum from notch to xiphoid. Divide the subcutaneous tissues down to the bone.
- Bluntly dissect in the substernal space immediately deep to the sternum from sternal notch to xiphoid to reduce the chance of underlying tissue damage from the sternal saw.
- While pulling upward with the sternal saw and deflating both lungs, divide the sternum in the midline from the xiphoid to the suprasternal notch. Take care to stay in the midline to optimize the strength of the sternal closure.
- Bleeding from the cut bone surface may be controlled with bone wax.
- Identify and protect the internal mammary arteries running under the chest wall just lateral to the sternum bilaterally.
- Place a sternal retractor and spread widely.
- Open the pericardium in an inverted T incision (vertical incision with horizontal incision at inferior portion of vertical incision) and tack the pericardium with suture to skin to facilitate exposure.
- Repair penetrating cardiac wounds with pledgeted sutures on a taper needle. Use a horizontal mattress suture on cardiac muscle. Note the location of the coronary vessels to avoid injuring or inadvertently ligating them (**FIGURE 6**).

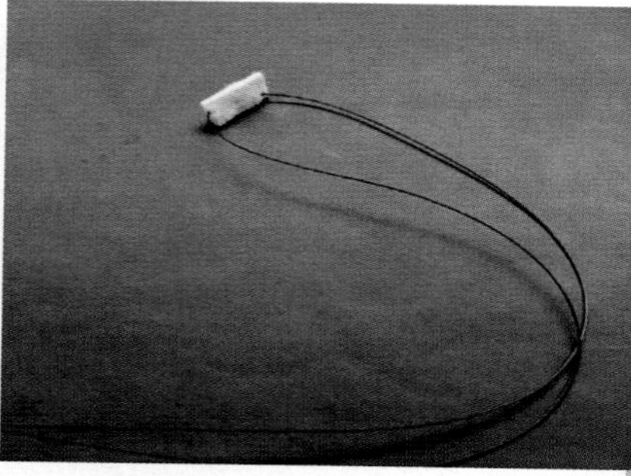
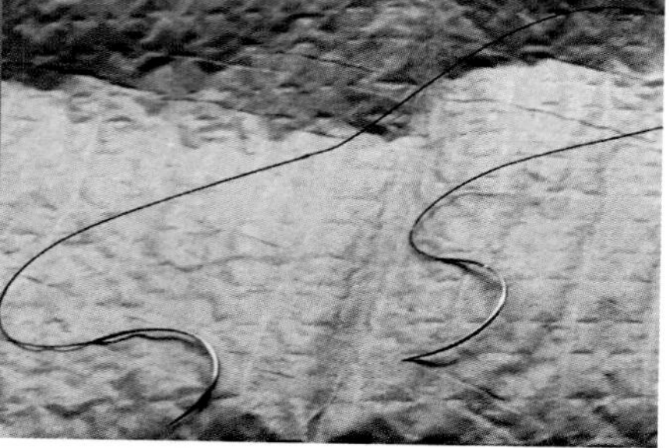

• Pre-pledget
• Double armed, 3-0 Prolene, MH needle
• Forehand, horizontal mattress
• Both throws though 2nd pledget, tie

FIGURE 6 ● After resuscitative thoracotomy: definitive cardiac repair. Repair cardiac injuries with a horizontal mattress suture using double-armed Prolene sutures with pledgets.

- Intraoperative transesophageal echocardiography may assist in the evaluation of septal, chordae, or valvular injuries.
- Once the repair is complete, leave a pericardial drain and leave the pericardium widely open to facilitate drainage.
- Close the sternum with sternal wires or sternal closure device.
- In damage control situations, the sternum may be left open and the incision temporarily closed with a vacuum device. Be conscious that doing so will alter pulmonary mechanics in the intensive care unit postoperatively.

POSTEROLATERAL THORACOTOMY[i]

- The anesthesia team should endotracheally intubate the patient with a double-lumen ETT. If bronchoscopy is required for intraoperative evaluation of the airways, intubate first with a single-lumen tube, perform bronchoscopy, and then change the tube to double-lumen ETT. Most standard bronchoscopes will not pass through the smaller lumen of a double-lumen ETT.
- Position the patient with the xiphoid at the break in the bed to facilitate full opening of the intercostal spaces once the patient is in lateral decubitus.
- Position the patient in lateral decubitus position with the operative site up and the arms supported either on pillows or with a device used to suspend the upper arm. Flex the bed at the break in the bed to open the intercostal spaces.
- Prep and drape to the spine posteriorly, the sternum anteriorly, the upper arm superiorly, and the anterior superior ischial crest inferiorly. Ensure electrocardiography (EKG) leads are moved out of the field.
- Identify the tip of the scapula and the costal margin.
- Make an incision in the skin overlying the sixth rib. Take the incision down through the subcutaneous fat to the muscle and divide the overlying muscles (latissimus dorsi, serratus anterior). When possible, attempt to split fibers rather than divide them.
- Divide the intercostal muscle, remembering that the intercostal neurovascular bundle is inferior to the rib.
    - If you are concerned for esophageal injury and considering the use of an intercostal muscle flap, preserve the intercostal muscle and divide it as anteriorly as possible for use as a flap.
- Open the pleura and enter the thoracic cavity.
- Place retractors to open the chest wall to visualize and address the injury:
    - Lung parenchyma—perform stapled wedge resection or tractotomy and oversew any injuries. Formal lobectomy is uncommonly indicated in the acute setting.
    - Esophagus—identify perforation and extend myotomy superiorly and inferiorly to visualize the full extent of mucosal injury. Repair the mucosal defect with running vicryl and muscular layers with interrupted silk suture. Buttress with an intercostal muscle flap, and widely drain.
    - Diaphragmatic injury—carefully inspect the diaphragm for injury and repair any defects. The presence of a diaphragmatic injury should alert the surgeon to the presence of a multicavitary injury involving both the thorax and the abdomen. After diaphragm repair, the potential for intra-abdominal injury should be addressed by operative abdominal exploration.
- Once the repair has been performed, place chest tubes to drain the thoracic cavity widely. Angled tubes drain the basilar space well; straight tubes drain the apices well. Clearly mark all chest drains and tubes.

[i]Presented for "completeness sake," but in reality, seldom indicated for initial operative management after trauma. Clinicians must be mindful that valuable patient access to the abdomen, pelvis, portions of the thorax, and extremities will be lost when placing patients in this position. Only consider this approach after complete examination and workup of patients with isolated injuries amenable to this incision, provided they maintain normal hemodynamics.

SUBXIPHOID PERICARDIAL WINDOW

- Make a vertical incision over the xiphoid process down to bone.
  - Excision of the xiphoid tip may be necessary to facilitate exposure.
- Dissect immediately deep to the xiphoid, maintaining careful hemostasis until the pericardium is encountered to avoid contamination of pericardial fluid with blood from the operative field and a falsely positive pericardial window.
- Placing the patient in steep reverse Trendelenburg positioning while an assistant retracts the sternum/costal margin anteriorly and superiorly greatly aids in exposure.
- Grasp the pericardium between two long Allis clamps. After ensuring complete hemostasis, incise the pericardium between clamps and assess the nature of the pericardial fluid.
  - If the fluid is nonbloody, the pericardial window is negative—proceed with any other indicated procedures.
  - If the fluid is bloody, perform median sternotomy to evaluate for cardiac injury.

LEFT SECOND INTERSPACE OR "HIGH" ANTEROLATERAL THORACOTOMY

- This incision may be used either in isolation or in conjunction with other incisions to improve exposure to the great vessels and specifically the left subclavian artery (**FIGURE 4**), which comes off of the aortic arch very posteriorly and is therefore difficult to access via median sternotomy.

SUPRACLAVICULAR INCISION (FIGURE 7)

- This incision may be used either in isolation or in conjunction with median sternotomy to improve exposure to the great vessels (specifically, the right subclavian artery).
- Make an incision above the clavicle on the side of the injury.
- Divide the sternocleidomastoid and scalene muscles at their insertion into the medial portion of the clavicle.
- Consider resecting the head of the clavicle and extension to an infraclavicular incision to improve exposure.

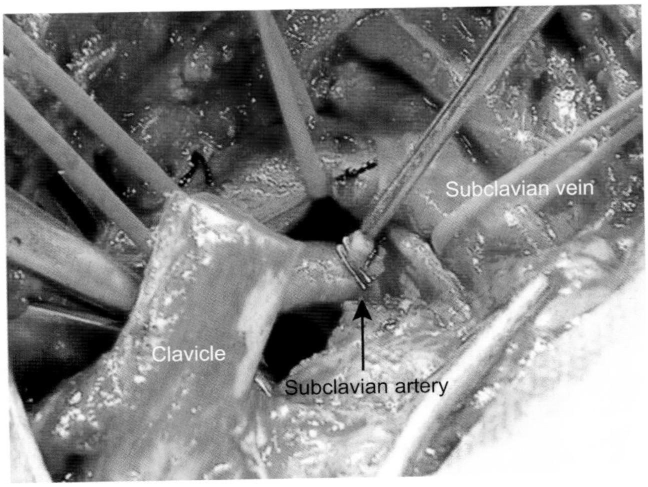

FIGURE 7 ● Exposure of left subclavian artery via left supraclavicular incision (clavicular head resected). A supraclavicular incision may be used to expose the proximal left subclavian artery. Full exposure may require resection of the head of the clavicle. (Reprinted with permission from Seamon MJ, Choudry R, Santora T, et al. Thyrocervical trunk transection: A rare cause of massive hemothorax. *J Trauma*. 2007;62:1534.)

INFRACLAVICULAR INCISION

- An infraclavicular incision may be used to obtain distal control of the proximal subclavian artery, axillary artery, or proximal control of a proximal brachial artery injury.
- Make an infraclavicular incision starting at the inferior edge of the center of the clavicle and running laterally in the deltopectoral groove.
- Split and retract the fibers of the pectoralis major muscle without dividing them if able.
- Divide the pectoralis minor muscle with electrocautery over a large clamp or Army-Navy retractor.
- The axillary artery with surrounding nerves should be visualized at the base of the wound.
- Avoid injury to the brachial plexus when isolating the axillary artery.

PEARLS AND PITFALLS

Pulseless patient	■ Resuscitative thoracotomy allows temporization of cardiac or great vessel injuries, open cardiac massage, and placement of descending thoracic aortic cross-clamp. Make sure each step is performed to maximize outcomes. ■ Quickly assess whether injuries are salvageable by direct inspection to avoid unwarranted potential occupational exposures or wasteful blood product resuscitation. ■ After injuries are temporized and perfusing rhythm is achieved, clamp and ligate each end of severed internal mammary arteries to avoid rebleeding. ■ Once the patient is resuscitated and injuries are controlled, warn the anesthesia team before removing the aortic cross-clamp. Remove it slowly—one "click" at a time to avoid reperfusion injury and hemodynamic collapse.
Patient in shock	■ In patients with isolated thoracic injury, assume cardiac or great vessel injuries are present until proven otherwise. ■ Utilize incisions that allow for adaptability along with proximal and distal control. ■ Continuously reassess the patient's hemodynamics and injury burden.
Hemodynamically normal patient	■ A proper workup can often eliminate nontherapeutic operations or incorrect initial surgical incisions. ■ In patients with normal hemodynamics, additional imaging and diagnostic adjuncts will facilitate and focus necessary operative care.

POSTOPERATIVE CARE

- Postoperatively, patients require excellent pain control and pulmonary toilet.
- Patients who remain intubated should be ventilated using standard ventilator strategies to reduce barotrauma.
- Patients who are extubated and awake should be instructed in the use of an incentive spirometer and encouraged to use it frequently and document improvements in vital capacity. They should be encouraged to utilize available analgesics to ensure that pain does not limit their ability to take deep breaths. Poor pain control results in decreased tidal volumes, atelectasis, and the development of pneumonia.
- Multimodal analgesia is important to ensure adequate pain control. Regional or epidural analgesia should be considered in all patients, but particularly in those with limited pulmonary reserve (eg, patients with older age, history of lung disease such as chronic obstructive pulmonary disease or asthma, prior lung surgery, comorbidities such as obesity, diabetes, or patients who are chronically immunosuppressed) or those whose injuries are severe or incisions extensive.
- Thoracic and mediastinal chest drains should be monitored for output quantity and quality and presence/absence of air leak.

COMPLICATIONS

- Characteristics of thoracic and mediastinal drainage tubes and presence/absence of air leak provide important information to guide the assessment of complications following thoracic surgery.
  - Ongoing bleeding should be addressed promptly and may mandate a return to the operating room after rewarming and coagulopathy is corrected. Thromboelastography and coagulation parameters may help guide ongoing optimization of coagulation status.
  - Volume overload is common in postoperative thoracic patients, and high-volume serous output from thoracic or mediastinal drains may reflect ongoing third-spacing of intravascular fluids. Consider diuresis.
  - Bronchopleural fistula may occur particularly in the setting of concomitant lung injury and may be identified as a persistent air leak. Typically, these heal with nonoperative measures but require ongoing evacuation of air from the pleural cavity via chest tube. It is important not only to minimize suction and/or positive end-expiratory pressure on these fistulae to avoid stenting them open but also to ensure that air is efficiently evacuated from the pleural space to allow for full lung inflation.
  - Chyle leaks may present with milky output from thoracic or mediastinal drains. The diagnosis may be confirmed by measuring fluid triglycerides in chest tube effluent. Chylothorax is managed by pleural drainage for symptom relief and to quantify the volume of drainage. Low-volume drainage is typically managed medically with a low-fat diet and somatostatin analogue. In patients with high-volume drainage or low-volume drainage who fail conservative therapy, the thoracic duct may be embolized or surgically ligated to reduce drainage.[9]
- Cardiac arrhythmias are common following thoracic surgery, and atrial fibrillation is among the most common.[10] Ensure electrolytes are normalized, obtain an EKG and CXR, and consider diuresis as volume overload can precipitate new-onset postoperative atrial fibrillation in patients following thoracic surgery.
- Retained hemothorax is common in the setting of injury to the thoracic cavity or mediastinum. Early (within 7 days), low-volume retained hemothorax may respond adequately to drainage without requiring subsequent operative drainage. Higher-volume or delayed (after 7 days) retained hemothoraces may require decortication via video-assisted thoracoscopic surgery or open thoracotomy. Decortication and evacuation of delayed hemothorax has been conditionally

recommended over thrombolytic therapy to reduce hospital length of stay and need for additional operative intervention. Over a quarter of patients may require more than one operative intervention to evacuate retained hemothorax.[11,12]

- Nerve injuries may occur in the setting of thoracic trauma. The phrenic nerve runs parallel to the aorta along the pericardium and may be injured when the pericardium is opened. This will result in paralysis of the ipsilateral diaphragm. The vagus nerve runs in the posterior mediastinum and gives rise to bilateral recurrent laryngeal nerves (RLNs). The right RLN loops around the subclavian artery, and the left RLN loops around the aortic arch lateral to the ligamentum arteriosum before running superiorly in the tracheoesophageal groove. Injury to either may lead to hoarseness; injury to both may lead to airway compromise requiring tracheostomy. Injury to the vagus nerve below the RLN takeoffs is less clinically concerning.[13] Injuries to the brachial plexus surrounding the subclavian and axillary arteries are also common in the setting of injury to these vessels.
- Delayed or missed aerodigestive injuries can lead to catastrophic outcomes including sepsis and death. It is imperative to look early for these potential injuries by performing an UGI, EGD, and bronchoscopy, as initially patients with these injuries are often asymptomatic.[8]

REFERENCES

1. Merrick C, ed. *American College of Surgeons Committee on Trauma. Advanced Trauma Life Support (ATLS)*. 10th ed. American College of Surgeons; 2018.
2. Seamon MJ, Haut ER, Van Arendonk K, et al. An evidence-based approach to patient selection for emergency department thoracotomy: a practice management guideline from the Eastern Association for the Surgery of Trauma. *J Trauma Acute Care Surg*. 2015;79(1):159-173.
3. Taghavi S, Jayarajan SN, Ferrer LM, et al. "Permissive hypoventilation" in a swine model of hemorrhagic shock. *J Trauma Acute Care Surg*. 2014;77(1):14-19.
4. Dumas RP, Jafari D, Moore SA, et al. Emergency department versus operating suite intubation in operative trauma patients: does location matter? *World J Surg*. 2020;44(3):780-787.
5. Dumas RP, Chreiman KM, Seamon MJ, et al. Benchmarking emergency department thoracotomy: using trauma video review to generate procedural norms. *Injury*. 2018;49(9):1687-1692.
6. Schellenberg M, Inaba K. Critical decisions in the management of thoracic trauma. *Emerg Med Clin North Am*. 2018;36(1):135-147.
7. DuBose JJ, Morrison J, Moore LJ, et al. Does clamshell thoracotomy better facilitate thoracic life-saving procedures without increased complication compared with an anterolateral approach to resuscitative thoracotomy? Results from the American Association for the Surgery of Trauma aortic occlusion for resuscitation in trauma and acute care surgery registry. *J Am Coll Surg*. 2020;231(6):713-719.e1.
8. Asensio JA, Chahwan S, Forno W, et al. Penetrating esophageal injuries: multicenter study of the American Association for the Surgery of Trauma. *J Trauma*. 2001;50(2):289-296.
9. Riley LE, Ataya A. Clinical approach and review of causes of a chylothorax. *Respir Med*. 2019;157:7-13.
10. Vaporciyan AA, Correa AM, Rice DC, et al. Risk factors associated with atrial fibrillation after noncardiac thoracic surgery: analysis of 2588 patients. *J Thorac Cardiovasc Surg*. 2004;127(3):779-786.
11. Patel NJ, Dultz L, Ladhani HA, et al. Management of simple and retained hemothorax: a practice management guideline from the Eastern Association for the Surgery of Trauma. *Am J Surg*. 2021;221(5):873-884.
12. DuBose J, Inaba K, Demetriades D, et al. Management of post-traumatic retained hemothorax: a prospective, observational, multicenter AAST study. *J Trauma Acute Care Surg*. 2012;72(1):11-22; discussion 22-24; quiz 316.
13. Auchincloss HG, Donahue DM. Prevention and management of nerve injuries in thoracic surgery. *Thorac Surg Clin*. 2015;25(4):509-515.

Chapter 11 Pericardial Window: Subxiphoid, Parasternal

Christofer B. Anderson and Sharven Taghavi

DEFINITION

- Pericardial window (PCW) is defined as the creation of an opening in the pericardium to allow drainage of pericardial fluid or blood via a catheter or into the pleural space.
- In trauma, a PCW is used to determine if there is a cardiac injury. A PCW that is positive for blood necessitates a sternotomy or thoracotomy to expose the heart.

DIFFERENTIAL DIAGNOSIS

- Thoracic trauma may be associated with injury to any of the contents within the thorax; hemorrhage may be secondary to injury to the lungs or mediastinal contents (heart, great vessels). The reported incidence of cardiac injury following penetrating thoracic trauma in those who undergo thoracotomy is 10% to 37% for gunshot wounds and 16% to 52% for stab wounds.[1,2]
- Penetrating chest trauma may be associated with intraperitoneal injury in up to 20% of patients.[3]

PATIENT HISTORY AND PHYSICAL FINDINGS

- History is often limited in the patient with penetrating chest trauma; however, the mechanism of gunshot vs stab wound should be elucidated. Initial assessment of the patient should follow the standardized approach outlined by the Advanced Trauma Life Support (ATLS) algorithm. The primary survey Airway, Breathing, Circulation, Disability, and Exposure (ABCDE) allows for rapid identification of penetrating chest injury. The airway should be secured and resuscitation with blood products begun for the hemodynamically unstable patient. Evidence of decreased or absent breath sounds or tracheal deviation in the unstable patient warrants immediate placement of tube thoracostomy on the affected side.
- External wounds within the "cardiac box," defined as the sternal notch superiorly, midway between the xiphoid process and umbilicus inferiorly and midclavicular line (nipples) laterally should raise suspicion for penetrating cardiac injury (PCI), but any wound to the thorax puts the heart at risk (**FIGURE 1**). Traditional physical examination findings of PCI are pulsus paradoxus and Beck's triad of muffled heart sounds, jugular venous distension, and hypotension; however, in those found to have a cardiac injury, only 10% display these findings.[4]

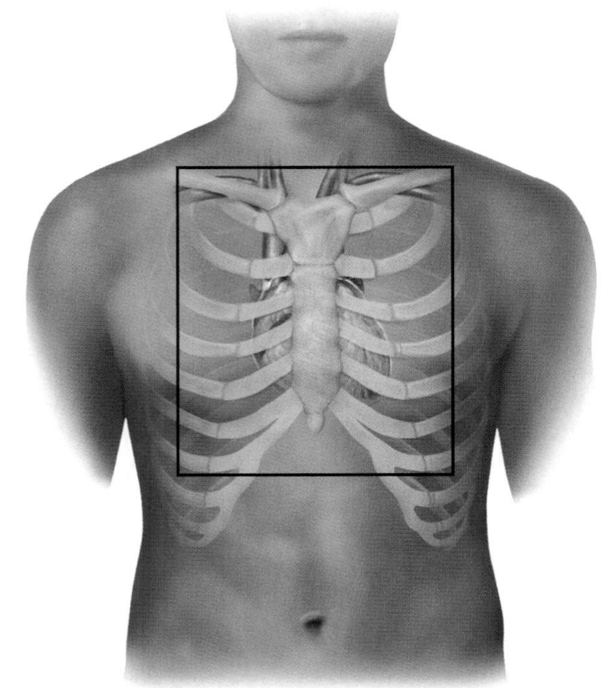

FIGURE 1 ● Cardiac box. Defined by sternal notch superiorly, midway between the xiphoid and umbilicus inferiorly and midclavicular lines laterally.

- If during the primary survey cardiopulmonary arrest occurs in the patient with penetrating thoracic trauma, emergency department resuscitative thoracotomy is performed.[5]

IMAGING AND OTHER DIAGNOSTIC STUDIES

- After completion of the primary survey, a chest X-ray and a focused assessment with sonography for trauma (FAST) are performed as part of the workup (**FIGURE 2**). Chest X-ray findings suggestive of pericardial effusion include an enlarged cardiac silhouette, but have poor sensitivity and specificity. Chest X-ray can also be important to discern the trajectory of bullets and to determine the risk of cardiac injury.

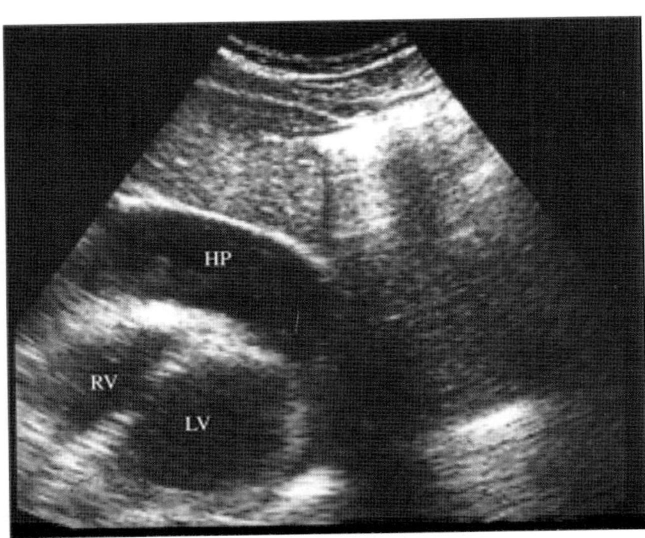

FIGURE 2 ● Focused assessment with sonography for trauma (FAST) demonstrating hemopericardium. RV, right ventricle, LV, left ventricle, HP, hemopericardium. (Reprinted with permission from Cardozo A, Peurta F, Valencia L. E-FAST: A propos of hemopericardium in the Emergency Department. *J Acute Dis.* 2016;5(3):260-263.)

- The role of PCW in the diagnosis of suspected PCI has diminished with the institution of FAST. FAST examines the hepatorenal recess (Morrison pouch), pericardium, splenorenal recess, and pelvis (Pouch of Douglas) for the presence of fluid. FAST can allow for detection of hemopericardium prior to decompensation secondary to tamponade physiology. Successful utilization of FAST is operator dependent. However, when performed by experienced users, in patients with PCI, the sensitivity of FAST for detection of hemopericardium has been reported to be as high as 100% with a specificity of 96.9%.[6] Small case series have demonstrated that PCI with a concomitant laceration to the pericardial sac allows for decompression of the cardiac injury into the thoracic cavity, resulting in a false-negative FAST examination.[6,7] However, a positive FAST examination demonstrating pericardial effusion in the setting of penetrating thoracic trauma and hemodynamic instability mandates operative intervention via sternotomy or thoracotomy.[8] In the hemodynamically stable patient in which the FAST examination is negative, but concern for PCI is present based on mechanism and location of injury, computed tomography angiography (CTA) should be performed and may exclude cardiac or great vessel injury.[3] However, PCW is a useful adjunct when the diagnosis of PCI remains in question in the setting of a hemodynamically stable patient with penetrating thoracic injury and/or massive hemothorax with an equivocal or negative FAST examination and/or CTA.

SURGICAL MANAGEMENT

Preoperative Planning

- After the decision is made to do PCW, the patient is transferred to the operating room. In the event that return of blood is noted, conversion to sternotomy or anterolateral thoracotomy must be performed. The operating room and staff must have the necessary equipment to perform a sternotomy or thoracotomy quickly, if necessary.
- Adequate large bore intravenous access should be obtained and type and cross match should be performed. If there is a high index of suspicion for cardiac injury, blood products should be immediately available. The blood bank should be notified of the possibility of activation of massive transfusion protocol. The operating room should be prepared to utilize cell saver.
- Periprocedural antibiotics should be administered.

Positioning

- The patient should be placed supine with arms out.
- A standard trauma prep including the neck, entire thorax, and abdomen should be performed.
- If the patient is hemodynamically compromised or has evidence of tamponade on ultrasound, the patient should be prepped and draped prior to induction of anesthesia.

SUBXIPHOID APPROACH

Incision

- Identify the xiphoid process and costal margins by palpation.
- A scalpel is used to make an approximately 5 cm incision in the upper midline over the xiphoid process extending to the xiphisternal junction and carried down through the subcutaneous tissues.
- The linea alba attaches to the inferior portion of the xiphoid and is divided sharply or with electrocautery exposing preperitoneal fat with care taken to avoid entry into the peritoneal cavity. The rectus abdominis inserts on the anterior surface of the xiphoid and is also divided sharply or with electrocautery.
- The xiphoid is then grasped with a Kocher and elevated, posterior diaphragmatic attachments to the xiphoid are bluntly swept away. A Kittner can be helpful for this dissection. The xiphoid is excised using Mayo scissors (**FIGURE 3A**).

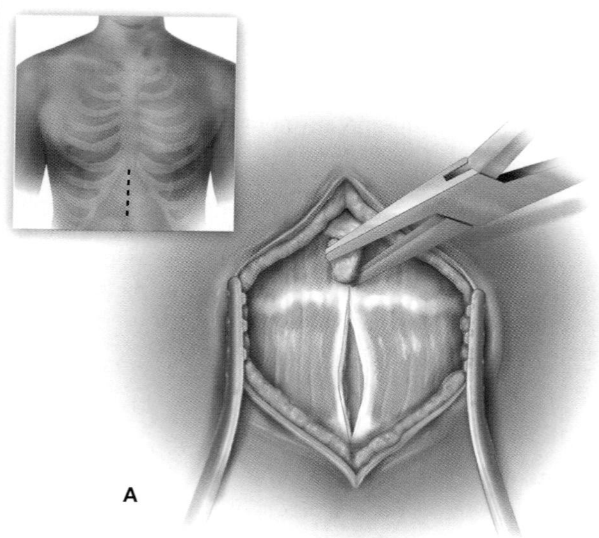

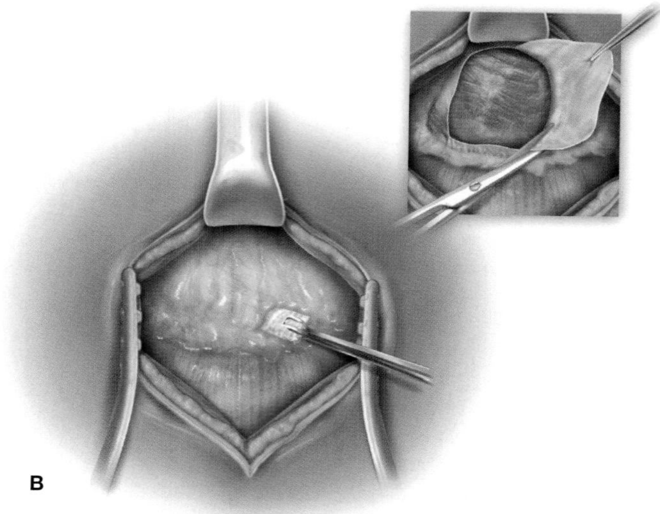

FIGURE 3 ● Subxiphoid pericardial window. **A,** Incision and exposure. **B,** Opening of pericardium. (Modified with permission from Asmat A, Rizk NP. Pericardial procedures. In: Kaiser LR, Kron IL, Spray TL, eds. *Mastery of Cardiothoracic Surgery*. 3rd ed. Wolters Kluwer; 2014:289-295. Figure 28.1.)

EXPOSURE OF THE PERICARDIUM

- A self-retaining retractor is placed within the incision and a small Richardson retractor is placed under the sternum displacing it anteriorly exposing the diaphragm and pericardium. The cardiophrenic fat pad is encountered; gentle palpation helps to identify the diaphragmatic and pericardial junction. The pericardial fat pad is bluntly swept away with a Kittner or sponge stick exposing the pericardium.
- Presence of a distended or tense pericardium with discoloration may be present, indicative of a potential cardiac injury.

OPENING THE PERICARDIUM

- The pericardium can then be grasped with small Allis or Kelly clamps and retracted inferiorly, gently.
- A second Allis or Kelly clamp is used to grasp the pericardium. It is important to gain meticulous hemostasis prior to opening the pericardium, to minimize the risk of a false-positive window.
- Metzenbaum scissors or a no. 15 blade is used to incise the pericardium between the two clamps (**FIGURE 3B**).

EVALUATION OF PERICARDIAL CONTENTS

- Evacuation of gross blood or clot indicates the presence of cardiac injury and the incision should be extended superiorly over the midline of the sternum to proceed with sternotomy. A left anterolateral thoracotomy at the 4th-5th intercostal space may also be performed depending on surgeon preference.
- Absence of gross blood with continued hemodynamic stability indicates a PCI is unlikely to have occurred. A pericardial drain or chest tube is not indicated if the PCW is negative. The linea alba is closed with interrupted monofilament such as PDS and the subcutaneous tissue and skin closed with absorbable suture or staples.

PARASTERNAL APPROACH

Incision

- The 4th-5th intercostal space is identified at the inframammary fold on the anterior chest wall, just lateral to the sternum.
- A scalpel is used to make an approximately 5 cm curvilinear incision beginning parasternal and curving laterally along the inframammary fold.

EXPOSURE OF PERICARDIUM

- The incision is carried through the subcutaneous fat and pectoralis major muscle, using electrocautery, until the 4th and 5th ribs are identified. The intercostal muscles of the 4th intercostal space are divided, transversely, staying close to superior border of the 5th rib to avoid the intercostal neurovascular bundle (**FIGURE 4A**).
- The parietal pleura is identified and divided, gaining access to the thorax. A pediatric Finochietto rib spreader is inserted into the 4th intercostal space and gently opened, exposing the anterior surface of the pericardium.

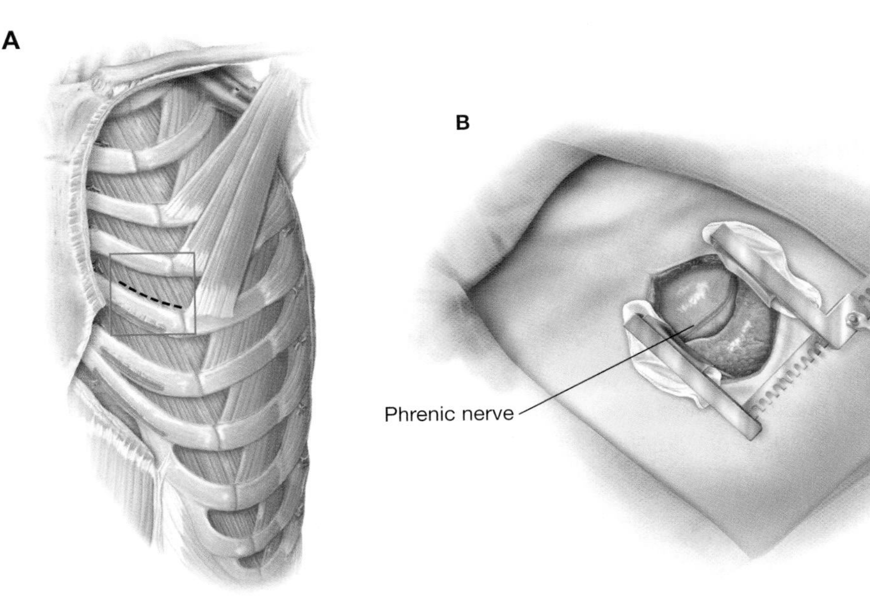

FIGURE 4 ● **A,** Division of intercostal muscles exposing the parietal pleura. **B,** Identification and opening of pericardium.

OPENING THE PERICARDIUM

- The anterior surface of the pericardium is bluntly dissected using a Kittner.
- The pericardium is gently grasped with small Allis or Kelly clamps and retracted ventrally.
- Care should be taken to preserve the phrenic nerve, laterally.
- Metzenbaum scissors or a no. 15 blade is used to sharply enter the pericardium.
- A 2-cm square of pericardium is excised (**FIGURE 4B**).

EVALUATION OF PERICARDIAL CONTENTS

- Evacuation of gross blood or clot indicates the presence of cardiac injury and the incision should be extended to perform a traditional anterolateral thoracotomy in the 4th-5th intercostal space. A large bore thoracostomy tube should be placed through a separate incision at the mid- to anterior axillary line in the intercostal space either above or below the existing incision, if not already done so for a previously identified hemo/pneumothorax.
- The fascia of the pectoralis major muscle is re-approximated with a running 0-Vicryl suture and the subcutaneous tissue and skin of the parasternal incision is then closed in a standard fashion with absorbable suture or staples.

PEARLS AND PITFALLS

Indications	■ PCW should be considered in the patient with penetrating thoracic injury and massive hemothorax with an equivocal or negative FAST examination that is hemodynamically stable. ■ Hemodynamic instability with a positive FAST examination mandates median sternotomy or anterolateral thoracotomy if there is suspicion of cardiac injury.
Incision	■ When performed under general anesthesia, the patient should be prepped and draped prior to induction in the event that hemodynamic collapse occurs due to tamponade physiology compounded by the progressive loss of venous return with the positive pressure of intubation.
Conversion to median sternotomy or thoracotomy	■ The presence of gross blood on PCW mandates conversion to median sternotomy or anterolateral thoracotomy to identify and repair PCI. ■ A clamshell thoracotomy may be necessary to improve exposure of the heart.
Associated intra-abdominal injury	■ As many as 20% of patients with penetrating thoracic injury may have an associated intra-abdominal injury.[3]

POSTOPERATIVE CARE

- For a negative subxiphoid or PCW, tube thoracostomy is not necessary.
- Patients can be discharged the same day if they have no other injuries after recovering from anesthesia.
- Chemical deep venous thrombosis prophylaxis should be initiated as early as possible.

COMPLICATIONS

- Bleeding
- Surgical site infection
- Postpericardiotomy syndrome
- Phrenic nerve injury with parasternal PCW
- Traumatic chylothorax
- Occult diaphragmatic injury

REFERENCES

1. Karmy-Jones R, Jurkovich GJ, Nathens AB, et al. Timing of urgent thoracotomy for hemorrhage after trauma: a multicenter study. *Arch Surg*. 2001;136(5):513-518.
2. Karmy-Jones R, Nathens A, Jurkovich GJ, et al. Urgent and emergent thoracotomy for penetrating chest trauma. *J Trauma*. 2004;56(3):664-668.
3. Renz BM, Cava RA, Feliciano DV, Rozycki GS. Transmediastinal gunshot wounds: a prospective study. *J Trauma*. 2000;48(3):416-421; discussion 421-422.
4. Trinkle JK, Toon RS, Franz JL, Arom KV, Grover FL. Affairs of the wounded heart: penetrating cardiac wounds. *J Trauma*. 1979;19(6):467-472.
5. Burlew CC, Moore EE, Moore FA et al. Western Trauma Association critical decisions in trauma: resuscitative thoracotomy. *J Trauma*. 2012;73(6):1359-1363; discussion 1363-1364.
6. Rozycki GS, Feliciano DV, Ochsner MG, et al. The role of ultrasound with possible penetrating cardiac wounds: a prospective multicenter study. *J Trauma*. 1999;46:543-552.
7. Ball CG, Williams BH, Wyrzykowski AD, et al. A caveat to the performance of pericardial ultrasound in patients with penetrating cardiac wounds. *J Trauma*. 2009;67:1123-1124.
8. Karmy-Jones R, Namias N, Raul C, et al. Western trauma association critical decisions in trauma: penetrating chest trauma. *J Trauma Acute Care Surg*. 2014;77(6):994-1002.
9. Cardozo A, Peurta F, Valencia L. E-FAST: a propos of hemopericardium in the Emergency Department. *J Acute Dis*. 2016;5(3): 260-263.

Chapter 12 Repair of Cardiac Injury

Zoë Maher, Valeda Yong, and Jessica H. Beard

DEFINITION

- Repair of cardiac injury is a surgical procedure in which a partial or full thickness injury of the heart is definitively closed.

DIFFERENTIAL DIAGNOSIS

- The clinical presentation of a patient with cardiac injury is highly variable, ranging from asymptomatic with normal vital signs to cardiac arrest. Low-grade, partial thickness injuries can be present in patients without hemodynamic sequelae. Patients with high-grade, full thickness injuries can present with shock or in cardiac arrest due to cardiac tamponade, hemorrhage, or both.
- A high index of suspicion for cardiac injury must be maintained for all patients with thoracic or thoracoabdominal penetrating trauma and for patients with significant blunt-force mechanism.

PATIENT HISTORY AND PHYSICAL FINDINGS

- Penetrating injury within the "cardiac box" has traditionally been associated with an increased risk of cardiac injury. The box is defined superiorly by the clavicles, laterally by the mid-clavicular lines and inferiorly by the costal margins. The clinical utility of the cardiac box has been challenged recently, with reports indicating that injury mechanism is an important consideration in determining risk for cardiac injury.[1,2]
- Patients with penetrating cardiac injury may present in shock due to cardiac tamponade. Physical examination findings of cardiac tamponade include Beck triad of sinus tachycardia, elevated jugular venous pressure, and pulsus paradoxus, though the latter two findings may not be immediately evident in the trauma bay. Sinus tachycardia and hypotension will be present in the majority of patients with cardiac tamponade, and volume loading early in the resuscitation can be effective in prevention of cardiac arrest in this patient population.
- Patients with cardiac injury decompressing into the thoracic cavity will likely have hemorrhagic shock refractory to volume loading. These patients can present with or quickly decompensate into cardiac arrest.
- In terms of mechanism, cardiac tamponade is classically seen with precordial stab wounds to the heart, while massive hemothorax may be the presenting finding of a transthoracic or thoracoabdominal gunshot or stab wound resulting in cardiac injury.
- Patients with blunt cardiac injury (BCI) will most commonly be asymptomatic. High-grade BCI, including The American Association for the Surgery of Trauma grades III–V, may present in shock due to cardiac tamponade from cardiac chamber rupture, cardiac failure from myocardial contusion or coronary artery injury, pericardial injury leading to cardiac herniation, or valvular injury. It is very uncommon for BCI to mandate surgical intervention.[3]

IMAGING AND OTHER DIAGNOSTIC STUDIES

- The Focused Assessment with Sonography for Trauma (FAST) exam is extremely useful in the initial evaluation of the patient with suspected cardiac injury.[4] Pericardial fluid seen on the subxiphoid view is diagnostic of a cardiac injury in the setting of penetrating trauma (see ▶ **Video 1**). The absence of pericardial fluid does not rule out cardiac injury, especially in a patient with concomitant hemothorax, as cardiac hemorrhage may decompress into the thoracic cavity without accumulation of hemopericardium.[5]
- In the setting of blunt trauma, consideration should be given to physiologic or nontrauma–related pericardial effusion in the stable patient with a positive pericardial FAST. Though assessment of cardiac performance is not a component of the FAST examination, cardiac ultrasound can be useful to detect findings of cardiac failure due to BCI. These findings may include depressed ejection fraction, valvular insufficiency, or regional wall motion abnormality.
- Chest x-ray is a useful adjunct in the assessment of the patient with cardiac injury. The absence of hemothorax with a negative pericardial FAST greatly reduces the suspicion for high-grade cardiac injury. The presence of hemothorax with a negative pericardial view does not eliminate the possibility of cardiac injury as described above. Hemothorax combined with pericardial effusion may influence the choice of operative incision.
- Chest computed tomography scan may help to clarify trajectory and evaluate for secondary findings of cardiac injury in stable patients with inconclusive physical examination or radiography.[6]

SURGICAL MANAGEMENT

- An unstable patient with cardiac injury diagnosed by physical examination, chest x-ray (hemothorax), and/or FAST exam should be managed in the operating room. A stable patient with a concerning penetrating trajectory and positive pericardial FAST should also receive operative intervention.

Preoperative Planning

- In patients with suspected cardiac injury and tamponade physiology, optimization of cardiac preload prior to intubation may prevent cardiac arrest at intubation. Anesthesia should be notified of the suspected cardiac injury as should the operating room staff. Prepping and draping the patient prior to induction should be considered in the hemodynamically acceptable patient with suspected cardiac injury.[7] A sternal saw should be available. The massive transfusion protocol should be initiated for patients with or at high risk of exsanguination, and cell saver should be considered if available.
- Patients with suspected cardiac injury who arrive in cardiac arrest with short prehospital times or who develop cardiac

arrest in the trauma bay should undergo left anterolateral thoracotomy with extension to clamshell thoracotomy as needed for exposure and control of the cardiac injury in the trauma bay.

Positioning

- The supine position is preferred for patients with suspected cardiac injury. Abduction of the arms can be helpful to open the rib spaces, improving exposure during any thoracotomy incision.

TECHNIQUES

INCISIONS

- The three incisions used to expose and repair a cardiac injury include median sternotomy, left anterolateral thoracotomy, and bilateral anterior "clamshell" thoracotomy (**FIGURE 1**).
- The median sternotomy incision is carried from the sternal notch to the xiphoid process taking care to remain in the midline of the sternum. Palpation of the intercostal spaces on either side of the sternum with marking of the center can be helpful to ensure midline entry. A window must be created superior to the sternal notch and inferior to the xiphoid to clear away the soft tissues and vasculature immediately deep to the sternum and prevent iatrogenic injury of these structures. A sternal saw may then be used to divide the sternum. Special caution should be used to avoid injury to the right ventricle in patients with prior sternal incisions or cardiac surgery. The Finochietto retractor is placed with the bar oriented caudally (**TABLE 1**). The mediastinal fat and anterior pericardium are incised widely to permit delivery and exposure of the heart. Tamponade will be relieved upon entry of the pericardium.
- The left anterolateral thoracotomy incision is carried from the right of the sternum at the level of the fourth or fifth intercostal space and is curved up into the axilla following the angle of the rib (**FIGURE 1**). Care should be used to avoid

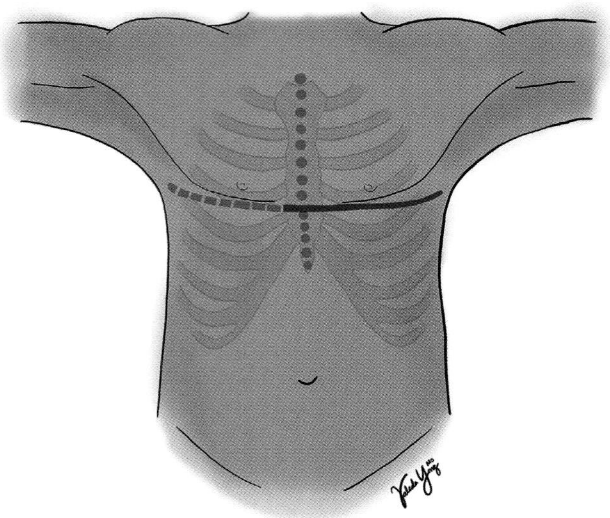

FIGURE 1 ● Incisions used to expose and repair a cardiac injury include the median sternotomy (red dotted line), left anterolateral thoracotomy (blue solid line), and bilateral anterior "clamshell" thoracotomy (green dashed line and blue solid line). (Courtesy of Valeda Yong, MD.)

Table 1: Essential Instruments and Supplies Used to Expose and Repair Cardiac Injuries

	Instrument name	Uses/tips
	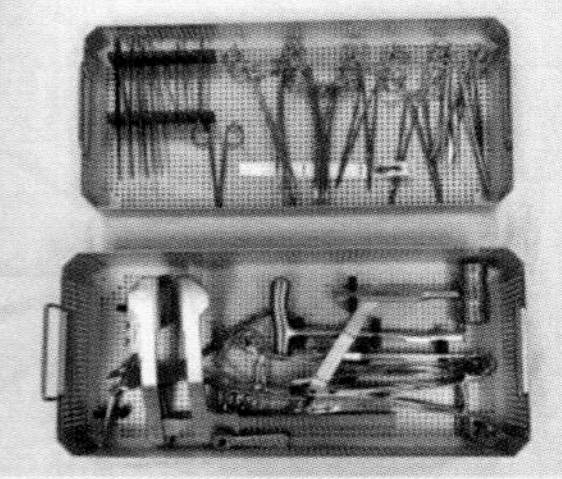	
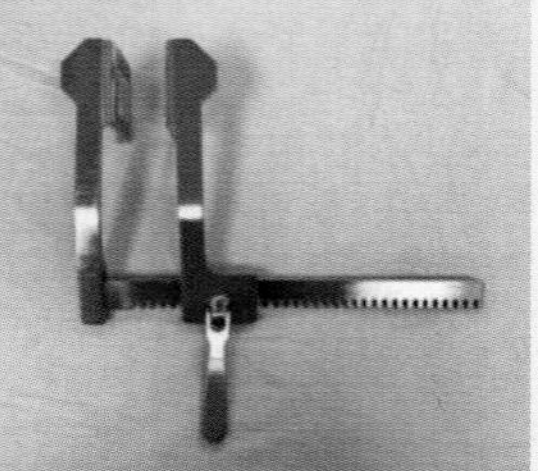	Finochietto retractor	• To spread the ribs during thoracotomy and/or median sternotomy • Turn handle counterclockwise to open • Orient the bar toward the bed for left anterolateral thoracotomy
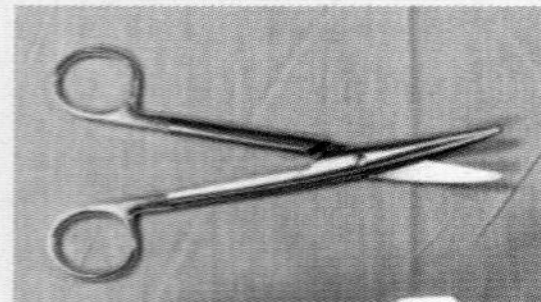	Curved Mayo scissors	• To incise the intercostal muscles

Table 1: Essential Instruments and Supplies Used to Expose and Repair Cardiac Injuries ***(continued)***

	Instrument name	Uses/tips
	Lebsche sternal knife and mallet	• To divide the sternum during clamshell thoracotomy • Hold mallet perpendicular to Lebsche knife • Hook Lebsche knife under sternum and apply upward traction prior to activating the mallet
	Toothed forceps	• To grasp the pericardium
	Metzenbaum scissors	• To incise pericardium anterior and parallel to the phrenic nerve • For tense hemopericardium, incision with a scalpel is preferred
	Debakey aortic clamp	• To cross-clamp the aorta
	Satinsky clamp	• To control a cardiac atrial injury
	Top picture from left to right: • Needle holder • 3-0 double-armed Prolene suture on MH needle • Debakey forceps **Bottom picture:** • Loading pledgets onto 3-0 polypropylene suture	• Cardiac injury should be repaired with 3-0 nonabsorbable monofilament suture on a large tapered needle • Atrial injuries may be sutured in a running fashion under a vascular clamp • Ventricular injuries should be reinforced with pledgets to prevent tearing

unnecessary division of the latissimus dorsi musculature laterally as this will increase postoperative bleeding risk without improving exposure. The intercostal muscles are divided with curved Mayo scissors on the cephalad aspect of the rib to avoid injury to the inferiorly running intercostal neurovascular bundle (**TABLE 1**). Medially, the left internal mammary artery must be ligated and divided. The Finochietto retractor is then placed with the bar oriented laterally toward the bed (**TABLE 1**, **FIGURE 2**).

- The clamshell thoracotomy incision is an extension of the left anterolateral thoracotomy (**FIGURE 1**). It is indicated for increased exposure of right-sided cardiac injuries or when there is concomitant right-sided thoracic injury as evidenced by right-sided hemothorax on chest tube placement. The incision should be extended onto the right chest either at the same rib space or at the rib space cephalad and curved up into the right axilla following the angle of the rib. It is critical that sufficient sternum remains at the caudal aspect of the

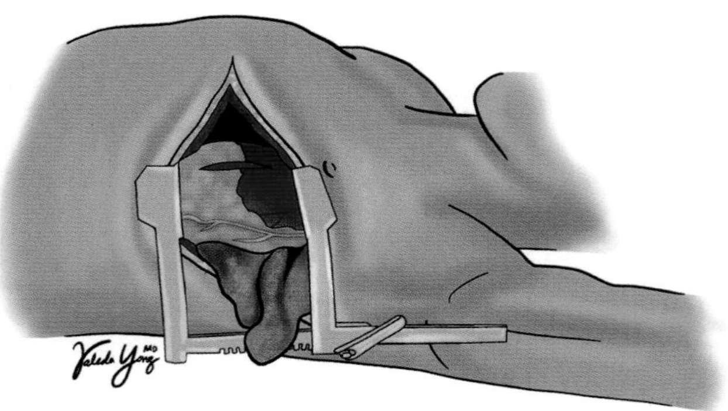

FIGURE 2 ● The left anterolateral thoracotomy incision and exposure. The pericardial incision should be made longitudinally and anterior to the phrenic nerve (yellow structure). The Finochietto retractor is placed between the ribs with the bar oriented laterally. (Courtesy of Valeda Yong, MD.)

incision to permit closure at the end of the case. Extension across the sternum is performed with either a sternal saw or Lebsche knife and mallet. The image and description in **TABLE 1** demonstrates the correct handling of these instruments. As in the left anterolateral thoracotomy, the intercostal muscle should then be divided on the cephalad aspect of the rib to avoid injury to the inferiorly running intercostal neurovascular bundle. The left and right internal mammary arteries should be identified, ligated, and transected, ideally prior to division of the sternum. In the hemodynamically unstable patient, this step can be delayed until after the compelling injury is addressed. The Finochietto retractor may be moved to the middle of the incision with the bar placed laterally or two Finochietto retractors may be placed (one in each chest cavity) for optimal exposure (**FIGURE 3**).

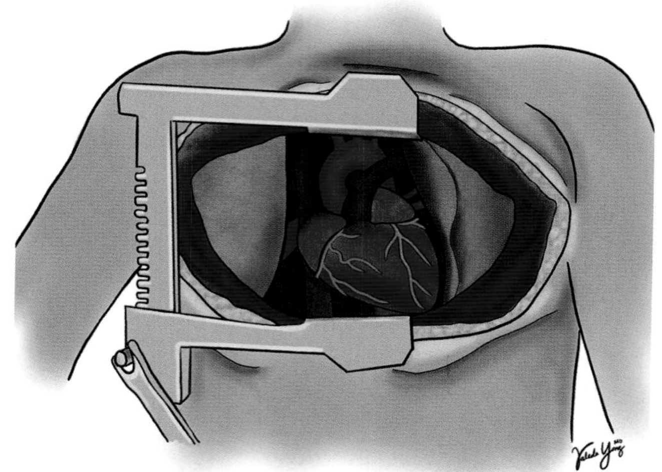

FIGURE 3 ● The bilateral anterior "clamshell" thoracotomy provides optimal exposure for all types of cardiac injuries as well as the anterior mediastinum and bilateral hemithoraces. This is our preferred incision for cardiac injuries resulting from gunshot wounds. (Courtesy of Valeda Yong, MD.)

- We advocate against the using the posterolateral thoracotomy for any suspected cardiac injury, as patient positioning and exposure are extremely limited.

EXPOSURE

- Median sternotomy is the incision of choice for isolated precordial stab wounds with suspected cardiac injury. This incision provides ideal exposure to the anterior heart and the thoracic outlet. It is challenging to evaluate and repair posterior cardiac injuries utilizing this incision. If a posterior cardiac wound is encountered through a median sternotomy, a cardiac suction elevator, typically used for cardiac stabilization, can be employed to assist with exposure. Median sternotomy does not permit exposure of the bilateral hemithoraces or posterior mediastinum and therefore should not be utilized when injuries in these locations are suspected.
- Left anterolateral thoracotomy permits exposure to the left ventricle, left atrium, and left hemithorax (**FIGURE 2**). Extension across the sternum with a sternal saw or Lebsche knife can be utilized as an adjunct to permit wider exposure for injuries in these locations and to improve exposure to the right ventricle, right atrium, superior vena cava, and inferior vena cava.
- Clamshell thoracotomy is required to optimally expose most injuries to the right ventricle as well as injuries to the superior and inferior vena cava and right atrium (**FIGURE 3**). This incision provides excellent exposure for the structures of the mediastinum. Of all the incisions mentioned, we consider the clamshell thoracotomy to be the optimal incision for gunshot wounds to the chest with suspected cardiac injury as it provides the most versatile exposure of all potentially injured structures in the chest and mediastinum.

ANATOMY

- A thorough understanding of cardiac anatomy is imperative to sound operative decision-making in the repair of cardiac injury. Entry into the pericardium should be performed anteriorly to avoid the phrenic nerve, which runs along the bilateral posterolateral aspects of the pericardium with the pericardiophrenic artery and vein (**FIGURE 2**).
- The surface anatomy of the heart can be used to define the anatomical location of the cardiac injury. Identification of the left anterior descending (LAD) artery provides a quick visual separation of the chambers of the left and right heart, with the right heart to the right of the LAD and the left heart to the left of the LAD (**FIGURE 4**). The right ventricle is the anterior most chamber of the heart and the right atrium is cephalad and to the right of the ventricle, separated by the right coronary artery. The left ventricle is positioned to the left of the LAD and is surprisingly posterolateral. Relative to the left ventricle, the left atrium is cephalad, separated by the circumflex branch of the left coronary artery.

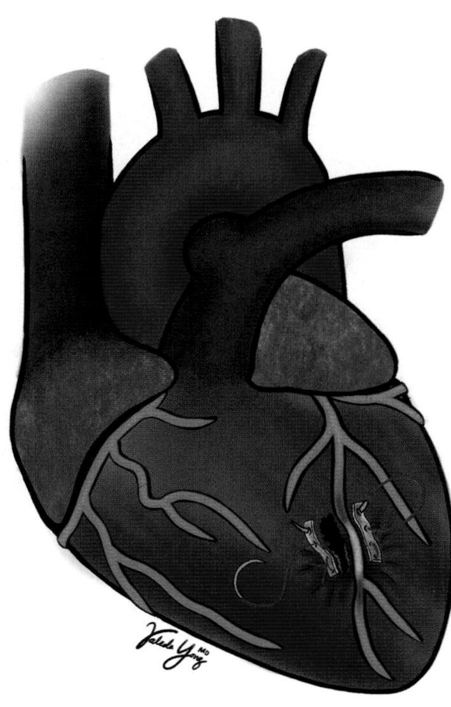

FIGURE 4 ● The surface anatomy of the heart can help identify the anatomic location of a penetrating cardiac injury. Injuries adjacent to coronary vessels, like the left anterior descending (LAD) artery pictured here, may be safely repaired with pledgeted horizontal mattress sutures placed under the vessel. (Courtesy of Valeda Yong, MD.)

CONDUCT

- Pericardiotomy should be performed sharply with either a toothed forceps and Metzenbaum scissors or with a scalpel (**TABLE 1**). In the case of tense hemopericardium, it may be impossible to elevate the pericardium with toothed forceps; therefore, the pericardium should be incised with a scalpel and the opening extended inferiorly and superiorly utilizing Metzenbaum scissors. The pericardiotomy should be large enough to permit complete delivery of the heart and to avoid ventricular outflow tract obstruction during evaluation and repair.
- Digital pressure for ventricular injuries and vascular clamp application (eg, Satinsky clamp) for atrial injuries are our preferred methods of temporary control of cardiac injuries prior to definitive repair (**TABLE 1**, **FIGURE 5**). Rapid, non-pledgeted suture repair of either the atria or the ventricle can be an effective method of temporary control in the case of a large cardiac injury. Temporary control of ventricular injuries can also be achieved with the use of staples or the application of a vascular clamp, especially if the injury is too long to permit digital control, as is often the case in gunshot wounds. Wounds necessitating temporary control by any of the above methods will be at risk for tearing adjacent to the injury, particularly if the injury is controlled prior to achieving return of spontaneous circulation. We advocate against the use of Foley catheter control of these injuries, as we have found that this technique is prone to dislodgement, inadequate control of blood loss, and increasing the size of the cardiac defect.
- Definitive cardiorrhaphy for ventricular injuries should be performed using horizontal mattress sutures buttressed with polytetrafluoroethylene (eg, Teflon) to prevent tissue tearing. **Video 2** demonstrates the closure of a gunshot wound to the left ventricle using this technique. In **Video 3**, the

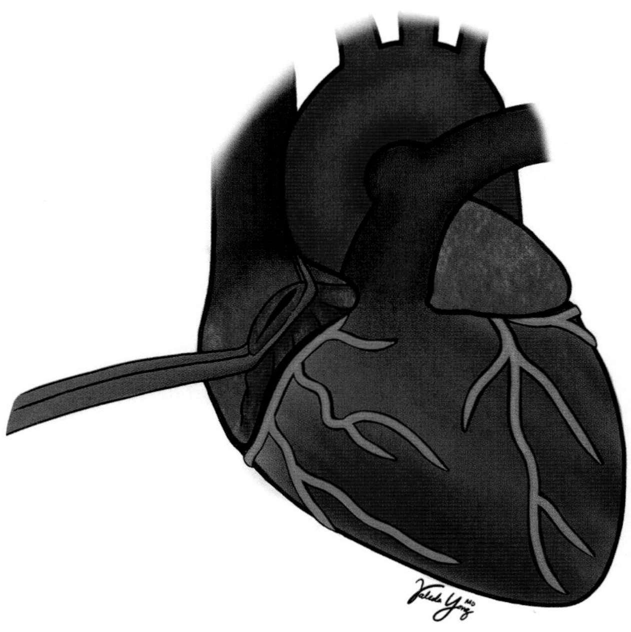

FIGURE 5 ● A Satinsky clamp can be used to control a right atrial injury. Atrial injuries do not routinely require pledgeted repairs. Instead, the 3-0 polypropylene suture may be used to repair the injury under the clamp with the clamp in situ. (Courtesy of Valeda Yong, MD.)

completed repair with two pledgeted horizontal mattress sutures can be seen.

- In the case of atrial injuries, a Satinsky clamp may be used to control the injury in the trauma bay or prior to repair in the operating room (**FIGURE 5**). If the cardiac injury has been temporarily controlled with a vascular clamp, definitive closure can be performed by running the suture under the clamp in situ. Pledgets are generally not necessary for the thinner-walled atria.
- Injuries adjacent to coronary vessels should be repaired with a horizontal mattress suture placed under the vessel to avoid injury to the vessel (**FIGURE 4**).
- Commercially available pledgets are generally precut and sized for standard nontrauma cardiac surgery applications. When possible, we advocate the use of larger polytetrafluoroethylene pledget material that may be cut-to-size based on the morphology of the individual cardiac injury as is shown in **FIGURE 6**. The pericardium may also be used as a pledget. The pericardium is trimmed to the desired length and width based on the size and morphology of the cardiac injury. It is then deployed in the same fashion as a synthetic pledget.
- We utilize a 3-0 polypropylene suture on a large tapered needle (eg, 3-0 Prolene MH double-armed) for definitive cardiac repair (**TABLE 1**). The needle is large enough to permit extension across both sides of a cardiac gunshot wound and shaped to permit reapproximation of smaller cardiac stab wounds. The double-armed suture is especially helpful if pledgets are being placed. We do not close the pericardium after cardiac injury repair.
- Though nearly all cardiac injuries occur by penetrating mechanism, there are rare exceptions. Blunt atrial blowout injuries should be managed in the same fashion as a penetrating atrial injury. As described above, Satinsky clamp may be used to control the injury in combination with Allis clamps to elevate the full thickness of the cardiac wall on either side of the injury (**FIGURE 5**). Repair should then be performed using a 3-0 polypropylene suture on a large tapered needle either single or double-armed in a running fashion under the clamp.
- Complex cardiac injuries, such as those that involve coronary vessels, valves, septum, or multiple chambers, require special attention. Distal coronary artery injuries can be ligated. Patients managed with coronary ligation must be closely monitored for evidence of cardiac arrhythmia, hypokinesis, or congestive heart failure. Proximal coronary injuries often require cardiopulmonary bypass, and for this, we request assistance from cardiac surgery. Intraoperative transesophageal echocardiogram (TEE) is a valuable tool for the detection of suspected valvular or septal injuries, and ideally intraoperative TEE is performed on all patients with cardiac injury. When diagnosed, consideration should be made for concurrent or future repair of valvular or septal injuries with input from cardiac surgery. Most commonly, these can be safely managed in a delayed fashion, provided the patient is hemodynamically acceptable.

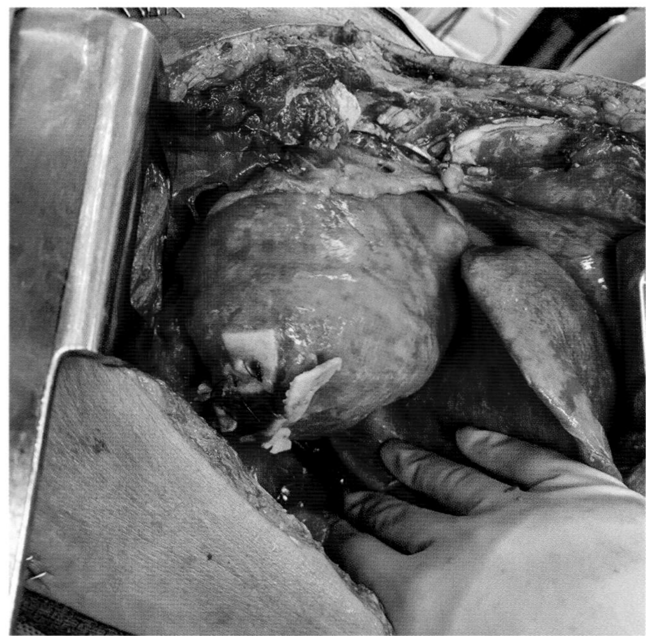

FIGURE 6 • Left ventricular stab wound repaired with polytetrafluoroethylene pledget material that has been cut-to-size to approximate the length of the injury. (Courtesy of Zoë Maher, MD.)

CLOSURE

- Meticulous technique during closure of the chest should be maintained to prevent serious morbidity from wound complications.
- Following median sternotomy, hemostasis at the sternal edge is achieved with cautery and/or bone wax. A chest drain (eg, 28 Fr Chest tube) to water seal is placed under the sternum, and the sternum is closed with five or six simple, single or double looped steel wires using a heavy needle driver. The presternal fascia is closed with absorbable running sutures (eg, 2-0 polyglactin).
- Following left anterolateral thoracotomy, one or two large chest tubes (eg, 36 Fr) should be placed. We orient one straight chest tube toward the apex and another curved chest tube toward the base of the thoracic cavity. The ribs are reapproximated with heavy absorbable figure of eight pericostal sutures with care to avoid injury to the neurovascular bundle traveling at the inferior edge of each rib. Our preferred suture for rib reapproximation is the #2 polyglactin suture on a large taper needle (eg, #2 Vicryl on CTX). The chest wall musculofascial layers are then reapproximated using running absorbable sutures (eg, 0 polyglactin).
- The clamshell thoracotomy is closed in a similar fashion to that described for the anterolateral thoracotomy. To reapproximate the sternum, we place two vertically oriented, simple, single steel wires through the sternum prior to closing the thoracic cavity. We do not routinely drain the mediastinum following clamshell thoracotomy.

PEARLS AND PITFALLS

Diagnosis	■ Cardiac injury should be considered in any gunshot wound to the thorax. ■ Hemothorax on chest X-ray or ultrasound may represent decompression of a cardiac injury into the chest, even with a negative pericardial FAST.
Clinical manifestations	■ Patients with penetrating cardiac injuries present on a clinical spectrum from asymptomatic to cardiac arrest. ■ Cardiac tamponade and hemorrhage (or both) are the likely causes of shock following cardiac injury.
Incision	■ A median sternotomy should only be used for an isolated stab wound to the precordium. In the case of gunshot wounds involving the thoracic cavity, we recommend anterolateral thoracotomy or clamshell thoracotomy, to allow access for identification and repair of noncardiac intrathoracic injuries.
Technical conduct	■ For a patient in cardiac arrest, the cardiac injury should quickly be controlled prior to administration of ACLS. ■ In the ED, judicious clamping of low pressure atrial injuries or finger occlusion of high pressure ventricular injuries is preferred to Foley placement, suturing, or stapling.
Closure	■ The pericardiotomy should be opened widely and left open at the completion of the procedure to prevent accumulation of pericardial effusion and pericarditis. ■ The internal mammary arteries ***MUST*** be identified and ligated prior to the closure of the chest. Following sternotomy, check for bleeding under the sternum after removing the retractor.
Concomitant injury	■ Valvular or septal injury must be considered, especially in patients with isolated cardiac injury and ongoing shock following repair. Intraoperative transesophageal echocardiography (TEE) and cardiac surgery consult should be considered in cases of suspected valvular or septal injury.

ACLS, advanced cardiac life support; ED, emergency department.

POSTOPERATIVE CARE

- All patients with cardiac injury should receive a postoperative transthoracic echocardiography (TTE) with consideration of bubble study.
- Lung protective ventilation and avoidance of acute hypercapnia are critical in the postoperative setting. Beta blockade may mitigate postoperative catecholamine surge and reduce the risk of dysrhythmias, which are rare but can be life threatening.
- Postoperative pericarditis is common and diagnosed by exam (chest pain, pericardial friction rub) along with characteristic ST segment elevation across all leads with PR depression on electrocardiography. Pericarditis may be treated with nonsteroidal anti-inflammatory drugs and colchicine, and patients should be monitored for pericardial effusion with follow-up echocardiography.

COMPLICATIONS

- Echocardiography is the cornerstone for the diagnosis of secondary complications following cardiac injury. We recommend obtaining a TTE for all patients prior to discharge with follow-up TTE on a case-by-case basis. Most secondary complications can be managed expectantly; when complications require surgical repair, outcomes are generally good.
- Transient congestive heart failure is common following repair of cardiac injury. In the acute postoperative period, depressed left ventricular function can be successfully managed with ionotropic vasopressors (eg, epinephrine), while right ventricular function is supported with pulmonary vasodilatory agents (eg, inhaled epoprostenol or nitric oxide). Persistent heart failure following repair is less common, though more likely in the setting of an injured coronary vessel, valve, or septum or in the case of a large cardiac injury with disruption of normal cardiac electrical activity.
- Postoperative bleeding is a potential complication, and unligated internal mammary (IMA) or intercostal arteries (ICAs) should be considered as sources. When patients with cardiac injury are in extremis, the IMA or ICA may not bleed or be easy to identify. Once the patient has stabilized, the proximal and distal ends of the internal mammary and any transected ICAs must be identified and ligated.
- Wound complications range from superficial skin infections to deep space infections like mediastinitis and empyema. A high index of suspicion must be maintained for infectious complications and aggressive treatment with antibiotics and drainage (including surgical drainage) should be undertaken. Sternal wound complications include sternal wound infection and dehiscence. Physical examination of the sternotomy is critical to detect early wound complications which may present as a sternal "click." In cases where sternal wound reconstruction is required, sternal plating should be considered.[8]

OUTCOMES

- For patients who survive penetrating cardiac injury without coronary or valvular injury, long-term outcomes are excellent.

REFERENCES

1. Jhunjhunwala R, Mina MJ, Roger EI, et al. Reassessing the cardiac box: a comprehensive evaluation of the relationship between thoracic gunshot wounds and cardiac injury. *J Trauma Acute Care Surg*. 2017;83(3):349-355.
2. Kim JS, Inaba K, de Leon LA, et al. Penetrating injury to the cardiac box. *J Trauma Acute Care Surg*. 2020;89(3):482-487. doi:10.1097/TA.0000000000002808
3. Schultz JM, Trunkey DD. Blunt cardiac injury. *Crit Care Clin*. 2004;20(1):57-70.

4. Rozycki GS, Feliciano DV, Ochsner MG, et al. The role of ultrasound in patients with possible penetrating cardiac wounds: a prospective multicenter study. *J Trauma*. 1999;46(4):543-551.
5. Ball CG, Williams BH, Wyrzykowski AD, Nicholas JM, Rozycki GS, Feliciano DV. A caveat to the performance of pericardial ultrasound in patients with penetrating cardiac wounds. *J Trauma*. 2009;67(5):1123-1124. doi:10.1097/TA.0b013e3181b16f30
6. Strumwasser A, Chong V, Chu E, Victorino GP. Thoracic computed tomography is an effective screening modality in patients with penetrating injuries to the chest. *Injury*. 2016;47(9):2000-2005.
7. Dumas RP, Jafari D, Moore SA, Ruffolo L, Holena DN, Seamon MJ. Emergency department versus operating suite intubation in operative trauma patients: does location matter? *World J Surg*. 2019;18.
8. Tang AL, Inaba K, Branco BC, et al. Postdischarge complications after penetrating cardiac injury: a survivable injury with a high postdischarge complication rate. *Arch Surg*. 2011;146(9):1061-1066. doi:10.1001/archsurg.2011.226

Chapter 13

Surgical Management of Lung Trauma: Tractotomy, Wedge Resection, and Lobectomy

Arvin C. Gee and Karen J. Brasel

DEFINITION

- Tractotomy is an operative technique to divide the lung parenchyma following the injury tract in the parenchyma created by a penetrating injury in order to expose areas of deep hemorrhage and air leakage. Tractotomies are nonanatomic in nature but generally do not result in loss of lung volume.
- A wedge resection is technique for nonanatomic resection of lung parenchyma. This is generally used for injuries to the peripheral lung parenchyma that are not amenable to primary repair and often lead to a loss of lung volume, albeit usually small.
- A lobectomy is an anatomic resection of a lung lobe. In the setting of a traumatic injury, lobectomies are generally reserved for severe lobar damage or injury to the lobar vessels with uncontrollable hemorrhage or unrepairable lobar bronchial injury.
- The goal of these three techniques, and of all lung surgery in trauma, is to control hemorrhage and air leaks.

DIFFERENTIAL DIAGNOSIS

- Lung parenchymal injuries will often present with a pneumothorax or a hemothorax. A pneumothorax can also be due to tracheal or esophageal injuries, but these patients will often have pneumomediastinum as well. Hemorrhage that presents as a hemothorax can also be from a cardiac injury or from an injury to any blood vessel within the chest.

PATIENT HISTORY AND PHYSICAL FINDINGS

- Patients will present with a history of a traumatic injury. Lung parenchymal injuries can occur after penetrating or blunt trauma to the torso. Rib fractures are also very common in chest injuries, and the fractured rib(s) may be the cause of the direct injury to the lung parenchyma.
- The majority of these injuries will not require operative intervention beyond placement of a chest tube for pneumothorax or hemothorax evacuation. The chest tube allows for evacuation of the air or blood and affords time for the lung parenchymal injury to heal.
- Indication for an urgent thoracotomy is any hemodynamic instability that is attributed to an injury in the hemithorax. General guidelines are:
  - If a chest tube has been placed and ≥1500 mL of blood output occurs, immediately the patient should be considered for a thoracotomy, particularly if there is evidence of continuing intrathoracic hemorrhage.
  - In addition, if the chest tube has put out ≥200 mL/h of blood for several hours, then a thoracotomy is indicated.[1]
  - A common goal of any emergent operation for lung trauma is to minimize the amount of lung tissue removed.

IMAGING AND OTHER DIAGNOSTIC STUDIES

- Chest x-ray is the least user-dependent and most universally available imaging study that can be readily deployed for trauma patients while they are in the trauma bay. These are best obtained as single anteroposterior projections. They can be diagnostic for bony injury, pneumothorax, pleural effusion/hemothorax, parenchymal damage, or mediastinal injury.
- Ultrasound, specifically extended focused ultrasonography for trauma (eFAST), is different from a "standard" FAST examination in that it includes an examination of the bilateral anterior thoraces, specifically to evaluate for the presence of a pneumothorax. As with all ultrasonography, the sensitivity and specificity of eFAST is user dependent. On eFAST, a pneumothorax is diagnosed by the lack of lung sliding, which happens when there is air between the visceral and parietal pleura. The lack of sliding is unfortunately a nonspecific sign and can be seen in other conditions (eg, post pleurodesis), so it is important to interpret the eFAST findings in relation to the patient's past medical and surgical history.
- Computed tomography (CT) provides a very high-resolution image of the chest and aids in the diagnosis of lung parenchymal injuries along with abnormalities in the pleural space. A CT scan can help define the trajectory of a missile and in identifying injury; adding intravenous contrast can also help diagnose and localize areas of active hemorrhage. A significant downside of CT scans is that the patient needs to be relatively stable due to the need to transport the patient out of the resuscitation area (see **FIGURES 1** and **2**).

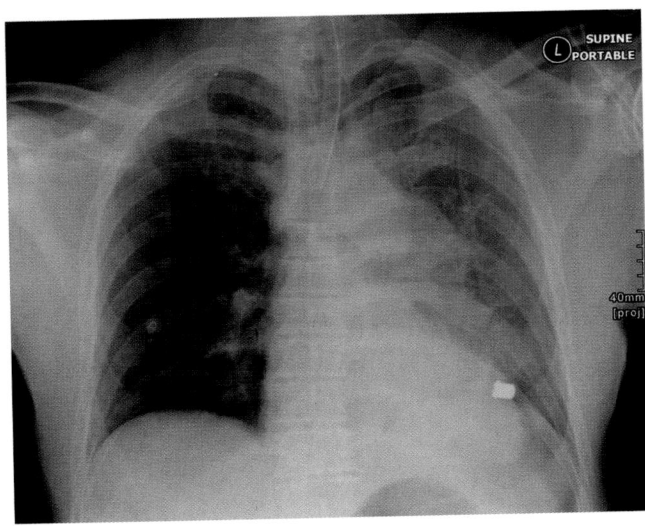

FIGURE 1 ● Chest X-ray following a gunshot wound to the left hemithorax. The radiodense bullet can be seen in the lower left chest.

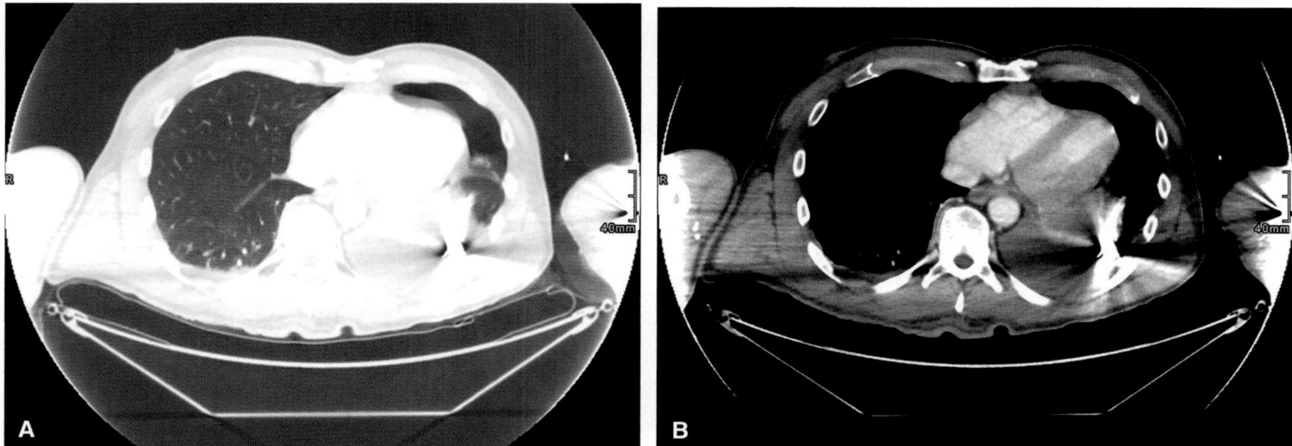

FIGURE 2 ● CT scans of the chest of the same patient seen in **FIGURE 1**. **A**, CT scan windowed to show the lung parenchyma, and a pneumothorax and the bullet are visible on the left. **B**, CT scan windowed for the soft tissues and a hemothorax is more easily seen in this image.

SURGICAL MANAGEMENT

Exposure

- When operating in the chest, particularly when operating on the lungs, it is important to discuss with the anesthesiology team the approach to intubation and lung isolation. Lung isolation allows for the selective ventilation of the lung that is not being actively operated on and can be achieved with three different techniques. Isolation of the operative lung allows for improved visualization, exposure, and manipulation of the lung.
- A single-lumen endotracheal tube can be advanced into the left or right main stem bronchus, and the contralateral lung is thereby not ventilated. A double-lumen endotracheal tube or bronchial blocker can be placed so that the left and right lungs can be independently ventilated. Each approach has advantages and disadvantages, but a discussion of the specifics is beyond the scope of this chapter.
- Both hemithoraces can be accessed through four incisions: a median sternotomy, an anterolateral thoracotomy, a transverse thoracosternotomy (commonly called a "clamshell" incision), or a posterolateral thoracotomy. Each of these four approaches carry advantages and disadvantages in terms of operative exposure of the lung parenchyma with sufficient access to repair or resect the lung. However, most trauma patients require supine positioning because of hemodynamic instability or other concomitant injuries that preclude a lateral decubitus position. With supine positioning both the left and right chest can be accessed through separate anterolateral thoracotomy incisions. The mediastinum can also be accessed by converting an anterolateral thoracotomy incision into a transverse thoracosternotomy or by combining a median sternotomy with a thoracotomy incision. These thoracic incisions are separately covered in Part 7, Chapter 10, Thoracic Incisions: Median Sternotomy, Anterolateral Thoracotomy, Bilateral Thoracotomy, Posterolateral Thoracotomy.

Lung Parenchyma Injury

- It is uncommon to need to resect lung parenchyma in the traumatically injured patient, and it is generally needed only if the lung tissue is injured beyond repair, there is nonrepairable pulmonary vascular injury, or there is an injury to the airway that is not amenable to repair. Fortunately, most lung injuries are amenable to direct repair and can therefore be addressed with "lung-sparing" techniques. In addition, there are data from several studies that show that formal lobectomies and pneumonectomies generally result in higher mortality.[2-4] These data, however, are confounded by their retrospective nature, and the occasional lobectomy or pneumonectomy may still be required. In such situations, the decision to do so should be made quickly.

TECHNIQUES

SUTURE PNEUMORRHAPHY

- If the lung injury is on the periphery of the lung and easily accessible from the surface, the lung parenchyma can be repaired with a simple suture repair along with ligation of visible intraparenchymal blood vessels. The edges of the lung wound are retracted apart to expose any bleeding vessels or open bronchi. The peripheral nature of these vessels and bronchi allows both to be suture ligated using absorbable suture without compromising the blood flow or aeration to the remainder of the lung. A 4-0 monofilament suture on a tapered needle can then be used to reapproximate the lung tissue to further buttress the repair. While there are case reports of permanent suture leading to granuloma formation, it is generally safe to use either absorbable or permanent suture. In addition, it can be helpful to ask the anesthetist to reinflate the lung when reapproximating the lung tissue as this will aid in setting the correct tension on the suture (see **FIGURE 3**).

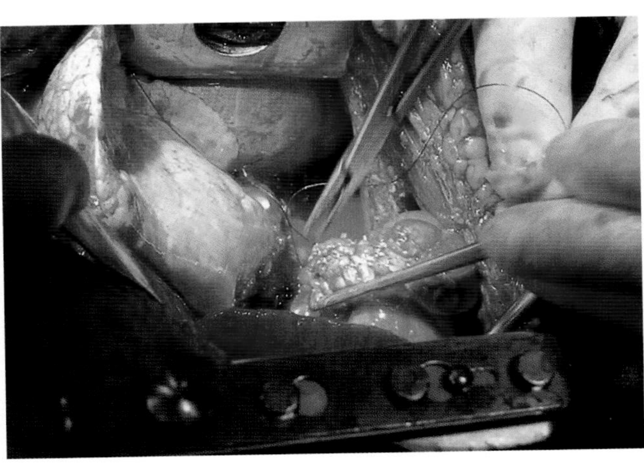

FIGURE 3 ● Suture pneumorrhaphy of a bleeding vessel in the lung parenchyma.

PULMONARY TRACTOTOMY

- As defined at the beginning of this chapter, a tractotomy is the division of the lung tissue to open up a penetrating injury tract to expose the injured deep lung parenchyma. This can be with a linear surgical stapler or with long surgical clamps. However, if a stapler is available, it is recommended to use one to minimize the operative time required to address the lung injury.
- For a stapled approach, the superficial portions of the injury tract are first identified and the lung tissue on either side of the tract to be opened is stabilized with Duval lung clamps or suture (**FIGURE 4A**). Next, one jaw (usually the anvil) of a linear laparoscopic or open GIA stapler (2.5-3.5 × 60-80 mm stapler, depending on the thickness of the lung and length of tract) is then placed into the tract while the second jaw is on the surface of the lung.
- Using staples that are too short in height can lead to the staples being pulled through the lung parenchyma when the lung is reinflated and can lead to prolonged air leaks. Therefore, it is important to use staple loads with appropriate thickness. Stapler devices designed for laparoscopic operations are helpful in this setting as they are easier to manipulate through a thoracotomy incision and keep the surgeons' hands outside of the chest cavity to improve visualization. The laparoscopic staples also have the advantage that the jaws can be articulated and can allow for more precise placement of the stapler in the desired position. Once the stapler is in position, it is closed down and fired. GIA staples have the advantage of laying down multiple rows of staples and dividing the tissue between the staple rows. Depending on the length of the tract and the length of the stapler used, multiple stapler firings may be required to fully open the tract and expose the injured deep lung parenchyma. Use of commercially available staple line reinforcement materials may help reduce the incidence of prolonged postoperative air leaks. Discussion of the available materials is beyond the scope of this chapter.
- Once the tract is opened, bleeding vessels and open bronchi are then ligated with absorbable suture. Air leaks can be identified by pouring a small volume of water into the opened tract to look for bubbles while the lung is ventilated. Any significant air leaks can be closed with suture. This same technique should be used to check the staple line for air leaks. Suture closure of the air leaks helps to minimize any prolonged air leaks. The lung that was divided with the stapler can then be reapproximated with suture as is done for any suture pneumorrhaphy, although this step is not absolutely necessary. The original superficial openings to the tract should be left open to minimize risk of developing an abscess or fluid collection within the lung (see **FIGURE 5**).

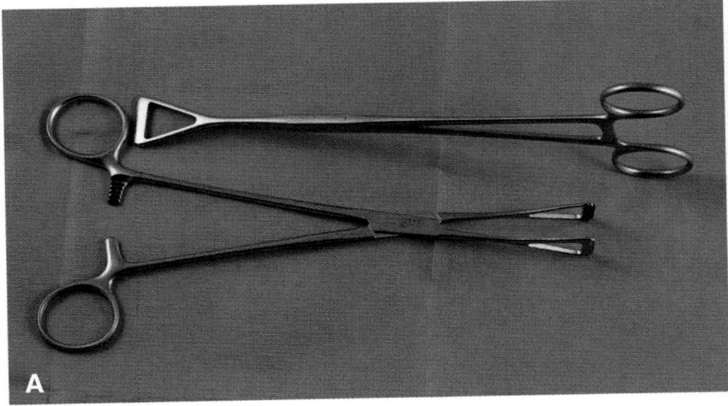

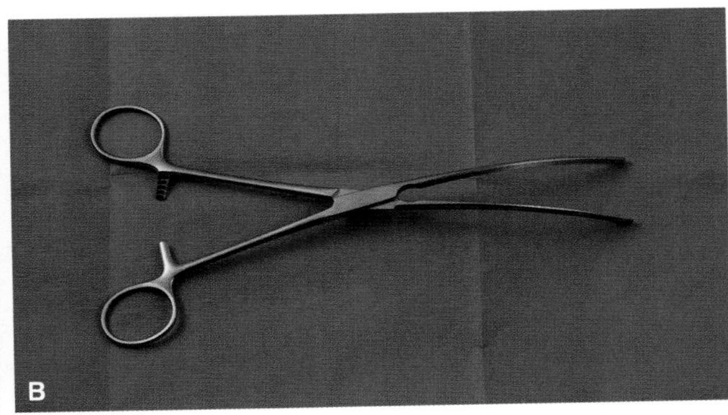

FIGURE 4 ● **A,** Duval lung clamps; **B,** Doyen atraumatic clamps.

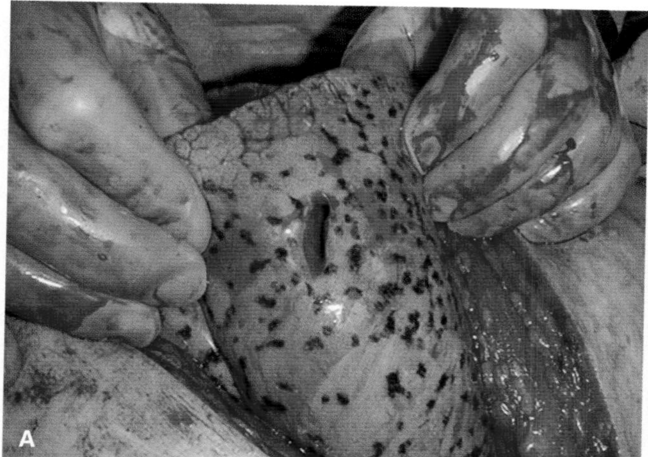

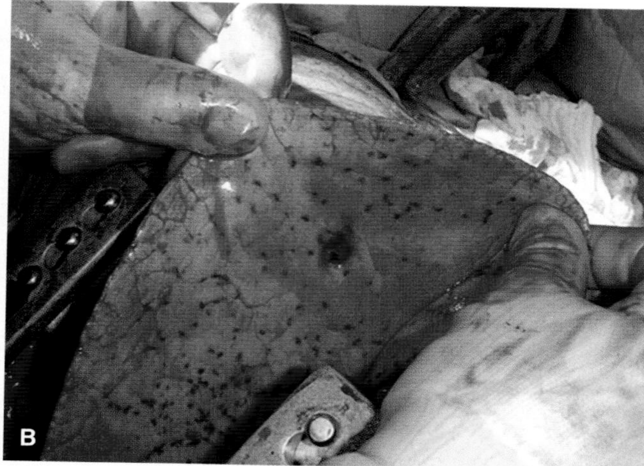

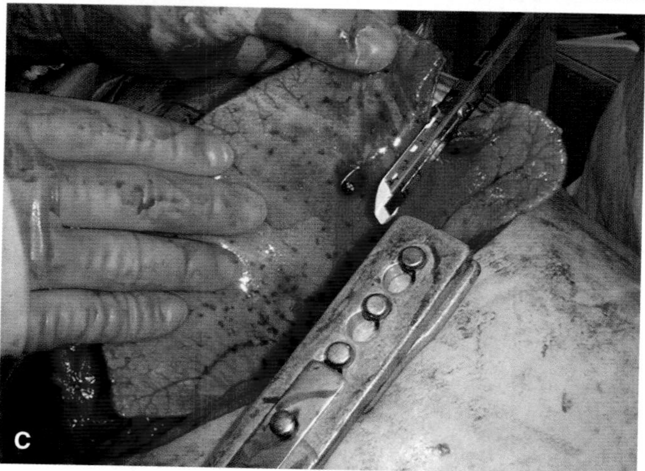

FIGURE 5 • **A** and **B,** The two sides of the penetrating injury to the center of the lung lobe. **C,** A laparoscopic linear stapler used to create the tractotomy through a sequential firing (the figure shows the second firing)

- Clamps can be used to perform the tractotomy as well, if a GIA stapler is not readily available. Atraumatic long-jawed clamps (eg, Doyen clamps) are ideally used to minimize further crushing injury to the already traumatically injured lung (**FIGURE 4B**). The lung is stabilized as is done with a stapled approach, and two clamps are placed into the injury tract and each clamp is positioned so that one jaw is in the tract and the other jaw on the lung surface. The lung tissue between the clamps is then divided sharply. The now-exposed injured vessels and bronchi are again controlled with suture ligation. The lung tissue within each clamp will usually need suture ligation and repair to control hemorrhage and air leaks within the clamped tissue. The lung tissue can then be reapproximated in a similar fashion as was described above for stapled tractotomies.[5]

PULMONARY WEDGE RESECTION

Nonanatomic Resections

- This technique can be used for injuries that are relatively peripheral on the lung lobes and away from the major pulmonary vasculature and larger bronchi. Generally, it is reserved for a discrete section of a lobe that is devitalized or otherwise too injured to be salvaged. This procedure is most easily performed with the aid of a linear stapler. To do the resection, the injured area that is to be resected is grasped with Duval clamps and elevated to allow a stapler to come across the lung. A GIA stapler is placed on healthy lung tissue just beyond the injured area and is used to staple and divide the lung.
- As with tractotomies, the staples should be 2.5 to 3.5 mm in thickness (or longer if the lung to be stapled is thicker) and the staple cartridge should be 60 to 80 mm long.
- Again, either laparoscopic or open GIA staplers can be used for this, but, as previously noted, the laparoscopic staplers may provide some advantage in ease and precision of stapler placement.
- Multiple staple reloads may be required to fully transect the lung parenchyma to release the injured segment. Reinforced staple loads are usually not required nor is it necessary to oversew the staple line with suture, but it is important to have the staple line solidly on healthy lung tissue (see **FIGURE 6**).

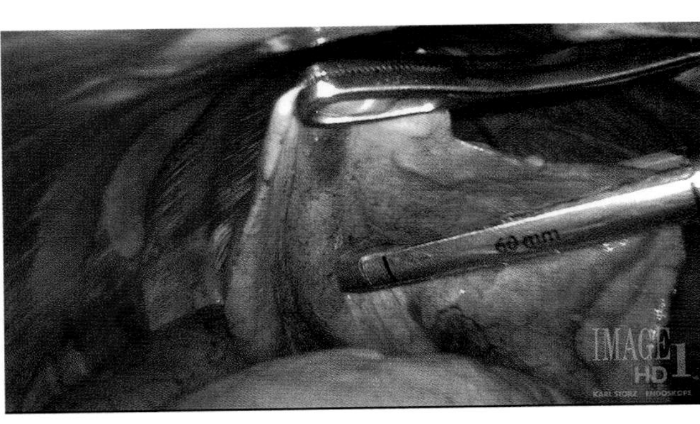

FIGURE 6 ● A thoracoscopic wedge resection. Notice the peripheral nature of the resection and small volume of resected lung.

PULMONARY LOBECTOMY

- Generally, this is reserved for injuries that have created significant tissue destruction in a lung lobe and is deemed not to be amenable for repair or a nonanatomic resection. This is the only anatomic lung resection that is done for traumatic injuries. Sleeve lobectomies or segmentectomies are generally not recommended due to the increased complexity, operative time, and lack of improved outcomes for trauma. As previous noted, lobectomies for traumatic injuries carry a higher mortality rate than do wedge resections or tractotomies. This mortality rate difference may simply be a function of the larger injury and blood loss that required a lobectomy and that was not amenable to simpler repair.[6] If a lobectomy or pneumonectomy is deemed necessary, it is important to try to obtain expert assistance as early as possible.
- A formal lobectomy for trauma is done in a similar fashion to lobectomies done in elective lung resections, but the anatomy in the traumatically injured patient is usually quite altered by the tissue injury. In addition, the loss of clear tissue planes from hemorrhage can make the usual landmarks difficult to discern. If a formal lobectomy is to be attempted, the lobectomy is conducted in the same fashion as is done in the elective setting. Single lung ventilation is necessary to complete a lobectomy as a ventilated lung greatly increases the difficulty of the hilar dissection required for a lobectomy. Another challenge of a lobectomy in the trauma setting is that the patient is usually in the supine position and the lung is exposed through an anterolateral thoracotomy. The usual landmarks and orientation of intrathoracic structures will be in different positions than when performing a lobectomy through a posterolateral thoracotomy incision.
- The inferior pulmonary ligament is divided with cautery or sharply with scissors up to the inferior pulmonary vein and the mediastinal pleura is opened over the hilum. It is important to identify and avoid the phrenic nerve during this step of the dissection. This initial dissection allows for full mobilization of the lung and access to the hilum for vascular control. At this point, if there is significant hemorrhage from the injured lung a large atraumatic vascular clamp can be used to clamp the lung hilum en masse to obtain proximal vascular control. Large Satinsky or other large vascular clamps can be useful for this maneuver. If the hilum is clamped, it is important to communicate this with the anesthesiology team as this will immediately increase right heart pressure and shunts all of the ventilator tidal volume to one lung (see **FIGURE 7**).
- The lobectomy is started by approaching the hilum by opening up the fissures adjacent to the lobe being resected. This is done with electrocautery and sharp dissection as the fissures are usually not completely separated. On the right, the upper and middle lobes are separated by the horizontal fissure and the middle and lower lobes are separated by the oblique fissure. On the left, the upper and lower lobes are separated by the oblique fissure. On the left, the lingua is analogous to the middle lobe of the right lung but is generally part of the upper lobe rather than being a separate lobe.
- The fissure dissection is carried lateral to medial until the fissure dissection is connected with the previously opened

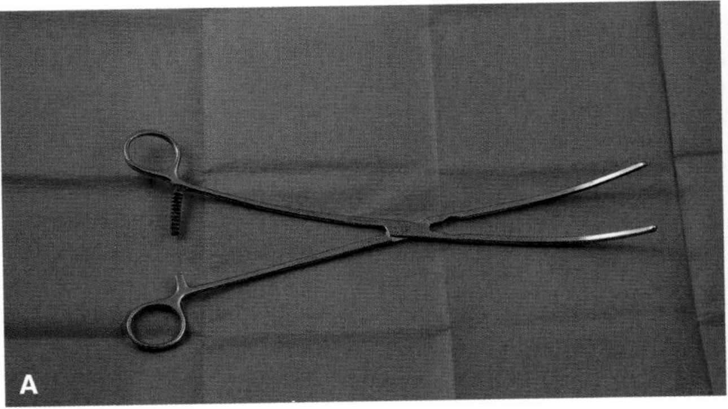

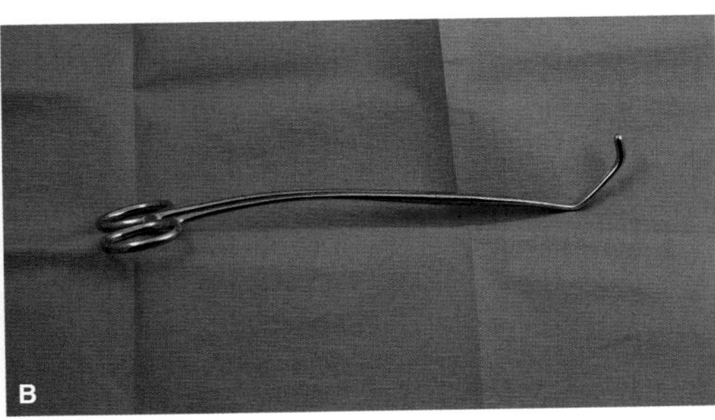

FIGURE 7 ● **A,** Aortic clamp; **B,** large Satinsky clamp.

mediastinal pleura along the anterior hilum. This approach opens up the anterior perivascular plane and provides exposure to the pulmonary artery and its lobar branches. Once the pulmonary artery branches to the target lobe are identified and isolated, they can be divided by suture ligation with permanent suture or with a linear surgical stapler with vascular staples. Division of these branches then exposes the pulmonary vein branches that lay immediately posterior to the pulmonary arterial vessels. These are isolated and divided in a similar fashion.

- After the pulmonary arteries and veins to the lobe are ligated and divided, the lobar bronchus is then exposed. The bronchi are ideally divided with a surgical stapler. If a stapler is not available, then the bronchi can be cut and closed with permanent suture. To do this, a clamp is placed a few millimeters distal to the point of resection and the lobe is then resected by dividing the bronchus just distal to the clamp. A suture ligature is placed around the bronchus proximal to the clamp, then the clamp is removed and the cut end of the bronchus is closed with interrupted braided polyester suture. Air leaks in the divided bronchi can be detected by reinflating the lung. Once there are no air leaks identified and the divided vessels are hemostatic, the remaining lobes should be sutured to one another and to the chest wall to minimize the risk of torsion of the lobes.
- In the trauma setting it may be more expeditious to perform nonanatomic (subtotal) lobectomies. These are essentially large wedge resections. The disruption of anatomic planes from the injury and from hemorrhage increases the difficulty of dissecting out the hilar vessels and bronchi, particularly for trauma and general surgeons who may not routinely perform formal lobectomies. Nonanatomic lobectomies are performed in the manner previous described for wedge resections, but the total volume of resected lung parenchyma is greater. One risk of nonanatomic lobectomies is developing a segment of lung that is not aerated and thereby creating a V/Q mismatch.

CLOSURE

- Once the lung injury has been repaired or resected, the lung should be inspected for hemorrhage and air leaks. The chest should then be irrigated with sterile saline. Chest tubes should be placed into the chest through separate incisions away from the thoracotomy incision, and these incisions should be sited in locations where the patient is not likely to lay on them to minimize discomfort and pressure injury to the soft tissues. Generally, the chest tubes should be 24 to 30 French in diameter. There is no benefit to placing larger-diameter chest tubes. At least one chest tube should be placed to the apex and ideally posteriorly to help with evacuation of both air and fluid. If a second chest tube is placed, a right-angled tube can be used to position the tube in basilar aspect of the hemothorax. The thoracotomy or sternotomy incision is closed in the usual fashion.
- At the completion of the operation, the patient should be returned to dual lung ventilation. If a double-lumen endotracheal tube was used for the operation and if the patient is not to be extubated, the tube should be exchanged for a single-lumen tube.

PEARLS AND PITFALLS

Indication for chest exploration	▪ Initial chest tube placement with ≥1500 mL of blood output or ≥200 mL/h of continued blood output from the chest tube.
Incision	▪ An anterolateral thoracotomy is going to be the incision for unstable trauma patients as it allows the patient to remain supine and for the surgeon to be able to extend the incision across the midline as a clamshell incision to access both pleural cavities and the mediastinum. Extending an anterolateral thoracotomy with a median sternotomy allows for access to the mediastinum and access to the hilar vessels in the pericardial space.
Damage control	▪ The injured lung should be repaired or resected to control hemorrhage. Utilizing linear stapler devices designed for laparoscopic or thoracoscopic operations can make it easier to position and use on lung tissue. Use of staplers can reduce operative time as compared with clamp and suture techniques. ▪ Chest incisions can be closed temporarily with a negative pressure dressing if needed for a planned second look or if the patient is too unstable to tolerate a definitive closure.
Definitive procedures	▪ Formal anatomic lung resections can be difficult and challenging in the trauma setting and should be avoided if possible.
Prolonged airleaks	For patients who are expected to require prolonged mechanical ventilation or those with significant injury, decreasing ventilator driving pressure and moving the chest tube drainage devices to water seal from suction can help facilitate "sealing" of the sites of air leakage. If the leak is large and persistent, it is important to consider that this may be from a tracheobronchial injury. If this is suspected, it is important to obtain expert consultation early.

POSTOPERATIVE CARE

- Initially, chest tubes should be placed to −20 cm of water suction via a three-chambered chest drainage system. These can be changed to water seal or maintained to suction after the effluent volume or air leak has stabilized.
- Typically, chest tubes can be removed when there is no air leak and the effluent is serous and less than 200 to 250 mL in a 24-hour period. Chest tubes can be removed if on suction or on water seal. If more than one chest tube is placed, they are removed sequentially rather than simultaneously.

COMPLICATIONS

Prolonged Air Leak

- This is one of the most common complications after lung resection surgery and is estimated to occur in 7% to 15% of elective lung resection patients. Generally, air leaks should seal within a week of an operation/injury. These can be managed with prolonged chest drainage, but this can also increase the risk of developing an empyema. Pleurodesis can also be done with sclerosing compounds such as talc, tetracycline, or doxycycline, but these can cause severe scarring and is generally very painful and best done under general anesthesia.[7] Pleurodesis can also be done with an autologous blood patch but if the blood is not completely drained it can result in an empyema. More recently fresh frozen plasma has been used for pleurodesis with a good efficacy at resolving prolonged air leaks.[8] If there is a large persistent air leak, a bronchopleural fistula must be considered.

Empyema

- Many of the injuries leading to destructive lung injury are penetrating in nature and by definition contaminates the chest cavity. The bleeding that occurs with injury and with operative intervention can lead to the development of a hemothorax, and the blood provides an excellent growth medium for bacteria. It is important to full drain out the chest at the end of the operation. If an empyema does form, it is important to treat it aggressively with antibiotics and drainage. Reoperation may be necessary to clear the infection, and lytic therapy may be contraindicated after a recent thoracotomy.

REFERENCES

1. Karmy-Jones R, Jurkovich GJ, Nathens AB, et al. Timing of urgent thoracotomy for hemorrhage after trauma: a multicenter study. *Arch Surg*. 2001;136(5):513-518. doi:10.1001/archsurg.136.5.513
2. Martin MJ, McDonald JM, Mullenix PS, Steele SR, Demetriades D. Operative management and outcomes of traumatic lung resection. *J Am Coll Surg*. 2006;203(3):336-344. doi:10.1016/j.jamcollsurg.2006.05.009
3. Aiolfi A, Inaba K, Martin M, et al. Lung resection for trauma: a propensity score adjusted analysis comparing wedge resection, lobectomy, and pneumonectomy. *Am Surg*. 2020;86(3):261-265.
4. Huh J, Wall MJ Jr., Estrera AL, Soltero ER, Mattox KL. Surgical management of traumatic pulmonary injury. *Am J Surg*. 2003;186(6):620-624. doi:10.1016/j.amjsurg.2003.08.013
5. Wall MJ Jr., Hirshberg A, Mattox KL. Pulmonary tractotomy with selective vascular ligation for penetrating injuries to the lung. *Am J Surg*. 1994;168(6):665-669. doi:10.1016/s0002-9610(05)80141-2
6. Jones WS, Mavroudis C, Richardson JD, Gray LA Jr, Howe WR. Management of tracheobronchial disruption resulting from blunt trauma. *Surgery*. 1984;95(3):319-323.
7. Dugan KC, Laxmanan B, Murgu S, Hogarth DK. Management of persistent air leaks. *Chest*. 2017;152(2):417-423. doi:10.1016/j.chest.2017.02.020
8. Moon Y. Treatment of postoperative air leak with fresh frozen plasma. *J Thorac Dis*. 2019;11(12):5655-5657. doi:10.21037/jtd.2019.12.77

Chapter 14 Pneumonectomy for Trauma

Lars Ola Sjoholm, Craig J. Profant, and Thomas A. Santora

DEFINITION

- Injury to the chest can result from any traumatic insult, the most common being blunt mechanisms as a consequence of motor vehicle crashes, falls, assaults, or crush and penetrating wounds from gunshot or stabbing.
- Chest injury can result in bleeding from the chest wall, the lung, or mediastinal structures such as the heart or great vessels.
- Injury to the airway, lung parenchyma, or open violation of the chest wall can lead to pneumothorax.

DIFFERENTIAL DIAGNOSIS

- Isolated chest injury does occur but is frequently associated with injures to the head/neck and abdomen.
- It is imperative to have a global view of the potential of all injuries and to approach discovery of those injures in a systematic fashion as outlined in the advance trauma life support (ATLS) course.[1]

PATIENT HISTORY AND PHYSICAL EXAMINATION

- Injury of the chest can present in a protean manner—essentially asymptomatic to extremis from shock physiology that can result from hemorrhage or obstructive mechanisms (cardiac tamponade or tension pneumothorax). The systematic evaluation taught in the ATLS course using the primary survey that assesses Airway-Breathing-Circulation-Disability-Exposure is the basis for rapid assessment and treatment of the injured patient.
- Chest injury can manifest with complaints of shortness of breath, increased work of breathing, diminished breath and/or heart sounds, or abnormal neck anatomy such as shift of the trachea from midline or distended neck veins. Especially when these findings occur with a plausible traumatic mechanism (ie, penetrating chest wound), the surgeon must intervene in attempt to rapidly mitigate this altered physiology without the aid of supportive imaging. Placement of needle thoracostomy followed by tube thoracostomy can be lifesaving in the evolution of tension pneumothorax. Tube thoracostomy allows the surgeon a means to better understand the presence of significant intrathoracic bleeding, usually considered to be approximately 1500 mL initially or a rate of chest tube output greater than 200 mL for the next several hours. In the vast majority of chest injuries, tube thoracostomy is the only invasive procedure needed for treatment.

IMAGING AND OTHER DIAGNOSTIC STUDIES

- The most common imaging used in trauma patients is the chest X-ray (CXR). It allows detection of chest injury such as hemothorax, pneumothorax, and/or rib fractures. In situations requiring interventions such as endotracheal intubation or tube thoracostomy, the CXR allows assessment of the proper positioning of these interventions as well as the effectiveness of evacuation of hemo/pneumothorax. In penetrating chest wounds, if markers such as paperclips are used at the external wounds, the CXR can allow better appreciation of the likely injuries along the trajectory (**FIGURE 1**).

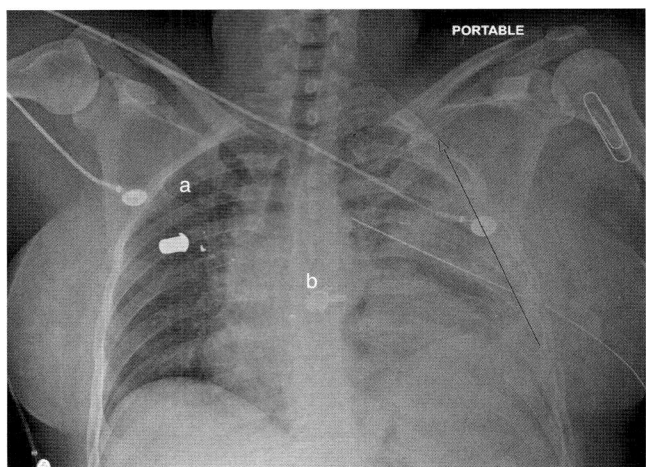

FIGURE 1 ● A chest X-ray demonstrating multiple gunshot wounds to the chest. A paperclip is taped to the patient's skin prior to the x-ray to mark the site of an external wound. Two retained missiles (a) (b) can be seen. Arrow points to large bore central venous access.

- The Extended Focused Assessment with Sonogram for Trauma (eFAST) examine has become an essential tool for the trauma surgeon in the evaluation of the trauma patient, especially those patients that present with shock physiology. In the hands of an experienced operator, eFAST allows rapid detection of fluid (always assumed to be blood in a "shock" patient) in the abdomen, pericardium, and the pleural cavities, as well as the presence of pneumothorax. In those patients with the potential for multicavitary injury, the eFAST can assist the trauma surgeon with determining which site is likely to be the major contribution to the shock state and thus should be addressed first with operative interventions.
- Computed tomography (CT) is helpful to determine the full extent of the injuries to the torso and should be obtained in those trauma patients that have likelihood of multiple injures based on mechanism. As useful as CT is in the management of trauma patients, its use following initial trauma bay evaluation requires that the patient's hemodynamics are stable enough to tolerate the time needed to accomplish the studies. When performed with intravenous contrast, ongoing bleeding can be detected with demonstration of a "contrast blush" at the site of injury.

PULMONARY ANATOMY AND PHYSIOLOGY

- The need for pneumonectomy (removal of the entire lung) after traumatic injury is uncommon. When performed, it is associated with a mortality of over 50% due to the devastating hemodynamic effects it has on the heart, especially in the setting of hemorrhagic shock.[2-6] Less aggressive surgical solutions should always be sought first, but if a pneumonectomy is found necessary, it needs to be carried out without delay.

Anatomy

- The left lung is smaller in volume than the right. The right lung has three lobes—superior, middle and lower. The left lung has two lobes—upper and lower. The lung is enveloped with a visceral pleural covering that fuses with the mediastinal pleura at the hilum and extends caudally to become the inferior pulmonary ligaments. The right lung contributes to a slightly larger portion of the total lung function, approximately 55%, but this does not seem to significantly affect long-term function after right pneumonectomy.[6] The phrenic nerve runs anterior to the fused hilar pleura on both sides.
- The hilum consists of the pulmonary artery—usually located anterior and superior to the bronchus which is located most dorsally. The pulmonary vein is usually located slightly dorsal and caudal to the pulmonary artery but still anterior to the bronchus (**FIGURE 2A-D**).

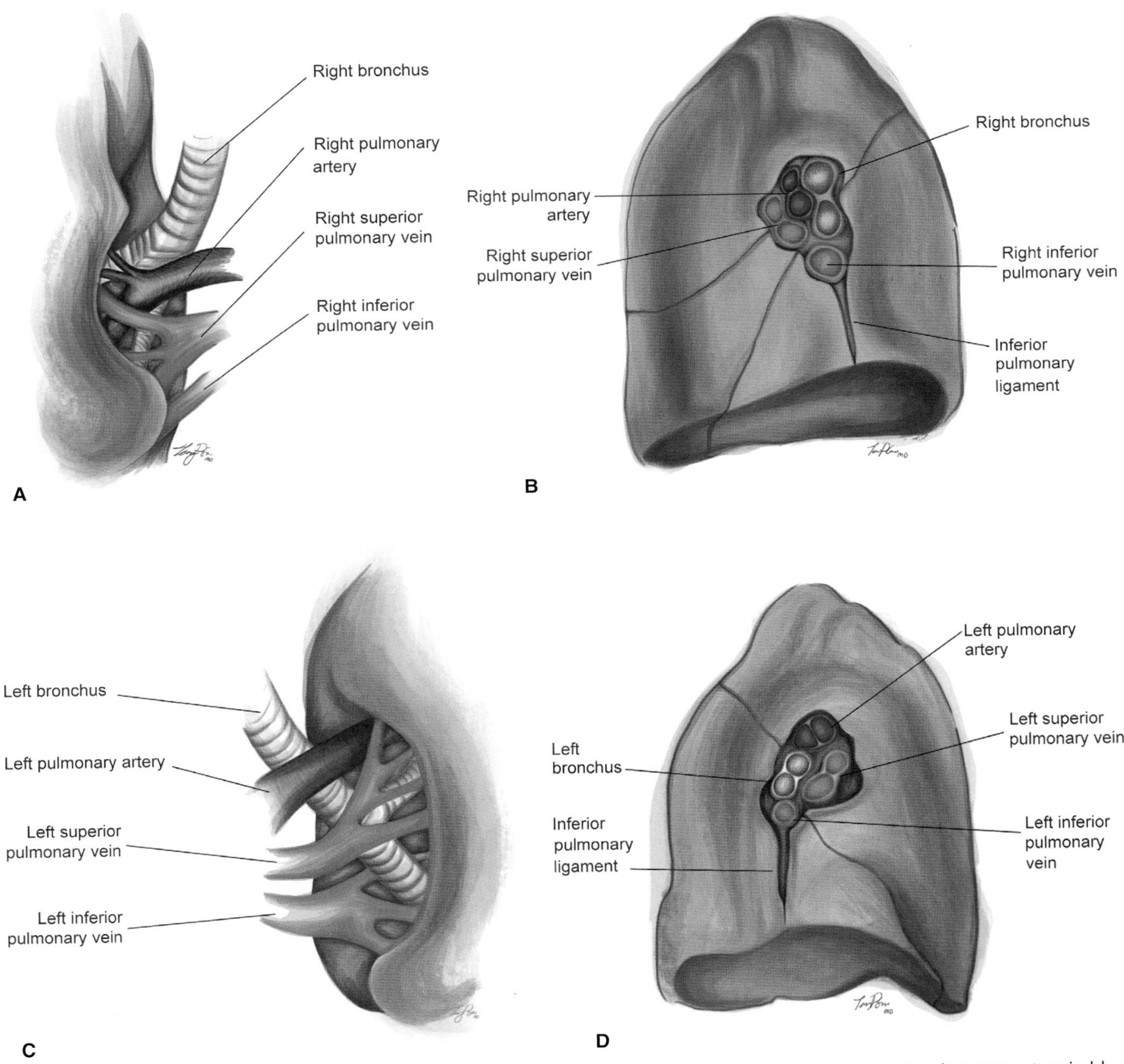

FIGURE 2 • **A,** Hilar structures of the right lung, coronal view. Superior and inferior pulmonary veins in red, pulmonary artery in blue. **B,** Hilar structures of the right lung, sagittal view. **C,** Hilar structures of the left lung, coronal view. Superior and inferior pulmonary veins in red, pulmonary artery in blue. **D,** Hilar structures of the left lung, sagittal view. (Courtesy of Terry P. Gao, MD.)

Physiology

- The pulmonary circulation, which is part of the oxygenation process, represents about 80% of the lung blood flow, but only contributes 20% of the oxygen to the lung.
- Bronchial arterial circulation, originating from the aorta on the left side and the intercostal arteries on the right side, usually represents 20% of the lung blood flow but provides 80% of the oxygen delivery to the lung parenchyma.[7]
- The lung receives all the cardiac output, and at any given time about 10% of the blood volume is within the lungs. The blood volume going through each lung is approximately the same.
- Pneumonectomy has an immediate effect on the hemodynamics. There is an acute increase in pulmonary vascular resistance (PVR) commonly leading to right ventricular failure/dysfunction, manifest as acutely decreased RV ejection fraction. The increase in PVR seen in pneumonectomy is sustained in the presence of significant hemorrhage and transient in its absence.[8]
- After pneumonectomy, there is a long-term beneficial compensating hyperinflation in the remaining lung. There is also gradual deterioration of the lung function, but most can adjust to a life with one lung.[9]

SURGICAL MANAGEMENT

Indication

- Indication for operative management of chest injury is dealt with in other chapters of this textbook. Indication for pneumonectomy is an intraoperative decision. Pneumonectomy for traumatic injuries should only be done if there are no other available options to obtain hilar hemorrhage control or repair of the main stem bronchial injury. As important as it is to be conservative, the decision to proceed with a pneumonectomy needs to be timely. The deeper and longer the patient is in hemorrhagic shock, which is a common scenario in these patients, the worse the outcome.

Positioning

- The patient is placed in a supine position and standard trauma preparation should be undertaken. The skin preparation is done from the chin to the knees. When time permits, ideally, the skin preparation and draping can occur prior to induction of anesthesia; this allows for rapid entry into the chest in the event of cardiovascular collapse from either induction agents, positive pressure ventilation, or both.

TECHNIQUES

INCISION

- Given the uncertainties of the extent of torso injuries in blunt trauma and the wounding trajectories in penetrating trauma, the most versatile incision is the anterolateral thoracotomy with the patient in the supine position. This position allows ready access to the abdominal cavity through the midline celiotomy incision. If wider thoracic exposure is needed, extension across the sternum into the contralateral chest, the so-called clamshell thoracotomy, can also be readily accomplished from this position.
- The incision should start from the ipsilateral sternal border along the curvature of the ribs in the fourth intercostal space, or just caudal to the inframammary fold in females, avoiding the pectoral muscle, and extends to the level of the anterior aspect of the latissimus dorsi muscle (**FIGURE 3**). If the incision is not curved up toward the axilla laterally, the exposure may be limited by the serratus anterior muscle. It is imperative that the entry into the ipsilateral chest is made at this level for two primary reasons: (1) the chest will be opened overlying the hilar structures—thus allowing ready exposure for control, if needed; (2) in the event a transverse sternotomy for increased exposure is needed, the division of the sternum will be done between rib spaces and across the bony sternum. The clamshell thoracotomy exposure necessitates division of both the right and left internal mammary vessels which require control both proximally and distally. If this sternotomy is done too low, costal cartilage and intercostal vessels will be divided requiring more vessels to control and limiting the quality/stability of the distal sternum available for chest closure.
- The intercostal muscle and the pleura are divided along the superior aspect of the rib. The rib spreader is placed with the crossbar/opening ratchet handle laterally oriented toward the axilla. Once in the thoracic cavity, rapid assessment of bleeding sites is undertaken. Chest wall bleeding can be temporarily packed. Lung bleeding can be controlled with direct pressure or with instruments such as Duval clamps. Circumferential control of the hilum should be avoided unless absolutely necessary as this is generally not well tolerated by patients in hemorrhagic shock. The surgeon should keep an open line of communication to the anesthesia team, discuss hemodynamic status, potential need for endotracheal techniques for lung isolation, or need for ancillary supportive interventions (see section that follows).

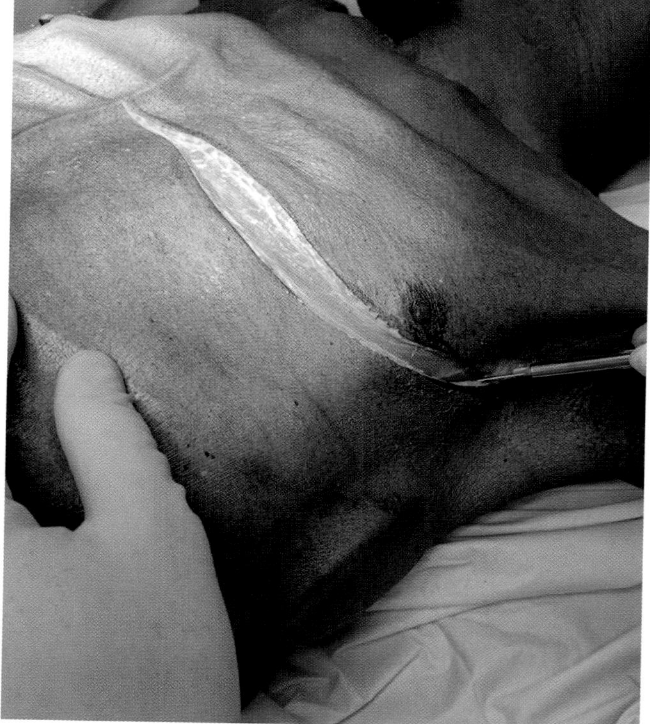

FIGURE 3 ● The patient is positioned supine with the ipsilateral arm externally rotated and extended, maximizing lateral exposure of the chest and facilitating extension of the incision into the axilla. The incision is made within the fourth intercostal space, along the superior margin of the fifth rib.

AIRWAY CONTROL

- In most emergent situations with hemodynamic instability, the patient is intubated with a regular endotracheal tube. If work is needed within the lung to control injury other than simple application of staplers, deflation of the lung is extremely helpful. Left lung isolation can be accomplished most easily by advancement of the endotracheal tube into the right mainstem bronchus. Right-sided isolation requires placement of an endobronchial blocker or replacement of the existing endotracheal tube with a double lumen endotracheal tube. Switching to a double lumen endotracheal tube should only be considered in a stable patient, which is rarely the case when trauma pneumonectomy is being contemplated.

HILAR CONTROL

- If bleeding is arising centrally in the area of the hilum, definitive hilar control may be necessary. Rapid temporary control can be obtained with the surgeon's hand compressing the hilar structures (**FIGURE 4A-C**)[8].
- This control will allow the inferior pulmonary ligament to be divided from the mediastinal pleural margin at the caudal aspect of the lower lobe cephalad up to just below the inferior pulmonary vein (**FIGURE 5**).
- Once divided, a large vascular (Satinsky or aortic) clamp can be placed across the entire hilar structures en bloc (**FIGURE 6A** and **B**) for more stable control.
- Another option for temporary control is to twist the lung 180° (**FIGURE 7**).[10] This serves the same purpose and can be a useful maneuver especially if proper surgical instruments are not readily available. Once the bleeding is controlled, exploration of the hilar area is undertaken to determine if repair is possible or resection is needed for definitive control.

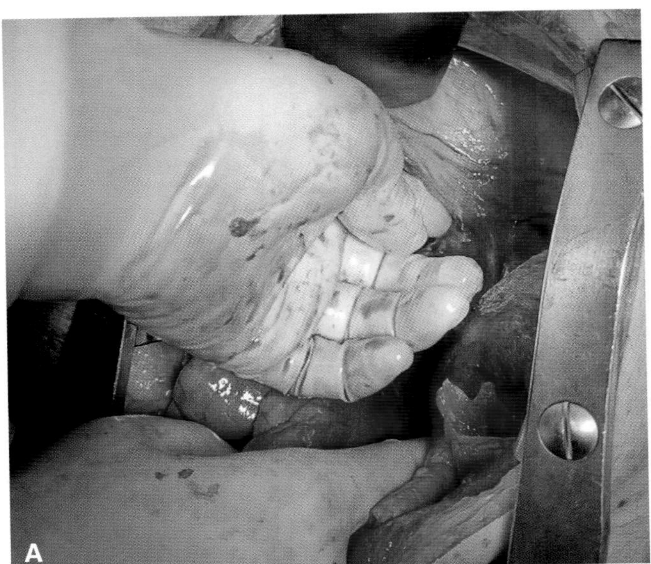

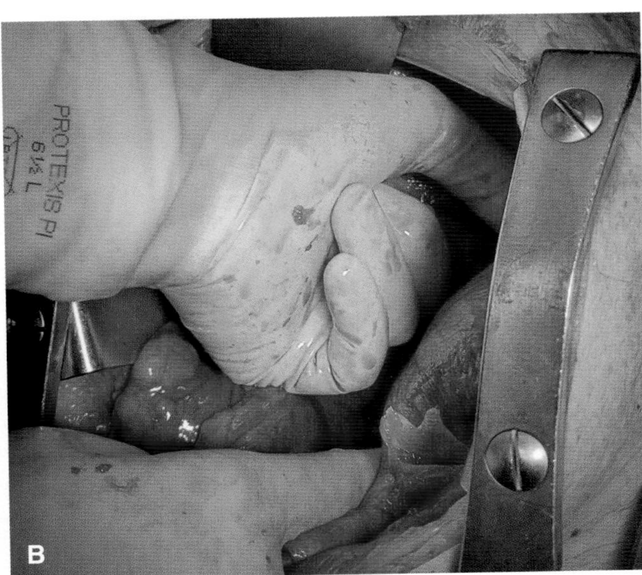

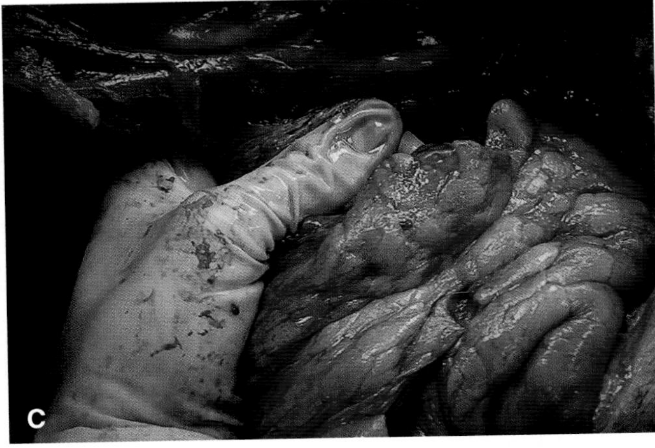

FIGURE 4 ● **A,** Left anterolateral thoracotomy. The surgeon's index finger is inserted behind the left hilar structures. **B,** With the index finger inserted behind, the surgeon's thumb is used to compress the hilar structures anteriorly. **C,** Right anterolateral thoracotomy. Digital compression of the right hilar structures.

- If pneumonectomy is deemed necessary, prompt definitive control should be undertaken to limit persistent or recurrent hemorrhagic shock. There are two general approaches to pneumonectomy:
  1. Individual control of the pulmonary artery and vein with standard vascular techniques coupled with staple closure of the bronchus[11,12] (**FIGURE 8A-C**); see **Video 1**.
  2. En bloc staple control of the hilum[13,14] (**FIGURE 9**); see **Video 2**.
- We prefer the staple technique because it is easy and quick; a TA stapler with a 60 to 90 mm length, 3.5 mm staple load is our stapler of choice. The size of the TA staple load should be predicated on the height and thickness of the hilar structures. It is important to leave room on the remaining hilar structures for stay sutures or Allis clamps to be placed at the cephalad and caudal aspects of the hilum (**FIGURE 10**); these interventions allow control to prevent retraction of the hilum once the stapler is removed in case there is residual bleeding that needs to be oversewn. Another strategy to secure control of the hilum involves two firings of the TA stapler.[13]
- In the event that hilar control is too close to the pericardium to allow safe definitive control with either technique, the pulmonary artery and vein can be controlled and divided within the pericardium (**FIGURE 11**). This exposure is easier on the left than the right due to the length of the respective vessels within the pericardium.

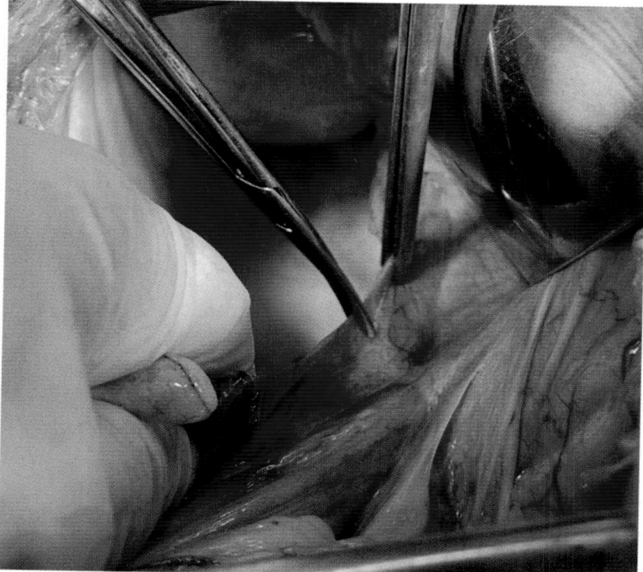

FIGURE 5 ● Incising the left inferior pulmonary ligament up to the caudal edge of the inferior pulmonary vein. Division of the inferior pulmonary ligament will facilitate circumferential dissection of the hilar structures in preparation for definitive clamp control.

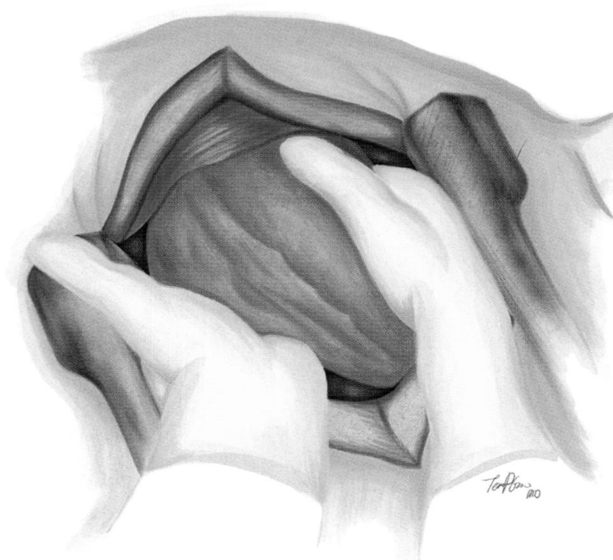

FIGURE 7 ● The left lung is controlled between both hands and twisted 180° along the axis of the hilum. (Courtesy of Terry P. Gao, MD.)

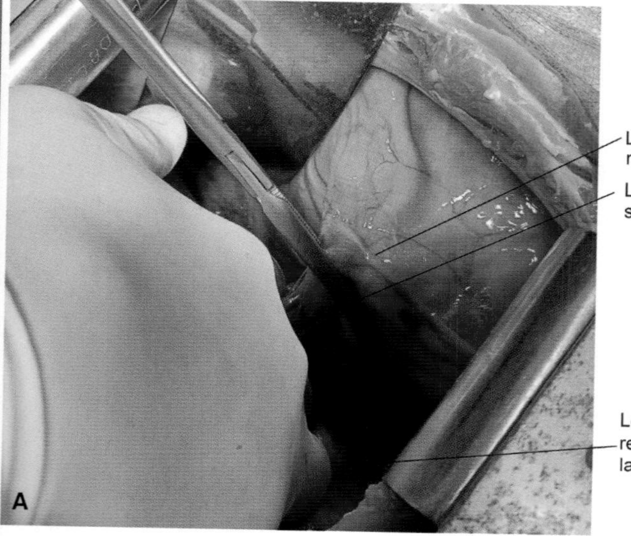

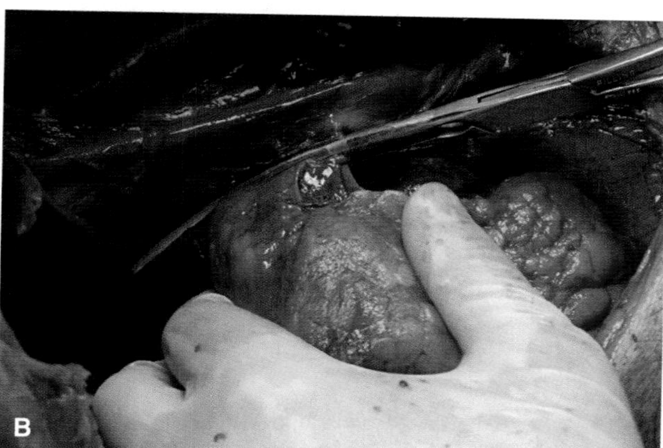

FIGURE 6 ● **A,** Left hilum. Large vascular clamp placed across hilar structures, en bloc. **B,** Right hilum. Large vascular clamp placed across hilar structures, en bloc.

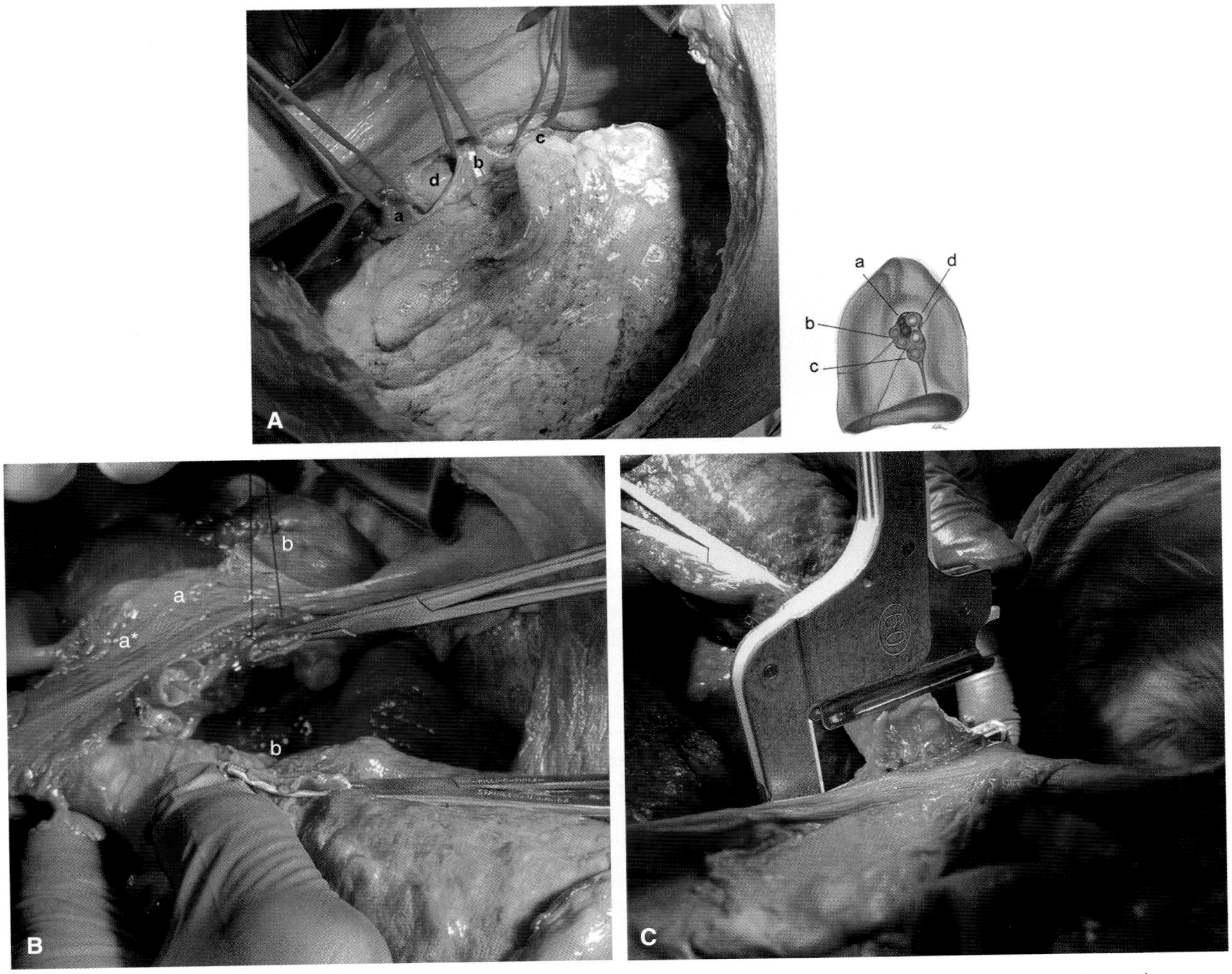

FIGURE 8 ● **A,** Right hilum. (a) Main pulmonary artery, (a*) truncus anterior of pulmonary artery, (b) superior pulmonary vein, (c) inferior pulmonary vein. **B,** Right hilum. (a) Divided pulmonary artery, (a*) truncus anterior, and (b) superior pulmonary vein. (d) right bronchus. Not pictured: (c) inferior pulmonary vein ligated and retracted out of view. **C,** Right hilum. Medial to lateral view. Staple closure of the bronchus. The bronchial division should be done without much dissection to minimize potential devascularization of the staple line. The bronchus should be controlled as distal as possible, leaving viable bronchial length in the event revision is needed.

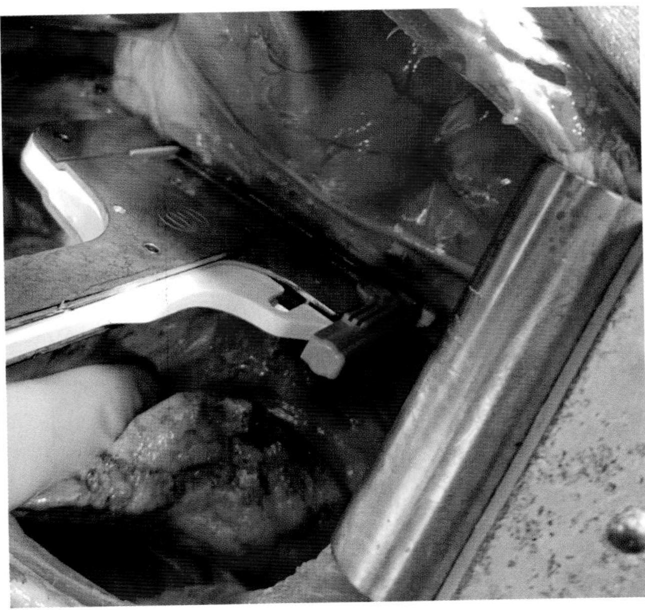

FIGURE 9 ● Left hilum. Lateral to medial view. En bloc stapling of hilar structures. Linear noncutting stapler with 3.5 mm staples, 60 mm length.

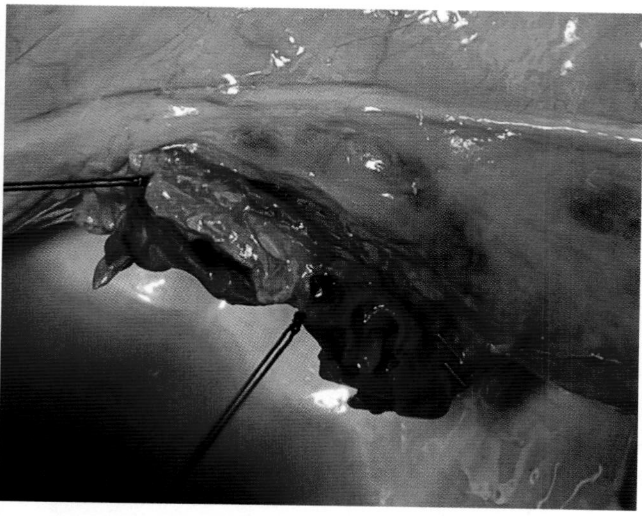

FIGURE 10 • Left hilum. Stay sutures in the stump of the hilar structures to maintain control and visualization in the event of medial retraction after stapler removal.

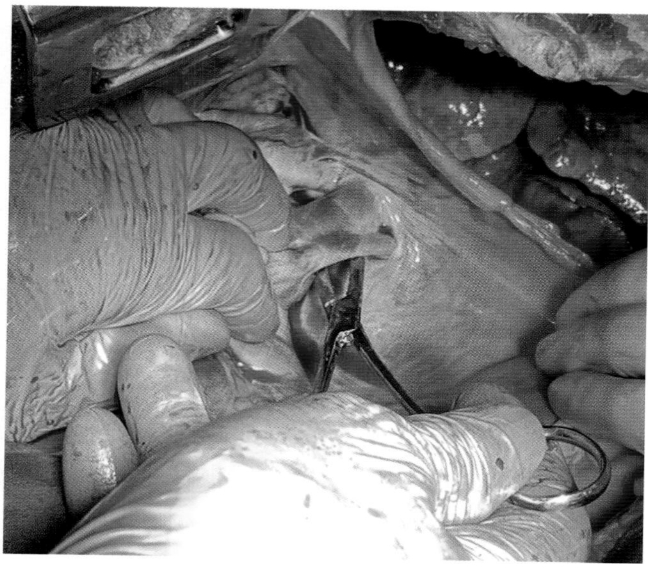

FIGURE 11 • Exposure for left intrapericardial pneumonectomy.

PEARLS AND PITFALLS

Hilar clamping	▪ Hilar clamping is poorly tolerated in patients in hemorrhagic shock due to the sudden increase in the pulmonary vascular resistance and the effect it has on the right ventricle. ▪ Once it is recognized that a pneumonectomy is necessary and performed, every effort to reduce the right ventricular afterload has to be undertaken.
Ancillary interventions	▪ Ancillary interventions (like vasodilators and ECMO) should be considered and readily available for use in the OR or immediate thereafter as conditions dictate.
Vasodilators	▪ In our experience, the best way to achieve reduced afterload in a hemodynamically unstable patient is the use of inhaled vasodilators (inhaled NO, prostaglandins). They have very little negative hemodynamic consequences compared to other pulmonary artery vasodilators.[15] These treatments can easily be started in the operating room and often need to continue postoperatively. Follow-up echocardiogram is advised while weaning the drugs.
Extracorporeal membrane oxygenation (ECMO)	▪ ECMO via veno-venous (VV) cannulation is another supportive adjunct that can be very valuable both intra- and/or postoperatively, as a rescue intervention for profound pulmonary dysfunction, to give the patient time to acclimate to the altered hypoxic/ventilatory changes that can result following pneumonectomy. ECMO use has been reported in a case series[16] following pneumonectomy with survival of two of the three patients treated. Although the literature for ECMO use as an adjunct after pneumonectomy is limited to this isolated report, ECMO use in traumatized patients who develop ARDS physiology has shown promise.[17] ▪ These above treatments need to be considered and initiated promptly as there is very little margin for delay.

POSTOPERATIVE CARE

Chest Tube Management

- After pneumonectomy, chest tube management is very different from when less extensive surgery is performed.[18] In pneumonectomy for trauma, a chest tube is usually placed to monitor for early complications of bleeding or failure of the bronchial stump closure. The pneumonectomy chest tube has to be off suction so as to not displace the heart and mediastinum into the empty pleural space, which can have a significant negative effect on the hemodynamics. The tube should be removed as soon as possible to minimize the risk of postpneumonectomy empyema.
- All postop CXRs should be obtained in the upright position, especially after the chest tube is removed, as this allows assessment of the air–fluid level that will exist in the post-pneumonectomy space until the entirety of the pleural space fills with fluid, ultimately resulting in a fibrothorax over time. If the space fills too rapidly, concern for intrathoracic bleeding should be entertained. In contrast, if the air–fluid level decreases, fluid has escaped the ipsilateral pleural space and evaluation for bronchial stump breakdown should be

undertaken. This is especially concerning if the patient reports a productive cough of serous material or develops acute respiratory distress with associated infiltrates in the contralateral lung. In this latter scenario, the patient should be promptly positioned with the pneumonectomized side down, obtain airway control if needed to support gas exchange, and prepare patient for return to operating room to address control of the bronchial stump breakdown. Details of this operative management are beyond the scope of this chapter but generally involve reclosure of the stump in a well-vascularized area and coverage with a vascularized flap.

Ventilator Management

- There is no difference in ventilator management, but there must be strict adherence to lung protective measures to reduce the risk of ventilator-induced lung injury in the remaining lung. Use of low tidal volumes, control of plateau pressures, and minimal FiO_2 settings constitute the mainstay of ventilator management in these patients.

Fluid Management

- While the patient is actively bleeding, blood loss should be replaced by blood products according to hemostatic resuscitation guidelines. After the acute bleeding phase, it is important to avoid fluid overload as this significantly contributes to ALI/ARDS in the remaining lung. Postpneumonectomy pulmonary edema (PPPE) has been reported[19] as high as 7% with mortality greater than 80%.

COMPLICATIONS

- Overall, complications are relatively common after pneumonectomy for trauma.
- Arrhythmias are more common after pneumonectomy than after other types of lung resections. Atrial fibrillation is the most frequent. It usually occurs during the first postoperative week. The mechanism is unclear but likely due to a combination of vagus nerve dysfunction, hypoxia, pulmonary hypertension, and right ventricle strain. It is managed in the usual fashion with rate control, cardioversion, and anticoagulation.[19]
- Empyema has been reported in 2% to 16% of patients following trauma pneumonectomy.[6,20] It usually results from bronchial breakdown and development of bronchopleural fistula. Polymicrobial infection is common with *Staphylococcus* and *Pseudomonas* species predominating. Early treatment is chest tube drainage, antibiotics, and possible consideration of vascularized flap coverage of the bronchial stump, but may ultimately require an Eloesser flap for chronic pleural packing.
- Postpneumonectomy syndrome,[6,19,20] a rare complication results from a shift or twist of the mediastinal structures as a consequence of unequal pleural pressures. This usually manifests as dyspnea. This syndrome seems to be more prevalent after right pneumonectomy and is thought to be due to compression of the left mainstem bronchus on the spine. Younger patients with more compliant bronchial tissues may be more prone to develop this condition. Treatment is equalization of the pleural pressures to return mediastinal structures to their normal position. Noninvasive ventilation can temporize until pleural pressures are equalized.
- Cardiac herniation after pneumonectomy is uncommon.[20,21] It is associated with a very high mortality. Pericardiotomy is performed in the majority of pneumonectomies done for trauma. If the heart is not dilated at time of completion of the operation, the pericardium should be closed; otherwise the pericardium is deliberately left open in most cases to accommodate the severely dilated heart that frequently follows pneumonectomy. To leave the pericardium widely open may not completely eliminate clinically significant rotation or luxation of the heart, but alternative practical options are limited. Cardiac herniation should be suspected in patients with sudden onset of hypotension and superior vena cava syndrome.

REFERENCES

1. ATLS. *Advanced Trauma Life Support*. 10th ed. 2018.
2. Phillips B, Turco L, Mirzaie M, Fernandez C. Trauma pneumonectomy: a narrative review. *Int J Surg*. 2017;46:71-74.
3. Matsushima K, Aiolfi A, Park C, et al. Surgical outcomes after trauma pneumonectomy. *J Trauma Acute Care Surg*. 2017;82(5):927-932.
4. Homo RL, Grigorian A, Lekawa M, et al. Outcomes after pneumonectomy versus limited lung resection in adults with traumatic lung injury. *Updates Surg*. 2020;72(2):547-553.
5. Halonen-Watras J, O'Connor J, Scalea T. Traumatic pneumonectomy: a viable option for patients in extremis. *Am Surg*. 2011;77(4):493-497.
6. Kopec SE, Irwin RS, Umali-Torres CB, et al. The postpneumonectomy state. *Chest*. 1998;114(4):1158-1184.
7. Craft RC (ed). Thoracic cavity. In: *A Textbook of Human Anatomy*. 3rd ed. Wiley Medical Publishing; 1985:217-218.
8. Cryer H, Mavroudis C, Yu J, et al. Shock, transfusion, and pneumonectomy. *Ann Surg*. 1990;212(2):197-201.
9. Deslauriers J, Ugalde P, Miro S, et al. Adjustments in cardiorespiratory function after pneumonectomy: results of the pneumonectomy project. *J Thorac Cardiovasc Surg*. 2011;141(1):7-15.
10. Wilson A, Wall MJ, Maxson R, Mattox K. The pulmonary hilar twist as a thoracic damage control procedure. *Am J Surg*. 2003;186(1):49-52.
11. de la Torre M, Fieira EM, Paradela M. Right pneumonectomy. In: Gonzalez-Rivas D, Rocco G, D'Amico T (eds.) *Atlas of Uniportal Video Assisted Thoracic Surgery*. Springer;2019:169-173. https://dpo.org/10.1007/978-981-13-2604-2_27
12. Dexter EU, Demmy TL. Thoracotomy pneumonectomy. In: Dienemann H, Detterbeck F (eds.) *Chest Surgery. Springer Surgery Atlas Series*. Springer; 2014:137-146. doi:10.1007/978-3-642-12044-2_14
13. Martin MJ, Meyer MS, Karmy-Jones R. Lung injuries in combat. In: Martin M, Beekley A, Eckert M (eds.) *Front Line Surgery*. Springer; 2017:261-280. doi:10.1007/978-3-319-56780-8_15
14. Wagner JW, Obeid FN, Karmy-Jones RC, Casey GD, Sorensen VJ, Horst HM. Trauma pneumonectomy revisited. *J Trauma Inj Infect Crit Care*. 1996;40(4):590-594.
15. Lubitz AL, Sjoholm LO, Goldberg A, et al. Acute right heart failure after hemorrhagic shock and trauma pneumonectomy—a management approach. *J Trauma Acute Care Surg*. 2017;82(2):243-251.
16. Robba C, Ortu A Bilotta F, et al. Extracorporeal membrane oxygenation for adult respiratory distress syndrome in trauma patients: a case series and systematic literature review. *J Trauma Acute Care Surg*. 2017;82(1):165-173.
17. Swol J, Cannon JW, Napolitano L. ECMO in trauma: what are the outcomes? *J Trauma Acute Care Surg*. 2017;82(4):819-820.
18. Rammohan KS, Pai VB, Treasure T. Management of the pleural space early after pneumonectomy. In: Ferguson MK (ed.) *Difficult Decisions in Thoracic Surgery*. Springer-Verlag; 2011;161-164. doi: 10.1007/978-1-84996-492-0_17
19. Grillo HC, Shepard JO, Mathisen DJ, et al. Postpneumonectomy syndrome: diagnosis, management, and results. *Ann Thorac Surg*. 1992;54:638-651.
20. Kazior MR, Streams JR, Dennis BM, et al. Pulmonary complications after trauma pneumonectomy. *J Cardiothorac Vasc Anesth*. 2020;34(7):1952-1961.
21. Deiraniya AK. Cardiac herniation following intrapericardial pneumonectomy. *Thorax*. 1974;29:545-552.

Chapter **15**

Arterial: Subclavian, Thoracic Aorta, Endovascular

Lisbi del Valle Rivas Ramirez, Natalie M. Wall, and Paula Ferrada

DEFINITION

- Thoracic vascular injury can result from both blunt and penetrating trauma, most common being the latter. Blunt thoracic vascular trauma is rare, contributing less than 5% of traumatic vascular injuries. While penetrating trauma can involve a multitude of arterial structures within the chest, blunt thoracic vascular trauma most commonly affects the aorta and innominate arteries.[1]
- Blunt thoracic aortic injury (BTAI) accounts for 1.5% of all thoracic trauma and is associated with high prehospital mortality. For those patients who survive to hospital arrival, mortality nears upward of 50%.[2-4] Mechanism of BTAI involves substantial high-impact force, most commonly an abrupt deceleration resulting in vascular injury at the level of the aortic isthmus.[2,5] Blunt injury sustained by such force typically leads to compromise and subsequent tearing of the vessel's intima and media, resulting in formation of a dissection plane along the artery. As the intimal injury progresses to involve the vessel's adventitia, pseudoaneurysm or free rupture can occur.[2] It is this reported mechanism of injury that must make the clinician mindful of elevated mean arterial pressures and aggressive fluid resuscitation, both of which may expedite this process and ultimately worsen outcomes.
- Much like blunt aortic injury, penetrating injury to the thoracic great vessels is associated with high prehospital mortality, nearing 50%. The literature places operative mortality between 5% and 40%, dependent on factors such as initial patient acuity and concomitant injuries.[6]

PATIENT HISTORY AND PHYSICAL FINDINGS

- Workup for blunt thoracic arterial injuries should begin with an examination performed in accordance with advanced trauma life support guidelines, with initial focus on performing a thorough primary survey, ensuring adequate airway, breathing, and circulation. Indicators of major chest trauma in the setting of high-velocity impact such as steering column markings on the chest, massive hemothorax, diaphragmatic injury, pulse discrepancies between upper and/or lower extremities, tracheobronchial or esophageal injuries, and fractures of the first or second rib, manubrium, and scapula should heighten suspicion of blunt aortic injury.[2,4] Chief complaints associated with major chest trauma are nonspecific and may not necessarily be present upon patient arrival. Likewise, up to 50% of hemodynamically stable patients may have no initial physical examination evidence of blunt thoracic vascular injury.[4]
- In the case of penetrating thoracic arterial injury, physical examination findings may include overt external hemorrhage through an obvious penetrating tract or internal hemorrhage leading to hemothorax, hematoma, or cardiac tamponade. Much like in the case of blunt trauma, these patients may also present with pseudoaneurysms or intimal flaps indicative of arterial compromise. While distal pulses may be absent, the presence of such does not exclude severe arterial injury and impending catastrophe.[7]

DIFFERENTIAL DIAGNOSIS

- Chest radiograph may demonstrate widened mediastinum, absence of aortic knob, apical cap, loss of aortopulmonary window, left hemothorax, tracheal deviation, or fractures of the bony structures noted above.[2,4] While chest radiograph may provide further evidence of suspicion, the gold standard of diagnosis remains computed tomography angiography (CTA) for the clinically stable patient.[2-4] Transesophageal echocardiogram may be performed to aid in diagnostic confirmation.[2] CTA is a useful adjunct in further identifying injury pattern and structural involvement. Patients with hemodynamic instability are taken directly to the operating room for surgical exploration.[6]
- The surgical approach is largely dependent on which anatomical structure(s) is/are involved in the injury. Given this, structural assessment with radiographic evaluation is preferable to aid in operative planning if the patient's hemodynamics allow for such.

SURGICAL MANAGEMENT

Approach

- Management of thoracic vascular injury can vary from nonoperative management to open or endovascular approach. The preferred method depends on clinical presentation, type of injury, hemodynamic stability, among other factors. Nonoperative management can be done in hemodynamically stable patients with small intimal injuries. Endovascular repair is a suitable option if the patient is stable and angiography is readily available, whereas in unstable patients, open repair is the best option.

SUBCLAVIAN INJURY

- Exposure of the subclavian artery is challenging for many reasons: its location in a very small space, proximity to other important neurovascular structures, and presence in a confined bony thorax. Exposure can also take a significant amount of time when the patient is hemorrhaging, and it can require very morbid incisions. The open approach to the subclavian artery injury depends on the side of the injury and location. Supraclavicular or infraclavicular incisions are often necessary. For proximal control of the right subclavian artery injury, median sternotomy is the best approach. The left subclavian artery can be approached from a high (2nd-3rd intercostal space) left anterior thoracotomy. Claviculectomy is rarely necessary and carries significant morbidity[8] (**FIGURE 1**).
- A combination of clavicular incision with a median sternotomy is often necessary for more proximal injuries to the subclavian vessels.

Supraclavicular Incision

- On the left side the subclavian artery courses posterior and deep; therefore, this incision works better for the right subclavian.
- Incision is made parallel to the medial half of the clavicle, 1 cm above.
- The platysma and the sternocleidomastoid attachment to the clavicle are divided to expose the internal jugular vein.
- The anterior scalene muscle is exposed identifying and preserving the phrenic nerve, which runs anterior to the muscle.
- The anterior scalene muscle is divided 1 cm above the clavicle to expose the subclavian artery.

Infraclavicular Incision

- Incision starts at the inferior border of the center of the clavicle and runs lateral in the clavipectoral groove.
- The pectoralis major muscle is exposed after the incision goes through the skin and subcutaneous tissue. The muscle is then either split along its fibers' direction or divided 2 cm from its humeral insertion. If the exposure seems to be adequate we avoid dividing the muscle.
- The pectoralis minor is divided exposing the subclavian/axillary artery. The brachial plexus is in close relationship with the artery, and the vein runs inferior to the artery (**FIGURE 2**).

"Trapdoor" Incision

- For injuries of the left subclavian artery a "trapdoor" incision is described.
- It is a combination of a supraclavicular incision, a midline sternotomy across the manubrium and upper portion of the sternum, and an anterior left thoracotomy on the 3rd or 4th intercostal space (**FIGURE 3**).

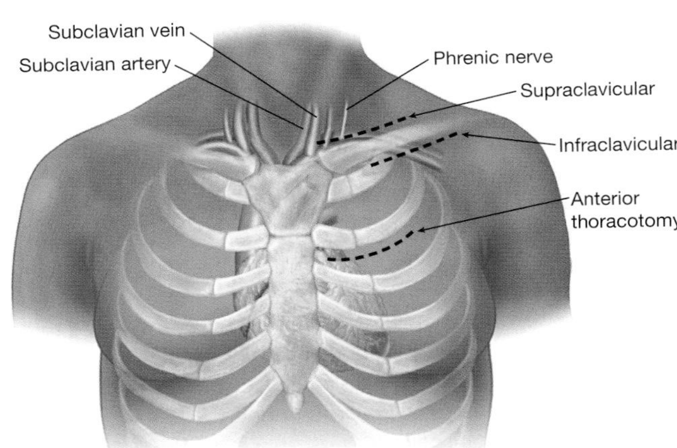

FIGURE 1 ● Subclavian vessels exposure.

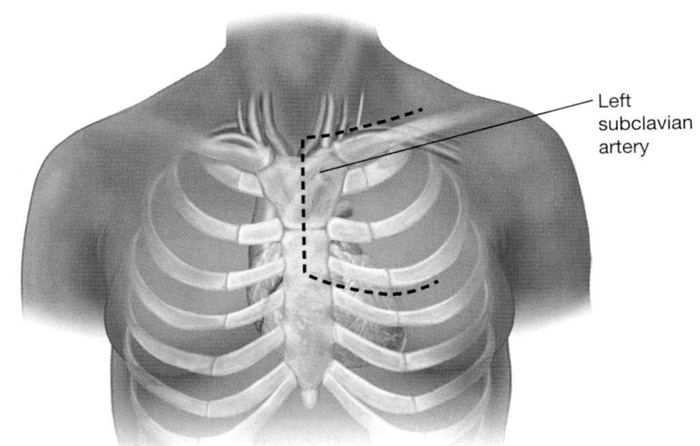

FIGURE 2 ● Infraclavicular exposure.

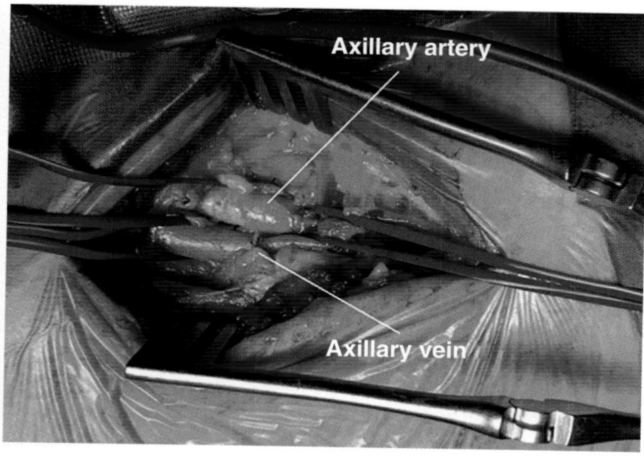

FIGURE 3 ● "Trapdoor" incision.

BLUNT AORTA INJURY

- Classification of blunt aortic injury is noted in **TABLE 1**.
- While the traditional approach to operative management of blunt thoracic arterial injury involved open repair, endovascular management has replaced this as the gold standard of care.[9] Data demonstrate lower mortality associated with endovascular vs open repair of BTAI.[2,3] Open repair with systemic anticoagulation is associated with mortality rates ranging from 24% to 42%. While the risk of paraplegia, a feared complication of open repair, decreased with routine use of cardiopulmonary bypass (3% vs 7%), studies noted a subsequent increase in hemorrhagic complications given systemic anticoagulation required for circuit initiation. The benefits of endovascular repair compared with open repair for blunt aortic injury include the absence of a thoracotomy incision and its associated recovery, no single-lung ventilation requirement, less systemic anticoagulation, no cross-clamping, and markedly less estimated blood loss.[3,10]
- Initial medical management consists of blood pressure and heart rate control, allowing for "permissive hypotension" as to not expedite aortic injury and potential catastrophe.[2] Esmolol is the first-line drug of choice for blood pressure management given its quick time of onset and short half-life allowing for easy titration.
- When operative repair is indicated, understanding of the patient's anatomy is essential for an endovascular approach. A small aortic arch can pose a challenge, specifically in young patients when this is the most common. Volume depletion can also lead to undersizing the graft, which can be helped by using intravascular ultrasound. Arterial access is obtained in the common femoral arteries percutaneously or by cutdown or iliac conduit. Aortogram is performed to confirm the anatomy and define the landing zones for the device. The endograft is advanced into approximate position over a stiff wire, and the position is confirmed with repeat angiography. The device is deployed at that time with subsequent completion aortogram performed to confirm that the injury has been excluded. The left subclavian artery may need to be covered by the graft for an adequate landing zone, depending on the location of the lesion. When this is the case, it will need to be determined preprocedure if the patient possesses a dominant left vertebral artery circulation.[11]

Table 1: Blunt Aortic Injury Grading Scale

Grade		Management
GRADE 1	Intimal tear	Can be managed nonoperatively, tends to resolve on own
GRADE 2	Intramural hematoma	Medical vs operative, if imaging demonstrates advancement of injury > delayed repair
GRADE 3	Pseudoaneurysm	Endovascular repair (endografting); delayed repair > immediate if stable
GRADE 4	Free rupture	Immediate repair, most do not survive to hospital

OUTCOMES

- There is growing evidence about the use of endovascular techniques in the management of vascular injuries, particularly interesting in the management of subclavian injuries.[12] A recent multicenter review showed that management of subclavian arterial injuries still requires a wide variety of open exposures, especially for the control of active hemorrhage. Endovascular repair was used in a small percentage of cases, who were hemodynamically stable, with the most common injury type being intimal tear and pseudoaneurysm.[13]
- Outcomes between open and endovascular management of subclavian injuries has been compared. Endovascular repair, when feasible, was associated with improved mortality and lower complication rates. Long-term outcomes were not reported.[14]

REFERENCES

1. Mattox KL, Feliciano DV, Burch J, Beall AC, Jordan GL, Debakey ME. Five thousand seven hundred sixty cardiovascular injuries in 4459 patients: epidemiologic evolution 1958 to 1987. *Ann Surg*. 1989;209(6):698-707. doi:10.1097/00000658-198906000-00007
2. Mouawad NJ, Paulisin J, Hofmeister S, Thomas MB. Blunt thoracic aortic injury - concepts and management. *J Cardiothorac Surg*. 2020;15(1):1-8. doi:10.1186/s13019-020-01101-6
3. De Mestral C, Dueck A, Sharma SS, et al. Evolution of the incidence, management, and mortality of blunt thoracic aortic injury: a population-based analysis. *J Am Coll Surg*. 2013;216(6):1110-1115. doi:10.1016/j.jamcollsurg.2013.01.005
4. Mattox KL. Thoracic vascular trauma. *J Vasc Surg*. 1988;7(5):725-729. doi:10.1016/0741-5214(88)90031-6
5. Sevitt S. The mechanisms of traumatic rupture of the thoracic aorta. *Br J Surg*. 1977;64(3):166-173. doi:10.1002/bjs.1800640305
6. O'Connor JV, Scalea TM. Penetrating thoracic great vessel injury: impact of admission hemodynamics and preoperative imaging. *J Trauma Inj Infect Crit Care*. 2010;68(4):834-837. doi:10.1097/TA.0b013e3181b250df
7. Wall J, Granchi T, Liscum K, Mattox KL. Penetrating thoracic vascular injuries. *Surg Clin North Am*. 1996;76(4):749-761. doi:10.1016/s0039-6109(05)70478-3
8. McKinley AG, Abdool Carrim AT, Robbs JV. Management of proximal axillary and subclavian artery injuries. *Br J Surg*. 2000;87(1):79-85. doi:10.1046/j.1365-2168.2000.01303.x
9. Scalea TM, Feliciano DV, DuBose JJ, Ottochian M, O'Connor JV, Morrison JJ. Blunt thoracic aortic injury: endovascular repair is now the standard. *J Am Coll Surg*. 2019;228(4):605-610. doi:10.1016/j.jamcollsurg.2018.12.022
10. Takagi H, Kawai N, Umemoto T. A meta-analysis of comparative studies of endovascular versus open repair for blunt thoracic aortic injury. *J Thorac Cardiovasc Surg*. 2008;135(6):1392-1395. doi:10.1016/j.jtcvs.2008.01.033
11. Farber MA, Mendes RR. Endovascular repair of blunt thoracic aortic injury: techniques and tips. *J Vasc Surg*. 2009;50(3):683-686. doi:10.1016/j.jvs.2009.01.009
12. White R, Krajcer Z, Johnson M, Williams D, Bacharach M, O'Malley E. Results of a multicenter trial for the treatment of traumatic vascular injury with a covered stent. *J Trauma Inj Infect Crit Care*. 2006;60(6):1189-1195. doi:10.1097/01.ta.0000220372.85575.e2
13. Walker PA, May AC, Mo J, et al. Multicenter review of robotic versus laparoscopic ventral hernia repair: is there a role for robotics? *Surg Endosc*. 2018;32(4):1901-1905. doi:10.1007/s00464-017-5882-5
14. Branco BC, Boutrous ML, DuBose JJ, et al. Outcome comparison between open and endovascular management of axillosubclavian arterial injuries. Presented at the 2015 Vascular Annual Meeting of the Society for Vascular Surgery, Chicago, Ill, June 17-20, 2015. *J Vasc Surg*. 2016;63(3):702-709. doi:10.1016/j.jvs.2015.08.117

Chapter 16

Thoracic Vascular Injury—Venous: Brachiocephalic Vein, Subclavian Vein

Michael A. Vella, Michael J. Nabozny, Adam Joseph Doyle, and Nicole A. Stassen

DEFINITION

- Injuries to the brachiocephalic vein (BCV) and subclavian vein (SCV) result most commonly from penetrating mechanisms. Blunt injuries can occur and are often related to hyperextension/traction, shearing, and compression, which ultimately lead to wall disruption, avulsion, and/or occlusion.[1]
- Mortality and need for blood transfusion appear to be higher for venous injuries, likely related to absence of vasospasm, high flow rates, and risk of air embolism.[2-4]
- Injuries to the BCV/SCV are associated with other significant thoracic and extrathoracic trauma, including injuries to the other thoracic great vessels and brachial plexus, depending on mechanism.[1]
- The American Association for the Surgery of Trauma (AAST) classifies injuries to the BCV/SCV as grade II vascular injuries.[5]

DIFFERENTIAL DIAGNOSIS

- Differential diagnosis of suspected BCV/SCV injuries should include injuries to the heart and vasculature of the chest, neck, and proximal upper extremities.

PATIENT HISTORY AND PHYSICAL FINDINGS

- Initial evaluation of any trauma patient, including those with suspected BCV/SCV injuries, should follow ATLS principles of primary and secondary surveys along with adjuncts.[6]
- It is important to understand that history and physical examination findings may be subtle in patients with BCV/SCV injuries, especially in the absence of a concomitant arterial injury.[7]
- Patients with SCV/BCV injuries who are able to communicate may complain of chest, shoulder, or arm pain depending on associated injuries. Neurologic complains (weakness, numbness) in the ipsilateral upper extremity may suggest a brachial plexus injury, which is associated with injuries to the adjacent subclavian vessels.
- Physical examination may reveal penetrating wounds to the chest, neck, axilla, or proximal upper extremity. There may be bruising and/or crepitus over the sternum or clavicle indicating a potential fracture.
- Hemodynamic instability or "hard signs" of vascular injury (expanding hematoma or active bleeding from the retroclavicular area) suggest a major vascular injury. Pulse discrepancy may suggest a subclavian artery injury. (See Part 7, Chapter 15.)
- Neurologic deficits may indicate an associated brachial plexus injury. We find that having a patient perform "rock, paper, scissors" easily evaluates the radial, median, and ulnar nerves, respectively.

IMAGING AND OTHER DIAGNOSTIC STUDIES

- Initial imaging evaluation of a hypotensive blunt trauma patient should include a FAST examination and plain films of the chest and pelvis.
- For patients with penetrating injuries, a thorough physical examination evaluating for ballistic wounds will determine what imaging evaluation is needed for trajectory analysis. Wounds should be marked with radiopaque markers. Plain films of the chest, abdomen, pelvis, head/neck, and extremities are obtained as clinically appropriate in order to identify wound trajectories. A cardiac ultrasound is used to evaluate for pericardial fluid in patients with penetrating anterior or posterior thoracic injuries as well as those with injuries to the epigastrium and thoracoabdominal regions.
- Findings on chest radiograph that suggest a possible BCV/SCV injury include widened mediastinum, hemothorax, and/or apical cap (**FIGURE 1**).
- In general, injuries to the BCV/SCV will not result in hemopericardium on ultrasound unless there is an associated injury to the heart or intrapericardial great vessels.
- Patients who are hemodynamically normal without another indication for urgent operative intervention should undergo computed tomography (CT) angiography of the chest. If a venous injury is suspected, a concomitant CT venogram can be helpful, although most venous injuries will be identified on arterial phase imaging.[7] It is vital that intravenous access is obtained and contrast is administered via the contralateral arm (away from site of potential injury) to avoid contrast artifact.

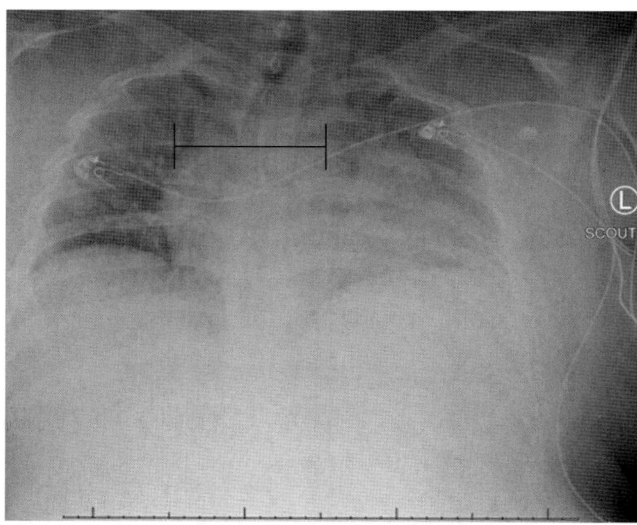

FIGURE 1 ● Chest X-ray showing widened mediastinum, which can be seen in thoracic vascular injury.

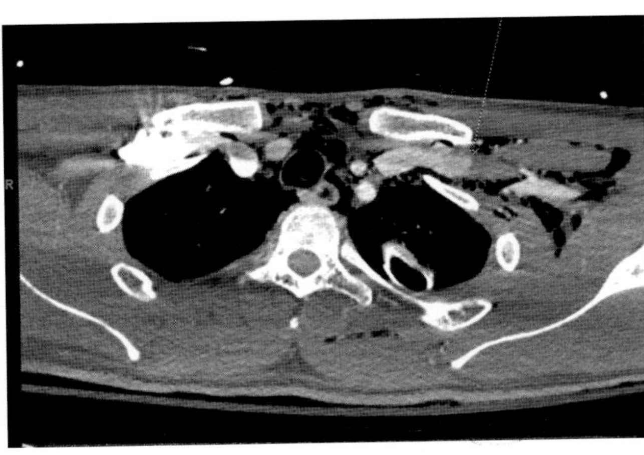

FIGURE 2 ● *Arrow* indicating injury to left subclavian vein as a result of blunt trauma. Contrast was injected in contralateral arm.

- Direct signs of injury on CT include thrombosis/occlusion, avulsion/complete tear, rupture, active extravasation, and pseudoaneurysm. Indirect signs include perivascular hematoma, fat stranding, and vessel wall irregularities[7] (**FIGURE 2**).
- Arterial pressure indices can be obtained if there is concern for arterial injury.

SURGICAL MANAGEMENT

General Considerations

- Nonoperative management of BCV/SCV injuries in hemodynamically normal patients with no other indication for operative exploration is feasible and should occur in a monitored setting.[8] However, the data to guide this practice are limited.
- Overall management of BCV/SCV injuries is based on patient hemodynamics, injury mechanism, concomitant injuries, surgeon experience, and local resources.

Preoperative Planning

- The preoperative management of those with suspected or confirmed BCV/SCV injury should follow the principles of the ATLS primary and secondary surveys.[6]
- Intubation should be considered in patients with immediate airway compromise and in those who are not breathing or are hypoxemic. Intubation in the emergency department should be avoided in penetrating trauma patients with a palpable pulse who are spontaneously breathing and maintaining an appropriate oxygen saturation in order to avoid cardiovascular collapse. Consideration should be given to intubating these patients after surgical prepping and draping is complete. A single-lumen tube is sufficient in most cases.
- Thoracostomy tubes should be placed in patients with suspected or confirmed pneumothorax/hemothorax.
- External junctional hemorrhage related to SCV injury may be temporarily controlled with hemostatic gauze packing. Foley balloon tamponade has also been described for retroclavicular bleeding.[3]
- A brief neurological examination should be performed along with complete exposure of the patient.
- Avoidance of crystalloid in favor of balanced (1:1:1 ratio of packed red blood cells:plasma:platelets) or whole blood resuscitation along with activation of a massive transfusion protocol is recommended. Consideration should be given to the administration of tranexamic acid depending on local practice.
- Preoperative antibiotics and tetanus should be administered.

Positioning/Equipment

- In general, patients should be supine with arms outstretched at 30° if there is concern for SCV injury.
- Prep should include the neck, entire chest, abdomen, and bilateral groins as well as proximal upper extremities.
- Equipment should include thoracotomy/sternotomy and vascular instruments as well as a sternal saw and appropriate lighting. Intraoperative blood salvage equipment should be readily available.

Procedure Descriptions

General Exposure

- The appropriate incision is primarily based on hemodynamic status and location of wounds in penetrating trauma.
- Moribund patients and those in cardiac arrest should undergo left anterolateral thoracotomy with or without extension to a right anterolateral thoracotomy ("clamshell") if presenting signs of life within 15 minutes in penetrating thoracic trauma or witnessed loss of pulses in blunt trauma.[9] This incision may also be of benefit in patients with lateral thoracic penetrating wounds with concern for lung injury.

BRACHIOCEPHALIC VEIN

Incision

- Exposure to the BCV is most often achieved through a median sternotomy.
- A skin incision is made from the suprasternal notch to the xiphoid process (**FIGURE 3**). Dissection is carried down through the presternal fascia, taking care to stay in the midline.
- The interclavicular ligament at the superior aspect of the incision is divided with cautery and blunt dissection and the posterior aspect of the sternum is cleared at the suprasternal notch and under the xiphoid. Respirations are held and a sternal saw (or Lebsche knife) is used to divide the sternum using a steady upward pressure, taking care to stay in the midline. This exposes the underlying pericardium.
- A Finochietto retractor is placed in the upper aspect of the incision with handle directed away from any area that requires additional exposure (ie, direct away from the abdomen if the abdomen may require exploration).

Identification of the Left Brachiocephalic Vein

- The pericardium is entered sharply and incised in the cranial and caudal direction. The remnant thymus tissue/fat is identified in the superior mediastinum anterior to the BCV.
- The crossing left BCV is identified and bluntly separated from surrounding tissue (**FIGURE 4A**).

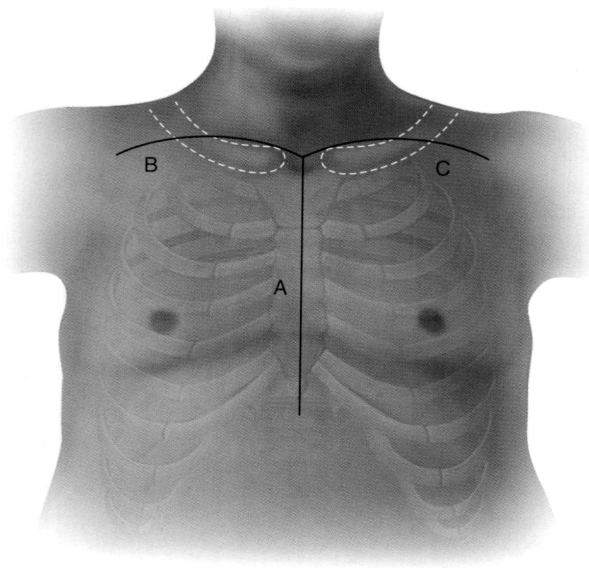

FIGURE 3 ● Recommended incisions for exposure of the thoracic vessels. **(A)** Median sternotomy for exposure of the brachiocephalic veins and **(B and C)** clavicular incisions for exposure of the bilateral subclavian veins. Median sternotomy and clavicular incisions can be combined for exposure of the proximal subclavian veins. Dotted lines indicate position of clavicles.

- At this point bleeding can be controlled with silastic vessel loops or vascular clamps (**FIGURE 4B**).

Brachiocephalic Vein Injury Management

- Data from the cardiac literature suggest that ligation of the left BCV is well tolerated without significant long-term morbidity due to the presence of venous collaterals.[10-14] Ligation has historically been the most common method of injury management; outcomes are similar between ligation and repair for venous injuries in general[12,14,15] (**FIGURE 4C**).
- We advise ligation in patients who are hemodynamically unstable, require repair beyond simple venorrhaphy, and/or require interventions in multiple cavities. Otherwise, repair (lateral venorrhaphy) can be achieved using fine monofilament suture (5-0 polypropylene) as long as this results in <50% vessel stenosis.

Incision Closure

- Bleeding from the sternal edge is controlled with cautery and bone wax as needed.
- A mediastinal tube is placed. Thoracostomy tubes should be placed if the pleura was entered.
- The sternum is closed with wires (we prefer two in the manubrium and five to close the sternum).
- The presternal fascia and subcutaneous tissues are closed in layers and the skin is closed with staples or running absorbable monofilament suture.

A

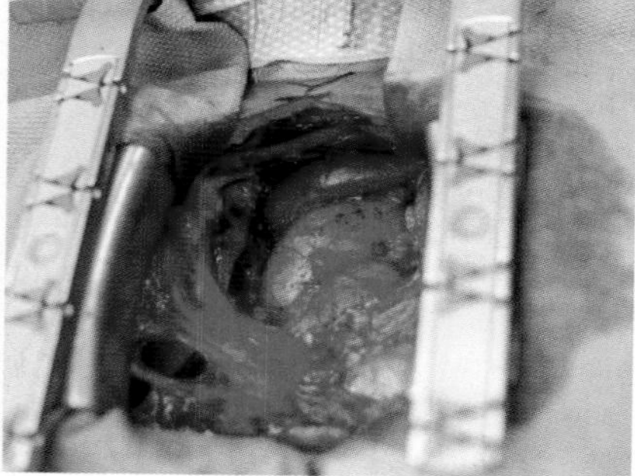

B

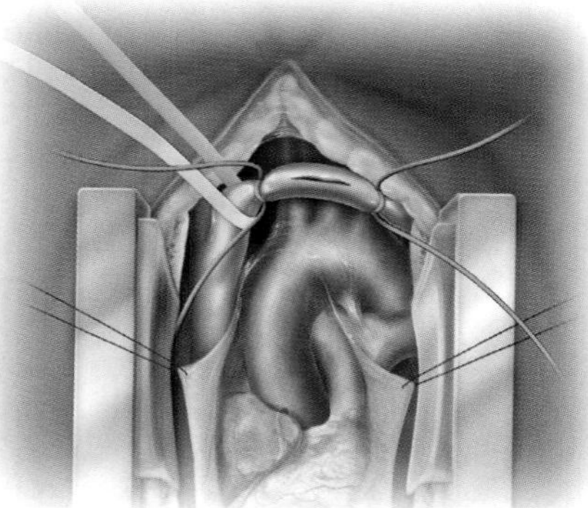

C

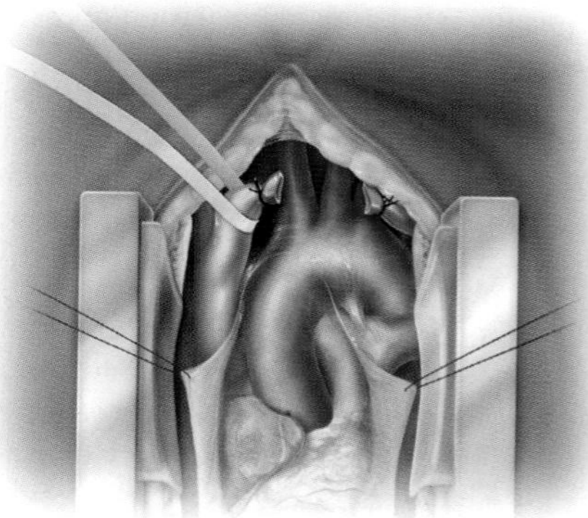

FIGURE 4 ● **A,** Median sternotomy has been performed, pericardium opened, and remnant thymic tissue cleared from the brachiocephalic vein, which is seen crossing the aortic arch at the cranial aspect of the wound. **B,** The left brachiocephalic vein has been identified and injury controlled with silastic vessel loops. **C,** The injured brachiocephalic vein injury is suture ligated. (B and C, Reprinted with permission from Lee WA, Kulik A. Arch and great vessel reconstruction with debranching techniques. In: Mulholland MW, Hawn MT, Hughes SJ, et al, eds. *Operative Techniques in Surgery*. Wolters Kluwer; 2015:1804-1809. Figure 2.)

SUBCLAVIAN VEIN

Incision

- The SCV can be accessed through a variety of incisions. We prefer a clavicular incision (with clavicular transection) with extension to a median sternotomy if required. The clavicular incision allows for excellent exposure of the mid and distal SCV with median sternotomy allowing for more proximal access on either side. The incision starts at the sternal notch, is carried over the clavicle, and is extended into the deltopectoral groove (**FIGURE 3**).
- Dissection is carried down through the subcutaneous tissue and platysma muscle until the clavicle is encountered.

Exposure of Subclavian Vein

- The proximal aspect of the clavicle is cleared of all muscular attachments.
- The clavicle is divided near the sternoclavicular junction and distal aspect retracted superiorly. Alternatively, the clavicle

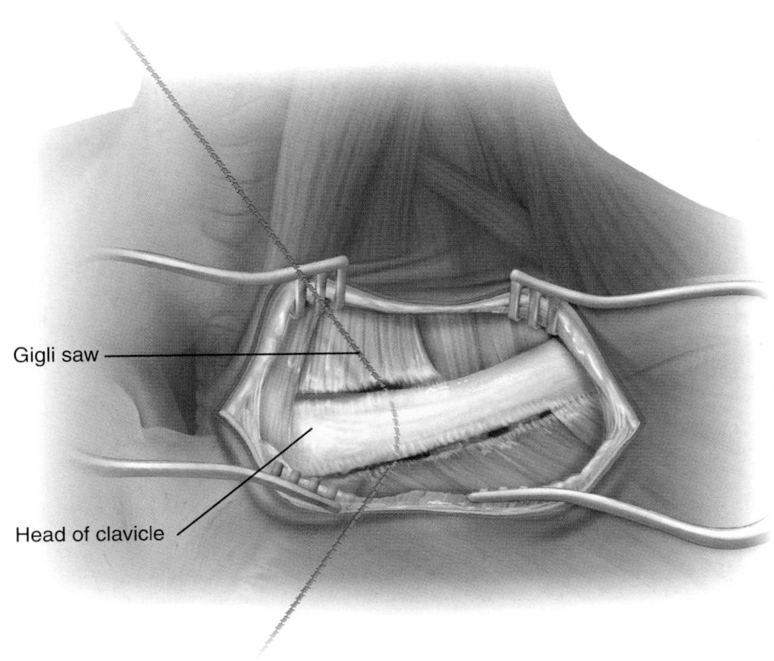

FIGURE 5 ● The skin, subcutaneous tissue, and platysma have been divided and clavicle cleared of muscular attachments. A Gigli saw is used to transect the clavicle. Alternatively, a segment of clavicle can be excised.

can be retracted without division, although the exposure is not as good with this approach. A medial claviculectomy (resection of the medial 2/3 of the clavicle) can also be performed and does not require bone reconstruction (FIGURE 5).

- The SCV is the first vessel encountered as it is anterior to the artery and anterior scalene muscle. Note that the phrenic nerve courses posterior to the SCV in the medial aspect of this exposure (FIGURE 6A and B).

Management of Subclavian Vein Injury

- The vein can be encircled with silastic vessel loops or bleeding controlled with vascular clamps.
- Management is similar to that of BCV injuries. Ligation is well tolerated and should be performed in patients who are critically ill or have other management priorities. Lateral venorrhaphy with fine monofilament suture (5-0 polypropylene) can be performed if repair results in less than 50% stenosis. Complex repairs as well as venous shunting should generally be avoided in our opinion[3,4,14,15] (FIGURE 7A-D).

Incision Closure

- If the clavicle was divided, it can be reapproximated with wire or plate (FIGURE 8).
- The platysma muscle and subcutaneous tissues are closed in layers with absorbable suture. The skin is closed with staples or monofilament suture.
- Median sternotomy, if performed, is closed as previously described.

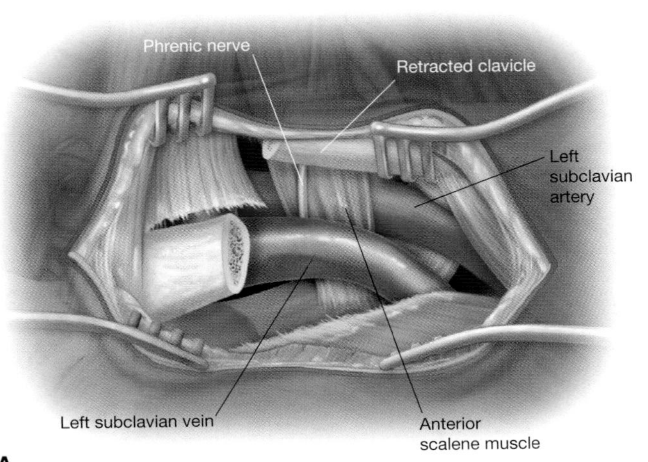

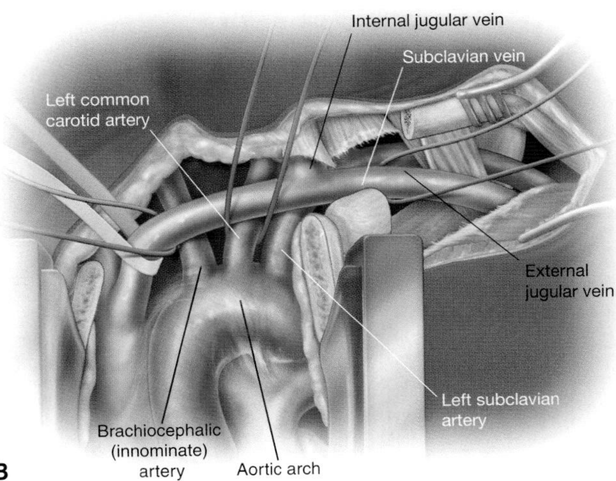

FIGURE 6 ● **A,** The clavicle has been transected and retracted upward. The subclavian vein, artery, and phrenic nerve are seen. **B,** Exposure of the proximal left subclavian vein after combined median sternotomy and left clavicular incision.

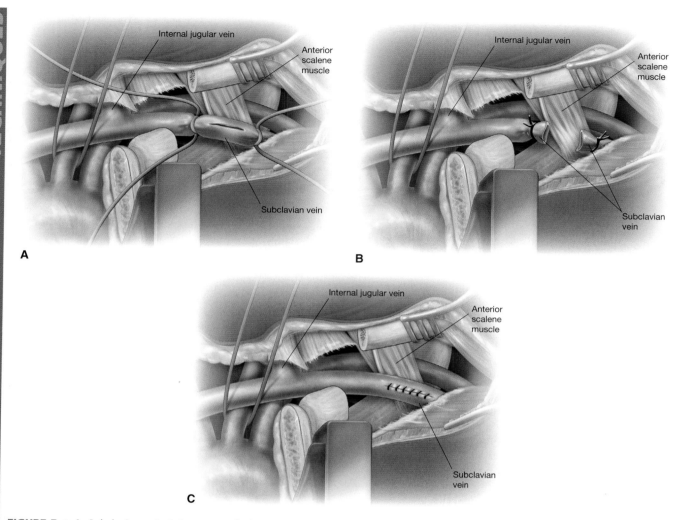

FIGURE 7 ● **A,** Subclavian vein injury controlled with silastic vessel loops. **B,** Subclavian vein injury managed with suture ligation. **C,** Subclavian vein injury managed with venorrhaphy.

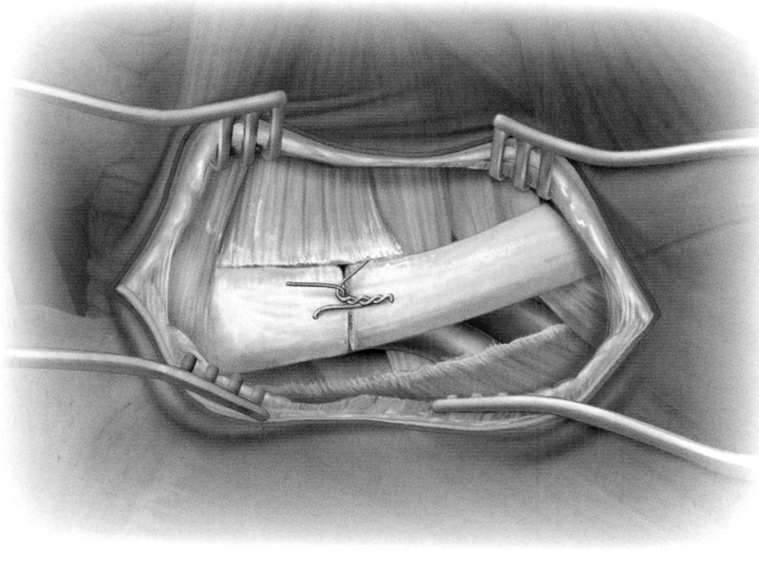

FIGURE 8 ● Reapproximation of the transected clavicle with wire.

ROLE OF ENDOVASCULAR MANAGEMENT

- Endovascular management should have a limited role in the treatment of these injuries. Those without active bleeding can typically be managed nonoperatively, and those that are bleeding are usually treated with ligation/or primary repair via appropriate exposure.
- There is limited literature to support the use of covered stents in traumatic venous injuries. Stents are more typically used in the setting of iatrogenic trauma (ruptured central vein during venoplasty in the treatment of central venous stenosis for example) with good effect.

DAMAGE CONTROL

- Patients with severe physiology derangement (acidosis, coagulopathy, hypothermia, hypocalcemia, shock) and/or injuries in multiple cavities may benefit from an abbreviated damage control procedure.
- BCV/SCV injuries can be ligated and the sternotomy/thoracotomy and/or clavicular incisions packed open for delayed return to the operating room following physiologic restoration.
- For temporary chest closure (sternotomy or thoracotomy), we employ a surgical towel covered on one side with a transparent iodine-impregnated dressing to cover the thoracic viscera following placement of thoracostomy tubes (**FIGURE 9**). A transparent dressing can then be used to cover the wound.

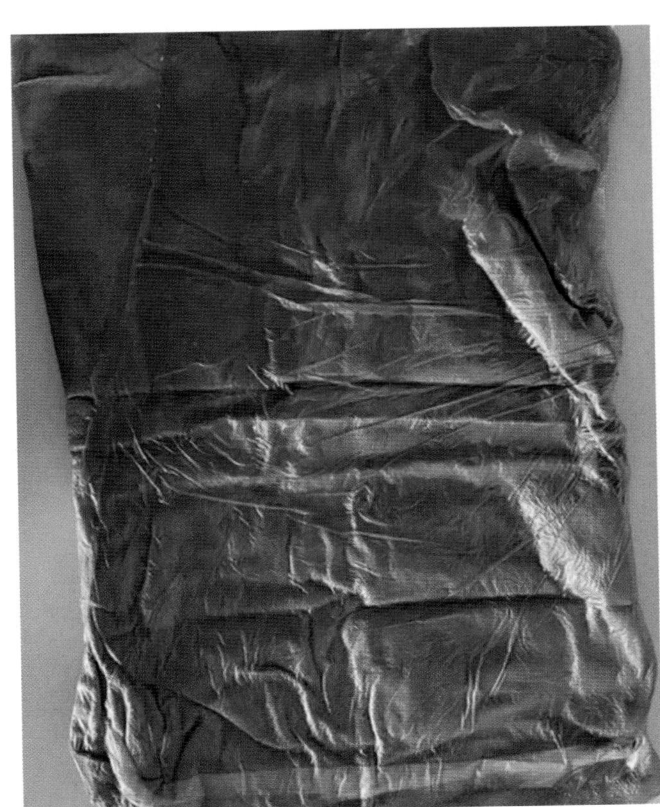

FIGURE 9 ● Surgical towel wrapped on one side with iodine-impregnated dressing, which is used to cover the intrathoracic viscera following damage control operation.

PEARLS AND PITTFALLS

Initial evaluation	■ Failure to recognize subtle signs of BCV/SCV injury ■ Failure to recognize associated injuries
Initial airway management	■ Recognize that intubation can lead to cardiovascular collapse in patients with thoracic venous injuries
Operative management	■ Understand the various utility incisions and how these can be extended to achieve additional exposure ■ Avoid complex BCV/SCV repairs, especially in critically ill patients
Postoperative care	■ Failure to start venous thromboembolism (VTE) prophylaxis

POSTOPERATIVE CARE

- Patients with BCV/SVC injuries are generally admitted to the intensive care unit postoperatively.
- The ipsilateral extremity should be elevated over several days to mitigate edema. Most upper extremity edema appears to be transient.[3]
- Serial upper extremity examinations should be performed to monitor for compartment syndrome (tense compartments, pain out of proportion to examination, paresthesia, etc.).
- Chemical VTE prophylaxis should be started immediately if there is no contraindication (ie, traumatic brain injury), as there appears to be an association between venous injury and VTE regardless of method of repair or ligation. In addition, withholding postoperative prophylaxis following venous injury repair has been shown to correlate with increased risk of VTE.[16]
- The need for full anticoagulation following nonoperative and operative repair of venous injuries as well as the role of screening venous duplex ultrasounds require further investigation.

COMPLICATIONS

- Air embolism
- Injury to the phrenic nerve or brachial plexus
- Upper extremity edema
- Upper extremity compartment syndrome
- VTE
- Malunion/osteomyelitis following clavicular division
- Sternal wound infection

REFERENCES

1. O'Connor JV, Byrne C, Scalea TM, Griffith BP, Neschis DG. Vascular injuries after blunt chest trauma: diagnosis and management. *Scand J Trauma Resusc Emerg Med*. 2009;17:42.
2. Demetriades D, Chahwan S, Gomez H, et al. Penetrating injuries to the subclavian and axillary vessels. *J Am Coll Surg*. 1999;188(3):290-295.
3. Sciarretta JD, Asensio JA, Vu T, et al. Subclavian vessel injuries: difficult anatomy and difficult territory. *Eur J Trauma Emerg Surg*. 2011;37(5):439.
4. Iscan S, Etli M, Gursu O, Eker E, El Kilic H. Isolated subclavian vein injury: a rare and high mortality case. *Case Rep Vasc Med*. 2013;2013:152762.
5. Moore EE, Malangoni MA, Cogbill TH, et al. Organ injury scaling. IV: thoracic vascular, lung, cardiac, and diaphragm. *J Trauma*. 1994;36(3):299-300.
6. American College of Surgeons. *Advanced Trauma Life Support Student Course Manual*. 10th ed. 2018.
7. Holly BP, Steenburg SD. Multidetector CT of blunt traumatic venous injuries in the chest, abdomen, and pelvis. *Radiographics*. 2011;31(5):1415-1424.
8. Madsen AS, Bruce JL, Oosthuizen GV, Bekker W, Laing GL, Clarke DL. The selective non-operative management of penetrating cervical venous trauma is safe and effective. *World J Surg*. 2018;42(10):3202-3209.
9. Seamon MJ, Haut ER, Van Arendonk K, et al. An evidence-based approach to patient selection for emergency department thoracotomy: a practice management guideline from the Eastern Association for the Surgery of Trauma. *J Trauma Acute Care Surg*. 2015;79(1):159-173.
10. Sai Sudhakar CB, Elefteriades JA. Safety of left innominate vein division during aortic arch surgery. *Ann Thorac Surg*. 2000;70(3):856-858.
11. McPhee A, Shaikhrezai K, Berg G. Is it safe to divide and ligate the left innominate vein in complex cardiothoracic surgeries? *Interact Cardiovasc Thorac Surg*. 2013;17(3):560-563.
12. Quan RW, Adams ED, Cox MW, et al. The management of trauma venous injury: civilian and wartime experiences. *Perspect Vasc Surg Endovasc Ther*. 2006;18(2):149-156.
13. Feliciano DV. Pitfalls in the management of peripheral vascular injuries. *Trauma Surg Acute Care Open*. 2017;2(1):e000110.
14. Nair R, Robbs JV, Muckart DJ. Management of penetrating cervicomediastinal venous trauma. *Eur J Vasc Endovasc Surg*. 2000;19(1):65-69.
15. O'Connor JV, Scalea TM. Penetrating thoracic great vessel injury: impact of admission hemodynamics and preoperative imaging. *J Trauma*. 2010;68(4):834-837.
16. Frank B, Maher Z, Hazelton JP, et al. Venous thromboembolism after major venous injuries: competing priorities. *J Trauma Acute Care Surg*. 2017;83(6):1095-1101.

SECTION V: Injury to the Neck

Chapter 17 Incisions: Anterior Sternocleidomastoid Incision, Collar Incision

Scott A. Zakaluzny and Joseph M. Galante

DEFINITION

- Injuries to the neck are approached via a unilateral sternocleidomastoid incision, a collar incision, or a combination of bilateral sternocleidomastoid and collar incisions. These approaches are the same used for elective procedures such as carotid endarterectomy or thyroid surgery.

DIFFERENTIAL DIAGNOSIS

- Airway injury: thyroid complex, proximal trachea
- Nasopharyngeal injury
- Esophageal injury
- Nerve injury—most notably the spinal cord or one of the recurrent laryngeal nerves
- Vascular injury—most notably the carotid artery and the internal jugular vein

PATIENT HISTORY AND PHYSICAL FINDINGS

- The mechanism of injury is an important factor in the determination of management of neck trauma, with penetrating trauma more likely requiring operative exploration and intervention.[1,2]
- Key physical exam findings include the following:
  - Patient's ability to phonate and whether their voice is altered from baseline;
  - Presence of marks, abrasions, ecchymosis, or open wounds;
  - Any swelling or asymmetry;
  - Presence of a hematoma or other signs of a potential vascular injury (active bleeding, expanding hematoma);
  - Ability to move extremities suggestive of a spinal cord injury or carotid injury;
  - Blood in the airway;
  - Air bubbling from any wounds or subcutaneous emphysema;
  - Presence of a bruit or thrill; and
  - Cranial nerves and nerves of the brachial plexus should also be evaluated.[1]
- A patient with hard signs of a vascular injury, pulsatile bleeding, expanding hematoma, or signs of compromised distal perfusion need not have any further workup and should go directly to the operating room for exploration and control of bleeding. Otherwise, the patient, if stable, can either have their airway controlled, if indicated, or simply proceed to imaging workup.

IMAGING AND OTHER DIAGNOSTIC STUDIES

- Classic teaching for penetrating neck trauma was based on the three zones of the neck. This is due to the surgical inaccessibility of structures at the thoracic inlet and the base of the skull. However, the wound on the outside does not dictate the possible trajectory a penetrating object takes, with the potential for injuries in more than one zone and wide spread access to high-quality imaging; this classification system is primarily of historical value or clinical reference to describe external wounds.
- In the absence of hard signs of vascular injury, preoperative imaging is most often obtained and consists of computed tomography (CT) angiography of the neck, which images the aortic arch and takes off vessels through the thoracic inlet and neck. This is most sensitive for arterial injuries.[3] Contrast should be injected on the contralateral side of suspected or potential injuries to avoid contrast artifact.
- Direct or fiberoptic laryngoscopy can assist with the evaluation of the pharynx and hypopharynx.
- An esophagogastroduodenoscopy, or more rarely rigid esophagoscopy, can be used to evaluate the esophagus.[4] Although highly sensitive, negative endoscopy should be followed by contrast swallow studies based on the level of suspicion to prevent missed injury.[4]

SURGICAL MANAGEMENT

Preoperative Planning

Ensure access to the following:

- Appropriate equipment for endoscopy
- Vascular
  - Instruments
  - Sutures
  - Shunts
  - Vessel loops
  - Heparinized saline
- Sternal saw or Lebsche knife with mallet
- Rib spreader
- Blood and blood products
- Bougie
- Penrose drain
- Various sized tracheostomy tubes

Positioning

- Supine
- In penetrating trauma, if the patient was neurologically intact or you have a normal CT scan of the cervical spine, it is safe to turn the neck.[5] Additionally, a shoulder roll allows for mild extension of the neck.
- The arms, which are typically out for trauma, will likely be in the way, so placing the right arm at the patient's side is helpful but avoid tucking to allow anesthesia access.
- A standard trauma prep should be done—chin to knees and table to table. This prep allows access to the chest if there is a need for extension to a median sternotomy or resuscitative thoracotomy as well as bilateral groins for harvesting saphenous vein for use in a vascular repair. Most of the body can be covered to help prevent hypothermia.

ANTERIOR STERNOCLEIDOMASTOID INCISION

- The incision is made from the mastoid process just posterior to corner of the mandible to the sternal notch along the *anterior* boarder of the sternocleidomastoid muscle—this can be performed on either the left or right side of the neck. This incision can be extended to a sternotomy or connected to a collar incision with or without a mirror incision on the opposite side of the neck.
- Carry incision through the platysma to find the sternocleidomastoid muscle (**FIGURE 1**).
- Retract the sternocleidomastoid muscle posterior lateral (**FIGURE 2**).
- The proximal carotid sheath can be exposed further by dividing the omohyoid muscle (**FIGURE 3**).
- The bifurcation of the carotid artery is exposed by ligating the facial vein (**FIGURE 4**) The carotid sheath can be opened, revealing the anatomical relationship of the structures within the sheath—the internal jugular vein lateral, the carotid artery medial, and the vagus nerve between but somewhat posterior to the artery and vein (**FIGURES 5** and **6**).
- The distal internal carotid artery can be difficult to access. First, divide the posterior belly of the digastric muscle. Be cautious of the hypoglossal nerve anterior and the vagus nerve posterior, and avoid cutting during your dissection. Next, have an assistant use two "army-navy" retractors to provide retraction on the mandible from the opposite side of the table. If a lumen can be seen, a Fogarty catheter can be inserted into the distal internal carotid artery to achieve control. If a larger defect needs to be filled to compress the vessel, a Foley balloon can be inflated in the space.

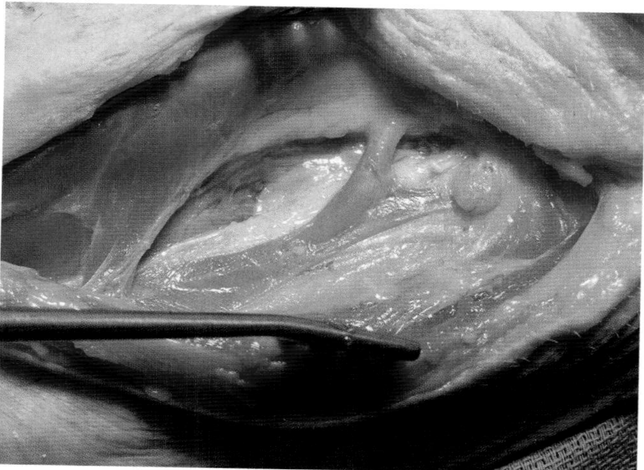

FIGURE 2 ● Image of left neck with head to right. The sternocleidomastoid muscle is retracted; the facial vein in the superior aspect of the incision and the omohyoid muscle in the inferior aspect of the incision can be seen.

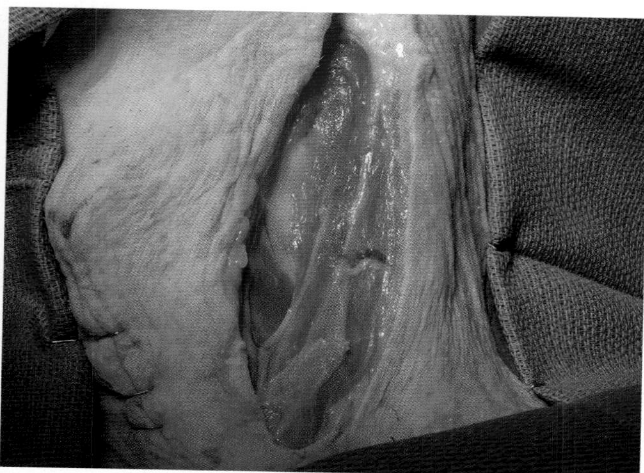

FIGURE 1 ● An incision made from the angle of the mandible to the sternoclavicular joint along the anterior border of the sternocleidomastoid muscle on either side of the neck is the most common incision for exposing the structures of the neck.

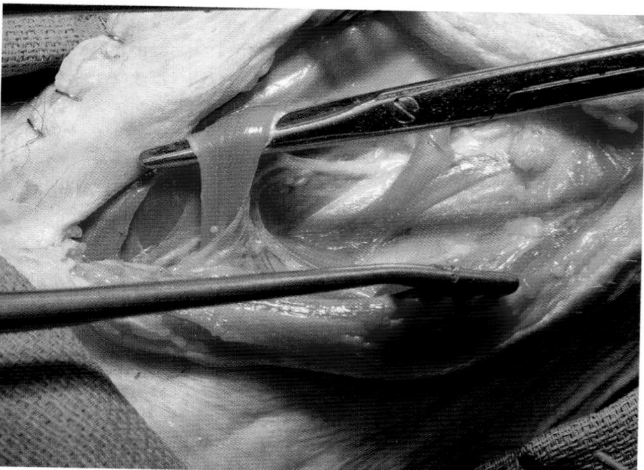

FIGURE 3 ● Image of left neck with head to right. The omohyoid muscle can be divided for proximal exposure of the common carotid artery in the neck.

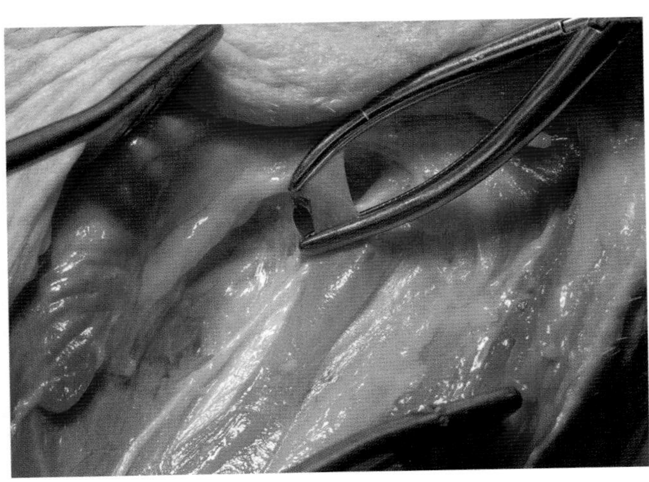

FIGURE 4 ● The facial vein can be divided to expose the carotid bifurcation.

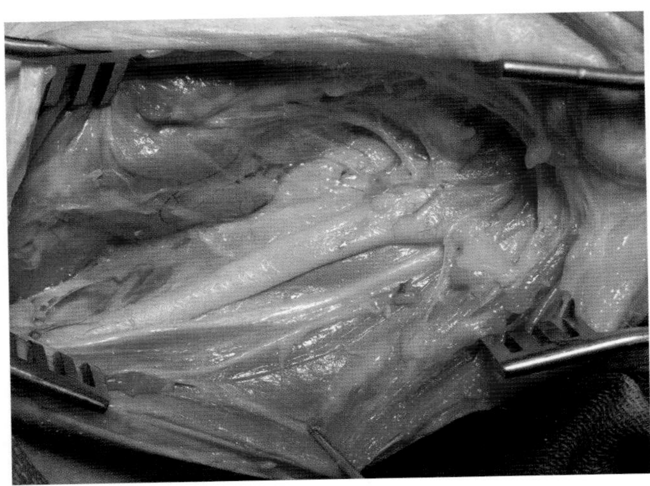

FIGURE 5 ● The facial vein and omohyoid muscle are divided, the carotid sheath is opened to expose the common carotid and its bifurcation in the neck.

- The esophagus is typically accessed from the left neck; but can be accessed from the right if necessary. It is exposed by retracting the carotid sheath contents laterally and the thyroid and thyroid cartilage medially. You may need to divide the middle thyroid vein and inferior thyroid artery. The esophagus lies posterior to the airway and anterior to the cervical spine. Identification can be facilitated by the placement of a nasogastric tube or a bougie. It can be encircled with a Penrose drain to provide retraction (**FIGURES 7** and **8**).

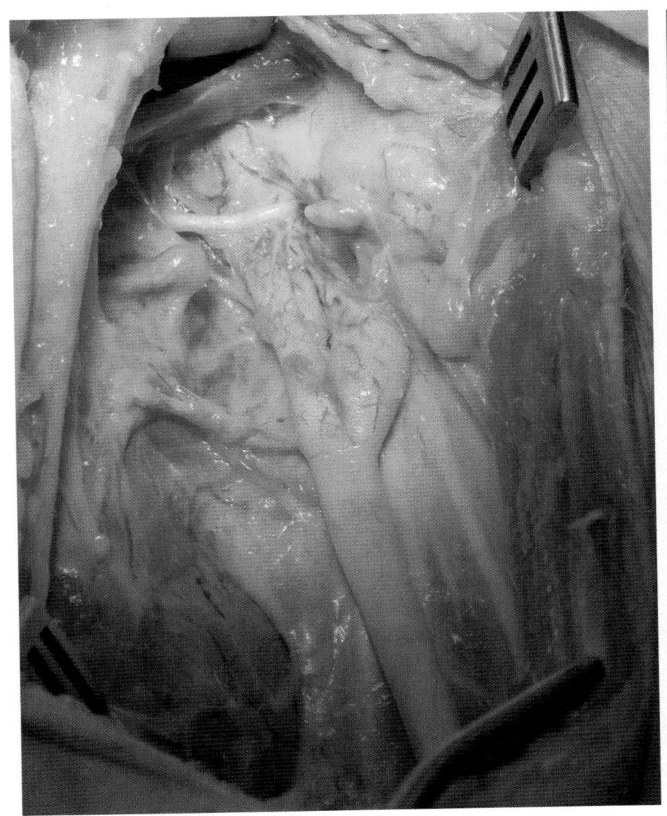

FIGURE 6 ● The carotid bifurcation is dissected free with the hypoglossal nerve running across the internal carotid artery.

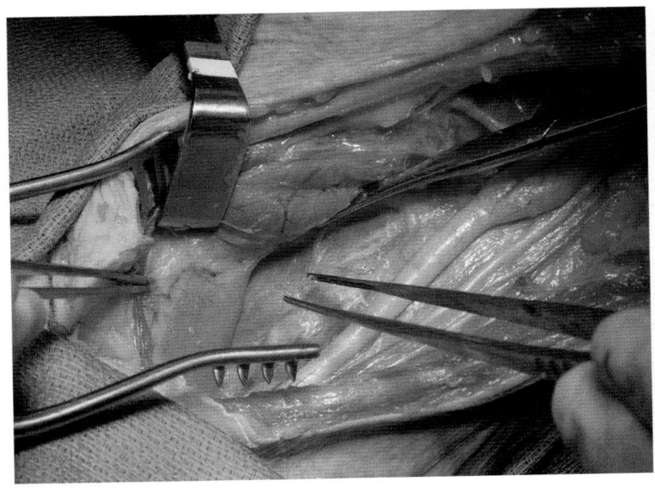

FIGURE 7 ● The esophagus is accessed by retracting the thyroid anterior medial.

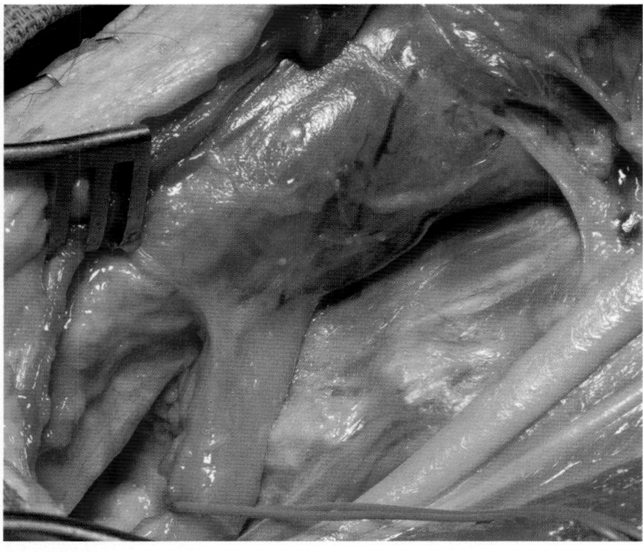

FIGURE 8 ● The esophagus dissected free and encircled with a vessel loop.

COLLAR INCISION

- Transverse incision is made approximately 2 to 3 finger breadths above the sternal notch. The incision can extend as far as the anterior border of the sternocleidomastoid muscle on either side of the neck as needed (**FIGURE 9**).
- The incision is carried through the platysma muscle. To optimize exposure, subplatysmal flaps can be created.
- The thyroid and airway complex are approached through a longitudinal dissection plane (perpendicular to transverse skin incision) by dividing the strap muscles in the midline along a natural raphe.
- A plane under the strap muscles can be developed as needed for exposure.
- The incision may be extended along the anterior boarder of either or both sternocleidomastoid muscles for further exposure. The combination of bilateral sternocleidomastoid and a collar incision with generous subplatysmal flaps gives access to virtually any structure in the anterior neck and bilateral carotid sheaths. Connecting this incision with a vertical incision to create a "T" allows further exposure of the trachea or for a sternotomy.

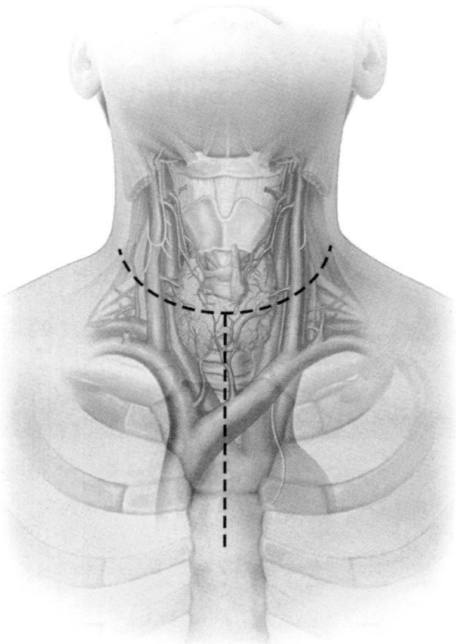

FIGURE 9 ● A collar incision can be used to access the anterior neck. This can be extended on to either or both sides of the neck via a sternocleidomastoid incision. Additionally, it can be extended inferiorly as a "T" with a median sternotomy.

PEARLS AND PITFALLS

Assessment	■ Any identified injury should prompt a thorough assessment for a second injury to the same structure, ie., anterior/posterior.
Airway repairs	■ The airway should be repaired with *absorbable* sutures. Small injuries can be adequately treated if needed by the use of an endotracheal tube with the cuff distal to the injury.
Operative pearls	■ Bleeding from the vertebral arteries within the transverse spinal foramen is controlled with bone wax and packing for tamponade and/or interventional radiology. ■ The external carotid artery (ECA) can be ligated for uncontrolled facial hemorrhage in the absence of interventional radiology. Be reminded, the ECA has branches where the internal does not. ■ Caution should be taken in isolating the esophagus so as not to injure the recurrent laryngeal nerve in the tracheoesophageal groove. ■ In combination with aerodigestive and/or vascular injuries, the repairs should be separated by a viable muscle flap, usually of strap muscle. ■ Drain all esophageal repairs; consider draining all neck explorations for the potential of a small missed esophageal or oropharyngeal injury.

POSTOPERATIVE CARE

- The decision to extubate should depend on the patient's general medical condition, airway edema, and stability, and typically is not based on the need for any type of repair.

COMPLICATIONS

- Leaks of repairs are the most common and feared complication.
  - Vascular repair failure typically requires urgent/emergent intervention, often associated with a missed oropharyngeal injury that leaks saliva into the wound
  - Esophageal or oropharyngeal injuries are best managed by washout and drainage
  - Airway—least common, manage by assuring control of distal airway, control of infection
- Thrombosis of arterial repair with associated stroke

REFERENCES

1. Demetriades D, Ali S, Brown C, Martin M, Rhee P. Neck injuries. *Curr Probl Surg*. 2007;44(1):13-85.
2. Asensio JA, Chahwan S, Forno W, et al. Penetrating esophageal injuries: multicenter study of the American association for the surgery of trauma, *J Trauma Inj Infect Crit Care*. 2001;50(2):289-296.
3. Madsen AS, Kong VY, Oosthuizen GV, Bruce JL, Laing GL, Clarke DL. Computed tomography angiography is the definitive vascular imaging modality for penetrating neck injury: a South African experience. *Scand J Surg*. 2018;107(1):23-30.
4. Arantes V, Campolina C, Valerio SH, et al. Flexible esophagoscopy as a diagnostic tool for traumatic esophageal injuries. *J Trauma Inj Infect Crit Care*. 2009;66(6):1677-1682.
5. Connell RA, Graham CA, Munro PT. Is spinal immobilisation necessary for all patients sustaining isolated penetrating trauma? *Injury*. 2003;34(12):912-914.

Chapter 18

Upper Aerodigestive Tract Injury: Trachea

John Andrew Harvin and Rushabh Prakash Dev

DEFINITION

- Tracheal injuries are defined as injury to the cervical or thoracic trachea. They are infrequent; however, they can be life threatening in the setting of trauma.
- The adult trachea is between 10 to 13 cm in length and 2 to 2.5 cm wide. It is a centrally located, flexible hollow organ. The cervical portion of the trachea begins at the level of the sixth vertebral body. Superiorly, it is supported by the thyroid cartilage and circumferential cricoid cartilage. About 15 to 20 incomplete anterior cartilaginous rings support the body of the trachea caudally. The trachea is nearly cylindrical in cross section with posterior flattening. The flattening is the membranous portion that is posterior to the opening of each C-shaped anterior tracheal ring. This posterior wall is made of dense longitudinal folds of tracheal smooth muscle overlong the esophagus.
- The cervical trachea is the most superficial and the surgically accessible portion is between the thyroid cartilage and sternal notch. The thoracic portion of the trachea begins as it traverses the neck at the sternal notch at the level of the second thoracic vertebrae. It enters the superior mediastinum and terminates with the carina at the bifurcation of the right and left bronchi at the fourth and fifth thoracic vertebrae. The blood supply of the distal trachea receives contributions from the subclavian, intercostal, internal thoracic, and bronchial arteries.
- The cervical trachea is supplied by the inferior thyroid artery from the thyrocervical trunk, and the thoracic trachea is supplied by bronchial arteries coming off the aorta. In both cases, the arterial blood supply is segmental in that it enters the trachea laterally. This is important during dissection; mobilization of the trachea for repair should be limited to only what is needed to avoid ischemic complications of tracheal repair.

DIFFERENTIAL DIAGNOSIS

- Tracheal trauma can be associated with neck and thoracic injury. Penetrating injuries most commonly involve the cervical trachea. While not the topic of this chapter, penetrating laryngeal injuries are more common than cervical tracheal injuries.[1]
- The skin, subcutaneous tissue, strap muscles, thyroid isthmus, and pretracheal fascia overlay the cervical trachea. The thyroid, anterior jugular veins, and recurrent laryngeal nerves border the trachea laterally, with the esophagus posteriorly. The innominate artery crosses to the right at a variable level, often between the level of the sixth to tenth tracheal ring. Blunt injuries typically involve the intrathoracic trachea, with the right main-stem bronchus being the most commonly involved segment.[2] Often trauma to intrathoracic organs such as heart, vessels (aorta, superior, and inferior vena cava), esophagus, lungs, and diaphragm must be ruled out.

PATIENT HISTORY AND PHYSICAL FINDINGS

- Injuries to the cervical trachea are often obvious. Air bubbling through a neck wound is considered pathognomonic for airway injury. This could be accompanied by subcutaneous emphysema. Endotracheal intubation for isolated cervical tracheal injuries can often be delayed until the patient is in the operating room and is typically performed with minimal difficulty. However, the addition of respiratory distress, unstable hemodynamic status, altered mental status, size and site of hematoma, and injury can make endotracheal intubation more urgent and complex.
- Distal thoracic trachea or proximal bronchial injuries typically present with large and persistent pneumothorax with associated air leak despite tube thoracostomy placement. In this setting endotracheal intubation is straightforward followed by evaluation with fiberoptic bronchoscopy to identify the location of the injury. The majority of distal tracheal injuries occur within 2 cm of the carina.

IMAGING AND OTHER DIAGNOSTIC STUDIES

- Flexible fiberoptic bronchoscopy should be considered when major airway and tracheal injury is suspected. Bronchoscopy allows for blood, tissue, and secretions to be cleared in order to assess the entire circumference of the airway.
- Thin-slice multidetector computed tomography can be employed in stable patients with injury to the trachea, and when the penetrating trajectory is far from the trachea, injury can be effectively ruled out. Although three-dimensional formatting of the trachea is possible and can assist in evaluating tracheal injury, a negative study does not rule out injury. Therefore, bronchoscopy remains the gold standard for identifying the location and extent of the injury.
- Direct laryngoscopy and video laryngoscopy will provide additional information, as well as aid at the time of intubation. However, its use is typically dictated by the skill of the provider, type of injury, and impeding airway loss.

SURGICAL MANAGEMENT

Positioning

Cervical Trachea

- In a patient with isolated neck and no cervical spine injury, it is ideal to place a bump or shoulder roll underneath the upper back to allow head extension and flexion during the case. This will open the neck for improved exposure by elevating the trachea and allowing for more distal access above the sternal notch. If there is a known cervical spine injury, the neck should be kept neutral and straight.

CERVICAL TRACHEA

Incision

- The choice of incision depends on the location and associated injuries.

Collar Incision and Exposure

- For anterior injuries, a low transverse collar incision is made two finger breadths above the sternal notch with extension to the medial borders of the sternocleidomastoid muscles. After creating a collar incision, the platysma is incised and subplatysmal flaps are created superiorly and inferiorly exposing the strap muscles. The strap muscles are divided by incising the median raphe to expose the trachea, larynx, and thyroid. The thyroid isthmus can be divided with electrocautery to fully expose the first through third tracheal rings.

Sternocleidomastoid Incision and Exposure

- For injuries to the esophagus or major vessels, an incision is made over the corresponding anterior border of the sternocleidomastoid that is then extended across the midline two finger breadths above the sternal notch. If incorporating a single or bilateral sternocleidomastoid incisions, respectively, this creates a J- or U-type incision. The platysma is divided and the sternocleidomastoid is retracted laterally to expose the carotid sheath. Division of the facial vein superiorly and the omohyoid muscle inferiorly will allow exposure to the carotid artery, jugular vein, and esophagus (on the left). The lateral trachea can be exposed by retracting the carotid sheath laterally.

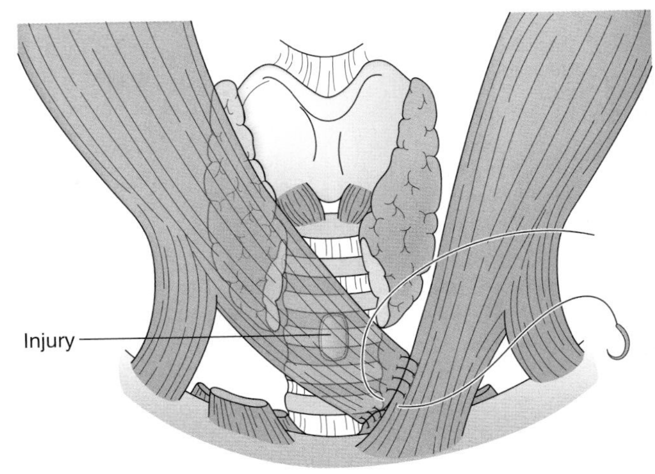

FIGURE 1 ● Divided strap muscle utilized to buttress tracheal injury/repair. (Reprinted with permission from Bruns BR, Scalea TM. Neck Injuries. In: Dimick JB, Upchurch GR Jr, Alam HB, et al, eds. *Mulholland & Greenfield's Surgery Scientific Principles and Practice*. 7th ed. Wolters Kluwer; 2021:362-369. Figure 23.5.)

Repair

- Most injuries without significant tissue loss can be managed by primary repair. Debridement should be minimal. Lacerations are closed and large fragments of tracheal rings secured with 3-0 or 4-0 absorbable suture.
- If the injury is not amenable to primary repair, then tracheal resection and anastomosis is performed. The endotracheal tube should be advanced passed the injury or a reinforced endotracheal tube inserted into the defect on the operating field.
- The injured trachea is resected. The superior and inferior portions of the trachea are mobilized to both minimize devascularization of the trachea and avoid injury to the recurrent laryngeal nerve. Lateral traction sutures are placed on either side of the injury and used to pull the superior and inferior edges together. If there is tension a suprahyoid laryngeal release can be performed, although this is not commonly needed in the setting of trauma. The anastomosis is performed with interrupted 3-0 or 4-0 absorbable suture with the knots oriented on the outside of the lumen.
- The endotracheal tube cuff should be advanced distal to the repair and inflated until the end of the operation. If there is concern for direct exposure of the suture line to vessel or concomitant esophageal injury, care must be taken to buttress the repair with viable tissue from strap muscle (**FIGURE 1**). Place a drain and bring it out anteriorly without crossing the carotid sheath. Reapproximate the platysma and close the skin.
- While some anterior injuries can simply have a tracheostomy placed through them, we prefer repair and extubation. Immediate tracheostomy is associated with an increased risk of surgical site infection, a complication that can range from minor to devastating for the patient.

THORACIC TRACHEA

Incision

- The proximal thoracic trachea can be exposed from a supine position and collar incision ± median sternotomy (**FIGURE 2**).
- A right posterior lateral thoracotomy at the 5th intercostal space can expose the distal trachea, right main stem bronchus, and proximal left main stem bronchus. A left lateral decubitus can expose the distal left main stem bronchus.

Exposure

- The proximal thoracic trachea as discussed previously can be exposed through a collar incision; if the injury is out of reach of the collar incision, a median sternotomy can be performed to allow access. The distal trachea, right main stem bronchus, and proximal left main stem bronchus are approached through a right posterolateral thoracotomy. The distal left main stem bronchus is exposed via left thoracotomy. While a double-lumen endotracheal tube will facilitate better exposure, often times it does not allow for placement. The endotracheal tube can be advanced and manually guided past the injury, including intubation of the contralateral bronchus and single lung ventilation.

Repair

- Repair of the thoracic trachea is done in a similar fashion as the cervical trachea. However, the repair should be buttressed with an intercostal muscle flap, a pericardial flap, or a pleural flap.

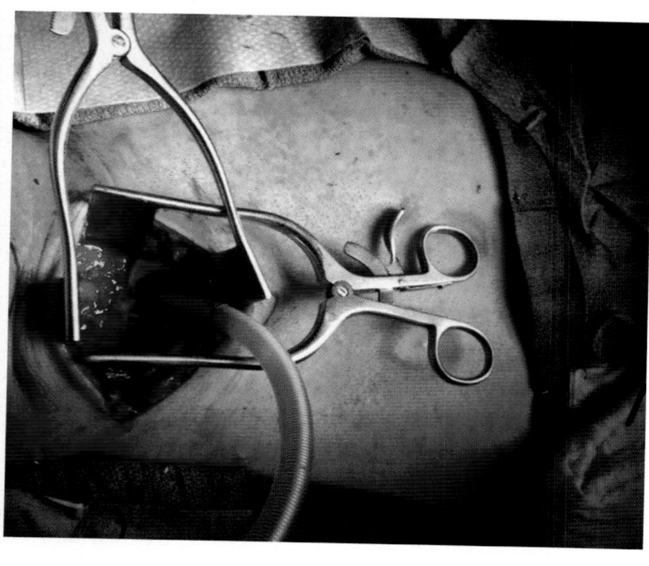

FIGURE 2 • Intubation of a distal tracheal transection in the neck. (Reprinted with permission from Bruns BR, Scalea TM. Neck Injuries. In: Dimick JB, Upchurch GR Jr, Alam HB, et al, eds. *Mulholland & Greenfield's Surgery Scientific Principles and Practice*. 7th ed. Wolters Kluwer; 2021:362-369. Figure 23.2.)

PEARLS AND PITFALLS

Spontaneous breathing	▪ Spontaneous breathing should be maintained and bag-mask ventilation minimized until the team is prepared to obtain a secured airway. Depending on the expertise of the team, awake intubation with sedation is preferable to paralysis during rapid sequence intubation. Direct or video laryngoscopy is recommended to assess for laryngeal obstruction or airway distortion, therefore facilitating endotracheal intubation and providing information if a surgical airway is indicated. Furthermore, direct laryngoscopy can safely facilitate intubation through the injury via a cervical wound if indicated.
Surgical options	▪ If endotracheal intubation fails, there are two surgical options. First, if the cervical skin wound is large and the tracheal injury is visible, the side of the trachea can be grasped with an instrument and the distal trachea intubated with a 6.0 endotracheal tube (**FIGURE 3**). Second, a cricothyroidotomy can be performed above the injury. A tracheotomy in an uninjured trachea should be avoided if possible as it complicates the repair of the actual tracheal injury.

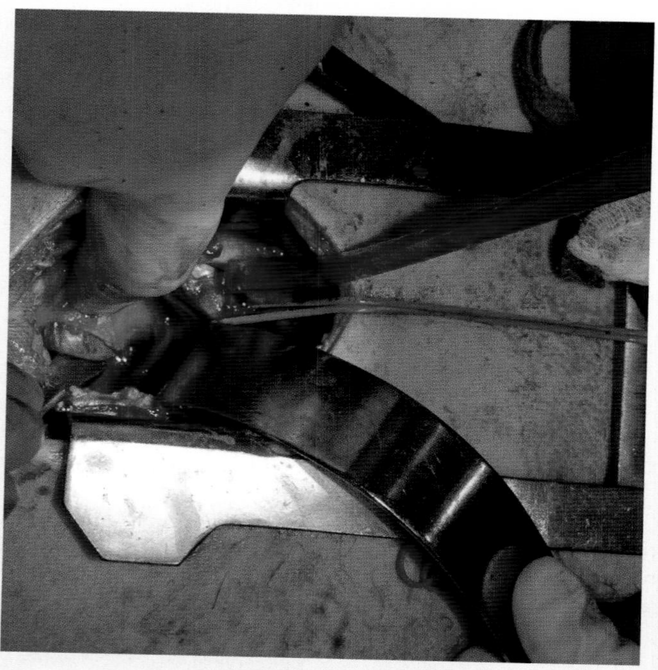

FIGURE 3 • Partial sternal split for evaluation of tracheal injury. The endotracheal tube balloon is visualized within the lumen of the injured trachea. (Reprinted with permission from Bruns BR, Scalea TM. Neck Injuries. In: Dimick JB, Upchurch GR Jr, Alam HB, et al, eds. *Mulholland & Greenfield's Surgery Scientific Principles and Practice*. 7th ed. Wolters Kluwer; 2021:362-369. Figure 23.4.)

Complications	■ If evaluation of trachea is complicated by blood and secretions, then the endotracheal tube is advanced past the injury. Blood and secretions are suctioned from the airway and the endotracheal tube is then carefully withdrawn keeping the bronchoscope distal to the end of the endotracheal tube to obtain complete visualization. In some cases, the actual injury cannot be wholly delineated outside of blood and air emanating from a suspect area.

POSTOPERATIVE MANAGEMENT

- Following tracheal repair, the location and extent of injury and, more importantly, concomitant injuries will dictate immediate postoperative management. For cervical injuries repaired primarily or reconstructed tracheal injuries without significant tension, immediate or early extubation is recommended if not precluded by concomitant injuries (eg, traumatic brain injury or spinal cord injury). Immediate or early extubation is recommended with thoracic tracheal injuries to avoid positive pressure on the suture line.

COMPLICATIONS

- Immediate tracheostomy is associated with increased risk of surgical site infection, which can increase the risk of tracheal complications postoperatively. When concomitant injuries require tracheostomy, we recommend delayed tracheostomy 3 to 7 days after repair.
- Tracheoesophageal fistula, although rare, occurs in the setting of concomitant injury to the esophagus. Suture lines are typically opposed to each other when this injury occurs. A fistula is avoided by interposing vascularized tissue, such as strap muscle between suture lines.
- Tracheal stenosis is rare and presents with wheezing through an obstructed airway. Diagnosis and identification are made by bronchoscopy or computed tomography. Treatment is initially performed by control of the airway. Subsequent therapy is directed by balloon dilation and/or stent placement vs surgical resection and primary anastomosis.

REFERENCES

1. Cameron JL, Cameron AM. *Current Surgical Therapy*. 13th ed. Elsevier; 2020:889-893.
2. Burke JF. Early diagnosis of traumatic rupture o the bronchus. *JAMA*. 1962;181:682-686.

Chapter 19

Surgical Management of Injuries to the Cervical Esophagus

James P. Byrne and Patrick M. Reilly

DEFINITION

- Injury to the cervical esophagus is defined as injury to the esophagus in the neck due to blunt or penetrating trauma. Anatomically, the cervical esophagus extends from the cricopharyngeus muscle, which forms the upper esophageal sphincter, to the sternal notch. Esophageal injuries, including those in the neck, are described along a spectrum of organ injury severity (**TABLE 1**).[1] While these injuries are relatively rare, morbidity and mortality are high particularly if diagnosis is delayed. Therefore, early recognition is a cornerstone of effective management.

DIFFERENTIAL DIAGNOSIS

- Trauma to the neck presents a unique challenge due to proximity of several critical structures in a confined anatomic region. These include aerodigestive structures (trachea and esophagus), carotid artery and jugular vein, and the spinal column including spinal cord and vertebral arteries. Multiple concomitant injuries are commonly present and it is often difficult to determine which structures are involved from mechanism or physical examination alone. High degree of suspicion for esophageal injury must be maintained.

PATIENT HISTORY AND PHYSICAL FINDINGS

- Injuries to the cervical esophagus are most commonly caused by penetrating mechanisms (60%-90%),[2,3] two-thirds of which are due to firearm injury.
- Rapid evaluation of the ABCs in keeping with ATLS should be prioritized.
- An early logroll with careful inspection of the head and neck (in addition to the rest of the body) must be performed to identify penetrating wounds. Where feasible, wounds should be marked with radio-opaque markers (eg, taped paperclips) for X-ray identification to aid in determining trajectories (**FIGURE 1**).
- Where hard signs of airway injury are present (respiratory distress, hemoptysis, or bubbling from wounds), early intubation should be performed with a surgeon at standby to perform a surgical airway procedure if required.
- Where there are hard signs of vascular injury (expanding hematoma or active bleeding), direct finger pressure should be applied. Adjunctive maneuvers such as placing a Foley catheter into the wound followed by insufflation of the balloon can help to achieve temporary hemostasis.
- While dysphagia, odynophagia, bloody secretions, or subcutaneous emphysema could reflect esophageal injury, these findings are not pathognomonic and are neither sensitive nor specific.

IMAGING AND OTHER DIAGNOSTIC STUDIES

- Plain film X-rays: These are an essential adjunct to the primary survey in the trauma bay. In patients with gunshot wounds, X-rays should encompass the body compartments at risk for injury. For patients with gunshot wounds to the neck we advocate obtaining X-rays of the head (so-called "big head"), neck, and chest. Retropharyngeal air or pneumomediastinum raise concern for esophageal injury and warrant further investigation (**FIGURE 1**).
- Computed tomographic angiography (CTA): CTA has become the diagnostic modality of choice in patients with

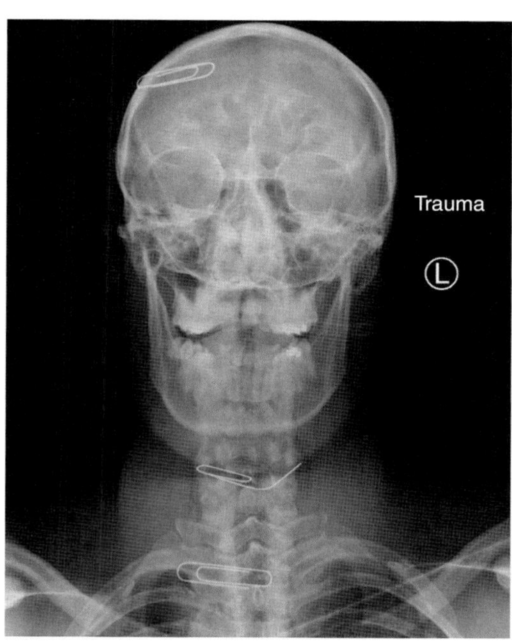

FIGURE 1 • "Big head" X-ray demonstrating use of radio-opaque markers (in this case, paperclips) to mark gunshot wounds. Closed paperclips denote anterior injuries, while bent paperclips denote posterior injuries. No retained projectiles are seen. Findings in this patient are clearly concerning for transcervical trajectory. Gas in the deep tissue planes of the neck raise concern for aerodigestive injury. The scalp wound was tangential and did not penetrate the skull.

Table 1: Grading of Esophageal Injuries

Grade	Description of injury
I	Contusion/hematoma or partial thickness laceration
II	Laceration <50% circumference
III	Laceration >50% circumference
IV	Segmental loss or devascularization <2 cm
V	Segmental loss or devascularization >2 cm

Advance one grade for multiple injuries up to grade III

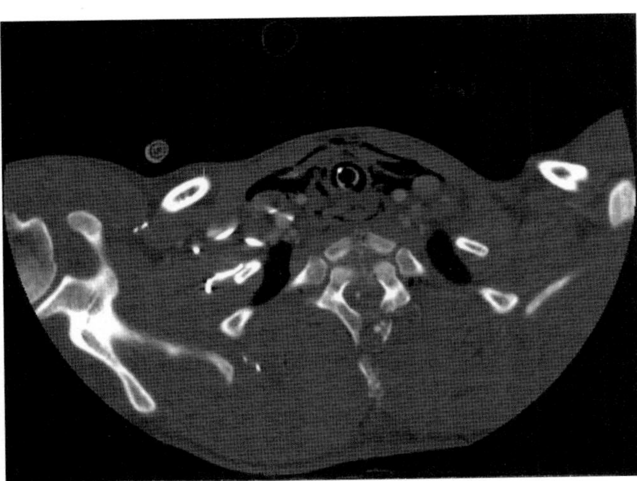

FIGURE 2 • Computed tomographic angiography of the neck of patient with anterior cervical gunshot wound. Extensive subcutaneous emphysema and gas in the paratracheal and paraesophageal spaces raise high concern for tracheal and esophageal injuries. Combined with trajectory showing cervical spinal column injury, operative exploration was clearly indicated.

neck trauma where immediate operative exploration is not indicated by hemodynamic instability or hard signs. CTA should be performed in all stable patients with penetrating injuries to the neck, with the rare exception of asymptomatic patients with trajectories that are clearly low risk. In patients with penetrating injury, CTA is highly sensitive (100%) and specific (97.5%) for aerodigestive and vascular injury (FIGURE 2).[4] However, sensitivity for detecting esophageal injury might be lower in stab wounds.[5] In patients with blunt trauma, CTA is indicated based on history of trauma to the neck, external signs of injury (such as seatbelt sign), or the presence of soft signs such as nonexpanding hematoma, dysphonia, dysphagia, odynophagia, or subcutaneous emphysema.

- Esophagography: Gastrografin or thin barium esophagography is a helpful imaging modality in stable patients where CTA is nondiagnostic for esophageal injury. Patients undergoing esophagography must be able to sit up and follow instructions to swallow contrast material. The decision to pursue esophagography must also take into consideration the timing and availability of this resource since the diagnosis of esophageal injury should not be delayed.
- CT esophagography: It is possible to evaluate the cervical esophagus with contrast esophagography using CT. This can be challenging, however, requiring an alert patient capable of following instructions to swallow a bolus of contrast with precise timing while supine. Therefore, this test is often not useful in the acute phase of care, and more reliable diagnostic approaches, such as flexible endoscopy, are favored.
- Flexible esophagoscopy: Esophagoscopy is a resource that can be readily mobilized to the bedside or the operating room (OR) in real time. In one series of patients with esophageal injuries, predominantly in the neck, flexible esophagoscopy diagnosed the injury with a sensitivity of 96%.[6] Therefore, esophagoscopy is an extremely helpful modality in patients where there is diagnostic uncertainty and esophagography is not readily available.

SURGICAL MANAGEMENT

Indications

- Patients with hard signs of aerodigestive or vascular injury require operative exploration.
- In patients with esophageal injury identified on CTA, esophagography, or flexible esophagoscopy, prompt surgical intervention is the safest decision to avoid the increased morbidity and mortality associated with delays in treatment.

Preoperative Planning

- Early communication with the OR and anesthesia teams is essential prior to transporting the patient to the OR. Information regarding the patient history and current status, the planned operation and positioning, expected blood loss, and transfusion requirements should be given.
- Specific equipment needs should be relayed. These might include flexible endoscope and bronchoscope, vascular shunts, and feeding tubes not typically stored in the OR.

Positioning

- The patient is positioned on the operating table supine with arms out. A rolled sheet or inflatable support is placed transversely under the patient's upper back to hyperextend the neck. The bed is placed in reverse Trendelenburg or flexed at its midpoint to elevate the patient's head, neck, and chest.
- Where there is concern for unstable cervical spinal column injury, which is unlikely in the setting of penetrating trauma, the decision to limit neck extension while maintaining inline stabilization is made in selected patients.
- The patient should be prepped and draped from the chin to the knees. Access to the chest is important should proximal arterial injury in the neck or thoracic vascular injury necessitate median sternotomy or thoracotomy. At least one lower extremity should be prepped to allow for harvest of a saphenous vein graft. Prepping the abdomen reserves the option of placing a gastrostomy tube if long-term need for enteral access is predicted.

SKIN INCISION

- The incision of choice for suspected injury to the cervical esophagus is a left-sided oblique cervical incision (**FIGURE 3**). This incision follows a line along the anterior border of the sternocleidomastoid muscle (SCM) from the mastoid to the sternal notch. This approach is chosen because the esophagus in the neck lies to the left of midline posterior to the trachea.
- Depending on the burden of injury suspected, extension of this incision across the midline into a modified collar incision, or into bilateral oblique incisions, might be required for adequate exposure of associated injuries.

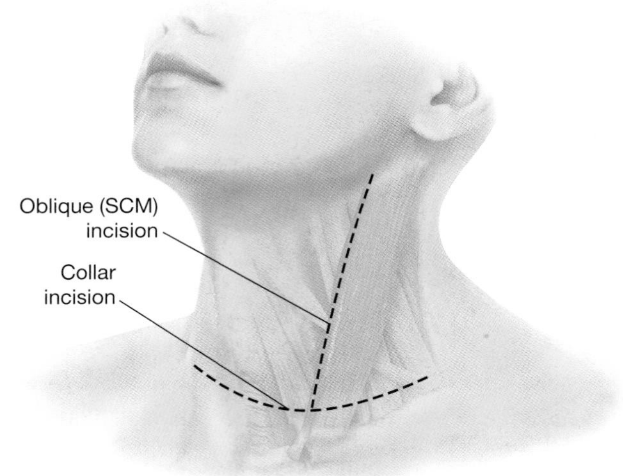

FIGURE 3 ● Depiction of incisions for surgical exposure of the neck. The esophagus is best exposed through a left oblique incision, along the anterior border of the sternocleidomastoid muscle (SCM). Where broader exposure to the bilateral neck is required, the collar incision or bilateral oblique incisions can be used.

EXPOSURE AND EVALUATION OF THE ESOPHAGUS

- Through a left-sided oblique cervical incision, the platysma is divided and the SCM is retracted laterally. This exposes the underlying strap muscles and carotid sheath (**FIGURES 4** and **5**).
- Omohyoid, the lateral-most strap muscle belly, is divided to provide exposure of the deep structures in the neck.
- The carotid sheath is retracted laterally with SCM, while trachea with thyroid gland are retracted medially, to expose the length of the esophagus in the neck. A blunt Weitlaner self-retaining retractor can be placed to maintain this exposure (**FIGURE 6**).

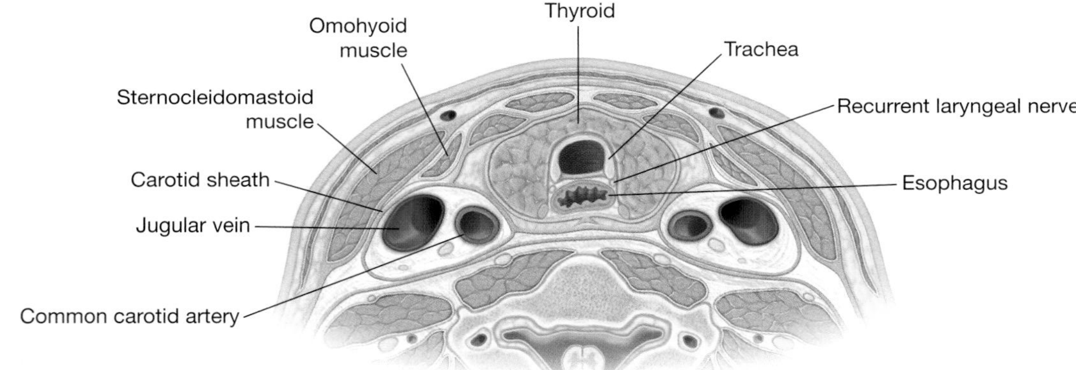

FIGURE 4 ● Cross section of the neck at the level of C6 or C7. The relationship between the sternocleidomastoid and strap muscles, the carotid sheath, and the trachea and esophagus is shown.

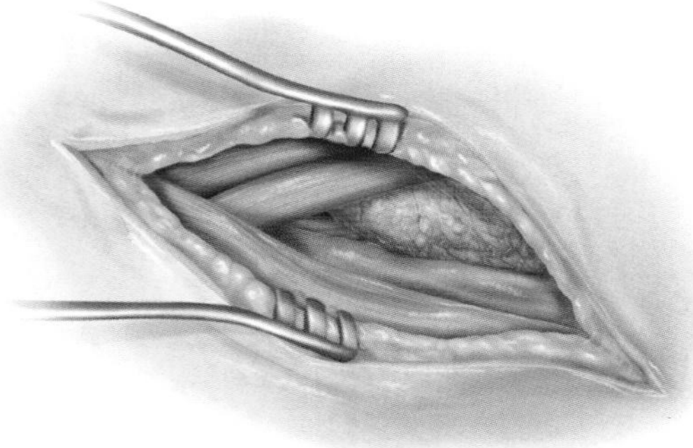

FIGURE 5 ● Left oblique neck incision with retraction of the sternocleidomastoid muscle laterally exposes sternothyroid and omohyoid strap muscles and the carotid sheath. The omohyoid must be divided to provide access to the trachea and esophagus.

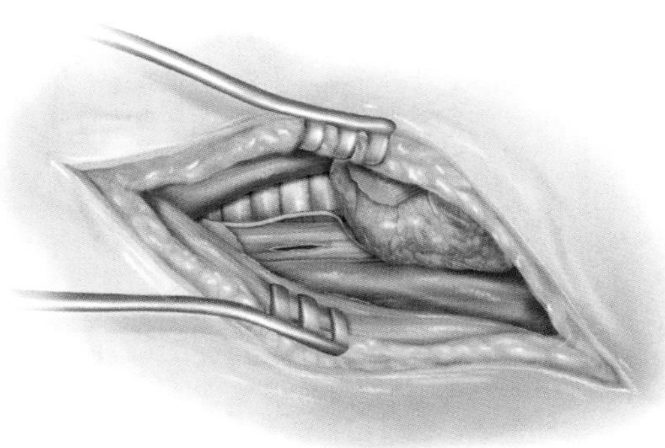

FIGURE 6 ● With omohyoid divided, a blunt Weitlaner retractor is used to retract sternocleidomastoid muscle laterally to expose the trachea and esophagus.

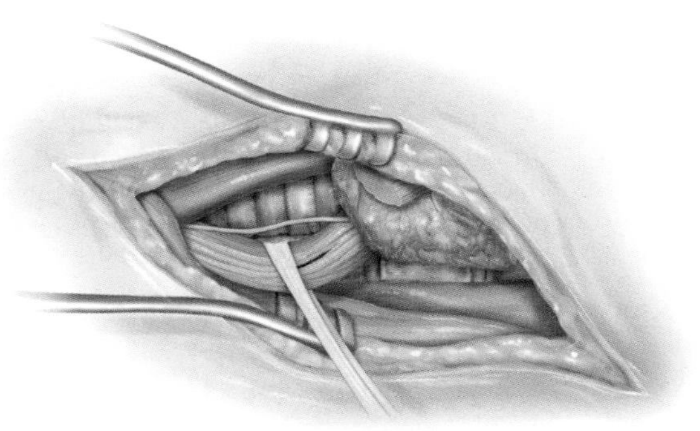

FIGURE 7 ● After bluntly separating the esophagus from the anterior surface of the spinal column, a Penrose drain is placed around it for the purpose of mobilization and inspection.

- The recurrent laryngeal nerve should be identified running in the tracheoesophageal groove with the purpose of protecting it during further dissection.
- A nasogastric tube (NGT) should be gently passed to aid in palpating the esophagus.
- Blunt finger dissection posterior to the esophagus can now be performed to separate it from the prevertebral fascia and anterior surface of the vertebral column. The prevertebral fascia may need to be incised first. With a hooked finger, the esophagus is mobilized circumferentially. Care to avoid injury to the overlying trachea is critical.
- A Penrose drain is placed around the esophagus for manipulation. With this control the surgeon can now inspect the length of mobilized esophagus for injury (**FIGURE 7**).
- Areas of questionable injury or hematoma should be gently explored with Metzenbaum scissors.
- If there remains question of injury, the cervical esophagus can be tested for leak. The NGT is withdrawn to the level of the esophagus in the neck. The esophagus is occluded distally at the thoracic outlet. With the neck incision filled with saline, the esophagus is gently insufflated with air via the NGT by the anesthesia team. Bubbling indicates a full-thickness injury. Alternatively, methylene blue dye injected by NGT can be used to identify full-thickness perforation.

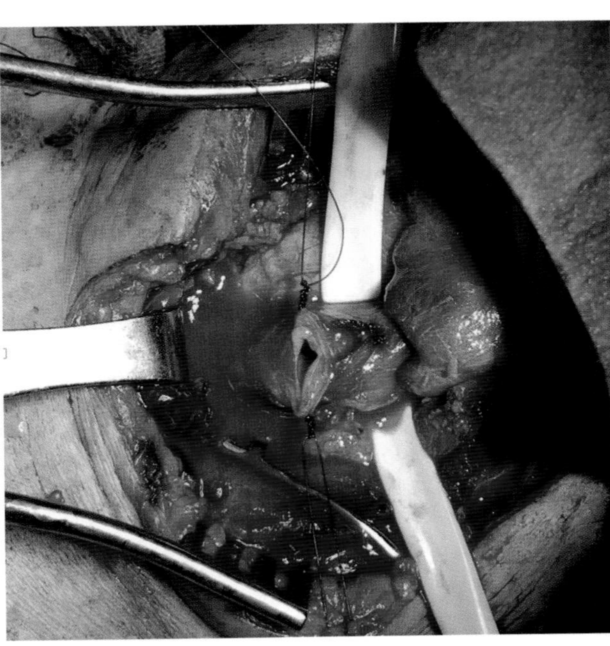

FIGURE 8 ● Esophageal injury exposed through left oblique neck incision. Penrose is in place. The thyroid is cranial (right in picture) and the trachea to the right (top of picture) of the injury. The edges of the mucosal defect are seen well exposed with use of stitches placed at the apices of the planned closure.

Esophageal Repair

- Once an injury is identified, care must be taken to delineate the full extent of the mucosal defect. This might require enlarging the muscular defect to achieve. Devitalized tissue is debrided.
- Repair is performed in a two-layer tension-free fashion.
- The inner mucosal layer is approximated using a 3-0 absorbable suture (eg, Maxon, PDS, or Vicryl).
- The outer muscular layer is closed using 3-0 nonabsorbable suture (eg, silk).
- Using the long tail of suture from the apex of the injury, the margins of the defect can be brought outward under subtle tension to better expose the edges of the injury and make placement of suture bites easier (**FIGURE 8**).
- The inner layer should carefully reapproximate the mucosal edges to achieve water-tight closure in running fashion. This is particularly important to the integrity of the repair because the esophagus lacks serosa.
- The outer layer of the repair reapproximates the muscular layer over the inner repair in running or interrupted fashion.

VASCULARIZED MUSCLE FLAP

- In the setting of concomitant injuries to the trachea or carotid artery, a vascularized muscle flap should be positioned to separate the repairs.
- Use of the sternal head of the SCM has been classically described. The mobilized end of the muscle is placed in position to separate the esophageal repair from repairs of the trachea or carotid (**FIGURE 9**).
- Because the SCM receives blood supply at multiple levels from the occipital, superior thyroid, and suprascapular arteries, variations of well-vascularized SCM flaps can be fashioned by mobilizing the muscle from above or below.
- In young or well-nourished patients, the strap muscles are often robust enough to provide an adequate alternative to the SCM for buttressing repairs.

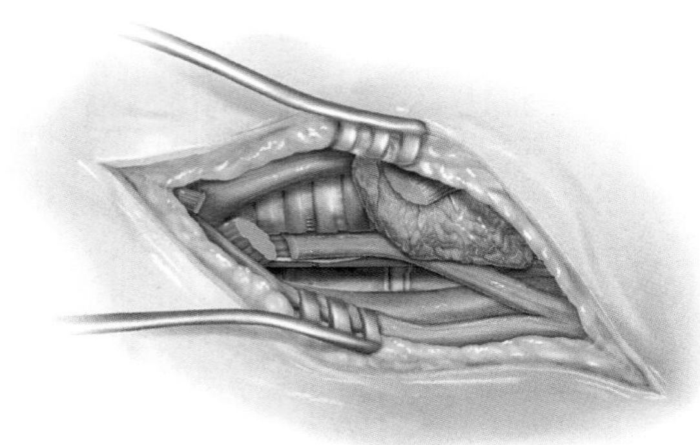

FIGURE 9 ● If needed after repair of concomitant tracheal and esophageal injuries, the sternal head of the sternocleidomastoid muscle can be separated from its insertion and mobilized as a vascularized muscle flap. This is placed between the tracheal and esophageal repairs as a buttress.

DRAINAGE

- Because leak rates are high, a drain should be placed adjacent to the repair and exiting the skin away from the surgical incision at the base of the neck.
- Open (eg, Penrose) or closed (eg, Jackson-Pratt or Blake) drain systems can be used depending on surgeon preference.
- The drain should not be left in direct contact with the carotid artery out of concern for risk of erosion into the vessel.

DAMAGE CONTROL

- Where injury to the esophageal wall is too extensive, or local sepsis due to a delayed diagnosis makes primary repair not feasible, a cervical esophagostomy should be created. This is performed by exteriorizing the site of perforation as a "blowhole" esophagostomy, loop esophagostomy, or double-barreled esophagostomy.

ENTERAL ACCESS FOR NUTRITION

- We recommend leaving an NGT in place at the time of surgery, initially for gastric decompression, but also to allow for feeding in the early postoperative period. This tube should be bridled to the nasal septum before leaving the OR (this can be done tying the large-bore NGT to a small-bore feeding tube bridle using 0 silk suture). Clear signage in plain view should be left at the bedside in the intensive care unit (ICU) stating that only the surgical team should manipulate this tube.
- Open surgical gastrostomy tube placement is reasonable if a patient is expected to be unable to eat for a prolonged period. Examples are patients with complex esophageal injuries, concomitant tracheal or spinal cord injuries, or anticipation of prolonged mechanical ventilation.

PEARLS AND PITFALLS

Indications for surgery	■ Hemodynamically unstable patients and those with hard signs of aerodigestive or vascular injury should undergo urgent operative exploration, bypassing CT scan.
Incision	■ The left-sided oblique incision provides the best exposure of the cervical esophagus. ■ If exposure is difficult, do not struggle. Extend the incision across the midline into a "modified collar" incision or bilateral oblique incisions for better exposure.
Mobilization of the esophagus	■ Finger dissection is used to separate the esophagus from the anterior surface of the spinal column. A hooked finger is then used to mobilize the esophagus along its full length in the neck. ■ This step is easiest with an NGT present.

Identifying the injury	■ If suspicion for injury exists, persistence is required to thoroughly evaluate the cervical esophagus. ■ Inspect the full circumference of the esophagus and examine areas of hematoma. ■ Test for full-thickness perforation by distending with air or using methylene blue dye. ■ Use flexible endoscopy. ■ Where a single penetrating injury is seen, examine for a paired through-and-through injury.
Muscle flaps	■ The SCM receives blood supply from multiple levels and can therefore be mobilized in either direction to achieve a tension-free flap. ■ Strap muscles are a viable alternative if sized and placed appropriately.
Enteral access for nutrition	■ Always consider need for durable access for feeding. ■ Leave an NGT. ■ Bridle the NGT to the nasal septum yourself before leaving the OR. This can be done using a bridle designed for a small-bore feeding tube (Dobhoff tube). The large-bore NGT is tied to the bridle using an 0 silk tie. ■ Leave a sign in the ICU stating that this tube should be manipulated only by the surgical team.

POSTOPERATIVE CARE

- Postoperative care begins in the ICU. Due to a high frequency of concomitant injuries (75%), patients remain mechanically ventilated for a median of 4 days. Median ICU length of stay is 6 days.[2]
- Patients with esophageal repair should remain nil per os (NPO) in the early postoperative period. We recommend that patients remain NPO for 7 days. A contrast esophagogram on day 7 is performed to evaluate for signs of leak (**FIGURE 10**). If this study is negative, the patient can be advanced to oral intake.
- Enteral feeding, by NGT or gastrostomy tube, should begin early while the patient is NPO.
- Drains left at the time of surgery should be monitored for volume and character of output. These are removed after the patient has progressed to oral intake and output is negligible.

COMPLICATIONS

Leak

- The most frequent complication specific to cervical esophageal injury is leak, most often following attempted primary repair. In one multi-institutional study, the rate of leak following intervention for cervical esophageal injury was approximately 29%.[3] Half of leaks were uncontained and all required subsequent intervention. One-fifth of leaks persisted despite subsequent intervention. An important predictor of esophageal injury-related complications such as leak is delayed recognition and treatment,[7] reinforcing that high index of suspicion and expeditious treatment are essential.

Infectious Complications

- Patients with cervical esophageal injuries are high risk for septic complications, due to breakdown of repair or failure of drainage, often in the setting of multiple injuries. Infectious complications of some kind (eg, pneumonia, mediastinitis, sepsis, esophageal fistula) arise in 14%-37% of patients.[2,3]

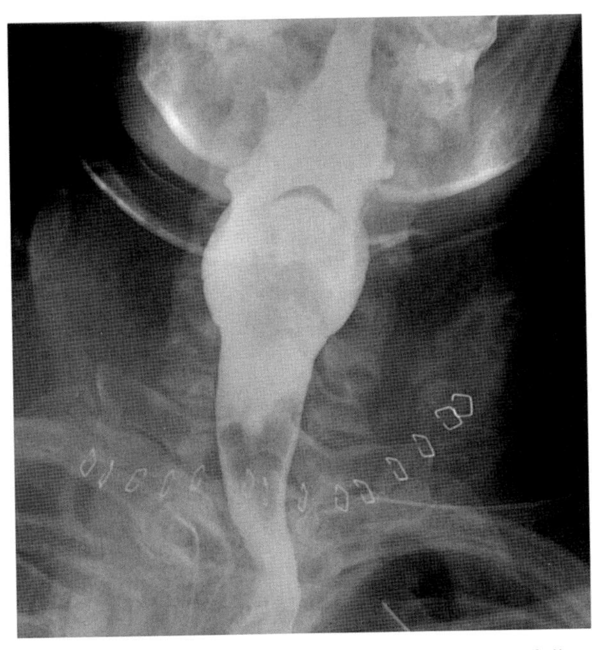

FIGURE 10 ● Barium swallow on postoperative day 7 following primary repair of a cervical esophageal injury. No leak is seen.

Mortality

- While lower than mortality observed following thoracic esophageal injury (13%), mortality following cervical esophageal injury remains relatively high (8%-9%).[2,3]

REFERENCES

1. Moore EE, Jurkovich GJ, Knudson MM, et al. Organ injury scaling. VI: Extrahepatic biliary, esophagus, stomach, vulva, vagina, uterus (nonpregnant), uterus (pregnant), fallopian tube, and ovary. *J. Trauma*. 1995;39(6):1069-1070.
2. Aiolfi A, Inaba K, Recinos G, et al. Non-iatrogenic esophageal injury: a retrospective analysis from the National Trauma Data Bank. *WJES*. 2017;19(12):19. doi:10.1186/s13017-017-0131-8

3. Raff LA, Maine RG, Jansen J, et al. Contemporary management of traumatic cervical and thoracic esophageal perforation: the results of an Eastern Association for the Surgery of Trauma multi-institutional study. *J Trauma Acute Care Surg*. 2020;89(4):691-697.
4. Inaba K, Branco BC, Menaker J, et al. Evaluation of multidetector computed tomography for penetrating neck injury: a prospective multicenter study. *J Trauma Acute Care Surg*. 2012;72(3):576-584.
5. Gonzalez RP, Falimirski M, Holevar MR, Turk B. Penetrating zone II neck injury: does dynamic computed tomographic scan contribute to the diagnostic sensitivity of physical examination for surgically significant injury? A prospective blinded study. *J. Trauma*. 2003;54(1):61-64.
6. Arantes V, Campolina C, Valerio SH, et al. Flexible esophagoscopy as a diagnostic tool for traumatic esophageal injuries. *J. Trauma*. 2009;66(6):1677-1682.
7. Asensio JA, Chahwan S, Forno W, et al. Penetrating esophageal injuries: multicenter study of the American Association for the Surgery of Trauma. *J. Trauma*. 2001;50(2):289-296.

Chapter 20

Repair of Internal and External Carotid Injury

Melike N. Harfouche and Rosemary A. Kozar

DEFINITION

- Penetrating neck trauma is classified into zones, traditionally applied to anterior wounds of the neck.
- Zone I is defined as any injury from the sternal notch to the cricoid cartilage, zone II is any injury from the cricoid cartilage to the angle of the mandible, and zone III is any injury from the angle of the mandible to the base of the skull[1] (**FIGURE 1**).
- Blunt cerebrovascular injuries can occur to either the carotid artery or the vertebral arteries and develop from intimal trauma due to rapid acceleration/deceleration injuries or direct blunt force injury to the neck.
- In these cases, injury to the carotid artery usually occurs in the region in proximity to the petrous portion, where the artery is relatively fixed.
- Blunt carotid injury rarely requires operative intervention, and if so, it is usually treated with an endovascular approach. On the other hand, penetrating injuries to the carotid artery frequently mandate operative exploration.

DIFFERENTIAL DIAGNOSIS

- Penetrating trauma to the neck can involve vascular structures, but it can also involve the aerodigestive tract. It is important to consider laryngeal, tracheal, and esophageal injuries in the differential diagnosis.

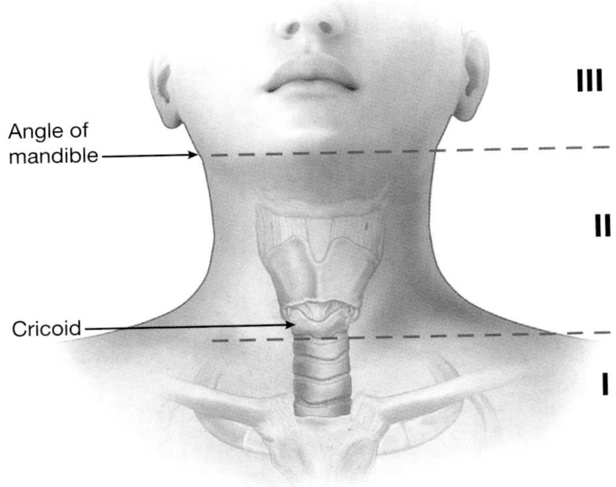

FIGURE 1 ● Zones of the neck. The neck is divided into three zones: Zone III is above the angle of the mandible, Zone II is between the angle of the mandible and the cricoid cartilage, and Zone I is below the cricoid cartilage. (Reprinted with permission from Roon AJ, Christensen N. Evaluation and treatment of penetrating cervical injuries. *J Trauma*. 1979;19(6):391-397.)

- Injuries to the thoracic inlet (zone I) can involve other vascular structures, namely the subclavian arteries and veins and the innominate artery and veins.
- Injuries to the base of the skull can extend into intracranial structures.
- Missiles carry more kinetic energy than stab wounds and travel further distances. In these cases, it is important to have a wide differential diagnosis as to the body cavities and associated structures that may be injured, as they may not be limited to the structures within the neck.[2]

PATIENT HISTORY AND PHYSICAL FINDINGS

- Clinical findings of vascular injury to the neck are divided into hard signs and soft signs (**TABLE 1**).
- Hard signs of vascular injury mandate operative exploration; the surgical approach is dictated by the zone of injury (see below).
- Soft signs of vascular injury require investigation with imaging modalities, namely computed tomography angiography (CTA) or digital subtraction angiography (DSA).
- Crepitus in the neck is usually indicative of a tracheal injury, which may also present with severe hypoxia and rapid decompensation requiring orotracheal intubation or a surgical airway.
- Esophageal injuries rarely present with crepitus and are usually insidious. In some cases, hematemesis may occur.

IMAGING AND OTHER DIAGNOSTIC STUDIES

- In the absence of penetration of the platysma and no soft signs of vascular injury, no further imaging and a short period of observation is appropriate.
- A plain anteroposterior X-ray of the neck can be performed in the trauma bay to evaluate for subcutaneous emphysema. A lateral X-ray can provide additional information regarding missile trajectory.
- In the absence of hard signs of vascular injury mandating direct operative exploration, patients with soft signs of vascular injury should have further imaging.
- Traditionally, the gold standard test to evaluate for vascular injury in the neck was DSA; however, due to improvements in CT technology and speed of performance, CTA has largely replaced DSA as the imaging modality of choice to evaluate for vascular injury in the neck.[3] It has a sensitivity of 79%-100% and a specificity of 61%-100%.[4] **FIGURE 2** demonstrates a penetrating injury to the carotid artery at the thoracic inlet.
- Bronchoscopy can be performed to evaluate for injuries to the trachea or main bronchi. If this is being performed on an intubated patient, the endotracheal tube must be withdrawn

to the level of the vocal cords to adequately assess the entire trachea.

SURGICAL MANAGEMENT

- Patients with vascular injuries to the neck can deteriorate rapidly and require emergent intubation.
- It is important to anticipate potential airway loss and intubate patients prophylactically rather than wait for deterioration. Remain vigilant and communicate clearly with your anesthesiology and/or emergency room staff to ensure the patient is intubated safely and appropriately.
- Be prepared to perform emergent cricothyroidotomy if orotracheal intubation cannot be achieved.

Preoperative Planning

- Injuries to vascular structures within the thoracic inlet (Zone I) usually require sternotomy or thoracotomy to provide adequate exposure.
- Injuries to zone III are rarely amenable to direct surgical exploration and usually require endovascular techniques.
- Injuries to zone II can be exposed directly through a neck incision.

Table 1: Hard and Soft Signs of Vascular Injury to the Neck

Hard signs	Soft signs
Active bleeding	Neurologic deficit
Expanding or pulsatile hematoma	Nonpulsatile hematoma or venous oozing
Thrill/bruit	History of significant bleeding

- Communicate the planned procedure to the operating room staff, including surgical approach and any additional equipment that may be required.
- Consider requesting a bronchoscopy and/or endoscopy cart.
- Ask for blood products to be immediately available.

Positioning

- Patients should be placed supine with the neck rotated 45° away from the side of injury. Cervical spine injuries resulting from blunt trauma should be ruled out prior to neck rotation. If a cervical spine fracture is present, the neck should be immobilized in a midline position.
- A towel or padding underneath the shoulders may assist with improved exposure of the neck structures.
- Both arms should remain extended away from the body, to allow for access to the chest if needed, and the patient should be placed in a sitting position to bring the operative field closer.

Setup

- In general, the entire chest and neck should be prepped into the field to allow for sternotomy or thoracotomy if needed. If additional injuries have not been ruled out, a wide prep of chin to knees should be performed.
- If there is a documented zone II injury based on preoperative imaging, the entire neck from slightly above the angle of the mandible to the upper sternum should be prepped. If there is any concern for esophageal or tracheal injury, both sides should be prepped in the event an extension anteriorly needs to be performed or the contralateral side needs to be explored.
- The upper sternum, earlobe, and jaw should be draped into the field.

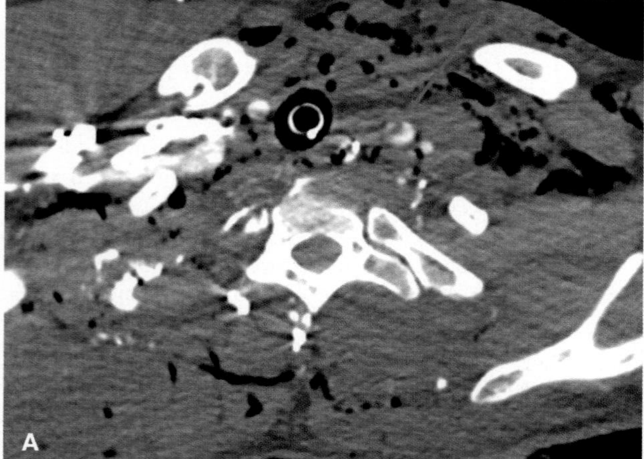

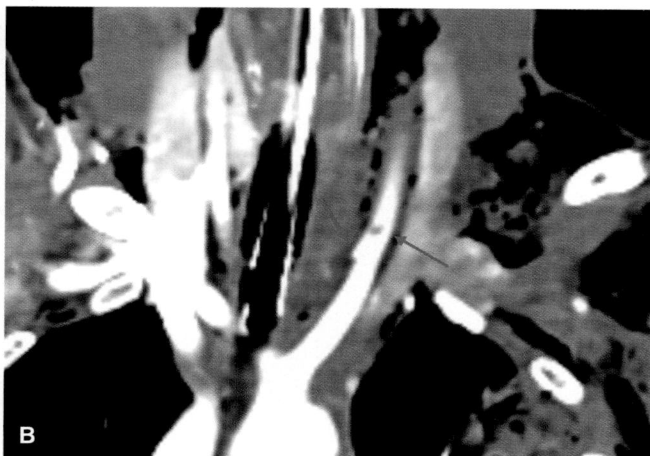

FIGURE 2 ● Computed tomography scan of the neck demonstrating injury to the common carotid artery. Gunshot wound to the left neck, resulting in injury to the common carotid artery at the thoracic inlet, as well as an injury to the upper left lobe of the lung and an esophageal injury. **A,** The vascular injury is demonstrated by an intimal flap on the axial view (*red arrow*). **B,** The coronal view demonstrates an associated pseudoaneurysm (*blue arrow*) and an intimal flap (*red arrow*).

INCISION

- Mark out the angle of the mandible to the sternal notch (**FIGURE 3**).
- The incision should be made anterior to the sternocleidomastoid muscle (SCM), extending from the angle of the mandible to the sternal notch. The incision should be generous, to allow for adequate exposure for both proximal and distal control of the carotids.

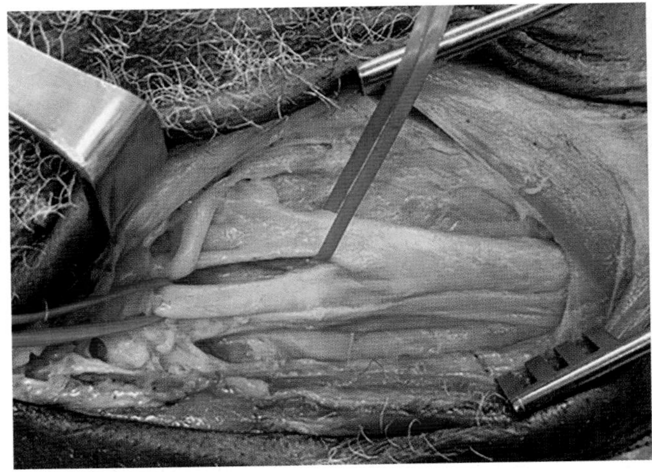

FIGURE 3 ● Incision for neck exploration. The incision should typically extend from the angle of the mandible to the sternal notch.

EXPOSURE OF THE NECK

- The dissection should proceed through the platysma muscle, below which the SCM is visible.
- Continue the dissection anterior to the SCM, taking care to protect the parotid gland which is located at the superior most border of the incision. The first structure to be identified is the internal jugular vein, located lateral and superficial to the carotid sheath (**FIGURE 4**). A small venous branch crossing medially from the internal jugular vein is the facial vein, which can be ligated and transected. This vein usually lies immediately anterior to the bifurcation of the carotid artery. This will expose the carotid sheath, a thin structure overlying the carotid artery.

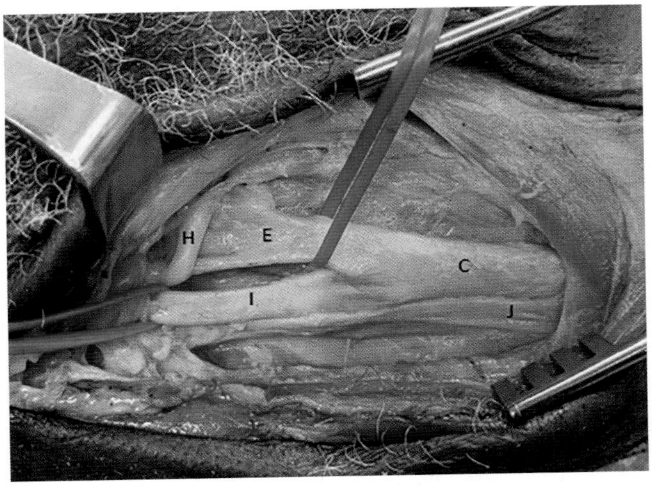

FIGURE 4 ● Exposure of the carotid artery. Shown in this figure is the common carotid as it branches into the internal and external carotid. Also shown are the internal jugular vein and the hypoglossal nerve.C, common carotid artery; E, external carotid artery; H, hypoglossal nerve; I, internal carotid artery; J, internal jugular vein.

- Continue dissection through the carotid sheath, exposing the common carotid artery (CCA) (**FIGURE 4**). Dissect the CCA circumferentially and encircle it with a vessel loop, attaining proximal control. If there is significant bleeding preventing adequate visualization, direct pressure can be applied over the area of maximum bleeding while proximal control of the CCA is achieved.
- Identify and protect the vagus nerve (**FIGURE 5**), which is located in the carotid sheath and runs along the CCA. As dissection is continued cranially, the bifurcation of the internal carotid artery (ICA) and the external carotid artery (ECA) will be identified, the latter of which courses medially and gives off the superior thyroidal artery as its first branch (**FIGURE 4**). Circumferentially dissect and encircle each branch with a vessel loop. Take care to identify and preserve the hypoglossal nerve, which crosses transversely over the internal and external carotid arteries (**FIGURE 4**).

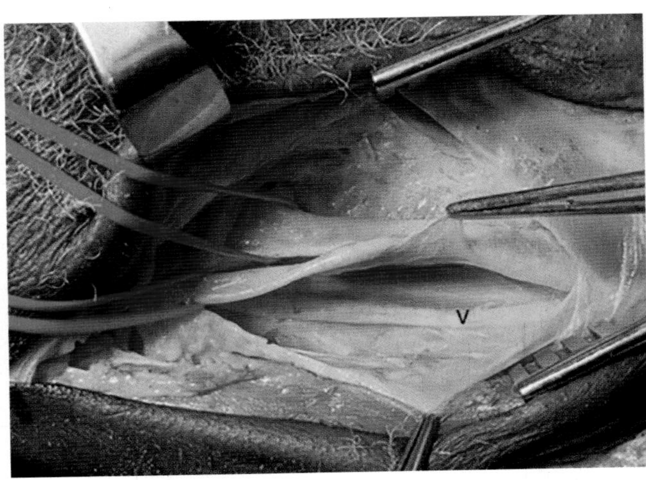

FIGURE 5 ● Vagus nerve.

MANAGEMENT OF THE VASCULAR INJURY

- The use of systemic unfractionated heparin is generally recommended for complex repairs if not prohibited by associated injuries.
- Management of the vascular injury is dictated by the extent of the injury and the physiologic status of the patient. If the patient is hypothermic, coagulopathy, and acidotic (pH < 7.2), then damage control surgery should be performed. In this case, the fastest method that can achieve hemorrhage control should be performed.
- A small laceration of the CCA can be repaired with either a continuous or interrupted 5-0 Prolene suture. Larger injuries may need to be controlled with a temporary shunt if expedient hemorrhage control is required in an unstable patient as part of damage control surgery (**FIGURE 6**). In stable patients with brisk back bleeding, routine shunting is generally not needed. Although any tubular structure can serve as a shunt, commonly used shunts for the carotid artery are Argyle, Javid, and Pruitt-Inahara shunts. Once the physiologic derangements have been corrected, the patient should be taken back to the operating room for definitive repair (**FIGURE 7**).
- A similar approach can be used for repair of the ICA. In rare cases where gaining control of the ICA distal to the injury cannot be achieved due to its anatomic location, subluxation of the mandible can be performed to gain better exposure. However, this maneuver will only expose an additional 1-2 cm of vessel. If distal control cannot be achieved, temporary insertion and inflation of a Fogarty balloon into the injury tract can control bleeding.
- If primary, tension-free repair of either the ICA or CCA injury cannot be achieved, a saphenous vein or bovine pericardial patch can be applied to bridge the defect. If the artery must be replaced due to extensive tissue loss, a 6-mm polytetrafluoroethylene (Gore-Tex) graft or saphenous vein can be used as a conduit depending on vessel size. In these cases, an end-to-end interposition of the conduit should be performed.
- Simple injuries to the ECA can be repaired primarily, but in cases of complex injuries the artery can be ligated without consequence. Prior to ligation, ensure that the vessel is the ECA by identifying the presence of branches, which the ICA does not have.

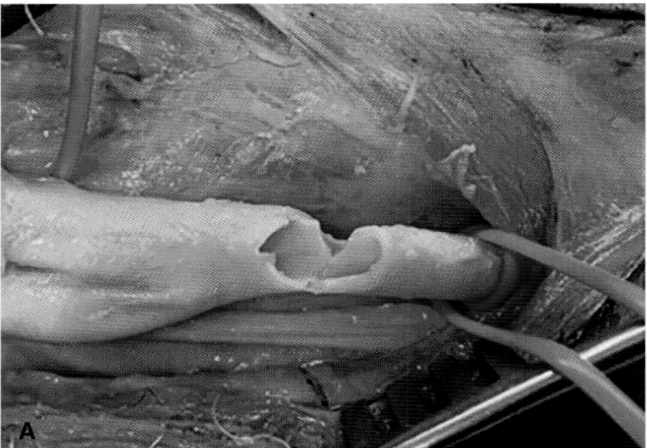

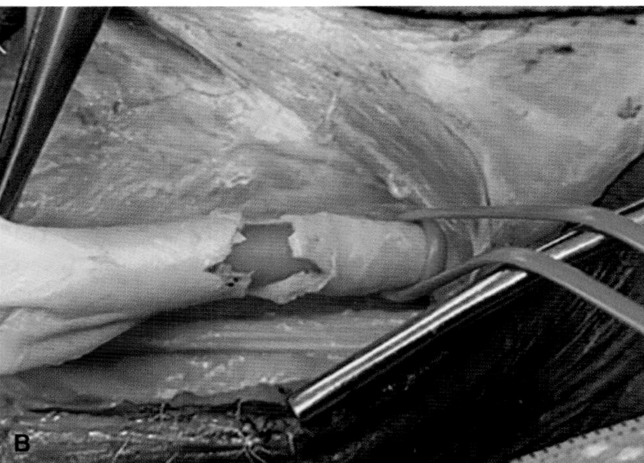

FIGURE 6 ● Injury to common carotid artery. The left image **(A)** shows a large injury to the common carotid artery. The right image **(B)** shows temporary control with a shunt.

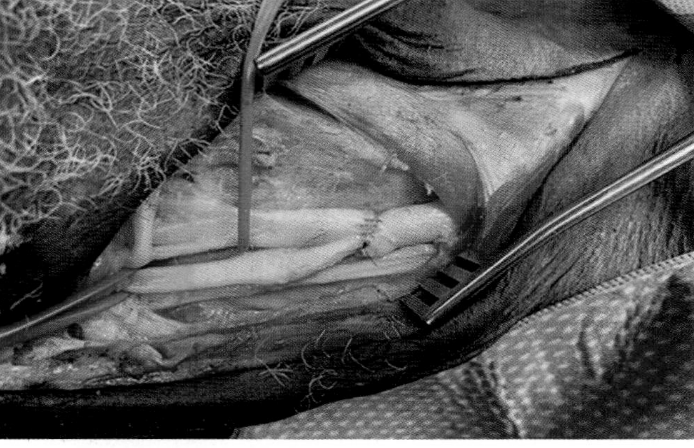

FIGURE 7 ● Definitive repair of an injury to the common carotid artery.

PEARLS AND PITFALLS

- Patients with zone II injuries and hard signs of vascular injury (pulsatile bleeding, expanding hematoma) should proceed directly to the operating room.
- Principles of proximal and distal control pertain to the carotid arteries.
- Obtaining proximal and distal control prior to opening a hematoma is the preferred approach.
- When in doubt, the chest and bilateral neck areas should be included in the operative field. Prep out the contralateral neck if there is concern for aerodigestive tract injury that might require bilateral neck exploration.

POSTOPERATIVE CARE

- Patients should be closely monitored for the first 24 hours after surgery, preferably in an intensive care unit. Cross-clamping of the carotid artery places the patient at risk for cerebral ischemia.
- Once the patient is awake, a full neurologic assessment should be performed and documented.

COMPLICATIONS

- **Nerve injury:** Injuries to the vagus nerve may cause vocal cord dysfunction but will likely not impede breathing unless bilateral injury occurs. Patients with hoarseness postoperatively should be monitored closely for airway compromise and intubated early if there are any concerns.
- **Bleeding:** Patients should be monitored closely for evidence of ongoing bleeding, including hematoma development, shunt dislodgement, or missed injuries. As the patient is rewarmed and the acidosis corrected, vessels that were previously under vasospasm may relax and start bleeding. If this occurs, the patient should be taken back to the operating room expediently.
- **Stroke:** This is uncommon in most patients with penetrating injury to the carotid arteries but can occur in patients who have atherosclerotic carotid disease resulting in plaque dislodgement, or those who have little to no contralateral cerebral flow from the circle of Willis causing abrupt cessation of flow when the carotid artery is clamped. Stroke rate is higher in ICA injuries compared to CCA injuries.[5] In order to reduce the risk of stroke, minimize manipulation of the carotid artery and duration of clamp time.

REFERENCES

1. Roon AJ, Christensen N. Evaluation and treatment of penetrating cervical injuries. *J Trauma*. 1979;19(6):391-397.
2. Low GM, Inaba K, Chouliaras K, et al. The use of the anatomic "zones" of the neck in the assessment of penetrating neck injury. *Am Surg*. 2014;80(10):970-974.
3. Inaba K, Munera F, McKenney M, et al. Prospective evaluation of screening multislice helical computed tomographic angiography in the initial evaluation of penetrating neck injuries. *J Trauma Inj Infect Crit Care*. 2006;61(1):144-149.
4. Ibraheem K, Wong S, Smith A, et al. Computed tomography angiography in the "no-zone" approach era for penetrating neck trauma: a systematic review. *J Trauma Acute Care Surg*. 2020;89(6):1233-1238.
5. Ramadan F, Rutledge R, Oller D, Howell P, Baker C, Keagy B. Carotid artery trauma: a review of contemporary trauma center experiences. *J Vasc Surg*. 1995;21(1):46-55; discussion 55-56.

Chapter 21

Vascular Injury—Neck: Internal Jugular Vein

Jennifer E. Reid and Deborah M. Stein

DEFINITION

- Traumatic injury to the internal jugular vein (IJV) is most commonly the result of penetrating trauma to the neck and rarely the result of blunt injury.

DIFFERENTIAL DIAGNOSIS

- When a patient presents with a projectile or stab wound injury to the neck, rapid evaluation of the patient's hemodynamic and neurovascular status and knowledge of the complex anatomy of the neck is important to determine the next steps in management.
- Zone I injuries are located between the clavicle and the cricoid cartilage. Important structures contained within this zone include the thoracic outlet vessels, the proximal common carotid arteries, IJVs, vertebral vessels, subclavian vessels, and the trachea.[1]
- Zone II injuries lie between the cricoid cartilage and the angle of the mandible. This zone includes the internal and external carotid arteries, jugular veins, trachea, esophagus, and the recurrent laryngeal nerves.[1]
- Zone III injuries are located between the angle of the mandible and base of the skull and contain the distal portions of the extracranial internal carotid and vertebral arteries, the most superior portions of the jugular veins, and cranial nerves[1] (**FIGURE 1**).
- As you can imagine, the next steps in management will be different for a zone I injury with concern for damage to the thoracic outlet vessels vs an anterior zone II injury with concern for tracheal injury, for example. Also, one should be particularly aware, if an injury crosses midline an aerodigestive injury becomes more likely. Therefore, physical examination becomes extremely important in neck injuries.

PATIENT HISTORY AND PHYSICAL FINDINGS

- In a patient presenting with a traumatic injury to the neck, physical examination is extremely important, as delay in management can result in not only hemorrhagic shock but also rapid airway compromise or neurologic deficits.
- As with any patient presenting with traumatic injuries, these patients should first be assessed using the standard "airway, breathing, circulation" method to determine hemodynamic stability and establish the next steps required for intervention.
- Airway management is of utmost importance in patients with neck injury.
- "Hard signs" of vascular injury within the neck, meaning those that are highly suggestive of vascular injury, include active hemorrhage, pulsatile or expanding hematoma, hematemesis/hemoptysis, audible bruit, palpable thrill, or neurologic deficits.[2]
- However, with isolated jugular venous injuries, the vessel usually tamponades or occludes without any hard signs ever being present since it is a low-pressure venous system.[2] Therefore, most isolated injuries can go unrecognized and can progress without any clinical significance.
- However, given the close proximity to other structures within the neck, damage to which usually warrants surgical intervention, IJV injuries are usually diagnosed during exploration for an arterial injury that presents with hard signs of vascular injury or aerodigestive injury.

IMAGING AND OTHER DIAGNOSTIC STUDIES

- Traditionally, management of penetrating injuries to the neck would have been dictated based on zone. However, these practices have evolved to include selective use of imaging,

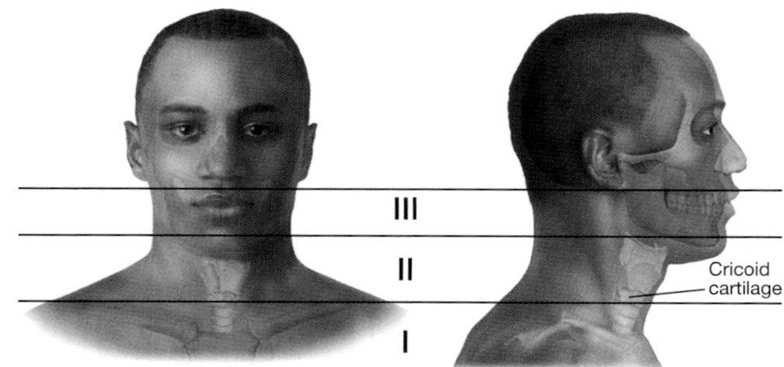

FIGURE 1 ● Entry zones for penetrating injury to the neck.

observation, and endoscopy in patients without hard signs of vascular injury dictating emergent surgical exploration for injuries to all three zones.[3]

- Duplex ultrasonography can be performed rapidly at the bedside and is very useful in settings where computed tomographic imaging is not readily available. When color flow duplex and spectral waveform analysis are combined, ultrasound can provide critical information. However, use and interpretation of ultrasound images require sufficient training, and hematoma or soft tissue or bony injuries may obscure vascular injuries; therefore, its use may be limited in the acute setting for penetrating injury to the neck.[4]
- Computed tomographic angiography should be used routinely in patients without any other clear indications for surgical exploration including hard signs of cerebrovascular injury or signs of injury to the aerodigestive tract including stridor or clinically apparent air leak. This use of imaging has resulted in more frequent identification of isolated internal jugular injury, which would have likely otherwise gone undiagnosed.[3]

SURGICAL MANAGEMENT

Selective Nonoperative Management

- In patients with isolated IJV injury diagnosed on imaging, who are hemodynamically stable, nonoperative management is considered safe.[3] Neck exploration is necessary if nonoperative management fails or when other cervical injuries are suspected based on physical examination or diagnostic imaging.

Preoperative Planning

- The patient should undergo the necessary active resuscitation dictated by their clinical status while the operating room is being prepared.
- If available, the surgeon may consider performing the exploration in an operating room that has angiographic capabilities as to have the option for endovascular exploration should the trajectory of injury travel into zone III of the neck and become surgically inaccessible.

Positioning

- Prepare and position the patient in standard fashion with the patient prepped and draped sterilely from chin to knees. In the presence of isolated neck injury, it may be preferable to keep the arms tucked at the patient's sides. Although the injury is to the neck, the surgeon must be prepared if the saphenous vein is required for arterial reconstruction of an arterial injury (discussed elsewhere in this text) discovered during exploration. In addition, the surgeon must be prepared if the trajectory of the projectile dives down into the chest requiring sternotomy.
- The patient's head should be turned away from the side of the injury.

SETUP

- In general, the surgeon should be prepared with the necessary equipment to explore all three zones of the neck, as projectile trajectory is often unpredictable, even if preoperative imaging was obtained.
- Therefore, operative setup for a neck exploration should include vascular instruments, as well as a sternal saw, should proximal control of the great vessels become necessary.
- Bronchoscopy and endoscopy equipment should also be available should there be concern for an occult airway or esophageal injury that cannot be visualized during operative exploration.

INCISION

- Exploration for a presumed IJV injury should begin with an incision at the anterior border of the sternocleidomastoid muscle.
- This anterolateral neck incision can be extended down to the sternal notch or up to the ear if necessary for improved exposure[1] (**FIGURE 2**).
- The incision is carried through the subcutaneous tissue, and the platysma is divided to expose the underlying vessels.

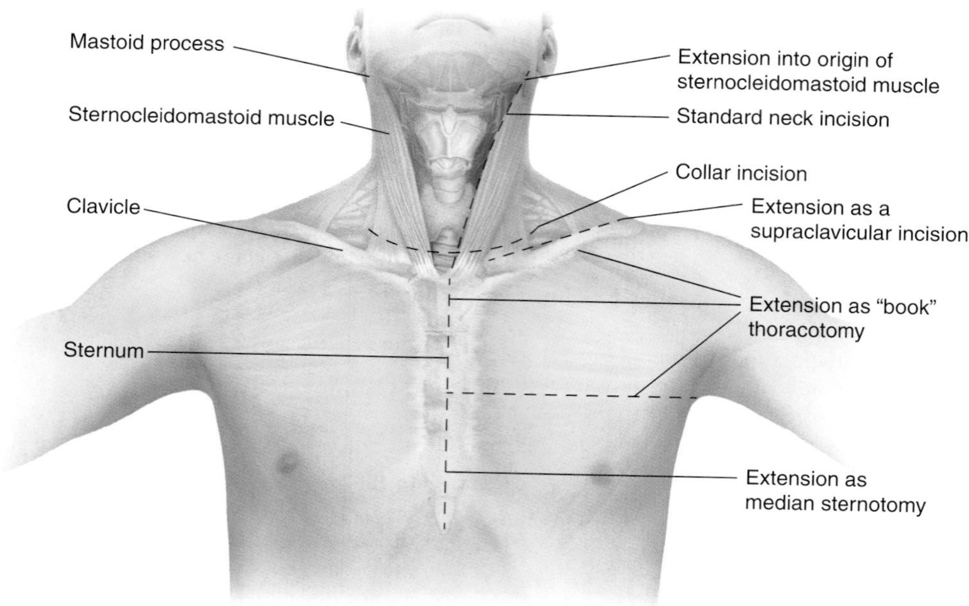

FIGURE 2 ● Incisions for exposure of penetrating neck injuries. (Reprinted with permission from Fischer J. *Fischer's Mastery of Surgery*. 7th ed. Wolters Kluwer; 2019. Figure 35.5.)

EXPLORATION

- After making incision and dividing the platysma, there is usually a significant hematoma that distorts the anatomy, especially if there is concomitant carotid or vertebral artery injury.
- Evacuate the hematoma to gain adequate visualization of the trajectory of the injury and to identify structures that lie within the tract.
- Dissect along the plane between the IJV and the carotid to gain full visualization of the area. Use vessel loops if needed for gentle retraction of the vessels.
- Identify the trachea and the esophagus and explore for injury. Further discussion regarding injury to the aerodigestive tract is discussed elsewhere (**FIGURE 3**).
- Once an IJV injury is identified the next steps are determined based on the extent of the injury and the clinical status of the patient.

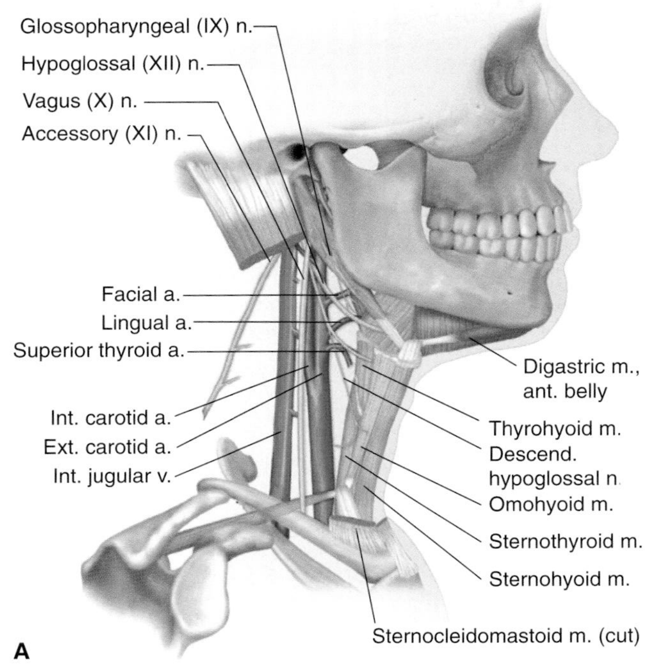

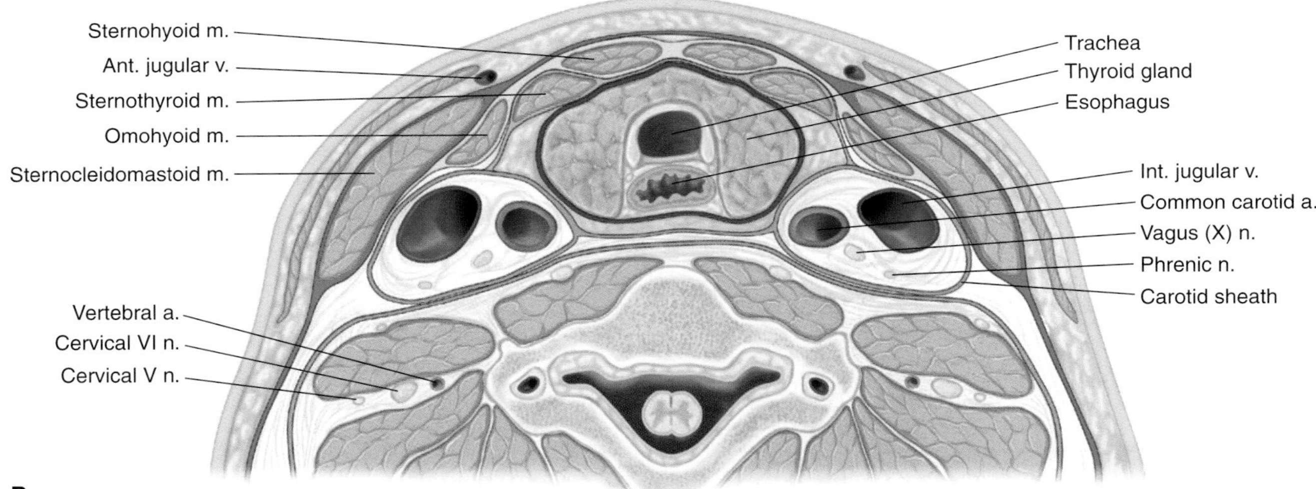

FIGURE 3 • **A,** Anatomy of the neck demonstrating the important structures in the neck exploration. **B,** The cross section shows the carotid sheath and its contents and the anatomy of the trachea and esophagus. (Reprinted with permission from Britt LD, Peitzman AB, Barie PS, et al. *Acute Care Surgery*. 2nd ed. Wolters Kluwer; 2019. Figure 11.2.)

LIGATION

- Ligation of a unilateral IJV is acceptable if repair is difficult or would result in significant stenosis, or if the patient is hemodynamically unstable, or if there are concomitant life-threatening injuries that need to be addressed (**FIGURE 4**).
- Ligation can be performed simply by using a nonabsorbable tie or suture ligation technique.

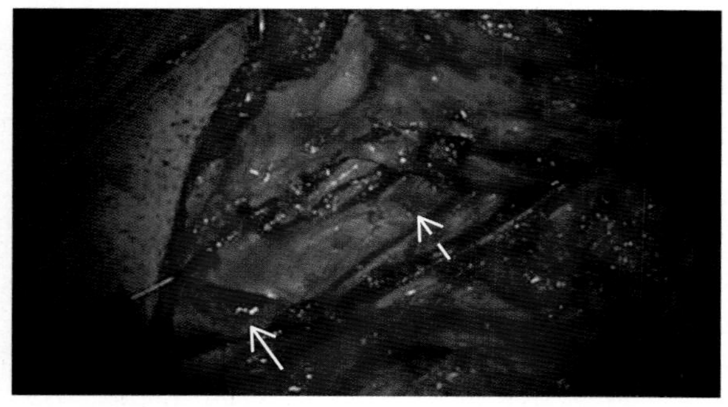

FIGURE 4 ● Neck dissection—the carotid artery and the ligated IJV (*arrows*). (Reprinted with permission from Roland, JT Jr. *Master Techniques in Otolaryngology – Head and Neck Surgery*. Wolters Kluwer; 2019. Figure 27.5.)

REPAIR

- At least one IJV should be repaired when there are bilateral injuries to the veins. This is due to a concern that bilateral ligation can result in cerebral venous congestion, which is associated with high mortality.[4]
- Primary repair with lateral venorrhaphy for lateral wall defects to the IJV can be performed using nonabsorbable, monofilament suture in a running fashion with care to not narrow the vessel.
- Vein patches can also be used to repair large defects. The saphenous vein is a good choice for patch repair.

COMPLETION OF THE PROCEDURE

- The procedure is completed once all of the injuries have been addressed and hemostasis has been achieved.
- A muscle flap, most commonly the strap muscles, should be mobilized and placed between the artery and vein in cases of concomitant vein and artery repair as to prevent arteriovenous fistula formation.
- The platysma can be reapproximated and the incision can be closed in layers.
- The placement of a drain can be done at the discretion of the surgeon.

PEARLS AND PITFALLS

Ligation	■ The IJV can typically be ligated without consequence.
Repair	■ Repair of the IJV is associated with a high rate of thrombosis, which leaves the patient at risk of pulmonary emboli.
Nonoperative management	■ When proceeding with nonoperative management, missed aerodigestive injury is a concern, and therefore, endoscopic/bronchoscopic evaluation or exploration may be considered.
High IJV injury	■ Bleeding from the IJV at the base of the skull is best managed by direct pressure.
Concomitant carotid injury	■ The IJV can be used as a patch for arterial reconstruction.

POSTOPERATIVE CARE

- Postoperative care is guided by severity of other injuries and the stability of the patient.
- Most patients with penetrating neck trauma will likely require care in a monitored setting.
- These patients may need to stay intubated to monitor for swelling or hematoma development depending on the extent of injury and other related cervical structure injuries. For example, if a patient had a repair of a destructive airway injury, they may need to stay intubated to allow for healing of the repair.

COMPLICATIONS

- Air embolism
- Vagus nerve or other cranial nerve injury
- Arteriovenous fistula
- Stenosis leading to cerebral venous congestion

REFERENCES

1. Le Roux D, Veller M, Grant I. Carotid, jugular and vertebral blood vessel injuries. In: Velmahos GC, Degiannis E, Doll D, eds. *Penetrating Trauma*. Springer; 2017:257-264. doi:10.1007/978-3-662-49859-0_33
2. Rowe VL, Petrone P, García-Núñez LM, Asensio JA. Carotid, vertebral artery, and jugular venous injuries. In: Petrone P, García-Núñez LM, Asensio JA eds. *Current Therapy of Trauma and Surgical Critical Care*. Mosby; 2008:203-206.
3. Inaba K, Munera F, McKenney MG, et al. The nonoperative management of penetrating internal jugular vein injury. *J Vasc Surg*. 2006;43(1):77-80.
4. Teixeira PGR, DuBose J. Surgical management of vascular trauma. *Surg Clin N Am*. 2017;97:1133-1155.

SECTION VI: Traumatic Injury to the Gastrointestinal Tract

Chapter 22 Trauma Laparotomy

S. Ariane Christie and Andrew B. Peitzman

DEFINITION

- Trauma laparotomy encompasses a vast array of general surgery techniques, the details of which are covered comprehensively in other sections this book. This chapter will provide a framework for thinking through trauma laparotomy in the context of the overall treatment and resuscitation of the critically ill and often multiply injured patient. In particular, we will emphasize perioperative planning, intraoperative decision making, and taking a systematic, step-up approach to the repair of specific intra-abdominal injuries while balancing the patient's overall physiology and injury burden.

DIFFERENTIAL DIAGNOSIS

- Patients may require abdominal exploration for penetrating, blunt, blast, or combined trauma mechanisms. Common indications for trauma laparotomy include peritonitis, hemodynamic instability with positive Focused Assessment with Sonography for Trauma (FAST), positive diagnostic peritoneal aspirate (DPA), or computed tomography (CT) findings of free abdominal fluid without solid organ injury, penetrating injury extending through the fascia, or thoracoabdominal penetrating injury with trajectory concerning for diaphragmatic injury (laparoscopy is an option in these circumstances). The essential decision is whether the trauma patient requires laparotomy and not identification of specific organ injuries (**FIGURES 1** and **2**). Delay to hemorrhage control will result in avoidable morbidity and mortality.

PATIENT HISTORY AND PHYSICAL FINDINGS

- Regardless of injury mechanism or severity, trauma resuscitation follows the Advanced Trauma Life Support guidelines beginning with the primary survey and treatment of immediately life-threating conditions. Vascular access ideally consists of two large-bore intravenous (IV) catheters. Supradiaphragmatic IV access is preferred for abdominal

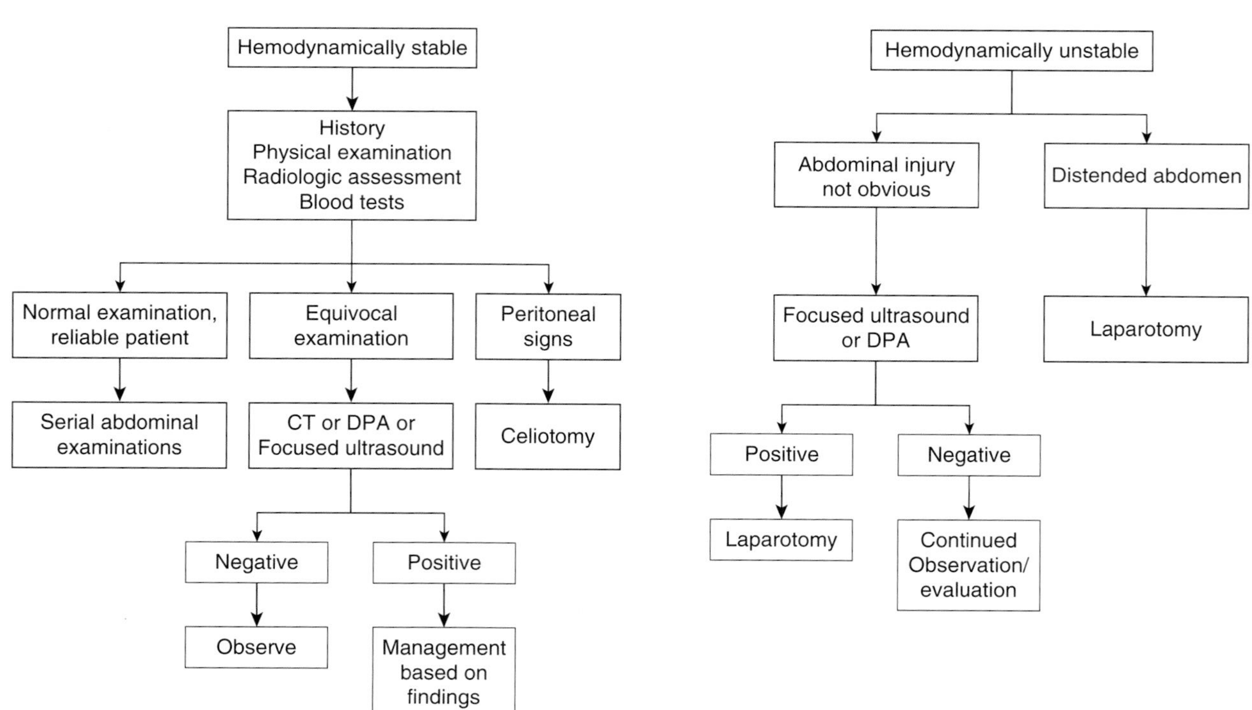

FIGURE 1 ● Algorithm for management of blunt abdominal trauma. (From Peitzman AB, Yealy DM, Fabian TC, et al. *The Trauma Manual*. 5th ed. Wolters Kluwer; 2020:426. Figure 37.1.)

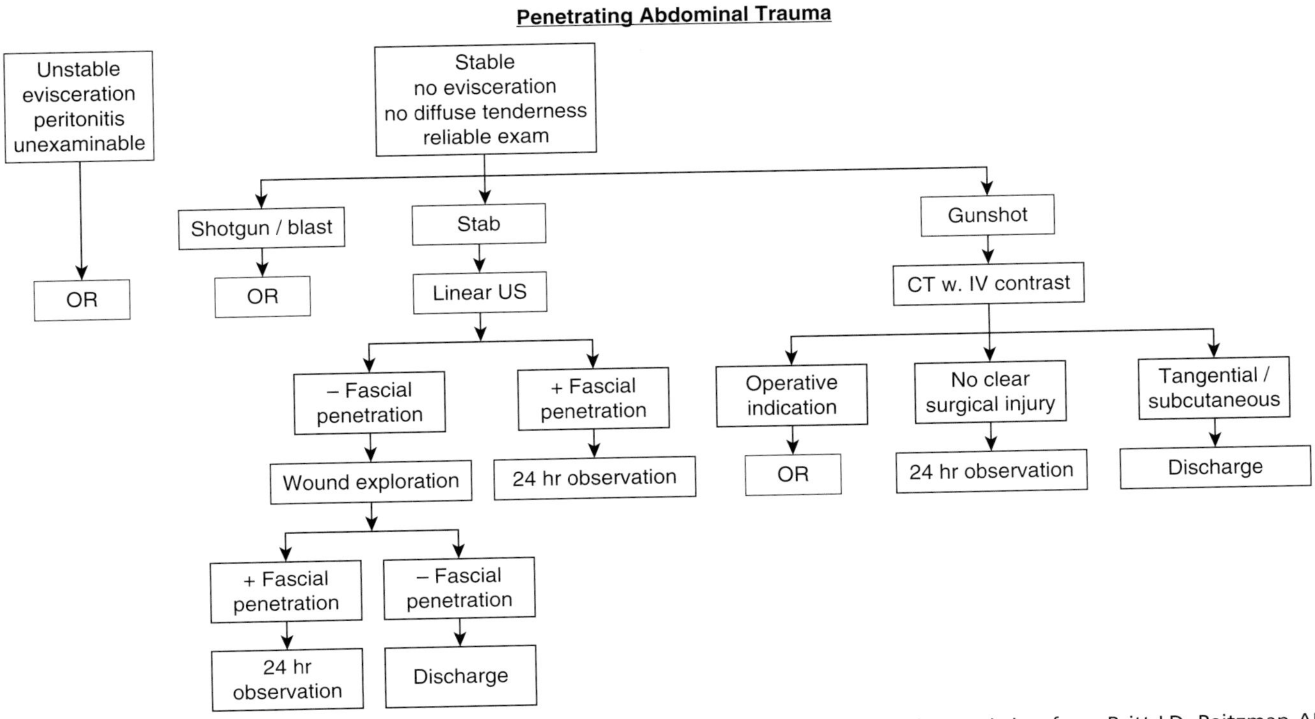

Penetrating Abdominal Trauma

Unstable
evisceration
peritonitis
unexaminable
→ OR

Stable
no evisceration
no diffuse tenderness
reliable exam

Shotgun / blast → OR

Stab → Linear US
- – Fascial penetration → Wound exploration
  - + Fascial penetration → 24 hr observation
  - – Fascial penetration → Discharge
- + Fascial penetration → 24 hr observation

Gunshot → CT w. IV contrast
- Operative indication → OR
- No clear surgical injury → 24 hr observation
- Tangential / subcutaneous → Discharge

FIGURE 2 ● Algorithm for management of penetrating abdominal trauma. (Reprinted with permission from Britt LD, Peitzman AB, Barie PS, et al. *Acute Care Surgery*. 2nd ed. Wolters Kluwer; 2019:450. Algorithm 36.1.)

injury. With uncertain penetrating trajectory, obtain IV access above and below the diaphragm. Address hypotension rapidly with transfusion of whole blood[1,2] or a balanced 1:1:1 resuscitation strategy.[3,4] Additional resuscitation is guided by functional coagulation assays such as thromboelastography. The CRASH-2 trial was a randomized international clinical trial supporting early administration of tranexamic acid to patients at elevated risk of hemorrhagic shock. Notably, outcomes are best when tranexamic acid is administered within the first 3 hours of injury, ideally within the first hour.[5,6]

IMAGING AND OTHER DIAGNOSTIC STUDIES

- FAST is routinely performed in the trauma bay as part of the initial assessment and resuscitation of injured patients. Positive findings of fluid in the right upper quadrant, left upper quadrant, or pelvic windows are presumed to be blood until proven otherwise.
- If the patient is hemodynamically stable, obtaining cross-sectional imaging using multidetector CT provides valuable information regarding burden and severity of injury to guide operative strategy. However, unstable patients with clear operative indications should transfer to the operating room (OR) promptly and not be delayed to obtain cross-sectional imaging.[7]
- Patients with polytrauma and physiologic derangement require damage control planning and staged repair. Obtain consultation with neurosurgical, orthopedic, interventional radiology, and other services early.
- Most adjunctive tests and procedures beyond those performed in the ABCDE assessment are also better performed once the patient has been taken to the operating theater.

SURGICAL MANAGEMENT

Preoperative Planning

- The general operative strategy outlined here specifically addresses exploratory laparotomy for trauma. However, the following approach is equally applicable to any "crash" abdominal operation or emergency surgery. Acting in accordance with a few key principles greatly aids efficiency to gain and maintain control of complex injuries while minimizing collateral and iatrogenic injury. Plan for what you expect. Equally, anticipate and prepare for the unexpected.
- Conduct of the lead surgeon[8]
  - The comportment of the lead surgeon sets the tempo for the operating team and facilitates optimal communication and performance.
  - The lead surgeon should
    - Maintain situational awareness; quickly assess the OR when entering by obtaining a concise report from the other team members.
    - Control the room; maintain composure, communicate calmly. The commanding voice need not be the loudest. Request necessary actions or equipment in sequence, rather than issuing multiple requests at once. Be explicit to whom each request is made.
    - Encourage and reassure the team members; reserve constructive criticism for after the operation.
    - Perform deliberate, progressive maneuvers, without wasted movement or time.
    - Control bleeding rapidly, reconstruct deliberately. Control bleeding digitally; do not clamp or suture haphazardly. Repair correctly on the first attempt.

GENERAL OPERATIVE APPROACH

- The trauma laparotomy is systematic (**FIGURE 3**). The primary goals are to control hemorrhage and gastrointestinal contamination. Only after these goals are achieved should one begin a systematic search for all injuries.
- Recognize early when a patient requires damage control approach: either preoperatively or early in the laparotomy. Convey that decision to the entire OR team.[9,10]
- **Utilize a "step-up" approach**: Patients may have many intra-abdominal injuries. Begin with the most life-threatening; stabilize using the least invasive strategy. For bleeding, apply well-directed pressure. Packing may be effective damage control management of solid organ or pelvic bleeding. Although definitive repairs are tempting, hasty moves result in iatrogenic injury or "burning bridges" before the full extent of the problem is recognized. If conservative strategies fail to temporize the problem, proceed with stepwise escalation. Minor injuries should not distract from getting the patient off the operating table.[11,12]
- **Maintain a list of injuries**: Keep track of the patient's overall trauma burden to guide operative decisions. Definitive repair of an isolated bowel perforation is appropriate in a stable healthy patient but is poorly tolerated in an elderly patient with multiple injuries. Keep a mental (or physical) list of suspected and confirmed injuries and refer to this throughout the operation and resuscitation.[13]
- **Physiological embarrassment supersedes surgical repair.** Critically injured patients can withstand only a limited time for operative repair. Two hours has been suggested as a time benchmark, but physiologic embarrassment may occur sooner in patients with multiple injuries or shock, or in older or chronically ill patients. Do not truncate the operation until *surgical bleeding* is controlled. Temporize quickly and transfer the patient to the intensive care unit (ICU) to avoid the "deadly terrible triad" of acidosis, hypothermia, and coagulopathy. Keep track of operative time, physiologic metrics (blood transfused, temperature, pH, and thromboelastography), and clinical indicators of physiology such as "oozing" from the operative field (*medical bleeding*).[14]
- **Communication is essential**: Resuscitation and surgery require the coordinated interaction of a care team including the emergency room physicians and staff, anesthesia team, scrub and circulating nursing staff, blood bank, and surgeons and operative team. Without constant, ongoing communication, the patient will not have a successful outcome. Use a directed, closed-loop communication strategy with all members of the team empowered to share information and raise concerns.
  - Setting and instrumentation: The surgeon leads the resuscitative, nursing, and anesthesia teams in preparing the patient for a successful operation. Consider the operative setting and potential intraoperative adjuncts.
    - Where major vascular injury is expected, use a room with hybrid capabilities for digital subtraction angiography to expand options for bleeding control.
    - Call for endoscopy and bronchoscopy or proctoscopy equipment early.
    - Laparoscopy equipment is uncommonly indicated in trauma, and never when the patient is hemodynamically unstable.
  - A standard major basic set will suffice for most trauma laparotomies, with a major vascular set kept on hand. Also, have equipment available for median sternotomy or thoracotomy.
  - The set should include essential equipment only; keep instruments to the minimum required. If the likelihood of major vascular injury is high, the circulating staff should prepare heparin flushes, Fogarty balloons, and shunts of various sizes. A headlight and surgical loupes improve visualization and forestall delays. Consider monopolar and bipolar thermocoagulating instruments including Bovie electrocautery, LigaSure, Argon beam, and Aquamantys. Separate patient circuits and priming may be necessary to allow concomitant use. A list of standard equipment and recommended adjuncts for surgical laparotomy is given in **TABLE 1**.

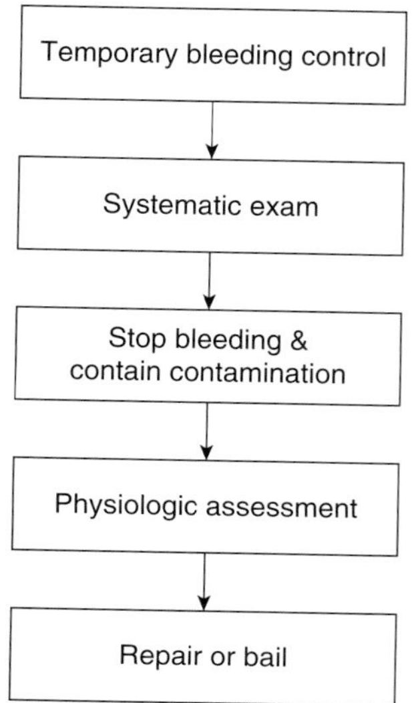

FIGURE 3 ● Systematic approach to abdominal exploration for trauma.

Table 1: Instrumentation for Trauma Laparotomy

Standard	Major basic set
Adjuncts	Major vascular set
	Self-retaining retractors: Balfour Thompson Bookwalter Omni
	Headlight Surgical loupes
	Proctoscope Vaginal speculae Endoscope Bronchoscope
	Thermocautery devices *(consider separate energy source)* LigaSure Aquamantys Argon beam

- Prepare to cross between body cavities during the operation, as injuries are often not fully delineated preoperatively (**FIGURE 4**). Drape from chin to knees and table to table laterally to allow extensile exposures and maximize reconstruction opportunities. A towel covering the genitals exposes the bilateral groins for potential REBOA (Resuscitative Endovascular Balloon Occlusion of the Aorta) access and the medial thighs for potential saphenous harvest. The patient's arms should be well padded and secured on arm boards abducted just under 90° to prevent neuropraxia. If there is a high suspicion of rectal or perineal injury, position the patient in lithotomy on an operating table with a removable or retractable footplate.

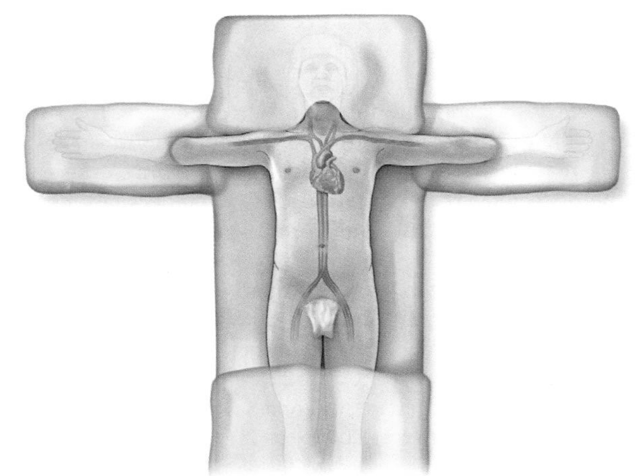

FIGURE 4 ● Extensile exposures in trauma.

TRAUMA EXPLORATORY LAPAROTOMY: STEPS

Open the Abdomen

- Particularly in instances of severe injury and hemodynamic instability, induction should be postponed until the operating team is ready to make incision. We routinely prep and drape the patient prior to inducing anesthesia. Be ready with a #10 blade and two working suctions. The back table should have ready buckets for removal of clot, large handheld retractors, and a minimum of 20 to 30 laparotomy pads, rolled or unrolled according to the surgeon's preference.
- Make a midline incision with one pass of the knife from just below the xiphoid inferiorly to the lower abdomen and with a smooth transition around the umbilicus. A second pass of the knife should expose the linea alba, and a third the preperitoneal fat. In the unstable patient, do not be distracted by cauterizing subcutaneous and skin bleeding. In patients with intra-abdominal bleeding the peritoneum will often be dark and tented. This finding should be clearly communicated with the anesthesia team, as tamponade release may lead to hemodynamic instability and potential cardiac arrest. If possible, a large amount of uncross-matched blood product should be in the room and a rapid infusion system should be prepared before proceeding.
- The preperitoneal fat and peritoneum can be grasped with a forceps and opened with a Mayo scissors. The surgeon's nondominant hand should protect the intestine and other viscera, taking care to avoid injury to the liver, bowel, or bladder. The peritoneum should be opened completely for the length of the incision, regardless of the patient's physiologic response to tamponade release.

Stop Exsanguinating Hemorrhage

- As the surgeon is opening the abdomen, the assistant should help with counter-tension and begin evacuating clot. Once the peritoneum is fully opened, clot should be scooped into a bucket for removal from the field and liquid blood should be suctioned.
- The initial exploration should begin with the most compelling bleeding. The assistant should retract the sidewall, allowing the surgeon to tamponade any bleeding by packing laparotomy pads using a "hand-over-hand" approach. Once accomplished, the next quadrant should be addressed, proceeding in either a clockwise or counterclockwise fashion until all quadrants are packed and exsanguinating bleeding is controlled. Take care not to overpack and impair venous return. Special consideration should be taken in the right upper quadrant, where the surgeon may need to manually reconstitute the liver. With severe hepatic injury, compress the hemilobes of the liver together with your hands, then push the liver posteriorly to slow retrohepatic bleeding. If successful, then pack above and below the liver, restoring normal anatomy. Do not pack within the hepatic injury as this may exacerbate parenchymal bleeding. In the left upper quadrant, packing should similarly extend posterolaterally to the spleen. Take care to avoid iatrogenic injury to the liver, spleen, and other organs from forceful retraction or packing.
- If systematic packing fails to control the hemorrhage, a useful next step is to gently eviscerate the small bowel and reattempt packing. Effective packing will significantly attenuate bleeding from liver, spleen, mesentery, and retroperitoneal hematomas from blunt injury but will not stop hemorrhage from vascular lacerations. If specific bleeding vessels are visualized, targeted manual compression can control bleeding while preparations are made for vascular isolation, ligation, or repair. If major venous bleeding is identified within the abdomen, instruct the anesthesia team to stop any infusion through femoral or lower extremity intraosseous IV access.
- If the patient arrests or audible arterial bleeding is encountered, transition from packing to obtaining inflow control with supraceliac aortic compression. To accomplish this, the assistant should gently retract the left lobe of the liver to facilitate entry through the gastrohepatic ligament.

Bluntly enter the bare area of the gastrohepatic ligament and retract the esophagus laterally, revealing the anterior surface of the aorta, which should be firmly compressed against the spine with fingers or a sponge-stick. This should rapidly decrease arterial bleeding and allow the anesthesia team to resuscitate. If desired, the crural muscles can be dissected off the anterior aorta to allow placement of a vascular clamp. In an emergent setting where an aortic cross-clamp must be applied, a combination of blunt and sharp dissection can be used to define the periaortic space for clamp placement. Once established, confirm that the clamp is completely across the aorta by manually feeling that the posterior extent of the clamp continues at least to the posterior borders of the aorta. Finally, mark the start time of the aortic cross-clamp, as it is essential to unclamp within a 45-minute period to prevent irreversible visceral ischemia and metabolic acidosis.

- Increasingly, REBOA is utilized to gain rapid control of exsanguinating hemorrhage. Many centers routinely place REBOA in the resuscitation bay, particularly when the cause of bleeding is suspected to be a pelvic fracture. Our approach is (1) to prioritize prompt transfer of the hypotensive patient to the OR, (2) to routinely obtain femoral arterial access in all hypotensive patients either in the resuscitation bay or in the OR, and (3) to selectively utilize REBOA in the setting of a major pelvic fracture or zone I hematoma with a suspected vascular injury.

Perform a Systematic Examination of the Abdomen

- Once temporary hemorrhage control has been achieved, the next step in the trauma laparotomy is to perform a systematic survey to control other points of bleeding and identify and control sources of gross contamination.
- Exposure
  - Anatomic exposure can be optimized while the anesthesia team catches up on resuscitation efforts. Depending on the injury, it may be useful to extend the abdominal incision either cephalad to the xiphoid or caudally toward the symphysis pubis. Further exposure can be gained by excising the xiphoid process with a Mayo scissors or electrocautery.
  - To free up hands, place a self-retaining retractor. Retractor selection depends on both injury and surgeon comfort. The Bookwalter retractor is a good general abdominal retraction device, whereas the Thompson and Omni retractor systems are well suited for upper abdominal and liver injuries.
- Systematic examination of the abdomen
  - Begin removing abdominal packing starting from the least injured area and work toward the sites of the most severe injury. If removal results in hemorrhage, replace the packs until control is regained. Often, leaving packing in place is the most appropriate hemostatic option in an initial damage control laparotomy.
  - The abdominal cavity can be considered as two compartments separated by the transverse colon.
    - The supramesocolic compartment contains the stomach, spleen, liver, and gallbladder and is explored by gently retracting the transverse colon caudally.
    - The inframesocolic compartment contains the small bowel, colon and rectum, bladder, uterus, and pelvis and can be explored by gently retracting the transverse colon cephalad.
    - Careful visual inspection of all surfaces of the solid and hollow viscera and mesentery are required for adequate exploration. A two-person, hand-to-hand technique should be used to carefully inspect the small bowel and colon. In general, any structures that are found to have bruising or hematomas or those located close to a missile trajectory should be fully mobilized and carefully examined for injury.
    - Notable sites of missed intra-abdominal hollow viscus injury include the esophagogastric junction, the ligament of Treitz, the small bowel along the mesenteric border, the posterior stomach, the transverse colon, and the extraperitoneal rectum. Pancreatic or posterior diaphragmatic injury is also commonly missed. Missing injuries in these areas leads to considerable morbidity and may contribute to higher rates of mortality.
- Retroperitoneal exploration (**FIGURE 5**): In addition to the supramesocolic and inframesocolic intraperitoneal compartments, examine all three retroperitoneal compartments.
  - Zone I—The central/medial zone. All hematomas and injuries require surgical exploration regardless of mechanism. To evaluate, open the lesser sac by widely incising the gastrocolic ligament to ensure

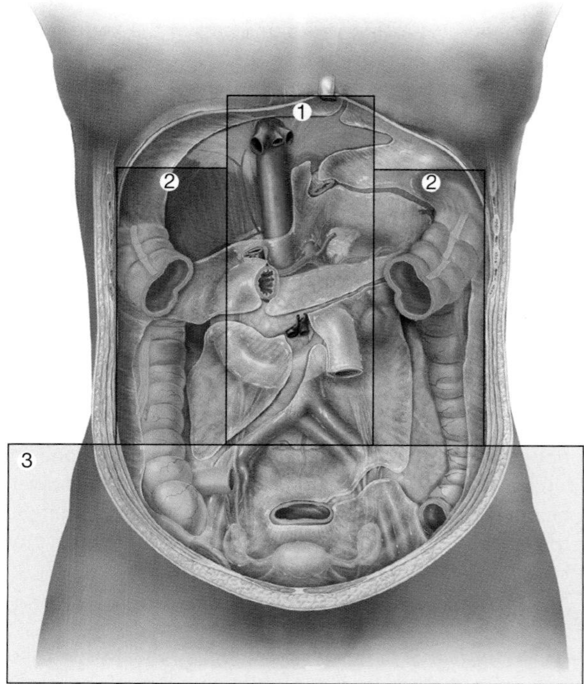

FIGURE 5 • Zones of the retroperitoneum. (From Peitzman AB, Yealy DM, Fabian TC, et al. *The Trauma Manual*. 5th ed. Wolters Kluwer; 2020:426. Figure 38.1.)

that there is no hematoma overlying or underlying the pancreas. Suspected injury to the pancreas should be evaluated by visual inspection and mobilization for bimanual palpation (see Part 7, Chapter 27).

- Zone II—The lateral retroperitoneal zone. Zone II injuries are managed differently based on mechanism. All penetrating injuries to zone II with hematomas should be surgically explored. Blunt injuries with *expanding* hematomas should be surgically explored, while those with stable hematomas can generally be observed.
- Zone III—The pelvic retroperitoneal zone. Management of pelvic retroperitoneal injuries also takes into account mechanism. Penetrating injuries should be explored. Blunt injuries are often amenable to endovascular intervention for angiographic management of bleeding, ideally in a hybrid OR.

- Surgical access to the retroperitoneum—In general, exposure of the retroperitoneum involves rotating overlying structures medially (**FIGURE 6**). The following specific approaches can be used to evaluate retroperitoneal structures:
- Left-to-right medial visceral rotation
  - This approach will expose zone I injuries to the suprarenal aorta and its visceral branches (eg, celiac artery, superior mesenteric artery, left renal artery) and can be extended to access the inframesocolic aorta and the aortic bifurcation with the left common iliac artery.
  - Begin by gently retracting the left colon toward the right to incise the white line of Toldt. Colonic mobilization is extended to the splenic flexure and continued lateral to the spleen. The dorsum of the surgeon's hand rests along the posterior abdominal musculature behind the spleen, left kidney, and pancreatic tail and provides anterior tension. Divide the avascular plane behind these organs, progressively rotating these structures medially to the diaphragmatic hiatus. Often, the hematoma in this region will have already performed much of the dissection maneuver. Alternatively, the left kidney may be left on the retroperitoneal musculature with the dissection plane proceeding anteriorly.
  - Potential pitfalls include iatrogenic splenic injury or avulsion of lumbar veins.
- Right-to-left visceral medial rotation
  - This approach will expose zone I injuries to right-sided structures, including the intrahepatic inferior vena cava (IVC), the right kidney, the right renal hilum, and the right common iliac artery and can be extended to the bilateral iliac structures.
  - There are three steps to this exposure.
    - Step 1: Kocherization of the duodenum and the hepatobiliary structures. Mobilize the right colon and hepatic flexure off the duodenum. Incise the peritoneum just lateral to the C-loop of the duodenum and begin to retract the duodenum and pancreatic head medially. Using a combination of blunt and sharp dissection free the avascular plane behind the common bile duct and the superior mesenteric vein (SMV) to reveal the IVC to the left renal vein. Avoid avulsion to the right gonadal vein as it dives into the IVC at this level.

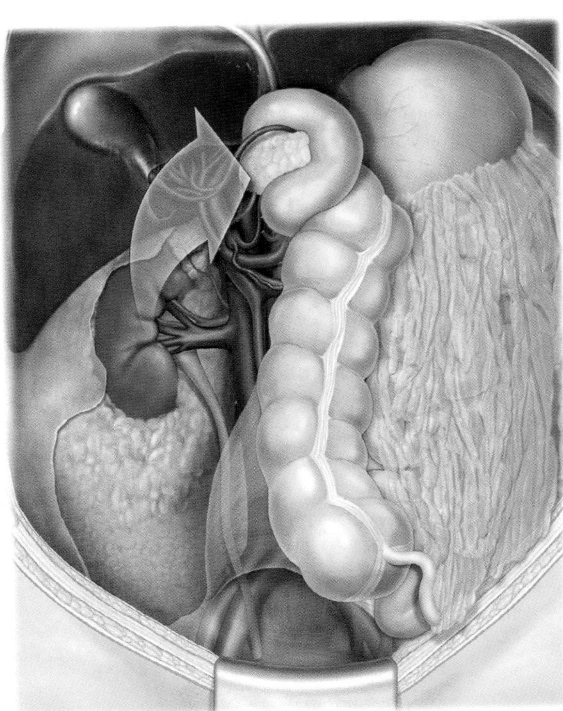

A. Right to left medial visceral rotation

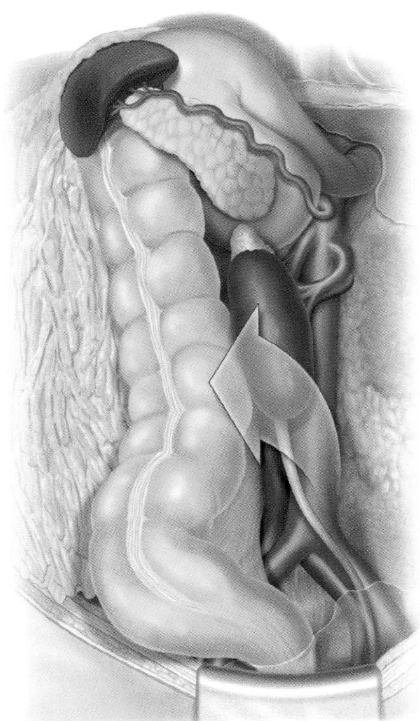

B. Left to right medial visceral rotation

FIGURE 6 ● **A,** Right and **(B)** left medial visceral rotation.

- Step 2: Right colonic mobilization. Continue mobilizing proximally from the hepatic flexure by incising the white line of Toldt and medializing the right colon.
- Step 3: Superior-medial extension. Extend mobilization of the avascular plane behind the cecum and the distal ileum. Retract the small bowel toward the liver and incise the peritoneum along the small bowel mesentery from medial to the cecum to the ligament of Treitz. This will allow the small bowel, mesentery, and right colon to be retracted superiorly, revealing the widest exposure of the retroperitoneal vascular structures available. This exposure will gain access to the inframesocolic retroperitoneum and direct visualization of the infrarenal aorta, IVC, bilateral renal arteries and veins, bilateral common iliac arteries, third and fourth portions of the duodenum, and SMV.

- Potential pitfalls include injury to the right gonadal vein during kocherization and injury to the SMV at the root of the mesentery with undue traction or avulsion of the right colon vein off the SMV.
- Surgical treatment of pelvic hematoma: Temporize hemodynamically significant pelvic hematomas from blunt trauma with preperitoneal packing of the pelvic space (see Part 7, Chapter 33).
    - Access the preperitoneum through the inferiormost aspect of a mid-line laparotomy or, ideally, through a separate incision above the symphysis pubis.
    - Dissect between the rectus and the peritoneum; avoid entering the peritoneal space. Bluntly dissect the avascular plane behind the rectus posterolaterally until the peritoneum is pushed medially and your knuckles are resting on the inside of the pelvis. Pack this space "hand over hand" until adequate compression is attained (often three per side).
- Repairs of specific abdominal injuries including the spleen, liver, duodenum, pancreas, biliary tree, and urinary tract as well as detailed management of retroperitoneal injuries are addressed directly in other sections of this text.

Approach to Stopping Surgical Bleeding

- As discussed previously, begin with the least invasive method possible to achieve hemostasis. At a minimum, direct manual pressure or packing is often required to prevent hemorrhage during additional dissection to facilitate safe definitive treatment. However, in many cases of small vessel, venous, or organ parenchymal bleeding, continued compression will apply sufficient tissue apposition and coagulation to stop bleeding.
- Initial manual control is often achieved with a hand or finger but can be exchanged for a less space-occupying and lower-profile instrument, such as a sponge-stick or a dissecting peanut.
- Clamping can cause injury if not performed judiciously. Clamping "blindly" may result in iatrogenic injury to the vessel or other adjacent structures. Only apply a clamp if the transected end of the vessel is entirely visible or the clamp can be passed cleanly around the vessel. Clamp application damages the endothelium; close clamps only to the setting necessary to stop bleeding.
- Although a basic surgical concept, suturing *well* on an actively bleeding vessel requires consideration and skill. Envision the axis along which the bleeding vessel runs. Place the initial needle pass on one side of the bleeding point, cross beneath the bleeding point without avulsion exiting the tissue several millimeters past the other side of the bleeding point. Gently hold up the suture to visualize the direction of ongoing bleeding relative to your suture. Place the next throw deep to this in the opposite direction, ideally creating a figure eight around the bleeding. Success is determined by pulling gently up upon the suture and surveying the results. Even if some bleeding persists, it is usually diminished, and another throw can be planned, again systematically in the direction toward the bleeding opposite the last throw.
- The importance of adequate exposure by the assistant during suturing cannot be overstated. Retraction should be maintained at all costs, and successful exposure may entail brief periods of allowing a vessel to bleed with well-targeted suctioning near, but without obstructing, the bleeding point. The suction itself is often best used as a combined suction device and retractor.
- Needle selection is also important. Take into consideration the suspected depth and location of the bleeding. Use a large, tapered needle such as a CT or SH needle. In a deep hole with a narrow aperture such as the pelvis, use a hemicircular needle such as an SH or CT-3 to allow smooth collection of the suture. With very deep bleeding and a narrow aperture consider using a UR-6 or tailor the needle carefully using two needle drivers.
- *Vascular ligation*
    - In general, any vein distal to the renal vessels can be ligated if necessary. Still, it is useful to know the general risk involved in ligation (**TABLE 2**). Sacrificing the common and external iliac veins portends a high risk of venous insufficiency. In these cases, consider four-compartment fasciotomy on the ipsilateral limb. Portal vein ligation can lead to massive intestinal edema and warrants a scheduled second-look laparotomy to examine intestinal viability.
    - Ligation can be performed in several ways. Clamping both ends of a vessel and tying around each with an appropriately sized silk tie remains the gold standard. Electric bipolar cautery devices such as the LigaSure can provide secure hemostasis of vessels up to 7 mm

Table 2: Ligation of Abdominal Vascular Structures

May ligate	Attempt repair if possible	Repair
Celiac artery	Common iliac artery	Aorta
Hypogastric artery	External iliac artery	Suprarenal IVC
Any vein below renal veins	Infrarenal IVC	Superior mesenteric artery
Inferior mesentery artery	Common iliac vein	Superior mesenteric vein
Inferior mesenteric vein	External iliac vein	
	Portal vein	
	Proper hepatic artery	

in diameter. Notably, the LigaSure device does not function where staples or other metal clips have been deployed and may melt monofilament suture. Suture ligate or oversew arterial and high-pressure venous vessels. Finally, vascular staplers can control large and small vascular pedicles and can be maneuvered into difficult-to-access areas. Although beyond the scope of this chapter, vascular staplers facilitate good hemostasis with minimal dissection in hepatic resections (Part 7, Chapter 34).

- Named arteries and proximal veins should be repaired in the stable patient if possible. Begin by obtaining proximal and distal control with a combination of pressure, clamps, or obstructive balloons. Debride the vessel to healthy endothelium proximally and distally. Although systemic heparin is often not needed, a Fogarty catheter should always be passed proximally and distally until one clean Fogarty pass is performed without extracting clot. Dilute local heparin can also be infused.
- Depending on patient stability, proceed with shunting or definitive repair techniques.[15]
  - **Shunting**: Shunt vessels in unstable patients to maintain distal flow or when significant orthopedic reconstitution may change the geometric layout of the anastomosis. We typically use an Argyle shunt; however, any appropriately sized sterile plastic tubing can be passed from the proximal to distal ends and secured in place with a tie or a plastic band. In general, systemic heparinization is not necessary with arterial repairs as brisk flow remains the best anticoagulant. Shunting preserves perfusion and allows delayed repair when the patient has been stabilized.[16,17]
  - **Primary Repair**: Reserve primary repair for injuries where the vessel can be adequately mobilized to allow tension-free repair after debridement. Select a monofilament suture of appropriate size (for example, a 4-0 Prolene for aorta or IVC). Close partial defects transversely to avoid narrowing. Large venous repairs (such as the IVC) are tolerant of some narrowing, but attempt to maintain greater than 50% of the original lumen size. For smaller venous repairs, use an interrupted suture technique or a running technique leaving a slight air knot to allow for venous re-expansion. If it is not possible to perform a primary repair without tension or without significantly narrowing the lumen of the vessel, another approach should be considered.
  - **Patching**: Patch if a portion of the vessel wall remains uninjured but primary closure would result in significant narrowing of the vessel. Options for patch material include synthetic materials (such as Dacron), bovine pericardial patches, or portions of autologous vein cut to size. Patching decreases the risk of vessel narrowing but is more time consuming than primary repair.
  - **Interposition grafting**: Interposition grafting remains the gold standard for transected vessels where primary repair would lead to tension on the anastomosis. Options for conduit include synthetic materials such as PTFE and Dacron. However, synthetic materials should not be used where there is contamination from either enteric spillage or from the injury itself. In these instances, autologous vein is the conduit of choice. Options include the greater and lesser saphenous veins, the arm veins, the external jugular vein, and the internal iliac (or hypogastric) vein. Harvesting and repair can be time consuming. Shunt in the unstable or multiply injured patient. Where more conduit length is necessary, creating spiral vein grafts remains an option but this is beyond the scope of this chapter.

Contain Contamination

- The secondary objective of the trauma laparotomy is containment of gross contamination. Injured segments of hollow viscera should be identified and isolated.[18,19] Soft bowel clamps such as Doyen or intestinal clamps can be employed for temporary control and defects closed with a whip or baseball stitch. A GIA blue or purple load stapler can be used to contain spillage; black load staplers are similarly useful on the proximal stomach or other thick tissue. In patients who are stable, proceed with formal repair or resection and anastomosis. Unstable patients should be left in discontinuity and moved to the ICU for resuscitation.[20,21] Irrigation with warm sterile fluid should be performed to clear gross contamination. Neither copious irrigation nor antibiotic-impregnated fluid has been demonstrated to reduce surgical site infection rates.[22]

Physiologic Assessment and Planning

- Once bleeding has been controlled and contamination contained, make a physiologic assessment of the patient considering the overall burden of injury, time already spent on the operating table, blood products infused, and other needed procedures and operations.
- Physiologic criteria for damage control laparotomy in trauma include pH < 7.2, temperature <35 °C, and coagulopathy.[23] In many cases, the safest thing to do is to place a temporary abdominal closure and bring the patient to the ICU for the next steps in their care. Currently, there are many proprietary and bespoke methods to establish temporary abdominal closure.
  - Cut small perforations in a sterile, plastic, fluid impermeable drape to allow fluid egress, and place around the abdominal viscera. Place an overlying sponge or series of towels in the wound on top of the plastic drape. Place flat 19-Fr Jackson-Pratt drains over this layer and secure to the abdomen with Ioban drape or another adhesive fluid-impermeable dressing. Apply gentle wall or vacuum-monitored suction.[24,25]
  - The Abthera wound vac system is a proprietary system specifically designed to accommodate application to an open abdomen. To apply, a large premade plastic drape is tailored to the size of the abdominal cavity. Premade perforations in the drape allow passage of fluid while providing relative protection for the underlying bowel.

Definitive Closure

- Only leave the abdomen open when necessary. In stable patients with intra-abdominal injuries, primary fascial closure after all repairs have been completed is preferable at the index operation. Fascial closure should conform to general guidance regarding secure closure technique including 0.5-cm bites and distance from fascial edges, utilization of a 4:1 suture to wound length, and use of an absorbable synthetic suture. Large abdominal wall defects can be managed either in a single stage or multiple stages, depending on the patient's anatomy, associated comorbidities, and recovery of the surrounding injuries in a polytrauma patient.[26] With gross intraperitoneal contamination or profound hemorrhagic shock, the skin should not be closed.

PEARLS AND PITFALLS

Pearls	■ Position the patient to allow extensile exposure and consider use of a hybrid room. ■ Decide early if the laparotomy will demand a damage control approach. ■ Keep a mental injury list. ■ Use a step-up approach to hemorrhage control. ■ Get the patient off the operating table before physiologic embarrassment.
Pitfalls	■ Failure to communicate with the anesthesia and nursing teams. ■ Iatrogenic injuries from excessive force or retraction while opening and packing. ■ Failure to systematically examine the abdomen resulting in missed injuries. ■ Performing extensive repairs at the index operation in a critically ill patient.

POSTOPERATIVE CARE

- Wait 24 to 48 hours to return to the OR in critically ill patients, if possible. Wait to perform bowel anastomoses or ostomies until the patient no longer requires high-dose vasopressor support.
- Abdominal packing should be removed gently using copious warm fluid to minimize distraction of clot or iatrogenic injury to the viscera. If bleeding occurs, repack.
- Consider the need for future abdominal procedures prior to definitive closure; these may include feeding gastrostomy or jejunostomy creation, drain placement for pancreatic or duodenal injury, ileo- or colostomy creation to divert stool from perineal injuries, and on-table endoscopic retrograde cholangiopancreatography to access the biliary tree. A gastropexy for possible endoscopic gastrotomy at later time is also useful.

COMPLICATIONS

- The multiply injured and critically ill patient often receives massive fluid and blood product resuscitation leading to considerable fluid shifts and volume overload following injury. Furthermore, exposure to the environment with the open abdomen leads to intestinal swelling and third spacing, which may preclude early fascial closure. Premature closure can lead to abdominal compartment syndrome and relaparotomy. Monitor closely for signs and symptoms of compartment syndrome including oliguria, rising peak pressures, CO_2, difficulty ventilating, or new-onset respiratory failure. Measure bladder pressure as a vital sign. Critically, compartment syndrome can occur in patients with Abthera or other wound vacs or with skin-only closure. In all cases, the abdomen must be fully reopened to avoid morbidity.
- Options for interim closure of the abdomen include skin-only closure,[27,28] interposition of absorbable mesh or biologic mesh, and rarely closure by secondary intention. Generally, successful abdominal closure utilizes temporary closure, which combines a vacuum suction system and a method to maintain tension on the fascia (to avoid retraction). We plan repeated trips to the OR over the first week and progressive closure of the midline fascia to avoid the long-term risks of the open abdomen. In the patient on whom fascia cannot be closed, apply a split-thickness skin graft as soon as the tissue bed appears ready. Patients who survive their injuries may go on to have component separation and formal hernia repair months to years later.

REFERENCES

1. Murdock AD, Berséus O, Hervig T, Strandenes G, Lunde TH. Whole blood: the future of traumatic hemorrhagic shock resuscitation. *Shock*. 2014;41(suppl 1):62-69.
2. Strandenes G, BerséusO, Cap AP, et al. Low titer group O whole blood in emergency situations. *Shock*. 2014;41(suppl 1):70-75.
3. Holcomb JB, del Junco DJ, Fox EE, et al. The prospective, observational, multicenter, major trauma transfusion (PROMMTT) study: comparative effectiveness of a time-varying treatment with competing risks. *JAMA Surg*. 2013;148:127-136.
4. Holcomb JB, Tilley BC, Baraniuk S, et al. Transfusion of plasma, platelets, and red blood cells in a 1:1:1 vs a 1:1:2 ratio and mortality in patients with severe trauma: the PROPPR randomized clinical trial. *JAMA*. 2015;313:471-482.
5. CRASH-2 trial collaborators; Shakur H, Roberts I, Bautista R, et al. Effects of tranexamic acid on death, vascular occlusive events, and blood transfusion in trauma patients with significant haemorrhage (CRASH-2): a randomised, placebo-controlled trial. *Lancet*. 2010;376:23-32.
6. Li SR, Guyette F, Brown J, et al. Early prehospital tranexamic acid following injury is associated with a 30-day survival benefit: a secondary

analysis of a randomized clinical trial. *Ann Surg*. 2021;274(3):419-426. doi:10.1097/SLA.0000000000005002
7. Neal MD, Peitzman AB, Forsythe RM, et al. Over reliance on computed tomography imaging in patients with severe abdominal injury: is the delay worth the risk? *J Trauma*. 2011;70:278-284.
8. Moeng MS. *Visceral Trauma Surgery – Under Pressure—My Top 5 (Leadership) Tips to Regain Control in a Crisis*. 2021.
9. Stone HH, Strom PR, Mullins RJ. Management of the major coagulopathy with onset during laparotomy. *Ann Surg*. 1983;197:532-535.
10. Rotondo MF, Zonies DH. The damage control sequence and underlying logic. *Surg Clin*. 1997;77:761-777.
11. Sugrue M, D'Amours SK, Joshipura M. Damage control surgery and the abdomen. *Injury*. 2004;35:642-648.
12. Roberts DJ, Bobrovitz N, Zygun DA, et al. Indications for use of damage control surgery in civilian trauma patients: a content analysis and expert appropriateness rating study. *Ann Surg*. 2016;263:1018-1027.
13. Shapiro MB, Jenkins DH, Schwab CW, Rotondo MF. Damage control: collective review. *J Trauma*. 2000;49:969-978.
14. Moore EE, Burch JM, Franciose RJ, Offner PJ, Biffl WL Staged physiologic restoration and damage control surgery. *World J Surg*. 1998;22:1184-1190. discussion 1190-1191.
15. Davis TP, Feliciano DV, Rozycki GS, et al. Results with abdominal vascular trauma in the modern era. *Am Surg*. 2001;67:565-570. discussion 570-571.
16. Reilly PM, Rotondo MF, Carpenter JP, Sherr SA, Schwab CW. Temporary vascular continuity during damage control: intraluminal shunting for proximal superior mesenteric artery injury. *J Trauma*. 1995;39:757-760.
17. Ball CG, Feliciano DV. Damage control techniques for common and external iliac artery injuries: have temporary intravascular shunts replaced the need for ligation? *J Trauma*. 2010;68:1117-1120.
18. Behrman SW, Bertken KA, Stefanacci HA, Parks SN Breakdown of intestinal repair after laparotomy for trauma: incidence, risk factors, and strategies for prevention. *J Trauma*. 1998;45:227-231. discusion 231-233.
19. Torba M, Gjata A, Buci S, et al. The influence of the risk factor on the abdominal complications in colon injury management. *G Chir*. 2015;36:57-62.
20. Ott MM, Norris PR, Diaz JJ, et al. Colon anastomosis after damage control laparotomy: recommendations from 174 trauma colectomies. *J Trauma*. 2011;70:595-602.
21. Ordoñez CA, Pino LF, Badiel M, et al. Safety of performing a delayed anastomosis during damage control laparotomy in patients with destructive colon injuries. *J Trauma*. 2011;71:1512-1517. discussion 1517-1518.
22. Georgoff P, Perales P, Laguna B, et al. Colonic injuries and the damage control abdomen: does management strategy matter? *J Surg Res*. 2013;181:293-299.
23. Asensio JA, McDuffie L, Petrone P, et al. Reliable variables in the exsanguinated patient which indicate damage control and predict outcome. *Am J Surg*. 2001;182:743-751.
24. Barker DE, Green JM, Maxwell RA, et al. Experience with vacuum-pack temporary abdominal wound closure in 258 trauma and general and vascular surgical patients. *J Am Coll Surg*. 2007;204:784-792. discussion 792-793.
25. Brock WB, Barker DE, Burns RP. Temporary closure of open abdominal wounds: the vacuum pack. *Am Surg*. 1995;61:30-35.
26. Jernigan TW, Fabian TC, Croce MA, et al. Staged management of giant abdominal wall defects: acute and long-term results. *Ann Surg*. 2003;238:349-355. discussion 355-357.
27. Acker A, Leonard J, Seamon MJ, et al. Leaving contaminated trauma laparotomy wounds open reduces wound infections but does not add value. *J Surg Res*. 2018;232:450-455.
28. Seamon MJ, Smith BP, Capano-Wehrle L, et al. Skin closure after trauma laparotomy in high-risk patients: opening opportunities for improvement. *J Trauma Acute Care Surg*. 2013;74:433-439. discussion 439-440.

Chapter 23 Gastric and Small Bowel Injury: Primary Repair, Resection, Anastomosis, Wedge Resection

Alex Helkin and Carrie Sims

DEFINITION

- Gastric and small bowel injuries can be defined as direct damage to the organ resulting in contusion, hematoma, laceration, or completed transection requiring repair or reconstruction. Indirect injury may also occur to the mesentery or other vasculature, resulting in devascularized segments at risk for ischemia.

DIFFERENTIAL DIAGNOSIS

- Generating a differential diagnosis for trauma patients is focused on determining the most likely injuries based on the presenting mechanism.
- Abdominal stab wounds most commonly injure the liver, with small bowel being the second most likely organ to be injured. Estimates of incidence range from 30% to 80%, whereas in abdominal gunshot wounds, small bowel is the most likely organ to be injured.[1,2]
- Blunt hollow viscus injuries (HVIs) are rare compared to solid organ injuries, occurring in an estimated 5%-15% of blunt traumas. Small bowel injuries account for approximately 90% of HVI. High energy impacts and deceleration injuries, such as motor vehicle and bicycle accidents, falls, crush injuries, assaults, and the concussive force of explosions are the leading mechanisms of blunt HVIs.[3,4] The mobility and relatively elasticity of the bowel provides some protection. As a result, small bowel perforation is rare and occurs in only 1%-3% of blunt trauma.
- Blunt trauma resulting in gastric perforation is also uncommon, due to the stomach's thick walls, distensible nature, and relatively protected location in the abdomen. True gastric perforation from blunt trauma is estimated to occur with an incidence ranging from 0.02% to 1.7%. Anterior perforations are the most common.[5,6]
- Shear forces will localize to tethered points along the bowel including the ligament of Treitz, small bowel mesentery, ileocecal valve, and adhesions secondary to prior surgery. A full stomach or inappropriately place lap belt can also contribute to blunt gastric and small bowel injuries.

PATIENT HISTORY AND PHYSICAL FINDINGS

- Indications for laparotomy in search of gastric and small bowel injuries remain the same as in other instances of penetrating trauma. Hemodynamic instability, obvious evisceration or impalement, or peritonitis necessitate emergent progression to the operating room for exploration. Exploration is also indicated in hemodynamically stable patients with penetrating wounds suspected to violate the peritoneal cavity due to the likelihood of intra-abdominal injury.
- Indications for exploration in blunt trauma also include peritonitis, evidence of free intra-abdominal air on imaging, and hemodynamic instability with positive focused assessments with sonography (FAST). Patients who are hemodynamically stable and those with equivocal physical examinations on presentation provide a greater diagnostic challenge.

IMAGING AND OTHER DIAGNOSTIC FINDINGS

- Abdominal radiographs obtained in the trauma bay to evaluate for pelvic fracture may show air under the diaphragm indicative of bowel perforation. However, these films are typically taken with the patient supine, and absence of free intraperitoneal air does not rule out gastrointestinal injury.
- FAST examination performed in the trauma bay may demonstrate free intraperitoneal fluid; however, it is not sensitive for bowel injury.
- Computed tomography (CT) is the diagnostic modality of choice in hemodynamically stable patients. Although evidence of blunt HVI may be subtle, CT findings including mesenteric fat stranding, bowel wall thickening (4-5 mm), or mesenteric hematomas are suggestive of a small bowel injury.[7]
- Peritoneal free fluid in the absence of solid organ injury is the most commonly reported CT finding associated with blunt bowel injury; however, it remains nonspecific. Even in a large multicenter investigation, only 9% of patients with free peritoneal fluid and no solid organ injury on CT had true small bowel injury.[8]
- Blunt HVI is still possible even with negative CT (ie, no abnormal findings). Early reports have indicated a missed injury rate as high as 13%; however, newer studies have showed improvement to about a 4% missed injury rate, largely secondary to improved CT scan quality over the past 2 decades.[9]
- Providers should have a higher index of suspicion of blunt HVI in cases of high energy blunt trauma mechanisms, such as motor vehicle collisions, but also in relation to concomitant injuries such as thoracic or lumbar spine fracture, seat belt signs, direct abdominal wall injury, or evidence of other high shear force injuries, such as aorta dissection.
- Hemodynamically stable patients with equivocal physical examinations found to have free intraperitoneal fluid on CT should be admitted for monitoring and serial abdominal examinations. Repeat imaging or diagnostic laparoscopy may also be considered.

SURGICAL MANAGEMENT

Preoperative Planning

- Early identification and control of hemorrhage is the initial priority during trauma laparotomy, followed by the control of gastrointestinal contamination, identification of all injuries, and finally reconstruction.
- Early placement of a nasogastric tube by anesthesia providers can aid exposure by decompressing intraluminal air, fluid

contents, and to identify intraluminal bleeding. However, oftentimes trauma patients will have full stomachs of solid content, making it difficult to decompress the stomach by nasogastric tube.

- Broad-spectrum preoperative antibiotics are recommended with guidance from local antibiograms and antibiotic stewardship protocols.
- The role of diagnostic laparoscopy remains controversial in the evaluation of abdominal trauma. While contraindicated in the setting of hemodynamic instability, laparoscopic exploration may be useful in hemodynamically stable patients to rule out penetrating abdominal injuries or to evaluate abdominal pain following blunt injury. Evaluation of the gastrointestinal tract in its entirety, solid organs, and the diaphragm can be performed adequately, and repairs performed based on comfort and skill of the surgeon.[10]

POSITIONING

- Standard supine trauma positioning with arms extended for use during resuscitation should be used. Preparation with betadine or chlorhexidine/alcohol from chin to knees is the standard preparation for trauma patients and can facilitate additional procedures such as sternotomy or thoracotomy, if needed.

EXPOSURE

- Due to the intrathoracic abdominal location of the stomach, midline laparotomy beginning in the subxyphoid area is ideal for exploration of gastric and small bowel injuries and facilitates a complete abdominal exploration. Self-retaining retractors are crucial to maintain exposure, allowing for the examination of the entire stomach from gastroesophageal junction to pylorus.
- Caudal retraction of the transverse colon will aid in examining the anterior surface of the stomach, with care taken to avoid traction injuries to the greater curvature and underlying gastroepiploic arteries and arterial branches to the greater omentum.
- Division of the gastrohepatic ligament may be necessary to provide exposure to the lesser curvature and gastroesophageal junction. The vagus nerve or smaller braches, as well as an anomalous left hepatic artery may traverse this area and could be injured in the exposure.
- Additional exposure of proximal stomach injuries may be obtained by encircling the intra-abdominal esophagus with a Penrose drain to provide caudal traction.
- Exposure of the posterior stomach is an essential step in evaluating gastric injury, especially in penetrating injury mechanisms where through-and-through injuries are more likely to occur. We also recommend examination of the posterior stomach during exploration for blunt HVIs.
- The posterior stomach can be accessed by opening the avascular portion of the gastrocolic ligament, with care taken to avoid injury to the gastroepiploic vessels. The transverse colon is retracted caudally and the posterior gastropancreatic attachments carefully dissected to allow visualization as cranially as the lesser curvature.
- Accessing the posterior stomach in patients with a shortened transverse colon mesentery or a thick greater omentum may be facilitated by a lateral approach higher on the greater curvature by first ligating the short gastric vessels with an energy device.
- The small bowel examination, commonly called "running the bowel," should be performed from the duodenojejunal origin, at the ligament of Treitz, to the cecum. The ligament of Treitz can be located by lifting the transverse colon and tracing its mesentery posteriorly. A hand placed in the abdomen will palpate the left lateral border of the spine and moving anteriorly will locate the duodenojejunal junction coursing inferiorly, fixed at the ligament of Treitz. The bowel should be meticulously examined for injury on all surfaces including the associated mesentery.

INJURY GRADING

- Once gastric or small bowel injuries are identified, we recommend review of the American Association for the Surgery of Trauma (AAST) grading systems, to identify severity of injury and recommendations for reconstruction (**TABLES 1** and **2**).[11]

Table 1: AAST Stomach Injury Scale

Stomach injury scale

Grade[a]	Description of injury	ICD-9	AIS-90
I	Contusion/hematoma	863.0/0.1	2
	Partial thickness laceration	863.0/0.1	2
II	Laceration <2 cm in GE junction or pylorus	863.0/0.1	3
	<5 cm in proximal 1/3 stomach	863.0/0.1	3
	<10 cm in distal 2/3 stomach	863.0/0.1	3
III	Laceration >2 cm in GE junction or pylorus	863.0/0.1	3
	>5 cm in proximal 1/3 stomach	863.0/0.1	3
	>10 cm in distal 2/3 stomach	863.0/0.1	3
IV	Tissue loss or devascularization <2/3 stomach	863.0/0.1	4
V	Tissue loss or devascularization >2/3 stomach	863.0/0.1	4

[a]*Advance one grade for multiple lesions up to grade III. GE, gastroesophageal.*
Reprinted with permission from Moore EE, Jurkovich GJ, Knudson MM, et al. Organ injury scaling. VI: Extrahepatic biliary, esophagus, stomach, vulva, vagina, uterus (nonpregnant), uterus (pregnant), fallopian tube, and ovary. J Trauma. 1995;39(6):1069-1070. Table 3.

TECHNIQUES

Table 2: AAST Small Bowel Injury Scale

Small bowel injury scale				
Grade[a]	**Type of injury**	**Description of injury**	**ICD-9**	**AIS-90**
I	Hematoma	Contusion or hematoma without devascularization	863.20	2
	Laceration	Partial thickness, no perforation	863.20	2
II	Laceration	Laceration <50% of circumference	863.30	3
III	Laceration	laceration ≥50% of circumference without transection	863.30	3
IV	Laceration	Transection of the small bowel	863.30	4
V	Laceration	Transection of the small bowel with segmental tissue loss	863.30	4
	Vascular	Devascularized segment	863.30	4

[a]*Advance one grade for multiple injuries up to grade III.*

Reprinted with permission from Moore EE, Cogbill TH, Malangoni MA, et al. Organ injury scaling, II: Pancreas, duodenum, small bowel, colon, and rectum. J Trauma. 1990; 30(11):1427-1429. Table 3.

GASTRIC INJURY

Primary Gastric Repair

- The stomach is a thick-walled, highly vascular organ, and as such, even long lacerations (>10 cm) can be primarily repaired without need for resection. In the setting of partial thickness injuries, hematomas should be opened to assess mucosal injury and repaired. We recommend two-layer closure with full-thickness 2-0 polyglactin 910 suture and a second 3-0 silk layer in the Lembert fashion to ensure hemostasis.

Wedge Gastric Resection

- Wedge resection of gastric trauma, such as isolated anterior or greater curvature stab wounds, may be performed as a primary repair instead of suture repair; however, little data exist to suggest superiority of either method in trauma. Staple height chosen should be appropriate for tissue thickness as guided by manufacturer instructions for the stapler chosen. We recommend staple heights of at least 1.5 mm to accommodate tissue thickness without ischemia.

Resection for Devastating Injury

- Gastric injuries resulting in tissue loss or devascularization are rare and typically associated with hemorrhagic shock due to solid organ and vascular injuries. Such injuries may require distal or total gastrectomy and a complex subsequent reconstruction dictated by the anatomy and viability of remaining bowel. These complex reconstructive surgeries should be deferred until the patient's physiology has normalized.

Intraoperative Leak test

- Intraoperative tests of gastric repairs are commonly conducted via insufflation of the stomach via nasogastric tube, or esophagogastroduodenoscopy, after filling the peritoneal cavity with saline. Leaks are indicated by bubbles emerging from the distended, submerged stomach. Alternatively, one ampule of methylene blue dye diluted into 200 cc saline may be administered via the nasogastric tube for identification of additional injuries or leaks in the current repair. This is commonly not necessary since the gastric repair is usually under no tension, due to its size and abundant vascular supply. The risk of leak is low as long as good technique is used.

SMALL BOWEL INJURY

Primary Small Bowel Repair

- For injuries less than 50% of the total circumference of the bowel, primary repair is often a viable option. We recommend two-layer closure with an inner layer of 3-0 polyglactin 910 suture consisting of full-thickness bites and a secondary layer utilizing silk suture in a Lembert fashion to cover the inner suture line. Care is taken to repair in a transverse fashion, so as not to narrow the bowel.

Resection

- Resection is advised for lacerations greater than 50% of the bowel circumference, complete transections, multiple injuries in close proximity (where primary closure would result in luminal narrowing or kinking), or devastating mesenteric injuries resulting in a devascularized segment.

Technique

- Create small window in mesentery of normal appearing bowel proximal and distal to injury (**FIGURE 1**).

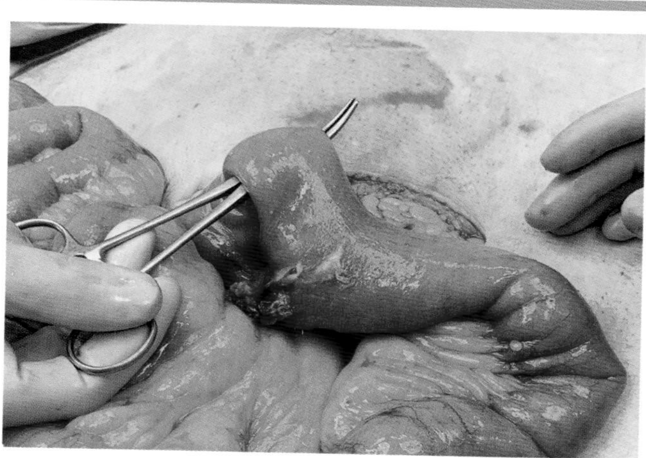

FIGURE 1 ● Windows in the mesentery should be made close to the bowel with care taken to not injure either the bowel or vessels in the mesentery. The clamp can be left in place to assist guiding the stapler in place.

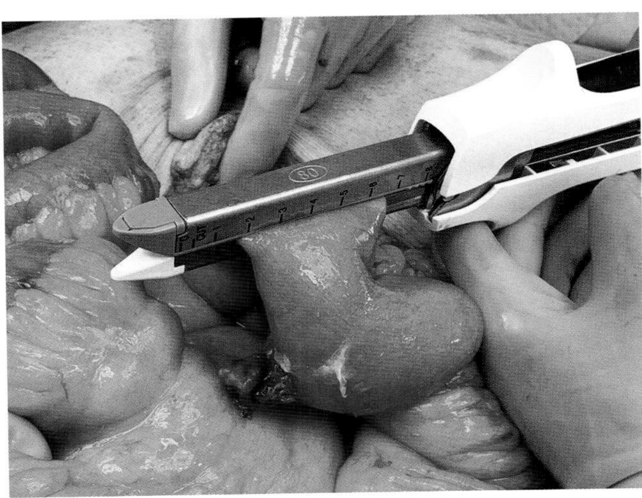

FIGURE 2 ● A linear cutting stapler allows quick transection with control of enteric contents. Ensure that the staple load length is adequate for complete transection.

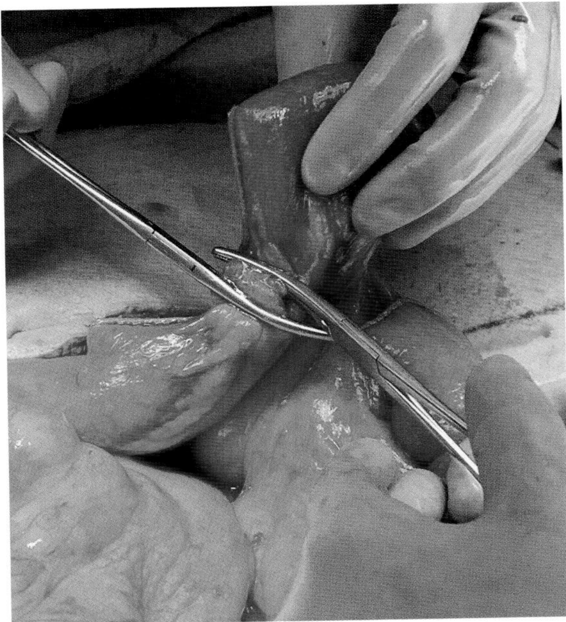

FIGURE 3 ● For nononcologic resection such as during trauma, the mesentery may be taken close to the bowel as long as it is otherwise uninjured. Care must be taken to preserve the mesentery to the cut edges of bowel to provide adequate perfusion to the anastomosis. Here, the "clamp-and-tie" method is used; however, vessel-sealing energy devices are also acceptable.

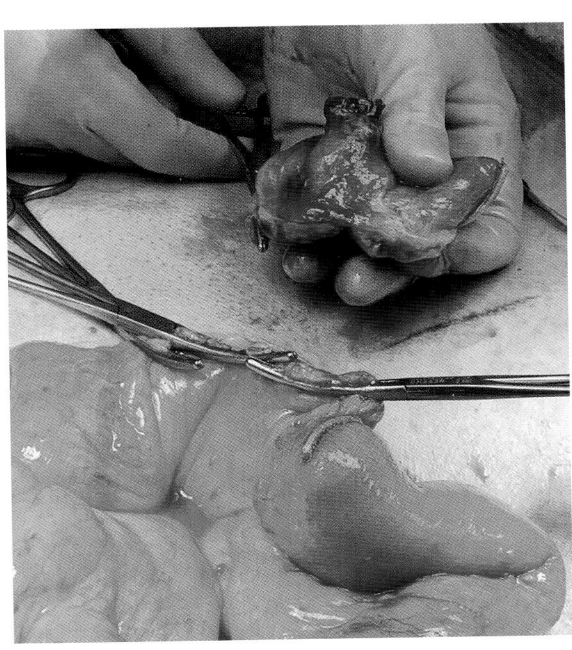

FIGURE 4 ● Resected bowel segment with small edge of mesentery.

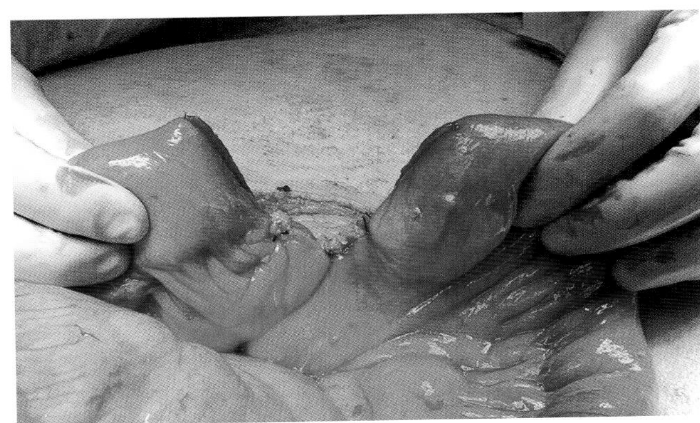

FIGURE 5 ● The cut edges of bowel should be inspected for viability. Active bleeding from the staple line may be controlled with 3-0 polyglactin 910 suture. Cut edges with signs of ischemia (ie, dusky color or necrosis, or failure to hold staples) should be resected back to healthy appearing bowel.

- Apply stapler in a mesenteric to antimesenteric direction (or bowel clamps) and transect bowel (FIGURE 2).
- Ligate mesentery close to bowel with sequential clamps and ties or an energy device (FIGURES 3 and 4).
- Inspect the cut edges for viability (FIGURE 5).

ANASTOMOSIS

- Anastomoses in trauma surgery should follow the same principles as during elective surgery, with respect given to blood supply, tension, orientation, contamination, and condition of the bowel as well as overall condition of the patient. Patient with highly contaminated wounds, severe septic or hemorrhagic shock, acidosis, and associated coagulopathy may benefit from temporary abdominal closure and anastomosis after resuscitation.
- Consideration must be given to the total number of repairs and anastomoses to minimize opportunities for leaks and breakdown. In some cases, resection of a longer segment of bowel, incorporating multiple injuries, may be advantageous to serial repairs.

- The use of stapled vs handsewn small bowel anastomoses in trauma continues to be controversial, as no controlled trial specific to trauma patients has been performed. One prospective AAST multicenter trial, performed in emergency general surgery patients, demonstrated similar complication rates between stapled and handsewn anastomoses (12.5%), agreeing with prior data from emergency and elective general surgery settings showing no significant difference between the two techniques.[12] Certainly, surgeon judgment should dictate technique choice based on bowel wall edema, bowel size mismatch, mesentery orientation, etc., as well as equipment availability and surgeon comfort.

Stapled Small Bowel Anastomosis

- Align the bowel such that the anastomosis can be created on the antimesenteric borders of the proximal and distal segments of the bowel. Place stay sutures beyond the extent of the planned staple line to maintain alignment and reduce tension (**FIGURE 6**).
- Cut a small area off the corner of the staple line to accommodate the stapler. Care must be taken to ensure this results in a full-thickness enterotomy for the stapler to pass into the lumen and not dissect into the bowel side wall (**FIGURE 7**).
- Pass the stapler into the enterotomies, aligning the antimesenteric border inward and check to ensure that nothing has slipped between the bowel before firing the stapler (**FIGURE 8**).
- Carefully withdraw the stapler and inspect the interior staple line for continuity and hemostasis. Align the common enterotomy with Allis clamps (**FIGURE 9**).
- Close the common enterotomy with a linear noncutting stapler (**FIGURE 10**). Ideally, the staple lines should be arranged

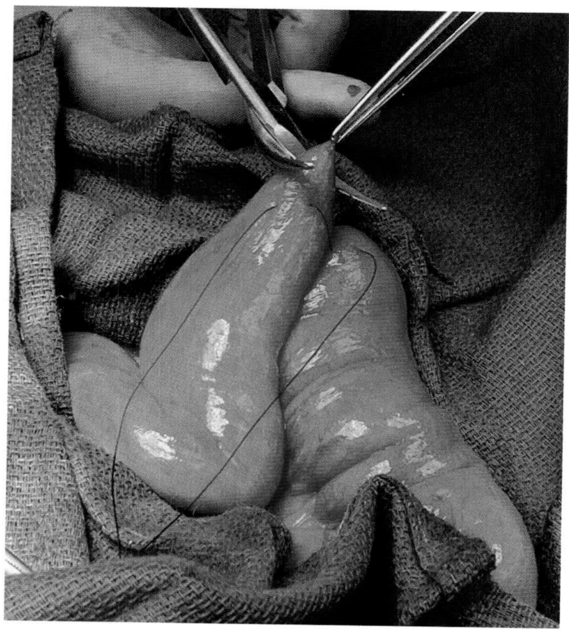

FIGURE 7 ● Heavy curved scissors are used to cut the antimesenteric corner off the staple line from the proximal and distal bowel loops. The resulting enterotomies should be full thickness and allow a hemostat or other clamp to pass easily, or else introducing the staple could dissect along the bowel wall. The enterotomy should also not be too big, as this would allow enteric contents to spill into the field.

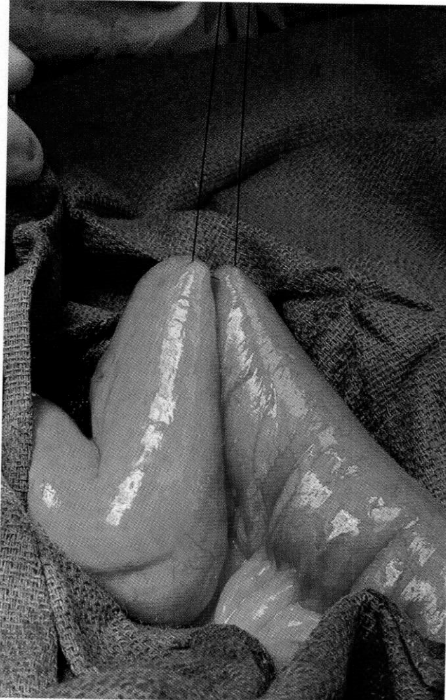

FIGURE 6 ● Braided silk stay sutures placed on the antimesenteric wall near the cut edge of bowel and distally allow for easier alignment during anastomosis creation.

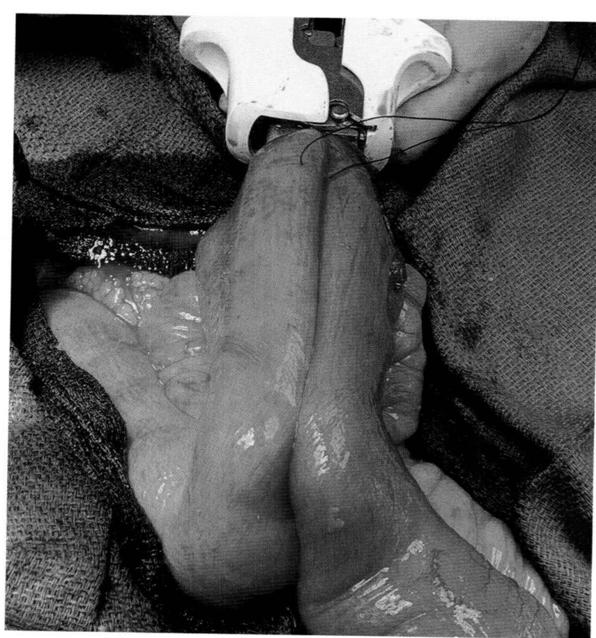

FIGURE 8 ● Gently advance each half of the stapler into the enterotomies. Attention must be paid to the stapler angle to avoid perforating the bowel distally or misaligning the bowel before the anastomosis is created. The stay suture is useful here to uniformly advance the bowel up the stapler. The mesentery is then fanned out laterally to align the antimesenteric borders and ensure no bowel or other structures have slipped into the stapler trajectory.

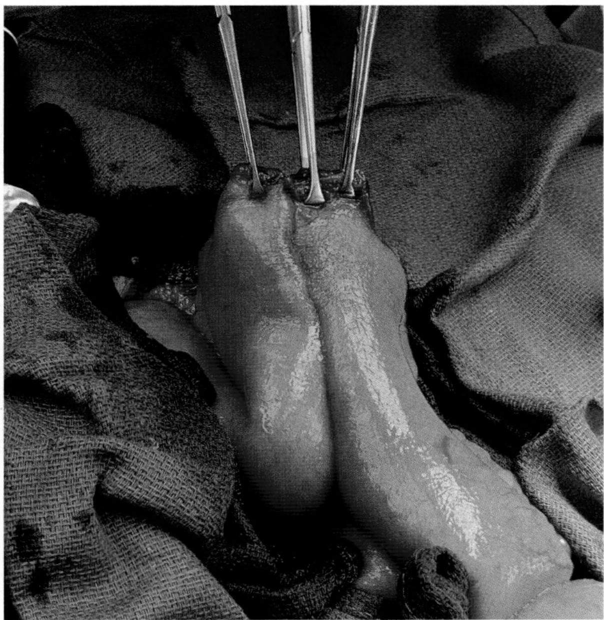

FIGURE 9 ● After the stapler is withdrawn, a clamp or ringed forceps can be used to gently open and inspect the anastomosis for bleeding. A 3-0 polyglactin 910 suture could be used to internally suture ligate any active bleeding, should an area be found. After inspection, the common enterotomy is aligned with Allis or Babcock clamps with the staple line slightly offset to prepare for stapled transection.

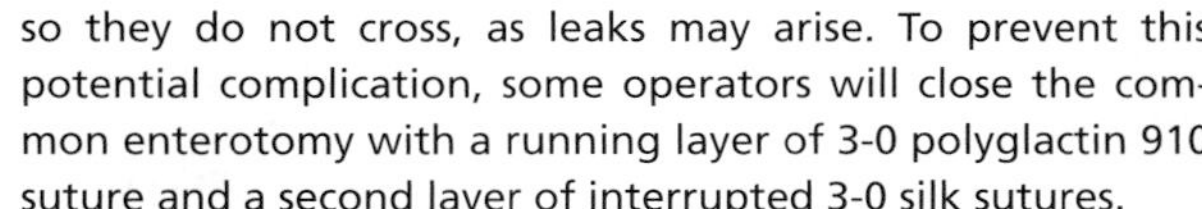

so they do not cross, as leaks may arise. To prevent this potential complication, some operators will close the common enterotomy with a running layer of 3-0 polyglactin 910 suture and a second layer of interrupted 3-0 silk sutures.

- Inspect the staple lines for hemostasis (**FIGURE 11**).

Handsewn Anastomosis

- Align the bowel such that the anastomosis can be created on the antimesenteric borders of the proximal and distal small bowel segments. Place silk stay sutures beyond the extent of the planned anastomosis to maintain alignment and reduce tension (**FIGURE 12**).
- Place posterior row of interrupted silk seromuscular sutures (ie, Lembert sutures). It is critical to place these sutures at a 90° angle to the bowel wall in order to avoid skiving the tissue which can lead to ischemia and anastomotic breakdown (**FIGURE 13**).
- Create 4-5 cm parallel enterostomies. Care should be taken to create the enterostomies with reasonable distance from the posterior row such that those sutures are not incorporated into the posterior row of the anastomosis (**FIGURE 14**).
- Starting at the midpoint of the anastomosis, begin a bidirectional posterior layer of polyglactin 910 suture. Full-thickness bites are taken to align the mucosal layers and ensure the posterior silk suture line is excluded. Approaching the corners, we recommend transition to Connell sutures to avoid foreshortening when the suture is tightened (**FIGURE 15**). It is also critical to pull the suture through on the mucosal side in order to invert the serosa.

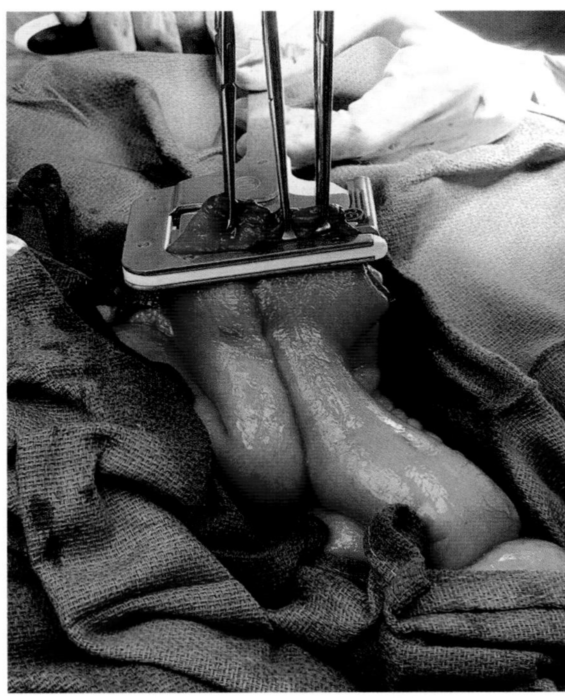

FIGURE 10 ● A noncutting linear stapled is positioned just below the Allis clamps to close the common enterotomy. Cutting linear staplers may also be used, though leaks will occur if the staple lines are crossed.

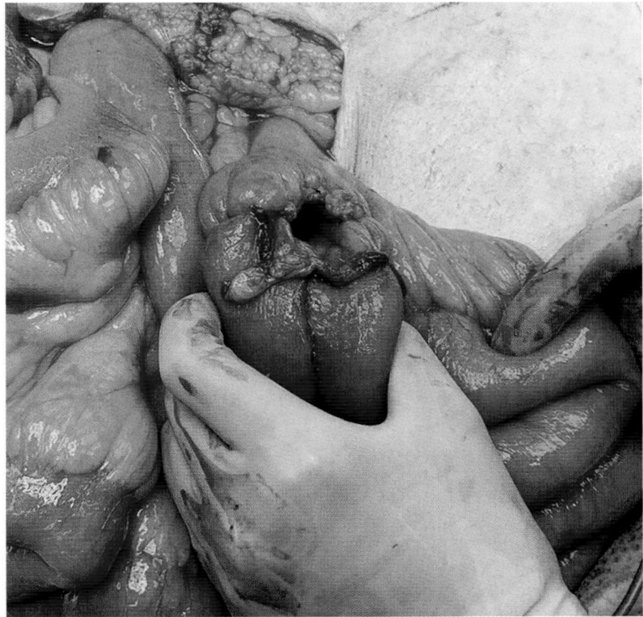

FIGURE 11 ● Areas of active bleeding can be suture ligated with interrupted or "figure-of-eight" 3-0 polyglactin 910 sutures. Some operators will choose to oversew and imbricate the staple line with polyglactin 910 and a second layer of braided silk sutures in a Lembert pattern.

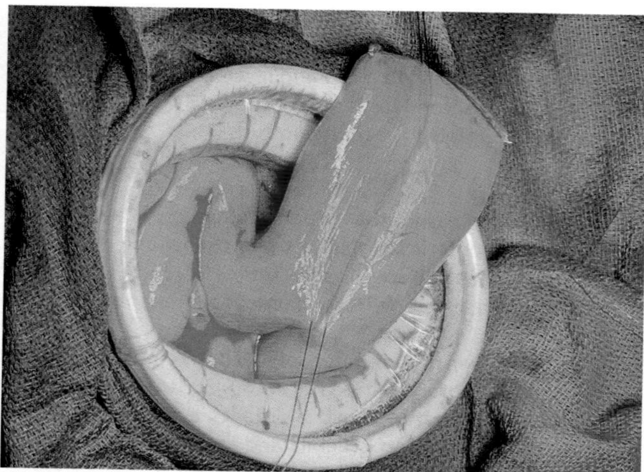

FIGURE 12 ● The bowel is aligned, as above, with silk stay sutures placed near the bowel cut edge and again distally, approximately 6-7 cm to accommodate a 5-cm anastomosis. The anastomosis above is aligned in the antiperistaltic fashion, as in the stapled anastomosis in the prior example, but may be aligned in the isoperistaltic fashion, depending on which orientation is favorable and tension-free.

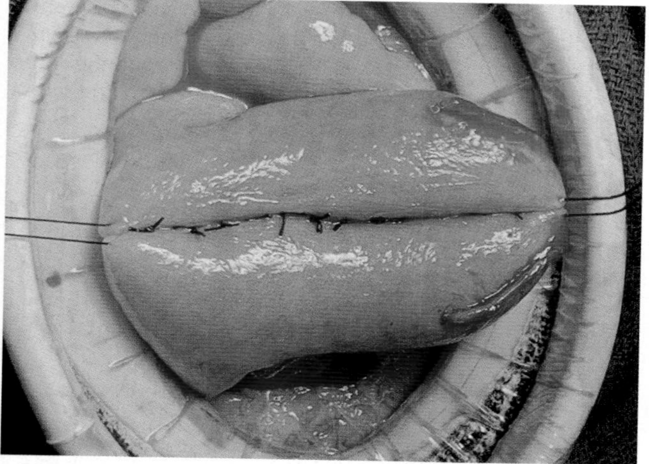

FIGURE 13 ● The posterior wall is created with seromuscular interrupted braided silk sutures. Care must be taken not to skive on each needle pass, as an area of ischemia could result in anastomotic leak.

Pulling the suture to advance the stitch on the serosal side causes the mucosa to evert.

- After rounding the corner in the first direction and approaching the anterior layer, begin suturing the posterior layer in the opposing direction. When completing the anterior layer, care should be taken not to grab the back wall with suture (**FIGURE 16**).

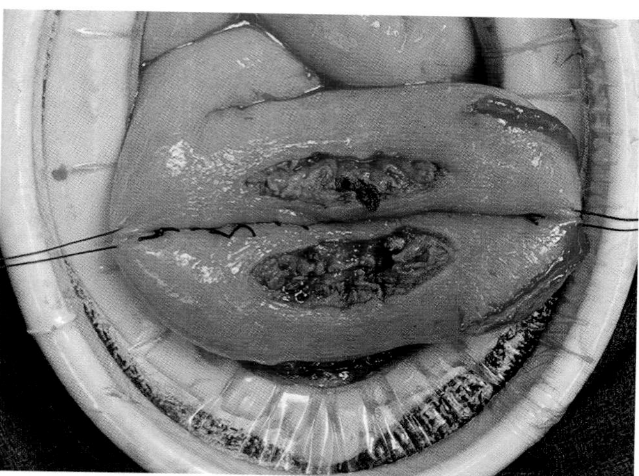

FIGURE 14 ● At the completion of the posterior layer, enterotomies are then created parallel to the posterior layer, sharply or with electrocautery. Care should be taken to allow a few millimeters distance from the posterior layer of sutures, so it is not inadvertently incorporated in inner layer of suture.

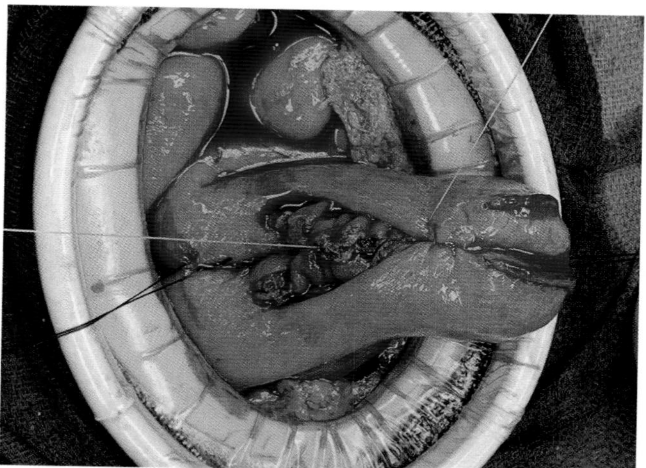

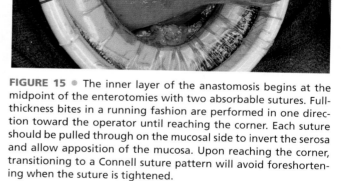

FIGURE 15 ● The inner layer of the anastomosis begins at the midpoint of the enterotomies with two absorbable sutures. Full-thickness bites in a running fashion are performed in one direction toward the operator until reaching the corner. Each suture should be pulled through on the mucosal side to invert the serosa and allow apposition of the mucosa. Upon reaching the corner, transitioning to a Connell suture pattern will avoid foreshortening when the suture is tightened.

- Complete the anterior layer (**FIGURES 17** and **18**).
- Finally, perform anterior layer of interrupted seromuscular silk Lembert sutures to cover the polyglactin 910 layer to complete the anastomosis (**FIGURE 19**).

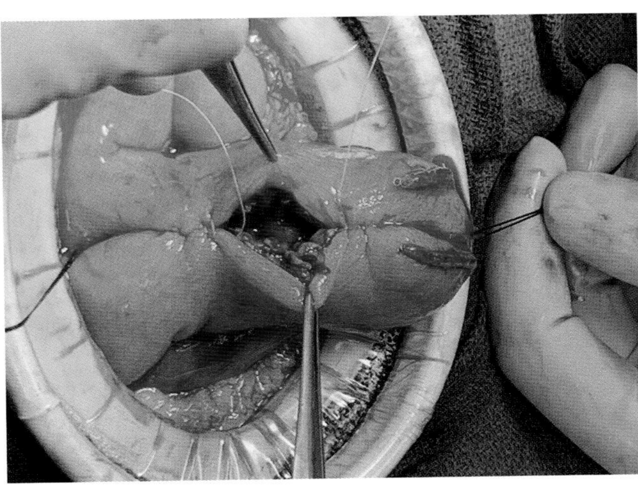

FIGURE 16 ● The initial corner suture is progressed until it is rounded and advanced to the anterior bowel layer. The posterior layer is then completed with the remaining suture in the same fashion and transitioning to a Connell suture to round the corner. Again, care must be taken not to foreshorten the anastomosis.

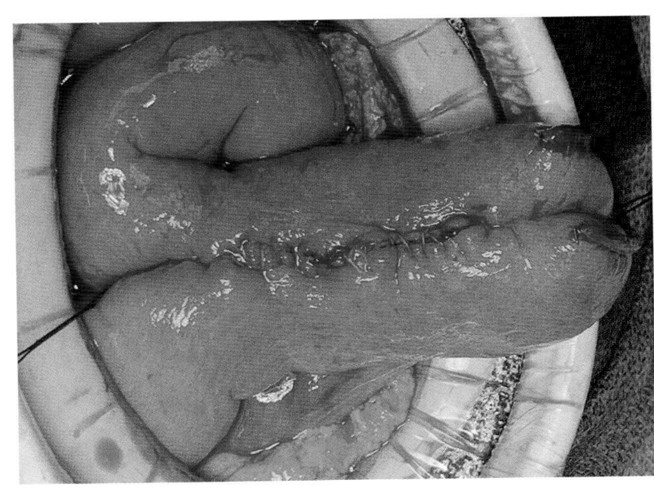

FIGURE 18 ● The inner layer is completed by tying the two operating sutures together at the midpoint of the anastomosis.

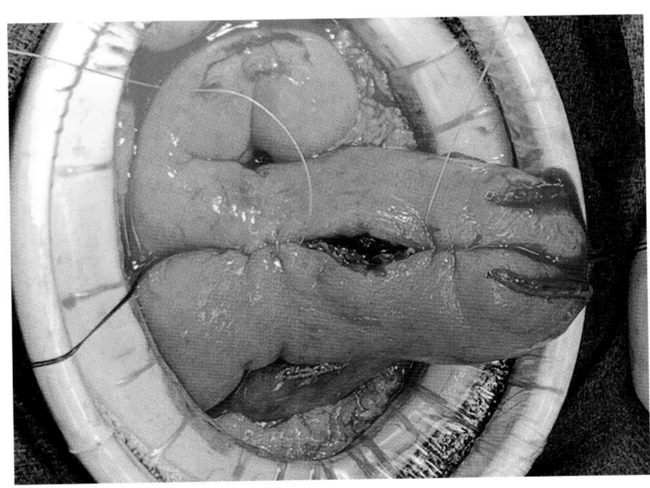

FIGURE 17 ● The anterior layer may be completed with a Connell suture pattern or transitioned back to a simple running pattern. Be sure to examine each needle pass exiting and entering the mucosa to avoid inadvertently suturing to the back wall of the bowel.

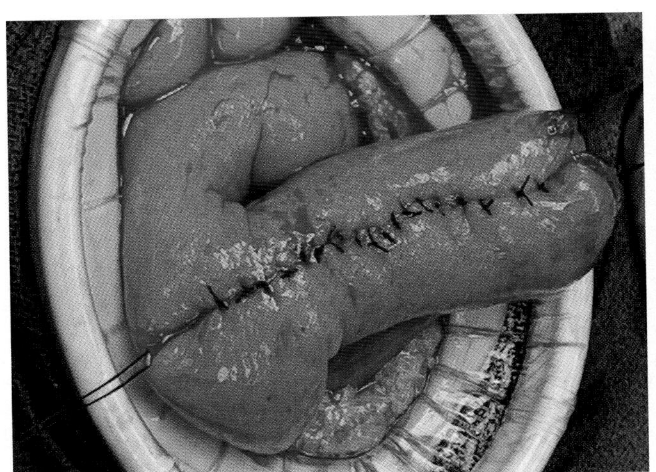

FIGURE 19 ● The completed inner layer is imbricated with interrupted silk sutures in a Lembert pattern.

PEARLS AND PITFALLS

- CT is the diagnostic modality of choice for HVI; however, most findings are nonspecific and may be normal in 4% of patients with true injury.
- Blunt HVIs are present in 1%-3% of blunt trauma patients, with most (90%) occurring in the small bowel.
- Patients with deceleration injuries should raise suspicion for concomitant HVIs.
- Anterior gastric injuries necessitate dissection and examination of the posterior stomach.
- The decision for resection vs repair of small bowel injuries should aim to reduce the total number of repairs and anastomoses, while preserving bowel length.
- Superiority of stapled vs handsewn small bowel anastomosis remains controversial.

POSTOPERATIVE CARE

- In cases of gastric or small bowel injury with limited contamination, antibiotics are not required beyond 24 hours. Delayed presentation of injury (>12 hours) or cases with severe contamination may require an extended course.[13]
- Routine use of nasogastric tubes following abdominal surgery has not been shown to hasten return of bowel function or reduce anastomotic leaks. However, placement of a nasogastric tube intraoperatively or postoperatively remains common practice and may be left to surgeon discretion.[14,15]
- Nutritional support should begin as soon as clinically feasible, with preference for gastric or enteral nutrition over parenteral.

COMPLICATIONS

- Missed intra-abdominal injury
- Postoperative ileus
- Postoperative bleeding
- Anastomotic leak
- Intra-abdominal abscess
- Surgical site infection
- Enterocutaneous fistula
- Internal hernia
- Small bowel obstruction
- Short gut syndrome

REFERENCES

1. Bloom MB, Ley EJ, Liou DZ, et al. Impact of body mass index on injury in abdominal stab wounds: implications for management. *J Surg Res*. 2015;197(1):162-166.
2. Salim A, Teixeira PGR, Inaba K, et al. Analysis of 178 penetrating stomach and small bowel injuries. *World J Surg*. 2008;32:471-475.
3. Mathonnet M, Peyrou P, Gainant A, Bouvier S, Cubertafond P. Role of laparoscopy in blunt perforations of the small bowel. *Surg Endosc*. 2003;17(4):641-645.
4. Watts DD, Fakhry SM. Incidence of hollow viscus injury in blunt trauma: an analysis from 275,557 trauma admissions from the East multi-institutional trial. *J Trauma*. 2003;54(2):289-294.
5. Tejerina Alvarez EE, Holanda MS, López-Espadas F, Dominguez MJ, Ots E, Díaz-Regañón J. Gastric rupture from blunt abdominal trauma. *Injury*. 2004;35(3):228-231. doi:10.1016/s0020-1383(03)00212-2. PMID: 15124787.
6. Oncel D, Malinoski D, Brown C, et al. Blunt gastric injuries. *Am Surg*. 2007;73:880-883.
7. Atri M, Hanson JM, Grinblat L, et al. Surgically important bowel and/or mesenteric injury in blunt trauma: accuracy of multidetector CT for evaluation. *Radiology*. 2008;249(2):524-533.
8. Livingston DH, Lavery RF, Passannante MR, et al. Free fluid on abdominal computed tomography without solid organ injury after blunt abdominal injury does not mandate celiostomy. *Am J Surg*. 2001;182:6-9.
9. Fakhry SM, Allawi A, Ferguson PL, et al. Blunt small bowel perforation (SBP). *J Trauma Acute Care Surg*. 2019;86:642-650.
10. Bain K, Meytes V, Chang GC, Timoney MF. Laparoscopy in penetrating abdominal trauma is a safe and effective alternative to laparotomy. *Surg Endosc*. 2019;33(5):1618-1625.
11. Moore EE, Jurkovich GJ, Knudson MM, et al. Organ injury scaling. VI: Extrahepatic biliary, esophagus, stomach, vulva, vagina, uterus (nonpregnant), uterus (pregnant), fallopian tube, and ovary. *J Trauma*. 1995;39:1069-1070.
12. Bruns BR, Morris DS, Zielinski M, et al. Stapled versus hand-sewn: a prospective emergency surgery study. An American Association for the Surgery of Trauma multi-institutional study. *J Trauma Acute Care Surg*. 2017;82:435-443.
13. Goldberg SR, Anand RJ, Como JJ, et al. Prophylactic antibiotic use in penetrating abdominal trauma: an Eastern Association for the Surgery of Trauma practice management guideline. *J Trauma Acute Care Surg*. 2012;73:S321-S325.
14. Cheatham ML, Chapman WC, Key SP, Sawyers JL. A meta-analysis of selective versus routine nasogastric decompression after elective laparotomy. *Ann Surg*. 1995;221:469.
15. Sapkota R, Bhandari RS. Prophylactic nasogastric decompression after emergency laparotomy. *J Nepal Med Assoc*. 2013;52(191):437-442.

Chapter 24

Colon and Rectal Injury: Primary Repair, Resection and Anastomosis, Colostomy

Louis Jude Magnotti, Devanshi D. Patel, and Martin A. Croce

DEFINITION

- Colon and rectal injuries can follow either penetrating or blunt trauma. The former results from direct penetration of the bowel. The latter is secondary to high-pressure force/compression to the bowel and/or supporting mesenteric blood supply. Both types of injuries can result in partial tears limited to the serosa, full-thickness injuries, or devascularizing injuries leading to bowel ischemia and eventual necrosis.

DIFFERENTIAL DIAGNOSIS

- High suspicion must be maintained when evaluating patients following either penetrating or blunt trauma for associated injuries. Depending on the mechanism, location and trajectory of the inciting injury, solid organs such as the liver, kidney, pancreas, spleen, aorta, or spine may also be affected. Injuries localized to the pelvic region should raise suspicion for concomitant genitourinary injuries.

PATIENT HISTORY AND PHYSICAL FINDINGS

- Any number of signs and symptoms can be present during the initial evaluation of the trauma patient. Complaints of abdominal pain coupled with physical examination findings suggestive of colon or rectal injury can include abdominal tenderness or distention, ecchymosis, rectal wall defect, or blood on digital rectal examination. Hemodynamic instability, peritonitis, or positive adjunct procedures such as focused assessment with sonography for trauma (FAST) or diagnostic peritoneal lavage are indications for exploratory laparotomy.

IMAGING AND OTHER DIAGNOSTIC STUDIES

- Ultrasound or, more specifically, the FAST examination can be utilized for patients with both penetrating and blunt trauma. However, for practical purposes, FAST should be reserved for the evaluation of blunt-injured patients. The perihepatic, perisplenic, and pelvic views are identified and evaluated for free fluid in the evaluation of patients with potential colorectal injuries. A positive finding can aid in decision for operative intervention; however, it is nonspecific for source of injury and should only prompt immediate exploration in the hemodynamically unstable patient.
- Computed tomography (CT) is indicated in the hemodynamically stable patient with signs and symptoms of abdominal injury. The clinician should be looking for findings such as pneumoperitoneum, intramural air, bowel wall thickening, bowel wall enhancement, mesenteric infiltration or stranding, arterial extravasation, fat pad injury, and free fluid in the intra- or retroperitoneal spaces. CT findings of blunt bowel and/or mesenteric injuries can be subtle so all studies must be reviewed with a high degree of suspicion in order to avoid missed injuries and delay intervention.
- CT with administration of rectal contrast (in addition to intravenous) can increase specificity of detecting rectal wall injuries. This technique can be performed quickly and does not significantly distract from further evaluation and treatment.
- Both rigid and flexible proctosigmoidoscopy can aid in identification of both intra- and extraperitoneal rectal injuries. Areas of bleeding, mucosal contusion, or mucosal defect should raise concern for injury and prompt additional intervention.

SURGICAL MANAGEMENT

Preoperative Planning

- Patients with hemodynamic instability, peritonitis, or evisceration require little preoperative planning and should proceed directly to laparotomy.

Positioning

- Patients should be placed in the supine position and with both arms out and prepped from nipples to knees. For suspected rectal injuries, patients may be placed in the lithotomy position to allow for examination under anesthesia and rigid or flexible proctosigmoidoscopy prior to laparotomy as long as the patient remains hemodynamically normal.
- Remove patient from lithotomy and place patient in the supine position prior to laparotomy.

OPERATIVE EXPOSURE AND ASSESSMENT FOR INJURY

- Begin with "running the bowel."
- Identify the terminal ileum.
- Inspect the colon and rectum for injury, from the ileocecal valve to the distal intraperitoneal rectum.
- Simultaneously evaluate the mesentery for injury.
- Maintain a high suspicion for missed injury in patients with an odd number of full-thickness penetrating injuries (particularly gunshot wounds).
- Injuries may be subtle, particularly at the mesenteric border.
- Closely inspect even the smallest hematomas for underlying injury.

REPAIR OF COLORECTAL INJURIES

Mesenteric Injuries

- Avoid mass ligation of the mesentery, which may result in bowel ischemia.
- Identify, isolate, and individually ligate bleeding vessels.
- For smaller vessels 4-0 silk ties or suture ligatures are the best.
- For larger vessels 2-0 or 3-0 silk may be used.
- Closely assess bowel surrounding areas of mesenteric injury for vascular compromise.
- In most cases, bowel viability can be determined by visual inspection.
- If bowel viability is in doubt, adjunctive measures may be used.
- Handheld Doppler is preferred because of its ease of use and ready availability in most operating rooms.
- Bowel viability is reliably confirmed by the presence of an audible Doppler signal from the antimesenteric surface of the bowel in question.
- After bleeding is controlled, close the mesenteric defect to prevent internal herniation.
- For devitalizing injuries, perform bowel resection with anastomosis.
- Anastomoses may be stapled or hand-sewn.

Serosal (Partial-Thickness) Injuries

- Repair with interrupted 3-0 silk sutures.
- Orient repairs transversely to minimize luminal narrowing.

Full-Thickness Injuries

- Babcock or other intestinal clamps should be applied to minimize spillage.
- Sharply debride wound margins to remove devitalized tissue if necessary.
- Primary closure is appropriate provided the bowel lumen is not significantly narrowed and the injury encompasses <50% of the bowel circumference.
- If the above is not possible, segmental resection and anastomosis should be performed.
- Orient repairs transversely to minimize luminal narrowing.

TYPES OF REPAIR

Primary Repair

- Closure is performed with either a two-layered repair with an inner layer of 3-0 absorbable suture and outer layer of interrupted 3-0 nonabsorbable suture (silk preferred) or a single layer of full-thickness 3-0 silk interrupted sutures (**FIGURE 1**). (Some surgeons choose a two-layer closure with Vicryl and silk or absorbable and nonabsorbable.)
- Each bite should include a generous portion of serosa with a small portion of mucosa to result in an inverted suture line—an easy way to remember this is to say to oneself—"a good bite of serosa and an Angstrom of mucosa."
- Primary repair of multiple low-grade small bowel injuries is usually preferred because it preserves intestinal length.
- If multiple injuries are contained within a short segment of bowel, resection and anastomosis should be performed instead.

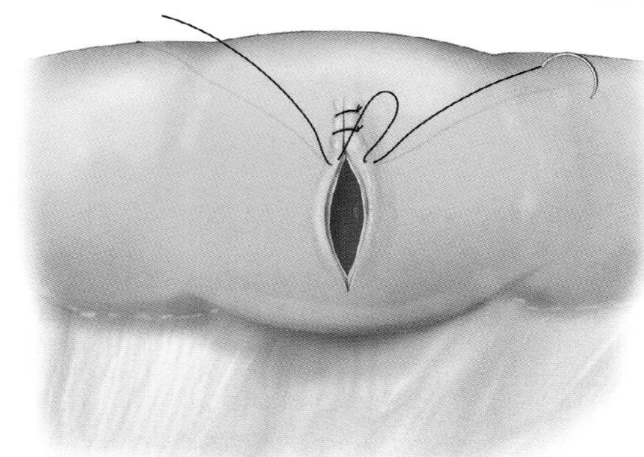

FIGURE 1 ● Primary repair of full-thickness colon injury. (Redrawn from Dr. Devanshi D. Patel.)

COLORECTAL RESECTION WITH ANASTOMOSIS

Dividing the Bowel

- Determine the segment to be resected.
- Identify avascular windows in the mesentery at the proximal and distal margins of the segment to be resected.
- Pinch the mesentery bordering the bowel between the surgeon's thumb and index finger.
- Using a small hemostat, create a window in the mesentery by spreading parallel to the mesenteric vessels so as not to create iatrogenic vascular injury.
- Divide the bowel with a linear cutting stapler.
- Make sure the stapler is oriented parallel to mesentery and angled toward the antimesenteric surface of the bowel that is to remain in situ.

CREATING THE ANASTOMOSIS

Side-to-Side Isoperistaltic (Bayonet) Colocolonic or Colorectal Anastomosis

- Orient the two ends of bowel in an isoperistaltic fashion—antiperistaltic orientation should be avoided as it is nonanatomic and can lead to unintended kinking of the bowel in the postoperative period.
- Near the mesenteric border of the bowel, 3-0 silk stay sutures are placed at the proximal and distal margins of the planned anastomosis.
- Continue with interrupted 3-0 silk suture placement to complete the "back wall" (**FIGURE 2A**).
- Create colotomies parallel to the back row of seromuscular sutures (**FIGURE 2B**).
- The anastomosis should be patulous, but one to two seromuscular stitches should remain distal to each end of the enterotomies to alleviate tension.
- A 3-0 absorbable suture on a tapered needle is used to create the inner layer of the anastomosis.
- Posteriorly, this is done with a running, full-thickness stitch, typically begun at the midpoint of the posterior wall (**FIGURE 2C**).
- The transition from the posterior to the anterior wall of the anastomosis is completed by continuing alternating "inside out" to "outside in" (**FIGURE 2D**).
- After this transition is completed, the above process is completed for the other half of the anastomosis with a second 3-0 absorbable suture until the entire posterior wall of the anastomosis is completed and both stitches are "around the corners."
- The anterior wall is completed with either a simple continuous stitch, a baseball stitch, or a Connell stitch according to the surgeon's preference.
- The key is to ensure mucosal apposition and suture line inversion.
- After this is completed, the two ends of absorbable suture are tied together.
- Complete the anterior second layer by placing interrupted 3-0 silk seromuscular sutures.
- The stay sutures are then tied down.
- Palpate the anastomosis to ensure adequate size.
- Close the mesenteric defect with braided 3-0 absorbable or permanent suture to prevent internal herniation.
- Be careful not to injure the mesenteric vasculature during the mesenteric closure.
- Antiperistaltic colocolonic anastomoses should be avoided as they can be bulky, leading to unwanted kinking of the bowel postoperatively.

End-to-End Colocolonic or Colorectal Anastomosis

- After resection of the injured segment, align the proximal end of the distal bowel with the distal end of the proximal bowel.
- While it is the authors' preference to perform a hand-sewn anastomosis, a side-to-side stapled colonic anastomosis may be performed.
- Regardless of the repair method, enough mobilization of the colonic segments must be performed to ensure a tension-free anastomosis.
- Ensure that the serosa near the mesenteric border on both ends of the bowel has been adequately cleaned to allow for ease of suture placement without compromising anastomotic blood supply.
- Seromuscular 3-0 silk stay sutures are placed at the lateral and medial margins of the planned anastomosis.
- Continue with interrupted 3-0 silk suture placement to complete the "back wall" oriented between both stapled resection lines.
- Create colotomies by removing the stapled resection lines, either sharply or with electrocautery, parallel to the back row of seromuscular sutures.
- As above, ensure that the anastomosis is patulous to prevent stricture.
- A 3-0 absorbable suture on a tapered needle is used to create the inner layer of the anastomosis.
- This is done with a running, full-thickness stitch, typically begun at the midpoint of the posterior wall.
- The transition from the posterior to the anterior wall of the anastomosis is completed by continuing alternating inside out to outside in as one approaches the stay sutures.

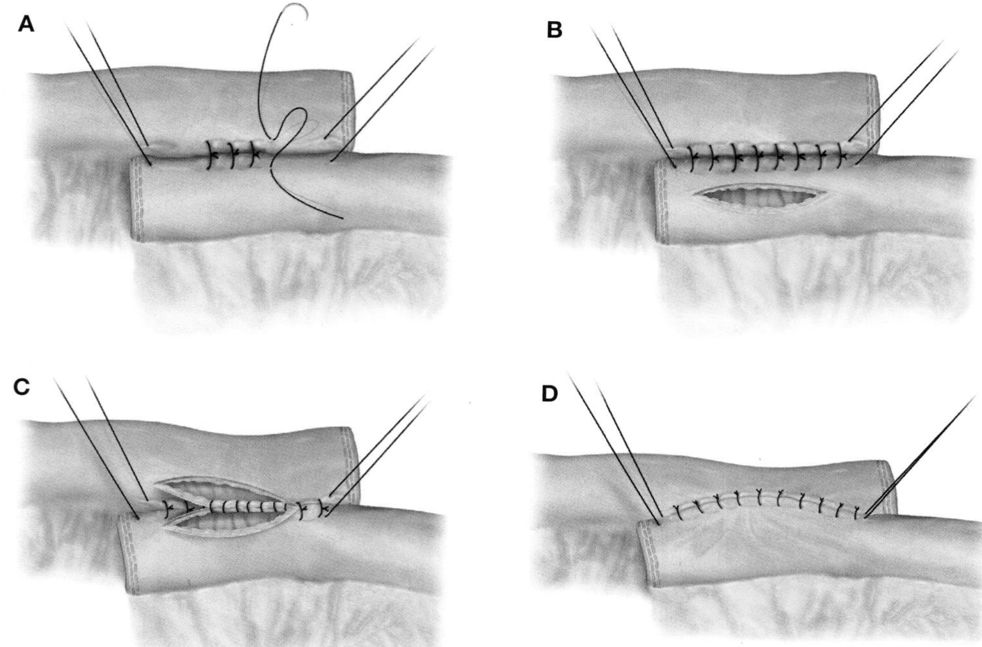

FIGURE 2 ● **A,** Securing the posterior wall. **B,** Creating colotomies. **C,** Inner layer secured with running full thickness stitch. **D,** Conversion to outside-in stitch ("baseball" stitch). (Redrawn from Dr. Devanshi D. Patel.)

- After this transition is made, the above process is completed for the other half of the anastomosis with a second 3-0 absorbable suture until the entire posterior wall of the anastomosis is completed and both stitches are around the corners.
- The anterior wall is completed with a simple continuous stitch, a baseball stitch, or a Connell stitch according to the surgeon's preference.
- The key is to ensure mucosal apposition and suture line inversion.
- After this is completed, the two ends of the absorbable suture are tied together.
- Complete the anterior second layer by placing interrupted 3-0 silk seromuscular sutures.
- The stay sutures are then tied down.
- Palpate the anastomosis to ensure adequate size.
- Close the mesenteric defect with braided 3-0 absorbable or permanent suture to prevent internal herniation.
- Be careful not to injure the mesenteric vasculature during the mesenteric closure.

End-to-Side Colorectal (Baker) Anastomosis

- After resection of the injured segment, mobilize sufficient proximal colon along the white line of Toldt such that the colon easily reaches into the pelvis to the rectal stump.
- Clear any additional fatty tissue from the side of the proximal colon.
- The side of the proximal colon should lay tension free against the rectal stump.
- A layer of seromuscular interrupted silk sutures (3-0) should be placed as the back row, below the rectal staple line and below the tinea of the proximal colon.
- The rectal staple line is removed and a colotomy is created on the proximal colon through the tinea (**FIGURE 3A**).
- A running absorbable 3-0 suture is used for the inner layer—full thickness bites, typically performed with two sutures run in opposite directions, with a running Connell for the top layer (**FIGURE 3B** and **C**).
- The anastomosis is then oversewn with 3-0 seromuscular interrupted silks (**FIGURE 3D**).

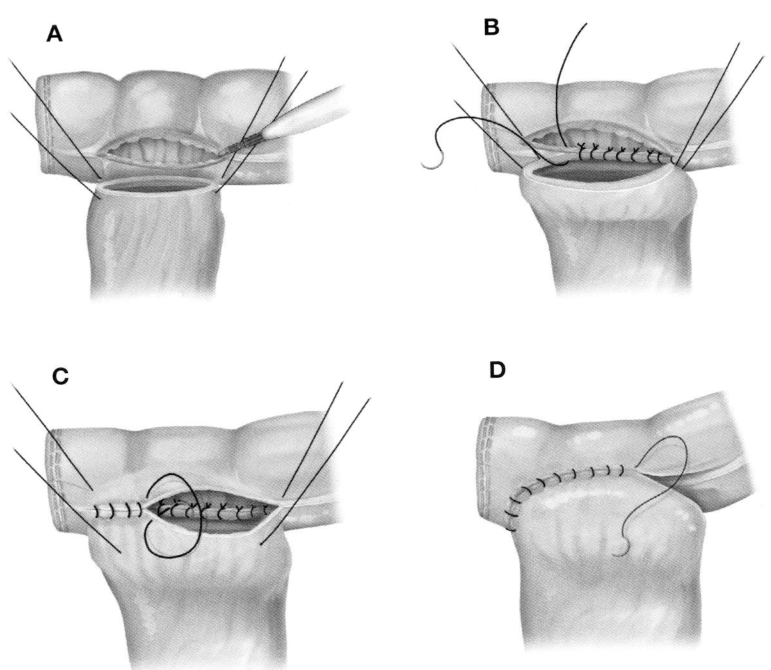

FIGURE 3 ● **A,** Removal of rectal staple line and colotomy creation. **B,** Inner layer secured with running full thickness stitch. **C,** Outer layer running Connell stitch. **D,** Seromuscular 3-0 silk interrupted sutures. (Redrawn from Dr. Devanshi D. Patel.)

COLOSTOMY CREATION

- After resection of the distal colon, mobilize sufficient proximal colon along the white line of Toldt such that the colon easily reaches above the skin level without tension.
- Identify target ostomy location on the abdominal wall, typically either above or below the umbilicus at the level of the rectus.
- Create a circular incision at the chosen ostomy site on the abdominal wall down to the level of the anterior rectus sheath (**FIGURE 4A**).
- Incise the anterior rectus sheath in a cruciate fashion.
- Bluntly separate the rectus muscle using a Kelly clamp and handheld retractors.
- Similar to the anterior rectus sheath, incise the posterior rectus sheath in a cruciate fashion.
- Three fingers should easily pass through the intended ostomy site.
- Grasp the resected end of the colon with a Babcock clamp and pull through the abdominal wall in a retrograde fashion (**FIGURE 4B**).
- Care must be taken to maintain proper orientation of the colon so there are no twists in the colon and mesocolon.
- Close the midline fascia in standard fashion.
- If there was any fecal contamination from the injury, the skin should be left open.
- Be sure to protect the skin incision prior to ostomy maturation.
- Remove the staple line from the resected end of the colon with electrocautery (**FIGURE 4C**).
- Mature the colostomy with interrupted full-thickness bites of colon at the edge of the colotomy (small amount of mucosa relative to large seromuscular bite), securing it to the dermis with an absorbable suture (**FIGURE 4D** and **E**).

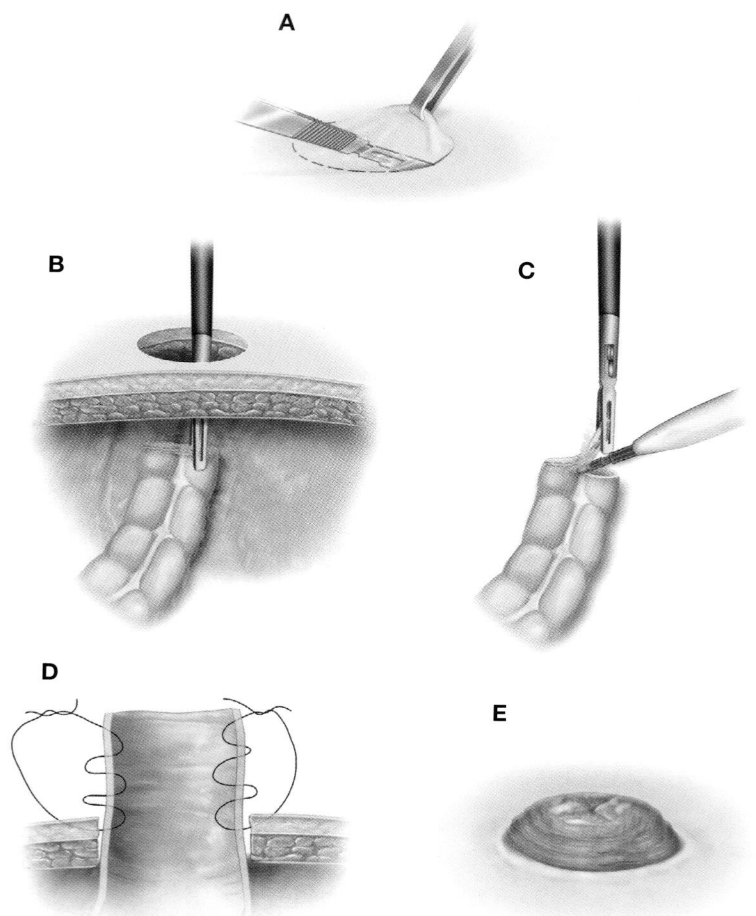

FIGURE 4 ● **A,** Circular incision at ostomy site. **B,** Introduction of colon through ostomy site. **C,** Removal of staple line. **D,** Interrupted full thickness sutures through dermis, colon, and colonic end. **E,** Matured colostomy. (Redrawn from Dr. Devanshi D. Patel.)

PEARLS AND PITFALLS

Indications for exploratory laparotomy	■ Hemodynamic instability, evisceration, and peritonitis are clear indications for urgent operative intervention.
Incision	■ Midline laparotomy provides maximum exposure and provides ease of access to evaluate for other sources of solid organ and/or associated injuries.
Damage control	■ Consideration for diversion or second look laparotomy should be based on the patient's hemodynamic status, temperature, pH, blood transfusion requirements, comorbidities, and associated injuries.
Resuscitation	■ Ongoing resuscitation is critical prior to, during, and after the operative period, especially when considering new anastomosis creation.
Definitive procedures	■ Definitive procedures can be performed in the hemodynamically stable patient without significant comorbidities or concern for bowel compromise. Strong consideration for end ostomy vs anastomosis plus proximal diversion (loop ostomy) should be given to those patients with significant pre- and intraoperative transfusion requirements and/or significant medical comorbidities. Ostomy reversal should be delayed until at least 3 months after creation for proximal diversion and up to 6 months for an end ostomy.

POSTOPERATIVE CARE

- Resuscitation should be continued in the postoperative setting until the patient stabilizes—from a hemodynamic, temperature, and pH standpoint. Nasogastric suction can be utilized until return of bowel function. Early mobilization and enteral feeding should be advanced as appropriate.

OUTCOMES

- Patients who present with hemodynamic instability or with significant comorbidities are at higher risk for increased mortality or morbidity. Overall, most patients can return to normal function preinjury functional status, similar to routine abdominal surgery.

COMPLICATIONS

Anastomotic Leak or Suture Line Failure

- Trauma patients are at increased risk of anastomotic leak or suture line failure. Continued resuscitation plays a vital role in the maintenance of the anastomosis as poor blood flow can severely compromise this portion of the bowel. Careful consideration should be placed on patient selection for definitive repair during the index case.

Intra-Abdominal Abscess

- Multiple factors—mechanism of injury, hemodynamic status, medical comorbidities, age, and sex—contribute to an increased risk of infection in the trauma patient. Contamination of the peritoneal or retroperitoneal space can lead to abscess formation. This should be appropriately and promptly managed with antibiotics and either interventional or operative drainage. A single dose of appropriate prophylactic antibiotic administered prior to operative intervention has been shown to decrease development of intra-abdominal infections.

Fistula

- A fistula is defined as an abnormal passage between two epithelial surfaces and can be a difficult problem to manage postoperatively for both the clinician as well as the patient. Factors that contribute to formation include large bowel resection, large volume resuscitation, and requirement of multiple operations. Management includes treatment of sepsis if present, maximizing nutrition, correcting fluid and electrolyte abnormalities, and prevention of further wound breakdown. Fistulas can spontaneously close; however, they may require further operative intervention.

Bowel Necrosis

- Unidentified or iatrogenic devitalization of colon or rectal blood supply can result in bowel ischemia and ultimately lead to full-thickness necrosis. Periods of postoperative hypotension increases the risk of bowel compromise. Patients may present with septic shock, and repeat laparotomy is required with likely diversion.

SUGGESTED READINGS

1. Baker JW. Low end to side rectosigmoidal anastomosis; description of technic. *Arch Surg*. 1950;61(1):143-157.
2. Bradley MJ, DuBose JJ, Scalea TM, et al. Independent predictors of enteric fistula and abdominal sepsis after damage control laparotomy: results from the prospective AAST open abdomen registry. *JAMA Surg*. 2013;148(10):947-955. doi:10.1001/jamasurg.2013.2514
3. Burch JM, Brock JC, Gevirtzman L, et al. The injured colon. *Ann Surg*. 1986;203(6):701-711.
4. George SM, Jr., Fabian TC, Voeller GR, Kudsk KA, Mangiante EC, Britt LG. Primary repair of colon wounds. A prospective trial in nonselected patients. *Ann Surg*. 1989;209(6):728-733; 33-4.
5. Gonzalez RP, Turk B. Surgical options in colorectal injuries. *Scand J Surg*. 2002;91(1):87-91.
6. Nakada I, Kawasaki S, Sonoda Y, Watanabe Y, Tabuchi T. Abdominal stapled side-to-end anastomosis (Baker type) in low and high anterior resection: experiences and results in 69 consecutive patients at a regional general hospital in Japan. *Colorectal Dis*. 2004;6(3):165-170.
7. Sharpe JP, Magnotti LJ, Fabian TC, Croce MA. Evolution of the operative management of colon trauma. *Trauma Surg Acute Care Open*. 2017;2(1):e000092.
8. Trust M, Veith J, Brown C, et al. Traumatic rectal injuries: is the combination of computed tomography and rigid proctoscopy sufficient? *J Trauma Acute Care Surg*. 2018;85(6):1033-1037.
9. Weinberg JA, Fabian TC, Magnotti LJ, et al. Penetrating rectal trauma: management by anatomic distinction improves outcome. *J Trauma*. 2006;60(3):508-513; discussion 13-14.

Chapter 25

Extraperitoneal Rectal Injury: Colostomy, Presacral Drains

Anne H. Warner and Kevin M. Bradley

DEFINITION

- Extraperitoneal rectal injury is defined as an injury to the distal two-thirds of the rectum from the peritoneal reflection to the anus.
- In most patients, the total length of the rectum is 10 to 12 cm and anus is 3 to 4 cm starting at levator ani muscles of the pelvic floor.
- Injuries to the proximal third of the rectum are intraperitoneal as the rectum at this level is covered anteriorly and laterally by the peritoneum.
- Proximal-third rectal injuries are treated as any colon injury and are outside the scope of this chapter.
- The extraperitoneal rectum is closely associated with the sacrum posteriorly, the bladder outlet anteriorly and the vagina in females and urethra and prostate in males.

DIFFERENTIAL DIAGNOSIS

- A high index of suspicion for extraperitoneal rectal injury should be maintained in cases where there is penetrating trauma to the pelvis, gluteal regions, lower abdomen with a trajectory crossing into the pelvis, perineum, and scrotum or any patient presenting with bleeding per rectum after a trauma. Blunt rectal injuries are rare but can occur with complex displaced pelvic fractures, true open pelvis fractures associated with perineal lacerations, and straddle-related injuries. They may be asymptomatic at first. Injuries can be partial or full thickness. Associated injuries to pelvic bones, bladder, prostate, vagina, or pelvic vascular injuries should be assessed given the convergence of these nearby structures within the pelvic outlet. Other associated injuries within the peritoneal and retroperitoneal space should be considered with blunt and penetrating mechanisms.
- The majority of extraperitoneal rectal injuries occur as a result of penetrating trauma, namely, low-velocity gunshot wounds. Additional mechanisms of injury include iatrogenic (surgery, colonoscopy, enemas), blunt mechanisms related to complex pelvic fractures, straddle injury, watercraft injury, and related to foreign bodies placed during intercourse. Patients may present immediately or in more delayed fashion depending on the mechanism and associated symptoms. They may be hemodynamically stable or unstable. In military combat casualty settings, high-velocity and caliber gunshot wounds and blast injuries may cause extraperitoneal rectal wounds.

STAGING

- Rectal injuries are staged by severity with the American Association for the Surgery of Trauma scale: stage I are hematomas/contusions or partial-thickness lacerations, stage II are lacerations less than 50% of the circumference, stage III are lacerations 50% or greater circumference, stage IV extend to the perineum, and stage V are devascularized segments[1] (**TABLE 1**).

Table 1: AAST Rectal Injury Grading[1]

11. AAST grade of rectal injury	Injury severity
I	Hematoma, contusion, partial thickness
II	Laceration <50% of circumference
III	Laceration ≥50% of circumference
IV	Extend to perineum
V	Devascularized segment

Reprinted with permission from Moore EE, Cogbill TH, Malangoni MA, et al. Organ injury scaling, II: Pancreas, duodenum, small bowel, colon, and rectum. J Trauma. *1990;30(11):1427-1429. Table 5.*

PATIENT HISTORY AND PHYSICAL EXAMINATION FINDINGS

- If the patient is alert, a history should be obtained, noting any complaints of rectal bleeding, pain, and the mechanism of injury.
- Prehospital providers play an important role in providing added information with mechanism and history.
- Evaluation of any trauma patient follows the standard format outlined in advanced trauma life support (ATLS) of primary and secondary surveys with evaluation of airway, breathing, circulation, disability, and exposure, followed by a head-to-toe physical examination.
- A complete trauma examination should include an examination of the perineum and external genitalia, examination of the bony pelvis, and digital rectal examination assessing for the presence of blood, palpable rectal wall injuries, and anal sphincter tone.

IMAGING AND OTHER DIAGNOSTIC STUDIES

- Adjunctive studies such as plain **x-rays** in patients with blunt and penetrating trauma, especially pelvis x-ray, and extended focused assessment with sonography for trauma (FAST) examination should be performed in all patients.
- Additional computed tomography (**CT**) imaging is obtained if the patient is hemodynamically stable, responsive to resuscitation, and without peritonitis on examination.
- CT with intravenous contrast and rectal contrast can be done in a hemodynamically stable patient to assess for injury. Signs of injury include direct trajectory through the rectum, associated free air or perirectal free fluid, adjacent air within the perirectal fat, and rectal wall thickening (**FIGURE 1**). CT will also give information on associated injuries. This can be done postoperatively if the patient needs immediate surgery (**FIGURE 2**).
- If feasible, administration of rectal water-soluble contrast may help to define rectal mucosal irregularities, location of injury, and degree of injury. A discussion of the procedure should be done with the patient prior to administration and should be administered by a skilled provider.
- **Rigid proctoscopy/flexible sigmoidoscopy** can be done in the emergency department or in the operating room, depending on the patient condition and presence of any indications for immediate operation. Digital rectal examination should

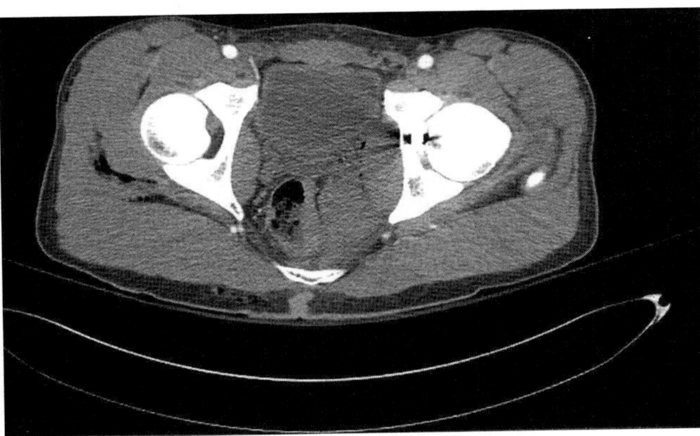

FIGURE 1 ● Preoperative CT image of a Hemodynamically Stable Patient. This is an 18-year-old man with multiple gunshot wounds including three to the right buttock and two to the right thigh with left acetabular missile who had left acetabular fracture, extraperitoneal rectal injury, and sacral hematoma. The missile is visible as well as hematoma to the left of the rectum, and subcutaneous air in the right gluteal region indicates where the missile entered the patient. The extraperitoneal rectum is clearly in the middle of this trajectory.

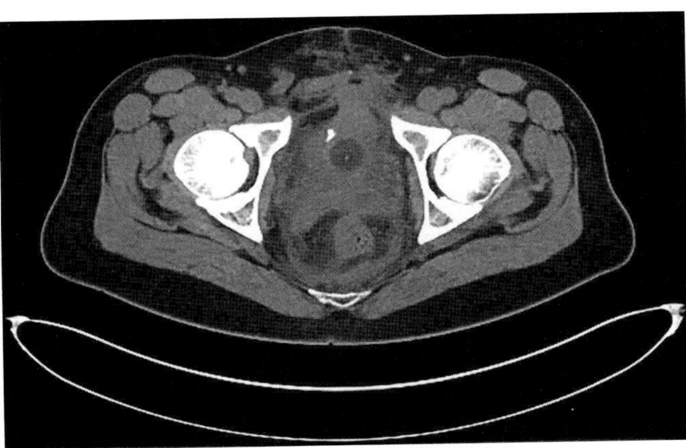

FIGURE 2 ● Postoperative CT image of Extraperitoneal Rectal Injury. This is a 35-year-old man with injuries to the right posterolateral rectal wall, posterior bladder, destroyed left ureteral orifice who underwent exploratory laparotomy with diverting colostomy for his rectal injury and had postoperative CT imaging. Hematoma is visible anterior to the rectum.

be done prior. During lighted proctoscopy, any visible stool should be removed to allow mucosal assessment, which can be aided by use of a large cotton swab placed through the channel of the proctoscope. Systematic assessment of mucosa should be done to look for any injuries or blood, and the approximate location and degree of injury should be noted relative to the anal verge.

- A multicenter trial was conducted by the The American Association for the Surgery of Trauma (AAST) looking retrospectively at full-thickness rectal injury diagnosis from 2004 to 2015. Thirty-four percent had positive CT findings and 94% had positive rigid proctoscopy findings and the combination was 97% sensitive.[2] All the patients with negative rigid proctoscopy had intraperitoneal injuries. This study points to the importance of a complete workup and utility of proctoscopy in these injuries.

SURGICAL MANAGEMENT

- Rectal injury management was historically based on care of the wartime patient in World War II and Vietnam. These injuries were high-velocity penetrating injuries, as seen with military weaponry. Historically, management included the combination of the "4 Ds" of Direct repair, Diversion, Distal rectal washout, and presacral Drains, and this was initially advocated for by Levenson and Cohen in 1971.[3] Since that time, there have been multiple retrospective studies, one prospective study, and much discussion over which aspects of management are needed in the civilian trauma population where injuries are more frequently caused by lower-velocity gunshots and cared for in modern trauma centers. No clear evidence-based consensus exists at this time, and approach should be based on patient's specific injury location, degree of tissue injury, hemodynamic status, and surgeon gestalt; however, more recent conditional recommendations have been made.
- The only randomized trial related to rectal injuries was published in 1998 and consisted of 25 patients managed without presacral drainage and 23 patients managed with presacral drainage at a single level 1 trauma center. All of the patients underwent proctoscopy and exploratory laparotomy where injuries were closed if exposed in the course of the exploration, loop or end colostomy with mucous fistulas was performed, the abdomen was washed out with 10 L of irrigation, and skin was left open to heal by secondary intention. No rectal washouts were done. At this point, they were randomized to presacral drainage or not. There were no significant differences in rate of complications between the groups. Two patients (8%) in the drain group had perirectal and perivesicular abscesses treated with CT-guided drain placement, and one (4%) in the nondrain group developed a rectocutaneous fistula related to a retained missile, which healed once it was removed.[4]
- The AAST Contemporary Rectal Injury Injuries Study Group also looked retrospectively in a multicenter trial of 785 patients managed from 2004 to 2015 at 22 trauma centers and found that those with diverting colostomy, presacral drains, or washout all had more abdominal complications and after multivariate analysis, both distal washout and presacral drains increased the risk of abdominal complications threefold.[5] The Eastern Association for the Surgery of Trauma has conditionally recommended diversion without presacral drainage or distal rectal washout in their 2016 management guidelines for extraperitoneal rectal injury.[6] A retrospective review of the US National Trauma Data Bank from 2013 to 2014 including 494 patients with isolated extraperitoneal rectal injuries found that 63.5% were managed by repair/resection alone with less morbidity (12.7% vs 30.2%, $P = .009$) and shorter length of stay (14 vs 23 days, $P < .001$) than those who had repair/resection with a stoma (36.5%).[7] One small study was done from 2003 to 2005 of 14 patients with extraperitoneal injuries <25% of circumference who did not undergo repair, diversion or washout and all had normal barium enemas by postinjury day 10 (range of 5-10 days postinjury study with one patient having extravasation on day 5 and resolution by day 10).[8] The Memphis group describes repair of extraperitoneal injuries in the proximal two-thirds of the rectum with or without diversion by surgeon discretion and repair of distal one-third injuries with diversion, and diversion and drainage if inaccessible for repair.[9] Use of this

anatomic-based pathway reduced infectious complications from 31% before the pathway to 13% afterward.[9] Resection and repairs were used for patients receiving >6 units of packed red blood cells or with comorbidities. LA County's retrospective review of extraperitoneal gunshot wound injuries showed no difference in complications between those who underwent diversion alone, repair and diversion, and diversion and presacral drains.[10]

- Unfortunately, without large prospective studies and with a large diversity of patient illness, even after many years, there is yet to be a clear consensus on the management of individual patients. Available techniques are therefore described.

Preoperative Planning

- Informed consent should be obtained if the patient is alert and hemodynamically stable. This should include discussion about potential need for an ostomy.
- Perioperative antibiotics should be given to cover gastrointestinal organisms to include gram negatives and anaerobes, typically cephazolin and metronidazole intravenously, just before the start of the procedure.

Positioning

- Lithotomy should be used for those patients who have isolated rectal injuries. This facilitates on table digital rectal examination, proctoscopy, and access to perineum.
- Care should be taken to carefully position the legs, particularly in elderly or obese patients to avoid tension on the knee joints and pressure on the common peroneal nerves posteriorly at the knee.
- If a prolonged case is expected or additional procedures are required, the patient can be positioned for proctoscopy either in lithotomy or in lateral decubitus position and then repositioned supine for laparoscopy or laparotomy.

TECHNIQUES

TECHNIQUE AND STEPS

- **Direct repair**:
  - Direct repair of the rectal extraperitoneal injury can be done transanally for distal accessible injuries below the peritoneal reflection with use of a side viewing Hill Ferguson anoscope or trans peritoneally for intraperitoneal high rectal injuries.
  - Excessive dissection to find and repair the injury can be detrimental and should be avoided.
  - If the injury is not accessible and is nondestructive, it can be left alone without further dissection or repair.
  - Those injuries within view should be debrided back to healthy edges and any nonviable tissue excised.
  - Repair should be done in two layers with inner PDS suture (3-0 or 4-0) and outer PDS or Vicryl or silk suture in lambert fashion.
- **Diversion with loop colostomy or end colostomy**
  - This is the mainstay of treatment of extraperitoneal rectal injuries.
  - This can be done laparoscopically or in an open fashion.
  - If an exploratory laparotomy is done to assess or treat additional injuries, this can be done in an open fashion.
  - The sigmoid colon should be able to reach the left lower quadrant abdominal wall without tension.
  - In instances of short or fatty mesentery, thick abdominal wall, or prior surgery where there is tension, the colon can be mobilized at the white line of Toldt until it can be brought up without tension to the abdominal wall.
  - More proximal colon can be utilized if needed.
  - The colon should be brought through the left lower quadrant of the abdominal wall mid-rectus muscle in the ostomy triangle (midpoint between the anterior superior iliac spine, pubic tubercle, and umbilicus).
  - If this portion of the abdominal wall is injured or has excessive thickness, or more proximal colon is mobilized for the ostomy, this could be done in the left upper quadrant of the abdomen.
  - A small ellipse of skin should be excised sharply at the chosen site of the ostomy. Subcutaneous fat dissection should be continued bluntly down to the anterior fascia, which may be aided with use of hand-held Army-Navy or small Richardson retractors. Excessive removal of subcutaneous fat at the stomal site should be avoided. A cruciate incision should be made in the fascia with cut mode of cautery enough to include two to three fingerbreadths, the rectus muscle should be bluntly retracted medially and laterally along its fibers with an Army-Navy retractor. Care should be taken to avoid the inferior epigastric vessels. The peritoneum should be opened in a similar cruciate fashion while protecting the underlying intra-abdominal cavity, with care not to injure intra-abdominal structures. The colon should be gently delivered through the stomal tract, which may be aided by use of a Babcock clamp applied to colon tinea (or divided edge of bowel if an end colostomy is chosen). Great care should be used to avoid excessive traction on the stoma, and to assure the colon is not under tension, constricted heavily by the stomal opening, and the mesentery is not twisted.
  - The colon can be matured as a loop colostomy with use of a bridge.
  - If a colon resection is done for additional injuries, an end colostomy can be made instead, with or without a mucous fistula, depending on the location after addressing facial closure.
  - If surgery is performed as part of a damage control procedure, the colon can be stapled off at an appropriate site to avoid ongoing contamination of the extraperitoneal space, and the colostomy matured at a subsequent staged operation.
  - If done laparoscopically, the abdomen should be assessed for any additional injuries. The colon should be grasped atraumatically with two graspers and brought up to the lower abdominal wall. Mobilization should occur if needed laparoscopically along the white line of Toldt. Once confirmed that the colon will reach the correct position without tension, make an opening in the abdominal wall as in the open procedure and then pass the colon through it with graspers. Make sure the

mesentery is properly positioned with direct visualization prior to removal of trocars. The ostomy should be matured after closure of incisions.

- Maturation of the ostomy should be done in a modified Brooke fashion. Using electrocautery on cut mode, open the colon on the antimesenteric side along a tineal edge and place four sutures through full thickness of bowel wall, seromuscular layer several centimeters closer to the fascia, and through deep dermal layer of the skin. Tie down after placing all four corner sutures while your assistant everts the mucosal layer to form a rosebud. Use 3-0 or 4-0 Vicryl or chromic sutures. Place additional sutures from the bowel wall to the deep dermal layer to close any gaps where stool could leak into the subcutaneous tissue around the ostomy.

PRESACRAL DRAINS

- Drains are placed less often in the presacral space than in the historic past.
- With the patient in lithotomy position a curved incision is made with No. 15 scalpel posterior to the anal margin skin and anterior to the coccygeal bone.
- Using cautery, the space is entered and guided by digital assistance by feel and use of a hand-held retractor, the post anal and rectal space is entered close to the presacral fascia.
- Penrose open drains or closed suction Blake or Jackson-Pratt drains can be left in situ and secured to skin with 3-0 Nylons.
- The skin is then loosely closed near the drains with similar Nylons in a simple interrupted fashion.
- This procedure can be used in cases of abscesses that do form postoperatively wherein drains have not been left or can be supplanted by use of interventional CT-guided drains for this region.

DISTAL RECTAL WASHOUT

- Initially described for washout of stool from rectum after injury.
- No longer generally recommended.
- Could consider if large amount of stool in rectum preventing adequate visualization on rigid proctoscopy.
- Remove any foreign bodies or large bullet fragments that may promote infection, fistula formation, or delayed healing.

PEARLS AND PITFALLS

- Stomal retraction
- Stomal necrosis
- Failure to recognize pelvic sepsis/the missed injury

POSTOPERATIVE CARE

- Postoperative care is focused on typical advancement of diet following bowel recovery.
- In those patients who are diverted, attention to ostomy viability, stomal appliance fit and function is routine.
- The stoma with delayed function can be carefully digitized by the experienced surgical team member.
- Ostomy appliance teaching should be provided prior to discharge.
- If a bridge was left in place for a loop colostomy for diversion, it may safely be removed by postoperative days 5 to 14 (depending on discharge timing, surgeon preference, and patient body habitus).
- Attention to abdominal wound care is otherwise aimed at monitoring for signs of infection and fascial dehiscence in cases of open surgery.
- Monitoring for signs of pelvic sepsis marked by persistent fevers, tachycardia, leukocytosis, and possible delay of bowel recovery should prompt use of empiric broad-spectrum antibiotics and a low threshold to obtain CT imaging of the abdomen and pelvis with intravenous contrast to assess for intra-abdominal or perirectal abscesses.
- In the diverted patient, a discussion on stomal reversal may be had prior to discharge to assist in managing patient expectations.
- In rare instances wherein presacral drains are placed, these may be removed following full resumption of diet and absent any signs of systemic toxicity provided the drain character is nonpurulent.

Reversal

- The timing of reversal depends on full patient recovery, healing of midline abdominal wounds, and adequate nutritional intake and weight maintenance.
- An assessment of anal continence should be done by history of prior continence issues prior to injury sustained.
- Digital rectal examination should be done assessing for tone.
- If there are any questions in this regard, full anal manometry can be done to confirm anal continence.
- Patients who are otherwise debilitated and nonambulatory for any reason should be rendered with a permanent stoma and are not candidates for reversal.

- Acceptable candidates can undergo barium enema to ensure injury is healed and consider colonoscopy based on patient age and history for preoperative colon cancer screening.

COMPLICATIONS

- The feared complication of rectal injuries is pelvic sepsis, related to abscess formation, sacral osteomyelitis, or fistulas from the rectum to adjacent organs or skin.
- In patients with large perineal wounds, debridement of all nonviable tissue is needed at initial case and may require repeated debridements until clean followed by various closure techniques.
- With any ostomy, there can be retraction, necrosis, or parastomal hernia formation. These complications can be minimized by making sure that the mesentery is in correct orientation, there is not excessive tension on the ostomy, and the fascia opening is big enough to not constrict the ostomy or its blood supply but only large enough to emit the colon.

REFERENCES

1. Moore EE, Cogbill TH, Malangoni MA, et al. Organ injury scaling II: pancreas, duodenum, small bowel, colon and rectum. *J Trauma*. 1990;30:1427-1429.
2. Trust MD, Veith J, Brown CVR, et al; AAST Contemporary Management of Rectal Injuries Study Group. Traumatic rectal injuries: is the combination of computed tomography and rigid proctoscopy sufficient? *J Trauma Acute Care Surg*. 2018;85:1033-1037.
3. Lavenson GS, Cohen A. Management of rectal injuries. *Am J Surg*. 1971;122:226-230.
4. Gonzalez R, Falimirski ME, Holevar MR. The role of presacral drainage in the management of penetrating rectal injuries. *J Trauma*. 1998;45:656-661.
5. Brown CVR, Teixeira PG, Furay E, et al; AAST Contemporary Management of Rectal Injuries Study Group. Contemporary management of rectal injuries at Level 1 trauma centers: the results of an American Association for the Surgery of Trauma multi-institutional study. *J Trauma Acute Care Surg*. 2018;84:225-233.
6. Bosarge PL, Como JJ, Fox N, et al. Management of penetrating extraperitoneal rectal injuries: an Eastern Association for the Surgery of Trauma practice management guideline. *J Trauma Acute Care Surg*. 2016;80:546-551.
7. Gash KJ, Suradkar K, Kiran RP. Rectal trauma injuries: outcomes from the U.S. National trauma Data Bank. *Tech Coloproctol*. 2018;22:847-855.
8. Gonzalez RP, Phelan H, Hassan M, et al. Is fecal diversion necessary for nondestructive penetrating extraperitoneal rectal injuries? *J Trauma*. 2006;61:815-819.
9. Weinberg JA, Fabian TC, Magnotti LJ. Penetrating rectal trauma: management by anatomic distinction improves outcome. *J Trauma*. 2006;60:508-514.
10. Velmahos GC, Gomez H, Falabella A, Demetriades D. Operative management of civilian rectal gunshot wounds: simpler is better. *World J Surg*. 2000;24:114-118.

SECTION VII: Traumatic Injury to the Duodenum and Pancreas

Chapter 26 Operative Management of Duodenal Injury

David I. Hindin and David A. Spain

DEFINITION

- Both penetrating and blunt injuries to the duodenum are rare. Overall, less than 2% of all abdominal traumas involve duodenal injury, and among patients who receive a laparotomy following abdominal trauma, a duodenal injury is appreciated in less than 2% of patients with stab wounds, 5% to 6% of patients with blunt trauma, and 10% to 11% of patients with gunshot wounds.[1,2]
- Despite the rarity of these injuries, duodenal trauma remains the subject of much focus, in part due to the risk of associated major vascular injury, as well as the challenges presented by the complexity of pancreaticoduodenal anatomy. Injuries to the duodenum are most commonly graded by using the AAST Organ Injury Scale (**TABLE 1**).[3]

PATIENT HISTORY AND PHYSICAL FINDINGS

- As with all trauma patients, the initial assessment and management should follow the established protocols defined by the American College of Surgeons Advanced Trauma Life Support (ATLS) guidelines.[4] The patient's airway should be assessed and, if necessary, secured. Breathing, ventilation, and adequate oxygenation must all be confirmed. Hemodynamic status should be evaluated, with consideration that in the earliest stages of hemorrhagic shock, tachycardia may be present in the absence of hypotension.
- Relevant information to collect for blunt trauma patients includes the mechanism of injury (deceleration vs assault), whether the patient sustained a handlebar-type injury, and the estimated speed at impact. Among patients presenting after motor vehicle collisions, additional pertinent details include whether the patient was wearing a seatbelt at the point of impact, whether there was airbag deployment in the vehicle, and whether the patient had to be manually extricated from the vehicle following the incident. If the patient was seated in the driver's seat, information regarding the status of the steering wheel (ie, whether this was damaged during the collision) can also be useful.
- Among patients arriving to the trauma bay after sustaining stab wounds, information about the size and length of knife involved may be helpful. For patients who have sustained gunshot wounds, any available details regarding the direction and source of gunfire may be useful in seeking to understand potential missile trajectories and their associated injuries.
- During physical examination, the surgeon should seek to determine whether the patient exhibits frank peritoneal signs, whether there is evidence of abdominal bruising or abrasion (including the so-called "seatbelt sign"), and for patients of penetrating trauma, whether there is obvious visible violation of fascia. Other more subtle findings may include isolated right upper quadrant tenderness or tenderness localized to the epigastrium.
- A thorough accounting should be made of all stab wounds or gunshot wounds, taking care to recognize that penetrating trauma which is not immediately overlying the abdomen (including the back, chest, and legs) may ultimately result in an intra-abdominal trajectory. Among hemodynamically

Table 1: Duodenum Organ Injury Scale

Grade[a]	Type of injury	Description of injury	AIS-90
I	Hematoma	Involving single portion of duodenum	2
	Laceration	Partial thickness, no perforation	3
II	Hematoma	Involving more than one portion	2
	Laceration	Disruption <50% of circumference	4
III	Laceration	Disruption 50%-75% of circumference of D2	4
		Disruption 50%-100% of circumference of D1, D3, D4	4
IV	Laceration	Disruption >75% of circumference of D2	5
		Involving ampulla or distal common bile duct	5
V	Laceration vascular	Massive disruption of duodenopancreatic complex	5
		Devascularization of duodenum	5

AIS, abbreviated injury score; D1, first portion of duodenum; D2, second portion of duodenum; D3, third portion of duodenum; D4, fourth portion of duodenum.
[a]Advance one grade for multiple injuries up to Grade III.
Reprinted with permission from Moore EE, Cogbill TH, Malangoni MA, et al. Organ injury scaling II: pancreas, duodenum, small bowel, colon, and rectum. J Trauma. 1990;30:1427-1429. Table 2.

stable patients with an odd number of gunshot wounds, it is a helpful practice to briefly gather plain films within the trauma bay to determine the location of retained missiles.

- A key determination during the physical examination is whether to proceed directly to the operating room or not. Penetrating trauma patients who are hemodynamically unstable should be brought directly to the operating room for exploration, as should those with frank abdominal tenderness or obvious fascial violation. Among hemodynamically stable patients who have sustained penetrating trauma, lack abdominal tenderness, and have unclear fascial violation, computed tomography (CT) imaging may be obtained, with variable use of oral and per-rectum contrast, before determining whether to proceed to diagnostic laparoscopy.
- A point-of-care ultrasound (focused assessment with sonography in trauma, or FAST) examination may be helpful in determining the presence of intra-abdominal fluid and the role for operative exploration in hemodynamically unstable blunt trauma patients. Among hemodynamically unstable blunt trauma patients who have an equivocal FAST examination, some clinicians may elect to perform a diagnostic peritoneal lavage in determining whether to proceed to operative exploration.

IMAGING AND OTHER DIAGNOSTIC STUDIES

- The majority of traumatic duodenal injuries following penetrating trauma are discovered at the time of laparotomy: often, these patients have not undergone preoperative imaging. However, among penetrating trauma population with duodenal injuries that are captured on CT, a variety of findings may suggest the diagnosis. It should be noted that whenever possible, CT imaging for patients with potential duodenal injury should include both oral and intravenous (IV) contrast.
- A duodenal hematoma may be suggested by the presence of isolated wall thickening. In the case of perforation, oral contrast extravasation may be observed either into the retroperitoneum or the general intraperitoneal space. Extravasation of IV contrast may be seen as well, immediately adjacent to the site of injury. Due to the partially retroperitoneal nature of the duodenum, injury may be exhibited as isolated retroperitoneal air—or, in contrast, free air within the abdomen.[5]
- CT findings consistent with blunt duodenal injury may include the above findings, as well as wall thickening or a "coiled spring" sign suggestive of intramural hematoma within D2 or D3. These injuries can also be associated with a flexion/distraction fracture of L1-L2 (so-called "Chance fracture") which may be seen on imaging, as well.[6,7]
- With the exception of frank extravasation of contrast from the duodenum, no imaging finding is pathognomonic for duodenal injury; a high index of suspicion is therefore paramount.

SURGICAL MANAGEMENT

- The patient is positioned supine on the operating room table. Broad-spectrum antibiotics are administered. Anesthesia is induced, and the patient is intubated. A Foley is placed. Both arms are left out, and the patient is prepped and draped from the chin to knees in standard trauma fashion. Some practitioners advocate lithotomy positioning if a rectal injury is suspected.
- A generous midline incision is carried out from xiphoid to pubis. A Bookwalter or other self-retraining retractor is inserted. All four quadrants of the abdomen are packed with rolled laparotomy pads. Zones of the retroperitoneum are assessed for overt injury or hematoma. Laparotomy pads are gradually removed from each quadrant, evaluating for bleeding after each quadrant before proceeding to the next.
- In patients with concern for duodenal injury, exposure of the duodenum (inframesocolic Zone I) is carried out, typically beginning with a right medial visceral rotation, or Cattell-Braasch maneuver.[8] The colon is mobilized along the white line of Toldt, followed by the hepatic flexure. Right colon and small bowel are mobilized medially. A Kocher maneuver is now performed to fully expose the duodenum (**FIGURE 1**).
- At this point, an assessment of overall injury burden and the patient's hemodynamic status is carried out, in addition to evaluation of the specific duodenal injury. For patients with hemodynamic instability, ongoing transfusion and/or pressor requirement, significant base deficit, or multiple comorbid injuries, a damage control procedure with temporary abdominal closure is performed and the patient is transferred to intensive care unit (ICU) for further resuscitation.
- For patients with isolated injury to the duodenum, a variety of techniques may be used depending on injury grade, surgeon preference, and patient anatomy. These techniques include primary repair, resection and anastomosis, pyloric exclusion, jejunal serosal patch, and use of a jejunal Roux limb.

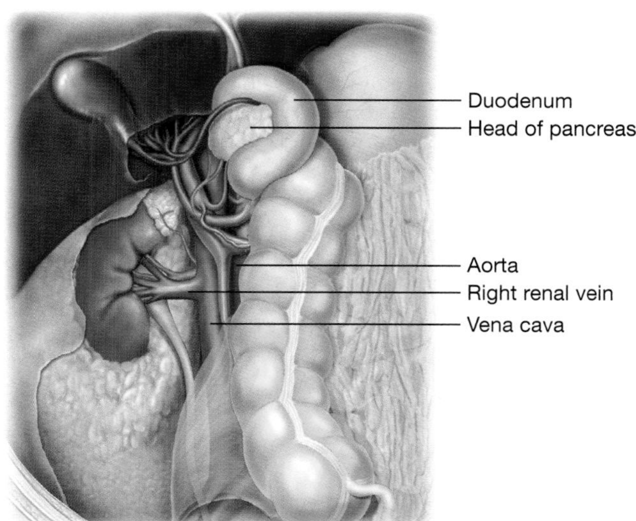

FIGURE 1 • Right medial visceral rotation.

PRIMARY REPAIR

- Patients with Grade II (laceration <50% of circumference) injuries and some Grade III injuries (laceration of 50%-75% of circumference of D2, or 50%-100% of circumference of D1, D3, D4) may be amenable to primary repair.
- An inner layer of interrupted, 3-0 absorbable suture is used to close the defect in transverse fashion. This is followed with an outer layer of interrupted 3-0 silk suture. One layer closure using 3-0 PDS is an option as well. Some surgeons also advocate mobilizing a flap of omentum to cover this repair.[7] In distal D2 or proximal D3 injuries, it is critical to ensure the major papilla has not been involved with the injury. For these defects, the papilla should be palpated and examined for injury prior to addressing the defect. In situations when it is difficult to locate the papilla, some surgeons will perform an open cholecystectomy and pass a small catheter through the common bile duct (via the cystic duct) to aid in localizing the papilla.

RESECTION AND ANASTOMOSIS

- For injuries distal to D3 and D4 that are not amenable to primary repair, resection and anastomosis may be considered.
- An intestinal load GIA stapler is used (two rows of titanium staples, closed staple size 1.5 mm) to divide proximal and distal to the defect.
- Intervening mesentery is divided with a vessel-sealing device, completing the resection.
- The ends are brought side by side. A seromuscular fixation stitch is used along the adjacent antimesenteric borders.
- A small corner of the staple line along each antimesenteric border is now excised from each end.
- Another intestinal load GIA stapler is now inserted and fired, creating a common channel. A TIA stapler can be used to complete the anastomosis or it can be oversewn (**FIGURE 2**).

A

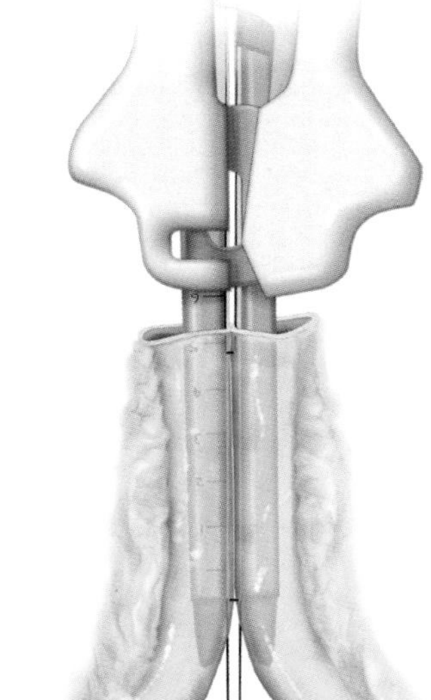

B

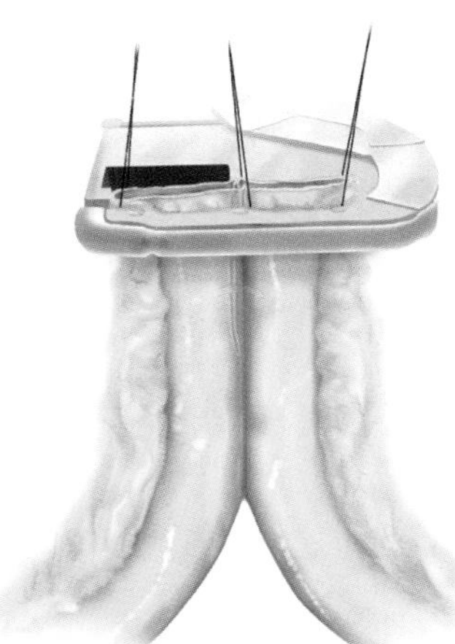

FIGURE 2 ● Duodenal anastomosis following resection. **A,** A GIA stapler is inserted and fired, creating a common channel. **B,** A TIA stapler is shown completing the anastomosis.

JEJUNAL SEROSAL PATCH

- In defects of the duodenum that have too much tissue loss to consider primary repair but are not amenable to resection and anastomosis, a jejunal serosal patch can be a useful option.[9]
- The defect is debrided to healthy tissue. An adjacent loop of distal jejunum is now brought antecolic and positioned to lie adjacent to the defect. Interrupted, serosa-to-serosa sutures are used to close the defect.
- Typically, a drain is left adjacent to this repair. Jejunal serosal patches are less commonly performed in recent years, with a Roux limb of jejunum (see section that follows) increasingly being used to address similar defects (**FIGURE 3**).

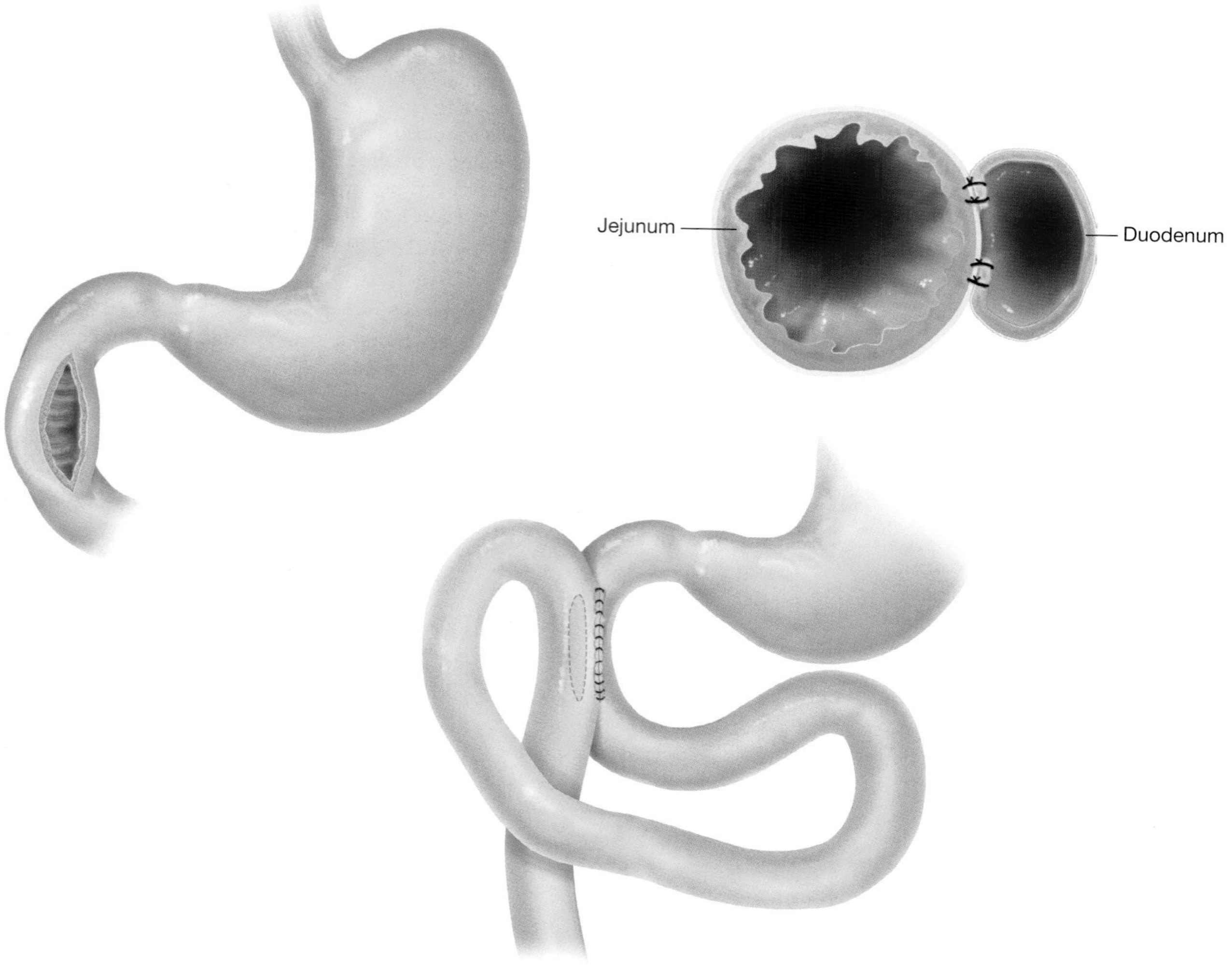

FIGURE 3 ● Jejunal serosal patch.

JEJUNAL ROUX LIMB REPAIR

- For a large duodenal defect that does not involve the papilla, but is not amenable to primary repair, addressing the defect with a jejunal Roux limb is increasingly gaining popularity. This is also seen as a useful adjunct to address narrowing of the duodenum caused by a primary repair carried out at the index damage control laparotomy.[2]
- Edges of the duodenal defect are debrided to healthy tissue. A 40-cm Roux limb of jejunum is created and passed through a defect in the transverse mesocolon. The hood of this Roux limb is now brought over the duodenal defect. A two-layer, side-to-end duodenojejunostomy is carried out, using 3-0 absorbable suture for the inner mucosal layer and an outer layer of interrupted 3-0 silk. An end-to-side jejunojejunostomy is now performed, once again with an inner layer of 3-0 absorbable suture and an outer layer of interrupted, 3-0 silk (**FIGURE 4**).

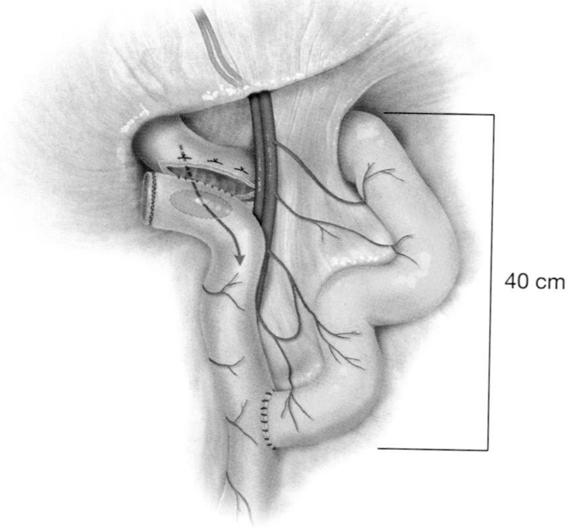

FIGURE 4 ● Roux-en-y duodenojejunostomy.

PYLORIC EXCLUSION

- Pyloric exclusion is considered when an existing duodenal repair is felt to be at risk for narrowing or potential breakdown (and risk for subsequent duodenal fistula). In these scenarios, a pyloroplasty may be performed, along with a diverting gastrojejunostomy.
- A portion of the greater curvature of the stomach is cleared of tissue and the overlying short gastric vessels or branches of gastroepiploic vessels are divided. A dependent gastrotomy is carried out and the pyloric muscle is grasped with babcocks and pulled toward the gastrotomy. A series of #1 polypropylene sutures are used to oversew the pylorus. In an alternative stapled approach, the pylorus may instead be closed by firing a single staple load (typically a TA-50) across the pylorus, followed by gastrojejunostomy creation (see section that follows).
- Next, a loop of jejunum is brought antecolic and positioned to lie adjacent to the gastrotomy. If the pylorus was closed with a stapled approach, a gastrostomy is made along the greater curvature of the stomach. A gastrojejunostomy is created, with an inner layer of 3-0 resorbable suture and an outer layer of 3-0 silk suture. The site of the duodenal repair is drained widely. Some surgeons elect to leave a drain adjacent to the gastrojejunostomy, as well (**FIGURE 5**). A second option for pyloric exclusion is to fire a TA-30 stapler distal to the pylorus

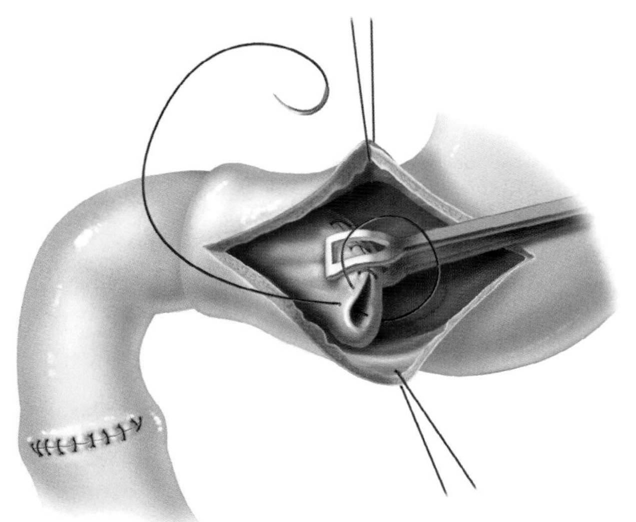

FIGURE 5 ● Pyloric exclusion.

FEEDING JEJUNOSTOMY TUBE

- As described in the previous secions, the initial operation for some patients with duodenal trauma may be a damage control procedure with temporary abdominal closure only.
- At the time of definitive repair however, a feeding jejunostomy tube is frequently placed.

PEARLS AND PITFALLS

Pearls	■ For any major duodenal repair, enteral access must be a consideration. Whether this is a feeding jejunostomy, a nasogastric tube, etc., a surgeon should not leave the operating room following definitive repair without a plan in place for enteral access. ■ Less is often better. In general, the minimum repair is typically the safest. When an isolated duodenal injury is amenable to primary repair, for instance, this is often the best approach. ■ In contrast, a complex repair, such as a trauma pancreaticoduodenectomy, should almost never be attempted in the acute setting.
Pitfalls	■ Inadvertently narrowing the duodenum during primary repair. ■ Inadequate drainage of duodenal repair. ■ Not securing enteral access at time of definitive repair. ■ Doing too much: in an unstable patient, the focus should be on damage control with prompt transfer to the ICU for further resuscitation. ■ Attempting a complex reconstruction in the acute setting leads to increased risk of morbidity and mortality.

POSTOPERATIVE CARE

- Postoperatively, patients are kept NPO on IV fluids, with a nasogastric tube in place until demonstrated return of bowel function.

COMPLICATIONS

- Missed enterotomy
- Missed pancreatic injury
- Risk of duodenal leak and fistula

REFERENCES

1. Malhotra A, Biffl WL, Moore EE, et al. Western trauma association critical decisions in trauma: diagnosis and management of duodenal injuries. *J Trauma Acute Care Surg*. 2015;79(6):1096-1101.
2. Feliciano DV. Abdominal trauma revisited. *Am Surg*. 2017;83(11):1193-1202.
3. Moore EE, Cogbill TH, Malangoni MA, et al. Organ injury scaling II: pancreas, duodenum, small bowel, colon, and rectum. *J Trauma*. 1990;30:1427-1429.
4. Henry S. *ATLS Advanced Trauma Life Support, 10th Edition Student Course Manual*. 10th ed. American College of Surgeons; 2018.
5. Jayaraman MV, Mayo-Smith WW, Movson JS, Dupuy DE, Wallach MT. CT of the duodenum: an overlooked segment gets its due. *Radiographics*. 2001;21 Spec No:S147-S160.
6. LeBedis CA, Anderson SW, Soto JA. CT imaging of blunt traumatic bowel and mesenteric injuries. *Radiol Clin North Am*. 2012;50(1):123-136.
7. Scalea TM, Feliciano DV. *The Shock Trauma Manual of Operative Techniques*, 2nd ed. Pancreas and Duodenum Injuries: Techniques. Springer, 2021; Vol 13: 339-351.
8. Cattell RB, Braasch JW. A technique for the exposure of the third and fourth portions of the duodenum. *Surg Gynecol Obstet*. 1960;111:378-379.
9. McKittrick JE. Use of a serosal patch in repair of a duodenal fistula. clinical application of an experimental method. *Calif Med*. 1965;103(6):433.

Chapter 27

Pancreas: Drainage, Distal Pancreatectomy/Splenectomy

Kojo Wallace, Randi N. Smith, and Christopher J. Dente

DEFINITIONS

- Blunt and penetrating abdominal trauma can be associated with injuries to the pancreas.
- While nonoperative management of minor pancreatic injuries is generally straightforward, the management of major pancreatic injuries which involve the pancreatic duct often requires more complex surgical intervention.
- For major injuries outside the head of the pancreas, both simple pancreatic drainage and resection in the form of distal pancreatectomy are surgical options for management.
- For the latter technique, both splenectomy and splenic preservation have been described.

INDICATIONS

- While there are multiple considerations in the management of distal pancreatic injuries, the two most important are the presence of pancreatic duct disruption and the hemodynamic status of the patient. For patients in extremis or with multiple injuries, pancreatic drainage is an option for all grades of injury, although this will likely commit the patient to a pancreatic fistula. Therefore, distal pancreatectomy for AAST Grade III and higher injuries is generally preferred (**TABLE 1**).
- Preservation of the spleen may be considered in the setting of trauma, assuming the patient's injury is relatively isolated and the patient's hemodynamic status is reasonable. Preservation of the spleen adds a layer of technical difficulty and a significant amount of time to the procedure. In a patient with multiple injuries that require active management and those who are requiring ongoing resuscitation, a splenectomy is indicated. In adults, the risk of overwhelming postsplenectomy infection (OPSI) is sufficiently low to warrant this life saving maneuver.

PATIENT HISTORY, PHYSICAL FINDINGS, AND DIAGNOSIS

- A high index of suspicion is required for diagnosis given the significant morbidity of a missed injury.
- With penetrating trauma, pancreatic injury is generally diagnosed on laparotomy. A thorough examination of the lesser sac is imperative during exploration. After blunt injury, diagnosis may be made during emergent operative intervention or on cross-sectional imaging as discussed below. Generally, direct, high-energy transfer to the upper abdomen is the typical cause of injury to the pancreas, given its relatively protected retroperitoneal location.
- Once pancreatic injury is identified, either on imaging or during laparotomy, the surgeon must next determine the integrity of the pancreatic duct. Pancreatic duct disruption is best treated with resection if the injury is to the left of the superior mesenteric vein. This is discussed further below.
- Physical examination findings may include abdominal bruising such as "seatbelt sign," peritonitis, and hemodynamic instability.

IMAGING AND OTHER DIAGNOSTIC STUDIES

- Computed tomography (CT) with intravenous (IV) contrast is generally a reliable study for intraperitoneal or retroperitoneal injuries and is indicated in stable patients who do not require immediate surgical exploration. However, this modality may miss minor pancreatic injuries[1]; clues such as air and fluid collections in the lesser sac may aid in diagnosis (**FIGURE 1**). Major pancreatic injuries are generally visualized as pancreatic parenchymal lacerations with surrounding free fluid.
- Ultrasound/E-FAST examinations are commonly performed in initial trauma evaluations but are not useful to identify injuries to the pancreas, due to its retroperitoneal location.
- As mentioned earlier, the intraoperative evaluation of ductal integrity is one of the key aspects that determine management. Examination of the injury may allow a surgeon to determine an obvious injury to the duct (eg, complete transection of the parenchyma). Further examination under loupe magnification in a stable patient may allow for identification of clear pancreatic fluid drainage from the injured organ. Unfortunately, intraoperative pancreatography is often impractical during laparotomy for trauma. Either endoscopic or direct transduodenal ampullary cannulation may be considered in a hemodynamically stable patient but these are often difficult to organize and, in the latter case, require an otherwise unnecessary enterotomy. Finally, a needle cholecystocholangiogram

Table 1: Pancreatic Grading System and Recommended Management

Grade	Findings	Treatment
1	Superficial laceration or small hematoma without injury to pancreatic duct	Drainage
2	Major laceration or contusion without injury to pancreatic duct	Drainage
3	Distal parenchymal injury with injury to pancreatic duct	Distal pancreatectomy
4	Proximal parenchymal injury involving pancreatic duct	Distal pancreatectomy if left of superior mesenteric vein (SMV) Closed suction drainage if right of SMV
5	Extensive injury of pancreatic head	Drainage with or without pyloric exclusion Pancreaticoduodenectomy

Reprinted with permission from Moore EE, Cogbill TH, Malangoni MA, et al. Organ injury scaling, II: Pancreas, duodenum, small bowel, colon, and rectum. J Trauma. 1990;30(11):1427-1429. Table 1.

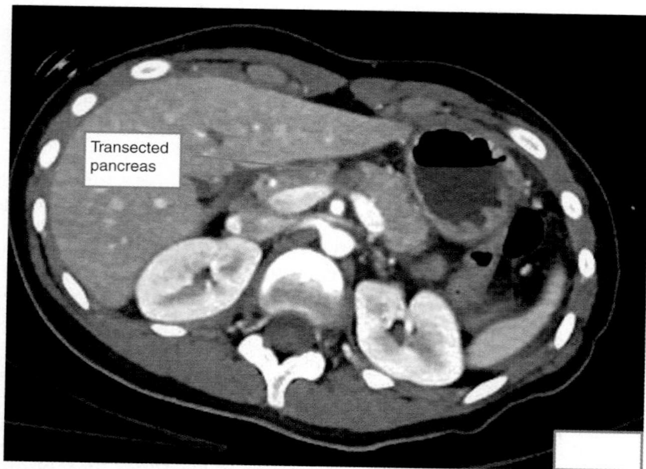

FIGURE 1 ● Computed tomography scan image of a transected pancreas. This modality may miss minor pancreatic injuries; clues such as air and fluid collections in the lesser sac may aid diagnoses in such cases.

is another described and simpler technique, but often does not visualize the pancreatic duct.

- Postoperative MRCP and/or ERCP may be used if there is concern about a missed pancreatic ductal injury, such as in a patient with persistent abdominal pain, elevated pancreatic enzymes, and nonspecific CT findings. It may also be used to determine the extent of known injury or provide a therapeutic option for patients with persistent pancreatic fistulas.

SURGICAL MANAGEMENT

Preoperative Management

- The suspected injury, anticipated procedure, need for special equipment such as stapling devices, potential need for transfusion, and/or imaging should be communicated with the operating room team and anesthesiologists.

Positioning

- The patient should be supine with both arms extended to allow access for IVs; they should also be exposed and prepped from the chin to knees as per trauma protocols.

STEPS

- Exploratory laparotomy is indicated for patients with suspected pancreatic injury; this is performed through a generous midline incision in the acute setting; however, an upper midline incision may be considered with caudal extension of the incision as indicated. In the acute setting, all quadrants of the abdominal cavity are inspected on entry—per trauma protocols—to identify and control other potential causes of instability/peritonitis such as hemorrhage or leakage from a hollow viscus.
- The pancreas is located in the lesser sac; it must be completely exposed to perform adequate evaluation for potential injury. The gastrocolic ligament inferior to the gastroepiploic vessels is divided to enter the lesser sac; this is facilitated by elevating and retracting the stomach and transverse colon to place tension on the gastrocolic ligament (**FIGURE 2**). A relatively thinned portion of the ligament is usually a safe entry point and can be extended to widely open the lesser sac. The anterior surface of the pancreas and the borders of the body and tail can then be visualized. Any posterior adhesions between the posterior wall of stomach and the anterior surface of pancreas may be lysed, and a malleable retractor may be used to facilitate anterior retraction of the stomach.
- The splenic vessels may be quickly accessed at this point in the procedure, as needed, along the superior border of the pancreas.
- A generous Kocher maneuver will allow complete visualization of the pancreatic head and uncinate process. This should be performed to confirm there is no associated pancreatic head injury. In some instances, mobilization of the hepatic flexure may be indicated to achieve this goal.
- Exposure of the splenic hilum and subsequent medial mobilization allows visualization of both spleen and posterior aspect of the pancreatic tail. Alternatively, if pancreatic injury is obvious, transection of the pancreas may be performed prior to splenic mobilization.
- If a splenectomy is to be performed, mobilization of this organ proceeds with division of the gastrosplenic ligament and short gastric vessels, as well as the splenocolic, splenorenal, and splenodiaphragmatic ligaments. These vessels may be clamped and tied and or controlled with a vessel sealing

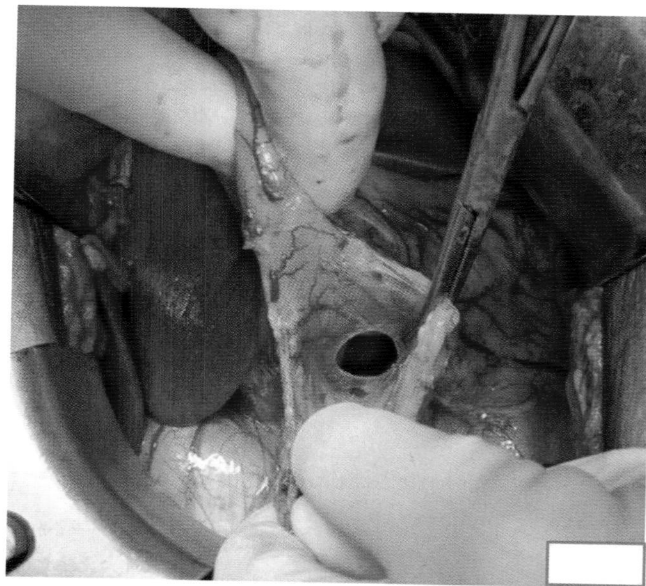

FIGURE 2 ● The gastrocolic ligament inferior to the gastroepiploic vessels is divided to enter the lesser sac; this is facilitated by elevating and retracting the stomach and transverse colon to place tension on the gastrocolic ligament.

device. After traumatic injury, a dissecting hematoma along this plane may facilitate relatively rapid blunt dissection; this can be achieved by "cupping" along superolateral border of the spleen and gently pulling it inferiorly.

- At this stage, if there is no concern for a ductal injury (Grade 1 or 2), management consists of hemostasis and closed suction drainage (**FIGURE 3**).
- The superior mesenteric vessels are located posteriorly and are a landmark defining the junction of the pancreatic head and body and, thus, the proximal and distal pancreas (**FIGURE 4A**). The surgeon is usually able to slide their fingers posterior to the pancreas at this location, elevating pancreas from the major vessels and demarcating a point of resection. This can be facilitated by dissecting along the avascular inferior border of pancreas to get into posterior plane behind the gland.

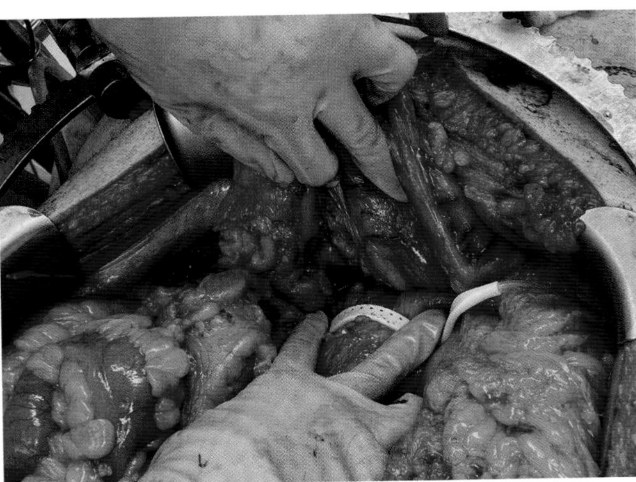

FIGURE 3 ● Closed suction drain is placed in lesser sac, anterior to the pancreas, to drain any accumulated pancreatic fluid or blood.

- When the spleen is to be preserved, fine ties and clips may be used to ligate pancreatic branches of these major vessels as dissection is carried toward the splenic hilum, at which point the pancreatic tail is removed. The IMV has a somewhat variable location and may be ligated if found lateral to the location of injury/lesion; otherwise, it should be preserved.
- The pancreas may be transected with a GIA or TA stapler or may simply be divided sharply and the raw end oversewn. A stapling device transects and closes the parenchyma in one step and is probably a simpler technique (**FIGURE 4B**). Sharp transection requires interlocking full thickness "U" stitches with nonabsorbable sutures to close the parenchyma (**FIGURE 4C**). With either technique the pancreatic duct should be identified and suture ligated as well if possible (**FIGURE 4D**). Unfortunately, the distal pancreatic duct in a normal pancreas is oftentimes not well visualized. Leak rates are equivalent with either technique. The splenic artery and vein are typically stapled prior to pancreatic resection.
- Additional buttressing with omentum or surgical glue has failed to show any benefit in leak rates, which approach 20% regardless of technique.[2] Therefore, routine drainage is recommended. Once resection is complete, a final check for hemostasis should be performed. Postoperative bleeding complications are most common from the short gastric vessels if splenectomy has been performed.

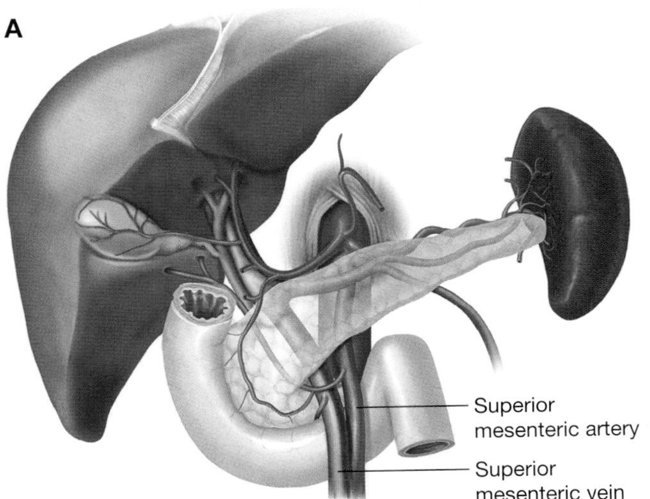

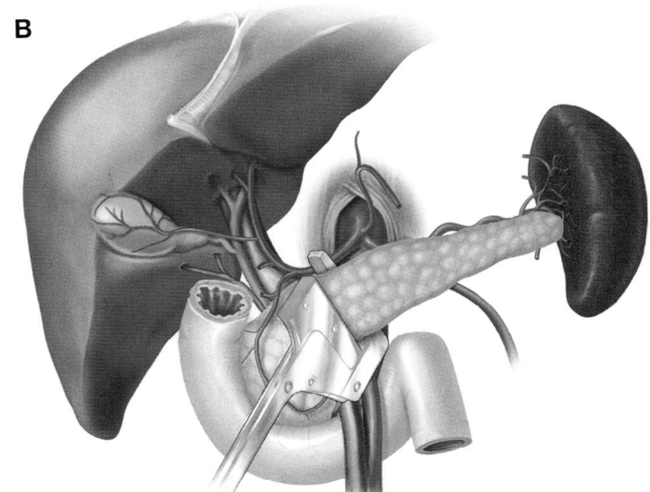

FIGURE 4 ● **A,** The superior mesenteric vessels are located posterior to the pancreas and are a landmark defining the junction of the pancreatic head and body and, thus, the proximal and distal pancreas. **B,** A "TA stapler" may be used to transect the pancreas. This may be a simpler technique, as parenchyma is transected, and edges approximated in one step.

PEARLS AND PITFALLS

- The most important determinations of treatment of distal pancreatic injuries are the presence or absence of pancreatic duct injury and the patient's hemodynamic status.
- Resection for injuries left of the SMV is indicated whenever pancreatic ductal injury is discovered or strongly suspected.
- Splenic preservation is desirable if possible, but commonly splenectomy is performed to expedite patient management.
- Complete exposure of the pancreas should be performed to decrease incidence of missed injury.
- Closed suction drains are important in the management of pancreatic injuries, whether or not resection is performed, as fistula rates are high. Fistulas, should they occur, are most often self-limited.
- Carefully examine the short gastric vessel ligations to prevent postoperative hemorrhage. Consideration of using Lembert sutures to invaginate the vessel stumps into the stomach wall is recommended.
- Postsplenectomy vaccinations should be administered in effort to mitigate OPSI (if splenectomy is performed).

POSTOPERATIVE CARE

- Standard post laparotomy care is indicated. Gastric dilatation early after injury may contribute to postoperative short gastric hemorrhage and should be avoided.
- Drain care: Drain is usually kept for 7 to 10 days to monitor for leaks; it may also be kept until the patient is tolerating a diet. Drain amylase is measured on day 3 for evidence of a leak; defined by drain amylase >3× serum level.[3]
- Vaccinations: If splenectomy is performed, vaccinations for encapsulated bacteria are performed 2 weeks after surgery or at discharge.

COMPLICATIONS

- A fistula is the most common complication following pancreatic injury, with studies citing an incidence range of 5% to 37%.[4] These are usually minor and self-limited. A closed suction drain aids in diagnosis and may be the only treatment required.
- Abscess formation may cause significant morbidity and may be more likely in the setting of associated hollow viscus injuries.
- Acute pancreatitis occurs uncommonly and is usually self-limited.
- Secondary hemorrhage may occur in the setting of infections, abscess, or inadequate drainage; these bleeding complications may be amenable to IR embolization, but may require reexploration.
- Pseudocysts may form and require internal drainage and/or ERCP.

REFERENCES

1. Phelan HA, Velmahos GC, Jurkovich GJ, et al. An evaluation of multidetector computed tomography in detecting pancreatic injury: results of a multicenter AAST study. *J Trauma*. 2009;66:641Y64.
2. Peck GL, Blitzer DN, Bulauitan CS, et al. Outcomes after distal pancreatectomy for trauma in the modern era. *Am Surg*. 2016;82(6):526-532. PMID: 27305885.
3. International Study Group on Pancreatic Surgery (ISGPS); Bassi C, Marchegiani G, Dervenis C, et al. The 2016 update of the International Study Group (ISGPS) definition and grading of postoperative pancreatic fistula: 11 Years after. *Surgery*. 2017;161(3):584-591. doi:10.1016/j.surg.2016.11.014. Epub 2016 Dec 28. PMID: 28040257.
4. Agarwal H, Gupta A, Kumar S. An overview of pancreatic trauma. *J Pancreatol*. 2020;3(3):139-146. doi:10.1097/JP9.0000000000000044

SECTION VIII: Traumatic Injury to the Spleen and Liver

Chapter 28 Splenic Injury: Splenectomy and Splenorrhaphy

Lucy Ruangvoravat and Kimberly A. Davis

DEFINITION

- Splenic injury can be blunt or penetrating and involve injury to either the splenic parenchyma or hilar vessels.
- These injuries can cause hemorrhage and hematoma formation. Injuries are graded on a scale of severity and may require repair, splenectomy, or occasionally damage control techniques.
- Many splenic injuries may be managed nonoperatively or in conjunction with angioembolization depending on the hemodynamic status of the patient. However, on average, 30% of patients with splenic trauma will present with hemorrhagic shock and require urgent splenectomy.

DIFFERENTIAL DIAGNOSIS

- Splenic injury may be present any time there is impact to the torso with blunt trauma, often in association with left-sided rib fractures.
- Splenic injury also can be present in penetrating injuries with thoracoabdominal trajectory.

PATIENT HISTORY AND PHYSICAL FINDINGS

- Traumatic splenic injury can present in isolation or in combination with other solid organ injury such as the liver, kidney, or pancreas.
- The spleen is contained within the lower portion of the ribs and fractures of the lower left ribs should increase suspicion for splenic injury in blunt or penetrating mechanisms.
- Depending on the extent of hemorrhage, patient vital signs may be variable. However, tachycardia and hypotension should prompt a rapid evaluation for clinically significant hemorrhage.
- The abdominal examination is a crucial step in assessing for splenic injury. Tenderness in the left upper quadrant should increase suspicion. Peritonitis can be present due to bleeding from the splenic parenchyma or hilum but is absent in 30% of patients with hemoperitoneum. Physical examination cannot differentiate peritonitis from hemoperitoneum due to perforated viscus, however.

IMAGING AND OTHER DIAGNOSTIC STUDIES

- Ultrasound is often the first imaging modality utilized in splenic injury due to its ability to be performed at the bedside. This is typically within the focused assessment with sonography for trauma (FAST) examination, which assesses for free fluid within the peritoneum in four views. Any blunt injury patient with hemodynamic instability who has free fluid present within the abdomen should proceed to laparotomy without delay or further imaging.[2] If no signs of shock are present, patients with hemoperitoneum can undergo further workup prior to determining whether laparotomy is indicated. The presence of hemoperitoneum may be from a broad array of injuries, and further diagnostic testing is needed to determine the source of abdominal hemorrhage.
- Cross-sectional imaging with computed tomography (CT) imaging allows for the diagnosis and grading of splenic injuries (**TABLE 1**). CT is indicated in patients with abdominal pain or tenderness, patients who cannot participate in an abdominal examination, stable patients with blunt injury and free fluid seen on FAST examination, or patients who have penetrating wounds to the left thoracoabdominal area without other clear need for immediate laparotomy. Evaluation of splenic injury, as with all blunt injuries, is augmented with the use of arterial contrast to assess for active bleeding. If extravasation of contrast is present or a parenchymal pseudoaneurysm (**FIGURE 1**) is identified, angioembolization should be considered as a therapeutic modality (**TABLE 2**).

CT Image of Grade V Splenic Injury

- Angiography with embolization is utilized when the patient is hemodynamically normal and does not have other injuries that require immediate laparotomy.
- Angioembolization allows the patient to keep the immune function of the spleen. Nonoperative management has a reported success rate of >92% in the literature.[2] Failure of nonoperative management may occur in a small percentage of patients who will go on to require splenectomy (**FIGURE 2**).[3,4]

Table 1: American Association for the Surgery of Trauma Splenic Injury Scale

AAST grade	AIS severity	Imaging criteria
I	2	• Subcapsular hematoma <10% surface area • Parenchymal laceration <1 cm depth • Capsular tear
II	2	• Subcapsular hematoma 10%-50% surface area, intraparenchymal hematoma <5 cm • Parenchymal laceration 1-3 cm depth
III	3	• Subcapsular hematoma 10%-50% surface area, intraparenchymal hematoma ≥5 cm • Parenchymal laceration >3 cm depth
IV	4	• Any injury in the presence of a splenic vascular injury or active bleeding confined within splenic capsule • Parenchymal laceration involving segmental or hilar vessels producing >25% devascularization
V	5	• Any injury in the presence of splenic vascular injury with active bleeding extending beyond the spleen into the peritoneum • Shattered spleen

AAST, American Association for the Surgery of Trauma; AIS, Adjusted Injury Score.
Adapted from Kozar RA, Crandall M, Shanmuganathan K, et al. Organ injury scaling 2018 update: spleen, liver, and kidney. J Trauma Acute Care Surg. 2018;85(6):1119-1122.

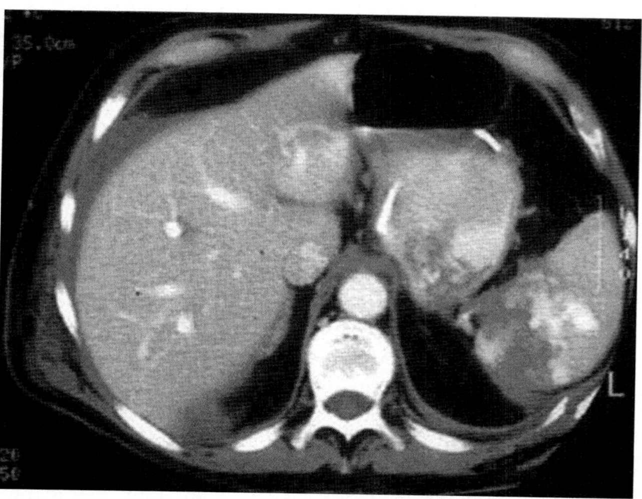

FIGURE 1 ● Pseudoaneurysm.

Table 2: Predictors of Failure of Nonoperative Management on Cross-Sectional Imaging

Imaging finding	Failure rate (%)
Large hemoperitoneum	22.3
Moderate hemoperitoneum	19
Small hemoperitoneum	6
Pseudoaneurysm[5]	6
Arteriovenous fistula[6]	40

Adapted with permission from Peitzman AB, Heil B, Rivera L, et al. Blunt splenic injury in adults: multi-institutional study of the eastern association for the surgery of trauma. J Trauma. 2000;49(2):177-189.

SURGICAL MANAGEMENT

Preoperative Planning

- All patients should have an active type and crossmatch to facilitate rapid transfusion if needed.
- A nasogastric or orogastric tube should be placed for gastric decompression.
- The operating room should be prepped for a patient who may become unstable at any point.
- Nonoperative management of higher grade splenic injuries is feasible but mandates the immediate availability of a surgical team. Hospitals with limited access to operating rooms at night or on the weekend may consider a more liberal surgical approach to splenic injury, specifically for higher grade injuries.

Positioning

- Patient should be positioned supine with arms extended to allow for placement of self-retaining retractor posts and surgical team members. This also allows the anesthesia team to perform venous or arterial cannulation as needed.

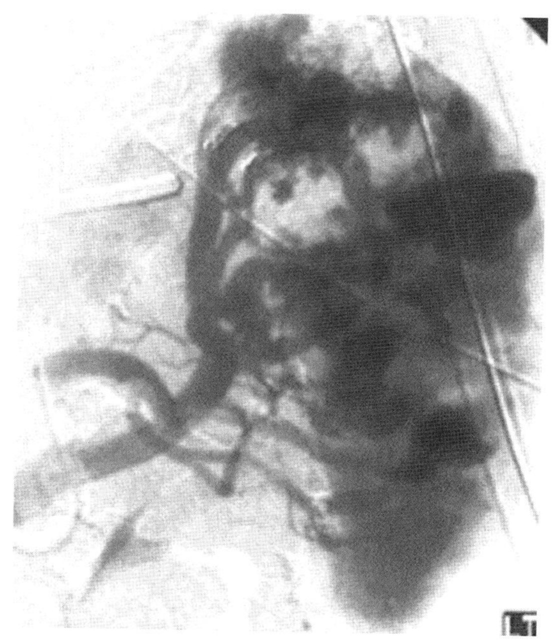

FIGURE 2 ● Computed tomography image of Grade V splenic injury.

SKIN INCISION

- Laparotomy is performed through a midline incision.
- Elective splenectomy is sometimes performed through left subcostal incision, but this does not provide adequate flexibility for laparotomy in trauma as it may impede the management of associated intra-abdominal injuries.
- A midline incision can be extended to the xyphoid for better splenic exposure or inferiorly as needed for evaluation of the entire abdomen and pelvis.

EXPLORATION

- Exploration of the abdomen should be carried out in a systematic fashion to assess for sources of bleeding or contamination. Hemoperitoneum should be evacuated to facilitate visualization. Laparotomy pads should be packed in all four quadrants. These pads should be placed above and below the injured spleen to facilitate tamponade. Specifically for effective splenic packing, pads should be seated firmly between the spleen and both the diaphragm and abdominal sidewall. While these are in place, the bowel can be assessed for injury.
- If significant splenic injury is suspected, pads effectively providing tamponade in the left upper quadrant should be left in place until all others have been removed and injury in other quadrants evaluated. Conversely, if the left upper quadrant is not hemostatic while fully packed, splenectomy should be expedited.

SPLENIC MOBILIZATION

- The spleen sits against the diaphragm deep to the stomach in the abdomen. Avascular attachments suspend the spleen in its anatomic position: the splenophrenic and splenocolic ligaments. The splenocolic ligament attaches the spleen to the splenic flexure of the colon and merges with the splenophrenic as a thin attachment of the spleen to the lateral abdominal wall.
- The surgeon, standing at the patient's right, can use their right hand to slide up the left upper quadrant wall of the abdomen, encountering the spleen (**FIGURE 3**). From here it can easily be delivered toward the surgical field with the surgeon's right hand providing traction for cautery of those attachments if needed. After lateral attachments have been mobilized, there should be an avascular plane which can be manually dissected between the posterior spleen and the retroperitoneum, sometimes referred to as the splenorenal ligament.
- Once those attachments are divided, either with cautery or by finger fracture, the spleen should be mobile within the abdomen. Gentle retraction of the colon caudally and the stomach medially is helpful in these maneuvers.

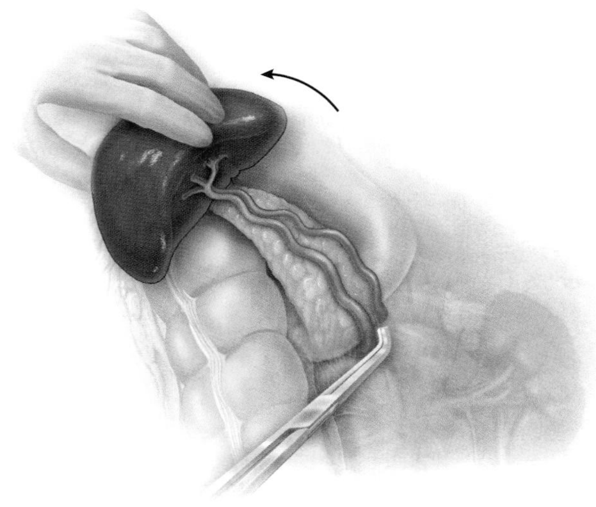

FIGURE 3 ● Mobilization of the spleen from the left upper quadrant to the midline.

SPLENECTOMY

- Once the spleen has been mobilized up and into the midline wound, it can be better visualized and assessed. In cases of ongoing hemorrhagic shock with active splenic hemorrhage, manual compression should be applied to the splenic hilum at the organ's medial aspect to facilitate hemostasis. This will allow some time for resuscitation before the splenectomy is carried out.
- Ligation of the splenic artery can then easily be performed. Care should be taken to avoid the superior border of the pancreas.
- After ligation of the artery, the splenic vein can be ligated at the inferior border of the pancreas. Individual ligation of the vessels is preferred to decrease the theoretical risk of arteriovenous fistula formation.
- At this point the spleen will have the gastrocolic ligament as its remaining attachment. A clear area along the greater curve of the stomach can be identified and entered with cautery. Any visible short gastric vessels should then be divided, completing the splenectomy.
- There are several methods for vascular control. Clamps and ties have traditionally been used but often an energy device or vascular stapler is more efficient in dividing these vessels.

Care should be used to avoid the stomach wall and ensure adequate ligation, particularly along the more proximal portions of the stomach approaching the diaphragm. Here there is less anatomic space. Adequate ligation is necessary to prevent postoperative bleeding.

- The splenic bed should be inspected for hemostasis. The border of the stomach and pancreas should also be reinspected for injury. It is not our practice to leave any drains after splenectomy if there is no suspected pancreatic injury. However, if vessel ligation is proximate to the tail of the pancreas, or there is evidence of associated pancreatic contusion, drain placement is indicated. Inspection of the diaphragm should also be performed to avoid missed injury (**FIGURE 4**).

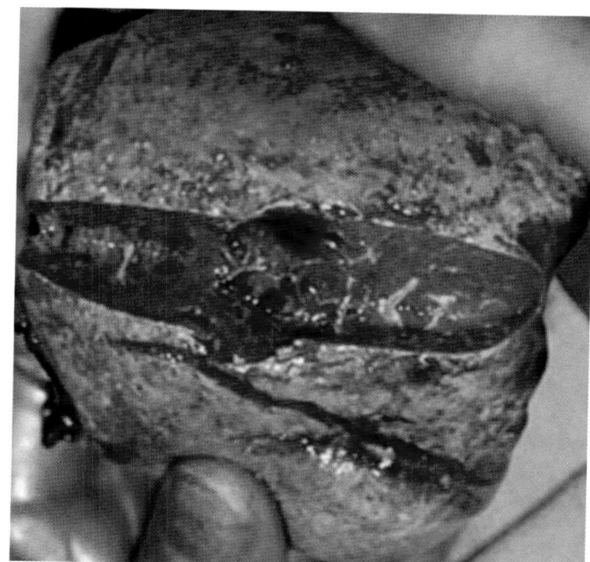

FIGURE 4 ● Pathology specimen: Spleen with traumatic lacerations.

SPLENORRHAPHY

- Particularly in blunt trauma there may be multiple solid organ injuries contributing to hemorrhage. Local control of bleeding from a splenic laceration can be performed in less severe injuries which are not the primary hemorrhage source, provided the patient has reasonable coagulation capabilities. Topical hemostatic agents, cautery, and argon beam can be utilized. These can be augmented by compression with laparotomy pads while resuscitation is ongoing and other bleeding or contamination is addressed.
- If only a pole of the spleen is injured, partial splenectomy can be performed. In this case, the branches of the splenic artery leading to the affected pole are dissected out and individually ligated. Once the injured portion of the spleen is devascularized, it can be resected with either an energy device or a stapler.
- Splenorrhaphy with pledgeted sutures can rarely be carried out for injuries in an isolated pole of the spleen but we find little utility for this in the trauma patient (**FIGURE 5**).
- Mesh splenorrhaphy involves wrapping the injured spleen tightly in absorbable mesh and leaving a keyhole for the splenic artery and vein (**FIGURE 6**). This allows hemostasis via compression from the mesh and reapproximation of the lacerated parenchyma. This technique, however, is time-consuming and can be cumbersome. It is not commonly performed.
- In all cases, if hemorrhage is persistent despite splenic salvage maneuvers or if no other source of bleeding is identified in a patient with signs of hemorrhagic shock, splenectomy should be performed.

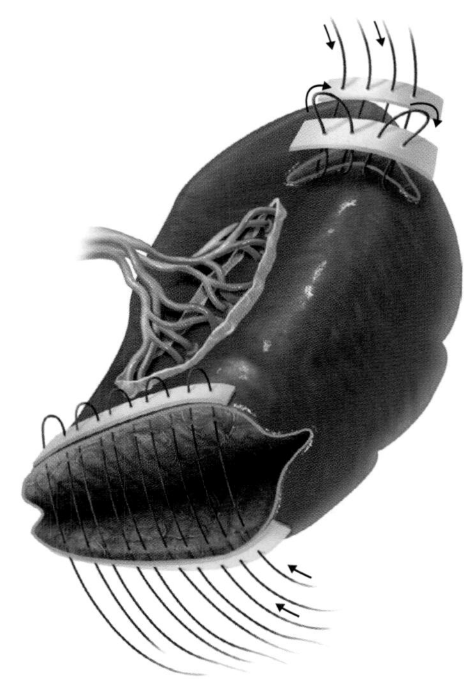

FIGURE 5 ● Splenic repair using pledgets after splenic resection.

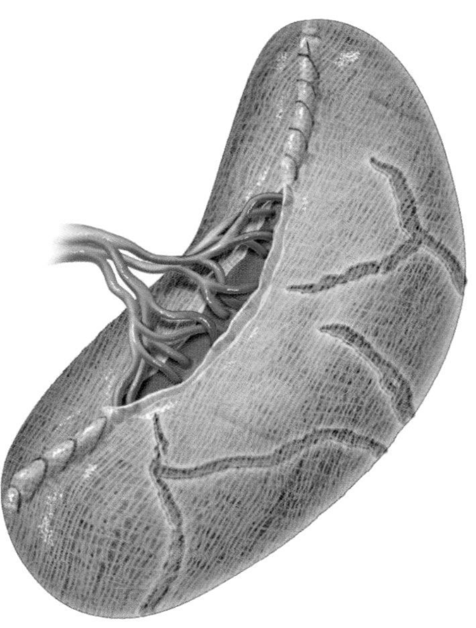

FIGURE 6 ● Mesh splenorrhaphy.

PEARLS AND PITFALLS

- The patient in shock should immediately be taken for laparotomy. If the patient is hemorrhaging from the spleen, then splenectomy should be performed without hesitation or attempts at splenorrhaphy.
- Care should be taken to identify the pancreas. If there is a question of pancreatic injury, a drain should be left.
- Short gastric vessels should be re-examined for hemostasis prior to abdominal closure as they can be a source of postoperative bleeding and return to the operating room.

Postoperative Care

- Patients with splenic injury should be monitored for adequacy of resuscitation. Thrombocytosis due to splenectomy is normal.
- Splenectomy patients who do not have other contraindications can typically have chemical prophylaxis for venous thromboembolism begun within 24 to 48 hours after splenectomy.
- Ileus, particularly gastric, can be common in these patients and patients should be monitored for aspiration risk.
- Early mobilization should be carried out in splenectomy patients to mitigate against both ileus and thromboembolism as well as pulmonary compromise.[7]
- Postsplenectomy patients also need to receive immunizations against pneumococcus, meningococcus, and *Haemophilus influenzae* per CDC guidelines.[8] Common practice in the setting of trauma is to give the initial vaccines prior to the patient's discharge from the hospital.

Complications

- Overwhelming postsplenectomy sepsis is a much-feared complication in asplenic patients, although with low incidence after splenectomy for trauma. It most frequently does not occur for at least 2 years after splenectomy.[9] Risk is minimized by adherence to vaccination schedule and early recognition of asplenia in patients with upper respiratory tract infections.
- Postoperative bleeding after splenectomy should initially be treated with resuscitation and correction of coagulopathy in stable patients. Patients with hemodynamic compromise or lack of response to resuscitation should be returned to the operating room. Short gastric vessels can often be the culprit in postop bleeding secondary to vasodilation associated with postoperative gastric distension.
- Due to its close association with the splenic vessels, any fluid collection in the splenic cavity should raise concern for pancreatic tail injury. Percutaneous image-guided drainage of the collection can be performed. Pancreatic duct stenting has a role in the management of persistent or high-volume pancreatic fistulae.

REFERENCES

1. Kozar RA, Crandall M, Shanmuganathan K, et al. Organ injury scaling 2018 update: spleen, liver, and kidney. *J Trauma Acute Care Surg*. 2018;85(6):1119-1122. doi:10.1097/TA.0000000000002058
2. Requarth JA, D'Agostino Jr RB, Miller PR. Nonoperative management of adult blunt splenic injury with and without splenic artery

embolotherapy: a meta-analysis. *J Trauma.* 2011;71(4):898-903. doi:10.1097/TA.0b013e318227ea50

3. Rowell S, Biffl W, Brasel K, et al. Western trauma association critical decisions in trauma. *J Trauma Acute Care Surg.* 2017;82(4):787-793. doi:10.1097/TA.0000000000001323
4. Peitzman AB, Heil B, Rivera L, et al. Blunt splenic injury in adults: multi-institutional Study of the eastern association for the Surgery of trauma. *J Trauma.* 2000;49(2):177-189. doi:10.1097/00005373-200008000-00002
5. Haan J, Biffl W, Knudson M, et al. Splenic embolization revisited: a multicenter review. *J Trauma Inj Infect Crit Care.* 2004;56(3):542-547. doi:10.1097/01.TA.0000114069.73054.45
6. Davis KA, Fabian TC, Croce MA, et al. Improved success in non-operative management of blunt splenic injuries: embolization of splenic artery pseudoaneurysms. *J Trauma.* 1998;44(6):1008-1015. doi:10.1097/00005373-199806000-00013
7. Fair KA, Connelly CR, Hart KD, Schreiber MA, Watters JM. Splenectomy is associated with higher infection and pneumonia rates among trauma laparotomy patients. *Am J Surg.* 2017;213(5):856-861. doi:10.1016/j.amjsurg.2017.04.001
8. "*CDC Recommendations for Vaccinations in Adults: Asplenia.*" Published May 2, 2016. Accessed September 2, 2021. https://www.cdc.gov/vaccines/adults/rec-vac/health-conditions/asplenia.html
9. Cullingford GL, Watkins DN, Watts AD, Mallon DF. Severe late postsplenectomy infection. *Br J Surg.* 1991;78(6):716-721. doi:10.1002/bjs.1800780626

Chapter 29 Surgical Management of Hepatic Trauma

Walter L. Biffl

DEFINITION

- Hepatic trauma is defined as injury to the liver. It may be associated with hemorrhage, bile leak and bile duct injury, or devitalized tissue. There is a spectrum of severity of liver trauma (**TABLE 1**),[1,2] and a broad range of techniques may be employed to manage various injuries.[2-5]

DIFFERENTIAL DIAGNOSIS

- Abdominal trauma can be associated with injuries to any abdominal organ. Major sources of hemorrhage include solid organs (eg, liver, spleen, kidneys) and blood vessels in the retroperitoneum (eg, aorta, inferior vena cava [IVC], renal vessels) or mesentery. Peritonitis may result from any injury to a hollow viscus (eg, bowel, biliary tree, pancreas), including bile leak from a liver injury.

PATIENT HISTORY AND PHYSICAL FINDINGS

- Liver injuries may occur following either blunt (eg, motor vehicle crash, fall) or penetrating (eg, gunshot or stab wound) trauma to the abdomen.
- The liver is one of the most commonly injured organs following blunt trauma, usually following impact to the lower right chest or the abdomen. Any high-energy mechanism should raise concern of intra-abdominal injury.
- The liver, due to its large surface area, is frequently injured in penetrating abdominal or lower thoracic trauma. The path of gunshot wounds to the torso cannot be determined based on physical examination alone.
- Abdominal pain or tenderness on examination raise concern for abdominal injury; however, patients may have significant liver injuries in the absence of pain or tenderness. Vital signs are a critical component of the assessment of trauma patients, and the decision to proceed with surgical (vs nonoperative) management is primarily based on the physiologic condition of the patient. The large majority of liver injuries are managed nonoperatively.

IMAGING AND OTHER DIAGNOSTIC STUDIES

- Ultrasound—in particular, the extended-focused abdominal sonographic examination for trauma (E-FAST)—is commonly used as an initial triage tool in trauma patients. Following blunt trauma, the finding of free fluid in the abdomen in the presence of shock is an indication to proceed to exploratory laparotomy (LAP) without delay. On the other hand, free fluid in a hemodynamically normal patient does not mandate LAP, as many solid organ injuries will stop bleeding spontaneously and do not require any intervention.
- The E-FAST examination is less useful in penetrating trauma victims. Patients with abdominal gunshot wounds should generally undergo immediate LAP. Those with stab wounds should undergo LAP if they exhibit shock, evisceration, or peritonitis. Otherwise, they should be admitted for serial clinical assessments to detect ongoing hemorrhage or hollow viscus injury. The finding of free fluid on FAST does not mandate LAP in stab wound victims.
- Computed tomography (CT) with intravenous contrast is currently the best diagnostic tool for hepatic injury (**FIGURE 1**). CT is indicated in any patient with major abdominal blunt trauma mechanism, abdominal pain or tenderness, hemoperitoneum on E-FAST examination in a stable patient, pelvic fractures, or the potential for abdominal trauma and the inability to clinically assess the abdominal

Table 1: Grading of Liver Injuries

Grade		Injury description
I	Hematoma	Subcapsular, <10% surface area
	Laceration	<1 cm parenchymal depth
II	Hematoma	Subcapsular, 10%-50% surface area; intraparenchymal, <10 cm diameter
	Laceration	1-3 cm parenchymal depth, <10 cm length
III	Hematoma	Subcapsular, >50% surface area or expanding; intraparenchymal, >10 cm diameter or expanding, or ruptured
	Laceration	>3 cm parenchymal depth
IV	Laceration	Parenchymal disruption involving 25%-75% of hepatic lobe or 1-3 Couinaud segments in a single lobe
V	Laceration	Parenchymal disruption involving >75% of hepatic lobe or >3 Couinaud segments in a single lobe
	Vascular	Juxtahepatic venous injuries
VI	Vascular	Hepatic avulsion

Advance one grade for multiple injuries up to grade III.
Reprinted with permission from Moore EE, Cogbill TH, Jurkovich GJ, et al. Organ injury scaling: spleen and liver (1994 Revision). J Trauma. 1995;38:323-324.

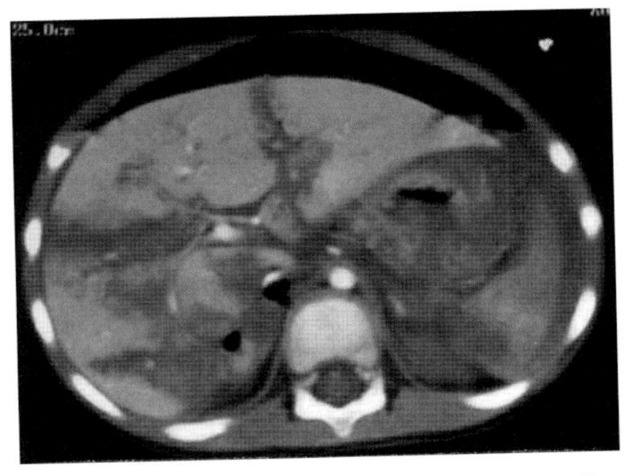

FIGURE 1 • CT scan image of a grade IV liver injury. Despite the extensive injury to the liver, note the relative paucity of blood surrounding the liver. This is a pitfall of FAST ultrasonography, as it detects primarily free fluid. It also speaks to the lack of sensitivity of FAST for individual organ injuries. It detects blood but not the source of the bleeding.

examination (eg, a patient with severe traumatic brain injury following motor vehicle crash).

- The identification of intravenous contrast extravasation on CT warrants consideration of interventional treatment regardless of physiologic condition.
- Arteriography with embolization may be selectively employed as a primary treatment in a stable patient without other indications for LAP. It may also be used as an adjunct to surgical management of liver lacerations with arterial hemorrhage.
- Cholangiography is sometimes useful to determine whether there is biliary injury and ongoing bile leak. This is generally performed later in the postinjury course. The presence of a biliary injury and bile leak generally calls for either surgical or endoscopic intervention.
- Magnetic resonance imaging has little role in the early management of liver trauma.

SURGICAL MANAGEMENT

- Severe abdominal pain or tenderness, peritonitis, evisceration, or shock with a presumed abdominal injury warrant LAP.
- Following stab wounds, the presence of shock, evisceration, or peritonitis is a clear indication for LAP. Gunshot wound to the abdomen, given its high association with significant injury, is an indication for LAP regardless of the initial physical findings. While some centers report reasonable success rates with nonoperative management of isolated penetrating liver injuries, it can be difficult to definitively exclude injuries to the colon, duodenum, gallbladder, or diaphragm without exploration.

Preoperative Planning

- Prior to taking the patient to the OR, the surgeon should communicate with the OR team regarding the suspected diagnoses and planned interventions, anticipated blood loss and transfusion requirements, positioning and incisions, extent of skin preparation, the need for imaging, and any special equipment needs. In a trauma center with a hybrid OR, it may be wise to utilize the room for major abdominal trauma in case angioembolization is necessary. In particular, a patient with abdominal trauma and hemorrhagic shock may prove to be a candidate for adjunctive hepatic artery embolization.

Positioning

- The patient should be positioned supine. It is best to leave both arms out to allow the anesthesiologist's access for venous and arterial catheterization and sampling.

TECHNIQUES

SKIN INCISION

- Exploratory LAP for trauma should be performed through a generous midline abdominal incision. Although it may not initially extend from the xiphoid to pubis, as is classically suggested, once a major liver injury is identified, extension up to the xiphoid process is recommended to afford optimal exposure. Some elective liver surgery is performed through right or bilateral subcostal incisions, with or without cephalad extension in the midline. This may be chosen if the operation is performed later in the patient's clinical course for complications of liver injury, such as hepatic necrosis or bile leak. However, this approach limits access to the lower abdomen. If a midline incision has been made, the surgeon should not hesitate to extend the incision to the right if necessary. Adequate exposure is critical to repairing major hepatic injuries.

ABDOMINAL EXPLORATION

- The initial objective of trauma LAP is to determine if there is exsanguinating hemorrhage and from where it emanates. Blood must be evacuated and the source identified. Primary culprits are solid organs, retroperitoneal blood vessels, and mesentery. The surgeon should be able to rapidly assess the liver for major lacerations, by inspecting it and palpating its surface.

MANUAL COMPRESSION

- The first step in hepatic hemorrhage control is manual compression (**FIGURE 2**). This should be able to control the majority of liver bleeding. The importance of simultaneous aggressive hemostatic resuscitation cannot be overemphasized. Restoration of blood volume and maintenance of tissue perfusion, correction of coagulopathy, and active warming of the patient are critical to avoid the "bloody vicious cycle" that can lead to early mortality.

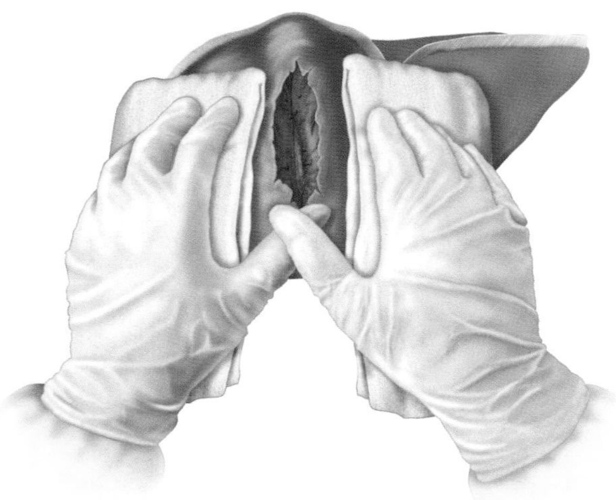

FIGURE 2 • Manual compression of the liver is performed to restore the normal anatomic contour of the liver and tamponade bleeding. This maneuver can control hemorrhage while planning packing or definitive interventions.

PERIHEPATIC PACKING

- Perihepatic packing should be performed in such a manner to maintain hemostatic compression on the liver (**FIGURE 3**). The supporting ligaments of the liver are left intact at the initial stage, as they may provide tamponade of venous bleeding. However, should the patient have stellate lacerations or extensive subcapsular injury, one should not hesitate to mobilize the suspensory ligament of the falciform or the right and left triangular ligaments to allow better exposure. Packing should be performed in a systematic fashion, placing packs between the liver and the abdominal wall, diaphragm, and retroperitoneum.

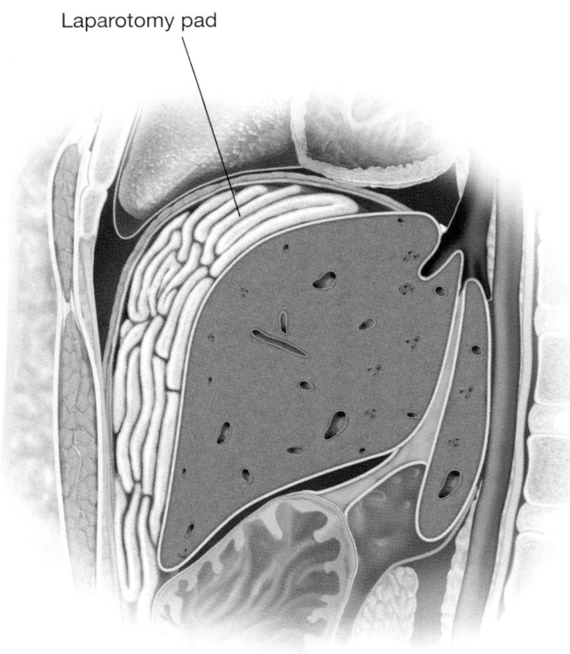

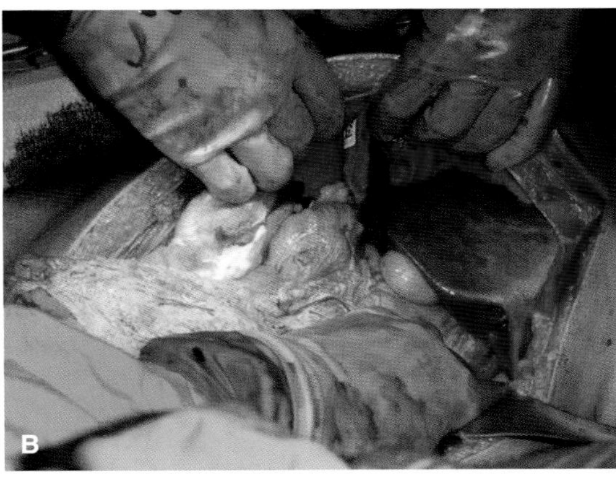

FIGURE 3 • The liver is packed with LAP pads to provide compression against the abdominal wall, diaphragm, and retroperitoneum. **A,** In the sagittal view, packs are present between the liver and the diaphragm and abdominal wall. **B,** In the photograph, the right lobe is compressed by packs.

TOPICAL HEMOSTASIS

- Grade I and II lacerations (see **TABLE 1**) may stop bleeding spontaneously or after a short period of packing (**FIGURE 4**). Ongoing hemorrhage can usually be controlled with electrocautery or argon beam coagulation, with or without application of topical hemostatic agents such as microcrystalline collagen, fibrin glue, or other agents (**FIGURE 5**).

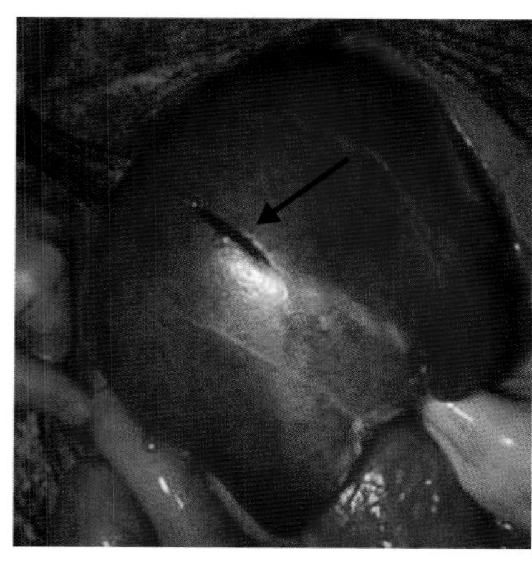

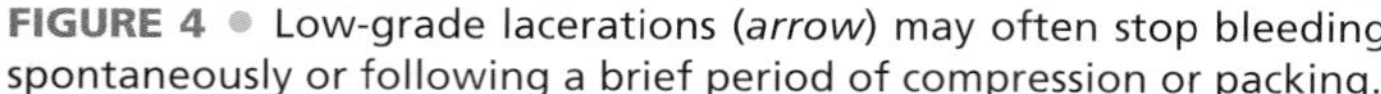

FIGURE 4 ● Low-grade lacerations (*arrow*) may often stop bleeding spontaneously or following a brief period of compression or packing.

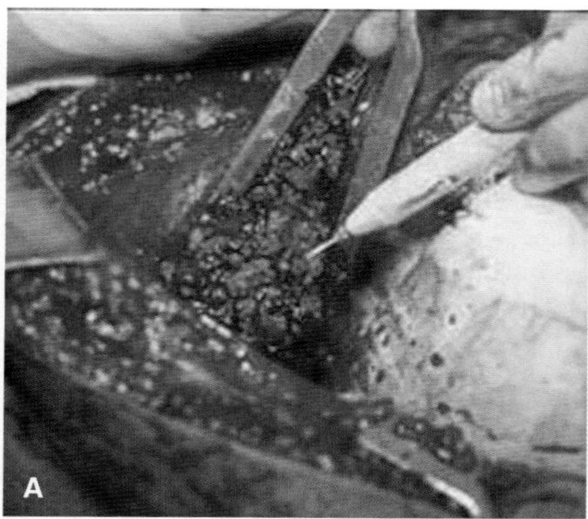

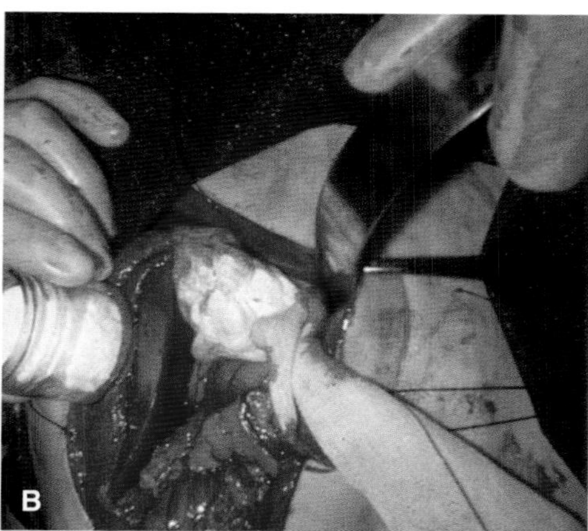

FIGURE 5 ● Low-grade injuries with persistent bleeding may be treated by topical hemostatic techniques such as argon beam coagulation **(A)** or microcrystalline collagen application **(B)**.

DAMAGE CONTROL

- In the physiologically compromised patient, the decision to pursue damage control must be made early in order to optimize the patient's chance of survival. Time-consuming efforts to stop relatively minor bleeding should not distract the surgeon from the primary objective. The liver should be packed quickly and other damage control maneuvers completed prior to a temporary abdominal closure. In order to facilitate later pack removal without disrupting clot, a nonadherent plastic drape such as a 3M 1010 Steri-Drape may be spread over the liver surface, with the packs placed on top of the plastic.

DEEP PARENCHYMAL HEMORRHAGE CONTROL

- If the patient's condition allows, the liver should be examined to determine the extent of the injury. Grade II and III lacerations should be inspected to determine whether a discrete vessel may be ligated (**FIGURE 6**). Bleeding can generally be controlled by packing the wound with an omental pedicle or a plug of topical hemostatic agents such as absorbable gelatin sponge wrapped in oxidized regenerated cellulose (**FIGURE 7**). Suture hepatorrhaphy is an option, but one must avoid leaving a large dead space and avoid devitalizing tissue or lacerating vessels or bile ducts. Extensive lacerations may need to be explored to control major vessels. The finger fracture technique allows one to reach major vessels for ligation (**FIGURE 8**). Stapling devices can also be useful in dividing the hepatic parenchyma to reach deep vessels (**FIGURE 9**).

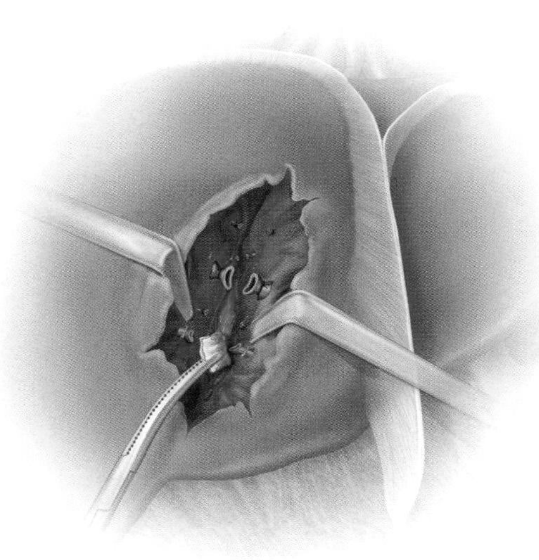

FIGURE 6 ● The laceration should be explored to identify discrete vessels to ligate.

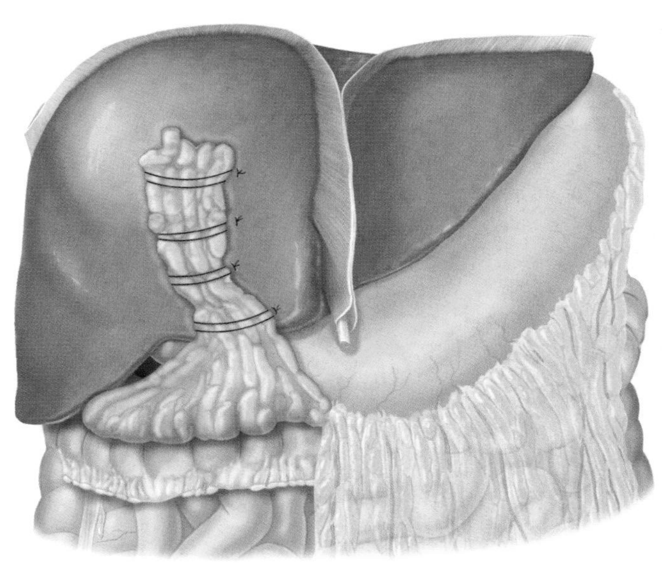

FIGURE 7 ● Omental pedicle packing may provide hemostasis for deeper injuries.

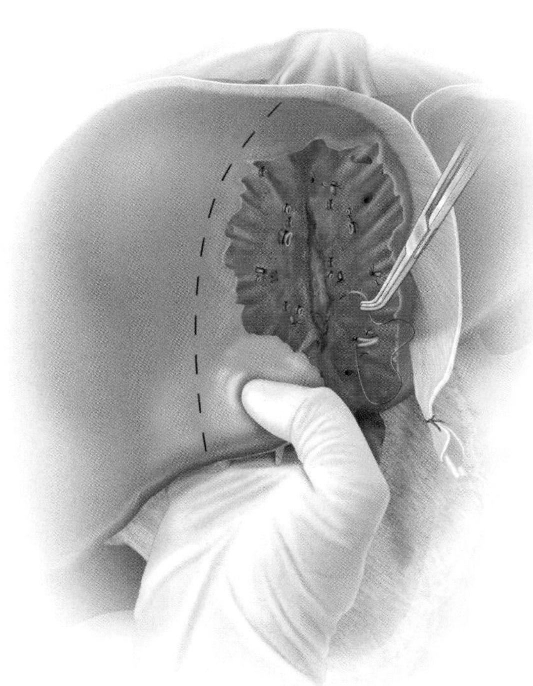

A

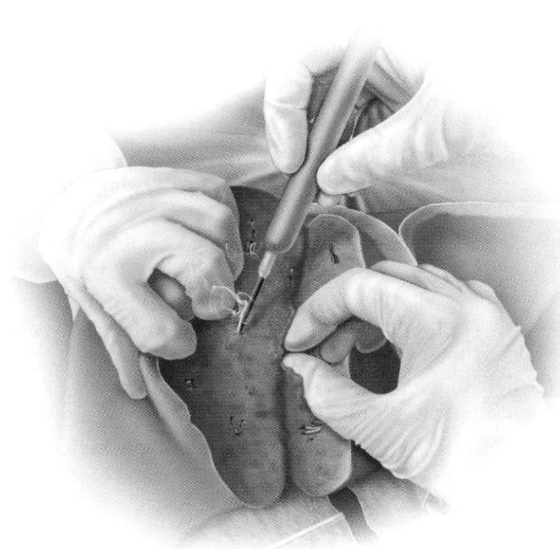

B

FIGURE 8 ● Finger fracture of liver parenchyma **(A)** can provide exposure for clipping or suture ligation of lacerated vessels **(B)**.

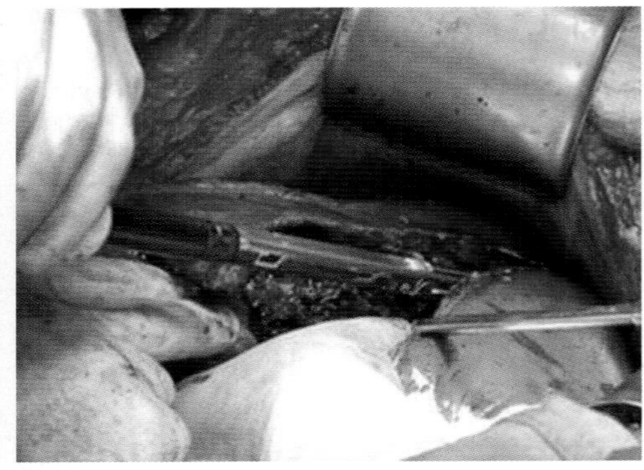

FIGURE 9 • Surgical staplers may be used to divide liver parenchyma to reach bleeding vessels.

BALLOON TAMPONADE

- Transhepatic penetrating wounds may leave a long intracavitary defect that is difficult to access for vascular control. Balloon tamponade may be accomplished by a device originally described by Poggetti and colleagues.[6] This may be fashioned by ligating a 1-in Penrose drain at one end. A red rubber catheter is inserted into the open end and secured with a second ligature. The Penrose drain is pulled through the wound, with the red rubber catheter and drain exiting the abdominal wall. The balloon is inflated with saline to achieve tamponade (**FIGURE 10**).

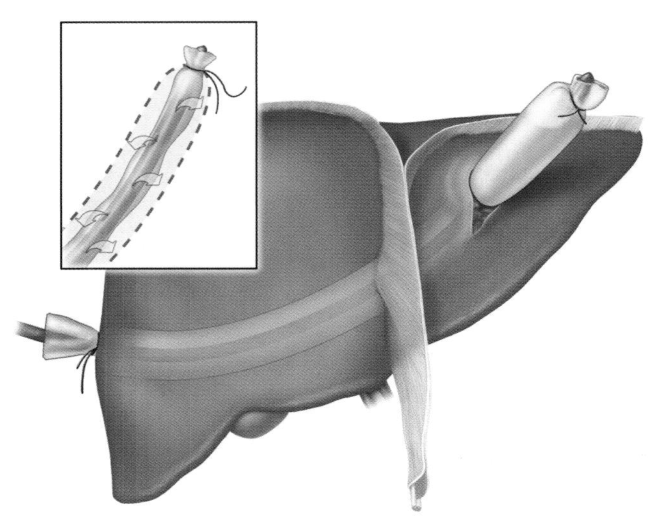

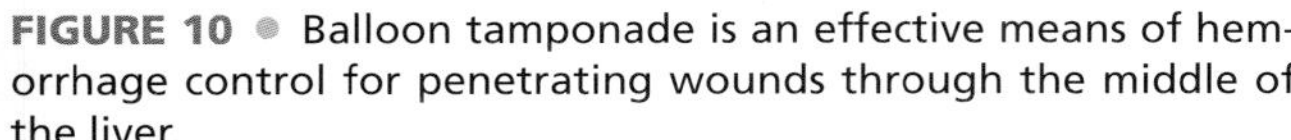

FIGURE 10 • Balloon tamponade is an effective means of hemorrhage control for penetrating wounds through the middle of the liver.

PRINGLE MANEUVER

- Bleeding that persists despite packing may be arterial in origin. The Pringle maneuver—that is, control of the hepatoduodenal ligament with a Rumel tourniquet or vascular clamp—should be employed (**FIGURE 11**). If this controls hemorrhage, it is likely that the bleeding is from either a hepatic arterial branch or major branch of the portal vein. This cannot be left in place for a prolonged period. Intermittent unclamping decreases the degree of ischemia/reperfusion injury. Definitive maneuvers must be undertaken and the clamp should be released within 60 minutes if possible. Ligation of the right or left hepatic artery may control the bleeding. Alternatively, in the appropriate setting, the patient may undergo arterioembolization.

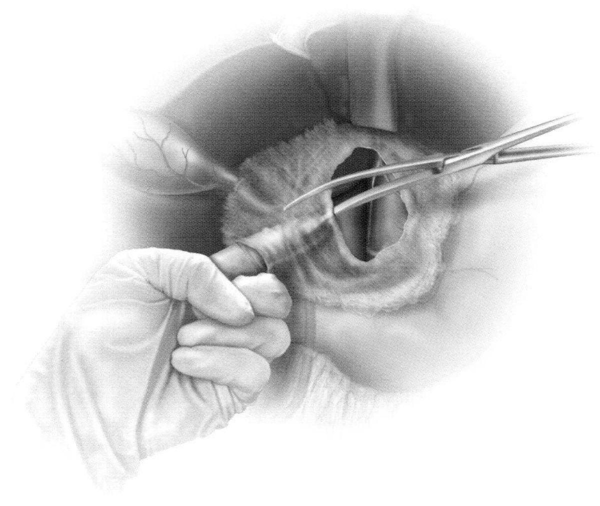

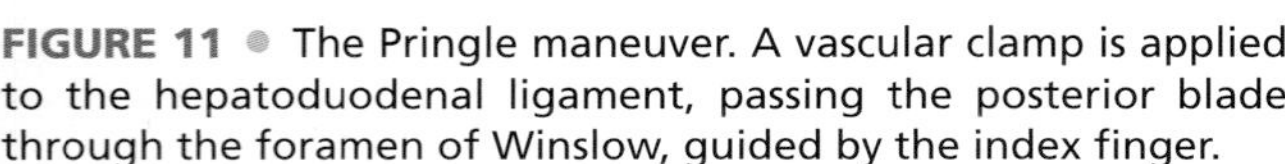

FIGURE 11 • The Pringle maneuver. A vascular clamp is applied to the hepatoduodenal ligament, passing the posterior blade through the foramen of Winslow, guided by the index finger.

HEPATIC RESECTION

- Resection of devitalized tissue may be performed at the initial operation; in the damage control setting, however, this is reserved for subsequent LAP. The extent of devitalized tissue is generally readily apparent (**FIGURE 12**). Resection may be necessary to control major vascular or biliary structures. Again, in the patient who is severely compromised physiologically, this is best done after resuscitation.

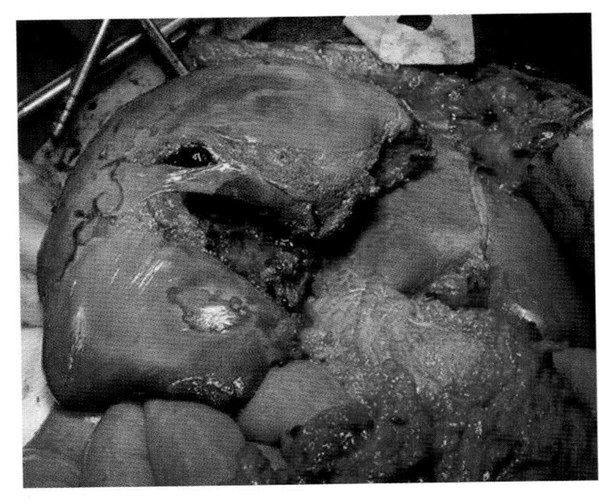

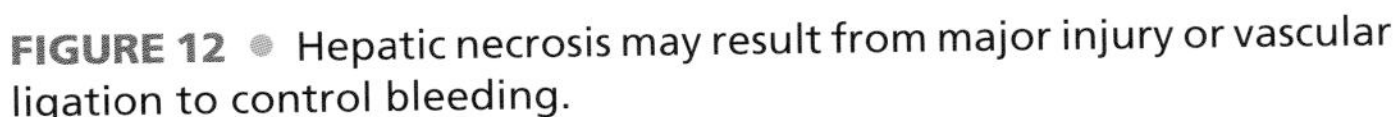

FIGURE 12 ● Hepatic necrosis may result from major injury or vascular ligation to control bleeding.

HEPATIC VASCULAR ISOLATION

- Bleeding that persists despite the Pringle maneuver is likely from the hepatic veins. Hepatic vascular isolation with or without venovenous bypass should be considered (**FIGURE 13**).[7] This entails control of the suprarenal IVC, the suprahepatic IVC, and a Pringle maneuver. If the interruption of venous return results in cardiovascular collapse, the aorta may need to be cross-clamped while venovenous bypass is established. The suprahepatic clamp may be placed below the diaphragm, but this is not ideal. The clamp optimally should be placed within the pericardium. This can be accomplished from within the abdomen, but the exposure is markedly improved by median sternotomy (**FIGURE 14**).

FIGURE 13 ● Hepatic vascular isolation and venovenous bypass is performed by clamping the suprarenal IVC, the suprahepatic IVC, and a Pringle maneuver. Venous cannulae are positioned in the femoral vein and superior mesenteric vein, and blood is shunted into the internal jugular vein.

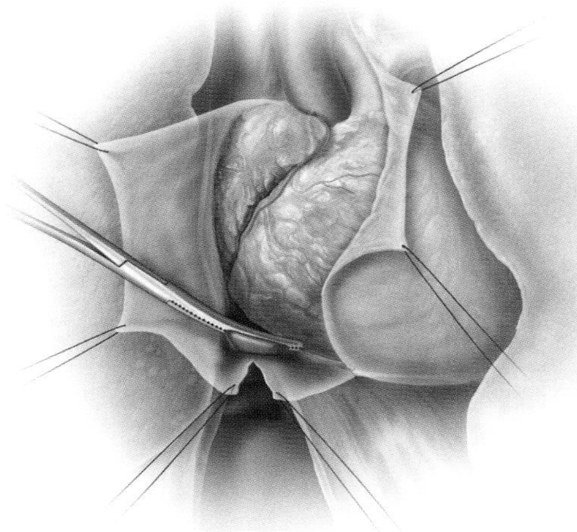

FIGURE 14 ● Combining a median sternotomy with a midline LAP incision provides exposure to the hepatic veins and retrohepatic vena cava while avoiding injury to the phrenic nerves. The pericardium and diaphragm can be divided down the center toward the IVC.

TECHNIQUES

CLOSURE

- If the liver is to remain packed, a temporary abdominal closure should be performed. Goals are rapid closure, containment of abdominal viscera, prevent bowel from adhering to fascial edges, allow room for swelling of abdominal viscera, provide a means for egress of ascites, maintain sterility of the abdominal cavity, avoid damage to fascia and skin edges, and minimize cost. The "Vac-Pack" dressing satisfies all of these requirements (**FIGURE 15**). A plastic sheet is draped over the bowel and extended to the paracolic gutters to keep the bowel from adhering to wound edges. Slits are cut in the sheet to allow egress of ascites. A towel is placed over the sheet to prevent suction drains from adhering to bowel through the slits. Drains are placed on top of the towel. An adhesive drape is placed over the entire wound. Definitive closure may be achieved by simple running fascial suture (eg, no. 2 nylon) and skin staples.

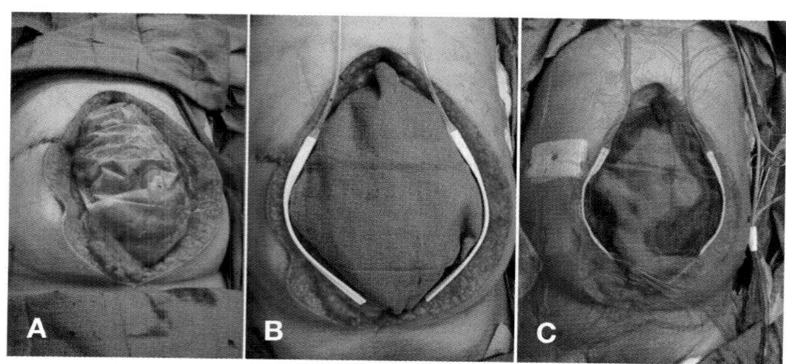

FIGURE 15 ● Temporary closure of the abdomen entails covering the bowel with a fenestrated plastic drape **(A)**, placement of closed suction drains and a blue towel **(B)**, followed by an adhesive occlusive dressing **(C)**.

PEARLS AND PITFALLS

Indication for LAP	■ Unstable patients should go to the OR promptly. Pursuing angioembolization in an unstable patient is not advisable and may prove disastrous.
Incision	■ A midline incision is the best choice in an unstable trauma patient. The surgeon should not hesitate to extend the incision rightward or into the chest in order to gain exposure and control. Median sternotomy markedly improves exposure for retrohepatic venous repairs.
Damage control	■ The decision to pack the liver should be made very quickly, as should the decision to adopt a "damage control" strategy.
Resuscitation	■ Ongoing resuscitation is critical during the operative phase.
Definitive procedures	■ Avoid major definitive procedures at the first operation, if the patient's condition warrants damage control.

POSTOPERATIVE CARE

- Trauma patients should be monitored for response to resuscitation. Patients who have extensive transfusion may benefit from viscoelastic assays such a thromboelastography (TEG) or rotational thromboelastometry (ROTEM), in order to target coagulation defects and limit unnecessary blood product transfusion. Once resuscitated, postoperative care is routine for abdominal surgery, with provision of diet as tolerated and early ambulation.

OUTCOMES

- Severe liver injuries may be associated with high morbidity and mortality rates. However, patients who survive without significant complications should be expected to have normal life span and functional status vis-à-vis the liver injury.

COMPLICATIONS

Hemorrhage

- Postoperative bleeding is not common outside of the damage control setting. Bleeding may continue despite liver packing. In this setting, TEG or ROTEM may be helpful in identifying coagulation abnormalities. In this case, depending on the patient's condition, angioembolization may be reasonable to control arterial hemorrhage. On the other hand, if the patient is physiologically compromised, it is prudent to return to the OR to control surgical hemorrhage while resuscitating the patient.

Abdominal Compartment Syndrome

- The abdominal compartment syndrome refers to intra-abdominal hypertension that is associated with organ dysfunction. It is often seen in association with damage control surgery in the presence of liver packing. The accumulation of ascites and retroperitoneal edema, coupled with bowel swelling, lead to a progressive rise in abdominal pressure. Patients may develop abdominal compartment syndrome in spite of an open abdomen, so the intra-abdominal pressure and organ function should be monitored.

Bile Leak

- This is the most common major complication of liver injury. Leaks may come from any biliary repair or anastomosis. They may also originate from peripheral biliary radicals. If a bile duct repair has leaked, it may be managed via endoscopic means (eg, stenting). Peripheral leaks usually spontaneously seal, but occasionally, leakage persists. This may be managed by endoscopic stenting. Bile collections should be drained.

Hemobilia

- Generally caused by injuries to an adjacent hepatic artery and bile duct, hemobilia is heralded by right upper quadrant pain, jaundice, and falling hemoglobin level. A more dramatic presentation may be upper gastrointestinal hemorrhage, as blood enters the duodenum via the common bile duct. Endoscopy can make the diagnosis, as blood is seen exiting from the ampulla of Vater. Angioembolization of the involved artery may be definitive treatment, but occasionally, drainage and/or debridement of a large hematoma/biloma cavity is needed.

Bilhemia

- Bilhemia results from a biliovenous fistula. Bilirubin levels can rise dramatically. Endoscopic biliary stenting may facilitate resolution, but hepatic resection may be required.

Hepatic Necrosis

- Although this may result from the initial injury, ligation or embolization of major vascular branches may also result in hepatic necrosis. This generally requires operative debridement or resection.

REFERENCES

1. Moore EE, Cogbill TH, Jurkovich GJ, et al. Organ injury scaling: spleen and liver (1994 Revision). *J Trauma*. 1995;38:323-324.
2. Coccolini F, Coimbra R, Ordonez C, et al. Liver trauma: WSES 2020 guidelines. *World J Emerg Surg*. 2020;15:24.
3. Kozar RA, Feliciano DV, Moore EE, et al. Western Trauma Association critical decisions in trauma: operative management of adult blunt hepatic trauma. *J Trauma*. 2011;71:1-5.
4. Pachter HL. Prometheus bound: evolution in the management of hepatic trauma—from myth to reality. *J Trauma*. 2012;72:321-329.
5. Peitzman AB, Marsh JW. Advanced operative techniques in the management of complex liver injury. *J Trauma Acute Care Surg*. 2012;73:765-770.
6. Poggetti RS, Moore EE, Moore FA, et al. Balloon tamponade for bilobar transfixing hepatic gunshot wounds. *J Trauma*. 1992;33:694-697.
7. Biffl WL, Moore EE, Franciose RJ. Venovenous bypass and hepatic vascular isolation as adjuncts in the repair of destructive wounds to the retrohepatic inferior vena cava. *J Trauma*. 1998;45:400-403.

Chapter 30 Genitourinary Injury—Kidney: Renorrhaphy, Nephrectomy

Denise Torres, Claire Lauer, and Christopher Thacker

DEFINITION

- Renal trauma presents up to 5% of all trauma patients and most commonly occurs worldwide in blunt injury (80%).[1] Penetrating injuries more likely require operative intervention.[2] Renal trauma occurs more commonly in males in a ratio of 3:1. There is a spectrum of the severity of renal trauma that is described in **TABLE 1**.[3] The classification is based on the degree of renal parenchymal injury, blood vessel rupture, and the extent of the subscapular or perirenal hemorrhage found on computed tomography (CT), in the operating room (OR), or on pathology.[1]
- Renal injury can be identified and graded with imaging or found intraoperatively in damage control surgery. Injury can occur to the renal parenchyma, renal hilum including arteries and veins, as well as the collecting system, all which can require different forms of management.
- Despite renal injury in trauma being common, the role of operative intervention has decreased significantly over time, and nonoperative management has become the standard for hemodynamically stable patients.[2] In addition, when intervention is required, angioembolization is often the preferred method.[3-5] Despite these changes in management, surgical intervention is still required at times, and the trauma surgeon must be prepared for operative exploration when necessary.[4,5]

Table 1: Renal Injury Scale

American association for surgery of trauma renal injury scale

Grade	Type	Description
1	Contusion	Microscopic or gross hematuria. Urological studies normal.
	Hematoma	Subcapsular, nonexpanding without parenchymal laceration.
II	Hematoma	Nonexpanding peri-renal hematoma confined to renal retroperitoneum.
	Laceration	<1.0 cm parenchymal depth of renal cortex with no urinary extravasation.
III	Laceration	>1.0 cm parenchymal depth of renal cortex w/out collecting system rupture or urinary extravasation.
IV	Laceration	Parenchymal laceration extending through renal cortex, medulla, and collecting system.
	Vascular	Main renal artery or vein injury with contained hemorrhage.
V	Laceration	Completely shattered kidney.
	Vascular	Avulsion of renal hilum that devascularizes kidney.

Reprinted from Heller MT, Schnor N. MDCT of renal trauma: correlation to AAST organ injury scale. Clin Imaging. 2014;38(4):410-417. Copyright © 2014 Elsevier. With permission.

DIFFERENTIAL DIAGNOSIS

- Renal injury should be suspected in patients presenting with signs and symptoms of abdominal trauma, specifically in patients with evidence of bloody urine, or zone II hematomas. In addition, they can be found alongside many other intra-abdominal injuries, resulting in complex and mixed presentations in the setting of multiorgan system trauma.

PATIENT HISTORY AND PHYSICAL EXAM FINDINGS

- Renal injury can occur after blunt (eg, fall, crush injury, motor vehicle crash) or penetrating (eg, stab or gunshot wound) trauma mechanisms.
- Patients undergoing a rapid deceleration event or direct blow to the flank should be suspected of having a renal injury.
- Findings on physical examination that may indicate significant renal injury include rib fractures, significant flank ecchymosis, and penetrating wounds of the flank, abdomen, and lower chest.[6]
- Hematuria is the most sensitive clinical sign of renal injury, yet the degree does not predict the injury severity.[6] In addition, hematuria can also result from lower genitourinary injuries, so it is not specific.
- Vital signs should be closely monitored. While imaging plays the largest role in diagnosis, the hemodynamic status of the patient will dictate the management (operative vs nonoperative).

IMAGING AND OTHER DIAGNOSTIC STUDIES

- Patient's presenting with trauma should undergo standard evaluation according to Advanced Trauma Life Support guidelines. Initial ABC evaluation is usually followed by a FAST exam (Focused Abdominal Sonography for Trauma), especially in the setting of hypotension or tachycardia. A positive FAST is not specific but is concerning for renal injury and or other solid or hollow viscus organ injury.
- In patients that are hemodynamically stable, CT imaging with IV contrast is the gold standard for imaging. In renal trauma, arterial and venous phase CT scan allows for the diagnosis of injuries. Delayed images (excretory phase) help to evaluate for urinary extravasation.
- CT scanning is useful to evaluate the grade of injury (**FIGURE 1**). The American Association of Surgery for Trauma Organ Injury

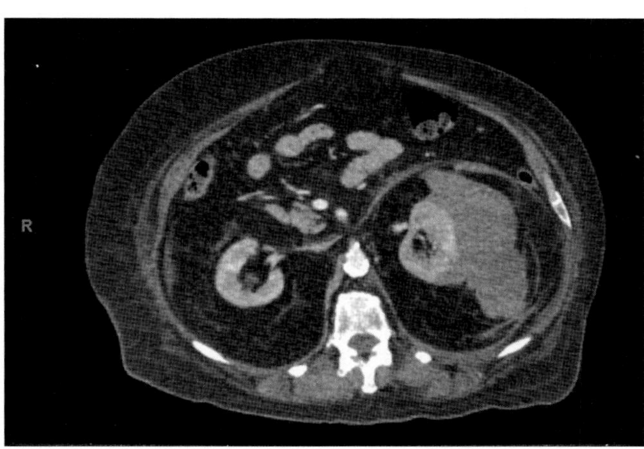

FIGURE 1 ● CT images of a grade 4 kidney laceration with surrounding hematoma after fall from standing.

Scale (OIS) for the kidney was most recently updated in 2018.[1,7] Both the OIS and the World Society for Emergency Surgery guidelines can be used to direct management, based on imaging findings and hemodynamic stability (**TABLE 1**).[7]

NONOPERATIVE MANAGEMENT

- Management of blunt renal injury is dependent primarily upon hemodynamic stability, and the safety and feasibility of pursuing nonoperative management. Due to the availability of CT scans and treatment with interventional radiology, operative intervention for blunt renal trauma has decreased significantly. While penetrating abdominal trauma such as a gunshot wound or a stabbing involving the kidney can necessitate exploration, trauma nephrectomy is extremely rare.[8]
- For patients hemodynamically stable enough to be observed, rates of conversion to operative management are extremely low.[9] Endovascular management with selective angioembolization is often a first step prior to attempting operative intervention.
- In general, hemodynamically compromised Grade IV and V renal injuries are most likely to require operative intervention, often only after failure of endovascular management.[8,9]
- CT scans can be used to identify patients that are at high risk of failing nonoperative management. These CT findings include contrast blush, perirenal hematoma >3.5 cm, medial laceration with significant medial urinary extravasation, and lack of contrast in the ureter, suggesting a complete ureteropelvic junction disruption. Patients with a moderate or severe renal injury with two or more of these findings have a high failure rate of nonoperative management (**FIGURE 1**).[7]
- Recent studies have found that upwards of 90% of renal injuries are now managed nonoperatively.[1,4,5] In addition, the role of interventional radiology has continued to grow, such that angioembolization is frequently used even in high OIS grade injuries if the patients are volume responsive during resuscitation.[9] Despite advancements in nonoperative and minimally invasive methods, operative intervention in trauma is still the treatment for complex abdominal and renal trauma resulting in hemodynamic instability.
- In penetrating trauma, all patients who are hemodynamically unstable, have peritonitis, evisceration, hematemesis, or gross blood per rectum or nasogastric tube should require operative exploration.
- Patients who are stable should be evaluated for peritoneal violation via local wound exploration (stab wounds), ultrasound or CT imaging, or diagnostic laparoscopy.
- Patients with abdominal stab wounds who remain stable, have no immediate indications for exploration, or findings on imaging that require exploration such as hollow viscus injury or active bleeding can be closely observed and treated nonoperatively.[7]

SURGICAL MANAGEMENT

Preoperative Planning

- Patients with penetrating abdominal injuries with hemodynamic instability and evidence of free fluid on FAST exam or other imaging require operative intervention.
- Patients taken to the OR for planned exploratory laparotomy should, if possible, be taken to a hybrid OR suite where endovascular intervention could be performed simultaneously if needed. The OR team should be made aware of potential interventions, transfusion requirements, and special requests.

Positioning

- Patient should be placed in the supine position with arms out. The patient should be prepped and draped fully exposing the chest and abdomen, so that the incision can be extended past the abdomen into the chest for further exposure. Consideration should also be given to bilateral groin exposure for endovascular access.

INCISION

- A midline abdominal incision should be made from xiphoid to the pubis.
- Then place a large abdominal wall retractor to aid with exposure. The retroperitoneum must be visualized in order to assess possible injury.

ABDOMINAL EXPLORATION

- The initial goal is to stop all ongoing hemorrhage. If major hemorrhage is encountered, all four quadrants should be packed. Packs should be systematically removed.
- All retroperitoneal zones of the abdomen should be visualized to determine the site of bleeding.
- Zone I is the central retroperitoneum. It consists of the aorta, IVC, pancreas, lesser sac, and the retroperitoneal duodenum. Zone I hematomas are divided into supramesocolic or inframesocolic.

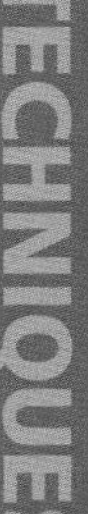

- Zone II is lateral to Zone I and occupies the flanks. Zone II is composed of the kidney, hilar structures, ureter, and psoas muscle. Zone II is visualized by moving the colon medially.
- Zone III occupies the pelvis. It is composed of the iliac vessels and pelvic organs.
- The absolute indications for renal exploration include hemodynamic instability, expanding or pulsatile hematoma, and injury to the renal pelvis or ureter.[10] Penetrating renal trauma resulting in disruption of Gerota fascia and intra-abdominal hemorrhage, as well as injury resulting in uncontrollable blood loss through the collecting system, can also require exploration.[7]
- Zone II retroperitoneal hematomas, found after blunt trauma, that are stable and not expanding, can be observed. Exploration increases the possibility of a nephrectomy. Once Gerota fascia is entered, its tamponading effect is lost and surgical repair may be required.[11,12]
- In patients with penetrating trauma, most Zone II hematomas should be explored, unless it is a lateral hematoma where the risk of injury to the renal vasculature and ureter, all medial structures, is low. If the hematoma is not explored, postoperative CT evaluation should be performed to define the full extent of injury.[13]

Renal Exploration

- Prior to exploring the kidney, it is best practice to confirm the presence of a contralateral kidney. If preoperative imaging was not performed, ideally this is done before entering the retroperitoneum to explore an expanding Zone II hematoma. The gold standard is a "one-shot" intravenous pyelogram.[14,15] This is performed by injecting 1-2 mL/kg of iodinated contrast and obtaining a 10-minute delayed, single-view abdominal radiograph to view the excretory phase. Another option is to palpate the contralateral kidney to confirm its presence.[8]
- The colon is mobilized by incising the peritoneal reflection along the white line of Toldt and reflecting it medially. On the right side of the abdomen, the duodenum will need to be mobilized as well (Cattel-Braasch maneuver). On the left side of the abdomen, the descending colon, spleen, and tail of the pancreas can be mobilized (Mattox maneuver).
- Exploration is carried out through an anterior vertical incision in Gerota fascia.
- There is controversy whether primary vascular control (PVC) should be obtained prior to opening Gerota fascia.[4] Previously in a large retrospective series, McAninch reported a reduced nephrectomy rate if PVC is obtained (56% vs 18%).[16]
- PVC can be obtained by opening the posterior peritoneum over the aorta medial to the inferior mesenteric vein (**FIGURE 2**). Renal vessels are then dissected and isolated with vessel loops (**FIGURE 3**).
- It has been reported that PVC can add 10 to 15 minutes to the procedure.[13]
- An alternative method to PVC of the renal hilum is to mobilize the left colon and reflect it medially (**FIGURE 4**). If there is significant bleeding, the renal hilum can then be clamped with a noncrushing vascular clamp.
- When visualizing the kidney, the whole kidney should be mobilized to allow for complete inspection. This requires delivery of the kidney out of Gerota fascia.

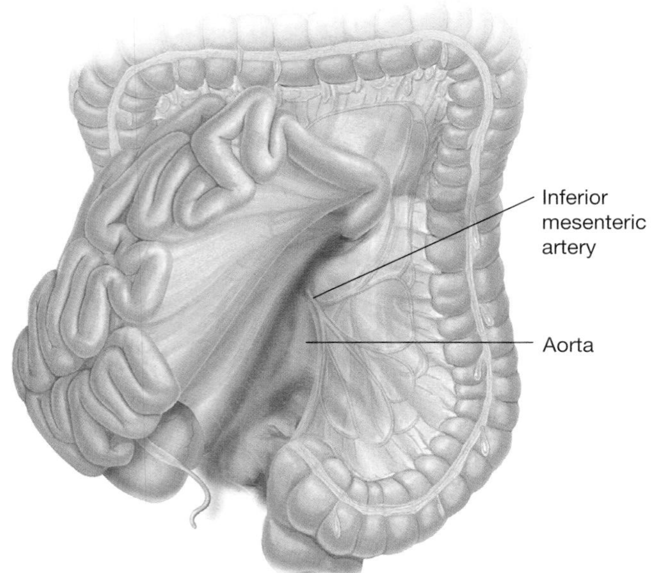

FIGURE 2 ● Surgical approach to the renal vessels and kidney. The retroperitoneal incision is made over the aorta medial to the inferior mesenteric vein. (Redrawn from McAninch JW. Surgery for renal trauma. In: Novick AC, Steem SB, Pontes JE (eds.), *Stewarts's Operative Urology*. Williams &Wilkins; 1989:234-239.)

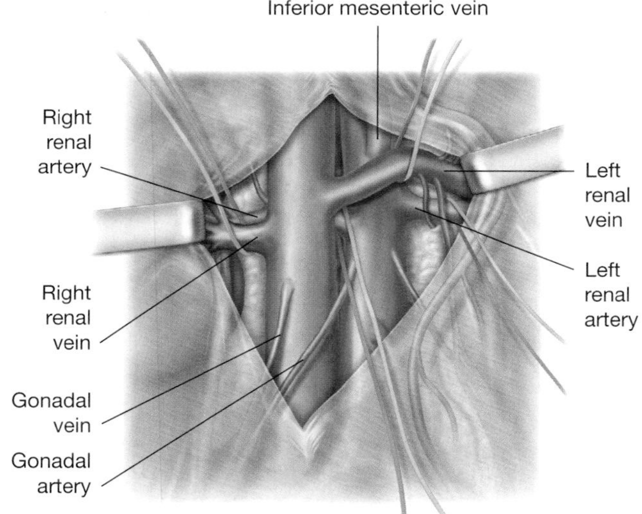

FIGURE 3 ● Anatomic relationship of the renal vessels. (Redrawn from McAninch JW. Surgery for renal trauma. In: Novick AC, Steem SB, Pontes JE (eds.), *Stewarts's Operative Urology*. Williams &Wilkins; 1989:234-239.)

Hemostatic Agents and Cautery

- Digital pressure and compression can first be used to control parenchymal bleeding.
- All small vessels can be ligated with 3 to 0 or 4 to 0 absorbable suture.
- If suture ligation and digital pressure are not sufficient and there is ongoing bleeding from superficial parenchyma or small lacerations, cautery as well as hemostatic agents can be

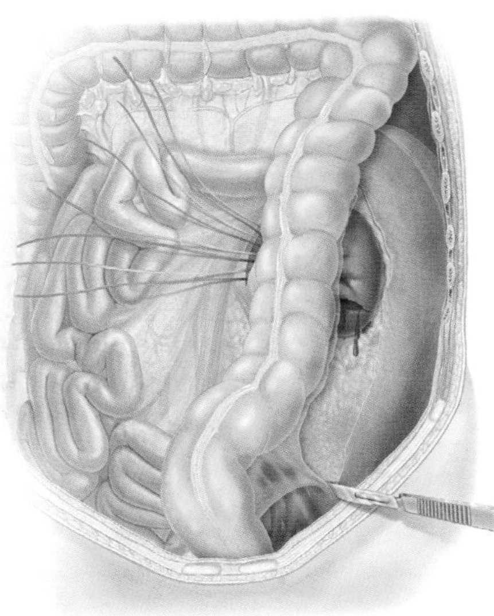

FIGURE 4 ● Retroperitoneal exposure of the kidney lateral to the colon. (Redrawn from McAninch JW. Surgery for renal trauma. In: Novick AC, Steem SB, Pontes JE (eds.), *Stewarts's Operative Urology*. Williams &Wilkins; 1989:234-239.)

helpful. Given that many of these patients are coagulopathic in the setting of trauma and active bleeding, standard electrocautery is often not sufficient.

- More recent developments in cautery include options such as Argon Plasma Coagulation, and the Aquamantys device which is a disposable bipolar irrigated sealer.[17] Both options are able to generate greater energy and therefore hemostasis and can be considered an option when standard electrocautery is not sufficient.
- Mechanical hemostatic agents can also be applied as they work to create a structure for clot formation with platelet aggregation and fibrin production.[18]

Renorrhaphy

- Ideally renal salvage is the preferred operative technique if the injury and situation allows.[8]
- The decision to proceed with renal salvage is one that should be based on the following: patient's hemodynamic status, the degree of injury to the parenchyma, vascular structures, and collecting system, as well as the ability to reconstruct the kidney.
- If the decision to proceed with renorrhaphy is made, first evacuate the hematoma.
- The renal capsule should be preserved for closure after renal reconstruction.
- Lacerated, devitalized parenchyma should be sharply debrided.
- Small intrarenal vessels can be controlled with absorbable 3 to 0 or 4 to 0 sutures.
- Open collecting system defects should also be closed with absorbable sutures. Absorbable suture is used for intrarenal suturing, as permanent suture may be a nidus for renal stone formation if there is contact with the collecting system.
- Topical agents may be placed in the parenchymal defect to aid in hemostasis.
- The capsule is then closed with a 0-chromic blunt-tipped liver suture. Pledgets may be used to help bolster the repair to help prevent further tearing. Gelfoam or surgicel can be used to create pledgets. This will help to aid in hemostasis (**FIGURE 5**).[7,12]
- Perinephric suction drain is placed away from the repair and removed once drainage subsides.
- If there is concern for a postoperative urine leak, the effluent can be sent for creatinine concentration. A positive leak will have a level that is higher than serum creatinine.

Trauma Nephrectomy

- For patients with uncontrollable bleeding or if the kidney is felt to be unable to be reconstructed, nephrectomy is the best surgical option for treatment.

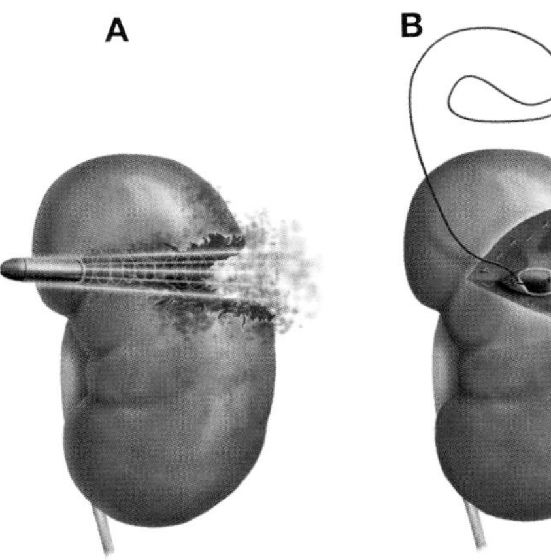

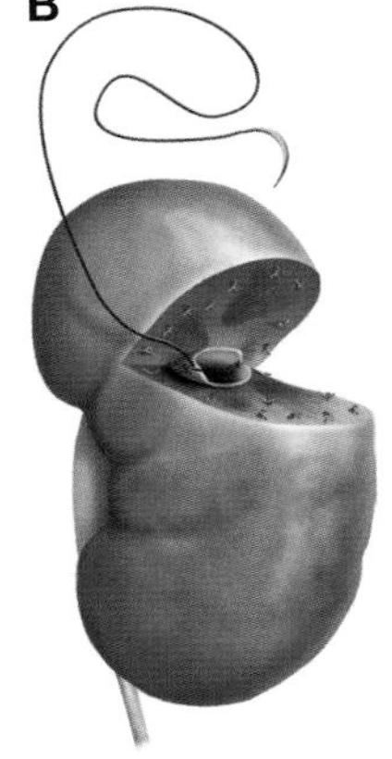

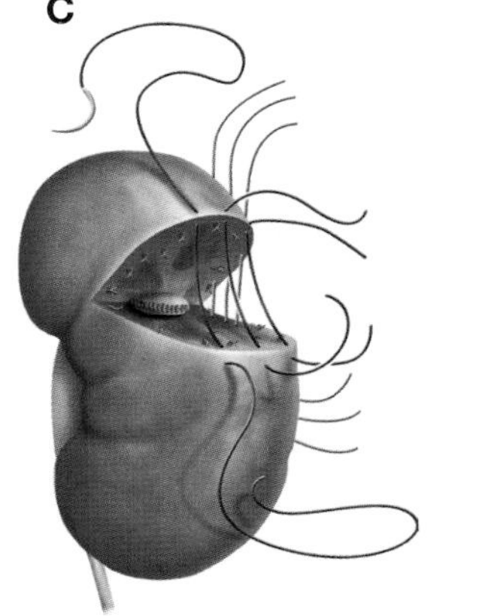

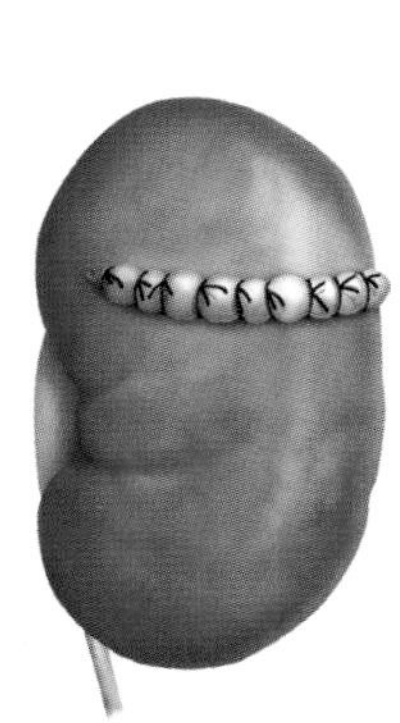

FIGURE 5 ● Techniques of renorrhaphy. (Redrawn from McAninch JW. Surgery for renal trauma. In: Novick AC, Steem SB, Pontes JE (eds.), *Stewarts's Operative Urology*. Williams & Wilkins; 1989:234-239.)

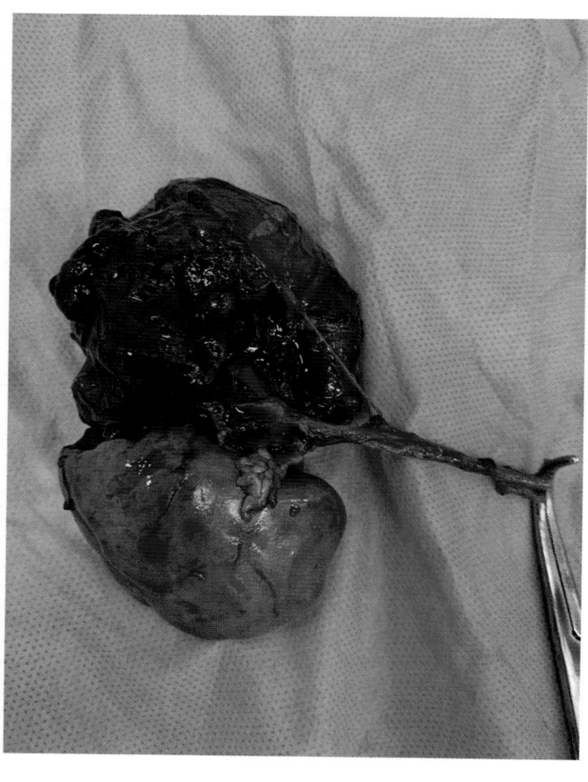

- Ideally, the renal artery and vein should be ligated individually to avoid the potential for arteriovenous formation.
- Vascular structures may be sutured-ligated, clipped, or stapled.
- Once the vascular structures are secured, elevate the kidney to allow for better visualization of the ureter to allow for ligation.
- The right renal vein usually receives its tributaries from the kidney, where the left renal vein receives tributaries from the left gonadal vein, inferior phrenic vein, and left adrenal vein. Attempts to save the tributaries should be made if possible.
- The ureter and vessels, including the tributaries, if needed should be ligated close to the kidney (**FIGURE 6**).

Vascular Injury

- Renal injury can be associated with vascular injury at the level of the hilum.
- Endovascular intervention in these cases can be beneficial. Performing these cases in hybrid ORs is helpful if available.
- Temporary deployment of REBOA (resuscitative balloon occlusion of the aorta) device within Zone II of the aorta at the level of the renal vessels can be used as an adjunctive means of controlling hemorrhage long enough to obtain vascular control.[19]

FIGURE 6 • Nephrectomy after high speed motor vehicle accident. Devascularization of upper renal pole.

PEARLS AND PITFALLS

Patient history and findings	▪ Patient with hemodynamic instability and abdominal trauma require exploration. ▪ Patients that are hemodynamically stable can be closely observed if they do not have a clear indication for surgery.
Intraoperative pearls	▪ Intraoperatively all expanding hematomas need to be explored. ▪ Intraoperative central Zone II hematomas from penetrating trauma should be explored.
Patient position and preparation	▪ Widely prep as always for trauma: chin to knees.
Incision	▪ Initially a larger incision may significantly help your exposure and dissection.
Technique	▪ Individually ligate the renal artery and vein to prevent postoperative arteriovenous fistulae. ▪ Left renal vein has additional nonrenal tributaries that should be preserved if possible.
Time and resuscitation	▪ In the operating room, be mindful of giving anesthesia time to catch up once hemostasis has been achieved.

POSTOPERATIVE CARE

- Patients should continue to be resuscitated postoperatively including correcting for any possible coagulopathy.
- Routine postoperative care for abdominal surgery: diet as tolerated, early ambulation, and local wound care.
- Monitor drain output. If there is concern for a urine leak, drain output can be sent for serum creatinine levels. Drain creatinine will be significantly higher than serum creatinine in the presence of a leak. Additional testing may be warranted to identify the source of the leak.

COMPLICATIONS

Acute Kidney Injury

- In general, risk for significant acute kidney injury (AKI) is greater with operative management than nonoperative management of renal trauma.[5]

- Patients with renal trauma should have their kidney function watched closely.

Urinoma

- Posttraumatic urinoma is generally managed nonoperatively.
- Indications for intervention of a known urinoma include signs of developing sepsis, in which case drainage is recommended, usually by interventional radiology.
- If drainage of the collection alone is not sufficient, additional placement of nephrostomy tubes can be considered, or ureteral stenting.

Page Kidney

- On the rare occasion, compression on the kidney by hematoma or fluid accumulation can result in a page kidney.
- The pathophysiology of the page kidney is thought to be due to activation of the Renin–Angiotensin–Aldosterone system due to the external compression. This causes significant secondary arterial hypertension and can also result in AKI.[20]
- Treatment for page kidney has evolved over time, and radical nephrectomy is now rarely indicated. First steps should include drainage procedures to evacuate the compressing collection or hematoma, or event endoscopic or laparoscopic management.

Arteriovenous Fistula and Pseudoaneurysm

- Although rare, arteriovenous fistula and pseudoaneurysm occasionally occur after high-grade renal trauma.
- These can have extremely deleterious effects, and attempted ligation or endovascular exclusion is recommended.

REFERENCES

1. Kozar RA, Crandall M, Shanmuganathan K, et al. Organ injury scaling 2018 update: spleen, liver, and kidney. *J Trauma Acute Care Surg*. 2018;85(6):1119-1122. doi:10.1097/TA.0000000000002058
2. Petrone P, Perez-Calvo J, Brathwaite CEM, Islam S, Joseph DK. Traumatic kidney injuries: a systematic review and meta-analysis. *Int J Surg*. 2020;74:13-21. doi:10.1016/j.ijsu.2019.12.013
3. Moore EE, Shackford SR, Pachter HL, et al. Organ injury scaling: spleen, liver, and kidney. *J Trauma*. 1989;29(12):1664-1666.
4. Gonzalez RP, Falimirski M, Holevar MR, Evankovich C. Surgical management of renal trauma: is vascular control necessary? *J Trauma*. 1999;47(6):1039-1042. doi:10.1097/00005373-199912000-00008
5. El Hechi MW, Nederpelt C, Kongkaewpaisan N, et al. Contemporary management of penetrating renal trauma—a national analysis. *Injury*. 2020;51(1):32-38. doi:10.1016/j.injury.2019.09.006
6. Morey AF, Broghammer JA, Hollowell CMP, McKibben MJ, Souter L. Urotrauma guideline 2020: AUA guideline. *J Urol*. 2021;205(1):30-35. doi:10.1097/JU.0000000000001408
7. Coccolini F, Moore EE, Kluger Y, et al. Kidney and uro-trauma: WSES-AAST guidelines. *World J Emerg Surg: WJES*. 2019;14:54. https://pubmed.ncbi.nlm.nih.gov/31827593 https://www.ncbi.nlm.nih.gov/pmc/articles/PMC6886230/. doi:10.1186/s13017-019-0274-x
8. Heiner SM, Keihani S, McCormick BJ, et al. Nephrectomy after high-grade renal trauma is associated with higher mortality: results from the multi-institutional genitourinary trauma study (MiGUTS). *Urology*. 2021;157:246-252. doi:10.1016/j.urology.2021.07.033
9. Colaco M, Navarrete RA, MacDonald SM, Stitzel JD, Terlecki RP. Nationwide procedural trends for renal trauma management. *Ann Surg*. 2019;269(2):367-369. doi:10.1097/SLA.0000000000002475
10. Martin M, Brown C, Shatz D, et al. Evaluation and management of abdominal stab wounds: a Western Trauma Association critical decisions algorithm. *J Trauma Acute Care Surg*. 2018;85(5):1007-1015. doi:10.1097/TA.0000000000001930
11. Keane T. *Glenn's Urologic Surgery*. 8th ed. Lippincott Williams & Wilkins; 2016. http://www.r2library.com/resource/title/9781451191462.
12. Rostas J, Simmons JD, Frotan MA, Brevard SB, Gonzalez RP. Intraoperative management of renal gunshot injuries: is mandatory exploration of gerota's fascia necessary? *Am J Surg*. 2016;211(4):783-786. doi:10.1016/j.amjsurg.2015.09.023
13. Brown CVR, Alam HB, Brasel K, Hauser CJ, de Moya M, Martin M, Moore EE, Rowell S, Vercruysse G, Inaba K. Western trauma association critical decisions in trauma: management of renal trauma. *J Trauma Acute Care Surg*. November 2018;85(5):1021-1025.
14. Oakland CDH, Britton JM, Charlton CAC. Renal trauma and the intravenous urogram. *J R Soc Med*. 1987;80(1):21-22. doi:10.1177/014107688708000109
15. McAninch JW, Carroll PR. Renal trauma: kidney preservation through improved vascular control-a refined approach. *J Trauma*. 1982;22(4):285-290.
16. Taheri A, Mansoori P, Sandoval LF, Feldman SR, Pearce D, Williford PM. Electrosurgery. *J Am Acad Dermatol*. 2013;70(4):591.e1-591.e14. https://www.clinicalkey.es/playcontent/1-s2.0-S0190962213010529. doi:10.1016/j.jaad.2013.09.056
17. Patrizi A, Jezequel C, Sulpice LL, Meunier BB, Rayar M, Boudjema K. Disposable bipolar irrigated sealer (aquamantys®) for liver resection: use with caution. *Updates Surg*. 2016;68(2):171. doi:10.1007/s13304-016-0367-y
18. Tompeck AJ, Gajdhar AUR, Dowling M, et al. A comprehensive review of topical hemostatic agents: the good, the bad, and the novel. *J Trauma Acute Care Surg*. 2020;88(1):e1-e21. https://www.ncbi.nlm.nih.gov/pubmed/31626024. doi:10.1097/TA.0000000000002508
19. Halvachizadeh S, Mica L, Kalbas Y, et al. Zone-dependent acute circulatory changes in abdominal organs and extremities after resuscitative balloon occlusion of the aorta (REBOA): an experimental model. *Eur J Med Res*. 2021;26(1):10. doi:10.1186/s40001-021-00485-y
20. Izekor BE, Odigwe C, Goraya N, Duran PA. Page kidney from a subcapsular urinoma following contralateral radical nephrectomy. *Cureus*. 2021;13(6):e15639. doi:10.7759/cureus.15639

Chapter 31 Genitourinary Injury—Bladder: Extraperitoneal, Intraperitoneal

John Donkersloot and Pauline K. Park

DEFINITION

- Trauma patients may sustain injury to the intraperitoneal or extraperitoneal urinary bladder. The extent of injury is graded based on the type, location, and size (**TABLE 1**). Full-thickness disruption of the bladder wall results in extravasation of urine, either into the peritoneal cavity or into the extraperitoneal space. Prompt diagnosis and control via catheter drainage and/or operative repair is warranted depending on the location, extent of injury, and presence of associated injuries.

DIFFERENTIAL DIAGNOSIS

- The hallmark of genitourinary injury is the presence of blood in the urine. The differential diagnosis includes injury to the kidney, ureters, bladder, and urethra. Injury to the lower tracts should be suspected with the findings of gross hematuria and abdominal, suprapubic, or pelvic pain. Penetrating injury with a trajectory through the pelvis should also raise suspicion for bladder injury, in addition to visceral and vascular injury.

PATIENT HISTORY AND PHYSICAL FINDINGS

- Genitourinary injury is present in less than 1% of all trauma patients; however, the morbidity related to a missed bladder injury mandates thoughtful evaluation. Bladder injury is most commonly seen following blunt rather than penetrating trauma (65% vs 35%).[1]
- Anatomically, the bladder is largely protected by the bony pelvis. Although the vast majority of pelvic fractures do not have associated bladder injury, conversely, bladder injuries are most commonly associated with pelvic ring fracture.
- When gross hematuria is present with pelvic fracture, the incidence of bladder injury is 29%.[2] More than 90% of bladder ruptures present with gross hematuria in the setting of a pelvic ring fracture, with a limited number presenting with microscopic hematuria (.6%-5.0%).[3]

Table 1: AAST Grading of Bladder Injuries

Grade[a]	Injury type	Description of injury
I	Hematoma	Contusion, intramural hematoma
	Laceration	Partial thickness
II	Laceration	Extraperitoneal bladder wall laceration <2 cm
III	Laceration	Extraperitoneal (≥2 cm) or intraperitoneal (<2 cm) bladder wall laceration
IV	Laceration	Intraperitoneal bladder wall laceration ≥2 cm
V	Laceration	Intraperitoneal or extraperitoneal bladder wall laceration extending into the bladder neck or ureteral orifice (trigone)

[a]Advance one grade for multiple lesions up to grade III.

Reprinted with permission from Moore EE, Cogbill TH, Jurkovich GJ, et al. Organ injury scaling. III: Chest wall, abdominal vascular, ureter, bladder, and urethra. J Trauma. 1992;33(3):337-339.

- Bladder injury in absence of pelvic fracture is associated with a distended bladder with the application of sudden, significant force, such as deceleration from high speed.
- Physical examination findings include suprapubic pain or tenderness, abdominal distention, and peritonitis, although these findings are neither sensitive nor specific enough to make definitive diagnosis of bladder injury.
- Other indicators of potential bladder injury include inability to void, decreased urine output, scrotal swelling, unexplained shock, and the presence of low-density free fluid on cross-sectional imaging (urinary ascites).[3]
- If blood is present at the urethral meatus, blind placement of a Foley catheter is discouraged and retrograde urethrography should be performed to exclude urethral injury prior to further manipulation.[3]

IMAGING AND OTHER DIAGNOSTIC STUDIES

- Hemodynamically unstable patients undergoing emergent laparotomy should undergo evaluation for bladder injury during operative exploration.
- Imaging is reserved for hemodynamically stable patients.
  - The presence of gross hematuria, particularly in association with pelvic fractures, should be evaluated by retrograde cystography.[4]
  - Microscopic hematuria in the setting of pelvic fracture does not mandate retrograde cystography, but certain fracture patterns (including pubic symphysis diastasis and obturator ring fracture >1 cm) have been shown to be associated with bladder injury[3] and cystography should be considered in these cases.[4]
  - Microscopic hematuria alone is not an indication for retrograde cystography.[4]
  - During evaluation of penetrating injury of the perineum, buttock, or pelvis, any degree of hematuria should prompt consideration for retrograde cystography.
- Both plain film and computed tomography (CT) retrograde cystography have excellent sensitivity and specificity for bladder injury; CT cystography is increasingly performed in the context of other 3D imaging. Visualization of the bladder on CT scan with intravenous contrast alone, without retrograde instillation of contrast, is insufficient.
  - Technique: 300 to 350 mL of water-soluble contrast material is instilled by gravity through the Foley catheter and the catheter is clamped.
  - For plain film cystography, a set of anterior-posterior and oblique views are obtained with the bladder filled with contrast and a second set following drainage. For CT retrograde cystography, imaging is performed after filling the bladder with contrast. See **FIGURES 1** to **3**.
- Laboratory studies, other than urinalysis for microscopic hematuria, are of limited use in the diagnosis of acute bladder injury. In the setting of an unrecognized bladder injury, a

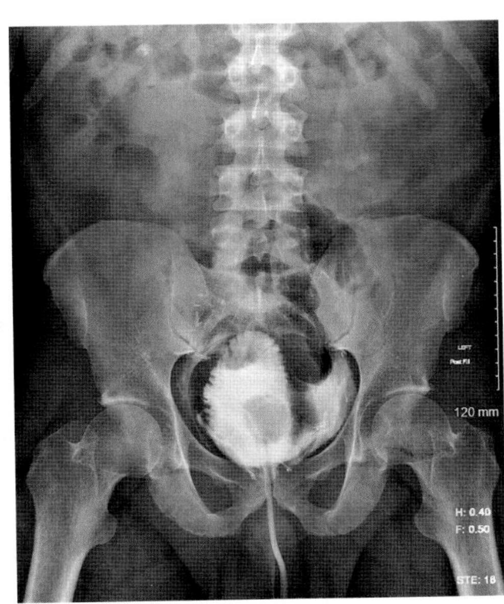

FIGURE 1 ● Retrograde cystography showing intraperitoneal perforation, with extravasated contrast outlining loops of bowel.

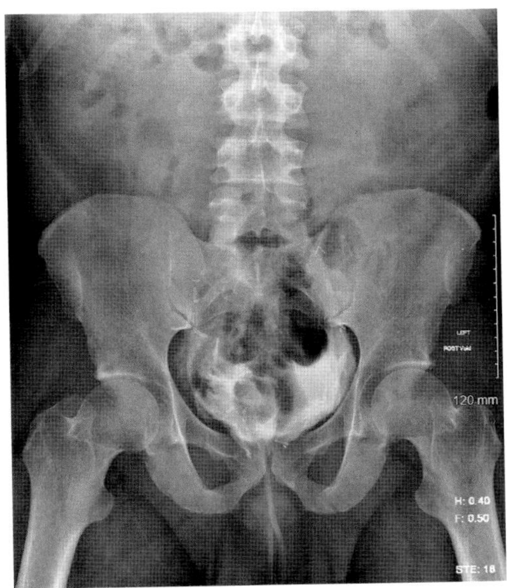

FIGURE 2 ● Contrast extravasation persists following drainage of the bladder.

late finding may be a rise in serum BUN/creatinine and electrolyte abnormalities due to absorption from urine within the peritoneal cavity.

SURGICAL MANAGEMENT

Preoperative Planning

- Following the diagnosis of a bladder injury, the decision to operate depends on the location and nature of the injury. Roughly 60% of bladder injuries are extraperitoneal, 30% are intraperitoneal, and 10% are mixed.[3]

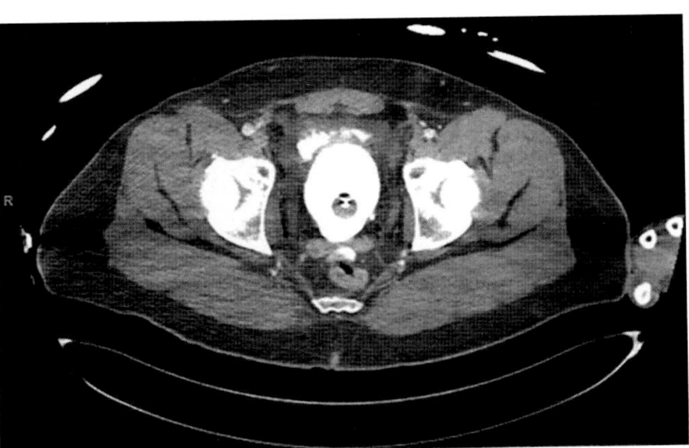

FIGURE 3 ● CT retrograde cystography showing intraperitoneal perforation with extravasation of contrast.

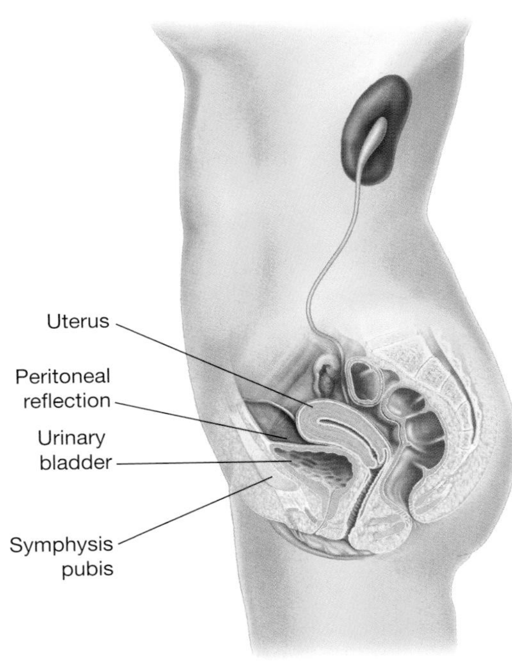

FIGURE 4 ● Anatomy of the female bladder.

- Anatomy
  - In women, the bladder lies behind the symphysis pubis, anterior to the uterus. The cervix, vagina, and extraperitoneal bladder lie below the peritoneal reflection (**FIGURE 4**).
  - In men, the bladder lies behind the symphysis pubis, directly anterior to the rectum. The prostate, prostatic urethra, and extraperitoneal bladder lie below the peritoneal reflection (**FIGURE 5**).
  - Coronal section through the male bladder demonstrates the internal anatomy. The trigone, ureteral orifices are posterior and retroperitoneal (**FIGURE 6**).
- Intraperitoneal bladder injuries
  - Intraperitoneal bladder injuries warrant operative repair.[4]

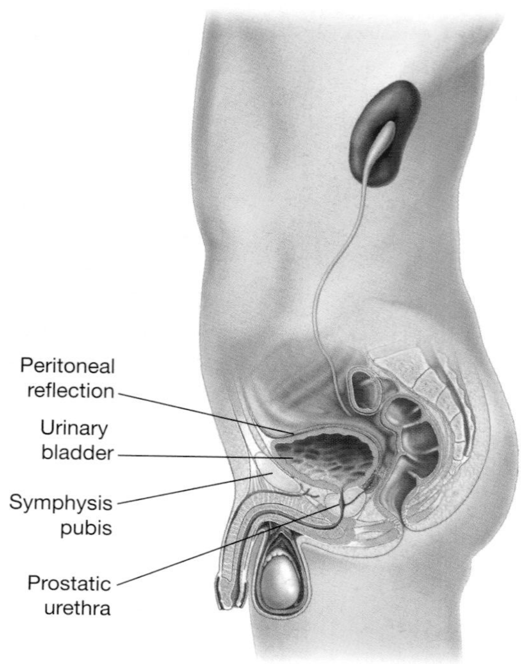

FIGURE 5 ● Anatomy of the male bladder.

- Extraperitoneal bladder injuries
  - Uncomplicated extraperitoneal bladder injuries are expectantly managed with Foley catheter drainage for 7 to 14 days. The majority will heal without operative intervention.
  - Complicated extraperitoneal bladder injuries may warrant operative repair. These include concurrent vaginal or rectal laceration, bladder neck injuries, pelvic fractures with fragment penetration into the bladder lumen, and bladder injuries in the presence of anterior pelvic ring fractures that require open reduction internal fixation,[5] due to the potential for hardware infection. Close communication with orthopedic trauma is mandatory as the presence of extraperitoneal bladder injuries can impact operative planning.
  - In the presence of complicated extraperitoneal bladder injury involving the bladder neck, urologic consultation is advised due to potential involvement of the trigone and potential need for complex reconstruction.
  - If the patient has another indication for laparotomy and an extraperitoneal bladder injury is present, repair can be considered, but is not mandatory.

Positioning

- The patient should be positioned for standard trauma laparotomy, in the supine position with the arms untucked.

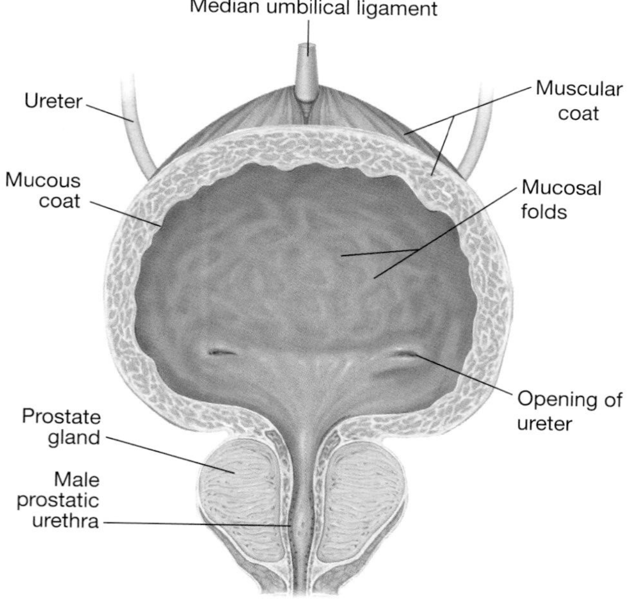

FIGURE 6 ● Internal anatomy of the bladder (male).

INCISION AND EXPOSURE

- The most common approach to the repair of bladder injury is a midline laparotomy with adequate infraumbilical length for exposure of the bladder.
- Exploration of the abdomen is performed to identify and prioritize other injuries. For the bladder repair, exposure is facilitated by Trendelenburg position with the abdominal contents packed away cephalad with radiopaque towels. A self-retaining retractor is placed to maintain adequate exposure to the pelvis and bladder. The size of the injury is characterized and inspected to ensure that it does not involve the trigone of the bladder (**FIGURES 7** and **8**).
- In the setting of orthopedic repair of pelvic fractures, a midline laparotomy or an extraperitoneal approach via a Pfannenstiel incision may be used.

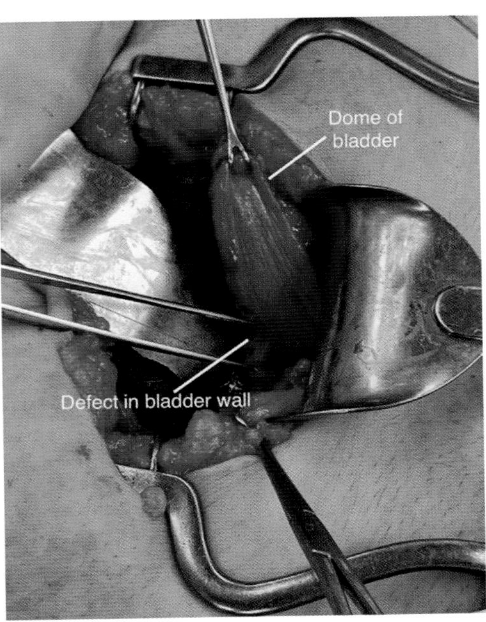

FIGURE 7 ● The dome of the bladder is elevated to expose the site of injury.

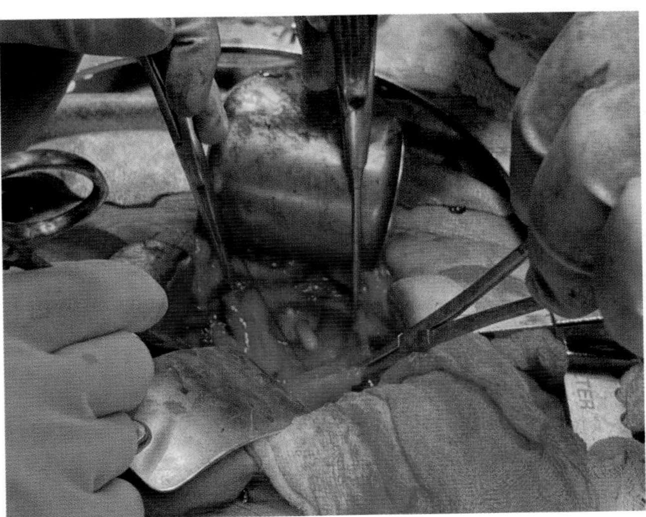

FIGURE 8 ● The bladder opening is exposed within the pelvis, with the Foley catheter balloon visualized within and a guidewire placed within the left ureteral orifice. Note the mucosal and detrusor muscle layers.

REPAIR OF INTRAPERITONEAL BLADDER INJURY

- The bladder is debrided back to healthy-appearing tissue. Prior to closing the cystotomy, inspection of urinary efflux from the ureteral orifices and examination of the interior surface of the bladder is indicated.[6] Stay sutures are placed on either end of the cystotomy to align the tissues for repair. The injury is then closed in two layers (see **FIGURE 9**).
- Following repair of the inner layer, a second layer closure including the outer muscular layer and peritoneum is performed with absorbable sutures in a running fashion (see **FIGURE 10**).
- Following repair, a leak test is performed by instilling 300 to 400 mL of saline via the Foley catheter to evaluate the integrity of the repair. The Foley catheter should remain in place.
- With both layers closed, the repair is completed (see **FIGURE 11**).
- In the setting of a posterior injury combined with a rectal injury, an omental pedicle flap can be placed between the rectal and bladder suture lines to reduce the potential for fistula formation.

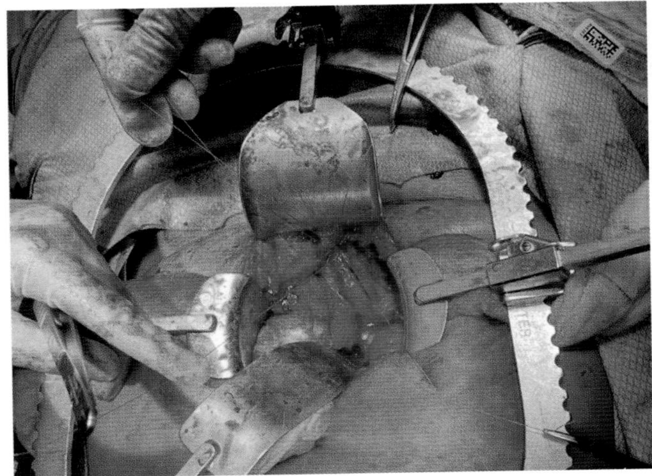

FIGURE 9 ● Stay sutures are placed at each end of the defect to facilitate alignment for closure. A running or locked running absorbable suture is used to close the mucosa and detrusor muscle.

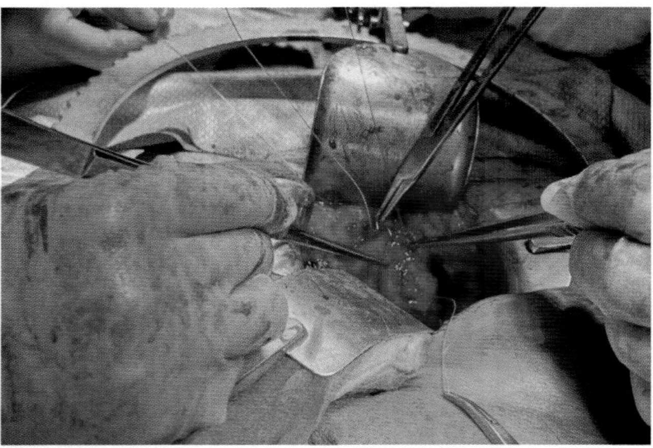

FIGURE 10 • A running or locked running absorbable suture is used to close the bladder muscle over the inner layer.

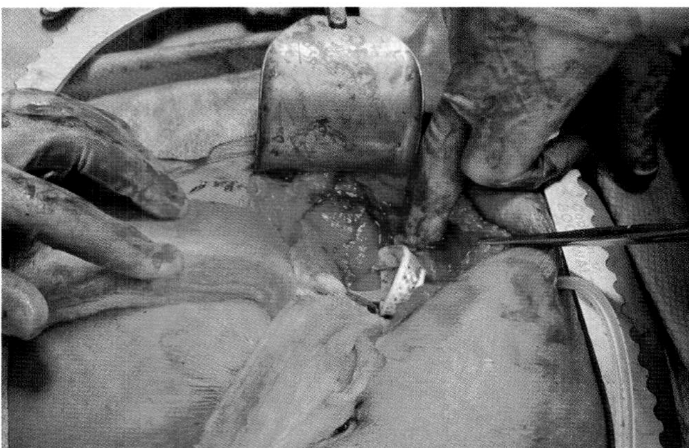

FIGURE 11 • A closed suction drain is placed adjacent to the repair.

REPAIR OF COMPLEX EXTRAPERITONEAL BLADDER INJURY

- The repair may be approached extraperitoneally. The space of Retzius is entered behind the symphysis pubis and the bladder mobilized to expose the preperitoneal space and the extraperitoneal anterior wall of the bladder.
- Anterior injuries may then be closed under direct visualization, in a two-layer fashion similar to intraperitoneal repair.
- Posterior extraperitoneal injuries may be approached from within the bladder. The anterior bladder wall is opened and the incision carried is caudad beyond the pubic symphysis to allow exposure and inspection of the intravesical aspect of the injury. A self-retaining retractor may be placed inside the bladder to improve exposure. The ureteral orifices are identified, and, if visualization is difficult, indigo carmine or fluorescein may be given intravenously to facilitate identification. Primary repair is then performed from the inside of the bladder, starting with closure of the outer muscular layer using absorbable suture, followed by closure of the inner seromuscular layer using 3-0 absorbable suture. Surgical knots should be tied on the outside of the suture line to avoid creating a nidus for stone formation.
- If the injury involves the trigone or the ureteral orifices, consideration should be given to intraoperative urologic consultation for assistance in reconstruction.[7]
- The Foley catheter should remain in place postoperatively.
- A closed suction drain should be left near the repair to monitor for the presence of a leak of urine.

PEARLS AND PITFALLS

Patient history and findings	■ Delayed diagnosis of bladder injury with uncontrolled urinary extravasation is a cause of significant morbidity and mortality. ■ The presence of gross hematuria in a trauma patient should prompt immediate evaluation for a bladder injury with retrograde cystography.
Surgical management	■ Intraperitoneal bladder injuries require operative repair. Confirmation of a watertight repair with a leak test should be performed after closure. ■ The majority of extraperitoneal bladder injuries may be managed with catheter drainage alone. ■ Complicated extraperitoneal bladder injury should be repaired operatively. A low threshold for intraoperative urology consultation should be maintained if there is a potential need for ureteral reconstruction.
Catheter management	■ Suprapubic cystostomy is rarely indicated; Foley catheter drainage alone is usually sufficient.

POSTOPERATIVE CARE

- Routine perioperative antibiotics should be administered.
- Prior to removal of the drain, a creatinine level can be checked to assess for the presence of a urine leak.
- Foley catheter drainage.
  - For operatively repaired intraperitoneal bladder injuries, the catheter should remain in place for 7 to 14 days following repair. For simple repairs, repeat imaging is not mandatory prior to catheter removal, but is often performed to confirm that there is no urinary extravasation. For complex repairs, retrograde cystography should be performed prior to catheter removal.
  - For nonoperatively and operatively managed extraperitoneal bladder injuries, the catheter should remain in place for 7 to 14 days. Prior to catheter removal, retrograde cystography is performed to confirm that the extraperitoneal bladder leak has resolved.[4]
- If persistent extravasation is noted on postoperative cystography, continued catheter drainage is indicated, with repeat imaging to confirm resolution of the leak prior to catheter removal.

COMPLICATIONS

- Unrecognized urinary leak.
  - Delayed recognition of bladder injury may lead to septic complications, electrolyte abnormalities from peritoneal urinary reabsorption, pelvic osteomyelitis, and prolonged hospitalization.[3]
- Fistula.
  - Patients who have concomitant injuries to the rectum and bladder are at risk for suture line breakdown and fistula formation, which may be minimized by placing a tongue of omentum between the repairs at the time of surgery.
- Postoperative urinoma or abscess.
  - Urinary leak following intraperitoneal bladder repairs are rare and generally can be managed with Foley catheter drainage and percutaneous drainage of collections.
- Persistent urinary leak.
  - Persistent urinary leak following repair is infrequent (<3%) and may resolve with a longer period of catheter drainage. Rarely, delayed operative intervention may be required.

REFERENCES

1. Terrier JE, Paparel P, Gadegbeku B, et al. Genitourinary injuries after traffic accidents: analysis of a registry of 162,690 victims. *J Trauma Acute Care Surg*. 2017; 82(6):1087-1093. doi:10.1097/TA.0000000000001448. PMID: 28328677.
2. Mahat Y, Leong JY, Chung PH. A contemporary review of adult bladder trauma. *J Inj Violence Res*. 2019;11(2):101-106. doi:10.5249/jivr.v11i2.1069
3. Morey AF, Broghammer JA, Hollowell CMP, et al. Urotrauma guideline 2020: AUA guideline. *J Urol*. 2021;205(1):30-35. doi:10.1097/JU.0000000000001408. PMID: 33053308.
4. Yeung LL, McDonald AA, Como JJ, et al. Management of blunt force bladder injuries: a practice management guideline from the Eastern Association for the Surgery of Trauma. *J Trauma Acute Care Surg*. 2019;86(2):326-336. doi:10.1097/TA.0000000000002132. [published correction appears in *J Trauma Acute Care Surg*. 2019;87(2):511].
5. *Calling the Urologist: Considerations in Intraoperative Consultations. American Urological Association Update Series*. 2020. Accessed January 20, 2021. https://auau.auanet.org/content/update-series-2020-lesson-11-calling-urologist-considerations-intraoperative--consultations
6. Morey AF, Zhao LC. Genital and lower urinary tract trauma. In: Partin AW, Dmochowski RR, Kavoussi LR, et al., eds. *Campbell-Walsh-Wein Urology*. 12th ed. Elsevier; 2021.
7. Moore EE, Cogbill TH, Jurkovich GJ, et al. Organ injury scaling. III: Chest wall, abdominal vascular, ureter, bladder, and urethra. *J Trauma*. 1992;33(3):337-339. PMID: 1404499.

Chapter 32 Ureter: Proximal Third, Middle Third, Distal Third

Irma J. Lengu, Esther S. Tseng, and John J. Como

DEFINITION

- Ureteral injury occurs when there is partial or complete damage to any portion of the ureter due to external trauma (blunt or penetrating) or, more commonly, iatrogenic causes. In this chapter, we will focus on the diagnosis, treatment, and sequela of ureteral injury incurred from external traumatic causes, both blunt and penetrating.
- Treatment of ureteral injuries depends on the grade and location of the injury, as well as the hemodynamic status of the patient (**TABLE 1**).[1]
- Ureteral trauma is rare, with the vast majority, 95%, due to penetrating trauma.[2] Traumatic ureteral injuries are associated with high mortality rates, with the mortality almost always due to associated injuries. Although they are uncommon, it is important to recognize and promptly address ureteral injuries, as delays in diagnosis or treatment can lead to significant complications including abscess formation, urinomas, strictures, fistulas, and even loss of the ipsilateral kidney.[3]
- Ureteral injuries are generally identified intraoperatively during trauma laparotomy for hemodynamic instability or peritonitis. In the setting of blunt trauma, ureteral injuries tend to occur in high-energy impacts. More than 90% of patients with ureteral injuries have other concurrent abdominal or retroperitoneal injuries.[4,5]

Table 1: Grading of Ureteral Injuries

Grade of injury	Type	Description
I	Hematoma	Contusion or hematoma. No devascularization
II	Laceration	<50% transection
III	Laceration	≥50% transection
IV	Laceration	Complete transection with <2 cm devascularization
V	Laceration	Avulsion with >2 cm devascularization

From Moore EE, Cogbill TH, Jurkovich GJ, et al. Organ injury scaling. III: Chest wall, abdominal vascular, ureter, bladder, and urethra. J Trauma. 1992;33(3):337-339.

PATIENT HISTORY AND PHYSICAL EXAMINATION

- The patient is evaluated per Advanced Trauma Life Support protocol. In cases of peritonitis or hemodynamic instability with an abdominal source, the patient is urgently explored in the operating room. Bullet trajectory and injury of organs in proximity to the ureter should raise suspicion for ureteral injury. In such cases, the ureter is meticulously explored.

IMAGING AND OTHER DIAGNOSTIC STUDIES

- For stable blunt trauma patients, computed tomography (CT) of the abdomen and pelvis with intravenous contrast, with delayed images, is obtained. Positive findings of ureteral injury include delayed urinary excretion, urinoma, hydronephrosis, or extravasation of intravenous contrast. CT is not an option in hemodynamically unstable patients, who may require urgent laparotomy. At laparotomy, if concern for ureteral injury persists despite an exhaustive attempt at direct visualization, we have administered intravenous methylene blue to assist in excluding injury to the ureter.

SURGICAL MANAGEMENT

- Penetrating wounds to the abdomen with peritonitis or hemodynamic instability require abdominal exploration. Unstable blunt trauma patients with hemoperitoneum should also undergo laparotomy. As part of a comprehensive abdominal exploration, ureteral injury should be excluded by direct inspection.

Positioning

- Trauma patients are generally positioned supine with arms extending outward for vascular access and exposure of the abdomen. A urinary catheter is placed. If bladder or ureteral injuries are known or highly suspected prior to exploration, consideration should be given to prepping the external genitalia into the operative field. Bloody output from an indwelling urinary catheter is suggestive of genitourinary tract trauma. A normal urinalysis, however, does not rule out injury to the ureter.[3]

ABDOMINAL EXPLORATION

- Exploratory surgery is done through a generous midline abdominal incision, as with any trauma laparotomy. Control of bleeding is performed first, followed by control of and repair of hollow viscus injuries. The ureters are visualized as part of the comprehensive laparotomy.
- It is important to note that observing peristalsis of part of the ureter and blind palpation are not reliable tools to rule out ureteral injury. With careful exploration, ureteral injuries are unlikely to be missed. Kunkle et al noted that out of 429 ureteral injuries, there was a 11% miss rate at the time of initial laparotomy.[3]

TREATMENT

- The treatment of ureteral injuries is dependent on the extent and location of the injury, as well as the hemodynamic status of the patient at the time of repair. In this chapter, we will describe treatment options based on the location of the injury (**FIGURE 1**). The location of ureteral injuries due to trauma is roughly evenly distributed between the upper, middle, and lower thirds of the ureter.[3]
- No matter the location, the principles of repair are the same.

Tension-Free Anastomosis

- The ureter must be mobilized carefully, sparing the adventitia and maintaining the blood supply. This lowers the risk of urine leak and eventual stricture of the ureter. Care should be taken to ensure that the anastomosis is tension-free to reduce the possibility of urine leak or eventual stricture.

Spatulation of the Ureter

- Spatulation provides a relatively large diameter at the repair site, thereby reducing the risk for eventual stricture of the ureter at this site.

Ureteral Stenting

- Placement of a ureteral stent decreases both the hydrostatic pressure transmitted to the renal pelvis and the incidence of urinoma.

Watertight Anastomosis

- Generally, a 5-0 absorbable suture is utilized to perform a watertight anastomosis; we prefer 5-0 polydioxanone (PDS).

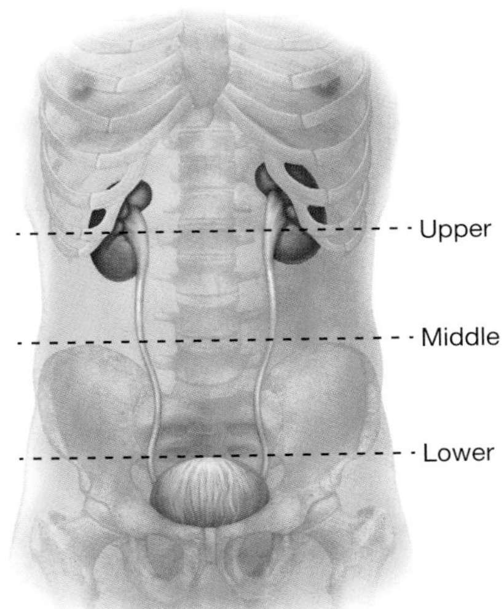

FIGURE 1 ● Anatomical division of the ureter into upper, middle, and lower thirds. (Redrawn from Pereira BMT, Ogilvie MP, Gomez-Rodriguez JC, et al. A review of ureteral injuries after external trauma. *Scand J Trauma Resusc Emerg Med*. 2010;18:6.)

External Closed Suction Drain Placement

- External drainage prevents the development of urinoma and allows for rapid diagnosis of urine leak.

PROXIMAL THIRD URETERAL INJURY REPAIRS

Ureteropelvic Junction Injuries

- Ureteropelvic junction injuries occur from high-velocity blunt deceleration trauma as well as from penetrating trauma. These injuries are generally managed by performing a dismembered pyeloplasty, which is defined as reimplantation of the injured ureter into the renal pelvis. This requires mobilization and debridement of the ureter, which is then spatulated laterally.
- The anastomosis is completed using 5-0 PDS suture in a running fashion, taking care not to narrow the lumen. A stent is placed after the posterior half of the anastomosis is completed. The anterior portion is then approximated similarly over the stent (**FIGURE 2**).

Ureterocalicostomy

- In cases of severe renal pelvis injury, there may not be sufficient pelvis to complete an anastomosis. In such a situation, if the patient is stable, a ureterocalicostomy may be indicated.
- In this procedure, the lower pole calyx is exposed by excising the lower pole and attaining access to the lower pole calyx. The first suture is placed over the apex of the spatulated ureter and the lateral portion of the calyx. The rest of ureter is then anastomosed using the same principles of a stented, tension-free, watertight, and spatulated anastomosis (**FIGURE 3**).

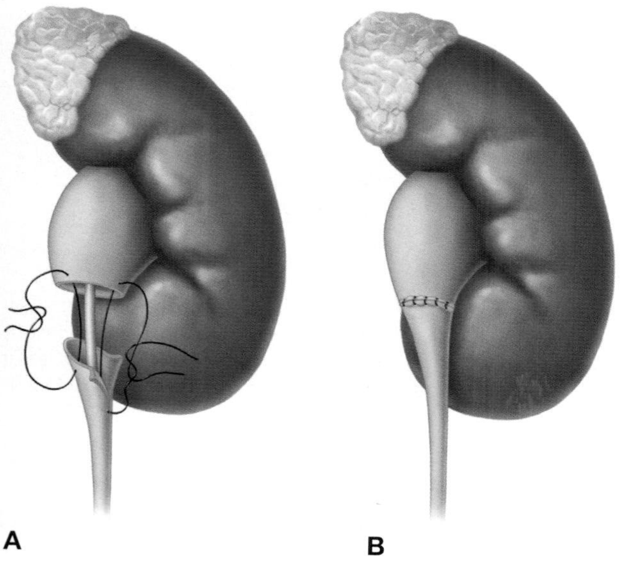

FIGURE 2 • Pyeloplasty. The injured ureter is debrided and spatulated. The ureter is anastomosed to the renal pelvis with absorbable suture over a stent **(A)**. The anastomosis is completed in a single, full thickness layer with absorbable, running suture in a watertight manner **(B)**. (Redrawn from Partin AW, Dmochowski RR, Kavoussi LR, Peters CA. *Management of upper urinary tract obstruction*. In: *Campbell-Walsh-Wein Urology*. 12th ed. Elsevier; 2021:1953.)

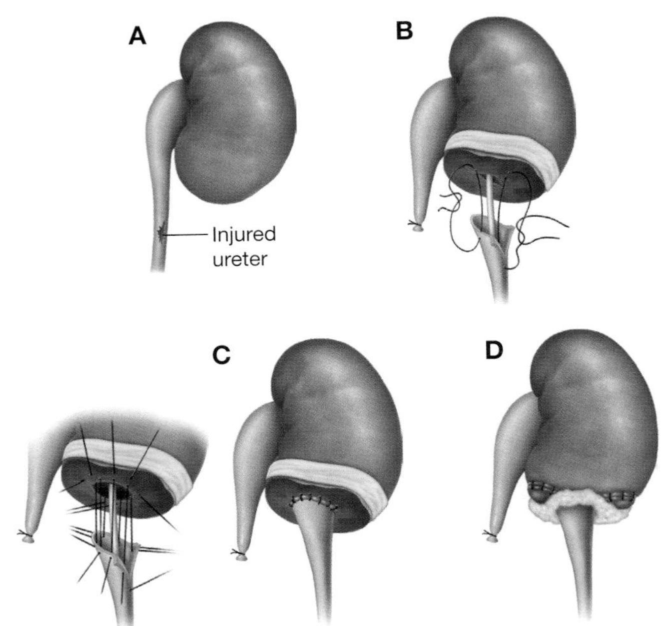

FIGURE 3 ● Ureterocalicostomy. The injured ureter is debrided. The proximal end is ligated **(A)**. The distal ureter is spatulated and the lower pole is resected to reveal the lower pole calyx. Stay sutures are placed at the apex **(B)**. The ureter is anastomosed to the lower pole calyx in interrupted absorbable suture in a full thickness, watertight fashion over a stent **(C)**. The anastomosis is covered with perinephric fat **(D)**. (Redrawn Partin AW, Dmochowski RR, Kavoussi LR, Peters CA. *Management of upper urinary tract obstruction*. In: *Campbell-Walsh-Wein Urology*. 12th ed. Elsevier; 2021:1962.)

MIDDLE THIRD URETERAL INJURY REPAIRS

Ureteroureterostomy

- The ureteroureterostomy is best reserved for short defects of the upper or middle portions of the ureter. In cases of penetrating trauma due to a gunshot wound, devitalized tissue and an adjacent segment of ureter that appears to be normal should be debrided to minimize the risk for delayed ischemic injury or stricture of the ureter.
- Once this has been accomplished, both ends of the ureter should be carefully mobilized, preserving the adventitia. Each end is spatulated 180° apart. Anastomosis is completed with 5-0 PDS in interrupted fashion, over a stent.[5] Omental or retroperitoneal fat can be used to wrap the ureteral anastomosis (**FIGURE 4**).

Transureteroureterostomy

- When end-to-end anastomosis is not technically possible due to loss of tissue, consideration should be given to transureteroureterostomy (TUU).[5] The only absolute contraindication to TUU is insufficient length to reach the contralateral ureter. Relative contraindications would include history of nephrolithiasis, urothelial cancer, and chronic pyelonephritis. It should be recognized that this repair may jeopardize the noninjured renal unit. In this procedure, the affected ureter is mobilized and the end to be anastomosed is thoroughly debrided. If the distal end of the damaged ureter is seen, it can be ligated. If the distal end cannot be identified, it is acceptable to leave it without ligation as the incidence of reflux is low.
- The contralateral colon is mobilized, and the recipient ureter is identified and then mobilized only minimally to preserve

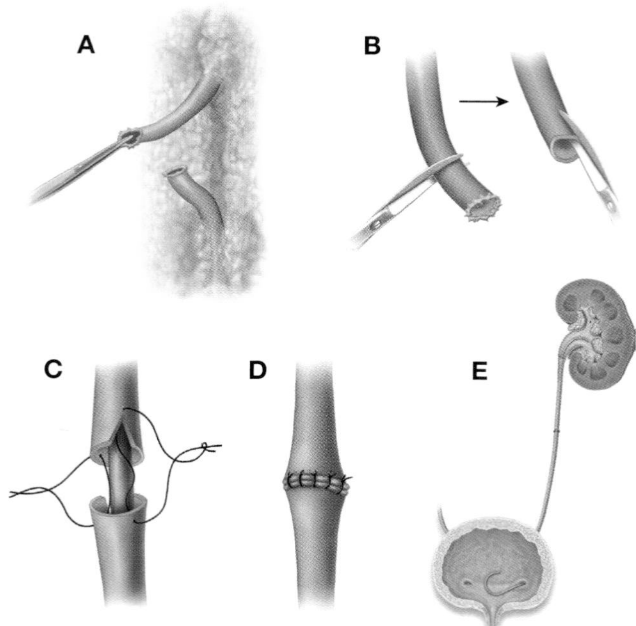

FIGURE 4 ● Ureteroureterostomy. The injured ureter is debrided to bleeding edges **(A)**. Each end is spatulated in the opposite direction **(B)**. Stay sutures are placed at each spatulated location **(C)**. The anastomosis is completed, full thickness, using absorbable suture in a watertight fashion **(D)**. This is completed over a stent **(E)**. (Redrawn from Partin AW, Dmochowski RR, Kavoussi LR, Peters CA. *Upper ureteral trauma*. In: *Campbell-Walsh-Wein Urology*. 12th ed. Elsevier; 2021:1996.)

the integrity of its blood supply. Generally, the recipient ureter is exposed about 5 cm proximal to the end of the affected ureter. The affected ureter is tunneled under the mesentery, proximal to the inferior mesenteric artery, to prevent tethering of the ureter by the vessel.

- The injured ureter is spatulated and a ureterotomy is made on the anteromedial portion of the recipient ureter. The end-to-side anastomosis is completed, using the same principles as previously discussed, with 5-0 absorbable suture in an interrupted fashion. Prior to the completion of the anastomosis, a stent is passed on the injured side (**FIGURE 5**).

Bowel Interposition

- Although bowel interposition is commonly utilized in the elective or chronic setting, this procedure is rarely employed in acute traumatic ureteral injuries. Cases of ileal and appendiceal interposition have, however, been reported after trauma.[6,7]

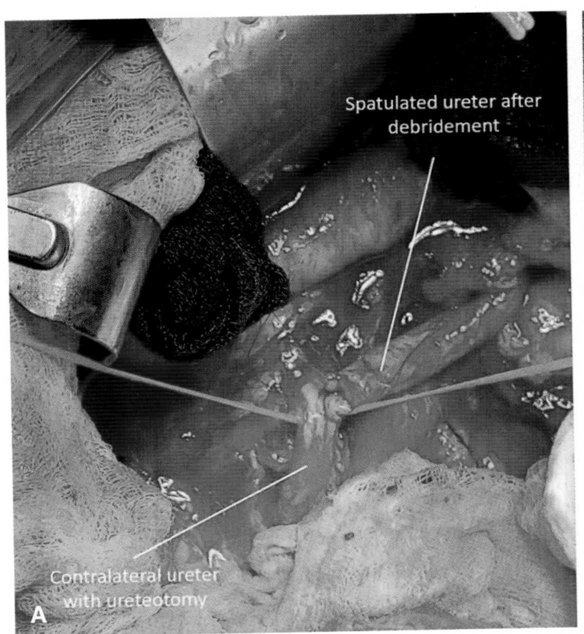

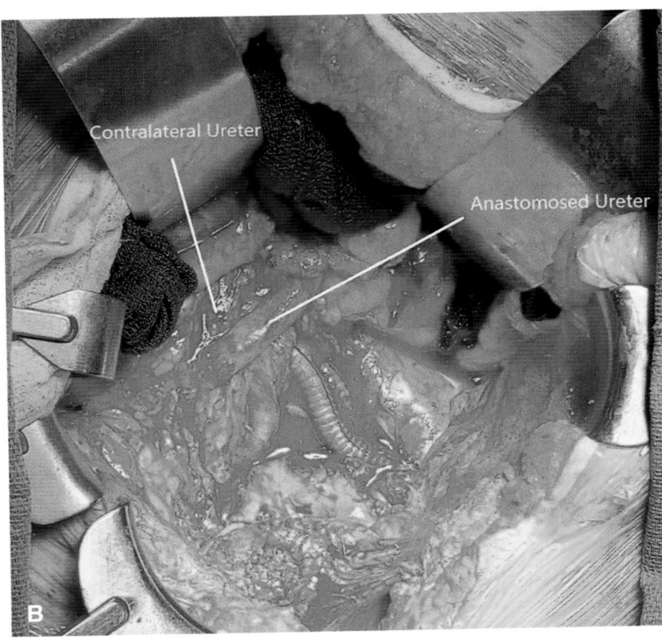

FIGURE 5 ● Transureteroureterostomy. The contralateral ureter is identified and ureterotomy is made. The injured ureter is debrided to bleeding edges and spatulated **(A)**. The anastomosis is completed, full thickness, using absorbable running suture over a stent **(B)**.

DISTAL THIRD URETERAL INJURY REPAIRS

Ureteroneocystostomy

- Ureteroneocystostomy, which is the reimplantation of the ureter into the bladder, works best for injuries affecting the distal 4 cm of the ureter. The ureter is most easily identified at its crossing over the iliac vessels.
- The ureter is mobilized and debrided. If able to complete a tension-free anastomosis, then a cystotomy is made. The ureter is spatulated and anastomosed to the cystotomy using 5-0 PDS suture. This is performed in a nontunneled extravesical fashion (**FIGURE 6**).
- If this is technically impossible, a more complex reconstruction, such as a psoas hitch or Boari flap, will be necessary. Although these are excellent options for the repair of distal ureteral injuries, they are complex and should be performed in conjunction with urologic consultation.

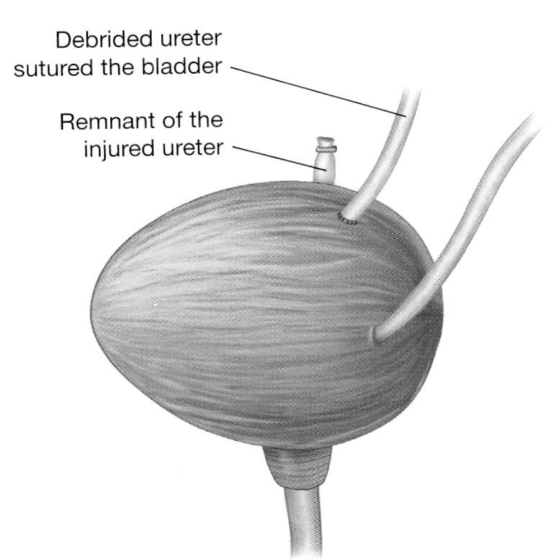

FIGURE 6 ● Ureteroneocystostomy. The injured ureter is debrided to bleeding edges and spatulated. The remnant ureter may be ligated if visible. A cystotomy is made and stay sutures are placed to anchor the ureter to the bladder. The anastomosis is completed using absorbable suture in a running or interrupted watertight fashion over a stent. (Redrawn from Partin AW, Dmochowski RR, Kavoussi LR, Peters CA. *Bladder surgery for benign disease*. In: *Campbell-Walsh-Wein Urology*. 12th ed. Elsevier; 2021:3023.)

Psoas Hitch

- The psoas hitch was first described by Zimmerman et al[8] It is used to aid in the repair of injuries located in the distal third of the ureter that cannot be repaired with simple ureteroneocystostomy. It can provide as much as 5 cm of additional length.[9]
- Once the ureter and bladder are sufficiently mobilized, a small cystotomy is made posteriorly at the site of reimplantation. A stay suture is placed on the ureter, which is used

to aid in the delivery of the ureter into the bladder lumen. The ureter is spatulated and anastomosed to the bladder in an interrupted tension-free fashion, using 5-0 PDS suture (**FIGURE 7**). A stent is placed prior to completion of the anastomosis.

- The dome of the bladder is then "hitched" to the psoas minor tendon or the psoas major muscle using 2-0 PDS suture. Care should be taken not to injure the genitofemoral nerve, which lies on the surface of the psoas muscle, or the femoral nerve, located deeper. The bladder is then closed in two layers with absorbable suture.

Boari Flap

- If a psoas hitch does not provide adequate length for tension-free reimplantation of the ureter, then a Boari flap may be considered to aid in the repair. The Boari flap is utilized for defects in the distal ureter that are greater than 5 cm and are often used for large gaps of 10 to 15 cm. Boari first described this technique in a canine model in 1894, it was described in humans in 1947 by Ockerblad, and it has been described in many series since.[10,11]
- In this procedure, the bladder is mobilized and opened obliquely in order to form a flap, to which the ureter is reimplanted. Subsequently, the flap is tubularized over a stent (**FIGURE 8**).
- The base of the flap should be at minimum 4 cm wide with the tip being about 3 cm wide. The length of the flap should be at least the length of the ureteral defect.
- Once the flap is created and the bladder is opened, a cystopexy is performed, suturing the distal tip of the flap to the psoas muscle as described for the psoas hitch. A small opening is created in the posterior portion of the flap. The ureter is spatulated and an anastomosis is performed as in the psoas hitch. A stent is placed, and the bladder is closed as above.

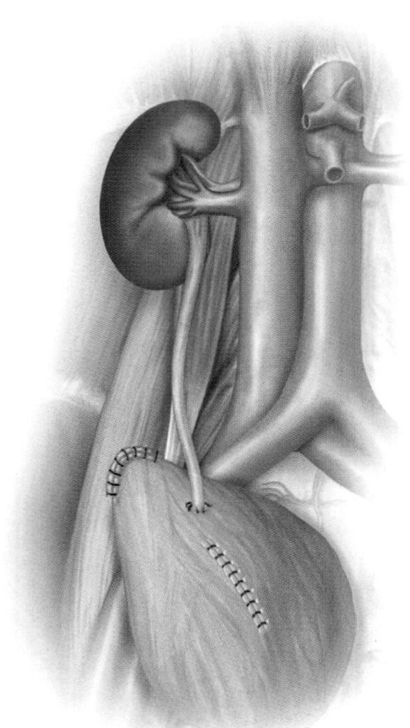

FIGURE 7 ● Psoas hitch. The ureter is debrided to bleeding edges and spatulated. The bladder is mobilized, and if needed, the contralateral superior vesical artery and vas deferens (or round ligament in women) are ligated and divided. A generous cystotomy is made anteriorly, a second smaller cystotomy is made, and the spatulated ureter is delivered into the bladder. The anastomosis is completed using interrupted absorbable suture and a stent is placed. The dome of the bladder is sutured to the ipsilateral psoas. The cystotomy is closed in two layers using absorbable suture. (Redrawn from Pereira BMT, Ogilvie MP, Gomez-Rodriguez JC, et al. A review of ureteral injuries after external trauma. *Scand J Trauma Resusc Emerg Med*. 2010;18:6.)

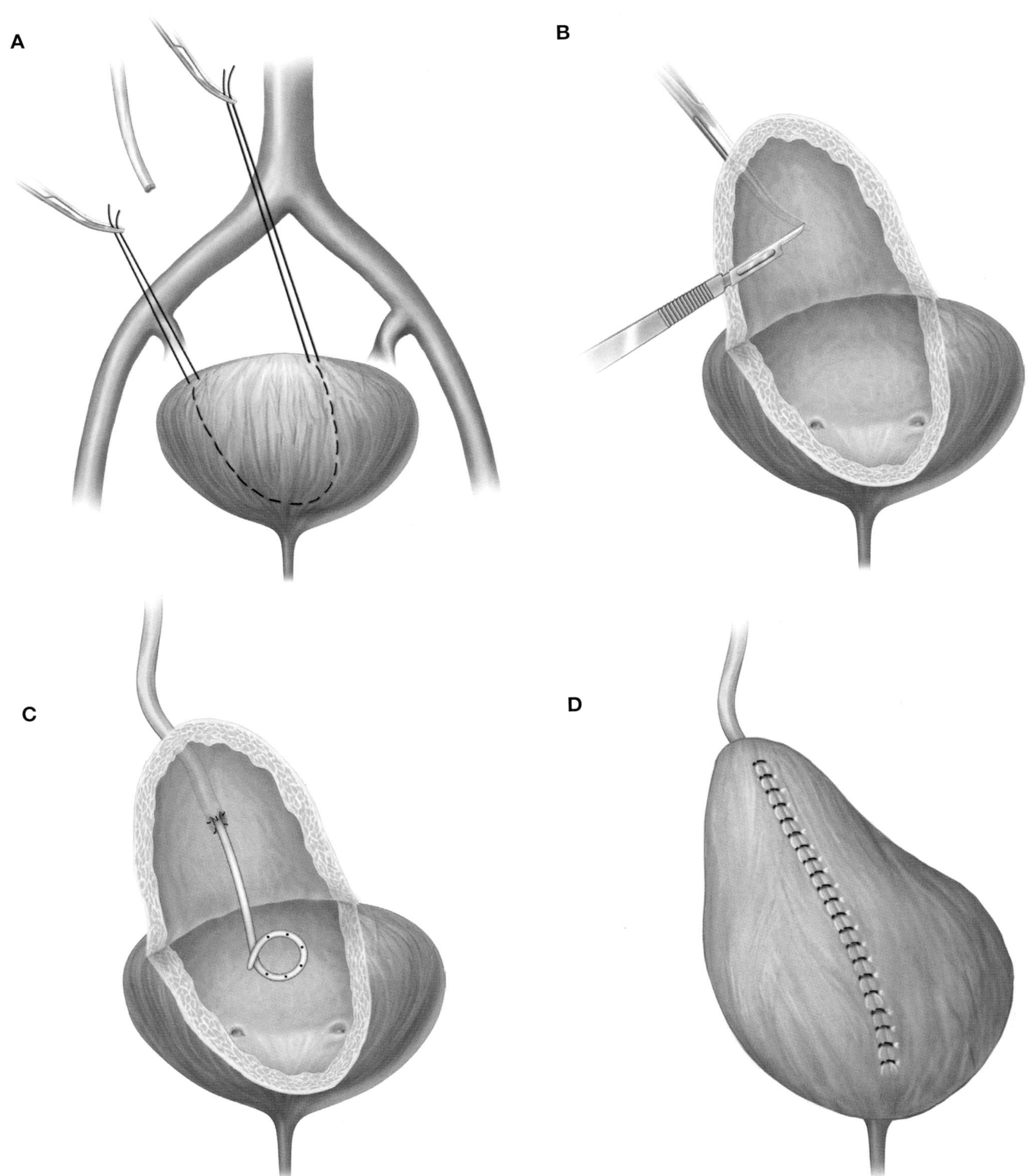

FIGURE 8 ● Boari flap. The bladder flap is marked and stay sutures are placed **(A)**. The flap is developed and a cystotomy is made on the flap preparing the reimplantation of the ureter **(B)**. The ureter is debrided and spatulated. The ureter is anastomosed to the flap with absorbable suture, over a stent **(C)**. The flap is tubularized and the cystotomy is closed **(D)**. (Redrawn Smith JA, Howards SS, Preminger GM. *Bladder Flap Repair (Boari)*. In: *Hinman's Atlas of Urologic Surgery*. 3rd ed. Elsevier Saunders; 2012:733-734.)

PEARLS AND PITFALLS

Treatment	■ The treatment of ureteral injuries depends on the extent and location of the injury, as well as the hemodynamic status of the patient at the time of repair. ■ The principles of repair are (1) tension-free anastomosis, (2) spatulation of the ureter, (3) ureteral stenting, (4) watertight anastomosis with 5-0 absorbable suture, and (5) placement of external closed suction drains.
Ureteral blood supply	■ Ureteral blood supply is delicate and easily disrupted. Preserving the ureteral adventitia is critical to decrease the risk of urine leak or ureteral stricture.
Technique	■ If a ureteral anastomosis is not tension free despite mobilization of the ureter, the bladder and/or the kidney should be mobilized. If this is not sufficient, more complicated procedures such as the psoas hitch or Boari flap should be considered. ■ Spatulation of the ureter should always be done to decrease the risk of stricture.
Unstable patient	■ In an unstable patient, ligation of the ureter and eventual nephrostomy tube placement may be necessary to provide renal preservation until definitive repair can be performed.
Consultation	■ When available, urological consultation should be considered, especially if the trauma surgeon has limited experience treating ureteral injuries.

- Debridement of the ureter should be significant enough to ensure bleeding edges but minimal enough to preserve length.

POSTOPERATIVE CARE

- External drains are generally removed in 24 to 48 hours if no urine leak is noted. For a procedure requiring a cystotomy, we maintain bladder drainage with a urinary catheter for 2 weeks and obtain a cystogram prior to removal. Stents are removed in the outpatient setting 4 to 6 weeks after repair.
- In cases of proximal ureteral repairs, if urine leaks are persistent, a urinary catheter is placed and maintained until resolution of the leak. The vast majority of leaks resolve without intervention, but should a leak be persistent, consideration may be given to nephrostomy tube drainage in addition to ureteral stenting and urinary catheter drainage. If a urinoma is noted, this can be drained percutaneously.
- We routinely obtain a follow-up CT urogram to evaluate the urinary tract about 4 to 6 weeks after the removal of any stents or nephrostomy tubes.

Damage Control

In damage control laparotomy for massive blood loss after trauma, patients may be too unstable for definitive repair of a ureter injury. In this situation, the priority is control of bleeding and contamination. Once these have been controlled, a tube may be placed in the proximal ureter and brought out through the skin. No attempt is made for ureteral reconstruction.[12] There is no need to identify the distal ureter at this time. Alternatively, the proximal ureter may be tied off with nonabsorbable suture for later identification. Generally, in such cases, a nephrostomy tube is placed by Interventional Radiology in 24 to 48 hours, assuming the patient is stable enough to tolerate this procedure. These patients generally have the abdomen packed open and are brought to the intensive care unit for resuscitation.

Once the patient's acidosis, coagulopathy, and hypothermia have been corrected in the intensive care unit, the patient may be taken back to the operating room 24 to 48 hours later for definitive ureteral repair utilizing one of the techniques described above, whichever is most appropriate given the pattern and location of the ureter injury and the hemodynamic status of the patient.

COMPLICATIONS

Missed Injuries

- Ureteral injuries missed at the time of initial presentation, as well as complications from disrupted ureteral anastomoses, can lead to short- and long-term complications.[3] Such complications can include development of urinoma, hydronephrosis, stricture, sepsis, renal failure, or even loss of the kidney. Patients often present with fever, peritonitis, or an elevated creatinine. CT urogram is the preferred imaging study to evaluate the kidneys and the ureters.
- Once the ureteral injury has been identified, the patient should undergo prompt drainage. A retrograde pyelogram and attempted stenting are preferred to establish continuity of the ureter whenever possible.[13] The stent is generally maintained for 6 weeks or until definitive repair, should additional reconstruction be needed. If a stent cannot be placed, then a nephrostomy tube should be placed for drainage. This is maintained until final reconstruction. In cases of urinoma, CT-guided drainage is utilized.

REFERENCES

1. Moore EE, Cogbill TH, Jurkovich GJ, et al. Organ injury scaling. III: Chest wall, abdominal vascular, ureter, bladder, and urethra. *J Trauma*. 1992;33(3):337-339.
2. Presti JC Jr., Carroll PR, McAninch JW. Ureteral and renal pelvic injuries from external trauma: diagnosis and management. *J Trauma*. 1989;29(3):370-374.
3. Kunkle DA, Kansas BT, Pathak A, et al. Delayed diagnosis of traumatic ureteral injuries. *J Urol*. 2006;176(6 Pt 1):2503-2507.
4. Campbell EW Jr., Filderman PS, Jacobs SC. Ureteral injury due to blunt and penetrating trauma. *Urology*. 1992;40(3):216-220.
5. Pereira BMT, Ogilvie MP, Gomez-Rodriguez JC, et al. A review of ureteral injuries after external trauma. *Scand J Trauma Resusc Emerg Med*. 2010;18:6.
6. Bhandari M, Mufti GR, Singh SM. Ileal replacement for gunshot injury to the ureter. *Aust N Z J Surg*. 1977;47(4):523-525.

7. Medina JJ, Cummings JM, Parra RO. Repair of ureteral gunshot injury with appendiceal interposition. *J Urol*. 1999;161:1563.
8. Zimmerman IJ, Precourt WE, Thompson CC. Direct uretero-cystoneostomy with the short ureter in the cure of ureterovaginal fistula. *J Urol*. 1960;83:113-115.
9. Kishev SV. Psoas-bladder hitch procedure: our experience with repair of the injured ureter in men. *J Urol*. 1975;113(4):772-776.
10. Ockerblad NF. Reimplantation of the ureter into the bladder by a flap method. *J Urol*. 1947;57(5):845-847.
11. Konigberg H, Blunt KJ, Muecke EC. Use of Boari flap in lower ureteral injuries. *Urology*. 1975;5(6):751-755.
12. Ball CG, Hameed SM, Navsaria P, et al. Successful damage control of complex vascular and urologic gunshot injuries. *Can J Surg*. 2006;49(6):437-438.
13. Sclafani SJA, Goldstein AS, Lipkowitz GS. Radiologic management of a disrupted ureteral anastomosis and infected urinoma after gunshot wound. *J Trauma*. 1984;24(12):1060-1062.

SECTION X: Pelvic Fracture/Retroperitoneal Hematoma

Chapter 33 Preperitoneal Pelvic Packing

Kaitlin A. Ritter and Clay Cothren Burlew

DEFINITION

- Preperitoneal pelvic packing (PPP) is a surgical procedure that opens the anatomic preperitoneal, paravesical plane in the pelvis for the purposes of exposing bilateral retroperitoneum for subsequent packing and tamponade of bleeding. It is a technique used in trauma populations to control life-threatening hemorrhage within the pelvis from traumatic vascular and bony injuries.
- First described in Europe in the early 1990s,[1] modifications in the United States utilized a different anterior suprapubic approach and added the use of concomitant external pelvic fixation. Outcomes reported to date demonstrate shorter time to intervention with PPP and lower mortality in patients with life-threatening hemorrhage from pelvic fractures.[2]

DIFFERENTIAL DIAGNOSIS

- Multiply injured patients often present as polytraumas, and it is critically important to perform a full evaluation on these patients to identify other sources of shock. Common sites for large-volume hemorrhage outside of the pelvis including the chest, abdomen, extremities, or on-scene losses due to lacerations causing external bleeding should be assessed.
- Mechanism of injury and injury patterns should be considered when evaluating for nonhemorrhagic shock, such as blunt cardiac injuries causing myocardial stunning and diminished perfusion or neurogenic shock secondary to traumatic cord injury and paralysis.
- Patients presenting in shock with multiple potential etiologies may still benefit from pelvic packing if it is felt pelvic hemorrhage is at least partially contributing to the patient's hemodynamic instability.

PATIENT HISTORY AND PHYSICAL FINDINGS

- Patients with pelvic fractures and hemorrhage severe enough to require PPP are often the result of high-speed injury mechanisms. Scene reports of high-speed vehicles, significant vehicular intrusion/destruction, persons thrown a distance, falls from a height, or pelvic crush injuries should heighten concern for potential pelvic bleeding.
- Low-energy mechanisms, such as ground-level falls, can also lead to pelvic hemorrhage, but this typically presents in elderly and frail patients. The increased use of vitamin K antagonists, novel oral anticoagulants/antiplatelet medications, and atherosclerotic disease impairing vasospasm are thought to contribute to the development of hemodynamically significant hemorrhage in some of these injuries.[3]
- Additional clinical history such as patient's ambulatory status on scene, pelvic or lower back pain, inability to void, numbness, and lower extremity weakness may suggest the presence of pelvic fractures. Reports of hematuria, rectal or vaginal bleeding, and bowel/bladder incontinence should also be noted as these may be indicative of concomitant intrapelvic injuries that may need to be addressed intraoperatively when pelvic packing is performed.
- Identification of other potential injuries is also a critical element of management for any multiply injured patient. Gathering a concise history of mechanism, field reports of injuries/deficits, and patient symptoms can assist in clinical planning, simultaneous workup, and management of the whole patient.
- Not all patients with pelvic fractures and bleeding require PPP; packing should be reserved for patients with evidence of ongoing hemorrhagic shock. Patients with hemodynamic instability, ongoing blood transfusion requirements, or evidence of end-organ perfusion should be evaluated for surgical intervention.
- Refractory shock, defined as "persistent hypotension despite two units of RBC transfusion," has been utilized as the trigger for PPP at several centers because this was historically utilized for the decision to pursue angioembolization prior to the adoption of PPP as the primary hemorrhage control technique.[1-4]
- Physical examination of the pelvis including palpation of bony landmarks, the pubic symphysis, and ring stability assessment should be part of the evaluation for any trauma patient. In situations of suspected pelvic fractures, care must be taken with anterior-posterior and lateral compression as overly zealous palpation may result in worsening misalignment of unstable fractures leading to further damage and bleeding. "Rocking" of the pelvis should be avoided; instead, a single posterior compression overlying bilateral iliac crests should provide sufficient feedback regarding ring stability.
- A pelvic examination including evaluation of the skin, soft tissue and rectal and genitourinary systems should be performed looking for blood, mucosal laceration, or bony fragments, which may indicate an open component of the fracture.
- Blood at the urethral meatus, hematuria, a high riding prostate, or perineal hematoma should raise concern for a urogenital injury, and appropriate evaluation should be

initiated. Concomitant genitourinary injuries occur at a rate of 4.6% with the highest risk in male pelvic fractures.[5] It is important that injury to the rectal or genitourinary system be identified early as repair of these injuries may need to occur concurrently with operative PPP.

- Patients arriving with an in-field pelvic binder should have the binder removed to allow for complete assessment of the bony structures of the pelvis in addition to the overlying skin, soft tissues, and genitourinary organs. Once the physical examination is completed a binder may be placed or reapplied if the patient becomes hemodynamically unstable.
- Pelvic binder should be applied so that it rests over the greater trochanters of the femurs to close down the pelvic space. Application too high or too low can paradoxically widen this space and result in worsening hemorrhage.
- It is also important to ensure the pelvic binder is applied with appropriate tension. Overly tightened binders can cross the pelvis or close the anterior fractures while opening the posterior elements and can exacerbate difficult to control venous bleeding.
- The pelvic binder is not a definitive treatment; therefore, once applied, rapid evaluation and determination of injuries and a decision regarding necessary interventions should be made so that the binder may be removed. All efforts should be made to remove the pelvic binder as soon as clinically feasible, optimally within 1 to 2 hours of application, as prolonged application increases the risk of skin, soft tissue, muscle, and nerve injury.[6]
- A complete physical examination of all patients should be performed in accordance with Advanced Trauma Life Support (ATLS) protocols. Special attention should be paid to other potential areas of hemorrhage in addition to identifying other nonpelvic injuries that may require intervention.

IMAGING AND OTHER DIAGNOSTIC STUDIES

- Standard trauma laboratory tests, including a complete blood panel, basic metabolic panel, venous or arterial blood gas, lactate, and coagulation labs including partial thromboplastin time and international normalized ratio, and a thromboelastogram (TEG), should be obtained. Base deficit and lactate provide indices regarding the severity of shock, and TEG is helpful in guiding blood component resuscitation in patients at high risk for coagulopathy of trauma and need for massive transfusion.
- A chest radiograph (CXR) should be performed in the trauma bay allowing for rapid assessment of the pulmonary fields for hemothorax and pneumothorax as a contributing factor to the patient's shock. CXR also permits evaluation for diaphragm rupture requiring need for concurrent exploratory laparotomy.
- A focused assessment with sonography in trauma (FAST) examination should also be performed in the trauma bay evaluating for clinically significant blood within the abdominal cavity. In patients for whom cross-sectional imaging is deferred due to hemodynamic instability, the FAST examination can determine if an abdominal exploration in addition to PPP is necessary.
- A single view anterior-posterior pelvic radiograph in the trauma bay is an essential step in the planning for PPP. Pelvic fractures come in a variety of injury patterns with risk of hemorrhage loosely correlated with specific fracture types with anterior-posterior compression and open pelvic at the highest risk.[7] Radiographic evaluation of pelvic injuries also allows for orthopedic assessment and planning to reestablish pelvic stability, a critical element to the success of PPP.
- Cross-sectional imaging does not play a role in the standard algorithms for PPP, and in cases with concern for significant pelvic hemorrhage, operative interventions should not be delayed for computed tomography (CT) imaging.

SURGICAL MANAGEMENT

Preoperative Planning

- Assessment of hospital resources and ability to support patients with complex pelvic fracture requiring PPP is crucial. While PPP requires no specialized equipment, availability of surgical subspecialists such as orthopedic surgery and urology, intensive care unit (ICU) capabilities, and operating room (OR) support staff should all be accounted for prior to operative intervention.
- Early involvement of orthopedic surgery and application of an external fixator prior to packing is critical for success of PPP. The external fixator stabilizes the pelvis and provides a framework against which the pelvic packs can be pushed causing a tamponading effect. In emergent situations where orthopedic surgery is unavailable a pelvic binder low across the greater trochanters may be utilized in lieu of the external fixator, but this is associated with much lower success in hemorrhage control.
- Tranexamic acid (TXA) while utilized as part of the resuscitation algorithm for pelvic hemorrhage at some institutions[8] is not part of our PPP algorithm.[2] We feel prompt intervention and reestablishment of the pelvic framework results in a larger effect than TXA as pelvic hemorrhage is due to mechanical disruption as opposed to a hematologic disturbance.
- Resuscitation in line with ATLS principles should be continued through evaluation and en route to OR. Two large-bore intravenous (IV) catheters should be placed for volume resuscitation and IV access should be above the level of the pelvis, as the risk of a concomitant vascular injury is possible and femoral cannulations may result in transfusion of blood products directly into the pelvic hematoma.
- Hand off of resuscitation to the OR/anesthesia team should include clear communication of the patient's hemodynamics, clinical parameters of shock, resuscitation efforts, and operative plan. The anesthesia team should then take over the resuscitation allowing the surgical team to direct their focus to procedural planning.
- In these often severely injured patients, a clear operative plan should be established prior to incision. Many patients may need concurrent operations including thoracotomy, craniotomy, orthopedic/vascular repair, or exploratory laparotomy. Having a clear plan and coordinating with the various surgeons can facilitate a multisystem approach.

Positioning

- Patients should be positioned supine on the operating table, with arms out at 90°, and should be prepped from neck to

knees allowing for PPP and any additional required procedures. The operating table should allow for C-arm utilization by the orthopedic surgery team.
- Placement of the external fixator should be discussed to avoid overlap with the planned surgical incision site. If the anticipated procedures include an exploratory laparotomy in addition to PPP, the external fixator bar is ideally placed lower on the pelvis. For isolated PPP the bar should be placed higher above the level of your PPP incision, at the level of the umbilicus.

INITIAL PLACEMENT

- After external fixation has been performed, we begin our packing with a 6 to 8-cm lower midline incision starting at the pubic symphysis and moving cephalad. Electrocautery is used to divide the subcutaneous tissues down to the level of the midline fascia. See **FIGURE 1**.
- The midline fascia is divided with Bovie taking care to leave the peritoneum intact. At this point the pelvic hematoma is typically encountered welling up from the paravesical and retroperitoneal compartments.
- The preperitoneal plane is then bluntly entered with clearance of a U-shaped space extending around the bladder from the midline back toward the psoas muscle. Often the hematoma will have already dissected out this space and minimal further blunt dissection will be required and the hematoma will be evacuated concurrently with packing. See **FIGURE 2**.
- Preperitoneal packing is then performed using three standard surgical laparotomy pads on each side of the true pelvis. The packs should be placed systematically utilizing a ring forceps to place the first pack deep and posteriorly onto the sacrum. Two additional laparotomy pads are placed, one anteriorly to the first pack, which is lateral to the bladder, and the third just behind the pubic symphysis. The bladder does not need to be fully mobilized and instead can simply be retracted toward the contralateral side as all packs are being placed. The identical process is repeated on the opposite side. See **FIGURE 3**.
- In rare cases the pelvis may require an additional seventh pack. This occurs very infrequently and should be done cautiously as overpacking of the pelvis can result in compression of major venous structures. If significant space remains after the placement of the six packs, investigation of the external fixator should be performed to ensure the pelvic space has been appropriately closed down.

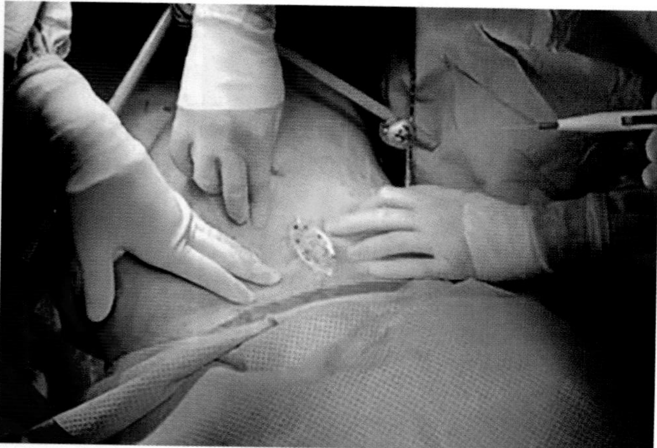

FIGURE 1 ● Incision is begun with a 6-8-cm lower midline cut just above the pubic symphysis. At the time of placement external fixator bars are positioned out of the planned surgical field.

- Pediatric patients require fewer laparotomy pads, and the exact number depends upon the age and size of the child.[9]
- Prior to closing the overlying fascia, any required urologic interventions should be completed. Even in the absence of a bladder or urethral injury, the bladder must be drained. This can be accomplished with a simple Foley catheter, or for more complex injuries placement of a suprapubic tube may be required. If needed, the suprapubic tube should be placed through a separate incision from the packing site. See **FIGURE 4**.
- The midline fascia is then closed with a running O-PDS suture, and the overlying skin is stapled closed. See **FIGURE 5**.

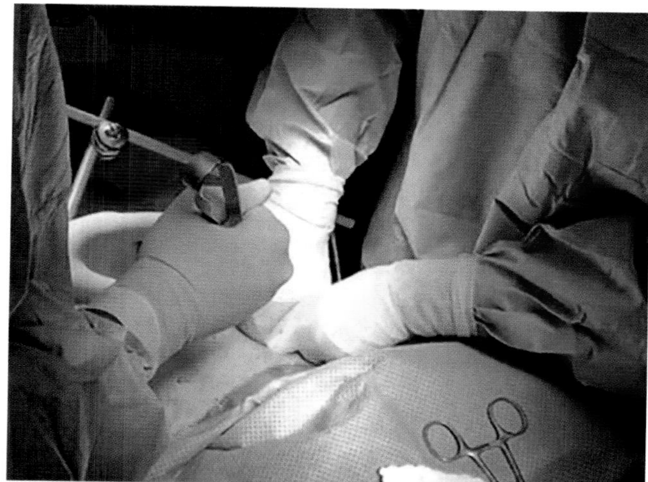

FIGURE 2 ● Opening of the paravesical and preperitoneal spaces can be accomplished with blunt hand dissection and adequate lateral retraction of the skin, subcutaneous tissues, and muscle.

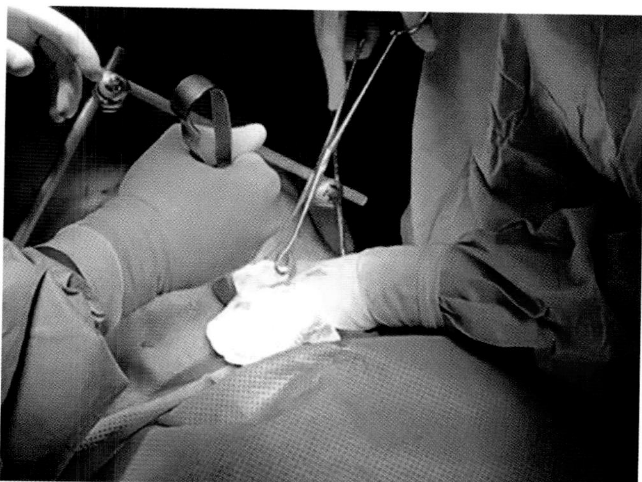

FIGURE 3 ● Standard surgical laparotomy pads are placed utilizing a ring forceps to direct the pack posteriorly onto the sacrum. Caution must be taken not to tear or damage the peritoneum.

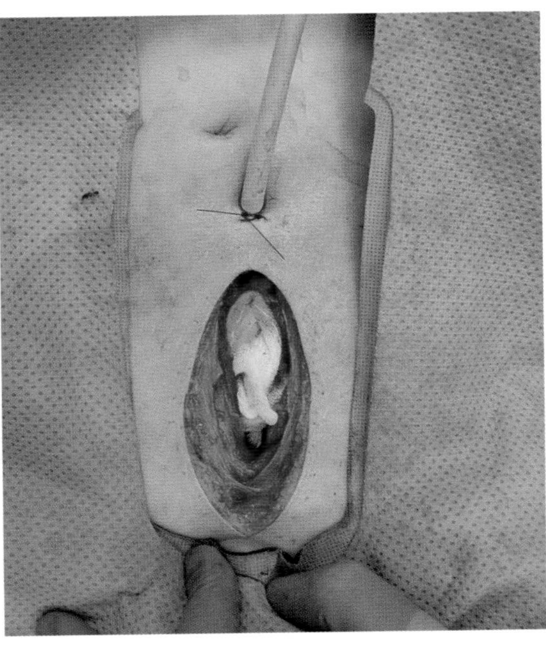

FIGURE 4 ● Placement of the suprapubic tube through a separate stab incision is important for the stability of the catheter and maintenance for long-term use.

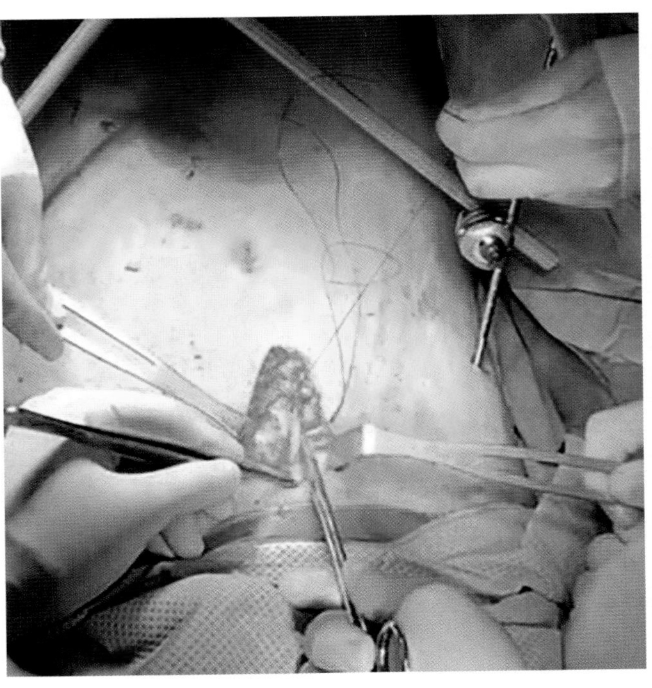

FIGURE 5 ● Once packed the midline fascia is closed with a running O-PDS suture and the skin is stapled closed.

PACK REMOVAL

- After 24 to 48 hours when the patient's hemodynamics have stabilized, the coagulopathy is corrected, and there is no further evidence of ongoing pelvic bleeding, the patient should return to the OR for pack removal.
- The skin staples are removed, the running O-PDS is cut, and the midline fascia is reopened.
- Using a bulb syringe, gently wet the laparotomy packs as they are removed from the pelvis to prevent tearing or dislodgement of formed clot. See **FIGURE 6**.
- The preperitoneal space is then gently suctioned and inspected for any evidence of ongoing bleeding. See **FIGURE 7**. Vicryl sutures and surgical clips can be utilized to control small vessel bleeding, and minor raw surface bleeding can be treated with topical hemostatic agents. See **FIGURE 8**.
- Repacking of the pelvis should be avoided due to unacceptably high infectious complications. In one study, patients who required pelvic repacking had a 47% infection rate vs 6% for those who had a single packing.[2] Pelvic infection risk is also increased in patients with open pelvic fractures and concurrent urogenital injuries.[10] Empiric antibiotics are not routinely used.
- Once satisfied with hemostasis, the midline fascia is again closed with a running O-PDS suture and the overlying skin is stapled closed for the final time.

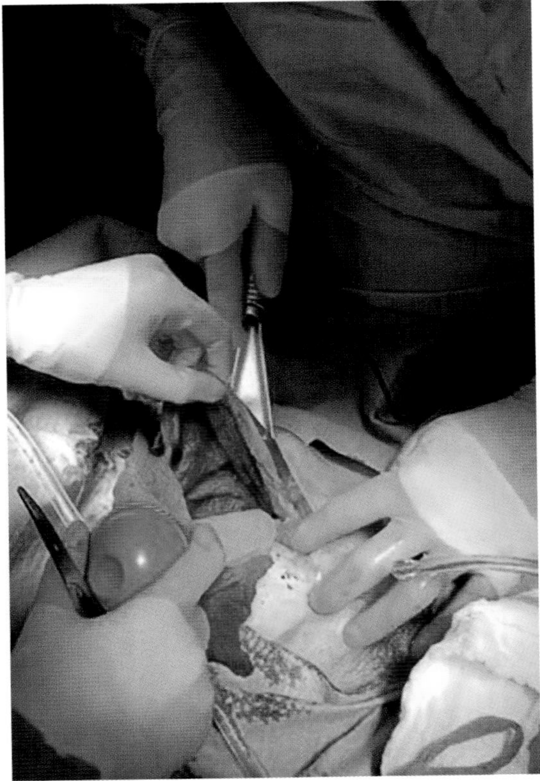

FIGURE 6 ● Pack removal is accomplished by moistening and gently removing each pack individually.

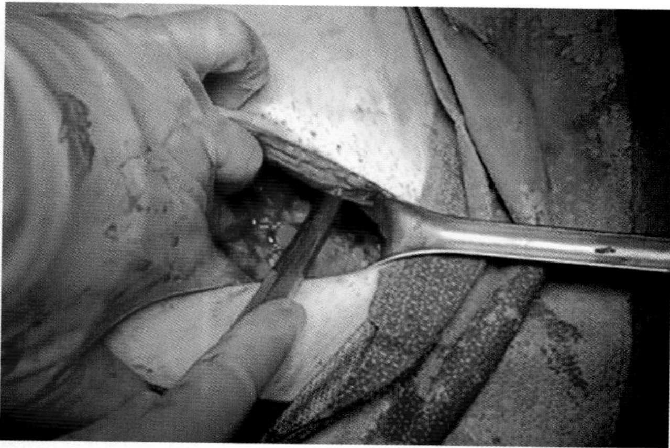

FIGURE 7 ● The pelvis is inspected for further areas of bleeding, and remaining hematoma is removed via suction.

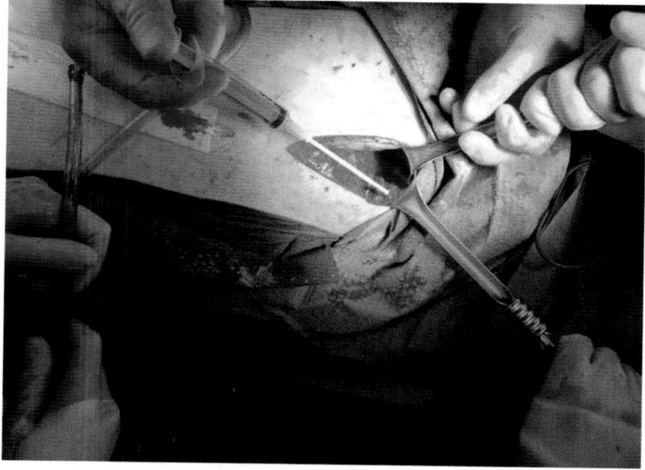

FIGURE 8 ● Application of topical hemostatic agents can assist in minor raw surface bleeding.

PEARLS AND PITFALLS

Peritoneal violation	■ Important to the success of pelvic packing is maintenance of an intact peritoneum. This tissue works to contain the hematoma within the true pelvis and as a layer to pack against. If the peritoneum is grossly violated, free hemorrhage into the abdominal activity can occur, limiting the efficacy of the pelvic packs.
Laparotomy	■ If a laparotomy is required for management of intra-abdominal injuries, care should be taken to keep the two incisions separated, ideally with a supraumbilical laparotomy. See **FIGURE 9**. If the exploratory laparotomy requires extension below the level of the umbilicus and entry into the pelvic hematoma occurs, it is possible to suture close this section of fascia reseparating the two spaces to facilitate packing. 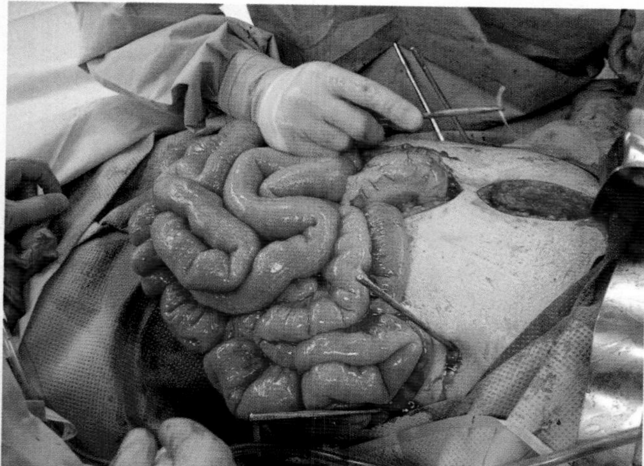 **FIGURE 9** ● Separate incisions should be utilized for laparotomy and pelvic packing to maintain the integrity of the preperitoneal space and containment of the hemorrhage.
Bladder drainage	■ Bladder drainage is required prior to leaving the operating room. This can be achieved via Foley catheterization or a suprapubic tube placement. Decompression of the bladder allows for easier access to the pelvis, reduces bleeding from bladder distention/manipulation, and protects the preperitoneal space from contamination in the event of an unidentified bladder or urethral injury.

Persistent shock	■ Following PPP, the vast majority of patients achieve a degree of hemodynamic stability in the operating room. Persistent hypotension may be as a result of inadequate resuscitation, and an assessment of the patient's volume status should be performed. If appropriate resuscitation has been performed and the patient still remains hypotensive, a search for other sources of ongoing bleeding should be performed. ■ Abdominal bleeding not seen on an emergency department FAST or bleeding into the chest can easily be evaluated by a repeat CXR or FAST in the operating room. In addition, large-volume hemorrhage and subsequent resuscitation can result in significant third spacing of fluid and place the patient at risk for abdominal compartment syndrome. Examination of urine output and peak airway pressures may help guide decision making and the role of decompressive laparotomy. ■ While most pelvic bleeding is venous in nature, an arterial injury warranting angioembolization is present in ~15% of patients.

POSTOPERATIVE CARE

- Following completion of PPP (and any concomitant operations), the disposition of the patient should be based upon their hemodynamic status following packing, the need for any further interventional procedures, or cross-sectional imaging. Most patients achieve some degree of hemodynamic stability following pelvic packing, which may allow for direct transport for CT imaging.
- If a patient has ongoing clinical parameters of shock, the patient should proceed directly to the ICU for ongoing resuscitation with goal optimization in 1 to 2 hours for CT imaging transport. It is our standard practice that all patients with PPP go to the ICU for close monitoring in the 24 to 48 hours following surgery. If hospital resources are limited, arrangements should be made for transfer of the patient to a higher level of care.
- While in the ICU ongoing resuscitation should continue with careful attention for signs of recalcitrant pelvic bleeding in addition to evaluation, assessment, and management for other associated injuries.
- Despite effective PPP, a small percentage (12%-15%) of patients will have continued arterial bleeding best managed with angioembolization. We utilize transfusion of greater than 4 units of packed red blood cells from a pelvic source in 12 hours once a normal coagulation profile is achieved as our threshold for angiographic pelvic interrogation.
- Patients should have a planned return to the OR within 24 to 48 hours after initial packing. Exact timing will be determined by stabilization of the patient's hemodynamics, normalization of their coagulation profile, and no evidence of ongoing pelvic bleeding. If concerns exist, angioembolization should be considered.

COMPLICATIONS

- Deep vein thrombosis (DVT) is a known complication of PPP with reported rates as high as 23% and an 8% incidence of pulmonary embolism.[11] We recommend early initiation of DVT prophylaxis if concurrent injuries permit.
- As part of our pelvic packing algorithm, all patients with packs undergo DVT duplex screening ultrasound to check for the presence of thrombus prior to their planned return to the OR. If the ultrasound demonstrates a DVT, patients receive an inferior vena cava filter prior to reexploration to minimize the effects of potential clot dislodgement with pack removal.

REFERENCES

1. Pohlemann T, Gansslen T, Bosch A, Tscherne U. The technique of packing for control of hemorrhage in complex pelvic fractures. *Tech Orthop*. 1994;9:267-270.
2. Burlew CC, Moore EE, Stahel PF, et al. Preperitoneal pelvic packing reduces mortality in patients with life-threatening hemorrhage due to unstable pelvic fractures. *J Trauma Acute Care Surg*. 2017;82(2):233-242.
3. Krappinger D, Zegg M, Jeske C, El Attal R, Blauth M, Rieger M. Hemorrhage after low-energy pelvic trauma. *J Trauma Acute Care Surg*. 2012;72(2):437-442.
4. Chiara O, di Fratta E, Mariani A, et al. Efficacy of extra-peritoneal pelvic packing in hemodynamically unstable pelvic fractures, a propensity score analysis. *World J Emerg Surg*. 2016;11:22.
5. Bjurlin MA, Fantus RJ, Mellett MM, Goble SM. Genitourinary injuries in pelvic fracture morbidity and mortality using the National Trauma Data Bank. *J Trauma Acute Care Surg*. 2009;67(5):1033-1039.
6. Suzuki T, Kurozumi T, Watanabe Y, Ito K, Tsunoyama T, Sakamoto T. Potentially serious adverse effects from application of a circumferential compression device for pelvic fracture: a report of three cases. *Trauma Case Reports*. 2020;26:100292.
7. Costantini TW, Coimbra R, Holcomb JB, et al. Pelvic fracture patterns predicts the need for hemorrhage control intervention—Results of an AAST multi-institutional study. *J Trauma Acute Care Surg*. 2017;82(6):1030-1038.
8. Chiara O, di Fratta E, Mariani A, et al. Efficacy of extra-peritoneal pelvic packing in hemodynamically unstable pelvic fractures, a propensity score analysis. *World J Emerg Surg*. 2016;11:22.
9. Burlew CC, Moore EE, Smith WR, Morgan SJ. Preperitoneal pelvic packing in the child with an unstable pelvis: a novel approach. *J Peds Surg*. 2006;41(4):e17-e19.
10. Stahel PF, Moore E, Burlew CC, et al. Preperitoneal pelvic packing is not associated with an increased risk of surgical site infections after internal anterior pelvic ring fixation. *J Ortho Trauma*. 2019;33(12):601-607.
11. Heelan AA, Freedberg M, Moore EE, et al. Worth looking! Venous thromboembolism in patients who undergo preperitoneal pelvic packing warrants screening duplex. *Am J Surg*. 2020;220(6):1395-1399.

SECTION XI: Vascular Injury—Abdominal

Chapter 34 Zone I Injuries

Caroline Park and Joseph P. Minei

DEFINITION

- Zone I injuries carry a high mortality up to 60% due to the consequences of massive hemorrhage.[1]
- Injuries in the abdomen and pelvis can be classified by zone, including Zone I, Zone II, and Zone III (**FIGURE 1**). Zone I injuries are defined as an injury to the inferior vena cava or abdominal aorta within the retroperitoneum. The superior boundaries include the diaphragm, the inferior portion to the bifurcation of the iliac vessels, and the lateral borders, including the proximal renal vessels. Zone II injuries include the kidneys, spleen, adrenal glands, and may include ascending or descending colon. Zone III injuries encompass the inflow and outflow of the pelvis, including the common iliac vein and artery and internal and external iliac veins and arteries.
- Zone I injuries can be further divided into supra and inframesocolic, a border defined by the mesentery of the transverse colon. This is an important distinction that may influence the surgeon's operative approach.

DIFFERENTIAL DIAGNOSIS

- Patients presenting with blunt trauma carry a high probability of concurrent injuries given the severe mechanism of injury, including solid organ (liver, spleen, kidney) and hollow viscus injuries. Patients with penetrating trauma may also present with solid organ and hollow viscus injuries associated with the path of the missile or other object, and can include the duodenum, esophagus, stomach, pancreas, and colon (**FIGURE 2**).
- Hemorrhagic shock must be excluded first before investigating other types of shock, including spinal, neurogenic, or cardiogenic shock.

PATIENT HISTORY AND PHYSICAL FINDINGS

- Initial workup includes the primary survey to assess the airway, breathing, and circulation. Patients in hemorrhagic shock may be obtunded and require a definitive airway;

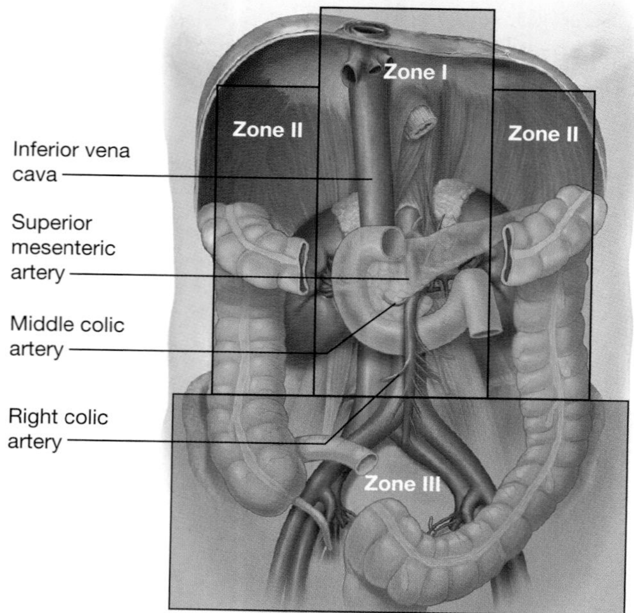

FIGURE 1 ● Zone I, II, and III injuries. (Modified with permission from Fischer J. *Fischer's Mastery of Surgery*. 7th ed. Wolters Kluwer; 2019. Figure 231.1.)

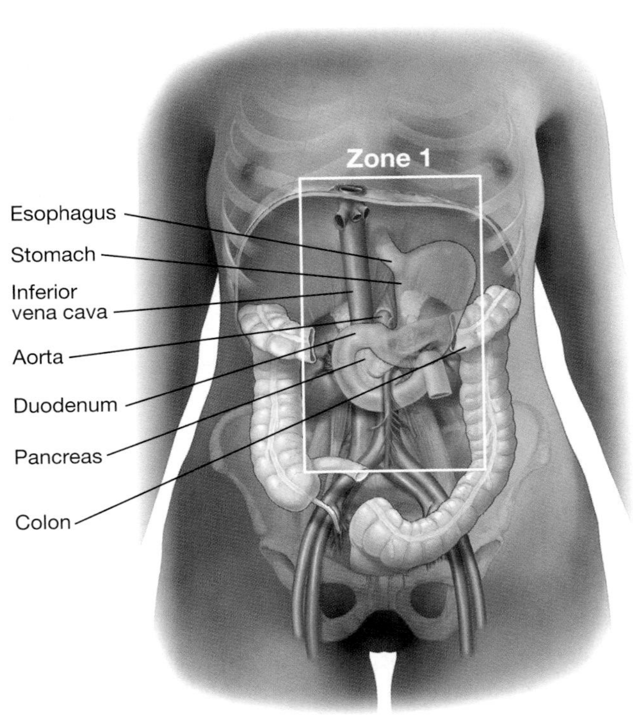

FIGURE 2 • Zone I and its relation to the abdominal organs and pelvis. Note the relation to the lesser curvature of the stomach and pancreas.

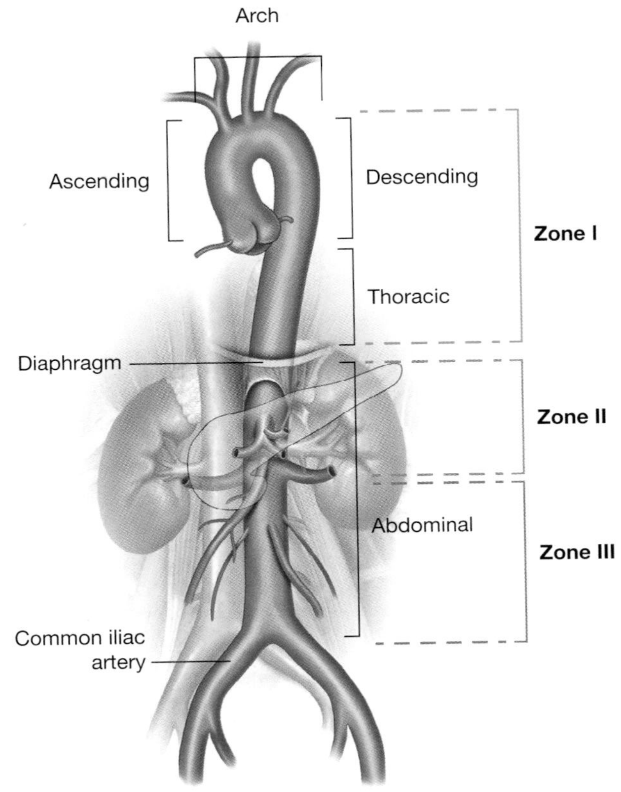

FIGURE 3 • Aorta, thoracic, and abdominal portions. Zone I = distal to the subclavian artery to the celiac trunk. Zone II = celiac trunk to the lowest renal artery. Zone III = just below the renal arteries to the bifurcation of the common iliac arteries. (Modified with permission from Kawamura D, Nolan T. *Abdomen and Superficial Structures*. 4th ed. Wolters Kluwer; 2018. Figure 4.1.)

however, if the patient is able to be bag-valve masked with satisfactory oxygenation, large-bore intravenous access should be obtained first with transfusion of blood prior to intubation.[2]

- Resuscitating the patient is critical prior to intubation to avoid precipitating cardiovascular collapse. If there is a suspicion for abdominal or pelvic hemorrhage, access should be secured above the heart (subclavian, internal jugular, or upper extremities).
- Injuries to the inferior vena cava and aorta often present with classic signs of hemorrhagic shock, including tachycardia, hypotension, and narrowed pulse pressure. Other signs or symptoms of shock may include diminished pulses, cool, clammy skin, confusion, or obtunded state in more severe cases. Patients with retroperitoneal hemorrhage may have bruising of the flank, "Grey Turner sign"; however, this is classically seen in more acute-on-chronic presentations and is not a reliable sign in the patient presenting acutely with hemorrhagic shock.

IMAGING AND OTHER DIAGNOSTIC STUDIES

- Injuries to the retroperitoneum are difficult to diagnose on primary and secondary survey and plain films, including chest X-ray, abdominal X-ray, or pelvis X-ray. Plain films should be utilized for blunt torso trauma for cavitary triage, to rule out hemothorax, pneumothorax, or pelvis fracture. Focused Assessment with Sonography in Trauma exam may be helpful to triage the abdomen for intraperitoneal fluid, but is not sensitive in detecting retroperitoneal injuries.[3]
- Computed tomography is reserved for patients who are otherwise stable and should be performed with contrast in both arterial and delayed phases to evaluate for active extravasation.

SURGICAL MANAGEMENT

Preoperative Planning and Equipment

- Patients with zone I injuries requiring operative intervention will often present with hemodynamic instability and may transiently respond to blood transfusions. Two large bore IVs in the bilateral arms are sufficient for rapid administration of blood and medications. If a multiple-access catheter or percutaneous sheath introducer is required, consider placing a subclavian or internal jugular venous catheter as femoral venous catheters may directly drain through an inferior vena cava (IVC) injury. However, these injuries are often recognized in the operating room, in which case a femoral line should be discontinued and switched to venous drainage above the heart.
- Resuscitative Endovascular Balloon Occlusion of the Aorta (REBOA)[4] is a minimally invasive technique to occlude the inflow of blood into the chest, abdomen, and pelvis based on zone of deployment (**FIGURE 3**—aorta and its zones). It has

been compared to the traditional resuscitative thoracotomy in occluding inflow to areas of hemorrhage and diverting blood to the heart and brain during a traumatic arrest with disputed outcomes.[5]

- This endovascular technique is minimally invasive and less painful and morbid than a thoracotomy incision, which is not without its own occupational hazards. The catheter can be delivered through a 7-Fr sheath in the common femoral artery and the balloon inflated to obtain partial or full occlusion to decrease blood loss (reference). For intra-abdominal bleeding, the catheter should be inflated at zone I.
- These catheters however are not without their own risks, including access problems (dissection, thrombosis), rupture of the iliac artery, aorta, or common femoral artery, and are generally not recommended for use in a patient with suspected thoracic aorta or cardiac injury, as this can potentially propagate the injury.

SURGICAL APPROACH

Positioning

- Patients should be prepped widely from chin to knees for maximum exposure and placed supine with the arms out for the anesthesiologists to access and administer anesthesia, products, and medications. Patients in extremis should be prepped awake and transfusions continued from the trauma bay. Excellent and timely communication with the anesthesiology team is paramount during intubation, as entering the abdomen and releasing any tamponade effect of a retroperitoneal hematoma could precipitate a traumatic arrest.

EXPLORATION

- A generous midline laparotomy incision from xyphoid to pubis is made and all hematoma evacuated, and all four quadrants packed with laparotomy pads. A quick survey and palpation of the spleen and liver can rule out injury that requires compression and packing. Any enteric violation should be quickly stopped with sutures or Babcock clamps. Next the zones of the abdomen should be explored.

ZONE I—ABDOMINAL AORTA AND INTRA-ABDOMINAL CONTROL

- Abdominal aortic injuries can be classified by region, including diaphragmatic, suprarenal, and infrarenal.
- Zone I injuries are most easily identified by mobilizing the left hepatic ligament, retracting on the body of the stomach, entering pars flaccida medial to the lesser curvature, and examining the hiatus where the esophagus and aorta exit the thoracic cavity (**FIGURE 4**).
- Once pars flaccida is opened, the left and right crura are identified and spread away from the aorta (**FIGURE 5**).
- Zone I injuries can also be grossly evaluated by lifting the transverse colon out of the abdomen and onto the chest—the middle colic vein and artery drain down through the transverse mesocolon and join the superior mesenteric artery and vein. However, massive injuries to zone I may result in large hematomas that track to zone II; thus, it is imperative to explore these injuries in the setting of hemorrhage shock.
- If the surgeon suspects an injury to the inferior vena cava, obtaining proximal aortic control may still be required to mitigate ongoing bleeding while determining which—or if both—has been injured.

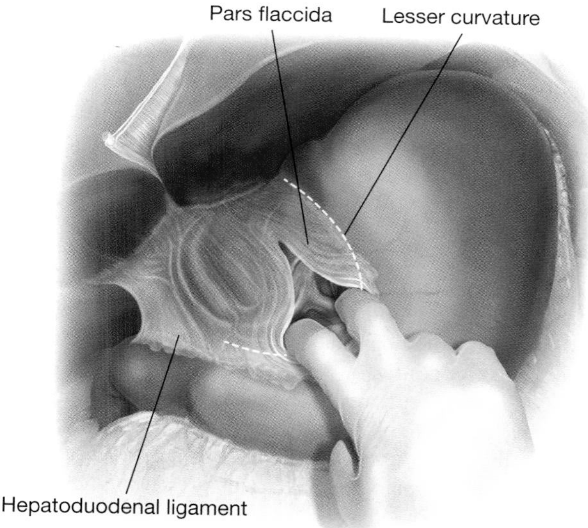

FIGURE 4 ● Surgeon dissecting the pars flaccida along the lesser curvature of the stomach. (Modified with permission from Britt LD, Peitzman AB, Barie PS, et al. *Acute Care Surgery*. 2nd ed. Wolters Kluwer; 2019. Figure 11.12A.)

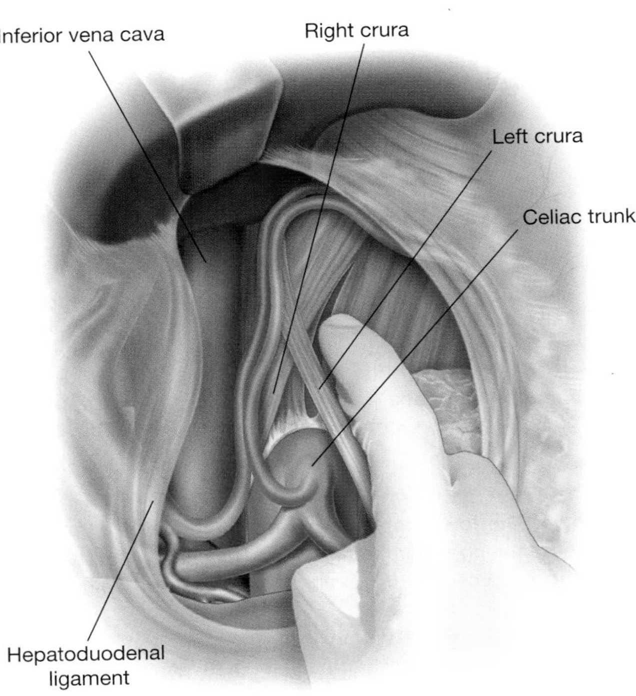

FIGURE 5 ● Left and right crura of the diaphragm are identified above the celiac trunk. (Modified with permission from Britt LD, Peitzman AB, Barie PS, et al. *Acute Care Surgery*. 2nd ed. Wolters Kluwer; 2019. Figure 11.12B.)

MANUAL COMPRESSION AND OCCLUSION

- A sponge stick can also be placed in this area and pressed along the spine to obtain immediate proximal control while waiting for an aortic clamp. The celiac trunk is also accessible in this space (**FIGURES 6** and **7**).

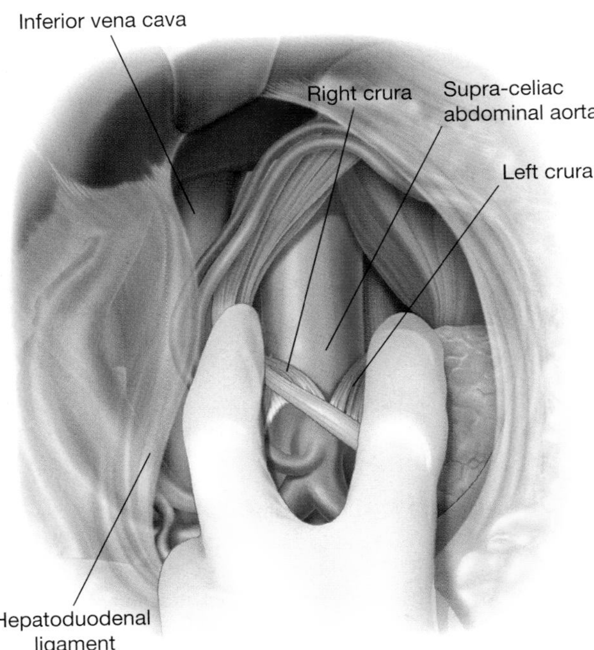

FIGURE 6 ● The crura are spread away from the abdominal aorta, freeing up space for a clamp or sponge stick. (Modified with permission from Britt LD, Peitzman AB, Barie PS, et al. *Acute Care Surgery*. 2nd ed. Wolters Kluwer; 2019. Figure 11.12C.)

- If aortic bleeding is identified below the celiac trunk, a sponge stick or an aortic clamp should be applied and ischemic time noted. The surgeon should take care to place this clamp cephalad to maximize space for exploration in the abdomen. Oftentimes the patient in extremis and in hemorrhagic shock or arrest may have a weakly palpable pulse. Defining the aorta from the esophagus may be challenging in this situation. An orogastric tube should be placed to palpate the esophagus, encircle it with a Penrose drain, and retract it aside to accurately identify and place a clamp on the aorta (**FIGURE 8**).

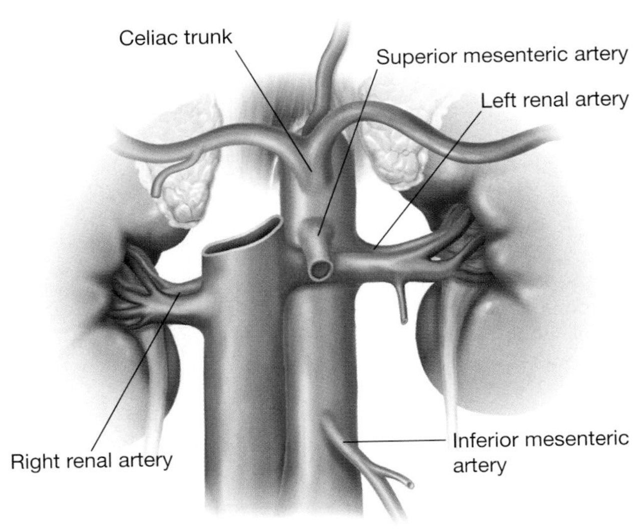

FIGURE 7 ● Relation of the celiac trunk and its proximity to the diaphragm, superior mesenteric artery, left and renal arteries.

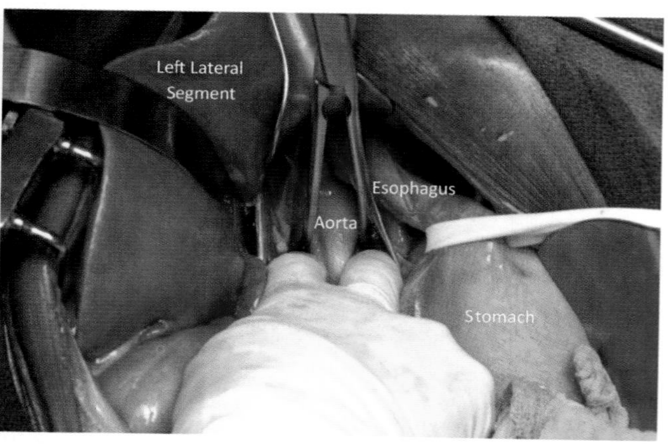

FIGURE 8 ● Spreading the crura away from the abdominal aorta and placement of a clamp for aortic occlusion. Penrose encircles the distal esophagus/gastroesophageal junction laterally. (Used with permission by Cambridge University Press, from Teixeira P, Magee G, Rowe V. Abdominal aorta and splachnic vessels. In: Demetriades D, Inaba K, Velmahos G, eds. *Atlas of Surgical Techniques in Trauma*. Cambridge University Press; 2020:268-285.)

PROXIMAL ABDOMINAL AORTIC INJURIES—APPROACH FROM THE LEFT CHEST

- If the abdominal aortic injury is at or above the celiac trunk, then a left anterolateral thoracotomy should be performed to access the thoracic aorta. The inferior pulmonary ligament tethers the left lower lobe to the diaphragm and is taken down. The lower lobe can then be retracted cephalad to expose the posterior mediastinum. The pleura over the aorta is incised above the diaphragm, taking care to avoid the left inferior pulmonary vein.
- An orogastric tube within the esophagus can help guide delineation between the thin plane between the esophagus and aorta. The thoracic aorta should be cross-clamped as low as possible to avoid injury to the hilar structures.

ZONE I—INTRA-ABDOMINAL AORTA, INJURIES, AND EXPOSURES

- The abdominal aorta is best exposed by a left medial visceral rotation, or a Mattox maneuver, although a retroperitoneal approach can also provide an unparalleled view of the abdominal aorta (**FIGURE 9**).
- In a trauma laparotomy, however, a left medial visceral rotation is most practical and efficient given the risk of concomitant intraperitoneal injury.

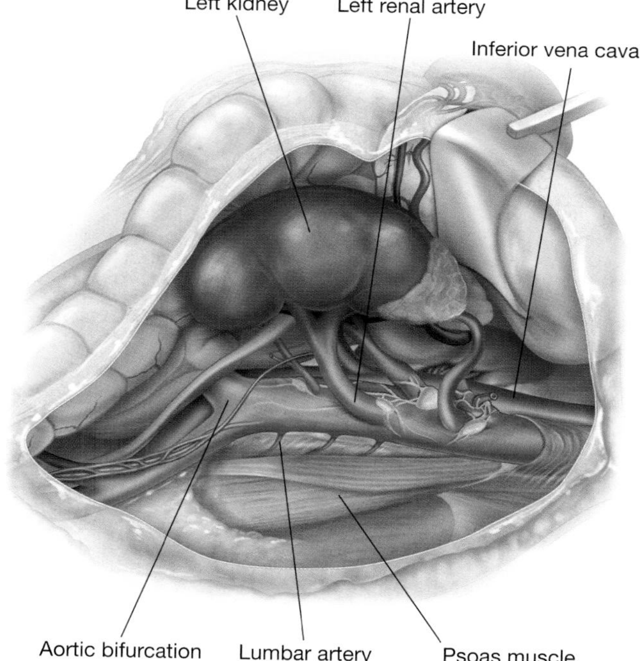

FIGURE 9 ● Exposure of the abdominal aorta through a retroperitoneal approach. Note the spleen, pancreas, and left kidney are all mobilized medially, exposing the abdominal aorta and psoas muscle.

LEFT MEDIAL VISCERAL ROTATION

- In this exposure, the descending colon is taken down at the peritoneal reflection, and cephalad toward the splenic flexure. The splenic flexure is taken down, taking care to avoid injury to the spleen. The spleen and all of its attachments, including the gastrosplenic, splenocolic, phrenocolic, and splenorenal ligaments, are taken down. In a complete left medial visceral rotation, the left kidney, including the hilum and ureter, is mobilized off the peritoneum and rotated medially.

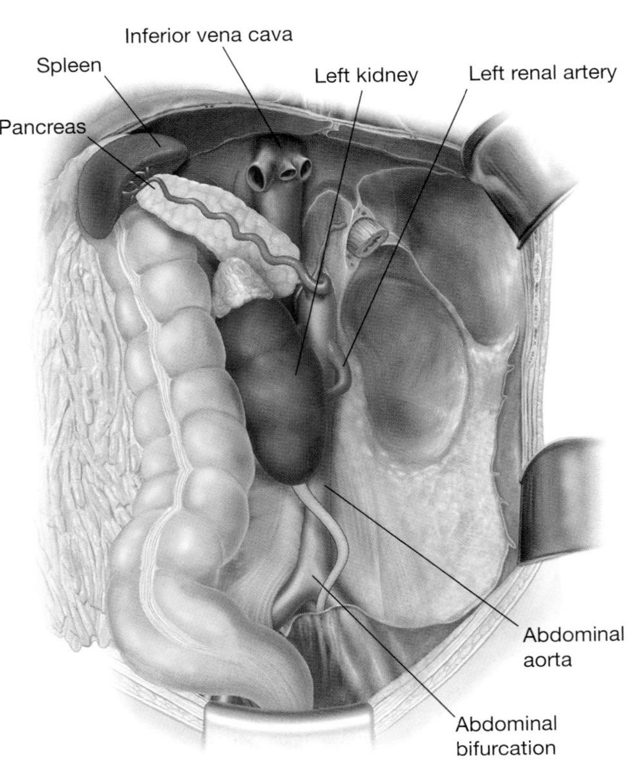

- This exposure will provide access to the abdominal aorta and bifurcation of the common iliac arteries. The left common iliac artery and vein can also be accessed through this exposure (**FIGURE 10**).
- In a modified Mattox maneuver, the left kidney remains in the retroperitoneum and Gerota fascia left intact. The surgeon should take care to avoid traction injuries when mobilizing the viscera to avoid avulsing the left renal vein (**FIGURE 11**).

FIGURE 10 ● Left medial visceral rotation. Full rotation of the spleen, pancreas, left kidney, and colon. (Modified with permission from Fischer J. *Fischer's Mastery of Surgery*. 6th ed. Wolters Kluwer; 2012. Figure 254.2.)

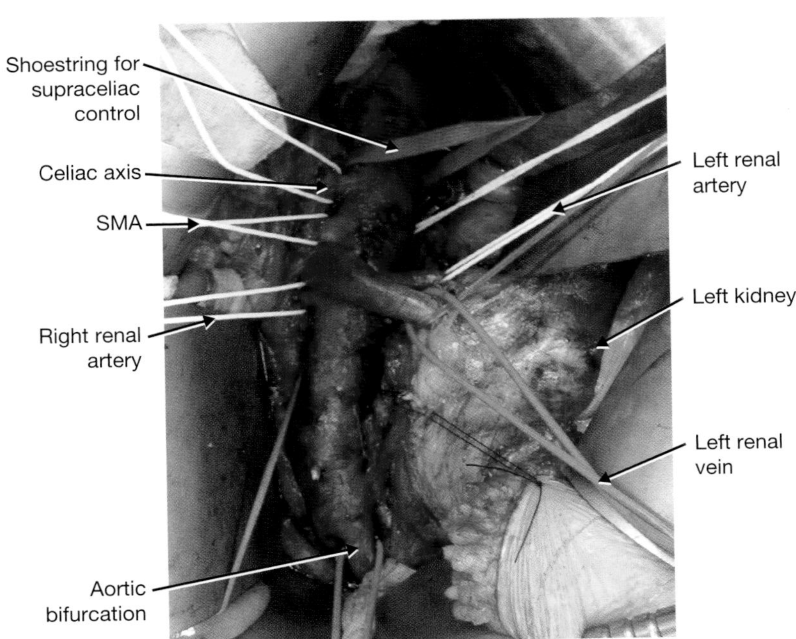

FIGURE 11 ● Modified Mattox maneuver with left kidney and renal vein/artery down. Abdominal aorta from above the celiac access to the bifurcation is exposed. Note the length of the left renal vein as it crosses over the aorta and its relation to the renal artery. (Reprinted with permission from Dalman R. *Operative Techniques in Vascular Surgery*. Wolters Kluwer; 2016. Figure 22.10.)

ZONE I—ISOLATED INJURIES TO ABDOMINAL AORTA

- Injuries to the infrarenal aorta can be better localized by mobilizing the fourth portion of the duodenum medially and incising the peritoneum over the aorta and IVC. This exposure allows to maintain the integrity of Gerota fascia of the left kidney and examine the left renal vein, inferior mesenteric artery, aorta, and some parts of the IVC. This maneuver may be helpful when encountering and controlling aortoduodenal fistulae (**FIGURE 12**).
- Penetrating injuries to the infrarenal aorta are in several ways easier to manage than venous injuries as the location is noted by pulsatile bleeding and can be controlled

immediately with the surgeon's finger. If the patient's condition allows, systemic heparinization should be administered prior to clamping for proximal and distal control, either with vessels loops, Rummel tourniquets, or vascular clamps (**FIGURE 13**).

- The most expeditious way to approach an infrarenal aorta injury includes a left medial visceral rotation and clamps proximal and distal to the injury. In penetrating injuries, it is critical to evaluate the posterior wall of the aorta for a concomitant injury. In **FIGURE 13**, the infrarenal aorta is controlled with vascular clamps. For a small injury that can be repaired primarily, a patch repair with bovine pericardium or primary repair may be sufficient. One must ensure there is brisk inflow and back-bleeding prior to definitive repair.

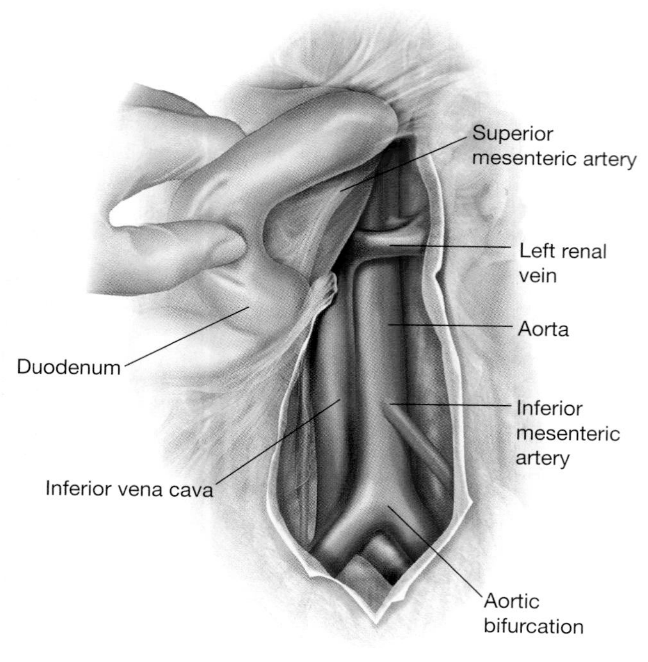

FIGURE 12 ● Alternative approach to injuries to the infrarenal aorta. (Modified with permission from Upchurch, GR Jr. *Clinical Scenarios in Vascular Surgery*. 2nd ed. Wolters Kluwer; 2016. Figure 36.3.)

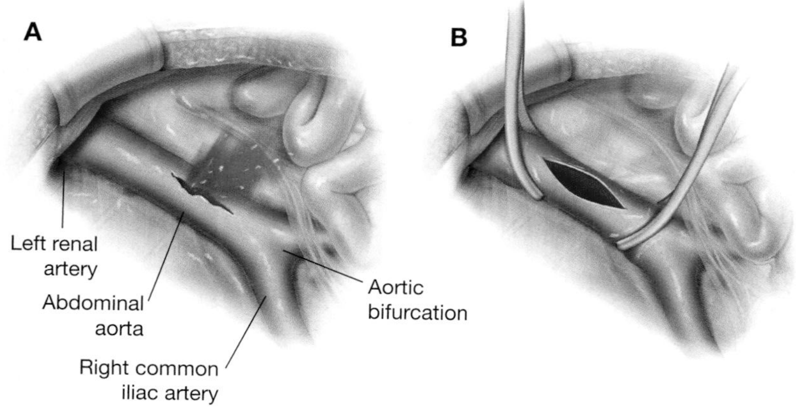

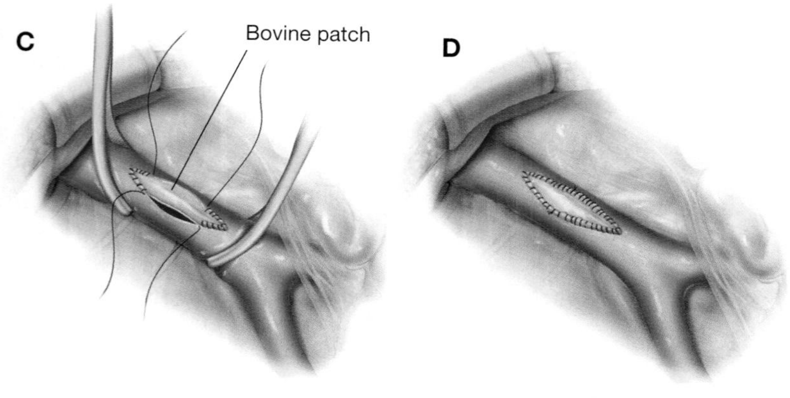

FIGURE 13 ● Contained rupture of aortic aneurysm. Proximal and distal control of an aortic repair with vascular clamps, followed by bovine patch placement. **A-D**, Obtaining proximal and distal control of an infrarenal aortic injury using vascular clamps, followed by bovine patch placement.

ZONE I—INTRA-ABDOMINAL AORTA AND JUNCTIONAL INJURIES

- Junctional injuries involving the iliac artery and vein can also be approached by a left medial visceral rotation. It is important to note that the right common iliac artery crosses over left common iliac vein. Careful use of dissection is warranted when encircling the common iliac artery to avoid injury to the iliac vein, which can precipitate massive bleeding. The ureter crosses over the common iliac artery before the bifurcation of the external and internal iliac arteries and is a reliable landmark if one needs to identify and ligate the internal iliac arteries for massive pelvic bleeding (**FIGURE 14**).
- Synthetic grafts or autologous conduits can be used, favoring the latter for contaminated cases (**FIGURES 15** and **16**).

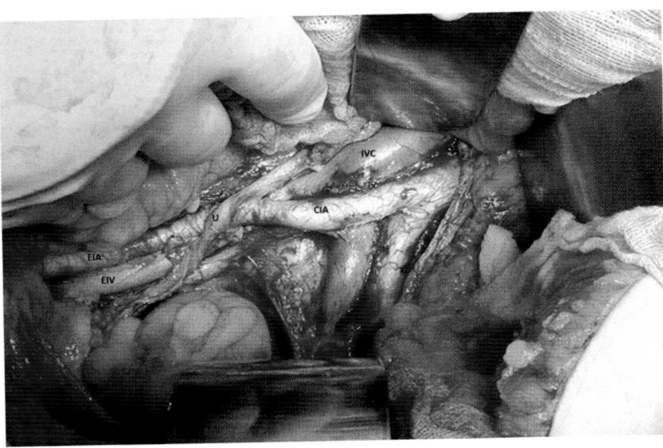

FIGURE 14 ● Intraoperative photo of IVC and aortic bifurcations and relation to ureter. CIA, common iliac artery; EIA, external iliac artery; EIV, external iliac vein; IVC, inferior vena cava; U, ureter. (Reprinted with permission from Dimick JB, Upchurch, GR Jr, Sonnenday CJ, Kao LS. *Clinical Scenarios in Surgery*. 2nd ed. Wolters Kluwer; 2019. Figure 21.3.)

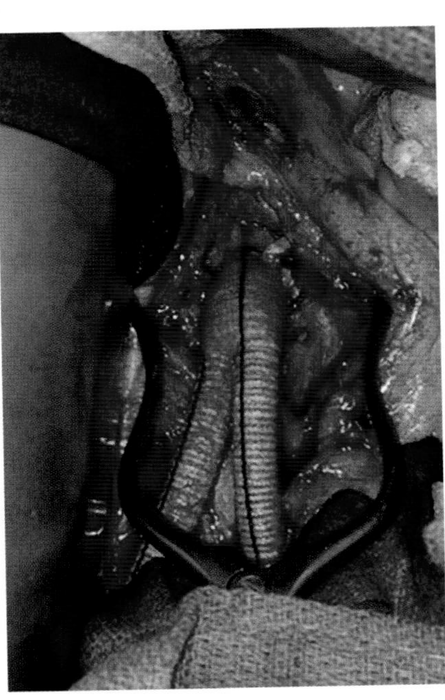

FIGURE 15 ● Infrarenal aortic synthetic graft. (Courtesy of Michael Siah, MD, University of Texas Southwestern Medical Center, Division of Vascular Surgery.)

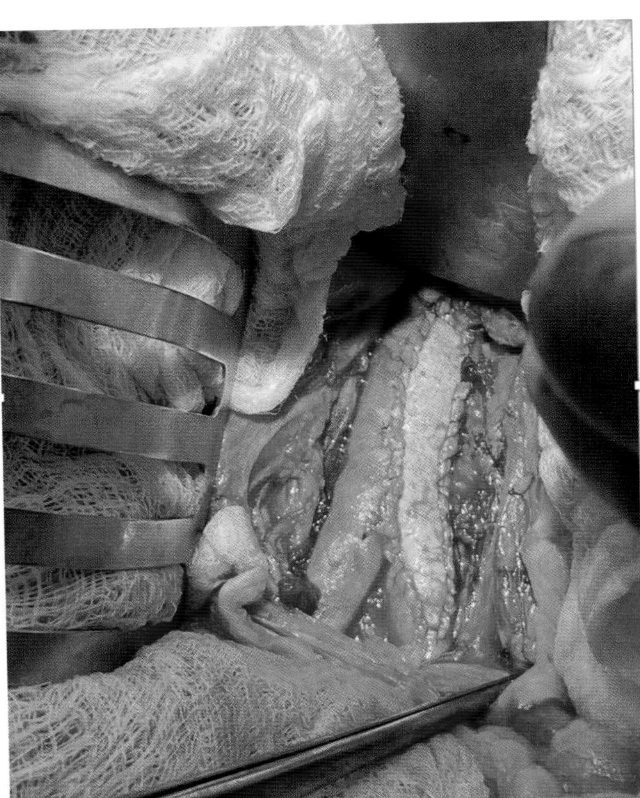

FIGURE 16 ● Bovine pericardium patch of aortoiliac vessels. (Courtesy of Michael Siah, MD, University of Texas Southwestern Medical Center, Division of Vascular Surgery.)

ZONE I—INFERIOR VENA CAVA AND INITIAL HEMORRHAGE CONTROL

- The inferior vena cava drains the common iliac veins, lumbar veins, renal, adrenal, hepatic veins, and phrenic veins before it drains into the suprahepatic IVC and right atrium (**FIGURE 17**). The retrohepatic vena cava, though it spans a short distance behind the liver, is the most difficult portion to access if injured (**FIGURE 18**).
- Massive IVC injuries often present with an expanding zone I hematoma, and in penetrating injuries can be devastating if the tamponade effect within the retroperitoneum is lost. Securing IV access, notably access above the heart (internal jugular vein, subclavian vein), is critical to prevent ongoing losses within the abdomen.
- Aortic occlusion should be obtained by the steps outlined previously in this chapter OR by endovascular occlusion with a REBOA catheter, keeping in mind the inherent risks of catheter placement with an existing aortic injury.

Injuries to the Inferior Vena Cava—Exposure

Right Medial Visceral Rotation

- A complete right medial visceral rotation offers the best approach to the infrahepatic IVC. The ascending colon is taken down along the peritoneal reflection, including the hepatic flexure. The avascular fusion plane between the small bowel mesentery and posterior peritoneum is scored to lengthen this plane. The duodenum is reflected medially via Kocher maneuver to include the head of the pancreas. This complete maneuver should allow for small bowel evisceration onto the patient's chest (**FIGURE 19**). Be wary of the inferior mesenteric vein, which can be avulsed in this maneuver.
- Once this is complete, the infrahepatic inferior vena cava and hepatoduodenal ligament are readily exposed.

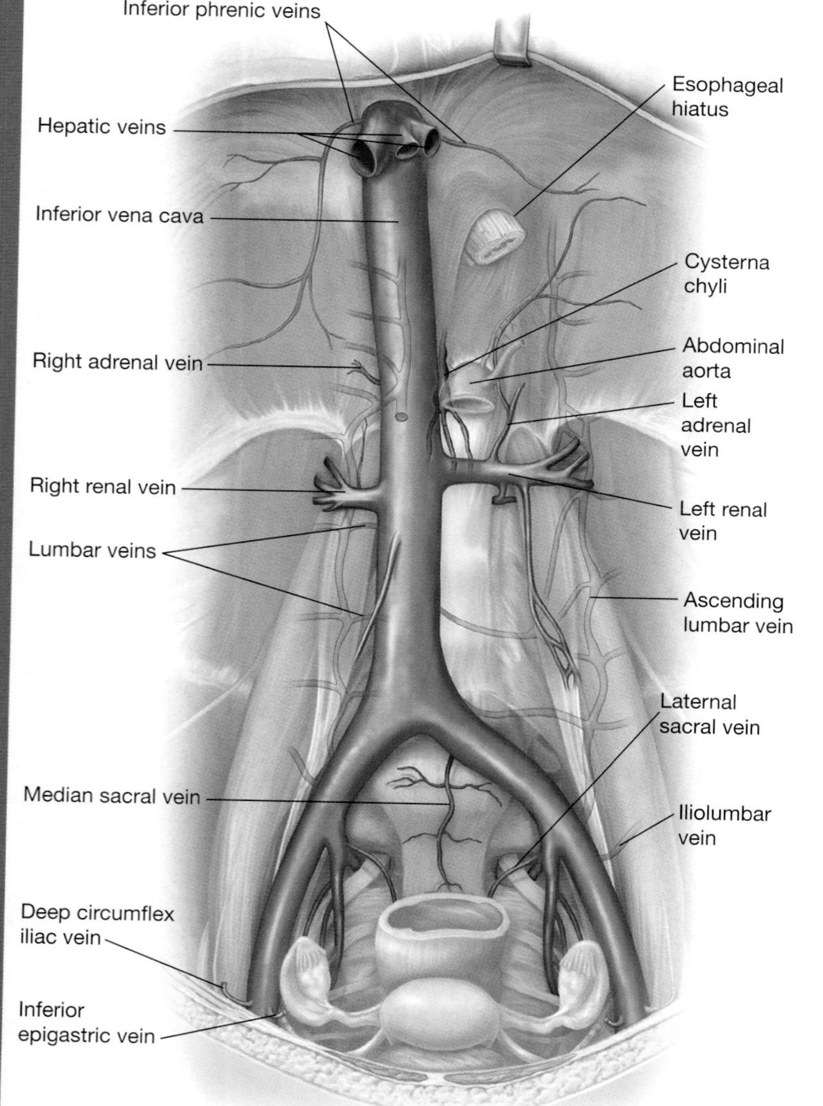

FIGURE 17 ● Inferior vena cava and its drainage.

- The right renal vein can be seen anteriorly draining the kidney, but the left renal vein, which typically drains into the inferior vena cava slightly more superior, should also be exposed and visualized (**FIGURE 20**). This is important to identify if an inferior vena cava injury is so destructive that it requires ligation.

Control of Hemorrhage

- Venous injuries are typically more difficult to control given the large volume but low pressure system. Oftentimes there is significant hemorrhage with poor visualization. Sponge sticks should be readily available and applied with direct compression above and below the injury. Vascular clamps can also be applied (**FIGURE 21**).
- Expanding Zone I injuries necessitate exploration. Both the posterior and anterior walls of the inferior vena cava should be explored.

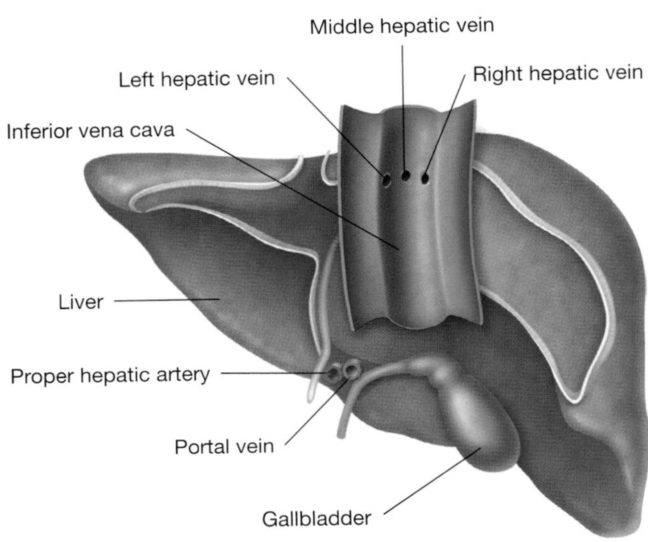

FIGURE 18 ● Retrohepatic inferior vena cava and its relation to the hepatic veins (posterior view). (Reprinted with permission from Olinger AB. *Human Gross Anatomy*. Wolters Kluwer; 2016. Figure 2.86c.)

Anterior, Posterior Injuries

- The back wall or posterior aspect of the inferior vena cava should be repaired primarily first prior to repairing the anterior wall using prolene suture (**FIGURE 21**). Be wary of severe stenosis or narrowing of the inferior vena cava. (If the inferior vena cava is so significantly narrowed with "waisting" (>40% narrowing), the incidence of deep venous thrombosis is predictably greater in patients after ligation. The risk of pulmonary embolus is unclear between patients who undergo ligation vs repair.[6])

Complete Laceration

- If the inferior vena cava is completely disrupted, it is unlikely to be approximated without significant tension. The tissue is usually tenuous and will not allow for a primary repair. An interposition graft is a suitable conduit in a stable patient without massive contamination (**FIGURE 22**). Otherwise, the infrarenal inferior vena cava can be ligated if the patient is in hemorrhagic shock and repair cannot be attempted. These patients are at high for massive swelling of the lower extremities and compartment syndrome. Prophylactic bilateral four-compartment fasciotomies may be necessary to mitigate the risk of ischemia.

Suprarenal and Retrohepatic Inferior Vena Cava Injuries—Approach

- Suprarenal inferior vena cava injuries can still be accessed by a right medial visceral rotation. Injuries in this area carry a high

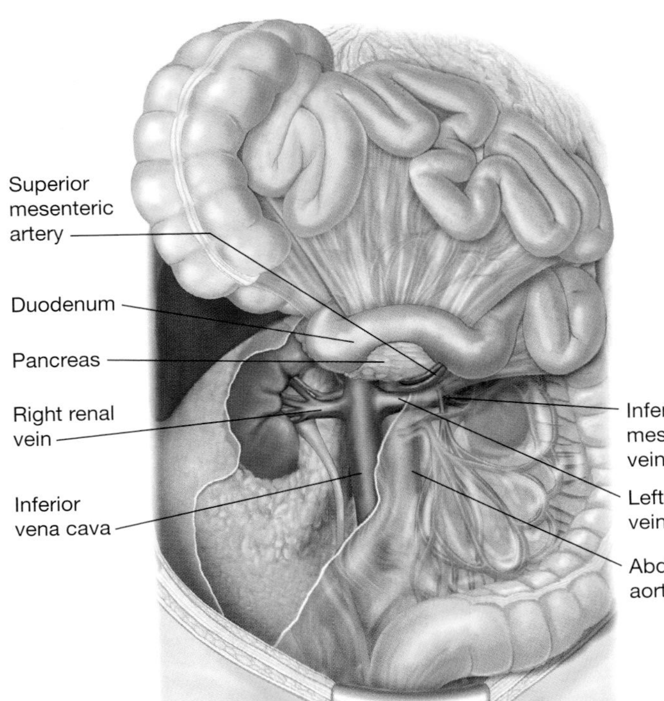

FIGURE 19 ● Right medial visceral rotation, or Cattell-Braasch maneuver to access the inferior vena cava.

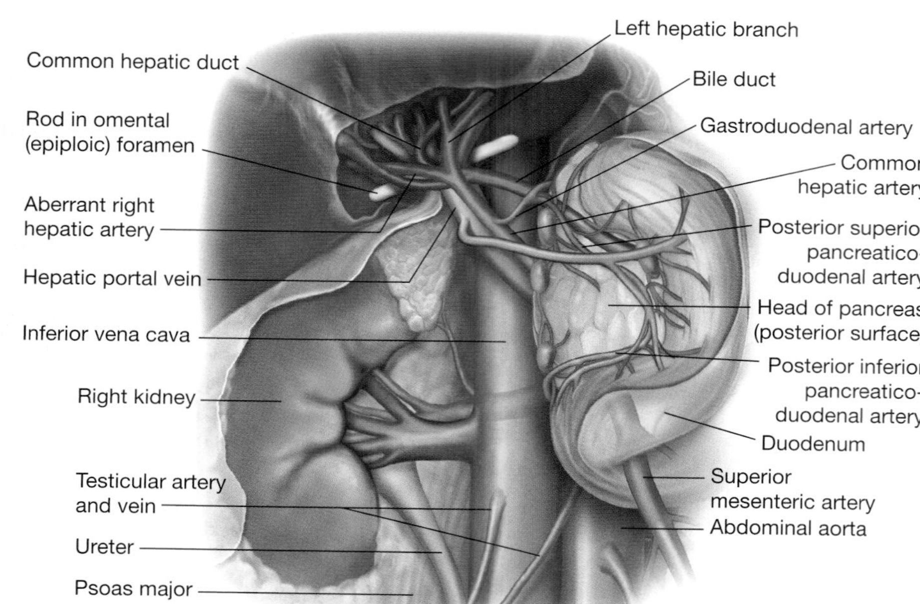

FIGURE 20 • Exposure of the infrahepatic inferior vena cava after right medial visceral rotation. Note the hepatoduodenal ligament and relation to the head of the pancreas and inferior vena cava.

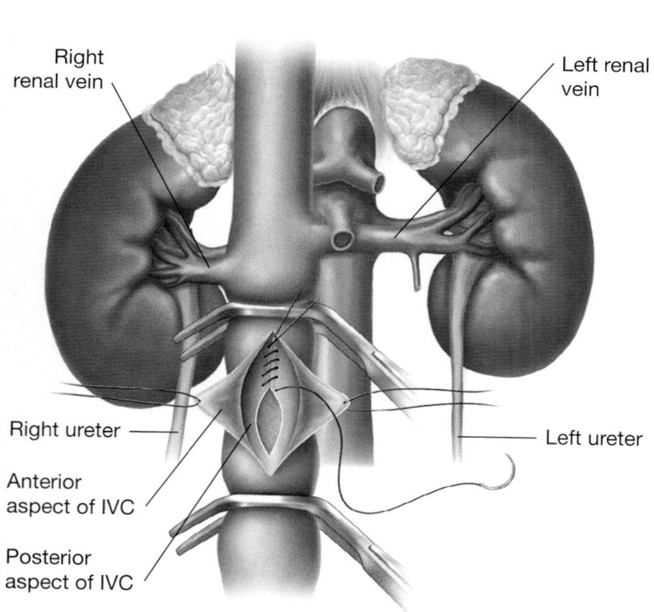

FIGURE 21 • Occlusion of the infrahepatic inferior vena cava and suture repair of a posterior inferior vena cava injury.

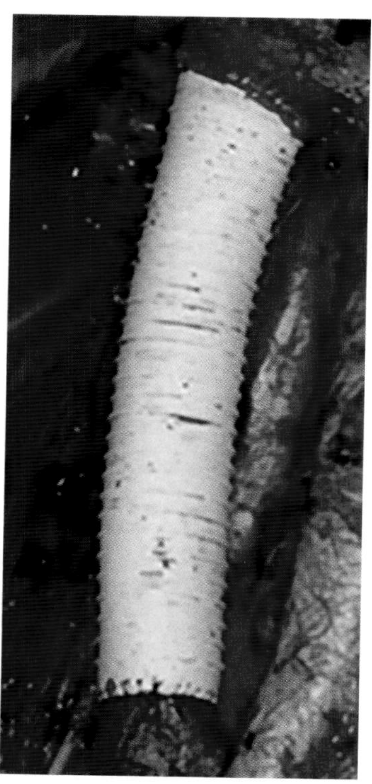

FIGURE 22 • Inferior vena reconstruction with synthetic graft. (Courtesy of Michael Siah, MD, University of Texas Southwestern Medical Center, Division of Vascular Surgery.)

risk of injury to the renal hilum, adrenal glands, aorta, duodenum, pancreas, and portal triad. Surgeons should take note of the anterior position of the renal veins and the length of the left renal vein as it crosses over the aorta (**FIGURES 23** and **24**).

Retrohepatic Inferior Vena Cava Injuries—Approach

- Retrohepatic caval injuries are the perhaps the most dreaded vascular injuries given their inaccessibility and associated

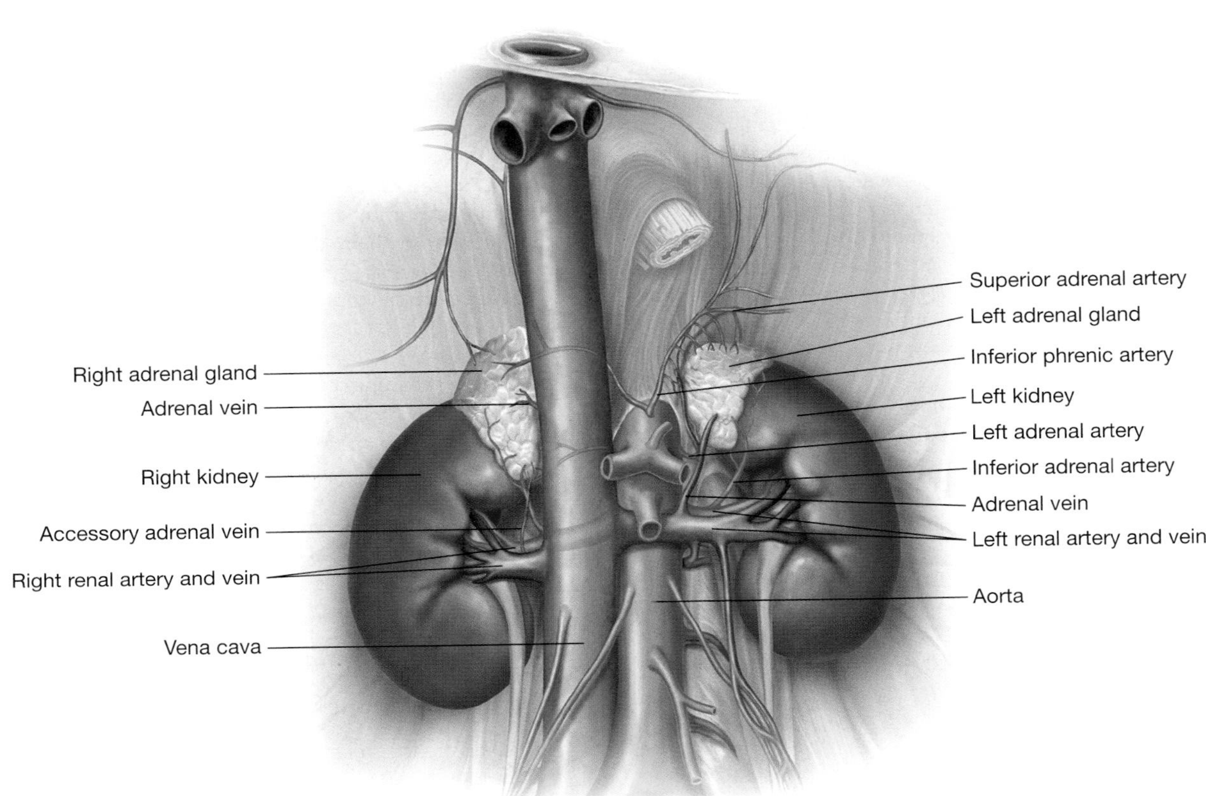

FIGURE 23 ● Inferior vena cava and relation to the renal hilum, aorta, and adrenal glands.

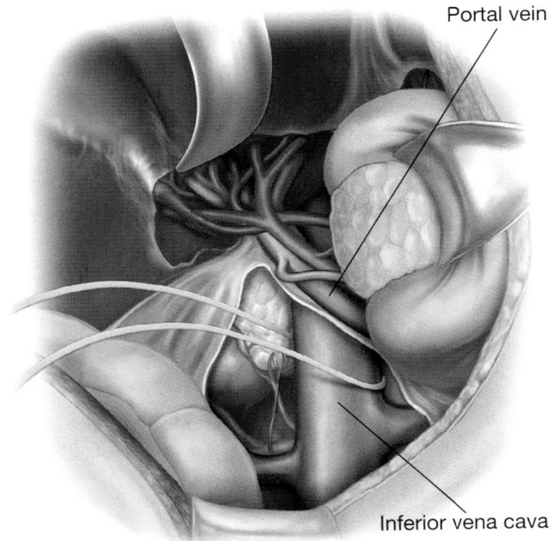

FIGURE 24 ● Suprarenal inferior vena cava and relation to renal veins and portal veins. (Modified with permission from Fischer J. *Fischer's Mastery of Surgery*. 7th ed. Wolters Kluwer; 2019. Figure 130.7.)

mortality. The dictum has classically been to "pack and not look." Mobilizing the ligaments, including the right triangular ligament, can release any tamponade effect and precipitate torrential bleeding.

- Measures to exclude other types of bleeding, including hepatic veins and arteries should be excluded by packing and compression above and below the liver, and a Pringle maneuver by encircling the hepatoduodenal ligament with a Rummel tourniquet.
- Total hepatic vascular isolation is the second to last alternative to an atriocaval shunt and entails clamping of the suprahepatic inferior vena cava, followed by the infrahepatic inferior vena cava, and a Pringle maneuver.
- If these measures are exhausted, and if the injury is suprahepatic, the last consideration should be toward mobilization of the liver and preparation for an atriocaval shunt.
- Prior to mobilizing the liver, it is critical to communicate with the anesthesiologist on the anticipated blood loss and to secure the following equipment prior to shunting the retrohepatic inferior vena cava:
  - Sternal saw or Lebsche knife
  - 28-Fr chest tube with created perforations
  - Rummel tourniquets or umbilical tape
  - Kelly Clamp

Obtaining Proximal Control

- The right triangular ligament is taken down and the right liver medialized. Multiple short veins to the inferior vena cava should be clipped and divided (**FIGURE 25**). Sponge sticks should be placed directly above and below the injury to temporize massive bleeding.

Securing Distal Control

- The intrapericardial inferior vena cava can be accessed above the liver and through the diaphragm, through the right chest or via median sternotomy.
- The central tendon is divided to access the intrapericardial inferior vena cava, taking care to avoid any injury to either one.
- The intrapericardial inferior vena cava can also be accessed through a right anterolateral thoracotomy; however, the most efficient way to approach the intrapericardial inferior vena cava is through a sternotomy, opening up the pericardium and clamping the inferior vena cava before it drains into the right atrium. Occluding the inferior vena cava can precipitate cardiovascular collapse; thus, the abovementioned equipment is critical to have stand-by.
- The thoracostomy tube should be prepared in advance by creating separate side holes that can drain into the right atrium and cut to length. The right atrial appendage should be elevated with an Allis clamp and a pursestring placed with prolene. The appendage should be opened readily clamped down to avoid ongoing blood loss.
- This extremely rare procedure requires the coordination of at least two surgeons placing the thoracostomy tube in through the injury of the inferior vena cava and the other anticipating its exit through the right atrial appendage. Once the thoracostomy tube stents open the right atrium and inferior vena cava, the pursestring suture should be tied down around the right atrial appendage and Rummel tourniquets tied down below the level of the injury and at the level of the atrial appendage. The thoracostomy tube will now act as stent to divert most of the blood from the abdomen to the heart to allow for next steps (**FIGURE 26**).

Superior Mesenteric Artery and Vein, Hepatic Artery and Portal Vein Injuries—Approach

- Injuries to the mesenteric vessels, notably the superior mesenteric vein and artery and portal vein, are commonly associated with injuries to the small and large bowel and pancreas.

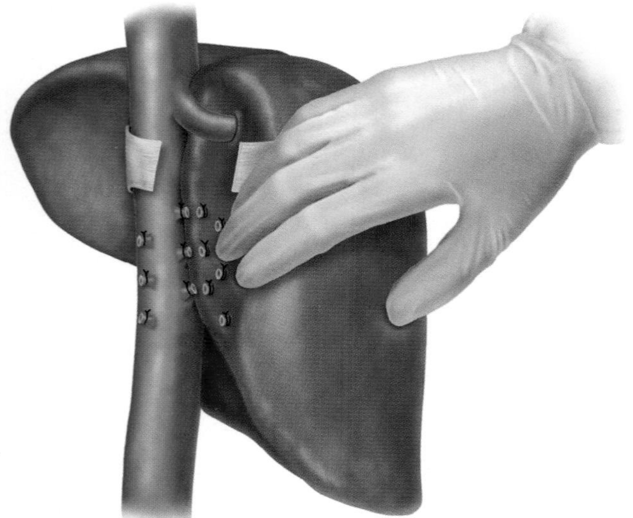

FIGURE 25 • Medializing the right liver lobe to visualize and ligate short veins of the retrohepatic vena cava. (Reprinted with permission from Dimick JB. *Mulholland & Greenfield's Surgery*. 7th ed. Wolters Kluwer; 2022. Figure 37.9.)

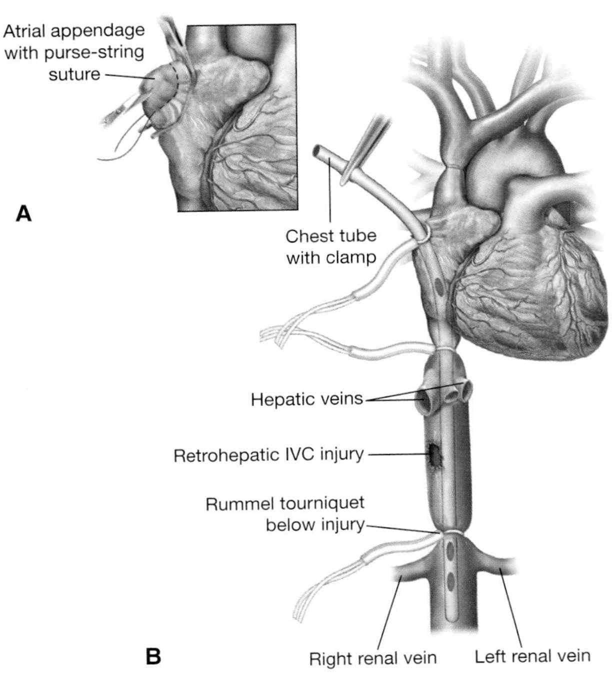

FIGURE 26 ● Atriocaval shunt for retrohepatic inferior vena cava injuries.

- The hepatic flexure is taken down and the duodenum medialized. A Pringle maneuver and clamping with a Rummel tourniquet can temporize bleeding from injuries toward the liver.
- Depending on whether the injury is on the left or right, a medial visceral rotation can improve visualization of the superior mesenteric artery and vein. Destructive injuries to either can cause massive small bowel ischemia with overall increased morbidity and mortality. Restoration of flow should be attempted, either with primary repair, patch angioplasty, or interposition graft.

PEARLS AND PITFALLS

Zone I—Abdominal	■ The aorta can be occluded by a clamp or by endovascular approach. Take note of the ischemic time, particularly if above the mesenteric or renal vessels. ■ Consider using a shunt (large Argyle or thoracostomy tube) in damage control situations. ■ Avoid the use of synthetic grafts in cases with massive contamination due to the risk of graft infection and pseudoaneurysm. If a graft is used, consider rifampin-soaked grafts after a thorough wash-out and cover with peritoneum to exclude from the abdomen.
Zone I—Inferior vena cava and initial hemorrhage control	■ In cases with massive contamination, and injuries requiring resection that cannot be brought together without tension, a synthetic graft is usually discouraged due to the risk of seeding and infection. Autologous graft (internal jugular vein, saphenous vein) and bovine pericardium may be used. ■ Infrarenal inferior vena cava injuries: The infrarenal vena cava can be ligated but may cause massive swelling of the extremities, warranting prophylactic bilateral lower extremity fasciotomies. Avoid narrowing the inferior vena cava >40% due to the risk of venous thromboembolism. ■ Suprarenal inferior vena cava injuries: One may consider using a large shunt (thoracostomy tube) in a damage control situation and returning for definitive repair with synthetic graft.

POSTOPERATIVE CARE

Zone I—Abdominal

- Patients after aortic repair should be followed with serial abdominal, neurovascular examinations, and laboratory studies as CBC, chemistry, and lactate. Patients with prolonged ischemic time, massive transfusion, and hypotension are at risk for mesenteric ischemia and renal failure.
- Systematic heparinization is typically not necessary given the large diameter and high-pressure state.
- Damage control surgery and resuscitation should be considered in patients in hemorrhagic shock requiring massive transfusion with subsequent acidosis, hypothermia, and coagulopathy. A second look within 24 hours is warranted to evaluate for ischemic bowel.

Zone I—Inferior Vena Cava and Initial Hemorrhage Control

- All patients are at risk for venous thromboembolism and should be on chemoprophylaxis. Patients who undergo repair with narrowing are also at risk for pulmonary embolus. Both lower extremities should be wrapped and elevated to decrease swelling.
- Patients are at risk for mesenteric ischemia from prolonged clamp time, hypotension, and possible venous congestion and should be followed with serial exams, complete blood county (including WBC), and lactate.

COMPLICATIONS

Zone I—Abdominal

- Graft infection: Patients presenting with concomitant bowel injury and vascular injuries requiring bypass are at risk for graft infection. Synthetic grafts typically carry a higher risk of infection compared to autologous tissue. Any signs of infection, flank pain, change in neurovascular status, or change in hemoglobin should prompt a computed tomography angiography (CTA) to evaluate for graft infection.
- Thrombosis: thrombosis of an arterial graft is rare but may be related to kinking, compression, dissection, infection, or hematologic disorders. CTA should be performed to evaluate for these complications and systemic anticoagulation initiated while planning next steps for revision, endovascular approach for thrombectomy, etc.
- Mesenteric ischemia: Patients may develop ischemia in watershed areas, develop lower gastrointestinal bleeds, or pain from ischemia. Early endoscopy is critical to diagnosis and treatment.
- Pseudoaneurysm: Be suspicious for pseudoaneurysm in the setting of back pain, bleeding, or change in vascular exam and image with CTA. Treatment will likely require endovascular treatment with stenting and coil embolization.

Zone I—Inferior Vena Cava and Initial Hemorrhage Control

- Complications of inferior vena cava injuries relate to drainage of the venous system, including thromboembolism and compartment syndrome.
- Surgeons should maintain a low threshold to perform fasciotomies in the presence of pain out of proportion and swelling. Loss of pulses and neurologic changes are very late signs of ischemia.
- Patients with suprarenal inferior vena cava injuries are at risk for acute renal injury and failure from hypotension and possible thrombus secondary to occluded inflow; thus, it is important to monitor urine output and creatinine.

REFERENCES

1. Kobayashi LM, Costantini TW, Hamel MG, Dierksheide JE, Coimbra R. Abdominal vascular trauma. *Trauma Surg Acute Care Open*. 2016;1(1):e000015.
2. Ferrada P, Callcut RA, Skarupa DJ, et al. Circulation first – the time has come to question the sequencing of care in the ABCs of trauma; an American Association for the Surgery of Trauma multicenter trial. *World J Emerg Surg*. 2018;13:8.
3. Rozycki GS, Ochsner MG, Feliciano DV, et al. Early detection of hemoperitoneum by ultrasound examination of the right upper quadrant: a multicenter study. *J Trauma*. 1998;45(5):878-883.
4. Stannard A, Eliason JL, Rasmussen TE. Resuscitative endovascular balloon occlusion of the aorta (REBOA) as an adjunct for hemorrhagic shock. *J Trauma*. 2011;71(6):1869-1872.
5. DuBose JJ, Scalea TM, Brenner M, et al. The AAST prospective Aortic Occlusion for Resuscitation in Trauma and Acute Care Surgery (AORTA) registry: data on contemporary utilization and outcomes of aortic occlusion and resuscitative balloon occlusion of the aorta (REBOA). *J Trauma Acute Care Surg*. 2016;81(3):409-419.
6. Byerly S, Cheng V, Plotkin A, Matsushima K, Inaba K, Magee GA. Impact of inferior vena cava ligation on mortality in trauma patients. *J Vasc Surg Venous Lymphat Disord*. 2019;7(6):793-800.

Chapter 35 Abdominal Vascular Injury Zone II

Melike N. Harfouche and David T. Efron

DEFINITION

- An abdominal vascular injury is defined as any injury to abdominal vascular structures located primarily in the retroperitoneal space. They are traditionally separated into three zones—I, II, and III. Zone I refers to the midline retroperitoneal vessels—the aorta and the inferior vena cava (IVC). Zone II refers to the lateral, upper retroperitoneal vessels, namely, the renal hilar vessels, and zone III refers to the pelvic vessels—the iliac artery and vein and their branches.

DIFFERENTIAL DIAGNOSIS

- Patients with abdominal vascular injury can have several concomitant injuries, depending on the mechanism. Abdominal vascular injuries from a blunt mechanism are very rare and can present more insidiously if the vascular injury is limited to the intima or contained by surrounding structures. In these cases, associated solid organ injuries affecting the liver, spleen, and/or kidney can also result in significant hemorrhage and may be the primary indication for operative intervention. Penetrating trauma more commonly results in abdominal vascular injury, with an acutely bleeding patient in hemorrhagic shock. In these cases, associated hollow viscus injuries are common, but the primary aim of operative intervention is expedient hemorrhage control.

PATIENT HISTORY AND PHYSICAL FINDINGS

- Patients with abdominal vascular injuries often present with hypotension and tachycardia, although this may not be present if the injury is incomplete, a clot has formed overlying the injury, or tamponade has been provided by surrounding structures; the absence of abnormal vital signs does not rule out abdominal vascular injury.
- A distended abdomen can also indicate retroperitoneal vascular injury, although this finding has a wide differential diagnosis in the setting of penetrating abdominal trauma.
- Injuries to the renal hilar structures often involve the collecting duct and/or the renal parenchyma, which can be seen as hematuria upon Foley insertion.

IMAGING AND OTHER DIAGNOSTIC STUDIES

- A foreign body series should be obtained in the trauma bay for all patients with penetrating injuries. The portable x-rays should include skin and soft tissue borders to ensure that all ballistic fragments are identified, and usually extend from the chest down to the pelvis. Defining the trajectory of penetrating wounds early in the trauma assessment is key to identifying potential injuries.
- A Focused Assessment with Sonography in Trauma (FAST) examination should be performed in all patients with blunt mechanism of injury and hemodynamic instability; it can be performed selectively in other groups (penetrating trauma, normal vital signs).
- A positive abdominal FAST is usually absent in isolated zone II injuries but may be seen if intraperitoneal structures are bleeding or the retroperitoneal hematoma is no longer contained within the retroperitoneum.
- Patients with stable vital signs without other indications for laparotomy (peritonitis, evisceration, clear intraperitoneal trajectory) should proceed to computed tomography (CT) of the abdomen and pelvis with intravenous contrast. Rectal contrast can be administered to increase detection of retroperitoneal colon injuries. Images should include both an arterial and venous phase to allow for identification of venous injuries and to distinguish the presence of pseudoaneurysms from active arterial extravasation. A 5-minute delayed phase can also be obtained to identify collecting duct and ureteral injuries.

SURGICAL MANAGEMENT

- In general, all patients with penetrating zone II abdominal vascular injury should undergo operative exploration. However, patients with stable vital signs who undergo CT scan demonstrating grades I to IV renal parenchymal injury can undergo selective nonoperative management (SNOM) based on clinician discretion.[1]
- Patients with blunt zone II abdominal vascular injuries identified on CT scan can be observed if they are hemodynamically stable. If a zone II injury is identified at the time of laparotomy, operative exploration of the retroperitoneum is indicated in the setting of hemodynamic instability and/or an expanding perinephric hematoma.
- Hemodynamically stable individuals with renal injury who undergo SNOM can be managed with angioembolization in cases where active bleeding is identified, and long-term complications of urinoma and/or urine leak can be managed with percutaneous drainage and/or ureteral stent placement.[2]

Preoperative Planning

- It is imperative to communicate with the OR staff regarding the planned procedure to ensure all necessary equipment is available.
- Patients presenting with signs of shock should have a massive transfusion protocol initiated, with blood product available in the operating room. Cell saver should be requested in settings where significant blood loss is anticipated.

Positioning

- Patients should be positioned supine, with both arms extended away from the body at 90°. This allows access to the chest cavity if necessary.

SETUP

- Skin preparation should extend from the chin to the knees, and down toward the operating table laterally. This ensures that additional procedures, if required, can be performed without breaking sterility.

INCISION

- The skin incision for all emergent trauma laparotomies should be generous, extending from below the xyphoid to the pubis.

EXPOSURE OF ZONE II

- Once the decision has been made to explore a zone II abdominal vascular injury, the first step consists of medial mobilization of the colon.
- On the right, medial mobilization of the colon should be initiated by identifying the avascular plane tethering the cecum to the retroperitoneum known as the white line of Toldt (**FIGURE 1**). Once this plane is entered, it can be extended cephalad along the right retroperitoneum toward the hepatic flexure of the colon. It is important to remain close to the colon during this dissection to prevent inadvertent injury to the ureter (**FIGURE 2**). As one extends toward the hepatic flexure, the retroperitoneal portions of the duodenum course very closely to the ascending colon and should be protected by ensuring the surgeons fingers dissect immediately posterior to the border of the colon (**FIGURE 3**).
- Immediately posterior to the duodenum lies the infrahepatic portion of the IVC and further cephalad the right renal vein can be identified (**FIGURE 4**). The kidney lies within Gerota fascia and can be challenging to fully expose due to its retrohepatic location (**FIGURE 5**).
- On the left, medial mobilization of the colon is similarly initiated at the left paracolic gutter by entering the avascular plane along the line of Toldt and extended cephalad, taking care to protect the ureter. The left kidney lies considerably lower than on the right, making it easier to expose (**FIGURE 6**).

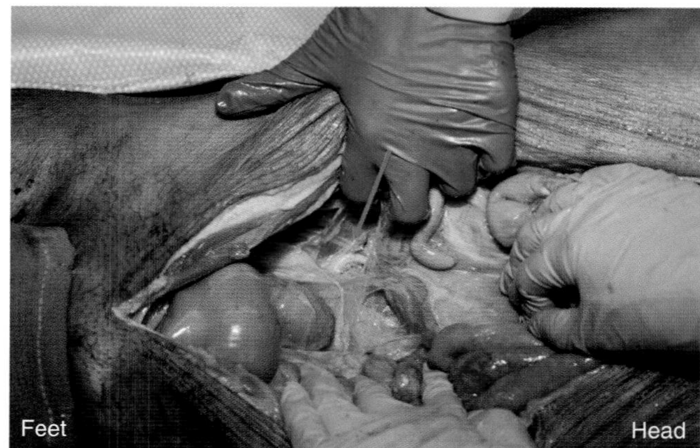

FIGURE 2 ● With the cecum retracted superiorly the ureter is identified in the retroperitoneum as it crosses the iliac vessels. *Red arrow* = ureter.

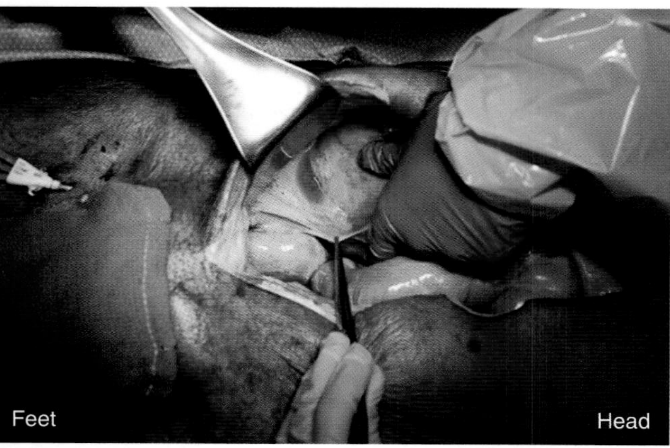

FIGURE 1 ● Line of Toldt to begin colon mobilization for access to the kidney in the retroperitoneum.

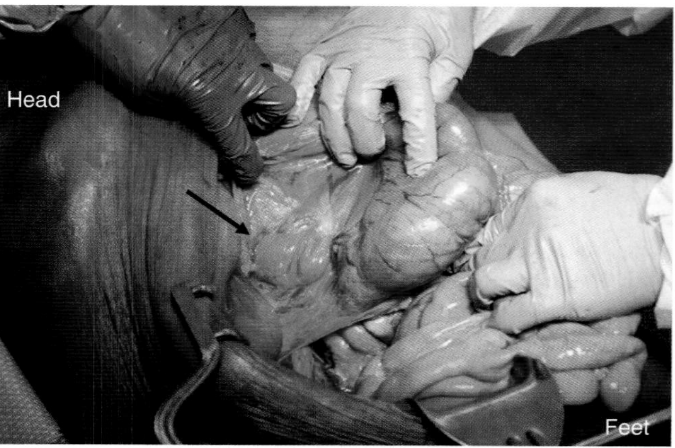

FIGURE 3 ● The retroperitoneal portions of the duodenum course very closely to the posterior border of the colon and should be protected. *Black arrow* = duodenum.

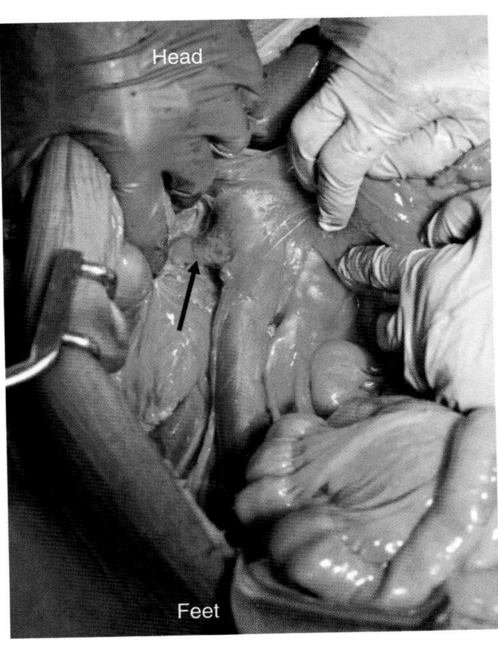

FIGURE 4 ● Further cephalad dissection along the inferior vena cava will reveal the right renal vein (*black arrow*). The kidney itself is obscured by the right lobe of the liver.

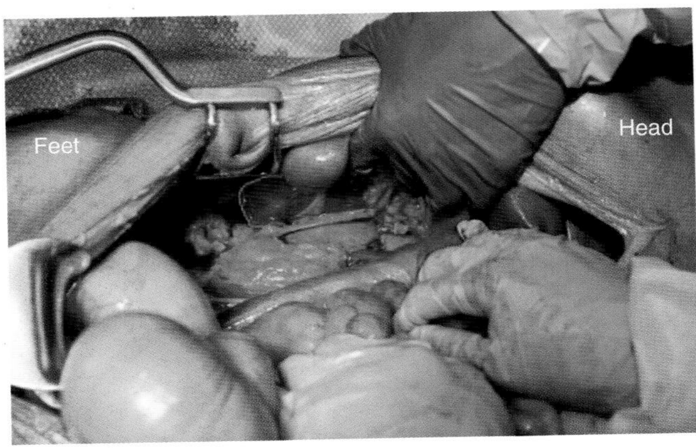

FIGURE 5 ● Right kidney visible within Gerota fascia rests underneath the right lobe of the liver (*red outline*).

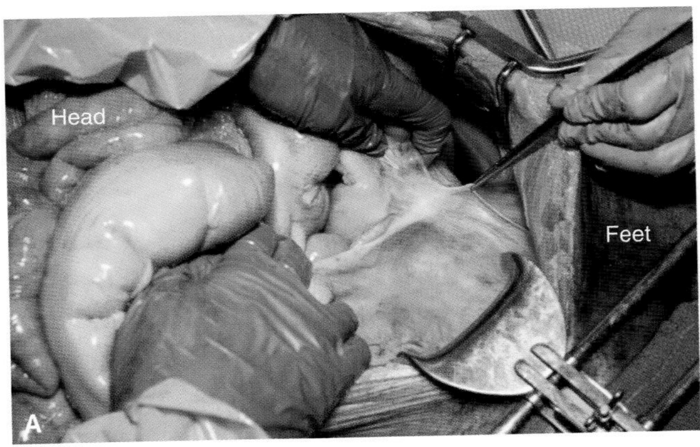

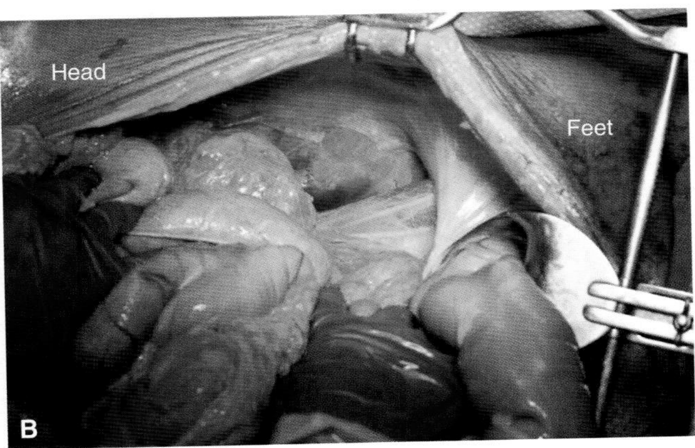

FIGURE 6 ● Mobilization of the line of Toldt **(A)** along the left paracolic gutter reveals the left kidney **(B)**, which sits considerably lower than the right kidney.

MANAGEMENT OF RENAL HILAR INJURY

- Exploration of zone II injuries often results in nephrectomy, which is most expediently performed by medial mobilization of the kidney to the midline, followed by hilar control. Experienced surgeons may prefer to obtain hilar control first prior to mobilization of the kidney at the risk of prolonging operative time.[3]
- Once the kidney is elevated and mobilized to the midline, the renal artery and vein can be identified and individually ligated. In a damage control setting, they can be ligated en bloc, with a low risk of long-term development of arteriovenous fistulae. As shown in **FIGURE 7**, several variants of renal hilar vasculature can exist with paired veins and/or paired arteries. The ureter can be traced to the pelvic brim and ligated to reduce the likelihood of development of urothelial cancer, although this is not necessary.

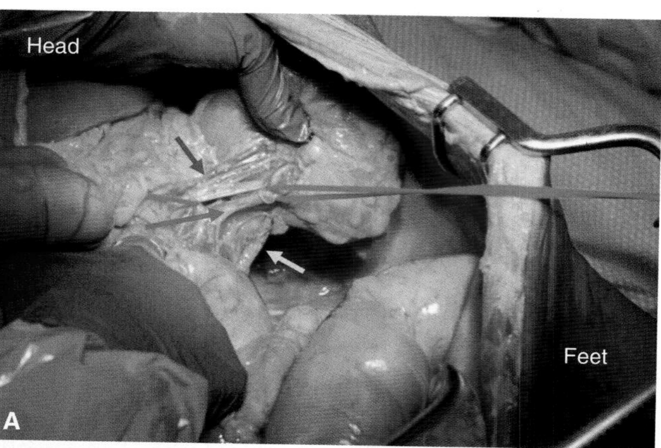

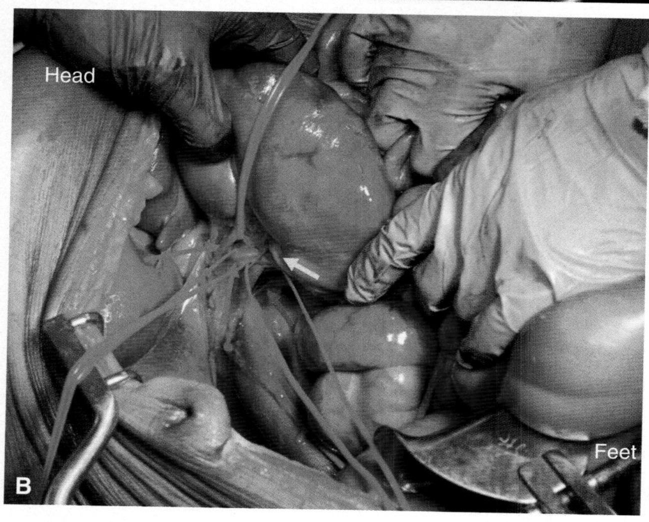

FIGURE 7 ● Hilar control of renal vessels of the left kidney from an anterior view **(A)** and right kidney from a posterior view **(B)**. *Red arrows* point to the renal arteries, blue arrows point to the renal veins, and yellow arrows point to the ureters.

PEARLS AND PITFALLS

Partial nephrectomy	■ Partial nephrectomy should only be performed in the hemodynamically stable patient with an isolated injury to upper or lower pole of the kidney; most zone II injuries mandating operative intervention will result in nephrectomy.
Contralateral kidney	■ Palpation of the contralateral kidney prior to proceeding with nephrectomy can be performed to determine if renal salvage should be attempted; in cases of damage control surgery (DCS), the absence of a contralateral kidney should not preclude life-saving procedures such as nephrectomy.
Endovascular approach	■ In hemodynamically stable patients with blunt renal trauma, an endovascular approach can be utilized for repair of intimal injuries to the renal artery to prevent development of renal ischemia and infarction.

POSTOPERATIVE CARE

- Patients should be monitored closely for evidence of ongoing bleeding or missed injuries, as right renal hilar injuries are also associated with pancreatic and duodenal injuries. Missed injuries often present in the first 24 hours with worsening hypotension, fever, and signs of peritonitis.
- DCS can be performed if patients have had massive blood loss, with evidence of coagulopathy (INR > 2), acidosis (pH < 7.2), or hypothermia (T < 34 °C). During DCS, an abbreviated surgery aims to control bleeding and hollow viscus injury, followed by temporary abdominal closure and planned return to the operating room in 48 to 72 hours.

COMPLICATIONS

- Urine leaks/urinomas can be managed effectively with percutaneous drainage.
- Endovascular coil embolization or deployment of a covered stent can be performed to treat the development of arteriovenous fistulae between the renal artery and vein.
- The risk of delayed bleeding and/or abscess formation increases with the presence of hollow viscus or pancreatic injury. In these cases, pancreatic injuries should be well drained and bowel anastomoses should be isolated from renal hilar vascular structures.

REFERENCES

1. Schellenberg M, Benjamin E, Piccinini A, Inaba K, Demetriades D. Selective nonoperative management of renal gunshot wounds. *J Trauma Acute Care Surg*. 2019;87(6):1301-1307.
2. Keihani S, Xu Y, Presson AP, et al. Contemporary management of high-grade renal trauma: results from the American association for the surgery of trauma genitourinary trauma study. *J Trauma Acute Care Surg*. 2018;84(3):418-425.
3. Gonzalez RP, Falimirski M, Holevar MR, Evankovich C. Surgical management of renal trauma: is vascular control necessary? *J Trauma*. 1999;47(6):1039-1042; discussion 1042-1044.

Chapter 36 Abdominal Vascular Injury Zone III

Elizabeth Dauer and Abhijit S. Pathak

DEFINITIONS

- Zone III of the retroperitoneum extends from the bifurcation of the aorta and confluence of the inferior vena cava to the level of the inguinal ligament and pelvic floor.
- The vascular structures in zone III are (**FIGURE 1**):
  - Common iliac artery and vein
  - External iliac artery and vein
  - Internal iliac artery and vein and its branches
  - Sacral venous plexus
  - Distal portions of the gonadal vessels

DIFFERENTIAL DIAGNOSIS

- Injuries to the vascular structures in zone III that require surgical management are most often associated with penetrating injuries, with missile injuries being the most common and outnumbering stab wounds. Blunt mechanisms and crush injuries of the pelvis are less common. These injuries are usually identified during exploration of the abdomen and present as retroperitoneal hematomas in zone III, which may or may not be contained. They are commonly associated with other visceral injuries including the ureter, bladder,

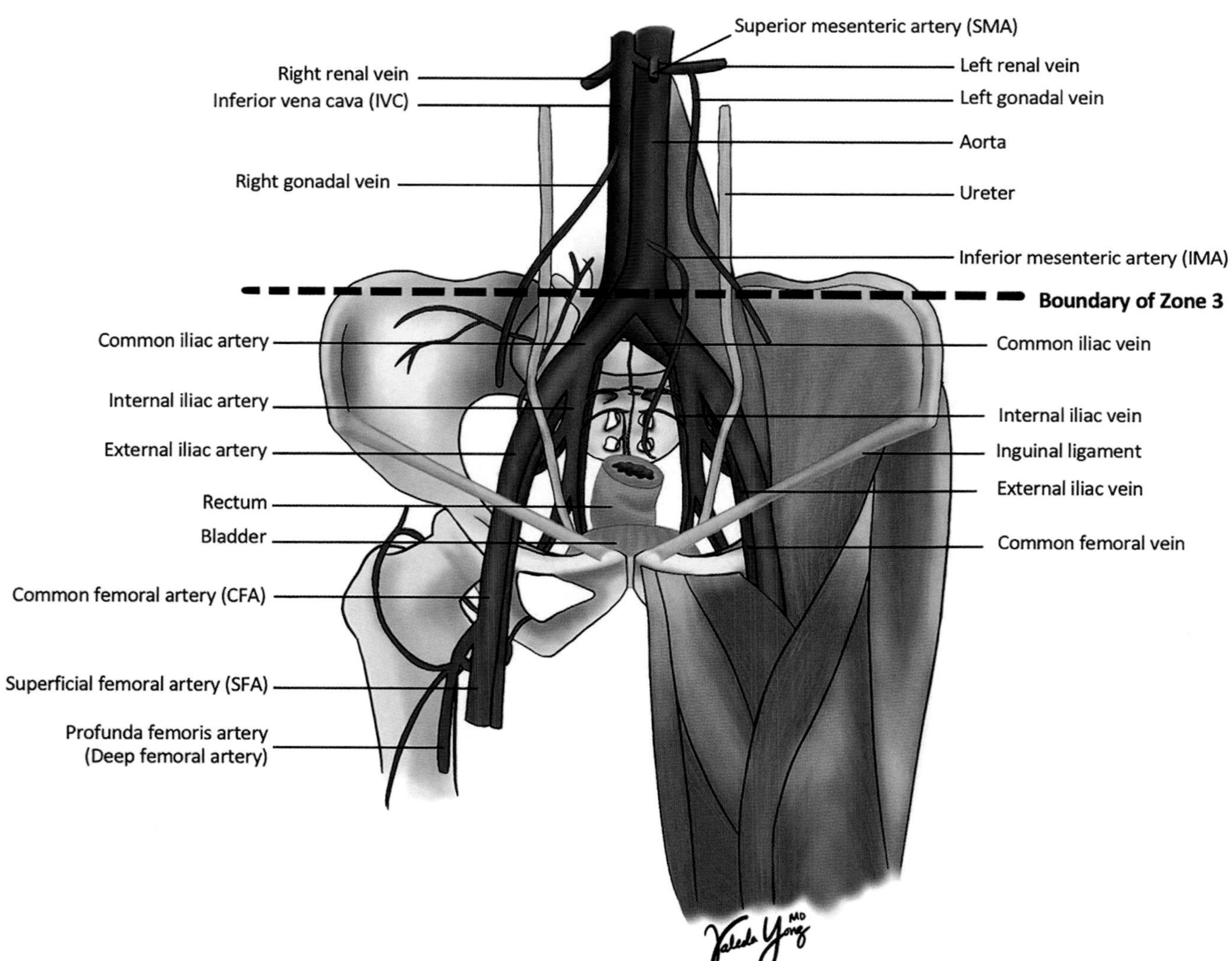

FIGURE 1 ● Vascular structures of zone III. (Courtesy of Valeda Yong, MD.)

rectum, small bowel, and colon. Furthermore, a diagnosis of zone III vascular injuries preoperatively requires a high index of suspicion based on the evaluation of the patient and the mechanism of injury. For instance, a gunshot wound to the abdomen or pelvic region with transpelvic trajectory as determined by clinical examination and plain radiographs along with hypotension may signify an iliac vascular injury.

PATIENT HISTORY AND PHYSICAL FINDINGS

- The patient history and physical examination may be limited depending on the severity of injury, the mechanism, and other associated injuries. The history should be focused on the mechanism of injury, forces that may have been applied due to that mechanism, and areas of perceived pain. Blunt mechanisms that should raise concern for bleeding from structures in zone III are those that are associated with high-energy forces and the development of pelvic fractures. These include fall from a significant height, pedestrian struck, high-speed motor vehicle collisions, and significant crush injury to the pelvic region. In penetrating trauma, zone III vascular injuries are considered when the estimated trajectory takes a course through the lower abdomen and pelvic region.
- Physical examination findings include:
  - Evidence of hemorrhagic shock: tachycardia, hypotension, poor distal perfusion, widened pulse pressure, altered mental status
  - Pulse discrepancy on palpation of the femoral pulses
  - Lack of dorsalis pedis or posterior tibial pulse or Doppler signals with concern for intracavitary injury
  - Abdominal tenderness or peritoneal signs on abdominal examination
  - Concerning penetrating injury trajectory
  - Significant bleeding from a penetrating wound
  - Pelvic instability or pelvic fracture on imaging
  - Scrotal/perineal hematoma

IMAGING AND OTHER DIAGNOSTIC STUDIES

- The focused assessment with sonography in trauma (FAST) examination may provide evidence of intra-abdominal or pelvic hemorrhage that can occur with zone III vascular injuries. The patients may have a positive FAST examination in the pelvis, right upper quadrant, or left upper quadrant views with zone III injuries; however, a negative FAST does not preclude injury. In a systemic review of randomized controlled trials from 1965 through 2009, Quinn et al found that FAST examination had a high specificity (94%-100%) and low sensitivity (28%-100%) in determining intra-abdominal hemorrhage after penetrating torso trauma. They concluded that a positive FAST examination should prompt exploratory laparotomy but a negative FAST examination should prompt further investigation through available diagnostic modalities.[1]
- The presence of a pelvic fracture on pelvic radiograph may suggest bleeding in the area of zone III, particularly if an open book pelvic fracture exists. Also, pelvic radiographs may give insight to missile trajectory in penetrating trauma, and if both a lateral and anteroposterior view of the pelvis is obtained, cavitary violation may be able to be excluded based on the location of the wounds and any retained foreign bodies.
- Computed tomography (CT) scan can be used to assess for zone III injury in patients who are hemodynamically acceptable to undergo CT scan imaging. CT scan can provide valuable diagnostic information with regards to vessel injury, areas of active hemorrhage, penetrating trajectory, and associated injuries. Active contrast extravasation on CT scan has been shown to be the most reliable indicator of significant arterial bleeding identified on subsequent angiography and can provide a roadmap for interventional radiologist to more accurately and expeditiously localize the site of bleeding.[2]
- Angiography can serve as both a diagnostic and therapeutic imaging modality. It can assess for ongoing arterial bleeding, pseudoaneurysm formation, or abrupt vessel cutoff, which is indicative of potential vessel injury. Angiographic embolization is a safe and effective tool for control of hemorrhage in surgically difficult areas such as deep in the pelvis (**FIGURES 2-4**).[3]

SURGICAL MANAGEMENT

- In patients with blunt trauma and potential pelvic bleeding, the decision for operative intervention may not always be clear. The patient's hemodynamics and other associated injuries must be taken into consideration when deciding how to proceed after the initial trauma assessment. In addition, simultaneous management of associated injuries, such as pelvic fractures, may be indicated in order to stabilize the patient.
- In the case of complex pelvic ring injuries with widening of the pubic symphysis, placement of a pelvic binder to decrease the volume of the pelvis may assist in creating tamponade for pelvic bleeding. It is imperative that these devices be placed correctly, in order to approximate the pubic symphysis without causing widening of the posterior elements of the pelvis. A sheet or a commercially available pelvic binder

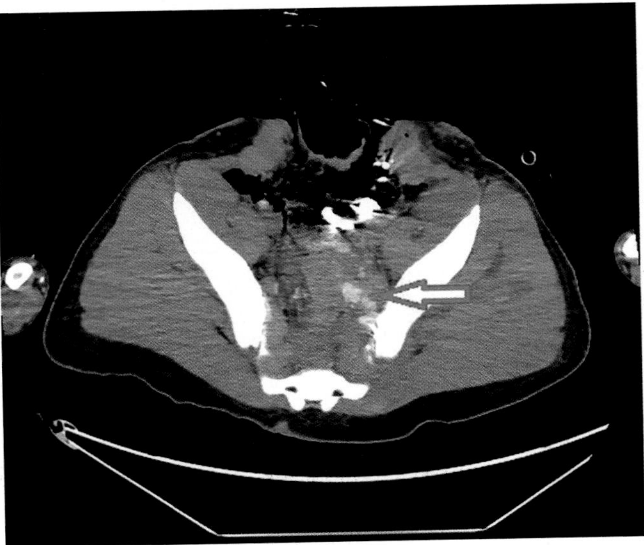

FIGURE 2 ● Postoperative computed tomography angiography demonstrates contrast blush from distal left internal iliac artery branches (*arrow*).

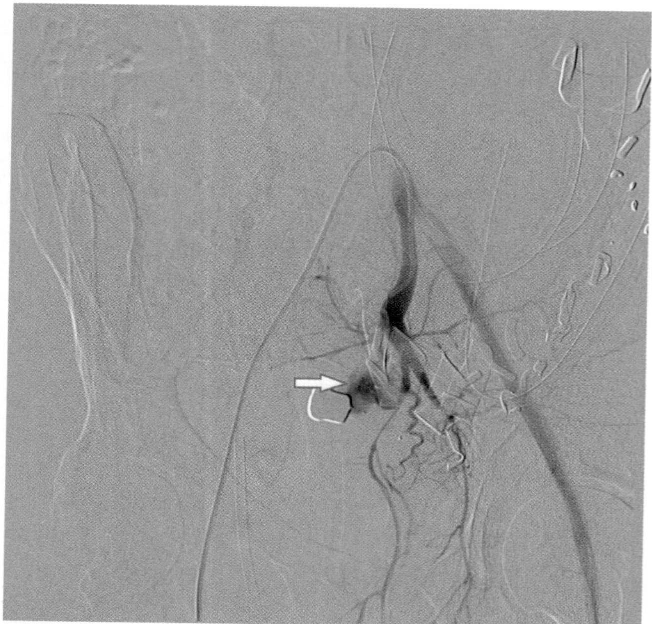

FIGURE 3 ● Angiogram demonstrates injury with blush/pseudo-aneurysm from distal left internal iliac artery branches (*arrow*).

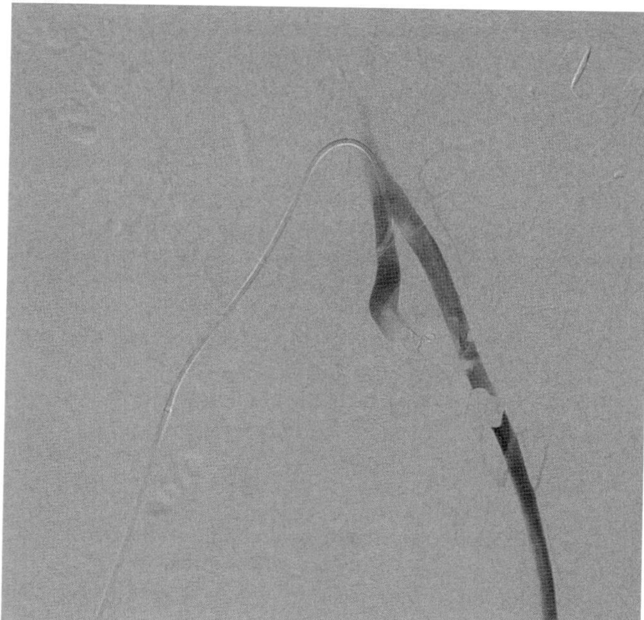

FIGURE 4 ● Gelfoam embolization of the distal left internal iliac artery performed with cessation of flow into the distal injured branch.

may be used to accomplish this task and should be placed at the level of the greater trochanters of the femurs to allow for proper reapproximation of the pubic symphysis. Blunt iliac artery injuries associated with pelvic fractures are rare; however, when they do occur they have a high complication and mortality rate.[4]

TECHNIQUES

- In blunt trauma, injury to the large pelvic vessels, including the common iliac artery and external iliac artery are rare but can range from small intimal irregularities to complete transection. These injuries are associated with severe pelvic fractures, hypotension, genitourinary injury, and bowel injury and have a high overall risk of morbidity and mortality.[4]
- When proceeding to the operating room for suspected zone III vascular injury, the patient should be placed supine on the operating room table in order to allow access to both the abdomen and thighs in the event it is necessary to gain vascular control at the level of the femoral vessels or if greater saphenous vein needs to be harvested to use as a conduit in the management of a vascular injury.
- A generous midline laparotomy incision should be used and taken caudally to the level of the pubic symphysis in order to provide the widest exposure of the pelvic structures as possible. The abdomen is packed tightly to allow for tamponade of bleeding, for placement of the self-retaining retractor for exposure, and for the anesthesiologists to properly resuscitate the patient prior to opening any retroperitoneal hematomas that may result in copious hemorrhage.
- In penetrating trauma, injury to the vascular structures of zone III must be in the differential diagnosis for every patient with a trajectory that enters the lower abdomen and pelvis. All zone III hematomas from penetrating injury obligate exploration for a source of hemorrhage, whereas, in blunt trauma, the presence of a zone III hematoma does not mandate exploration, as up to 85% of pelvic bleeding is venous.[5] Exploration of a zone III hematoma in blunt trauma risks release of tamponade and exsanguinating hemorrhage from the pelvic venous plexus. In the absence of significant ongoing major arterial injury, these injuries are better treated with a combination of preperitoneal packing, angiographic embolization, and pelvic stabilization. When major vascular injury is suspected, the basic tenets of vascular surgery with obtaining proximal and distal control should be followed to limit hemorrhage and to provide appropriate exposure of the injury.
- Based on trajectory and location of the zone III hematoma, the approximate level of the injury should be able to be estimated to help the surgeon determine where to gain control of the vasculature. If bleeding is significant and precluding identification of the structures, sponge sticks placed both proximally and distally or direct manual compression can be used to control bleeding and improve visibility in order to gain proximal and distal control of the vessels.
- To gain proximal control, a right medial visceral rotation (see **FIGURE 5**) is performed to expose the aorta and inferior vena cava at the level of the aortic bifurcation. This maneuver ensures the ability to isolate the arterial and venous structures at their most cranial extent, if necessary. If there is significant ongoing bleeding, the aorta can then be compressed or a vascular clamp applied at this level to greatly diminish inflow to the area. Also, the right medial visceral rotation

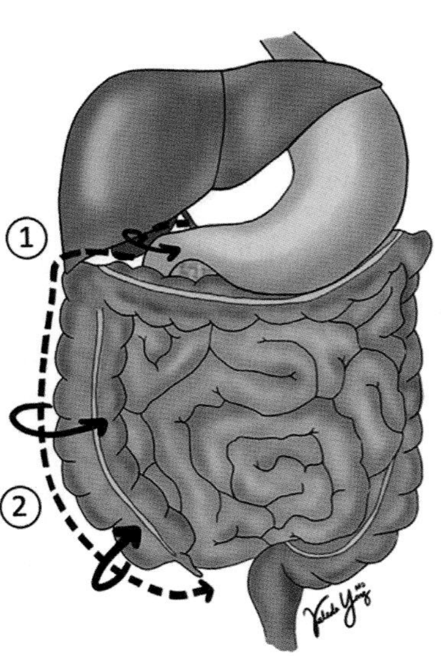

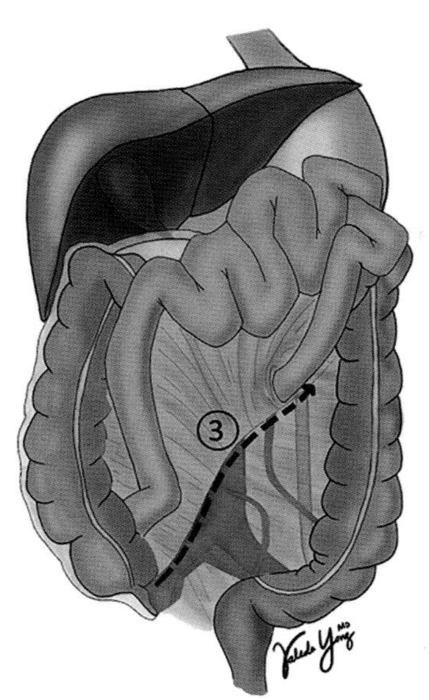

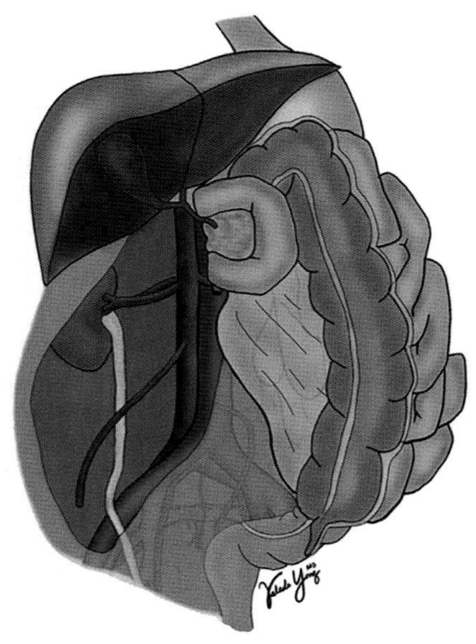

FIGURE 5 ● Right-sided medial visceral rotation (Cattell-Braasch-Kocher maneuvers). This maneuver involves mobilization of the right colon including the hepatic flexure (Cattell)[2] and mobilization of the small bowel (Braasch)[3] along the avascular plane between the small bowel mesentery and the posterior peritoneum. This will allow access to the subhepatic inferior vena cava and aorta, to the entirety of the right iliac vessels and the proximal left iliac vessels. (Courtesy of Valeda Yong, MD.)

provides optimal exposure for the right-sided iliac vessels. The most proximal portion of the left-sided iliac vessels can be accomplished in this way; however, the bifurcation of the left common iliac vessels is covered by the sigmoid and descending colon mesentery. To expose this area, the left colon and sigmoid colon should be released from its lateral attachments to the abdominal wall and be reflected medially to expose the left iliac vessels all the way to the level of the inguinal ligament. Depending on the assumed level of the injury, a vessel loop can be placed to encircle both the artery and vein or, alternatively, a vascular clamp applied on the side of injury at this time. Gaining control of the common iliac vein can prove to be challenging as it sits posterior to the common iliac artery on the right and posterior and medial to the common iliac artery on the left. It may be necessary to transect the right common iliac artery in order to gain access to a right common iliac vein injury, although this is rarely needed and, if performed, will necessitate reconstruction or placement of a temporary vascular shunt in order to ensure distal flow. In addition, it may be necessary to gain control of the internal iliac artery and internal iliac vein. The takeoff of the internal iliac artery and vein usually occurs at the level of the fourth lumbar vertebra, and the vessels course posteromedial and inferior to supply the pelvic structures. the internal iliac artery and vein can be ligated to control hemorrhage or to facilitate repair of the common or external iliac vessels if the injury spans the bifurcation of the common iliac artery and the confluence of the internal and external iliac veins. If this is done, the patient should be carefully monitored for the development of gluteal compartment syndrome on the effected side. If bilateral internal iliac vessels are ligated, the patient can develop ischemia or necrosis to the pelvic structures.

- To gain distal control, the external iliac artery and vein can be encircled below the suspected level of injury. For injuries occurring just before or at the level of the inguinal ligament, a counter incision can be made in the groin to isolate the common femoral artery and vein to gain distal control. The inguinal ligament can be divided to expose injuries at the level of the inguinal ligament. The most distal extent of the external iliac artery and vein and the most cranial extent of the common femoral artery and vein give rise to the circumflex vessels, which may need to be ligated to limit ongoing back bleeding into the surgical field.
- Once vascular control has been obtained, the injury can be exposed in its entirety. The vessels should be inspected circumferentially to ensure identification of all injuries as well as the extent of the injury as blast effect can lead to a larger area of injury than first appreciated (**FIGURE 6**).
- Management of arterial injuries to the common iliac artery and external iliac artery is determined based on the extent of the injury, available conduits, and clinical stability of the patient. Injuries that involve less than 50% circumference of the vessel can be considered for primary repair if no evidence of intimal injury or blast injury exists. The wound edges should be debrided and closed transversely to avoid narrowing of the vessel, which may impede distal flow. For larger injuries, the vessels should be debrided back to healthy tissue with excision of the edges and can be repaired primarily in an end-to-end fashion provided there is not a significant defect in length (usually <1 cm) or tension. If there is a significant resultant segmental defect then using a graft to span the vessel defect will be necessary. An interposition graft using autologous vein using polypropylene suture is ideal; however, a polytetrafluoroethylene prosthetic conduit may be necessary if no suitable autologous vein using polypropylene suture is available. If able, the retroperitoneum should be closed over the graft to isolate it from the intra-abdominal contents. The placement of either autologous or

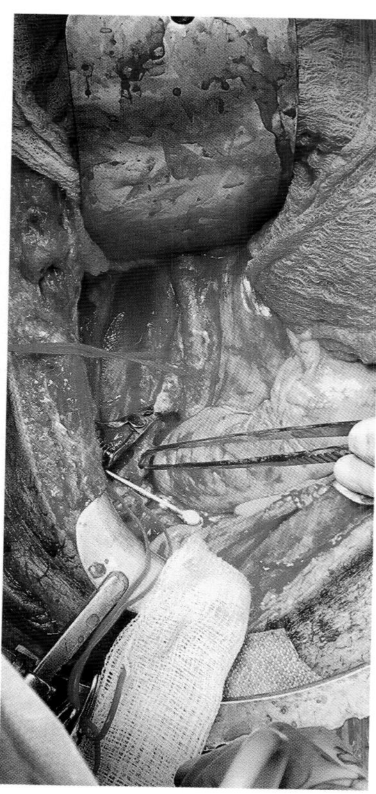

FIGURE 6 ● Injury to the right external iliac artery with proximal control at the right common iliac artery and distal control at the right external iliac artery with vessel loops and vascular clamps used immediately proximal and distal to the injury.

prosthetic graft in a grossly infected field from spillage of bowel contents remains a serious problem due to concern for graft infection. Development of graft infection can lead to anastomotic pseudoaneurysm formation, recurrent bacteremia and sepsis, and even graft blowout, which can lead to life-threatening bleeding. Owing to these potential complications, some have advocated the use of iliac artery ligation with reconstruction using extra-anatomic bypass to restore flow to the lower extremity in extreme circumstances,[6] but this has not gained widespread acceptance.

- In damage control situations, the use of a temporary intravascular shunt (TIVS) can be used to restore flow and abbreviate operating room time to allow for resuscitation and rewarming in the intensive care unit. There are a large number of commercially available vascular shunts that can be used in this situation. The shunt chosen should be an appropriate size match for the vessel and should be adequately secured to prevent dislodgement. The use of TIVS in damage control situations is not related to increased shunt-related complications in comparison with nondamage control use, and there is no attributable mortality to the shunt procedure itself in reported series.[7,8]
- The use of systemic anticoagulation during these procedures remains controversial. In a multicenter retrospective review of 323 patients, Maher et al found that the use of systemic anticoagulation during the repair of major arterial injuries was associated with better arterial patency without an increase in bleeding complications.[9] The surgeon must weigh the risks of arterial clot formation with the risk of ongoing bleeding to determine the utility of intraoperative systemic anticoagulation in each clinical situation.
- Venous injuries to the iliac vessels can be managed via ligation or repair. When comparing ligation vs repair in patients with isolated iliac vein injuries, Magee et al. found that patients who underwent ligation had increased mortality in comparison with those who had repair; however, rates of venous thromboembolism, fasciotomy, amputation, and acute kidney injury were comparable.[10] Venous repair is a viable option in injuries that are small or easily approximated; however, it may not be feasible in destructive venous injuries or if the patient is in extremis and the injury needs to be managed expeditiously. Also, the surgeon must have the experience and surgical expertise in order to perform the repair. Different repair strategies have been used including simple lateral venorrhaphy, vein patch, and interposition grafts. When looking at venous repair patency, early patency rates are approximately 60% to 70% with less early extremity edema, but long-term extremity morbidity is similar.[11,12] Hence, complex venous repairs or reconstruction should be avoided.
- Once hemorrhage control has been achieved and the vascular injuries managed with either definitive repair or damage control techniques, the abdomen should be thoroughly inspected for other associated injuries. Care should be taken to identify the trajectory of penetrating injuries to allow for meticulous assessment of the structures within that path. Specific attention should be paid to evaluation of the ureters as they cross the external iliac vessels below the level of the iliac bifurcation.
- After the intra-abdominal injuries and other major associated injuries are managed, the need for adjunctive procedures should be determined. The risk of ischemia and reperfusion to the lower extremity after injury to the iliac vessels, particularly in the setting of hemodynamic instability and massive resuscitation, is of great concern. Performance of four-compartment lower extremity prophylactic fasciotomy in this setting should be considered, and the decision to proceed should be based on the injury complex, the patient's clinical status, existing evidence of compartment syndrome in the operating room, and ability to effectively monitor the patient in the postoperative setting for the development of compartment syndrome. Prophylactic thigh fasciotomy is rarely performed and should be considered on a case-to-case basis. Early fasciotomy and the judicious use of crystalloid resuscitation has been associated with a decrease in amputation rates after vascular injuries effecting the lower extremity.[13,14]
- Patients who require ligation of the internal iliac vasculature, especially if needed bilaterally, can develop gluteal compartment syndrome over time. Routine prophylactic gluteal fasciotomy is unwarranted, but serial gluteal compartment checks should be performed to assess the need for compartment release.

PEARLS AND PITFALLS

Patient presentation	■ Any patient presents with a penetrating mechanism to the abdomen and pelvic region with associated abdominal tenderness and hypotension should go to the operating room. Diagnostic imaging studies should only be undertaken in those patients who are hemodynamically acceptable without concern for intracavitary injury that would require operative intervention.
Preoperative planning	■ The patient should be prepped from the chin to both knees and from table to table on either side in order to access the chest, abdomen, and both proximal extremities. A midline incision extending from the xiphoid to the pubis is the most versatile in an unstable trauma patient in order to access all regions of the peritoneal cavity and retroperitoneum. An inadequate incision will lead to difficulty in exposure of the injuries and may prolong time to hemorrhage control.
Operative pearls	■ Once the peritoneal cavity is entered, remove clots and free blood and then pack the abdomen. Inspect all retroperitoneal zones. Properly identifying the presence of and location of a retroperitoneal hematoma will dictate the next steps in the conduct of the exploration. All zone III hematomas from a penetrating injury should be explored. Proximal control to the iliac vessels is obtained via a right medial visceral rotation. The sigmoid and left colon will need to be mobilized medially to access the left iliac vessels. If necessary, a groin incision or splitting of the inguinal ligament can be undertaken to obtain distal control. Use sponge sticks or manual pressure to control any hemorrhage until proximal and distal vascular control is achieved.
Hemodynamic stability	■ The patient's identified injuries and hemodynamic stability should dictate the management strategy at the time of the initial operative intervention. Injuries to the common or external iliac arteries should be repaired or managed via temporary intravascular shunt in damage control situations. Ligation of these vessels leads to ischemia distally and the need for above-knee amputation or hip disarticulation. Iliac vein injuries can be ligated to shorten operative time in damage control scenarios. Avoid complex venous repairs in these circumstances. Consider lower extremity fasciotomies, especially in patients with both arterial and venous injuries.

POSTOPERATIVE CARE

- The general postoperative care is similar to that of any trauma patient who has undergone an exploratory laparotomy or damage control laparotomy. They should be monitored for any signs of bleeding, as well as frequent vascular examinations of the lower extremities should be done to monitor for any change. If the patient has undergone damage control laparotomy and has a temporary shunt in place, it is crucial to monitor the lower extremity by vascular examination for any signs that the shunt may have thrombosed. In addition, patients should be monitored for the development of compartment syndrome of the gluteal region, thigh, and lower leg. Patients should return to the operating room (OR) for pack removal and definitive management of their injuries as well as abdominal closure once their metabolic failure has been corrected.

COMPLICATIONS

- Postoperative bleeding is a true concern with these injuries since it is not only the main iliac vessels that may be injured but also other smaller distal branches in the pelvis as well as the presacral venous plexus. These patients can continue to bleed even after definitive control and may mandate damage control with packing and temporary abdominal closure. Even with packing, these patients may continue to bleed especially in the setting of metabolic failure, which should be aggressively corrected. Despite this, these patients may require a return to the OR for hemorrhage control. Delayed hemorrhage with significant bleeding can occur and is usually associated with pelvic sepsis, many times when there is a concomitant bowel injury with a leak from a repair or anastomosis. This can result in an anastomotic failure of a vascular repair/graft with pseudoaneurysm formation or graft blow out. Many times, the first indication of this complication is a herald bleed with new blood present in intra-abdominal drains placed for intra-abdominal infection or from an unexplained drop in hemoglobin or hematocrit levels. Depending on the time period from the index operation, the subsequent management of the abdomen, and perceived risk for reoperation in a "hostile" pelvis, this can be managed with endovascular techniques or a combination of endovascular techniques and extra-anatomic bypass on a case-by-case basis (**FIGURES 7-9**).

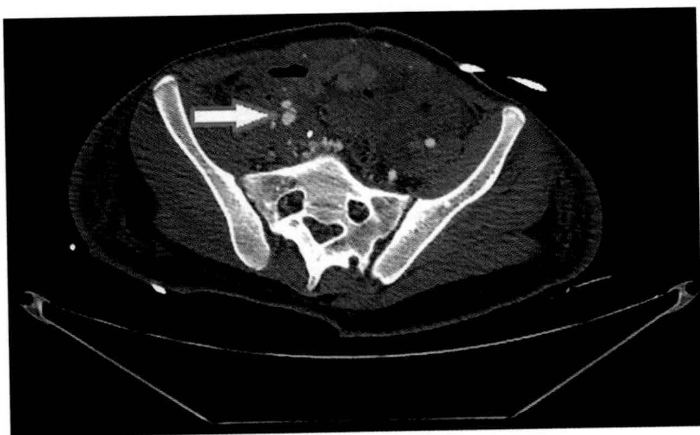

FIGURE 7 ● Computed tomography angiography demonstrates pseudoaneurysm from the proximal right iliofemoral bypass graft (*arrow*).

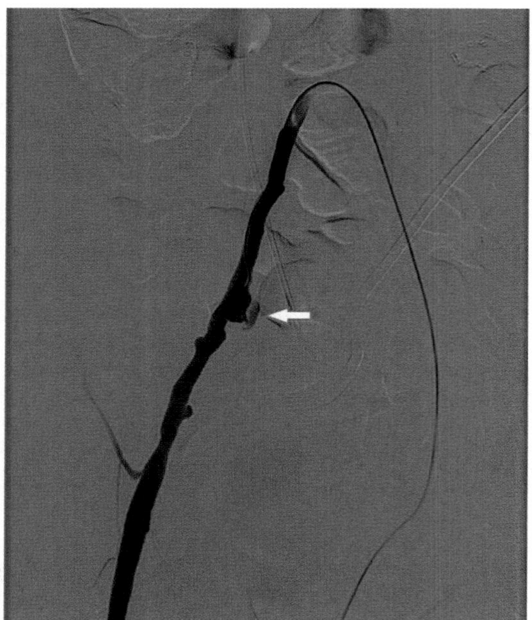

FIGURE 8 ● Angiogram demonstrates pseudoaneurysm from the proximal right iliofemoral bypass graft (*arrow*).

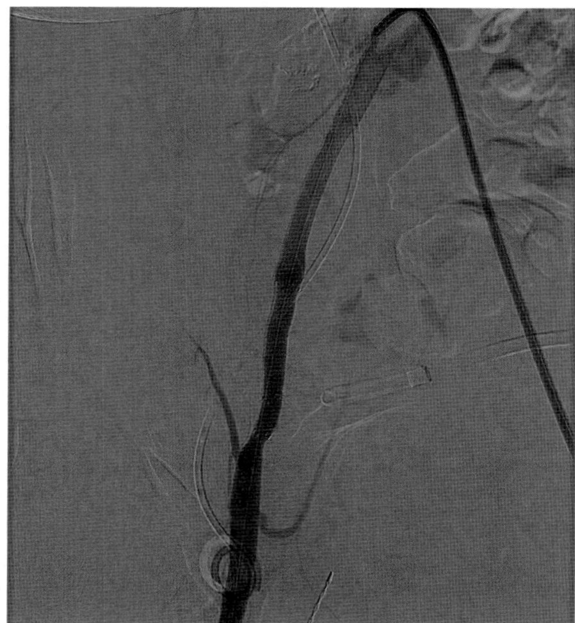

FIGURE 9 ● A covered endovascular stent was placed from the right common iliac artery to the right common femoral artery with resolution of the pseudoaneurysm.

- Patients may develop gluteal, thigh, or lower leg compartment syndrome, which is related to the ischemia and reperfusion injury to the affected extremity depending on the level of the vascular injury. If prophylactic fasciotomies had not been performed, one must be vigilant to monitor for its occurrence and proceed with early fasciotomy as indicated.
- Abdominal compartment syndrome can develop even in association with damage control surgery especially in the setting of intra-abdominal packing. There can be an accumulation of ascites, retroperitoneal edema, and/or blood and bowel edema, which can lead to increased intra-abdominal pressures. Patients should be monitored for intra-abdominal hypertension and development of abdominal compartment syndrome even in the setting of an "open" abdomen.
- Serial vascular examinations of the lower extremities after any repair or shunt are paramount. Any change in the examination may signify a concern for thrombosis. If there is any concern then prompt reexploration in the early operative period is the best chance for limb salvage. Delayed thrombosis can also occur and is usually associated with pelvic sepsis, many times due to a concomitant bowel injury with a leak from a repair or anastomosis. Depending on the time period from the index operation, the subsequent management of the abdomen, and perceived risk for reoperation in a "hostile" pelvis, this can be managed with endovascular techniques or a combination of endovascular techniques and extra-anatomic bypass on a case-by-case basis.

REFERENCES

1. Quinn AC, Sinert R. What is the utility of the Focused Assessment with Sonography in Trauma (FAST) exam in penetrating torso trauma? *Injury*. 2011;42(5):482-487.
2. Yoon W, Kim JK, Jeong YY, et al. Pelvic arterial hemorrhage in patients with pelvic fractures: detection with contrast-enhanced CT. *Radiographics*. 2004;24:1591-1605.
3. Velmahos G, Toutouzas K, Vassiliu P, et al. A prospective study on the safety and efficacy of angiographic embolization for pelvic and visceral injuries. *J Trauma*. 2002;53(2):303-308.
4. Cestero R, Plurad D, Green D, et al. Iliac artery injuries and pelvic fractures: a national trauma database analysis of associated injuries and outcomes. *J Trauma*. 2009;67(4):715-718.
5. Huittinen VM, Slatis P. Postmortem angiography and dissection of the hypogastric artery in pelvic fracatures. *Surgery*. 1973;73:454-462.
6. Feliciano D. Approach to major abdominal vascular injury. *J Vasc Surg*. 1988;7(5):730-736.
7. Tung L, Leonard J, Lawless R, et al. Temporary intravascular shunts after civilian arterial injury: a prospective multicenter Eastern Association for the Surgery of Trauma study. *Injury*. 2021;52(5):1204-1209.
8. Inaba K, Aksoy H, Seamon M, et al. Multicenter evaluation of temporary intravascular shunt use in vascular trauma. *J Trauma Acute Care Surg*. 2016;80(3):359-364.
9. Maher Z, Frank B, Salliant N, et al. Systemic intraoperative anticoagulation during arterial injury repair. *J Trauma Acute Care Surg*. 2017;82(4):680-686.
10. Magee G, Cho J, Matsushima K, et al. Isolated iliac vascular injuries and outcome of repair versus ligation of isolated iliac vein injury. *J Vasc Surg*. 2018;67(1):254-261.
11. Meyer J, Walsh J, Schuler J, et al. The early fate of venous repair after civilian vascular trauma. A clinical, hemodynamic, and venographic assessment. *Ann Surg*. 1987;206(4):458-464.
12. Agarwal N, Shah P, Clauss R, et al. Experience with 115 civilian venous injuries. *J Trauma*. 1982;22(10):827-832.
13. Farber A, Tan T, Hamburg N, et al. Early fasciotomy in patients with extremity vascular injury is associated with decreased risk of adverse limb outcomes: a review of the National Trauma Data Bank. *Injury*. 2012;43(9):1486-1491.
14. Dauer E, Yamaguchi S, Yu D, et al. Major venous injury and large volume crystalloid resuscitation: a limb threatening combination. *Am J Surg*. 202;219(1):38-42. doi:10.1016/j.injury.2011.06.006.

Chapter 37

Lower Extremity Vascular Trauma—Femoral and Popliteal With Infrapopliteal Fasciotomy

Kelly M. Sutter and Christine T. Trankiem

DEFINITION

- Lower extremity trauma is defined as trauma to an extremity below the inguinal ligament. Specifically, this includes trauma to all vessels distal to the iliofemoral junction, including the common femoral artery, superficial femoral artery, femoral vein, greater saphenous vein, and tibial artery.

DIFFERENTIAL DIAGNOSIS

- When a patient presents with hemorrhage from the lower extremity or with a tourniquet in place, named blood vessels are frequently not the culprit of bleeding.
- Venous bleeding can be exacerbated secondary to tourniquet placement and resultant venous congestion.
- Muscular bleeding, particularly hematomas resulting from muscular injury, can raise concern for serious vascular trauma.
- Motor deficits and sensory changes, harbingers for acute limb ischemia or compartment syndrome, may result from direct traumatic injury to the nerve.
- Vasospasm can mimic arterial injury, especially on imaging.

PATIENT HISTORY AND PHYSICAL FINDINGS

Presentation

- Lower extremity vascular trauma can result from both blunt and penetrating trauma.
  - Penetrating trauma to a blood vessel can be more easily identifiable than blunt injury because of the penetration defect. However, given the sometimes unpredictable ballistic or stab trajectory, it is important to examine the patient completely.
    - Overall, penetrating lower extremity trauma is more common in military settings. The majority of proximal lower extremity vascular injuries are penetrating, whereas distal lower extremity trauma is equally associated with penetrating and blunt mechanisms.[1]
    - Blunt vascular injury may be more challenging to diagnose as a patient may present with a constellation of injuries in multiple anatomic regions.
    - A commonly missed musculoskeletal injury is posterior knee dislocation. This can be seen in patients whose knees strike the dashboard during a motor vehicle collision or who fall on their knee; this injury is often associated with popliteal artery injury.
    - Additional orthopedic injuries associated with lower extremity vascular injury are tibial plateau fracture (popliteal artery injury) and femoral shaft fracture (superficial femoral artery injury).

Exam Findings

- Vascular injuries are typically assessed with respect to HARD and SOFT signs.
  - Hard signs in penetrating trauma usually require emergent intervention, while soft signs can provide time for diagnostic tests.
    - Hard signs: Pulsatile bleeding, expanding hematoma, thrill at injury site, pulseless limb
    - The "6 Ps" seen in advanced acute limb ischemia or compartment syndrome also fall into this category—Pain, Pallor, Paresthesia, Paralysis, Pulseless, and Poikilothermia
  - Soft signs: bleeding in transit, unexplained hypotension, injury near a major vessel, nonexpanding hematoma, or nonpulsatile bleeding.
- Patients who are in shock should be taken to the operating room for exploration, irrespective of hard or soft signs of vascular injury.

IMAGING AND OTHER DIAGNOSTIC STUDIES

- In any patient with lower extremity trauma, whether it is penetrating or blunt (dislocation, fracture, or contusion), it is important to complete a thorough neurovascular exam of the affected extremity. Commonly, palpable pulses on exam are thought to obviate the need for further workup, but this can be misleading, especially in a healthy, hemodynamically normal patient.
- In vascular trauma, the management algorithms are often geared toward whether to proceed directly to operation or whether to image first. Imaging has been linked to delay in management, which in the case of limb ischemia can lead to tissue loss, compartment syndrome, or even limb loss. When appropriate, the following image modalities are recommended.

Ankle-Brachial Index

- Historically, the ankle-brachial index (ABI) was used to determine the necessity of angiography in occult vascular injuries; that is, vascular trauma without hard signs.
  - Current guidelines recommend that patients who meet this demographic should undergo computed tomography (CT) angiography if ABI <0.9. ABIs of <0.9 are 95% sensitive and 97% specific in diagnosing clinically significant vascular trauma.[2] There is increasing literature that supports lowering the ABI threshold to avoid unnecessary radiation in both blunt and penetrating trauma.[3]
  - In cases of unilateral extremity trauma, some institutions advocate the use of the ankle-ankle index (also known as the Injury Extremity Index), comparing the systolic blood pressure of the normal extremity to that of the affected limb; if the ankle-ankle ratio is <0.9, the patient is sent for CT angiography.

CT Angiography

- In its 2020 guidelines for evaluation of lower extremity trauma, the American Association for the Surgery of Trauma recommends CT angiography as the preferred modality in evaluating lower extremity vascular trauma as compared with conventional angiography.[4]
- CT scan is convenient in most large centers and is much less invasive than traditional angiography. CT angiography can be used to evaluate both the arterial and venous injuries. The former is used to identify active arterial bleeding by demonstrating active extravasation, disruption of arterial flow, and intimal dissection and flaps, and the latter to identify injury to large veins, hematomas, or other less brisk sources of bleeding.
- When a patient cannot tolerate obtaining an ABI due to pain, has a mangled extremity, or when there are multiple possible sources of vascular injury, we recommend forgoing the ABI and sending the patient straight to CT for angiography.
- CT can also help guide operative management of concomitant injuries.

Mangled Extremity Severity Score

- In 1990, Johansen et al introduced a scoring system to assist in the decision to amputate in patients with severe lower extremity injuries.[5] A mangled extremity is, by definition, an extremity with injury to a combination bone, soft tissue, nerves, or blood vessels.[6]
- High-energy trauma, shock, increased age, and advanced signs of limb ischemia have been associated with higher rates of amputation (see **TABLE 1**). Given the advances in vascular and orthopedic surgery and in imaging since 1990, there is new literature to support utilizing mangled extremity severity score (MESS) with caution. Importantly, Loja et al in the AAST PROOVIT study showed that in their patient population, a MESS of 8 predicted in-hospital amputation in only 43.2% of patients,[7] compared with 100% of patients in Johansen's 1990 study.
- In mass casualty or limited resource settings, MESS can be considered for use as a triage tool. However, in advanced trauma centers, functionality, quality of life, and limb salvage options should be discussed in a multidisciplinary setting with input from the trauma, vascular, plastic, and orthopedic surgery teams prior to proceeding to amputation, regardless of MESS.

Table 1: MESS Scoring System

Skeletal/Soft-Tissue Injury	
Very high energy (high energy + contamination)	4
High energy (military GSW/close range GSW)	3
Medium energy (open fracture)	2
Low energy (stab, simple fx, civilian GSW)	1
*Limb Ischemia**	
Cool, paralyzed, numb, insensate	3
Pulseless, paresthesia, slow capillary refill	2
Diminished pulse, normal perfusion	1
*Double score if ischemia time > 6 h	
Shock	
Persistent hypotension	3
Transiently hypotensive	2
Systolic > 90 mm Hg	1
Age	
>50	3
30-50	2
<30	1

SURGICAL MANAGEMENT

Preoperative Management

- The management of the patient prehospital and preoperatively will play a large part in determining the appropriate operation.
- Use of tourniquets is widely advocated at most major trauma centers, prehospital (**FIGURE 1**), in the trauma bay, and intraoperatively (**FIGURE 2**). Historically, there had been concerns that tourniquet use could propagate limb ischemia and cause nerve injury. However, in recent years, tourniquet use has become more prevalent. Studies have shown that use of tourniquets in lower extremity trauma has both a mortality benefit[8] and a reduction in shock and blood product use in the hospital.[9]
- The life-saving yet basic principles of hemorrhage control in the prehospital setting have propelled an initiative by the American College of Surgeons Committee on Trauma through the **Stop the Bleed®** program. This program encourages both clinicians and nonhealth care workers to become trained in **Stop the Bleed®** so that the community can be armed in putting a stop to preventable death by hemorrhage.
- In addition to hemorrhage control, ischemia time is a factor that is integral to outcomes following lower extremity trauma, regardless of operative technique. For several decades, 6 hours has been used as the threshold for irreversible ischemia in lower extremity vascular trauma.
  - Alarhayem et al performed a retrospective review of 4406 patients who sustained lower extremity trauma between the years 2012 and 2015. The amputation rate overall was 11.3% but decreased to 6% when revascularization was done within 1 hour of injury. Increased amputation risk was associated with blunt trauma, nerve injury, corresponding lower extremity fractures, popliteal injury, age, and Injury Severity Score.[10] It is therefore imperative that revascularization be performed as soon as it is safe and reasonable to do so.

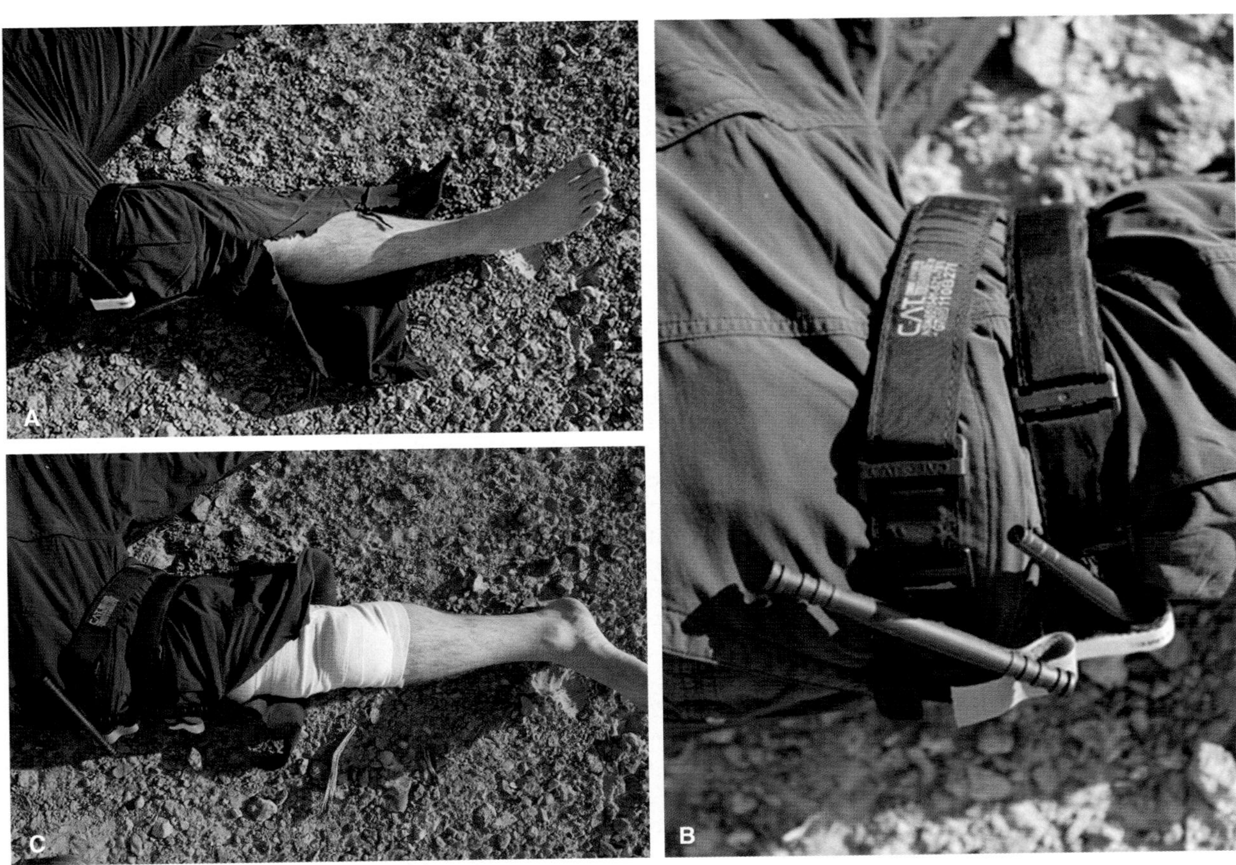

FIGURE 1 ● Tourniquet conversion. **A,** The original tourniquet in place proximal to the site of injury. **B,** First, place a second tourniquet in addition to the original, but do not tighten. This is in case bleeding cannot be controlled and the first tourniquet breaks as it is being retightened. **C,** Slowly release the tourniquet while evaluating the wound for bleeding, attempt to control with direct pressure or pressure dressing if needed. If hemorrhage is controlled, leave tourniquets in place in the event that severe bleeding resumes. If hemorrhage is not controlled, tighten tourniquet and reassess at a later time, if possible. (Courtesy of Matthew Horbal. Reprinted with permission from: Hawkins SC. Wilderness EMS. Wolters Kluwer; 2018. Figure 21.1C.)

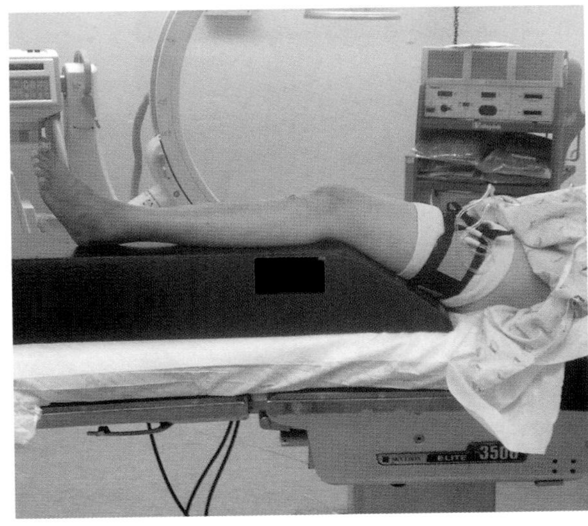

FIGURE 2 ● Supine positioning of the injured ankle. A thigh tourniquet is applied, a rolled sheet bump is placed under the hip to internally rotate the leg so the patella is pointed directly anterior, and the ankle is elevated on an inclined bump (foam bump or sheets) to allow for lateral fluoroscopic images without moving the ankle. (Used with permission from Wiesel SW, Albert T. *Operative Techniques in Orthopaedic Surgery*. 3rd ed. Wolters Kluwer; 2022. Part 2 Figure 24.4.)

OPERATIVE TECHNIQUES

- We will discuss operative techniques in lower extremity trauma, organized from proximal to distal

COMMON FEMORAL/SUPERFICIAL FEMORAL ARTERY

Prepping and Draping

- As with all lower extremity traumas, we recommend prepping and draping the patient from at least the chin to the knees including the groins and genitalia, with Foley catheter placement. It is important to prep in the contralateral groin and extremity for consideration of saphenous vein harvest (**FIGURE 3A-C**). The contralateral vein is preferable so that venous outflow in the affected (injured) extremity is not compromised, especially in the setting of undiagnosed deep venous injury.

Incision—Proximal and Distal Control of Hemorrhage

- One of the principal tenets of vascular trauma is obtaining control of hemorrhage proximal and distal to the injury. Preoperatively and intraoperatively, tourniquet use may be helpful in obtaining proximal control while the surgeon continues exploration of the involved vascular structures. Trauma involving the iliofemoral junction can be challenging to obtain proximal control of hemorrhage.
  - External control of hemorrhage using a tourniquet or direct pressure may not be possible in this region so expedient management is key.
  - Resuscitative endovascular balloon occlusion of the aorta (REBOA) use may be considered for proximal control in select patients.[11]
- We recommend first creating an incision spanning from the anterior posterior iliac spine to the inguinal canal and caudally (distal to the injury). If it is possible to obtain proximal control below the inguinal ligament, the artery can be controlled with an iliac clamp or a bulldog clamp. If control is required proximal to the inguinal ligament, the surgeon can perform a low midline incision in the abdomen, and isolation

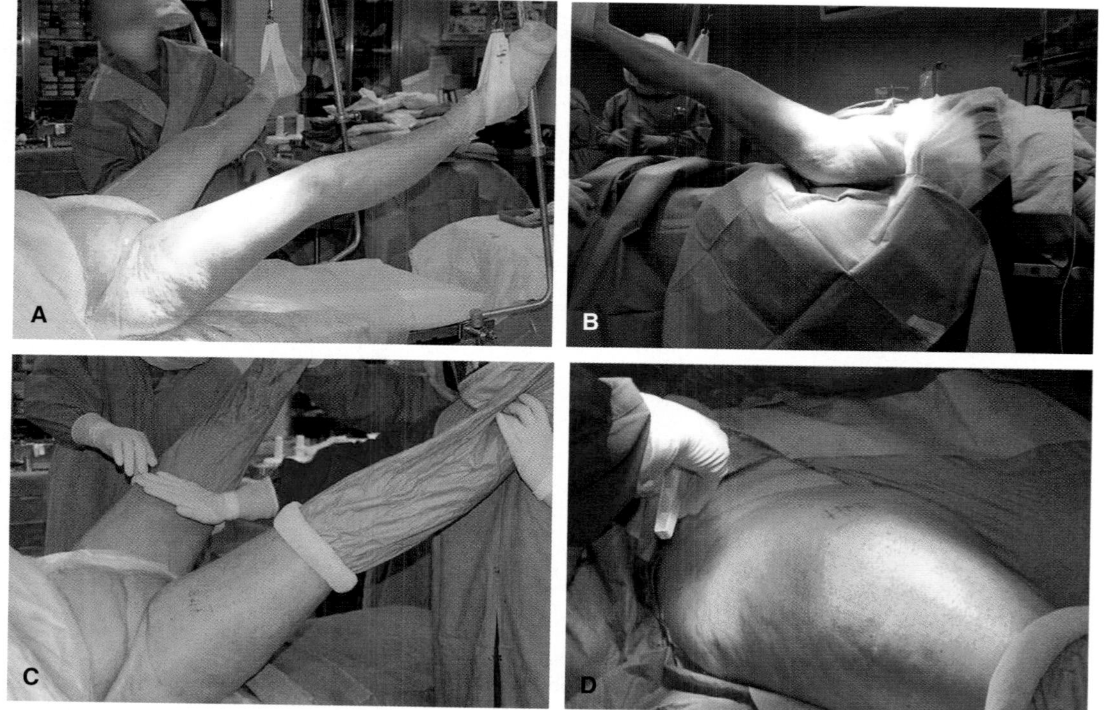

FIGURE 3 ● **A,** Both legs prepped. **B,** First sterile U-drape. **C,** Bilateral stockinettes. **D,** Operative side isolated. (Used with permission from Wiesel SW, Albert T. *Operative Techniques in Orthopaedic Surgery*. 3rd ed. Wolters Kluwer; 2022. Part 3 Tech Figure 18.1.)

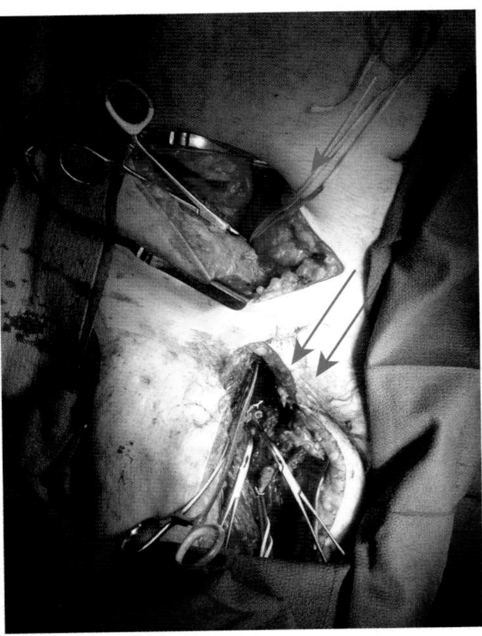

FIGURE 4 ● Retroperitoneal exposure for proximal control (*arrow*). Standard femoral exposure for the distal control (*double arrow*). (Reprinted with permission from Upchurch GR, Henke PK. *Clinical Scenarios in Vascular Surgery.* 2nd ed. Wolters Kluwer; 2016. Figure 124.1.)

of the external iliac vessels either via a peritoneal or retroperitoneal approach (**FIGURE 4**).

- We recommend whichever approach facilitates the safest and quickest control; this is often achieved with laparotomy. Takedown of the inguinal ligament may be required for adequate exposure; we recommend overcoming any hesitation in dividing this structure in the face of life- or limb-threatening bleeding.

- In the instance where injury prohibits ready access to the proximal aspect of the injured artery, a Fogarty balloon can be inserted and the balloon inflated to control hemorrhage. Distal control is usually more easily achieved via the superficial femoral artery with a vascular clamp (**FIGURE 5**). It is acceptable to make an initial or additional incision(s) away from the site of injury (in "virgin" territory) if this will facilitate or expedite control of hemorrhage.

Shunting

- In extremity trauma, it is particularly important to balance control of hemorrhage with ischemia time. Hemorrhage control is always the priority; however, once control is obtained, a focus on establishing distal perfusion should be the next step. In the setting of multiple injuries such as orthopedic trauma or severe hemorrhage shock, a shunt can be placed in the area of injury as a damage control measure.
- Shunts temporarily restore blood flow, allowing the patient to undergo additional resuscitation or other prioritized procedures prior to definitive vascular repair, such as reduction or external fixation of fractures. There are many commercial shunts available in the civilian setting; 14F chest tubes can also be used as a shunt in resource-limited situations. A shunt is used in **FIGURE 6**, for a patient who sustained a popliteal artery injury.

Primary Repair

- Once the patient is in an acceptable physiologic condition, the options for definitive repair must be addressed. Partially injured femoral arteries (<50%) can be debrided and repaired primarily or with a patch. Patch is favored to avoid narrowing of the vessel unless the injury is punctate, in which case a primary repair can be performed. Patch repair can be used with vein, biologic, or synthetic material and is usually not appropriate in smaller vessels.
- In patients with a transected common femoral or superficial femoral artery, end-to-end anastomosis is an option provided there is enough length after debridement of the vessel. Typically, a 2-cm defect can be resected with enough mobilization to perform a tension-free anastomosis. Primary anastomosis typically requires mobilization of both the distal and proximal ends of the artery.
- While all efforts are made to preserve arterial branches, however, a tension-free repair takes priority. Bridging veins may also need to be ligated; however, care should be taken to avoid ligating named veins if possible.

Interposition Graft

- It is when there is an injury prohibiting primary anastomosis that the surgeon will need to decide on the appropriate conduit for the patient (**FIGURE 7**). There is a paucity of current literature which discusses outcomes in civilians with synthetic grafts vs autologous vein grafts in the proximal lower extremity. In the military setting, synthetic graft infections are prevalent and vein graft is highly recommended if it meets size criteria. Feliciano et al found that in noncontaminated wounds, the infection rate and patency of synthetic grafts are comparable to vein grafts, especially when the conduit is >6 mm in diameter (which is usually the case with proximal lower extremity arteries) and in a noncontaminated setting.[12]
- In the civilian setting, ringed polytetrafluoroethylene (PTFE) is readily available and can save operative time compared to harvesting the saphenous vein. This is a major consideration in the polytrauma patient who may require multicavity surgery.

Extraanatomic Bypass

- Bypass, particularly in the thigh, is less frequently used in trauma. There is no particular size defect which mandates bypass. The main reason for bypass in most cases is inadequate, necrotic, or infected soft tissue over the area of defect. If there is no adjacent muscle or soft tissue to cover the vessels, then bypass must be considered to mitigate infection risk of the repaired vessel.

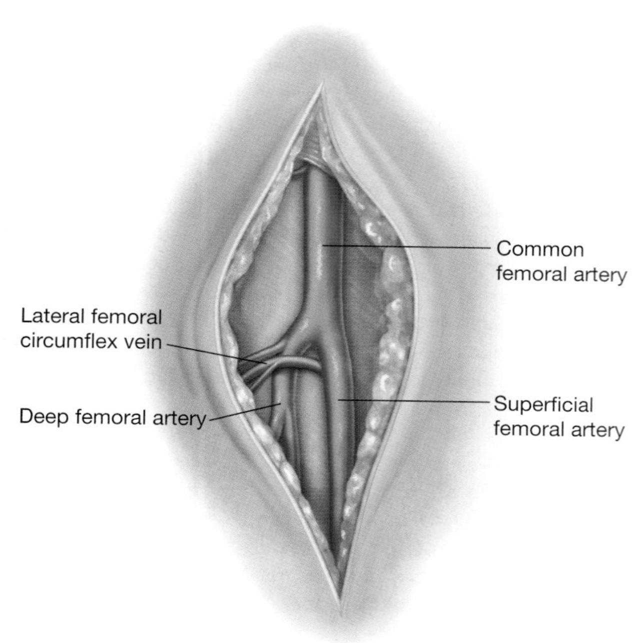

FIGURE 5 ● The deep femoral artery normally arises laterally off the common femoral trunk about 3.5 cm distal to the inguinal ligament. Its origin is crossed by the lateral femoral circumflex vein. (Reprinted with permission from Wind GG, Valentine RJ. *Anatomic Exposures in Vascular Surgery*. 3rd ed. Wolters Kluwer; 2014. Figure 15.21.)

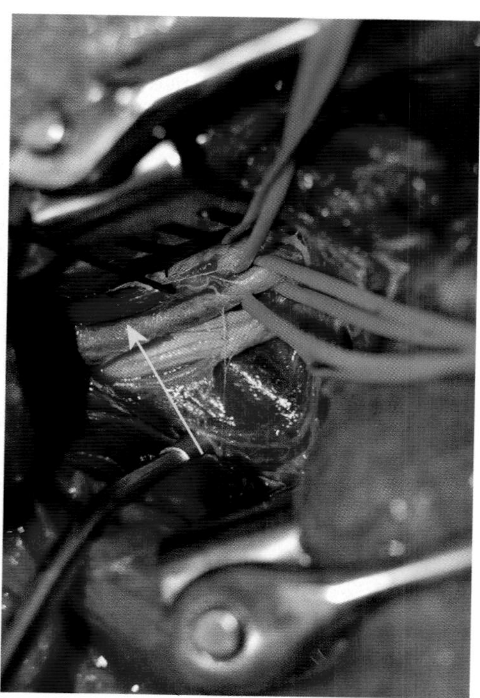

FIGURE 6 ● A close view of the structures of the below-knee popliteal space including the popliteal artery with a patent vascular shunt in place, the popliteal vein, and the tibial nerve. In this case, the popliteal vein was uninjured and has been dissected free from the medial portion of the artery and encircled with a blue vessel loop to allow retraction away from the artery. (Yellow arrow points to the popliteal arterial shunt and its securement by a silk suture.) (Reprinted with permission from Upchurch GR, Henke PK. *Clinical Scenarios in Vascular Surgery*. 2nd ed. Wolters Kluwer; 2016. Figure 122.4.)

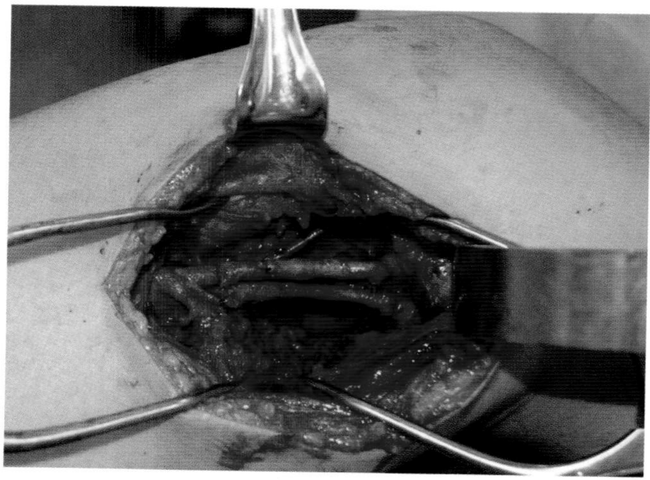

FIGURE 7 ● Operative photograph showing an interposition vein graft repair of the left proximal popliteal artery and vein. The interposition greater saphenous vein grafts were harvested from the right (contralateral) leg and performed following removal of the temporary vascular shunts. (Reprinted with permission from Dimick JB. *Mulholland & Greenfield's Surgery*. 7th ed. Wolters Kluwer; 2022. Figure 27.7.)

Technique

- From a technical standpoint, vascular anastomoses follow similar steps once exposure has been obtained:
  - Proximal and distal control of the injured vessel should be obtained using vessel loops or vascular clamps/bulldog clamps.
  - The ends of the artery should be debrided to expose healthy intima. Regardless of conduit, the ends should be spatulated to allow for expansion of the graft since

many vessels will be in significant vasospasm from injury.

- A Fogarty catheter should be passed at least twice distally and proximally to ensure no clot or occlusion of the injured vessel.
- Systemic heparinization or regional heparinized saline can be administered; the latter is typically favored in trauma due to the high bleeding risk.
- Using a 5-0 or 6-0 nonabsorbable monofilament suture, bites should be taken from internal to external on the artery in order to secure the intima using a double-armed needle. The suture is then run at 3 o'clock or 9 o'clock posteriorly and then anteriorly. It is often preferred to start posteriorly as this is the more technically challenging angle.
- Prior to securing the suture, the vessel will be flushed with additional heparinized saline while unclamping the vessels in each respective direction to ensure patency and remove debris.
- With the proximal clamp or loop reapplied, the distal clamp is left open to evaluate for backflow. This is universally used as a sign of distal patency. Distal pulses should be obtained before closure of the repaired vessel. If angiography is available, on-table angiogram is the best method to confirm distal patency. The suture can then be tied.

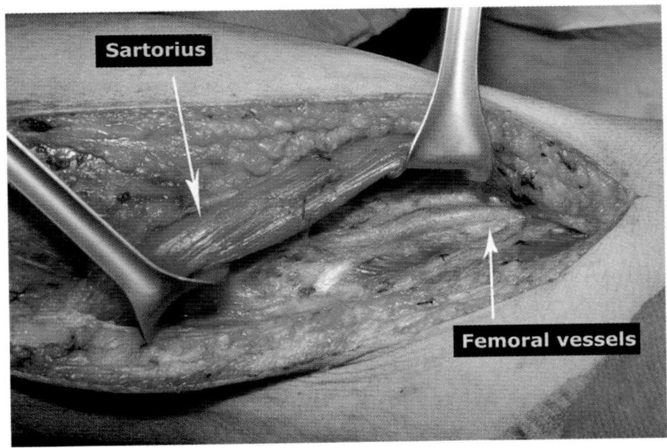

FIGURE 8 ● In the proximal thigh, retracting the sartorius anterior and lateral allows exposure of the femoral vessels, all the way to the inguinal ligament if necessary. (Used with permission from Wiesel SW, Albert T. *Operative Techniques in Orthopaedic Surgery*. 3rd ed. Wolters Kluwer; 2022. Part 5 Tech Figure 25.1E.)

- If possible, a muscle flap should be placed over the vessel to protect the vessel from contamination (**FIGURE 8**).
- Evaluate need for fasciotomy (discussed later in this chapter).

POPLITEAL ARTERY

Prepping and Draping

- The posterior location along the knee joint of the popliteal artery makes this arterial injury more challenging to manage than the femoral vessels. The patient should be prepped in the same manner as described above and positioned with the hip abducted and externally rotated in the "frog-leg" position.
- A blanket or sterile towels (a "bump") can be used under the thigh to improve exposure. If a tourniquet is in place, this can be prepped in the field and can be useful as a method of proximal control during dissection.

Incision—Proximal and Distal Control of Hemorrhage

- A medial approach is typically taken (see **FIGURE 9**). Incision is made posterior to the distal femur, spanning the knee joint down to the tibia. The distal femoral artery and proximal popliteal artery are in Hunter canal within the adductor magnus. An incision over the sartorius is made. In order to best expose the popliteal vessels, take down of the sartorius, semimembranosus, and semitendinosus muscles is often necessary; this transection can be achieved most efficiently with cautery. A clean transection of these muscles (as time allows) will allow a sounder reconstruction which will play a role in the recovery and function of the limb.
  - Care must be taken to avoid injury to the greater saphenous vein which often underlies the sartorius. Depending on the level of the injury, the two heads of the gastrocnemius may need to be taken down as well with the soleus muscle to obtain distal control.
- Once the popliteal fossa has been exposed, the tibial nerve will be the most superficial structure. Care should be taken to identify and carefully retract this nerve out of the field of view, typically with a vessel loop. The popliteal vein will be superficial and slightly lateral to the artery. This should be skeletonized and controlled with vessel loops proximally and distally to obtain better exposure of the artery. Once the artery is in view, the tourniquet may be relaxed to identify the area of injury and then reinflated as needed. Proximal and distal control should then be obtained with vessel loops.
  - The geniculate vessels should not be ligated unless they are contributing to hemorrhage; collateralization from these vessels is important in perfusing the leg, especially in the setting of injury to the popliteal artery.

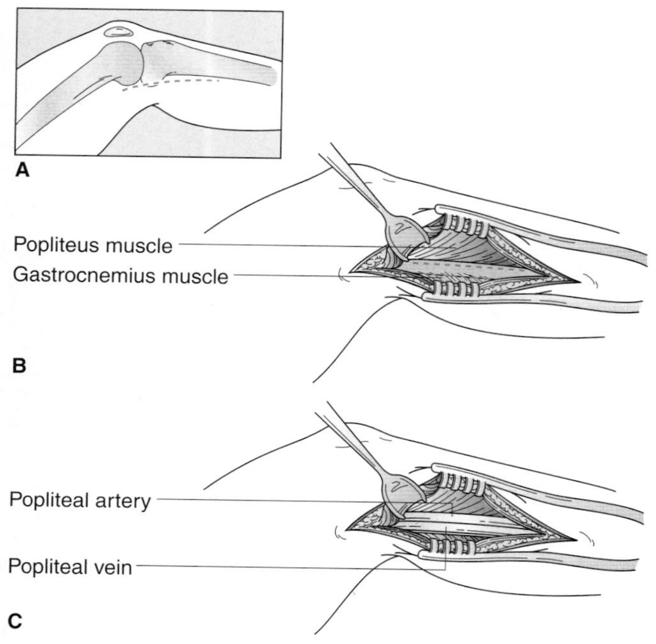

FIGURE 9 ● Exposure of the popliteal artery below the knee. The medial incision is made directly overlying the course of the greater saphenous vein **(A)**, with posterior retraction of the gastrocnemius muscle **(B)**, to reveal the popliteal vessels in the popliteal fossa **(C)**. (Reprinted with permission from Dimick JB. *Mulholland & Greenfield's Surgery*. 7th ed. Wolters Kluwer; 2022. Figure 91.8.)

Primary Repair

- As described in the above section, repair will depend on the nature of the injury. Popliteal artery injuries have a higher incidence of amputation than femoral vessel injuries; this is due to its association with blunt polytrauma and undiagnosed arterial injury.[13]
- For injuries <30% circumference of the vessel, primary repair can be considered. However, primary repairs are more prone to failure as the caliber of the vessel is smaller than that of the femoral vessels. To mitigate risk of stenosis, an alternative to primary repair is to excise the lesion and perform an end-to-end anastomosis or perform a patch repair.

Interposition Graft

- A tension-free end-to-end anastomosis becomes more challenging to achieve beyond 2 cm, and therefore, interposition graft (bypass) is typically the next best step in management. As with all vascular surgeries, the choice of conduit and technical approach will be integral in determining patency of the repair. Interposition graft is usually recommended in popliteal artery trauma with exceptions outlined below.
- Autologous vein graft is the preferred conduit at or below the knee. Historically, synthetic grafts were avoided overall due to findings that PTFE in popliteal artery injury has worse outcomes and inferior patency to autologous vein.[14] However, synthetic graft is often necessary in patients in whom suitable vein is not available (small caliber, diseased or injured vein). In fact, there is emerging literature that supports use of PTFE as a below the knee conduit, showing no difference in secondary amputation rate, wound infection, or graft infection.[15]
- We recommend using the largest caliber ringed PTFE graft available for interposition popliteal grafts to the extent that a size mismatch does not undermine the integrity of the repair. As described above, spatulation of the graft is important to accommodate the change in caliber of the vessel after reperfusion.

Alternative Revascularization Methods

- As with femoral artery injuries, extraanatomic bypass of the injury is typically reserved in patients whose native artery site is destroyed or at risk of severe contamination (eg, severe soft tissue or orthopedic injury resulting in an inability to cover the vessel with viable tissue postoperatively).
- In patients with small popliteal artery injuries or pseudoaneurysms, endovascular stenting has been suggested as a bridge to definitive repair, especially in patients with significant soft tissue and bone trauma. Specifically, endovascular therapy has been shown to be the safe alternative to open repair in patients with greater injury severity scores and blunt polytrauma.[16]

VENOUS INJURIES

- In patients with venous extremity trauma, the general trend in these patients is to ligate veins. In concomitant arterial injury or soft tissue injury, it is important to consider the importance of venous drainage. In the event of an isolated venous injury, however, repair may not prove as beneficial as ligation. Military literature has shown that repair of venous injury is associated with a lower amputation rate than ligation.[17] Therefore, if the patient's clinical status allows time for repair, it may be worth pursuing venous repair in instances of multivessel trauma or significant soft tissue damage.
- When a vein is ligated, it is important to remember that while collateralization may allow the patient to compensate for its lost drainage, in the immediate postoperative period, impaired venous drainage can result in DVT and/or significant edema. It is for this reason that in the acute setting, ligation of named veins is usually best accompanied by fasciotomy. Additionally, the lower extremity should be wrapped ankle to thigh and elevated above the heart to aid in adequate venous drainage.

BELOW KNEE FASCIOTOMY

- It is important to have a low threshold to perform fasciotomy in the trauma setting, especially when risk of compartment syndrome is high, such as with mangled extremities, venous injury, crush injury, reperfusion, etc.

Prepping and Draping

- The authors favor the standard approach to four-compartment fasciotomy, using two longitudinal incisions at the medial and lateral aspects of the calf. The patient's lower extremity from above the knee and including the foot should be prepped and draped.

Incision

- The medial incision is used to release the superficial and deep posterior compartments. An incision is made one fingerbreadth posterior to the palpable tibia and should be carried along the gastrocnemius muscles to 2 fingerbreadths/3 cm superior to the medial malleolus (**FIGURE 10A**).
  - Once the skin is incised, care should be taken to avoid the saphenous vein. Skin flaps can be raised several centimeters anteriorly and posteriorly, exposing the fascia. An incision should be created in the fascia and continued longitudinally overlying the gastrocnemius muscles for the entire length of the incision. This will open the superficial posterior compartment.
  - To ensure entry into the posterior compartment which contains the popliteal vessels and nerve, the soleus muscle should be taken down from its tibial attachments and the neurovascular bundle visualized (**FIGURE 10E**).
- The lateral incision is used to release the anterior and lateral compartments. The incision will start proximally two fingerbreadths below the fibular head and carried distally to 2 fingerbreadths/3 cm superior to the lateral malleolus. Once the skin is incised, care should be taken to avoid the superficial peroneal nerve. Skin flaps can be raised several centimeters anteriorly and posteriorly, exposing the fascia.
  - In order to eliminate the risk of missing a compartment, a transverse incision should be created in the fascia; once this is done, visualization reveals the following from anterior to posterior: anterior compartment, fascial septum separating anterior and lateral compartments, lateral compartment, fascial septum separating lateral and superficial compartments, and superficial posterior compartment.
  - Two incisions should be created in the fascia and continued longitudinally for the entire length of the incision, one releasing the anterior compartment and one releasing the lateral compartment.
  - Lateral fascial incisions create the risk of transecting superficial vasculature and the superficial peroneal nerve, so care must be taken to evaluate the anatomy prior to incision (**FIGURE 11**).
- Once fasciotomy is complete, the wounds can be covered with saline moistened gauge (**FIGURE 12A**) or petrolatum dressing covered with a dry gauze dressing and evaluated on a twice or once daily basis. Once the initial edema appears to have stabilized, return to OR should be planned for closure. A staged closure with a Jacob ladder technique (**FIGURE 12C**), negative pressure wound therapy (**FIGURE 12B**), or a combination (**FIGURE 12D**) of the two may be required. In the case of loss of domain, skin grafting may be considered. If only one incision can be closed under minimal to no tension, we advise that the lateral incision closure be prioritized for cosmetic reasons.

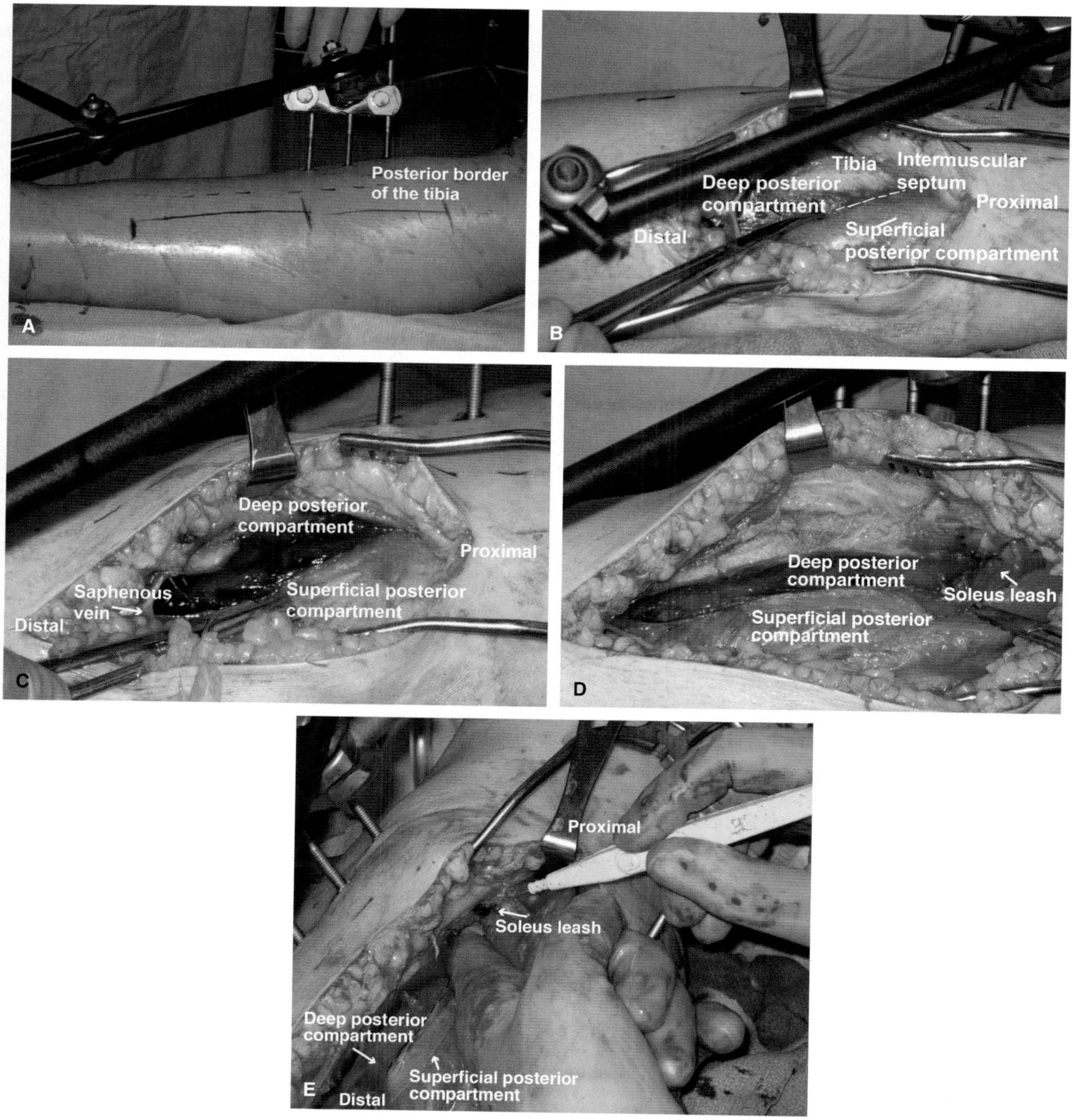

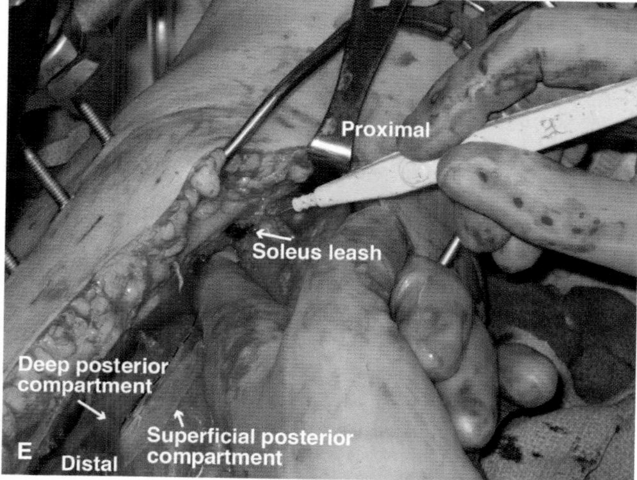

FIGURE 10 ● Medial incision of the two-incision technique. **A,** The medial incision lies approximately 2 cm posterior to the posterior tibial margin. **B,** Care is taken to avoid injury to the saphenous vein. The picture shows the posterior border of the tibia exposed along with the deep and superficial posterior compartments. The tips of the dissecting scissors lie on the deep posterior compartment. **C,** A small transverse incision is made to identify the intermuscular septum between the deep and superficial posterior compartments. Dissecting scissors are used to release the fascia over the deep posterior compartment proximally and distally. Proximally, the fascia is released under the soleus bridge. Scissors are shown under the fascia of the superficial posterior compartment. **D,** The deep and superficial compartments are released. The superficial posterior compartment looks healthy, whereas the deep posterior compartment is dusky. The tips of the clamp lie under the soleus bridge, which also needs to be released from its origin on the tibia. **E,** The surgeon releases the soleus bridge using electrocautery, taking care to protect the deep structures. (Used with permission from Wiesel SW, Albert T. *Operative Techniques in Orthopaedic Surgery*. 3rd ed. Wolters Kluwer; 2022. Part 2 Tech Figure 22.2.)

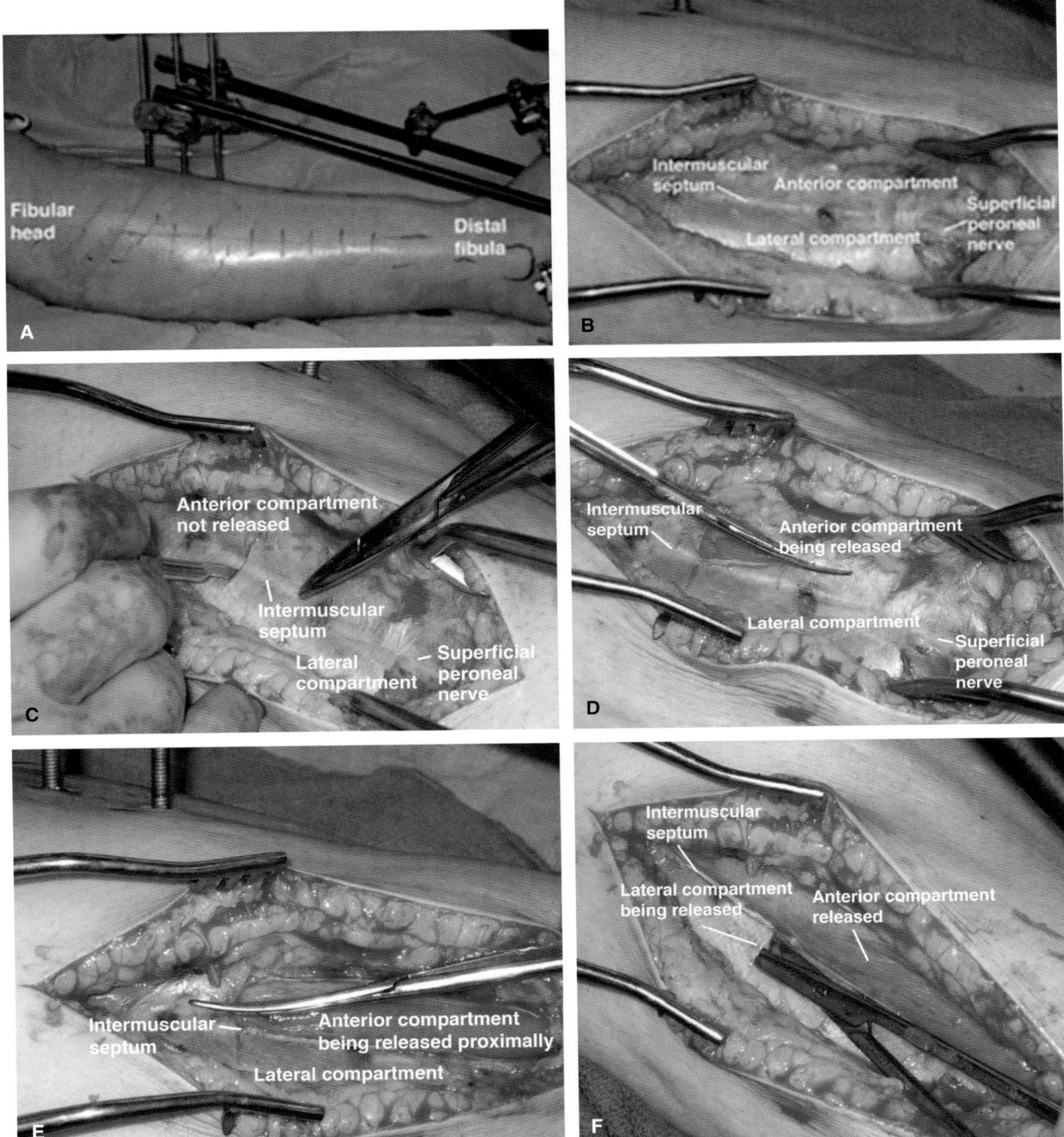

FIGURE 11 ● Lateral incision of the two-incision technique. **A,** The anterolateral incision is made halfway between the fibula and the tibial crest overlying the intermuscular septum dividing the anterior and lateral compartments. **B,** Close-up picture of the fasciotomy site after skin incision before the fascia is open, showing the intermuscular septum between the lateral and anterior compartments and the course of the superficial peroneal nerve. **C,** With a knife, a small transverse incision is made over the intermuscular septum. Care is taken to avoid injury to the superficial peroneal nerve. **D,** The surgeon inserts the tips of the scissors into the small rent in the fascia, and keeping the tips of the scissors up and away from the superficial peroneal nerve, the surgeon incises the fascia over the anterior compartment distally. **E,** The scissors are turned with the tips proximally, and the fascia of the anterior compartment is released proximally. **F,** The tips of the scissors are then inserted into the rent created in the fascia of the lateral compartment. Keeping the tips of the scissors up and away from the superficial peroneal nerve, the surgeon releases the fascia over the lateral compartment proximally and distally. (Used with permission from Wiesel SW, Albert T. *Operative Techniques in Orthopaedic Surgery*. 3rd ed. Wolters Kluwer; 2022. Part 2 Tech Figure 22.1.)

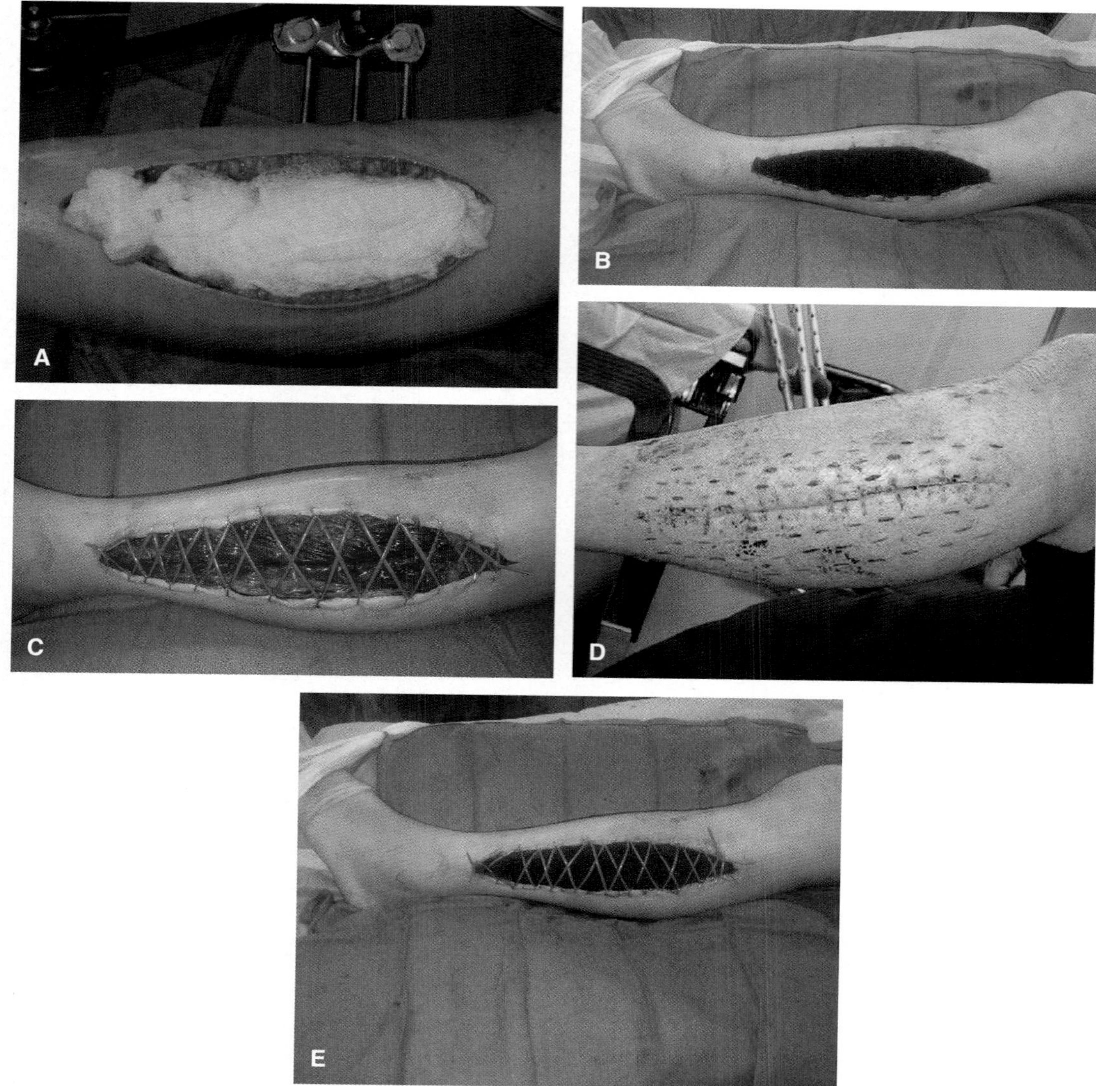

FIGURE 12 ● Closure of fasciotomies. **A,** Moist dressings covering the fasciotomy wound. **B,** Sterile vacuum system applied to the fasciotomy site. **C,** Bootlace technique for approximating the edges of a fasciotomy wound. **D,** Small relaxing incisions made around the fasciotomy site to release tension and allow easier closure. **E,** Bootlace technique combined with sterile vacuum system. (Used with permission from Wiesel SW, Albert T. *Operative Techniques in Orthopaedic Surgery*. 3rd ed. Wolters Kluwer; 2022. Part 2 Tech Figure 22.4.)

PEARLS AND PITFALLS

Prepping and draping	■ Prepare contralateral groin and lower extremity for potential vein harvest.
Leg fasciotomy	■ Be sure to take down the soleus muscle fibers from the tibia and visualize the neurovascular bundle to ensure the deep compartment is entered and decompressed.
Timely diagnosis	■ Have a high index of suspicion for vascular injury in all patients with extremity trauma. ABIs remain useful.
Exposure in junctional vasculature injuries	■ Do not be afraid to divide the inguinal ligament or perform laparotomy in order to obtain proximal control.
Document vascular exam	■ Be sure to document vascular exam immediately following revascularization ("index exam"). Communicate this clearly to the care team. Should the exam change, consider imaging vs return to OR.

POSTOPERATIVE CARE

- Following vascular surgery, it is most important that the patient undergoes frequent (hourly) neurovascular checks.
- Postoperative anticoagulation or antiplatelet therapy may not be indicated following vascular surgery for trauma and may be contraindicated in the setting of polytrauma and hemorrhagic shock.
  - In many cases, traumatized vessels will not have baseline disease and therefore do not require additional treatment. This contrasts with more elective vascular surgery in patients with atherosclerotic disease whose pathology originates from plaque build-up and embolic disease.
  - Recent evidence from the AAST's PROOVIT registry demonstrated that there was no difference in outcomes in anticoagulated patients compared with nonanticoagulated patients following traumatic vascular surgery; other than that the anticoagulated patients required more blood products than the latter group.[18]

COMPLICATIONS

- Complications from traumatic vascular surgery have primarily been highlighted in each of the sections above but the following are the most devastating:
  - **Compartment syndrome**—Lower extremity compartment syndrome can occur as a result of reperfusion after a period of ischemia, swelling from injury alone, or edema secondary to venous injury. There should be a low threshold to perform preemptive fasciotomy in patients who have sustained vascular trauma.
  - **Graft failure**—In the immediate postoperative period, graft failure is a technical complication. This can be avoided by shunt placement to reduce ischemia time. Some may consider intraoperative vascular surgery consultation; new data demonstrates noninferiority for extremity vascular repairs by trauma surgeons compared to vascular surgeons.[19]

REFERENCES

1. Kauvar DS, Sarfati MR, Kraiss LW. National trauma databank analysis of mortality and limb loss in isolated lower extremity vascular trauma. *J Vasc Surg*. 2011;53(6):1598-1603.
2. Fox N, Rajani RR, Bokhari F, et al. Evaluation and management of penetrating lower extremity arterial trauma. *J. Trauma and Acute Care Surgery*. 2012;73(5):315-320.
3. Hemingway J, Adjei E, Desikan S, et al. Re-evaluating the safety and effectiveness of the 0.9 ankle-brachial index threshold in penetrating lower extremity trauma. *J Vasc Surg*. 2020;72(4):1305-1311.
4. Kobayashi L, Coimbra R, Goes AMO, et al. American association for the surgery of trauma—World Society of emergency surgery guidelines on diagnosis and management of peripheral vascular injuries. *J Trauma Acute Care Surg*. 2020;89(6):1183-1196.
5. Johansen K, Daines M, Howey T. Helfet D, Hansen S. Objective criteria accurately predict amputation following lower extremity trauma. *J Trauma Inj Infect Crit Care*. 1990;30(5):568-572.
6. Prasarn ML, Helfet DL, Kloen P. Management of the mangled extremity. *Strategies Trauma Limb Reconstr*. 2012;7(2):57-66.
7. Sriussadaporn S, Pak-art R. Temporary intravascular shunt in complex extremity vascular injuries. *J Trauma Inj Infect Crit Care*. 2002;52(6):1129-1133.
8. Texiera P, Brown CVR, Emigh B, et al. Civilian prehospital tourniquet use is associated with improved Survival in patients with peripheral vascular injury. *J Am Coll Surg*. 2018;226(5):769-776.
9. Smith A, Ochoa JE, Wong S, et al.. Prehospital tourniquet use in penetrating extremity trauma: decreased blood transfusions and limb complications. *J Trauma Acute Care Surg*. 2019;86(1):43-51.
10. Alarhayem AQ, Cohn SM, Cantu-Nunez O, Eastridge BJ, Rasmussen TE. Impact of time to repair on outcomes in patients with lower extremity arterial injuries. *J Vasc Surg*. 2019;69(5):1519-1523.
11. Bulger EM, Perina DG, Qasim Z, et al. Clinical use of resuscitative endovascular balloon occlusion of the aorta (REBOA) in civilian trauma systems in the USA, 2019: a joint statement from the American College of surgeons committee on trauma, the American College of emergency physicians, the national association of emergency medical Services physicians and the national association of emergency medical technicians. *Trauma Surg Acute Care Open*. 2019;4(1):e000376.
12. Feliciano D. For the patient—evolution in the management of vascular trauma. *J Trauma Acute Care Surg*. 2017;83(6):1205-1212.
13. Mullenix P, Steel S, Anderson C, Starnes B, Salim A, Martin MJ. Limb salvage and outcomes among patients with traumatic popliteal vascular injury: an analysis of the National Trauma Data Bank. *J Vasc Surg*. 2006;44(1):94-100.
14. Feliciano DV, Mattox KL, Graham JM, Bitondo CG. Five-year experience with PTFE grafts in vascular wounds. *J Trauma*. 1985;25(1):71-82.
15. Rehman Z. Outcomes of popliteal artery injuries repair: autologous vein versus prosthetic interposition grafts. *Ann Vasc Surg*. 2020;69:141-145.
16. Worni M, Scarborough JE, Gandhi M, Pietrobon R, Shortell CK. Use of endovascular therapy for peripheral arterial lesions: an analysis of the National Trauma Data Bank from 2007 to 2009. *Ann Vasc Surg*. 2013;27(3):299-305.
17. Rich NM, Hobson RW, Collins GJ Jr., Andersen CA. The effect of acute popliteal venous interruption. *Ann Surg*. 1976;183(4):365-368.
18. Loja MN, Galante JM, Humphries M, et al. Systemic anticoagulation in the setting of vascular extremity trauma. *Injury*. 2017;48(9):1911-1916.
19. Parihar S, Benarroch-Gampel J, Teodorescu V, Ramos C, Minton K, Rajani RR. Vascular surgeons carry an increasing responsibility in the management of lower extremity vascular trauma. *Ann Vasc Surg*. 2021;70:87-94.

Chapter 38

Upper Extremity: Axillary, Brachial, Radial/Ulnar Fasciotomy

Brian K. Yorkgitis, Jeanette Zhang, and Matthew P. Kochuba

DEFINITION

- The content discussed in the following text assumes the reader has familiarity with standard upper extremity arterial anatomy and its most common variations along with the general principals of trauma evaluation and management. Management of traumatic vascular injury includes restoration of the distal circulation, and should be prioritized based on other injuries the patient may have sustained.
  - Upper extremity traumatic vascular injury accounts for close to 30% of all traumatic vascular injuries, with the majority being from a penetrating mechanism. Fractures and/or dislocation can injure neighboring vessels by direct laceration or stretch on the vessel.[1]
  - Vascular injury can be divided into five different types[2]
    - Intimal injuries
    - Vessel wall defect with bleeding, hematoma, or pseudoaneurysm
    - Transection with bleeding and/or occlusion
    - Arteriovenous fistula
    - Spasm
  - Concomitant injury to nerves that accompany arteries is common[3]

DIFFERENTIAL DIAGNOSIS

- Arterial injuries as described previously
- Compartment syndrome
- Venous injuries
- Fracture(s)
- Thrombosis/embolus from other conditions or injuries

PATIENT HISTORY AND PHYSICAL FINDINGS

- Assessment of extremity injury should take place within the context of overall Advanced Trauma Life Support (ATLS) resuscitation. Consideration should be given to the mechanism of injury, whether blunt, penetration, hyperextension, crush, or avulsion, as it can inform on the likely nature of the resulting arterial pathology.[4]
- Hemorrhage from upper extremity vascular injury can affect circulation that needs to be addressed in the "C" section of the Primary Survey. Strategies for hemorrhage control, in order of preference, include direct pressure, application of a commercial tourniquet, or direct clamping of a visible vessel. Blind clamping is discouraged as it is more likely to cause additional injury than control bleeding.[5]
- In the absence of ongoing bleeding, assessment of the extremity takes place during the Secondary Survey. Thorough vascular, sensory, and motor exams should be completed. Specifically, pulses palpated or signals achieved via Doppler, capillary refill, color, and temperature of the extremity should be checked and compared to the contralateral uninjured limb. If there are obvious fractures or dislocations, exams should be documented both before and after reduction or realignment.[6]
- Physical exam findings concerning for arterial injury have traditionally been categorized into "hard signs" or "soft signs" of injury. Hard signs include active hemorrhage, a large, expanding or pulsatile hematoma, any of the 6 "Ps" classically associated with arterial occlusion (pulselessness, pallor, paresthesias, pain out of proportion, paralysis, and poikilothermia), and a palpable thrill or audible bruit. Patients presenting with these findings are typically managed with immediate operation. Soft signs include a history of arterial bleeding at the scene or in transit, proximity of a penetrating wound or blunt injury to an artery, small nonpulsatile hematoma over an artery, and neurologic deficit in a nerve adjacent to a named artery. Further diagnostic studies may be necessary in these patients to evaluate for vascular injury.[2]
- Recent literature has questioned the focus on hard vs soft signs of injury, arguing that the defined hard signs are limited in their ability to characterize injuries. They argue that categorizing exam findings into hemorrhagic or ischemic signs provides a more clinically relevant paradigm.[7] For instance, those presenting with hemorrhagic signs were more likely to have arterial transection, while those with ischemic signs were more likely to be due to occlusive injury. This can have implications for the mode of diagnosis and subsequent management options, especially considering advances in and increased utilization of endovascular or hybrid approaches.
- Evaluation for compartment syndrome is needed as this can lead to a pulseless extremity or could result from ischemic insult. The forearm is comprised of four compartments: superficial and deep volar, dorsal, and the mobile wad of Henry. The interosseous membrane of the radius and ulna divides the dorsal and volar compartments. Compartment syndrome is largely a clinical diagnosis. The etiology of forearm compartment syndrome includes fractures (18%), soft tissue trauma without fracture (23%), along with vascular injuries, ischemia with reperfusion injury, rhabdomyolysis, burn/electrical injury, bleeding/hematoma, IV extravasation, insect bites, constricting bandage/splint, and infection. Timely diagnosis and treatment are needed to avoid sequelae.[8,9]
- Fractures and dislocations can be associated with vascular injury. For shoulder dislocation the rate of axillary artery injury is close to 1% and for elbow dislocations injury to the brachial artery is close to 0.5%.[10]

IMAGING AND OTHER DIAGNOSTIC STUDIES

- Adhering to principles of ATLS when obtaining imaging is important to not miss life-threatening conditions. Chest radiograph can assist in identifying pneumothorax, hemothorax, or signs suggesting injury to great vessels.[4]

- Radiographs of the injured extremity can identify fractures and/or dislocations that can be the etiology of vascular compromise. After any reduction maneuvers, repeat imaging should be obtained.[4]
- In patients presenting with soft signs of vascular injury, an Ankle or Brachial/Brachial Index (ABI or BBI = systolic blood pressure in extremity distal to the area of injury/systolic blood pressure in brachial artery of uninjured upper extremity) or Arterial Pressure Index (API = Doppler arterial pressure distal to injury/Doppler arterial pressure in uninvolved upper extremity) can be performed. A value of ≤0.9 or a difference between the extremities of >0.1 is considered abnormal, and is diagnostic or suspicious of an arterial injury and warrants further investigation.[4] However, normal ABI may be present in a subclavian or axillary injury due to its rich collaterals.
- Computed tomography angiography (CTA) in the hemodynamically stable patient can assist in the identification of vascular injury or abnormality. This is a readily available test that can assist with diagnosis of vascular injuries along with any associated injuries. In upper extremity and lower extremity vascular injuries, CTA has a sensitivity and specificity of 95% to 100% and 87%, respectively.[11] A single-institution prospective study found CTA to have 100% sensitivity and specificity in detecting clinically relevant vascular injury and was associated with favorable cost profile compared to conventional angiography.[12] Limitations include proximity of shrapnel and difficulty differentiating spasm from occlusion.
- Emergent diagnostic angiogram can be performed in select situations if the CTA was nondiagnostic (ex. secondary to artifact from shrapnel). It may also be used as a primary modality in the operating room (OR) in localizing an injury in a patient who is unable to undergo CTA.[1,2]
- Duplex ultrasonography can be used to identify arterial injury. The major limitation is having experienced staff to obtain and interpret the study. The specificity has been reported as high as 95%, but the sensitivity ranges from 50% to 100%.[1,2]

SURGICAL MANAGEMENT

Preoperative Planning

- Assuring adequate volume resuscitation with evidence-based strategies and availability of blood products is crucial to the patient's outcome. This requires good communication with the anesthesia team and blood bank.
- It is important to identify all life-threating injuries the patient may have sustained to assist the surgical team in the conduct of operative procedures. Often hemorrhage from extremities can be controlled by methods listed previously. Torso hemorrhage, on the other hand, is difficult to control without operative intervention and should be addressed expeditiously. Concomitant suspected or confirmed neurotrauma presents a challenge and spinal motion restriction should be maintained as able, and discussion with neurotrauma colleagues about any neurologic monitoring needed is crucial.[4]
- Perioperative antibiotics should be given. In the event of an open fracture, antibiotic selection and duration should be guided by the Gustilo-Anderson classification.
- Surgical management of the arterial injury will depend on patient acuity, mechanism of injury, and other traumatic injuries. Early discussion with orthopedic surgery should address any skeletal fixation that is needed for fractures of the upper extremity.[2,5,13] Restoration of arterial flow should be prioritized over skeletal fixation to minimize ischemic time. Temporary shunting allows for stabilization of unstable fractures or dislocations when not easily reduced prior to definitive repair, whereas immediate definitive repair can be performed when the skeletal injury is not significantly displaced. Fasciotomies should be performed early in combined vascular-skeletal injuries. Inspection of the vascular repair should be performed at the conclusion of skeletal fixation.
- Axillary artery exposure is dependent on the area of the injury along the course of the artery. The proximal artery is typically exposed via a transverse infraclavicular incision. Exposure of the second portion is approached through a deltopectoral incision and the third portion through axillary approach. In traumatic axillary artery injuries, exposure of the entire artery may be needed for injury identification and proximal and distal control.[14]
- The brachial artery is relatively superficial at the antecubital fossa, making it vulnerable to injury. Most injuries to the brachial artery are from penetrating trauma. Posterior elbow dislocations and supracondylar fractures may cause injury requiring inspection of the injured segment for intimal disruption or thrombosis.[15]
- The ulnar artery at the wrist is the dominant hand artery in the majority of patients. Achieving or maintaining sufficient arterial outflow at the wrist is essential to the hemodynamic and clinical success of the management of arterial injury to the radial and/or ulnar arteries. The status of both the radial and ulnar arteries at the wrist should be confirmed in the course of evaluating all patients for upper extremity revascularization options. An Allen test utilizing a Doppler on the palmar arch can assist in identification of flow into the hand.[16]
- Systemic intraoperative anticoagulation (SIAC) during traumatic vascular repair should be used with caution if the patient has trauma-induced coagulopathy, suspected, or confirmed additional sources of hemorrhage including the torso or central nervous system. There is varying literature on its efficacy. In a recent study examining mostly gunshot wounds, SIAC utilization experienced better arterial patency without additional bleeding complications.[17] In another study, SIAC was not associated with a difference in repair thrombosis or limb loss but increased blood product utilization and hospital length of stay.[18] The decision to use SIAC should be driven by the surgical team's risk–benefit analysis. Local heparin flushing (50units/mL), 20 to 25 mL into the injured artery proximal and distal to repair, is commonly used.[19]
- Temporary vascular shunts are used to establish arterial flow in a damage control setting. Plastic commercially available intraluminal shunts are available in a variety of sizes and configurations. Scenarios for consideration of a temporary shunt include patient hemodynamic instability, coagulopathy, acidosis, hypothermia, unstable skeleton, major wound contamination/infection, defects in soft tissue impeding wound coverage, need to address other life-threatening injuries, and austere environment with limited resources.[5]

Operating Room Setup

- Trauma patients may have multiple injuries and the ability to address the burden of injuries should guide the OR setup.

Ideally, a hybrid room or an OR equipped with radiolucent operating table, arm/hand table, and fluoroscopic equipment, preferably with digital subtraction angiography and last-image hold capabilities, is necessary.

- In trauma patients, general anesthesia is usually preferred, as regional anesthesia hampers neurologic examination of the upper extremity.
- For the majority of upper extremity vascular procedures, the affected limb is typically abducted 90°. To avoid stretch on the brachial plexus, care should be taken to avoid hyperabduction and extension of the limb. The operative field should take into account other injuries the patient may have sustained to the torso. In isolated upper extremity injuries, the operative field should include the ipsilateral axilla, chest, and neck.[14] The head should be rotated and extended to the contralateral side if no spinal trauma is suspected. A shoulder roll may be used under the ipsilateral shoulder to assist with neck and shoulder extension if able (**FIGURE 1**). For access to the deltopectoral region of the axillary artery, the arm can be externally rotated and abducted 30° relative to the lateral chest.
- In situation where a venous conduit may be needed, a lower extremity should be appropriately prepared into the surgical field to allow access for vein harvesting. The vein, if needed, should be harvested from the least affected lower extremity.

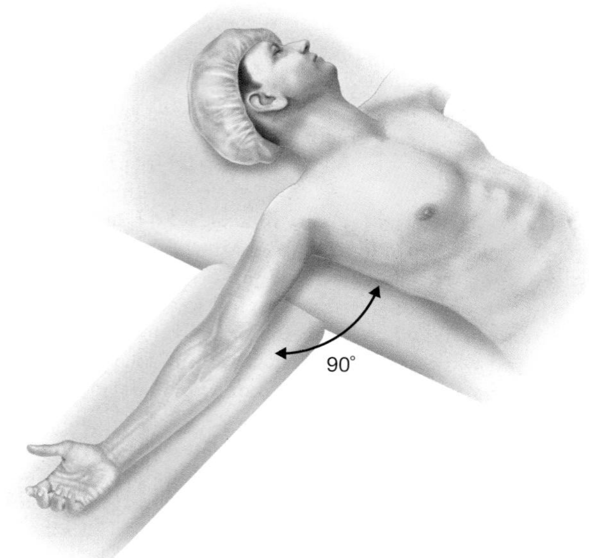

FIGURE 1 • With the patient supine, the arm of interest is pronated and extended at 90° relative to the chest. The head is externally rotated to the contralateral side to expose the ipsilateral neck segment.

TECHNIQUES

PROXIMAL AXILLARY ARTERY

First Step

- An approach to the proximal (first) portion of the axillary artery can be performed through an infraclavicular incision one fingerbreadth below the middle third of the clavicle and can extend to the deltopectoral groove when needed (**FIGURE 2A**). This may be needed to assist with delineation of tissue planes in an injured field.
- The pectoral fascia is opened longitudinally. The pectoralis major muscle is divided with a muscle-splitting incision if able. Otherwise the muscle should be divided approximately 2 cm from its attachment to the humerus to better access the vessel in traumatic injuries with significant hematoma or hemorrhage. The clavipectoral fascia is then divided to expose the proximal axillary sheath. Lateral retraction or division of the pectoralis muscle near its insertion on the coracoid process may be needed to aid in exposure.
- The arm may need to be repositioned to reduce position-related anatomic alteration.

Second Step

- Delicate dissection is performed to expose and control the axillary artery deep to the clavipectoral fascia. Care must be taken with dissection and retraction to minimize injury to the cords of the brachial plexus that surround the artery. The lateral pectoral nerve and proximal cephalic vein must be identified to avoid injury during dissection or traction from retraction (**FIGURE 2B**).

Third Step

- The axillary vein lies anteromedial to the artery and partially overlaps the artery. Retraction of the vein in a caudal direction with a vessel loop or small retractor is often needed to access the artery. Ligation of venous tributaries and the thoracoacromial artery and vein may be required. Again, care is needed to prevent injury to the lateral pectoral nerve.

Fourth Step

- Proximal and distal control of the injured segment of the axillary artery is achieved with vessel loops once circumferential dissection and exposure is obtained. If vascular clamps are used, assure nerve structures are not included when applying the clamp to the artery. Examination of the injured artery should be performed to identify the extent of the injury. If the patient is unstable or other injuries need to be addressed, consider temporary vascular shunt placement.

Fifth Step

- If the injury is small without significant vessel destruction, simple repair or debridement back to healthy intima and end-to-end anastomosis can be performed using nonabsorbable permanent monofilament, such as polypropylene (Prolene, Johnson & Johnson, New Brunswick, NJ, USA), suture.
- Gunshot wounds usually require a more extensive debridement and interposition. When performing interposition grafting, the damaged artery is transected and removed. The proximal and distal arterial segments should be examined for trauma, dissection, or thrombus formation. Repair of traumatic injuries should follow basic principles

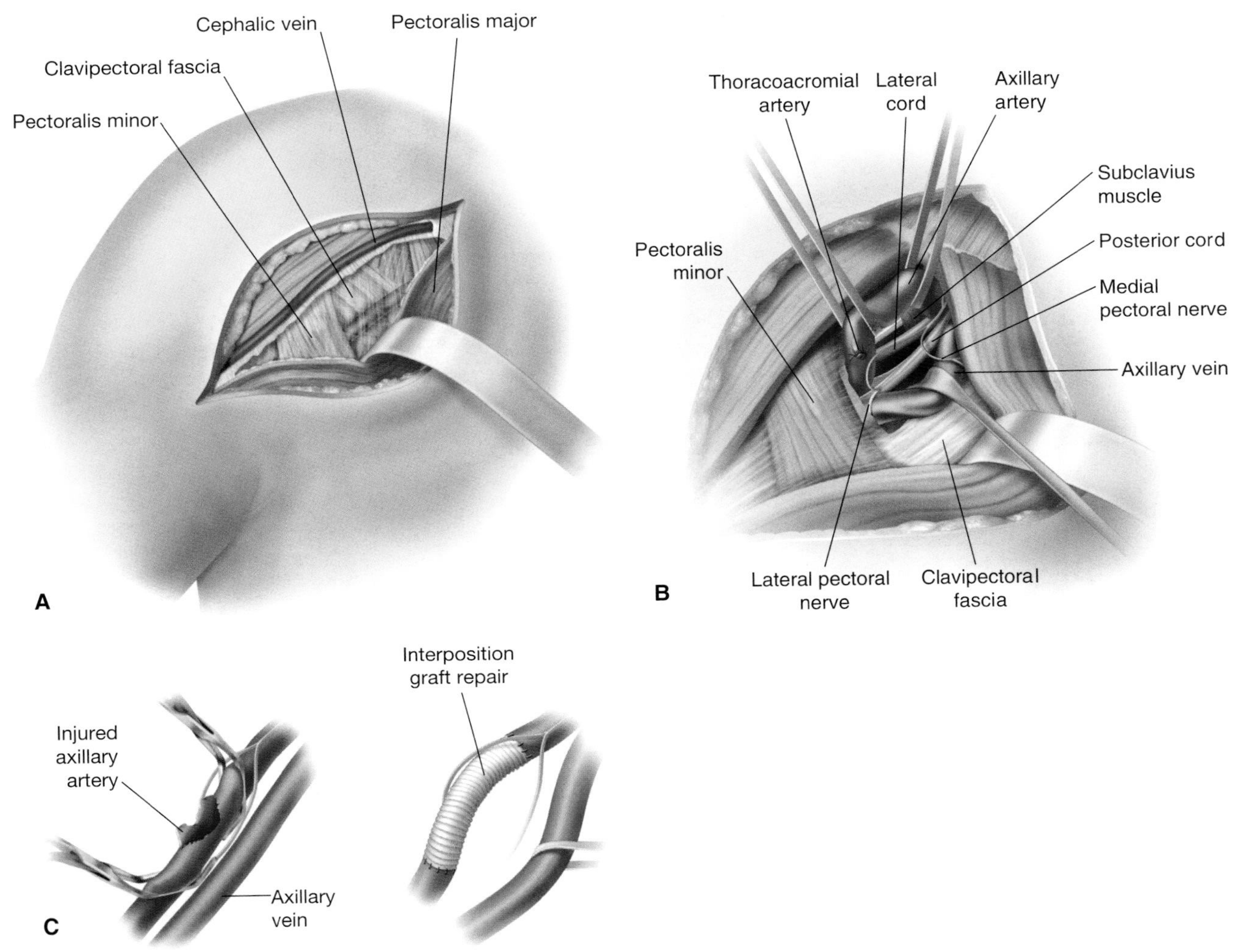

FIGURE 2 ● **A,** Infraclavicular exposure of the proximal axillary artery. **B,** Components of the infraclavicular axillary sheath. **C,** Interposition graft repair of a proximal axillary artery traumatic partial transection.

of vascular repairs, beginning with minimal debridement back to healthy intima. The vessel can be flushed with heparinized saline.

- Autologous vein is the preferred conduit if bypass is required and is harvested from the least injured extremity, typically the saphenous veins. Prosthetic material for the conduit may be needed. The use of stretch polytetrafluoroethylene can prevent excessive traction on the anastomosis with arm movement (**FIGURE 2C**). Appropriate length of the conduit should be confirmed to prevent kinking with arm motion.
- Proximal and distal anastomoses are performed in an end-to-end or end-to-side fashion depending on respective diameters of the inflow and outflow segments.
- Catheter embolectomy should be employed as needed if concern for thrombus exists. Imaging guidance can be used to assist in the decision and performance of this step.
- Performance of a completion angiogram may be performed to evaluate the graft and its flow.
- Venous injury repair should be attempted if quick and feasible. Otherwise, ligation results in limited long-term morbidity.

MID-DISTAL AXILLARY ARTERY

First Step

- Exposure of the mid-distal axillary artery can be performed through an axillary incision or deltopectoral incision. An incision through the posterolateral border of the pectoralis major muscles allows for partial mobilization and medial retraction to access the artery (**FIGURE 3A**).
- In a deltopectoral exposure, dissection is carried along the anterior border of the deltoid muscle extending through the subcutaneous tissue in the deltopectoral groove. Medial retraction of the pectoralis major muscle exposes the clavipectoral fascia, under which the neurovascular bundle lies.

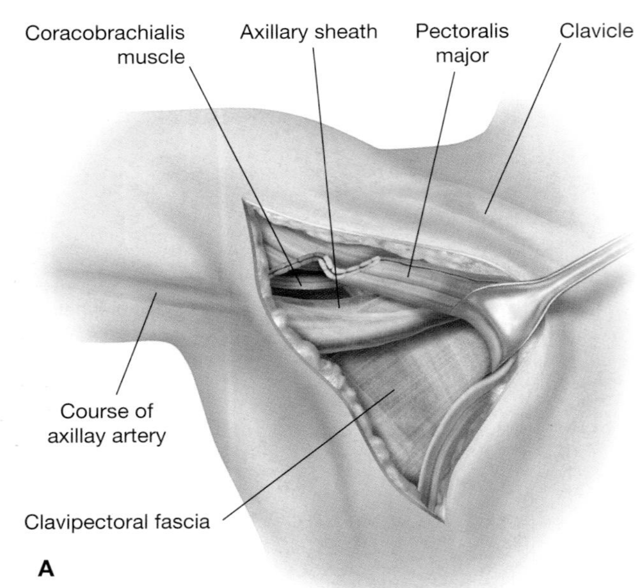

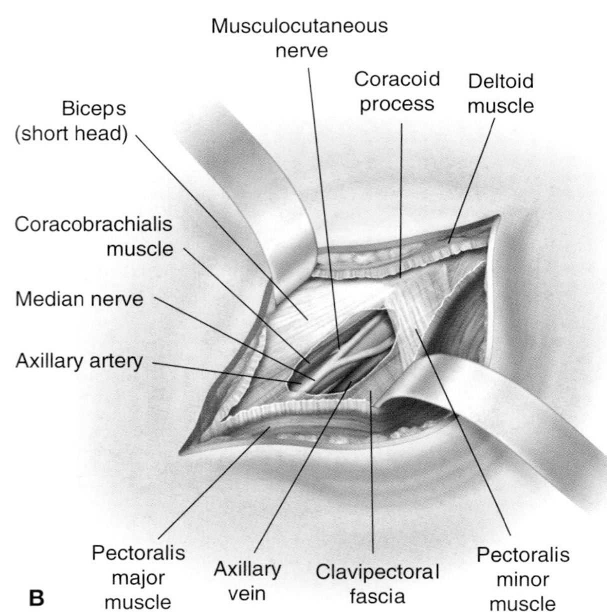

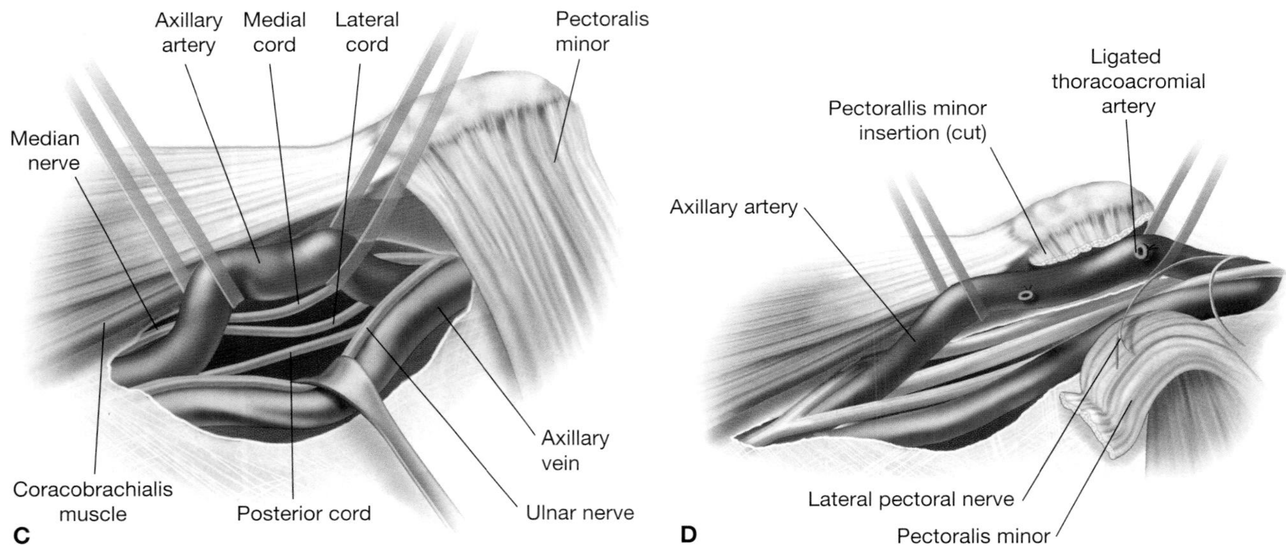

FIGURE 3 ● **A,** Axillary exposure of the mid-distal axillary artery. **B,** Deltopectoral exposure of a long segment of axillary artery. **C,** Exposure of the distal axillary artery and associated axillary sheath structures. **D,** Exposure of the midaxillary artery via reflection of the pectoralis minor muscle.

Second Step

- Inside the axillary sheath, the artery is under the median nerve (**FIGURE 3B**). The medial and lateral cords form the median nerve lateral to the border of the pectoralis major muscle. The ulnar nerve lies inferoposterior to the border of the axillary artery in this area. Identification of these surrounding structures is important to minimize risk of damage.
- Vessel loops can be applied proximal and distal to the injury. If vascular clamps are used, assure nerve structures are not included when applying the clamp to the artery. Caudal traction can be applied to the vessel loops to augment exposure and reduce the risk of injuring adjacent nerves (**FIGURE 3C**).

Third Step

- The pectoralis minor muscle can be divided with care to prevent injury to the lateral pectoral nerve when further exposure is needed.
- The second portion of the axillary artery is surrounded by brachial plexus nerves on all sides but the anterior surface. To allow circumferential exposure, the thoracoacromial artery can be ligated and divided at its origin (**FIGURE 3D**).

Fourth Step

- Addressing the injured artery follows the steps previously described through careful inspection and reconstruction.

BRACHIAL ARTERY

First Step

- Exposure of the brachial artery is best accomplished by making a longitudinal incision over the bicipital sulcus between the biceps and triceps muscles (**FIGURE 4A**).
- As dissection is carried out through the subcutaneous tissue, care should be taken to visualize the basilic vein. The vein can be retracted. Branches of the vein can be ligated and divided to facilitate artery exposure or if they are damaged from the trauma. If the vein is heavily damaged, it may require ligation and resection.

Second Step

- The deep fascia is incised at the medial border of the biceps. The neurovascular bundle is then encountered. The median nerve will be the first structure encountered in the brachial sheath. To allow gentle retraction of the nerve, wide mobilization should be performed to access the artery (**FIGURE 4B**).
- Branches of the brachial artery may require control during exposure. The deep brachial artery arises from the posteromedial surface of the brachial artery just distal to the lateral border of the teres major muscle. The superior and inferior ulnar collateral arteries are found in the distal upper arm arising from the brachial artery.
- To access the artery in the distal upper arm, the bicipital aponeurosis may need to be divided to obtain maximal exposure of the artery. At the level of the antecubital fossa, the incision should make a laterally oriented S curve to allow access to the bifurcation and to prevent joint contracture (**FIGURE 5A**). The median nerve is found posteromedial to the brachial artery in this location and care should be taken to avoid injury (**FIGURE 5B**).

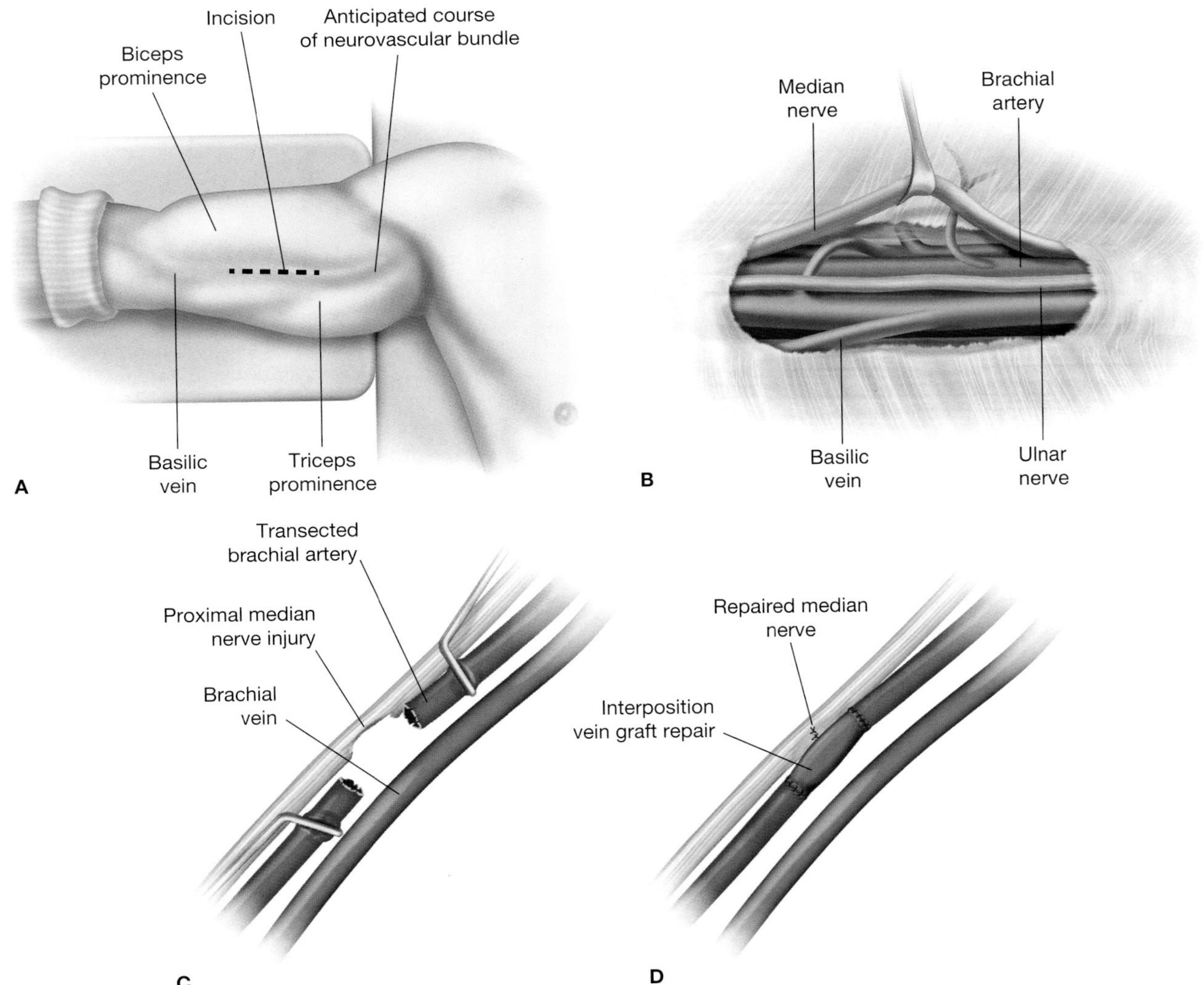

FIGURE 4 ● **A,** Incision created for exposure of the proximal brachial artery in the upper arm. **B,** The brachial artery in the upper arm is adjacent to the median and ulnar nerves. **C,** Traumatic transection of the brachial artery with associated intimal damage, along with partial injury to the median nerve. Subsequent repair is performed with a brachial artery interposition graft using a vein conduit and median nerve repair **(D)**.

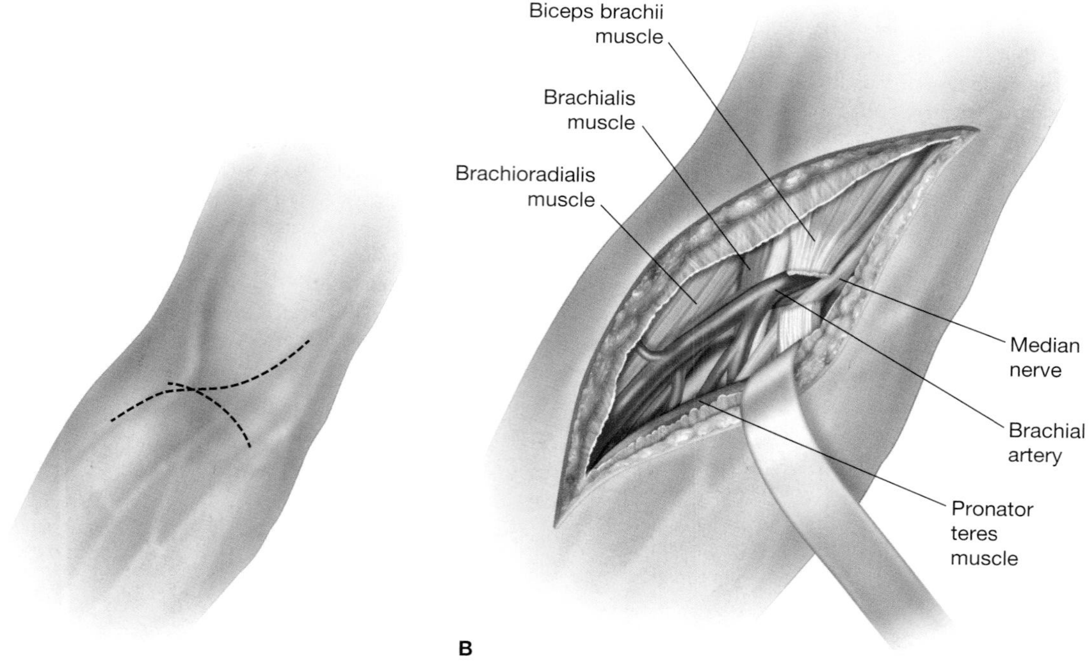

FIGURE 5 ● **A,** Typical incisions used for exposure of the distal brachial artery and proximal radial and ulnar arteries at the antecubital fossa. **B,** Relative anatomy of the brachial, radial, and ulnar arteries and adjacent median nerve.

Third Step

- Proximal and distal control must be obtained with vessel loops or vascular clamps. Examine the injured vessel to identify the extent of trauma (**FIGURE 4C**).
- Repair of traumatic arterial injuries should follow basic principles of vascular repairs, beginning with minimal debridement back to healthy intima. Small wounds of the artery may be repaired primarily or with debridement and reapproximation. Larger injury to the vessel and partial transections may be amenable to patch angioplasty. For destructive wounds often seen with gunshots, interposition grafting is recommended. Autologous vein is the preferred conduit harvested from the least injured extremity, typically the saphenous veins (**FIGURE 4D**). If the patient is unstable or other injuries need to be addressed, consider temporary vascular shunt placement.
- Ensure appropriate length to allow elbow motion without traction on the anastomosis. Kinking is reduced by reconstructing other injured structures in the area to limit graft motion during elbow flexion.
- Proximal and distal anastomoses are performed in an end-to-end or end-to-side fashion depending on respective diameters of the inflow and outflow segments.
- Catheter embolectomy should be employed as needed if concern for thrombus exists. Imaging guidance can be used to assist in the decision and performance of this step. This should be carried out in an antegrade fashion and may require a proximal incision if concerns about the proximal artery exist to avoid emboli into the systematic circulation.
- Performance of a completion angiogram may be done to evaluate the graft and its flow.

RADIAL ARTERY

First Step

- Direct exposure of the radial artery can be performed along the length of the forearm. Exposure needs to be adequate to achieve control proximal and distal to the injury.
- The brachial artery bifurcates into the radial and ulnar arteries at the level of the radial tuberosity (**FIGURE 5B**). Some patients may have high bifurcation, and in these cases, the radial artery originates proximal to the antecubital fossa.
- The proximal radial artery can be exposed via a transverse incision approximately two fingerbreadths distal to the antecubital crease. If distal brachial artery exposure is needed or the antecubital fossa is crossed, an alternate approach is a "lazy-S" incision beginning at the medial aspect of the biceps tendon, crossing the midpoint of the antecubital fossa, and extending toward the lateral aspect of the volar forearm.
- The mid- and distal radial artery is exposed via longitudinal incision over the course of the vessel. After emerging from the brachioradialis muscle, the radial artery travels between the brachioradialis and flexor carpi radialis muscles. Distally,

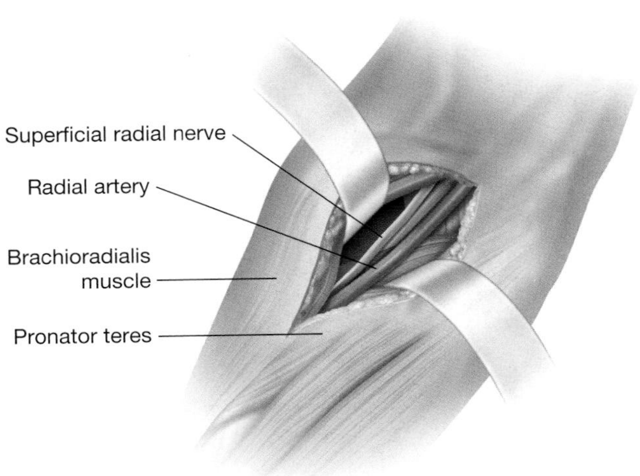

FIGURE 6 ● Exposure of the radial artery in the proximal forearm.

it is found between the flexor pollicis longus and lateral border of the radius until it passes behind the flexor retinaculum into the hand.

Second Step

- The radial artery is covered by antebrachial fascia, and therefore, this must be incised along the length of the incision. The brachioradialis muscle can then be retracted laterally to expose the radial artery (**FIGURE 6**).
- Paired radial veins travel with the radial artery along its course in the forearm. The superficial branch of the radial nerve can also be found laterally in closeness, proximity to the mid- and distal radial artery. Care should be taken not to injure these associated structures.

Third Step

- Isolated injury to the radial artery, in the presence of intact ulnar artery flow and complete palmar arch, is unlikely to result in ischemia to the forearm or hand. Repair is not mandatory and ligation is a reasonable approach.
- Repair of traumatic transections should follow basic principles of vascular repairs, beginning with minimal debridement back to healthy intima. Stab wounds are more likely to have minimal surrounding damage, whereas ballistic wounds with associated blast injury are more likely to result in more extensive tissue loss. Depending on the degree of tissue loss, an end-to-end anastomosis or interposition graft can be completed.

ULNAR ARTERY

First Step

- Similar to the radial artery, the ulnar artery can be exposed via an S-shaped incision at the antecubital fossa or via longitudinal incision over its course along the forearm.
- Proximally, the ulnar artery lies on the brachialis muscle, then the flexor digitorum profundus distally. It is deep to the pronator teres, flexor carpi radialis, and flexor digitorum superficialis. The distal ulnar artery emerges between the flexor digitorum superficialis and the flexor carpi ulnaris (FCU).
- The ulnar nerve lies just medial to the artery distally, and care should be taken not to injure this (**FIGURE 7**).

Second Step

- As with radial artery injuries, isolated ulnar artery injury is also unlikely to result in distal ischemia. The ulnar artery is more often the dominant inflow to the hand, and therefore in instances where both forearm vessels are injured, ulnar artery repair is preferred.
- Repair of injuries once again begins with debridement to healthy intima, followed by end-to-end anastomosis or interposition graft.

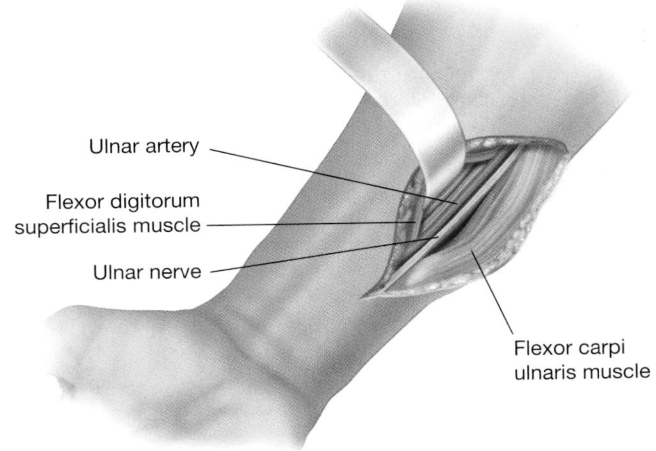

FIGURE 7 ● Exposure of the proximal midulnar artery in the forearm.

TEMPORARY VASCULAR SHUNT

First Step

- Expose the proximal portion of the injured artery. Then, locate the distal end of the injured artery. Control the ends of the vessel with a vessel loop using a double pass around the vessel tagged with a hemostat that is used to provide tension to occlude the vessel or a Rummel tourniquet.

Second Step

- Inspect the ends of the injured vessel and locate the true lumen. Debridement may be needed in heavily damaged vessels to locate the lumen.

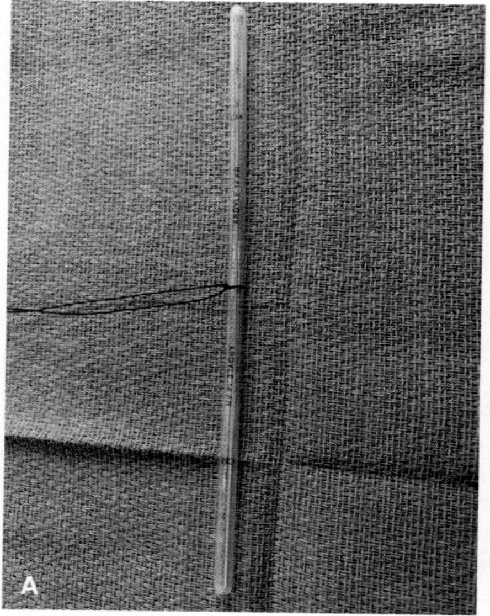

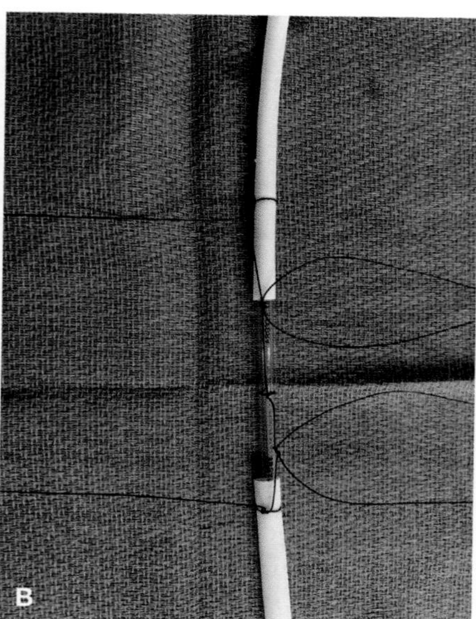

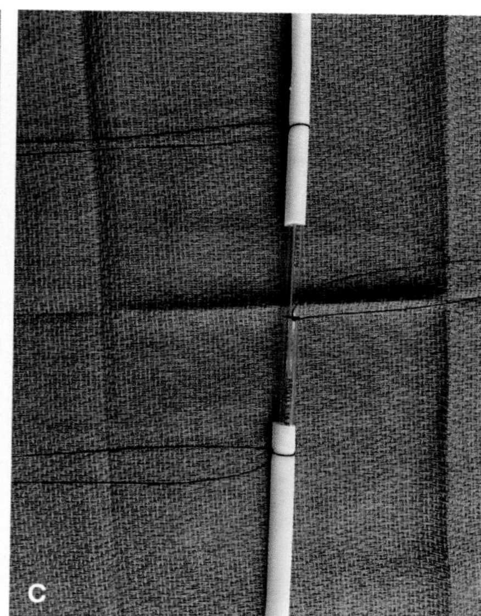

FIGURE 8 ● **A,** Commercial intraluminal shunt. **B,** Shunt in proximal and distal artery. **C,** Shunt and artery secured with suture.

Third Step

- Commercially available plastic intraluminal shunts are selected of appropriate size that closely mirrors the size of the injured vessel (**FIGURE 8A**). Flush the selected shunt with heparinized saline.

Fourth Step

- Place the shunt into the lumen of the proximal and distal segments of the injured vessel. Care is needed to avoid any further injury to the arterial lumen when inserting the shunt. Assure adequate shunt length of several centimeters inside each end of the injured vessel to prevent dislodgement. Secure the shunt by placing silk suture tied around the vessel over the shunt (**FIGURE 8B**). These sutures can then be tied together and around the mid-portion of the shunt to protect against dislodgement (**FIGURE 8C**).

Fifth Step

- A Doppler device can be used to assess the shunt through evaluation of signal presence. Assure patency of the shunt through palpation of distal artery pulsation or the use of a Doppler device to detect distal signals. If flow is not detected, thrombectomy with an embolectomy balloon catheter may be needed for the injured vessel and/or the shunt itself. If not contraindicated, systemic heparin can be administered to facilitate shunt flow. Assure flow periodically by palpation or Doppler device. If skeletal stabilization is needed after perfusion is restored, monitor the flow and shunt position (if able) prior to, during, and after stabilization maneuvers.

FOREARM FASCIOTOMIES

First Step

- The volar compartment is usually addressed first as it is most susceptible to ischemic and compressive injury due to fascial boundaries that limit expansion of the muscle bellies' swelling. An incision is planned over the volar forearm proximally, medial to the antecubital fossa and ends distally on the ulnar side of the wrist in a curvilinear fashion (**FIGURE 9A**). Several other incisions have been used including a zig-zag incision, ulnar- or radial-based single incision that extends proximally and distally, or separate radial- and ulnar-sided incisions (**FIGURE 9B**). No matter the incision selected, avoiding orthogonal incisions over the elbow and wrist joint is suggested. Adequate skin flap should allow coverage of the median nerve- and radial-sided neurovascular structures. The incision can be extended to perform a carpal tunnel release if needed.
- A skin incision is made over the planned path. A small fascial incision is made. If able, blunt dissection is performed below the fascia to protect underlying structures as the fasciotomy is performed. The fascia is released distally to the wrist and proximally to the lacertus fibrosis covering the FCU.

Second Step

- After decompression of the superficial compartment, the deep volar compartment should be assessed and decompressed if needed. Retraction of the FCU ulnarly and the flexor digitorum superficialis medially allows access to the deep compartment. Incise and open the deep fascia for its entire length with caution to avoid injury to underlying structures. Epimysiotomy of individual muscle bellies is done if muscles look pale and tense after fasciotomy. Particular attention is needed for the pronator quadratus as controversy remains over whether it is contained in its own compartment.
- If needed, the carpal tunnel and Guyon canal can be released through the volar approach by extending the distal incision over the transverse carpal ligament. Careful planning of the incision to be no further radially than the mid-axis of the ring finger or ulnar side of the palmaris longis is essential to

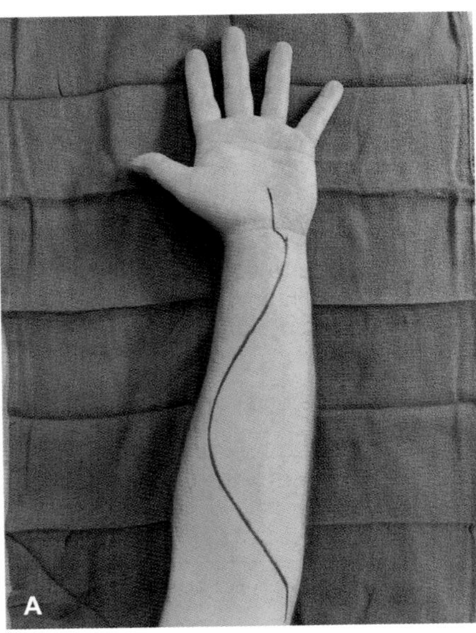

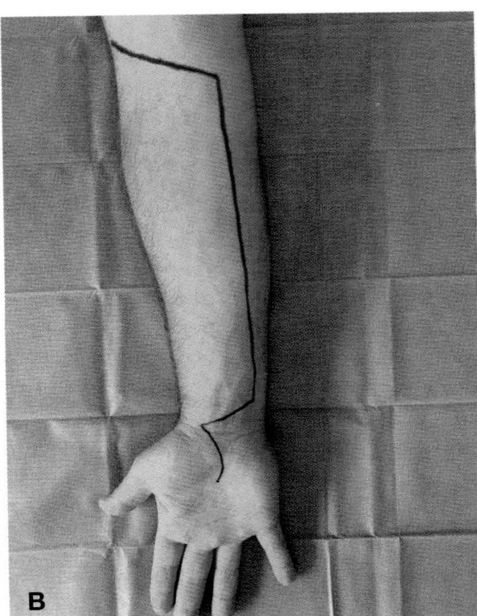

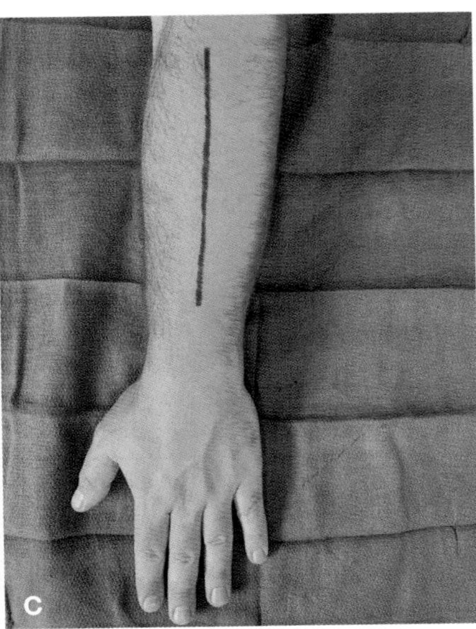

FIGURE 9 ● **A,** Volar forearm curvilinear fasciotomy incision. **B,** Volar forearm ulnar based fasciotomy incision. **C,** Dorsal forearm fasciotomy incision.

avoid injury to the recurrent motor and superficial palmar branches of the median nerve.

- After all volar compartments have been released adequately, inspection for necrotic muscle and debridement if present is performed. Inspection of the anatomy including nerves, blood vessels, and musculoskeletal structures should be performed to identify any injuries.

Third Step

- Assessment of the dorsal compartment is undertaken. Decompression of the volar compartment may provide adequate relief of the dorsal compartment. If dorsal compartment fasciotomy is needed, it is accomplished through a single midline incision (**FIGURE 9C**).

Fourth Step

- The incision is planned several centimeters distal to the lateral epicondyle extending to several centimeters proximal to the midline of the wrist.
- The skin incision is carried out over the planned path. A small fascial incision is made. If able, blunt dissection is performed below the fascia to protect underlying structures as the fasciotomy is performed. Divide the dorsal fascia. The dorsal muscles often are contained in separate fascial septae that will need to be decompressed individually.
- After the dorsal compartment has been released adequately, inspection for necrotic muscle and debridement if present is performed. Inspection of the anatomy should be performed to identify any injuries.

Fifth Step

- After adequate decompression of the compartments, inspection of anatomic structures and debridement of necrotic tissue within the wound is done.
- The wounds are often left open. Some surgeons advocate the use of retention sutures to assist with closure. The wound can be dressed with sterile wet-to-dry dressing or negative pressure wound therapy (NPWT). The dressing should be applied carefully to allow for further swelling as this is common in the first 24 to 48 hours.

Sixth Step

- The arm should be inspected regularly to assess swelling and neurovascular status. The patient typically returns to the OR every 48 to 72 hours to examine the wound and debride any further necrotic tissue. The wound can be closed once the swelling subsides. NPWT can assist with decreasing edema and facilitating wound closure. If wound closure cannot be achieved, the use of skin grafting can be employed.

PEARLS AND PITFALLS

Identification of injuries	Following standard evaluation of the trauma patient using ATLS principles assists in identifying injuries rather than focusing on the upper extremity injury.
Upper extremity nerve injuries	Upper extremity arterial injuries often are associated with concomitant nerve injuries. Early recognition and diagnosis of nerve injuries is important to long-term functional outcome. Consultation at the time of identification or suspected nerve injury with specialist trained in management of these injuries is prudent.
Iatrogenic nerve injury during axillary artery exposure	Whenever possible, axillary exposure proximal to the axilla should be obtained as proximal as possible, to limit the risk of nerve injury as the cords of the brachial plexus become more intimately related to the axillary artery as it proceeds laterally from the clavicle. Far proximal anastomotic positioning of the axillary artery minimizes artery displacement and traction with arm movement. The preferred choices for axillary artery exposure are proximal or distal to the second portion of the axillary artery unless repair requires deltopectoral exposure.
Arterial repair following segmental resection	The extent of injury to the artery should be delineated prior to attempts at reconstruction. Failure to identify the extent of injury will lead to complications of the repair.
Inflow assessment	Prior to completion of an arterial repair, the surgeon must ensure adequate inflow. A preoperative CTA can be reviewed if available or intraoperative angiogram can be performed.
Outflow assessment	Adequate arterial outflow is paramount to maintain patency of proximal repairs to reduce potential extremity ischemic symptoms. Intraoperative outflow assessment should be performed in circumstances where the distal vascular examination is abnormal following revascularization.
Compartment syndrome	Injury to the arm induces tissue edema, bleeding, and possibly ischemia. These factors can lead to compartment syndrome particularly if there is prolonged ischemic times (>4-6 hours). Early consideration for fasciotomy of the extremity is warranted. The carpal tunnel may need to be released if median nerve dysfunction is suspected or confirmed. Consultation with a specialist versed in compartment syndrome of the hand may be warranted if decompression of the hand is being considered.
Spasm	Spasm often occurs after injury. Restoration of normal hemodynamics, correction of hypothermia, and topical warming of the injured extremity may reverse spasm. In patients with limb-threatening arterial spasm intra-arterial injection with papaverine with or without infusion. Additionally, other vasodilators can be administered to attenuate spasm if the patient is stable to tolerate.

POSTOPERATIVE CARE

- Motor, sensory, and pulse status (including a Doppler and pulse examination) should be performed immediately postoperatively to determine the new baseline for subsequent serial examinations and to document improvement.
- Observation should be performed for bleeding, hematomas, or change in serial neurovascular status, as well as development of compartment syndrome.
- Antithrombotic medications should be considered for arterial repair or reconstruction. In a meta-analysis, the use of anticoagulation following vascular trauma reduced the risk of amputations and reoperative events.[20] Often aspirin 81 mg or 162 mg orally daily is recommended with reconstruction or concerns about distal runoff when concern for other etiologies of bleeding is tempered.[19]
- Patients with combined vascular injury with musculoskeletal injuries, nerve injuries, or large wound burdens may require a multidisciplinary discussion on further reconstructive procedures as well as the possibility of amputation.[1,5,19]

COMPLICATIONS

- Intraoperative arterial vasospasm or occlusion
- Missed concomitant venous or nerve injuries
- Iatrogenic brachial plexus, median, or ulnar nerve injuries from intraoperative electrocautery, traction, or accidental transection
- Arterial repair or bypass graft stenosis or thrombosis
- Bleeding
- Wound or graft site infection
- Compartment syndrome

REFERENCES

1. Huber GH, Manna B. Vascular extremity trauma. *STATPearls*. 2021. Available at: https://www.ncbi.nlm.nih.gov/books/NBK536925/
2. Feliciano DV, Moore FA, Moore EE, et al. Western Trauma Association/critical decisions in trauma evaluation and management of peripheral vascular injury. Part 1. *J Trauma*. 2011;70(6):1551-1556.
3. Shaw AD, Milne AA, Christie J, et al. Vascular Trauma of the upper limb and associated nerve injuries. *Injury*. 1995;26:515-518.
4. American College of Surgeons Committee on Trauma. *Advanced Trauma Life Support: Student Course Manual*. 10th ed. American College of Surgeons; 2018.
5. American College of Surgeons Committee on Trauma. *Management of Complex Extremity Trauma*. 2005. Available at: https://imsva91-ctp.trendmicro.com:443/wis/clicktime/v1/query?url=http%3a%2f%2fjasoncartermd.com%2fems%2fmedia%2fpdf%2facs%2fmancompexttrauma.pdf&umid=01BE9A7D-E350-8A05-A962-F45AD0ED0D29&auth=f717728ea12e7e4b3bc261b22673ae-2801b01ac9-068020fc621ee86617f9a8de50a828c791ed6729

6. Mavrogenis AF, Panagopoulos GN, Kokkalis ZT, et al. Vascular injury in orthopedic trauma. *Orthopedics*. 2016;39(4):249-259.
7. Romagnoli AN, DuBose J, Dua A, et al. Hard signs gone soft: a critical evaluation of presenting signs of extremity vascular injury. *J Trauma Acute Care Surg*. 2020;90(1):1-10.
8. Prasan ML, Ouellette EA. Acute compartment syndrome of the upper extremity. *J Am Acad Orthop Surg*. 2011;19:49-58.
9. Kistler JM, Ilyas AM, Thoder JJ. Forearm compartment syndrome evaluation and management. *Hand Clin*. 2018;34:53-60.
10. Pillai L, Luchette FA, Romano KS, Ricotta JJ. Upper-extremity arterial injury. *Am Surg*. 1997;63:224-227.
11. Miller-Thomas MM, West OC, Cohen AM. Diagnosing traumatic arterial injury in the extremities with CT angiography: pearls and pitfalls. *Radiographics*. 2005;Suppl 1:S133-S142.
12. Seamon MJ, Smoger D, Torres DM, et al. A prospective validation of a current practice: the detection of extremity vascular injury with CT angiography. *J Trauma*. 2009;67:238-244.
13. Wahlgren CM, Riddez L. Penetrating vascular trauma of the upper and lower limbs. *Curr Trauma Rep*. 2016;2:11-20.
14. Demetriades D, Asensio JA. Subclavian and axillary vascular injuries. *Surg Clin North Am*. 2001;81(6):1357-1373.
15. Degiannis E, Levy RD, Silwa K, et al. Penetrating injuries of the brachial artery. *Injury*. 1995;26(4):249-252.
16. Thai JN, Pacheco JA, Margolis DS, et al. Evidence-based comprehensive approach to forearm arterial laceration. *West J Emerg Med*. 2015;165(7):1127-1134.
17. Maher Z, Frank B, Saillant N, et al. Systemic intraoperative anticoagulation during arterial injury repair: implications for patency and bleeding. *J Trauma Acute Care Surg*. 2017;82(4):680-686.
18. Loja MN, Galante JM, Humphries M, et al. Systemic anticoagulation in the setting of vascular extremity trauma. *Injury*. 2017;48(9):1911-1916.
19. Feliciano DV, Moore FA, Moore EE, et al. Western Trauma Association/critical decisions in trauma evaluation and management of peripheral vascular injury. Part II. *J Trauma*. 2013;75(3):391-397.
20. Khan S, Elghazally H, Mian A, Khan M. A meta-analysis on anticoagulation after vascular trauma. *Eur J Trauma Emerg Surg*. 2020;46(6):1291-1299.

SECTION XIII: Trauma in Pregnancy

Chapter 39 Trauma Cesarean Section

Tracey A. Dechert, Tejal Sudhirkumar Brahmbhatt, and Aaron Powel Richman

DEFINITION

- The perimortem cesarean, or resuscitative hysterotomy, is the rapid delivery of the fetus from a pregnant woman during or after cardiopulmonary arrest. It is performed with the primary goal of increasing the chance of successfully resuscitating the mother and, potentially, improving fetal survival.
- Perimortem cesarean delivery is recommended in the event of a failure to achieve return of spontaneous circulation with standard of care within 4 minutes of arrest onset and if the uterine fundus is at or above the umbilicus in maternal cardiac arrest.[1,2]

DIFFERENTIAL DIAGNOSIS

- Sudden cardiac arrest in pregnancy can be due to conditions that are a direct result of pregnancy such as pulmonary/amniotic fluid embolism, hemorrhage, sepsis, cardiomyopathy, stroke, preeclampsia, and eclampsia.[3] Nonpregnancy causes include complications of preexisting medical conditions, anesthesia, and trauma.[4]

PATIENT HISTORY AND PHYSICAL EXAM FINDINGS

- Ongoing cardiopulmonary resuscitation with high quality chest compressions and following the "American Heart Association Guidelines for CPR and ECC".[5]
- Reversible causes for cardiac arrest have been assessed and are actively being addressed.
- The uterine fundus on physical exam is at or above the umbilicus. This indicates a gestation of about 20 weeks.
- Cardiopulmonary compromise continues despite appropriate leftward uterine displacement; the compressive effect of the gravid uterus is compressing the inferior vena cava and restricting thoracic compliance which may prevent effective resuscitative efforts.
- In spite of all maneuvers and resuscitative efforts, the patient has not demonstrated return of spontaneous circulation within 4 minutes of initiation of resuscitation.

IMAGING AND OTHER DIAGNOSTIC STUDIES

- There are no recommended imaging or diagnostic studies warranted to initiate perimortem cesarean section.
- Point-of-care echocardiography and thoracic/pulmonary ultrasound are a quick and reliable modality to assess for potential causes of arrest from a cardiac and pulmonary standpoint. The presence of free fluid in the peritoneal cavity on ultrasonography can provide additional clues as to the cause of the patient's arrest.

SURGICAL MANAGEMENT

Preoperative Planning

- Much like the resuscitative thoracotomy, the resuscitative hysterotomy should take place as soon as the patient meets the criteria for the procedure. As mentioned above, if there is failure to achieve return of spontaneous circulation with standard of care resuscitative measures within 4 minutes of cardiac arrest onset in a patient with her uterine fundus at or above the umbilicus, perimortem cesarean delivery is recommended.
- Moving the patient to the operative theater or delivery room delays definitive intervention and therefore is not recommended.
- The surgeon should communicate the plan to the remaining members of the team and ensure the appropriate resources are engaged to continue resuscitation as the procedure is performed. This should include the pediatric or neonatal ICU team to attend to the fetus after delivery.[6]

Positioning

- The patient should be placed supine with arms extended if possible. Leaving the arms extended allows the remainder of the resuscitation team to obtain venous and arterial access.
- Placement of a urinary catheter is helpful to facilitate visualization and to protect the bladder from injury. However, the procedure should not be delayed completing this.

ABDOMINAL INCISION

- A longitudinal, low-midline laparotomy incision allows for rapid access to the abdomen with minimal extraneous blood loss from the subcutaneous tissues. Although many techniques for cesarean delivery have been described, care of the pregnant patient in extremis demands simplicity and speed. The midline incision can also be easily extended to access the remainder of the abdomen in cases of traumatic circulatory arrests.
- The skin is incised with a scalpel from the umbilicus to the pubic symphysis. The incision should be of sufficient length (12-14 cm) to allow for broad visualization and easy fetal delivery. A complete laparotomy incision from xiphoid to pubic symphysis will allow for complete abdominal exploration once the fetal delivery is complete. Dissection is continued through the subcutaneous tissue down to the fascia with a combination of blunt and sharp dissection.
- The midline fascia is elevated and sharply incised to allow a finger into the peritoneum. A scissor is then used to complete the fascial incision cephalad and caudal. The bladder is retracted and protected inferiorly along the pubic symphysis exposing the uterus (see **FIGURE 1**).

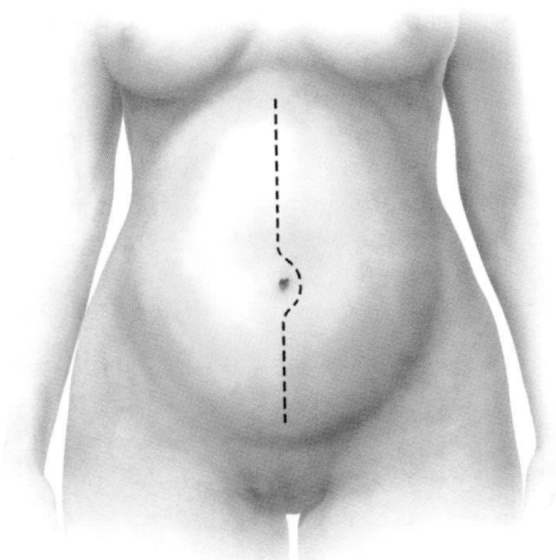

FIGURE 1 ● Abdominal incision. Standard midline laparotomy incision running from xiphoid to pubic symphysis. Allows for full access and visualization of the peritoneal cavity.

HYSTEROTOMY

- A longitudinal or "classical incision" should be used. This incision provides greater flexibility than the low-transverse technique. It is easy to enlarge, if necessary, without inadvertent extension into the laterally positioned uterine arteries. The myometrium is sharply incised approximately 6 cm in the upper uterine segment. The incision is deepened with the scalpel or electrocautery.
- Final entry into the uterine cavity can be made by bluntly dissecting the final layers of the uterine wall with the surgeon's finger to protect the underlying fetus from injury.
- If the placenta is encountered anteriorly, it can be divided to facilitate rapid entry (see **FIGURE 2**).

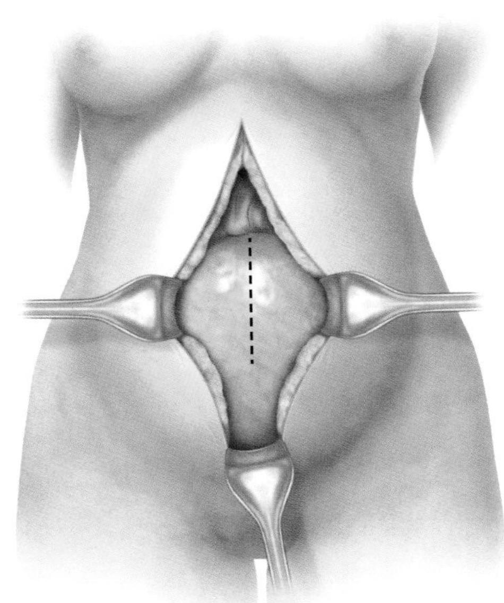

FIGURE 2 ● Hysterotomy. A longitudinal, midline or "Classical" uterine incision avoids the lateral uterine vessels to minimize hemorrhage

FETAL AND PLACENTAL DELIVERY

- In most cases, the fetus rotates, and the head engages in the pelvis late in the third trimester. To facilitate delivery, the surgeon's hand slides into the hysterotomy down toward the pelvis with palm and fingers curving around the fetal head. The fetal head is elevated cephalad and disengaged from the pelvis then anteriorly out of the hysterotomy. Pressure on the fundus can aid with delivery of the fetal body.
- For a transverse or breech presentation, the order of delivery is often reversed. The operator must find the feet of the fetus caudally within the uterus and then, using gentle traction, deliver the body and finally the head through the uterine incision. The cord is clamped, divided, and the infant passed off for evaluation and resuscitation.
- The placenta is delivered with steady traction on the cord. The delivered placenta should be inspected, and the uterine cavity manually explored to ensure complete evacuation of all products of conception (see **FIGURE 3**).

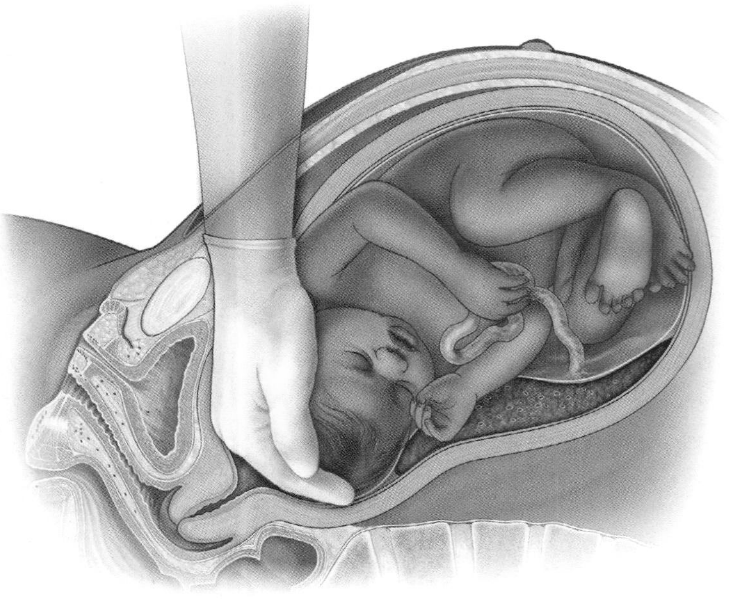

FIGURE 3 ● Fetal delivery. The surgeon's hand reaches into the pelvis to elevate the head out of the pelvis and then anterior to facilitate delivery.

CLOSURE

- Closure of the hysterotomy and the abdomen depends on the condition of the patient. Resuscitative efforts should continue based on the mother's primary pathology. In cases of abdominal trauma, the abdomen can be explored and packed as indicated. If spontaneous circulation resumes, the uterus can be rapidly closed using a full thickness running absorbable suture. A locking stitch technique can be used to aid with hemostasis. A temporary vacuum closure typical of damage control surgery can then be used to facilitate transfer of the patient for definitive management of the cause of her arrest. Once the patient is stabilized, definitive fascial closure can then be completed.
- In cases of maternal demise, an approximating aesthetic closure of the skin is sufficient.[7,8]

PEARLS AND PITFALLS

Hemostatic Adjuncts	■ Administration of tranexamic acid (10 mg/kg Intravenous) as an antifibrinolytic and hemostatic agent has demonstrated improvement in maternal blood loss during elective cesarean deliveries and should be considered in resuscitative hysterotomy.
Placental position	■ Knowledge of the placental position and fetal presentation can help with operative decision-making. An anteriorly placed placenta may be inadvertently lacerated with the hysterotomy causing fetal hemorrhage. If possible, care should be taken to avoid this. ■ Similarly, knowing the position of the fetus in the uterus can facilitate delivery. Unfortunately, these details are often difficult to obtain in these cases.
Uterotonic agents	■ Uterotonic agents can be used to help uterine contraction after delivery and mitigate uterine hemorrhage. Oxytocin IV infusion is the most common first-line agent.

POSTOPERATIVE CARE

- After delivery, postoperative care should focus on reversing the cause of the mother's cardiac arrest. For traumatic arrests, a complete exploration of the abdomen should be completed to evaluate other sources of hemorrhage. In medical arrest cases, resuscitative efforts should follow Advanced Cardiac Life Support and Advanced Life Support in Obstetrics guidelines.

COMPLICATIONS

- As the trauma cesarean section or resuscitative hysterotomy is a final maneuver for patients in extremis, the outcomes of this procedure are typically poor. Maternal survival rates in cases requiring perimortem cesarean section are reported between 34% and 54%. Fetal survival ranges from 61% to 80%.[9] Salvage of the fetus depends upon the gestational age and the expediency of delivery. The neonate is at risk for postdelivery cardiorespiratory failure as well as anoxic neurologic injury. Appropriate management of these issues requires a skilled neonatal care team.
- Like other emergent procedures, resuscitative hysterotomy carries an increased risk for wound complications like infection, fascial dehiscence, and hernia. Visceral injury to the bladder, ureter, and bowel is also more common. Venous thromboembolism rates are increased in pregnant patients and increase with emergent cesarean deliveries.
- Long-term risks include higher rates of uterine rupture or placental abnormalities in subsequent pregnancies.[10]

REFERENCES

1. Jeejeebhoy FM, Zelop CM, Lipman S, et al. Cardiac arrest in pregnancy: a scientific statement from the American Heart Association. *Circulation.* 2015;132(18):1747-1773. doi:10.1161/CIR.0000000000000300
2. Soar J, Perkins GD, Abbas G, et al. European Resuscitation Council Guidelines for Resuscitation 2010 Section 8. Cardiac arrest in special circumstances: Electrolyte abnormalities, poisoning, drowning, accidental hypothermia, hyperthermia, asthma, anaphylaxis, cardiac surgery, trauma, pregnancy, electrocution. *Resuscitation.* 2010;81(10):1400-1433. doi:10.1016/j.resuscitation.2010.08.015
3. Suresh MS, Latoya Mason C, Munnur U. Cardiopulmonary resuscitation and the parturient. *Best Pract Res Clin Obstet Gynaecol.* 2010;24(3):383-400. doi:10.1016/J.BPOBGYN.2010.01.002
4. Rose CH, Faksh A, Traynor KD, Cabrera D, Arendt KW, Brost BC. Challenging the 4- to 5-minute rule: from perimortem cesarean to resuscitative hysterotomy. *Am J Obstet Gynecol.* 2015;213(5):653-656, 653.e1. doi:10.1016/j.ajog.2015.07.019
5. Panchal AR, Bartos JA, Cabañas JG, et al. Part 3: Adult Basic and Advanced Life Support—2020 American Heart Association Guidelines for Cardiopulmonary Resuscitation and Emergency Cardiovascular Care. *Circulation.* 2020;142(16_suppl_2):S366-S468. doi:10.1161/CIR.0000000000000916
6. Baskett TF. Preparedness for emergency "crash" caesarean section. *J Obstet Gynaecol Can.* 2015;37(12):1116-1117. doi:10.1016/s1701-2163(16)30078-0
7. Gosset M, Ilenko A, Bouyou J, Renevier B. Emergency caesarean section. *J Visc Surg.* 2017;154(1):47-50. doi:10.1016/j.jviscsurg.2016.09.012
8. Lanoix R, Akkapeddi V, Goldfeder B. Perimortem cesarean section: case reports and recommendations. *Acad Emerg Med.* 1995;2(12):1063-1067. doi:10.1111/j.1553-2712.1995.tb03151.x
9. Drukker L, Hants Y, Sharon E, Sela HY, Grisaru-Granovsky S. Perimortem cesarean section for maternal and fetal salvage: concise review and protocol. *Acta Obstet Gynecol Scand.* 2014;93(10):965-972. doi:10.1111/aogs.12464
10. Yang XJ, Sun SS. Comparison of maternal and fetal complications in elective and emergency cesarean section: a systematic review and meta-analysis. *Arch Gynecol Obstet.* 2017;296(3):503-512. doi:10.1007/S00404-017-4445-2/TABLES/3

Chapter 40 Cricothyroidotomy

Bennett J. Berning and Marc Anthony de Moya

DEFINITION

- When orotracheal intubation is not possible or multiple attempts have failed, cricothyroidotomy is performed as a rescue procedure for emergent airway access. Although this procedure is never a first-line option for airway management, all emergency providers must be confident in performing the procedure in a time of need. Traditionally, an open technique has been used to perform this procedure. More recently, percutaneous options have become available. Both the open and percutaneous approaches will be discussed in this chapter.

INDICATIONS

- Owing to the high-stakes nature of emergent airway management, the decision to perform the cricothyroidotomy is often more difficult than the procedure itself. Emergent cricothyroidotomy is performed when ventilation and oxygenation become difficult to maintain and after attempts at orotracheal intubation have failed. Severe facial trauma, upper airway obstruction, and intrinsic patient factors, such as body habitus or anomalous facial anatomy, pose difficult conditions for effective airway management. Difficult airways should be identified early, and the approach should follow a difficult airway algorithm with an experienced person doing the procedure. The number of attempts depends upon the circumstances but should follow an escalation process with either different techniques or more experienced personnel.
- In ideal circumstances (which is often not the case), one should avoid performing cricothyroidotomy during episodes of severe desaturations, which may result in bradycardia or even asystole. Basic adjuncts to airway management such a jaw-thrust maneuver, bag-mask ventilation, use of oropharyngeal/nasopharyngeal and laryngeal mask airways can help as you prepare to perform a cricothyroidotomy.
- There are limited data to support the use of an open approach for cricothyroidotomy vs a percutaneous technique. The type of cricothyroidotomy performed is based largely on the resources available and provider experience.

PATIENT HISTORY AND PHYSICAL FINDINGS

- Patients who present after head and neck trauma pose a particular challenge due to suboptimal airway exposure. The need to maintain in-line cervical stabilization and/or the presence of facial injuries with bleeding from the sinuses into the nasopharynx make direct laryngoscopy difficult.
- If a difficult airway is anticipated, one should prepare for cricothyroidotomy, even if the procedure is ultimately not performed.
- Unfortunately, a formal history and physical examination is limited due to the emergent nature of the procedure. A quick and focused physical examination should include an assessment of the patient's neurologic status and facial and airway anatomy. A baseline Glasgow Coma Scale can be obtained, along with identification of any focal neurologic deficits. This will help one better understand potential head or spine injuries, which will in turn affect how the airway is managed.
- Face and neck anatomy should be quickly assessed. Patient factors that predict a difficult airway include a short neck, morbid obesity, inability for neck extension, or tracheal deviation. The use of the 3-3-2 rule (3-finger-breath distance between the upper and lower incisors, 3-finger-breath distance between the hyoid bone and the chin, 2-finger-breath distance from the thyroid cartilage to the floor of the mouth) is a helpful method to help anticipate airway difficulties.[1]
- Head and neck trauma results in a potential challenge for airway management. Both blunt and penetrating trauma to the head and neck region can result in severe hemorrhage and anatomic deformities. Prompt airway assessment to determine the security of the airway is essential. If a definitive airway is needed, preparation for emergent cricothyroidotomy should be made if intubation is unsuccessful.
- With the rise of the coronavirus (COVID-19) pandemic, special consideration has been made weighing the benefit of definitive surgical airway and the risk of personnel exposure. Now, more than ever, proper personal protective equipment (PPE) and abidance to special airway protocols have become of upmost importance. For patients known to be infected, the use of a highly specialized team minimizes the number of personnel exposed.[2]

IMAGING AND OTHER DIAGNOSTIC STUDIES

- Owing to the emergent nature of the procedure, no imaging or diagnostic studies are required prior to performing cricothyroidotomy. During the initial trauma resuscitation, a chest radiograph is often obtained, which can provide some insight into the status of the airway. This may include tracheal deviation, subcutaneous emphysema, and pneumothorax or hemothorax.

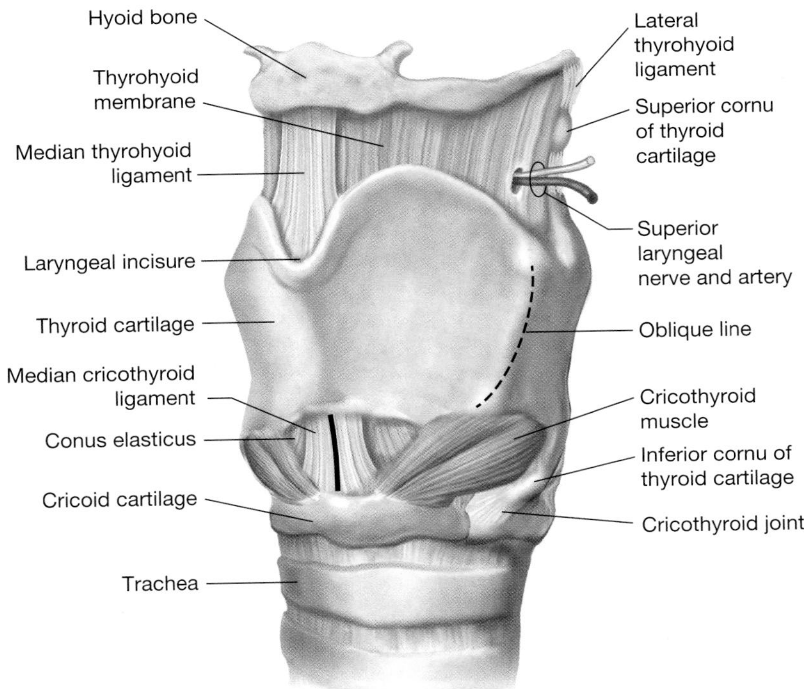

FIGURE 1 ● Laryngeal anatomy.

SURGICAL MANAGEMENT

Preoperative Planning

- The most common setting where a cricothyroidotomy is performed is in the emergency department, followed by the intensive care unit (ICU) and operating room (OR). However, they can occur anywhere in the hospital and therefore minimal equipment needed should be included in hospital code carts.
- A dedicated surgical airway team, often the trauma or surgical ICU team, is also a helpful way of stat paging a team that is prepared to perform the procedure particularly outside the emergency room (ER) or the OR.
- Obtaining equipment and prepping the neck should begin after the first attempt at direct laryngoscopy has failed. If significant desaturation occurs, preparation for emergent cricothyroidotomy should be expedited.
- Direct laryngoscopy can be continued after the cricothyroidotomy has begun but should not delay starting the procedure.
- The anatomy should be palpated and understood (see **FIGURE 1**).

Positioning

- The patient should be in the supine position with the neck slightly hyperextended with shoulder roll if possible (see **FIGURE 2**).

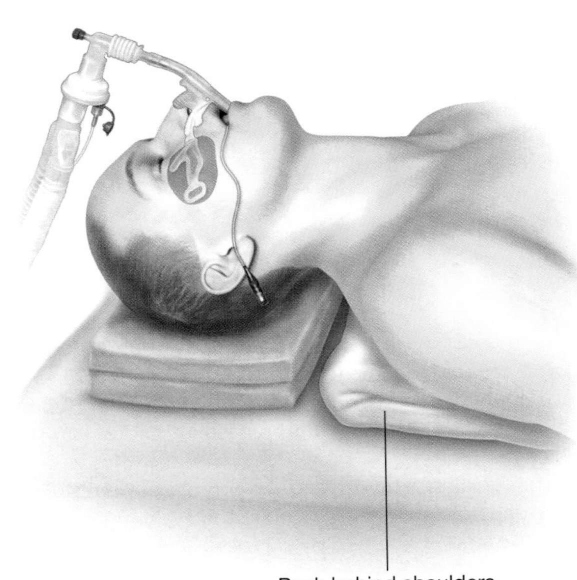

FIGURE 2 ● Hyperextension of neck for positioning.

- If there is concern for or confirmed cervical spine injury, inline stabilization with the neck in a neutral position must be maintained. An assistant can be placed at the head of the bed to ensure restriction of the patient's cervical motion.

OPEN CRICOTHYROIDOTOMY

- Don all appropriate PPE. Given the aerosolizing nature of the procedure, an N95 mask is recommended if COVID status is unknown.
- Surgically prepare the neck with chlorohexidine or Betadine scrub. Anesthetize the area locally if the patient is conscious.
- Palpate the thyroid cartilage, cricoid cartilage, and sternal notch for orientation. Stabilize the thyroid cartilage with the nondominant hand, and maintain stabilization until the trachea is intubated.
- Make a 4- to 5-cm generous midline vertical skin incision (**FIGURE 3**) over the cricothyroid membrane. Some may use a transverse incision; however, these authors find there is less bleeding with a midline incision and it may always be extended cranially or caudally if necessary.
- If the patient has a large neck it may not be possible to palpate the landmarks easily. If that occurs do not panic; just make the midline incision and cut through the anterior neck fat pad. Then palpate again and you will be able to identify the anatomical landmarks more easily.
- Confirm the anatomy again and incise the cricothyroid membrane transversely. Of note, once you enter the airway there will be bubbling out of the wound.
- Insert a hemostat, finger, or tracheal spreader to dilate the opening. These authors prefer the index finger, which is usually just bigger than the tube used for the airway.
- Insert a properly sized, cuffed endotracheal tube or tracheostomy tube (usually a size 5-6 mm) through the cricothyroid membrane incision directing the tube distally into the trachea. The distance from the cricothyroid membrane to the carina is only approximately 8 to 10 cm, so be careful not to intubate the right main stem. One only needs to have the cuff of the tube in the trachea and no further.
- Inflate the cuff and ventilate. Observe lung inflation and auscultate the chest to confirm bilateral breath sounds. Confirm the presence of end tidal CO_2.
- Secure the endotracheal or tracheostomy tube to the patient to prevent dislodgement (**FIGURE 4**). If an endotracheal tube is used then prepare for the patient to be transported to the OR to exchange it for a tracheostomy tube no larger than 6.5 mm.
- Obtain a chest x-ray to confirm appropriate positioning of the tube, rule out pneumothorax, and evaluate for bronchial obstruction.

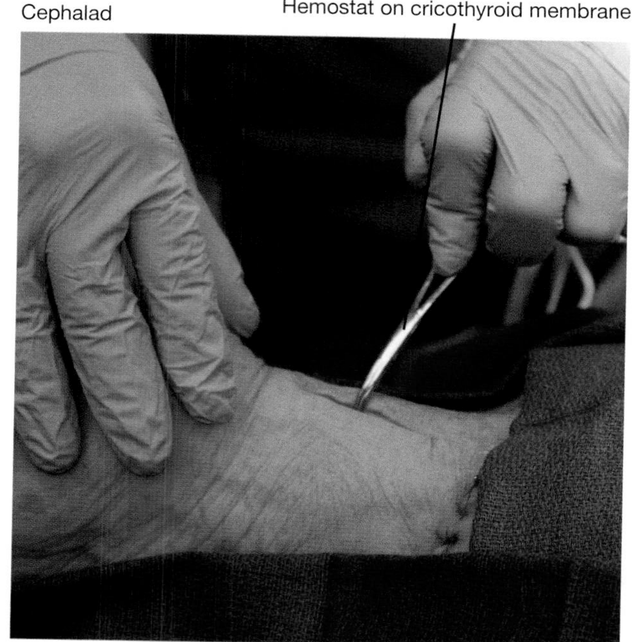

FIGURE 3 • Midline vertical incision.

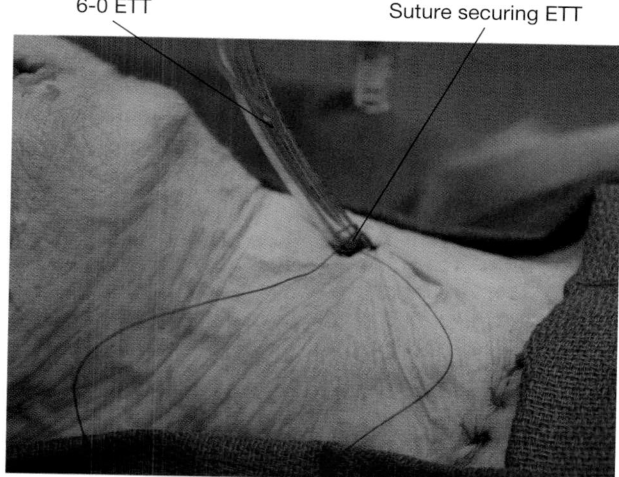

FIGURE 4 • Secure the airway.

PERCUTANEOUS CRICOTHYROIDOTOMY[3]

- A variety of percutaneous cricothyroidotomy kits exists. It is important to familiarize yourself with the kit your specific institution has available. In general, similar steps are used to successfully perform a cricothyroidotomy via the percutaneous approach no matter which kit is used.
- Don all appropriate PPE. Given the aerosolizing nature of the procedure, an N95 mask is recommended.
- Surgically prepare the neck with chlorohexidine or Betadine scrub. Anesthetize the area locally if the patient is conscious.
- Palpate the thyroid cartilage, cricoid cartilage, and sternal notch for orientation. Stabilize the thyroid cartilage with the nondominant hand, and maintain stabilization until the trachea is intubated.
- Make a 2- to 3-cm midline vertical skin incision over the cricothyroid membrane and reconfirm your landmarks. Again, if there is a large fat pad dissect through the fat pad with knife and bluntly with finger to ensure proper landmarks are felt.
- Insert the guide needle, with saline-containing syringe attached, at a 45° angle in the caudal direction through the cricothyroid membrane. Keep back pressure on the syringe as the needle is advanced.

- As you pass through the cricothyroid membrane, air will enter the syringe and bubble in the saline. It is important to not advance the needle further after the trachea is accessed.
- If a catheter is being used, the catheter is advanced into the airway and the needle is removed. A guidewire is then threaded through the needle or catheter into the trachea. The needle or catheter is then removed, leaving the guidewire in place.
- The blunt dilatator and tracheostomy tube are advanced together as a unit over the guidewire using the Seldinger technique. If resistance is encountered, use gentle and steady force. The tracheostomy should be fully inserted with the flange of the airway flush against the skin.
- The dilatator and the guidewire are then removed together, keeping the tracheostomy in place.
- Inflate the cuff and ventilate. Observe lung inflation and auscultate the chest to confirm bilateral breath sounds. Confirm the presence of end tidal CO_2.
- Secure the tracheostomy tube to the patient to prevent dislodgement.
- Obtain a chest x-ray to confirm appropriate positioning of the tracheostomy tube, rule out pneumothorax, and evaluate for bronchial obstruction.

PEARLS AND PITFALLS

Open and percutaneous techniques	▪ For both the open and percutaneous techniques, a vertical incision is preferable to avoid the anterior jugular veins, leading to significant bleeding and impeding visualization.
Open cricothyroidotomy	▪ While performing an open cricothyroidotomy, if the handle of the scalpel is used to dilate the tract, one must be careful not to injure themselves from the blade, particularly if the handle is short. These authors do not suggest using the blade handle to dilate the cricothyroidotomy due to this concern, better to use your finger to dilate.
Operative pearls	▪ Care must be taken to not cut the cricoid and/or thyroid cartilages. The transversely made incision of the membrane helps to avoid this injury. ▪ A bougie can be inserted into the trachea to aid in final tube placement. A bougie does not have to be used, but once in place, it maintains control of the airway and facilitates the introduction of the ETT. Do not advance the bougie more than 10 cm given the proximity to the carina. ▪ If an endotracheal tube is used, advance only until the cuff is no longer visible to avoid right mainstem intubation.

POSTOPERATIVE CARE

- Conversion to a tracheostomy tube (stiff plastic tube with flange) is always needed if not done at the initial cricothyroidotomy.
- Traditionally, conversion from cricothyroidotomy to formal tracheostomy within 48 hours was preformed to minimize risk of long-term complications of tracheal stenosis. More recent evidence does not support this practice. The risk associated with the prolonged use of a cricothyrotomy tube, particularly that of airway stenosis, may be much lower than previously believed.[4] Conversion to a formal tracheostomy is only needed if it is anticipated that the patient will be mechanically ventilated for a prolonged period of time (>7 days). If the patient has a more rapidly reversible cause of airway compromise (angioedema), one can wait several days for edema to resolve and then simply decannulate the patient.

COMPLICATIONS

- Short term[5,6]
  - Incorrect execution of the cricothyroidotomy
  - Injury to the cartilaginous structures
  - Failure to obtain a secure airway
  - Hemorrhage
  - Pneumothorax
  - Subcutaneous and mediastinal emphysema
  - Endotracheal tube dislodgement
  - Pressure ulceration
- Long term[6,7]
  - Tracheoinnominate fistula
  - Tracheoesophageal fistula
  - Tracheocutaneous fistula
  - Subglottic and tracheal stenosis
  - Dysphagia
  - Dysphonia
  - Parastomal infection
  - Tracheomalacia

REFERENCES

1. Sharma S, Patel R, Hashmi MF, et al. *3-3-2 rule*. In: *StatPearls [Internet]*. StatPearls Publishing; 2021. https://www.ncbi.nlm.nih.gov/books/NBK493235/
2. Hashimoto DA, Axtell AL, Auchincloss HG. Percutaneous tracheostomy. *N Engl J Med*. 2020;383(20):e112.
3. Chappell B. *How to Do a Percutaneous Cricothyrotomy-Critical Care Medicine*. Merck Manuals Professional Edition; 2020. Accessed June 23, 2021. https://www.merckmanuals.com/professional/critical-care-medicine/how-to-do-other-airway-procedures/how-to-do-a-percutaneous-cricothyrotomy
4. Talving P, DuBose J, Inaba K, Demetriades D. Conversion of emergent cricothyrotomy to tracheotomy in trauma patients. *Arch Surg*. 2010;145(1):87-91.
5. Durbin CG Jr. Early complications of tracheostomy. *Respir Care*. 2005;50(4):511-515.
6. DeVore EK, Redmann A, Howell R, Khosla S. Best practices for emergency surgical airway: a systematic review. *Laryngoscope Investig Otolaryngol*. 2019;4(6):602-608.
7. Epstein SK. Late complications of tracheostomy. *Respir Care*. 2005;50(4):542-549.

Chapter 41 Tracheostomy: Open and Percutaneous

Bennett J. Berning and Marc Anthony de Moya

DEFINITION

- A tracheostomy is the surgical creation of a communication between the anterior neck and trachea. This is considered definitive airway for the management of critically ill patients in need of prolonged ventilatory support.

DIFFERENTIAL DIAGNOSIS

- Tracheostomy should be considered if the patient has required prolonged mechanical ventilation or proven to be difficult to wean from ventilatory support. In addition, tracheostomy should be considered in cases of upper airway obstruction caused by neoplasm, infection, or vocal cord paralysis and in patients who have sustained severe traumatic brain injury or high cervical spinal cord injury resulting in paralysis.[1]
- Prolonged oral endotracheal intubation increases the risk of subglottic tracheal stenosis, although this risk has decreased with the use of high-volume, low-pressure cuffed endotracheal tubes.[2]
- Several studies have been performed to assess the benefit of early tracheostomy in critically ill patients. In mechanically ventilated adult patients, there is no 30-day or 2-year mortality benefit from performing an early tracheostomy. In addition, there was no difference in intensive care unit (ICU) length of stay.[3] For patients who experience trauma, early tracheostomy (<7 days) decreases the total days of mechanical ventilation and ICU length of stay in patients with head injuries. Early tracheostomy may also decrease the total days of mechanical ventilation and ICU length of stay in trauma patients without head injuries. Early tracheostomy may decrease the rate of pneumonia in trauma patients, although the evidence supporting this is limited. Because of these findings, it is recommended that early tracheostomy should be considered in all trauma patients who are anticipated to require mechanical ventilation for 7 days.[4]
- There are no absolute contraindications for tracheostomy placement. Relative contraindications include difficult or aberrant anatomy (inability to hyperextend neck, morbid obesity, thyroid pathology, atypical vasculature), unstable cervical spine injury, uncontrolled coagulopathy, significant problems with gas exchange (positive end-expiratory pressure [PEEP] greater than 10 or FiO_2 greater than 0.6), inability to tolerate transient hypoxemia or hypercarbia, elevated intracranial pressures, and evidence of infection in the soft tissue of the neck at the insertion site.[1]
- Neither previous tracheostomy nor other types of neck surgery are a contraindication for the tracheostomy placement. In fact, percutaneous tracheostomy may be preferred in patients whose surgical planes have been distorted.
- The percutaneous approach for tracheostomy placement has emerged as the procedure of choice if no obvious contraindications exist. Evidence suggests that percutaneous tracheostomy performed in the ICU results in reduced wound infection, favorable scaring patterns, reduced cost, and decreased procedural time. No difference between the open or percutaneous approach was seen with regards to creation of a false passage due to a misplaced tracheostomy tube, hemorrhage, subglottic stenosis, and mortality. Percutaneous tracheostomy did result in higher rates of unplanned decannulations and airway obstructions.[5,6]

PATIENT HISTORY AND PHYSICAL FINDINGS

- The need for tracheostomy is rarely urgent, allowing for a thorough history and physical examination to be performed.
- In the setting of trauma, the history should include the mechanism of trauma and all injuries present. If facial trauma is present, an understanding of the possible need for operative interventions in the future may lead to earlier tracheostomy. The need for early tracheostomy holds true for patients with severe traumatic brain injury because of the likely need for prolonged ventilatory support. The presence of cervical spine injuries will necessitate the need for strict spinal immobilization throughout the procedure.
- An understanding of chronic medical conditions is important. For example, ankylosing spondylitis may cause positioning issues due to the inability to lay flat or extend the neck.
- One should be aware of any difficulty with previous intubations, failure of previous extubation, previous neck surgery (thyroidectomy), previous surgical airways, and past radiation therapy to the head or neck.
- The physical examination should focus on the patient's body habitus, ability for neck extension, presence of a cervical collar, wounds/scars, and enlargement of the thyroid gland (goiters or masses). The neck should be palpated near the sternal notch to identify the pulse of a high-riding innominate artery.
- With the rise of the coronavirus (COVID-19) pandemic, special consideration has been made weighing the benefit of definitive surgical airway and the risk of personnel exposure. Now, more than ever, proper personal protective equipment (PPE) and abidance to special airway protocols have become of upmost importance. The use of complete neuromuscular blockade to prevent the cough reflex and apnea pauses while the ventilatory circuit is open may help prevent the aerosolizing of secretions. For patients known to be infected, the use of a highly specialized team minimizes the number of personnel exposed.[7]

IMAGING AND OTHER DIAGNOSTIC STUDIES

- Cross-sectional imaging (although not required) will allow for the identification of any anatomic variances. Specifically, tracheal deviation, low riding or enlarged thyroid, thyroid goiter, or high riding innominate artery.

- Preoperative laboratory studies should be obtained, paying attention to clotting parameters. If derangements exist, these should be investigated and optimized.

SURGICAL MANAGEMENT

Preoperative Planning

Open Tracheostomy

- The placement of a tracheostomy is unlikely an emergent procedure. This offers the luxury of time and preparation.
- It is important to take into consideration the patient's current ventilatory support. If the patient requires high ventilator settings (PEEP or FiO_2) the placement of a tracheostomy should be delayed until less ventilatory support is required.
- If the patient is being therapeutically anticoagulated, it should be held for the appropriate period prior to placing the tracheostomy. Prophylactic doses of anticoagulation (subcutaneous heparin or Enoxaparin) should not be held. Anticoagulation can be safely restarted after the tracheostomy is complete.[8]
- Periprocedural antibiotics should be administered.[9]
- To perform this procedure safely and efficiently, it is imperative all members of the team are prepared and understand the critical steps. Strong closed-loop communication between the surgical and anesthesia teams is imperative.
- Depending on the circumstance, various tracheostomy types and sizes should be considered. Traditionally, a size 8 cuffed tracheostomy tube is used for initial insertion with the plan to downsize to a size 6 when the patient's condition improves. Placement of a size 6 cuffed tracheostomy tube initially improves patient comfort but may have its disadvantages especially if secretion management is an issue requiring bronchoscopy. In addition, longer tracheostomy tubes are available. These come in two forms, proximal and distal, and are used in a variety of circumstances.

Percutaneous Tracheostomy

- The most important component to safely performing a percutaneous tracheostomy is preparation and setup.
- Percutaneous tracheostomies can be performed at bedside in the ICU or the operating room. If done in the ICU it is recommended that two physicians be present (one to perform the procedure and one managing sedation). An additional provider will need to be present to perform the bronchoscopy. A respiratory therapist and critical care nurse should both be available as part of the preoperative planning and setup portions of the procedure.
- Bronchoscopic guidance is highly recommended.
- Medications for the procedure consist of an anxiolytic, a narcotic pain medication, and a neuromuscular paralytic.
- An intubation/airway tray with associated equipment should be at the bedside should reintubation or emergent airway be needed.

Positioning

Open Tracheostomy

- The patient should be in the supine position with neck slightly hyperextended with shoulder roll if possible (see Part 7, Chapter 40, Figure 2). The patient's arms should be tucked to ensure access to the neck bilaterally. The procedure can be performed on the hospital bed if adequate positioning and exposure can be achieved.
- If there is a confirmed cervical spine injury, inline stabilization with the neck in a neutral position must be maintained.
- Reverse Trendelenburg.

Percutaneous Tracheostomy

- The patient should be placed supine in a slight reverse Trendelenburg position (30°). The neck should be slightly hyperextended with a shoulder roll if possible. The reverse Trendelenburg position decreases the central venous pressure in the neck and can decrease any bleeding that may occur.
- The patient's arms should be placed at the patient's side to ensure access to the neck bilaterally. The procedure can be performed on the hospital bed if adequate positioning and exposure can be achieved. The bed needs to be positioned to allow for access to the head of the bed so that translaryngeal reintubation can be performed if needed.
- If there is concern for or confirmed cervical spine injury, inline stabilization with the neck in a neutral position must be maintained.
- For right-handed surgeons, the bronchoscopy cart is generally placed on the patient's left with the person performing the tracheostomy on the patient's right. The respiratory therapist should be at the head of the bed with easy access to the patient's airway. A second person will be at the head of the bed performing the bronchoscopy. The patient's nurse needs to have easy access to the patient's IV in order to administer medications in a timely manner, and the monitor with vital signs and pulse oximetry with audio is easily visible to all.
- **FIGURE 1** provides a picture of the required percutaneous equipment.

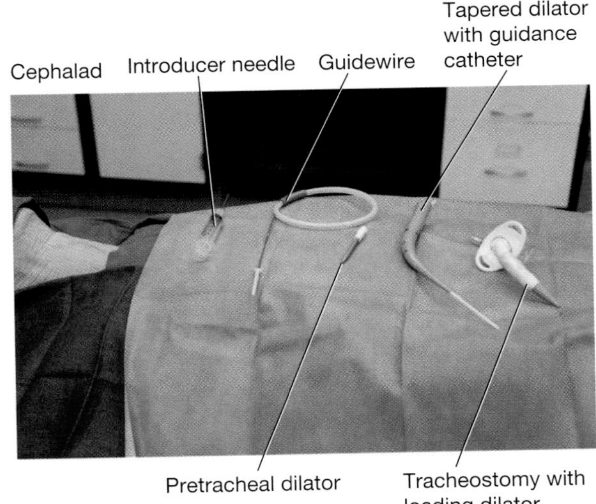

FIGURE 1 ● Tools for percutaneous tracheostomy.

OPEN TRACHEOSTOMY

- Don all appropriate PPE. Standard sterile surgical technique should be implemented.
- Surgically prepare the neck and upper chest with chlorohexidine skin prep. Standard sterile technique and draping should be performed. Consideration for easy access for the anesthesia provider to allow for easy airway exchange after the tracheostomy is placed.
- Palpate the neck to identify relevant anatomy. This should include the thyroid cartilage, cricothyroid cartilage, trachea, and sternal notch for orientation. At this point the thyroid gland can likely be palpated and consideration should be made if an enlarged thyroid or goiter is present.
- Using a #15 scalpel, make a horizontal 3- to 5-cm incision at level 1 cm below the cricoid cartilage or 3- to 4-cm vertical midline incision overlying the trachea. These authors prefer the vertical incision owing to less bleeding (**FIGURE 2**). However, either incision is acceptable.
- Continue the dissection with electrocautery through the platysma and between the strap muscles. The median raphe of the strap muscles is carefully opened craniocaudally and retracted laterally to aid in exposure of the thyroid isthmus and trachea. The anterior jugular veins may be encountered if using a horizontal incision. These can be preserved by retracting laterally or tied off without any undue harm.
- At this point the isthmus of the thyroid should be visualized. It is safe to divide the isthmus of the thyroid using electrocautery or suture ligation to assist in obtaining adequate exposure of the trachea (**FIGURE 3**). On occasion, tracheal exposure can be achieved by simply retracting the thyroid cephalad.
- Using electrocautery or careful blunt dissection, a plane is developed between the pretracheal tissue and the trachea anterior and anterior lateral on each side of the trachea. Meticulous hemostasis is of utmost importance. After the trachea is entered, one should not use electrocautery due to the increased risk of a surgical fire due to the use of a high percentage of FiO_2.
- Once adequate exposure of the trachea has been obtained, a 2-0 Prolene suture with a small tapered needle (RB-1) is placed around the 3rd tracheal ring laterally on each side as a stay suture. The endotracheal cuff should be briefly deflated as each stitch is placed so as not to incorporate the cuff with the suture.
- After the endotracheal cuff is deflated, a #11 or #15 blade is used to make an incision through the third tracheal ring creating a sideways "H-shaped" opening in the trachea. A Kelly clamp or tracheal spreader is then inserted, dilating the opening. Careful attention is needed to ensure only the anterior surface of the trachea is incised. If division of the 3rd ring is not possible with a scalpel, curved Mayo scissors can be used.
- The endotracheal tube is then slowly withdrawn by the anesthesia provider until the tip is just proximal to the tracheotomy site. The tracheostomy tube with stylet is inserted into the trachea under direct visualization at a 90° angle to the trachea to ensure that pretracheal placement is avoided.
- The stylet is removed and the inner cannula is placed into the tracheostomy tube and connected to the ventilator. The cuff should be inflated and proper placement confirmed by the presence of end-tidal carbon dioxide.
- The tracheostomy tube is secured with tracheal ties or collar. If the surgeon decides to keep the stay sutures in place, the ends should be tied together to form a loop of suture on either side to prevent them from being inadvertently removed. Each loop can be secured to the skin with Steri-Strips. This keeps the stay sutures out of the way and secured.

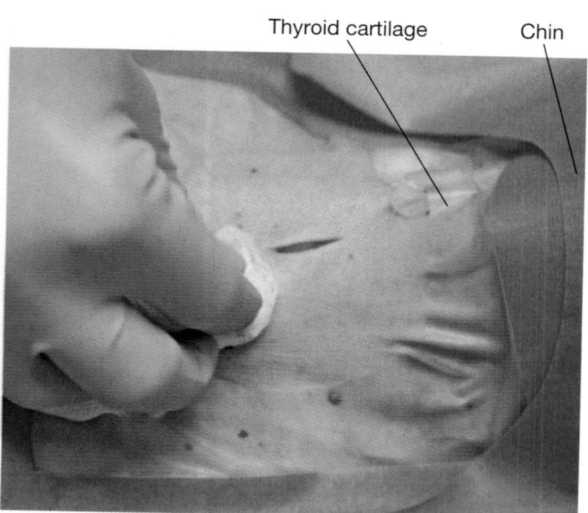

FIGURE 2 ● Midline vertical incision.

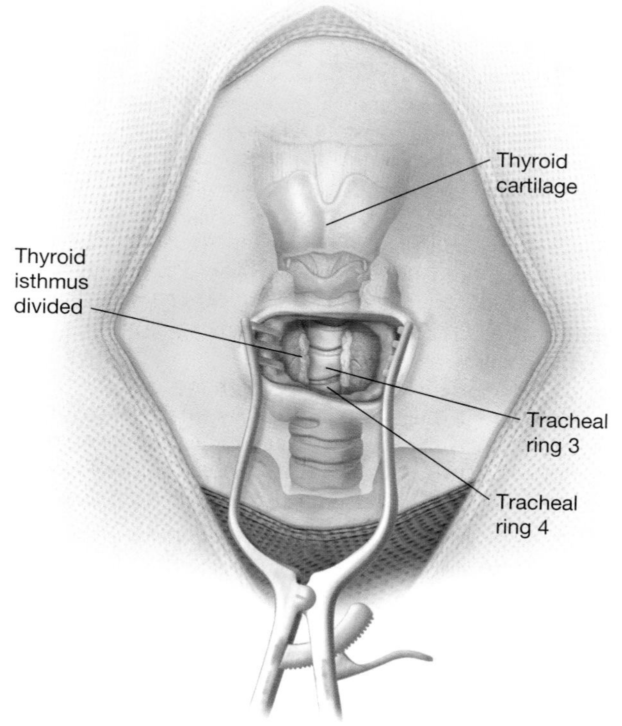

FIGURE 3 ● Isthmus of thyroid is divided.

- Suturing of the flange to the skin should be avoided given the high incidence of ulcerations from the flange. The tracheal ties or collar is adequate, but care must be taken to ensure proper tightness. With the neck flexed you should only be able to insert two fingers under the tracheal tie.
- Obtain a chest x-ray postoperatively to assess distance of tracheostomy tube tip to carina. Although rare, one must ensure no pneumothorax has developed during the operation.

PERCUTANEOUS TRACHEOSTOMY

- Set the ventilator to deliver a set volume and rate with 100% FiO_2 to preoxygenate the patient. The ICU monitor should be set so that the pulse oximeter is audible. Continuous hemodynamic monitoring should be achieved with electrocardiogram and arterial line or frequent blood pressure cuff monitoring.
- Adequate sedation should be achieved with anxiolytic and narcotic pain medications. This is followed by paralysis.
- Palpate the neck to identify relevant anatomy. Ideal location for placement of the tracheostomy is between the 2nd and 3rd tracheal ring.
- Don all appropriate PPE. Standard sterile surgical technique should be implemented.
- Surgically prepare neck and upper chest with chlorohexidine skin prep. Standard sterile technique and draping should be performed. Consideration for easy access to the endotracheal tube to allow for easy airway exchange after the tracheal tube is placed.
- Anesthetize the skin and subcutaneous tissue with lidocaine with epinephrine.
- Using a #15 scalpel, make a 2- to 3-cm vertical, midline incision approximately 40 mm cephalad (1-2 finger breaths) to the sternal notch and just below the cricoid cartilage. If an anterior jugular vein is encountered in the incision (even if no injury is suspected), consider ligation proximally and distally as this is easiest to perform before the tracheostomy tube has been placed.
- Using a hemostat, bluntly dissect the subcutaneous tissue and muscle in the midline down to the pretracheal tissue along the length of the incision in order to better palpate the trachea to determine the point of entry. The degree of dissection should be directly correlated to the thickness of the neck. The thicker the neck the more dissection should occur to ensure easy passage of the tracheostomy tube.
- With the bronchoscope adaptor in place, advance the bronchoscope into the airway. Inspect the trachea and bronchial trees and clear any secretions.
- There are two techniques frequently used.
    - (1) The authors of this chapter prefer the following: The surgeon palpates the cricoid cartilage and ensures they can palpate the trachea approximately one finger breadth below the cricoid. That position will place the needle approximately 2 to 3 rings below the cricoid. With the fingers removed from the wound the introducer needle is placed into the wound at an angle that is perpendicular to the trachea. The dominant finger is then placed over the needle to ensure that again it is one finger breadth below the cricoid and in the midline. Anesthesia is asked to deflate the cuff. With saline in the syringe connected to the needle one should aspirate while applying force until the trachea is entered and one confirms bubbles are aspirated into the partially filled syringe (**FIGURE 4**).
    - The wire is then threaded into the needle (**FIGURE 5**) and visualized bronchoscopically to course into the trachea usually seen going down the right main-stem bronchus (**FIGURE 6**).
    - The introducer needle is then removed over the wire while leaving the wire in place.
    - The small blue dilator is introduced over the wire and the initial dilation is performed (**FIGURE 7**).

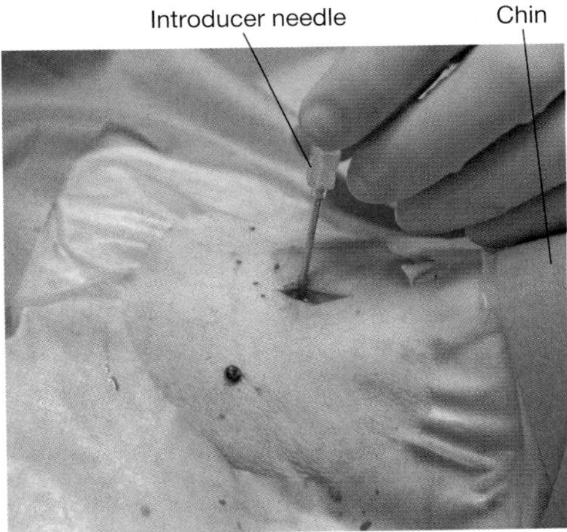

FIGURE 4 • Needle placed into midline into trachea.

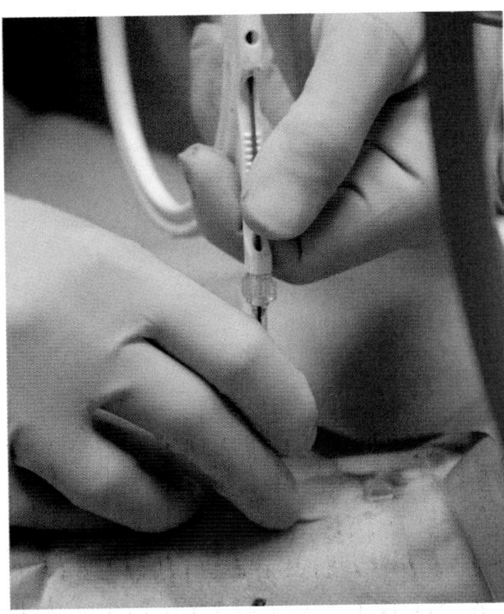

FIGURE 5 • Wire is introduced through needle.

- With the small blue dilator in place the bronchoscope is placed at the end of the endotracheal tube so as to visualize both the tracheal lumen and the end of the tube. The endotracheal tube is then withdrawn until the entry point of the blue dilator is in view. The endotracheal tube withdrawal is stopped to ensure the patient is not prematurely extubated.
- The initial small blue dilator is then removed.

- (2) The other commonly described way is the following: With the assistance of the respiratory therapist, while keeping the bronchoscope at the end of the endotracheal tube, retract both the endotracheal tube and bronchoscope simultaneously until the subglottic structures are visualized and one can see the anterior wall of the trachea being palpated by the surgeon. The bronchoscope should be kept within the endotracheal tube at all times during this portion of the procedure in order to maintain control of the airway and ensure that the bronchoscope is not damaged.
  - An introducer needle is used to enter the anterior portion of the trachea between the 2nd and 3rd tracheal rings (approximately one finger breadth below the cricoid cartilage). With the bevel of the needle facing downward, the guidewire is passed into the trachea. Visualization of the guidewire going in the direction of the carina is required. Advance the guidewire slightly passed the carina into the right or left mainstem bronchus.
  - The initial small blue dilator is placed over the wire and then removed.
- Using the Seldinger technique, with constant bronchoscopic visualization and control of the wire within the trachea, the trachea is dilated with the tapered larger dilator (**FIGURE 8**). The handle is hydrophobic, which makes it less likely to slip in a wet environment while the actual dilating portion is hydrophilic, which only requires water/liquid to be lubricated. Markings on the side of the progressive dilator guides the depth to which it is inserted (**FIGURE 9**). All catheters (pretracheal dilator, tapered dilator, and guiding catheter) should enter perpendicular to the trachea as to prevent pretracheal dissection or false passage.
- The tapered dilator is removed from the guiding catheter and the guidewire, leaving the guiding catheter and the guidewire in place. If there is a longer distance between the tracheal surface and the skin surface, a finger can be used to dilatate the tract to help facilitate placement of the tracheostomy during the next step.
- Next, an appropriately sized (usually 8 mm) and well-lubricated tracheostomy tube with introducer is advanced over the wire and guiding catheter into the trachea (**FIGURE 10**). The wire, guiding catheter, and loading introducer is then removed, keeping the tracheostomy in place.
- Inflate the tracheostomy cuff, insert the inner cannula, and connect the tracheostomy to the ventilator circuit. The presence of end-tidal carbon dioxide after ventilation resumes confirms placement in the airway (**FIGURE 11**).

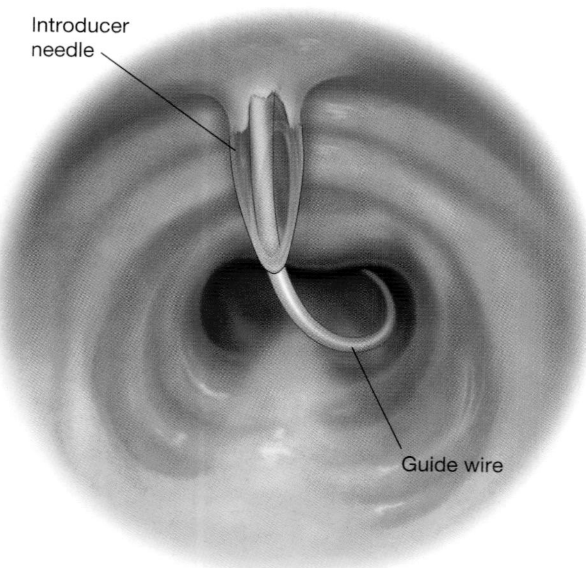

FIGURE 6 ● Wire visualized usually down right main stem.

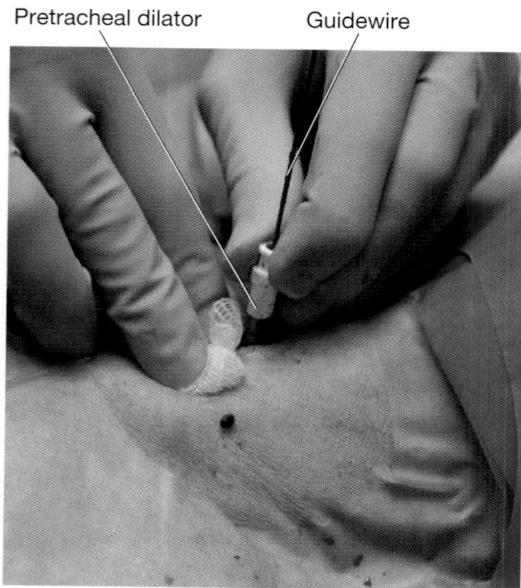

FIGURE 7 ● Small firm dilator inserted over wire.

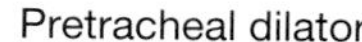

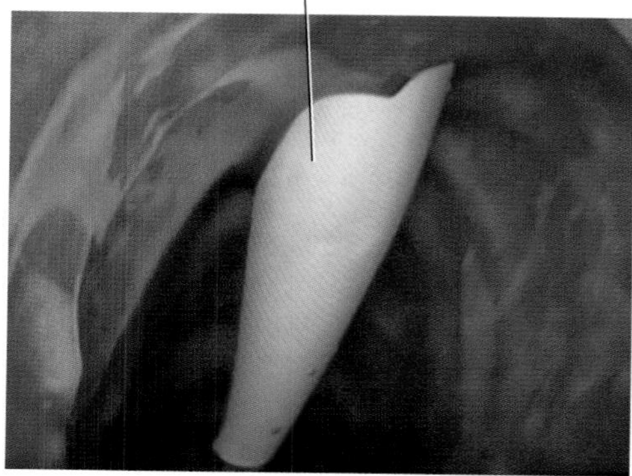

FIGURE 8 ● Tapered dilator inserted while being visualized.

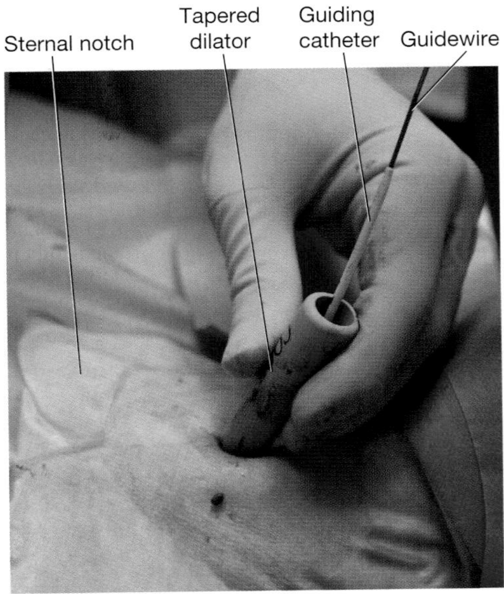

FIGURE 9 ● Markings on dilator guide surgeon to stop.

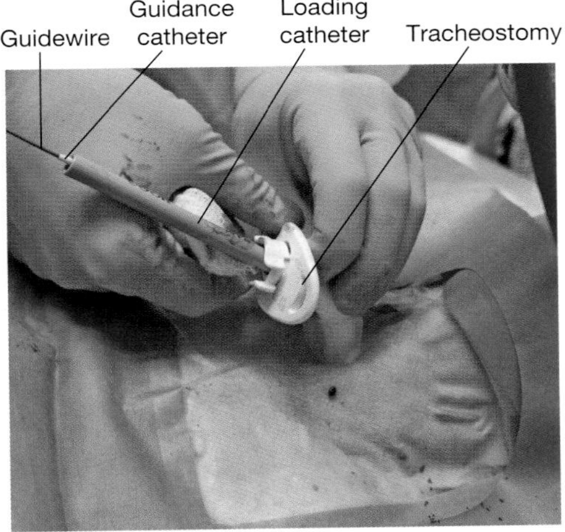

FIGURE 10 ● Appropriately sized tracheostomy is inserted with its introducer.

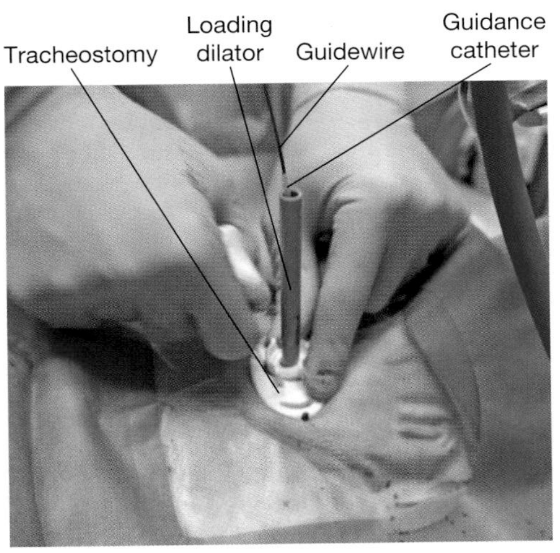

FIGURE 11 ● Tracheostomy in place.

- A bronchoscopy should be performed through the newly placed tracheostomy to visually confirm that it is within the trachea in proper position. Only remove the endotracheal tube (ETT) after placement of the tracheostomy tube within the trachea is confirmed.
- The tracheostomy is secured with a tracheostomy collar or ties to help prevent accidental dislodgement and provide time for adequate tract formation. Sutures are avoided to prevent skin ulceration.
- Obtain a chest x-ray to confirm appropriate positioning of the tracheostomy tube, rule out pneumothorax, and evaluate for bronchial obstruction.

PEARLS AND PITFALLS

Open tracheostomy	■ Surgical fires are a "never event" in medicine. Airway fires have been encountered with the use of electrocautery to enter the trachea or to control hemorrhage. Sharp entry with a scalpel is the safest means to enter the trachea. ■ Tracheal stay sutures allow for lateral traction making placement of tracheostomy less difficult, particularly for high-risk anatomy. The sutures also allow for reinsertion of the tracheostomy tube in the case of accidental dislodgement before a tract has formed. ■ It is important to maintain the position of the endotracheal tube just past the cords until confirmation of proper tracheostomy tube placement. Should malposition occur, the oral endotracheal tube can be advanced past the tracheotomy, allowing for adequate ventilation and oxygenation before a second attempt at tracheostomy placement is performed. ■ Avoid suturing the tracheostomy flange to the skin due to the higher incidence of skin pressure necrosis. Suturing the flange should only be done in the highest-risk patients with tenuous airways.

Percutaneous tracheostomy	■ It is critical to avoid damaging the balloon on the oral endotracheal tube. In the event that the patient's condition becomes clinically unstable or there is difficulty performing the tracheostomy, as long as the balloon is intact, the oral endotracheal tube is simply advanced to its original location and normal ventilation is resumed. ■ The trachea should be stabilized with the nondominant hand while the dominant hand is used to pass the needle into the midline of the trachea; this helps prevent the needle from sliding off the lateral wall of the trachea. The guidewire should pass easily through the introducer needle into the trachea; however, at times it can get caught between the side of the ETT and the mucosa of the trachea and requires some slight back and forth motion to finally advance the wire. ■ For patients with low tracheas, particularly patients with kyphosis where the cricoid cartilage sits close to or even deep to the sternal notch, placing a tracheal hook under the cricoid cartilage or placing a fingertip under the cartilage may be helpful to elevate the cartilage and therefore the trachea. By elevating the cricoid cartilage one further exposes the trachea to ensure it is well above the sternal notch and provides an opportunity for a more perpendicular angle of entry. A more perpendicular entry angle into the trachea can improve the ease by which the tracheostomy tube enters. ■ During the bronchoscopy through the tracheostomy tube, visualize the tracheostomy within the trachea with the patient's head in both flexion and extension. This can ensure the tracheal tube is the appropriate length extending no closer than 2 cm from the carina and the balloon of the tube is well within the trachea. Occasionally you may need to replace the initial tracheostomy with an extra-long tracheostomy. There are two varieties available, one with an extra-long distance from the skin (proximal) to the tracheotomy and another with the more distal length from the elbow of the tracheostomy to the distal end. The type used is dictated by the anatomy of the patient.

POSTOPERATIVE CARE

- Following tracheostomy placement, standardized tracheostomy care bundles should be implemented. These protocols include steps to ensure the tracheostomy is secure, suctioning techniques, daily stoma hygiene, and knowledge of emergency protocols should the newly placed airway be compromised. Special attention should be given to prevent pressure ulceration, particularly along the inferior aspect of the tracheostomy faceplate, especially if the flange is sutured to the skin.
- The tracheostomy tube should be exchanged no sooner than postoperative day 7. The Prolene stay sutures, if they remain, can be removed after the first tracheostomy tube exchange.
- Once the patient is liberated from the ventilator and secretions are reasonably managed the process of tracheostomy tube downsizing can occur. The downsizing of the tracheostomy tube allows for improved patient comfort and the ability to participate in speech therapy.
- After the tracheostomy is no longer necessary, the patient can be decannulated. The stoma is covered with a sterile occlusive dressing, which generally closes within 2 to 4 days.

COMPLICATIONS

- Short term[10]
  - Wound infection
  - Postoperative hemorrhage is usually self-limiting and able to be controlled at bedside with pressure and hemostatic agents
  - Tracheostomy dislodgement
  - Pressure ulceration
  - Airway obstruction
- Long term[11]
  - Tracheoinnominate fistula
  - Tracheoesophageal fistula
  - Tracheocutaneous fistula
  - Tracheal stenosis
  - Tracheomalacia

REFERENCES

1. Cheung NH, Napolitano LM. Tracheostomy: epidemiology, indications, timing, technique, and outcomes. *Respir Care*. 2014;59(6):895-915. discussion 916-919.
2. Dorris ER, Russell J, Murphy M. Post-intubation subglottic stenosis: aetiology at the cellular and molecular level. *Eur Respir Rev*. 2021;30(159):200218.
3. Young D, Harrison DA, Cuthbertson BH, Rowan K; TracMan Collaborators. Effect of early vs late tracheostomy placement on sur- vival in patients receiving mechanical ventilation: the TracMan randomized trial. *JAMA*. 2013;309(20):2121-2129.
4. Holevar M, Dunham JC, Brautigan R, et al. Practice management guidelines for timing of tracheostomy: the EAST Practice Management Guidelines Work Group. *J Trauma*. 2009;67(4):870-874.
5. Delaney A, Bagshaw SM, Nalos M. Percutaneous dilatational tracheostomy versus surgical tracheostomy in critically ill patients: a systematic review and meta-analysis. *Crit Care*. 2006;10(2):R55.
6. Higgins KM, Punthakee X. Meta-analysis comparison of open versus percutaneous tracheostomy. *Laryngoscope* 2007;117(3):447-454.
7. Hashimoto DA, Axtell AL, Auchincloss HG. Percutaneous tracheostomy. *N Engl J Med*. 2020;383(20):e112.
8. Pasin L, Frati E, Cabrini L, et al. Percutaneous tracheostomy in patients on anticoagulants. *Ann Card Anaesth*. 2015;18(3):329-334. doi: 10.4103/0971-9784.159802
9. Sittitrai P, Siriwittayakorn C. Perioperative antibiotic prophylaxis in open tracheostomy: a preliminary randomized controlled trial. *Int J Surg*. 2018;54(pt A):170-175.
10. Durbin CG Jr. Early complications of tracheostomy. *Respir Care*. 2005;50(4):511-515.
11. Epstein SK. Late complications of tracheostomy. *Respir Care*. 2005;50(4):542-549.

Index

Note: Page numbers followed by"*f*" indicate figures and "*t*" indicate tables.

G

H

J

R

S